THIRD EDITION

Critical Care Transport

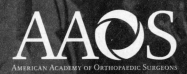

AAOS
AMERICAN ACADEMY OF ORTHOPAEDIC SURGEONS

AAOS Series Editor:
Alfonso Mejia, MD, MPH, FAAOS

Lead Editors:
Mike McEvoy, PhD, NRP, RN, CCRN

Jeffrey S. Rabrich, DO, FACEP, FAEMS

Sean M. Kivlehan, MD, MPH, FACEP

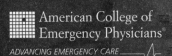

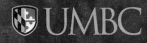

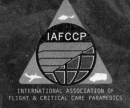

INTERNATIONAL ASSOCIATION OF
FLIGHT & CRITICAL CARE PARAMEDICS

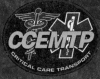

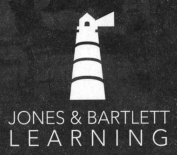

JONES & BARTLETT
LEARNING

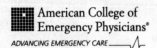

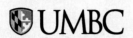

Jones & Bartlett Learning books and products are available through most bookstores and online booksellers. To contact the Jones & Bartlett Learning Public Safety Group directly, call 800-832-0034, fax 978-443-8000, or visit our website, www.psglearning.com.

Substantial discounts on bulk quantities of Jones & Bartlett Learning publications are available to corporations, professional associations, and other qualified organizations. For details and specific discount information, contact the special sales department at Jones & Bartlett Learning via the above contact information or send an email to specialsales@jblearning.com.

Production Credits
Vice President, Product Management: Marisa R. Urbano
Vice President, Content Strategy and Implementation: Christine Emerton
Director, Product Management: Cathy Esperti
Director, Product Management: Laura Carney
Director, Content Management: Donna Gridley
Manager, Content Strategy: Tiffany Sliter
Developmental Editor: Mike Boblitt
Content Coordinator: Mark Restuccia
Director, Project Management and Content Services: Karen Scott
Manager, Project Management: Kristen Rogers
Project Manager: Kelly Mahoney
Senior Digital Project Specialist: Angela Dooley
Director of Marketing: Brian Rooney

Vice President, International Sales, Public Safety Group: Matthew Maniscalco
Director of Sales, Public Safety Group: Brian Hendrickson
Content Services Manager: Colleen Lamy
Vice President, Manufacturing and Inventory Control: Therese Connell
Composition: S4Carlisle Publishing Services
Cover Design: Scott Moden
Text Design: Scott Moden
Senior Media Development Editor: Troy Liston
Rights & Permissions Manager: John Rusk
Rights Specialist: Liz Kincaid
Cover Image (Title Page): Courtesy of Staff Sgt. Kevin Iinuma/US Air Force photo
Printing and Binding: LSC Communications

Library of Congress Cataloging-in-Publication Data
Names: McEvoy, Mike, editor. | Kivlehan, Sean, editor. | Rabrich, Jeffrey S., editor. | American Academy of Orthopaedic Surgeons, issuing body.
Title: Critical care transport / edited by American Academy of Orthopaedic Surgeons ; lead editors, Mike McEvoy, Sean Kivlehan, Jeff Rabrich.
Description: Third edition. | Burlington, MA : Jones & Bartlett Learning, [2023] | Includes bibliographical references and index.
Identifiers: LCCN 2021043628 | ISBN 9781284236347 (paperback)
Subjects: MESH: Transportation of Patients | Critical Care | Patient Transfer | Emergency Medical Services
Classification: LCC RA996.5 | NLM WX 215 | DDC 616.02/8--dc23
LC record available at https://lccn.loc.gov/2021043628

6048

Printed in the United States of America
26 25 24   10 9 8 7 6 5 4 3

Brief Contents

Contents

Skill Drills

Acknowledgments

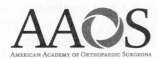
AMERICAN ACADEMY OF ORTHOPAEDIC SURGEONS

The American Academy of Orthopaedic Surgeons, American College of Emergency Physicians, and Jones & Bartlett Learning would like to acknowledge the editors, authors, and reviewers of previous editions who were involved in the development of this textbook.

Editorial Board

Mike McEvoy, PhD, NRP, RN, CCRN
EMS Coordinator
Saratoga County, New York
Cardiovascular Surgery Nurse Clinician
Albany Medical Center
Albany, New York

Jeffrey S. Rabrich, DO, FACEP, FAEMS
Senior Regional Medical Director
Envision Healthcare Northeast
Parsippany, New Jersey

Sean M. Kivlehan, MD, MPH, FACEP
Department of Emergency Medicine
Brigham and Women's Hospital
Boston, Massachusetts

Alfonso Mejia, MD, MPH, FAAOS
Program Director, Orthopedic Surgery Residency
  Program
Vice Head, Department of Orthopedic Surgery
University of Illinois College of Medicine
Medical Director
Tactical Emergency Medical Support Physician
South Suburban Emergency Response Team
Chicago, Illinois

Authors

Chapter 1
Introduction and Overview of Critical Care Transport

Mike McEvoy, PhD, NRP, RN, CCRN
EMS Coordinator
Saratoga County, New York
Cardiovascular Surgery Nurse
  Clinician
Albany Medical Center
Albany, New York

Chapter 2
Medical-Legal Issues

Matthew R. Streger, Esq., MPA, NRP
Partner, Keavney & Streger, LLC
Princeton, New Jersey

Chapter 3
Patient Safety

Jeffrey S. Rabrich, DO, FACEP, FAEMS
Senior Regional Medical Director
Envision Healthcare–Northeast
Parsippany, New Jersey

Chapter 4
Aircraft Fundamentals and Flight Physiology

Paul M. Mazurek, MEd, RN, NRP, CCRN, CFRN, CHSE, I/C
Educational Nurse Coordinator
University of Michigan Survival
  Flight
Ann Arbor, Michigan

Chapter 5
Patient Assessment

Kevin Collopy, MHL, NRP, FP-C, CMTE
Clinical Outcomes and
  Compliance Manager
Novant Health AirLink & VitaLink
Wilmington, North Carolina

Vahé Ender, NRP, FP-C, C-NPT
Critical Care Transport Paramedic
Boston MedFlight
Bedford, Massachusetts

Chapter 6
Respiratory Emergencies and Airway Management

Lauren M. Maloney, MD, NRP, FP-C, NCEE
Clinical Assistant Professor of Emergency Medicine
Stony Brook Medicine
Stony Brook, New York

Rudolph Princi, Jr, MA, EMT-P, TP-C, NCEE, CIC
Emergency Medical Services Educator
Northeast Regional Course Director
The Difficult Airway Course: EMS
Stony Brook University Hospital
Stony Brook, New York

Chapter 7
Ventilation

Michael Schauf, RRT-NPS
Flight Respiratory Therapist
AirMed International
Birmingham, Alabama
Neonatal/Pediatric Transport Team
Albany Medical Center
Albany, New York
Global Medical Response
Clinical Education Specialist
Englewood, Colorado

Chapter 8
Critical Care Pharmacology

Zlatan Coralic, PharmD, BCPS
Emergency Medicine Clinical Pharmacist
Associate Clinical Professor
Departments of Pharmacy and Emergency Medicine
University of California San Francisco
San Francisco, California

Mike McEvoy, PhD, NRP, RN, CCRN
EMS Coordinator
Saratoga County, New York
Cardiovascular Surgery Nurse Clinician
Albany Medical Center
Albany, New York

Chapter 9
Laboratory Analysis and Diagnostic Studies

Gregory Peters, MD
Resident Physician
Department of Emergency Medicine
Brigham and Women's Hospital
Boston, Massachusetts

Christopher J. Hanowitz, MD
Assistant Clerkship Director, MSIV Critical Care
Assistant Professor of Emergency Medicine and Surgery
Divisions of Critical Care, Trauma, and Emergency Ultrasound
Albany, New York

Chapter 10
Resuscitation, Shock, and Blood Products

Amar Deshwar, MD
Department of Emergency Medicine
Brigham and Women's Hospital
Boston, Massachusetts

Sean M. Kivlehan, MD, MPH, FACEP
Department of Emergency Medicine
Brigham and Women's Hospital
Boston, Massachusetts

Chapter 11
Trauma

Christopher J. McLaughlin, MD, MBA, NRP
Resident Physician, Department of Surgery
Pennsylvania State University, College of Medicine
Hershey, Pennsylvania

Chapter 12
Neurologic Emergencies

Heidi Hutchison, MBBS
Emergency Medicine and EMS Physician
Central Coast Emergency Physicians
San Luis Obispo County, California

Chapter 13
Burns

Jeremy Lacocque, DO
Assistant Clinical Professor
UCSF Department of Emergency Medicine
Zuckerberg San Francisco General Hospital
Medical Director
San Francisco Fire Department
San Francisco, California

Chapter 14
Electrophysiology, Pacemakers, and Defibrillators

Mike McEvoy, PhD, NRP, RN, CCRN
EMS Coordinator
Saratoga County, New York
Cardiovascular Surgery Nurse Clinician
Albany Medical Center
Albany, New York

Chapter 15
Hemodynamic Monitoring

Mike McEvoy, PhD, NRP, RN, CCRN
EMS Coordinator
Saratoga County, New York
Cardiovascular Surgery Nurse
  Clinician
Albany Medical Center
Albany, New York

Chapter 16
Mechanical Circulatory Support

William David Sadler, MS, RN, NRP, CCRN, CFRN
Flight Nurse/Paramedic
Survival Flight, Michigan
  Medicine
Ann Arbor, Michigan

Johnnie Peoples, BSN, EMT-P
Flight Nurse
Survival Flight, Michigan
  Medicine
Ann Arbor, Michigan

William Hallinan, MSBA, RN
Trauma Program Manager
University of Rochester Medical
  Center
Rochester, New York

Chapter 17
Gastrointestinal and Genitourinary Emergencies

Lorenzo Albala, MD, MS
Emergency Medicine Physician
Massachusetts General Hospital
Boston, Massachusetts

Sean M. Kivlehan, MD, MPH, FACEP
Department of Emergency
  Medicine
Brigham and Women's Hospital
Boston, Massachusetts

Chapter 18
Endocrine Emergencies

Eric Silverman, MD, MPH
University of California, San
  Francisco, Assistant Clinical
  Professor of Emergency
  Medicine
Zuckerberg San Francisco
  General Hospital, EMS Base
  Hospital, Associate Medical
  Director
King-American Ambulance
  Company Medical Director
San Francisco, California

Chapter 19
Environmental Emergencies

David Fifer, MS, NRP, FAWM
Assistant Professor of Emergency
  Medical Care
Eastern Kentucky University
Richmond, Kentucky

Michael Murphy, RN, EMT-P
Chief of Operations (ret.)
Rockland Paramedic Services
Chestnut Ridge, New York

Chapter 20
Infectious and Communicable Diseases

Robert P. Holman, MD
Medical Director
District of Columbia Fire and
  EMS
Washington, DC

Ryan Gerecht, MD, FACEP
Assistant Medical Director
District of Columbia Fire and
  EMS
Washington, DC

Chapter 21
Toxicologic Emergencies

Jason Chu, MD
Assistant Professor of Emergency
  Medicine
Columbia University Medical
  Center
Department of Emergency
  Medicine
New York, New York

Theodore C. Bania, MD, MS
Director of Toxicology
Mount Sinai West, Mount Sinai
  Morningside
Department of Emergency
  Medicine
Icahn School of Medicine at
  Mount Sinai
New York, New York

Chapter 22
Obstetric and Gynecologic Emergencies

Kathleen A. Kerrigan, MD, FACEP, FACOG
Cape Cod Hospital
Hyannis, Massachusetts

Adrianne Wurzl, DO
Emergency Medicine Resident
Baystate Medical Center
Springfield, Massachusetts

Chapter 23
Neonatal Emergencies

Patricia R. Chess, MD, MSEd
Professor of Pediatrics
  (Neonatology)
Golisano Children's Hospital
University of Rochester School of
  Medicine
Rochester, New York

Yogangi Malhotra, MD, FAAP
Director, Pediatric Quality and
  Safety
Lewis M. Fraad Department of
  Pediatrics
New York City Health +
  Hospitals/Jacobi
Associate Professor
Albert Einstein College of
  Medicine
Bronx, New York

Nirupama Laroia, MD
Professor, Pediatrics/
  Neonatology
University of Rochester Medical
  Center
Neonatologist, Golisano
  Children's Hospital
Rochester, New York

Chapter 24
Pediatric Emergencies

**Matthew Harris, MD, FAAP,
FAEMS**
Pediatric Emergency Medicine
  Attending
EMS and Disaster Medicine
  Fellow
New Milford, New Jersey

Chapter 25
**Bariatric and Special
Situations**

Bariatric Patients section:

**Peter I. Dworsky, MPH, NRP,
CEM**
Paramedic/Consultant
Outcome Solutions
Edison, New Jersey

Excited Delirium section:

Eric Silverman, MD, MPH
University of California, San
  Francisco, Assistant Clinical
  Professor of Emergency
  Medicine
Zuckerberg San Francisco
  General Hospital, EMS Base
  Hospital, Associate Medical
  Director
King-American Ambulance
  Company Medical Director
San Francisco, California

**Children With Special Health
Care Needs section:**

Lindsay Riedl Jaeger, MD
EMS Medical Director
University of Chicago Comer
  Children's Hospital
Chicago, Illinois

Emily Kivlehan, MD, MS
Pediatric Rehabilitation Medicine
  Fellow
Spaulding Rehabilitation
  Hospital
Boston, Massachusetts

Supplemental Content

Katherine Dickerson, MD, PhD
Resident Physician
Department of Emergency
  Medicine, Brigham and
  Women's Hospital
Boston, Massachusetts

Ancillary Contributors

**Richard J. Pryor, MD, ABEM,
FACEM**
Emergency Medicine Consultant
Wollongong, New South Wales,
  Australia

**William David Sadler, MS, RN,
NRP, CCRN, CFRN**
Flight Nurse/Paramedic
Survival Flight, Michigan
  Medicine
Ann Arbor, Michigan

**Sean G. Smith, MSc, BBA, BSN,
RN, NRP, C-NPT, FP-C/CCP-C,
CFRN/CTRN, CCRN-CMC**
Smith's Critical-Care/
  Critical-Care Professionals
  International
Durham, North Carolina;
  Philadelphia, Pennsylvania

Susan Truba, NRP, CCP-C
Ashburn, Virginia

Josh Weiner, FP-C, CCP-C
Flight Paramedic
Minneapolis, Minnesota

Reviewers

Jonathan A. Alford, NRP, CCEMTP
Virginia Commonwealth
    University, School of Medicine
Center for Trauma and Critical
    Care Education
Richmond, Virginia

Angela M. Atwood, MSN, RN, CFRN
Global Medical Response
Salt Lake City, Utah

Alan M. Batt, PhD, MSc, PGCME, CCP, FHEA
Fanshawe College
London, Ontario, Canada

Jason Baumgartner, RN, NRP/CCEMTP
Nicolet College
Rhinelander, Wisconsin

Jason Brooks, EdD, NRP
University of South Alabama
Mobile, Alabama

Jansen D. Casscles, EMT-P
Manlius Fire and EMS
Manlius, New York

Ann Crawford, PhD, MSN, RN, CNS, CEN, CPEN
University of Mary Hardin-Baylor
Belton, Texas
Baylor Scott & White Health
    McLane Children's Medical
    Center
Temple, Texas

Kevin Curry, NRP/CCEMTP
United Training Center
Lewiston, Maine

Adam C. Fritsch, NRP, CCP
Advanced Professional
    Healthcare Education LLC
Delafield, Wisconsin

Rudy Garrett, AS, NR-P, FP-C
Air Methods
Somerset, Kentucky

Mat Goebel, MD, MAS, NRP
Baystate Medical Center
Springfield, Massachusetts

James E. Gretz, MBA, NRP, CCP-C
JeffSTAT, Jefferson Health
Philadelphia, Pennsylvania

Kevin M. Gurney, MS, CCEMT-P, I/C
Delta Ambulance
Waterville, Maine

Kirk Hallett, RN, NREMT-P, CCT
Richmond, Virginia

Paul Hitchcock, NRP
Department of Homeland
    Security
Herndon, Virginia

Troy Hoover, NRP, CCP-C, FP-C
Air Idaho Rescue
Idaho Falls, Idaho

Timothy M. Kimble, BA, AAS, NRP, CEM
Washington Township
Waynesboro, Pennsylvania

Blake E. Klingle, MS, RN, CEN, CCEMT-P
Waukesha County Technical
    College
Pewaukee, Wisconsin

Karen "Keri" Wydner Krause, RN, EMT-P, CCRN
Lakeshore Technical College
Cleveland, Wisconsin

Monica Malec, MD
University of Chicago
Chicago, Illinois

Amanda McDonald, MA, NRP
University of South Alabama
Mobile, Alabama

Nicholas Miller, MS, NRP
EMS World and EMS Expo
St. Louis, Missouri

Charles Murphy, MS, NRP
National EMS Academy
Lafayette, Louisiana

Sue L. Parrigin, MSN, RN, NRP, CFRN
Global Medical Response
Hewitt, Texas

David S. Pecora, MS, PA-C, NRP
Bemidji EMS
Bemidji, Minnesota

Ernest K. Ralston, PhD
Center for Asymmetric
    Emergency Medicine
Centreville, Virginia

Wanda Roberts, RN, EMT-P
Rochelle, Georgia

Sean G. Smith, MSc, BBA, BSN, RN, NRP, C-NPT, FP-C/CCP-C, CFRN/CTRN, CCRN-CMC
Smith's Critical-Care/
    Critical-Care Professionals
    International
Durham, North Carolina;
    Philadelphia, Pennsylvania

Stephen Trala, RN, MPH, MSN, CFRN, NRP
The University of Vermont Health
    Network
Burlington, Vermont

Thomas (Tom) F. Watson, AS, AAS, Paramedic
Thomas Nelson Community
    College
Hampton, Virginia

Michael H. Wilhelm, DNP, APRN, CRNA
UConn Health, John Dempsey
    Hospital
Farmington, Connecticut

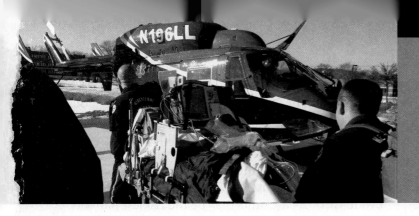

Chapter 1

Introduction and Overview of Critical Care Transport

Mike McEvoy, PhD, NRP, RN, CCRN

OBJECTIVES

After completing this chapter, you will be able to:

1. Define the terms *critical care, critical care transport, critical care patient,* and *critical care transport professional* (p 2).
2. Differentiate between interfacility and specialty care transport (p 2).
3. Describe the composition of the critical care transport team (p 3).
4. List the qualifications of members of a critical care transport team (pp 3–4).
5. Identify the modes of transportation used during critical care transports, including mobile (ground) units, rotor-wing aircraft, and fixed-wing aircraft (p 5).
6. Discuss the differences between the modes of transportation (p 5).
7. Discuss the advantages and disadvantages for each mode of transportation (pp 9–10).
8. Describe the role of dispatch in determining the mode of transportation (pp 5–7).
9. Describe the steps involved in the transport process (pp 7–9).
10. Discuss how the decision for ground transport versus air transport is made (p 9).
11. Describe the role of medical control in the critical care transport environment (pp 10–11).
12. Discuss state and national standards for critical care transport (pp 11–12).
13. Discuss reimbursement criteria and their relevance to critical care transport (p 12).
14. Identify sources of stress specific to the critical care transport professional and their signs (pp 12–14).
15. Discuss ways to ensure safety for both critical care transport professionals and their patients (p 14).
16. Discuss the importance of interpersonal communications with the patient and family members (pp 14–15).
17. Explain the process of quality assurance and improvement, and understand the importance of maintaining skills and knowledge (p 15).
18. Summarize the history of critical care transport, including both air and ground transport (pp 15–20).

Introduction
Trends in Patient Transportation

The continued evolution of health care has dramatically affected patient transportation. Notably, in recent times the emphasis on efficiency and cost containment has altered referral patterns and increased utilization of specialty centers. Payers and providers are increasingly referring patients with urgent conditions to alternative destinations such as clinics and freestanding emergency centers. Nurses, paramedics, and physicians routinely visit patients in their homes. Use of telemedicine skyrocketed during the coronavirus disease 2019 (COVID-19) pandemic, not only facilitating virtual house calls but also providing ready access to consultation by health care providers in the field or outlying facilities. Treatment of patients with costly and more complex conditions is being migrated to increasingly sophisticated specialty centers. As these facilities become more advanced, they are absorbing the workload of lower-volume specialty centers, many of which are closing because they were not designed for today's high patient volumes or cutting-edge procedures. Rural hospitals are also closing their doors, unable to cope with the regulatory burden of the 21st-century health care system.

Emergency medical services (EMS) are experiencing shifts in call types as more Americans obtain health insurance and their payers prioritize destinations for their care other than emergency departments (EDs). Closer scrutiny of costs and billing practices has also significantly curtailed ambulance and ambulette transport of patients for routine tests and procedures. At the same time, health insurance plans and accountable care organizations have a significant financial incentive to transport their insured patients back to contracted health care centers when they become injured or seriously ill outside of their home networks.

Even as emergency and routine ambulance and ambulette transports continue to decline, critical care transport (CCT) volumes have increased—and will continue to increase—exponentially. Moreover, the field of critical care has become increasingly complex. Critical care is intensive care and monitoring provided to patients with life-threatening conditions that require constant monitoring and treatment with drugs and equipment.

Despite our best intentions, health care is not always safe for the critical care patient. Unintentional harm and unnecessary deaths continue to occur at alarming rates. The larger the number of medications and the more complex the equipment being used, the greater the likelihood of an adverse event. Critical care units may be the riskiest patient care environments for patients. Because it lacks many of the common safety practices and technologies employed in critical care units, such as barcoded medication administration, independent double-checks, and readily accessible intensive care physicians (to name a few), the CCT setting may have an even greater potential for errors leading to patient harm. Indeed, significant adverse events—such as hypothermia, hypotension, drug errors, procedure errors, loss of vascular access, and ventilator and oxygen system malfunctions—frequently occur during these transports.

Transports once managed exclusively by physicians and nurses now rely on emergency medical technicians (EMTs) and paramedics to conduct them. Use of specialized teams with CCT training has been shown to decrease rates of adverse events in the transport of children and neonates. A growing body of evidence indicates that specialized CCT teams can also offer more competent and safer care to critically ill adults during transport. This text provides a core curriculum for the specialized and additional education needed to aid providers in bridging the gap from their respective educational foundations to the level of critical care transport professional (CCTP).

Definitions

The terms interfacility transport (IFT) and specialty care transport (SCT) are often used interchangeably when, in fact, they represent different types of CCT. IFT is the transport of a patient between two health care facilities. For health insurance billing claim purposes, definitions of facilities are typically obtained from the Centers for Medicare and Medicaid Services (CMS), because other health insurance plans in the United States often adopt CMS rules and definitions in administering their own plans. Health care "facilities," as defined by CMS, include skilled nursing facilities and hospitals that participate in the federal Medicare program. IFT, then, may involve transport between hospitals, between clinics and hospitals, between hospitals and reha-bilitation facilities, or between hospitals and long-term care facilities.

CMS defines SCT as the interfacility ground transport of a critically ill or injured patient, includ-ing provision of medically necessary supplies and services that are beyond the paramedic scope of practice. SCT is necessary, according to CMS, when a patient's condition requires ongoing care from providers in a specialty area such as emergency or critical care nursing, emergency medicine, respi-ratory care, or cardiovascular care, or from a para-medic with additional training. For a service to bill CMS for SCT, three conditions must be met: (1) the patient must be critically ill or injured, (2) the trans-port must be interfacility, and (3) the care provided must be beyond the scope of a paramedic. Thus, merely putting a nurse aboard an ambulance does not turn that transport into SCT, nor does moving a stable ventilator-dependent patient from a skilled nursing facility to a hospital meet the definition of SCT.

Setting the CMS definitions aside, CCT is a transport level of care provided to a patient with immediate life threats from injury or illness. Unlike the CMS definition of SCT, which specifies ground transport, the definition of CCT does not designate a specific mode of transportation. CCT requires a specialized body of knowledge and skills, an envi-ronment with the proper equipment, and ability above and beyond the intensive care unit (ICU) environment to address the specific challenges en-countered during transport.

This curriculum recognizes that CCT team composition varies considerably from one area to another and with respect to the resources and skills needed to transport each patient. Team members may include almost any health care provider with an expertise in caring for a particular CCT patient.

Critical Care Team Composition and Qualifications

Crew Configurations

The most common CCT crew configurations used in the United States employ various combinations of EMTs, paramedics, registered nurses (RNs), and respiratory therapists (RTs). Crew configurations

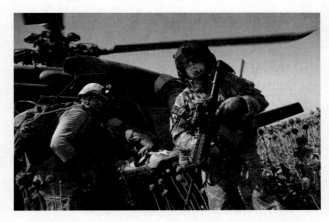

FIGURE 1-1 The CCT team composition varies depending on staffing policies, state requirements, scopes of practice, and patient needs.
© Kevin Frayer/AP/Shutterstock.

depend largely on the staffing policy of the organi-zation, state requirements, scopes of practice, and patient needs **FIGURE 1-1**. Additional crew mem-bers, including perfusionists, surgeons, neonatolo-gists, or pediatric intensivists, may be required for certain patient transports.

A three-member team configuration is some-times used, but is less common than the two-member crew because of the increased costs associated with adding a third staff member as well as the space and weight limitations of some transport vehicles. Most patients requiring CCT do not have a condition that necessitates a third team member.

Educational Qualifications

Just as crew configurations vary, so do the recom-mended educational qualifications for each team member. CCTPs must be able to provide care at the same, or higher, level than their non-CCT counter-parts. In addition, they must be educated and profi-cient in the following skills:

- Advanced practice procedures, such as man-aging surgical airways or performing an escharotomy
- Management of chest tubes
- Blood product administration
- Intracranial pressure monitoring
- Mechanical circulatory support
- Central line management
- Invasive arterial and cardiac pressure monitoring

- Interpretation of lab test results and diagnostic imaging
- Use and troubleshooting of ventilators
- Use of a variety of invasive catheters, tubes, and drains
- Management of pacemakers
- Use of portable ultrasonography

Many of these devices and procedures may not be covered by CCTPs' formal medical education.

Because critical care medicine is a dynamic, ever-changing science, CCTPs must be lifelong learners. Most CCT programs require CCTPs to complete frequent continuing professional education classes, which exceed the requirements to maintain the state or national certification and/or licensure necessary for employment. Most CCT services hold a variety of mandatory educational and competency training days each year. Objectives of these sessions include reviewing uncommonly used advanced procedures, validating skills and competencies, simulating case-based scenarios, and disseminating cutting-edge clinical information.

Types of CCTPs

Emergency Medical Technicians

An EMT is trained at the basic life support level and frequently operates the emergency transport vehicle. This position requires completion of an EMT course and current EMT certification by the state in which the person practices. Under the current National EMS Education Standards, most EMT courses require roughly 148 hours to complete. Employers and states may mandate additional requirements. Because the EMT role involves driving the CCT team, training in the form of an emergency vehicle operator course (EVOC) is highly recommended. Like all health care providers, an EMT should maintain current certification and proficiency in cardiopulmonary resuscitation (CPR).

Paramedics

Paramedics are trained at the advanced life support level. They may be the primary CCTP, or they may work with an RN or another paramedic-level provider. This position requires completion of a paramedic course and current paramedic certification in the state in which the person is practicing. Some states require certification by the National Registry for EMTs as a Nationally Registered Paramedic (NRP) to attain state paramedic certification. Most paramedic courses meeting the current National EMS Education Standards encompass some 1,200 hours of didactic and clinical time, in addition to demonstrating competency. Beginning in 2013, paramedic program graduates seeking National Registry of EMTs certification must have graduated from a program that is approved by their state and accredited by the Commission on Accreditation of Allied Health Education Programs (CAAHEP). Not all states require their approved paramedic programs to be accredited by the CAAHEP. Given that many CCTP programs desire paramedics with NRP certification, however, prospective CCTP candidates should verify that the paramedic program they apply to is CAAHEP accredited.

Many programs require paramedic CCTPs to have at least 5 years' experience in a busy 9-1-1 EMS system and hold specialty certifications in basic, advanced, pediatric, and neonatal life support, as well as basic and prehospital trauma life support. In addition, they should have successfully completed a sanctioned CCT course of training.

Registered Nurses

RNs are licensed health care providers. In a CCT service, RNs may be the primary CCTP, or they may work with another RN or paramedic provider. This position requires completion of a state-approved nursing program and licensure by the state in which the person is practicing. Obtaining licensure requires successful completion of the National Council Licensure Examination for Registered Nurses (NCLEX-RN), which is administered by the National Council of State Boards of Nursing.

Programs frequently require RN CCTPs to have at least 5 years' experience in a combination of the following areas: critical care, emergency nursing, and prehospital care. They should also hold specialty certifications in basic, advanced, pediatric, and neonatal life support; have completed an advanced trauma nursing course; and preferably hold an emergency, flight, ground transport, or critical care nursing specialty certification. Many CCTP programs desire or require CCTP RNs to have paramedic certification as well, since paramedics' training and scope of practice differ significantly from those of nurses.

Respiratory Therapists, Perfusionists, and Physicians

When patient needs dictate their inclusion, RTs, perfusionists, and advanced providers such as nurse practitioners or physician assistants, physicians, or surgeons may be members of the CCT team. Rarely are these providers permanent members of the CCT team; instead, they typically join the CCT crew on an as-needed basis. The institutions or practices that employ these providers credential them, verify their education and licensing, and often monitor their practice. It is important to remember that non-CCTP providers accompanying a CCT team on transport are likely clinical experts in management of a specific patient problem or technology but rarely have equivalent experience operating in the harsh and often adverse transport environment. They typically require assistance in preplanning for anticipated complications related to transport.

Modes of Transportation

Modes of transportation vary widely from agency to agency and by region of the country. The optimal transportation mode is dictated by patient acuity, distance between the sending and receiving facilities, ability of the transport service to respond, weather conditions, and the topography of the region. The standard types of mobile intensive care units used for CCT include ground units, rotor-wing aircraft, and fixed-wing aircraft. Commonalities among these transportation modes include availability of standard equipment, adequate room for specialty equipment and providers to deliver patient care, compliance with safety standards, electrical power, adequate lighting systems, and reliable communication systems with redundant backup.

Equipment

States have specific equipment requirements for transport vehicles, and professional organizations interested in CCT publish lists of recommended additional equipment. The additional and specialty equipment carried on a CCT vehicle must fit the mission profile of the CCT service. It is particularly important that electrical power systems such as generators or inverters are readily accessible for troubleshooting should power issues arise during transport.

Mobile Units

Mobile (ground) units, commonly referred to simply as ambulances, are typically used to transport critically ill or injured patients for distances of up to 50 miles (80 km). They may be used for greater distances when the transport is not time critical. A ground unit may also be used when a patient has contraindications to air transport. Ground units are available in a wide variety of configurations, body types, and sizes to suit the needs of the specific provider.

Rotor-Wing Aircraft

Rotor-wing aircraft, commonly called helicopters, are used to transport critically ill and injured patients in rural and difficult-to-access settings; they can travel for distances of up to 150 miles (240 km). A wide variety of helicopters are available for use, including the BK 117, Bell Model 220/230, Sikorsky S-76, AgustaWestland AW109, and Dauphin **FIGURE 1-2**. These helicopters can be single- or twin-engine models. Depending on the design, patients may be loaded from the side or the rear of the aircraft. As with ambulances, the size and type of helicopter varies by program needs and the area serviced.

Fixed-Wing Aircraft

Fixed-wing aircraft, or planes, are typically used to transport critically ill or injured patients for distances of 150 miles (240 km) or more. These aircraft are often used in combination with mobile critical care units, which transport patients to the aircraft take-off site **FIGURE 1-3**.

For further discussion of the types of aircraft used in CCT, see Chapter 4, *Aircraft Fundamentals and Flight Physiology*.

The Transport Process
Dispatch

Dispatch is the first point of contact for the CCT team. The dispatch center may reside within a hospital, in a 9-1-1 center, or at a remote, independent site. Regardless of its location, the initial triage process starts with the dispatch center's call taker. The call taker typically follows a standard question template to obtain information

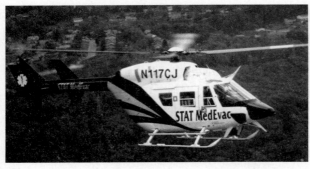

A

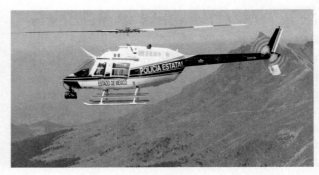

B

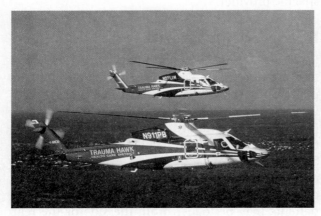

C

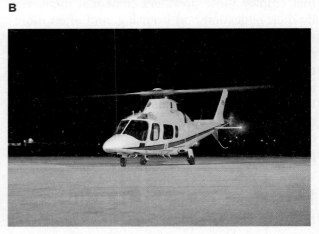

D

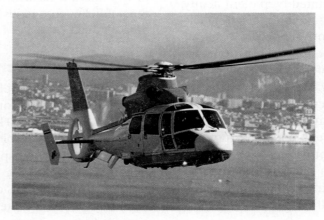

E

FIGURE 1-2 The various types of helicopters used for CCT include some of those shown here. **A.** BK 117. **B.** Bell Model 206. **C.** Sikorsky S-76. **D.** AW109. **E.** Dauphin.

about the patient and their condition from the referring facility. Call-taking checklists ensure dispatchers cover all relevant information so providers can arrive fully prepared, but also so the sending facility can properly prepare the patient for transport. Pertinent information that should be obtained from the referring facility includes the following:

- Patient age
- Patient weight
- Diagnosis

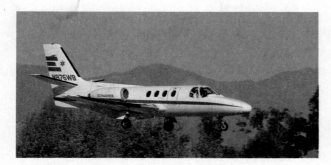

FIGURE 1-3 Fixed-wing aircraft are used for longer transports.

© Ralph Duenas/www.jetwashimages.com.

- Number and type of infusions
- Most recent vital signs
- Level of consciousness
- Airway status (patent or intubated)
- Presence of mechanical ventilation
- Presence of mechanical circulatory support devices

Although this list is not all-inclusive, it does provide dispatch center personnel with adequate information for making the proper decisions. Once this information is obtained, a clinical supervisor or algorithm should be used to help select the most appropriate crew configuration and mode of transportation. Often, the attending physician and staff at the referring facility suggest a particular mode of transportation. Many CCT services honor these requests, whereas others make their own determination based on the patient report provided.

Dispatch centers should also be cognizant of certain equipment, medications, or infusions described when taking IFT calls. The following information should raise a flag for the call taker that the transport likely requires a CCT team:

- Mechanical ventilation
- Infusions running into vascular access devices
- Vasoactive medications
- Blood or blood product infusions (eg, blood, plasma, platelets, cryofibrinogen)
- Mechanical circulatory support devices (eg, intra-aortic balloon pump, extracorporeal membrane oxygenation, ventricular-assist device)
- Patient instability requiring frequent interventions such as sedation, paralytics, or analgesia

Transport Choreography

Communication breakdowns are the root cause of many, if not most, adverse outcomes for patients during CCT. Communication begins with the receipt of a request for transport. Dispatch center staff talk directly with a referral source to obtain medical details, insurance information, and demographic information needed to prioritize the request, determine patient acuity, and assign appropriate resources (equipment and personnel) to the transport.

Transport choreography starts on receipt of a request for transport. Just as it is inadvisable to respond to a 9-1-1 call without knowing the location and type of call, it is inadvisable to roll into a hospital without obtaining details about the patient and equipment needed in advance. Knowing what you are walking into helps you prepare for that situation. A well-choreographed approach to each transport will make the move safer and improve patient outcomes.

Time Frame

The response following the receipt of a request for CCT may vary depending on the circumstances. Some contracts between transport services and referring hospitals specify response times, whereas other facilities rely on the availability and staffing of the service to meet their needs. In general, the critically ill nature of the typical CCT patient suggests a need for the CCT team to arrive within 60 minutes from the time of request. Referring facilities, however, may request a longer or shorter interval depending on patient needs, tests or procedures in progress, and the receiving facility's availability to accept the patient.

The generally accepted time frame for a CCT team to receive the report from the handoff team, package the patient, and begin moving the patient to the transport vehicle is 20 minutes. In situations where additional interventions or procedures are needed to stabilize or prepare the patient for transport, bedside times may be longer. Evidence suggests that extended bedside times are associated with worse patient outcomes. Meeting the 20-minute standard is no easy feat when a complex critical care patient is attached to a variety of medical devices and equipment. It takes practice and skill to achieve this goal.

Planning for the Patient Transfer

Planning should begin on arrival at the referring facility. Always maintain situational awareness of the ingress and egress pathways at this facility, and later at the receiving facility. Failure to plan for the dimensions of these pathways could result in problems with equipment or machinery accompanying the patient not fitting through doorways, preventing you from smoothly exiting the referring facility and accessing your transport vehicle.

Handoff Considerations

Handoff refers to the brief report that staff at the sending facility—generally the bedside nurse, physician, or care provider currently responsible for the patient—submits to the CCTP team when they arrive to accept responsibility for the patient's care. There is no standardized handoff practice between hospital staff and CCTPs; however, safety experts and accreditation bodies recommend that agencies and providers incorporate standardized practices into their routines, including use of checklists. Equipment checklists help avoid omissions so providers will have all the tools and supplies required to manage the patient's condition during transport.

Communicating With Hospital Personnel

It cannot be overemphasized that the worlds of CCT and EMS are far removed from those of the ED and inpatient hospital practitioners. While the medications and care provided are similar, the equipment and practices employed by CCTPs are as unfamiliar to hospital personnel as hospital practices are to CCTPs.

The handoff should include medical records from the sending facility and physician orders for the patient during transport, which are usually accompanied by a physician certification statement (PCS) that documents the reasons for transfer, the potential risks and benefits of the transfer, and the patient's current condition(s). Medical records from the sending facility are sent not only for reference by the receiving facility, but also so the CCTP can confirm the information presented during handoff

and answer specific questions not addressed during the handoff that may arise during transport.

Your CCTP team must quickly make two determinations during the handoff: (1) Are the patient's needs within your scope of practice? and (2) Will you be able to safely manage this patient during transport? Certain red flags may become evident during the initial report, warranting further questioning and planning:

- The referring provider tells you that other transport services refused the transfer.
- The medications or equipment required are beyond your training, experience, or scope of practice.
- There is no recent charting on the patient by nursing or medical staff.
- The sending providers seem unfamiliar with the patient.
- Inconsistencies exist between the dispatch information and the information provided during the handoff.
- The patient appears much sicker than described during dispatch, possibly even too sick to move.

In any of these situations, you should consult with not only the sending physician but also your own online medical control/consultation (OLMC) before moving the patient. The two most common sources of poor patient outcomes and resulting litigation involving CCT are failure to consult OLMC and inability of the CCTP to recognize or manage patient deterioration during transfer.

Initiating Transport

Once a cursory handoff has been accomplished, the crew can meet the patient/family and begin transferring care. Typically the equipment and stretcher are prepared and the patient is moved to the transport stretcher before transferring the ventilator, infusions, and other devices to the transport equipment. This approach allows all providers to continue discussing and assessing the patient's status while the patient is still attached to hospital equipment. Thus, hospital staff or CCTPs can properly position the patient and administer any necessary sedatives or analgesics needed to maintain the patient's current level of comfort. Once the patient is comfortable and stable, the ventilator, infusions, and other machinery attached to the patient can be assessed, prepared, and transferred to the equivalent transport devices. CCTP providers must remember that once they begin transferring hospital equipment, machinery, and infusions to their transport devices, they have assumed responsibility for the patient.

To avoid errors, two providers should check ventilator or respiratory device settings and compare these settings to both the transfer orders and the hospital's settings at the time of transfer. A CCTP should read the labels on each IV being infused, trace the infusion line toward the patient, and label the distal end with the name of the medication or fluid. Providers should conduct a "pull-away" test in which they move the transport equipment 1 or 2 feet and carefully examine all tubing, plugs, and cables to ensure everything previously connected to hospital equipment has been successfully reconnected to the transport devices.

As noted earlier, problems occur quite frequently during CCT. Anticipating those problems and being prepared to address them require interpersonal as well as technical skills. During handoff, ask the hospital providers about any anticipated issues during transfer. Personnel caring for the patient want to see the good care they have provided continued and the best possible patient outcomes achieved. They may offer valuable insights into titration of infusions, positioning, and management of the patient, based on their experiences caring for this person. Make your best calculations about necessary oxygen, medications, fluids, electrical needs, and battery power. Any shortages can lead to poor patient outcomes. Anticipate and plan for equipment failures or accidental dislodgements of tubes, drains, venous access, or other lines. Subsequent chapters will address specific concerns associated with ventilators, pacemakers, and mechanical circulatory support devices during transport.

Transporting by Ground Versus Air

Each mode of transporting critically ill and injured patients has its own set of advantages and disadvantages. **TABLE 1-1** lists some of the advantages and disadvantages of each mode.

The decision to transport a patient by ground ambulance or helicopter should be made as rapidly as possible. In most cases, the CCT patient needs expedient transport to a tertiary care center that can provide care not available at the present location. Helicopters allow for more rapid transport than ground vehicles because they can bypass vehicular traffic, intersections, and traffic signals, which might otherwise delay the total transport time. Nevertheless, even though a helicopter travels much faster than a ground ambulance, it is not always the most practical solution for transporting a patient to a tertiary care center. Helicopters are usually strategically located throughout a geographic area. Depending on the location of the referring hospital, a helicopter may have a lengthy travel time to reach the patient. At times, a helicopter may already be committed to another mission, significantly extending the response time. In such situations, a critical care ground ambulance may be significantly closer; thus, the most reasonable solution may be ground transportation.

Patient acuity is another major determinant of whether to transport by ground or by air. The referring physician, who remains responsible for the patient until care is transferred to the CCTP team, typically makes this decision. Time-sensitive conditions that may require air transport include the following:

- Acute myocardial infarction
- Acute cerebrovascular accident
- Severe traumatic injury
- Acute intracranial hemorrhage
- Surgical emergency (eg, acute aortic dissection, amputation requiring limb reattachment)
- Major burns

This list is not all-inclusive, and many other conditions and situations are particularly relevant when selecting the transportation mode. Each case must be evaluated individually, and a determination made after all data have been reviewed.

Because practical considerations might preclude use of the preferred transportation mode, an alternative transport method must be identified to ensure the patient will arrive at the accepting facility within a reasonable time frame. For example, a clinical coordinator could decide to transport a patient by helicopter or fixed-wing service, but bad weather might rule out flight. Sending a ground unit may be more harmful to the patient due to the extended time needed to reach the accepting facility. In most such cases, providers opt to wait for the weather to

TABLE 1-1 Advantages and Disadvantages of Transportation Modes

Transportation Mode	Advantages	Disadvantages
Mobile (ground) unit	• Large interior • Quieter than aircraft • No special vehicle housing needed • Less expensive to operate and maintain • Less specialized training needed to operate vehicle (emergency vehicle operator course) • Multiple provider capabilities • Less weather dependent • Fewer height and weight limitations • Fewer adverse effects on patient and crew	• Usually limited to single-patient transport • Slower than aircraft • Limited travel distance
Rotor-wing aircraft (helicopter)	• Speed (100–180 mph) • Specialized personnel and technology needed or provided • Few altitude ramifications below 2,000 ft (610 m) • Can service a larger catchment area • Two-patient capabilities	• Restricted by weather conditions • Interior space limitations • Expensive to operate and maintain • Special landing requirements • Need for FAA communications • Adverse effects on crew members and patients • Expensive for patient • Requires special vehicle housing • Limited space for providers and equipment • Weight limitations
Fixed-wing aircraft (plane)	• Speed • Multiple-patient capabilities • Capable of traveling great distances • Specialized personnel and technology needed or provided • No weight limitations • Instrument-assisted flying	• Adverse altitude considerations • Adverse effects on patient and crew • Need for FAA communications • Expensive for patient • Expensive to operate and maintain • Can serve only a small portion of the community • Requires special vehicle housing • Special landing requirements

Abbreviation: FAA, Federal Aviation Administration

© Jones & Bartlett Learning.

improve and launch the aircraft as soon as is practical. When the distance from the sending facility to the accepting facility is not lengthy, the CCTP team may choose to complete the mission by ground.

Helicopter Shopping

Helicopter shopping, a practice defined by the Federal Aviation Administration (FAA) as "the practice of calling, in sequence, various operators until an operator agrees to take a flight assignment, without sharing with subsequent operators the reasons the flight was declined by previously called operators," is often cited as a contributing factor in fatal air medical crashes.

Medical Oversight

The complexities encountered in CCT patients require a very sophisticated level of care and an equally high level of medical direction. It is imperative that the service medical director has an active role in all aspects of the service that relate to patient care. In addition to a comprehensive set of triage, treatment, and transport protocols that include standing orders for the CCT team, OLMC must be available to CCTPs at all times **FIGURE 1-4**. OLMC can be helpful when CCTPs find it necessary to exceed or deviate from written protocols or standing orders; when unforeseen or unpredictable situations arise during CCT; in situations where patient complexity exceeds

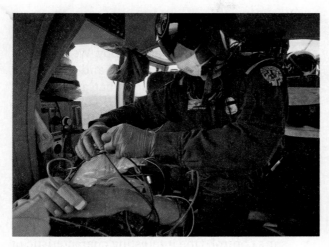

FIGURE 1-4 Online medical control involves working directly with a medical control physician via phone or radio.
© Mark C. Ide.

that ordinarily encountered; and in circumstances where CCTPs are unable to reach agreement with a sending or accepting provider regarding orders for patient care during transport.

While EMS physicians typically serve as medical directors for transport services, CCT may require expertise and experience outside the scope of an EMS-trained physician's practice. Depending on the breadth of services delivered and the equipment used, CCT services may require intensive care physicians (intensivists), critical care physicians, surgeons, or anesthesiologists to assist in providing medical control and oversight of their transports. Often, several physicians may need to work collaboratively to provide CCT medical control and oversight. Medical oversight is equally important in examining outcomes, the effects of care provided, the efficiency and compliance with processes in place, and all aspects of the service's quality assurance and improvement programs.

State and National Standards

In the United States, standards for CCT vary considerably from state to state. Most CCT programs follow national standards for training and equipment issued by professional organizations with an interest in CCT. As mentioned previously, the CMS describes SCT as requiring care beyond the paramedic's scope of practice.

Although individual states may define the specific training required for a paramedic to qualify

as a CCT provider, not all states have such requirements. In the absence of state requirements, CMS relies on regional and sometimes even agency-level requirements. Some states, such as Maryland, require any air medical service that operates in the state to be certified by the Commission on Accreditation of Medical Transport Systems (CAMTS). In most states, however, a state organization governs the licensure or certification of air medical services and their practitioners. For example, in Pennsylvania, the Department of Health licenses air medical transport services and prehospital care providers.

A CCTP's scope of practice may also vary according to their level of certification and the state in which they practice. For example, RNs may administer nearly any medication ordered by a licensed prescriber, whereas paramedics are often restricted to medications approved and listed in their protocols or their state's prehospital formulary. The most accurate information on regulations governing organizations and scope of practice is available from the state agency responsible for EMS accreditation and licensure.

The National EMS Scope of Practice Model outlines a framework under which all EMS providers, including CCTPs, operate. There are four elements in this model:

- **Education.** Cognitive, psychomotor, and affective learning that a person must undergo to act as a provider
- **Certification.** External verification of competencies that a provider has achieved through examination
- **Licensure.** Legal authority granted to an individual by the state to perform certain activities
- **Credentialing.** Clinical determination from a physician medical director that a provider is authorized to perform a skill or role

By the time EMS providers become CCTPs, they have already completed this process for their paramedic and/or nursing licensure, but they must continue to engage in professional development throughout their career. Sometimes a person might move from one state to another and need to become licensed there, or the person was credentialed to perform a certain procedure for a former employer, through the medical director, but is not credentialed at a new service. Providers must embrace education and training throughout their career.

There are no national consensus standards on CCT training courses, likely owing to the wide variation in CCT practices. The scope of services can range from transporting a mechanically ventilated patient with an arterial line and chest tube and several intravenous (IV) infusions to transporting a patient on extracorporeal membrane oxygenation with a dozen IV infusions. The typical level of care provided drives the additional training that CCTPs undergo. In general, a basic course covering the fundamentals of CCT requires at least 80 hours of additional training.

Reimbursement

Ambulance transport is expensive, and air medical transport is *very* expensive. CCT is even more costly than routine transport. In many cases, insurance reimbursement does not adequately cover transport costs, especially when overhead and operational expenses are factored in. The complexities of reimbursement, from determining the need for CCT to selecting the closest appropriate receiving facility and beyond, exceed the scope of this clinical text. Suffice it to say that health care reimbursement is undergoing a major shift from paying for care delivered to paying for health outcomes achieved. It is only a matter of time before quality and outcomes measures are connected to CCT reimbursement.

Well-Being

Well-being, according to the Centers for Disease Control and Prevention, is "a positive outcome that is meaningful for people and for many sectors of society, because it tells us that people perceive that their lives are going well"; it indicates that people are comfortable, healthy, and happy. Well-being is also a course component in EMT and paramedic programs, and the same tenets that apply to patients apply to the CCTP.

Resilience, a person's ability to withstand negative pressure, or "bounce back" from difficulties, is associated with maintaining well-being. The three key determinants of personal resilience are thought to be biology (genetics), attachment, and control.

- *Genetics* is a component of a person's biologic makeup and generally is not under the person's control. One interesting characteristic of CCTPs, which is shared by paramedics and the nurses and physicians who work in ICUs, is the tendency for other family members to work in the same or similar high-stress occupations. This familial connection suggests there is a genetic predisposition toward resilience.
- *Attachment* refers to a person's capacity to bond or form significant relationships with others. Associated with this aspect of personal resilience is the capacity for empathy, a characteristic commonly seen in CCTPs.
- *Control* refers to the degree of mastery a person feels over their environment, social competence, self-esteem, autonomy, and sense of purpose in life.

Providers can maintain and even improve their sense of wellness by supporting these foundations of resilience. Encouraging the development of these building blocks in coworkers, patients, and children helps to facilitate resilience in others as well.

Stress

Stress is often defined as the reaction of the mind or body to a demand for change. Stress is both physical and psychological; that is, physical stress such as that resulting from a traumatic injury always has a psychological component. Conversely, psychological stress, such as that resulting from an argument with a coworker, invariably has a physical component.

We obviously need some level of stress to remain alive, and virtually any stressor will affect people differently. There is a tendency, especially among people in high-stress occupations, to associate stress with negative happenings. This is an incorrect assumption: Social scientists have long known that joyous life events, such as getting married, getting a new job, buying a new home, and celebrating holidays, are just as stressful as unpleasant events, such as death of a spouse, termination from a job, jail sentence, or traffic crash. The need to assess all life events for their stress-inducing value is important for CCTPs, whose role entails unpredictable events that could be significant stressors. Managing life stress by spreading out controllable events such as job changes, marriage, home buying, and vacations can allow leeway for managing the stress associated with these unpredictable job-related events. Focusing on such cumulative stress is important for each of us, as stress tolerance varies from person to person.

Stress in the CCTP most likely encompasses a combination of the same stressors seen in field EMS providers and the stressors most often reported by ICU personnel. The most frequently reported stressor by field EMS providers is poorly managed organizations. Critical care nurses most commonly cite negative interactions with coworkers.

Curiously, people who choose to work in high-stress occupations—such as CCTPs, paramedics, ICU nurses, surgeons, and airline pilots—have key personality differences from the average citizen. The primary difference is an innate addiction to the hormone adrenaline, or a sense of happiness resulting from events that elevate blood levels of adrenaline. Most people, when experiencing high levels of adrenaline, become anxious, fearful, and uneasy; they are often terrified, in fact—quite the opposite of happiness. Therein lies a character insight that few appreciate: Not every person is suited to work in a high-stress occupation. Indeed, many people are unable to perform in a fast-paced, high-stress environment. The relatively few members of a society who enjoy the stress associated with the release of catecholamines (such as adrenaline) are the same people who tend to be successful at high-stress occupations, such as CCTPs.

CCTPs need a solid personal stress management program and resources they can avail themselves of when they encounter extremely stressful situations at work. Some suggestions for a personal stress management program include the following:

- *Condition your mind and body.* Maintaining a healthy weight and diet, including participation in a regular exercise program, helps avert injury in the very physically demanding job of a CCTP. Moreover, it induces a mental feeling of well-being that correlates with good physical health and fitness.
- *Listen to your inner voice.* In his book *The Gift of Fear*, Gavin de Becker interviewed survivors of violent crimes and concluded that they, like most members of society, had learned to suppress intuitive thoughts that could have alerted them to danger. Becoming more in touch with their inner voice helps alert CCTPs to potential stressors and helps them avoid bad situations before they become worse.
- *Never stop growing and learning.* Critical care is a constantly changing and evolving science and art. Staying current with trends and new technologies helps CCTPs achieve a sense of mastery over their work. They are present at the darkest moments of other people's lives—an experience that few others are privileged to have. CCTPs can glean life lessons from these experiences, if they choose to.
- *Be positive.* Interactions with others often affect the CCTP's mood. Likewise, how the CCTP interacts with others has a greater influence on the overall work environment than the CCTP might imagine. Spoken words can be either positive or negative. Positivity and a sense of humor create a highly desirable work environment.
- *Have a life outside of your work.* Balance is important in any profession, but it is particularly important in high-stress professions. Activities and friendships outside of work help CCTPs relax and view the world from a different perspective.

Recommendations for acute stress situations involving emergency responders such as CCTPs have evolved considerably over the years. **Critical incident stress debriefing (CISD)**—an approach favored since the 1980s to manage the psychological aftereffects in emergency personnel after particularly distressing responses—has now been largely replaced by the principles of **psychological first aid (PFA)**. CISD requires a specially trained team and has the potential to create iatrogenic harm from mandatory attendance, practitioner error, mixing of groups, and a variety of preexisting conditions that may unknowingly be present in participants. In contrast, PFA is implemented within the workplace by management and coworkers with an emphasis on encouraging personal resilience.

Unquestionably, every emergency responder and CCTP should have access to professional assistance with stress management. Every CCTP program should have a protocol for action following a serious event, availability of an employee assistance program (EAP) for employees and their families, a department chaplain, screening tools that supervisors and coworkers can use to assess employees when a concern arises, and educational resources for employees and their families on dealing with acute stress situations. The ready availability of EAP services is crucial. CCTPs are not immune to routine life stressors or personal difficulties such as marriage, family, financial, or substance use problems, all of which may considerably impair their ability to function in this high-stress occupation.

Safety

Personal safety is a crucial issue for all CCTPs, and one that feeds directly into well-being. CCTPs may work in a variety of hazardous environments, either in the external environment or within the confines of the transport vehicle. Consequently, appropriate safety gear and clothing are necessities for every member of the CCT crew. CCTPs should ensure that they properly and consistently wear the appropriate safety gear (eg, personal protective equipment [PPE], N95 mask) and clothing **FIGURE 1-5**. At a minimum, safety gear should meet the following criteria:

- Clothing should fit properly, and flight clothing should be flame retardant. Clothing should include a uniform or flight suit, outerwear such as a coat or vest, and undergarments. Clothing should never be tight or loose fitting.
- Clothing should be layered for proper ventilation and heat regulation. Long-sleeved shirts and pants limit water loss and reduce the potential for exposures.
- Head and eye protection should fit snugly and meet or exceed Occupational Safety and Health Administration (OSHA) specifications.
- Leather boots should be worn to protect feet against the elements and fire. Flame-retardant gloves should be available to protect hands against the elements and fire.
- Uniforms should have reflective materials or striping to increase nighttime visibility of CCTPs at crash scenes or when it becomes necessary to exit the transport vehicle on a roadway.

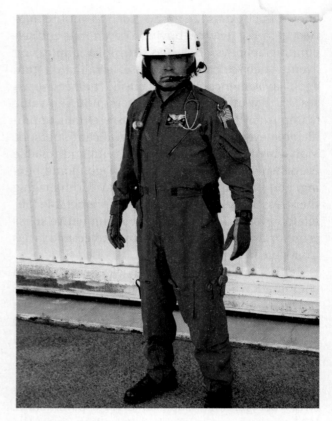

FIGURE 1-5 Proper safety gear and clothing, including snug-fitting head and eye protection, leather boots, and flame-retardant gloves. Layers should be worn underneath the uniform and for additional protection. If involved in scene transports, the CCTP uniform should also include reflective material or striping.

© Jones & Bartlett Learning.

Interpersonal Communication

Communicating effectively with patients, families, and other health care providers may be the most important determinant of how competent and capable a CCTP is perceived to be. Rarely, if ever, does a patient survey praise a provider's evident proficiency in starting an IV line or safely drawing up and administering a medication. Instead, compliments, and indeed criticisms, most often center on how personable, concerned, friendly, and communicative a provider or CCTP team was (or was not) with the patient, family, and others. No matter how acutely ill a patient is, members of the CCT team must make every effort to communicate their assessment of the situation and plan of care to the patient and family.

Communication starts with an introduction of each team member. These simple introductions help comfort patients and families. When family members desire, they should be in the room when the team assesses the patient.

When preparing to depart with the patient, providers should give family members time to speak briefly with the patient and should answer any questions they have. Requests for a brief prayer by members of the clergy or others should be honored. Although every second counts when transporting critically ill or injured patients, such brief moments spent supporting family involvement have positive effects that words cannot describe.

Quality Assurance and Improvement

A quality assurance and improvement (QA&I) program is an essential part of the overall health care system in the United States. The primary function of such a program is to generate data that are then used to improve the quality of service provided. Thus, a QA&I program is an integral component of a successful CCT program. CCTPs regularly provide advanced care to the "sickest of the sick," often in uncontrolled, unpredictable environments. An effective QA&I program serves as a checks-and-balances system to protect stakeholders.

Once financial and human resources are devoted to a QA&I program, the first step is to define quality. Many CCT programs use their mission statement to define what quality means to their stakeholders. Once this definition is in place, measurable indicators of quality must be established and baseline data must be obtained.

The second step is to collect and analyze data. Data can be obtained from various sources. Most CCT programs obtain data, at a minimum, from patient charts, dispatch records, and customer feedback surveys. Once obtained, these data must then be analyzed for meaning and application to the program's goals, objectives, and indicators of quality.

The third step in the QA&I process focuses on improving quality, which requires use of the data analysis results and development of an understanding of underlying issues. For example, if an audit of patient charts reveals that several CCTPs are incorrectly documenting the use of transport ventilators, and analysis of the reason for the incorrect documentation reveals a lack of knowledge, a continuing professional education course on effective documentation for ventilator-dependent patients can be conducted. The QA&I program should direct the continuing professional education for transport program staff.

Benchmarking is a popular concept in quality circles and has considerable value to any CCT program. It is extremely helpful for an agency to participate in shared databases and to seek out opportunities to compare the service's own data against the data from other CCT programs. Without the ability to compare and contrast findings to others in the industry, the QA&I program will operate in a vacuum and might venture off on the wrong track.

Two sets of metrics widely used by CCT programs are the Ground Air Medical qUality Transport (GAMUT) database and the National EMS Quality Alliance (NEMSQA) statistics. GAMUT is a free resource for transport teams offered by the GAMUT Quality Improvement Collaborative. NEMSQA publishes quality metrics specific to EMS. Both gather and analyze quality-related data from a broad sample of the CCTP community, then disseminate metrics based on these data that individual services can use to benchmark themselves against other services.

Since 2007, quality activities across the health care spectrum have been driven by the Triple Aim framework developed by the Institute of Healthcare Improvement. The three aims for optimizing health care system performance are improving the patient care experience, improving the health of the population, and simultaneously reducing per capita health care costs. Quality metrics, increasingly tied to reimbursement, are often organized around this framework.

The History of CCT

To fully appreciate the current state of CCT, it is important to recognize how this industry evolved over time. Methods for transporting critical care patients have evolved from horse-drawn carts in the 17th century, to the use of hot-air balloons, to the use of ground, rotor-wing, and fixed-wing vehicles today. As transport methods and equipment advance, it becomes possible to safely move increasingly sicker patients between health care facilities. The skills and equipment used by CCTPs are sometimes requested for 9-1-1 scene responses, recognizing that critically ill patients are not just confined to health care facilities but can be encountered anywhere an EMS system responds. Additionally, routine transfers of patients with high-technology home-based or skilled-nursing medical devices such as ventilators and infusion pumps often fall within the purview of the CCTP. These calls not only help to maintain the CCTP's proficiency, but also provide for greater patient safety, as they tend to be high-risk, low-frequency patient encounters for the non-CCTP.

Ground Transport

Early methods of patient transportation were developed out of necessity to reduce the high rates of morbidity and mortality among soldiers. Later, the same modes of transportation were used to move critically ill and injured patients to facilities that could provide more definitive care. The first record of moving injured patients was in the 11th century during the Crusades by the Knights of St. John. The Knights of St. John treated and transported injured soldiers after learning about first aid procedures from Arab and Greek physicians—a service that is considered the birth of the first emergency medical providers. At the same time, any soldier who carried an injured comrade to receive medical treatment would receive a small monetary reward.

Ground transportation was first used to evacuate injured soldiers in 1792, during the French Revolution. A surgeon in the French army, Dominique Jean Larrey, noticed that many of his countrymen lay wounded on the battlefield for as long as 36 hours until they were evacuated by fourgons, or multihorse wagons **FIGURE 1-6**. This delay in transport resulted in the death and disability of many soldiers, which Larrey found unacceptable.

Larrey designed and produced several two- and four-wheeled carts called *ambulance volantes* (flying ambulances), which were both fast and maneuverable **FIGURE 1-7**. These carts were used to transport surgeons and equipment to the battlefield to give first aid and then return the wounded to nearby field hospitals. Larrey's flying ambulance was the first recorded use of an evacuation system to help improve the survival rates of soldiers. He is also credited with creating the first official army medical corps using stretchers, handcarts, and wagons as a means of transporting injured patients.

The surgeon Jonathan Letterman instituted the first US ambulance service in 1862 during the Civil War at the Battle of Antietam. As director of the Army of the Potomac, Letterman developed a plan for an integrated medical treatment and evacuation system with its own vehicles, facilities, and personnel **FIGURE 1-8**. This system, which became known as the Ambulance Corps, was the basis of Army medical doctrine. On June 23, 1917, the US Army Ambulance Service was established as a descendent of the initial Ambulance Corps. During this time, the use of train ambulances, steamboat hospitals, and car or trolley ambulances was popular in some cities.

In 1869, Bellevue Hospital established the first US city ambulance service in New York City **FIGURE 1-9**. The hospital's Center Street Branch dispatched ambulances via telegraph and was staffed

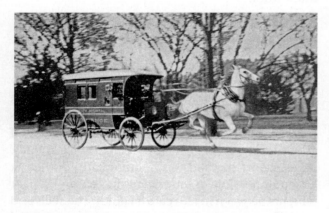

FIGURE 1-6 The first vehicles used for transport of casualties were horse-drawn wagons.

© National Library of Medicine.

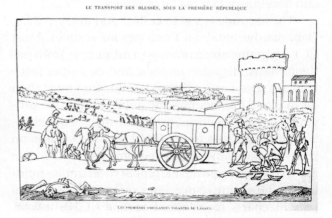

LE TRANSPORT DES BLESSÉS, SOUS LA PREMIÈRE RÉPUBLIQUE

LES PREMIÈRES AMBULANCES VOLANTES DE LARREY.

FIGURE 1-7 The *ambulance volante* (flying ambulance), shown here, was a two- or four-wheeled cart that transported surgeons and equipment to the battlefield.

© National Library of Medicine.

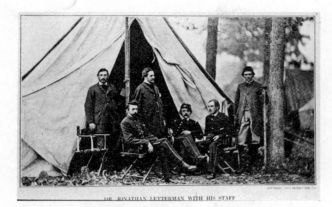

FIGURE 1-8 The first integrated treatment and evacuation system was established by surgeon Jonathan Letterman in 1862 during the Civil War at the Battle of Antietam.

© National Library of Medicine.

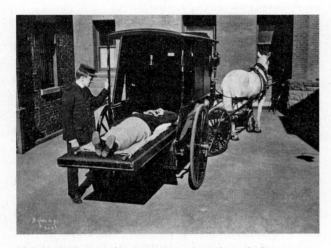

FIGURE 1-9 One of New York City's early ambulances.

© National Library of Medicine.

with physicians or surgeons from the hospital. Incredibly, the ambulance responded to more than 1,800 calls throughout the city of New York that first year. As the call volume increased, it became more difficult to staff the ambulances without decreasing the number of physicians in the hospital; in response to this problem, the hospital began placing orderlies or kitchen or janitorial staff on the ambulance. Because these employees had little or no medical training, responded without equipment, and frequently arrived at the scene hours after being dispatched, the mortality rate of seriously ill and injured patients increased dramatically. The continued population growth and the Industrial Revolution fueled the need for better training and

easier access to rapid prehospital emergency medical care.

In 1899, a group of businessmen developed the first motorized ambulance in Chicago and donated it to the Michael Reese Hospital. This vehicle weighed 1,600 pounds and could travel at speeds up to 16 miles per hour. In the early 1900s, ambulance crews evolved to include a driver and a person responsible for patient care, but generally the crews only picked up and delivered the patient to a base hospital.

The next milestone for prehospital care came in 1966 in Dublin, Ireland, with the provision of prehospital coronary care by physicians. Research by Francis Pantridge, a physician, indicated that most patients experiencing treatable ventricular fibrillation developed this fatal arrhythmia outside the hospital. Pantridge advocated for portable, lightweight, battery-driven defibrillators to be carried as part of the rapid response system he had developed. His foresight was the driving force for the current use of defibrillators by paramedics on mobile coronary care units and the automated external defibrillators (AEDs) used by the lay public.

Prehospital defibrillation was not used in the United States until 1969, shortly after the Miami, Florida, Fire Department, under the direction of Eugene Nagel, MD, instituted the nation's first paramedic program. Physicians in Los Angeles, California; Seattle, Washington; and Columbus, Ohio, followed Nagel's lead and began paramedic programs in their states, hoping that such prehospital emergency care would reduce preventable deaths. Today, prehospital and interfacility transports are accomplished not only by ground, but also by air.

Air Transport

After witnessing balloon flight demonstrations by the Montgolfier brothers in 1784, physicians began to consider the benefits that flight could bring to their patients. However, it was not until 1870 that the first documented case of air medical transport took place during the Prussian Siege of Paris, when 160 wounded soldiers and civilians were transported from the battlefield by hot-air balloons. At the time, this method was considered a radical means of transport and was met with harsh criticism; improvements were subsequently made. During the period between 1890 and 1910, M. de Mooy, chief of the Dutch Medical Service, pursued the idea of using litters suspended from balloons to transport patients.

On December 17, 1903, Orville Wright climbed into the plane he and his brother Wilbur built for the second attempt at flying a motorized plane. The site was Kill Devil Hills, North Carolina, and the Wright brothers' plane stayed airborne for 12 seconds and flew for 120 feet before landing under the power of its pilot, making history as the first pilot-operated airplane.

In 1909, Captain George Groaman of the US Army Medical Corps built a plane specifically designed to carry patients; unfortunately, it crashed during testing and never received government approval. The first successful use of a motorized aircraft for transporting patients occurred 8 years later, when a plane named the French Dorand AR II served as an air ambulance, transporting patients. During the next several decades, the air medical transport industry grew, predominantly as part of the military. In 1914, Igor Sikorsky invented the first helicopter to fly for more than just a few seconds, which the military later used to transport wounded soldiers from the battlefield to facilities offering definitive medical care.

After World War I, the US Army took a new interest in the development and use of air ambulances. The chief surgeon of the Army proposed modifications to the de Havilland aircraft, making it capable of transporting a pilot, a medical officer, and two patients. This arrangement became the standard for the evacuation of injured soldiers during wartime. Further advancements continued to be made, however, and in the 1930s, air ambulances were specifically designed with multiple engines, heated cabins, and short runway capability.

During the next decade, the push to create helicopters capable of transporting patients continued. On April 23, 1944, several wounded airmen were transported via helicopter in Burma during World War II. This event is thought to be the first time wounded soldiers were transported via this means, marking a new era of air medical transport. After the war, the military determined that air evacuation of wounded patients from battlefields would be a major goal. The first official military rescue evacuation was made on August 4, 1950, one month after the start of the Korean War. Wounded soldiers

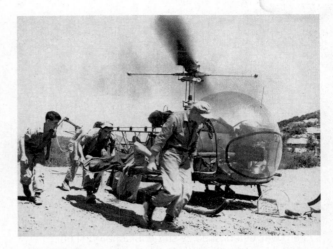

FIGURE 1-10 Soldiers wounded during the Korean War were sometimes evacuated on litters strapped to the skids of aircraft.

Courtesy of Bell Helicopter, a Texatron Company. Used with permission.

were transported to mobile army surgical hospital (MASH) units on cots fitted on the skids of Bell-47 and Sikorsky S-51 helicopters **FIGURE 1-10**. The drop in the mortality rate during this war was directly attributed to the use of helicopters to rapidly evacuate wounded soldiers from combat and deliver them to surgical care.

The Vietnam War brought a significant change in the removal of wounded patients from the front lines. The majority of battlefield rescues, stabilizations, and evacuations were carried out by a much larger helicopter, the Bell UH-1 (Huey), code-named *Dustoff* **FIGURE 1-11**. This helicopter, which was capable of carrying more patients and personnel, could accommodate patients inside the aircraft, where they could receive medical care en route to the receiving facility. The Vietnam War ultimately saw the transport of more than 800,000 patients to specialty care facilities. The marriage of rapid air transport to specialty care facilities proved successful and kindled interest in similar services in the civilian arena.

Medical evacuation (medevac) helicopter transport during the Vietnam War emphasized speed with little standardization or enhancement of care during transport.

The Vietnam model met with significant challenges in Iraq and Afghanistan owing to far more extensive evacuation times, typically averaging 2 hours. Tail-to-tail flights were often needed to

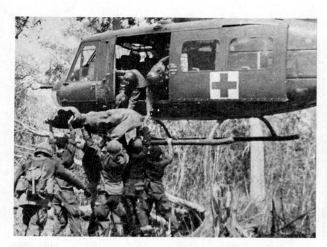

FIGURE 1-11 The Bell UH-1 helicopter, code-named *Dustoff*, evacuated patients during the Vietnam War.

Courtesy of Bell Helicopter, a Texatron Company. Used with permission.

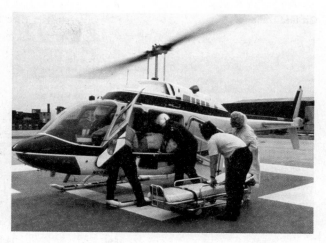

FIGURE 1-12 The Bell JetRanger helicopter was used for the first public service medevac program.

© MIEMSS. Used with permission.

keep medevac crews in their assigned areas. To facilitate better care, the Army deployed UH-60 Black Hawk helicopters staffed by flight medics, most of whom had extensive experience as civilian paramedics. The improved survival observed with this configuration led to enhanced training of military flight medics, equivalent to that of their civilian counterparts.

In 1958, Bill Mathews, a northern California businessman who lived in the small town of Etna, became the first person to organize a civilian air medical service. His idea initially met with skepticism from the town's 700 residents. Fortunately, Granville Ashcroft, the area's only physician, began using the helicopter to transport patients. Soon the town druggist also started using the helicopter to deliver medications during emergencies.

Later, during the 1960s, European countries instituted helicopter programs that were dedicated to patient care and transport. In that same period, the United States saw the emergence of several civilian- and government-funded helicopter projects. These projects sought to study the feasibility of using helicopters to transport patients in the civilian arena. In 1966, the National Institutes of Health and National Academy of Sciences published *Accidental Death and Disability: The Neglected Disease of Modern Society*, a report that paved the way for the initiation and growth of civilian air medical transportation programs; it

recommended the development of a system designed to transport patients via air ambulances based on the successful military model.

In 1969, the state of Maryland received a grant to purchase a Bell JetRanger helicopter and instituted the nation's first public service medevac program **FIGURE 1-12**. The four helicopters, staffed with paramedics, were part of the Maryland State Police and were strategically stationed throughout the state so that they could provide quick responses to emergencies. When the helicopters were not being used for medical emergencies, they could be used for law enforcement missions.

In 1972, the first hospital-based air medical transport program was established at St. Anthony's Hospital in Denver, Colorado. Following continued skepticism about the civilian use of helicopters for medical transports, the National Highway and Transportation Safety Administration (NHTSA) released a study titled *Helicopters in Emergency Medical Systems: Experience to Date*. This study suggested that the use of helicopters in urban settings was not realistic and offered little or no advantage over ground-based EMS systems. In 1981, the NHTSA released a second report titled *Air Ambulance Guidelines*, in which Willis Winert, MD, indicated that air ambulances were improperly equipped to handle critically ill or injured patients and were nothing more than flying taxis with removable seats. This statement prompted the FAA

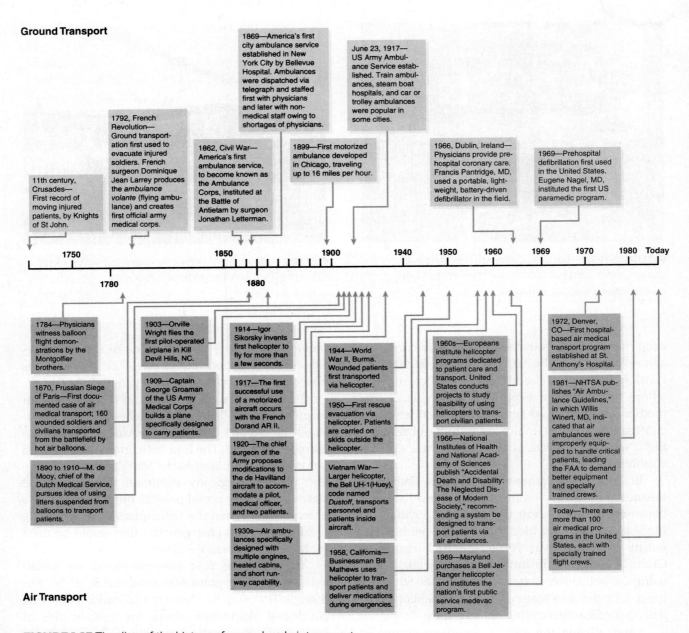

FIGURE 1-13 Timeline of the history of ground and air transport.

© Jones & Bartlett Learning.

to demand better equipment and specially trained crews for air ambulances.

The industry responded to these criticisms by developing the educational programs and specialty certifications mentioned earlier in this chapter. Today, there are more than 100 air medical programs in the United States, each with specially trained flight crews. **FIGURE 1-13** outlines the history of ground and air transport.

Summary

Much attention has been focused on specialty care and CCT since reimbursement fees for such services were established by the CMS and subsequently offered by other insurers. As the health care system continues to evolve, the need to relocate critically ill patients has increased. The sophistication of both CCTPs and the agencies, providing CCT has had to evolve to keep pace with the continued demand. Today, a variety of ground units, fixed-wing aircraft, and rotor-wing aircraft are used for CCT, and specialty certifications and educational programs are required for the personnel who staff them.

Despite the high degree of specialized training required for CCT teams, clinical care is but one aspect evaluated when assessing the quality of clinical care transports. Excellence in clinical care is not a "nice to have," but rather an expectation in today's health care environment. CCTPs must remember that an incident that they consider a "routine trauma case" is most likely a life-changing event for patients and their families. With this in mind, CCTPs must look and act in a professional manner at all times, even as they manage their own stress levels and ensure the safety of both themselves and their patients. In addition, CCTPs need highly effective communication skills for their interactions with patients, families, and other health care providers.

Case Study

Your CCT team is called to a community hospital to transfer a 34-year-old woman with end-stage (Class 4) pulmonary arterial hypertension to a tertiary medical center for specialized care and management. The patient presented to the local hospital during a blinding snowstorm with acute shortness of breath. Her family, who accompanied her, were unable to drive the 90 minutes to the tertiary center where she usually receives her care. Her medications include home oxygen, sildenafil, calcium channel blockers, and a continuous infusion of IV epoprostenol.

The nurse attending the patient indicated that she appeared to have pulmonary edema on arrival at the ED, some 2 hours previously. The patient was treated aggressively with high-flow oxygen and diuretics, and her symptoms improved. The nurse seems unfamiliar with the oxygen device the patient is currently using, which you recognize as a high-flow nasal cannula (HFNC) at 40 L/min with a fraction of inspired oxygen (F_{IO_2}) level of 1.0. You review the transfer orders and note that they call for oxygen by nonrebreathing mask, cardiac monitoring, and continuation of the IV epoprostenol.

When you quickly assess the patient, you note that she remains tachypneic, with a respiratory rate of 34 breaths/min; she has some slight intercostal retractions, crackles in the bases of both lungs, and an oxygen saturation of 93% on the HFNC. There is no central or peripheral cyanosis, but the patient appears to have a moderately increased work of breathing. She tells you that she has been intubated multiple times in the past for pulmonary edema and was concerned that this episode would also result in intubation. Her breathing seemed markedly improved once the HFNC was applied, some 30 minutes prior to your arrival.

You recognize that the HFNC is probably delivering a low level of positive end-expiratory pressure and, in conjunction with 100% oxygen, providing a higher level of respiratory support than the nonrebreather prescribed in your transfer orders. You locate the sending ED physician and explain that the patient is currently on HFNC at 40 L/min. A 40 L/min flow, during transport through a major snowstorm that might take twice as long as the usual 90-minute trip, would consume multiple on-board tanks of oxygen, which is much more than is carried on the ambulance. The physician is dismissive of your concerns, insists that her orders for a nonrebreathing mask are sufficient, and encourages you to expeditiously transfer the patient. The RT attending to the patient suggests that adding a nasal cannula under a nonrebreathing mask might be similar to the oxygen concentration provided by the high-flow setup.

Concerned that you may not be able to safely manage this patient during transport, you contact your OLMC for consultation. You review options with your medical control physician, including intubation and noninvasive ventilation. After some discussion with your patient and medical control, you elect to place the patient on bilevel positive airway pressure (BPAP) using your transport ventilator while monitoring end-tidal carbon dioxide ($ETCO_2$) using a nasal capnography cannula. Medical control also orders an additional dose of IV diuretics.

The patient remains comfortable on BPAP with settings of 8/4, and you are able to lower the FIO_2 from 1.0 to 0.7 during transport, with oxygen saturations remaining at 95%. The $ETCO_2$ level is initially 48 mm Hg and stabilizes at 40 mm Hg during transport, which takes a total of 2 hours. The patient's respiratory rate declines to 28 breaths/min and remains there during transport. The patient relates that she feels her breathing has improved, and you note the previously observed intercostal retractions are no longer present.

You arrive at the tertiary receiving hospital, provide your report to the team receiving the patient in the pulmonary ICU, and transfer care to their providers.

1. Who is responsible for deciding whether a patient is stable for transfer?
2. What situations warrant consult with OLMC?
3. When does responsibility for patient care transfer from hospital personnel to the transport team?

Analysis

This case study illustrates an interfacility transfer that could have gone terribly for the patient and transport crew had the CCTP team not consulted OLMC. Initially, the physician caring for the patient is responsible for arranging transfer and stabilizing the patient for transport. Ultimately, however, the CCTP responsible for the patient during transport must decide whether the patient's care needs are within the CCTP's scope of practice and whether the CCTP can safely manage

the patient during transfer. It is important to understand that the CCTP is responsible, and likely liable, for adverse outcomes that occur during transport. In any transport, the CCTPs should be confident that the patient's needs are within their scope of practice and that they will be able to manage foreseeable adverse events during transfer. If that is not the case, they should discuss their concerns with OLMC and consider not accepting the transport.

The worlds of prehospital care and CCT differ dramatically from those of the ED and ICU. In any situation where disagreement arises about patient care or physician orders, CCTPs should discuss the issue with the sending providers and clarify orders with the prescriber. If residual concerns or unaddressed needs remain, CCTPs should contact OLMC for clarification. Likewise, when CCTPs are concerned about the stability of a patient for transfer, they should consult with OLMC. Communication is key to safe transfers and good patient outcomes. The time to speak with medical control is prior to a patient decompensating, not after decompensation occurs.

On arrival at the sending facility, the CCTP team should gather information from the sending provider(s). This handoff report, coupled with a cursory assessment of the patient, should allow the team to quickly determine the complexity of the transport, the necessary equipment, and their ability to proceed. Responsibility for patient care transitions from the sending providers to the CCTP team once the patient is transferred to the transport stretcher, which should occur prior to transferring infusions, ventilation equipment, and other devices. This transition is important because it demarcates the point at which the patient has physically moved from the hospital to the EMS or transport environment. It is precisely the same choreography that occurs when EMS providers deliver a 9-1-1 patient to the ED: The moment the patient is moved from the ambulance gurney to a hospital stretcher, the patient becomes the responsibility of ED providers.

Prep Kit

Ready for Review

- Critical care is intensive care and monitoring provided to patients with life-threatening conditions who require constant monitoring and treatment with drugs and equipment to sustain life.
- CCT is the provision of medical care to a critically ill or injured patient during ground or air transport.
- Interfacility transport (IFT) and specialty care transport (SCT) are distinctly different entities. IFT is the transport of a patient between two health care facilities. SCT, as defined by the Centers for Medicare and Medicaid Services, is the interfacility ground transport of a critically ill or injured patient, including provision of medically necessary supplies and services that are beyond the scope of practice of paramedics.
- CCTPs may include EMTs, paramedics, nurses, physicians, and specialty health care personnel such as RTs and perfusionists.
- CCTPs must be able to provide care at the same level, or sometimes a greater level, than their non–critical care counterparts.
- CCTPs must be educated and skilled in the use of advanced practice procedures that may fall outside of their formal medical education. They must be lifelong learners who pursue continuing education to keep up to date with changes in clinical practice.
- Crew configurations vary as much as the types of ambulances and helicopters. The configuration depends on the staffing policy of the organization. The most common configurations are nurse and paramedic, nurse and RT, and nurse and physician.
- Additional crew members, including perfusionists and neonatal or pediatric intensivists, may be required for transport of certain patients.
- Modes of transportation may vary widely by agency and by region of the country. Possible modes of transport include ground units, rotor-wing aircraft, and fixed-wing aircraft.
- The transportation mode to be used is dictated by patient acuity, the distance between the sending and receiving facilities, the weather conditions, and the topography of the region.
- Mobile, or ground, units (ambulances) are generally used to transport critically ill and injured patients up to distances of 50 miles (80 km) from the patient's location to the receiving facility.
- Rotor-wing aircraft (helicopters) are used to transport critically ill and injured patients in rural settings and can travel distances of up to 150 miles (240 km).
- Fixed-wing aircraft (airplanes) are typically used to transport critically ill and injured patients for distances of 150 miles (240 km) or more.
- Communication breakdowns are the root cause of many adverse patient outcomes during CCT.
- When a transport is requested, dispatch personnel obtain pertinent information about patients and their condition from the referring facility. A clinical supervisor or algorithm should be used to determine the appropriate crew configuration and mode of transportation.
- A CCT team should be dispatched and used for patients who meet any of the following criteria: mechanical ventilation, vasoactive medications, blood product infusions, mechanical circulatory support devices, and unstable conditions requiring frequent interventions such as sedation, paralytics, and/or analgesia.
- The generally accepted time frame for an CCT team to receive the report from the handoff team, package the patient, and begin moving the patient to the transport vehicle should not exceed 20 minutes. In situations where additional interventions or procedures are needed to stabilize or prepare the patient for transport, bedside times may be longer.

Prep Kit Continued

- On arrival at the sending facility, the CCT team must quickly determine whether the patient's needs are within their scope of practice and whether they can safely manage the patient during transport.
- In situations where concerns arise, the CCT team should discuss these issues with the sending providers and, if not completely resolved, consult with their OLMC.
- Although a helicopter travels much faster than an ambulance, in some cases a ground ambulance may be located significantly closer to the patient and, therefore, is the preferred transportation mode.
- Patients with the following time-sensitive conditions are typically transported by air; these conditions include acute myocardial infarction, acute cerebrovascular accident, severe trauma, acute intracranial hemorrhage, the need for emergency surgery, and major burns.
- Weather issues may prohibit a flight from taking place. Usually, a decision is made to wait for the weather to improve and launch the aircraft as soon as practical.
- The basic concept of a CCT service is to rapidly transport CCTPs to a patient, stabilize the patient's condition, and transport the patient to the receiving facility as quickly as possible.
- Medical control within CCT systems includes protocols and OLMC. Protocols in a CCT setting are typically much more aggressive than those found in other aspects of prehospital care.
- Standards for CCT services vary from state to state; however, most CCT programs follow national standards. Usually, a state organization governs the licensure of air medical services and their practitioners.
- A CCTP's scope of practice varies according to their level of certification and the state in which they practice.

- Health care reimbursement is undergoing a major shift from paying for care delivered to paying for health outcomes achieved, and it is only a matter of time before quality and outcomes measures are connected to CCT reimbursement.
- Resilience, defined as a person's ability to withstand negative pressure or "bounce back" from difficulties, affects the well-being of both CCTPs and their patients. The three key determinants of personal resilience are thought to be biology (genetics), attachment, and control.
- CCTPs, like anyone else working in a high-stress profession, need not only a solid personal stress management program, but also resources they can avail themselves of when they encounter extremely stressful situations at work.
- Appropriate safety gear and clothing are necessities for every member of the CCT crew. They include layered clothing with reflective materials and flame resistance, head and eye protection, and leather boots.
- Interpersonal communication is as important in CCT as it is in other health care settings. CCTPs should introduce themselves to patients and family members and maintain both their professionalism and a caring demeanor.
- Quality assurance and improvement programs are an essential part of the overall health care system. Most CCT programs obtain data from patient charts, dispatch records, and process customer feedback surveys, which they can then use to inform their QA&I programs.
- Ground and air transport have evolved along with changes in transportation and technology. Since its earliest days of removing soldiers from the battlefield for treatment, CCT has become a sophisticated endeavor that combines a solid health care knowledge base with use of advanced medical technology and excellent interpersonal skills.

Prep Kit Continued

Vital Vocabulary

Benchmarking The process of comparing an organization's processes and performance to those of the overall industry or the best practices from other companies.

critical care Constant, complex, detailed health care as provided in various acute life-threatening conditions; the ability to deal with such situations rapidly and with precision using various advanced machines and devices for treating and monitoring the patient's condition.

critical care patient Any patient who experiences an actual or potential life-threatening illness or injury that requires continual monitoring and care by a specially trained physician, registered nurse, or paramedic.

critical care transport (CCT) The transport of a patient from an emergency department, critical care unit, or incident scene during which the patient receives the same level of care as was provided in the hospital or originating facility.

critical care transport professional (CCTP) A health care professional who has successfully completed a recognized critical care program and meets the minimum qualifications set forth by the employing transport program.

critical incident stress debriefing (CISD) An approach favored since the 1980s to manage the psychological aftereffects in emergency personnel after particularly distressing responses; it requires a specially trained team and has the potential to create iatrogenic harm.

dispatch The person or organization that receives the request for critical care transport and contacts the critical care transport team with the details of that request to ascertain the team's availability.

fixed-wing aircraft A transportation mode typically used to transport critically ill and injured patients distances of 150 miles (240 km) or greater; also called airplanes.

handoff The brief report that staff at the sending facility—generally the bedside nurse, physician, or care provider currently responsible for the patient—submits to the CCTP team when they arrive to accept responsibility for the patient's care.

interfacility transport (IFT) The transport of a patient between two health care facilities.

medical director A physician who provides guidance and oversight for the practice of a critical care transport service's personnel.

mobile intensive care units Ambulances or helicopters that are used only for maintaining specialized or intensive care treatment; they are used primarily for interfacility transports.

morbidity An illness or an abnormal condition or quality; the rate at which an illness occurs in a particular area or population.

mortality The condition of being subject to death; the number of deaths per unit of population in any specific region, age group, disease, or other classification.

online medical control/consultation (OLMC) Immediate medical direction provided to critical care transport professionals in outlying locations by a physician; a system in which field personnel contact an emergency department physician via telephone or radio for a consult.

perfusionists Highly trained technicians who are intimately familiar with the operation of intra-aortic balloon pumps and adult and pediatric extracorporeal membrane oxygenation machines, and who may assist during any medical situation, including critical care transports, in which it is necessary to support or temporarily replace a patient's circulatory or respiratory function.

psychological first aid (PFA) An evidence-based approach to managing psychological aftereffects in emergency personnel after particularly distressing responses that relies on the concept of human resilience.

quality assurance and improvement (QA&I) program A program that seeks to generate data that are then used to improve the quality of service provided.

Prep Kit Continued

resilience A person's ability to withstand negative pressure or "bounce back" from difficulties.

rotor-wing aircraft A transportation mode used to transport critically ill and injured patients in rural settings distances of up to 150 miles (240 km); also called helicopters.

specialty care transport (SCT) The interfacility ground transport of a critically ill or injured patient, including provision of medically necessary supplies and services that are beyond the scope of practice of a paramedic; a term used by the Centers for Medicare and Medicaid Services

in determining whether transport charges are reimbursable.

stress The reaction of the mind or body to a demand for change; it can have either positive or negative effects.

well-being "A positive outcome that is meaningful for people and for many sectors of society, because it tells us that people perceive that their lives are going well" (Centers for Disease Control and Prevention); a state of being comfortable, healthy, and happy.

References

Aeromedical evacuation in World War I. http://www.olive-drab .com/od_medical_evac_fixedwing_ww1.php. Accessed May 18, 2021.

Balka E, Tolar M, Coates S, Whitehouse S. Socio-technical issues and challenges in implementing safe patient handovers: insights from ethnographic case studies. *Int J Med Informatics*. 2013;82:e345-e357.

Bellis M. Ambulance history. http://theinventors.org/library /inventors/blambulance.htm. Accessed June 5, 2021.

Blakeman TC, Branson RD. Inter- and intra-hospital transport of the critically ill. *Respir Care*. 2013;58:1008-1023.

de Becker G. *The Gift of Fear*. New York: Random House; 1997.

Delgado MK, Staudenmayer KL, Wang E, et al. Cost-effectiveness of helicopter versus ground emergency medical services for trauma scene transportation in the United States. *Ann Emerg Med*. 2013;62:351.e19-364.e19.

Department of Health and Human Services, Centers for Medicare and Medicaid Services. *CMS Manual System: Pub 100-02. Medicare Benefit Policy, Transmittal 68: Ambulance Fee Schedule—Ground Ambulance Services—Revision to the Specialty Care Transport (SCT) Definition*. March 30, 2007.

Department of Health and Human Services, Centers for Medicare and Medicaid Services. *CMS Manual System: Pub 100-02. Medicare Benefit Policy, Transmittal 130: Definition of Ambulance Services*. July 29, 2010.

Ground Air Medical qUality Transport Quality Improvement Collaborative. The GAMUT database. http://gamutqi.org /index.html. Accessed May 23, 2021.

McEvoy M. *Straight Talk About Stress: A Guide for Emergency Responders*. Quincy, MA: National Fire Protection Association; 2004.

Morganti KG, Alpert A, Margolis G, Wasserman J, Kellermann AL. Should payment policy be changed to allow a wider range of EMS transport options? *Ann Emerg Med*. 2014;63:615.e5-626.e5.

National Association of State EMS Officials. *National EMS Scope of Practice Model 2019* (Report No. DOT HS 812-666). Washington, DC: National Highway Traffic Safety Administration. https://www.ems.gov/pdf/National_EMS _Scope_of_Practice_Model_2019.pdf. Accessed May 19, 2021.

National EMS Quality Alliance. Establishing quality measures for patient care. https://nemsqa.org/. Accessed May 23, 2021.

National Highway Traffic Safety Administration. *Guide for Interfacility Patient Transfer*. Washington, DC: National Highway Traffic Safety Administration; April 2006.

Parmentier-Decrucq E, Poissy J, Favory R, et al. Adverse events during intrahospital transport of critically ill patients: incidence and risk factors. *Ann Intens Care*. 2013;3(1):10.

Singh JM, MacDonald RD, Ahghari M. Critical events during land-based interfacility transport. *Ann Emerg Med*. 2014;64:15.e2.

The history of the air ambulance and Medevac. https://www .mercyflight.org/history-of-ems/. Accessed May 18, 2021.

The history of EMS: milestones in EMS. http://warhammer .mcc.virginia.edu/cars/milestones.html. Accessed May 18, 2021.

The IHI Triple Aim Initiative. Institute for Healthcare Improvement website. www.ihi.org/Engage/Initiatives/TripleAim /Pages/default.aspx. Accessed May 23, 2021.

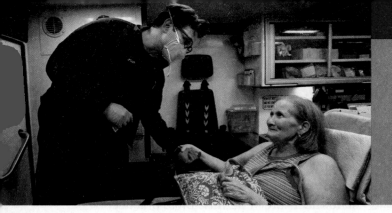

Chapter 2

Medical-Legal Issues

Matthew R. Streger, JD, MPA, NRP

OBJECTIVES

After completing this chapter, you will be able to:

1. Describe the basic concepts of negligence and the four findings required to establish an act of negligence (pp 28–29).

2. Explain the laws that determine whether a health care provider can be found responsible for an injury (pp 28–29).

3. Describe the concept of *respondeat superior* and the conditions under which providers may not be protected by their employer's liability insurance (pp 29–30).

4. Describe the legal principle of consent and the concepts of informed, expressed, and implied consent (pp 30–31).

5. Discuss how competence and decision-making capacity (DMC) are assessed in establishing consent (pp 30–31).

6. Explain the importance, from a legal standpoint, of proper documentation in the patient care report (p 32).

7. Discuss the Emergency Medical Treatment and Active Labor Act (EMTALA), its implications for critical care transport, and the potential consequences of violating the law (pp 32–33).

8. Discuss the general concepts established by current EMTALA case law (p 33).

9. State the major steps and pertinent issues in accepting a patient transfer (pp 33–34).

10. State the responsibilities of critical care transport professionals during transport (pp 37–38).

11. Explain the role of other health care providers who accompany the patient during transport (pp 38–39).

12. Discuss the ways in which communications capabilities and agreements about medical direction affect medical decision making in the transport environment (p 39).

13. State the major steps and pertinent issues in transferring care to the receiving facility (pp 39–40).

14. Describe how risks can be minimized in the critical care transport environment (p 40).

15. Explain accurate and complete documentation for a transport, including its critical nature in protecting against liability claims (pp 39–40).

Introduction

Of all the areas in which health care providers operate, the legal world can be the most unfamiliar and uncertain. EMS providers often have little training and experience in this area, where the consequences of errors or inaction can be damaging both for the provider individually and for the EMS agency as a whole. The education that providers do receive in regard to legal issues is often intermingled with bad information shared through anecdotal stories and misunderstandings. A shortage of subject-matter experts in the medical-legal realm with EMS or health care experience makes it all the more difficult to ensure providers are receiving sound information.

Health care providers, including EMS professionals, must familiarize themselves with legal concepts and terms to operate effectively and protect themselves in this area. They must understand the laws that apply where they practice, know the local protocols and their limitations, have appropriate documentation skills, and maintain proper communications and interpersonal dynamics with other providers and other health care professionals, patients, and family members.

This chapter examines the real-world issues facing critical care transport professionals (CCTPs), including civil liability, and specific laws such as EMTALA and HIPAA. Of course, this is an ever-evolving area of practice, and CCTPs should continually monitor changes in the law, including relevant legal cases that are binding on their practice. Throughout this chapter, we will look for best practices and ways to limit risk and ensure regulatory compliance.

General Concepts of Liability

Any discussion of legal issues associated with the transportation of critically ill or injured patients must start with an understanding of the basic concepts of negligence. **Negligence** is an area of civil **tort** law—that is, the law that deals with harm rendered by one person or entity against another **TABLE 2-1**. Negligence's foundations largely lie in **common law**, which is case law established by prior disputes, in court, that is published to guide future proceedings. However, certain aspects of negligence law originate in **statutes**. Usually, cases brought in negligence law are state-law cases, and for this reason each state has its own independent body of law in this area.

While the basic concepts may be related, certain details, such as statutes of limitations, comparative negligence, and immunity laws, can vary widely in different jurisdictions. Health care providers also may have criminal liability for some improper acts or may have administrative liability related to their state's licensure or permission to practice.

Negligence Law

A finding of negligence requires that four criteria be met **FIGURE 2-1**:

1. The health care provider had a **duty to act**.
2. The provider committed a **breach of duty to act**.

TABLE 2-1 Areas of Law
• **Criminal law.** Wrongs against the rules of the "state"
• **Civil law.** Wrongs between people or entities
• **Administrative law.** Wrongs committed by people who are granted permission to practice by the state

© Jones & Bartlett Learning.

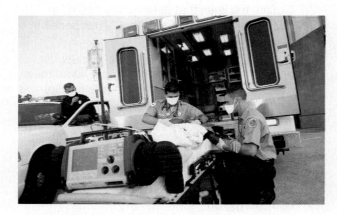

FIGURE 2-1 Four criteria are considered when determining whether a provider has behaved negligently. Consider a scenario in which a paramedic has intubated a patient in respiratory failure. The paramedic has been called to respond to a respiratory emergency (1: duty to act). He must confirm correct placement of the endotracheal tube. His EMT partner suggests that the tube may not be placed correctly because there is no chest rise with ventilations. The paramedic does not attach end-tidal capnography (even when suggested by his partner) to confirm tube placement, and the tube was placed incorrectly (2: breach of duty to act). The patient, who was awake and alert prior to intubation, remains comatose and is discharged to a long-term care facility (3: damages to patient). The paramedic would be guilty of negligence because the consequences of an unrecognized esophageal intubation are foreseeable (4: proximate causation).

© Thinkstock Images/Stockbyte/Getty Images.

3. The patient suffered damages as a result of the breach of duty.
4. The damages were proximally caused (foreseeable) from that breach of duty.

The breach of duty can be either an act of omission, which means not doing something that should have been done, or an act of commission, which means doing something that should not have been done or doing something improperly. If any of these elements is missing or cannot be proven, then there will be no finding of negligence.

The most critical point regarding negligence is that there is no requirement of intent to cause harm. A finding of intent changes the nature of the charges; it can lead to punitive damages awarded to the plaintiff in a civil lawsuit or to criminal charges against the defendant. Negligence is simply a mistake that leads to harm, and the law provides that the person who injures someone else through a mistake should compensate the victim.

Negligence cases must be brought within a set time, called the statute of limitations; after that time limit expires, the plaintiff will be unable to file a lawsuit. The statute of limitations is usually 2 years but varies from state to state. It may be longer if the patient is a minor (the clock does not start until the patient is 18 years of age) or if the patient did not know they were the victim of negligence, called the discovery rule. However, the discovery rule does not apply if the patient should have known that the negligent act occurred. For example, if the patient experiences pain or limitation after the adverse event but delays investigating the cause, the discovery rule will not apply. In many administrative matters (ie, instances where providers have a duty to act), there is no statute of limitations.

Other Standards and Immunity Laws

Negligence is not the only standard that can apply to health care providers. Some laws apply a higher standard that must be reached to find a health care provider responsible for an injury. One of these standards is reckless conduct, which is a more serious finding than typical negligence. Often termed *gross negligence*, it involves consciously disregarding the known risks of a course of action. Another standard is willful and wanton misconduct, which usually requires an intentional act of misconduct. Many state immunity statutes provide for one of these higher standards to be applied in EMS provider cases, and they often look more closely at the specific type of action being performed. For example, clinical judgment errors often require a higher standard to find the provider liable, whereas improper vehicle operations are usually evaluated based on a negligence standard.

Another type of immunity often afforded EMS providers is sovereign immunity, which covers only governmental entities. This immunity can align with the reckless or willful and wanton requirements, or it can differentiate between ministerial acts and discretionary acts. Ministerial acts are those that require a specific act given a set of circumstances, whereas discretionary acts are those in which the provider has some latitude in decision making. Sovereign immunity usually protects providers in the case of discretionary acts, because the law wants to encourage people to make necessary decisions without fear of reprisal; however, it does not offer protection for ministerial acts, for which people need not use their judgment. In terms of clinical protocols, judgment regarding a differential diagnosis or hospital destination choice would be covered under immunity, because it involves a discretionary act, but failure to follow a mandatory protocol element (eg, verifying endotracheal tube placement) would not be covered by immunity.

Insurance

Most CCTPs are covered by their employer's professional liability insurance, or other insurance, owing to *respondeat superior*—the legal concept that an employer is responsible for the acts of its agents. There are two limitations of this type of insurance coverage: (1) The act in question must occur while the person is employed and (2) it must be within the person's scope of practice and reason for employment. An employer who believes the employee has acted beyond their authority may decline to cover the employee for a bad act, leaving that person responsible for paying for the costs of their legal defense and any damages. Needless to say, these costs can be substantial. Often, for these reasons, employers will not pay for a defense involving criminal or administrative wrongdoing; thus, it is important that providers stay within their practice boundaries.

Finally, providers must remember that their employer will not cover them for acts they undertake while they do not have a duty to act, such as rendering aid as a bystander. Good Samaritan statutes often confer immunity to bystanders who render aid, but this is not always the case. Even if providers render assistance while they have no duty to act, they must act reasonably and competently as another reasonable off-duty CCTP would.

Many people question the need to obtain private malpractice insurance, often fearing that they will be sued in civil court because they have "deep pockets." This is a misinformed fear, as plaintiffs' counsel typically will not know about insurance coverage until after a lawsuit is filed. Moreover, private insurance may cover administrative or licensure actions where an employer may not.

The Patient's Right to Decide

The right to bodily integrity is well established in law. Numerous court cases have affirmed the right of individuals to determine what can be done with their body, subject to various limits, and many states have established stronger protections for individual autonomy. Various court cases have interpreted and limited these protections, so each jurisdiction may have different laws. One protection is especially common, however: the basic right for adult patients to consent to medical care. This right relates to all aspects of care, including the physical assessment, any aspect of treatment, and transport decisions, including destination choice.

Competence and Consent

Several legal aspects must be considered in determining consent. First is the presence of legal competence, which is typically found when a person reaches the age of majority, commonly 18 years old. Certain factors may lower this age, such as being pregnant, being legally emancipated, or serving in the military. Local laws may lower this age as well, such as when a patient is seeking reproductive treatment or treatment for drug or alcohol addiction. Finally, a court may change this factor by determining that a patient is not legally competent, thereby removing a person's right to make decisions and vesting that right with another person, usually called a guardian. A person may sign an agreement that gives another person the right to make health care decisions for them under certain circumstances. These designations are often called a health care power of attorney or a health care proxy. A living will, which may take the form of a do not resuscitate (DNR) order or physician orders for life-sustaining treatment (POLST), is a legal document that establishes in advance what care a person wants, and does not want, in the event that they are found to lack competence.

Clearly, the determination of competence does not rest with health care providers, including CCTPs. The provider's analysis in the context of critical care transport focuses on assessing a person's decision-making capacity (DMC). The determination of DMC is not a simple task, and there is no clearly established legal guideline for making this decision. CCTPs must instead analyze the totality of the circumstances and decide if a patient's brain is functioning well enough to process information.

Decision-Making Capacity

Determining decision-making capacity typically includes an assessment of:

- Orientation
- Substances that can alter mentation
- Clinical conditions that can alter mentation, such as hypoxia, hypovolemia, hypoglycemia, and seizures
- Environmental factors, such as language barriers and people in the environment of care

DMC starts with orientation, but it does not end there. While a patient who is not fully oriented almost certainly does not have DMC, a person can be alert and fully oriented and yet not have DMC. As an example, consider alcohol intoxication. Picture a person who has been out drinking and is clearly intoxicated to the point of having slurred speech and unsteady gait, but who can still answer the basic questions about orientation to person, place, and time. This person most likely is impaired to the point of not having the capacity to process information about health care decision making.

Other factors can also impact a patient's DMC. Countless medical conditions can prevent a person's brain from effectively processing information;

examples include hypoxia, hypoglycemia, hypothermia, seizures, and sepsis. Similarly, environmental factors can impact a person's ability to make decisions about their health care; for example, an abusive person at the scene may influence the patient's decision making.

Determining a patient's DMC is simply a matter of making sure the "computer" in the person's head is turned on and booted up, has input/output devices installed, and is ready to process.

Consent and Refusal

Once the patient's "computer" is working properly, you must give it the information to process. Informed consent is the process of proposing to the patient a course of action (assessment, treatment, transport), the risks associated with that action, the benefits associated with the action, and any reasonable alternatives, and then allowing the patient to decide if they want you to proceed with the action. Consent is ideally obtained in writing, and confirmed with a patient's signature. Nevertheless, the most important element of informed consent is not the signature, but rather the risk/benefit discussion you have with the patient and their clear confirmation of understanding.

Expressed consent is consent that is clearly communicated by the patient after having been properly informed. This type of consent is required by law unless an exception applies. It is often established by a physician, but CCTPs may obtain expressed consent from the patient under certain circumstances, most notably when the patient is directly under the CCTP's care.

Picture, however, a patient who is so sick that they cannot provide you with informed consent. Perhaps the patient lacks DMC, is unconscious, or is not legally competent to make decisions (often the case with minors when no parent is available). The law generally assumes that a person would want life-saving treatment if offered it, so under these circumstances the doctrine of implied consent applies. It is expected that the patient would give expressed consent if able to do so. In most jurisdictions, implied consent applies only when the patient has an emergency medical condition that is serious enough to risk life or disability.

Refusal of any aspect of medical care, most notably transport, is simply an expression of a patient

TABLE 2-2 Actions to Deal With Patient Refusal to Consent
• Is the patient legally permitted to refuse care?
• Make multiple, sincere attempts to convince the patient to accept care.
• Enlist the help of others (such as the patient's family or friends) to convince the patient to accept care.
• Make sure the patient is informed in their decision.
• Attempt to get someone to stay with the patient.
• Thoroughly document the situation.

© Jones & Bartlett Learning.

(who has DMC) refusing to consent to care that is being offered after an informed consent discussion. When faced with a person who is refusing care that you believe is in their best interests, you should use all available tools at your disposal to convince the patient to accept your offer. You can try restating your suggestion in clearer terms or with a greater sense of urgency, appealing to friends or family who are present, or enlisting the help of online medical control **TABLE 2-2**. Contacting medical control may strengthen your documentation because those calls are often recorded for later use. Finally, remember that a patient may accept your care in part and refuse it in part, and may revoke their consent at any time.

Risks of Failing to Assess DMC and Obtain Consent

CCTPs who fail to assess DMC and obtain informed consent risk liability on several fronts. As previously discussed, the primary risk is negligence. In addition, other significant risks may arise from these failures.

Touching a patient without the patient's consent is called battery. Battery is a civil tort, but also may be a crime. Criminal battery involves some aspect of intent to harm, and the specifics of battery vary from state to state. Technically, both the tort and the crime of assault simply refer to placing a person in imminent fear of battery. Battery can occur by performing an action or transporting a patient against their will. Abandonment is the civil tort associated with terminating a clinical relationship without obtaining informed consent and without transferring care to a clinically appropriate provider; thus, it is the flip side of battery.

CCTPs may also be subject to civil and criminal penalties for violations of federal law, specifically 42 U.S.C. 1983, for compelling transportation against a patient's will. It is often stated that health care providers are not sued for "wrongful life" (a play on the legal ruling of "wrongful death"), but this is simply not the case. Legal cases are often brought against providers for forcing medical care and/or transportation when consent was not granted.

Any of these circumstances can also give rise to investigations and actions by local and state licensing authorities.

Documentation of Competence

All aspects of the assessment of competence, including any associated documents, DMC, and informed consent or refusal, should be objectively documented on your patient care report. This documentation should always use clear, concise, and objective language in reciting the facts that established the patient's DMC, and specifying exactly what risks and benefits were explained to the patient leading to the patient's consent or refusal. It is a wise practice to have patients explain back, in their own words, what you have offered and what you said will happen if they accept or refuse your suggestion.

Case Scenario

In *Lemann v Essen Lane Daiquiris, Inc.* 923 So. 2d 627 (2006), paramedics were called to a bar by police officers to evaluate an intoxicated man for a hand injury. They were told it was a nonemergency call, with no life-threatening injuries. When they arrived at the scene, the patient, 21-year-old Parker Lemann, reportedly told the paramedics he was under arrest, although the paramedics stated that police did not confirm this claim. No witnesses to the altercation were present for police to interview.

Mr. Lemann was able to answer paramedics' questions without difficulty and told them he got into a fight and punched someone and that his hand was hurting. The paramedics found that he was alert, and Mr. Lemann told them he had no other complaints. His vital signs were all normal. His pupils were equal and reactive to light. He denied any loss of consciousness, and a physical examination, which included his head, revealed no injuries other than an abrasion to his hand.

The paramedics at the scene offered twice to take Mr. Lemann to the hospital; both times he refused to go to the hospital. Mr. Lemann then signed a form acknowledging his refusal of transport.

Police officers took Mr. Lemann home. Several hours later, he was found unconscious by neighbors. He was then transported to a hospital and diagnosed with a fractured skull and a subdural hematoma. He died 2 days later.

Mr. Lemann's parents filed a lawsuit against the paramedics and their employer. They argued that paramedics should have taken Mr. Lemann to the hospital despite his lack of consent to be transported. The paramedics responded that Mr. Lemann must have suffered injuries subsequent to their evaluation of him and that he did not have the visible injuries to his head that were noted after his death.

The court ruled that the paramedics were not required to take Mr. Lemann to the hospital because he had the right to refuse transportation. The court further found that "the EMS personnel must balance fulfilling a person's emergency medical needs with respecting a person's wish not to be treated or transported to the hospital." In this case, the court said, paramedics did not observe a head injury while assessing Mr. Lemann, so they acted properly in respecting his refusal of transport to the hospital. The court granted judgment for the paramedics.

Although the published legal decision in this case does not discuss the patient care report, there appears to be no issues or questions surrounding those facts. The paramedics' documentation of Mr. Lemann's clinical presentation, DMC, and refusal of care held up to legal scrutiny, a major reason why the paramedics were able to prevail.

Emergency Medical Treatment and Active Labor Act

The Emergency Medical Treatment and Active Labor Act (EMTALA) is a federal law passed by the US Congress in 1986, with the primary goals of ensuring that all patients who need emergency medical care at an emergency department (ED) receive it, and of preventing hospitals from transferring patients to other facilities regardless of their insurance status or ability to pay for services. Even though this law has now been in force for several decades, there are still misunderstood provisions that apply to CCTPs. Because CCTPs primarily transport patients between facilities, several key provisions of EMTALA apply to their everyday practice.

EMTALA Requirements

EMTALA has two main obligations that involve ambulances. The first normally applies to patients who seek treatment for an emergency medical condition in the ED of a hospital that accepts Medicare for payment (which is virtually every ED in the United States). Any person who presents for treatment for an emergency medical condition must receive a medical screening exam and stabilization to the extent of the hospital's capabilities without consideration for the patient's ability to pay. This provision typically applies to ambulances that operate in the 9-1-1 system, or equivalent, and the hospital ED. EMTALA includes many details about how and when these requirements apply, including the requirement for "presentation" on hospital property and the immediate surrounding area, but most of them are not relevant to the CCTP.

However, the use of landing facilities for air medical units at hospitals is directly relevant to the CCTP. Current Medicare guidelines provide that EMTALA requirements are not triggered if a ground ambulance and crew are using the hospital's landing facilities as the facility of convenience; in this case, the patient is not considered to be presenting to the hospital for treatment for an emergency medical condition, and EMTALA obligations are therefore not triggered. However, if the CCTP requests any assistance from the hospital's personnel, then the EMTALA transfer obligations discussed next apply.

Medical Screening Exams

When a patient presents to the hospital for treatment of an emergency medical condition, the medical screening exam and stabilization requirements are triggered. An emergency medical condition is defined by the Centers for Medicare and Medicaid Services (CMS), in part, as "a condition manifesting itself by acute symptoms of sufficient severity [including severe pain] such that the absence of immediate medical attention could reasonably be expected to result in . . . serious jeopardy to the health of a patient, including a pregnant woman or a fetus."

The medical screening exam is not a triage exam. It must be performed by a physician, physician assistant, or nurse practitioner and is limited by the capabilities of the hospital. If the hospital does not have a particular diagnostic capability, it is not held responsible for not performing that study. The medical screening exam should include (1) a triage record; (2) initial vital signs; (3) oral history; (4) physical examination; (5) use of appropriate diagnostic resources to determine if an emergency medical condition exists; (6) use of on-call physicians, if necessary; and (7) discharge vital signs.

The medical screening exam requirement is triggered when the patient is within 250 yards of the hospital, or on hospital property, and is seeking treatment for an emergency medical condition. Thus, a patient who presents to the front door of a hospital rather than the ED entrance is considered to have presented for purposes of EMTALA. Also note that many critical care ambulances and air medical units are hospital-owned, making them "hospital property" for purposes of EMTALA. This does not mean that all patients in a hospital-owned vehicle must be transported back to the owning hospital, but it does mean that the patient must receive a screening exam; failure to ensure it happens may constitute an EMTALA violation.

Finally, stabilization means that within a reasonable degree of medical certainty, no "material" deterioration should occur from or during the transfer. In the case of a pregnant woman having contractions, stabilization is defined as delivery of the baby (or babies) and placenta.

Transfer Obligations

CCTPs typically deal with the EMTALA transfer obligations on a daily basis. The sending facility is responsible for arranging safe transport, including ensuring that qualified personnel and appropriate equipment are used. The receiving facility may actually perform the transport with its CCTP team, but that does not absolve the sending facility of its responsibilities. It is also the sending facility's responsibility to ensure that informed consent is obtained from the patient, or from a legally valid representative, prior to transport. The sending facility is also responsible, under EMTALA, for sending the medical records with the patient and ensuring that the receiving facility has space for the patient, has qualified personnel for managing the patient's medical condition, and accepts the patient. The records must also include a transfer form and certificate of medical necessity for Medicare patients.

In regard to the stabilization requirement, it is understood that many patients transported by CCTPs are not "stable." In fact, the very lack of stabilization is often the reason for the transport. For unstable patients, the sending physician must certify that the medical benefit outweighs the risks of transport, with that risk/benefit analysis and certification being clearly documented in the records.

The receiving hospital does not have to facilitate a "bed-to-bed" transfer but must have capacity for the patient. Capacity for the receiving hospital can be established in any way that that facility has established capacity in the past. For example, if the hospital admits patients through the ED, and typically holds overflow patients there, then the hospital must do that for any requested EMTALA transfer. It is an EMTALA violation, sometimes called "reverse dumping," for a hospital to refuse a patient if it has the specialty services that the patient requires and has the capacity to accept the patient.

A sending facility must receive agreement from a physician at the receiving facility to accept the incoming patient, and this acceptance must be documented; however, it does not have to be accomplished by physician-to-physician contact. This acceptance may not be delayed while the accepting physician receives approval from the hospital's administration. Furthermore, on-call physicians must come to see a patient at either the sending facility or the receiving facility, respond in a timely manner, and provide services if they ordinarily do so. The failure to provide any of these elements that leads to a patient transfer is an EMTALA violation.

EMTALA Violations

EMTALA is geared toward hospital and physician conduct; it was never intended to apply to the EMS community. If a hospital or physician is found to have violated the provisions of this law, several possible penalties may be imposed:

- A hospital may be fined between $25,000 and $50,000 per violation.

- A physician may be fined up to $50,000 per violation.
- A hospital or physician may be terminated from the Medicare and Medicaid programs.
- A patient may seek **civil damages** against a hospital or physician for injuries arising out of an EMTALA violation.

The fact that a non–hospital-based ambulance service may not be subject to the provisions of EMTALA does not mean that you or your service is absolved from all liability under this law. Although you cannot be held accountable for injuries arising out of an EMTALA transfer, the patient, or the patient's family, may file a lawsuit alleging malpractice or negligence against anyone involved.

EMTALA Case Scenarios

Many EMTALA cases have bearing on critical care transport. Specific judgments made in particular EMTALA cases include the following findings:

- EMTALA is not a substitute for malpractice action.
- Emergency stabilization prior to transport does not guarantee against patient deterioration en route.
- A patient can be transferred, even if unstable, if the benefits of transfer outweigh the risks.
- Stabilization relates to available capabilities.
- The patient must present to the ED or be on a hospital campus to trigger EMTALA coverage.
- Admission to inpatient care ends the EMTALA medical screening exam process (unless admission is used to avoid EMTALA requirements).
- An inpatient who becomes unstable and requires transfer is covered by EMTALA.
- The patient must have an emergency medical condition for EMTALA to apply.
- The physician has an obligation to "certify" transfer.
- Active labor requires treatment.

These examples of lessons learned from EMTALA cases give CCTPs an idea of the implications of EMTALA and suggest how this law might be applied in the critical care transport setting. The following are examples of the specific judgments in the preceding list.

Transfer Benefits Versus Risks

In *Heimlicher v Steele*, 615 F Supp 2d 884 (ND Iowa 2009), Ms. Heimlicher was an expectant mother who came to the hospital after experiencing severe pain and bleeding. An ED physician, Dr. Steele, failed to properly diagnose her condition. Dr. Steele ordered the transfer of Ms. Heimlicher to a hospital 100 miles away.

A nurse sent the ultrasonogram to a radiologist who was on call, who told her the images showed mass versus hemorrhage versus fibroid. Dr. Steele testified that he had never been advised of these findings, and if he had been informed he would have ordered an immediate cesarean section.

During transport, Ms. Heimlicher "almost immediately began experiencing too-rapid contractions, profuse vaginal bleeding, and severe pain in her abdomen," and the fetal monitor showed that the baby was in distress. The ambulance did not turn back, but rather continued to transport Ms. Heimlicher to the second hospital. The baby was stillborn.

The court found that there are three circumstances under which the hospital would have been justified in transferring Ms. Heimlicher and not been liable under EMTALA: "(1) her emergency medical condition was stabilized (EMTALA § (c)(1)); (2) her emergency medical condition was not stabilized, but she requested transfer to another hospital (EMTALA § (c)(1)(A)(i)); or (3) her emergency medical condition was not stabilized, but a physician signed a certification that the medical benefits reasonably expected from medical treatment at another hospital outweighed the increased risks to her and her unborn child from the transfer (EMTALA § (c)(1)(A)(ii))."

The court concluded that Ms. Heimlicher had not been stabilized and had not requested transfer. It also found that Dr. Steele failed to properly weigh the risks and benefits. Under these circumstances, the court found that the hospital had violated EMTALA. The court did not find the transport service had any liability under EMTALA.

In *Ramos-Cruz v Centro Medico del Turabo*, 642 F.3d 17 (1st Cir. 2011), Jose Ramos Lopez presented to the ED at Centro Medico del Turabo (CMDT) with a history of abdominal problems and experiencing abdominal pain. The ED physician diagnosed him with upper gastrointestinal bleeding.

CMDT did not have a gastroenterologist available to treat Mr. Lopez, so Dr. Ramon, the treating physician, arranged to have him transferred to San Juan Medical Center (SJMC) for treatment by a gastroenterologist there. Dr. Ramon signed a certification at the time of transfer stating that the benefits of transfer were greater than the risks. However, in the section titled "explain why the benefits of transfer for the patient . . . are greater than the risks, if any, for the transfer," Dr. Ramon documented simply "gastroenterologist." Mr. Lopez was treated for his bleeding ulcer at SJMC, but he began bleeding again later and physicians were unsuccessful in saving his life.

The family sued CMDT under EMTALA, claiming that Mr. Lopez had been improperly transferred. The First Circuit court found that EMTALA was a "limited anti-dumping statute, and not a federal malpractice statute." It also found that by entering only "gastroenterologist," Dr. Roman was making a "summary statement of a more explicit explanation that Mr. Lopez needed a gastroenterologist, none was present at the hospital and, therefore, he needed to be transferred because the benefits of a gastroenterologist outweighed the dangers of transportation." This summary statement alone was enough for the court to find that the hospital had not violated EMTALA.

Stabilization as It Relates to Available Capabilities

In *Cherukuri v. Shalala (DHHS)*, 175 F.3d 446 (6th Cir. 1999), five patients were brought by ambulance to the ED at Appalachian Regional Hospital (ARH) in Williamson, Kentucky. Two had serious internal injuries and head injuries. The hospital had no trauma center or equipment for monitoring anesthesia during brain surgery and had a long-standing policy of not performing neurosurgery on brain injuries. ARH had always transferred patients with these types of injuries to larger hospitals with the expertise to deal with them.

Dr. Cherukuri, a general surgeon, was on call. He arrived and treated the five patients for several hours. After stabilizing their blood pressure and other vital signs, he transferred the two seriously injured patients to the hospital. One patient died during the transfer, and the other survived.

The Department of Health and Human Services (DHHS) fined Dr. Cherukuri $50,000 for each of the two transfers. They claimed Dr. Cherukuri could have performed surgery and stabilized the patients' conditions because an anesthesiologist was willing to "put the patients to sleep." Dr. Cherukuri appealed the decision; DHHS denied the review. He then appealed the decision to the Sixth Circuit Court of Appeals.

The Circuit Court dismissed the fine and all EMTALA charges against Dr. Cherukuri. In doing so, the Court of Appeals looked to the act, which states that a patient whose condition has not been stabilized may be transferred (1) only on "a certification that based upon the information available at the time of transfer, the medical benefits reasonably expected from the provision of appropriate medical treatment at another medical facility outweigh the increased risk to the individual . . . from effecting the transfer" and (2) only if "the receiving facility . . . has agreed to accept the transfer of the individual and to provide appropriate medical treatment."

The court found that Dr. Cherukuri did not violate the stabilization provision of EMTALA. Stabilization requires an objective standard of reasonableness based on the situation at hand and "requires merely that a hospital stabilize patients within the staff and facilities at the hospital." The patient must be evaluated and, at a minimum, provided with whatever medical support services and transfer arrangements are consistent with the capabilities of the institution and the well-being of the patient.

Health Insurance Portability and Accountability Act

The **Health Insurance Portability and Accountability Act (HIPAA)** was originally passed in 1996, with the first set of regulations established in 2003. The HITECH Act, which updated HIPAA for a health care world that transitioned to electronic medical records (EMRs), was passed in 2009, with those regulations taking effect in 2013.

The original goals of HIPAA were many, including to allow people to take their health insurance from one employer to another, to create medical spending accounts, and, most importantly, to safeguard the privacy and security of patients' health care information. Despite these seemingly clear objectives, HIPAA's legal implications are frequently misunderstood and the act is often used in a manner inconsistent with its intent and provisions. Understanding HIPAA starts with defining some basic terms and concepts.

Definitions

Protected health information (PHI) refers to health data created or shared by HIPAA-covered entities and their business associates in the course of providing health care and paying or billing for health care services. The key points about PHI are that it must be created by a covered entity; must be related to health status, health care, or payment; and must be linked to a specific individual.

A **covered entity** under HIPAA is one of three things: a health care provider, a health plan (eg, HMO, insurance company), or a health clearinghouse. These entities must transmit health information in electronic form in connection with a transaction covered by HIPAA (payment or administrative) to qualify. Ambulance providers of all kinds are explicitly included in the definition of a covered entity. A **business associate** is a person or entity, other than a covered entity, who performs activities on behalf of, or provides services to, a covered entity that involves access to PHI. Examples of services performed by a business associate include claims processing, quality improvement, practice management, and legal services. Covered entities must have a written agreement with business associates under which all of the standard HIPAA provisions are extended to the business associate.

HIPAA Privacy Rule

The HIPAA Privacy Rule addresses when a covered entity is permitted to use PHI. The default rule under HIPAA is that no party may use or disclose PHI without the patient's (or their representative's) written consent. However, HIPAA provides for numerous exceptions to the default rule.

First, and most importantly, providers may use or disclose PHI to accomplish the three main goals of health care: treatment, payment, and operations (TPO). Treatment is the provision, coordination, and management of health care providers. Payment is the reimbursement for treatment. Operations refers to administrative, financial, legal, or quality improvement services. A covered entity may disclose PHI without the patient's (or representative's) written consent to TPO entities; however, for payment and operations, the covered entity may disclose only the minimum necessary information to accomplish the stated goal. For example, providers may not disclose an entire health record just to accomplish payment, if a "face sheet" will do in that circumstance.

Many other disclosures are permitted under HIPAA without the patient's consent, including those related to public health activities, health oversight, end-of-life matters (funeral directors, coroners, medical examiners), organ and tissue donation, research activities, essential government functions, worker's compensation activities, and prevention of a serious imminent threat to health and safety. Specific disclosures to law enforcement are also permitted, such as identifying a specific person, providing information about a crime victim, and alerting law enforcement to a suspicious death. Likewise, a disclosure would be permitted when required by another specific law, such as reporting gunshot wounds or dog bites. Finally, PHI may be disclosed any time it is required by a judicial order.

HIPAA Security Rule

The HIPAA Security Rule addresses preventing unauthorized use of or access to PHI. HIPAA requires numerous levels of safeguards to protect patient information. Administrative safeguards include policies, authorization, training, and audits. Physical safeguards include hardware and software security, access limits, locks, and cameras. Technical safeguards include authentication and encryption of data.

Other HIPAA Requirements

HIPAA has other relevant provisions, such as the requirement to provide a notice of privacy practices at the time of services or when the emergency is over. It also allows for the correction of errors in PHI and requires that covered entities disclose PHI when requested by the patient within 30 days in the manner in which the patient requests it. This final provision is a common source of HIPAA violations.

HIPAA Violations

The Department of Health and Human Services, Office of Civil Rights, has exclusive jurisdiction over HIPAA violations. There is no private right for people to sue for HIPAA violations, although negligence claims can be brought using HIPAA as the default standard of care.

HIPAA violations range from a $100 fine for a violation that happened without the covered entity's knowledge and where reasonable diligence could not have prevented the violation, to willful neglect that goes uncorrected, which has a $50,000 minimum fine per violation. For offenses such as knowingly obtaining or disclosing PHI, using false pretenses to obtain PHI, or using PHI for personal gain or malicious harm, criminal penalties may potentially apply as well.

Legal Considerations During Transport Operations

Organizing the Personnel

CCTP qualification requirements are an issue that starts with the state licensing authority. State statutes and regulations will determine what each level of provider can do, and what levels of providers are necessary for certain types of transportation.

EMTALA requires the sending physician to specify the qualifications of personnel accompanying the patient during transport. To determine the level of personnel necessary to care for the patient and manage specialized equipment during transport, the physician should consider that personnel aboard local transport vehicles (ground and air) may be trained in a variety of skill levels, ranging from EMT to paramedic. Some systems also staff transport vehicles with nurses and physicians. Those personnel will be functioning under medical direction that provides protocols, including standing orders, for prehospital providers within their system. It is also important that all necessary and appropriate equipment, medications, and supplies that are within the scope of practice of the personnel onboard and that may be required by the patient be available in sufficient quantities. It is your responsibility to ensure the transport vehicle is adequately stocked **FIGURE 2-2**.

If the patient's current condition and all reasonably foreseeable complications can be managed within the licensure, training, and capability of the crew on the transfer vehicle, the patient may be transferred without being accompanied by ancillary personnel. However, when faced with the need to provide care beyond your scope of practice, you should request additional personnel for the transport.

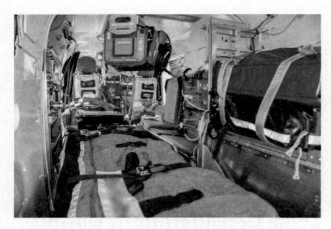

FIGURE 2-2 The critical care transport professional is responsible for making sure the vehicle is adequately stocked.

© VanderWolf Images/Shutterstock.

Ancillary personnel may have specialized skills (eg, a balloon pump technician or a perfusionist) or may assume overall responsibility for care (eg, a neonatologist for a neonatal intensive care patient). Whenever ancillary personnel assume ultimate responsibility for the care of the patient, you should provide support to them as needed. If the sending facility provides ancillary personnel and special equipment, it is that facility's responsibility to maintain the special equipment and provide for its return.

Preparing for Transfer

In preparation for transport, obtain the pertinent patient information, including the following:

- Reason for transfer
- Name of the receiving hospital and/or physician
- Level of care the patient needs during transport
- Treatment provided at the sending facility
- Medical treatment and drug orders for the duration of the transfer
- Any devices, such as ventilators or infusion pumps, that are necessary
- Complications to anticipate

In addition, obtain the name of the receiving physician before transport to avoid an unnecessary delay, embarrassment, and potential conflict at the receiving facility.

Review the transport orders for treatment *before* leaving the sending facility. Ensure those orders do not exceed your scope of practice. If they do, talk with the sending physician to modify the plan of care. If the plan cannot be modified, the sending facility must provide additional personnel to accompany you and facilitate the provision of needed care.

Communicating With the Health Care Team

When preparing for a transport, you should make every effort to communicate effectively, professionally, and succinctly with other members of the health care team. In some rare cases, conflict may arise between you and the sending physician regarding the interventions needed before transport. If this happens, state your concerns clearly and professionally. If there is still disagreement, contact the receiving facility's physician to attempt a cooperative resolution. If the situation cannot be resolved, contact the critical care transport agency's medical director for assistance. The ultimate decision may be to refuse to transport, but it should be carefully considered. Use extreme care and make sure your decision is reasonable and in the patient's best interests.

Some requests for transport may originate in a physician's office or clinic. The physician in this setting may not be familiar with your local protocols. In this situation, you should thoroughly communicate your capabilities and limitations to the sending physician. A plan of care that is within your scope of practice must be developed. If the physician is unwilling to help you develop such a plan, politely insist that the sending physician accompany the patient to the receiving facility **FIGURE 2-3**. If the

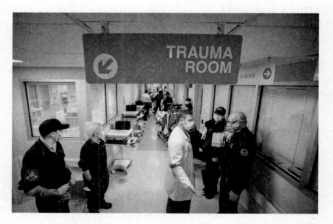

FIGURE 2-3 The critical care transport professional must work with the sending physician to develop an appropriate plan of care.

© Jeffrey Basinger/Newsday LLC/Getty Images.

sending physician is unwilling to do so, proceed as outlined in the preceding paragraph or contact medical control for assistance in resolving the conflict. Also consider having the sending physician speak directly with medical control to develop a plan of care for transport. In many circumstances involving conflict, you may become the mediator, with the goal of making sure the patient gets the best care. If you keep this objective in mind, you will be in the right almost every time!

Working With Medical Direction

During transport, you will usually operate with off-line medical direction using established written protocols or standing orders. If treatment beyond protocol is indicated or consultation is needed, establish contact with medical control and proceed under online medical direction. Make sure that online medical direction will be readily available before you begin the transport. Also, confirm that the sending and receiving physicians understand who will provide medical direction and that this may necessitate an alteration in the established plan of care. Sometimes the distance ranges of communications equipment may require shared responsibility between the sending and receiving physicians or even with the transport agency's medical director.

Protocols should include appropriate actions for cases in which communication with the established medical director is not possible. When continuous communications are not available, transport orders should enable you to respond appropriately to medical crises and changes in the patient's status. Standing orders or protocols may be developed to meet these needs.

You may need to remind the sending physician that prehospital protocols for EMS systems do not automatically apply in the interfacility transport environment. Prehospital protocols may be limited to use in specified environments by personnel who are described under state rules for the EMS system; hospital personnel who accompany the patient usually do not fall under these protocols and often are not familiar with them. When sending physicians write transport orders, they should designate the protocols by name in the transport orders, write pertinent sections into the orders, or attach a printed copy.

Completing the Transport

On arrival at the receiving facility, you must ensure continuity of care by giving a report to the designated receiving care provider. This report should include the following information:

- Patient's name, age, and sex
- Names of sending physician and facility
- Reason for the transfer
- Brief review of body systems
- Patient's history
- Medications administered
- Fluid intake
- Summary of the patient's condition during and tolerance of the transport in a clear, concise, and logical format

Transfer specimens, records, and laboratory and radiography results to the receiving provider, and make yourself available to answer questions after the transfer of care.

Documentation

All health care personnel are taught the importance of documentation **TABLE 2-3**. At no time is accurate and complete documentation more important than when providing care for a patient who is seriously ill or in critical condition. When a patient's status changes rapidly and without warning, numerous interventions may be carried out and transfer orders may have to be modified during transport. It is often a challenge to maintain documentation during a transfer that requires your constant attention to the patient.

Good documentation serves as protection for EMS personnel, and a complete and accurate report is a reflection of good patient care. An accurate, complete, legible medical record implies accurate,

TABLE 2-3 Purposes of Documentation
• Provides a record of care for CCTPs
• Ensures continuity of care through the health care system
• Facilitates quality improvement efforts
• Provides a mechanism for reimbursement
• Satisfies regulatory requirements
• Ensures legal defensibility of the care provided

© Jones & Bartlett Learning.

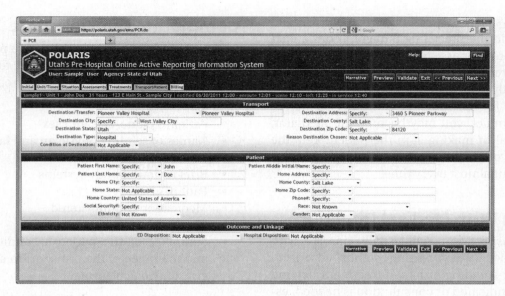

FIGURE 2-4 Electronic medical reports are the standard in EMS documentation.
Courtesy of the Utah Department of Health.

complete, organized assessment and management. If you make a mistake, document it. Include all requested information. If the information requested does not apply, include a "not applicable" or "N/A" note. If you look for something and it is not there, document its absence.

If the report is incomplete, others will assume the care was equally incomplete. The implementation of EMRs makes sloppiness a nonissue **FIGURE 2-4**, but that does not excuse the need for accuracy and completeness. Good documentation is a reflection of good patient care!

In the critical care transport setting, in which transfer often represents a team effort, it is important for team members to understand who has the responsibility for each aspect of documentation. When dealing with an acutely ill patient, it is easy to assume that the other team member may have documented an intervention or a set of vital signs, only to learn later that the documentation was not included in either report. Team members should work together at the conclusion of a run to ensure the documentation is accurate and complete.

It is particularly important to record certain essential elements of every transfer:

- Times of each set of vital signs and each assessment finding
- Details and times of each intervention (eg, drug doses and routes of administration)
- Patient responses to all interventions
- Untoward or adverse reactions
- Communications with medical control

- Deviation from transfer orders or standing orders
- Diversion to another hospital
- Refusal of treatment by the patient

If you must amend a run report following its submission to the receiving facility, make sure the amendment is done in accordance with local protocol.

Summary

The legal concepts described in this chapter may seem daunting at first, but are issues that CCTPs deal with every day. A basic understanding of the fundamentals of critical care transport laws can help guide your care and help you avoid negative legal consequences. Local laws vary, but general legal principles such as consent and negligence apply in all jurisdictions. Likewise, all transport providers are subject to, and should clearly understand, EMTALA and HIPAA. You should continue to learn about, become familiar with, and comply with these laws, regulations, and protocols as part of your continued growth as a CCTP.

Remaining calm, professional, and compassionate at all times will help you maintain the proper mindset to provide the best possible care for your patients. Further, it will engender in your patients and their families confidence that you have done your job well, thereby decreasing the likelihood they will file complaints or lawsuits if an adverse outcome occurs. Of course, ensuring that your documentation is clear and complete will go a long way toward protecting you as well.

Case Study

Your critical care transport team has been requested to provide an interfacility transport from a rural hospital. The patient is a 28-year-old woman at 29 weeks' gestation. She presented to the local ED around 2230 hours, reporting contractions every 10 minutes. ED staff placed the patient on a fetal monitor and confirmed their suspicions of preterm labor. The fetal monitor showed normal variability with no decelerations. The patient received a 0.25 mg subcutaneous injection of terbutaline prior to your arrival.

When you arrive, you find the patient in the ED. She has responded to the terbutaline, and her uterine contractions have slowed to 15 minutes apart and are less intense. The physician reports to you and your team that the fetal monitor has shown normal variability with no decelerations. You are assessing the patient and preparing her for transport when you realize that you accidentally left the transport fetal monitor in the ambulance. Given the transport time will be only 20 minutes, you decide not to go to the ambulance to retrieve the fetal monitor; instead, you plan to place the patient on the fetal monitor once you reach the ambulance.

During the short transfer time to the ambulance, the patient's contractions become more frequent. You load the patient into the ambulance and begin your transport. The patient's contractions have now increased to every 5 minutes. Your critical care protocols state to administer magnesium sulfate, with the initial loading dose of 4 to 6 g IV over 20 minutes, followed by a maintenance drip of 1 to 4 g/h. While you are mixing the loading dose, the patient is screaming and crying hysterically in pain. Your partner is attempting to calm her while you prepare the drip.

You place the magnesium sulfate on the transport infusion pump. The pump beeps, indicating that there is air in the line. You disconnect the drip, flush the line, and reattach it to the pump. The pump beeps again, indicating air in the line. You again disconnect the line in an attempt to flush it. The patient continues to scream in pain, and her contractions continue to increase

in frequency. You once again flush and reattach the line; the pump gives the green light indicating that it is functioning. Your ETA (estimated time of arrival) to the hospital is 5 minutes. You and your team reassess the patient and determine that the contractions are slowing in frequency.

As you and your team arrive at the receiving hospital, you realize that you forgot to attach the fetal monitor during the commotion. You quickly attach the fetal monitor without reviewing the strip. You unload the patient from the ambulance and transfer her to the obstetrics (OB) unit. You report to the staff that the patient was administered magnesium sulfate because of an increase in her contractions.

You and your team disconnect the patient from your equipment and transfer the patient to the hospital bed. The OB nurse attaches the patient to the hospital fetal monitor and becomes concerned with the fetal monitoring strip. She immediately calls for a physician. The fetal strip shows late deceleration. The nurse and physician ask to see the previous strip during the transport. You report that you forgot to place the patient on the monitor.

The patient is rushed to the operating room for immediate surgery. The infant is delivered with an Apgar score of 0 and requires full resuscitation efforts. The infant does not survive, despite the intense resuscitation efforts.

1. What actions on the part of the critical care transport team were responsible for the infant's outcome?
2. What factors would make this a case of negligence?
3. What has to be proven for a negligence lawsuit?
4. What should have been done to prevent this outcome?

Analysis

The symptoms of preterm labor include a contraction every 10 minutes or more, frequent pelvic pressure, lower back pain, and abdominal cramping. This patient was, indeed, in preterm labor.

Terbutaline is used to relax the smooth muscle of the uterus.

In this case, the critical care transport team's conduct was negligent, most certainly by not performing fetal monitoring during transport. The delay in administering magnesium could also qualify as negligence, depending on the circumstances.

Prep Kit

Ready for Review

- CCTPs must familiarize themselves with legal concepts and terms to operate effectively and protect themselves from charges of unlawful conduct. They must understand the laws where they practice and know the local protocols.
- CCTPs must understand the basic concepts of negligence and the following four findings, which are required to establish an act of negligence:
  1. A health care provider had a duty to act.
  2. The provider committed a breach of duty to act.
  3. The patient suffered damages as a result of the breach of duty.
  4. The damages were proximately caused (foreseeable) from that breach of duty.
- Providers may be protected from charges of negligence by laws and statutes requiring a higher standard be reached to find a health care provider responsible for an injury. These higher standards include reckless conduct and willful and wanton conduct.
- Although CCTPs are typically covered by their employer's professional liability insurance through the concept of *respondeat superior*, they may not be covered if they act beyond their scope of practice or if they provide care while off duty.
- Adult patients have a basic right to consent to medical care. Consent should be informed and may be either explicit or implicit.
- Providers must determine the patient's competence and decision-making capacity (DMC) in establishing consent. CCTPs who fail to assess DMC and obtain informed consent risk claims of liability that go beyond negligence, including battery and abandonment.
- All aspects of the assessment of competence, including any associated documents, DMC, and informed consent or refusal, should be objectively documented in the patient care report. This documentation should always use clear, concise, and objective language.
- CCTPs must understand the requirements defined by the Emergency Medical Treatment and Active Labor Act (EMTALA), including the medical screening exam and patient stabilization requirements, and the transfer requirements.
- Hospitals or physicians found in violation of the EMTALA provisions face several possible penalties, including fines, termination from Medicare and Medicaid programs, and civil litigation against the hospital and/or physician for injuries arising from an EMTALA violation.
- Current EMTALA case law has broad implications for interfacility transport, though it was originally developed simply to prevent hospitals from "dumping" patients because of inability to pay. Many EMTALA cases have a bearing on critical care transport, and as more cases are decided, their interfacility transport implications may become more far-reaching. This is a frequently changing area of the law through ongoing court cases.
- CCTPs must understand the purpose and requirements of the Health Insurance Portability and Accountability Act (HIPAA), especially including the concept of protected health information. They must adhere to the

Prep Kit Continued

guidelines, including the default conditions and the limited exceptions, under which they may share private patient information.

- In preparing for transport, you should communicate fully with the other members of the health care team at the sending and receiving facilities, and a plan of care should be developed that is within your scope of practice.
- In preparation for transport, you need to take the following actions:
  - Determine the reason for transfer.
  - Obtain the name of the receiving hospital and/or physician.
  - Determine whether a BLS, ALS, or CCT provider must accompany the patient and whether the sending facility plans to provide an escort.
  - Obtain information on the treatments provided at the sending facility, the treatments and drug orders for the duration of the transfer, and any potential complications that may arise during transport.
- The sending physician must send copies of medical records with the patient to the receiving facility that document the patient's current diagnosis and condition, symptoms the patient is experiencing, treatments given, results of tests conducted, written consent of the patient or a person with legal authority agreeing to the transfer, and the physician's verification that the benefits of transferring the patient outweigh the risks. The sending physician must also send samples of pertinent laboratory specimens.
- As a CCTP, you will typically operate with off-line medical direction using established written protocols. If treatment beyond those protocols is indicated or consultation is needed, you should establish contact with medical control and proceed under online medical direction.
- EMTALA requires the sending physician to designate the qualifications of personnel accompanying the patient during transport and to ensure that all necessary and

appropriate equipment, medications, and supplies that may be required by the patient are available in sufficient quantities and are within the scope of practice of the personnel accompanying the patient during transport.

- At the sending facility, you must assess the patient, discuss potential complications with the sending physician, and ensure the sending physician understands the capabilities and limitations of the transport team.
- During transport, you must monitor the patient's condition, provide the appropriate care within your scope of practice, inform medical control or the receiving facility of any changes in the patient's condition or any extenuating circumstances, and maintain thorough documentation.
- On arrival at the receiving facility, you must ensure continuity of care by giving a detailed report to the designated receiving care provider. This report must include all patient information, the names of the sending physician and facility, the reason for transfer, all documentation and records (including the patient's history, medications, fluid intake, condition during transport, and tolerance of transport), any transfer specimens from the sending facility, and any laboratory and/or radiography results from the sending facility.
- You should be available to answer questions from the receiving care provider after the transfer of care is complete.
- Documentation for every transfer should include the times of each set of vital signs and each assessment finding, the details and times of each intervention (such as drug doses and routes of administration), the patient's responses to all interventions and any adverse reactions, all communications with medical control, any deviations from the transfer or standing orders, any diversions to another hospital or facility, and any refusals of treatment by the patient.

Prep Kit Continued

Vital Vocabulary

abandonment The termination of the patient relationship without assurance that an equal or greater level of care will continue.

assault The unlawful act of placing a person in apprehension of immediate bodily harm without their consent.

battery The unlawful touching of another person without their consent.

breach of duty to act A case in which a health care provider does not conform to the standard of care by providing inappropriate care, failing to act, or acting beyond the scope of practice.

business associate As defined under HIPAA, a person or entity, other than a covered entity, who performs activities on behalf of, or provides services to, a covered entity that involves access to protected health information.

civil damages Monetary compensation awarded to a plaintiff in noncriminal court proceedings.

common law Case law established by prior disputes that is published to guide future proceedings.

competence A legal determination, through a statute or court proceeding, that a person is capable of making personal decisions, including about their health care.

consent Voluntary agreement by a patient with sufficient mental capacity to capably accept or refuse assessment, treatment, or transport offered by the care provider.

covered entity As defined under HIPAA, a health care provider, a health plan, or a health clearinghouse that must transmit health information in electronic form in connection with a transaction covered by HIPAA (payment or administrative) to qualify. Ambulance providers of all kinds are explicitly included in the definition of a covered entity.

damages In a legal context, harm that results from a breach of duty by a health care provider who is found negligent. Usually, the injury is physical.

decision-making capacity (DMC) The determination that a patient's brain is functioning well enough to process information and make health care decisions.

discovery rule A legal rule stating that the statute of limitations for filing a legal case does not begin until the injured party can reasonably be expected to know of the injury.

do not resuscitate (DNR) order A type of advance directive that describes which life-sustaining procedures should be performed if the patient suffers cardiopulmonary arrest.

duty to act A legal obligation of health care providers to render medical care to a certain level. When the duty to act applies varies from state to state.

emergency medical condition A condition manifesting itself by acute symptoms of sufficient severity (including severe pain) such that the absence of immediate medical attention could reasonably be expected to result in placing the individual's health (or the health of an unborn child) in serious jeopardy, serious impairment to bodily functions, or serious dysfunction of bodily organs.

Emergency Medical Treatment and Active Labor Act (EMTALA) A federal law passed by the US Congress in 1986, with the primary goal of preventing hospitals from failing to treat patients, or transferring patients to other facilities, based on their insurance status or ability to pay for services.

expressed consent A patient's voluntary verbal, nonverbal, or written agreement to consent to treatment or transport.

Health Insurance Portability and Accountability Act (HIPAA) A federal law enacted in 1996, providing for criminal sanctions and civil penalties for releasing a patient's protected health information in a way not authorized by the patient.

implied consent The legal assumption made on behalf of a person who is unable to give consent that they would give consent if able to do so.

Prep Kit Continued

informed consent The process of proposing to the patient a course of action (assessment, treatment, transport), the risks associated with that action, the benefits associated with the action, and any reasonable alternatives, and then allowing the patient to decide if they want the provider to proceed with the action.

medical control The oversight designed to ensure that actions taken by providers on behalf of patients are appropriate. It is divided into direct (online) medical control, which is available in real time via radio or mobile phone, and indirect (off-line) medical control, such as standing orders and protocols.

medical direction Supervision of medical care by a physician empowered to authorize and review CCTPs, usually through protocols, standing orders, education, and quality improvement efforts.

medical screening exam An exam that is legally required when the patient is within 250 yards of the hospital, or on hospital property, and is seeking treatment for an emergency medical condition; it must be performed by a physician, physician assistant, or nurse practitioner.

negligence Failure to provide the same quality of care (as defined by applicable standards) that is reasonably expected for a provider to give under similar circumstances. Negligence is established when the plaintiff proves four elements: duty to act, breach of the duty, injury to the patient, and the breach as the direct cause of the injury.

off-line medical direction Medical direction given through a set of protocols, standing orders, educational programs, policies, and/or standards.

online medical direction Medical direction in which the care provider is in direct contact with a physician, usually via two-way radio or telephone.

physician orders for life-sustaining treatment (POLST) A legal document that establishes in advance what care a person wants, and does not want, in the event that they are unable to consent to care at the time.

protected health information (PHI) Individually identifiable information (eg, name, Social Security number, and date of birth), health information (eg, laboratory results and medical history), and demographic information (eg, address and telephone number) that is protected by HIPAA.

proximally caused A legal term that describes damages that could have reasonably been anticipated before the breach of duty occurred.

reckless conduct A more serious finding than typical negligence; it involves consciously disregarding the known risks of a course of action. Also called gross negligence.

respondeat superior The legal concept that an employer is responsible for the acts of its agents.

scope of practice The body of knowledge, skills, and therapies that CCTPs can legally apply in patient care, based on training, certification, medical direction, and applicable law.

sovereign immunity A type of immunity often afforded EMS providers that is provided only to governmental entities. This immunity can align with the reckless or willful and wanton requirements, or it can differentiate between ministerial acts (those requiring a specific act given a set of circumstances) and discretionary acts (those in which the provider has some latitude in decision making).

statutes Formal laws passed by a legislative body and signed by an executive.

statute of limitations The time limit within which negligence cases must be filed; it is typically 2 years but varies from state to state and may be longer if the patient is a minor.

tort A wrongful act between people or entities that gives rise to a civil lawsuit.

willful and wanton A more serious finding than typical negligence misconduct; it usually requires an intentional act of misconduct.

Prep Kit Continued

References

Barstow C, Shahan B, Roberts M; Womack Army Medical Center, Fort Bragg, North Carolina. Evaluating medical decision-making capacity in practice. *Am Fam Physician*. 2018;98(1):40-46.

Emergency Medical Treatment and Active Labor Act. Centers for Medicare and Medicaid Services website. https://www.cms.gov/Regulations-and-Guidance/Legislation/EMTALA. Modified March 4, 2021. Accessed April 30, 2021.

EMTALA fact sheet: main points. American College of Emergency Physicians website. https://www.acep.org/life-as-a-physician/ethics--legal/emtala/emtala-fact-sheet. Accessed April 30, 2021.

Health information privacy. US Department of Health and Human Services website. https://www.hhs.gov/hipaa/index.html. Accessed April 30, 2021.

HIPAA basics. Office of the National Coordinator for Health Information Technology website. https://www.healthit.gov/topic/privacy-security-and-hipaa/hipaa-basics. Accessed April 30, 2021.

Lindberg J, Johansson M, Brostrom L. Temporizing and respect for patient self-determination. *J Med Ethics*. 2019;45(3):161-167.

Negligence. Legal Information Institute, Cornell Law School website. https://law.cornell.edu/wex/negligence. Accessed April 30, 2021.

Sovereign Immunity. Legal Information Institute, Cornell Law School website. https://law.cornell.edu/wex/sovereign_immunity. Accessed April 30, 2021.

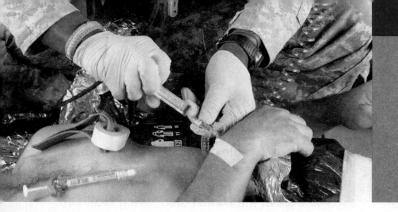

Chapter 3

Patient Safety

Jeffrey S. Rabrich, DO, FACEP, EMT-P

OBJECTIVES

After completing this chapter, you will be able to:
1. Recognize how health care quality has evolved and is measured (p 48).
2. Define patient safety (p 49).
3. Recognize the various levels of safety violations (pp 49–50).
4. Describe the elements of a safety culture, including a just culture and the characteristics demonstrated by highly reliable organizations (pp 50–51).
5. Identify the various types of errors that arise in health care, including medication and prescription errors, errors related to patient and procedure identification, and errors occurring during transitions of care and handoffs (pp 52–54).
6. Explain the systemic factors that contribute to health care errors (pp 54–55).
7. Describe the process for handling sentinel events (serious adverse events) (pp 55–57).
8. Summarize strategies and techniques to avoid errors, including Six Sigma, Lean, crew resource management, simulation training, and failure mode and effect analysis (pp 59–60).
9. Discuss key factors affecting quality in EMS settings (pp 60–63).

Introduction

The process of a patient entering the emergency medical services (EMS) system begins with the decision by the patient to seek care and ends when the patient is handed off to hospital personnel. Critical care transport (CCT) begins when a referring practitioner or a transfer call center contacts a CCT service with a request to move a patient. In an ideal EMS system (or any hospital setting), the correct medication is given via the correct route to the correct patient, the destination decision is always right, and the differential diagnosis is adequately considered. A patient's care process is very complex, including many separate components— clinicians, radiology, laboratory, transport, and prehospital care, among others—and all of these groups must coordinate their actions as part of the joint effort that makes up the health care organization. In fact, if one were to create a process map of the steps to safely move a patient from one care setting to another, it would undoubtedly contain hundreds of steps that must be flawlessly executed. In an ideal world, a patient moves seamlessly through the various departments from initial presentation to disposition. Of course, in the real world, the complexities of patient care, among other variables, present many opportunities for process failures, errors, and adverse outcomes. It is the goal of the patient safety organization or the highly reliable organization to reduce the chance of error as close to zero as possible.

History of Quality as a Health Care Discipline

Awareness of health care quality remained minimal and measurement of quality was a slow-moving process until the early 1990s, when several landmark papers on this topic were published. One of the earliest movements for quality began in the early 1900s with Dr. Ernest Codman, a surgeon at Massachusetts General Hospital. Codman was one of the first physicians to insist on recording and reporting on individual physician outcomes—that is, an "end-results system"—to monitor the quality of physician and hospital care. His work led to the establishment of the American College of Surgeons in 1913. Unfortunately, work in improving health care quality languished for much of the 20th century.

Scope of the Problem

In the early 1990s, the Harvard Medical Practice Study reported that almost 4% of hospitalized patients sustained significant adverse events during their care and nearly one-third of these events occurred secondary to human error. This study and others ultimately led the Institute of Medicine (IOM; now called the National Academy of Medicine) to investigate health care quality. The IOM's seminal report on this topic was published in 1999. Titled *To Err Is Human: Building a Safer Health System*, this report not only captivated the medical community, but also caused the media and the general public to become keenly aware of the issue of safety in health care and put this concern on the national agenda.

To Err Is Human reported in 1999 that almost 100,000 Americans were dying each year secondary to medical errors, citing these errors as the eighth leading cause of death in the United States. The major revelation in this report was the concept that failures or errors in care were frequently not the result of individual behaviors or decisions, but rather were often related to the intrinsic processes of care in the health care system. Thus, the IOM suggested, efforts to improve safety should address process-related errors rather than target individuals. Slowly, over time, the idea of system failure rather than human error as the key consideration gained credence within the health care community. Eventually, other organizations, such as the National Quality Forum, the Institute for Healthcare Improvement, and the

Agency for Healthcare Research and Quality, invested in efforts to decrease the frequency of medical errors.

Despite these efforts, an analysis published in 2016 suggests that medical errors may now be the third leading cause of death, claiming more than 250,000 lives in the United States each year. However, a more recent study, published by the Yale School of Medicine in 2020, suggests that the number of preventable hospital deaths may be grossly overestimated at 250,000, and is more likely closer to 22,000, with these deaths occurring mostly in patients with a life expectancy of 3 months. While 22,000 is still far too many preventable deaths, emphasis on patient safety and just culture appear to be helping reduce errors.

Quality of EMS Care

In 2007, the IOM published *Emergency Medical Services: At the Crossroads,* a comprehensive look at the current state of EMS at the time and the challenges and limitations of the modern EMS system in the United States. Among the information provided in this report was a review of safety and efficacy of EMS care. The IOM report noted that EMS providers face numerous challenges in delivering care:

> Prehospital emergency care services are delivered in an uncertain, stressful environment where the need for haste and other potential distractions produce threats to patient care and safety. In addition, shift work and around-the-clock coverage contribute to fatigue among EMS providers. Error rates for such procedures as endotracheal intubation are high, especially compared with the same procedures performed in a hospital setting.

Although this topic has not been studied extensively, the critical care transport professional (CCTP) likely encounters more critically ill patients and more complex patient care scenarios than a 9-1-1 responder simply because of the serious nature of an injury or illness that necessitates transfer. Hence, the likelihood of errors may be much greater in the CCT environment than in the usual EMS setting.

The *EMS at the Crossroads* report went on to discuss the six quality aims included in the IOM's *Crossing the Quality Chasm: A New Health System for the 21st Century* report, which had been published in 2001. Specifically, *Crossing the Quality*

TABLE 3-1 Six Quality Aims

- **Safety:** Avoid needless death, injury, pain, and suffering for patients and staff.
- **Timeliness:** Waste no one's time.
- **Effectiveness:** Provide care and service based on best evidence and informed by patient values and preferences.
- **Efficiency:** Remove all unnecessary processes or steps in processes; streamline all activities.
- **Equity:** Provide fair and equitable care and service; treat all patients equally.
- **Patient centeredness:** Honor individual patients— their values, choices, culture, social context, and specific needs.

Data from Institute of Medicine. *Crossing the Quality Chasm: A New Health System for the 21st Century.* Washington, D.C.: National Academy Press; 2001.

Chasm insisted that health care should be safe, effective, patient centered, timely, efficient, and equitable **TABLE 3-1**. Each of these characteristics is examined further in this chapter.

The six quality aims have some unique implications in the EMS field. Although EMS systems try to be patient centered and provide the appropriate resources to each patient at the appropriate time, numerous barriers to patient-centered care remain. Barriers include language and care of special populations such as geriatric patients, pediatric patients with and without special needs, and patients who have undergone bariatric surgery, to name a few. Chapter 25, *Bariatric, Psychiatric, and Special Situations,* discusses some of these special patient populations in more detail.

While many of the issues raised in the 2007 IOM report remain valid today, numerous advances have occurred since it was released. Research has increased dramatically in the prehospital field, the role of the EMS medical director has been given more weight, a medical subspecialty of EMS medicine has been created, and many large EMS agencies have devoted considerable time and personnel to safety and quality efforts. In 2012, the unique knowledge and skill set of EMS medicine was acknowledged when the American Board of Emergency Medicine recognized EMS as an official subspecialty. By creating a specialty certification in EMS medicine, a minimum standard for qualifications and training was established. Part of the core content for EMS medicine is quality improvement and medical oversight of agency quality programs.

In more recent years, several organizations have focused on disease-specific quality measures for EMS systems to ensure key measures are met. For example, the American Heart Association's Mission: Lifeline program recognizes EMS agencies and hospitals that have achieved excellence in caring for patients with ST-elevation myocardial infarction (STEMI). The American College of Surgeons has established trauma measures for EMS. The National Academies of Sciences, Engineering, and Medicine released a report in 2016 titled *A National Trauma Care System: Integrating Military and Civilian Trauma Systems to Achieve Zero Preventable Deaths After Injury,* which provides recommendations geared toward achieving zero preventable deaths.

What Is Patient Safety?

Defining patient safety has proved difficult for organizations, because it can be considered a philosophy, a discipline, or an attribute. The World Health Organization provides a fairly simple definition: Patient safety means freedom from unnecessary harm or potential harm associated with health care. The Agency for Healthcare Research and Quality (AHRQ) offers a more complex definition:

> Patient safety is a discipline in the health care sector that applies safety science methods toward the goal of achieving a trustworthy system of health care delivery. Patient safety is also an attribute of health care systems; it minimizes the incidence and impact of, and maximizes recovery from, adverse events.

In this chapter, patient safety is defined as the reduction of risk of unnecessary harm associated with EMS care to an acceptable minimum. The acceptable minimum is defined by the limits of the best available medical evidence, equipment, technology, and human skill.

Error Versus Harm

The impetus for patient safety programs is the body of evidence showing that adverse medical events are widespread and preventable, resulting in too much harm. Emergency medicine, EMS, and CCT are all fields characterized by the need for quick decision making using limited information, complex tasks, and long work hours. These characteristics mean that even the brightest and most conscientious clinician will at times make errors.

When thinking about adverse events, however, it is important to distinguish between the concepts of error and harm. A medical error is a preventable adverse effect resulting from care, whether or not it is evident or harmful to the patient. Harm is unintended physical injury resulting from or contributed to by medical care. Not all errors will reach patients and cause harm, but it is essential for organizations to study these errors and look for opportunities to improve the processes that allow them to happen. Errors that lead to serious patient harm are rarely the result of just one error involving just one person. Instead, they usually comprise a series of errors or breakdowns in processes, many of which have been occurring for some time, but not all at once. This multifaceted breakdown is often referred to as the Swiss cheese model (discussed later in the chapter) or, in aviation, as links in the accident chain.

Near Misses

Breakdowns in communication that almost led to errors or harm can be referred to as near misses or close calls. A near miss is an unplanned event that did not cause injury, illness, or damage, but had the potential to do so; it is indistinguishable from a full-fledged adverse event in all but the outcome. Near misses may occur many times before an actual harmful incident takes place, and provide opportunities to learn from the occasion and identify improvement options.

An example of a near miss is a provider ordering a medication without considering the patient's allergies; however, a nurse or paramedic checks for allergies and speaks with the provider before administering the prescribed medication. Thus, the provider's error is caught and the contraindicated medication is not given.

It is widely believed that near-miss events are heavily underreported. Often staff do not report these events because they fear they will be disciplined, they perceive a lack of support or caring by supervisors, or they believe it is unnecessary to report the incident if no patient harm occurred. In fact, near-miss events are among the most important to report, because they provide the organization with an opportunity to analyze its processes and improve safety. Moreover, talking about near misses can be easier for staff because there are fewer liability concerns when no one was harmed.

Medical Errors

Although the study of errors began in the early 1900s, it really took off when the safety of commercial aviation came under scrutiny. In this field, studies showed a system-level approach was the best way to detect and prevent errors. In other words, rather than looking at individuals and deeming every incident to be a single human failure, it was necessary to look deeper and see other confounding factors that may have set the stage for error.

Medical error can be defined as the failure of a planned action to be completed as intended, or the use of a wrong plan to achieve an aim related to health care. Such errors can be categorized as adverse drug events, wrong-site surgeries, falls, burns, pressure ulcers, and mistaken patient identities. High error rates with serious consequences are most likely to occur in the intensive care unit (ICU), operating room, emergency department (ED), and, in all likelihood, CCT. Every error represents an opportunity to improve a process, but to achieve this goal, these errors must be recognized and made known so they can be analyzed.

Safety Culture

Improving the culture of safety within health care is essential in preventing and reducing errors and improving quality of care. The safety culture is primarily a locally managed issue, as each hospital or transport service may vary in its perception of this culture and the programs it implements to manage safety concerns. A safety culture encompasses several key features:

- Acknowledging that organizations engage in high-risk activities and determining the importance of consistent safe operations to counteract these activities
- Supporting a blame-free environment where errors can be reported without fear of punishment
- Maintaining organizational commitment to address reported errors and safety concerns

Validated surveys given to providers through the AHRQ, including the Surveys on Patient Safety and the Safety Attitudes Questionnaire, can be used to measure an organization's safety culture. These surveys ask providers to rate the safety culture of their workplace and the organization in its entirety. The AHRQ provides yearly updated benchmarking data from the hospital survey, including assessments of specific activities, such as teamwork training, development of safety teams, and use of leadership WalkRounds (a concept developed by the Institute for Healthcare Improvement to encourage employees in leadership positions to regularly review safety matters with frontline staff). Such activities have been associated with some improvements in safety culture measurements but are not yet linked to lower error rates.

While hospitals that accept any federal payment are required to participate in the Surveys on Patient Safety on a regular basis, there is no such requirement for EMS organizations. Indeed, few EMS agencies seem to survey their providers regarding safety culture or attitudes regarding safety. To help address this problem, the Center for Patient Safety and the National Registry of EMTs developed a survey specific to EMS, called the EMS Patient Safety Culture Survey. This survey includes some components taken from the AHRQ's Surveys on Patient Safety.

Just Culture

Assigning blame for errors is not a panacea for a less-than-stellar safety culture. Don Norman, author of *The Design of Everyday Things*, highlights the futility of this blame game:

> People make errors, which lead to accidents. Accidents lead to deaths. The standard solution is to blame the people involved. If we find out who made the errors and punish them, we solve the problem, right? Wrong. The problem is seldom the fault of an individual; it is the fault of the system. Change the people without changing the system and the problems will continue.

A key element of an effective safety culture is the concept called just culture. A just culture focuses on identifying issues that lead to errors or unsafe behaviors, while still maintaining individual accountability for reckless behavior. It helps distinguish various types of errors, including human error (ie, slips), at-risk behavior (ie, taking shortcuts), and reckless behavior (ie, ignoring required safety steps). Humans are not perfect, so systems should anticipate some level of error; a mistake or lapse can happen to anyone. Human error is typically a product of the current system design and behavioral choices; therefore, it should not be viewed as a punishable action, but rather as an opportunity to improve the systems.

Highly Reliable Organizations

Another concept that contributes to an effective safety culture is the highly reliable organization (HRO). The airline and nuclear power plant industries are populated with HROs that share some common traits. For example, all HROs are preoccupied with failure, and there is an understanding in each organization's culture that failures will inevitably occur. HROs focus on managing these failures, however, so that a failure does not reach the public (the patient, in the health care industry). This drive has led to the redundancy in training, equipment, and maintenance seen in the airline industry. The airlines and nuclear power plants recognize that a person or piece of equipment may fail, so they have put considerable effort into ensuring that a single failure does not cause a catastrophic event (ie, plane crash, nuclear meltdown). In health care, an HRO would focus on double-checks (of high-alert medications, for example) and other systems to ensure that a single failure, which is inevitable, does not lead to patient harm.

Developing a Safety Culture in EMS

Many organizations involved in EMS care have recognized that the harm reductions seen in well-designed patient safety programs in hospitals need to be adapted and developed for EMS systems. EMS agency leaders and medical directors will be critical leaders in furthering this effort.

In 2014, two of the most prominent organizations involved in EMS and emergency care, the American College of Emergency Physicians (ACEP) and the National Association of EMS Physicians (NAEMSP), released a policy statement emphasizing the critical nature of a safety culture in EMS. The statement, which was revised in 2021, reads as follows:

The American College of Emergency Physicians (ACEP) and the National Association of EMS Physicians (NAEMSP) believe that safety must become a foundational component of every emergency medical services (EMS) system. Providing high-quality EMS requires understanding risk and embracing practices to prevent harm to patients, EMS professionals, and members of our communities. EMS physicians should lead development and support of a culture of safety in EMS systems.

We believe:

- EMS systems should partner with national organizations to increase safety in all aspects of EMS.
- EMS systems should support the development, implementation, and ongoing evaluation of comprehensive system-wide safety, quality, and risk management programs.
- EMS safety and comprehensive risk management should be emphasized in both initial and continuing education for all EMS professionals, including EMS physicians.
- EMS systems should implement and support the Just Culture approach to facilitate honest and prompt reporting of risk and error and to support analysis of near miss and adverse events in an environment of professionalism and accountability for systems and individuals.
- Integrated EMS safety data systems with mandatory reporting should be created to promote evaluation of safety programs and to promote research that advances understanding of safety for EMS professionals, systems, and patients.
- EMS physicians should advocate for EMS safety-related programs coordinated at the local, regional, state, and federal levels based on evidence-based practice and benchmarks.
- EMS physicians should evaluate technologies and equipment for improvements in safety for patients, EMS professionals, and the public.
- EMS physicians should support the development of and adherence to safety standards and guidelines based on the best available evidence.
- EMS physicians should integrate opportunities to limit risk and increase safety within protocols, policies, and standing orders.

A culture of safety in EMS systems. American College of Emergency Physicians website. https://www.acep.org/patient-care/policy-statements/a-culture-of-safety-in-ems-systems/. Revised April 2021. Accessed September 22, 2021.

Common Health Care Errors

Many types of errors can occur in health care. Perhaps most notable are medication and prescription errors, but other, less-common errors include wrong patient identification, transfusion errors, preventable suicides, falls, burns, wrong-side procedures, and errors in transition of care or handoffs. Lucian Leape has identified and categorized these errors **TABLE 3-2**, and some of the most important are discussed here.

Medication and Prescription Errors

Medication-related errors occur frequently in hospitals and to an unknown degree in EMS. Not all

TABLE 3-2 Types of Medical Errors

Error Category	Specific Errors
Diagnostic	Error or delay in diagnosis Failure to employ indicated tests Use of outmoded tests or therapy Failure to act on results of monitoring or testing
Treatment	Error in the performance of an operation, procedure, or test Error in administering the treatment Error in the dose or method of using a drug Avoidable delay in treatment or in responding to an abnormal test Inappropriate care
Preventive	Failure to provide prophylactic treatment Inadequate monitoring or follow-up of treatment
Other	Failure of communication Equipment failure Other system failure

© Jones & Bartlett Learning.

result in actual harm, but those that do can have devastating and costly consequences.

The process of a patient receiving a medication is complex and fraught with opportunities for error, including prescribing, dispensing, administering, and monitoring errors. One study conducted at two prestigious teaching hospitals found that almost 2% of admissions experienced a preventable adverse drug event, resulting in increased hospital costs amounting to approximately $2.8 million annually for a 700-bed teaching hospital.

Medication-related errors are studied by examining adverse drug event (ADE) incidence. The discussion in this chapter is related to the subset of ADEs considered to be preventable or to occur secondary to error.

Medication Errors in EMS Settings

Children are at higher risk of incorrect dosing for several reasons. Often estimations of children's weights can be significantly different from their actual weights due to EMS providers' inability to accurately estimate weight even when using length-based measuring devices such as the length-based assessment tape. Additionally, many more medication doses are based on weight in children than in adults, so they require weight-based calculations to arrive at the correct total dose—a process that is prone to calculation errors by providers. Adding to the dosing confusion, several medications, such as antibiotics and vasopressors, come in more than one concentration.

In general, each time a dose calculation (such as that based on weight) is performed, the chance of error increases. Additionally, the potential for medication-related errors increases as the average number of drugs administered increases.

Variations in product packaging and labeling increase the potential for medication errors in the EMS environment. Medication manufacturing shortages may compel EMS agencies to substitute medications with which CCTPs are less familiar, medications from different manufacturers that use different labeling or packaging, and medications used as therapeutic substitutions that may have different dosing regimens. For example, recent medication shortages have included $D_{50}W$ (dextrose 50% in water), sodium bicarbonate, dopamine, morphine sulfate, and glucagon. In a high-pressure, uncontrolled environment such as the back of a moving ambulance with a patient who is decompensating or going into cardiac arrest, it is very easy for medication errors to occur.

The EMS community has given much attention over the past 10 years to medication errors in the pediatric population and to addressing calculation errors in high-stress situations. Devices such as syringes with graduated stops, color coding, and other engineering controls have been designed to prevent calculation and administration errors, and smartphone apps are available to help guide and calculate pediatric dosing.

Look-Alike, Sound-Alike Medication Errors

One type of medical error that has been specifically targeted in recent years is prescribing and dispensing errors related to look-alike, sound-alike (LASA) medications. The Joint Commission highlighted the potential for LASA medication errors in a Sentinel Event Alert. As part of the effort to avoid such errors, hospitals are expected to maintain a list of these LASA medications. The Institute for Safe Medication Practices (ISMP) maintains a reference table of these drugs. In addition, the ISMP recommends the following processes to help avoid LASA errors:

- Use both the brand name and the generic name on prescriptions and labels.
- Note the medication's purpose on prescriptions.
- Configure selection options on computer screens so that look-alike names do not appear consecutively.
- Change the appearance of look-alike names to highlight their differences. For example, use tall-man, or mixed-case, lettering (eg, DOPamine versus DoBUTamine).

Additional recommendations include focusing on prescription legibility through improved handwriting or the use of electronic prescribing, and physically separating LASA medications in different storage areas.

Wrong Patient Identification/ Wrong-Side Procedures

Wrong patient identification is a potentially serious problem in health care that can easily lead to a medication administration error. Most commonly, this problem involves a nurse accidentally administering an intended medication to the wrong patient. Practice recommendations to rectify this error include always using multiple patient identifiers. Providers administering medications at the bedside should always use two patient identifiers, such as the patient's name and date of birth.

The confirmation of patient identity is particularly important for EMS crews picking up a patient for an interfacility transport or transport home. While the 9-1-1 EMS call for a single patient yields one obvious patient in most cases, it is entirely possible for a crew to pick up the wrong patient at a hospital or health care facility. This kind of error has occurred on several occasions, illustrating why a transport agency must employ the same safety measures, such as two patient identifiers, that the hospitals use.

Few medical errors are as terrifying as those related to surgery involving the wrong site, wrong patient, or wrong procedure. In the literature, this type of error is termed a **never event**, meaning it should never occur and indicates serious underlying safety problems. Fortunately, this type of event is exceedingly rare. Efforts to combat its occurrence include developing redundant mechanisms for identifying the correct site, procedure, and patient through initiatives where surgeons (and sometimes the patient) mark the site prior to the patient's arrival in the operating room.

Other protocols created to combat this problem focus on a **universal time-out**. The time-out is a planned pause before the beginning of a procedure that improves communication among all personnel in the room; it allows time for everyone to review important aspects of the procedure. This time-out concept has been proposed for the EMS environment as well. Examples include implementing an "EMS time-out" for trauma and other critical patients on EMS arrival so no key information is lost. While most 9-1-1 calls lead to procedures that are emergent, such that a pause is not feasible, an interfacility transport usually affords enough time for ensuring certainty.

Errors During Transitions of Care and Handoffs

Transitioning care is an integral part of care in an ED and prehospital care of a patient. Multiple handoffs may occur between various providers, including physicians, nurses, medics, and support staff, and errors during handoffs can easily occur.

Standardized approaches to transitions in care help prevent handoff errors. One method integrated in multiple health systems is the **situation, background, assessment, and recommendation (SBAR)** technique. This technique has become best practice in health care, effortlessly structuring critical information. The US Navy developed it as a communication technique for use in nuclear submarines, and it was introduced into health care in the 1990s.

The SBAR technique allows for a brief, yet concise and expected, handoff of information. Through this method, everyone involved in a handoff has a shared mental model, which improves the safety of these handoffs and transitions in care. The elements of the SBAR technique are summarized in **TABLE 3-3**.

Many EMS systems have implemented a standardized format for the handoff from the EMS crew to the hospital to ensure the transfer of critical information and completeness. One such format,

TABLE 3-3 Situation, Background, Assessment, and Recommendation (SBAR) Technique

Situation	Briefly describe the current situation. Give a clear, succinct overview of the pertinent issues.
Background	Briefly state the pertinent history. What got us to this point?
Assessment	Summarize the facts and give your best assessment. What is going on? Use your best judgment.
Recommendation	Which actions are you asking for? What do you want to happen next?

Courtesy of Michael Leonard, Doug Bonacum, and Suzanne Graham.

used for trauma patients, is MIST—an acronym that stands for Mechanism of injury, Injuries/Inspection, vital Signs, and Treatment. A study published in *Prehospital Emergency Care* in 2020 demonstrated an improved handoff experience between nurses and paramedics when using MIST; however, data on error reduction with this technique are limited.

Why Do Health Care Errors Occur?

Various factors have contributed to the epidemic of medical errors. One commonly cited problem is the decentralized and fragmented nature of the health care delivery system. Medicine has traditionally treated errors as a failure on the part of one person, reflecting inadequate knowledge or skill. Governmental agencies, which set the standards for much of US health care, no longer use this terminology; they believe that errors reflect the functioning of the entire health care system.

Systems Approach

The systems approach suggests that most human errors occur in the context of a poorly designed system. For example, lapses in human tasks may occur secondary to long work hours, and predictable mistakes occur when inexperienced staff members face complex cognitive decisions. Instead of punishing the person, the systems approach seeks to identify those situations that give rise to human error and remedy the underlying problem. This approach acknowledges the reality that most major accidents result from multiple, smaller mistakes in environments with serious underlying system flaws.

Swiss Cheese Model

A British psychologist, James Reason, pioneered the modern field of systems analysis and introduced the Swiss cheese model to address errors. In this model, people make errors that result in consequences because of flawed systems—the holes in the cheese. Imagine several slices of Swiss cheese lined up next to one another; usually the holes do not all line up. If you tried to thread a string through the holes in all the slices, one or more slices would probably act as a barrier to the string's passage. However, sometimes all the holes might line up, leading to catastrophic error **FIGURE 3-1**.

Reason also introduced the concepts of latent and active errors to distinguish between human and system errors. An active error usually involves frontline staff and occurs at a contact point between a staff member and some aspect of a larger system. A latent error is a mistake that is likely to occur secondary to organizational or design failures that allow the inevitable active errors to cause harm.

Another way to think about latent and active errors is to envision the sharp and blunt ends of something. The sharp end refers to an active error, such as when a frontline staff member makes

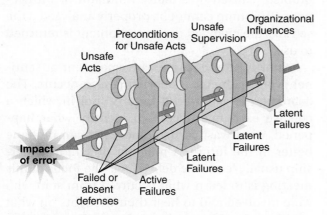

FIGURE 3-1 The Swiss cheese model of error.

Reproduced from Reason J. Human error: models and management. *BMJ*. March 18, 2000;320:768-770 with permission from BMJ Publishing Group Ltd.

an error in patient care—for example, a surgeon performing the wrong procedure. Active errors can further be classified as slips and mistakes. A slip refers to a lapse in concentration that occurs in the face of distractions, fatigue, or stress. An example of a slip would be if a CCTP accidentally pushed the wrong button on a piece of equipment or, because of a memory failure (lapse), failed to administer a medication. A mistake is when an action occurs as intended but is the wrong action; such an event often occurs secondary to lack of experience, insufficient training, or negligence. The blunt end refers to a latent error, which may be attributable to the complexity of the health care system and to those not in direct contact with patients who set policy and manage the overall system.

Handling Serious Errors

A sentinel event or serious adverse event (SAE) is a patient safety event in which an error reaches a patient and results in death, permanent harm, or severe temporary harm with interventions required to sustain life. Examples include wrong-site procedure, wrong procedure, retained foreign body, or medication error resulting in death. These events are considered sentinel because they trigger the need for immediate investigation and response by the health care system. Careful investigation of these events and corrective action plans can help to reduce further risk and prevent patient harm in the future. When such an event occurs, most hospitals activate a serious adverse event response system that includes a formalized notification chain and immediate huddle, shortly followed by a debriefing and root cause analysis (discussed in detail later in this chapter), with senior leadership endorsement and support of this process **TABLE 3-4**.

Effective communication to discuss patient safety events such as a sentinel event is vital to those participating in the aftermath of an event. Communicating effectively helps groups navigate competing priorities, overcome issues related to human factors, and reduce error. A huddle is a communication technique and event that often takes the form of a structured, short meeting in which patient care teams come together to talk about a patient, procedure, or situation. It can also be called on an ad hoc basis when a medical team needs to regroup and share concerns, discuss

TABLE 3-4 Example of a Serious Adverse Event Response System

	Huddle	Debriefing	Interview	RCA
Objective	Determine what happened Stabilize patient Address staff concerns Secure all equipment	Clarify timeline of event Assess ongoing safety risks Determine need for emotional support to staff, patient/family	Further investigation to obtain information/details not uncovered via debriefing	Determine root causes of event Use tools to depict standard process and redesigned process Determine system versus individual culpability
When?	Immediately (within 24 hours)	24–72 hours after event	Post debriefing, in preparation for root cause analysis	Within 2 weeks of event
Who participates?	Staff directly involved in event	Staff directly involved in event	Interviewer and staff involved in event	Frontline staff and local leadership *not* directly involved in event CMO Risk/QM content experts
Who leads?	Most-senior local staff members (*typically RN unit managers*)	CMO	Trained interviewer (typically QA/RM staff)	CMO or vice president/director for risk management
Training	RN unit managers, *or* supervisors, night/evening administrators Conducted internally by each facility	SAE workgroup to facilitate "cross-pollination" of expertise among CMOs	QA/RM QI nurses Conducted centrally by a risk management organization	SAE workgroup to facilitate "cross-pollination" of expertise among CMOs/RM

Abbreviations: CMO, chief medical officer; OR, operating room; QA, quality assurance; QI, quality improvement; QM, quality management; RCA, root cause analysis; RM, risk management; RN, registered nurse; SAE, serious adverse event

Prepared in accordance with New York State Public Heath Law 2805 j through m; New York State Education Law 6527; & Federal Law 109-4.

resource allocation, anticipate outcomes, and create contingency plans. After a serious adverse event, the medical team is advised to huddle and discuss the event that occurred (including the stabilization of the patient and situation), determine the facts of what happened, mitigate any ongoing harm, address staff safety concerns, secure equipment or materials, and alert others as deemed necessary by the senior staff member leading the huddle. The huddle is crucial to ensure that actual events, sequences, and timing are accurately recorded to aid in further analysis and corrective actions related to the situation. It is also the only opportunity to sequester equipment in the actual state when the incident occurred; for example, a problem caused by a faulty ventilator or intravenous (IV) pump cannot be properly analyzed if the settings are changed or the equipment is returned to use.

Shortly after a serious adverse event or sentinel event happens, a debriefing also occurs. The debriefing is a powerful inquiry tool in which a concise exchange occurs to identify what happened, what was learned, and what can be done better in the future. A member of senior leadership usually leads the debriefing. The focus of this meeting is to learn what occurred from staff who were involved and to hear their thoughts on what could or should have been done differently. The debriefing does not focus on system changes, as that is the role of the root cause analysis. During this meeting, it is important to obtain a timeline of the event. Additionally, the senior leadership should use the debriefing to provide emotional support to staff and/or family, determine reporting obligations, and perhaps visit the event site. Ideally, a debriefing is a nonjudgmental, nonpunitive investigation to determine what happened, looking at the process and system, and should not be used for disciplinary purposes.

The next step after an SAE or sentinel event is to complete a root cause analysis (RCA). The RCA is a systematic approach to understanding the causes of an SAE and identifying system flaws that can be corrected to prevent future harm. During the RCA, a team of mixed professionals from different specialties, who were not involved directly with the event, meet and discuss the event with senior administrative leadership.

There are six steps in most RCAs:

- **Step 1: Identify what happened.** This step is occasionally completed using a flowchart to depict each step accurately and completely.
- **Step 2: Determine what should have happened.** A flowchart can also be used in this step to identify the proper steps that should have been taken.
- **Step 3: Determine the cause.** In this step, the group members ask why the error occurred. When doing so, they should consider patient characteristics, task factors, individual staff members, team factors, work environment, organizational and management factors, and institutional context.
- **Step 4: Develop a causal statement.** In this step, a statement is made about the cause, the effect, and the event.
- **Step 5: Generate a list of recommended actions to prevent recurrence of the event.** These recommendations consist of suggested action plans that the group believes will help prevent the error from occurring in the future. Action plans are created to help eliminate or significantly reduce the likelihood of an SAE from happening again, control the root cause, or limit vulnerability. They vary widely, but can include actions such as standardizing equipment, educating staff, or developing new policies.

- **Step 6: Summarize the results.** A summary document is created reviewing all steps and action plans.

Under a system of just culture, an algorithm is applied during the RCA to determine if a similar person under similar conditions could or would take the same actions. If so, the event must be treated as a system failure and not as an individual failure **FIGURE 3-2**. Under a just culture, persons who demonstrate reckless or malicious behavior are still punished, but persons who engage in unintentional at-risk behaviors are coached and given additional training.

Tools to Identify Errors

Many hospitals and transport services expect staff to report near misses and medical errors. Such reporting systems are designed to reduce future risks for all patients, trigger improvements in weak areas of care processes, alert other providers to possible vulnerabilities and gaps, and contribute to planning and strategies to prevent harm. One example of an error-reporting system used by EMS agencies is the EMS Voluntary Event Notification Tool (EVENT). The National Association of Emergency Medical Technicians (NAEMT) launched EVENT in 2012 to provide a confidential, anonymous means for providers to report events without fear of punishment. Another such system is the US Food and Drug Administration's (FDA's) Adverse Event Reporting System (FAERS), which is used to report adverse medication reactions or device malfunctions. For example, if a defibrillator failed to charge or deliver a shock during a call, the provider or agency could report the event directly to the FDA. Alternatively, they could report the incident to the manufacturer, which is required to then notify the FDA.

In 2013, the National Highway Traffic Safety Administration (NHTSA), EMS for Children, and ACEP published "Strategies for a National EMS Culture of Safety." This document discusses the need for a secure national database to report and catalog adverse events in EMS in a way that could identify best practices and enhance patient safety nationally. Such a system could leverage the National EMS Information System database, which includes a wide array of data but lacks some specific information

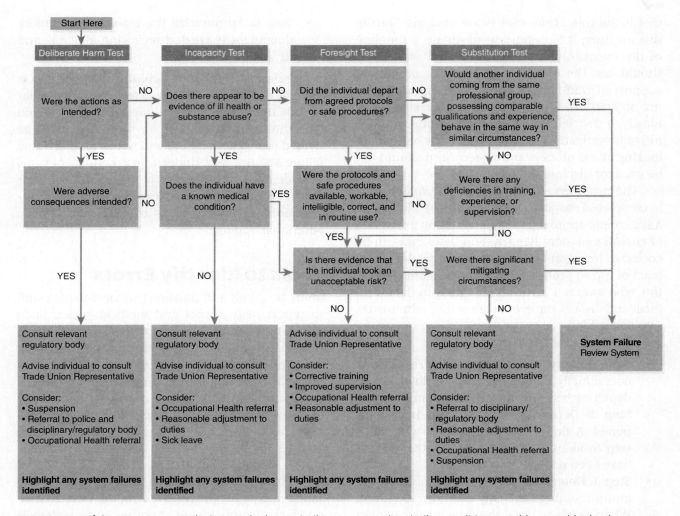

FIGURE 3-2 If the root cause analysis reveals that a similar person under similar conditions could or would take the same actions, the event must be treated as a system failure and not as an individual failure.

Courtesy of National Health Service and US Department of Health and Human Services. https://www.ahrq.gov/downloads/pub/advances/vol4/meadows.pdf.

that would be useful in identifying and mitigating patient and provider harm. To encourage voluntary reporting of near misses and adverse events, organizations must support a just culture and exhibit other traits of an HRO so that both patients and providers can trust that the outcomes of that reporting will be fair. An HRO focuses on managing its inevitable failures, so that a failure does not affect the patient or the customer.

According to the Institute for Healthcare Improvement, the use of *triggers* has reduced hospitals' reliance on employees' voluntary reporting:

> The use of "triggers," or clues, to identify adverse events (AEs) is an effective method for measuring the overall level of harm from medical care in a health care organization. Traditional efforts to

detect AEs have focused on voluntary reporting and tracking of errors. However, public health researchers have established that only 10 to 20 percent of errors are ever reported and, of those, 90 to 95 percent cause no harm to patients. Hospitals need a more effective way to identify events that do cause harm to patients, in order to select and test changes to reduce harm.

Trigger tools define events or rates of error that prompt a further evaluation of processes to improve error prevention.

A 2018 study by Howard et al. adapted the IHI Global Trigger Tool to an EMS system, with the researchers calling their adapted version the EMS Trigger Tool. Interestingly, they found that three events accounted for 93% of the triggers in the analysis: change in systolic blood pressure (BP) by greater than 20%, temperature greater than 38°C without reduction, and oxygen saturation of less than 94% without oxygen or less than 85% without assisted ventilation.

In addition to use of trigger tools, some organizations have developed specific quality measures for EMS. One organization, Ground and Air Medical Quality in Transport, looks specifically at performance and quality metrics across the industry and facilitates benchmarking against other services. Another organization, the National EMS Quality Alliance, has published specific quality metrics for EMS relating to topics such as pediatrics, trauma, stroke, and safety.

Strategies to Avoid Errors

Many strategies and techniques that have been used successfully in the manufacturing industry are now being applied to health care, along with safety techniques that have proven useful in aviation, such as checklists. Two of the most popular of these strategies are Six Sigma and Lean.

Six Sigma

Six Sigma is a disciplined, data-driven approach and methodology for eliminating defects in any process—from manufacturing to transactional processes, and from products to services. It was first introduced by Bill Smith while working at Motorola in 1986 and was a central tenet of Jack Welch's strategy at General Electric in the 1990s. Its name is derived from its goal of achieving reliability within six standard deviations between the mean and the nearest specification limit for the process to which Six Sigma is applied. Few industries have been capable of reaching Six Sigma reliability, which would result in a 99.99% nonfailure rate. Perhaps most notably, the aviation industry has achieved this goal.

Lean

Lean was developed by Toyota engineers in the mid-1990s. The Lean strategy looks at all processes and attempts to reduce waste and ensure all activities add value. It relies on a pull system and ideas such as just-in-time manufacturing to reduce waste. Lean focuses on the frontline worker and the work space (*gemba* in Japanese) to see all the steps involved. Once the process is fully understood, the team creates "standard work"—that is, the one standard way that all workers perform this task so as to reduce waste and the chance for error. These principles are being applied to health care; indeed, several hospitals and hospital systems have become "Lean hospitals" in the sense that they apply Lean culture to all aspects of hospital operations.

Crew Resource Management

In health care, one of the major sources of error is lack of effective communication and teamwork. The enormous risk associated with such problems became painfully apparent in the aviation industry in 1977: In Tenerife in the Canary Islands, two fully loaded 747 planes collided on the runway, resulting in the deadliest collision in aviation history; 583 people were killed. Analysis of this collision led to several alarming discoveries. The KLM captain involved in the collision was one of the most senior pilots in the company and had thousands of hours flying the aircraft. While the captain mistakenly believed the flight was cleared for takeoff, the first officer and flight engineer did not; however, they were unwilling to question the captain because the prevailing wisdom and culture at the time asserted that the captain knew best and was the ultimate authority. In that culture, it was considered wrong and detrimental to one's career to question a captain. This collision triggered major changes in the aviation industry, including the development of crew resource management (CRM). CRM emphasizes a culture of mutual support, teamwork, and the expectation and requirement that any crew member can and should voice a concern regarding the safe operation of the aircraft.

Many industries have adopted these lessons, including the military, nuclear industry, and now health care. The US Department of Defense, along with AHRQ, developed a program for health care providers and facilities called TeamSTEPPS (team strategies and tools to enhance performance and patient safety) that embraces the principles of CRM. TeamSTEPPS is being taught and employed across a wide variety of high-risk health care settings, such as the operating room, labor and delivery, and EDs. This course teaches tools and methods by which team members can safely raise concerns, challenge orders that are unclear, and if necessary "stop the line." Many malpractice insurance carriers are now encouraging or requiring their client hospitals to implement team training programs such as TeamSTEPPS.

Simulation Training

Another area of emphasis in team building is the rapidly expanding role of simulation training. Use of simulation allows health care providers to hone their skills in a safe environment without risk of patient harm and to work in teams to practice both procedures and communication skills. For example, it provides an opportunity to safely train for so-called HALO (high-acuity, low-occurrence) events such as surgical cricothyrotomy and needle decompression, and it enables the safe simulation of equipment failures (eg, ventilators, monitors) much in the same way that a flight simulator allows for pilot training.

Simulation training has been growing in popularity in many medical settings, such as trauma, obstetrics and gynecology, and ED care. In EMS, simulation training can range from very simple task trainers, such as cardiopulmonary resuscitation (CPR) manikins to full-scale, high-fidelity simulation manikins that can simulate numerous life-threatening situations and allow EMS providers to practice procedures and management techniques in a safe environment. For example, rhythm simulators are commonly used to practice management of the crashing cardiac patient. Simulation is also used in EMS driver training and retraining, as the emergency response environment can be simulated and hazards presented in a safe setting.

Failure Mode and Effect Analysis

An additional tool that is helpful in analyzing potential sources of error or patient harm is failure mode and effect analysis (FMEA). This process was developed by military engineers in the 1940s and further refined and used by NASA engineers working on the Mercury, Gemini, and Apollo space programs. More recently, this process has been applied to analyze the potential for health care failures.

To use FMEA, one constructs a risk matrix for each potential failure that incorporates the likelihood of that failure, the ability to detect the failure, and the potential harm, and assigns a risk score to

the event. An example is provided in **TABLE 3-5**. This process can help identify priorities in risk mitigation and process redesign.

Quality in EMS Settings

Methods for understanding and measuring patient safety and quality in the EMS environment are in their infancy, with only limited studies of these techniques having been conducted to date. Recently, greater interest has arisen in promoting patient safety concepts and quality measurements in EMS, with several organizations (eg, NAEMSP, ACEP, NHTSA, EMS Chiefs of Canada) leading the call for enhanced patient safety in EMS. The environment and conditions in which prehospital care is provided create significant safety challenges. More specifically, EMS care is often provided in a high-stress, limited-time situation in less than ideal conditions, such as low light, moving vehicles, noisy aircraft, or extremes of temperature. Many providers work long hours, sometimes for 24 hours straight, and often have more than one job, leading to fatigue, often compounded by disturbances of their circadian rhythm. Given these factors, EMS care is potentially more dangerous and less controlled than the same care provided in an inpatient environment or ED, yet patient safety strategies and team training are only now being incorporated into the EMS system. In addition, as the Patient Protection and Affordable Care Act matures, many hospitals are organizing into large hospital systems with site-specific specializations. This trend of consolidating hospital systems and specializations has greatly accelerated in the last few years, and the rate of critical care transports has increased proportionally.

One problem with assessing adverse events during EMS care and transport, and patient safety in EMS in general, is the lack of standard data definitions and event categories. Several organizations are currently working to create standard data definitions and data sets that will enable meaningful comparison across systems.

For example, in 2012, Bigham et al. conducted a systematic literature review on patient safety in EMS. Seven themes emerged across the articles they found in the literature:

- Clinical judgment
- Adverse events and error reporting
- Communications

TABLE 3-5 Sample Failure Mode and Effect Analysis: Analysis for Patient-Controlled IV Analgesia

Processes and Subprocesses	Failure Modes (What Might Happen)	Causes (Why It Happens)	Effects	Severity	Probability	Hazard Score	Actions to Reduce Failure Mode
Prescribing							
Assess patient	Inaccurate pain assessment	Cultural influences; patient unable to articulate	Poor pain control	2	4	8	Standard scale to help assess pain; training on cultural influences
Choose analgesic/ mode of delivery	Wrong analgesic selected	Clinical situation not considered (age, renal function, allergies, etc); tolerance to opiates not considered; standard PCA protocols not followed (or not available); concomitant use of other analgesics not considered; drug storage; knowledge deficit; improper selection of patients appropriate for PCA	Improper dosing; improper drug; allergic response; improper use of substitute drug	4	3	12	CPOE with decision support, clinical pharmacy program; standard PCA protocol with education on use; point-of-use access to drug information; feedback mechanism on drug shortages with information on substitute drugs available; selection criteria for PCA patients
Prescribe analgesic	Wrong dose (loading, PCA, constant, lock-out), route, frequency	Knowledge deficit; mental slip; wrong selection from list; information about drug not available	Overdose; underdose; ADR	4	3	12	CPOE with decision support; clinical pharmacy program; standard PCA protocols
	Proper patient monitoring not ordered	Knowledge deficit; mental slip	Failure to detect problems early to prevent harm	4	3	12	Standard PCA order sets with monitoring guidelines
	Prescribed to wrong patient	Similar patient names; patient identifier not clear; name does not appear on screen when ordering medications	Wrong patient receives inappropriate drug and dose; ADR; allergic response	3	3	9	Match therapy to patient condition; alerts for look-alike patient names; visible demographic information on order form or screen
	No order received	Unable to reach covering physician	Poor pain control	2	2	4	Proper physician coverage and communication channels

Abbreviations: ADR, adverse drug reaction; CPOE, computerized physician order entry; IV, intravenous; PCA, patient-controlled analgesia

Adapted from Institute for Safe Medication Practices.

- Ground vehicle safety
- Aircraft safety
- Interfacility transport
- Field intubation

These themes are helpful in understanding potential pitfalls and focusing safety efforts for providers and agencies. Field intubation is discussed in detail in Chapter 6, *Respiratory Emergencies and Airway Management.*

Clinical Judgment

Several studies have examined clinical decision making by EMS personnel and looked at paramedics' determination of medical necessity for transport, appropriate cancelation of advanced life support (ALS) calls, the effectiveness of paramedics' scope of practice, and other clinical issues. Collectively, they suggest that perhaps EMS providers are being asked to make decisions that they are not trained to make. Moreover, as procedures and tasks have been added to these providers' duties, a sort of "scope creep" may lead to providers making decisions that could harm their patients. While these observations point to an increased potential for error due to increasing demands on EMS providers' skills and decision making, no concrete recommendations have been proposed to remedy this problem. Nevertheless, it would seem likely that additional training in complex decision making; low-frequency, high-risk skills; and advanced equipment will be needed, as well as additional real-time support from medical control physicians.

Error Reporting

As stated previously, only limited data are available on adverse events, medication errors, and reporting in the EMS environment. There appear to be patterns of both underreporting and nonreporting of events, which survey data suggest may be due to both a fear of reporting and a lack of recognition of near-miss events and their significance.

Communications

Communications is another major theme in patient harm and the focus of considerable patient safety efforts in the hospital environment. Numerous studies of prehospital communications have examined handoffs between EMS and ED or hospital staff. This line of research has generally demonstrated a loss of key clinical information during these handoffs, such as changes in vital signs (eg, transient hypotension), medications administered, and changes in ventilator settings, which may sometimes lead to direct patient harm.

Vehicle and Provider Safety

The transport environment is associated with the unique requirement of preventing vehicular harm to both the patient and the provider. While a full discussion of vehicle safety practices, such as those covered in emergency vehicle operation course (EVOC) training and other operational safety programs, is beyond the scope of this chapter, the CCTP should be mindful of basic safety techniques when riding in the passenger compartment. Whenever possible, the provider should remain seated and secured during transport, and should ensure that all equipment is secured to minimize the risk of injury from loose equipment in the event of a collision. Transport agencies should establish policies and procedures to help the CCTP ensure maximal safety in the patient compartment.

Air Transport Safety

The air transport crew has an especially arduous task in ensuring safety. Given the noise level, limited space, and poor lighting in most rotor-wing aircraft, identifying adverse events is more difficult in this environment than in other patient care settings. The air transport crew needs to minimize risk (maximize risk reduction) by optimizing the patient's condition prior to flight and ensuring adequate monitoring equipment is in place. Additionally, using excellent CRM skills and making appropriate go/no-go decisions are critical to the safety of the patient and the crew.

Interfacility Transport
Adverse Events During Interfacility Transport

While critical events occur across all EMS settings, adverse events associated with interfacility transfers have recently drawn closer scrutiny. A recent Canadian study suggests that the event rate is lower when transports are staffed with specially trained CCTPs than with EMT-P personnel. Overall, the data indicate that 1 in 15 patients experienced one of several adverse events during transport, including hypotension, initiation of vasopressor therapy, and respiratory events. An analysis showed that hemodynamic instability requiring intervention such as fluids or vasopressors was by far the most common adverse event, followed by respiratory instability or hypoxia. Additionally, in-transit critical events were independently associated with mechanical ventilation and baseline hemodynamic instability.

Some problematic events have been identified in relation to specific types of transports. For pediatric transports, the most common adverse events noted were hypothermia, drug errors, tachycardia, procedure error, loss of IV access, and cyanosis. Of interest, the adverse event rate was lower in this population when specialized teams performed the transport.

Currently, there is no mandatory regulatory oversight for transport teams. The Commission on Accreditation of Medical Transport Systems is the only accrediting body, but accreditation is voluntary, and a recent study showed that only 20% of specialty teams have received accreditation. Nevertheless, the importance of specialty-trained teams in interfacility transport of complex cases is increasing as newer and more advanced therapies become more widely employed during transport, such as inhaled nitric oxide and extracorporeal membrane oxygenation.

Mitigation Strategies for Adverse Events During Interfacility Transport

While no large-scale trials have been conducted that demonstrate a clear benefit from the guidelines proposed by some organizations, many of these strategies have shown benefit in small observational studies or are recommended as expert opinion. In a review of adult transports, Ligtenberg et al. found that 70% of adverse events could have been avoided by better preparation prior to transport, communication between the sending and receiving facilities, and the use of checklists and protocols.

One of the best ways to mitigate the risk of adverse events en route is to ensure the correct crew configuration is available for the transport. While in most cases a single CCTP may be sufficient for stable patients, additional personnel should be considered as needed, such as a critical care nurse, respiratory therapist, or physician for more complicated transports, or advanced equipment such as an intra-aortic balloon pump or extracorporeal membrane oxygenation.

Additionally, specific checklists with sections for ventilator, IV pumps, and other equipment have been shown to decrease the risk of adverse events and errors of omission **FIGURE 3-3**. One study demonstrated a decrease in the overall rate of adverse events from 36% to 22% and a decrease in the serious adverse events rate from 9% to 5% with the use of checklists.

Another consideration is availability of appropriate equipment that has been properly maintained and checked. For example, IV pumps and ventilators have battery backup power supplies, and it is critical to ensure that all devices are in good working order with fully charged batteries prior to initiation of patient transport. Waveform capnography is critical for monitoring intubated patients during transport and must be considered a minimum standard of care. Likewise, monitor alarms are critical for alerting providers to unexpected changes in the patient's condition. Alarm limits and volumes must be set correctly prior to transport to ensure the CCTP is immediately made aware of any parameters that move out of range.

Summary

Patient safety and quality have become a major focus of both health care organizations and regulatory agencies such as The Joint Commission. While enhanced patient safety techniques and team-training skills are becoming standard in the hospital environment, EMS systems have only recently begun to address these issues. The ultimate goal is to ensure application of one high standard of care and quality across the health care setting. In this environment, both the CCTP and the transport agency are critical links in the patient safety chain from admission to discharge. Hospitals are organizing into large hospital systems with site-specific specializations, and the CCTP is being called on to carry out increasingly frequent and complex transfers. Ensuring the safety of these transfers is paramount for the CCTP.

Nursing - Prior to transport	RN Initials	RT Initials
RN given 45 minute notification from procedural area to prepare		
Oral contrast given or 20g IV in antecubital (AC) vein obtained (for CT PE protocol) (If no AC IV can be obtained, consider alternative of VQ scan)		
Upon notification of procedure, verify with MD that test is needed and consent obtained.		
IF NOT Vented: Full oxygen tank obtained. RN will bring ambu Vbag with mask.		
Transportation present		
All invasive lines assessed and secured. All IV fluids and drips assessed for adequate amount.		
If going to MRI: MRI checklist is completed. Retrieve MRI pump (from MRI; max 3 pumps available). Obtain MRI pump tubing for needed infusions and add to Baxter tubing. Prepare infusions on MRI pump.		
Portable monitor obtained for continued level of care monitoring. Alarms set as appropriate for patient.		
All equipment checked for function and battery length		
If chest tube present, can patient tolerate chest tube to H_2O seal during transport or at target site? Test patient on H_2O seal before transport as instructed below: *Suction available at target site: patient must tolerate H_2O seal twice the anticipated transport time.* *No suction available at target site: patient must tolerate H_2O seal twice the anticipated total time off suction.* *If air leak present and on mechanical ventilation: use portable suction during transport and at target site.*		
If the patient is in **PACU** and PACU nurse is transporting patient, Anesthesia faculty aware that nurse will be off the unit (Faculty:_____)		

Respiratory Therapy - Vented Patients - Prior to transport	RN Initials	RT Initials
Obtain ambu bag with face mask and PEEP valve. Oxygen tank is **FULL**. One disposable $ETCO_2$ check device available.		
Transport ventilator set up and trialed to assess patient tolerance and stability. *If PEEP ≤8 and FiO_2 ≤50%, MD approval and order may be obtained for transport via manual bag/valve ventilation in situations in which a delay may be incurred and a risk: benefit ratio has been evaluated.* Portable continuous $ETCO_2$ monitor in place.		

Nursing/Respiratory Therapy - At procedural site	RN Initials	RT Initials
Switch to procedural area monitor if available. Transport monitor plugged in and charging.		
Report given to procedural area RN (if ICU RN is not staying, and patient is going to anarea other than Cardiac Cath Lab or GI suite, physician order is required)		
RN confirms vital signs are stable prior to leaving patient		
RT places patient on procedural area ventilator		
RT and RN agree that patient's respiratory status is stable and RT may leave		
RT will stay with patient if patient remains on transport ventilator		

Weight limits: MRI 1,2,3 = 350 lbs with 60 cm (23.6 in) circumference. MRI 4 = 550 lbs with 70 cm (27.6 in) circumference. CT 1 & ER CT = 450 lbs with 55 cm (21.7 in) diameter. CT 3 = 600 lbs with 70 cm (27.6 in) diameter.

PATIENT DESCRIPTION	Circle answer If yes to any, complete column on right	ADDITIONAL TRANSPORT SAFETY REQUIREMENTS Complete entire column if any checked "yes" on left
Previous failed attempt to transport within the past 24 hours due to patient instability	Y/N	1. Physician faculty or chief must be aware of and approve the transport _____ (name of physician)
In the past 4 hours, there has been: 1.) addition of new vasopressors 2.) active increased titration of vasopressors 3.) sustained RASS +2-+4 despite medical management	Y/N	2.Call procedure area*. Provide information regarding patient acuity and any additional patient safety requirements for procedure area.
Patient actively requiring BiPAP	Y/N	_____ (name of person you spoke to)
Chest tube with active air leak & on mechanical ventilation	Y/N	*CT: Neuro CT: Ext. 24229
PEEP ≥8 and <10	Y/N	Body CT: Ext. 21760 After hours (1900): Ext. 23480 or 23473 *MRI: Ext. 20917
Patient's cardiac rhythm has high likeli-hood of requiring intervention	Y/N	Physician to accompany the team on transport and remain with the patient until the patient returns to the unit.
PEEP ≥10 (or) PaO_2/FiO_2 <100* (*on most recent ABG result)	Y/N	Call procedure area*. Provide information regarding patient acuity and any additional patient safety requirements for procedure area.
Rapid infuser is being utilized for fluid resuscitation	Y/N	_____ (name of person you spoke to)
Patient is receiving mechanical circulatory support (IABP, CPS, ECMO)	Y/N	*CT: Neuro CT: Ext. 24229 Body CT: Ext. 21760
Unstable cervical spine fracture	Y/N	After hours (1900): Ext. 23480 or 23473 *MRI: Ext. 20917

COMPLETE AT THE CONCLUSION OF TRANSPORT: Transport Start time:_____ End time: _____

Where did you transport your patient? ❏ CT Scan ❏ MRI ❏ Other: _____

Did your patient experience any complications during the transport? ❏ NO ❏ YES _____
(Complication defined as an unexpected event [eg hypotension, hypoxia] that required intervention to correct, either during or immediately after transport)

FIGURE 3-3 Adult critical care transport checklist from the University of Texas Medical Branch, Galveston, Texas.

Abbreviations: ABG, arterial blood gas analysis; BiPAP, bilevel positive airway pressure; CPS, cardiopulmonary support; CT, computed tomography; ECMO, extracorporeal membrane oxygenation; ER, emergency department; FiO_2, fraction of inspired oxygen; IAPB, intra-aortic balloon pump; MRI, magnetic resonance imaging; PEEP, positive end-expiratory pressure; RASS, Richmond Agitation Sedation Scale; Y/N, yes/no
SI conversion factor: to covert pounds to kilograms, multiply by 0.45.

Reprinted by permission of the Board of Regents of the University of Texas System, on behalf of the University of Texas Medical Branch at Galveston.

Case Study

Your critical care ground transport crew is called late in the afternoon to a rural hospital for a 37-year-old patient with suspected sepsis, hyperglycemia, and new-onset atrial fibrillation. This patient needs transport to a tertiary medical center where she can receive a higher level of care.

You arrive to find the patient in the ED appearing moderately ill. She presented to the hospital in the early morning with gastrointestinal distress, protracted vomiting, and fever. The ED providers administered fluids and antiemetics; obtained blood, urine, and sputum cultures; and obtained chest and abdominal radiographs, a 12-lead ECG, and chemistry and hematology lab studies. Empiric antibiotics and acetaminophen were also started.

The patient has a history of poorly controlled diabetes, hypertension, and obesity. She denies allergies and confirms the hospital note that she is currently taking an angiotensin-converting enzyme (ACE) inhibitor for BP control and uses both insulin glargine (Lantus) and insulin aspart

(NovoLog) but often has wide swings in her blood sugars. She denies any cardiac history and has never experienced palpitations or been told that her ECG was abnormal.

Lab studies were all normal except for a white blood count of 14,500 cells/mm^3, a serum lactate level of 4 mmol/L, and a serum glucose of 295 mg/dL. The patient's initial 12-lead ECG showed uncontrolled atrial fibrillation with a rate of 185 beats/min and no evidence of ischemia. The chest radiograph showed consolidation in the left lower lobe. The abdominal films were unremarkable. The patient's BP has remained normal to slightly elevated, and her fever has decreased from 102.8°F (39.3°C) on initial presentation to 99.5°F (37.5°C) 30 minutes prior to your arrival. Her heart rate did not decrease significantly with the lower temperature, so an infusion of diltiazem (Cardizem) was initiated at 5 mg/h, then decreased to 3 mg/h once her heart rate dropped to 100 beats/min. The patient's blood glucose continued to climb, so an insulin infusion was started and titrated to lower blood glucose to 150 mg/dL. The ED staff report that they turned the insulin infusion off 30 minutes prior to your arrival because the finger-stick blood glucose was 90 mg/dL.

While your partner finishes obtaining the report and copies of the transfer paperwork, you move the three IV pumps to your ambulance stretcher. You note that three medication bags are hanging: insulin, diltiazem, and piperacillin–tazobactam (Zosyn). The pump labeled insulin is on standby, the pump labeled diltiazem is running at 8 mg/h, and the pump labeled piperacillin–tazobactam is running at 12.5 mL/h, which you recognize will deliver the antibiotic over the usual 4-hour period. A cursory set of vital signs matches those taken by the ED staff 30 minutes earlier, except that the patient's heart rate has climbed from 105 beats/min to 148 beats/min. You note the rhythm remains atrial fibrillation, and you increase the rate on the diltiazem pump to 10 mg/h as you wheel the patient to the ambulance. The patient is alert and oriented and does not appear to be in acute distress. You talk with her family about the transfer plan, and they indicate that they will meet you at the receiving hospital.

Once in the ambulance and under way, you obtain a finger-stick glucose of 20 mg/dL and note that the patient is slightly obtunded. Her heart rate continues to climb despite your earlier increase in the diltiazem infusion rate. You decide to trace each of the infusions from the peripheral IV sites at which they are connected to back to the medication bags. All three are labeled at the tubing ends where they connect to the IVs and the pumps match the labels on the tubing. When you reach the medication bags, you discover that the diltiazem tubing and pump are actually infusing a bag of insulin and the insulin pump (currently on standby) is connected to a bag of diltiazem. You stop the pump labeled diltiazem, begin an infusion of 10% dextrose, and hang a new bag of diltiazem with new tubing on the diltiazem pump.

On arrival at the receiving facility, the patient's blood glucose has increased to 110 mg/dL, her heart rate has dropped to 120 beats/min with a 3 mg/h rate for the newly hung diltiazem drip, and the 10% dextrose infusion has been discontinued. The patient is alert and oriented.

1. How common are medication errors in critical care transport?
2. What were the causal factors that gave rise to this error?
3. What should the role of staff be with regard to reporting adverse events, and how should employers encourage and support reporting?
4. Which actions, including discipline, are appropriate in this case?

Analysis

Medication errors account for a significant percentage of medical errors. While there is little information specific to CCT medication errors, the literature suggests that at least 2% of hospitalized patients experience a medication error. Many safety professionals and risk managers believe the incidence of medication errors in hospitalized patients is significantly underreported and potentially unrecognized. Given the austerity of the CCT environment, the lack of independent double-checks, and the lack of the barcode technology used to reduce errors in the inpatient setting, the risk of medication errors during transport is probably significantly higher than that in the hospital setting.

The CCTPs reported this medication error using their service incident reporting system. The transport service risk managers categorized the error as an SAE, and an RCA was conducted. It was determined that both the diltiazem and insulin infusion bags ran out nearly simultaneously. The nurse caring for the patient ordered additional bags of both infusions in advance from the pharmacy, scanned them individually, and then proceeded to hang both bags, inadvertently connecting the insulin to the diltiazem tubing and the new bag of diltiazem to the insulin tubing. While the insulin was a high-alert medication, requiring an independent double-check by a second registered nurse, the transferring facility had in excess of 55 medication infusions on its high-alert list. Nurses merely scanned the badge of a coworker without actually conducting the independent double-check because they perceived the frequency of this process to be an annoyance.

The CCTP examined all three medication bags, confirming that they contained the medications and concentrations expected. He also examined the pumps but failed to follow the tubing from each medication bag to the corresponding pump and to the label on the distal end of the tubing. Had this been done with each infusion, the error would have been discovered prior to initiating transport. While hindsight is often 20:20, there was arguably a failure to carefully consider potential causes for the patient's increasing heart rate and decreasing blood glucose level.

Many employers expect team members to report adverse events in an effort to reduce future risk for all patients, trigger improvements in weak spots in processes of care, alert other providers to possible vulnerabilities and gaps, and contribute to planning and strategies to prevent harm. To encourage reporting, organizations must support a just culture and exhibit other traits of an HRO. When team members sense that reporting may result in disciplinary actions or a perceived lack of concern or even incompetence from their supervisors, they may downplay adverse events or fail to report them at all.

Using a systems approach and considering the just culture system, it is very likely that this error was a result of a poorly designed system rather than being caused by people. Within a just culture, if a similar person under similar conditions could or would take the same actions, the event must be treated as a system failure, rather than as an individual failure. Looking at the history of both the nurse and the CCTP, neither had similar experiences in the past, and neither seemed to exhibit reckless behavior. Both seemed to have made honest mistakes. The behavior of the nurse in bypassing the independent double-check was an action called **normalization of deviance**, in which a shift away from policies and practices becomes normative behavior. Both the nurse and the CCTP were able to learn from this experience. Neither was punished, but changes were made to policies and practices in an effort to prevent a recurrence of the same error in the future.

Prep Kit

Ready for Review
- The complexity inherent in an EMS system provides many opportunities for process failures, errors, and adverse outcomes.
- A series of reports published by the Institute of Medicine not only captivated the medical community, but also caused the media and general public to become aware of the issue of safety in health care and put this concern on the national agenda.
- The CCTP likely encounters more critically ill patients and more complex patient care scenarios than does a 9-1-1 responder, so the likelihood

Prep Kit Continued

- of errors may be significantly greater in the CCT environment than in the usual EMS setting.
- Quality goals suggest that health care should be safe, effective, patient centered, timely, efficient, and equitable; these quality aims may be difficult to achieve in an EMS environment owing to its time-limited nature and the critically ill nature of patients.
- Many definitions of patient safety have been proposed, including the World Health Organization's definition of freedom from unnecessary harm or potential harm associated with health care.
- Not all errors will reach patients and cause harm, but it is essential for organizations to study these errors and look for opportunities to improve the processes that allow them to happen before any true patient harm results.
- Errors that lead to serious patient harm are rarely the result of just one error involving one person, but rather usually involve a series of errors or breakdowns in processes.
- Breakdowns in communication that almost lead to errors or harm are referred to as near misses or close calls. They may occur many times before an actual harmful incident occurs.
- Many transport services expect staff to report near misses through a reporting system to reduce future risks for all patients, trigger improvements in weak spots in processes of care, alert other providers to possible vulnerabilities and gaps, and contribute to planning and strategies to prevent harm.
- A medical error is the failure of a planned action to be completed as intended or the use of a wrong plan to achieve an aim. Such errors may generally be categorized as adverse drug events, wrong-site surgeries, falls, burns, pressure ulcers, and mistaken patient identities.
- A safety culture encompasses several key features: (1) acknowledging that organizations engage in high-risk activities and determining the importance of consistent safe operations to counteract these activities; (2) supporting a

- blame-free environment where errors can be reported without fear of punishment; and (3) maintaining organizational commitment to address reported errors and safety concerns.
- A just culture focuses on blamelessly identifying issues that lead to errors or unsafe behaviors, while still maintaining individual accountability for reckless behavior.
- Highly reliable EMS organizations focus on managing failures, so that a failure does not affect the patient.
- Among the most notable errors in health care are medication and prescription errors. Other, less-common errors include wrong patient identification, transfusion errors, preventable suicides, falls, burns, wrong-side procedures, and errors in transition of care or handoffs.
- The process of a patient receiving a medication is complex and fraught with opportunities for error, including prescribing, dispensing, administering, and monitoring errors.
- Practice recommendations to rectify wrong-patient errors include always using multiple patient identifiers.
- The concept of the universal time-out has been proposed for the EMS environment, such as implementing an EMS time-out for trauma and other critical patients on EMS arrival to ensure that no key information is lost during handoff.
- Transitioning care is an integral part of the ED and prehospital care of a patient. The situation, background, assessment, and recommendation (SBAR) technique allows for a brief, yet concise and expected, handoff of information.
- The systems approach suggests that most human errors, including those in health care, occur in the context of a poorly designed system.
- In the Swiss cheese model, errors made by people result in consequences related to flawed systems.
- Active errors occur at a contact point between a staff member and some aspect of a larger

Prep Kit Continued

system; latent errors are mistakes that are likely to occur secondary to organizational or design failures that allow the inevitable active errors to cause harm.

- Active errors can be further classified as slips and mistakes: A slip is a lapse in concentration; a mistake is when an action occurs as intended but is the wrong action.
- A sentinel event or serious adverse event is a patient safety event in which an error reaches a patient and results in death, permanent harm, or severe temporary harm, such that interventions are often required to sustain life. It triggers the need for immediate investigation and response by the health care system.
- When a sentinel event occurs, most hospitals activate a serious adverse event response system that includes a formalized notification chain and immediate huddle, followed shortly by a debriefing and a root cause analysis, with senior leadership endorsement and support of the process.
- Many strategies and techniques that have been successful in the manufacturing industry, such as Six Sigma, Lean, and crew resource management (CRM), are now being applied to health care, along with safety techniques that have proved useful in aviation, such as checklists.
- EMS care is potentially more dangerous and less controlled than the same care provided in an inpatient environment or ED, yet patient safety strategies and team training are only now being incorporated into the EMS system.
- Key issues related to quality in EMS settings include clinical judgment, adverse event and error reporting, communications, ground vehicle safety, aircraft safety, interfacility transport, and field intubation.
- In some cases, EMS providers are being asked to make decisions that they are not trained to make; scope creep in their responsibilities may also lead to providers making decisions that could harm the patient.
- Underreporting and nonreporting of error events in the EMS setting may be due to both a fear of reporting and a lack of recognition of near-miss events and their significance.
- During the handoff between EMS and either ED or hospital staff, the loss of key clinical information may sometimes lead to direct patient harm.
- Whenever possible, the provider should remain seated and secured during transport, and should ensure that all equipment is secured to minimize the risk of injury from loose equipment in the event of a collision.
- The air transport crew needs to maximize risk reduction by optimizing the patient's condition prior to flight and ensuring adequate monitoring equipment is in place.
- One of the best ways to mitigate the risk of adverse events en route is to ensure the correct crew configuration is available for the transport.
- Prior to transport, appropriate equipment should be properly maintained and checked. Specific checklists with sections for ventilators, IV pumps, and other equipment have been shown to decrease the risk of adverse events and errors of omission.

Vital Vocabulary

active error An error that almost always involves frontline staff and occurs at a contact point between a staff member and some aspect of a larger system.

adverse drug event (ADE) An adverse reaction caused by taking a medication.

crew resource management (CRM) A safety-oriented program that emphasizes a culture of mutual support, teamwork, and the expectation and requirement that any team member can and should voice a concern regarding the safe operation of the team.

Prep Kit Continued

debriefing A powerful inquiry tool in which a concise exchange occurs to identify what happened, what was learned, and what can be done better in the future.

error A preventable adverse event in the delivery of care, whether or not it is evident or harmful to the patient.

failure mode and effect analysis (FMEA) A process that helps identify priorities in risk mitigation and process redesign.

harm Unintended physical injury resulting from or contributed to by medical care.

highly reliable organization (HRO) An organization that focuses on managing its inevitable failures, so that a failure does not affect the patient or the customer.

huddle A communication technique and event that often takes the form of a structured, short meeting in which patient care teams come together to talk about a patient, procedure, or situation.

just culture A system of beliefs and practices that focuses on blamelessly identifying issues that lead to errors or unsafe behaviors, while still maintaining individual accountability for reckless behavior.

latent error A mistake that is likely to occur secondary to organizational or design failures that allow the inevitable active error to cause harm.

Lean A strategy that looks at all processes and attempts to reduce waste and ensure all activities add value.

medical error The failure of a planned health care action to be completed as intended, or the use of a wrong care plan to achieve an aim.

mistake A situation in which an action occurs as intended but is the wrong action; it often occurs secondary to lack of experience, insufficient training, or negligence.

near miss An unplanned event that did not cause an injury, illness, or damage, but had the potential to do so; it is indistinguishable from a full-fledged adverse event in all but the outcome.

never event An event that should never occur and indicates a serious underlying safety problem.

normalization of deviance A process in which a shift away from acceptable policies and practices becomes the behavioral norm.

patient safety According to the World Health Organization, freedom from unnecessary harm or potential harm associated with health care.

root cause analysis (RCA) A systematic approach to understanding the causes of a serious adverse event and identifying system flaws that can be corrected to prevent future harm.

safety culture In an EMS organization, a system of beliefs and practices that includes acknowledging that organizations engage in high-risk activities and determining the importance of consistent safe operations to counteract these activities, supporting a blame-free environment where errors can be reported without fear of punishment, and maintaining organizational commitment to address reported errors and safety concerns.

sentinel event A patient safety event in which an error reaches a patient and results in death, permanent harm, or severe temporary harm such that interventions are required to sustain life.

serious adverse event (SAE) A sentinel event.

simulation A training technique that allows health care providers to hone their skills in a safe environment without risk of patient harm and to work in teams to practice both procedures and communication skills.

situation, background, assessment, and recommendation (SBAR) A technique that allows for a brief, yet concise and expected, handoff of information.

Six Sigma A disciplined, data-driven approach and methodology for eliminating defects in any process.

Prep Kit Continued

slip A lapse in concentration that occurs in the face of distractions, fatigue, or stress.

Swiss cheese model A model in which errors made by people result in consequences related to flawed systems.

TeamSTEPPS Team strategies and tools to enhance performance and patient safety; a program that embraces the principles of crew resource management and teaches tools and

methods by which team members can safely raise concerns, challenge orders that are unclear, and if necessary "stop the line."

universal time-out A planned pause before the beginning of a procedure that improves communication among all personnel in the room; it allows time for everyone to review important aspects of the procedure.

References

Bates DW, Spell N, Cullen DJ, et al. The costs of adverse drug events in hospitalized patients. *JAMA.* 1997;277(4):307-311.

Berwick DM. Errors today and errors tomorrow. *N Engl J Med.* 2003;348:2570-2572.

Bigham BL, Buick JE, Brooks SC, et al. Patient safety in emergency medical services: a systematic review of the literature. *Prehosp Emerg Care.* 2012;16(1):20-35.

Blakeman TC, Branson RD. Inter- and intra-hospital transport of the critically ill. *Respir Care.* 2013;58(6): 1008-1023.

Choi HK, Shin SD, Ro YS, et al. A before and after intervention trial for reducing unexpected events during the intrahospital transport of emergency patients. *Am J Emerg Med.* 2012;30(8):1433-1440.

Cone D, Brice JH, Delbridge TR, Myers JB, eds. *Emergency Medical Services: Clinical Practice and Systems Oversight.* Olathe, KS: National Association of EMS Physicians; February 2015.

Donabedian A. The quality of care: how can it be assessed? *JAMA.* 1988;260(12):1743-1748.

EMS Patient Safety Culture Survey. Center for Patient Safety website. https://www.centerforpatientsafety.org /emsforward/ems-safety-culture-survey/. Accessed May 20, 2021.

EVENT: EMS Voluntary Event Notification Tool. Center for Leadership, Innovation, and Research in EMS website. https://www.ruralcenter.org/sites/default/files /EVENT%20White%20Pape%206.29.11.pdf. Published June 29, 2011. Accessed May 20, 2021.

Folli HL, Poole RL, Benitz WE, et al. Medication error prevention by clinical pharmacists in two children's hospitals. *Pediatrics.* 1987;79(5):718-722.

Grissinger M. Oops, sorry, wrong patient! Applying The Joint Commission's "two-identifier" rule goes beyond the patient's room. *Pharmacy Therap.* 2008;33(11):625-651.

Haig KM, Sutton S, Whittington J. SBAR: a shared mental model for improving communication between clinicians. *Jt Commission J Qual Patient Saf.* 2006;32(3):167-175.

Henriksen K, Battles JB, Keyes MA, Grady ML. *Advances in Patient Safety: New Directions and Alternative Approaches.* Vol. 1: Assessment. Rockville, MD: Agency for Healthcare Research and Quality; 2008.

Howard I, Pillay B, Castle N, et al. Application of the emergency medical services trigger tool to measure adverse events in prehospital emergency care: a time series analysis. *BMC Emerg Med.* 2018;18(47). https://doi .org/10.1186/s12873-018-0195-0.

Institute of Medicine. *Crossing the Quality Chasm: A New Health System for the 21st Century.* Washington, DC: National Academies Press; 2001.

Institute of Medicine. *Emergency Medical Services: At the Crossroads.* Washington, DC: National Academies Press; 2007.

Kohn LT, Corrigan JM, Donaldson MS. *To Err Is Human: Building a Safer Health System.* Washington, DC: National Academies Press; 2000.

Kupas DF, Wang HE. Critical care paramedics: a missing component for safe interfacility transport in the United States. *Ann Emerg Med.* 2014;64(1):17-18.

Kwaan MR, Studdert DM, Zinner MJ, Gawande AA. Incidence, patterns, and prevention of wrong-site surgery. *Arch Surg.* 2006;141(4):353-357; discussion 357-358.

Leape L. Error in medicine. *JAMA.* 1994;272(23): 1851-1857.

Leape LL, Bates DW, Cullen DJ, et al. Systems analysis of adverse drug events. *JAMA.* 1995;274(1):35-43.

Leape LL, Berwick DM. Five years after "To Err Is Human": what have we learned? *JAMA.* 2005;293(19):2384-2390.

Leape L, Lawthers AG, Brennan TA, et al. Preventing medical injury. *Qual Rev Bull.* 1993;19(5):144-149.

Ligtenberg JM, Arnold LG, Stienstra Y, et al. Quality of interhospital transport of critically ill patients: a prospective audit. *Crit Care.* 2005;9(4):R446-R451.

List of confused drug names. Institute for Safe Medication Practices website. https://www.ismp.org /recommendations/confused-drug-names-list. Published February 28, 2019. Accessed May 20, 2021.

Prep Kit Continued

Maddry JK, Arana AA, Clemons MA, et al. Impact of a standardized EMS handoff tool on inpatient medical record documentation at a level I trauma center. *Prehosp Emerg Care*. 2020;1-8. doi:10.1080/10903127.2020.1824050.

Makary Martin A, Daniel M. Medical error—the third leading cause of death in the US. *BMJ*. 2016;353:i2139.

Norman DA. *The Design of Everyday Things*. New York, NY: Basic Books; 2002.

Singh JM, MacDonald RD, Ahghari M. Critical events during land-based interfacility transport. *Ann Emerg Med*. 2014;64(1):9-15.

Trigger tools. Institute for Healthcare Improvement website. http://www.ihi.org/Topics/TriggerTools/Pages /default.aspx. Accessed May 20, 2021.

World Health Organization. *WHO Patient Safety Curriculum Guide: Multi-Professional Edition*. Geneva, Switzerland: World Health Organization; 2011.

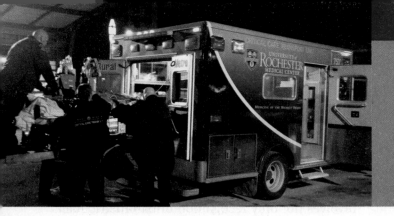

Chapter 4

Aircraft Fundamentals and Flight Physiology

Paul Mazurek, MEd, RN, NRP

OBJECTIVES

After completing this chapter, you will be able to:

1. Briefly discuss the emphasis of the air medical role in facilitating critical care transports (pp 74–75).
2. Describe the composition of the atmosphere (p 75).
3. List the three physiologic zones in the atmosphere (pp 76–77).
4. Discuss the primary gas laws affecting flight physiology (pp 77–81).
5. Summarize the advantages and disadvantages of the use of rotor-wing aircraft (pp 81–82).
6. Summarize the advantages and disadvantages of the use of fixed-wing aircraft (p 82).
7. Summarize the advantages and disadvantages of pressurized and nonpressurized aircraft (p 82).
8. Recognize the physical and physiologic effects of rapid cabin decompression (p 82).
9. List the primary stressors of flight and their physiologic impacts (pp 82–90).
10. Define the factors affecting tolerance of the stressors of flight (pp 90–92).
11. Define the effective performance time and the time of useful consciousness (pp 92–93).
12. Define the four types of hypoxia (pp 93–95).
13. Describe the four stages of hypoxia as they relate to altitude (pp 95–96).
14. Recognize the signs and symptoms of altitude-induced hypoxia and the appropriate treatment (p 97).
15. Identify different dysbarisms and trapped gas disorders (p 97).
16. Explain the role of the Commission on Accreditation of Medical Transport Systems and the concepts of visual flight rules, instrument flight rules, and a sterile cockpit (pp 99–100).
17. Discuss the concept of flight following (pp 100–101).
18. List standards created to enforce aircraft safety (pp 103–104).
19. Describe causes of air medical crashes, including human errors and risk factors (pp 102–103).
20. Summarize crew resource management (pp 104–106).
21. Summarize the Federal Aviation Administration guidelines that pertain to air medical transport (p 106).
22. Explain the importance of taking safety precautions as part of air medical programs (p 107).

Introduction

Many critical care transport professionals (CCTPs) will work in the aircraft environment in the course of their duties. Some CCTPs may be permanently assigned to an aircraft, whereas others may rotate to aircraft as part of their staffing assignments. The CCTP needs to be familiar with both rotor-wing (helicopter) and fixed-wing (airplane) operations. In the air medical environment, crew safety is always the top priority. Providers must never forget that safety is the most important part of patient care and an absolute requirement for successfully completing the mission.

The air medical environment is both complex and extremely dynamic. A thorough knowledge of flight physiology is essential to keep the flight crew airworthy and to prevent transport-related complications in critically ill and injured patients. CCTPs frequently encounter patients with comorbidities and patients who have experienced multiple traumas and are already in a severely compromised condition. Many of these patients' conditions will be exacerbated by changes in the barometric pressure that occurs at higher altitude. Likewise, the forces experienced during flight can have a significant effect on disease pathophysiology. For all these reasons, CCTPs must have a strong understanding of the effects of altitude on the body.

A number of gas laws are pertinent to flight medicine, and several common problems can occur as the result of changes in oxygen levels and barometric pressure during air transport. In addition to these issues, this chapter discusses the advantages and disadvantages of pressurized and nonpressurized aircraft and the effect of decompression at altitude. CCTPs must have a solid understanding of the potential catastrophic consequences that can be experienced with rapid cabin decompression.

Further, CCTPs must be aware of the primary stressors related to flight on the flight crew members and appreciate the factors that can affect tolerance of those stressors. Aircrew members need to be familiar with different illusions of flight and spatial disorientation, which can have disastrous consequences on flight operations. Some types of spatial disorientation can have negative effects on patients as well and can precipitate serious medical conditions.

Even providers whose responsibilities pertain almost exclusively to ground-based services must still have a comprehensive knowledge of flight physiology. They will frequently prepare patients for air transport and receive patients who have been flown to their destination. For this reason, they must have a thorough understanding of how flight dynamics affect their patients. Knowledge of flight physiology involves not only recognition of barometric maladies, but also (and more importantly) the prevention of such problems.

The Air Medical Role

The basic role of an air medical service is to rapidly transport CCTPs to a patient, stabilize the patient's condition, and transport that patient to a tertiary care center as quickly as possible. The patients who benefit most from air medical transport are those who are critically ill or injured or who would have a negative outcome with a prolonged transport.

Although air transport offers many benefits, as a CCTP you must weigh the potential advantages for the patient against the risks associated with the specific mode of transport. Before selecting this mode of transportation, patients should be evaluated and assessed for the effects of altitude and other forces that might adversely alter their condition en route. For example, patients who have cardiac conditions for which activity-sensing pacemakers have been implanted may experience severe complications if the pacemaker malfunctions because of flight vibrations.

Air medical transport may be relatively contraindicated for patients with the following conditions, requiring a careful risk–benefit analysis:

- Severe anemia
- Hemoglobinopathy
- Myocardial infarction (MI) within 10 days or complications in the 5 days before the flight (with the exception of a patient with an acute MI being flown to the catheterization lab, which is done routinely)
- Uncontrolled arrhythmia
- Pregnancies past 24 weeks' gestation
- Recent eye surgery affecting the globe
- Nonacute hypovolemia

If air medical transport is undertaken in such cases, special considerations, such as flying at a lower altitude than usual, may need to be taken to optimize the patient's outcome. Although patient conditions and possible complications must always be considered, the terrain, weather, and geographic location of the closest facility must also be factored into the decision-making process. In addition, it is important to recognize the transport crew's capabilities and to ensure crew members' safety.

Although there are certainly some drawbacks associated with air medical transport, history has shown that air medical transports decrease mortality rates and allow patients to have access to more specialized tertiary care facilities. Air medical transports may facilitate more rapid entry into the health care system, especially for patients who live in otherwise inaccessible areas. Such programs can be a major source of support for community hospitals and rural areas when they are confronted with critically ill or injured patients.

The Atmosphere

The atmosphere extends from the surface of the earth to an altitude of about 6,200 miles, which is the beginning of space **FIGURE 4-1**. This chapter focuses primarily on the components of the lower atmosphere, in which all aviation except

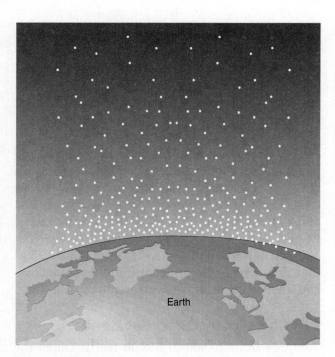

Earth

FIGURE 4-1 The density of the atmosphere decreases the farther you are from sea level.

© Jones & Bartlett Learning.

space exploration occurs. The atmosphere varies with time of day, season of the year, and latitude. Because of these variables, only averages are discussed in this chapter.

Atmospheric Composition

The composition of the atmosphere is constant and is defined in terms of percentages of gases. Although the percentage of gases is constant, the density of the atmosphere and its constituent gases vary with the altitude. Three gases—oxygen, nitrogen, and argon—constitute almost 99% of the atmosphere, which remains constant from the surface to altitudes of 250,000 feet.

- Oxygen makes up 21% of the atmosphere's volume. A by-product of photosynthesis, it is the most critical gas needed to sustain life.
- Nitrogen is the most abundant gas in the atmosphere, accounting for 78% of the total volume. This inert gas is odorless, colorless, and tasteless. While not readily used by humans, nitrogen is a critical element for life. It is present in the human body in abundant quantities and can be responsible for evolved gas disorders at altitude or after rapid ascent while scuba diving.
- Argon constitutes approximately 0.93% of the atmosphere's volume.

Other gases found in the atmosphere in trace amounts include carbon dioxide, neon, helium, methane, krypton, and hydrogen.

No matter the altitude, the percentage of the atmosphere consisting of oxygen will always be roughly 21%. During an ascent to higher altitude, the molecules of gases, including oxygen, spread out and become less numerous in each breath. This is why it can be difficult for human beings to breathe at high altitudes, such as at the top of Mount Everest.

Layers of the Atmosphere

Five distinct layers of the atmosphere have been identified based on thermal characteristics (temperature changes), chemical composition, movement, and density. The density of the atmosphere decreases with height because the weight of the molecules actually compresses its component gases near the earth's surface.

The first layer of the atmosphere is called the troposphere. The troposphere extends from sea level to about 26,000 feet (5 miles) over the poles and to nearly 52,000 feet (10 miles) above the equator. Virtually all weather occurs in the troposphere because of the presence of water vapor and strong vertical currents there. In this layer, clouds form, rain falls, wind blows, and humidity varies depending on the climate. The strong jet stream is located above 35,000 feet, with maximum winds in the jet stream averaging 200 mph at about 30° latitude north or south. The troposphere is also the densest portion of the atmosphere. Temperature in this layer varies from 62.6°F (17°C) to minus 68.8°F (minus 56°C) and decreases proportionately with increases in altitude.

The tropopause is the layer between the troposphere and the stratosphere, which is the next layer. The tropopause ranges in height from 30,000 feet at the poles to more than 60,000 feet at the equator. More solar energy is received by the earth near the equator, causing the air there to heat and expand. This expansion of rising air increases the height of the tropopause. Conversely, the cool air at the poles results in contraction and shrinkage of the air, resulting in a lesser height of the tropopause at these locations. The tropopause and the troposphere are collectively known as the lower atmosphere.

The layers above the tropopause include the stratosphere, stratopause, mesosphere, thermosphere, and exosphere, in that order. Critical care transports do not occur at these altitudes. **FIGURE 4-2** shows the layers of the atmosphere and indicates how they compare with the zones of the atmosphere (discussed next).

Physiologic Zones of the Atmosphere

The atmosphere is divided into three distinct zones that directly correlate to a human's response to hypoxia: the physiologic zone, the physiologically deficient zone, and the space equivalent zone.

Physiologic Zone

The physiologic zone is the area of the atmosphere that contains the oxygen and barometric pressure needed for a normal, healthy person to live. This zone extends from sea level to 10,000 feet. In this zone, the barometric pressure falls from 760 mm Hg

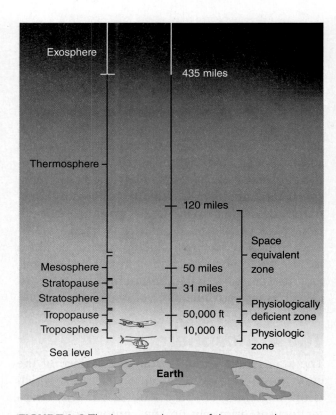

FIGURE 4-2 The layers and zones of the atmosphere.
© Jones & Bartlett Learning.

at sea level to 523 mm Hg at 10,000 feet. The pressure at 10,000 feet is still enough to maintain an adequate partial pressure of oxygen (arterial) (Pao$_2$) without the use of supplemental oxygen, pressurization, or protective equipment. Nevertheless, at 10,000 feet, many healthy people will begin to experience very mild effects of hypoxia (oxygen deprivation), such as a mild headache, and almost all patients with comorbidities will be hypoxic at this altitude. As will be discussed in more detail later, air medical transport providers are subject to Part 91 and/or Part 135 under Title 14 of the Code of Federal Regulations (14 CFR), often referred to as the Federal Aviation Regulations (FARs). Part 135.89 states that commercial pilots must use supplemental oxygen when flying at altitudes greater than 10,000 feet.

Physiologically Deficient Zone

The area from 10,000 to 50,000 feet is called the physiologically deficient zone. Above 10,000 feet, barometric pressure begins to decrease to levels that will result in hypoxic hypoxia (a state of oxygen deficiency caused by a decrease in the amount of oxygen in the blood), which is discussed later in this chapter. Barometric pressure at this level ranges from 523 mm Hg at 10,000 feet to 87 mm Hg at 50,000 feet. At these altitudes, the effects of trapped gases become more pronounced, and protective equipment, supplemental oxygen, and pressurized aircraft are necessary for transports.

Space Equivalent Zone

The space equivalent zone extends from 50,000 feet to 120 miles. At this point in the atmosphere, 100% supplemental oxygen is no longer adequate because of the minimal barometric pressure. Pressure suits and sealed cabins are also required. Two additional hazards can be present. First, exposure to atmospheric conditions could result in the boiling of body fluids as the fluids turn to a vapor. Second, personnel might be exposed to increased levels of radiation from the sun in this zone. Currently, no commercial aircraft used for air medical transport operate in this zone.

Barometric Pressure

Barometric pressure, also called atmospheric pressure, is a direct result of the weight of air. Barometric pressure varies with time and location because the amount and weight of air above the earth vary with time and location. This pressure is also related to the density of the air, which reflects the air temperature and height above the earth's surface. Thus, barometric pressure is the weight per unit area of all the molecules of the gas above the point at which the measurement was taken, with temperature and humidity as variables. It is also one of the most important factors that determines weather.

Barometric pressure is reported in a variety of units. Inches of mercury is the unit most commonly used in the United States, but millibars is used in most countries that use the metric system, such as most of Europe. It may also be measured in atmospheres (atm), although different scientific definitions of the atmosphere exist. The two most prevalent definitions are the US Standard Atmosphere and the International Standard Atmosphere. The US Standard Atmosphere has been recognized for the longest time, but the International Standard is now more widely recognized around the globe.

Gas Laws

CCTPs must have a thorough knowledge of the applicable gas laws as they relate to both flight and hyperbaric medicine (ie, medicine involving one or more gases at a greater than normal pressure). The various gas laws have an important role not only in patient care, but also in the overall safety of the flight crew. Several gas laws, some of which are interdependent, are integral to flight physiology.

Boyle's Law

Robert Boyle studied the relationship between the volume of a dry gas and its pressure. Boyle found that when he increased the volume of the gas, the pressure decreased. Conversely, a decrease in volume resulted in an increase in pressure. A practical example of this law's application is that as altitude increases, the atmospheric pressure decreases.

Boyle's law has numerous implications for aviation medicine. For example, any gas trapped in the chest, such as in a pneumothorax, will expand approximately 35% when going from sea level to 8,000 feet **FIGURE 4-3**. At 18,000 feet, a given volume of gas will expand to twice its size at sea level.

Several disease processes can have drastic effects with increasing altitude. An injury such as a pneumothorax can quickly become a tension pneumothorax as altitude increases. Patients with an open skull fracture are at risk for pneumocephalus because air becomes trapped inside the skull and expands with altitude, causing a significant increase in intracranial pressure. Patients with

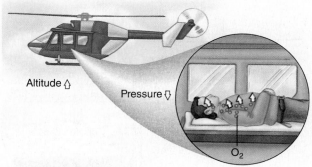

FIGURE 4-3 Boyle's law. As altitude increases, atmospheric pressure decreases, and gases inside the body expand.
Abbreviation: O_2, oxygen

© Jones & Bartlett Learning.

pneumoperitoneum (a collection of air within the peritoneum) or pneumomediastinum (a collection of air within the mediastinum) are also susceptible to worsening of their condition with increasing altitude. Although these disease processes might not cause a high-tension event within the body, they create significant discomfort for the patient.

Boyle's law also applies to the expansion of any trapped gas within the body, such as in the middle ear, sinuses, stomach, and intestines. Many pieces of medical equipment are also exquisitely sensitive to an increase or decrease in barometric pressure. The cuffed balloon on endotracheal tubes, for example, can double in size with a change in altitude from 5,000 feet to 10,000 feet, causing the balloon to rupture or triggering tissue necrosis if the balloon is allowed to remain hyperinflated for a significant length of time. Therefore, cuffed balloons should be filled with saline before flights planned at altitudes greater than 6,000 feet, or cuff pressure should be monitored and adjusted.

All patients who have a nasogastric or orogastric tube inserted should be transported on aircraft with the tube open or frequently vented. Patients with colostomy bags should frequently have the built-up gas "burped" to prevent overpressurization and failure of the colostomy bag.

Charles's Law

Discovered in 1787 by Jacques Charles, Charles's law states that the volume of a gas is directly proportional to the temperature, with the pressure remaining constant **FIGURE 4-4**. The practical application of this law is that as the air heats up, the volume increases, allowing the molecules to spread out and making the air less dense. Helicopters fly more easily in cold weather because gas molecules are more compressed and allow more lift as the rotor blades spin. In contrast, gas molecules are farther apart in hot weather and provide less lift. Therefore, a helicopter or airplane is able to carry a smaller amount of weight on a hot, humid day than on a cold, dry day.

Dalton's Law

In 1800, John Dalton postulated Dalton's law, which states that the total pressure of a gas mixture is the sum of the individual pressures. Simply put, all of the parts equal the whole. This law is also referred to as the law of partial pressures, where a partial pressure is the pressure of a single gas in the mixture.

Dalton's law illustrates that increasing altitude results in a proportional decrease in the partial pressures of the gases found in the atmosphere. Although the percentage concentrations of gases remain stable with increasing altitude, their partial pressure decreases in direct proportion to the total barometric pressure. Dalton's law is extremely important in critical care medicine because when supplemental oxygen is given, this law can be used to calculate the expected partial pressure of oxygen (Po_2) that should be obtained when arterial blood gas values are checked **FIGURE 4-5**.

Fick's Law

Fick's law, established by Adolph Fick in 1855, states that the diffusion rate of a gas is (1) proportional to

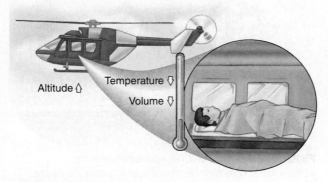

FIGURE 4-4 Charles's law. The volume of a gas is directly proportional to the temperature, with the pressure remaining constant.

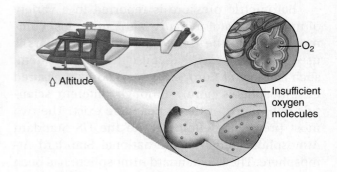

FIGURE 4-5 Dalton's law. The total pressure of a gas mixture is the sum of the individual pressures. Insufficient oxygen (O_2) molecules can lead to hypoxia.

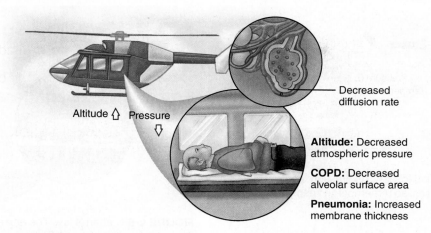

FIGURE 4-6 Fick's law. The diffusion rate of a gas is affected by atmospheric pressures, the surface area of the membrane, and the thickness of the membrane. A patient with chronic obstructive pulmonary disease (COPD) and pneumonia will have decreased gas exchange.

© Jones & Bartlett Learning.

the difference in partial pressure, (2) proportional to the area of the membrane, and (3) inversely proportional to the thickness of the membrane **FIGURE 4-6**. In practical terms, the rate of diffusion is affected by atmospheric pressures, the surface area of the membrane, and the thickness of the membrane. Fick's law is the primary gas law governing the diffusion of oxygen across the alveolar membrane. For example, an older adult with chronic obstructive pulmonary disease (COPD) who also has pneumonia will have decreased gas exchange at altitude because of the decreased partial pressure of oxygen at altitude, coupled with the decreased surface area of the alveoli and the increased membrane thickness secondary to the disease processes.

Henry's Law

In 1800, J. W. Henry postulated Henry's law, which states that the amount of a gas in a solution varies directly with the partial pressure of a gas over the solution. In other words, as the pressure of a gas over a liquid decreases, the amount of gas dissolved in the liquid will also decrease.

The effect of Henry's law in the body is seen in decompression sickness, which is discussed later in this chapter. In this case, inert gases in the body tissue (primarily nitrogen) are maintained in equilibrium with the partial pressures of the same gases in the atmosphere. As barometric pressure decreases, the partial pressure of nitrogen in the atmosphere decreases as well. As the body attempts

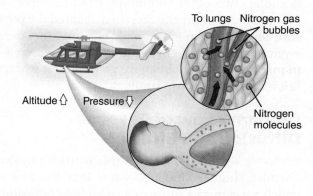

FIGURE 4-7 Henry's law. As the pressure of gas over a liquid decreases, the amount of gas dissolved in the liquid will also decrease. In decompression sickness, nitrogen saturates the tissues, then forms gas bubbles that travel to the lungs.

© Jones & Bartlett Learning.

to establish a new equilibrium, nitrogen comes out of solution in the form of gas bubbles and travels in the venous blood system to the lungs **FIGURE 4-7**.

Gay-Lussac's Law

In 1809, the French chemist Joseph Louis Gay-Lussac found that there is a correlation between the pressure and the temperature of a gas when its volume is constant. Gay-Lussac's law can be expressed as a ratio: If pressure increases, temperature increases, and vice versa **FIGURE 4-8**. As an example, think of a room full of people (molecules). As the room becomes smaller (pressure increases),

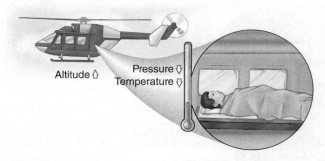

FIGURE 4-8 Gay-Lussac's law. As pressure decreases, temperature decreases, so remember to keep your patients warm.

© Jones & Bartlett Learning.

people will bump into each other, creating friction that will generate heat. As the room gets larger (pressure decreases), people no longer bump into each other and no heat is generated; thus, the room is cooler. Two other commonly cited examples of Gay-Lussac's law are the drop in measured tire pressure seen when an automobile sits outdoors overnight in a very cold environment and the increase in pressure observed in an oxygen cylinder when it is left out in very warm sunlight.

Graham's Law of Gaseous Diffusion and Effusion

Graham's law, formulated by the Scottish physical chemist Thomas Graham, states that the rate at which a gas moves through a small hole (effusion), avoiding interaction with other particles along the way, is inversely related to the square root of the mass of one mole of its molecules. In comparison, diffusion refers to particles moving from an area of high concentration to one of low concentration. When a gas is dissolved in liquid, its relative rate of diffusion is directly proportional to its solubility in the liquid. Both the effusion and diffusion concepts come into play when discussing the movement of oxygen and carbon dioxide between the alveolus and its capillary network.

A practical example of Graham's law is the ongoing process of diffusion of oxygen and carbon dioxide in the blood and transfer of oxygen from blood into the cells. Carbon dioxide molecules are much more massive than oxygen molecules (which would initially suggest a higher rate of effusion on the part of oxygen). However, carbon dioxide also has 22 times the solubility of oxygen, which

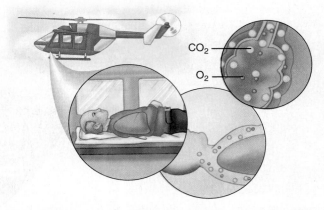

FIGURE 4-9 Graham's law. The rate at which a gas moves through a small hole is related inversely to the square root of the mass of one mole of its molecules. Diffusion of a gas in solution (eg, blood) is directly proportional to its solubility. Carbon dioxide (CO_2) diffuses more readily into the bloodstream than does oxygen (O_2) due to its higher solubility.

© Jones & Bartlett Learning.

mathematically means that carbon dioxide's diffusion rate is much faster than that of oxygen.

At altitude, with a lower barometric pressure and a greater overall volume of gas (particularly oxygen) in the atmosphere, the gas is less dense (ie, less concentrated) and the gradient for movement across the alveolar capillary membrane is altered. These dynamics can ultimately affect cellular respiration, leading to a reduction in movement of both oxygen and carbon dioxide. In short, oxygen is present, but there is not enough pressure to keep the molecules close enough together that a person can draw a meaningful breath. The CCTP must understand and remain mindful of this key concept **FIGURE 4-9**.

Formulas Based on the Gas Laws

The following formula, based on Henry's law, is used to determine how much additional oxygen will be needed to compensate for the altitude and barometric pressure changes. Fraction of inspired oxygen is indicated by F_{IO_2}.

$$\frac{\text{Initial } F_{IO_2} \times \text{Initial Barometric Pressure}}{\text{Baraometric Pressure at Cruising Altitude}} = \text{Adjusted } F_{IO_2}$$

If the barometric pressure is 760 mm Hg at sea level and 600 mm Hg at 6,000 feet above sea level, and if the patient's initial F_{IO_2} is 70%, the adjusted F_{IO_2} would be calculated as follows:

$$\frac{70\% \text{ Initial } F_{IO_2} \times 760 \text{ mm Hg}}{600 \text{ mm Hg}} = 88.7\% \text{ Adjusted } F_{IO_2}$$

To ensure that the patient continues to receive 70% F_{IO_2}, the ventilator would need to be adjusted to 88% F_{IO_2}.

Medical Transport Aircraft

As a CCTP, you need to be familiar with both rotor-wing (helicopter) and fixed-wing (airplane) operations. Transports via both types of aircraft have advantages and disadvantages. Nevertheless, they share many commonalities, including the four primary forces that constantly act on the aircraft in flight: lift, thrust, weight (gravity), and drag **FIGURE 4-10**. Lift counteracts weight, and thrust opposes drag. Essentially, greater amounts of thrust and lift allow an aircraft to take off. Conversely, greater amounts of drag and weight must exist for an aircraft to land. In straight and level flight, thrust equals drag and lift equals weight.

Rotor-Wing Transport

Rotor-wing transport, the means of transport that facilitates helicopter emergency medical service (HEMS), has the distinct advantage of vertical takeoff and landing, allowing the helicopter access to areas that may be inaccessible by ground vehicles or fixed-wing aircraft **FIGURE 4-11**. Rotor-wing aircraft generally have sustained speeds in excess of 150 mph, can operate at altitudes of less than 2,000 feet, and can move from point to point. (Depending on the local terrain, the altitude at which an aircraft will be able to fly may vary and is always at the discretion of the pilot-in-command.) Air medical providers who use such aircraft serve all types of population bases, from dense urban locations to extremely rural areas. A relatively small number of helicopters can serve a large population because of the quick turnaround time for most flights and their ability to cover distances quickly.

Rotor-wing transport has some disadvantages. Helicopters are more restricted than fixed-wing aircraft regarding weather limitations. They also have more stringent interior space limitations, which often make it difficult to perform complex patient-care procedures in the aircraft. For example, because of space constraints, when being transported by HEMS, a patient may be inaccessible from the waist down, or there may not be enough space behind the patient's head to allow intubation. These situations can have major ramifications for patient care.

Another limiting factor is the expense of helicopters compared to ground transport vehicles. A used helicopter may cost $2 million, and a new one may be closer to $20 million. There must be justification for the necessity of the helicopter to offset its increased costs relative to ground transport. HEMS is considerably more expensive than ground transport, averaging almost seven times the cost of an ambulance transport. (See Table 1-1 for further comparison of the advantages and disadvantages of different transportation modes.)

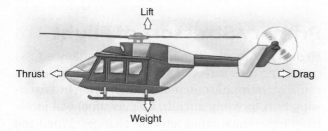

FIGURE 4-10 The forces of flight: weight, lift, drag, and thrust.

© Jones & Bartlett Learning.

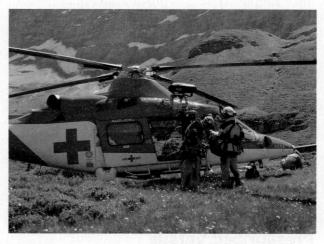

FIGURE 4-11 Helicopters can access locations that ground vehicles and fixed-wing aircraft cannot, making them ideal for certain situations.

Courtesy of Rega, Swiss Air-Rescue.

Helicopter transport is also subject to weight limitations. This concern becomes more problematic in the summer when the air is less dense, decreasing the amount of lift that the blades can achieve (ie, lift capacity). (Remember Charles's law?)

Fixed-Wing Transport

As a general rule, transport by fixed-wing aircraft is safer than transport by rotor-wing aircraft. Fixed-wing aircraft use established landing areas (airports) and fly at designated cruising altitudes that minimize their risk of colliding with human-made objects. The vast majority of fixed-wing air medical aircraft are certified to follow instrument flight rules (discussed later in the chapter) and fly with a two-pilot crew, further increasing safety.

Fixed-wing aircraft offer several advantages for medical transport. Two of their greatest advantages are their high speeds, ranging from 250 to 600 mph, and their ability to travel over greater distances. Some fixed-wing aircraft can carry multiple patients, ranging from two on smaller aircraft to hundreds on large military air medical aircraft. There are usually no weight limitations regarding patient size, and the aircraft can carry multiple medical crew members with a variety of equipment.

Nevertheless, fixed-wing aircraft have some distinct disadvantages, including the high cost of obtaining an aircraft for air medical purposes. Many air medical providers do not purchase or lease their own aircraft, but instead contract with various executive aircraft services to provide aircraft as needed. The cost of patient transport by fixed-wing aircraft can exceed $10,000 or more for short-distance flights and can exceed $100,000 for international flights. Most fixed-wing services secure reimbursement from patients or insurance companies prior to initiating a flight because of the high costs involved.

Fixed-wing aircraft must use maintained landing fields, and restrictions on runway length may apply, depending on the size of the aircraft. In addition, fixed-wing aircraft require hangars to house them on the ground, which increases their overall operating costs.

Pressurized Versus Nonpressurized Aircraft

The most effective method of protecting people from the physiologic effects of reduced barometric pressure is to pressurize the aircraft. This pressurization is accomplished by increasing the barometric pressure in the aircraft above the ambient pressure outside the aircraft. Two primary methods are used for pressurizing aircraft: the isobaric system and the differential control method for pressurization. The majority of civilian and military aircraft use isobaric systems for pressurization. The differential control (also known as conventional or isobaric-differential) method is designed primarily for military aircraft and has an aircraft cabin pressure that fluctuates with altitude.

Decompression at altitude is categorized as either slow or rapid. Rapid cabin depressurizations are dramatic events. With a loud explosion and numerous master caution warning horns sounding in the cockpit, it is quickly obvious to everyone that a major emergency has occurred. When rapid cabin depressurization occurs, the occupants of the aircraft are immediately exposed to the dangers of hypoxia, decompression sickness, gastrointestinal expansion, and hypothermia. Commercial pilots are extensively trained and tested on rapid decompression and emergency descent procedures.

A slow decompression, in contrast, can occur when a small leak develops in a pressurized aircraft. This type of decompression is dangerous because of its insidious onset and the undetectable loss of oxygen, which can lead to hypoxia and death if uncorrected.

If a loss of cabin pressure occurs, a descent must be made immediately to a level at which cabin altitude can be maintained at or below 10,000 feet. In addition, all occupants must use oxygen until the pilot-in-command indicates it is no longer necessary. As described later in this chapter, rapid cabin depressurization also dramatically affects the effective performance time and the time of useful consciousness, reducing these times by as much as one-half.

Primary Stressors of Flight

Flight crew members will experience many stressors during their career; however, some stressors may cause catastrophic outcomes. When flying in a fixed-wing or rotor-wing aircraft, all personnel will inevitably experience rapid altitude changes. When the body is exposed to significant altitude changes without the proper precautions, adverse outcomes may occur as the body attempts to maintain homeostasis.

Decreased Levels of Po$_2$

Decreased levels of Po$_2$ can quickly cause hypoxia in both the flight crew and passengers. At 15,000 feet, the barometric pressure is 429 mm Hg, and average values for a healthy patient would include an oxygen saturation of 80% (the body requires 87% to 97%) and a Pao$_2$ of 44 mm Hg (the body requires 60 to 100 mm Hg) **TABLE 4-1**. Remember that these values are averages for a healthy person; they are not representative of the patients who require critical care.

Barometric Pressure Changes

The greatest pressure change in an aircraft takes place from sea level to 5,000 feet. Therefore, problems associated with pressure must be considered even in nonpressurized aircraft that are not flying at altitudes requiring supplemental oxygen or cabin pressurization. During daylight hours for nonpressurized aircraft, 10,000 feet of altitude is the ceiling at which crew members must begin to use oxygen. Because the loss of night vision is one of the first symptoms of hypoxia, the ceiling drops to 8,000 feet for nighttime flight operations that exceed 1 hour in length. The alveolar Po$_2$ at 10,000 feet is approximately 61 mm Hg, which produces the maximum acceptable degree of hypoxia allowed. The upper limit for the indifferent stage of hypoxia (discussed later in this chapter) is 10,000 feet. However, deviation by only a few thousand feet for a short time will have little difference. For this reason, certain military operations are allowed at 13,000 feet as long as the duration of the flight is less than 3 hours.

In addition to causing hypoxia and malfunctioning pacemakers, ambient pressures and increasing altitudes can cause discomfort in air-trapped organs and sinuses (eg, the ears and gastrointestinal system).

Thermal Changes

Flight crew members are subjected to a variety of thermal extremes, ranging from the very cold to the very hot. Temperature changes increase the body's demand for oxygen and make the body less tolerant of the effects of hypoxia. Such changes can also cause the effects of hypoxia to become evident at lower altitudes than would normally be expected.

Temperature decreases as altitude increases. Specifically, temperature decreases by 3°F to 5°F per 1,000-feet gain in altitude, depending on the humidity. (At altitudes from 35,000 to 99,000 feet, the temperature remains relatively constant at minus 32°F [minus 50°C].) If the air conditioner cannot keep the cabin cool because of high ambient temperatures, rotor-wing aircraft may have the option to ascend and take advantage of the cooler temperatures at higher altitudes.

Flight personnel are often subjected to a wide range of ambient temperatures because of the geographic range of their aircraft. For example, flight crew assigned to rotor-wing aircraft may experience

TABLE 4-1 Partial Pressures of Oxygen at Various Altitudes					
Altitude (ft)	Atmospheric Pressure (mm Hg)	Pao$_2$ (mm Hg)[a]	Pvo$_2$ (mm Hg)	Pressure Differential (mm Hg)	Blood Saturation (%)[a]
Sea level	760	100	40	60	98
10,000	523	60	31	29	87
18,000	380	38	26	12	72
22,000	321	30	22	8	60
25,000	282	7	4	3	9
35,000	179	0	0	0	0

[a]These are average measurements for a healthy patient.

Abbreviations: Pao$_2$, partial pressure of oxygen (arterial); Pvo$_2$, partial pressure of oxygen (venous)

a temperature of 80°F (26.7°C) at their base but fly less than 1 hour into mountainous areas where the temperatures can be less than 40°F (4.4°C). Crews assigned to fixed-wing aircraft may see an even broader range of temperatures as they start in a northern climate in the snow and end in the hot sun in a southern climate.

A secondary hazard is the greenhouse effect, which results from radiant solar heat. This effect can increase the temperature in the cockpit or cabin of a small aircraft by as much as 50°F to 59°F.

Given the potential for such temperature changes, flight crews must be cognizant of the potential for heat stress. Core body temperatures that exceed 100°F (37.8°C) result in decreased short-term memory, degradation of motor skills, and a general decrease in performance. Heat stress also causes increased irritability and poor judgment, increases the propensity for motion sickness and hypoxia, and potentiates the effects of gravitational forces, which are discussed later in this chapter.

Vibration

Vibration is noted in all helicopters, most propeller-driven aircraft, and, minimally, jet-engine aircraft. Studies have found that vibrations between 1 and 12 Hz can cause significant effects on the body. Low-frequency vibrations can cause body discomfort, pain (usually in the abdomen or chest), decreased vision, and, most notably, fatigue. Excess vibration is an issue that must be addressed with aircraft mechanics and manufacturers. Nevertheless, some modifications can be made to reduce the effects of vibration. Increasing the cushioning on seats is one of the most important modifications, as is proper use of shoulder and lap belts, which reduces the transmission of vibrations.

Prolonged effects of vibration can increase the core body temperature as the body constantly tries to fight the effects of vibration and movement. As just mentioned, one of the most notable effects of vibration is fatigue. As the body becomes fatigued with prolonged exposure to vibration, it becomes more susceptible to the effects of vibration, which perpetuates the cycle.

To combat crew fatigue due to vibration, the amount of time a crew is allowed to fly on any given shift before resting is subject to restrictions. Preventive measures include prohibiting medical crew members from leaning against the airframe (to decrease vibration) and providing extra padding for patients so they are not leaning against the airframe.

Decreased Humidity

Humidity is the degree of moisture (water vapor) in the air; it is expressed as a percentage. The level of humidity is related to temperature: As temperature increases, so does humidity. Conversely, as temperature falls, so does the relative humidity. Because temperature falls with altitude, so does humidity. Given the relatively low altitudes at which they fly, rotor-wing and propeller aircraft tend to have higher humidity levels compared to jet aircraft. The air in a pressurized jet aircraft is also constantly being recirculated through filters, and any moisture is drawn off by the system. In high-speed, high-altitude, long-range flights, less than 5% humidity remains after 2 hours of flight and less than 1% remains after 4 hours of flight.

During a long flight, the dry air in the aircraft can cause dry, cracked mucous membranes, chapped lips, and sore throats; it can also lead to dehydration. This lack of humidity is why many people feel fatigued or jet-lagged after a long commercial flight. These problems can further be compounded in injured or ill patients, so it is important to consider patient hydration status before and during the flight **FIGURE 4-12**.

Patients who are receiving supplemental oxygen are at twice the risk of becoming dehydrated. If available, humidified oxygen should be used during air transports. The dry air in the aircraft can also cause

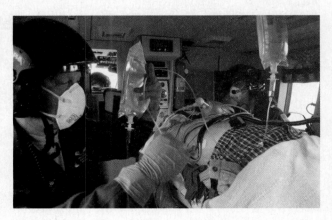

FIGURE 4-12 Proper hydration should be provided for all patients transported by air.
© Mark C. Ide.

drying of the cornea in unconscious or intubated patients if their eyes are not protected by taping or using artificial tears. In addition, owing to the relatively dry environment, consideration should be given to increasing the rate of intravenous (IV) fluids or providing additional oral hydration, if possible. To combat the effects of decreased humidity, crew members are encouraged to increase their fluid intake.

Noise

Noise is defined as any unwanted sound. Long exposure to noise can damage the soft tissues of the inner ear. The cells and nerves in the inner ear may be completely destroyed by continuous exposure to loud sounds. If enough cells are damaged, hearing is permanently damaged.

One of the biggest problems with damage caused by noise involves the subtle symptoms of hearing loss. Hearing loss usually manifests as feelings of pressure or fullness in the ears, muffled speech, or ringing in the ears. These symptoms may go away within minutes, hours, or days after the exposure or, depending on the damage, may never go away.

To determine how noise will affect hearing, three factors must be considered: loudness, pitch, and duration of exposure. It was once thought that only extremely high sound levels produce hearing loss; however, cumulative exposure to levels around 70 decibels from A-weighted noise-monitoring equipment (dBA) without protection have been shown to lead to irreversible hearing loss **TABLE 4-2**. Sound at 140 dB causes pain and indicates danger of immediate hearing loss.

Noise in the cabin of the aircraft can make it difficult for patients and care providers to communicate, which can lead to patient anxiety. The noise also makes it difficult for CCTPs to assess heart and lung sounds. Many monitoring errors and malfunctions can be attributed to the noise and vibrations associated with air medical transport. Assessment techniques such as pulse oximetry, capnography, and hemodynamic monitoring are less affected by noise and vibrations and help enable early recognition of complications.

To preserve the hearing of patients and accompanying family members, CCTPs must remember to provide them with appropriate hearing protection for the flight. In addition, CCTPs and other flight crew members must protect their own hearing.

TABLE 4-2 Noise Exposure Without Hearing Protection That Leads to Irreversible Hearing Loss

Sound	Decibel Level (dBA)[a]	Time of Exposure
Whispering	20	No limit
Normal conversation	60	No limit
Car	70	No limit
Diesel truck, jackhammer	100	2 h
Helicopter	105	1 h
Live rock music	90–130	8 h at 90 dB, but imminent hearing loss at 130 dB
Propeller aircraft	120	7 min
Jet aircraft	140	Imminent hearing loss at any length of exposure

[a]dBA refers to noise levels from the A-weighted noise-monitoring equipment used in noise studies to filter noises so they are more similar to how they would be interpreted by the human ear.

© Jones & Bartlett Learning.

Many employers require aircraft personnel to wear hearing protection to limit the effects of noise in the aircraft.

Crew members who work in the aircraft environment must be very attentive to the potential for hearing loss. They should be required to wear hearing protection approved by the American National Standards Institute whenever they are operating around an aircraft that is running.

All crew members working inside a rotor-wing aircraft should always wear hearing protection. Oftentimes this protection is accomplished by wearing a helmet with an internal communication system. Many crew members elect to wear soft hearing protection under their helmets as a secondary means of protection. Rotor-wing programs that do not use helmets should require use of headsets at all times. Not only do the helmets and headsets protect personnel from noise, but they also facilitate communication between crew members.

Crew members who operate on fixed-wing aircraft may or may not be required to have hearing protection inside the aircraft. Hearing protection depends on the type of aircraft (propeller versus jet) and the individual aircraft design. Generally speaking, larger aircraft will have better sound insulation and will not require the use of hearing protection inside the aircraft.

Fatigue

Fatigue involves much more than simply the lack of sleep; however, lack of sleep is the foundation for fatigue. Most physiologic problems encountered in the flight environment can cause significant fatigue, and their effects can quickly pile up when combined with a lack of restful sleep. Studies conducted by the **Federal Aviation Administration (FAA)** and the **National Transportation Safety Board (NTSB)** have noted that crew fatigue is often a contributing factor in aviation accidents and near misses.

Many flight crew members begin their shift already tired. Indeed, studies have shown that more than 50% of flight personnel are chronically fatigued because of long work hours. Air medical crew members most commonly work 12- or 24-hour shifts, but most pilots are limited by federal regulations to a maximum of 8 flight hours in any 24-hour period and are required to have at least 8 hours of uninterrupted rest. Most companies and flight crews do not rely on government agencies to police their duty time; instead, they impose more stringent requirements on themselves.

In addition to lack of sleep, three other factors contribute to crew fatigue: jet lag, vibration of the aircraft, and poor diet, which often includes missed meals due to the very nature of air medical transport. Jet lag is a factor leading to fatigue that is encountered in the fixed-wing environment, but not the rotor-wing environment. When flight crew travel across time zones, their bodies require time to adjust to the new time zone. Studies have shown that it takes 1 day for each hour of difference from the original time zone to reset the body's own circadian rhythm.

It is not uncommon for CCTPs to experience fatigue while flying, but the real challenge arises when CCTPs are required to maintain competency while caring for critically ill or injured patients during flights. Fatigue causes delayed reaction time, thereby increasing the risk of error. To minimize these risks, the Commission on Accreditation of Medical Transport Services emphasizes measures such as providing for crew rest and ensuring that duty days are not excessive. To avoid beginning another flight in a fatigued state, CCTPs should immediately request crew rest as soon as they feel fatigued. This request must be granted and typically lasts for 4 hours, occurring between flights. At the end of the 4 hours, a CCTP is reassessed to determine fitness for duty.

Gravitational Forces

The body's response to **gravitational forces** is affected by the intensity of the effect of acceleration, its direction, the length of time the body is subjected to stress, the time it takes for gravity's effects to appear, and the individual's unique physical makeup. Although this effect is termed gravitational force, it is actually rapid acceleration or deceleration, not gravity, that affects the body. One unit of gravitational force (informally referred to as *g*-force: 10*g*, for example) is equal to the weight of the object. The gravitational force experienced is multiplied by the person's weight to determine the actual force on the body. For example, a 100-pound (45.4-kg) person who experiences 10*g* will have 1,000 pounds (454 kg) of force on their body.

Two types of gravitational forces can be experienced. Negative gravitational forces result from a steep dive in an aircraft. Positive gravitational forces result from high-speed acceleration, climbs, or high-speed turns. Positive gravitational forces push blood away from the brain, whereas negative gravitational forces push blood toward the brain. Most humans can survive a greater degree of positive gravitational force than negative gravitational force.

Gravitational forces can have significant effects on the human body. The first physiologic sensation of gravitational force is the feeling of being pushed down in a seat or feeling weightless, depending on whether the aircraft is accelerating or decelerating. As the gravitational force increases, breathing becomes labored. Acceleration compresses the rib cage and lungs, making it difficult to draw in air or exhale and potentially resulting in exhaustion and air hunger. Hypoxia arises when gravitational force causes blood to leave the brain (eg, during a high-speed acceleration or turn) and move into the lower extremities. The body must then work much harder to circulate blood to the brain. Hypoxia can result in a loss of peripheral vision when the body is subjected to gravitational forces of 5g to 6g. As the gravitational force continues, tunnel vision develops, and eventually vision becomes gray (loss of color perception). Further exposure to acceleration stress will cause a person to experience blackout: a loss of all vision. During this time, the organs are displaced downward, significantly affecting blood flow. If the gravitational force continues, the flight crew member will lose consciousness (also called gravitational force loss of consciousness, or gravitational force–induced loss of consciousness). Other signs and symptoms include petechiae, rashes, and bruising; loss of consciousness with accompanying seizures, amnesia and confusion; and cardiac arrhythmias (tachycardia and bradycardia), heart blocks, and stress cardiomyopathy.

Several factors are known to decrease tolerance to positive gravitational force during acceleration. Age can play an important role in determining the extent to which a person may be affected by acceleration. People older than 60 years, for example, have a diminished tolerance for gravitational forces. Infection and illness, resulting in fever and dehydration, also increase the body's susceptibility to the effects of gravitational forces. A person with hypoglycemia will lose consciousness, under acceleration stress, 0.5g earlier than someone with a higher, normal blood glucose level. Alcohol consumption will cause a person to feel effects 0.1g to 0.4g sooner.

Spatial Disorientation and Illusions of Flight

A key concept in flight physiology is spatial orientation, which is the ability to use the senses to orient oneself to the surroundings. In flight, specific movements or situations may result in spatial disorientation, a condition in which the person has an incorrect understanding of their body's position with respect to the earth.

To maintain spatial orientation on the ground, three components come into play: effective perception; integration; and interpretation of visual, vestibular, and proprioceptive sensory information. Vestibular sensory information comes from the organs of equilibrium located in the inner ear. Proprioceptive sensory information is obtained from the skin, muscles, tendons, and joints. The brain recognizes changes in linear acceleration, angular

acceleration, and gravity and attempts to relate them to the visual input. In flight, spatial orientation is difficult to achieve because of conflicting sensory input. When visual, vestibular, and proprioceptive sensory stimuli provide conflicting information, a sensory mismatch occurs and results in illusions and spatial disorientation.

Of all of these senses and stimuli, visual reference provides approximately 90% of the information needed to maintain spatial orientation. This dominant source of input will overpower conflicting sensations from other systems, such that people seldom realize when the brain has received contradictory information. Learning not to rely on visual reference is an important factor for pilots who are flying by instruments. Indeed, a great deal of time during instrument training is spent convincing students to trust the instruments and not their senses. The senses may provide invalid information because the brain is convinced that "down" is the bottom of the aircraft, no matter the aircraft's actual position or angle.

All of the illusions discussed in this section result from vestibular ear disorders. As a consequence, these illusions can also cause significant nausea and vomiting, further debilitating the flight crew. According to the FAA, spatial disorientation is responsible for 5% to 10% of all general aviation crashes, and crashes resulting from spatial disorientation are usually fatal (90%).

Types of Spatial Disorientation

Spatial disorientation has been studied extensively by both military and civilian organizations. Spatial disorientation is divided into three types:

- Type I spatial disorientation occurs when the pilot does not notice that spatial disorientation is occurring because the senses confirm that the pilot's experience is real. A flight crew member who does not sense danger will not respond to the disorientation. This is a potentially deadly type of disorientation, because it can lead to a crash. A pilot experiencing type I spatial disorientation may fly directly toward the earth without realizing where the aircraft is headed.
- Type II spatial disorientation occurs when the pilot initially does not recognize the onset of spatial disorientation, but senses that something is wrong. Usually the pilot will misinterpret the problem as an instrument malfunction

and trust their own senses instead of relying on the instruments. For example, during gradual banking and descent, the pilot may sense the descent but not the bank and may attempt to gain altitude. The attempt to gain altitude actually increases the rate of the bank until the aircraft spirals out of control. Fortunately, such a graveyard spiral is a rare occurrence.

- **Type III spatial disorientation** occurs when the pilot is affected by the illusion of intense movement and is unable to regain spatial awareness. Usually when one person is affected this way, the other generally is not, and the correctly oriented person (the copilot) can steer the aircraft to safety.

Since John F. Kennedy, Jr.'s fatal crash in 1999, the FAA has revised several rules regarding recognition of and training for spatial disorientation. Currently, even initial private pilot applicants must receive at least 3 hours of instrument training and be taught recovery techniques, and most instructors include the topic of spatial disorientation during recurrent training.

Visual Illusions

The visual system can give deceptive signals to the brain, especially during instrument meteorological conditions, such as when flying in clouds or low visibility. These illusions can lead to misperceptions about location, altitude, distance away from other aircraft or objects, the rate of speed as the aircraft closes in on other objects, and attitude. For example, a **somatogravic illusion** is an error in perception that occurs with acceleration, as the otolith organs are displaced rearward, similar to when a person is looking up. This perception of a nose-up altitude may cause the pilot to push the nose of the aircraft down inappropriately at night or in unlit terrain. Flight crew members need to have a good understanding of such visual illusions to prevent and recognize potentially disastrous situations. These situations are potentially lethal but extremely rare.

Third Spacing

Third spacing, loss of fluids from the intravascular space into the tissues, became a factor in aviation at the end of World War II. The German Luftwaffe encountered this phenomenon after they developed the first jet-powered aircraft. It became evident that the human body was not designed for rapid acceleration and deceleration or for high-speed turns. Third spacing becomes a factor during high-speed turns because of the addition of centrifugal force in concert with the acceleration or deceleration of the aircraft. These forces actually began to push fluids (primarily plasma) from the intravascular space into the extravascular space, causing hypovolemia and potentiating hypoxia.

To counteract the effects of third spacing, the "g-suit" or military antishock trousers (MAST pants) were developed. The first g-suits were tightly laced suits that were similar to corsets. Aviators donned these suits and then tightened the laces to help counteract third spacing. Subsequent suits were designed to recognize high-gravitational-force maneuvers and automatically inflate to apply circumferential pressure on body tissues, thereby helping prevent plasma from leaching into the extravascular space. Today, in most aircraft that will experience high-gravitational-force maneuvers, the flight team is equipped with pressure suits and trained in techniques to prevent them from experiencing third spacing.

Flicker Vertigo

Flicker vertigo is defined by the Flight Safety Foundation as "an imbalance in brain cell activity caused by exposure to low-frequency flickering (or flashing) of a relative bright light." The effects of flicker vertigo may include nausea, vomiting, seizures, or fainting. These symptoms are usually mild and stop as soon as the source of the flickering is removed. This condition can be brought about by any bright light flickering at a frequency of 4 to 20 cycles per second (hertz [Hz]). Helicopter personnel are most often affected by flicker vertigo when natural light or reflections of anticollision strobe lights are distorted by the aircraft's rotor blades. This same phenomenon is possible in fixed-wing propeller aircraft. A rotating beacon can also cause flicker vertigo. If the propellers are the trigger for flicker vertigo, simply changing the revolutions per minute of the engine can often eliminate the symptoms; if strobe lights while in clouds are the cause, they can be turned off until the aircraft is in clear skies.

Fuel Vapors

Flight crew members and patients alike are exposed to the noxious odors of fuel vapors during air transport.

Most of this exposure occurs when the flight crew is loading or unloading a patient. The jet fuel odors can cause headaches and precipitate feelings of nausea, if prolonged. The flight crew is more susceptible to these effects than is the patient, because the crew has more prolonged exposure to them.

Weather

Weather can be an additional stressor. For example, rapidly worsening conditions or inadvertent flight into conditions that require the use of instrument flight rules cause stress. Transport programs that operate by visual flight rules (discussed in detail later) fly only in conditions that meet a visibility minimum of 3 miles (5 km) and appropriate clearance from clouds. Transport programs rated for instrument flight rules can fly in all but the worst of weather. The vast majority of rotor-wing programs operate under visual flight rules only because the pilots often must land the aircraft at unimproved sites (ie, sites that are not paved). Pilots undergo extensive training intended to ensure that they can quickly handle changing weather conditions.

Anxiety

Anxiety has a pivotal role in flight operations but is rarely addressed or discussed; it is often assumed to have been covered in the initial crew training. Several factors can cause anxiety. Numerous studies have shown that catecholamine release occurs in both flight crew members and patients during rotor-wing operations. Even among experienced flight crew members, a significant release of adrenaline, a catecholamine, occurs. This release of catecholamines can be advantageous to performance if it occurs in small quantities, but detrimental if large quantities flood the body.

For new flight nurses and paramedics, the learning curve related to air medical transport is exceptionally steep. These professionals must be adept at treating patients with the most critical conditions (traumatic and medical) and of all age ranges. Initially, all new flight crew members can be expected to have a high level of anxiety until they have gained experience transporting patients with a range of conditions during different types of flights.

Anxiety can occur in patients as well as the crew. Patients who express concern about the tight confines of the aircraft may be pretreated with anxiolytics **FIGURE 4-13**. Administration is based on individual protocols and patient presentation.

Night Flying

Crew members must be vigilant in assisting the pilot in scanning for other aircraft when able to do so, both at night and during the day. Fortunately, due to their lighting systems, aircraft are often easier to spot at night. Lights on airplanes indicate the direction of flight: From the seat of the aircraft being flown, the green light is on the right wing, the red light is on the left wing, and a white light is displayed to the rear. Because the positioning of lights on all aircraft adheres to this standard, it is easy to determine the direction of flight at night **FIGURE 4-14**.

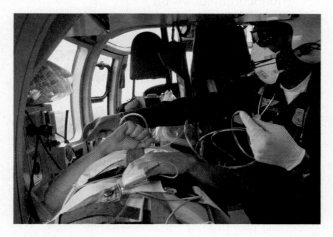

FIGURE 4-13 Aircraft cabins are very small, which can lead to anxiety on the part of patients and CCTPs.
© Mark C. Ide.

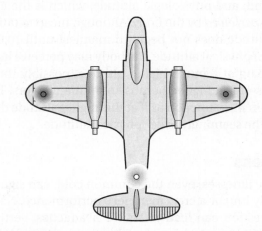

FIGURE 4-14 An aircraft's lights are set up in a standard format that makes it possible to determine the aircraft's direction of flight.
© Jones & Bartlett Learning.

For example, when pilots in an aircraft see another aircraft with a red light on the left, a green light on the right, and a white light in the middle, they know that the aircraft is moving away.

Crew members should reduce use of white light that may affect the pilot's night vision. Red lighting inside the aircraft is preferred.

The pilot and crew face other challenges in night flights. For instance, the crew has severely limited outside visibility. The pilot has the following disadvantages:

- Limited field of vision (reduced by 40% due to night-vision goggles, if used)
- Added weight stress from the helmet
- Loss of depth perception
- Monochromatic vision
- A reduced sense of speed

Factors Affecting Tolerance of the Physiologic Stressors of Flight

The primary human factors affecting the provider's tolerance of the stressors of flight can be remembered by the mnemonic IM SAFE, which stands for Illness, Medication, Stress, Alcohol, Fatigue, and Emotion. Other human factors, such as tobacco use and hypoglycemia, also affect stress tolerance and are important considerations in assessing flight fitness.

In flight medicine, there are two types of altitude: physical altitude, which is represented in feet above ground, and physiologic altitude, which is the altitude *perceived* by the body. Although incapacitation to altitude does not begin to manifest until 10,000 feet of physical altitude, the body may perceive itself as being at a much higher altitude, possibly thousands of feet higher, because of human factors. The person may function as if at this higher altitude despite the seemingly "safe" physical altitude.

Illness

Many illnesses, even the common cold, can significantly impair a crew member's performance. Nasal congestion can lead to severe headaches, vertigo, or nausea during pressure changes, such as during a rapid descent. All flight crew members should be cleared to fly by a physician during any period of illness.

Medications

The use of medications affects the tolerance of hypoxia. Over-the-counter (OTC) medications, although frequently considered benign, can result in incapacitation when their effects are combined with the effects of hypoxia. In addition, an underlying problem might go untreated because OTC medications can mask the problem. All flight crew members should follow approved lists for OTC medications before they fly, or consult with a flight surgeon or a physician knowledgeable in flight medicine, such as an aviation medical examiner, before taking any medications when they are scheduled to work.

The FAA has published a list of approved prescription and OTC medications that flight crew members are permitted to use. In 14 CFR Part 61, the FAA states that pilots assume responsibility for all medications they take and that if there is any doubt about the effect of the medication on the ability to fly, they must consult with a flight surgeon before flying. All flight crew members should be strongly cautioned against taking a medication for the first time when they are working because they cannot know how their body will react to the medication.

Stress

Most pilots and flight crew cannot simply "leave stress on the ground." Everyday stresses such as work, financial, and family issues can affect performance negatively and can lead to distraction and poor judgment. If crew members are experiencing high levels of stress, they should be encouraged to discuss this situation with members of management at their program. High levels of stress can cause inattentiveness and may have adverse effects on performance, including catastrophic effects in the aviation environment. If crew members recognize high levels of stress in their coworkers, they should take action to ensure the safety and effective operation of the program.

Alcohol

Alcohol can be a toxin in the body and can result in histotoxic hypoxia, inhibiting the use of available oxygen by hemoglobin and delaying metabolism at the cellular level. Research indicates that the intake of 1 ounce (30 mL) of alcohol is equivalent to

2,000 feet of physiologic altitude. Simply drinking two beers can add between 4,000 and 8,000 feet of physiologic altitude. Alcohol works by depressing the central nervous system and inhibiting judgment and coordination, further amplifying the effects of altitude. Part 91 of 14 CFR clearly addresses the topic of alcohol. It reads as follows:

a.   No person may act or attempt to act as a crewmember of a civil aircraft—
   (1)   Within 8 hours after the consumption of any alcoholic beverage;
   (2)   While under the influence of alcohol;
   (3)   While using any drug that affects the person's faculties in any way contrary to safety; or
   (4)   While having an alcohol concentration of 0.04 or greater in a blood or breath specimen. Alcohol concentration means grams of alcohol per deciliter of blood or grams of alcohol per 210 liters of breath.

Most aviation companies have a 12-hour "bottle to throttle" policy; however, all policies are underscored by the caveat that people who feel under the influence of alcohol, regardless of the time from the last drink, should not fly. Parts 91 and 135 of 14 CFR also state that all flight crew members are subject to random drug and alcohol tests at any time while on duty.

Regardless of whether the service's policy calls for maintaining 8 or 12 hours between drinking alcohol and flying, another significant hazard is the hangover, or post-alcohol impairment, associated with drinking. Physical and mental performance is still markedly reduced 14 to 24 hours after the blood alcohol level has returned to zero. One of the most dangerous problems during the hangover phase is the propensity for hypoglycemia and significant fatigue. Despite the frequent claims made about OTC medications, there is no simple remedy for hangovers.

Fatigue

Exhaustion and fatigue play important roles in an individual's ability to tolerate the effects of hypoxia. Shift work causes a tremendous disruption in the circadian rhythm, making it difficult for crew members to regulate their sleep at work and at home. Many air medical crew members also work second jobs during their time off and must be careful to allow for plenty of rest before the start of their flight shifts. Exhaustion can lead to errors in judgment, narrowed attention, uncharacteristic behavior, and falling asleep at work. Crew members who find that they need to use pharmacologic sleeping aids need to first have the medication approved by a flight surgeon. Frequent use of sleeping aids should be considered a flight safety issue and discussed in depth with a flight surgeon.

Emotion

Certain emotionally upsetting events, such as major arguments, a death in the family, and divorce, can significantly impair pilot and crew performance. Any pilot or crew member who experiences an intense emotional event should not fly until satisfactory resolution of that incident occurs.

Tobacco

An aviator who smokes risks incurring the effects of hypemic hypoxia, because carbon monoxide is 50 to 300 times more strongly attracted to hemoglobin than to oxygen. Hypemic hypoxia is caused by a decrease in the blood's oxygen-carrying capacity due to a reduced amount of hemoglobin in the blood or a reduced number of red blood cells. Research has shown that smoking 3 cigarettes in rapid succession or smoking 20 to 30 cigarettes in a 24-hour period can saturate 10% of the hemoglobin in the body. Consequently, at sea level, a regular smoker has a starting physiologic altitude of 3,000 to 8,000 feet, even before the aircraft takes off. Smoking also affects night vision; a regular smoker has already lost 20% of the night vision, even at sea level.

Hypoglycemia

A nutritious diet allows flight crew members to be much more tolerant of the effects of hypoxia. Poor diet and low blood glucose levels can cause nausea, headache, dizziness, shakiness, nervousness, and judgment errors. Also, not eating anything or eating foods high in sugar and fat or cooked in grease can precipitate the effects of motion sickness. A good way to prevent the effects of motion sickness is to eat several small meals or to regularly snack on healthy foods during the shift. A lack of food in the stomach can cause nausea and exacerbate motion sickness.

All flight team members should be encouraged to maintain a healthy weight. Obesity can cause many problems in the flight environment and can be detrimental to the overall safety and performance of the overweight flight crew member. In addition, most rotor-wing flight programs have a weight limit for crew members.

Additional Stressors

In addition to the aforementioned stressors, several others may affect crew members' effectiveness during air medical transport. Age is an important factor: As the body ages, its ability to compensate for stress declines. Good physical conditioning is also important for flight crew members. Physical exertion during flight significantly lowers the altitude at which evolved gas disorders occur. Physical exertion increases oxygen demand, increasing the risk for hypoxia. Maintaining good physical conditioning can help to increase this threshold.

Hypoxia

Hypoxia is a major hazard in aviation that can have catastrophic results. This physiologic effect can occur in otherwise healthy people at altitudes less than 10,000 feet, but can greatly affect patients with impaired pulmonary function at much lower altitudes.

A common misconception in aviation is that a person can readily recognize the early signs of hypoxia and take immediate corrective actions. This misconception is dangerous and can be deadly. In fact, one of the earliest effects of hypoxia is impaired judgment. This impaired judgment can limit flight crew members' ability to recognize hypoxia and, consequently, their ability to take immediate corrective actions. Numerous aircraft crashes have documented aircrews responding to hypoxic events with inappropriate and dangerous actions. Also, early hypoxia mimics fatigue and hypoglycemia, making it difficult to recognize. Fatigue and hunger contribute to hypoxia as well.

Effective Performance Time and Time of Useful Consciousness

There is a limit to how long a person can function with an inadequate level of oxygen. This limited span of time is called effective performance

TABLE 4-3 Relationship Between Effective Performance Time and Altitude

Altitude (ft)	Effective Performance Time (Standard Ascent Rate)	Effective Performance Time (After Sudden Decompression)
18,000	20–30 min	10–15 min
22,000	8–10 min	5 min
25,000	4–6 min	1.5–3.5 min
35,000	30–60 s	15–30 s
43,000	9–12 s	5 s
> 50,000	9–12 s	5 s

Data from Federal Aviation Administration.

time **TABLE 4-3**. In contrast, the time of useful consciousness is the period between a person's sudden deprivation of oxygen at a given altitude and the onset of physical or mental impairment to the point that deliberate function is lost.

The times in Table 4-3 are based on experiments conducted with healthy military volunteers in a standard altitude chamber. The effective performance time and time of useful consciousness will vary for each person and depend on individual tolerances, the method of hypoxia induction, and the environment before hypoxia. Any exercise will reduce these times considerably. For example, on exposure to hypoxia at 25,000 feet, the average person has a time of useful consciousness of 3 to 5 minutes. The same person, after performing 10 deep knee bends, will have a time of useful consciousness in the range of 1 to 1.5 minutes. Also, an aircrew member who was breathing 100% oxygen before the onset of hypoxia will have a longer period of compensation than an aircrew member who was breathing ambient air.

Rapid cabin depressurization also dramatically affects the effective performance time and the time of useful consciousness. When aircraft cabin decompression occurs above 33,000 feet, oxygen flow in the alveoli is immediately reversed. A higher Pao_2 in the pulmonary capillaries occurs, causing the oxygen reserves in the blood to become depleted and reducing the effective performance time by as much as one-half. The time of useful consciousness varies from 5 minutes to 1 minute; however, if the crew is subjected to rapid depressurization, this period may last only a matter of seconds. A **rapid decompression** can reduce the time of useful consciousness by as much as 50% because of the forced exhalation of the lungs during decompression or during an extremely rapid ascent.

Another common misconception regarding hypoxia is that individuals living at higher altitudes do not require supplemental oxygen to function effectively at more extreme heights. In reality, although these individuals may have adapted to their environment to some extent, the physiologic changes in their bodies do not afford the level of protection that most assume. Living at higher altitudes causes the body to produce red blood cells at a faster rate, facilitating oxygen transport. A slight physiologic advantage exists; however, an aircrew member who, for example, lives at 5,000 feet may be able to fly 1,000 to 2,000 feet above the 10,000-feet recommended ceiling without ill effects, but this tolerance is not extended to an additional 5,000 feet.

Types of Hypoxia
Hypoxic Hypoxia

Hypoxic hypoxia (also referred to as altitude hypoxia) results from inadequate respiration or a reduction in Po_2 and is characterized by a lack of oxygen entering the blood **FIGURE 4-15**. Hypoxic hypoxia can have a variety of causes, including lung disease, right-to-left shunt in the heart, airway obstruction, a reduction in gas exchange area in the alveoli, and a low Po_2. Increased altitude also leads to hypoxic hypoxia.

In the air medical environment, personnel will most likely encounter this condition as a result of reduced atmospheric pressure that causes a reduced alveolar Pao_2. Simply put, there is not enough oxygen available in an inspired breath at higher altitudes owing to decreased Po_2. Clinical hypoxia actually starts to develop within a few hundred feet from the ground; however, symptoms do not begin to manifest until the aircraft reaches an altitude above 5,000 feet.

Histotoxic Hypoxia

Histotoxic hypoxia is caused by the cell's inability to adequately use oxygen because of substances in the blood such as narcotics, alcohol, chewing tobacco, and other poisons. In such a case, plenty of oxygen is available, but the tissues cannot accept it, or oxygen cannot offload from the hemoglobin **FIGURE 4-16**. During histotoxic hypoxia, the venous hemoglobin oxygen saturation is higher than normal because the oxygen is not being unloaded to the tissues, a situation that arises because the tissues are unable to metabolize the delivered oxygen. This type of hypoxia is the most frequently encountered by aircrew members in flight.

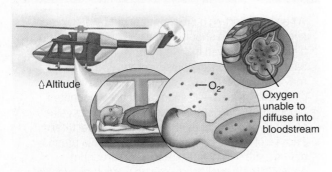

FIGURE 4-15 Hypoxic hypoxia results from a lack of oxygen or an inability of oxygen (O_2) to diffuse into the bloodstream.

© Jones & Bartlett Learning.

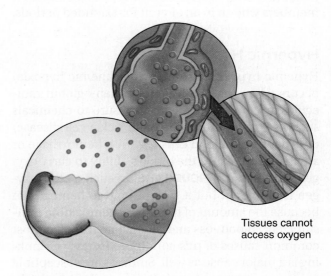

FIGURE 4-16 In histotoxic hypoxia, plenty of oxygen is available and can bind to the hemoglobin, but the tissues cannot access it.

© Jones & Bartlett Learning.

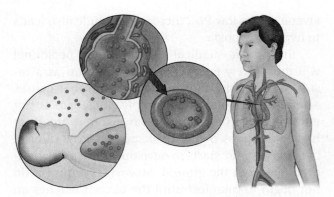

FIGURE 4-17 In stagnant hypoxia, there is a failure to transport oxygenated blood.

© Jones & Bartlett Learning.

Stagnant Hypoxia

Stagnant hypoxia occurs when there is failure to transport oxygenated blood. This form of hypoxia occurs when the flow of blood is reduced, but not necessarily completely stopped **FIGURE 4-17**. Outside of the aviation environment, this condition is frequently seen in patients with heart failure and major MIs. In flight medicine, stagnant hypoxia can result from venous pooling in the patient during accelerated maneuvers, such as steep turns and other maneuvers that increase the gravitational load on the aircraft. Another practical example is blood pooling in the lower extremities of patients and crew members who sit in an aircraft for extended periods.

Hypemic Hypoxia

Hypemic hypoxia (also known as anemic hypoxia) occurs when too few functional hemoglobin molecules are present (eg, with exposure to chemicals such as carbon monoxide or in sickle cell disease) or a lack of red blood cells (eg, with hemorrhage or anemia) diminishes the blood's ability to carry oxygen to the tissues **FIGURE 4-18**. In such a case, oxygen is abundant but it cannot bind to hemoglobin because the amount of functional hemoglobin is insufficient. Blood loss and anemia are the two most common causes of this condition. Excessive smoking is a major cause as well: Smokers are susceptible to hypoxia at lower altitudes compared to nonsmokers. The blood may be completely saturated with oxygen in hypemic hypoxia; however, it is insufficient to meet the metabolic demands of the body.

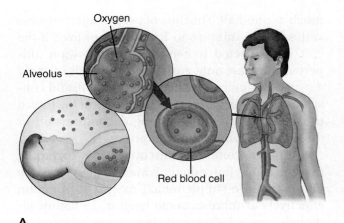

A

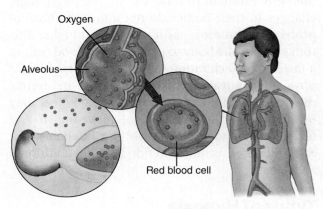

B

FIGURE 4-18 With hypemic hypoxia, the blood's ability to carry oxygen to the tissues is reduced. **A.** Impaired attachment of oxygen to hemoglobin. **B.** Reduced number of red blood cells.

© Jones & Bartlett Learning.

Special Populations

When transporting a pregnant patient by air, oxygen supplementation should always be provided at high altitudes. Even if a pregnant woman's oxygen saturation is 100% (by pulse oximetry), the fetus may still be compromised. The pregnant patient's circulatory system will shunt all richly oxygenated blood to her own vital organs, robbing the fetus and placenta of much-needed oxygen. A normal fetal Pao_2 level is approximately 45 mm Hg (in a pregnant patient with 90% to 100% Pao_2). If a pregnant patient's Pao_2 level decreases as a result of hypoxia, the oxygen status of the fetus can quickly become compromised, because the fetus has only limited reserves.

TABLE 4-4 Stages of Hypoxia

	Indifferent Stage	Compensatory Stage	Disturbance Stage	Critical Stage
Altitude (ft)	0–10,000	10,000–15,000	15,000–20,000	20,000–25,000
Oxygen saturation (%)	98–90	89–80	79–70	69–60
Symptoms	Decrease in night vision	Drowsiness Poor judgment Impaired coordination Impaired efficiency	Impaired flight control Impaired handwriting Impaired speech	Circulatory failure

© Jones & Bartlett Learning.

Four Stages of Hypoxia as They Relate to Altitude

The symptoms of hypoxia can be divided into four stages directly related to the altitude, approximate barometric pressure, and the oxygen saturation of the blood: the indifferent stage, the compensatory stage, the disturbance stage, and the critical stage **TABLE 4-4**. Symptoms of hypoxia are listed in **TABLE 4-5**.

Indifferent Stage

The indifferent stage is so named because of its minor physiologic effects on the body. This stage is typically experienced between sea level and 10,000 feet, but in some people it may manifest at altitudes as low as 5,000 feet. The mild hypoxia associated with the indifferent stage can cause night vision to deteriorate at altitudes above 5,000 feet. Recognizing this problem, the military requires fighter pilots to breathe oxygen from the ground up during night-flight operations. In addition, electrocardiographic changes have been known to occur at altitudes as low as 5,000 feet. Tachycardia is common in the indifferent stage, as is a slight increase in alveolar ventilation. Oxygen saturation in this stage varies from 98% to 87%.

Compensatory Stage

In the compensatory stage, the body is able to provide short-term physiologic compensation to counteract the effects of hypoxia. The extent of this compensation depends on the flight crew member's physical shape, physical activity level, and duration of exposure. In this stage, the respiratory rate and depth may increase and cardiac output increases. The compensatory stage is experienced between

TABLE 4-5 Symptoms of Hypoxia

Confusion/altered mental status
Fatigue
Headache
Changes in vision acuity • Tunnel vision • Blurred vision and/or inability to focus • Difficulty focusing from near to far • Loss of night vision
Euphoria
Tingling in the hands and feet
Feelings of air hunger
Tachypnea
Cyanosis of the skin
Irregular heart rhythms
Short-term memory loss
Decreased muscular coordination
Loss of hearing
Diminished sense of pain
Diminished sense of touch and feel
Difficulty speaking; stammering
Loss of self-criticism
Overconfidence
Overly aggressive behavior

© Jones & Bartlett Learning.

10,000 feet and 15,000 feet (between 39,000 feet and 42,000 feet if breathing 100% oxygen). Hemoglobin saturation in this stage varies from 87% to 80%.

Disturbance Stage

In the disturbance stage, which is experienced between 15,000 and 20,000 feet, the body's tissues can no longer depend on the physiologic compensatory mechanisms for sufficient oxygen supply. Hemoglobin saturation in this stage varies from 79% to 70%. This stage is characterized by subjective and objective symptoms of hypoxia. During altitude testing, some subjects did not experience the subjective symptoms before becoming unconscious from hypoxia. In the disturbance stage, the following aspects of body functioning can be affected by hypoxia: the respiratory system, senses, mental processes, manifestations of personality, and psychomotor functions.

Senses

Vision, hearing, and sense of touch are affected during the disturbance stage. Visual ability decreases as the eye muscles become weak and uncoordinated. Sensations of touch and pain become diminished and eventually are lost. Weakness and loss of muscular coordination are experienced and become worse with a greater degree of hypoxia. This loss of muscle coordination, in conjunction with confusion, quickly becomes a deadly combination.

Cognition

One of the most dangerous hallmarks of hypoxia is the early impairment of intellect that makes it impossible for people to comprehend their own disabilities. As the cerebrum becomes hypoxic, the victim loses the ability to make coherent judgments and calculations. Reaction time becomes slower, and short-term memory is severely impaired. All of these impairments prevent the person from recognizing the ongoing effects of hypoxia.

Personality Manifestations

Hypoxia can cause the emergence of symptoms similar to those a person may exhibit while under the influence of alcohol. These symptoms include the following:

- Aggressiveness
- Euphoria
- Irritability
- Overconfidence
- Depression

Psychomotor Functions

As hypoxia is induced, muscular coordination decreases. As hypoxia progresses, muscle coordination deteriorates to levels that are incompatible with coordinated activity. The first problems manifested are speech difficulty, illegible handwriting, and poor coordination in flying the aircraft. As the degree of hypoxia increases, delicate and fine muscular movements become impossible, and gross motor movements become significantly impaired. It is interesting to note that stammering and illegible handwriting are two of the hallmark signs of typical hypoxic impairment.

Critical Stage

The last stage of hypoxia, called the critical stage, occurs at 20,000 feet and above (44,800 feet and above with the use of 100% oxygen). Within 3 to 5 minutes of hypo-oxygenation, judgment and coordination deteriorate to the point of inadequate or inappropriate function. In this stage, mental confusion is quickly followed by incapacitation, unconsciousness, and death, if uncorrected. Hemoglobin saturation in the critical stage drops to less than 65%.

Hyperventilation Versus Hypoxia

Hyperventilation symptoms mimic those of hypoxia, so it is critical to first address the possibility of hypoxia before assuming that the problem is caused by hyperventilation. Hyperventilation and hypoxia result in confusion, poor judgment, and inappropriate corrective maneuvers.

Hyperventilation may be caused by the subconscious reaction to a stressful situation. This reaction is manifested by an abnormal increase in the volume of inspiratory and expiratory air and by tachypnea, which results in respiratory alkalosis as the carbon dioxide is blown off. This aberration in blood gases can have serious consequences. Normal control of respiration is mediated reflexively through the chemoreceptors in the aorta and the carotid artery by arterial oxygen deficiencies. In healthy people without a hypoxic drive, ventilation rate and depth are controlled by carbon dioxide and the acid–base balance of the blood circulating through the respiratory center in the medulla. Cellular activity, in turn, is dependent on proper acid–base balance. When the pH of the blood falls out of normal range, homeostasis is interrupted in the cell, and cellular activity quickly declines or stops.

Hyperventilation leads to several important physiologic changes that begin a cascade of events. As the minute volume (tidal volume × rate) increases, the partial pressure of carbon dioxide decreases, leading to an increase in the pH of the blood. The cerebral blood vessels respond to the decreased carbon dioxide pressure by demonstrating vasoconstriction, resulting in decreased cerebral perfusion. Unconsciousness quickly follows the induction of prolonged or significant hypoxia into cerebral tissues.

Hyperventilation can cause assorted symptoms, including the following:

- Light-headedness
- Feelings of suffocation
- Drowsiness
- Tingling in the extremities
- Painful muscle spasms
- Ataxia
- Disorientation
- Unconsciousness

One of the most disastrous effects of hyperventilation is that it produces panic in the person with this condition.

Recognition and Treatment of Altitude-Induced Hypoxia

The key to quickly recognizing altitude-induced hypoxia is a thorough knowledge base and understanding of basic flight physiology. As previously mentioned, many aviators have erroneously believed that they can recognize hypoxia as it is occurring and immediately correct the problem. To be sure, recovery from hypoxia is rapid when sufficient oxygen is supplied. People who are on the precipice of unconsciousness can regain their full mental abilities within 15 seconds after receiving high-flow oxygen. In fact, studies show that a hypoxic person who rapidly breathes in 100% oxygen may experience sudden dizziness, which is quickly resolved, followed by complete restoration of function.

Prevention is the key to treatment, and avoidance of hypoxia is the key to safety. If hypoxia is detected, the flight crew must immediately use supplemental oxygen and descend to an altitude below 10,000 feet. Hypoxia in crew members is a valid reason to declare an emergency with air-traffic control (ATC).

Supplemental Oxygen Requirements

Part 135.89 of 14 CFR governs the use of supplemental oxygen by pilots and provides rules for both pressurized and nonpressurized aircraft. In nonpressurized aircraft (including helicopters), at altitudes from 10,000 to 12,000 feet, each pilot must use oxygen continuously if the duration of flight at this altitude is longer than 30 minutes. Pilots must use oxygen at all times above 12,000 feet. In a pressurized aircraft when the cabin altitude exceeds 10,000 feet, the same rule applies. At altitudes from 25,000 to 35,000 feet, each pilot must use continuous oxygen unless the aircraft is equipped with an approved quick-donning–type mask. Pilots must wear an oxygen mask continuously above 35,000 feet. More stringent rules regarding oxygen use as altitude increases are mandated because of the dramatic decrease in time of useful consciousness as distance above sea level increases; above 35,000 feet, pilots will have mere seconds to respond to a sudden loss of cabin pressure.

Passengers must be provided with supplemental oxygen as well, in accordance with 14 CFR Part 91.211. At cabin altitudes above 15,000 feet, all occupants must be provided with supplemental oxygen. In a pressurized aircraft, a 10-minute supply of oxygen must be available for each occupant if the aircraft will operate above 25,000 feet. These rules for supplemental oxygen apply to crew and nonpatient passengers only: A sick or injured patient will likely need supplemental oxygen at all altitudes to prevent hypoxia.

Dysbarism and Evolved Gas Disorders

Several disorders are directly related to altitude. Barotrauma, for example, can result from gases expanding and contracting in the body, which causes pain, usually in the digestive tract, sinuses, teeth, middle ear, or lungs. Some illnesses, such as decompression sickness, are associated with symptoms that are not fully understood. Other illnesses, such as dysbarism, are directly related to the effects of altitude as described by the various gas laws. Dysbarism is a syndrome resulting from a difference between the barometric pressure and the pressure of gases within the body. As gases expand at altitude, they can cause pain in closed cavities.

Barotitis Media

Barotitis media affects the middle ear and is one of the most common trapped-gas problems. A flight team member who flies with a head cold can experience substantial pain. Barotitis media results from failure of the middle ear space to equalize pressures when going from low to high atmospheric pressure. In this situation, pressure in the middle ear becomes increasingly negative, and a partial vacuum is created. As the pressure increases, the tympanic membrane is depressed inward and becomes inflamed, and a petechial hemorrhage develops. Blood and tissue fluids are drawn into the middle ear cavity. The eardrum may rupture if the pressure does not equalize.

As the barometric pressure in the aircraft cabin decreases during ascent, the air trapped in the middle ear begins to expand, pushing the eustachian tube open **FIGURE 4-19**. Air escapes through the nasal passages, and the pressure is equalized. Normally, the eustachian tubes can be opened by swallowing, yawning, tensing the muscles in the throat, or pinching the nose and attempting to blow through the nostrils. On ascent, expanding trapped air usually escapes easily, with the eardrums equalizing the pressure, which is typically felt as popping in the ears. On descent, however, it becomes much more difficult for the negative pressure inside the middle ear to equalize. As the negative pressure continues to build, the affected individual experiences loss of hearing and pain. Any type of respiratory infection can make equalization in the eustachian tube difficult or impossible. If the eustachian tubes cannot equalize pressure on descent, profound pain may be felt, and hemorrhage may occur, indicating that the eardrum is about to burst or has already ruptured. To relieve the symptoms, the pilot should ascend until the pain is relieved and equalized, then take a very slow descent so the ears can slowly equalize.

Barosinusitis

Another risk to persons exposed to ambient pressure changes is barosinusitis, an inflammation of one or more of the paranasal sinuses resulting from a pressure gradient between the sinus cavity and atmosphere. Barosinusitis is relatively uncommon, generally affecting the frontal sinuses, and is not usually seen in children because the frontal sinus cavities are not fully mature until adolescence. Patients and providers with upper respiratory tract infections are at greater risk for barosinusitis because secretions associated with the infection tend to block the sinus ostia, interfering with pressure equalization.

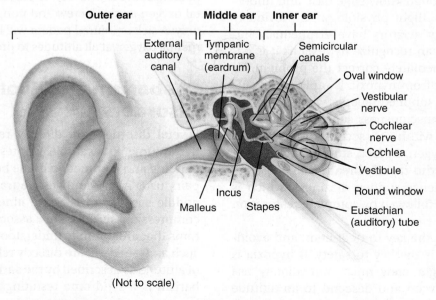

(Not to scale)

FIGURE 4-19 The inner ear, including the vestibular system. The otolith organs within the vestibular system are responsible for sensing equilibrium.

The clinical presentation of barosinusitis manifests during or very shortly after exposure to barometric pressure changes as unilateral sharp facial pain and headache. A pressure like sensation may be felt in the sinuses, and occasionally individuals exhibit epistaxis.

Treatment includes pain management and decongestants. Topical decongestants such as phenylephrine nasal spray or oral decongestants such as pseudoephedrine are effective. Antihistamines should be avoided, as they tend to dry the nasal mucosa and secretions, although if the underlying cause is poorly controlled allergies, antihistamines may have a preventive value.

Barodontalgia

Like barotitis media and barosinusitis, barodontalgia ("flyer's toothache") results from ambient pressure changes. The rarest of the three conditions, barodontalgia may be caused by gas bubbles trapped below the gums during restorative dental treatments, by periodontal cysts, or by abscesses. Symptoms include pain and pressure in or surrounding a tooth and usually resolve on return to sea level. Barodontalgia is most commonly seen among scuba divers and military pilots who experience extremely rapid changes in pressure. Most cases seem to be associated with dental disease and may be considered a symptom of such disease.

Decompression Sickness

Although decompression sickness is not the most frequently encountered dysbarism, it is the most widely recognized. Decompression sickness is explained by Henry's law: It occurs when inert nitrogen gas bubbles form at one or more locations in the body. The symptoms manifested depend on the location in the body in which the nitrogen bubbles form. This scenario is much more common in deep-water diving.

The tissues and fluid of the body typically contain approximately 1 to 1.5 L of dissolved nitrogen, depending on the barometric pressure of the atmosphere. As altitude decreases, nitrogen leaves the body in an attempt to reestablish equilibrium. Normally, the excess nitrogen diffuses into the capillaries in solution and is eliminated through the venous circulation. If a human body is subjected to a rapid decrease in atmospheric pressure, however, the capillaries become

TABLE 4-6 Symptoms of Decompression Sickness
Shortness of breath
Chest pain
Cough
Joint pain
Numbness and tingling of an arm or leg
Partial paralysis
Loss of speech
Loss of hearing
Vertigo
Visual disturbances (blind spots or the sensation of flashing or flickering lights)
Rashes
Itching of the skin

© Jones & Bartlett Learning.

supersaturated and nitrogen begins to leave as a gas instead of in a solution. In that case, nitrogen bubbles form in the tissue and blood. Fat is able to dissolve nitrogen five to six times more readily than blood can, so those tissues having the highest fat content are more likely to become saturated with nitrogen.

Decompression sickness can cause circulation problems and, in severe cases, even death because of the potential for nitrogen bubbles in the arterial circulation to cause an arterial gas embolism. Symptoms of decompression sickness are listed in **TABLE 4-6**.

Operational Issues Related to Medical Transport
Communications

The Commission on Accreditation of Medical Transport Services (CAMTS) is a program dedicated to ensuring high-quality patient care and safety within ground, rotor-wing, and fixed-wing medical transport services. CAMTS has established many communication standards to help improve the overall safety of most critical care transport systems. Much of its effort has focused on rotor-wing and fixed-wing divisions because proper communication procedures within the cockpit are important for ensuring the safety of both patients and crew.

Sterile cockpit is a term used by the pilot-in-command to describe the mode of operation during takeoffs, landings, and any other critical phase of flight. During this time, communication should be restricted to only what is necessary for the safety of the flight so as not to distract the pilot-in-command. Air carrier standards state that a sterile cockpit should be enforced at all altitudes less than 10,000 feet; however, most helicopters fly only between 2,000 and 5,000 feet. In such situations, the sterile cockpit times are determined by the pilot-in-command, but will always include takeoff, approach, and landing. Sterile cockpit times should be clearly defined by the pilot-in-command prior to flights. Once the rotor-wing aircraft has reached its cruising altitude and speed, the pilot-in-command will typically permit crew members to take part in casual conversation unless this interferes with other communications such as monitoring or discussing flight operations with ATC. Communications with operation centers and dispatchers should also be permitted during this phase of the flight process. The rule of thumb should be that communications to operation centers, such as those that give lift-off time and estimated time of arrival (ETA), should be relayed prior to lift-off, after the aircraft reaches its cruising altitude, or after the pilot declares a non-sterile cockpit.

Sterile cockpit procedures also apply to communications among the medical crew about patient care and communications with the patient. Most pilots have the option of "isolating" crews; that is, by flipping a switch in the cockpit, the pilot can take the crew out of the communication loop with ATC and ground units.

If, during flight, the pilot-in-command experiences a mechanical issue, it may be necessary to land short of the original destination. In most cases, when mechanical issues arise, the pilot-in-command seeks out the closest airport as a landing site. The crew should also be alert at all times for potential mechanical malfunctions such as smoke in the patient care area, abnormal odors, unusual vibrations not reported by the pilot, abnormal sounds, or fluids leaking into the patient bulkhead. Pilots may also choose to declare an emergency to ATC. This should immediately result in a sterile cockpit.

Instrument Flight Rules Versus Visual Flight Rules (Fixed-Wing and Rotor-Wing Operation)

In the aviation industry, all parties must be familiar with the two possible modes of flight: visual flight rules and instrument flight rules.

Visual flight rules (VFR) describe a mode of flight used when weather conditions are good, meaning there is generally good visibility and minimal cloud cover. A pilot can fly VFR in many areas without being in contact with ATC and is responsible for keeping the aircraft clear of clouds; however, in populated areas such as large cities, the pilot must be in contact with ATC even when flying VFR.

Instrument flight rules (IFR) describe a mode of flight used when minimum cloud clearance and visibility requirements cannot be met. During these conditions, the pilot may not be able to see outside the aircraft (eg, owing to clouds or fog) and must rely on the instruments inside the cockpit to maintain control and navigation of the aircraft **FIGURE 4-20**. A pilot flying IFR must receive an ATC clearance prior to takeoff and maintain contact with ATC during the flight, which will ensure the aircraft maintains the proper distance from other air traffic.

Initiating a Flight and Flight Following

A critical care transport is initiated when the communications center receives a request for service from an authorized agency such as local police, fire, emergency medical services (EMS), or a referring

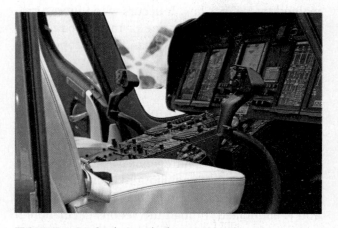

FIGURE 4-20 Cockpit with electronic instruments.
© Pavel L Photo and Video/Shutterstock.

hospital and then passes that request on to the flight team. The flight team then either accepts or declines the mission after reviewing the relevant factors, such as the weather, terrain, and nature of the patient's injury or illness. Some programs require that the pilot make the decision without any knowledge of the patient. This prevents pilots from being influenced by patient characteristics and taking on extra risk—for example, deciding to transport a pediatric patient when it is actually not safe to do so. Once the aircraft launches, the communications center and/or ATC remains in contact with the aircraft throughout the flight.

When a pilot is flying IFR, ATC is legally mandated to stay in contact with the aircraft to ensure it maintains a safe distance (ie, separation) from other IFR aircraft. When a pilot is flying VFR, a type of monitoring called **flight following**, or radar advisory service, may be provided by an authorized ATC facility **FIGURE 4-21**. This service consists of a controller notifying the aircraft about traffic in the area when the controller is available to do so.

When a pilot is flying VFR, it is good practice to maintain constant contact with other local traffic and ATC facilities in proximity of the aircraft. When a pilot is flying IFR, a filed flight plan, flight clearance, and ATC contact are mandatory.

When a pilot is flying VFR in a helicopter, contact is maintained with one of two entities: ATC and a communications center. If the pilot-in-command decides not to flight follow with ATC, the flight must be tracked by a communications center, either by a commercial flight-tracking system or by real-time radio contact with a communications center, with an update provided every 15 minutes.

Identifying Flight and Scene Locations

It is critical that the flight-following center use global positioning system (GPS) technology so that it can constantly track the aircraft's movement even when the pilot is not in radio contact with the center. Several commercial flight-tracking programs are available that use a GPS signal sent from the aircraft and received by the center. In the event of an in-flight emergency requiring an emergency landing, the center can use this signal to immediately determine the aircraft's last known position.

The flight-following center also needs to have computer software available that can allow for a physical address to be input and converted to GPS coordinates. In the rotor-wing environment, responders to the scene frequently use handheld GPS devices to obtain coordinates for the geographic location. These devices are extremely accurate: If the coordinates are properly read and relayed, they will lead the aircraft to within a few hundred yards of the scene. To prevent inaccuracies in the relayed coordinates, at least two sets of coordinates should be obtained for all scene flights.

Air Medical Safety

Air medical transport has inherent hazards but is rich with rewards. Providers working in this setting encounter a complex myriad of hazards. They are expected to launch quickly after a request has been made, placing stress on the flight crew to rapidly become airborne. Subsequently, their aircraft often lands at chaotic scenes where a hasty landing zone has been established and where a variety of emergency personnel are operating in close proximity to the landing zone. Air medical providers are also called to situations where patients are facing catastrophic injury or illness, requiring the flight crew to give maximum attention and apply expert decision-making abilities to treat the patient. Frequently the aircraft is called because the patient's condition is so serious that it has exceeded the capabilities of the medical

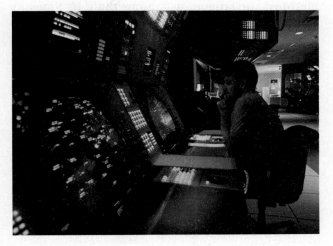

FIGURE 4-21 Flight following occurs when an air-traffic control center stays in contact with a pilot.
© Photodisc/Alamy Stock Photo.

personnel on the ground, putting additional stress on the aircrew. Finally, the aircraft environment is physically demanding and can induce heat illness, dehydration, motion sickness, and physical and mental exhaustion in air medical personnel after extended operations.

Air Medical Crashes

Annually, more than 1,000 helicopters are used to transport an estimated 400,000 patients in the United States. These numbers have been growing steadily since the inception of air medical flights, and as the total number of medical flights has increased, so has the total number of air medical crashes. From 1999 to 2018 in the United States, 206 EMS helicopter crashes occurred, representing about 10% of all helicopter crashes in that time. However, when analyzed according to crashes per 100,000 flight hours, rates have been declining in that time.

An unfortunate trend in EMS medical flight crashes continues to be the high fatality rates. Despite the overall improving safety of medical flights, when a crash occurs it has a far greater likelihood of being fatal when compared to non-EMS flights. From 1999 to 2018, in the United States, only 14% of non-EMS helicopter crashes involved at least one fatality, whereas 33% of EMS helicopter crashes involved a fatality. The primary factors in the higher fatality rates in the EMS crashes seem to be lack of a pilot with a first-class medical certificate and lack of a second pilot. Of note, per 100,000 hours flown, EMS flights have a much lower crash rate, at about 3% for EMS flights versus 6% for non-EMS flights. Further, the rate of fatal crashes does not differ between EMS and non-EMS flights. The concern lies in the disproportionate tendency of the EMS crash to be fatal.

Causes of Air Medical Crashes

The NTSB has found that aircraft crashes are rarely caused by a single event. Instead, they are the culmination of a series of factors that ultimately contribute to the final event. As FAA Advisory Circular Number 60-22 states, "One bad decision often leads to another. As the string of bad decisions grows, it reduces the number of subsequent alternatives for continued safe flight."

Because a crash may involve multiple factors, researchers attempt to cite all possible contributing or causal factors in each crash, which creates a complex picture in which certain factors appear with disproportionate frequency, although they may not in themselves have caused a crash. Any one of these factors may have prompted the next contributing factor to occur, which prompted the next, and so on, in what the NTSB terms "the accident chain."

When trying to appreciate the contributing factors most relevant to HEMS, a common approach is to compare EMS helicopter crashes to non-EMS helicopter crashes. The NTSB reports from 2008 to 2017 suggest that several factors are more likely to contribute to EMS crashes:

- Pilot incapacitation (10.54 times more likely in EMS crashes)
- Pilot inexperience (7.69 times more likely in EMS crashes)
- Visibility/darkness (5.18 times more likely in EMS crashes)
- Organizational compliance issues (4.91 times more likely in EMS crashes)
- Nonscheduled operations (4.55 times more likely in EMS crashes)
- Multiengine aircraft (3.76 times more likely in EMS crashes)
- Pilot decision-making or judgment issues (3.38 times more likely in EMS crashes)

Thus, pilot incapacitation, broadly defined as issues related to impairment, incapacitation, fitness, alertness, or fatigue, was more than 10 times as likely to factor into an EMS helicopter crash as it was a non-EMS crash.

When comparing EMS flights to non-EMS flights, it must be noted that EMS flights are much more likely to occur at night, with poor visibility being a significant risk factor. Other factors that complicate this comparison include the types of aircraft used, the types of equipment transported, and the inherent risks of on-scene responses.

When looking specifically at fatal EMS helicopter crashes from 2008 to 2017, the most common contributing factors, in order, were as follows:

- Pilot decision making
- Visibility or darkness
- Mechanical problems with the aircraft

- Pilot attention/orientation
- Organizational compliance
- Object/terrain encounter
- Pilot experience
- Pilot flight preparation

Two factors, pilot decision making and visibility, were associated with a much higher rate of fatality when compared to non-EMS helicopter crashes.

When assessing the role of weather in EMS helicopter crashes, the key issue is rarely the pilot's disregard for weather at takeoff, but rather encounters with unpredicted (inadvertent) **instrument meteorological conditions (IMC)**, such as cloudiness or low visibility, during flight. Weather is cited as a contributing factor in approximately 25% of crashes, but two-thirds of those crashes are fatal.

HEMS is an inherently dangerous form of aviation. Although risk can be mitigated in this setting, it can never be completely eliminated. Recognizing the factors that contribute to crashes is a key step in the ongoing effort to reduce risk. Specific safety initiatives are discussed later in this chapter.

Human Errors

Human factors contributing to error can be classified into three types: errors that involve skill deficiency, perception errors, and decision-making errors. Pilots and other members of the flight crew are expected to have the basic skills necessary to fly an aircraft safely. When there are deficiencies in these basic skills, a number of hazards can occur. Examples of these types of errors include losing control of the aircraft on the runway, flying at an improper speed, and not following standard operating procedures in the event of an emergency.

Errors in perception (discussed earlier in this chapter) involve spatial disorientation, a somatogravic illusion, or a mistake in judgment regarding distance, altitude, or airspeed. Spatial disorientation may occur during a flight that becomes out of control in midair. Errors in perception may also occur during nighttime landings and during landings that involve reduced visibility.

Errors in decision making may lead to an undesirable outcome as well. Decision-making errors include failing to choose the appropriate emergency procedure and failing to take corrective action when the aircraft is flying below the minimum altitude.

Areas Requiring Improvement

Retrospective studies of air medical crashes conducted by the NTSB, the FAA, and the **Air Medical Physician Association (AMPA)** have identified several areas within HEMS operations that need improvement:

- Weather forecasting
- Flight operations during instrument meteorological conditions
- Personnel training
- Design standards
- Crashworthiness
- Operations management

Other areas of HEMS operations identified as risk factors for air medical personnel include the following:

- Unprepared landing sites
- Complacency
- Additional stress of responding and caring for critical patients

Safety reports also indicate that communication problems with ATC and collision with ground objects are issues that warrant improvement.

Adding to the risk is the time-critical nature of the job. Because of the rapid preparation involved, crews do not have the luxury of conducting a leisurely preflight inspection of the aircraft, nor do they have plenty of time to check and recheck current and forecast weather reports. Instead, crews must move quickly to provide timely, life-saving care. Use of crew resource management has improved the decision-making process after receipt of a request. Most program policies have all flight crew members perform a quick walk-around the aircraft prior to initial startup. The rule of thumb is that three sets of eyes are better than one.

Making the Industry Safer

Within the industry, several solutions have been proposed to reduce the number of air medical crashes. Crew resource management training (discussed in the next section) for all flight team members is now the industry standard. All new flight team members are required to attend initial training, and most programs offer annual refresher training.

Another important safety measure is information sharing between competing agencies. In the air medical industry, the term helicopter shopping describes the practice of making sequential calls to numerous air medical providers in an attempt to find a service that will accept a mission request that has been declined by other services based on safety factors such as poor weather, limited landing zone availability, exceptional distances, or other factors. To prevent helicopter shopping, air medical providers should share their decisions to decline certain missions based on safety issues with surrounding air medical services, even if they are in direct competition with those services. Field providers, hospital personnel, and dispatch/referral centers may also shop for helicopters, and this dangerous referral pattern should be addressed and eliminated.

Air medical programs need full support from their organization's administration and the aircraft vendor when they choose to decline a mission. Some believe that stiff competition in the air medical industry prompts some services to take missions even when safety is in question. In the face of intense scrutiny of the air medical industry from the federal government, other oversight agencies, and the community, air medical services have implemented numerous guidelines to prevent flight crews from being pressured into taking questionable flights.

To facilitate cooperation among the various parties involved in the transport decision, joint agency training is encouraged between air medical providers and the various agencies with which they interact. Air medical providers should routinely train with other area HEMS programs, EMS agencies, fire departments, and hospital providers. This training should include aircraft familiarization, landing zone requirements, flight activation criteria, and flight request training.

Advanced technology that can increase the safety of flight operations is now available. Many HEMS programs use night vision goggles **FIGURE 4-22** on the aircraft. Unfortunately, implementation of this measure throughout the industry has been slow because of the cost of the equipment, required modifications to the aircraft cabin, and the need for extensive flight crew training.

Flight-tracking software is now used throughout the industry to assist with real-time tracking

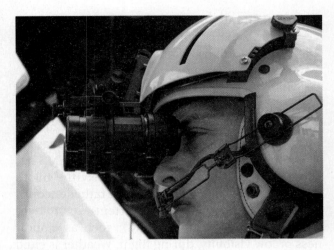

FIGURE 4-22 Night vision goggles.
Courtesy of Nivisys Industries, LLC.

of the aircraft at all times. The practice of flight following can help locate an aircraft that crashes or loses radio contact. Some air medical programs have also begun implementing ground-proximity warning systems and obstacle detection and alerting systems on their aircraft, also known as a terrain awareness and warning systems (TAWS).

Most rotor-wing aircraft do not have real-time weather data available in the aircraft. Instead, the pilot must rely on weather data obtained before launch as well as weather information given by the flight-following center. To provide for better in-progress forecasts, some aircraft now have weather display and alerting systems installed that can give pilots real-time weather data and warnings. Additionally, operational control centers (OCC) and flight dispatch and communications centers can monitor the weather and notify a pilot of changes in weather conditions.

Crew Resource Management

With the implementation of cockpit voice recorders and flight recorders in the 1960s and 1970s, investigators discovered that many crashes were not the result of mechanical or technical malfunctions of the aircraft or its systems, nor were they caused by poor piloting skills or lack of knowledge or experience from the crew. Instead, more than 80% of crashes involved human error—primarily related to the crew's inability to respond appropriately to the situations in which they found themselves.

Crew resource management evolved as a result of both that statistic and the KLM Royal Dutch Airlines/Pan American crash on Tenerife, Canary Islands, in 1977, in which two 747s collided on the runway. The deadliest crash in aviation history, this disaster was primarily attributable to unclear communication between the KLM pilot and the control tower regarding takeoff. The pilot understood that the aircraft was cleared for takeoff, but the control tower was only confirming position for takeoff, not actually clearing the flight for takeoff. The control tower made a clarifying statement, but the KLM pilot could not hear it because of interference. The Pan American aircraft was taxiing on the main runway when the KLM aircraft started to take off. The KLM flight engineer heard a transmission from the Pan American crew and asked the pilots if Pan American was clear of the runway; the KLM pilot assumed Pan American was clear and continued with takeoff. All KLM passengers and crew members died (248 total people) as well as most (335) of the 396 people on the Pan American flight.

In response to this crash and a series of alarming statistics, the National Aeronautics and Space Administration (NASA) held a workshop in 1979 focusing on ways to improve air safety. Before this workshop, the captain or pilot-in-command of the aircraft was considered to be the only person who was able to make decisions regarding the operations of the aircraft. The other crew members, including the first officer, had minimal input into the final decision that was made. The new procedure advocated as a means to overcome this reliance on only one person's judgment was called **crew resource management**, defined as "using all available resources—information, equipment, and people—to achieve safe and efficient flight operations." In air medical programs, this approach is often referred to as **air medical resource management (AMRM)**.

Crew resource management challenged the assumption that the pilot should make decisions alone. Flight crew members were encouraged to speak up when they did not agree with the pilot; pilots were encouraged to listen and take into account flight crew input. In short, the aviation industry learned to accept that human-to-human interactions are an integral part of any team performance.

Crew resource management is not concerned with the technical aspects of flying an aircraft. Instead, it focuses on the cognitive and interpersonal skills needed to successfully complete the flight:

- Cognitive skills take into account the mental processes needed to maintain situational awareness, make decisions, and solve problems.
- Interpersonal skills focus on individual and group behavior, communication, and teamwork.

Today, the **International Civil Aviation Organization (ICAO)** requires crew resource management for airlines in 185 countries. A study by the University of Texas Human Factors Research Project found that commercial airline flights experience an average of four threats per flight. Most of these threats or errors are caught through crew resource management and have no detrimental consequences.

Crew resource management allows for subordinate crew members to participate in the decision-making process, but it does not imply that all decisions are made by committee without considering rank. That is, the amount of participation by subordinate crew members depends on the situation. For the most part, your role as a medical crew member in crew resource management focuses on passive monitoring. You will not typically provide flight instructions to the pilot, nor will you be involved in technical decisions made in regard to operation of the aircraft. Instead, you are obligated to intervene if the level of skill displayed by the pilot falls below a safe standard (eg, if you notice that the aircraft is on an imminent collision course with a radio tower, or to advise the pilot of nearby air traffic).

One area of crew resource management in which all members of the crew should have equal empowerment is the decision of whether to accept a mission. In the past, it was often solely the pilot's decision to accept, decline, or abort a mission. More recently, this practice has been changed by the majority of air medical providers and replaced by the "all to go, one to say no" rule. Under this rule, every member of the crew, regardless of time or rank, has the power to decline a flight. Although the pilot does have the ultimate authority over all operations of the aircraft, if any crew member does not feel comfortable with a mission, the mission should be aborted.

Federal Aviation Administration Guidelines

All aircraft fall under one or both of the following guidelines set forth by the FAA:

- **Title 14 of the Code of Federal Regulations (14 CFR) Part 91** governs the operation of all aircraft within the United States, including the waters within 3 nautical miles (6 km) of the US coast. All aircraft must abide by this guideline. General aviation (private) aircraft operate under these less restrictive rules.
- **Title 14 of the Code of Federal Regulations (14 CFR) Part 135** governs the operations of all commuter or on-demand commercial operations. The guidelines for 14 CFR Part 135 operations are much stricter than those for 14 CFR Part 91 aircraft and apply to almost all air medical operators.

One of the significant differences between 14 CFR Part 91 and 14 CFR Part 135 is the minimum weather conditions in which the aircraft is allowed to operate. Under previous regulations, a pilot could potentially accept a mission under 14 CFR Part 91 weather requirements, fly to the scene, and then be under 14 CFR Part 135 weather requirements for the transport to the hospital. This discrepancy posed a major safety hazard, in that the aircraft would be allowed to launch under weather standards that were not conducive for patient transport with the hope that the weather would improve by the time the patient was loaded on the aircraft.

Only Part 135 is relevant to you as a CCTP: All commercial operators must abide by Part 135 regulations. Only a few government operators (such as law enforcement) can operate solely under Part 91.

Due to the high rate of accidents in air transport missions, air ambulance operations were placed on the NTSB's "Most Wanted Safety Improvements List" for 2014. In response to this and ongoing concerns, the FAA released updated rules aimed at increasing the safety of HEMS operations **TABLE 4-7**.

TABLE 4-7 FAA Helicopter Emergency Medical Services Regulations
Conduct all flights under Part 135 regulations when medical crew are on board
Install helicopter terrain awareness and warning systems (HTAWS) on all aircraft
Mandate that all pilots-in-command have instrument rating
Install a flight data monitoring system in all aircraft within 4 years (implemented as of 2018)
Utilize an FAA-approved preflight risk analysis tool
Increase VFR minimums for Part 135 operations
Permit IFR operations at airports without weather reporting systems
Establish guidelines for transitioning from IFR to VFR
Require life preservers to be worn by all crew members when conducting flights over water
Increase pilot training requirements for inadvertent instrument meteorological conditions
Require all aircraft to have a radio altimeter

Abbreviations: FAA, Federal Aviation Administration; IFR, instrument flight rules; VFR, visual flight rules

Data from Press Release— FAA Issues Final Rule to Improve Helicopter Safety. Federal Aviation Administration website. Published February 20, 2014. Accessed August 22, 2021.

Although not all of these rules were scheduled to take effect immediately, their implementation is intended to address the areas of greatest concern in air transport operations **TABLE 4-8**.

Weather-Related Issues

Weather has an obvious effect on the ability to accept and complete missions. Some mission requests result in a **weather decline**; that is, an air medical provider is requested, but the pilot and the flight team determine that the weather conditions do not meet established company or FAA guidelines for flight operations. In addition to visibility and ceilings, other considerations related to weather and flight include icing, thunderstorms, and high winds.

TABLE 4-8 Visual Flight Rules for Helicopter Emergency Medical Services: Ceiling and Flight Visibility Requirements

Location	Day		Night		Night (with NVIS or HTAWS)	
	Ceiling	Visibility[a]	Ceiling	Visibility	Ceiling	Visibility
Nonmountainous, local	800 ft	2 statute mi	1,000 ft	3 statute mi	800 ft	3 statute mi
Nonmountainous, nonlocal	800 ft	3 statute mi	1,000 ft	5 statute mi	1,000 ft	5 statute mi
Mountainous, local	800 ft	3 statute mi	1,500 ft	3 statute mi	1,000 ft	5 statute mi
Mountainous, nonlocal	1,000 ft	3 statute mi	1,500 ft	5 statute mi	1,000 ft	5 statute mi

[a]A statute mile equals 5,280 feet, or 1,760 yards (1.609 kilometers).

Abbreviations: HTAWS, helicopter terrain awareness and warning system; NVIS, night vision imaging system

Data from Federal Aviation Administration. Helicopter air ambulance, commercial helicopter, and Part 91 helicopter operations. Federal Register website. https://www.federalregister.gov/documents/2014/02/21/2014-03689/helicopter-air-ambulance-commercial-helicopter-and-part-91-helicopter-operations. Published February 21, 2014. Accessed August 22, 2021.

Crew Safety Precautions

CAMTS strongly emphasizes the need for adequate crew rest and ongoing safety precautions, both of which affect CCTPs and patients. The following are standards that CAMTS suggests for all CCTPs:

- Shifts longer than 24 hours are discouraged.
- Personnel should have at least 8 hours of rest before starting any shift longer than 12 hours.
- Personnel should not be on duty more than 16 hours within any 24-hour span.
- Crew members who must work longer than 16 hours must have the right to take an unscheduled break.

Other requirements have been adopted by CAMTS for pilots. Some CAMTS standards indicate that pilots must have the following qualifications:

- A minimum of 2,000 total flight time hours, with 1,500 of those hours in a helicopter
- 1,000 hours qualified as pilot-in-command time
- 200 hours of night flying
- A minimum of 500 hours of turbine time, with 1,000 hours encouraged
- 5 hours of geographic orientation with another pilot before accepting a mission alone

Summary

The air medical environment comprises a complex mix of aircraft operations and treatment of critically ill and injured patients. Medical crew personnel must have a strong knowledge base in both aircraft operations and critical care treatment. As a CCTP, you must have a thorough knowledge of flight physiology, not only for your patients, but also for yourself and your fellow flight team members. Even if you are ground based, you need to recognize the physiologic implications of flight because a large number of your patients will be prepared for flight or received from a flight. Because the majority of patients whom you will encounter have comorbid conditions or will have multiple traumatic injuries, the effects of altitude will be far more pronounced in these already vulnerable individuals.

The most important aspect of flight medicine is safety. The air medical environment is filled with risks, and providers must take every step possible to limit their exposure to danger. Many different agencies are actively working to reduce the risk of aircraft crashes, and flight team personnel are encouraged to become involved and aggressively work to make the industry safer. The air medical transport industry continues to grow, and flight team personnel must be ready to meet the myriad challenges they will inevitably face as air medical transport professionals.

Case Study

You and your partner are working for a small, rural air medical transport service located in southeastern West Virginia that operates an American Eurocopter H-135. The terrain to which you are accustomed is extremely mountainous, with elevations of more than 5,000 feet above sea level. Owing to the geographic layout of your service area, many of the flight legs are completed in mountainous terrain with limited signs of human population.

It is 1700 hours, and you are about halfway through your 24-hour shift when you are dispatched to a small community hospital 45 nautical miles (83 km) from your base. The requesting facility is asking your team to transport a patient via rotor-wing aircraft to a university hospital that is 2 hours away by ground and 25 minutes away by helicopter. Your pilot-in-command checks the local weather, and the decision is made to accept the flight. Once your pilot-in-command calls your operations center to confirm that the crew can accept the flight, you head to the aircraft and prepare for departure.

As soon as your aircraft reaches cruise altitude and speed, the communications center informs you that the patient is a 64-year-old man with respiratory failure caused by bilateral pneumonia and exacerbation of chronic obstructive pulmonary disease (COPD). The patient was admitted to the hospital 2 days ago with acute shortness of breath and required immediate ventilatory support, including endotracheal intubation. The patient's condition has been stable during the hospital stay, but the family is requesting transport to the university hospital for a second opinion. The patient is receiving a propofol infusion for sedation, normal saline, and ceftriaxone. The patient is being mechanically ventilated with the following ventilator settings: tidal volume, 750 mL; synchronized intermittent mandatory ventilation rate, 12 breaths/min; and F_{IO_2}, 70%.

When you reach the patient in the outlying hospital's intensive care unit, you are met by the staff nurse, who provides you with a more detailed patient report. During this report, the nurse tells you that the local pulmonologist has been weaning the patient's ventilator settings with the goal of extubation. You and the staff nurse review the results of the patient's laboratory studies, including blood gases. The most recent set of vital signs are as follows: blood pressure, 124/64 mm Hg; pulse rate, 84 beats/min; respiratory rate, 16 breaths/min (patient is breathing 4 breaths/min on his own); and pulse oximetry, 94%. The nurse tells you that a copy of the patient's chest radiograph and medical chart are in a folder for you to review and asks that you take them to the accepting hospital.

Once the patient assessment has been completed and the medications are transferred to your transport pumps, you secure the patient to your stretcher and prepare him for transport. You and your partner are concerned about his respiratory status owing to the bilateral pneumonia and are worried that he may not tolerate your transport ventilator as well as he did the hospital ventilator. You and your partner decide to perform a trial with the patient on your ventilator for at least 10 minutes before departing for your aircraft. The trial goes smoothly, and you proceed toward the aircraft.

During the initial phase of your flight to the university hospital, the patient remains adequately sedated and his vital signs remain unchanged. About 12 minutes into the flight, you notice that the patient's oxygen saturation readings are beginning to drop into the low 90% levels. After checking the patient and troubleshooting the ventilator and oxygen connections, you determine that ventilator settings are appropriate. You adjust the F_{IO_2} to 100%; within minutes of making this change, the pulse oximetry readings return to normal, at 99%. The remainder of the flight is unremarkable, and you give a full patient report to the nurse in the intensive care unit upon your arrival at the university hospital.

1. What is the most likely cause of the patient's hypoxia that arose during the flight?
2. Which type of changes would you expect to see, as a result of the barometric pressure

changes, with the IV solutions that you are infusing through the transport pump?

3. What are some common medical conditions that are typically worsened by altitude changes?

Analysis

It is important to first understand the critical state of a patient who has been diagnosed with bilateral pneumonia and has an underlying lung disease. Patients with these conditions often experience desaturation rather quickly with any change in position, altitude, or ventilator settings. In this particular case, flying at 6,000 feet above sea level over very mountainous terrain was required to get to the university hospital. In such situations, it is very important to understand Dalton's law, which states that the F_{IO_2} should be adjusted upward proportionate to the change in barometric pressure in the helicopter cabin. Because the barometric pressure in the hospital and the barometric pressure in the air are rarely available to CCTPs in advance, it is essential to recognize that increasing the F_{IO_2} en route may be necessary as altitude increases.

The second question asks which type of changes would be expected as a result of barometric changes when IV solutions are infused through the transport pump. The answer is none! As long as the infusions are being maintained on a pump, the barometric changes will not affect the flow rates. However, if the patient is receiving an infusion via gravity, the infusion rate will increase as the barometric pressure decreases, which occurs with increasing altitudes.

Pneumonia is one of the most common medical conditions that might require additional oxygen therapy to prevent worsening hypoxia. Other medical conditions that are adversely affected by altitude changes include COPD, asthma, coronary artery disease, pneumothorax, shock, and blood loss. Close attention should be given to patients with these conditions, and medical consultation should be obtained before departing the referring facility to discuss adaptive therapies that might be needed throughout the transport.

Prep Kit

Ready for Review

- As a CCTP, you must have a thorough understanding of flight physiology and its implications for both your patients and you. The medical environment during flight is complex and extremely dynamic, and the changes in barometric pressures and the forces experienced in flight can have a significant effect on disease pathophysiology.
- Critically ill or injured patients and those who would have a negative outcome with prolonged transport by ground units may benefit most from air medical transport.
- The earth's atmosphere contains several distinct layers. The first layer, called the troposphere, is located beneath the tropopause; together, these two layers constitute the lower atmosphere. Above the tropopause are the stratosphere, stratopause, mesosphere, and thermosphere, respectively. Critical care transports do not usually fly above the tropopause.
- The earth's atmosphere is divided into three distinct zones that directly correlate with a human's response to hypoxia. The physiologic zone extends from sea level to 10,000 feet; it contains the oxygen and has the barometric pressure needed for a healthy person to live. In the physiologically deficient zone (from 10,000 to 50,000 feet), the barometric pressure begins to decrease and protective equipment, supplemental oxygen, and pressurized aircraft are necessary. In the space equivalent zone

Prep Kit Continued

(from 50,000 feet to 120 miles), pressure suits and sealed cabins are required.

- Barometric pressure, also called atmospheric pressure, is a direct result of the weight of air. It is also influenced by air density, air temperature, height above the earth's surface, and weather.
- You need a thorough knowledge of several gas laws—Boyle's law, Charles's law, Dalton's law, Fick's law, Gay-Lussac's law, Graham's law, and Henry's law—that have integral roles in aviation medicine and flight physiology.
- Boyle's law states that as altitude increases, atmospheric pressure decreases, and the gases inside the body expand. Boyle's law also applies to the expansion of any trapped gas within the body (eg, in the chest, skull, middle ear, sinus, stomach, and intestines) and to situations characterized by increasing tension and pressure. Medical equipment and supplies can also be sensitive to changes in barometric pressure, including IV fluids, nasogastric and orogastric tubes, and colostomy bags.
- Charles's law states that the higher the altitude, the lower the pressure and the colder the temperature, which puts patients and crew members at risk for hypothermia.
- Dalton's law states that the total pressure of a gas mixture is the sum of the pressures of the individual gases in the mixture. At higher altitudes, oxygen molecules are less densely distributed; thus, at higher altitudes, the presence of an insufficient number of oxygen molecules can lead to hypoxia.
- Fick's law states that the rate of diffusion is affected by atmospheric pressures, the surface area, and the thickness of the membrane. This gas law governs the diffusion of oxygen across the alveolar membrane, and it means that patients with chronic obstructive pulmonary disease and pneumonia will have decreased gas exchange.
- Henry's law states that as the pressure of gas over a liquid decreases, the amount of gas

dissolved in the liquid will also decrease. Thus, as the barometric pressure decreases, nitrogen, which normally saturates the tissues in the body, will form gas bubbles that travel to the lungs.

- Gay-Lussac's law states that as pressure decreases, temperature decreases; thus it is important to keep patients warm.
- Graham's law states that if an existing permeable or semipermeable membrane separates regions of unequal pressure, the gas at higher pressure will diffuse through the membrane into the region of lower pressure.
- CCTPs need to be familiar with both rotor-wing (helicopter) and fixed-wing (airplane) operations.
- The four primary forces that act on all types of aircraft in flight are lift, thrust, weight (gravity), and drag, with lift counteracting gravity and thrust counteracting drag. In flight, thrust equals drag and lift equals weight. To take off, a greater amount of thrust and lift are needed, whereas a greater amount of drag and weight are required to land.
- Advantages of rotor-wing transport include vertical takeoff and landing (ability to access areas where other vehicles cannot) and ability to maneuver.
- Disadvantages of rotor-wing transport include weather limitations, interior space limitations, weight limitations, and cost.
- Advantages of fixed-wing transport include that it is generally safer than rotor-wing transport. In addition, fixed-wing aircraft are more often able to fly under instrument flight rules, to fly at high speeds, to travel great distances, and to carry multiple patients, and they have no weight limitations.
- Disadvantages of fixed-wing transport include the high cost of operating the aircraft, performing maintenance work, and maintaining a hangar for housing the aircraft.

Prep Kit Continued

- Pressurizing an aircraft, which is accomplished by increasing the barometric pressure inside the aircraft above the ambient pressure outside, is the most effective method of protecting people from the physiologic effects of reduced barometric pressure during flight.
- Aircraft decompression at altitude is categorized as either slow (eg, a small leak develops) or rapid (a dramatic event that occurs with a loud explosion). Decompression exposes the occupants of the aircraft to the dangers of hypoxia, decompression sickness, gastrointestinal expansion, and hypothermia.
- Flight crew members will experience many stressors during their career; however, some stressors may cause catastrophic outcomes.
- A decrease in the Po_2 can quickly cause hypoxia in flight crew members and passengers.
- The greatest change in barometric pressure occurs from sea level to 5,000 feet. Thus, problems associated with pressure may occur even in nonpressurized aircraft that are not flying at high altitudes at which supplemental oxygen or cabin pressurization is required.
- Flight crew members are subjected to a variety of extreme temperature changes as a result of changes in air temperature and altitude, as well as the greenhouse effect (radiant solar heat). These changes affect the metabolic rate and the oxygen demands on the body, while simultaneously making the body less tolerant of the effects of hypoxia.
- Vibration is noted in all helicopters, in most turboprop aircraft, and, minimally, in jet-engine aircraft. As the body becomes fatigued from prolonged exposure to vibration, the person becomes more susceptible to pain, decreased vision, and fatigue. Preventive measures to decrease vibration include not leaning against the airframe and providing extra padding for the patient.
- Humidity is the degree of moisture in the air and is relative to temperature. Humidity decreases during a long flight, and the dry air in the aircraft can cause cracked mucous membranes, chapped lips, and sore throats and lead to dehydration. To counteract these risks, crew members should increase their fluid intake, and all patients should be properly hydrated.
- Noise in the cabin of an aircraft can make it difficult for patients and care providers to communicate and for providers to assess patients' heart and lung sounds. Monitoring errors and malfunctions can be attributed to the noise and vibrations associated with air medical transport; however, pulse oximetry and hemodynamic monitoring can lessen these negative effects and help identify complications.
- Most physiologic problems encountered in the flight environment can cause significant fatigue and, when coupled with a lack of restful sleep, quickly become cumulative. Jet lag in the fixed-wing environment becomes another fatigue factor. While caring for critically ill or injured patients, you should request crew rest, up to 4 hours, when you feel fatigued.
- Gravitational forces can have a significant effect on the human body, including the feeling of being pushed down in the seat or feeling weightless, depending on whether the aircraft is accelerating or decelerating. As the gravitational force increases, other complications may arise, including difficulty breathing, hypoxia, loss of vision, loss of consciousness, petechiae, rashes, bruising, seizures, amnesia, confusion, and cardiac arrhythmias.
- Spatial disorientation is the state of having an incorrect understanding of the body's position in relation to the earth and can cause significant nausea and vomiting. The three components to maintaining spatial orientation on the ground are effective perception, integration, and interpretation of visual, vestibular (from the organs of equilibrium in the inner ear), and proprioceptive (from the

Prep Kit Continued

skin, muscles, tendons, and joints) sensory information.

- Third spacing is the loss of fluids from the intravascular space into the tissues, causing hypovolemia and potentially hypoxia. In the flight setting, it may result from high-speed turns in conjunction with acceleration or deceleration of the aircraft.
- Flicker vertigo is an imbalance in brain cell activity caused by exposure to low-frequency flickering or flashing or a relatively bright light that occurs when sunlight flickers through the rotor blades or propeller, at night by the anticollision lights reflecting off the clouds, or by rotating beacons or strobe lights. This condition may result in nausea, vomiting, seizures, or unconsciousness.
- Exposure to the noxious odors of fuel vapors occurs mostly when the flight crew is loading or unloading a patient; it can cause headaches and nausea if prolonged.
- Flight stressors include weather, anxiety, and night flying.
- Factors affecting tolerance of the stressors of flight can be remembered by the mnemonic IM SAFE, which stands for Illness, Medication, Stress, Alcohol, Fatigue, and Emotion. Other contributing factors, such as tobacco use and hypoglycemia, may also affect stress tolerance.
- Although incapacitation to altitude does not begin to manifest until 10,000 feet of physical altitude, the body may perceive itself as being at a much higher altitude, possibly thousands of feet higher, because of human factors.
- A major hazard in aviation is hypoxia (oxygen deprivation). Hypoxia mimics fatigue and hypoglycemia, making it difficult to recognize. In addition, one of the earliest effects of hypoxia is impaired judgment, which likewise limits an aviator's ability to recognize this condition.
- Effective performance time is the length of time a person can function with an inadequate level of oxygen. Time of useful consciousness

is the period between an individual's sudden deprivation of oxygen at a given altitude and the onset of physical or mental impairment to the point at which deliberate function is lost.

- Hypoxic hypoxia, which can be due to increased altitude, results from a lack of oxygen or an inability of oxygen to diffuse into the bloodstream. Its symptoms begin to manifest at heights greater than 5,000 feet.
- Histotoxic hypoxia arises when the cells are unable to adequately use oxygen, even though plenty of oxygen is available, because the tissues are not able to accept it or because the oxygen cannot detach itself from the hemoglobin.
- Stagnant hypoxia is the failure to transport oxygenated blood. In flight medicine, venous pooling during acceleration maneuvers can lead to a reduction of blood flow. Stagnant hypoxia can also result in blood pooling in the lower extremities of patients and crew members when they sit in aircraft for extended periods.
- Hypemic hypoxia, also known as anemic hypoxia, occurs when the blood's ability to carry oxygen to the tissues is reduced due to a lack of hemoglobin or red blood cells.
- The symptoms of hypoxia are divided into four stages—the indifferent, compensatory, disturbance, and critical stages—that are directly related to the altitude, approximate barometric pressure, and oxygen saturation of the blood.
- The indifferent stage is experienced between sea level and 10,000 feet but can occur at altitudes as low as 5,000 feet. At this stage, night vision begins to deteriorate; electrocardiographic changes, including tachycardia, are common; a slight increase in alveolar ventilation may be noted; and the oxygen saturation varies from 98% to 87%.
- In the compensatory stage, which occurs between 10,000 and 15,000 feet, the body is able to provide short-term physiologic

Prep Kit Continued

compensation against the effects of hypoxia, such that the respiratory rate and depth may increase and the cardiac output increases. At this stage, hemoglobin saturation varies from 87% to 80%.

- In the disturbance stage, which occurs between 15,000 and 20,000 feet, the physiologic compensatory mechanisms are no longer able to provide adequate oxygenation to the tissues. In turn, respiration, the senses, mental processes, personality manifestations, and psychomotor functions may all be affected. At this stage, hemoglobin saturation varies from 79% to 70%.
- The critical stage, occurring above 20,000 feet, is the last stage of hypoxia. Within 3 to 5 minutes of hypo-oxygenation, judgment and coordination deteriorate, and mental confusion is quickly followed by incapacitation, unconsciousness, and death, if the hypoxia is not corrected. At this stage, hemoglobin saturation is less than 65%.
- Recovery from hypoxia is rapid, and full mental abilities can be recovered within 15 seconds after receiving high-flow oxygen. Prevention and avoidance of hypoxia are key to safety, but if hypoxia is detected, immediate use of supplemental oxygen and descent to below 10,000 feet are necessary.
- Illnesses such as dysbarism (a condition that results from the difference between the barometric pressure and the pressure of gases within the body) are directly related to the effects of altitude as described by various gas laws. As gases expand at altitude, they can cause pain in closed cavities. Barotrauma can result from gases expanding and contracting in the body. This expansion causes pain, usually in the digestive tract, sinuses, teeth, middle ear, or lungs.
- Barotitis media results from the failure of the middle ear space to equalize pressures when going from low to high atmospheric pressure. As the pressure increases, the tympanic

membrane is depressed inward and becomes inflamed; petechial hemorrhage also develops. Blood and tissue fluids are then drawn into the middle ear cavity, and the eardrum may rupture if the pressure does not equalize.
- Although decompression sickness is not the most frequent dysbarism, it is the most commonly known.
- The Commission on Accreditation of Medical Transport Services (CAMTS) is a program dedicated to ensuring high-quality patient care and safety within ground, rotor-wing, and fixed-wing medical transport services. CAMTS has established many communication standards to help improve the overall safety of most critical care transport systems.
- The term "sterile cockpit" is used by the pilot-in-command to describe the mode of operation during takeoffs, landings, and any other critical phase of flight. During this time, communication should be restricted to only that necessary for the safety of the flight so as not to distract the pilot-in-command.
- Visual flight rules (VFR) are used when there is generally very good visibility and minimal cloud cover.
- Instrument flight rules (IFR) apply when adverse weather conditions exist, visibility is poor, or the cloud cover is low.
- An authorized air-traffic control (ATC) facility may provide flight following to aircraft flying VFR; in this process, the controller notifies the aircraft about traffic in the area.
- If a pilot flying VFR in a helicopter decides not to flight follow with ATC, real-time radio contact with a communications center must occur every 15 minutes.
- During fixed-wing operations, when a flight plan has not been filed, the pilot-in-command must make contact with ATC or a communications center every 30 minutes.
- Helicopter emergency medical services are consistently shown to be safer than non-EMS helicopter flights. However, the EMS

Prep Kit Continued

community must address a concerning reality: When an EMS helicopter crashes, the crash is more likely to be fatal.

- Aircraft crashes are never caused by a single event, but rather by a series of factors. Human error is the number one cause, and weather is the main contributing factor.
- Crew resource management was developed to address communication issues that resulted in fatal crashes.
- All members of the crew should have equal empowerment regarding whether to accept a mission. If any crew member does not feel comfortable with a mission, the mission should be aborted.
- Two Federal Aviation Administration guidelines apply to air medical operations: Title 14

CFR Part 91 and Title 14 CFR Part 135. The guidelines for 14 CFR Part 135 operations are much stricter than those for 14 CFR Part 91 aircraft and apply to almost all air medical operators.

- A weather decline occurs when an air medical provider refuses a mission because the weather does not meet established company or Federal Aviation Administration guidelines for flight operations.
- CAMTS publishes safety standards to which CCTPs and pilots should adhere. It strongly emphasizes the need for adequate crew rest and ongoing safety precautions, both of which affect CCTPs and patients.

Vital Vocabulary

Air Medical Physician Association (AMPA) An organization of physicians and air medical professionals that promotes safe patient transport.

air medical resource management (AMRM) The term used in air medical programs to denote the concept of crew resource management—an initiative designed to ensure all parties involved in an operation have decision-making input.

atmosphere Gases that extend from the earth's surface to space; composed primarily of nitrogen, oxygen, argon, and trace gases.

barodontalgia A condition caused by ambient pressure changes that may result from gas bubbles trapped below the gums during restorative dental treatments, from periodontal cysts or abscesses; previously referred to as flyer's toothache.

barometric pressure The weight per unit area of all the molecules of the gases above the point at which the measurement was taken.

barosinusitis An inflammation of one or more of the paranasal sinuses resulting from a

pressure gradient between the sinus cavity and atmosphere.

barotitis media Inflammation and possible petechial hemorrhage in the middle ear and possible rupture of the eardrum that results from the failure of the middle ear space to ventilate when going from low to high atmospheric pressure; also known as ear block.

Boyle's law A gas law stating that the volume of a gas is inversely proportional to the pressure to which it is subjected. Gases trapped in body cavities will expand with increases in altitude and will contract with decreases in altitude.

Charles's law A gas law stating that when pressure is constant, the volume of a gas is very nearly proportional to its absolute temperature. Thus, the volume is directly proportional to the temperature when it is expressed on an absolute scale where all other factors remain constant.

Commission on Accreditation of Medical Transport Services (CAMTS) An organization dedicated to improving the quality of patient care and safety of the transport environment for both

Prep Kit Continued

rotor-wing and fixed-wing providers. CAMTS also provides voluntary accreditation of critical care transport agencies.

compensatory stage A stage of hypoxia in which the physiologic adjustments that occur in the respiratory and circulatory systems are adequate to prevent the effects of hypoxia. Factors such as environmental stress and prolonged exercise can potentiate certain effects of hypoxia.

crew resource management A system that originated as the result of a National Aeronautics and Space Administration workshop in 1979 as a means to improve air safety. It incorporates equipment, procedures, and crew concerns to make the best decision during flight operations, focusing on interpersonal communication, leadership, and decision making.

critical stage The stage of acute hypoxia in which there is almost complete mental and physical incapacitation, resulting in rapid loss of consciousness, seizures, respiratory arrest, and death.

Dalton's law A gas law stating that the total pressure of a gas mixture is the sum of the individual or partial pressures of the gases in the mixture; also referred to as the law of partial pressure.

decompression sickness A condition resulting from exposure to low barometric pressure, causing inert gases normally dissolved in body fluids and tissue to come out of physical solution and form bubbles.

disturbance stage A stage of hypoxia in which physiologic responses are inadequate to compensate for the oxygen deficiency, and hypoxia is evident.

drag The resistance of an aircraft to forward motion, directly opposed to thrust.

dysbarism A condition resulting from the effects (excluding hypoxia) of a pressure differential between the ambient barometric pressure and the pressure of gases within the body.

effective performance time The amount of time an individual is able to perform useful duties in an environment of inadequate oxygen; also known as expected performance time.

Federal Aviation Administration (FAA) A US governmental agency within the Department of Transportation that regulates and oversees civil aviation within the United States; it established and enforces the Title 14 CFR that govern aircraft operation within the United States.

Fick's law A gas law stating that the net diffusion rate of a gas across a fluid membrane is proportional to the difference in partial pressure, proportional to the area of the membrane, and inversely proportional to the thickness of the membrane.

flicker vertigo An imbalance in brain cell activity caused by exposure to low-frequency flickering or flashing light. Light flickering from 4 to 20 times per second can precipitate reactions including nausea, migraines, unconsciousness, and seizures.

flight following A service in which an authorized air-traffic control facility maintains constant contact with aircraft to notify the crew about traffic in the area.

flight surgeon A physician who specializes in flight medicine and has been trained extensively in various aspects of aviation and the effects of flight on the human body; also specializes in working with pilots and flight crew members.

Gay-Lussac's law A gas law stating that the pressure of a gas when volume is maintained at a constant level is directly proportional to the absolute temperature for a constant amount of gas. Simply stated, as pressure increases, temperature increases.

Graham's law A gas law stating that the rate at which gases diffuse is related inversely to the square root of their densities.

gravitational forces Force changes that occur with acceleration and deceleration.

Prep Kit Continued

helicopter emergency medical service (HEMS) Use of a rotor-wing aircraft to deliver air medical service, for which the goals are to rapidly transport CCTPs to a patient, stabilize the patient's condition, and rapidly transport that patient to a tertiary care center.

helicopter shopping The practice of making sequential calls to numerous air medical providers in an attempt to find a service that will accept a mission request that has been declined by other services based on safety factors such as poor weather, limited landing zone availability, exceptional distances, or other factors.

Henry's law A gas law stating that the amount of gas dissolved in solution is directly proportional to the pressure of the gas over the solution.

histotoxic hypoxia Hypoxia caused by the inability of the tissues to use oxygen, usually as a result of poisoning by toxins such as carbon monoxide and cyanide.

humidity The degree of moisture in the air, expressed as a percentage.

hypemic hypoxia Hypoxia caused by a decrease in the blood's oxygen-carrying capacity due to a reduced amount of hemoglobin in the blood or a reduced number of red blood cells; also known as anemic hypoxia.

hypoxia A state of oxygen deficiency in the body, which is sufficient to cause an impairment of function. Hypoxia is caused by a reduction in the partial pressure of oxygen, inadequate oxygen transport, or an inability of the tissues to use oxygen.

hypoxic hypoxia Hypoxia caused by a decrease in the amount of oxygen in the blood due to a reduction in oxygen pressure in the lungs, a reduced gas exchange area, exposure to high altitude, or lung disease.

indifferent stage The stage of altitude hypoxia in which the body is able to compensate for the hypoxia induced by low barometric pressures.

instrument flight rules (IFR) A mode of flight used when adverse weather conditions exist, visibility is poor, or cloud cover is low. The pilot may not be able to see outside the aircraft, must rely on instruments, and must be in constant contact with an air-traffic controller who assists in maintaining proper separation from other air traffic.

instrument meteorological conditions (IMC) Weather conditions (eg, cloudiness or low visibility) in which a pilot must fly under instrument flight rules, depending on instruments to guide the aircraft.

International Civil Aviation Organization (ICAO) An agency of the United Nations that defines standards for international air navigation and, as part of its role in developing safe practices, requires crew resource management.

lift The upward force created by the wings moving through the air, which sustains the aircraft in flight.

National Transportation Safety Board (NTSB) An independent federal agency that promotes transportation safety, including aviation, railroad, highway, maritime, pipeline, and hazardous materials safety; it investigates transportation crashes to identify the cause and make safety recommendations.

partial pressure of oxygen (arterial) (Pao_2) The amount of the total pressure in the blood contributed by oxygen; a value measured when analyzing the arterial blood gas level.

physiologically deficient zone The zone that extends from 10,000 to 50,000 feet. Noticeable physiologic deficits occur above 10,000 feet. A decrease in barometric pressure results in oxygen deficiency, causing hypoxic hypoxia; the manifestation of trapped and evolved gases then occurs. The use of pressurized aircraft and/or supplemental oxygen is necessary in this zone.

physiologic zone The atmospheric zone that extends from sea level to 10,000 feet; the area of the atmosphere to which humans are well adapted. The barometric pressure is sufficient in this zone to facilitate adequate oxygenation. The changes in pressure encountered with rapid ascents or descents within this zone can produce ear or sinus trapped-gas problems.

pneumocephalus A condition in which air or gas accumulates within the cranial cavity.

pneumomediastinum The collection of air within the mediastinum (the space within the chest that contains the heart, major blood vessels, vagus nerve, trachea, and esophagus; located between the two lungs).

pneumoperitoneum The collection of air within the peritoneum (the membrane in the abdomen encasing the liver, spleen, diaphragm, stomach, and transverse colon).

proprioceptive Referring to information that comes from receptors located in the skin, muscles, tendons, and joints; this information helps a person know the position of their body.

rapid decompression A condition that occurs when a large leak or hole develops in a pressurized aircraft; it can result in hypoxia and injury to people inside the aircraft and catastrophic failure of the aircraft.

somatogravic illusion An error in perception that occurs with acceleration, as the otolith organs are displaced rearward, similar to when a person is looking up. This perception of a nose-up altitude may cause the pilot to push the nose of the aircraft down inappropriately at night or in unlit terrain.

space equivalent zone The atmospheric zone that begins at 50,000 feet. In this zone, 100% oxygen is not sufficient to prevent hypoxia without the use of a pressurized aircraft or suit. Unprotected personnel may experience boiling of body fluids at a level above 66,500 feet.

spatial disorientation An error in perception that may result from a person's inability to determine their position, altitude, and motion in relation to the surface of the earth or to a significant fixed object during flight.

stagnant hypoxia Hypoxia caused by a malfunction of the circulatory system resulting in a decrease in blood flow.

sterile cockpit The time when unnecessary communication that could distract the pilot is banned in the cockpit—usually during takeoffs, landings, and any other critical phase of flight at the discretion of the pilot-in-command.

third spacing A loss of fluids from the intravascular space into the tissues caused by an increase in intravascular pressures and/or increased permeability of the cell membranes. Physical stressors of flight such as temperature, vibration, and changes in gravitational force can cause or aggravate this condition.

thrust The force exerted by the aircraft engine, which pushes air backward with the objective of causing a reaction of the aircraft in the forward direction.

time of useful consciousness The time between a person's sudden deprivation of oxygen at a given altitude to the point at which deliberate function is lost. With the loss of effective performance during flight, a person is no longer capable of taking proper corrective or protective actions.

Title 14 of the Code of Federal Regulations (14 CFR) Part 91 A guideline established by the Federal Aviation Administration that governs the operation of all aircraft within the United States, including the waters within 3 nautical miles (6 km) of the US coast.

Title 14 of the Code of Federal Regulations (14 CFR) Part 135 A guideline established by the Federal Aviation Administration that governs the operations of all commuter or on-demand commercial operations.

tropopause The space between the troposphere and the stratosphere. It rises to 60,000 feet at the equator owing to the expansion of heated air masses and sinks to about 30,000 feet at the poles owing to contracting cold air masses.

troposphere A portion of the earth's atmosphere that extends from the surface of the earth to 5 to 10 miles (26,000 to 52,000 feet) high depending on the relation to the equator and the poles.

Prep Kit Continued

This layer is characterized by the presence of water vapors, a constant decrease in temperature with increasing altitude, and large-scale vertical currents.

Type I spatial disorientation A loss of positional awareness in which the pilot is unaware of becoming disoriented.

Type II spatial disorientation A loss of positional awareness in which the pilot is initially unaware of spatial disorientation, but senses that something is wrong.

Type III spatial disorientation A sudden incapacitating form of loss of positional awareness.

vestibular Related to the organs of equilibrium located in the inner ear.

visual flight rules (VFR) A mode of flight used when weather conditions are good, meaning there is generally very good visibility and minimal cloud cover; the pilot is responsible for maintaining separation from other aircraft.

weather decline A situation in which an air medical provider is requested, but the pilot and the flight team determine that the weather does not meet established Federal Aviation Administration guidelines and therefore decline to make the flight.

weight The downward force due to the weight (gravity) of the aircraft and its load; directly opposed to lift.

References

A history of helicopter emergency medical services. Airbus website. https://www.airbus.com/newsroom/stories /history-helicopter-hems.html. Published December 2020. Accessed August 22, 2021.

Baker SP, Grabowski JG, Dodd RS, et al. EMS helicopter crashes: what influences fatal outcome? *Ann Emerg Med.* 2006;47:351-356.

Baxt WG, Moody P. The impact of rotorcraft aeromedical emergency care service on trauma mortality. *JAMA.* 1983;249:3047-3051.

Baxt WG, Moody P, Cleveland HC, et al. Hospital-based rotorcraft aeromedical emergency care services and trauma mortality: a multicenter study. *Ann Emerg Med.* 1985;14:859-864.

Beckman IN, Syrtsova DA, Shalygin MG, Kandasamy P, Teplyakov VV. Transmembrane gas transfer: mathematics of diffusion and experimental practice. *J Membrane Sci.* 2020;601. https://doi.org/10.1016/j.memsci.2019.117737.

Benson NH, Hunt RC, Tolson J, Stone CK, Sousa JA, Nimmo NJ. Improved flight following through continuous quality improvement. *Air Med J.* 1994;13:163-165.

Better Hearing Institute. *Your Guide to Better Hearing.* Washington, DC: Better Hearing Institute; 1998.

Blumen IJ. *Principles and Direction of Air Medical Transport: Advancing Air and Ground Critical Care Transport Medicine.* 2nd ed. Salt Lake City, UT: Air Medical Physician Association; 2015.

Blumen IJ, UCAN Safety Committee. *A Safety Review and Risk Assessment in Air Medical Transport: Supplement to the Air Medical Physician Handbook.* Salt Lake City, UT: Air Medical Physicians Association; November 2002.

Bolen RL Jr. Flight physiology. *Duke LifeNet.* 2004;12(2):4-5.

Boyd DR, Cowley RA. Comprehensive regional trauma/ emergency medical services (EMS) delivery systems: the United States experience. *World J Surg.* 1983;7:149-157.

Branas CC, MacKenzie EJ, Williams JC, et al. Access to trauma centers in the United States. *JAMA.* 2005;293(21):2626-2633.

Code of Federal Regulations: Section 61.65. Federal Aviation Administration website. https://rgl.faa.gov/Regulatory_and _Guidance_Library/rgFar.nsf/FARSBySectLookup/61.65. Published April 12, 2016. Accessed August 19, 2021.

Collett H. Air medical helicopter transport. *Hosp Aviat.* 1998;7(7):5-7.

Cowley RA. Trauma center: a new concept for the delivery of critical care. *J Med Soc NJ.* 1977;74:979-987.

Disorientation. South African Civil Aviation Authority website. http://www.caa.co.za/Aviation%20Medicine%20 General%20Information/Disorientation.pdf. Accessed August 21, 2021.

Dodd RS. The cost-effectiveness of air medical helicopter crash survival enhancements: an evaluation of the costs, benefits and effectiveness of injury prevention interventions. *Air Med J.* 1994;13:281-293.

Eavis P. Air ambulances offer a lifeline, and then a sky-high bill. *New York Times* website. https://www.nytimes.com /2015/05/06/business/rescued-by-an-air-ambulance-but -stunned-at-the-sky-high-bill.html. Published May 5, 2015. Accessed August 21, 2021.

Electronic Code of Federal Regulations. https://www.ecfr.gov /cgi-bin/text-idx?tpl=/ecfrbrowse/Title14/14cfr135 _main_02.tpl. Accessed August 21, 2021.

Prep Kit Continued

FAA delays effective date for new air ambulance rule. Vertical Mag website. https://verticalmag.com/news/faadelays effectivedatefornewairambulancerule/. Accessed August 21, 2021.

FAA regulations. Federal Aviation Administration website. https://www.faa.gov/regulations_policies/faa_regulations/. Modified February 19, 2020. Accessed August 22, 2021.

Federal Aviation Administration. Helicopter air ambulance, commercial helicopter, and Part 91 helicopter operations; final rule. http://www.gpo.gov/fdsys/pkg/FR-2014-02-21/pdf/2014-03689.pdf. US Government Publishing Office website. Published February 21, 2014. Accessed August 21, 2021.

Green N, Gaydos S, Ewan H, Nicol E, eds. *Handbook of Aviation and Space Medicine*. Boca Raton, FL: CRC Press; 2019:35-41.

Greenhaw R, Jamali M. Medical helicopter accident review: causes and contributing factors. Federal Aviation Administration website. https://www.faa.gov/data_research/research/med_humanfacs/oamtechreports/2020s/media/202119.pdf. Published May 2021. Accessed August 22, 2021.

Holleran RS, Wolfe AC, Frakes MA, eds; Air and Surface Transport Nurses Association. *ASTNA Patient Transport: Principles and Practice*. 5th ed. New York, NY: Mosby; 2017.

Huber M. HEMS industry getting safer. Aviation International News website. https://www.ainonline.com/aviation-news/business-aviation/2016-12-22/hems-industry-getting-safer. Published December 22, 2016. Accessed August 30, 2021.

Making air travel safer through crew resource management. American Psychological Association website. http://www.apa.org/research/action/crew.aspx. Accessed August 21, 2021.

Mark R. NTSB adds helicopter ops to most wanted list. https://www.ainonline.com/aviation-news/2014-01-27/ntsb-adds-helicopter-ops-most-wanted-list. American International News website. Published January 27, 2014. Accessed August 21, 2021.

Military Assistance to Safety and Traffic. *Report of Test Program by the Interagency Study Group*. DHEW publication HSM-72-7000. Washington, DC: Department of Health, Education, and Welfare; 1970.

Occupational Safety and Health Administration. Commercial diving. US Department of Health website. https://www.osha.gov/commercial-diving. Accessed August 21, 2021.

Qureshi SM, Mustafa R. Measurement of respiratory function: gas exchange and its clinical applications. *Anaesthes Intens Care Med*. 2018;19(2):65-71.

Rash CE. Awareness of causes and symptoms of flicker vertigo can limit ill effects. Flight Safety Foundation website. https://flightsafety.org/hf/hf_mar-apr04.pdf. Published 2004. Accessed August 21, 2021.

Reinhart RO. *Basic Flight Physiology*. 3rd ed. New York, NY: McGraw-Hill Education; 2007.

Transport Canada Civil Aviation. *Handbook for Civilian Aviation Medical Examiners—TP 13312*. Government of Canada website. https://tc.canada.ca/en/aviation/publications/handbook-civil-aviation-medical-examiners-tp-13312. Accessed August 21, 2021.

Wynbrandt J. Spatial disorientation: confusion that kills. *Safety Advisor*. AOPA Foundation website. https://www.aopa.org/-/media/Files/AOPA/Home/Pilot-Resources/ASI/Safety-Advisors/sa17.pdf. Accessed August 21, 2021.

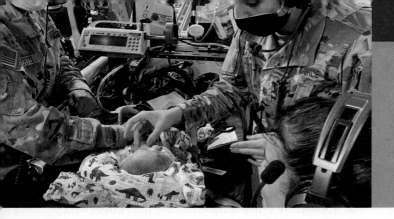

Chapter 5

Patient Assessment

Kevin Collopy, MHL, NRP

Vahé Ender, NRP, FP-C, C-NPT

OBJECTIVES

After completing this chapter, you will be able to:

1. Discuss the unique aspects of patient assessment as they relate to scene calls and interfacility transports, and modifications to assessments based on the individual transport setting (p 122).

2. Discuss the importance of critical thinking to clinical decision making and differential diagnosis (p 122).

3. Explain the necessity for the critical care transport professional to utilize physical and technological assessment findings to develop a clear clinical picture (p 122).

4. Identify similarities and differences in assessment as they relate to scene calls and interfacility transport (pp 122–125).

5. Explain the importance of reviewing all available information from the sending facility, including any available patient care records (pp 125–127).

6. Explain the assessment process used to establish the initial care plan, make appropriate treatment decisions, and assess the effects of treatments (pp 125–127).

7. Describe the SAMPLE approach used to determine the patient's history (pp 127–128).

8. Describe the ABCDE approach used to guide the primary assessment to evaluate organ systems and anatomy fundamentally necessary for life (p 129).

9. Describe the various elements of the primary assessment, including the following:
   - Airway assessment (pp 129–131)
   - Respiratory assessment (pp 131–132)
   - Circulatory assessment (pp 132–134)
   - Gastrointestinal assessment (pp 134–135)
   - Genitourinary assessment (p 135)
   - Assessment of bleeding control (p 134)
   - Neurologic assessment (pp 135–137)

10. Explain the importance of and safety considerations relating to patient exposure during the primary assessment (pp 139–141).

11. Describe the process of conducting a secondary assessment (p 141).

12. Discuss the inherent instability of the transport environment, and the potential need to adjust infusion settings, ventilator settings, and pain relief and/or sedation as the patient's condition demands (p 141).

13. Describe unique stabilization, packaging, and transport considerations for technology-dependent patients (pp 139–141).

14. Explain the importance of continuous assessment during transport, especially for technology-dependent patients (pp 144–147).

15. Discuss the elements of the patient handoff report necessary to assure continuity of care at the transport destination (p 147).

Introduction

A comprehensive patient assessment is one of the most important skills critical care transport professionals (CCTPs) perform. The assessment builds the foundation for the CCTP's treatment plan and helps guide which interventions may be performed before and during transport. Assessment of critical care patients differs from the traditional emergency medical services (EMS) field assessment in two respects: Critical care patients have often received significant treatment and stabilization prior to the CCTP's arrival, and sophisticated diagnostic information is often available. While this information provides invaluable insights into the patient's condition, prior assessments may not reflect the patient's current status; hence it is vital to confirm the information relayed to you and to conduct your own comprehensive assessment. Patients change over time, and your assessment may reveal new information related to the patient's condition.

While the assessment findings may be no different in a hospital intensive care unit (ICU) than in a wrecked car, patient acuity in the critical care transport (CCT) environment will generally be far higher. Critical care patients are also likely to be attached to invasive equipment. All equipment, from an intravenous (IV) line to an intraventricular drain, must be evaluated as a component of the patient assessment. CCTPs may also have the opportunity to integrate advanced technology, such as ultrasonography, into the assessment process, when these modalities were not available or employed prior to arrival. This equipment provides additional diagnostic information and helps develop a more comprehensive clinical picture. CCTPs must then employ critical-thinking skills to incorporate the information gained from these advanced assessments into problem lists and care plans.

Scene Versus Interfacility Transports

Scene Responses

While CCTPs do not primarily respond to prehospital scenes, operating in this environment does remain within their scope of practice. Critical care flight teams often complete scene flights, and many EMS systems use CCTPs in a dual role, assigning the CCTP to either 9-1-1 responses or high-acuity interfacility transports. CCTPs responding to an emergency scene ideally should be authorized to use their critical care equipment and medications, as appropriate. While the approach to such scenes is not significantly different than that employed in any other prehospital scene, the CCTP must realize that the patient may have received significant advanced life support (ALS) care by ground EMS crews prior to the CCTP's arrival. Moreover, the CCTP may not have the opportunity to survey the scene and the mechanism of injury directly, or have the opportunity to interview family members. Effective communication is paramount to a seamless and rapid transfer of care. Information can be lost during the transfer of care if clinicians are not diligent about asking questions and actively listening to answers.

On scene, the CCTP should query the first responders as to the exact nature of the patient's illness and/or mechanism of injury, assessment findings, interventions performed, and the patient's response to those interventions. Trust this information but verify it as much as you can through your own patient assessment. Prehospital scenes, by their very nature, are less controlled than a hospital emergency department (ED) or intensive care unit (ICU), and the interventions performed are done under austere conditions with a minimum of personnel. Expect devices to move or be dislodged during packaging and transfer to the ambulance or landing zone. For example, endotracheal (ET) tubes may become dislodged or pushed down into the right main stem; IV lines may get kinked or dislodged. Assess items before and after movement and have the necessary equipment ready to reapply dislodged devices.

Interfacility Transport Responses

Interfacility transports usually account for the majority of a CCTP's workload. The amount of information that is gathered and passed on to CCT teams at dispatch varies greatly among medical transportation systems. In some situations, the CCT team will know only basic details about the patient, such as name, sex, age, medical category, referring and receiving locations, and equipment needed. In other situations, a team member may participate in physician-to-physician conference calls during the referral process and have immediate access to electronic medical records; in this scenario, the team will have extensive information about the patient's condition and needs.

Whenever possible, the CCT team should use the response time to develop a plan that includes all members. Some systems use this time to phone the bedside nurse to obtain an updated patient report and provide an estimated time of arrival (ETA). Most interfacility transport responses occur without the use of red lights and siren. Limit emergency responses to situations when the patient has been diagnosed with a time-sensitive emergency that cannot be treated at the referring facility.

Four distinct variables influence interfacility transport planning:

- The reason for transport
- The type of originating facility and location within the origination facility
- The duration of transport
- The receiving facility type and destination bed

Understanding these variables helps the transport team frame the expectations for transport and the ongoing management plan.

Reason for Transport

Physicians ordering a patient transport are not making a benign decision. Patients who require interfacility transport for medical care tend to have longer length of stays and increased risk of morbidity and mortality compared to patients who are not transported.

The reason for transport will likely inform the anticipated patient care needs when planning interfacility transports. Patients who require services not available at the referring facility are at the greatest risk of needing urgent interventions and deteriorating. Patients transferred for the purpose of maintaining continuity of care may have specialized needs unrelated to the reason for admission or may be receiving ongoing care at the accepting facility. Examples include specialized oncology, cardiology, and neurology services. Bed capacity is a major health care issue, and calls to transport patients due to a lack of available beds within a hospital or a region are becomingly increasingly common. Bed capacity on a regional level also results in increased transportation distances.

Originating Facility and Patient Location

Patients are frequently transferred from critical-access hospitals, free-standing EDs, and smaller community hospitals in both urban and suburban settings. The type of facility from which the transfer originates influences the interventions patients may receive prior to transport. Critical-access and free-standing EDs typically have a limited number of ventilators and limited support staff, and are unlikely to have emergent surgical support services or access to sophisticated imaging. Community hospitals may have ICUs where patients receive invasive interventions, ongoing critical care management, and other forms of comprehensive care prior to transport. Tertiary care centers may transport patients to other tertiary or quaternary care centers, such as academic medical centers. These transports typically involve patients with complicated conditions who are transported for specialized care, such as burn treatment, extracorporeal membrane oxygenation, limb reattachment, or organ transplant.

Within facilities, patients may be transferred from the ED, a floor bed, an ICU, or a procedural area or operating room. The type of care the patient has been receiving will depend largely on the type of unit making the referral. The CCT team should consider this information in anticipating the patient's needs. The team should also consider the referring unit's location within the facility; a referring unit located deep within the facility may considerably extend or complicate the transport process.

Transport Length and Mode

While there is no standardized definition of short versus long transport, the length of transport influences how teams should approach patient care planning. Certainly a 15-minute transport from a free-standing ED to a tertiary care center is a short transport, whereas a trans-Atlantic flight is a long transport. As a general guideline, transports of less than an hour may be considered short. Transports lasting 1 to 3 hours may be considered medium or long transports, and those lasting more than 3 hours are certainly long.

Time is used when planning transport length because it is a consistent and reliable factor across transport modes. Mileage, in comparison, can have very different implications depending on the

Types of Medical Facilities

- **Critical-access hospitals**. The Centers for Medicare and Medicaid Services provides the *critical access* designation to hospitals that have 25 or fewer beds, are located more than 35 miles from another hospital, have an average length of stay of less than 96 hours, and provide 24/7 emergency medicine services. Critical-access hospitals are a lifeline and provide some level of medical access in rural communities, but offer very limited services. Most acutely ill or injured patients require transport to higher levels of care once stabilized.

- **Community hospitals**. Community medical centers offer emergency medicine and inpatient facilities. They may have standard consultant and specialist services. Community hospitals typically are not affiliated with graduate medical education (residency programs) and focus on providing general medical care. Some may offer limited specialty services such as low-risk labor and delivery management, pediatric care, critical care, cardiology, or neurology. Across the United States, most nonfederal acute care hospitals qualify as community hospitals.

- **Primary care centers** and **secondary care centers**. Primary care centers offer outpatient, routine family medicine services, including obstetrics and gynecology, geriatric care, and pediatric primary care. These centers are responsible for coordinating patient care with outpatient specialists as appropriate. Secondary care centers may offer primary care within the same facility but also offer outpatient specialties such as cardiology, neurology, nephrology, mental health, endocrinology, or oncology. Interfacility

transport teams in some systems may transport patients from primary or secondary care centers to hospitals when patients are directly admitted from their care center to a hospital bed.

- **Tertiary care centers**. Tertiary care centers offer highly specialized inpatient medical care, including advanced and complex medical interventions performed by specialty physicians. Examples of tertiary care include interventional cardiology and cardiothoracic surgery, neurosurgery, acute care surgery, pediatric surgery, inpatient dialysis, and orthopedic surgery. Tertiary care centers are often recognized as regional referral centers and are frequently associated with medical residency and fellowship programs or medical schools.

- **Quaternary care centers**. Centers offering highly specialized or novel interventional therapy are often referred to as quaternary care centers. These highly specialized tertiary care referral centers may be dedicated to advancing the clinical research of one or more areas of medicine and serving as academic medical centers. Quaternary care centers generally accept the most acutely ill patients whom physicians at tertiary care centers may infrequently treat or whose care is identified as too risky. Think of quaternary care centers as the specialty center for specialists. Examples include hospitals that place left ventricular assist devices or perform organ transplantation, cancer centers that offer bone marrow transplantation, and centers that offer experimental therapies.

transport mode. For example, a 100-mile (161-km) transport may take 2.5 hours by ground transport but only 45 minutes by helicopter; mileage, therefore, is not nearly as relevant in predicting the patient's needs as is time. As transport length increases, more planning is needed to determine strategies to care for a patient's medical and physical needs. Planning to turn and reposition a patient may be unnecessary on a 30-minute trip, but becomes imperative during a 3-hour transport.

Destination Facility

The destination facility may be considered a higher, equivalent, or lower level of care from the referring facility. In general, patients who require services that are unavailable at a referring facility or who

are transported due to bed capacity issues need to be transported to an equivalent or higher level of care facility. Most interfacility transports will be to a facility that offers a higher level of care, such as a tertiary or quaternary care center. A community hospital with an ICU may be a higher level of care when compared to a critical-access hospital but a lower level of care when compared to an academic medical center.

In some systems, CCT teams may be asked to transport patients to long-term acute care facilities if the patient is ventilator dependent, requires long-term physical therapy or rehabilitation, or has a chronic medical condition requiring long-term acute care. It is important that CCT teams continue the care plans implemented by the referring facility, which may involve careful forethought given the differences between transport-based equipment and hospital-based equipment, and the physiologic conditions of the transport itself.

Finally, patients can be transported to a variety of locations at referring facilities, including the ED, a flood bed, an ICU, or an interventional unit such as radiology or the operating room. It is important to confirm that the receiving staff are aware of the medications and equipment used to care for the patient and can accept and continue the same level of care. Although your interventions should never be based on the care that the destination unit will provide, it may become necessary to call an accepting facility and change destination units based on the care transport teams have provided.

Arrival and Planning

Upon arrival at the referring facility, introduce yourself to the patient's care team. Ask for a moment to review the chart and all available diagnostic information prior to taking a handoff report. This introduction serves the same purpose as it does on a prehospital scene: It lets caregivers know that you have arrived and are ready to render care.

Reviewing the chart prior to obtaining a handoff report and physically assessing the patient give you a general understanding of the patient's condition, allow you to focus your assessment accordingly, and avoid the likelihood of the hospital care team repeating information that is already readily available. The purpose of the handoff report from the treating nurse or physician is the same as it is when a 9-1-1 paramedic gives a handoff report to the ED staff: to fill in the blanks between the written patient care report and the prearrival notification. Do not be surprised if the nurse or physician giving the handoff report is not the person who has delivered most of the patient care. Transfers are often delayed while waiting for a bed at the destination facility to open up, and new care teams may be on duty by the time the transfer occurs.

When gathering information, immediately determine if the patient has a traumatic injury or is experiencing a medical illness, and adjust your questions appropriately. Identify the following key items when preparing to transport injured patients:

- Time of injury
- Mechanism of injury and speeds

- Whether the incident was accidental or deliberate
- Whether safety equipment was used
- Diagnosed injuries
- Applicable diagnostic tests that have been performed and their results, if available
- Diagnostic tests indicated but not yet performed

When transporting patients with a medical complaint, obtain the following details:

- Onset of symptoms (time)
- Time of arrival at the referring facility
- Symptom progression over time (improving versus deteriorating)
- Diagnostic tests performed and their results
- Differential diagnosis
- Presence or absence of complications
- Interventions and the patient's response to those interventions

For all patient transports, a wealth of information can be gleaned from the hospital patient care record. Indeed, the CCTP may be given a large amount of information, and must quickly separate necessary information from irrelevant information. Anticipated transport time is a critical variable in differentiating between the two. More information may be necessary to provide appropriate assessment and interventions for a longer transport.

The following items in the hospital patient care record are of particular note:

- Demographics
- Transfer order, including the sending and accepting physicians, the destination hospital and care unit, and contact information for each
- As-needed and standing orders for transport
- History and physical (H&P) examination findings **FIGURE 5-1**
- Physician notes
- Nursing notes and flow chart
- Medication administration record
- Lab values and results of diagnostic studies, including imaging copies (digital media)
- Physiologic scoring method results
- Advance directives
- Family and caregiver names and contact information

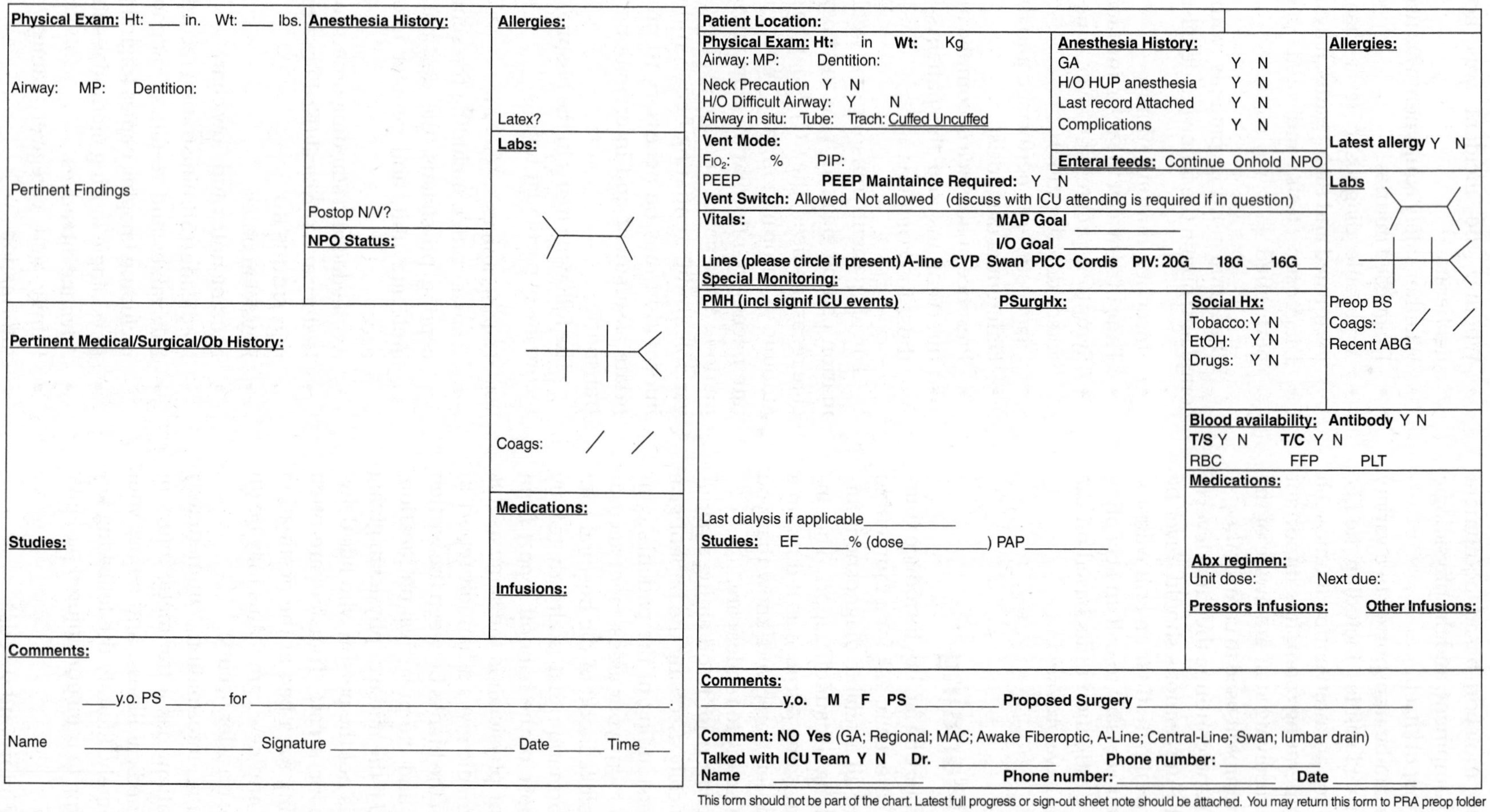

Patient Location:

Physical Exam: Ht: ___ in **Wt:** ___ Kg

Airway: MP: ___ Dentition: ___

Neck Precaution Y N

H/O Difficult Airway: Y N

Airway in situ: Tube: Trach: Cuffed Uncuffed

Vent Mode:

FiO₂: ___ %

PEEP ___ PIP: ___

Vent Switch: Allowed Not allowed (discuss with ICU attending is required if in question)

Vitals: **PEEP Maintaince Required:** Y N

MAP Goal ___

I/O Goal ___

Lines (please circle if present) A-line CVP Swan PICC Cordis PIV: 20G ___ 18G ___ 16G ___

Special Monitoring:

PMH (incl signif ICU events)

Anesthesia History:

GA   Y N

H/O HUP anesthesia   Y N

Last record Attached   Y N

Complications   Y N

Enteral feeds: Continue Onhold NPO

PSurgHx:

Last dialysis if applicable

Studies: EF ___ % (dose) ___) PAP ___

Allergies:

Latest allergy Y N

Labs

Preop BS ___

Coags: ___

Recent ABG ___

Social Hx:

Tobacco: Y N

EtOH: Y N

Drugs: Y N

Blood availability: Antibody Y N

T/S Y N   **T/C** Y N

RBC ___   FFP ___   PLT ___

Medications:

Abx regimen:

Unit dose: ___   Next due: ___

Pressors Infusions: ___   **Other Infusions:**

Comments:

___ y.o. M F PS ___ Proposed Surgery ___

Comment: NO Yes (GA; Regional; MAC; Awake Fiberoptic, A-Line; Central-Line; Swan; lumbar drain)

Talked with ICU Team Y N   Dr. ___ **Phone number:** ___

Name ___ **Phone number:** ___ **Date** ___

This form should not be part of the chart. Latest full progress or sign-out sheet note should be attached. You may return this form to PRA preop folder

---

Physical Exam: Ht: ___ in. **Wt:** ___ lbs.

Airway: MP: ___ Dentition: ___

Pertinent Findings

Postop N/V?

NPO Status:

Pertinent Medical/Surgical/Ob History:

Studies:

Comments:

___ y.o. PS ___ for ___

Name ___ Signature ___ Date ___ Time ___

Anesthesia History:

Allergies:

Latex?

Labs:

Coags:

Medications:

Infusions:

FIGURE 5-1 Assess each therapy the patient is receiving before and after making transfers to the transport equipment.

Careful review of the hospital patient care record, particularly the H&P report, physician notes, nursing notes, and medication administration record, may yield valuable clues as to the patient's condition and guide the CCTP's bedside assessment. The prehospital patient care record, if available, can also be a valuable source of information. The CCTP should note any details in these reports that suggest the patient has a time-sensitive injury or illness that requires immediate intervention. Time is of the essence when packaging patients with time-sensitive emergencies for transport, and scene time needs to be kept to a minimum.

Diversity and Cultural Considerations

Providing the right care to each patient means more than just following the clinically indicated evidence-based interventions. The right care is patient-centered care, which places patients at the center of the care team and embeds them in care planning. A simple and effective way to include patients in care planning is to ask them about their personal and cultural preferences. Determine patients' gender and address them as they would like to be addressed, which includes using the correct pronouns. Inquire about cultural preferences that may impact their care during transport and while hospitalized. For example, some cultures do not allow blood transfusions. Reviewing a patient's cultural preferences may also help identify social determinants of health, which are predictors of worsened health outcomes. Keep in mind that some cultures are distrustful of health care or follow practices that do not align with Western medicine practices. It is imperative to discuss your treatment plans with patients and align those plans with their cultural needs to the best of your ability.

SAMPLE History

SAMPLE is a familiar and useful acronym for remembering the pertinent details of a patient's history: Signs and symptoms, Allergies, Medications, Pertinent past medical history, Last oral intake, and Events leading up to the illness or injury. While CCTPs may use this framework to guide their history gathering, they should not think of it as a simple checklist; instead, they should strive to obtain in-depth details for each component.

Signs and symptoms continue to serve a vital role in the ongoing assessment. Determine how symptoms have changed over time, and use the detailed physical exam (discussed later in this chapter) to assess whether physical signs of injury/illness are improving or worsening.

Understanding the patient's allergies is critical. Try to determine whether the patient has medication, environmental, and food-based allergies. Food-based allergies are important because some medications are prepared using food derivatives.

The patient's medications include any over-the-counter and prescribed medications, recreational drugs, and herbal supplements and vitamins. You should also determine whether the patient has been complying with prescribed medications. Review any ordered medications that need to be continued or administered during transport. Consult medical direction if you believe an ordered medication may not be indicated. Do not delay administration of ordered medications on the assumption that the accepting facility will promptly administer them after arrival. Accepting facility staff will likely need to wait for a new physician evaluation and order before administering medications, which can result in significant delays.

While 9-1-1 providers focus on a *pertinent* past history, the CCTP should consider the patient's *entire* past medical history. Although some aspects of the history may seem unrelated to a current complaint, diseases are often interrelated, which may increase the risk of complications or influence drug administration decisions. For example, suppose a patient receiving transport for a fractured distal femur requires analgesia. This patient has never broken a bone before but has a history of atrial fibrillation and chronic kidney disease. The medications prescribed for these conditions place the patient at risk for increased hemorrhage, impaired compensation, and slow drug elimination.

Last oral intake actually means *last ins and last outs*. Yes, it is important to document whether a patient has a full or empty stomach, but this questioning falls short. In addition to documenting the last foods and liquids consumed (including time and quantity), CCTPs must document output. Output includes urine output, vomiting, blood loss, bowel movements, and each drain attached to the patient. In the context of the patient assessment, anticipate documenting how much of each output occurs per hour. Urine is the most frequently measured output and should be documented during every patient contact. Normal adult urine output is 0.5 to 1 mL/kg/h. Other drains should be labeled to assist in documenting output.

For the CCTP, *events* describe the context, including the mechanism of injury or nature of illness, leading up to the patient's hospital presentation, but also interventions and observations that have occurred since then. Although much of this information will be documented in a hospital record, there are two reasons to summarize this information in your records. First, doing so forces

Transport Paperwork

Paperwork is an essential component of safe, appropriate, and proper interfacility transports. In addition to the transport-specific patient care report, the CCTP must complete other important forms for each interfacility transport.

A *physician certification statement (PCS) form* is required by insurers for reimbursement. The PCS form, more aptly referred to as a medical necessity certification statement, documents the reason for transfer, the risks of transfer, the monitoring and treatment needed during transport, and the patient's physical condition at the time of transfer. As a CCT team member, you must ensure not only that the PCS form is completed but also that it accurately represents the patient at the time of transport and provides the necessary orders for care during transport. Inaccurate PCS forms delay reimbursement for transports and may expose the CCTP to liability for omissions or additions of care during transport.

All interfacility transports require a *patient consent form*. Often the consent is included in an ambulance assignment of benefits (AOB) form. This form states that the patient or their legal representative agrees to ambulance transport and authorizes the release of applicable health records to the ambulance service and the patient's insurer for the purposes of appropriate reimbursement. While it is a best practice to have the patient legibly sign the AOB, the patient's legal representative may also sign the form. When no legal representative is available and the patient cannot sign, this form must be signed by the receiving facility's medical staff to validate that no other appropriate party was available to sign for the patient and the patient arrived at the receiving facility.

each CCTP to obtain a complete understanding of the patient's current condition, which will improve critical thinking when determining treatment plans for the patient. Second, the interfacility transport record must stand as its own complete document for reimbursement and legal purposes.

Referring Facility Interventions

The patient's history includes the referring facility's management. Specifically, the CCTP should determine any diagnostic tests and imaging performed and their results, the differential diagnosis, and any interventions performed and the patient's response to them.

Tests may include blood samples and laboratory results, radiologic exams, and physical exams. Lab values should be assessed to recognize trends over time and responses to interventions (eg, transfusion, hyperkalemia treatment).

The differential diagnosis is the process of selecting the most likely underlying cause of the patient's condition by comparing multiple potential causes of the presenting signs and symptoms. For example, a patient may present with signs and symptoms suggestive of two different disorders, ST-segment elevation myocardial infarction and Takotsubo cardiomyopathy. Thus, these conditions would be included in the differential diagnosis. The actual diagnosis would not be determined until angiography is completed in the cardiac catheterization lab. As a CCTP, you may have access to that diagnosis if the patient is being transferred from a facility where the necessary diagnostic workup can be performed; however, you may be transferring the patient from a facility where such studies have not been completed. In that case, your care may be guided by a working diagnosis, which is based on the best information available in the differential diagnosis.

Finally, determine what interventions the referring facility has performed to manage both the patient's underlying problem and the patient's symptoms. These interventions may be separate from one another. For example, in septic shock, a vasopressor may be administered to treat the symptom of hypotension while antibiotics are given treat the underlying infection. CCTPs must understand the differences between interventions that treat symptoms and those that treat underlying problems and recognize when they need to be modified. Whenever possible, the CCTP's interventions should align with the receiving facility's definitive interventions. If the receiving facility has requested interventions that the sending facility has not yet performed, the CCT team should include these interventions in the transport treatment plan, provided they are indicated and within the CCTP's scope of care.

Primary Assessment

The primary assessment provides a brief glimpse into the patient's condition. During this assessment, providers place absolute priority on quickly identifying any acute life threats, doing so at the cost of thoroughness. This brief exam should seldom take more than 60 seconds, as acutely life-threatening problems require timely intervention. This survey involves a stepwise, rapid evaluation of organ systems and anatomy fundamentally necessary for life. Primary assessment is also used whenever sudden or unexpected patient deterioration occurs during transport.

Generally speaking, the provider completes the primary assessment while positioned at the patient's head, though many gross abnormalities, such as hemorrhage or pallor, can be noted at a glance from a distance.

While many abbreviations have been used to guide clinicians in carrying out a structured primary assessment, two have taken hold: MARCH and ABCDE. The MARCH acronym, introduced by the Committee on Tactical Combat Casualty Care (CoTCCC), lists assessment priorities in the following order:

- **M**assive hemorrhage
- **A**irway
- **R**espiration
- **C**irculation
- **H**ypothermia

The CoTCCC rightfully prioritizes massive hemorrhage, which is the primary cause of death in trauma. That said, seldom will a CCT team be the first-arriving responders at most incidents; exsanguinating injuries will have likely been addressed long before their arrival. Moreover, the work of a transport team spans all medical domains, and as such the MARCH acronym is likely too specific to trauma care to be the model framework proposed in this text.

The ABCDE abbreviation is preferred in this text. It prioritizes the assessment sequence as follows:

- **A**irway
- **B**reathing
- **C**irculation
- **D**isability
- **E**xposure

This abbreviation is already familiar to most providers and applies to the broad patient population seen by transport teams.

XABCDE and CABDE

The ABCDE mnemonic is sometimes adjusted during the primary survey in two scenarios. First, when life-threatening bleeding is present, the sequence may be described as XABCDE, where X represents eXsanguination (life-threatening bleeding). Second, when the patient appears lifeless and is in suspected cardiac arrest, the sequence is described as CABDE to prioritize circulation.

Airway Assessment

Understanding the human airway, including how it is supposed to function and what to do when normal functioning is impaired, is fundamental to patient care. A brief discussion of the airway, in the context of the decision making that occurs during the assessment of a patient in critical condition, is provided here; it is discussed in detail in Chapter 6, *Respiratory Emergencies and Airway Management*, and Chapter 7, *Ventilation*.

Much like other organ systems, the airway is a dynamic anatomic structure subject to change during the course of disease. An airway deemed adequate early in the patient's care may change over time, requiring intervention. Conversely, a threatened airway may become "safe" (meaning the airway is patent and ventilation appears to be effective) following the correction of a broader clinical illness; for example, a lethargic patient with sepsis may regain mentation, and thus airway control, after effective resuscitation.

Determining the Need for Airway Intervention

The first priority of the primary assessment is to determine whether the airway is safe in its current state or whether intervention is needed. This determination is best made collaboratively as a team, with clinical and logistical considerations being weighed to determine if, when, and where airway management should occur.

Anatomic evaluation of the airway is aimed at identifying pathology and diseases of the airway as well as factors associated with difficulty intubating the patient, if that step is required. The exam needs to be tailored to the patient's ability to follow commands. For example, while a Mallampati classification can yield useful information regarding intubation difficulty, the exam cannot be performed in a supine or obtunded patient. (The Mallampati classification is described in Chapter 6, *Respiratory Emergencies and Airway Management.*)

In transport medicine, several significant, inherent logistical factors can affect clinical decision making. Generally speaking, the most conservative airway plan will be the best and safest option. Intubation, including high-risk anesthesia, is best performed in the least chaotic environment. Providers should err on the side of caution by intubating the patient in the hospital or at the emergency scene prior to transfer. That said, in certain cases, it may be feasible to perform an elective in-transport intubation to mitigate delays to definitive care. In-transport intubation requires careful patient selection and screening, with only patients determined to be reasonably anatomically "easy" being selected. Most importantly, intubation en route requires prior practice and equipment configurations to ensure this intervention does not pose unreasonable risk. Some vehicle types may preclude or complicate intubation. The confined cabin of smaller single-engine aircraft may be a suboptimal environment for in-flight intubation, whereas a twin-turbine aircraft may offer more ample space. Finally, distance and transport time should be weighed when deciding whether to perform airway management. A patient with an already tenuous airway, who has a lengthy transport time, is at risk for requiring emergent intervention in transit.

Assessing the Intubated Patient

For patients with an artificial airway in place, such as a supraglottic or ET tube, the airway and respiratory exam should focus on immediate risks to the patient. The CCTP should consider the life-threatening sequelae of an inappropriately placed ET tube. Tube placement and positioning must be confirmed as part of the initial survey. The CCTP should visually inspect the ET tube, including its size and depth. Once ET tube size has been identified, appropriate depth can quickly be approximated by multiplying the tube size times three:

$$\text{ET tube size} \times 3 = \text{Tube depth}$$

Providers must perform auscultation to evaluate for signs of right main stem intubation. A patient with decreased lung sounds on the left side is presumed to have a right main stem placement until proven otherwise.

While physical examination is an important part of confirming ET tube placement, the gold standard in confirming placement is waveform capnography, which measure end-tidal carbon dioxide ($ETCO_2$) levels. A patient with an artificial airway must be placed on continuous $ETCO_2$ monitoring. When considering the often hectic, loud environment in which CCT teams often work, $ETCO_2$ monitoring is a standard of care essential to the safe transfer of an intubated patient.

Because CCT inherently involves relocating and repositioning the patient and medical apparatus, maintaining the security of the artificial airway is paramount. CCTPs must inspect the securing device to ensure it is adequately holding the ET tube in place and, just as importantly, to confirm the securing strap is correctly routed. The securing strap must be routed around the base of the skull, not the occiput. A strap that is secured high over the occiput could slide downward, rendering the device ineffective and threatening ET tube security.

Much like the natural airways of the human body, artificial airways are prone to becoming filled with secretions. Because sedation suppresses the cough reflexes, ET tubes can be blocked by mucus plugs or obstructions by other contaminants such as blood. Evidence of mucus plugging can present with high peak inspiratory pressures and decreased breath sounds. It is not unreasonable to perform a preventive suction maneuver during the initial assessment of the intubated patient. An added advantage of suctioning during the initial assessment is that it helps providers determine the adequacy of analgesia and sedative infusions. The stimulation that occurs during packaging and transport is similar to that resulting from suctioning an invasive airway. Thus, CCT teams should review the patient's suction needs during the transport planning stage. If a patient will need frequent suctioning, an in-line suction device should be placed and suction must be available during all phases of patient care.

Respiratory Assessment

Primary assessment of the respiratory system should focus on detecting any injury or illness that is directly affecting the respiratory system. This assessment takes into consideration evidence of illness by proxy, where the respiratory rate, effort, or breathing patterns may suggest underlying nonpulmonary pathology.

Frequently, the first harbinger of illness is a change in the respiratory rate, as this rate fundamentally serves as a compensatory mechanism. A patient with subtle tachypnea may have occult illness, and a patient with air hunger should be presumed to be critically unwell until proven otherwise. A cardinal finding, air hunger suggests dyspnea profound enough to trigger the primal instincts of survival: fear and anxiety. Additionally, a large tidal volume should be assumed to be an adaptive response to acidosis. This finding is particularly important if intubation and subsequent mechanical ventilation are required.

During assessment, it is paramount that providers carefully note the respiratory rate and effort. Establishing the patient's initial rate enables early detection of changes during the course of care. As with other vital signs, trending is more useful than a single value, so providers should repeat this evaluation.

Recognizing Indications of Specific Injuries

Certain respiratory patterns can suggest specific pathology, including diseases involving other organs (eg, metabolic or neurologic disorders). Chapter 6, *Respiratory Emergencies and Airway Management*, describes pathologic breathing patterns. Providers should consider any evidence of dyspnea.

Supraclavicular or intercostal retractions suggest an increase in *inspiratory* resistance. In comparison, abdominal "see-saw" breathing, in which the abdominal muscles forcefully contract during exhalation, is suggestive of *expiratory* resistance to flow. This finding may be seen in obstructive lung diseases, though it can also appear during severe dyspnea.

Palpation of the chest wall can provide valuable clues regarding injury burden that may be missed by other means. By placing their open palms over the patient's chest wall, the provider may detect clues that suggest injury, such as rib fractures, flail chest, or pneumothorax. Asymmetry in chest excursion, though subtle, can be seen in patients with significant pneumothorax. Note that this finding is seldom sensitive enough to rule out a collapsed lung and should be considered as part of a constellation of other findings suggestive of pneumothorax. Tactile crepitus over a specific area can indicate fracture of the chest wall; similarly, paradoxical movement of the chest wall can point to flail chest, a condition in which fractures over two points of a rib produce a free-floating segment that moves in the opposite direction as the rest of the chest.

Assessing the Patient on Mechanical Ventilation

This section briefly discusses how to integrate the assessment of mechanical ventilation into the broader patient assessment; a more thorough review of caring for patients on mechanical ventilation can be found in Chapter 7, *Ventilation*. As part of obtaining an initial "snapshot" of an intubated patient, mechanical ventilation parameters should be assessed, with a closer, more targeted assessment to follow.

First, during patient packaging, the CCTP should confirm the adequacy and safety of mechanical ventilation. *Safe* mechanical ventilation implies the patient is receiving ventilatory support that is both adequate and not injurious to the lungs. The first confirmatory steps should be aimed at assessing adequate tidal volume delivery. Providers may encounter a patient who, due to either inadequate sedation or mucus plugging, is not receiving adequate tidal volumes and thus is developing a respiratory acidosis. Alternatively, a patient on noninvasive mechanical ventilation could have declining mental status, resulting in inadequate ventilation.

Generally speaking, exhaled tidal volumes should be 5 to 8 mL/kg of ideal body weight. If the tidal volume is significantly above or below this approximation, further investigations should be made.

To determine whether ventilation is injurious to the lungs, peak inspiratory pressure levels should be evaluated. Though high peak inspiratory pressures are not direct evidence of barotrauma, they can be caused by high plateau pressures, which may result in lung injury. Plateau pressure should be maintained at less than 30 cm H_2O in patients with poor lung compliance. Before connecting the ventilator to the patient, a high-pressure alarm should be preset, either by measuring a baseline peak inspiratory pressure from the hospital ventilator or by starting at 30 to 35 cm H_2O and titrating accordingly. A peak inspiratory pressure greater than 35 cm H_2O should prompt further evaluation of ventilatory parameters. As part of the early formulation of the transport plan, the CCT team should review the fraction of inspired oxygen (FIO_2) level. This information will help providers determine anticipated oxygen consumption for transport and can also elicit useful information about the patient's condition. A patient with an oxygen saturation (SpO_2), as measured by pulse oximeter, less than 92% with an FIO_2 of 1.0 is exhibiting significant pulmonary dysfunction.

Teams should screen for patients at risk for hyperoxia, as this condition has clinical significance: A growing body of literature suggests significant patient harm is associated with hyperoxia. Given this risk, patients with SpO_2 levels of 100% with an FIO_2 of 1.0 should have their FIO_2 level down-titrated to an SpO_2 level of 93% to 97%.

Circulatory Assessment

Assessment of the circulatory system requires the collation of information from multiple diagnostic sources, including the physical exam, monitoring equipment, and other diagnostic tools. For the transport team, circulatory assessment may be complicated during ICU transfers by the presence of advanced monitoring tools. That said, the rapid assessment of patient acuity can be initially surmised by simple bedside examination.

Skin

Skin color, temperature, and condition can provide a valuable initial glimpse into illness severity. Pallor

in isolation, without associated diaphoresis (sweating), may indicate anemia, with its earliest manifestations being found in the mucosa of the eyelids. In conjunction with other skin findings, pallor is a sign of impaired cutaneous capillary perfusion. As part of the sympathetic response to an insult, whether from injury or illness, sweating of the brow or clammy skin is a cardinal sign of inadequate perfusion and increased sympathetic response. Cool skin temperature indicates vasoconstriction and directing of blood away from the superficial dermal layers toward the more essential organs necessary for survival.

Assessing Skin Pallor

The word *pale*, as used in this text, may apply to any patient whose skin presentation suggests reduced blood flow or oxygenation. In patients with light skin, pallor typically presents as unusual lightness compared with the person's baseline skin color. In patients with dark skin, pallor may appear as ashen or gray skin on general assessment. In general, the mucous membranes inside the inner lower eyelid and the oral mucosa will have a pink coloration in all healthy patients, regardless of baseline skin color; thus, a white or pale appearance of these areas in any patient suggests reduced blood flow or oxygenation.

Because providers do not necessarily know the patient's baseline skin color, they should consider the observations of friends or family members on scene. Simply asking, "Does her skin look like its usual color to you?" may produce useful insights into the patient's condition.

While it can be hard to quantify many physical findings, capillary refill time (CRT) of the nail bed can serve as a window into the state of peripheral perfusion. Many exam findings, such as the severity of pallor or pulse strength, are subject to the shortcomings of poor interobserver reliability. CRT can be a valuable exam finding that is reproducible by another clinician with reasonable accuracy. In the 2019 ANDROMEDA-SHOCK trial, CRT was found to be as reliable as serum lactate for guiding teams during the resuscitation of patients with sepsis. Considering its ease of use, reliability, and availability, CRT is likely underutilized during patient assessment.

Cold Shock Versus Warm Shock

Assessment of skin temperature may play an additional role in differentiating forms of shock. It has been theorized that "cold shock" suggests disorders resulting in a low cardiac output state. Patients with cold shock present with tachycardia, pallor, decreased peripheral pulses, and cold extremities—the last due to insufficient cardiac output to adequately perfuse the skin. This finding can be seen in cardiogenic shock and hypovolemic shock, both of which are associated with a low output state.

In contrast, "warm shock" suggests adequate cardiac output but vasodilation that is hindering systemic perfusion. The vasodilatory state causes a relatively warm skin condition and preserved or bounding pulse pressure. This finding is seen in patients with shock secondary to syndromes that cause a vasodilatory state, such as sepsis or anaphylaxis.

Vital Signs

Descriptions of how to obtain and interpret vital signs in specific CCT contexts are presented throughout this text. For the purposes of this chapter, it is worth noting some key insights relating to the use of vital signs during the primary patient assessment.

During the primary assessment, the evaluation of vital signs is limited to looking for evidence of acute instability. However, providers should keep in mind that their initial documentation establishes the reference point against which later vital signs recordings will be compared. Ongoing measurement of vital signs is a fundamental element in documenting trends and responses to interventions (eg, response to vasopressors, ventilatory changes).

In the CCT domain, vital signs serve as both a diagnostic tool and a threshold for intervention. It is essential for the CCTP to be familiar with the use of mean arterial pressure (MAP). While much of prehospital care focuses on systolic blood pressure (SBP) values, the MAP is a more physiologic representation of systemic blood flow.

Finally, CCTPs should remain mindful that vital signs, although an integral part of a patient assessment, are not without their limitations. For example, some types of medications can alter physiologic response (eg, beta blockers may suppress adaptive

tachycardia). Failure to consider this possibility could result in misinterpretation of the patient's condition.

Shock Index

The shock index, defined as heart rate divided by SBP, was first described in a Swiss paper in 1967 and was subsequently validated across multiple observational studies. These studies evaluated the use of the shock index to predict mortality and the need for transfusion. It is from these studies that a shock index threshold of 0.9 or greater was identified as being of clinical value in determining critical illness.

A limitation of these observational studies is the relatively young age of the patients included, largely a result of trauma historically being a disease disproportionately affecting the young. Basing the shock index threshold on this young trauma patient cohort leads to particular challenges when dealing with other patients at the extremes of age, including the pediatric and geriatric patient populations.

To account for the variable significance of hemodynamic derangements in the older patient, the age shock index was developed. This tool multiplies the conventional shock index by the person's age:

$$\text{Age} \times (\text{Heart rate} \div \text{SBP}) = \text{Age shock index}$$

It is reasonable to assume that a shock index of 1.2 would be of greater significance in a 70-year-old than in a 22-year-old. Thus, the age-adjusted shock index increases the accuracy with which we can predict mortality in an injured patient who is older than 55 years. A cutoff value of 50 is used to avoid arbitrarily high values.

Considering the significant variations in hemodynamics across age groups in children, the conventional shock index can be an unreliable tool for grading illness or injury severity in this population. The shock index pediatric-adjusted (SIPA) was derived to address this problem. It clusters heart rate and blood pressure (BP) values by age to establish thresholds for a shock index of statistical and clinical significance:

- 4 to 6 years: 1.2
- 6 to 12 years: 1
- >12 years: 0.9

Assessment of the Patient With Hemorrhage

As part of early assessment of the injured patient, providers must seek sources of hemorrhage. Life-threatening external hemorrhage should have already been controlled prior to the arrival of a CCT team. That said, an initial survey for external hemorrhage should be performed to ensure continued efficacy of the bleeding control interventions performed prior to arrival. Additionally, with the presence of a large distracting major hemorrhage, initial providers may miss other sources of bleeding. The occult oozing bleed, whether from a tourniquet or from a fracture site, can result in a significant amount of blood loss if left unaddressed.

Examination for external hemorrhage must be done early and in a systematic fashion. Extremity sweeps should be performed, including a review of the axillae, groin, and neck. From there, an inspection of the chest, abdomen, and back must be made. If a truncal injury is found, it is paramount to inspect both sides of the patient to avoid missing an associated exit wound. Extremity wounds should be packed, dressed, and splinted. If a tourniquet has been placed prior to the CCT team's arrival, its efficacy should be confirmed: The hemorrhage must be controlled and there must be no palpable distal pulse to the limb. Care should be taken to secure the tourniquet to avoid its accidental dislodgement or release during patient moves.

Signs of internal hemorrhage can be difficult to detect. Grey Turner sign (ecchymosis of the flanks) is a late finding, seldom seen during the initial transport phase, and should not be relied upon for early detection of internal bleeding. Instead, detection relies on thoughtful consideration of the mechanism of injury and detection of external signs of blunt trauma. Examination of the skin for abrasions and underlying contusions is helpful to guide assessment. From there, palpation may reveal point tenderness over solid organs. Seat belt sign is a significant finding, particularly in the patient with tenderness on exam, as the risk of organ injury can be high.

Evaluation of the pelvis is an important part of the exam of the major trauma patient. CCTPs should examine the pelvis for injury in patients who have experienced a significant mechanism of injury, including a vehicle rollover or ejection, significant fall, or vehicle–pedestrian collision. Through gentle palpation, providers should evaluate symmetry of the anterior-superior iliac spine. CCTPs should also review imaging studies conducted at the sending facility prior to their arrival.

Gastrointestinal Assessment

Inspection

A general overview of the oral mucosa and abdominal areas gives CCTPs general information about the gastrointestinal (GI) system. For example, the lips and mucous membranes should be moist and without lesions. Dry mucous membranes may indicate dehydration, and pale mucous membranes may indicate hypovolemia. A large abdomen may indicate ascites, especially if abdominal wall veins are noted. Hernias or masses may be visible. Bruising over the abdominal wall may indicate trauma or bleeding into the abdominal cavity.

Critical care patients often have GI bleeding as a secondary stress response to their illness. Stools should be assessed for color, consistency, and a foul odor. Upper GI bleeding is characterized by dark melena stools, and lower GI bleeding by stools mixed with bright red blood (although bright red blood may also suggest brisk bleeding from higher up). Either of these findings should be reported promptly.

Auscultation

In the GI assessment, auscultation of the abdomen should precede palpation or percussion of the abdomen. The rationale is that the CCTP may get a false-positive assessment for bowel sounds if manual manipulation of the intestines occurs first. Bowel sounds should be present in all four quadrants of the abdomen. These sounds may be hypoactive or hyperactive in various disease states. Nevertheless, there is great variation in bowel sounds with clinical conditions such as an ileus.

Auscultation of bowel sounds, if necessary, should be done in a quiet ICU or ED room. Bowel sounds auscultated during transport have a tendency to sound exactly like the engine of the transport vehicle.

Palpation

A CCTP typically uses palpation to document tenderness or rebound tenderness. Tenderness occurs with simple palpation; rebound tenderness occurs when the pain is reported as the pressure of palpation is removed. Rebound tenderness suggests peritoneal inflammation.

If a pelvic fracture is suspected, the pelvis should not be assessed for stability by every caregiver. Any hematoma that has formed to maintain hemostasis in such a case may be disrupted by the repeated palpation exams, inducing internal hemorrhage.

The Murphy sign is noted when the patient has severe right upper quadrant pain on deep palpation, which is often exacerbated by deep inspiration and associated with cholecystitis. Deep palpation is performed by applying firm pressure to the abdominal wall. The liver may also be palpated by placing the left hand behind the patient under the liver and applying firm pressure upward. The fingers of the right hand are placed on the right upper quadrant of the patient's abdomen, and the patient is asked to take a deep breath. The edge of the liver can be felt as it comes down to meet the examiner's fingers **FIGURE 5-2**. Next, the applied pressure is lightened and nodules or tenderness are noted as the liver slips under the fingers. Nodules of the liver may be related to a malignancy.

The spleen is generally not palpable. The right kidney may be palpated, but this examination is not of much clinical value. The kidney should never be palpated if the patient has a history of polycystic kidney disease.

Genitourinary Assessment

Assessment of the genitalia includes the mammary, testicular, and prostate glands. These assessments are limited to patients with specific needs, such as those with spinal cord injuries or trauma.

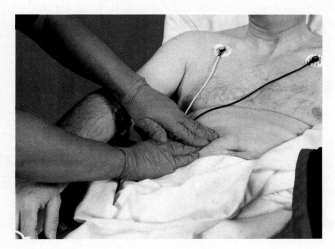

FIGURE 5-2 Palpation of the liver.
© Jones & Bartlett Learning.

In end-stage renal disease, patients may require peritoneal dialysis (PD) or hemodialysis. In PD, a catheter is placed in the peritoneum, and the peritoneum serves as the filter to remove waste from the peritoneal cavity using a dialyzing solution. Patients who rely on this type of dialysis are especially prone to peritonitis. Therefore, an aseptic technique is important when assessing or performing PD. Patients undergoing hemodialysis will often have an arteriovenous (AV) shunt in the forearm or thigh, or a tunneled dialysis catheter in the chest.

The AV shunt should be assessed for a thrill, which indicates that the shunt is patent and functioning normally. AV shunts should be used only for hemodialysis. In patients who have a central line and a tunneled line access for dialysis, these lines should not be accessed except in dire emergency and only while maintaining the strictest sterile technique possible. Additionally, these lines are typically heparin locked at the completion of treatments. Lines that contain heparin should not be flushed prior to aspiration of a significant amount of waste (a minimum of 10 mL per port).

Disability Assessment

The neurologic exam should be performed not only during initial survey, but also subsequently during transport to establish and monitor for trends. Neurologic emergencies can be dynamic, particularly in the acute phase, during which the CCT team may be involved in the patient's care. The exam can be tiered, with an initial exam focusing on identifying major neurologic pathology and a subsequent, more thorough exam focusing on detecting more subtle findings.

Neurologic Scoring

As part of the initial survey, the patient's level of consciousness should be determined. The most rudimentary means of assessment is to determine patient responsiveness to voice or pain using the AVPU scale **TABLE 5-1**. In the absence of sedatives, failure of the obtunded patient to respond to a painful stimulus is concerning for major intracranial pathology.

While the Glasgow Coma Scale (GCS) was initially developed and validated for the purpose of neurologic prognostication following traumatic brain injury, it has become the de facto means of measuring and conveying mental status across health care settings. Though it remains subject to poor interobserver reliability, this scoring tool is best applied in a structured fashion with the use of a reference guide, such as that shown in **TABLE 5-2**.

One of the most common errors made with the GCS is assuming that the tool's value lies in the total derived score. In reality, the tool more accurately conveys the patient's condition when each component's score is reported individually.

Another scale, useful for assessment of both agitation and sedation, is the Richmond Agitation–Sedation Scale (RASS). The RASS score is often used as a target for sedation. With an agitated patient, this score quantifies the severity of the agitation **TABLE 5-3**. To determine the RASS score, observe, but do not speak to or otherwise engage, the patient. Scores of +1 to +4 can be observed without interacting with the patient. If necessary, speak to the patient to determine the patient's response and thereby assign a score of 0 or –1. A score of –2 means the patient responds to verbal stimulation with eye contact lasting less than 10 seconds; a score of –3 indicates that a voice stimulus triggers a motor response other than eye opening; –4 means only physical stimulation elicits a response; and –5 signifies no response to any stimuli.

Focused Neurologic Assessment

Assessment of the patient with a suspected neurologic disorder includes efforts to identify signs of disease by proxy. During this assessment, examination of visual fields, sensation, or balance may provide outward evidence of dysfunction deep within the brain. As such, targeted neurologic assessments require careful attention to a broad list of findings.

For the CCT team, primary assessment of neurologic status should be envisioned as occurring at three phases of care: (1) prior to the event, (2) on initial presentation, and (3) on team arrival for transfer. This approach establishes a comprehensive baseline that will allow providers to note any trends and changes during transport.

It has been said that "the eyes serve as windows into the brain," as they provide valuable and early indications of neurologic disease. Beyond

TABLE 5-1 AVPU Scale
Awake: eyes open spontaneously
Verbal: arouses to stimulation by voice
Painful: purposeful movement to a painful stimulus such as a pectoral pinch
Unresponsive: not responsive to any stimuli

© Jones & Bartlett Learning.

TABLE 5-2 Glasgow Coma Scale						
Eye Opening		**Best Verbal Response**		**Best Motor Response**	
Spontaneous	4	Oriented conversation	5	Obeys commands	6
In response to sound	3	Confused conversation	4	Localizes to pressure	5
In response to pressure	2	Words	3	Withdraws from pressure	4
No response	1	Sounds	2	Abnormal flexion	3
		None	1	Extension	2
				No response	1

[a]Some systems use a "Not testable (NT)" score for any element that cannot be tested. Eye opening cannot be tested in a patient whose eyes are closed due to a local factor, such as swelling; verbal response cannot be tested in a patient who has a preexisting factor interfering with communication, such as mutism; and motor response cannot be tested in a patient who has preexisting paralysis or other limiting factor.

Score: 13–15 may indicate mild dysfunction, although 15 is the score a person without neurologic impairment would receive.

Score: 9–12 may indicate moderate dysfunction.

Score: 8 or less is indicative of severe dysfunction.

© Jones & Bartlett Learning.

TABLE 5-3 Richmond Agitation–Sedation Scale

Score	Classification	Description
Observation		
+4	Combative	Violent, immediate danger to staff
+3	Very agitated	Pulls or removes tube(s) or catheter(s); aggressive
+2	Agitated	Frequent nonpurposeful movements, fights ventilator
+1	Restless	Anxious but movements not aggressive, vigorous
0	Alert and calm	Spontaneously pays attention to caregiver
Verbal Stimulation		
−1	Drowsy	Not fully alert, but has sustained awakening (eye opening or eye contact) to voice (>10 seconds)
−2	Light sedation	Briefly awakening to voice with eye contact to voice (<10 seconds)
−3	Moderate sedation	Movement or eye opening to voice (but no eye contact)
Physical Stimulation		
−4	Deep sedation	No response to voice, but movement or eye opening to physical stimulation
−5	Unarousable	No response to voice or physical stimulation

© Jones & Bartlett Learning.

conventional pupillary assessment, there is great value in assessing visual fields and observing for nystagmus. The assessment of visual fields aims to identify lesions affecting the patient's ability to perceive objects within their field of view. Patients with medial or posterior cerebral artery occlusions can lose the ability to identify objects placed within the left or right side of their visual field. This exam can be performed by asking the patient to follow a fingertip that sweeps across their visual field, while encouraging them to keep their head midline. Inability to track objects across midline is suggestive of visual field hemianopia.

Gaze-induced nystagmus is also of diagnostic value, particularly when trying to identify posterior cerebral lesions. This finding can be detected by observing the patient's eyes during extraocular movements; nystagmus induced by gaze will become apparent when the eyes are moved laterally or upward and downward.

Pupil Assessment

Another neurologic indicator of great concern is the pupil assessment. Pupils are assessed bilaterally for size (1 to 6 mm), reactivity to light (direct and

TABLE 5-4 Pupil Response

Pupil Finding	Possible Etiology
Unilaterally dilated, fixed, and nonreactive	Increased intracranial pressure May be normal in some patients Brainstem herniation Impending death
Bilaterally dilated, fixed, and nonreactive	Hypoxia Severe brain damage at the level of the midbrain
Bilaterally pinpoint and nonreactive	Narcotic use Severe brain damage at the level of the pons Ischemia

© Jones & Bartlett Learning.

consensual), and shape. **TABLE 5-4** lists common pupil findings related to size and reactivity and their possible causes.

Pupil reactivity to light is described as brisk, sluggish, or nonreactive. Occasionally, a CCTP will note a pattern of response in which rapid constriction of the pupil in response to light is followed by dilation. This so-called hippus phenomenon may be a variant of normal, but it is also seen with compression of cranial nerve III. Anisocoria, or unequal pupil size bilaterally, is a normal variant and is seen in approximately 17% of the population.

Unexplained changes in pupil assessment findings should be reported immediately. Consideration must be given to medications the patient is receiving (such as narcotics or cholinergics), anxiety, and other extraneous influences on pupils.

Speech should be assessed for impaired ability to speak such as dysarthria and dysphasia. Following ischemic stroke, the loss of control of the muscles of the face, tongue, or larynx can lead to a muffled speech despite appropriate word choice.

Cranial Nerve Assessment

A cranial nerve assessment is valuable in a patient with a neurologic insult. Subtle changes may indicate impending herniation. Cranial nerve assessment is covered in detail in Chapter 12, *Neurologic Emergencies*.

Assessment of cranial nerve III (the oculomotor nerve) is especially helpful in caring for the patient with a neurologic insult. Changes in the extraocular movements and papillary response controlled by this nerve are often the first signs of an increase in intracranial pressure (ICP).

Exposure Assessment

After addressing the ABCD phases of the initial assessment, the CCTP should expose the patient to conduct a rapid head-to-toe, anterior and posterior, assessment of the entire patient. Exposure affords the CCTP the opportunity to make key observations, such as scars that may provide clues to remote history, pressure injuries, and items that have inadvertently slipped under the patient during resuscitation and must be removed to avoid pressure injuries during transfer.

Although exposing the patient inherently increases their risk of hypothermia, doing so is actually an important step in ensuring normothermia. Wet clothes should always be removed, because they significantly contribute to cooling and create an opportunity for skin breakdown during prolonged contact. Removal of clothing is also beneficial when pelvic binders are indicated because these devices are best placed on bare skin. Placement on bare skin

mitigates skin breakdown and, more importantly, avoids the need for subsequent loosening and removal of the splint before imaging is performed at the receiving hospital. Loosening the splint would result in a loss of hemostasis of underlying pelvic hemorrhage, undermining resuscitation efforts.

Open wounds should be evaluated for severity and continued bleeding. Open fractures should be splinted and bandaged. Contaminated wounds ideally should be irrigated to help mitigate the risk of infection. As a CCTP, your primary role may be ensuring that wound management performed prior to your arrival continues during transport to provide adequate hemorrhage control. In patients with major penetrating trauma, you may need to repack wounds.

CCTPs should also assess splinting efficacy, and replace any splints that do not adequately stabilize fractured limbs. Ensure that distal circulation is not compromised by the splint. Further, check for adequate padding under the patient, as inadequate padding can result in pressure injuries.

In the CCT setting, edema and pressure injuries are particularly relevant concerns given the increased likelihood that the patient has been bedbound for an extended time. When edema is present, its location and severity should be noted. Pedal edema is usually graded on a scale from trace to 3+ or 4+ pitting, depending on the scale used **FIGURE 5-3**. To evaluate pedal edema, press on the skin behind the medial malleolus, over the shin, and over the dorsum of each foot with the thumb and index finger for at least 5 seconds. Indentation can be noted by running the pads of the fingers over

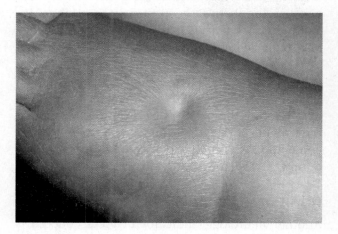

FIGURE 5-3 Pitting edema.

© Dr. P. Marazzi/Science Source.

the area pressed. A slight indentation that disappears in a short time is termed trace edema. Grade 3+ or 4+ (depending on the scale) is deep pitting that does not disappear readily. The location of the edema and the usual position of the patient should be noted to differentiate between dependent and nondependent edema. In ambulatory and seated patients, edema develops in their lower extremities, whereas patients confined to bed may have more edema in the sacral area.

As mentioned earlier, the exposed patient is at increased risk of hypothermia. Following exposure of the patient, a plan must be made to maintain normothermia. Considering that critical illness and injury as well as sedation suppress adaptive mechanisms to the cold, patients under the care of a CCT team are at risk for hypothermia. Patients should be covered with dry, warm blankets whenever possible. The use of moisture–vapor barriers such as blankets can also assist in maintaining patient warmth. Kits specifically designed to mitigate hypothermia provide excellent thermal insulation;

these kits are extensively used by the military but are also available in the commercial market. On the lower end of the cost spectrum, bubble wrap has been used by some mountain rescue teams to help stave off hypothermia.

SKILL DRILL 5-1 shows the steps for packaging patients for interfacility transports, which are also described here:

1. Transfer the patient to the transport ventilator, duplicating as many settings as possible. It may take a few minutes for the patient to become acclimated to the transport ventilator **STEP 1**.
2. Once monitoring equipment is in place, transfer any infusions to the transport unit infusion pumps. Consolidate infusions wherever possible. Use a nursing drug reference to confirm medication compatibility **STEP 2**.
3. Be certain to:
   - Read the labels of the medication bags **STEP 3**.

Skill Drill 5-1 Packaging Procedure for an Interfacility Transport

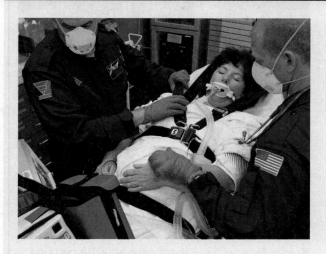

Step 1

Transfer the patient to the transport ventilator, duplicating as many settings as possible. It may take a few minutes for the patient to become acclimated to the transport ventilator.

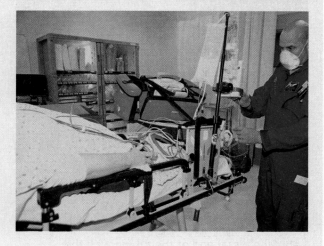

Step 2

Once monitoring equipment is in place, transfer any infusions to the transport infusion pumps. Consolidate infusions wherever possible. Use a nursing drug reference to confirm medication compatibility.

Continues

Skill Drill 5-1 Packaging Procedure for an Interfacility Transport (continued)

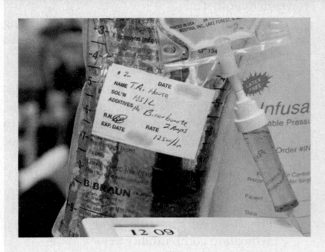

Step 3

Read the labels of the medication bags. Ensure you have sufficient supplies of infusions for the anticipated duration of transport.

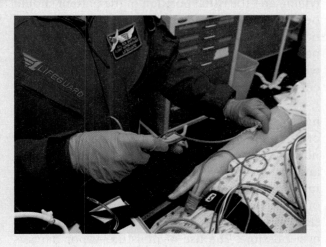

Step 4

Trace the infusion tubing completely between each bag and its connection to the patient.

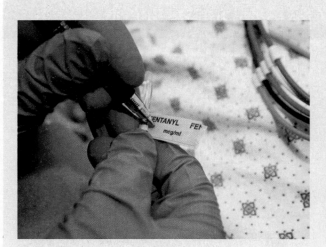

Step 5

Label the distal end of the tubing with the infusion name. Once all infusions have been transferred and are operational, reassess the patient's hemodynamic stability. Proceed to transfer the patient to the transport unit stretcher.

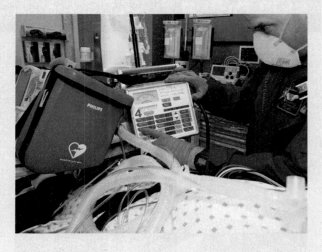

Step 6

Before leaving the patient care area, be certain that all necessary equipment adapters and connectors are with the patient. Ensure that family members have directions to the receiving facility. Provide the sending staff with contact information for follow-up. Show your appreciation for the care and assistance provided by the staff.

- Trace the infusion tubing completely between each bag and its connection to the patient **STEP 4**.
- Label the distal end of the tubing with the infusion name **STEP 5**.

4. Secure all equipment to the transport unit stretcher or carrier, bundle the patient as appropriate for the weather conditions, and reassess the patient to ensure that no change in their condition has occurred **STEP 6**.

5. Before leaving the patient care area, be certain that all necessary equipment adapters and connectors are with the patient, ensure that family members have directions to the receiving facility, and provide the sending staff with contact information should they want to follow up on the transport of the patient. Show your appreciation for the care and assistance provided by the staff in packaging and transferring the patient to your care.

Secondary Assessment

Begin the secondary assessment after completing the primary assessment and identifying and stabilizing immediate life threats and hemodynamic instability. The secondary assessment involves several components, including a detailed head-to-toe examination, a systems-based approach to specific diseases, and a complete evaluation of vital signs. Specific systems-based and disease-based assessments are detailed throughout this text. Every patient should receive a detailed physical exam, and a best practice is to perform the same head-to-toe exam on every patient. This discipline helps CCTPs master their understanding of "normal," which increases the likelihood of identifying subtle abnormal findings earlier.

Another key reason for the secondary assessment is to detect changes in the patient's condition. For example, following abdominal trauma, bruising may not develop for several hours; similarly, a flail chest may not become visually apparent until the thoracic muscles have become fatigued. Patients encountered later in their injury or disease process, the time when CCTPs are often involved in the patient's care, are likely to have different findings than those seen initially.

Finally, as a part of the secondary assessment, CCTPs must evaluate invasive equipment in use on each patient as well as any fluids infusing.

Vital Signs

Initial vital signs will nearly always be available from referring facilities and obtained during the primary assessment. Basic vital signs warranted for every patient include pulse rate, BP (including MAP), respiratory rate, pulse oximetry, mental state, and patient temperature. Single measurements of vital signs are rarely significant or helpful. Instead, the greatest value of vital signs comes from their ongoing monitoring and trending over time. Patients whose vital signs are unchanging are typically stable. Changing vital signs indicate the patient's condition is changing: The more rapidly the vital signs change, the more rapidly the patient's condition is changing.

Placing patients on a cardiac monitor for continuous monitoring is often appropriate. When patients do not require ongoing cardiac monitoring, the frequency with which vital signs are reassessed is somewhat debatable. The CCTP should determine an appropriate interval for this reassessment based on clinical findings, anticipated outcomes, and local practice protocols. Typically, reassessments are conducted every 5 to 15 minutes. Additional vital signs to consider include capnography, central venous pressures, ICP, airway pressures in intubated patients, and pulses in injured or cannulated extremities.

SpO_2 Versus SaO_2

The terms SpO_2 and SaO_2 are often erroneously interchanged.

- SpO_2, which stands for oxygen saturation as measured by pulse oximeter, measures the number of hemoglobin molecules passing the device's infrared light. Conventional pulse oximeters cannot distinguish when oxygen molecules, as opposed to other molecules, are saturating hemoglobin. Pulse oximeter readings are expressed as a percentage.

- SaO_2 stands for oxygen saturation as measured in the plasma by an arterial blood gas machine. Some point-of-care devices calculate SaO_2, in which case the value is expressed as $cSaO_2$.

Capnography

Capnography is a tool used to evaluate and monitor the respiratory carbon dioxide levels in critically ill

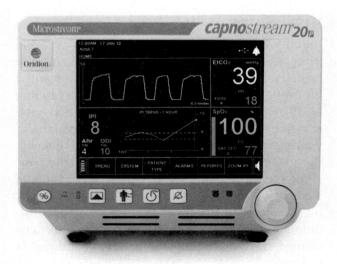

FIGURE 5-4 Capnography allows CCTPs to assess the respiratory status of critically ill patients by evaluating their respiratory carbon dioxide levels.

patients **FIGURE 5-4**. This reading may be obtained by measuring $ETCO_2$ via mainstream or side-stream sampling of exhaled gases, or by measuring the partial pressure of carbon dioxide (PCO_2) via blood gas sampling.

While there is little practical difference in mainstream and side-stream sampling, there is a difference between $ETCO_2$ and PCO_2 readings. $ETCO_2$ values will always be lower than PCO_2 values, as carbon dioxide diffuses from high-pressure to lower-pressure environments. Thus, for this gas to diffuse from the bloodstream to the lungs, the carbon dioxide concentration must always be higher in the bloodstream. The gradient between PCO_2 and $ETCO_2$ values in healthy patients is typically only 2 to 5 mm Hg. Because the normal PCO_2 level is 35 to 45 mm Hg, and given the small gradient between PCO_2 and $ETCO_2$ values, the same range is generally recorded for $ETCO_2$ even though it is expected to be slightly lower. However, in critically ill patients, particularly those with lung disease or a ventilation/perfusion mismatch, the gradient may be much larger. A focused review of critically ill patients being treated in ICUs found poor correlation between the two values and recommended against using $ETCO_2$ values as a surrogate for PCO_2 values. Thus, in critically ill patients, $ETCO_2$ is a reasonable tool to monitor for changes in their condition, but only PCO_2

should be used to monitor the ventilation strategy's effectiveness.

Evidence supports the use of $ETCO_2$ as an indicator of metabolic acidosis in critically ill patients with septic shock or diabetic ketoacidosis. $ETCO_2$ also represents cardiac output when ventilation and oxygenation are maintained at a steady state, which explains its use in monitoring the effectiveness of CPR.

Vital Signs as an Indicator of Underlying Diseases

When linked together, several groupings of vital signs can provide evidence for specific underlying disease states.

In *pulsus paradoxus*, the patient's BP declines by greater than 10 mm Hg during inspiration. In some patients, this condition may also be associated with the loss of peripheral pulses. Pulsus paradoxus needs to be considered within the overall context of the patient's clinical presentation and may indicate cardiac tamponade, advanced obstructive lung disease (chronic obstructive pulmonary disease and asthma), or croup; it occurs because of excessive pressures compressing the right side of the heart.

The *Beck triad* is the combination of three findings: hypotension or narrowed pulse pressure, muffled heart tones, and jugular venous distention. Beck triad is associated with pericardial tamponade, although studies have suggested it is actually present in fewer than 20% of these cases.

The *Cushing triad* is highly suggestive of increasing ICP and presents first with hypertension and tachycardia. Without intervention, it progresses to the classic findings of hypertension with a widened pulse pressure (declining diastolic BP), bradycardia, and abnormal respirations. While respirations are sometimes described as *decreased*, providers should look for abnormal breathing patterns such as Biot or Cheyne-Stokes respirations. Both of these patterns feature overall slow respirations, but the respirations are also highly irregular. Chapter 6, *Respiratory Emergencies and Airway Management*, further discusses breathing patterns.

Aortic dissections may be associated with different BP readings between the patient's right and left arms. The left arm often has a higher SBP, and a difference of greater than 20 mm Hg is suggestive of aortic dissection.

As patients progress through *hemorrhagic shock,* vital signs follow a predictable pattern. The body attempts to keep SBP at a normal level. As long as the body is compensating, SBP is relatively unchanged, while both pulse and respirations continuously increase. The more rapidly pulse and respirations are rising, the more quickly shock is progressing. Simultaneously, urine output decreases along with skin perfusion. Decompensated shock begins when both BP and mental state begin to decline.

Assessment of Severity

Many clinical scores are available to help clinicians objectively assess the severity of disease and injury. The CCTP must be proficient in selecting the correct assessment tool for the patient, administering it, and interpreting its results. It is often during the ongoing assessment phase, after the patient's most urgent needs have been addressed, that these tools come into play.

Assessment tools are often tailored to specific organ systems. For example, the Sequential [Sepsis-related] Organ Failure Assessment (SOFA) and quick SOFA (qSOFA) scores are used to rapidly identify life-threatening organ dysfunction caused by a dysregulated host response to infection, culminating in septic shock; these scores are discussed in detail in Chapter 10, *Resuscitation, Shock, and Blood Products.* Likewise, the shock index, which was discussed in the primary assessment portion of this chapter but is also applicable during the secondary assessment, is a predictor of post-intubation hypotension (score > 0.8) and cardiac arrest (score > 0.9).

Scales relating to pain and sedation tend to have wider application across patient encounters. Sedation scores should be obtained in all patients receiving ongoing sedation, including push-dose benzodiazepines. The most widely used ICU sedation score is the RASS score, introduced earlier in the chapter (Table 5-3). This scale has a range of +4 to −5. Patients with scores of +1 to +4 may require additional sedation, and those with a score of 0 are considered calm and alert. Providers sedating nonintubated patients should generally target a score of −1 or −2, whereas scores of −3 to −5 should be associated with only intubated patients during CCT.

Pain is a vital sign and should be monitored over time using validated pain scales. The perception and severity of pain are unique to each patient. Use a numeric pain scale of 0 to 10, where 0 is no pain and 10 is the worst pain the patient has ever experienced, when patients are at least 9 years of age and are able to communicate effectively with the transport team. The Wong-Baker FACES Pain Rating scale is appropriate for patients older than 3 years, including adults, who may have difficulty using a numeric scale **FIGURE 5-5**. Both the FLACC (Face, Legs, Activity, Cry, Consolability) scale **TABLE 5-5** and the CRIES (Crying, Requires oxygen, Increased vital signs, Expression [facial], and Sleeplessness) scale **TABLE 5-6** are validated scales for pediatric patients.

Reassess pain throughout transport, after analgesia, and following painful procedures. Premedicating patients with analgesia prior to painful procedures may be appropriate.

Wong-Baker FACES® Pain Rating Scale

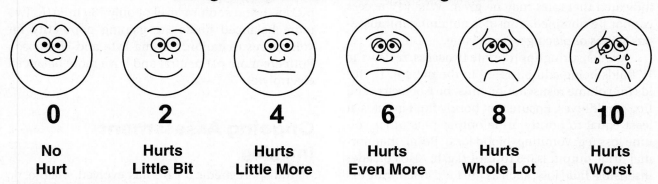

0	2	4	6	8	10
No Hurt	**Hurts Little Bit**	**Hurts Little More**	**Hurts Even More**	**Hurts Whole Lot**	**Hurts Worst**

FIGURE 5-5 The Wong-Baker FACES Pain Rating scale.

TABLE 5-5 FLACC Scale

Category	0	1	2
Face	Disinterested, no expression	Occasional grimace, withdrawn	Frequent frown, clenched jaw
Legs	No position or relaxed	Uneasy, restless, tense	Kicking or legs drawn up
Activity	Normal position, moves easily	Squirming, tense	Arched, rigid, or jerking
Cry	No crying	Moans or whimpers	Cries steadily, screams, or sobs
Consolability	Content, relaxed	Distractible	Inconsolable

Scores add up and range from 0 to 10.

© Jones & Bartlett Learning.

TABLE 5-6 CRIES Scale

Category	0	1	2
Crying	None	High-pitched	Inconsolable
Requires oxygen	None	<30% FIO_2 needed	>30% FIO_2 needed
Increased vital signs	Normal HR and BP	Increased HR and BP <20%	Increased HR and BP >20%
Expression	Normal	Grimace	Grimace and grunt
Sleeplessness	None	Wakes frequently	Awake constantly

Abbreviations: BP, blood pressure; FIO_2, fraction of inspired oxygen; HR, heart rate

© Jones & Bartlett Learning.

IV Access and Fluid Therapy

While completing your secondary assessment, ensure that the patient has appropriate IV access. Discuss your plan of care with the other team members, and review anticipated medication administrations. If the planned drugs are not compatible with each other, establish additional lines so that all indicated therapies may be given. When IV access cannot be obtained, consider obtaining intraosseous access or placing a central line.

After ensuring appropriate IV access, review the IV fluids being administered to the patient. IV fluids for volume resuscitation must be isoelectric and free of additives. Ensure that hourly fluid input is at least equal to hourly urine output plus other volume loss (eg, vomiting, blood loss). Recall that normal urine output is 0.5 to 1 mL/kg/h. Also consider insensible fluid loss, such as the fluid lost during exhalation—particularly when transporting pediatric patients. See Chapter 24, *Pediatric Emergencies*, for further details on the unique challenges of managing fluid volume in this population.

Different fluids can have different effects on patients; therefore, fluid selection must be carefully considered. Normal saline is actually hyperchloremic and has a pH of roughly 5.5. Lactated Ringer solution is more neutral, with a pH of 6.5; however, it is slightly hypotonic, with an osmolarity of 272 mOsm/L and sodium level of only 130 mEq/L. Two more balanced fluids are gaining popularity for volume resuscitation: Plasma-Lyte and Normosol. Both are more pH neutral and have more balanced electrolytes.

Ongoing Assessment
Imaging

As transport medical care has evolved, diagnostic tools previously available only within the confines of a hospital have been modified for use in the out-of-hospital setting. Imaging modalities such as ultrasonography, radiography, and computed tomography are increasingly available to CCT teams during patient transport. Imaging techniques are discussed broadly in Chapter 9, *Laboratory Analysis and Diagnostic Studies*, but also more specifically throughout this text in the context of specific injuries and illnesses.

In the context of the CCT team's assessment, providers will identify which imaging has been completed and why, determine which actions have been taken based on the imaging findings, and decide which additional imaging is still needed. The information gained from these studies can be indispensable in anticipating the patient's needs and monitoring the patient's ongoing condition and response to interventions. For example, ultrasonography provides a bedside assessment of cardiac status, allowing providers to grade the function and condition of the left and right ventricles; in effect, this tool provides rapid snapshots into cardiac output and thus a glimpse inside the patient's chest at the point of care.

Electrocardiography

Electrocardiography is a valuable tool to CCT teams, just as it is to their prehospital EMS counterparts. Beyond providing continuous monitoring of a patient undergoing transport, 12-lead electrocardiography is an essential diagnostic tool with innumerable uses, spanning the broad spectrum of patients seen by transport teams.

Twelve-lead electrocardiography can serve a purpose in settings other than the conventional cardiac transport. It can reveal useful information for patients with many disorders, including acute right ventricular failure, pulmonary embolism, metabolic disorders, and toxicologic issues. While Chapter 14, *Electrophysiology, Pacemakers, and Defibrillators*, provides a detailed review of the 12-lead electrocardiogram (ECG), CCTPs must be familiar with ECG findings associated not just with diagnostic criteria, but also treatment criteria. For example, a patient who has overdosed on tricyclic antidepressant (TCA) medication will present with ECG abnormalities associated with the resulting sodium channel blockade. ECG findings are routinely used as a treatment trigger, where widening QRS duration indicates sodium bicarbonate administration.

Electrocardiography is also valuable because it can be performed in a serial fashion. In the example of a TCA overdose, obtaining repeat 12-lead ECGs is necessary to monitor for worsening toxicity. Such monitoring is also important for patients with cardiac disorders, whereas a patient being transferred for non-ST-segment elevation myocardial infarction may develop ECG evidence of ST-segment elevation during transfer, prompting the need for emergent reperfusion therapy. Serial ECGs should be obtained whenever the patient's initial 12-lead ECG contained abnormal findings and following any change in the patient's condition.

Evaluating Tubes and Lines

Ongoing clinical care for many patients requiring interfacility transport involves insertion of invasive devices. CCTPs must recognize the indications for invasive equipment, assess each device's patency and effectiveness, and monitor for complications.

Gastric Tubes

Nasogastric and orogastric tubes may be placed to facilitate gastric decontamination, medication administration, or ongoing drainage of the upper GI system when treating bowel obstructions. In less common situations, a gastric tube may be placed to confirm a GI hemorrhage or to look for evidence of an esophageal rupture. Gastric tubes can help reduce the risk of aspiration but will not prevent it as a stand-alone intervention.

Nasogastric tubes are typically used unless a patient is unresponsive and intubated. When inspecting these tubes, ensure they are properly secured (ie, taped in place). Note the tube size and depth at the beginning and end of transports. The staff at the referring facility should have confirmed gastric tube placement via radiography before placing the tube on intermittent suction. When feasible, review the radiograph: Trace the gastric tube down the esophagus and observe the tip's position, which should be clearly visible below the diaphragm and at least 10 cm into the stomach. Although it is common to inject air into the stomach during gastric tube placement (listening for a "whoosh" sound), doing so is not an acceptable way of confirming placement. Observing gastric aspirate in the tube indicates that aspirate is being suctioned from the body, but it does not confirm where in the digestive tract the tube has been placed.

Once their placement is confirmed, gastric tubes are placed on low intermittent suction. It is reasonable to disconnect gastric tube suction while moving a patient to and from an ambulance; however, do not leave the tube capped throughout transport. Gastric tubes must continue to drain regularly to effectively remove the fluid developing within the upper GI tract.

Foley Catheters

A Foley catheter is indicated when patients have on-going incontinence or require accurate fluid output monitoring. Normal urine output is 0.5 to 1 mL/kg/h, but occasionally higher urine output is desired, such as in the treatment of rhabdomyolysis or fluid over-load. Foley catheters pose particularly high risk for infection, and the Centers for Medicare and Medicaid Services will not reimburse hospitals for infections associated with Foley catheter insertion. Thus, most health care systems will evaluate the need for continued Foley catheter use every 24 hours.

Begin assessing a Foley catheter by inspecting its entrance site. The site should be free of redness, drainage/discharge, and pain. Urine should be present in the catheter's tubing, and a small amount of blood is also occasionally present following insertion. Ensure the catheter's tubing is secured to the patient's leg with slack between the securing device and the urethra. Note the volume of urine, its color and clarity, and the presence/absence of any particulate matter or blood. Document these findings, and then drain the bag before departing the referring facility; beginning with an empty catheter bag makes it easier to document total output while the patient is your care.

Feeding Tubes

While feeding tubes are rarely placed in the emergency setting, they are used during prolonged hospitalizations to provide enteral nourishment directly into the GI tract. CCTPs may encounter feeding tubes during transfers between ICUs, during transfers to long-term acute care facilities, or when transporting a chronically ill patient experiencing decompensation or an acute illness. The types and purposes of feeding tubes are discussed in Chapter 17, *Gastrointestinal and Genitourinary Emergencies*.

To assess feeding tubes, begin by listening to the patient's bowel sounds. Palpate the patient's abdomen, noting rigidity or pain and tenderness; these signs or vomiting may indicate a feeding tube complication and the need to discontinue feedings. Inspect the stoma where the feeding tube enters the patient. The skin around this hole should not be inflamed or irritated, and there should be no discharge. When the tube is initially inserted, gauze is placed between the feeding tube's flange and the skin; replace this gauze if it is discolored, wet, or dirty.

All patients with a prepyloric tube (ie, a tube that enters the GI tract above the pyloric sphincter) must have their head elevated at least 30° to prevent aspiration; placing the patient supine, even for a short time, creates a risk that gastric contents will migrate up the esophagus and into the hypopharynx. When placing these patients supine, such as for lifting and moving, temporarily pause the feeding. Continue ordered feedings as soon as the patient's head is returned to its elevated position. Enteric nutrition mixes often contain only simple sugars; therefore, discontinuing feeding poses a risk of hypoglycemia. Note that when patients cannot reliably sit up, postpyloric tubes are useful, as they are less likely to be associated with aspiration. Be sure to document the total volume of nourishment administered during transport.

External Ventricular Drains

For the purposes of the secondary assessment, the CCTP must assess the functionality of, and patient's response to, any external ventricular drain (EVD). The management and monitoring of EVDs is discussed in great detail in Chapter 12, *Neurologic Emergencies*. Assessment of the EVD should occur upon patient contact and after all major patient movements, including when moving the patient from one bed to another, after loading the patient into the transport unit, and after unloading the patient at the destination facility.

To assess an EVD, first review the orders for ICP monitoring and cerebrospinal fluid drainage. After reviewing the orders, evaluate the system, beginning at the patient. Never advance or withdraw an EVD! Ensure the drain is properly secured and the tubing is not kinked. Trace the tubing to the ICP drain and confirm all connections are tight. Align the ICP drain with the foramen of Monro, which is roughly in line with the tragus of the ear.

Re-zero the drain once it is connected to the transport monitor and after all major patient movements. Air medical transport teams must re-zero the drain upon reaching cruising elevation and after descent.

Assembling the Assessed Information

After reviewing the written information received from the referring facility, the findings from the CCTP's own patient examination, current lab values, the patient's response to therapeutic interventions, and the patency of any invasive equipment, the CCTP should develop a problem list. A problem list is effectively a differential diagnosis that defines associated symptoms or concerns that may require management during transport. For example, the differential diagnosis for a patient with acute coronary syndrome may include non-ST-segment elevation myocardial infarction that is associated with hypertension and pain, both of which will require management. Identifying the anticipated problems allows the CCTP to prioritize interventions and prepare for potential complications during transport.

Life threats, including potentially impending life threats, should be managed before initiating transport. When these conditions cannot be stabilized by the referring facility or transport team, an emergency transport is likely indicated. Identified conditions with anticipated problems that are unlikely to develop for hours or days can be managed during transport. For example, if an open fracture is the identified condition, one problem the transport team can anticipate is infection. The team can reduce the risk of infection by administering antibiotics.

While it is reasonable for CCT teams to initiate new interventions to stabilize patients prior to transport, a caveat applies: As the number of on-scene interventions increases, so does the scene time. The need to treat the patient on scene must be weighed against delayed delivery to definitive care. Limit on-scene interventions to those addressing severe pain, major life threats, or deterioration from baseline. Otherwise, consider deferring new interventions until transport has been initiated.

Communications With Receiving Facilities

While it might seem counterintuitive that staff at a hospital that has accepted a transfer might not know what they will need to care for the patient, often acceptance of transport simply involves approval from a house supervisor, acceptance by a physician, and confirmation of an available bed. Particularly after long transports, the staff receiving a patient may have had no direct communication with the staff at the sending facility, a particularly common scenario after a shift change. To ensure the staff at the receiving facility are prepared to treat the patient, contact the facility 20 to 30 minutes prior to your anticipated arrival and provide an update to the nurse or clinical team who will be caring for the patient. If you anticipate that the initial bed destination may be inappropriate and an upgrade to an ICU bed may be indicated, contact the facility even earlier, because many hospitals have limited ICU beds availability.

Transferring care to a referring facility is a high-risk opportunity for loss of important information. To avoid the loss of critical information during a transfer of care, employ critical communication strategies during the handoff. Further, take the time during and after the transfer to ensure your written patient care report provides an accurate reflection of the quality care your team provided. These skills are discussed further in Chapter 2, *Medical-Legal Issues*, and Chapter 3, *Patient Safety*.

Summary

The patient assessment is an essential skill for CCTPs. A complete patient assessment creates the foundation for a differential diagnosis and problem list and enables teams to develop meaningful treatment plans. Assessments performed by CCT teams extend beyond scene size-up, safety, and primary and secondary assessments. The CCT assessment includes a thorough review of the originating facility reports, a verbal report from the referring staff, a comprehensive primary and secondary assessment, a review of interventions and invasive medical equipment as well as their impact on the patient, and a review of pertinent lab values. Your assessment may be supported by a variety of advanced technology.

Never rush or short-change a patient assessment; this process is critical in ensuring success for both the transport team and the patient. Taking the time to obtain a complete picture of the patient's condition and progression helps improve outcomes. Remember, patients will change over time.

Perform repeat assessments as necessary throughout the transport. Communicate early with receiving facilities to ensure they are prepared to treat the patient upon arrival, and use standardized communication strategies to help minimize the risk of information loss during the transfer of care.

Case Study

You and your CCT team are providing an interfacility transport of a 48-year-old man who presented to the ED with severe chest pain. The patient was diagnosed with acute myocardial infarction, and an intra-aortic balloon pump (IABP) was inserted. The patient was admitted to the ICU while awaiting transport to the specialty heart hospital.

En route to the hospital, your crew receives an update on the patient's condition. The patient's vital signs are as follows: blood pressure, 120/75 mm Hg; pulse rate, 110 beats/min; respiratory rate, 30 breaths/min; and pulse oximetry reading, 93%. The patient is on 4 L of oxygen by nasal cannula. He continues to report chest pain, rating his pain as an 8 on a scale of 1 to 10. He also reports severe back pain.

On your crew's arrival, you find the patient in the ICU. You and your team receive a report from the ICU nurse. She states that the patient presented to the ED this morning around 0830 hours, reporting severe chest pain. He was given an aspirin, started on a nitroglycerin drip, and administered a total of 5 mg of morphine. Blood was drawn for lab analysis. The ICU nurse hands you the lab results. You review the results and report the findings to the rest of your crew. The lab results were as follows:

- Calcium: 9.5 mg/dL (normal range, 8.2 to 10.2 mg/dL)
- Chloride: 100 mEq/L (normal range, 96 to 106 mEq/L)
- Magnesium: 2.0 mEq/L (normal range, 1.3 to 2.1 mEq/L)
- Potassium: 4.0 mEq/L (normal range, 3.5 to 5.0 mEq/L)
- Sodium: 142 mEq/L (normal range, 136 to 142 mEq/L)

- Hemoglobin: 14.4 g/dL (normal range, 14.0 to 17.5 g/dL)
- Hematocrit: 45% (normal range, 41% to 50%)
- White blood cell count: 10,400/μL (normal range, 4,500 to 11,000/μL)
- Platelet count: 210×10^3/μL (normal range, 150 to 350×10^3/μL)
- Creatine kinase-MB: 3.5 ng/mL (normal range, 0 to 7 ng/mL)
- Creatine kinase: 100 U/L (normal range, 40 to 150 U/L)
- Cholesterol: total, 198 mg/dL (normal range, 200 to 239 mg/dL); high-density lipoprotein, 278 mg/dL (normal range, 40 mg/dL); low-density lipoprotein, 32 mg/dL (normal range, 160 mg/dL); triglycerides, 205 mg/dL (normal range, 160 mg/dL)

The arterial blood gas measurement results were as follows:

- pH: 7.30 (normal range, 7.35 to 7.45)
- $Paco_2$: 55 mm Hg (normal range, 35 to 45 mm Hg)
- HCO_3^-: 25 mEq/L (normal range, 21 to 28 mEq/L)
- Po_2: 93 mm Hg (normal range, 80 to 100 mm Hg)

An ECG revealed sinus tachycardia with right axis deviation.

As you enter the patient's room, you find the patient lying supine, with 4 L of oxygen being delivered via nasal cannula. The patient is attached to the bedside cardiac monitor and the IABP. The cardiac monitor reveals a pulse rate of 130 beats/min, a blood pressure of 145/96 mm Hg, and a pulse oximetry reading of 93%. The patient is awake, is oriented, and follows all commands.

His skin is paler than his baseline color. His respiratory rate is 30 breaths/min.

Your patient assessment reveals the following:

- **Cardiopulmonary assessment:** The patient's airway is patent, with a slight decrease in chest rise on the right side. Breath sounds are present bilaterally, but slightly diminished on the right side. No wheezes, crackles, or rhonchi are noted. Respiratory effort is labored. No subcutaneous emphysema is noted on palpation. The patient's skin is pale and diaphoretic. Capillary refill is 4 s. No murmur, rubs, friction, or gallops are noted on auscultation of the heart. Pulses are equal in pattern, intensity, and quality in all four extremities. The ECG reveals sinus tachycardia with a rate of 133 beats/min. No pitting edema is noted in the extremities.
- **Neurologic assessment:** The patient has a GCS score of 15. He is able to move all four extremities without difficulty. His pupils are equal, round, and reactive to light. All cranial nerves are intact.
- **GI assessment:** No ascites or bruising is noted on inspection of the abdominal area. The abdomen is soft, with no tenderness or distention on palpation. No masses or hernias are noted. No rebound tenderness is present. Auscultation of the abdomen reveals hyperactive bowel sounds. The patient denies having vomited blood or blood with a coffee-ground appearance and also denies having had dark, tarry stools.
- **Musculoskeletal assessment:** The patient is able to move all four extremities without difficulty. All reflexes are intact. No swelling to extremities is present. Pulses are present in all extremities.

1. Which complications could be occurring with this patient?
2. What do the lab values, arterial blood gas results, and ECG reveal?
3. What is your general impression of this patient?
4. Which additional information should you request from the hospital? Would you request any other test(s) prior to transport of this patient?

Analysis

This patient presented with severe chest pain that started 2 hours prior to his arrival at the ED. The patient stated that the pain occurred suddenly and nothing he did relieved it. He described the pain as sharp, and originally rated it as a 10 on a scale of 1 to 10. The ED physician made a diagnosis of acute myocardial infarction based on borderline lab values. An IABP was inserted and arrangements were made to transport the patient to a specialty heart hospital. The transport crew received the update that the patient was having severe back and chest pain.

The crew's first concerns while en route to the patient included dissection of the aorta, which is a potential complication after an IABP insertion. The classic presentation of an aortic dissection is chest and back pain. The crew discovered that a chest radiograph had not been obtained and asked for an updated chest radiograph. A chest radiograph should be performed before and after IABP insertion.

The lab results and ECG in this case did not confirm the physician's diagnosis of a myocardial infarction. More testing is needed to confirm an accurate diagnosis. The general impression of this patient is that he is in respiratory distress. Further investigation is warranted because of the possibility of heart failure, respiratory infection, or pneumothorax. Assessment reveals the possibility of a pneumothorax, which must be investigated further—for example, with the chest radiograph already requested.

In addition to the chest radiograph, the CCTP should consider requesting a rapid (point-of-care) determination of the patient's troponin level. Troponin is a cardiac enzyme specific to injuries of the cardiac muscle. Physicians diagnose myocardial infarction based on several factors, including an ECG, lab values, and patient presentation.

In terms of assessment and treatment, the patient has diminished breath sounds on the right side of the chest. He has labored respirations, and arterial blood gas determinations revealed respiratory acidosis, which are all classic signs of a pneumothorax and possible tension pneumothorax. In situations in which you believe more testing should be done to determine the diagnosis, the members of the CCT team should discuss their assessment findings and ask whether a radiograph or other relevant test can confirm their assessment. Professional and nonconfrontational communication patterns are expected. Respectful behavior on the part of the CCTP, regardless of the situation, helps to promote positive working relationships, whereas disrespect or negativity may result in a referring facility no longer calling that particular CCT service. If the physician disagrees with your team, a team member should contact the medical director and have this person contact the sending physician to help determine the best course of action.

In this case, on the crew's arrival to pick up the patient, the relieving attending physician stated that chest radiography revealed a pneumothorax. After chest tube insertion, the patient was transported to the specialty facility and was evaluated.

No cardiac problems were found.

Prep Kit

Ready for Review

- A comprehensive patient assessment is one of the most important skills critical care transport professionals (CCTPs) perform. It builds the foundation for the treatment plan.
- Assessment of critical care patients differs from the traditional emergency medical services field assessment in two respects: Critical care patients have often received significant treatment and stabilization prior to the CCTP's arrival, and sophisticated diagnostic information is often available.
- As part of prearrival planning, the CCTP team should consider the reason for transport, the type of facility from which the transfer originates, the length and mode of transport, and the type of destination facility. All of these considerations provide valuable clues in anticipating the patient's needs.
- Upon arrival, the CCTP should carefully review all available information from the sending facility, including any available patient care records, and should take the time to understand the patient as a person, including cultural preferences.
- CCTPs should be familiar with the assessment process used to establish the initial care plan and have an understanding of pathophysiology and differential diagnosis so that they can make appropriate treatment decisions and assess the effects of treatments.

- The systems-based assessment approach recognizes that critical care patients are usually receiving treatment for problems involving multiple systems and interrelated complications.
- The SAMPLE approach can be used to establish the pertinent details of a patient's history—Signs and symptoms, Allergies, Medications, Pertinent past medical history, Last oral intake, and Events leading up to the illness or injury. Providers should strive to obtain in-depth details for each component.
- The patient's history includes the referring facility's management. Specifically, the CCTP should determine any diagnostic tests and imaging performed and their results, the differential diagnosis, and any interventions performed and the patient's response to them.
- During the primary assessment, providers place absolute priority on quickly identifying any acute life threats. This brief exam should seldom take more than 60 seconds, as acutely life-threatening problems require timely intervention.
- The primary assessment follows a stepwise, rapid evaluation of organ systems and anatomy fundamentally necessary for life. The ABCDE mnemonic, which stands for Airway, Breathing, Circulation, Disability, and Exposure, is often used to guide this process.

Prep Kit Continued

- The primary assessment of the airway involves determining whether the patient's airway is "safe," meaning the airway is patent and ventilation appears to be effective. If not, the team may need to establish an effective airway, possibly by correcting existing interventions (eg, correction of an inappropriately placed endotracheal tube).
- Primary assessment of the respiratory system involves detecting any injury or illness that is directly affecting the respiratory system. Providers must understand the implications of irregularity in the respiratory rate for other body systems and processes.
- When assessing mechanical ventilation, the CCTP must ensure the patient is receiving ventilatory support that is both adequate and not injurious to the lungs.
- Assessment of the circulatory system requires the collation of information from multiple diagnostic sources, including the physical exam, monitoring equipment, and other diagnostic tools. Skin color, temperature, and condition can provide a valuable initial glimpse into illness severity.
- During the primary assessment, the evaluation of vital signs is limited to looking for evidence of acute instability. However, providers should keep in mind that their initial documentation establishes the reference point against which later recordings will be compared.
- Blood pressure can be a valuable clinical parameter, but it is important to remember that normal blood pressure may differ for individual patients. A more objective means of assessing perfusion status is mean arterial pressure.
- Before transport, trends in blood pressure over time should be noted, especially in response to cardiogenic medications and interventions.
- How frequently vital signs are assessed is dictated by the patient's condition and may range from continuous to every 15 minutes.

- During assessment of the gastrointestinal system, examination of the oral mucosa and abdominal areas provides general information.
- In gastrointestinal assessment, auscultation of the abdomen precedes palpation and percussion.
- Palpation of the abdomen can determine tenderness and rebound tenderness.
- Genitourinary assessment includes assessments of the mammary, testicular, and prostate glands. Such exams are generally limited except in the case of trauma.
- During the primary assessment of a patient who has sustained traumatic injury, providers must seek sources of hemorrhage. Although life-threatening external hemorrhage will likely have been controlled before the transport team arrives, CCTPs must ensure continued efficacy of the bleeding control.
- Examination for external hemorrhage must be done early and in a systematic fashion. It includes an extremity sweep and inspection of the chest, abdomen, and back.
- Internal hemorrhage can be difficult to detect and requires thoughtful consideration of the mechanism of injury and detection of external signs of blunt trauma, such as skin abrasions and contusions. Palpation may reveal point tenderness over solid organs.
- Twelve-lead electrocardiography is an essential diagnostic tool. It can reveal useful information for patients with many disorders, including acute right ventricular failure, pulmonary embolism, metabolic disorders, and toxicologic issues.
- Before the critical care transport begins, a neurologic exam is necessary to establish the patient's baseline status for comparison with the findings from later examinations.
- Neurologic evaluations should be repeated frequently, noting relevant findings, such as the patient's level of consciousness, the Glasgow Coma Scale score, the Richmond Agitation–Sedation Scale score, cranial nerve assessment,

Prep Kit Continued

and pupil assessment, including size, reactivity to light, and shape.

- As the final step in the ABCDE approach to the primary assessment, the CCTP should expose the patient to conduct a rapid head-to-toe, anterior and posterior, assessment of the entire patient. Exposure enables the CCTP to more fully determine the severity of injuries, confirm ongoing effectiveness of wound management performed prior to the team's arrival, and assess the skin for edema and pressure injuries. Providers must guard against hypothermia in the exposed patient.

- The secondary assessment involves several components, including a detailed head-to-toe examination, a systems-based approach to specific diseases, and a complete evaluation of vital signs.

- The secondary assessment involves review of the basic vital signs (ie, pulse rate, blood pressure, respiratory rate, pulse oximetry, mental state, and temperature). Capnography is often used at this stage to evaluate and monitor the respiratory carbon dioxide levels in critically ill patients.

- A key reason for conducting the secondary assessment is to detect changes in the patient's condition. Typically, reassessments are performed every 5 to 15 minutes.

- During the secondary assessment, CCTPs may need to incorporate scales relating to pain and sedation. The CCTP must be proficient in selecting the correct assessment tool for the patient, administering it, and interpreting its results.

- CCTPs should prepare for the patient's medication needs before initiating transfer. They should examine any intravenous lines already started and ensure they will have the access needed for any medications they anticipate administering.

- Imaging modalities such as ultrasonography, radiography, and computed tomography are increasingly available to teams during patient transport. Providers will identify which imaging has been completed and why, determine which actions have been taken based on the imaging findings, and decide which additional imaging is still needed.

- The ongoing clinical care for many patients requiring interfacility transport involves insertion of invasive devices. CCTPs must recognize the indications for invasive equipment, assess each device's patency and effectiveness, and monitor for complications.

- Regardless of the patient's condition, CCTPs should always strive for compassionate and empathetic interactions with the patient and family, even in the face of critical illness.

- Assessment findings before transfer, en route, and after arrival at the destination facility (based on the acuity of the patient) should be documented.

- The medical record should include documentation of all assessment findings, as even subtle changes in an individual patient or an individual finding may be significant in critical-level patients.

Vital Vocabulary

ABCDE A mnemonic used to help providers remember the patient assessment sequence: Airway, Breathing, Circulation, Disability, and Exposure.

anisocoria A condition in which the pupils are not of equal size.

AVPU scale An evaluation tool used to determine patient responsiveness; stands for Alert, responds to Voice, responds to Pain, Unresponsive.

capillary refill time (CRT) The time it takes for baseline skin color to return to the nail bed after

Prep Kit Continued

being pressed by the provider; serves as a window into the state of peripheral perfusion.

community hospitals Community medical centers that offer emergency medicine and inpatient facilities but with limited inpatient specialists other than hospitalists and general surgery physicians.

critical-access hospitals As defined by the Centers for Medicare and Medicaid Services, hospitals that have 25 or fewer beds, are located more than 35 miles from another hospital, have an average length of stay of less than 96 hours, and provide 24/7 emergency medicine services. Most acutely ill or injured patients treated at these hospitals require transport to higher levels of care once stabilized.

differential diagnosis The process of selecting the most likely underlying cause of the patient's condition by comparing multiple potential causes of the presenting signs and symptoms.

Glasgow Coma Scale (GCS) An evaluation tool used to determine level of consciousness, which evaluates and assigns point values (scores) for eye opening, verbal response, and motor response, which are then totaled; effective in helping predict patient outcomes.

hippus phenomenon A pattern of pupil response to light in which rapid constriction of the pupil is followed by dilation; it can be normal or signify compression of cranial nerve III.

mean arterial pressure (MAP) The average arterial pressure during a single cardiac cycle.

Murphy sign A painful reaction elicited by asking the patient to take and hold a deep breath as the provider palpates the right subcostal area; if pain occurs on inspiration, when the inflamed gallbladder comes in contact with the provider's hand, Murphy sign is positive. May signal the presence of gallbladder problems.

pallor Skin presentation suggestive of reduced blood flow or oxygenation. In patients with light skin, paleness typically presents as unusual lightness compared with the person's baseline skin color. In patients with dark skin, pallor may appear as ashen or gray skin on general assessment. In general, the mucous membranes inside the inner lower eyelid and the oral mucosa will have a pink coloration in all healthy patients, regardless of skin color; thus, a white or pale appearance of these areas in any patient suggests reduced blood flow or oxygenation.

primary assessment A brief assessment of the patient's condition in which providers quickly identify any acute life threats. This survey follows a stepwise, rapid evaluation of organ systems and anatomy fundamentally necessary for life, often described as the ABCDE (Airway, Breathing, Circulation, Disability, and Exposure) approach.

primary care centers Medical centers that offer outpatient, routine family medicine services, including obstetrics and gynecology, geriatric care, and pediatric primary care, and that coordinate patient care with outpatient specialists as appropriate.

quaternary care centers Highly specialized tertiary care referral centers that may be dedicated to advancing clinical research in one or more areas of medicine.

rhabdomyolysis A condition in which damaged skeletal muscle tissue breaks down rapidly.

Richmond Agitation–Sedation Scale (RASS) An evaluation tool used to assess both agitation and sedation.

SAMPLE An acronym for the pertinent details of a patient's history: Signs and symptoms, Allergies, Medications, Pertinent past medical history, Last oral intake, and Events leading up to the illness or injury.

secondary assessment A patient assessment that occurs after completing the primary assessment and identifying and stabilizing immediate life threats and hemodynamic instability. The secondary assessment involves several components,

Prep Kit Continued

including a detailed head-to-toe examination, a systems-based approach to specific diseases, and a complete evaluation of vital signs.

secondary care centers Medical centers that may offer primary care within the same facility but also offer outpatient specialties such as cardiology, neurology, nephrology, mental health, endocrinology, or oncology.

sequelae Consequence of a previous disease or injury.

shock index An evaluation tool used to predict mortality and the need for transfusion in the trauma patient; defined as heart rate divided by systolic blood pressure.

tertiary care centers Medical centers that offer highly specialized inpatient medical care, including advanced and complex medical interventions performed by specialty physicians.

working diagnosis An assumed decision on the medical condition of a patient based on the preliminary investigation; assists in the provision of initial treatment and projection of further diagnostic testing requirements.

References

Acker SN, Ross JT, Partrick DA, et al. Pediatric specific shock index accurately identifies severely injured children. *J Pediatr Surg*. 2015;50(2):331-334.

Bickley LS. *Bates Guide to Physical Examination and History Taking*. 13th ed. Philadelphia, PA: Lippincott; 2020.

Collopy K, Langston B, Powers WF IV. Patient care alterations following point of care lab testing during critical care transport. *Air Med J*. 2016;35(5):285.

Eastman J, Allen D, Mumma K, et al. Point-of care laboratory data collection during critical care transport. *Air Med J*. 2020;40(1):81-83.

Hernández G, Ospina-Tascón GA, Petri Damiani L. Effect of a resuscitation strategy targeting peripheral perfusion status vs serum lactate levels on 28-day mortality among patients with septic shock: the ANDROMEDA-SHOCK randomized clinical trial. *JAMA*. 2019;321(7):654-664.

Hernandez-Boussard T, Davies S, McDonald K, Wang NE. Interhospital facility transfers in the United States: a nationwide outcomes study. *J Patient Safety*. 2017;13(4):187-191.

Hickey JV, Strayer AL. *The Clinical Practice of Neurological and Neurosurgical Nursing*. 8th ed. Philadelphia, PA: Lippincott; 2019.

Kreit JW. Volume capnography in the intensive care unit: potential clinical applications. *Ann Am Thorac Soc*. 2019;16(4):409-420.

Morton P, Fontaine D. *Critical Care Nursing: A Holistic Approach*. 11th ed. Philadelphia, PA: Lippincott; 2017.

Stolz L, Valenzuela J, Situ-LaCasse E, et al. Clinical and historical features of emergency department patients with pericardial effusions. *World J Emerg Med*. 2017;8(1):29-33.

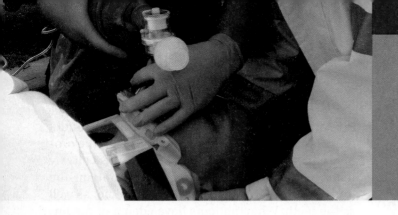

Chapter 6

Respiratory Emergencies and Airway Management

Lauren M. Maloney, MD, NRP, FP-C, NCEE

Rudolph Princi, BS, EMT-P

OBJECTIVES

After completing this chapter, you will be able to:

1. Summarize the anatomy and physiology of the respiratory system (pp 156–162).
2. Describe how ventilation and perfusion abnormalities affect blood gas values (pp 162–164).
3. Name the five requirements for normal ventilation and oxygenation (p 164).
4. Define tidal volume, vital capacity, and minute volume (pp 164–165).
5. Differentiate between obstructive and restrictive diseases (p 165).
6. Interpret normal and abnormal breath sounds (pp 166–168).
7. Describe particular clinical events that alter the functioning of the respiratory system in the critical care patient (pp 165–166).
8. Review the breath sound assessment technique used in critical care transport patients (pp 166–168).

9. Perform a basic respiratory assessment for adequacy of ventilation and oxygenation using inspection, auscultation, palpation, and noninvasive monitoring (pp 166–169).
10. Identify abnormal respiratory patterns (pp 169–171).
11. Assess a respiratory cycle (pp 164–171).
12. Identify the parameters measured in arterial blood gas monitoring and which parameter reflects the effectiveness of ventilation and oxygenation (p 172).
13. Discuss basic airway management strategies (pp 176–181).
14. Discuss advanced airway management strategies (pp 181–215).
15. Describe how pulse oximetry, capnometry, and capnography can be used to monitor respiratory function (pp 172–176).

Introduction

There is no more important—or controversial—skill associated with prehospital care than airway management. The ability to assess and manage the airway at the basic life support (BLS) level is the starting point in airway management. For advanced life support (ALS) providers, it is a standard to fall back on. This assessment will guide the critical care transport professional (CCTP) in developing a treatment plan that may be as simple as providing supplemental oxygen to a spontaneously breathing patient, or as complex as placing an artificial airway device or providing adequate ventilation with a bag-mask device or ventilator.

Ensuring the adequacy of ventilation and oxygenation in critically ill patients is one of the primary treatment goals of the CCTP. A thorough understanding of respiratory function and assessment is essential to meet this goal. The patient history and a focused physical exam, in conjunction with the analysis of hemodynamic parameters, laboratory values, and diagnostic imaging, all provide key information about the functioning of the patient's respiratory system. When respiratory compromise occurs during transport, time is critical, and you as a CCTP must be prepared to perform a rapid, accurate respiratory assessment followed by implementation of the appropriate intervention.

Anatomy and Physiology of the Respiratory System

An understanding of airway anatomy and physiology is essential to successful airway management.

Upper Airway Structures

Important airway structures of the upper airway include the nose, mouth, pharynx, and larynx, which contains the epiglottis.

Nose

The nose is a cartilaginous, bony structure in the midline of the face that warms and humidifies inspired air. It is lined with coarse hairs in the vestibular area, which act as a filter to trap small, inspired particles. Olfaction (sense of smell) also originates here via the first cranial nerve (olfactory nerve). The nasal cavities connect to the four sinuses: frontal, ethmoidal, sphenoidal, and maxillary. These sinuses are hollow chambers lined with membranes that secrete mucus into the nasal cavities. The nasal cavity subsequently opens into the nasopharynx.

The nose, which is extremely vascular, can be a significant source of epistaxis. Such bleeding may complicate airway patency and management.

Mouth

Primarily designed for phonation and mastication, the mouth begins at the lips and ends with the oropharynx. The size of the oral cavity can affect airway management **FIGURE 6-1**. The mouth contains the tongue, which is attached to the mandible, as well as the teeth. When patients have edema of the lingual or sublingual spaces, both of these structures can make airway management more difficult. Additionally, prominent central incisors (buck teeth) or conditions affecting the mandible's range of motion can make airway management more difficult, as they could interfere with insertion of the laryngoscope blade. Salivary glands continuously secrete saliva, which may make achieving topical anesthesia and visualizing airway structures difficult.

In the unconscious patient, the tongue is the most common cause of airway obstruction. A simple jaw-thrust maneuver may temporarily alleviate this airway obstruction and allow for effective bag-mask ventilation.

Pharynx

The pharynx is a U-shaped tube that begins at the base of the skull and extends to the lower border of the cricoid cartilage, a complete ring structure located at the level of C6, near the esophagus **FIGURE 6-2**. It is composed of three parts: the nasopharynx, the oropharynx, and the hypopharynx (or laryngopharynx):

- The nasopharynx extends from the posterior choana (the posterior portion of the nasal cavity) of the nose to the soft palate. It contains the adenoid tissue and the eustachian tubes.
- The oropharynx extends from the soft palate to the vallecula. It is the portion that is visible when the mouth is opened.
- The hypopharynx is the portion of the pharynx found inferior to the epiglottis.

The normal resting muscle tone of the oropharynx maintains upper airway patency. The ninth cranial nerve, the glossopharyngeal nerve, provides sensory innervation to many of the structures in this area (posterior tongue, valleculae, and parts of the epiglottis). The inferior portion of the pharynx ends with the entrance to both the trachea and the esophagus.

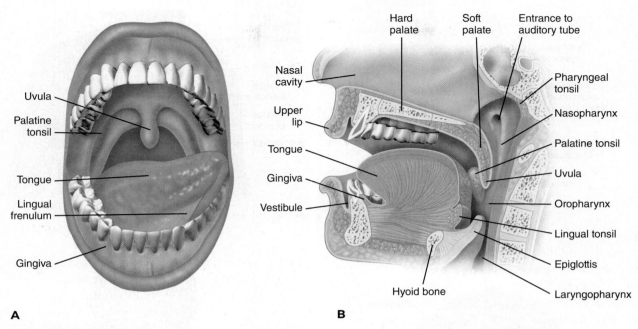

FIGURE 6-1 The oral cavity. **A.** Anterior view. **B.** Lateral view.

© Jones & Bartlett Learning.

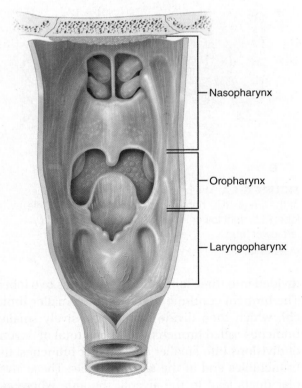

FIGURE 6-2 The pharynx.

© Jones & Bartlett Learning.

Larynx

The structures contained within the larynx consist of the thyroid cartilage, aryepiglottic folds, epiglottis, vallecula, and arytenoid cartilages **FIGURE 6-3**. The larynx is the final structure encountered before entering the trachea. The 10th cranial nerve, the vagus nerve, provides strong sensory innervation to the larynx. Overstimulation of the larynx during airway management may cause parasympathetic nervous system stimulation, resulting in significantly decreased heart rate and blood pressure, especially in the pediatric population. The cricothyroid membrane is also located here, extending from the lower surface of the cricoid cartilage to the upper border of the thyroid cartilage. In the adult patient, the cricothyroid membrane is approximately 6 to 8 mm from superior to inferior border.

Lower Airway Structures

Important structures of the lower airway include the trachea, right and left main stem bronchi, bronchioles, alveolar ducts, and alveolar sacs.

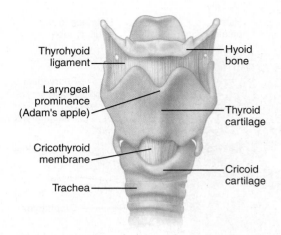

A

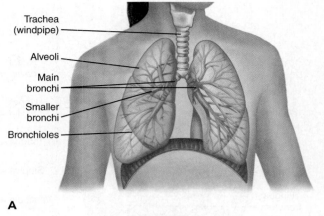

A

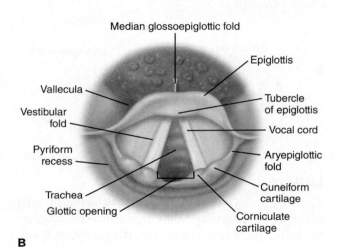

B

FIGURE 6-3 A. The larynx. **B.** The glottis and surrounding structures.

© Jones & Bartlett Learning.

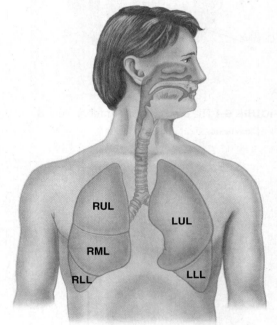

B

FIGURE 6-4 A. The respiratory system. **B.** The lobes of the lungs: RUL, right upper lobe; RML, right middle lobe; RLL, right lower lobe; LUL, left upper lobe; LLL, left lower lobe.

© Jones & Bartlett Learning.

Trachea

Beginning at the inferior border of the cricoid ring and ending at the carina, the trachea is approximately 9 to 15 mm in diameter and approximately 12 to 15 cm long. It is not cylindrical, but rather is composed of 16 to 20 C-shaped cartilaginous rings on the anterior portion, with the posterior portion consisting of fibrous tissue and muscular fibers. These rings help maintain luminal patency to allow unimpeded airflow. The trachea is larger in adult males than in adult females.

Lungs

The trachea divides into the right and left main stem bronchi, which lead to the right and left lobes of the lungs, respectively **FIGURE 6-4**. The right lung is

divided into three lobes; the left lung has two lobes. The bronchi continue to divide into smaller bronchi, which then divide into progressively smaller branches called bronchioles. After a total of dozens of divisions into smaller and smaller branches, the bronchioles end at the alveolar ducts. These alveolar ducts lead to the alveoli, the area where gas exchange occurs. The adult lung contains approximately 300 million alveoli, each one in contact with a pulmonary capillary. This interface is referred to as the alveolar-capillary membrane.

An alveolus is composed of type I and type II squamous epithelial cells. Type I cells are involved in gas exchange, whereas type II cells manufacture surfactant. Surfactant, a phospholipid, reduces the surface tension within the alveolus, preventing its collapse and making it easier for the alveolus to expand during inhalation. Without surfactant, the work of breathing would be significantly more difficult. A lack of surfactant is commonly found in premature neonates and is a leading cause of respiratory issues in this patient population. Another type of cell, the alveolar macrophage, is also present in the alveolus; its function is to help defend the body by ingesting inhaled particles.

The blood supply in the lung arises from the right ventricle. The pulmonary trunk then splits into the right and left pulmonary arteries. The pulmonary arteries contain deoxygenated blood that is high in carbon dioxide (CO_2). These arteries subdivide into the pulmonary capillaries.

The pulmonary vasculature is a low-pressure system. The pressure in the normal pulmonary artery is approximately 25/10 mm Hg, as compared with a normal systemic pressure of approximately 120/80 mm Hg. For gas exchange to occur, blood flow must be in contact with the alveoli, a relationship described by the $\dot{V}/\dot{Q}$ ratio. The normal ratio is 0.8 for the entire lung. This means that for every 4 L of air ($\dot{V}$), a blood flow ($\dot{Q}$) of 5 L is needed. Gravitational effects cause perfusion to be better in areas that are positioned lower (dependent areas) and ventilation to be better in higher (nondependent) areas. Changes in the $\dot{V}/\dot{Q}$ ratio are one of the most common causes of hypoxemia (low oxygen level). Disruptions in the respiratory system can include changes in gravity, pulmonary artery pressure, alveolar pressure, airway obstruction, and lung compliance. Many diseases can cause these changes, including chronic obstructive pulmonary disease (COPD), pulmonary embolism, heart failure (HF), and pneumonia, to name a few.

Pediatric Considerations

Several variations in airway anatomy occur that are specific to the pediatric patient. Newborns and infants, for instance, have a proportionally larger head with a prominent occiput. This may cause flexion of the airway and create difficulty in visualizing laryngeal structures unless proper positioning is maintained. For example, placing a towel under the infant's shoulders

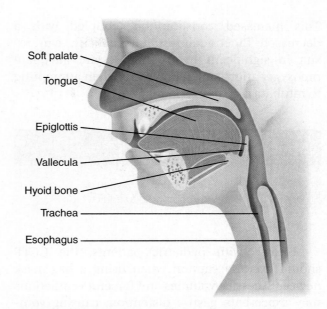

FIGURE 6-5 The child's epiglottis and surrounding structures.
© Jones & Bartlett Learning.

to raise the rest of the body to align the airway axes usually improves airflow and direct laryngoscopy visualization. Infants are also obligate nose breathers, and congestion may result in respiratory distress.

The tongue occupies a much larger proportion of the oropharynx in pediatric patients compared with adults. This difference in tongue size may result in airway obstruction in the unresponsive pediatric patient and make visualization of the glottis more difficult when performing laryngoscopy. The glottic opening is more cephalad and anterior in the pediatric patient **FIGURE 6-5**. A child's epiglottis is at a 45° angle to the anterior pharyngeal wall, whereas an adult's epiglottis lies parallel to the base of the tongue. In addition, the epiglottis is proportionally larger, floppier, and U-shaped in a child compared with an adult. This may necessitate using a laryngoscope blade tip to directly lift the epiglottis to improve visualization during laryngoscopy of a child.

The larger adenoidal tissue found in pediatric patients, and particularly in infants, may result in significant hemorrhaging if subjected to trauma. Additionally, the cricothyroid membrane is small in young children. For this reason, only needle (not surgical) cricothyrotomy is generally recommended in children younger than 10 years.

Furthermore, children have significantly higher oxygen consumption rates when compared with adults. Oxygen consumption in the pediatric patient is approximately double that of an adult.

This increased consumption, coupled with a decreased functional residual capacity, can result in significant hypoxemia despite adequate preoxygenation, a major concern when attempting to intubate a pediatric patient.

Special Populations

Children have significantly higher oxygen consumption rates as compared to adults.

Finally, with pediatric patients, the CCTP should exercise caution when using a bag-mask device. Excessive volumes and forceful ventilations may exacerbate gastric distention, causing vomiting; decrease lung compliance; and increase the risk of pneumothorax.

Physiology of the Respiratory System

Gas Exchange and Transport

Fick's law of diffusion states that the rate of diffusion of a gas across a semipermeable membrane is proportional to the surface area available for diffusion and the concentration gradient of gases on either side of the membrane, and inversely proportional to the thickness of the membrane. Simply stated, gas will move from an area of higher concentration to an area of lower concentration in an attempt to achieve equilibrium. The difference between the partial pressures of gases on each side of the membrane is the driving force for diffusion. In the lungs, gas exchange is caused by the pressure gradient and driving forces across the alveolar-capillary membrane **FIGURE 6-6**.

Partial pressure can be determined by applying Dalton's law, which states that a gas mixture's total pressure is equal to the sum of the component gases' partial pressures. At sea level, the atmospheric pressure of all mixed gases is 760 mm Hg. Oxygen accounts for 21% of this gas mixture. Thus, the partial pressure of oxygen in the atmosphere at sea level is 159.6 mm Hg (760 × 21%). In the capillary, the partial pressure of oxygen (P_{O_2}) is 40 mm Hg, whereas the partial pressure of carbon dioxide (P_{CO_2}) is 45 mm Hg. In the alveolus, the P_{CO_2} is 40 mm Hg

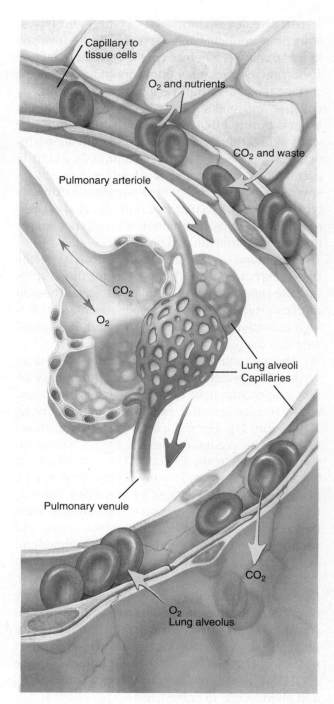

FIGURE 6-6 With diffusion, molecules of oxygen (O_2) move out of the alveoli and into the blood because there are fewer O_2 molecules in the blood. Similarly, molecules of carbon dioxide (CO_2) diffuse out of the blood and into the alveoli because there are fewer CO_2 molecules in the alveoli.

© Jones & Bartlett Learning.

and the P_{O_2} is 100 mm Hg. This difference in the partial pressures of oxygen between the capillary and the alveolus forms a gradient. If the capillary

Po_2 is 40 mm Hg and the alveolar Po_2 is 100 mm Hg, then the driving force of the oxygen molecule across the membrane is 60 mm Hg in the direction of the capillary. If the alveolar Pco_2 is 40 mm Hg and the capillary Pco_2 is 45 mm Hg, then the driving Pco_2 is 5 mm Hg in the direction of the alveolus. The result is that the blood returning to the left side of the heart via the pulmonary vein contains 100 mm Hg of oxygen and 40 mm Hg of CO_2; these are the normal arterial blood gas (ABG) values. Additionally, it is important to remember that carbon dioxide diffuses 20 times faster in the blood than does oxygen.

Factors that affect the diffusion of gases across the membrane may create a ventilation-perfusion ($\dot{V}/\dot{Q}$) mismatch. $\dot{V}/\dot{Q}$ mismatch can be caused by inadequate ventilation, perfusion, or both. Three types of $\dot{V}/\dot{Q}$ mismatch are possible: low, high, and silent.

- **Low $\dot{V}/\dot{Q}$ ratio.** Characterized by perfusion exceeding ventilation. The low ratio results in blood being shunted past the alveoli without adequate gas exchange taking place. A 20% shunting results in severe hypoxia. Causes may include pneumonia, atelectasis, tumors, and mucus plugs.
- **High $\dot{V}/\dot{Q}$ ratio.** Characterized by ventilation exceeding perfusion, resulting in dead space. In this case, the alveoli are inadequately perfused, preventing adequate gas exchange from occurring. Causes of high $\dot{V}/\dot{Q}$ ratio may include pulmonary embolus, pulmonary infarction, and cardiogenic shock.
- **Silent alveolar unit.** Characterized by decreased ventilation and perfusion, as is seen in patients with a pneumothorax and severe acute respiratory distress syndrome (ARDS).

Although it is common practice to assess oxygenation in terms of the partial pressure of (arterial) oxygen (Pao_2), it is important to remember that hemoglobin is the iron-containing protein found in erythrocytes that functions as the actual transporter of oxygen to tissues. The Pao_2 drives oxygen to be bound to hemoglobin, a relationship expressed in the oxyhemoglobin dissociation curve **FIGURE 6-7**.

The oxyhemoglobin dissociation curve is a graphical representation of hemoglobin's affinity for binding to oxygen molecules, as viewed from the perspective of oxyhemoglobin saturation (*y*-axis) compared to the partial pressure of oxygen

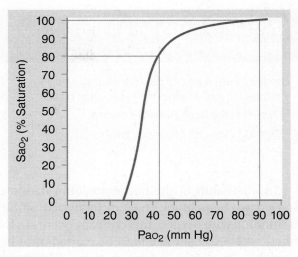

FIGURE 6-7 Oxyhemoglobin dissociation curve.
Abbreviations: Pao_2, arterial partial pressure of oxygen; Sao_2, arterial oxygen saturation
© Jones & Bartlett Learning.

(*x*-axis). At the base of the curve, oxygen is beginning to bind to hemoglobin. As the partial pressure of oxygen increases across the *x*-axis, oxygen saturation of the hemoglobin molecule (Spo_2) increases considerably, represented by the steep upslope on the graph. This increase in Spo_2 is directly related to hemoglobin's positive cooperativity with oxygen molecules. Positive cooperativity, in this case, refers to the heme molecule within the hemoglobin increasing its affinity for binding to oxygen molecules with each successive oxygen bond formed. When the curve becomes flat (plateaus), Spo_2 is not increasing significantly for a given increase in partial pressure. At this point, the oxyhemoglobin is nearly saturated.

The oxyhemoglobin dissociation curve can shift left or right respective to the baseline curve depending on changes in the patient's pH, temperature, and 2,3-diphosphoglycerate (2,3-DPG) level. A right shift in the curve represents a reduction in hemoglobin's affinity for binding with oxygen molecules, which typically occurs in tissue cells where oxygen needs to be delivered. In a right shift, for a given partial pressure of oxygen there will be a correlated reduction in the amount of hemoglobin saturated with oxygen due to the loss of hemoglobin's affinity for binding to oxygen. This shift may be caused by an increase in Pco_2, an increase in the number of hydrogen ions (therefore a decrease in pH), an increase in temperature, or an increase in 2,3-DPG.

In a left shift of the oxyhemoglobin dissociation curve, hemoglobin has an increased affinity for binding with oxygen; this typically occurs in the lungs, where oxygen needs to be loaded onto hemoglobin. In a left shift, for a given partial pressure of oxygen, there will be a correlated increase in hemoglobin saturated with oxygen due to hemoglobin's increased affinity for binding to oxygen. This shift may be caused by a decrease in the P_{CO_2}, a decrease in the number of hydrogen ions (an increase in pH), a decrease in temperature, or a decrease in 2,3-DPG.

When hemoglobin's ability to bind with oxygen is impaired, a patient can experience tissue hypoxia even though the Pa_{O_2} and Sp_{O_2} may be normal. Many substances can bind to hemoglobin and cause it to be dysfunctional. For example, carbon monoxide's affinity for hemoglobin is 240 times greater than oxygen's. When carbon monoxide binds to hemoglobin, it results in the formation of carboxyhemoglobin, which in turn prevents oxygen from being transported and released to the tissues. In addition, nitrite poisoning can result in the formation of abnormal hemoglobin. When nitrite binds to hemoglobin, it results in methemoglobinemia. This phenomenon also alters the oxygen-carrying capacity of the hemoglobin molecule and can result in hypoxia.

Mechanics of Ventilation

The mechanics and dynamics of breathing involve four key concepts: elastance, compliance, resistance, and pressure gradients. Lung parenchyma, the functional part of the lung involved in gas exchange, in an independent state would tend to collapse. This tendency is known as elastance. The construction of the bony thorax and ribs, however, creates an opposing force that prevents the lung tissue from collapsing completely.

The ease with which the thorax and lungs expand is referred to as compliance. If compliance is reduced, it becomes more difficult for the lungs to expand; therefore, any process that affects the integrity of this relationship results in increased work to expand the lungs. We can define compliance as a change in volume per unit of pressure: $\Delta V / \Delta P$. For example, if the chest wall becomes rigid due to pain, injury, or disease, its expansion becomes more challenging and breathing becomes more difficult. Likewise, if the lung parenchyma becomes diseased and grows stiffer, the work of breathing increases.

Resistance refers to the amount of force needed to move a gas or fluid through a single capillary tube. As defined by Poiseuille's law, viscosity, length of the tube, driving pressure, and radius of the tube contribute to the work required to move a liquid or gas through a tube. Of these conditions, the radius of the tube is the most important factor affecting airflow. If the radius of the tube is decreased by half, the work required to move air through it increases 16 times. This concept is crucial when selecting an endotracheal (ET) tube size; to minimize the work required for gas delivery, the CCTP should generally use the largest appropriate size of tube possible when intubating patients. The relationship described by Poiseuille's law is also important in bronchospasm: A decreased tube radius results in more resistance to flow of gases. Thus, even small amounts of swelling in a child's relatively narrow airway can cause significant distress. The decreased flow of gas results in a greater sense of respiratory distress, which then increases respiratory effort, and ultimately further increases the work of breathing. Increased mucus production, basal membrane edema, and artificial airways will also reduce airway diameter, increase resistance, and potentially result in increased work of breathing.

Pressure gradients allow for the bulk movement of gas into and out of the lungs. During the inspiration phase of a patient-initiated spontaneous ventilation, contraction of the chest muscles increases the size of the thorax **FIGURE 6-8**. The increased size of the thorax results in an increase in the volume contained within the thorax. The increased volume, in turn, results in a negative pressure within the thorax relative to the atmospheric pressure, causing air to move into the lungs. At the end of inspiration, the muscles relax, allowing the thorax to return to its original size. This decrease in

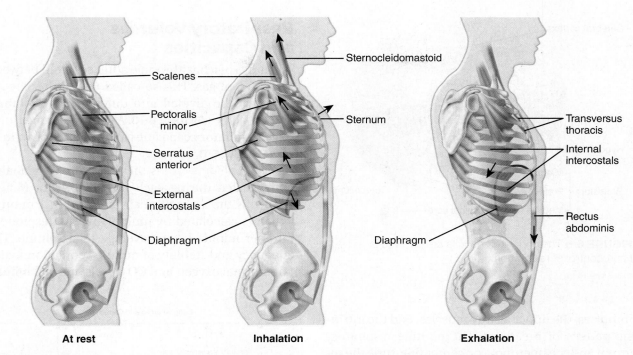

At rest	Inhalation	Exhalation

Scalenes

Pectoralis minor

Serratus anterior

External intercostals

Diaphragm

Sternocleidomastoid

Sternum

Transversus thoracis

Internal intercostals

Rectus abdominis

Diaphragm

FIGURE 6-8 The muscles involved in the mechanics of breathing. The arrows indicate the direction of muscle contraction during inhalation and the direction of muscle relaxation during exhalation.

© Jones & Bartlett Learning.

intrathoracic volume results in an increase in intrathoracic pressure, and exhalation occurs. Thus, spontaneous inspiration is an active process that requires work, whereas exhalation is usually a passive event.

In contrast to patient-initiated ventilation, mechanically assisted ventilation is driven by positive pressure, which is generated by a ventilator or a bag-mask device. Positive-pressure ventilation increases both airway and alveolar pressures, which may then reduce venous return to the heart, thereby reducing cardiac output. For further discussion of positive-pressure ventilation, see Chapter 7, *Ventilation*.

The thoracic expansion that begins the inspiratory cycle is driven by muscle contraction. The primary muscles used during inspiration are the diaphragm and external intercostal muscles. In times of increased stress, accessory muscles such as the pectorals, sternocleidomastoid, and scalenes may be used for thoracic expansion, though this process also increases oxygen use. Continued use of these muscles can quickly lead to muscle fatigue, hypercapnia, hypoxemia, and respiratory failure. Some muscles can augment exhalation in times of increased work of breathing, although exhalation

remains mostly a passive process. Specifically, if necessary, the intercostal and abdominal muscles can assist exhalation.

The stimulation and innervation of breathing is a complex process involving the pulmonary, cardiac, and neurologic systems. Normally, the drive to breathe comes from the need to eliminate CO_2. In the blood, CO_2 combines with water (H_2O) to form carbonic acid, which then dissociates into H^+ and HCO_3^- ions. Thus, as CO_2 increases, so does the level of H^+. Recall that pH is a function of H^+ concentration; that is, as H^+ increases, pH decreases. The effects of this change are transmitted across the blood–brain barrier and stimulate the respiratory centers in the brainstem. As a backup mechanism, chemoreceptors located in the aortic arch and carotid arteries are sensitive to changes in oxygen levels. When the Pao_2 level drops below 60 mm Hg, these receptors are subjected to their maximal stimulation and subsequently trigger increased breathing.

The body's respiratory centers are located in the medulla and pons areas of the brainstem **FIGURE 6-9**. In the medulla, the dorsal respiratory group regulates impulses to the diaphragm. The ventral respiratory group controls expiratory

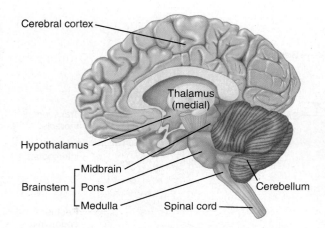

FIGURE 6-9 The pons and medulla are involved in neurocontrol of respiration.

© Jones & Bartlett Learning.

impulses, the upper airway muscles, and the intrinsic pattern of breathing. The pontine respiratory group and the pneumotaxic center fine-tune the respiratory pattern. The innervation of the diaphragm comes from the phrenic nerve, which branches from the spinal cord at the level of C3 to C5. Spinal cord injury near this level dramatically affects the ability to breathe adequately.

Putting It All Together

The proper functioning of the respiratory system can be explained by five factors:

- **Ventilation.** There must be an adequate bulk flow of gas into and out of the lung.

- **Distribution.** The gas must be delivered into the areas of the lung that are able to engage in gas exchange. Changes in compliance or resistance will send the gas to areas of the lung with an unsuitable V̇/Q̇ ratio.

- **Diffusion.** The alveolar-capillary membrane must be able to engage in gas exchange. Widening of the space (as in pulmonary edema) or disease (such as fibrosis) results in a decreased diffusion capacity.

- **Perfusion.** Blood flow through the pulmonary vasculature and contact with the alveolus is essential.

- **Circulation.** The heart must be able to not only pump blood to the lung, but also distribute blood through the systemic circulation. In addition, levels of hemoglobin must be adequate to ensure delivery of oxygen to the cells.

Respiratory Volumes and Capacities

The lungs of a healthy male adult can hold between 5 and 6 L of gas. This so-called total lung capacity (TLC) can be divided into different lung volumes and capacities **FIGURE 6-10**. A spirometer measures these respiratory capacities and volumes of air in liters **FIGURE 6-11**.

Tidal volume (V_t) is the amount of air inhaled and exhaled during each normal breath. Minute volume is the amount of air breathed in 1 minute, which is calculated by multiplying the respiratory rate per minute by the average tidal volume. The adequacy and stability of minute ventilation maintain normal oxygen and CO_2 levels; normal minute

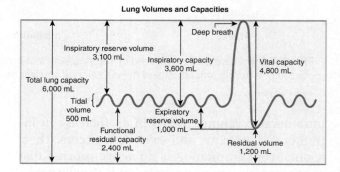

FIGURE 6-10 Respiratory cycle, capacities, and volume. The numbers are approximations.

© Jones & Bartlett Learning.

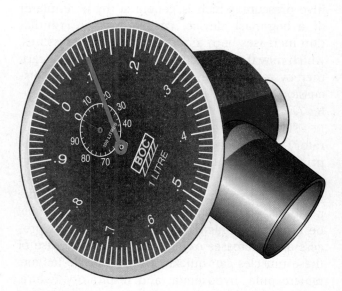

FIGURE 6-11 A spirometer.

Courtesy of Smiths Medical.

ventilation is 5 to 8 L/min. The amount of air that can be inhaled after tidal volume is inhaled is the **inspiratory reserve volume (IRV)**, whereas the air that can be expelled from the lungs after a normal exhalation is the **expiratory reserve volume (ERV)**. The **inspiratory capacity (IC)** is the sum of IRV and V_t. **Vital capacity (V_c)**, also known as the pulmonary reserve, represents the total amount of air that can be exhaled following a maximal inspiration. Normal V_c is 60 to 70 mL/kg of ideal body weight. This value varies with sex, age, and height: Women have a smaller V_c than men do, and V_c decreases with greater age (approximately 20 mL/kg per year for persons older than 20 years) and increases with greater height. A decrease in vital capacity to less than 10 to 15 mL/kg indicates poor pulmonary reserve and an inability to cough effectively. Persons with this condition almost always require some form of mechanical ventilation.

At the end of a maximal forced exhalation, the volume of air remaining in the lungs constitutes the **residual volume (RV)**. RV added to ERV gives the **functional residual capacity (FRC)**. The FRC allows for gas exchange between breaths; it is also targeted during the application of **positive end-expiratory pressure (PEEP)**. Specifically, applied PEEP recruits collapsed alveoli and stents them open. This expansion of the alveoli makes an increased surface area available for gas exchange, facilitating improved oxygenation and increased FRC.

One other volume of note is the **anatomic dead space (V_d)**. This space, found in the upper airway, comprises areas that do not participate in gas exchange. The volume in this space is normally approximately 2 mL/kg.

Pathophysiology: Obstructive and Restrictive Disease States

Respiratory disease states can be categorized in several ways. Disease states that make it more difficult to move air out of the lungs can be classified as **obstructive diseases**. These conditions, which include asthma, COPD, cystic fibrosis, and bronchiectasis, involve an increase in airway resistance. Diseases that result in difficulty moving air into the lungs are classified as **restrictive diseases**. These conditions result in the loss of chest or lung compliance, either individually or together. Restrictive diseases include occupational lung diseases

(asbestosis, mesothelioma), idiopathic pulmonary fibrosis, pneumonia, atelectasis, chest wall deformities and injuries, and the various neuromuscular diseases that affect breathing (eg, Guillain-Barré syndrome and amyotrophic lateral sclerosis).

Both diseases and temporary conditions can alter the $\dot{V}/\dot{Q}$ ratio. Ventilation that exceeds the capacity of blood flow to absorb the gases and carry them to the tissues creates a dead space effect, in which gas exchange is impaired (such as in tachypnea in the setting of a pulmonary embolism). Gas exchange is also impaired when blood flow is in excess of ventilation, as this condition creates a **shunt** effect. For example, in pneumonia, a lobe of the lung is perfused but not ventilated because of infection in the parenchymal air spaces. Anatomic shunts may also prevent blood from participating in gas exchange. Some anatomic shunts are congenital heart defects; others, such as those that involve the bronchial and thebesian veins, are normal and occur in the lung. The extent of the shunt effect (abbreviated Qt) varies: The normal Qt range is 3% to 5%, whereas a value greater than 20% indicates that the patient's condition is critical.

Because oxygen is vital to the life and metabolism of every cell in the body, evaluating the patient for the presence of hypoxia and treating this condition when it is identified are crucial. It is important to understand the mechanisms underlying hypoxia as well as the causes of hypoxemia:

- **Hypoxic hypoxia.** Defined as insufficient oxygen in the blood. It affects all of the body's tissues. It may be caused by hypovolemia, airway obstruction, decreased cardiac output, or coronary artery disease.
  - Low oxygen tension may occur in the alveolus itself, such that sufficient amounts of oxygen cannot diffuse across the alveolar-capillary membrane. This condition may be caused by hypoventilation, high altitude (low barometric pressure), and suffocation.
  - Diffusion defects may include fibrosis or edema.
  - Shunting can be intrapulmonary, as when it is caused by atelectasis, bronchospasm, and pneumonia, or extrapulmonary, as occurs with a congenital heart defect.
- **Anemic hypoxia (hypemic hypoxia).** Caused by a reduced level of hemoglobin or dysfunctional

hemoglobin. Hypemic hypoxia interferes with the transportation phase of respiration, causing a reduction in oxygen-carrying capacity. Specific causes of hypemic hypoxia include anemias, hemorrhage, hemoglobin abnormalities, use of certain medications (sulfa drugs), and intake of chemicals. It may also be caused by carbon monoxide poisoning. Carbon monoxide is present in exhaust fumes—from ambulances and both conventional and jet-engine aircraft—as well as in cigarette smoke.

- **Stagnant hypoxia.** Reduced cardiac output resulting in tissue hypoxia due to lack of circulation. Specific causes include heart failure, shock, continuous positive-pressure breathing, acceleration (*g* forces), and pulmonary embolism. A reduction in regional or local blood flow may be caused by extremes of environmental temperatures, postural changes, tourniquets, hyperventilation, embolism by clots or gas bubbles, and cerebral vascular accidents.
- **Histotoxic hypoxia.** Occurs when cells are unable to use oxygen due to inactivation or destruction of key enzymes, such as in cyanide and strychnine poisoning as well as in later stages of carbon monoxide poisoning.

Determining the mechanisms underlying hypoxemia can dramatically affect the course of the patient's treatment. Notably, simply providing supplemental oxygen may not always be sufficient in alleviating hypoxia.

Patient Assessment

Chapter 5, *Patient Assessment*, covers the techniques of inspection, auscultation, and palpation. This section covers respiratory-specific considerations during the assessment process.

Breath Sound Assessments

After an adequate airway is in place and secured, assessment of breath sounds is vital. Breath sounds are created as air moves through the tracheobronchial tree and the alveoli, and can be auscultated using a stethoscope. The size of the airway determines the type of sound that is produced. (Recall that there are significant differences in the proportional sizes of adult and pediatric airways.)

- The trachea and bronchi have large diameters, so the sound produced there is higher in pitch and is heard during inspiration and expiration. To hear the tracheal breath sounds (also called bronchial breath sounds), place the stethoscope diaphragm over the trachea or over the sternum. Assess breath sounds for duration, pitch, and intensity.
- Vesicular breath sounds are softer, muffled sounds and have often been described as wind blowing through the trees. The expiratory phase is barely audible. Breath sounds are heard over the majority of the chest, representing airflow in the alveoli.
- Bronchovesicular sounds are a combination of the tracheal and vesicular breath sounds. They are heard in places where airways and alveoli are found—that is, the upper part of the sternum and between the scapulae.

FIGURE 6-12 describes the normal breath sounds. The locations where these sounds may be heard are shown in **FIGURE 6-13**.

Bronchovesicular sounds should be assessed for duration, pitch, and intensity. *Duration* refers to the length of time for the inspiratory or expiratory phase of the breath. Normally, expiration is at least twice as long as inspiration. This relationship is expressed by the I:E ratio, where a normal I:E ratio is 1:2. When a patient's airway is obstructed and the patient has difficulty getting air out, the expiratory component is prolonged and may be four to five times as long as inspiration; in such a case, the I:E ratio would be 1:5. In patients who are tachypneic, the expiratory cycle is short and approaches that of inspiration, and the I:E ratio may be 1:1. During mechanical ventilation, manipulation of the I:E ratio (such that expiration is longer than inspiration, or inverse I:E) may be used to improve ventilation and hypoxemia in patients with severe lung injury. Extreme caution must be exercised when caring for this patient population.

Pitch of breath sounds is described as either higher or lower than normal, as in patients with stridor or wheezing. The intensity of sound depends on the airflow rate, the constancy of flow throughout inspiration, the patient's position, and the site selected for auscultation.

The thickness of the chest wall may affect the *intensity* of breath sounds. Sounds that are less intense are said to be diminished. A common error in assessing the intensity of breath sounds occurs when auscultation is performed over the patient's clothing.

"Normal" Breath Sounds

Tracheal. Inspiratory and expiratory sounds are both loud.

Bronchial. Inspiratory sounds are shorter than expiratory sounds, and both are loud.

Bronchovesicular. Inspiratory and expiratory sounds are about the same, and of medium intensity.

Vesicular. Inspiratory sounds last longer than expiratory sounds, and both are faint.

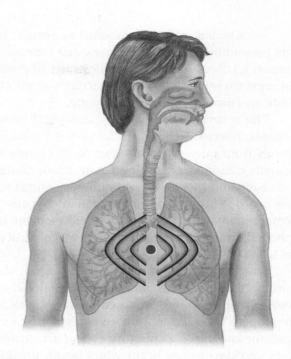

The thickness of the bars shows intensity (loudness) of the breath, and slope correlates with pitch (steeper slope, higher pitch).

FIGURE 6-12 Normal breath sounds are heard over different parts of the chest. As you move away from the largest airways, breath sounds become softer. The character of inspiration versus exhalation also changes.

© Jones & Bartlett Learning.

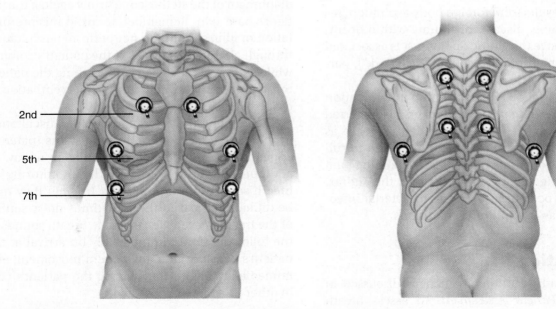

FIGURE 6-13 Commonly assessed auscultation sites, indicated by numbered intercostal spaces.

© Jones & Bartlett Learning.

Sounds that might be classified as normal, but are present in an unexpected area, can indicate an abnormal condition. For example, tracheal sounds in areas that should produce vesicular sounds may indicate consolidation or pneumonia.

The terminology regarding abnormal breath sounds, referred to as adventitious breath sounds, varies from one text to another. Such sounds are usually classified as continuous or discontinuous. Wheezes and rhonchi are continuous sounds that are heard as air flows through a constricted airway. Wheezes are usually high pitched. Rhonchi are low pitched, indicating the airway is not as obstructed as when wheezing is heard.

Crackles (formerly known as rales) occur when airflow causes mucus or fluid in the airways to move, such as when collapsed airways or alveoli pop open. These discontinuous sounds may occur early or late in the inspiratory cycle. Early inspiratory crackles usually occur when larger, proximal bronchi open; they are common in patients with COPD and tend not to clear with coughing. Late inspiratory crackles are heard when peripheral alveoli and airways pop open; these sounds are more common in the dependent lung regions. Late inspiratory crackles are common in patients with reduced lung volumes.

Stridor results from foreign body aspiration, infection, swelling, disease, or trauma within or immediately above the glottic opening. It is associated with a loud, high-pitched sound ("seal bark"), particularly in pediatric patients.

A pleural friction rub results from inflammation that causes the lung pleura to thicken, also referred to as pleurisy. The pleural space can decrease as a result, allowing the surfaces of the pleura to rub together. This decrease often creates stabbing pain with breathing or any movement of the thorax. Pleurisy can be caused by viral or bacterial infections as well as autoimmune conditions.

Auscultation

Baseline breath sound assessment is discussed in Chapter 5, *Patient Assessment*. To assess breath sounds in a patient with an invasive airway device, such as an ET tube or supraglottic airway (SGA), listen over the epigastrium and sternal notch **FIGURE 6-14**, over the six recommended sites on the anterior chest wall, and in the axillae (see Chapter 5,

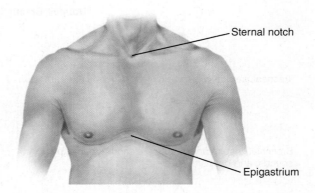

FIGURE 6-14 In patients with an invasive airway, listen for breath sounds over the epigastrium and sternal notch.
© Jones & Bartlett Learning.

Patient Assessment). Assess these areas for proper device placement and airflow. The baseline respiratory assessment establishes the standard against which subsequent assessments will be compared.

Breath sounds are best evaluated while the patient is taking slow, deep breaths through an open mouth and while seated in a semi-Fowler or high Fowler position. Because of clinical circumstances, however, such an assessment may not be possible. If the patient cannot be elevated, auscultate as many of the six recommended sites as possible. Place the diaphragm of the stethoscope firmly against the patient's bare skin. Remember, to avoid misinterpretation of lung sounds, do not perform auscultation through clothing. Be aware of the patient's comfort while assessing breath sounds. Rushing the patient through the process may cause hyperventilation or exacerbate existing dyspnea.

Document the sites chosen for auscultation in the patient care report and the status (patency, appearance, integrity) of any artificial airway. In addition to performing periodic monitoring of breath sounds during transport (though they may be difficult to hear in the sometimes-noisy setting of the transport vehicle), evaluate breath sounds at the following times: immediately on arrival at the patient's bedside, after any patient movement, and immediately before transferring the patient's care to other providers.

Palpation

Palpation of the patient's chest wall enables the CCTP to evaluate the status of the lungs, skin, and subcutaneous tissues and chest expansion. A snap, crackle, pop sensation indicates the presence of subcutaneous emphysema, in which air escapes from the pleural space and dissects through the subcutaneous tissues. Although subcutaneous emphysema itself is benign, its underlying cause may be life threatening. If subcutaneous emphysema is detected, it is important to inquire about recent trauma or invasive procedures (ie, intubation, central line placement) and to determine whether these are new findings.

When a person is speaking, the vibrations of the vocal cords are transmitted to the chest wall, a phenomenon called vocal fremitus. Vocal fremitus is assessed by performing tactile fremitus, which is done by placing the hands bilaterally on the upper thorax and asking the patient to say "ninety-nine." This procedure is repeated in a methodical way down the chest. An increase in the fremitus, or vibration, indicates that the underlying lung tissue is more solid (consolidated) and contains less air than normal, which may be attributable to pneumonia or atelectasis. In addition, if secretions are present in the airways, the vibrations will increase. This finding may indicate that the patient needs to cough or be suctioned. The procedures of vocal fremitus and tactile fremitus are useful in patient assessment but are usually not practical in the transport setting.

Ultrasonography

Point-of-care lung ultrasonography can be a useful assessment tool, especially in a patient with undifferentiated shortness of breath, as described in greater detail in Chapter 9, *Laboratory Analysis and Diagnostic Studies*. For example, lung ultrasonography can show the relationship of the parietal and visceral lung pleura. An absence of shimmering as these two layers slide past each other (sliding lung sign) suggests poor lung ventilation, which can be seen with a pneumothorax. Additionally, different acoustic artifacts can be used to distinguish well-aerated lungs (A lines) from lungs with alveolar-interstitial syndromes (B lines) such as pulmonary edema or pneumonia.

Normal and Abnormal Respiratory Patterns

When you are assessing respiratory patterns, consider three characteristics of the patient's respirations: rate, depth, and pattern.

Rate

Eupnea is normal breathing at a rate of approximately 12 to 20 breaths/min in the adult patient. Pediatric norms range from 30 to 50 breaths/min in the newborn to 12 to 20 breaths/min in the adolescent. A number of factors can cause tachypnea (an abnormally fast respiratory rate), including fever, pneumonia, metabolic acidosis, hypoxemia, some poisonings and drug uses (aspirin overdose, stimulant use), and lesions of the respiratory center in the brain. Stress, anxiety, and pain can also result in tachypnea. Although tachypnea is a compensatory mechanism, it has negative effects as well. Because rapid respiratory rates usually result in shallower breaths, the amount of alveolar ventilation (V_a)—that is, the volume of air that comes into contact with the alveolar-capillary membrane surfaces and participates in the exchange of gases between the lung and the blood—decreases in the patient with tachypnea. More muscle work is used to generate "wasted" ventilation, and the increased work also results in increased oxygen consumption.

Numerous factors can also lead to bradypnea (a slower than normal respiratory rate), including use of narcotic or sedative drugs, alcohol, metabolic disorders, respiratory system decompensation or fatigue (particularly in pediatric patients), and traumatic and nontraumatic central nervous system (CNS) lesions. Mild bradypnea is normal in certain stages of sleep.

Apnea, the absence of respiration, may be episodic or periodic. Periods of apnea longer than 15 seconds require immediate intervention. The patient with apnea may need ventilatory support or other resuscitative efforts.

Depth

In addition to measuring the respiratory rate, always assess the patient's depth of respiration. Assessment of depth can be achieved by direct observation or by palpation. Hyperpnea describes a deeper than normal breath, whereas hypopnea refers to a shallow breath. Hyperpnea can lead to low levels of CO_2, thereby increasing pH and resulting in respiratory alkalosis. Hypopnea can result in increased CO_2 levels, thereby decreasing pH and resulting in respiratory acidosis, as well as decreased oxygen values.

Pattern

Several abnormal respiratory patterns present with characteristic alterations of the respiratory rate, depth, or regularity **FIGURE 6-15**.

Cheyne-Stokes respiration features a cyclic pattern of increased respiratory rate and depth with periods of apnea. Following the apnea, the patient begins breathing with slow, shallow breaths that increase in rate and depth until apnea returns. This condition can be caused by increased intracranial pressure, renal failure, meningitis, drug overdose, or hypoxia secondary to congestive heart failure. Otherwise, healthy individuals may breathe in a Cheyne-Stokes pattern following exposure to altitude changes or with hyperventilation syndrome. Acidosis, particularly when caused by CO_2 levels, can also trigger Cheyne-Stokes respirations.

Cluster breathing is another abnormal respiratory pattern, in which a cluster of irregular respirations that vary in depth are followed by a period of apnea at irregular intervals.

Biot (ataxic) respiration is similar to Cheyne-Stokes respiration, but the pattern is irregular. While Cheyne-Stokes respiration features repeating patterns of gradual increases concluding with apnea, three patterns occur in Biot respiration: (1) slow and deep, (2) rapid and shallow, and (3) apnea

without any predictable pattern. Causes of Biot respiration may include meningitis, increased intracranial pressure, and central nervous system dysfunction. This condition often indicates the presence of lesions higher in the respiratory center in the brainstem than those that produce Cheyne-Stokes respirations.

Kussmaul respiration is fast and deep without periods of apnea. The rate and depth are greater than the normal rate expected for the patient's age group. Breathing is labored, with periods of deep breaths punctuated by sighs. The Kussmaul pattern may indicate metabolic acidosis, including diabetic ketoacidosis, or renal failure. It generally represents a compensatory mechanism to blow off CO_2 during conditions that cause severe acidemia, such as diabetic ketoacidosis.

Apneustic breathing indicates lesions in the respiratory center of the brainstem. The patient exhibits a prolonged, gasping inspiration, followed by an extremely short, ineffective expiration at a rate between 1 and 2 breaths/min. Over a period of several minutes of ineffective exhalation, the patient's lungs may hyperinflate. This pattern results in severe hypoxemia and, if uncorrected, rapid death.

Central neurogenic hyperventilation is a pattern of deep, rapid respirations at rates of 40 to 60 breaths/min. It is caused by a midbrain lesion or dysfunction. Patients exhibiting central neurogenic hyperventilation are generally comatose, with Glasgow Coma Scale scores of less than 8. These patients require intubation and ventilatory assistance to stabilize their ABG parameters.

Hyperventilation syndrome presents with increases in both the rate and depth of respiration. It can result from exertion, fear, anxiety, fever, hepatic coma, acid–base imbalance, or midbrain lesions. A respiratory rate between 20 and 30 breaths/min in the adult is classified as moderate hyperventilation. A prolonged respiratory rate greater than 30 breaths/min is considered severe, and ventilatory support is often necessary in such a case to prevent respiratory muscle fatigue. Use caution when assessing the underlying cause of hyperventilation before initiating any corrective treatment. Never withhold oxygen from a patient showing signs or symptoms of hypoxia.

A state of hyperventilation may also develop in a patient who is intubated or being ventilated. Closely monitor vital signs, pulse oximetry,

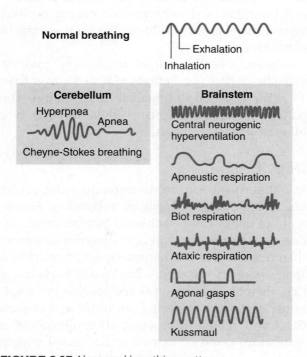

FIGURE 6-15 Abnormal breathing patterns.

© Jones & Bartlett Learning.

capnometry readings, end-tidal CO_2 ($ETCO_2$) levels, mental status, and skin color in any patient receiving ventilatory support.

Agonal respirations are also abnormal. This pattern of deep, slow, shallow, irregular, "all-or-none" breaths or occasional gasping breaths is accompanied by a slow respiratory rate.

Another abnormal respiratory pattern is seen in patients with obstructive diseases such as COPD and asthma. The pathology of these diseases leads to airway collapse and hyperinflation of the lungs. Affected individuals have difficulty exhaling completely, which leads to air trapping in the lungs and shallow compensatory respirations. To facilitate exhalation, these individuals exhale for longer periods and with the lips pursed. Pursed-lip breathing applies a back pressure to the airways in an effort to prevent airway collapse. This breathing technique represents an attempt to maintain PEEP (the amount of pressure above ambient pressure present in the airway at the end of the respiratory cycle). The I:E ratio in patients with obstructive disease is usually abnormal.

The appropriate level of intervention for patients with these breathing abnormalities is directly related to the work of breathing and the patient's ability to maintain that work. Remember that all muscle activity uses oxygen to metabolize glucose and manufacture adenosine triphosphate; CO_2, in turn, is produced as a waste product. This process increases the need for further ventilation, which may then exacerbate muscle fatigue. Remember also that the diaphragm is the most efficient of the respiratory muscles. By comparison, the accessory muscles (the scalene, sternocleidomastoid, and external intercostal muscles) use more oxygen. The patient's ability to maintain the increased workload associated with the use of the accessory muscles for breathing depends on age, physical conditioning, degree of cardiopulmonary reserve, and other combined medical conditions. Failure to adequately manage the work of breathing can lead to cardiopulmonary arrest.

Descriptions of Breathing

Do not confuse *shortness of breath* with *work of breathing*. Shortness of breath is a subjective complaint, whereas work of breathing is a physical exam finding.

Assessment in Preparation for Transport

Prior to transport, the CCTP should review the patient care report, noting any medications, disease processes, or trauma that might compromise ventilation. Also note the results of any lab or imaging studies, and review the patient's vital signs. Take special note of when the last ABG measurement was performed and whether the data are valid; for example, consider whether there have been any changes in patient status or interventions since the ABG analysis was performed. If an artificial airway is in place, note its size, type, and depth, and confirm its proper placement before continuing with transport. If the patient requires mechanical ventilation, note the ventilator settings and patient response. If any doubt arises about the placement of tracheal tubes, nasogastric (NG) tubes, orogastric (OG) tubes, or central lines, the CCTP should communicate these concerns to hospital personnel.

If the transport will take place by ground in a mountainous region or by air, remember that altitude-induced pressure changes can occur during travel by helicopter or fixed-wing aircraft. Remember Boyle's law: At a fixed temperature, the volume of a gas varies inversely with the pressure surrounding it. This relationship may cause air or gases within the body to expand as altitude increases (and barometric pressure decreases). Such pressure changes are particularly important for air within the pleural space (pneumothorax). In equipment with air-filled spaces, such as the balloon of an ET tube, the air may need to be replaced with fluid to prevent problems with expansion during ascent in an air transport. During these transports, monitor the patient closely for evidence of dyspnea or the development of an air embolus.

When assessing the respiratory system, begin with the basics:

1. Assess the ABCs.
2. Determine the stability of the airway.
3. Observe the rate, pattern, depth, and character of respiration.
4. Inspect the chest, looking for symmetric rise and fall with each respiratory cycle. Note any accessory muscle use. Note the presence of any central lines or Hickman catheters, nitroglycerin or other medication patches, or indwelling devices such as pacemakers, implanted defibrillators, chest tubes, or medication delivery devices.

5. Note any wounds, abrasion, or bruising. Note the presence and location of bony crepitus or subcutaneous emphysema.
6. Examine any dressings on the chest (eg, wounds, central venous access, chest tubes) and confirm that they are dry and intact.
7. Observe any drainage being collected and note its color and consistency.
8. Auscultate the chest, noting the presence or absence, quality, and type of breath sounds heard. Compare the breath sounds from one side of the chest to the sounds on the other side.
9. If the patient requires oxygen, assess the oxygen delivery device and confirm that the delivered fraction of inspired oxygen (FIO_2) meets the patient's needs and adequately maintains the desired SpO_2 as measured by pulse oximetry. Recall Henry's law about gas solubility and apply the following formula to determine the required oxygen adjustment for altitude changes:

$$P_1/A_1 = P_2/A_2$$

where P_1 is the partial pressure of gas overlying a solution initially, A_1 is the corresponding amount of gas dissolved in solution at that pressure, P_2 is the ratio of the same gas at a different pressure, and A_2 is the corresponding amount of dissolved gas at this new pressure. Because the two sides of the equation are set equal, a change in P_2 requires a corresponding change in A_2.

Because cardiac and respiratory functions are intimately linked, assess the patient's circulation to obtain a complete clinical picture. Check the patient's blood pressure, pulse rate, capillary refill time, skin color, and temperature. Mental status is another important consideration, because hypoxia directly affects mental status and level of consciousness.

ABG Monitoring

The gold standard for assessing the functioning of the respiratory system is an ABG measurement. In this procedure, using a heparinized syringe, blood is obtained from a superficial artery, such as a radial or brachial artery, or an arterial line. The blood is then analyzed for pH, $PaCO_2$, PaO_2, HCO_3^- (concentration of bicarbonate ion), base excess (BE, indicating whether the patient has acidosis or alkalosis), and SaO_2. The technique for obtaining an ABG

value is covered in Chapter 9, *Laboratory Analysis and Diagnostic Studies.*

The values for pH, FIO_2, and HCO_3^- are used to evaluate the patient's acid–base status. In contrast, $PaCO_2$ is an indicator of the effectiveness of ventilation. The PaO_2 and SpO_2 values are indicators of oxygenation. If an ABG sample cannot be obtained, a venous blood gas (VBG) analysis can be useful to assess pH, $PaCO_2$, and HCO_3^- (see **TABLE 6-1** for a comparison of values). Further discussion of blood gas interpretation and abnormalities appears in Chapter 7, *Ventilation;* Chapter 9, *Laboratory Analysis and Diagnostic Studies;* and Chapter 17, *Gastrointestinal and Genitourinary Emergencies.*

To maintain normal blood gas values, the appropriate relationship between alveolar ventilation and perfusion of the alveolar capillaries must be maintained. This relationship is expressed as the $\dot{V}/\dot{Q}$ ratio. Recall that $\dot{V}/\dot{Q}$ mismatch is the most common cause of hypoxemia.

Noninvasive Ventilatory and Oxygenation Monitoring

In addition to ABG analysis, continuous hemodynamic monitoring of critically ill patients, such as via pulse oximetry and capnography, is essential not only in evaluating the patient's current clinical status, but also in determining how the patient is responding to adjustments in treatments.

Pulse Oximetry

Pulse oximetry provides information about arterial SpO_2 and the pulse **FIGURE 6-16**. Normal pulse oximetry readings should be greater than 92%, but can vary with underlying diseases such as COPD.

All pulse oximetry models work on a similar principle. The machine's diode directs two wavelengths of light, red and infrared, through body tissues toward a photoreceptor. Bound hemoglobin alters light absorption; the degree of change in light transmission indicates the level of arterial SpO_2. Most detectors also supply the monitor with a pulsatile waveform that shows beat-to-beat changes in pulse amplitude and regularity. Commonly used monitoring sites include the finger, pinnae of the ear, toe, and forehead, and sometimes the bridge of the nose.

The pulse oximetry reading reflects the relationship between oxygen and hemoglobin in the

TABLE 6-1 Normal Blood Gas Values

Normal Arterial Values

pH	Paco₂	Hco₃⁻	O₂ Saturation	Pao₂	BE
7.35–7.45	35–45 mm Hg	22–26 mEq/L	96%–100%	80–100 mm Hg	−2 to +2 mmol/L

Abnormal Values

pH	Paco₂	HCO₃⁻	Acid–Base Imbalance
↓	↑	Normal	Respiratory acidosis
↑	↓	Normal	Respiratory alkalosis
↓	Normal	↓	Metabolic acidosis
↑	Normal	↑	Metabolic alkalosis
↓	↑	↑	Respiratory acidosis with metabolic compensation
↑	↑	↑	Metabolic alkalosis with respiratory compensation
↓	↑	↓	Metabolic and respiratory acidosis
↑	↓	↑	Metabolic and respiratory alkalosis

Normal Venous Values

pH	Paco₂	Hco₃⁻	O₂ Saturation	Pao₂	BE
7.32–7.43	38–50 mm Hg	22–29 mEq/L	60%–85%	40 mm Hg	0 to +4 mmol/L

© Jones & Bartlett Learning.

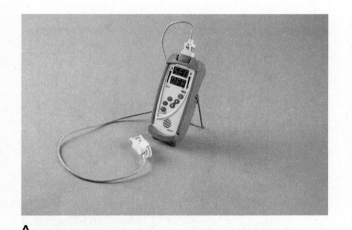
A

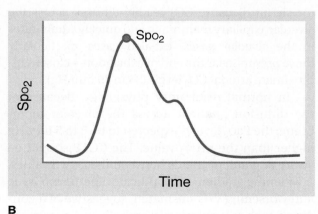
B

FIGURE 6-16 A. A pulse oximeter. **B.** The characteristic shape of the waveform when the pulse oximeter is properly sensing. Oxygen saturation (Spo₂) indicates the percentage of available hemoglobin that is saturated with oxygen.

© Jones & Bartlett Learning.

body. A number of factors can alter this relationship. Abnormal hemoglobin levels, such as are seen in conditions that produce carboxyhemoglobin, methemoglobin, and sulfhemoglobin, significantly reduce the reliability of pulse oximetry. Conventional pulse oximetry cannot differentiate between normal oxyhemoglobin and the dyshemoglobinemias. Because the dysfunctional hemoglobin is still bound, the pulse oximetry reading will be normal. A newer technology, pulse carbon monoxide oximetry, uses additional wavelengths of both infrared and visible light to measure and differentiate oxyhemoglobin, deoxyhemoglobin, carboxyhemoglobin, methemoglobin, and hemoglobin itself.

Decreased tissue perfusion (eg, hypotension, cardiogenic shock) to the periphery may also result in impaired light absorption and inaccurate pulse oximetry readings. Hypothermia may alter pulse oximetry readings because of peripheral vasoconstriction. Peripheral vascular disease (PVD) and vasopressor use may alter blood flow to the periphery and pulse oximetry readings.

Capnography

Capnography (a graphic representation of exhaled CO_2) and capnometry (a numeric value) are both essential adjuncts to determining airway patency and appropriateness of ventilation **FIGURE 6-17**. CO_2 is produced intracellularly as a by-product of cellular metabolism and is transported to the lungs for diffusion and subsequent ventilation. Capnography and capnometry devices monitor the CO_2 concentration within the patient's exhaled air by analyzing air samples obtained directly from the airway through nasal prongs in the spontaneously breathing patient or by insertion of a sampling port into the ventilator circuit. Because CO_2 readily diffuses across the alveolar-capillary membrane and quickly equilibrates in the alveolar gases, exhaled gases—particularly those present near the end of exhalation—closely approximate arterial CO_2 levels (35 to 45 mm Hg).

In normal respiratory physiology, because of the diffusion gradient across the alveolar membrane, the Pao_2 level is expected to be 2 to 5 mm Hg higher than the ETCO$_2$ value. The CCTP should be aware of gradient trends between these two values. A widening gradient may indicate a perfusion issue and worsening $\dot{V}/\dot{Q}$ mismatch, suggestive of a condition such as a pulmonary embolism. A narrowing gradient may indicate a ventilation issue and developing shunt pathology.

Waveform capnography morphology can inform the astute CCTP of changes in the patient's respiratory status and metabolism, provide diagnostic information, and help establish the differential diagnosis. Capnography will depict respiratory rate and tidal volume changes almost instantaneously,

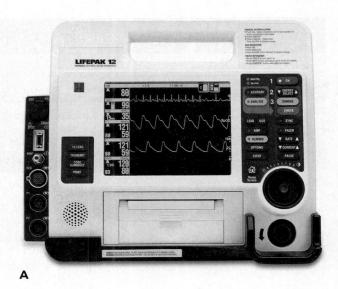

A

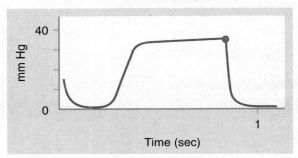

B

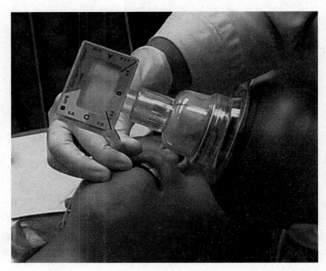

C

FIGURE 6-17 Patient monitor with capnometry capability. **A.** Capnometer. **B.** A normal capnogram waveform. **C.** An end-tidal carbon dioxide detector.

A. LIFEPAK® 12 defibrillator/monitor courtesy of Physio-Control; **B.** © Jones & Bartlett Learning; **C.** Courtesy of Marianne Gausche-Hill, MD, FACEP, FAAP.

compared to pulse oximetry, which is a lagging indicator of the patient's condition. The normal capnography waveform **FIGURE 6-18** is rectangular with rounded corners and is divided into four phases:

- Phase I (A–B) begins on inspiration, when there are low levels of CO_2. It is considered the baseline.

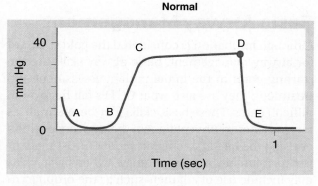

FIGURE 6-18 Normal capnographic waveform with points A through E shown.

© Jones & Bartlett Learning.

- Phase II (B–C) begins with the movement of PCO_2 from the anatomic dead space at the beginning of exhalation. It is represented by the first expiratory upstroke.
- Phase III (C–D) is the alveolar plateau. It ends with the last alveolar gas sampled, referred to as $PETCO_2$.
- Phase IV (sometimes referred to as phase 0; D–E) is depicted by the inspiratory downstroke. It is caused by the sudden reduction in PCO_2 on inspiration.

Given these phases, the capnograph reflects changes in PCO_2 over time during ventilation. If the normal flow of PCO_2 is disrupted, the capnography will display the abnormalities as a modified waveform. In cases involving obstructive pathology, PCO_2 becomes trapped in the alveoli, thereby causing prolonged exhalation. This prolongation would be represented on the capnograph in the phase II expiratory upstroke and the phase III plateau by curving the initial upward deflection, producing a characteristic shark-fin pattern **FIGURE 6-19. FIGURES 6-20** through **6-23** represent other abnormal capnographic waveforms.

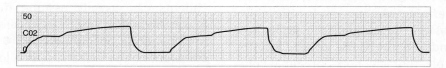

FIGURE 6-19 A shark-fin capnographic waveform indicates bronchospasm and incomplete alveolar emptying.

© Jones & Bartlett Learning.

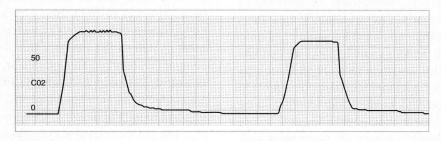

FIGURE 6-20 Capnographic waveforms caused by hypoventilation.

© Jones & Bartlett Learning.

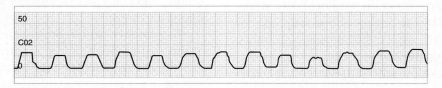

FIGURE 6-21 Capnographic waveforms caused by hyperventilation.

© Jones & Bartlett Learning.

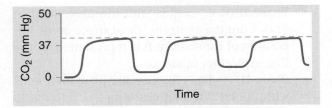

FIGURE 6-22 Capnographic waveforms caused by rebreathing.

© Jones & Bartlett Learning.

Waveform Morphology

When interpreting waveform morphology and trends in values, remember that capnography depends on cellular metabolism and patient ventilation.

Respiratory and Ventilation Abnormalities

Respiratory insufficiency is the inability of the respiratory system to keep up with the body's metabolic demands. Careful respiratory assessment can help the CCTP to determine whether the insufficiency stems from ventilation or oxygenation problems. Treatment depends on the cause of the insufficiency. For example, thoracic, head, or spinal cord injury; central nervous system depression; use of drugs; and conditions in which fatigue challenges the patient's ability to breathe normally may cause respiratory depression. Symptoms of respiratory depression consist of a low respiratory rate (less than 12 breaths/min in adults) for a prolonged time or hypoventilation. In this case, increasing ventilation will resolve the insufficiency. Oxygen therapy is indicated in those patients who cannot maintain normal Spo_2. In general, oxygen therapy should be titrated to a goal Spo_2 level of greater than 92%. Hyperoxygenation should be avoided because it may contribute to nitrogen washout and subsequent damage to alveolar cells, oxygenation toxicity leading to pulmonary dysfunction, and oxidative stress on tissues caused by the release of free radicals.

Respiratory failure occurs when the respiratory system fails to meet the body's metabolic needs. Respiratory failure can present with decreasing respiratory effort and depth. The patient may be anxious, confused, or obtunded. If not reversed, respiratory failure will lead to respiratory or cardiopulmonary arrest. Two basic types of respiratory failure are distinguished: oxygenation failure and ventilatory failure. Tachypnea is the hallmark of oxygenation failure. In this case, the ability to sustain a high respiratory rate is related to the amount of accessory muscle use the patient can endure before muscle fatigue occurs. The astute CCTP must intervene before the patient sustains an arrest. Ventilatory failure develops with increased arterial tension of CO_2.

Basic Airway Management

Although intubation is considered the gold standard for airway management, basic airway skills are the starting point in the initial patient assessment and treatment; they are also what CCTPs fall back on in difficult cases. These basic skills may be as simple as placing a nontrauma patient in the recovery position or using the head tilt–chin lift or jaw-thrust maneuver to maintain airway patency. Other basic skills may include use of adjuncts such as the oropharyngeal airway (OPA) or nasopharyngeal airway (NPA).

Positioning

Patients can usually assume the position that makes breathing easiest—typically, sitting upright in the sniffing position **FIGURE 6-24**. In most circumstances, the CCTP should allow the patient to assume this position or be prepared to assist the patient in doing so. Patients with spinal precautions and those with a diminished level of consciousness, however, may not be able to assume this position or adequately protect their airway. As the level of consciousness decreases, control of the muscles located within the oropharynx is lost, causing the tongue to contact the posterior pharyngeal wall or soft palate, which results in airway obstruction. Muscular control of the epiglottis may also be lost, leading to partial or total airway obstruction.

As a patient's level of consciousness diminishes, the ability to control secretions also decreases. This diminished control may result in significant aspiration, especially when patients are found unconscious and supine.

In patients undergoing resuscitation that requires supine positioning, manual airway maneuvers may be used to open the airway:

- **Head tilt–chin lift maneuver.** The most commonly known and used manual method of opening the airway in an unconscious,

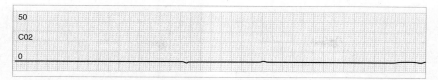

FIGURE 6-23 The complete loss of a capnographic waveform and end-tidal carbon dioxide reading in the intubated patient requires immediate attention.

© Jones & Bartlett Learning.

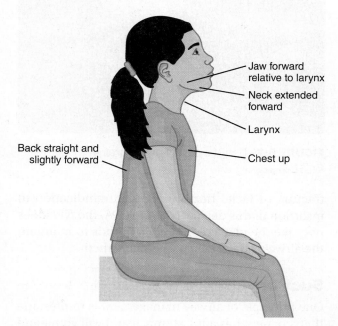

FIGURE 6-24 A patient seated in the sniffing position sits upright with the head and chin thrust slightly forward.

© Jones & Bartlett Learning.

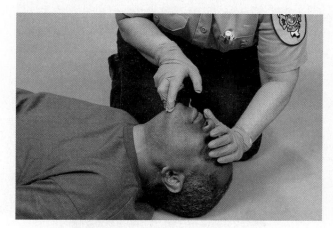

FIGURE 6-25 Head tilt–chin lift maneuver.

© Jones & Bartlett Learning.

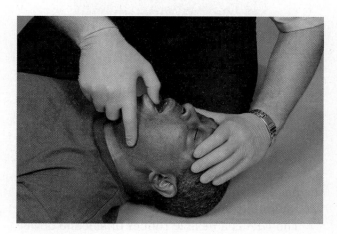

FIGURE 6-26 Tongue-jaw lift maneuver.

© Jones & Bartlett Learning.

nontrauma patient **FIGURE 6-25**. Evidence suggests the head tilt–chin lift maneuver is not as effective as the jaw-thrust maneuver.

- **Tongue-jaw lift maneuver.** Most commonly used to open and assess a patient's airway for foreign body obstruction. The patient cannot be ventilated while this maneuver is being used **FIGURE 6-26**.
- **Jaw-thrust maneuver.** Frequently used to ensure a patent airway and provide cervical spine protection in the unconscious trauma patient. In the nontrauma patient, the jaw thrust may be combined with a slight head tilt to provide a better airway opening **FIGURE 6-27**.

Airway Adjuncts

Both the OPA and the NPA are used along with manual airway maneuvers to provide a patent airway. In

the unconscious patient, neither can be used independently, as both adjuncts require maintaining manual airway maneuvers.

The OPA is a rigid device made of plastic or similar material that is placed in an unconscious patient's mouth **FIGURE 6-28**. An OPA can be inserted only when the patient does not have a gag reflex; if the gag reflex is working, the airway must be removed immediately because it will induce

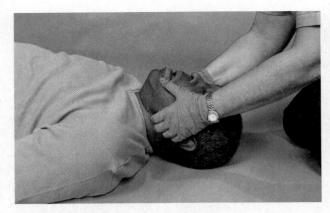

FIGURE 6-27 Jaw-thrust maneuver.

© Jones & Bartlett Learning.

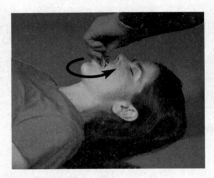

FIGURE 6-28 Use of an oropharyngeal airway.

© Jones & Bartlett Learning.

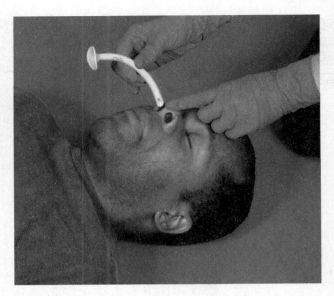

FIGURE 6-29 Use of a nasopharyngeal airway.

© Jones & Bartlett Learning.

vomiting. The appropriate size of airway is determined by measuring from the central incisors to the angle of the jaw. Insertion of an airway that is too small or too large will not provide for a patent airway and, in fact, may worsen an already compromised airway. Insertion of an OPA does not replace the need for manual methods to maintain the airway, but rather supplements them.

The NPA is a flexible rubber or silicone device that is placed in one of the nares and extends to the oropharynx **FIGURE 6-29**. It is better tolerated than the OPA in semiconscious patients. To select the appropriate size (length) of airway, measure from the tip of the patient's nose to the tragus of the ear. The diameter of the NPA should be the largest possible, but not large enough to cause blanching of the naris. Its placement should not be forced, as the mucosa of the nose is easily lacerated, which can lead to significant bleeding. Application of a non–petroleum-based lubricant might be helpful in inserting the NPA. Head trauma with evidence of basilar skull

fracture or facial fracture is a contraindication to insertion of this device. Like the OPA, the NPA does not take the place of manual methods to maintain the airway, but rather supplements them.

Suction

One principle of airway management is to presume that a patient has a full stomach and will vomit and potentially aspirate. The prehospital provider's ability to clear debris (eg, vomit, blood) from a patient's airway, while a basic skill, may be lifesaving. Clearing the airway can restore airway patency and minimize the potential for aspiration. In the context of upper airway suctioning, a large-bore suction apparatus can be used. There are various types of these devices, both fixed and portable. These suctioning devices use rigid suction catheters (Yankauer, tonsil tip, DuCanto) to remove debris. In a patient with large volumes of debris or vomit, turning the patient to their side while using a large-bore suction device works best **FIGURE 6-30**. Adequate suction should be immediately available during all airway procedures.

Flexible or soft suction catheters are used for suctioning the nasopharynx, oropharynx, and lower airways in patients with an artificial airway in place. These suction catheters, which are not designed to remove large volumes or large particulate matter, come in a variety of sizes, measured using the French scale.

Suctioning of the nasopharynx, oropharynx, and lower airway may cause hypoxemia and

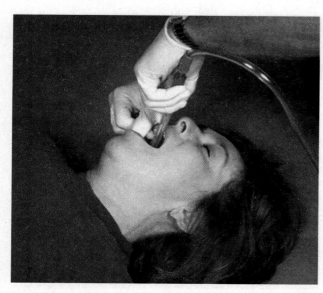

FIGURE 6-30 Suctioning.

© Jones & Bartlett Learning.

hemodynamic instability. Patients should be preoxygenated before suctioning begins, and suction attempts should be limited to 10 seconds or less while withdrawing the catheter. Patients should be oxygenated and ventilated if necessary between suction attempts.

In the critical care transport setting, you will often use suctioning while an ET tube is in place.

Indications for suctioning in this scenario include the following:

- Dyspnea
- Obstruction
- Excessive secretions

Several complications are possible with suctioning:

- Hypoxemia
- Cardiac arrhythmias
- Mechanical trauma
- Infection
- Increased intracranial pressure
- Inability to remove material due to a mucus plug or dried crusting

SKILL DRILL 6-1 shows the steps for suctioning a patient with an ET tube in place, which are also described here:

1. Choose an appropriate suction adjunct: a Yankauer or DuCanto catheter for larger objects, or a French ("whistle tip") catheter for fluid or ET tube obstructions.
2. Check, prepare, and assemble your equipment **STEP 1**.
3. Maintain universal precautions.
4. Use a sterile technique.
5. Lubricate the suction catheter **STEP 2**.
6. Preoxygenate the patient for 1 to 2 minutes with 100% oxygen **STEP 3**.

Skill Drill 6-1 Suctioning a Patient With an ET Tube in Place

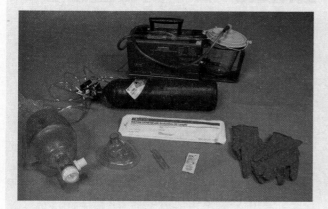

Step 1

Check, prepare, and assemble your equipment.

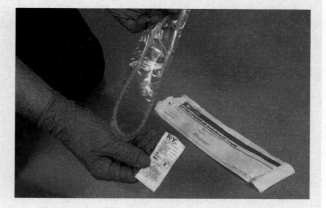

Step 2

Lubricate the suction catheter.

Continues

Skill Drill 6-1 Suctioning a Patient With an ET Tube in Place (continued)

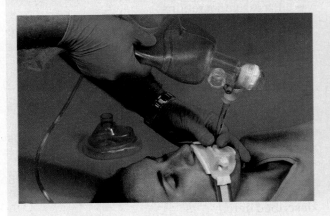

Step 3

Preoxygenate the patient.

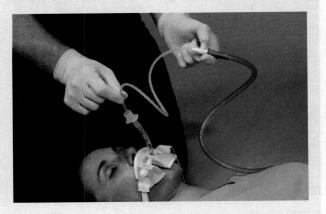

Step 4

Gently insert the catheter into the ET tube until the patient coughs.

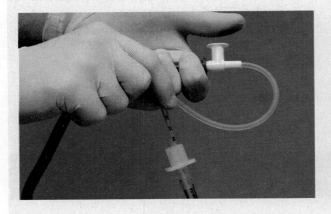

Step 5

Suction in a rotating motion while withdrawing the catheter. Monitor the patient's cardiac rhythm and Spo₂ during this procedure.

© Jones & Bartlett Learning.

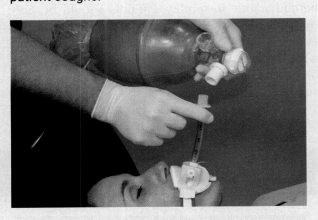

Step 6

Reattach the bag-mask device and resume ventilation and oxygenation.

7. Measure the suction catheter tip from the corner of the patient's mouth to the angle of the jaw or insert it through the ET tube until the patient coughs **STEP 4**.

8. Suction for no longer than 5 to 10 seconds as you remove the suction catheter with a twisting motion **STEP 5**.

9. Continuously observe the patient's response to suctioning (vital signs).

10. Rinse the catheter with sterile water.

11. Assess the airway, ET tube, and lungs to determine the effectiveness of the suctioning. Reattach the bag-mask device and resume ventilation and oxygenation **STEP 6**.

Oxygen Administration

Oxygen is the most commonly administered drug in the hospital and prehospital environments. Oxygen administration has potentially significant benefits when this therapy is used appropriately. As a general rule, hypoxic patients should receive supplemental oxygen to maintain an SpO_2 level of greater than 92%. Unnecessary oxygen administration, resulting in a supranormal SpO_2 level (hyperoxia), has been associated with increased morbidity and mortality in critically ill patients. Remember, it is possible for a patient to have an SpO_2 of greater than 92% and still be hypoxic at the cellular level.

Low-flow oxygen devices such as a nasal cannula can safely and comfortably deliver an FIO_2 up to approximately 40% **TABLE 6-2**. Flow rates ranging from 6 L/min up to a flush rate may be indicated for patients with apneic oxygenation during airway procedures. Patients in significant respiratory distress and those with significant hemodynamic instability require higher oxygen flow rates, usually through a nonrebreathing mask, which can deliver an FIO_2 closer to 1.0 (100%). Remember, with a critical patient, too much oxygen is better than too little oxygen.

The appropriate oxygen delivery device should be chosen based on the physical assessment of the patient. Patients in significant respiratory distress

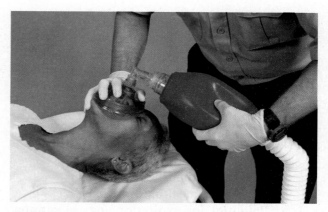

FIGURE 6-31 Use of a bag-mask device.
© Jones & Bartlett Learning.

require high-flow oxygen via a nonrebreathing mask or bag-mask device. Patients with agonal respirations or those who are apneic require bag-mask ventilation with supplemental high-flow oxygen. The device chosen must fit the patient's overall assessment.

When gas flow is inadequate, positive-pressure ventilation is required to ensure the patient is appropriately oxygenated. Indeed, delivery of positive-pressure ventilation when the patient's spontaneous respiration is inadequate may be life-saving care. A bag-mask device is commonly used to deliver supplemental oxygen via positive-pressure ventilation, and can be used in combination with a face mask or an invasive airway device such as a SGA or ET tube **FIGURE 6-31**.

Advanced Airway Management

Although basic airway maneuvers are a starting point in the CCTP's assessment and patient care, they are not considered to be definitive airway management. Instead, definitive airway management entails the placement of an ET tube or tracheostomy tube within the trachea. Insertion of such a tube facilitates adequate oxygenation and ventilation. Patients primarily require intubation for two reasons:

- Failure to maintain a patent airway
- Failure to adequately oxygenate or ventilate

When an ET tube is present in the trachea, the upper airway structures, such as the tongue and epiglottis, do not affect airway patency. With a cuffed

TABLE 6-2 Oxygen Versus Approximate FIO_2	
Oxygen, L/min	**Approximate FIO_2, %**
Nasal cannula	
1	24
2	28
3	32
4	36
5	40
6	44
Simple face mask, 10	40–60
Nonrebreathing mask, 12–15	80–100

Abbreviation: FIO_2, fraction of inspired oxygen

Data from Federal Aviation Administration.

ET tube, aspiration of upper airway secretions and vomitus is minimized, albeit not entirely prevented. A properly placed and maintained ET tube virtually ensures that the airway will remain patent. It also facilitates delivery of oxygen and adequate ventilation. Some indications for ET intubation are as follows:

- Diminished level of consciousness with loss of airway control
  - Absent or diminished gag reflex
  - Glasgow Coma Scale score of 8 or less
  - Potential for aspiration (eg, secretions, blood, vomitus)
- Respiratory failure (eg, hypoxemia, hypercarbia)
- Cardiac arrest, after adequate CPR or bag-mask ventilations have been provided

Predicting the Difficult Airway

In the prehospital environment, an estimated 20% of all emergency intubations are classified as difficult. In such a case, the prehospital provider has to decide how to accomplish airway management. Ask yourself, "Can I manage this airway at the BLS level? Can I intubate this patient's trachea?"

History is one factor to consider when treating a difficult airway. Anatomic findings suggestive of a difficult airway may include congenital abnormalities, recent surgery, trauma, infection, or neoplastic disease (cancer). Two commonly used mnemonics to guide assessment of the difficult airway are LEMONS and HEAVEN. The elements of LEMONS mnemonic are described here:

L Look externally
E Evaluate 3-3-2
M Mallampati
O Obstruction
N Neck mobility
S Saturation

As indicated by the *L* in the LEMONS mnemonic, simply looking at the patient may suggest the relative difficulty that may be encountered during airway management. Patients with short, thick necks may be difficult to intubate. Morbid obesity significantly complicates intubation. Dental conditions such as overbite, or buck teeth, may make intubation difficult.

The *E* stands for "evaluate 3-3-2." Three different anatomic measurements are assessed using the **3-3-2 rule FIGURE 6-32**. The first 3 refers to mouth

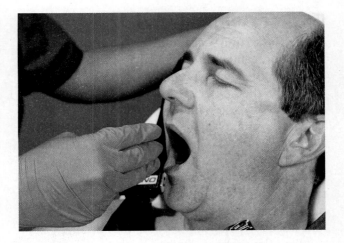

A

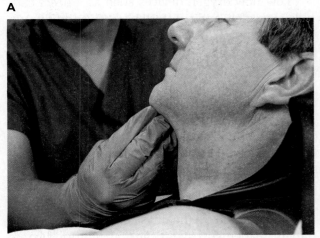

B

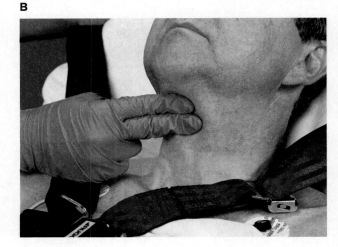

C

FIGURE 6-32 The 3-3-2 rule. **A.** The mouth should be at least three fingers wide when open. **B.** The space from the chin to the hyoid bone should be at least three fingers wide. **C.** The distance from the hyoid bone to the thyroid notch should be at least two fingers wide.

© Jones & Bartlett Learning.

opening. Ideally, a patient's mouth will open at least three fingerbreadths (approximately 5 cm) wide. Conversely, a width of less than three fingers indicates a possibly difficult airway. The second 3 refers to the length of the mandible, measured from the tip of the chin to the hyoid bone: At least three fingerbreadths is optimal. Smaller mandibles have less room for displacement of the tongue and epiglottis, which can make airway management more difficult. The 2 part of this rule refers to the ideal distance (two fingerbreadths) from the hyoid bone to the thyroid notch.

The *M* stands for Mallampati, an anesthesiologist who developed the Mallampati classification to predict the relative difficulty of intubation **TABLE 6-3**. This classification is based on the oropharyngeal structures visible in an upright, seated patient who can fully open their mouth. Although this system is an accurate predictor of difficult intubation, it has limited utility in unconscious patients and in patients who cannot follow commands. If a patient is cooperative and able to comply with this evaluation, emergent prehospital intubation is probably not necessary, but the evaluation is important in that it can provide useful information should intubation be needed.

The *O* represents obstruction. Anything that might interfere with visualization or tracheal tube placement should be noted. Foreign bodies, obesity, hematoma, and masses are all examples of obstructive situations that can create a difficult airway.

The *N* stands for neck mobility. The ideal position for visualization and intubation is the sniffing position, in which the adult head is slightly elevated and extended **FIGURE 6-34**. The two types of patients who most commonly have neck mobility problems are trauma patients (due to use of cervical collars and/or injury) and older patients (due to osteoporosis or arthritis). The inability to place the patient in the sniffing position can significantly impact the ability to visualize the airway.

The *S* in LEMONS stands for saturation or situation. Unlike the other components of this mnemonic, which assess anatomic features, the *S* reminds providers to consider the physiologic presentation.

TABLE 6-3 Mallampati Classification	
Mallampati Class	**Description**
I	Entire posterior pharynx fully exposed **FIGURE 6-33A**
II	Posterior pharynx partially exposed **FIGURE 6-33B**
III	Posterior pharynx cannot be seen; base of uvula exposed **FIGURE 6-33C**
IV	No posterior structures can be seen **FIGURE 6-33D**

© Jones & Bartlett Learning.

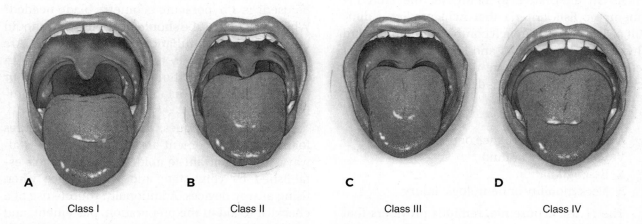

A	B	C	D
Class I	Class II	Class III	Class IV

FIGURE 6-33 Mallampati classification to predict the relative difficulty of intubation.

© Jones & Bartlett Learning.

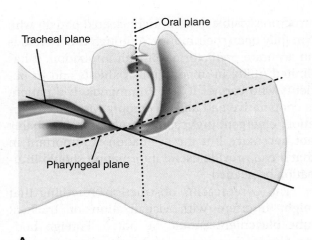

A

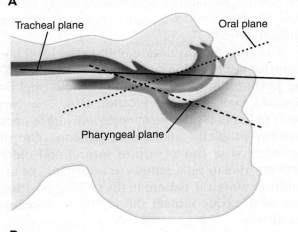

B

FIGURE 6-34 Sniffing position. **A.** The three axes of the airway (oral, pharyngeal, and tracheal) in the neutral position. **B.** The three axes in the sniffing position.

© Jones & Bartlett Learning.

As an alternative to LEMONS, the HEAVEN mnemonic lists criteria that help predict a difficult airway. This approach combines anatomic and physiologic assessments and suggests a course of action. It does not require the patient to be conscious. HEAVEN is described as follows:

H Hypoxemia
E Extreme of size
A Anatomic disturbance or obstruction
V Vomit, blood, or fluid
E Exsanguination
N Neck mobility or neurologic injury

The *H*, for hypoxemia, reminds providers that patients will desaturate rapidly during intubation if their initial oxygenation is low. Providers must maximize oxygenation before making any intubation attempt.

The first *E* stands for extreme of size. It includes pediatric patients younger than 8 years and adults who are clinically obese.

The *A* stands for anatomic disruption or obstruction. Such a finding may limit direct visualization during laryngoscopy. Consider nonintubation management and provide support to achieve oxygenation.

The *V* stands for vomit, blood, or fluid noted in the pharynx or hypopharynx before laryngoscopy. Suction clinically significant fluids before attempting intubation.

The second *E* stands for exsanguination. Blood loss raises concerns of anemia and reduced oxygen-carrying capacity. Consider not intubating such patients to reduce the apnea time for them.

Finally, the *N* stands for neck mobility or neurologic injury. Consider performing a hyperacute video laryngoscopy in patients with these issues.

Orotracheal Intubation

Once the decision to intubate a patient has been made, the CCTP needs to determine how to most effectively accomplish the procedure. The goal is to intubate the patient on the first attempt (first-pass success) without induction of hemodynamic compromise or aspiration. Important questions that must be answered before undertaking orotracheal intubation include the following: Does direct laryngoscopy or indirect (video) laryngoscopy offer the greatest chance of successful intubation on the first attempt? Which size of blade should be used? Is a hyperacute geometry blade needed? Which size of ET tube should be used? What should be done if the intubation is unsuccessful? Are medications necessary to facilitate intubation? In addition, the CCTP should consider LEMONS or HEAVEN criteria to help determine the best intubation approach.

Multiple techniques, devices, and procedures for airway management are discussed next. As always, it is important to abide by the protocols established by your state and your service when using airway devices. Additionally, routine use of a checklist to aid in the preparation, placement, and postprocedure care of advanced airways is highly recommended.

Equipment

The following equipment is needed to provide advanced, invasive airway management:

- Gloves, mask, and goggles
- ET tubes of various sizes
  - Usual size range of 2.0 to 9.0
  - Most adults accept a size 7.0 to 8.0
- Appropriate-size stylet (adult or pediatric)
- Appropriate-size laryngoscope handle and blades (Miller or Macintosh)
- Suctioning equipment
- 10-mL syringe
- Water-soluble lubricant
- Commercial tube-holding device
- Age- and size-appropriate bag-mask device with reservoir
- Supplemental oxygen
- Stethoscope
- Device able to perform continuous waveform
- Magill forceps
- Topical anesthetic spray (for nasotracheal intubation)
- Rescue airway device (King LT, laryngeal mask airway, i-gel)
- 20-mL syringe
- 40-mL syringe

The laryngoscope handles and blades must also be the appropriate size:

- Straight blades: sizes 00, 0, 1, 2, 3, 4
  - Miller
  - Wisconsin
- Curved blades: sizes 1, 2, 3, 4
  - Macintosh

Many believe the type of blade used can have a significant impact on the success of intubation. For many older children and adults, the choice of the blade is not as important as the comfort and experience of the CCTP with a particular blade type and the technique used in the intubation attempt. For smaller children, because of age-related anatomic differences, choosing a straight blade to actually pick up the epiglottis may facilitate successful intubation. Remember, the curved blade is placed in the vallecula, which is located at the base of the tongue and displaces the epiglottis indirectly via pressure on the underlying hyoepiglottic ligament. However, the curved blade may also be used to pick up the epiglottis to facilitate visualization.

Special Populations

In infants, children, and young adults, many methods may be used to estimate the appropriate size of ET tube for the patient.

- For children older than 1 year, calculate the appropriate size by adding 16 to the child's age in years, then dividing this number by 4:

  $$(16 + \text{Child's age in years})/4 = \text{ET tube size}$$

- Use the diameter of the child's pinky finger to estimate the diameter of the tube.
- Use a weight-based chart.

Orotracheal Intubation

Indications for orotracheal intubation include:

- Airway control following coma, respiratory arrest, and/or cardiac arrest
- Ventilatory support prior to impending respiratory failure
- Need for prolonged artificial ventilatory support
- Medication administration (atropine, epinephrine, naloxone)
- Impending airway compromise (burns, trauma)
- Expected complicated clinical course

Relative contraindications for orotracheal intubation include:

- Inability to open the mouth because of trauma, dislocation, or pathologic condition
- Epiglottitis
- Inability to see the glottic opening
- Copious secretions, vomit, or blood in the airway

Direct Laryngoscopy

Orotracheal laryngoscopy can be performed in two ways. The first, more traditional way is via direct visualization of the vocal cords by displacement of the tongue with a laryngoscope blade. Advantages of direct laryngoscopy include high success rates, low equipment cost, and reliability. Disadvantages include difficulty maintaining proficiency, anatomic limitations, and cervical motion restriction precautions.

This procedure begins with airway assessment, equipment preparation, oxygenation, and patient positioning. Each of these processes is key to achieving successful intubation. When performing direct laryngoscopy, the provider must align the oral, laryngeal, and pharyngeal axes to visualize the larynx. In patients without suspected cervical injury, placing the patient's ears level with the sternal notch, with the face parallel to the plane of the ceiling, may achieve this goal.

Once the patient is positioned, the provider inserts the laryngoscope blade into the oral cavity, sweeps the tongue to the left, and progressively advances the blade until the epiglottis is identified. At this point, if using a straight Miller blade, the provider would use the distal tip of the blade to directly elevate the epiglottis to expose the larynx and vocal cords. The Miller blade is generally preferred in the pediatric population because it allows for direct control of the epiglottis, which may be floppy and more challenging to manage in young patients as compared to adult patients. In the event that a curved Macintosh blade is selected, the tip is inserted into the vallecula to apply pressure to the hyoepiglottic ligament, which in turn lifts the epiglottis to expose the glottic opening.

The view obtained during laryngoscopy can be graded with the Cormack-Lehane system, which scores the view of the glottic opening:

- **Grade 1.** The entire glottic opening is visible.
- **Grade 2.** The arytenoid cartilages or the posterior portion of the glottic opening is visible **FIGURE 6-35**.
- **Grade 3.** Only the epiglottis is visible.
- **Grade 4.** Only the tongue and/or soft palate is visible.

Grade 3 on laryngoscopy can result in significant difficulty intubating the trachea due to the CCTP's inability to visualize any part of the glottic opening.

When visualization of the larynx is successful, an ET tube may be placed through the larynx and into the trachea. Following successful placement and verification of the ET tube, a small distal cuff is inflated to seal the airway. Note that microaspiration is still a risk even when this seal is in place. Monitor the ET tube's pilot balloon for proper inflation pressure, which ranges from 20 to 30 mm Hg. If ET tube cuff pressure exceeds the pressure within the superficial capillaries of the trachea (30 mm Hg), the resulting tissue ischemia can lead to tracheal stenosis. If the clinical condition permits, raising the head of the stretcher to 30° allows gravity to help reduce aspiration events.

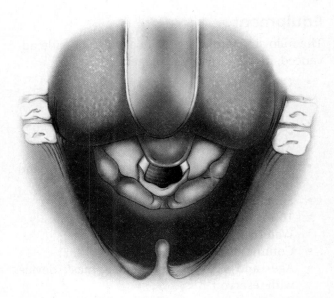

FIGURE 6-35 Laryngoscopic view of the vocal cords (white fibrous bands).

© Jones & Bartlett Learning.

Indirect (Video) Laryngoscopy

The second way to perform orotracheal intubation is via indirect visualization of the vocal cords using video laryngoscopy. The video laryngoscope provides for indirect viewing of the glottic opening via a video camera at the distal end of the blade, which sends a video feed to a screen that is either a separate handheld tablet **FIGURE 6-36** or attached to the handle of the device **FIGURE 6-37**. Advantages of video laryngoscopy include the ability to visualize the vocal cords without needing to align the airway axes, minimal need for significant tongue displacement, and, although somewhat device specific, often a greater distance between the CCTP's face and the patient's face. Disadvantages include the cost of purchasing and maintaining the devices, the need for space to store the device, and the potential for fluids in the airway to obscure the video camera. The use of video laryngoscopy has expanded exponentially in the past several years due to reduced unit costs, recognition of its effectiveness, and greater education on use of these devices.

Two distinct types of video laryngoscopes may be used: those with a **standard geometry blade** and those with a **hyperangulated blade**. The standard geometry blade is inserted using a similar technique as for its direct laryngoscope counterparts. As previously described, the procedure begins with airway

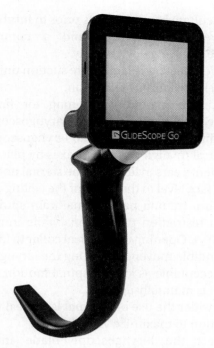

FIGURE 6-36 The GlideScope Ranger video laryngoscope.

Used with permission. © Verathon Inc.

assessment, equipment preparation, oxygenation, and patient positioning. Each of these processes is key to achieving successful intubation. Using the standard geometry video laryngoscope, the CCTP directly visualizes the blade entering the oral cavity, then transitions attention to the device monitor for indirect viewing of the larynx.

Video laryngoscopes often provide excellent visualization of airway structures, but this does not always translate to successful intubation. When using these devices, the CCTP should account for the delta blade angle and camera angle. The larynx should be positioned in the center upper half of the monitor and the blade should not be advanced farther when visualization is achieved. Once this view is obtained, an angulated **rigid stylet** may be necessary to pass the ET tube around the nondisplaced tongue. A Cormack-Lehane grade 2 view may be optimal to facilitate ET tube passage. If the patient has limited neck mobility, either from a preexisting condition or because of the current clinical need for spinal motion restriction, the use of a hyperangulated blade may be beneficial. This blade overcomes the need to align the airway axes due to its anterior viewing angle, but almost always requires the concurrent use of an angulated rigid stylet to guide ET tube advancement.

Bougie-Assisted Intubation

A bougie is a flexible 10–15 French, 60-cm, ET tube introducer with a distal coude tip **FIGURE 6-38**. Its tip angle of 30° to 40° allows this device to transmit a tactile sensation to the user as it passes the tracheal rings and encounters resistance as the airways narrow. This simple device allows the CCTP to perform laryngoscopy in difficult airways and may be considered for all intubations.

The bougie may be inserted blindly or when the larynx is visualized, at which point the bougie would be passed under the epiglottis. It is inserted from the side of the patient's mouth and rotated into the

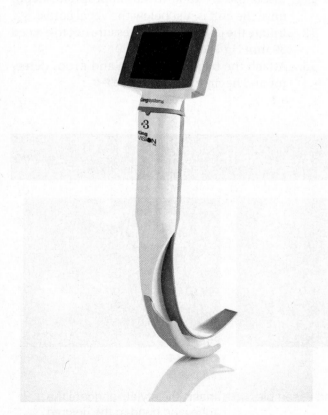

FIGURE 6-37 The King Vision video laryngoscope.

© Ambu.

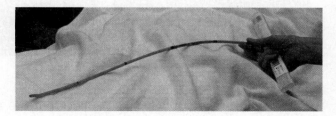

FIGURE 6-38 The bougie.

Courtesy of Marianne Gausche-Hill, MD, FACEP, FAAP.

trachea until gentle resistance is encountered. Next, an assistant places an ET tube onto the bougie and slides it down the introducer into the trachea. Alternatively, the bougie may be preloaded with the ET tube. The bougie may also be used during ET tube exchange and surgical airway placement.

Orotracheal Intubation With Direct Laryngoscopy

SKILL DRILL 6-2 shows the steps for orotracheal intubation, which are also described here:

1. Follow standard precautions.
2. Preoxygenate the spontaneously breathing patient for 3 minutes (eight vital capacity breaths) with high-flow oxygen or a nonrebreathing mask. Try to avoid bag-mask ventilations because these devices increase air insufflation of the stomach and, therefore, the potential for regurgitation and aspiration **STEP 1**.
3. Check, prepare, and assemble your equipment **STEP 2**.
4. Choose an appropriate-size tube, with the tube still in the package to maintain sterility. Check the cuff's integrity by inflating it and checking for leaks. Insert the stylet, lubricate the tube, and bend it to the desired position. It is also a good idea to have a tube of a slightly smaller diameter prepared, in case it is needed **STEP 3**.
5. Auscultate breath sounds prior to intubation.
6. Have Magill forceps and a commercial tube-securing device ready.
7. Have at least one large-bore suction unit at the patient's side and turned on.
8. Optimize patient positioning for first-pass success. When using direct laryngoscopy or a traditional geometry video laryngoscope, it is critical to align the airway axes by placing the patient's ears in line with the sternal notch and the face level to the plane of the ceiling **STEP 4**. With a trauma patient, maintain spinal motion restriction precautions while intubating **STEP 5**. Opening the cervical collar to facilitate mandible movement during the laryngoscopy is acceptable as long as spinal motion restriction is manually applied.
9. Consider the use of external laryngeal manipulation to maximize visualization.
10. Insert the laryngoscope blade into the right side of the patient's mouth, sweep the tongue to the left, and visualize the vocal cords **STEP 6**.
11. Insert the ET tube to the appropriate depth until the cuff is just below the vocal cords.
12. Inflate the cuff, with this pressure not to exceed 30 mm Hg **STEP 7**.
13. Attach the bag-mask device and ETCO$_2$ detector and begin to ventilate **STEP 8**.

Skill Drill 6-2 Performing Orotracheal Intubation

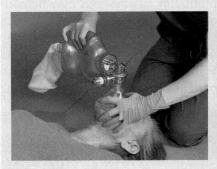

Step 1

Follow standard precautions. Preoxygenate the patient.

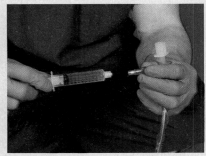

Step 2

Check, prepare, and assemble your equipment.

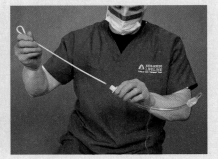

Step 3

Insert the stylet, lubricate the tube, and bend to the desired position. Auscultate breath sounds.

Skill Drill 6-2 Performing Orotracheal Intubation (continued)

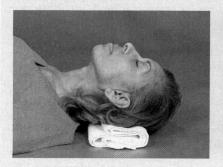

Step 4

Align the airway axes by placing the patient's ears in line with the sternal notch and the face level to the plane of the ceiling.

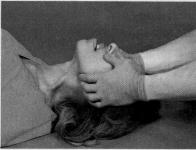

Step 5

With a trauma patient, maintain cervical spine immobilization while intubating.

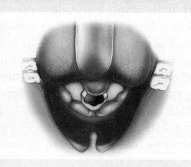

Step 6

Insert the laryngoscope blade into the right side of the patient's mouth, sweep the tongue to the left, and visualize the cords. Insert the ET tube to the appropriate depth until the cuff is just below the vocal cords.

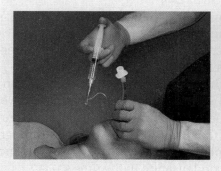

Step 7

Inflate the cuff with 10 mL of air and remove the syringe. Remove the stylet if applicable.

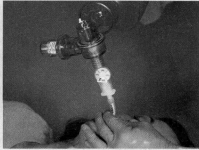

Step 8

Attach the bag-mask device and $ETCO_2$ detector and begin to ventilate. Verify correct tube placement by auscultating the epigastrium and bilateral chest.

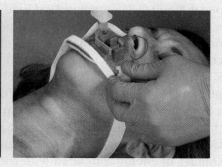

Step 9

Secure the ET tube with a commercial device or tape

All images © Jones & Bartlett Learning.

14. Verify correct tube placement by auscultating the patient's epigastrium and bilateral chest.
15. Observe for bilateral chest expansion, compliance of the bag-mask device, condensation in the tube, and the presence of continuous waveform end-tidal capnography.
16. Secure the ET tube with a commercial device or tape **STEP 9**.
17. Frequently verify placement of the ET tube, ideally with waveform capnography. If continuous waveform capnography is not available, the tube position should be verified, at a minimum, each time the patient is moved.

Flight Considerations

When you are performing tracheal intubation in the air medical environment, consider filling the cuff with water equivalent to the volume of air needed for a seal. Another consideration is using a cuff pressure manometer to monitor and adjust pressures as altitude changes, or using the minimal occluding technique. This technique involves placing the stethoscope over the laryngeal area while inflating the cuff until air leak is no longer present at peak inspiratory pressure. The goal is to keep cuff pressures at less than 20 to 30 mm Hg.

Nasotracheal Intubation

Nasotracheal (nasal) intubation was once the preferred airway management technique in patients suspected of having a spinal cord injury. With the advent of rapid sequence intubation (RSI), however, nasal intubation is now used relatively infrequently. Most patients who undergo nasotracheal intubation are receiving care in the prehospital environment where RSI may not be permitted or are spontaneously breathing but present the likelihood of a difficult airway, making RSI inadvisable.

Nasotracheal intubation requires a spontaneously breathing patient. The likelihood of success with this procedure may be enhanced by using ET tubes specifically designed for nasotracheal placement. Even so, this type of intubation carries a fairly high failure rate and takes longer to perform than intubation under direct laryngoscopy. It also frequently requires placement of an ET tube of a smaller diameter compared with the tubes placed during direct laryngoscopy.

Prolonged attempts at nasotracheal intubation may result in significant hypoxemia and glottic edema secondary to trauma. This procedure may also cause significant bleeding and vomiting. The risks of hypoxemia and hypercarbia in a patient with inadequate respirations must be weighed against the risks of performing nasal intubation. Combativeness, facial trauma with suspected basilar skull fracture, coagulopathy, and upper airway infection are a few of the relative contraindications to nasotracheal intubation.

Indications for nasotracheal intubation include the following:

- Patients who are awake and breathing but are in danger of respiratory failure

- Patients with a gag reflex
- Patients who are breathing but cannot open their mouth

Contraindications to nasotracheal intubation include the following:

- Apneic or near-apneic patients
- Inability to pass the tube through the nostril
- Blood clotting or anticoagulation therapy
- Severe nasal, facial, or basilar skull fractures

SKILL DRILL 6-3 shows the steps for nasotracheal intubation, which are described here:

1. Follow standard precautions (gloves and face shield).
2. Preoxygenate the patient whenever possible with 100% oxygen provided by an appropriate delivery device **STEP 1**.
3. Check, prepare, and assemble your equipment **STEP 2**.
4. Place the patient's head in a neutral position **STEP 3**.
5. Select the proper size of ET tube and form it into a circle **STEP 4**.
6. Apply topical anesthetic spray to the patient's nostrils and pharynx.
7. Lubricate the tip of the tube with a water-soluble gel **STEP 5**.
8. Release the circle from the ET tube and gently insert it into either nostril, with the bevel of the tube pointed toward the septum **STEP 6**.
9. Advance the tube until the tip passes through the nasopharynx. Listen for breath sounds and look for condensation in the tube **STEP 7**.
10. As the tube approaches the larynx, the patient's breath sounds will be amplified. Gently and evenly push the tube into the larynx during inspiration.
11. The 15-mm adapter should rest close to the nostril. Passing the tube through the trachea may stimulate the gag reflex, which could result in the patient coughing and bucking. Watch and monitor for vomiting.
12. Inflate the distal cuff with 5 to 10 mL of air and detach the syringe **STEP 8**.
13. Attach an ETCO$_2$ detector to the ET tube **STEP 9**.
14. Attach the bag-mask device and ventilate. Verify tube placement by auscultating the patient's chest bilaterally and over the epigastrium.
15. Secure the ET tube **STEP 10**.

Face-to-Face Intubation

Intubation may be performed with the provider's face at the same level as the patient's face when other positions are not possible, such as in the context of a motor vehicle crash where the patient is in a seated position or in a tight space where the space above the head cannot be accessed. This approach is called face-to-face intubation, or the tomahawk method. The procedure is the same as with orotracheal intubation, except for the following points:

- The patient's head cannot be placed in the sniffing position. It is manually stabilized by a second provider during the entire procedure.
- Hold the laryngoscope (with a Macintosh blade) in your right hand with the blade facing downward like a hatchet, while holding the ET tube in your left hand. Insert the laryngoscope blade into the right side of the patient's mouth, sweep the tongue to the patient's left, and visualize the vocal cords.
- Once the laryngoscope blade has been placed, the provider who is intubating the patient may slightly adjust the patient's head for better visualization by pulling the mandible forward while pressing down.

Skill Drill 6-3 Performing Nasotracheal Intubation

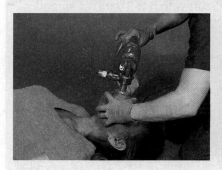

Step 1

Follow standard precautions (gloves and face shield). Preoxygenate the patient.

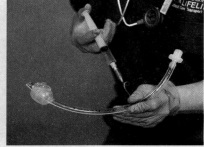

Step 2

Check, prepare, and assemble your equipment.

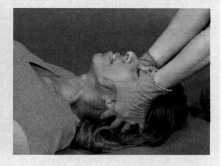

Step 3

Place the patient's head in a neutral position.

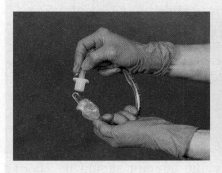

Step 4

Select the proper size of ET tube and form it into a circle.

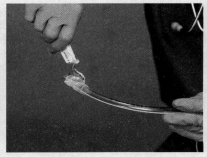

Step 5

Apply topical anesthetic spray to the patient's nostrils and pharynx. Lubricate the tip of the tube with a water-soluble gel.

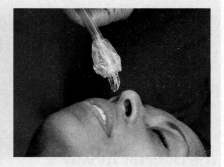

Step 6

Release the circle from the ET tube and gently insert it into either nostril, with the bevel of the tube pointed toward the septum.

Continues

Skill Drill 6-3 Performing Nasotracheal Intubation (continued)

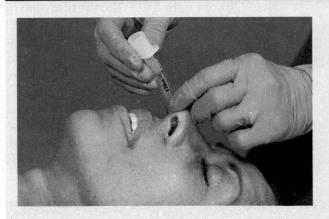

Step 7

Advance the tube until the tip passes through the nasopharynx. Listen for breath sounds and look for condensation in the tube.

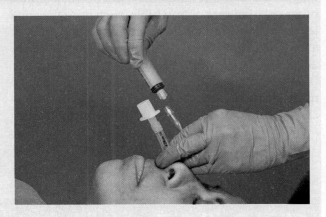

Step 8

Inflate the distal cuff with 5 to 10 mL of air and detach the syringe.

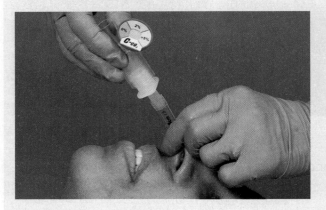

Step 9

Attach an ETCO$_2$ detector to the ET tube.

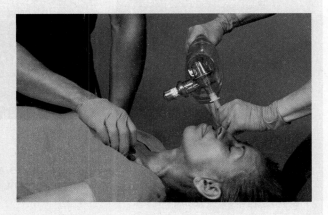

Step 10

Attach the bag-mask device and ventilate. Auscultate the chest bilaterally and over the epigastrium. Secure the ET tube.

© Jones & Bartlett Learning.

The Difficult Airway

Attempts at laryngoscopy should be limited to approximately 30 seconds or less, as lengthy attempts at intubation can result in significant hypoxemia, hypercarbia, and hemodynamic instability. Even a single episode of hypoxia may negatively affect the patient's outcome. If the patient is hypoxic or having clinically significant desaturation during a laryngoscopy, the attempt should be aborted and the patient immediately oxygenated. Remember that pulse oximetry is a lagging indicator, and the patient's Pao$_2$ may be lower than the displayed Spo$_2$.

The intubation strategy should be optimized to realize first-pass success. However, if you are attempting intubation and not visualizing what you need to proceed, stop, ventilate, and try something different. The patient's position is probably the most crucial aspect to reconsider.

1. Reposition the patient's head, if possible, to elevate the ear to the level of the sternal notch, with the face parallel to the ceiling. In some patients, achieving this position may require placing multiple blankets under the head and shoulders and/or elevating the head of the stretcher.
2. If spinal motion restriction precautions have been implemented, remove the front of the collar while maintaining manual spinal precautions to allow for increased mandibular displacement.
3. Consider performing external laryngeal manipulation. In this procedure, the provider uses the right hand to manipulate the larynx and improve the laryngeal view, and then has an assistant maintain this view while the provider passes the ET tube under direct visualization **FIGURE 6-39**.
4. Consider using a bougie or tracheal tube introducer.

Difficult Airway Versus Failed Airway

The Difficult Airway Course defines a failed airway as one that meets the following three criteria:

1. Failure to maintain an acceptable SpO_2 during or after one or more failed laryngoscopic attempts

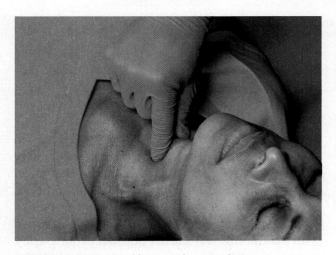

FIGURE 6-39 External laryngeal manipulation.

© Jones & Bartlett Learning.

2. Three failed attempts at orotracheal intubation by an experienced intubator, even when oxygenation can be maintained
3. The single "best attempt" at intubation fails in the "forced to act" situation

More simply, a failed airway can be defined as "a failure to oxygenate or ventilate the patient."

With a difficult airway, providers can predict complications that might occur while securing the patient's airway. For example, the CCTP can determine a difficult airway through assessment of the patient using the LEMONS or HEAVEN mnemonic. Both anatomic and physiologic indicators need to be considered in this assessment. Anatomic issues may be overcome with positioning and equipment, whereas physiologic issues may necessitate additional treatment of the patient, optimization, and resuscitation. Failing to predict the difficult airway is a leading cause of preventable airway failures. In other words, you must determine whether the patient will be difficult to ventilate via bag-mask device, whether the patient will be difficult to intubate, whether you can use an SGA, or whether a cricothyrotomy is likely. As emergency medical providers, CCTPs do not have the option of canceling a case due to a difficult or failed airway. Guidance for caring for patients with difficult and failed airways is described in the algorithms in **FIGURE 6-40** and **6-41**, respectively.

Special Populations

Pregnant patients have a four times higher rate of failed intubation as compared with nonpregnant patients. Keep the following facts in mind when you are treating a pregnant patient:

1. The airway in pregnant patients is usually more anterior.
2. The airway tissues of a pregnant patient are often friable and will bleed easily when manipulated.
3. Pregnant patients are at a high risk of aspiration secondary to release of the hormone relaxin.
4. Pregnant patients have more oral secretions and require more suctioning, even after being intubated.

Postintubation Management

Once the ET tube has been passed and the balloon inflated, correct tube placement should be

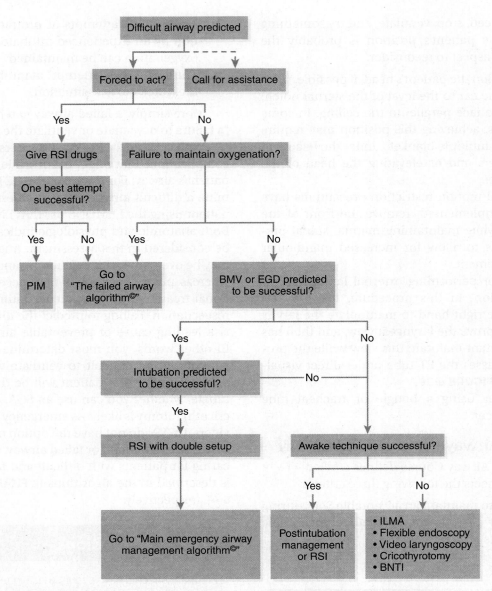

Abbreviations: BMV, bag-mask ventilation; BNTI, blind nasotracheal intubation; EGD, extraglottic device; ILMA, intubating laryngeal mask; PIM, Postintubation management; RSI, rapid sequence intubation

FIGURE 6-40 The difficult airway algorithm.

Brown CA, Sakles JC, Mick NW, eds. *The Walls Manual of Emergency Airway Management.* 5th ed. Philadelphia, PA: Wolters Kluwer; 2018:27-28.

confirmed through the use of continuous wave-form end-tidal capnography. Additionally, the chest should be auscultated to ensure the presence of bilateral lung sounds and the absence of epigastric sounds with ventilation. If breath sounds are heard for the right lung only and you believe the ET tube may have been placed too deep, consider deflating the cuff, withdrawing the ET tube slightly, reinflating the cuff, and repeating auscultation. Do not automatically assume the ET tube is too deep when you do not hear breath sounds on the left side of the chest. Other factors may be present that affect left-side breath sounds, including pneumothorax, pneumonia, atelectasis, and pneumonectomy.

If ET tube placement cannot be confirmed with continuous waveform end-tidal capnography, remove the ET tube and remove bag-mask device ventilation.

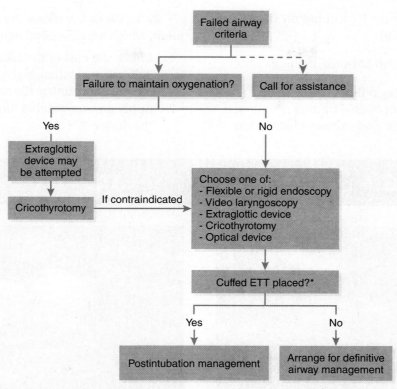

* In children under 8 years of age, an uncuffed or cuffed endotracheal tube may be placed. In neonates, uncuffed endotracheal tubes should be placed.

FIGURE 6-41 The failed airway algorithm.

Brown CA, Sakles JC, Mick NW, eds. *The Walls Manual of Emergency Airway Management*. 5th ed. Philadelphia, PA: Wolters Kluwer; 2018:27-28.

Once the patient is successfully intubated, provide postintubation analgesia and sedation per your local protocol. Ensure the tube is secured using a commercial tube holder and the patient is connected to the ventilator. If available, obtain a postintubation chest radiograph and ABG analysis. Finally, consider placing an orogastric tube to allow for stomach decompression.

Supraglottic Airways

Several SGAs are available that can be used as rescue airways if orotracheal intubation is unsuccessful or predicted to be difficult. These options include the laryngeal mask airway, King LT airway, and i-gel airway.

Laryngeal Mask Airway

The laryngeal mask airway (LMA) was designed for use as an alternative to mask ventilation and intubation in the operating room. The LMA has been advocated for use as a rescue airway in the setting of failed intubation in both the emergency and EMS environments. LMAs have various designs, some of which allow an ET tube to be passed through the airway or a tube to decompress the stomach. The basic design is similar to an ET tube at the proximal end, in that a standard adapter is present to allow ventilation. The distal end is equipped with an elliptical cuff, which, when inflated, covers the supraglottic area and allows ventilation.

An advantage of the LMA is ease of insertion—placement of the device does not require laryngoscopy. It also provides superior oxygenation and ventilation compared with bag-mask ventilation. Some disadvantages associated with LMA use are the risk of aspiration and difficulty with obtaining an adequate seal, allowing a loss of tidal volume and gastric insufflation.

Indications for LMA use include:

- Deep coma, cardiac arrest, and/or respiratory arrest

- Inability to perform ET intubation (including lack of equipment)

  Contraindications to LMA use include:

- Patients with a gag reflex
- Facial and/or esophageal trauma
- Suspected foreign body airway obstruction

SKILL DRILL 6-4 shows the steps for LMA placement, which are described here:

1. Check the cuff of the LMA by inflating it with 50% more air than is required for that size of airway. Then deflate the cuff completely **STEP 1**.
2. Apply a water-soluble lubricant to the base of the device **STEP 2**.

Skill Drill 6-4 LMA Insertion

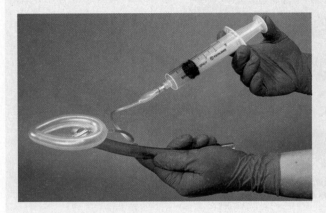

Step 1
Check the cuff of the LMA by inflating it with 50% more air than is required for that size of airway. Then deflate the cuff completely.

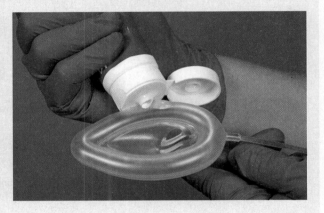

Step 2
Apply a water-soluble lubricant to the base of the device.

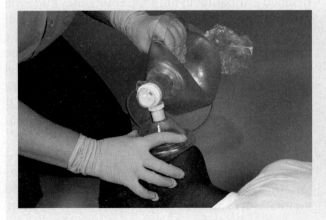

Step 3
Preoxygenate the patient. Ventilation should not be interrupted for more than 30 seconds to accomplish LMA placement.

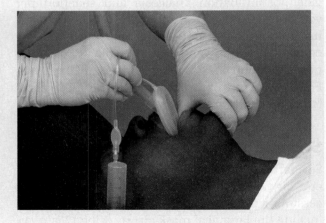

Step 4
Place the patient's head in the sniffing position. Insert your finger between the cuff and the tube. Place the index finger of your dominant hand in the notch between the tube and the cuff. Open the patient's mouth.

Skill Drill 6-4 LMA Insertion (continued)

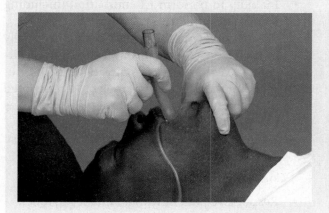

Step 5

Insert the LMA along the roof of the mouth, with the aperture of the mask facing the tongue and the back of the mask against the roof of the mouth.

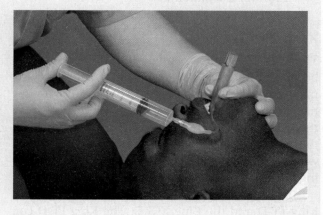

Step 6

Inflate the cuff with the amount of air indicated for that size of airway.

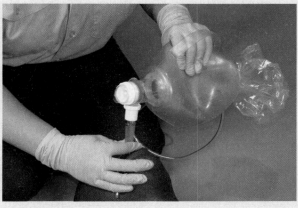

© Jones & Bartlett Learning.

Step 7

Attach the bag-mask device and begin to ventilate the patient. Check for chest rise and lung or epigastrium sounds.

3. Preoxygenate the patient with a bag-mask device and 100% oxygen. Ventilation should not be interrupted for more than 30 seconds to accomplish LMA placement **STEP 3**.
4. Assemble and check the equipment.
5. Place the patient's head in the sniffing position. Insert your finger between the cuff and the tube. Place the index finger of your dominant hand in the notch between the tube and the cuff. Open the patient's mouth **STEP 4**.

6. Insert the LMA along the roof of the mouth, with the aperture of the mask facing the tongue and the back of the mask against the roof of the mouth **STEP 5**. Use your finger to push the airway against the hard palate.
7. Blindly push until resistance is felt.
8. Ensure that the black line on the tube shaft is opposite the upper lip.
9. Inflate the cuff rim of the mask with the amount of air indicated for that size of airway **STEP 6**. Remove the syringe.

10. Attach the bag-mask device and begin to ventilate the patient. Check for chest rise and lung or epigastrium sounds **STEP 7**. Continuously monitor the patient.

King LT Airway

The King LT airway is a single-lumen SGA that may be placed blindly **FIGURE 6-42**. Placement occurs mostly within the esophagus. The King LT airway has not been proven to protect the airway from the effects of regurgitation and aspiration; thus, the risk of regurgitation and aspiration must be weighed against the potential benefit of establishing an airway.

Two types of King LT airway are available: the King LT-D and the King LTS-D. The King LT-D can be used in adults and children in the prehospital setting, whereas the King LTS-D is used only in adults. Five sizes of each type are available, with sizes based on the patient's height and/or weight. Each size has

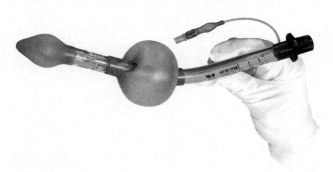

FIGURE 6-42 King LT airway.

Courtesy of Ambu and King Systems.

a different color of proximal connector and requires different cuff inflation pressures **TABLE 6-4**.

Indications for use of the King LT airway are:

- Inability to perform ET intubation (including lack of equipment).
- Rescue airway in failed intubation, especially in the setting of failed RSI. If the King LT airway is used as a rescue airway after RSI, remember that the patient must be kept sedated and paralyzed once proper placement has been verified.
- Deep coma, cardiac arrest, or respiratory arrest.
- To reduce the risk of gastric distention.

Contraindications are:

- Responsive patient with an intact gag reflex
- Upper airway obstruction
- Patient with known esophageal disease
- Patient who has ingested caustic substances

It is recommended that the patient be at least 35 inches (89 cm) tall or weigh at least 26 pounds (12 kg).

SKILL DRILL 6-5 shows the steps for placement of the King LT airway, which are described here:

1. Take standard precautions (glove and face shield) **STEP 1**.
2. Preoxygenate the patient with a bag-mask device and 100% oxygen **STEP 2**.
3. Gather your equipment **STEP 3**.
4. Choose the proper size of King LT airway for the patient. Test the cuff inflation system for leaks. Ensure that all air is removed from the cuffs before inserting the airway. Lubricate the

TABLE 6-4 King LT-D and LTS-D Sizes, Patient Criteria, and Cuff Volumes			
Size	**Connector Color**	**Height and Weight Criteria**	**Cuff Volume**
2	Green	35–45 in or 12–25 kg	25–35 mL*
2.5	Orange	41–51 in or 25–35 kg	30–40 mL*
3	Yellow	4–5 ft	LT-D (45–60 mL) LTS-D (40–55 mL)
4	Red	5–6 ft	LT-D (60–80 mL) LTS-D (50–70 mL)
5	Purple	>6 ft	LT-D (70–90 mL) LTS-D (60–80 mL)

*Sizes 2 and 2.5 are available only in the King LT-D.

Data from Ambu.

tip of the device with a water-soluble lubricant for ease of insertion and to minimize risk of airway damage.

5. Place the patient's head in a neutral position, unless contraindicated (use the jaw-thrust maneuver if trauma is suspected). In your dominant hand, hold the King LT at the connector. With your other hand, hold the

patient's mouth open while positioning the head **STEP 4**.

6. Insert the tip of the device into the corner of the mouth and continue to advance it behind the base of the tongue while rotating the device. When the rotation is complete, the blue line on the device should face the patient's chin.

Skill Drill 6-5 King LT Airway Insertion

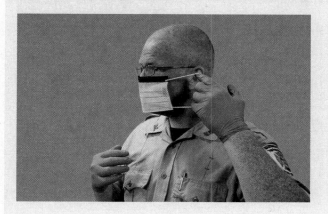

Step 1

Take standard precautions (gloves and face shield).

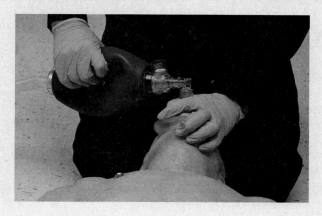

Step 2

Preoxygenate the patient with a bag-mask device and 100% oxygen.

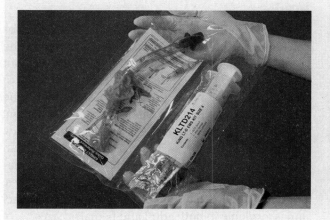

Step 3

Gather your equipment.

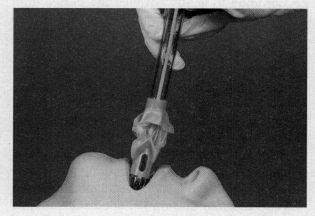

Step 4

Place the patient's head in a neutral position unless contraindicated. Open the patient's mouth and insert the King LT airway in the corner of the mouth.

Continues

Skill Drill 6-5 King LT Airway Insertion (continued)

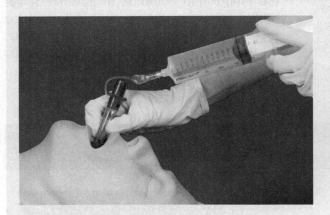

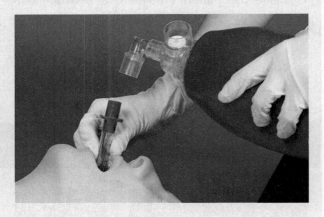

Step 5

Advance the tip behind the base of the tongue while rotating the tube back to midline so the blue line on the device faces the patient's chin. Gently advance the device until the base of the connector is aligned with the teeth or gums. Do not use excessive force. Inflate the cuffs with the recommended amount of air or enough to just seal the device.

© Jones & Bartlett Learning.

Step 6

Attach the tube to the bag-mask device and confirm tube placement by auscultating the lungs and epigastrium and attaching waveform capnography. While ventilating, gently withdraw the tube until ventilation becomes easy and free flowing (ie, good tidal volume with minimal resistance). Adjust the cuff inflation, if necessary, to maximize the airway seal.

7. Continue to gently advance the device until the base of the connector is aligned with the patient's teeth or gums. Do not use excessive force.

8. Inflate the cuffs with the recommended amount of air or enough to just seal the device **STEP 5**.

9. Attach the tube to the bag-mask device and confirm tube placement by auscultating the lungs and epigastrium and attaching waveform capnography **STEP 6**. While ventilating, gently withdraw the tube until ventilation becomes easy and free flowing (ie, good tidal volume with minimal resistance). Adjust the cuff inflation, if necessary, to maximize the airway seal.

10. Perform standard reassessment of lung sounds while continuing ventilation. Ensure appropriate capnography waveform is present, and consider securing the tube with tape or a commercial tube holder.

i-gel

The i-gel is an SGA that may be placed blindly. In contrast to other SGAs, this device does not require the use of an inflatable cuff or balloon. The i-gel has not been proven to protect the airway from the effects of regurgitation and aspiration; thus, these risks must be weighed against the potential benefits of establishing an airway. The i-gel is constructed of a medical-grade thermoplastic elastomer and is designed to create an anatomic seal of the pharyngeal, laryngeal, and perilaryngeal structures while avoiding compression forces. It includes an integral bite block and gastric channel and is available in both adult and pediatric sizes.

Indications for use of the i-gel airway are:

- Inability to perform ET intubation (including lack of equipment).
- Rescue airway in failed intubation, especially in the setting of failed RSI. If the i-gel airway is used for this purpose, remember that the

patient must be kept sedated and paralyzed once proper placement has been verified.

- Deep coma, cardiac arrest, and/or respiratory arrest.
- To reduce the risk of gastric distention during bag-mask device ventilations prior to ET intubation.

Contraindications are:

- Responsive patients with an intact gag reflex
- Upper airway obstruction
- Patients with known esophageal disease
- Patients who have ingested caustic substances
- Obstructive lesions below the glottis
- Trismus, limited mouth opening, pharyngo-perilaryngeal abscess, trauma, or mass
- Conscious or semiconscious patients with an intact gag reflex

SKILL DRILL 6-6 shows the steps for placement of the i-gel airway, which are described here:

1. Take standard precautions (glove and face shield).
2. Preoxygenate the patient with a bag-mask device and 100% oxygen **STEP 1**.

3. Gather your equipment and choose the proper size of i-gel airway for the patient.
4. Open the i-gel package and, on a flat surface, take out the protective cradle containing the device.
5. Lubricate the back, sides, and front of the cuff with a water-soluble lubricant for ease of insertion and to minimize the risk of airway damage **STEP 2**.
6. Place the patient's head in a sniffing position, unless contraindicated **STEP 3**. Use the jaw-thrust maneuver if trauma is suspected.
7. Grasp the lubricated i-gel firmly along the integral bite block. Position the device so that the i-gel cuff outlet is facing toward the patient's chin.
8. Gently press down the patient's chin to open the mouth.
9. Introduce the leading soft tip into the patient's mouth, directed toward the hard palate.
10. Glide the device downward and backward along the hard palate with a continuous but gentle push until a definitive resistance is felt **STEP 4**. The tip of the airway should be located in the upper esophageal opening and

Skill Drill 6-6 i-gel Airway Insertion

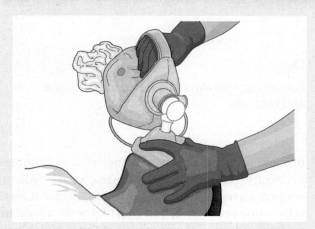

Step 1

Take standard precautions (gloves and face shield). Preoxygenate the patient with a bag-mask device and 100% oxygen.

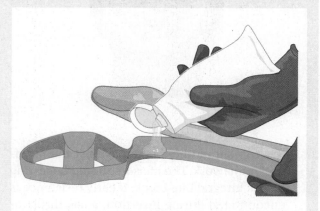

Step 2

Gather your equipment and choose the proper size of i-gel airway. Lubricate the back, sides, and front of the cuff with a water-soluble lubricant applied initially to the protective cradle.

Continues

Skill Drill 6-6 i-gel Airway Insertion (continued)

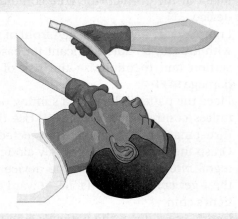

Step 3

Place the patient's head in a sniffing position, unless contraindicated. Use the jaw-thrust maneuver if trauma is suspected.

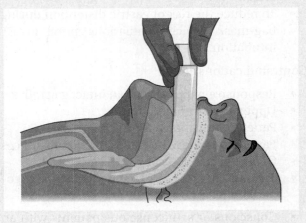

Step 4

Introduce the leading soft tip into the patient's mouth, directed toward the hard palate. Glide the device downward and backward along the hard palate with a continuous but gentle push until a definitive resistance is felt.

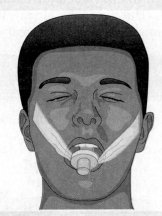

© Jones & Bartlett Learning.

Step 5

Secure the i-gel. Attach the bag-mask device and ventilate.

the cuff should be located against the laryngeal framework. The incisors should be resting on the integral bite block. If early resistance is encountered during insertion, a jaw thrust or insertion with deep rotation is recommended.

11. Tape down the i-gel from "maxilla to maxilla" **STEP 5**.

Surgical Airways

In case of a failed airway, meaning the patient cannot be oxygenated or ventilated despite maximization of the bag-mask device or advanced airways, placement of an airway by other means becomes necessary. This frequently means some type of surgical airway must be established. Before undertaking this procedure, you must have an adequate understanding of the anatomy of the anterior part of the neck.

The most prominent structure in the anterior part of the neck is the thyroid cartilage (Adam's apple). It is more easily palpable in males than in females. Directly inferior to the thyroid cartilage is the cricoid cartilage. The cricothyroid membrane lies between these two structures. A thin membrane covered only by skin, the cricothyroid membrane is an important landmark to identify in the setting of a surgical airway.

Equipment

The equipment needed to perform a surgical airway depends on the method used. This equipment may include:

- ET tube or tracheostomy tube (various sizes)
- Scalpel
- Bougie
- Curved hemostats
- Suction equipment
- 14-gauge or larger over-the-needle catheter
- ¼-inch tape
- 10-mL syringe
- Three-way stopcock
- Two pieces of standard oxygen tubing, 4 to 5 feet (1 to 2 m) each
- Y-connector
- Oxygen cylinder (coupled with a 50-psi step-down regulator and a needle flowmeter)
- Povidone-iodine swabs
- PPE, including sterile gloves
- Sterile fenestrated drape (hole in center)
- 4 × 4–inch gauze pads
- Bag-mask device
- Guide wire (28 inches [70 cm])
- Cotton tie or commercial tracheostomy tube holder

Needle Cricothyrotomy

A surgical airway is used to provide temporary oxygenation when intubation by other means is not possible. This type of airway may be needed in the unusual situation in which the patient cannot be intubated or ventilated. Needle cricothyrotomy may be performed in any patient but is the surgical airway of choice in the emergent setting for children younger than 10 to 12 years. In these patients, anatomic differences create a higher potential for damage to the larynx and surrounding structures when a formal cricothyrotomy is performed.

In a needle cricothyrotomy, a large-bore angiocatheter (14 to 16 gauge) is placed through the cricothyroid membrane into the trachea. A transtracheal jet ventilator may be used to provide temporary oxygenation through this catheter. Exhalation is passive and requires SGA patency.

Needle cricothyrotomy does not allow optimal ventilation—only oxygenation—so hypercarbia is an expected complication. It also does not protect the airway or allow suctioning. Instead, this surgical airway is simply a temporary measure intended to oxygenate the patient until a more definitive airway can be placed.

Indications for needle cricothyrotomy include:

- Intubation is not feasible.
- Intubation does not relieve obstruction.
- A field procedure is necessary to establish a temporary airway.

Contraindications to needle cricothyrotomy include severe airway obstruction below the site of the catheter insertion.

Complications of needle cricothyrotomy are:

- Hemorrhage
- Subcutaneous emphysema
- Infection
- Misplacement of the cannula
- Accidental removal
- Subglottic stenosis
- Mediastinal emphysema
- Tracheal and esophageal laceration
- Barotrauma

SKILL DRILL 6-7 shows the steps for needle cricothyrotomy, which are described here:

1. Follow standard precautions (gloves and face shield) **STEP 1**.
2. Attach a 14- to 16-gauge IV catheter to a 10-mL syringe containing approximately 3 mL of sterile saline or water **STEP 2**.
3. With the patient's head in a neutral position, palpate for and locate the thyroid cartilage, cricothyroid membrane, and suprasternal notch **STEP 3**.
4. Cleanse the area with an iodine-containing solution **STEP 4**.
5. Attach the syringe (if preferred) to the needle.
6. Stabilize the patient's larynx, and insert the needle into the cricothyroid membrane at a 45° angle toward the feet **STEP 5**.
7. Push the needle until it "pops" into the trachea. Aspirate with the syringe to determine correct catheter placement **STEP 6**.
8. Confirm correct tracheal placement by noting movement of air.
9. Advance the catheter over the needle until the hub rests against the skin **STEP 7**.

10. Place the syringe and needle in a puncture-proof container **STEP 8**.
11. Connect one end of the oxygen tubing to the catheter and the other end to the jet ventilator **STEP 9**.
12. Open the release valve on the jet ventilator, and adjust the pressure to provide adequate

chest rise **STEP 10**. If a jet ventilator is unavailable, temporary ventilation can be provided with a bag-mask device by attaching a 15-mm bag-mask device adapter from a 3-0 ET tube to the catheter, or by attaching a 3-mL syringe with the plunger removed and an adapter from a 7-0 tube.

Skill Drill 6-7 Performing Needle Cricothyrotomy

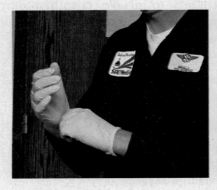

Step 1

Follow standard precautions (gloves and face shield).

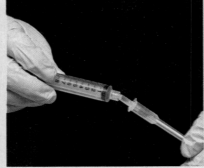

Step 2

Attach a 14- to 16-gauge IV catheter to a 10-mL syringe containing approximately 3 mL of sterile saline or water.

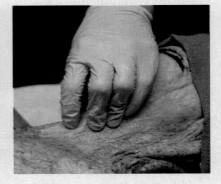

Step 3

With the patient's head in a neutral position, palpate for and locate the thyroid cartilage, cricothyroid membrane, and suprasternal notch.

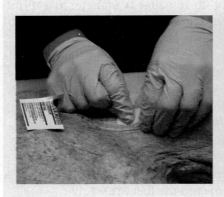

Step 4

Cleanse the area with an iodine-containing solution.

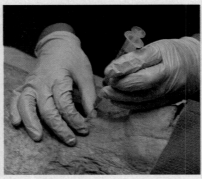

Step 5

Attach the syringe (if preferred) to the needle. Stabilize the patient's larynx, and insert the needle into the cricothyroid membrane at a 45° angle toward the feet.

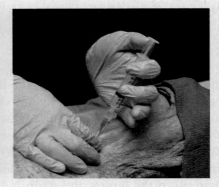

Step 6

Push the needle until it pops into the trachea. Aspirate with the syringe to determine correct catheter placement.

Skill Drill 6-7 Performing Needle Cricothyrotomy (continued)

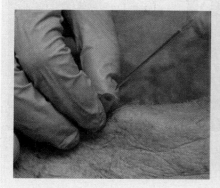

Step 7

While holding the catheter, slide the catheter off the needle until the hub of the catheter is flush with the patient's skin.

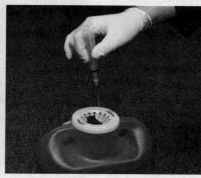

Step 8

Place the syringe and needle in a puncture-proof container.

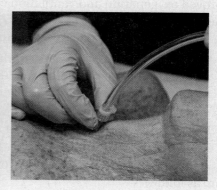

Step 9

Connect one end of the oxygen tubing to the catheter and the other end to the jet ventilator.

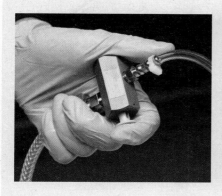

Step 10

Open the release valve on the jet ventilator and adjust the pressure to provide adequate chest rise.

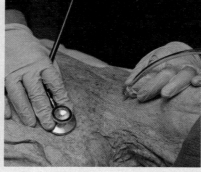

Step 11

Auscultate the apices and bases of both lungs and over the epigastrium to confirm correct catheter placement.

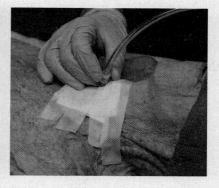

Step 12

Secure the catheter with a 4 × 4–inch gauze pad and tape. Continue ventilations while frequently reassessing for adequate ventilations and any potential complications.

All images © Jones & Bartlett Learning.

13. Auscultate the apices and bases of both lungs and over the epigastrium to confirm correct catheter placement **STEP 11**.

14. Secure the catheter with a 4 × 4–inch gauze pad and tape. Continue ventilations while frequently reassessing for adequate ventilations and any potential complications **STEP 12**.

Surgical Cricothyrotomy

Many techniques for performing a surgical cricothyrotomy have been developed, ranging from a fully open technique using only a scalpel, bougie, and 6.0 ET tube (scalpel–finger–bougie technique) to modified techniques using various premanufactured kits. The advantages of an open cricothyrotomy are the greater speed of insertion compared with formal tracheostomy and the improved oxygenation and ventilation compared with needle cricothyrotomy.

Indications for surgical cricothyrotomy include:

- Intubation is not feasible, in that the patient is unable to be ventilated and/or oxygenated.
- Intubation does not relieve the airway obstruction.
- A field procedure is necessary to establish a temporary airway.

Contraindications to surgical cricothyrotomy are as follows:

- Inability to identify anatomic landmarks, usually secondary to trauma.
- Pediatric patients younger than 10 years. Children younger than this age have a smaller cricothyroid membrane that generally cannot accept a larger-bore tube, making needle cricothyrotomy the preferred procedure in such patients.

Complications to surgical cricothyrotomy include the following conditions:

- Hemorrhage
- Infection
- Misplacement of the cannula/tube
- Accidental removal
- Subglottic stenosis
- Mediastinal emphysema
- Tracheal and esophageal laceration

Open cricothyrotomy involves incising the patient's skin and cricothyroid membrane with a scalpel and placing an ET tube or tracheostomy tube. Several commercial kits containing the equipment needed to perform a modified cricothyrotomy are available, many of which rely on a variant of the Seldinger technique to place the airway **FIGURE 6-43**. The Seldinger technique uses a needle and guide wire/guide catheter or tube placement in blood vessels or other hollow organs. Other devices for performing cricothyrotomy, such as the Nu-Trake and Pertrach, are commercially manufactured airway placement devices that may be used in the prehospital environment **FIGURE 6-44**. These devices do not use the Seldinger technique, but rather rely on a device that functions as both an introducer and an airway.

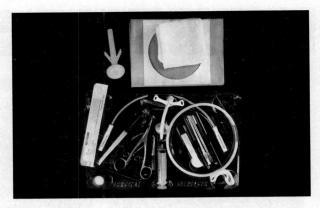

FIGURE 6-43 The Cook critical care Melker cricothyrotomy catheter kit.

Courtesy of Cook Medical.

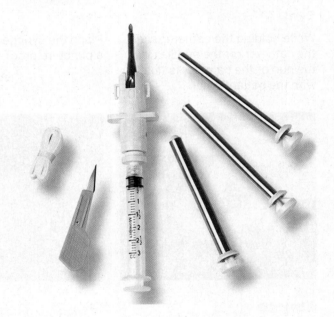

A

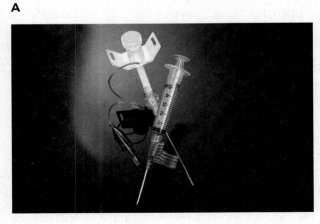

B

FIGURE 6-44 A. Nu-Trake kit. **B.** Pertrach kit.

A. Courtesy of Smiths Medical; B. Courtesy of Pulmodyne, Inc.

SKILL DRILL 6-8 shows the steps for one surgical cricothyrotomy technique, which are described here:

1. Follow standard precautions, including use of gloves and a face shield **STEP 1**.
2. Place the patient supine. Ventilate the patient.
3. Check, assemble, and prepare the equipment **STEP 2**.
4. Approach the patient from the left side of the neck. With the patient's head in a neutral position, palpate for and locate the cricothyroid membrane **STEP 3**.

Skill Drill 6-8 Performing Surgical Cricothyrotomy

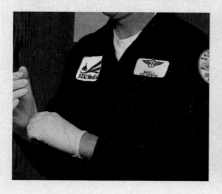

Step 1

Follow standard precautions, including use of gloves and a face shield.

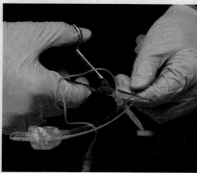

Step 2

Check, assemble, and prepare the equipment.

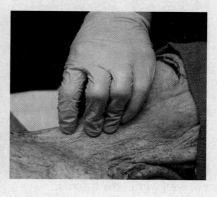

Step 3

Approach the patient from the left side of the neck. With the patient's head in a neutral position, palpate for and locate the cricothyroid membrane.

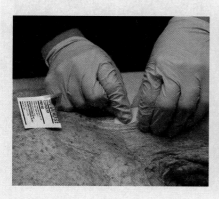

Step 4

Cleanse the anterior part of the neck from the laryngeal prominence to just below the cricoid ring and position a fenestrated drape.

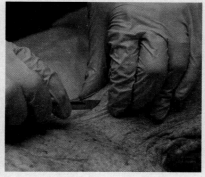

Step 5

With the scalpel in your dominant hand, make a 1- to 2-cm vertical skin incision over the cricothyroid membrane.

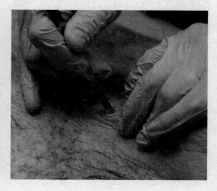

Step 6

Puncture the cricothyroid membrane and make a horizontal incision 1 cm in each direction from the midline (a shallow incision, so that the posterior tracheal wall is not injured).

Continues

Skill Drill 6-8 Performing Surgical Cricothyrotomy (continued)

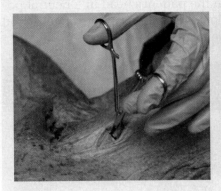

Step 7

Place a curved hemostat (pictured) or a tracheal hook through the incision before removing the scalpel. Open the hemostats, ensuring that the tips are well within the trachea.

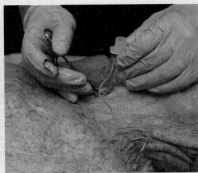

Step 8

With your free hand, insert the ET tube between the tips of the open hemostats, advancing the balloon about 1.0 to 1.5 cm below the lower margin of the incision.

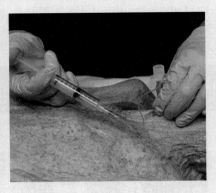

Step 9

Inflate the cuff on the tube with 8 to 10 mL of air and remove the syringe.

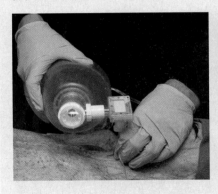

Step 10

Attach an ETCO$_2$ detector between the tube and the bag-mask device.

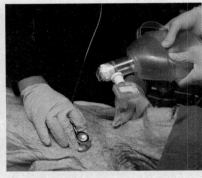

Step 11

Ventilate the patient and auscultate the chest bilaterally and over the epigastrium.

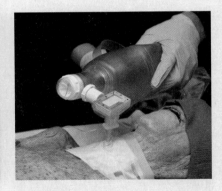

Step 12

Secure the tube to the neck and reconfirm correct tube placement. Continue to ventilate the patient.

All images © Jones & Bartlett Learning.

5. Cleanse the anterior part of the neck from the laryngeal prominence to just below the cricoid ring and position a fenestrated drape **STEP 4**.
6. Palpate the cricothyroid membrane.
7. Stabilize the thyroid cartilage with your non-dominant hand.
8. With the scalpel in your dominant hand, make a 1- to 2-cm vertical skin incision over the cricothyroid membrane **STEP 5**.

9. Puncture the cricothyroid membrane and make a horizontal incision 1 cm in each direction from the midline (a shallow incision, so that the posterior tracheal wall is not injured) **STEP 6**.
10. Place a curved hemostat through the incision *before* removing the scalpel. Open the hemostats, ensuring that the tips are well within the trachea **STEP 7**.

11. Remove the scalpel.
12. With your free hand, insert the ET tube between the tips of the open hemostats, advancing the balloon about 1.0 to 1.5 cm below the lower margin of the incision **STEP 8**.
13. Remove the hemostats.
14. Inflate the cuff on the tube with 8 to 10 mL of air and remove the syringe **STEP 9**.
15. Attach an ETCO₂ detector between the tube and the bag-mask device **STEP 10**.
16. Ventilate the patient and verify correct tube position by auscultating the chest bilaterally and over the epigastrium **STEP 11**.
17. Secure the tube to the neck and reconfirm correct tube placement. Continue to ventilate the patient **STEP 12**.

An alternative technique, commonly referred to as the scalpel–finger–bougie method, replaces the use of hemostats with the insertion of a fingertip into the incision to palpate the tracheal lumen. A bougie is then passed alongside the finger, and (generally) a 6.0 ET tube is subsequently passed over the bougie until the balloon is no longer visible, then inflated.

Rapid Sequence Intubation

Rapid sequence intubation (RSI) involves the rapid administration of sedative induction and neuromuscular blocking agents to produce a state of unconsciousness and paralysis in the patient and allow for tracheal intubation. RSI was originally developed to facilitate airway management in obstetric patients requiring intubation with a presumed full stomach.

The 7 Ps of RSI

1. Prepare
2. Preoxygenation
3. Preintubation optimization
4. Paralysis with induction
5. Positioning
6. Placement with proof
7. Postintubation management

The indications for performing RSI include many of the same indications for ET intubation, with one notable exception: Patients in cardiac arrest should not undergo medication-facilitated intubation. Remember, sedatives may eliminate the patient's ability to protect their airway and cause hemodynamic effects if the patient is catecholamine dependent. Paralytic agents will cause respiratory arrest, and the CCTP must be prepared to ventilate a patient who begins to desaturate. When these medications are administered, the CCTP *must* be able to successfully establish an airway on the first pass without inducing hypoxia or hypotension in the patient. RSI also assumes that patients have eaten prior to needing emergent intubation. When medications are administered during RSI to sedate and paralyze patients, the risks of regurgitation and aspiration are minimized but not eliminated.

The usual contraindications and complications for standard intubation also apply to RSI. Airway assessment and planning are essential. The most crucial contraindication is predicted inability to intubate. In this case, RSI should not be attempted; other airway management strategies, such as using an SGA or performing a cricothyrotomy, should be considered. The most devastating complication of RSI is not being able to oxygenate or ventilate the patient. This scenario will almost invariably result in a catastrophic patient outcome. Thus, the use of RSI requires careful assessment, planning, and preparation.

RSI consists of a series of steps to facilitate ET intubation following preoxygenation and patient optimization. It begins with preparation. All equipment necessary for intubation, rescue ventilation, and placement of a surgical airway must be available, checked, and working prior to use. At least one working intravenous (IV) or intraosseous (IO) access must be available—and preferably two, because one IV/IO line may infiltrate, fall out, or be pulled out inadvertently—for the administration of the appropriate medications.

The next step is preoxygenation. All patients undergoing RSI should be given oxygen prior to the CCTP beginning the procedure. In the patient who is breathing spontaneously with adequate tidal volumes, applying high-flow oxygen via a nonrebreathing mask *and* a nasal cannula running at the maximum flow rate is sufficient. The nasal cannula remains in place during laryngoscopy, allowing for passive apneic oxygenation and subsequent oxygen diffusion. (This process is now called apneic oxygenation, but has been described in the past as mass flow ventilation, diffusion respiration, or apneic diffusion oxygenation.) Once spontaneous breathing ceases, the nonrebreathing mask is removed to provide access for the intubation. Positioning of the patient before and during the apneic period should focus on maximizing upper airway patency. Bag-mask device ventilation with RSI prior to intubation should be used only when absolutely necessary, with attention paid to avoiding gastric insufflation and possible regurgitation.

The goals of preoxygenation are twofold: (1) to maximize the patient's oxygenation reserve and (2) to remove nitrogen from the lungs to prolong the safe apneic time. Preoxygenation with high-flow oxygen saturates the air remaining in the lungs after normal expiration (functional residual capacity, approximately 30 mL/kg) with 100% oxygen. Many RSI protocols recommend administering high-flow oxygen for at least 3 minutes, if possible. This will allow for a prolonged period of apnea without significant desaturation in most patients. Children and patients who are obese or pregnant tend to desaturate much more rapidly than do typical adults.

To reduce the changes of hypoxic injury or peri-intubation cardiovascular collapse, the CCTP must consider preintubation optimization to assess for potential hemodynamic stressors and take corrective actions to mitigate them. In the critical care transport setting, a patient requiring RSI often exhibits hypotension and respiratory failure, requiring positive-pressure ventilation to remedy these conditions. The confluence of these conditions coupled with the administration of induction agents with vasodilatory and cardiac depression effects may be a precursor to peri-arrest. In such a case, the CCTP should consider "resuscitation sequence intubation" and the physiologic *HOp* killers: *H*ypotension, *O*xygenation (hypoxemia), and *p*H and ventilation (metabolic acidosis). Mass hemorrhage, tension pneumothorax, cardiac tamponade, hypotension, and hypoxia should be corrected before RSI begins.

The medications used in RSI are classified into two broad categories: (1) sedative induction agents to induce unconsciousness and (2) neuromuscular blocking agents to induce paralysis. The combination of both types of medications is essential to successful RSI and intubation. For both types of medications, the ideal agent would have a rapid onset, a short duration of action, a stable hemodynamic profile, and few, if any, adverse side effects. Unfortunately, no such agent meets all of these criteria. Also, the use of these agents as single therapies

may result in adverse outcomes. That is, the use of sedative/induction agents alone frequently does not result in successful intubation secondary to intact airway reflexes. Conversely, the use of neuromuscular blocking agents alone may result in a paralyzed, yet awake, patient. The combination of both sedation/induction and neuromuscular blockade results in significantly greater intubation success with fewer complications.

SKILL DRILL 6-9 shows the steps for performing RSI, which are described here:

1. Prepare and assemble the equipment.
2. Preoxygenate with 100% oxygen **STEP 1**.
3. Administer medications to premedicate, sedate, and paralyze the patient. When premedicating:
   a. If your medical director or protocol recommends it, consider a defasciculating dose of a nondepolarizing neuromuscular blocking agent.
   b. Consider opiates to decrease the cardiovascular effects and elevations of intracranial pressure associated with upper airway stimulation.
   c. Consider atropine in pediatric patients to decrease the bradycardia associated with the administration of succinylcholine.
4. When sedating the patient, use an agent that induces sedation and amnesia, provided the patient is hemodynamically stable (systolic blood pressure >90 mm Hg).
5. Paralyze the patient using an appropriate agent.
6. Apply posterior cricoid pressure **STEP 2**.
7. Intubate the patient **STEP 3**.
8. Confirm correct ET tube placement.
9. Release the cricoid pressure.
10. Maintain paralysis and sedation.

As with non–medication-facilitated intubation, ET tube confirmation is crucial in RSI. Continuous waveform end-tidal capnography is considered the gold standard for confirming proper ET tube location. Pulse oximetry and a chest radiograph, if available, can also aid in confirmation. The ET tube should be secured in place. Subsequent placement of an orogastric tube to decompress the stomach should be considered as well. A ventilator should be attached with the proper settings, as described in Chapter 7, *Ventilation*.

Following RSI, postintubation sedation and analgesia should be ensured. If a long-acting paralytic

Skill Drill 6-9 Performing Rapid Sequence Intubation

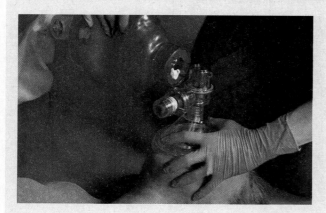

Step 1

Prepare and assemble the equipment. Preoxygenate the patient. Administer medications to premedicate, sedate, and paralyze the patient.

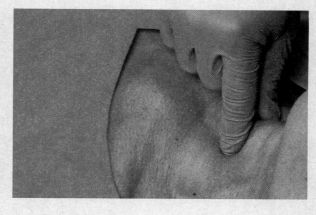

Step 2

Apply posterior cricoid pressure.

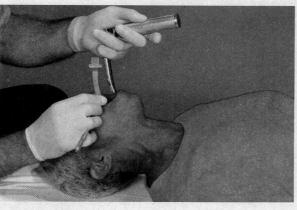

Step 3

Intubate the patient. Confirm correct ET tube placement. Release cricoid pressure.

All images © Jones & Bartlett Learning.

such as rocuronium is administered, it is crucial that appropriate sedation and analgesia be automatically provided to prevent the patient from having awareness during paralysis. Because the paralyzed patient will likely not exhibit signs of pain, strict attention to ongoing pharmacologic interventions is necessary.

Special Populations

Children and patients who are obese or pregnant desaturate much more rapidly than the typical adult patient.

Pharmacologic Agents Used in RSI

Sedative/Induction Agents. **TABLE 6-5** lists sedative/induction agents that may be used in RSI, and their doses, onsets, durations, advantages, and disadvantages. The induction agent chosen for use in RSI must be appropriate for the individual patient, preexisting comorbidities, acute clinical condition, and expected clinical course, including the anticipated success of the RSI.

Etomidate is a hypnotic with no analgesic properties. Due to its hemodynamic stability and cerebroprotective action, this agent is widely used in RSI. Etomidate's onset of action is 15 to 45 seconds,

TABLE 6-5 Sedative/Induction Agents

Drug Category	Drug Name	Dose	Onset	Duration	Advantages	Disadvantages
Benzodiazepines	Midazolam (Versed)	2–5 mg on induction; 5 mg as needed for sedation	30–60 s	15–30 min	Provide amnesia, hypnosis, sedation. Anticonvulsant properties.	Vasodilation, hypotension, myocardial depression.
	Lorazepam (Ativan)	0.03–0.06 mg/kg	1–2 min	1–2 h		
	Diazepam (Valium)	0.3–0.6 mg/kg	45–60 s	15–30 min		
Anesthetic agents	Etomidate (Amidate)	0.2–0.6 mg/kg	15–45 s	3–12 min	Usual induction dose is 0.3 mg/kg. Preferred induction agent for RSI secondary to its rapid onset, short duration, and stable hemodynamic profile. Cerebroprotective, reducing cerebral blood flow and metabolism in the setting of elevated ICP.	Injection site pain secondary to the diluent (propylene glycol). Myoclonic movements that may mimic seizure activity. Not FDA approved for use in pediatric patients, although many published reports in pediatric patients report no adverse effects. Plasma cortisol suppression has also been reported with long-term etomidate use in the ICU environment. Short-term use in RSI has not shown cortisol suppression.

Ketamine (Ketalar)	1–2 mg/kg	45–60 s	10–20 min	Phencyclidine derivative with analgesic, anesthetic, and amnestic properties. Also has a stable hemodynamic profile secondary to catecholamine release and stimulation of the sympathetic nervous system. Also a bronchodilator, making it an ideal induction agent in the setting of bronchospasm.	Emergence reactions are an occasional complication of ketamine administration. Reactions are rarely an issue when ketamine is used in the setting of RSI because the benzodiazepine used for post-RSI sedation attenuates this response.
Propofol (Diprivan)	1–2 mg/kg	15–45 s	5–10 min	Decreases cerebral oxygen demand and ICP.	Vasodilation and myocardial depression, which may result in hypotension and a subsequent reduction in CPP. Pain at injection site.
Opiates					
Fentanyl (Sublimaze)	2–3 µg/kg	3–5 min	30–60 min	Attenuation of the sympathetic response to laryngoscopy.	Hypotension and apnea. Potential for chest wall rigidity. May administer dose in fractional amounts. If rigidity occurs and paralysis is not indicated, treat with naloxone 1–10 µg/kg.

Abbreviations: CPP, cerebral perfusion pressure; FDA, Food and Drug Administration; ICP, intracranial pressure; ICU, intensive care unit; RSI, rapid sequence intubation

and patients have a rapid recovery. The induction dose should be reduced in hemodynamically compromised patients. Patients may exhibit myoclonic movement (which is not seizure activity) following administration of etomidate, though this movement should end with neuromuscular blockade.

The benzodiazepines midazolam, lorazepam, and diazepam have a slightly longer onset of action and a significantly longer duration of action, especially as compared to etomidate, which makes them less attractive as induction agents. They also have the ability to cause hypotension secondary to vasodilation. However, they are frequently used for sedation after intubation in hemodynamically stable patients.

Ketamine is a dissociative anesthetic agent with analgesic properties. Its onset of action is 45 to 60 seconds when given intravenously. It has minimal impact on respiratory drive, and its bronchodilatory properties make it an attractive induction agent in patients with reactive airway disease. Ketamine is also used for awake intubation and is increasingly being used in patients with head injury, despite previously noted concerns that it might increase intracranial pressure. Ketamine may increase secretions and can cause laryngospasm in rare cases.

Propofol is commonly used for induction in surgical cases, as well as for sedation of ventilated patients and for short painful procedures in the emergency department. However, its use as an induction agent in emergent situations is often limited by its tendency to produce vasodilation and hypotension.

Special Populations

Heightened vagal stimulation in pediatric patients can result in significant bradycardia. It is a good idea to administer atropine to children younger than 1 year who will be receiving succinylcholine and to have it available for children between 1 and 10 years old.

Neuromuscular Blocking Agents. Two types of neuromuscular blocking agents are distinguished: depolarizing and nondepolarizing. The depolarizing agents act by rapidly depolarizing the neuromuscular end plate, causing resistance to further stimulation. The nondepolarizing agents block the binding of acetylcholine to its receptors in the neuromuscular end plate. Both types of drugs result in paralysis. The only depolarizing neuromuscular blocking agent in use in the United States is succinylcholine.

Succinylcholine has a rapid onset of action and a short duration, which has made it a commonly selected paralytic agent for RSI in the EMS setting. However, this medication has several important absolute contraindications for its use. It should not be used in patients who have suspected or confirmed hyperkalemia, burns greater than 5 days old, denervation injury (stroke, spinal cord injury) greater than 5 days old until 6 months post injury, crush injuries, a history of malignant hyperthermia, or neuromuscular diseases (eg, amyotrophic lateral sclerosis [ALS], muscular dystrophy).

Several nondepolarizing neuromuscular blocking agents are used in RSI: vecuronium, pancuronium, rocuronium, atracurium, and cisatracurium. These agents primarily serve three purposes as a part of the RSI sequence:

- They may be used as pretreatment agents to prevent the fasciculations encountered with succinylcholine. The defasciculating dose range is 10% to 20% of the intubating dose. For vecuronium and pancuronium, the range is 0.01 to 0.02 mg/kg; for rocuronium, the dose is 0.06 mg/kg. The use of defasciculating doses is rare in the prehospital setting, however.
- They may be used as the primary paralytic agent in the face of contraindications to succinylcholine (hyperkalemia).
- They are used to maintain postintubation paralysis.

Recently, a reversal agent for rocuronium and vecuronium has been introduced into clinical practice. Sugammadex selectively binds to these neuromuscular agents in the blood plasma, thereby reducing the amount of paralytic molecules available to bind to receptors at the neuromuscular junction. Following administration of sugammadex, rocuronium and vecuronium cannot be readministered for 24 hours.

Neuromuscular blocking agents are summarized in **TABLE 6-6**.

TABLE 6-6 Neuromuscular Blocking Agents

Drug Category	Drug Name	Dose	Onset	Duration	Advantages	Disadvantages
Depolarizing neuromuscular blocking agents	Succinylcholine (Anectine, Quelicin)	1–2 mg/kg	<1 min	5 min	Rapid onset, short duration of action.	Fasciculations. Hyperkalemia. Increased intracranial pressure, increased intraocular pressure, and increased intragastric pressure. May cause or worsen bradycardia, particularly in pediatric patients. Has been implicated in malignant hyperthermia and may cause prolonged neuromuscular blockade.
Nondepolarizing neuromuscular blocking agents	Vecuronium (Norcuron)	For intubation: 0.15 mg/kg Postintubation paralysis: 0.01–0.1 mg/kg	90–120 s	60–75 min	Longer duration means that effects are less likely to wear off during transport.	Possible prolonged paralysis with long-term use; renal or hepatic dysfunction. Possible prolonged paralysis with concurrent use of corticosteroids. No effect on level of consciousness, so must be administered with adequate anesthesia, analgesia, or sedation. In patients with apnea, establish a patent airway prior to use.
	Rocuronium (Zemuron)	For intubation: 0.6–1.2 mg/kg Postintubation paralysis: 0.1–0.2 mg/kg	<2 min	30–60 min		
	Pancuronium (Pavulon)	For intubation: 0.1 mg/kg Postintubation paralysis: 0.015–0.1 mg/kg	1–2 min	45–60 min		
	Cisatracurium (Nimbex)	For intubation: 0.15–0.2 mg/kg Postintubation paralysis: 0.03 mg/kg	2–3 min	30–40 min		
	Atracurium (Tracrium)	For intubation: 0.5 mg/kg Postintubation paralysis: 0.5 mg/kg/h	2–3 min	45–60 min		

Tracheostomy Management

Patients receiving interfacility transport may already have a tracheostomy in place for a variety of reasons:

- Facial trauma
- Significant tracheal trauma
- Head injury
- Most commonly, failure to wean/long-term ventilator support

Contraindications to a tracheostomy include coagulopathy, neck tumor, and infection. These are relative contraindications, however, because the alternative is death.

Complications of a tracheostomy include:

- Accidental removal, particularly of a "fresh" or nonmature tracheostomy
- False passage or false tract
- Infection
- Hemorrhage
- Aspiration
- Mediastinal emphysema
- Tracheoesophageal fistula
- Tracheal stenosis
- Tracheomalacia
- Tracheoarterial fistula (frequently from a "low-lying" tracheostomy that erodes into the innominate artery)

Tracheostomy placement does not occur in the field, so it is usually not in the skill set of the prehospital provider. This procedure takes longer to perform than other surgical airways and requires equipment not typically found in the prehospital environment.

In general, patients with long-term tracheostomy devices can easily remove and replace them. In the acute setting, it is common hospital policy to have a spare tracheostomy at the bedside. For the CCTP, it is recommended to carry that spare tracheostomy during the transport. If necessary, ET tubes can be placed into a tracheotomy stoma if a device cannot be replaced or is malfunctioning. In addition, if a patient with a tracheostomy goes into acute respiratory failure, deep suctioning, such as with a red rubber suction catheter, should be performed immediately, as tracheostomies can be susceptible to formation of mucus plugs.

A false passage may occur when moving a patient on transport. Signs of this event include the patient appearing air hungry, the vent alarm signaling high or low pressure, subcutaneous emphysema, or crepitus in the upper chest and neck area. Measures to prevent dislodgement include keeping the tracheostomy securing devices tight and midline while monitoring frequently. In a patient who needs positive-pressure ventilation, the cuff on a tracheostomy device should be inflated or replaced with a cuffed ET tube if ventilation is inadequate.

Summary

Assessing the respiratory system of a critical care transport patient involves a thorough physical assessment and a review of the patient's history and care chart. Obtaining a thorough report from the transferring personnel will help establish the clinical picture before the transport begins.

Establishing a baseline assessment and being able to differentiate normal and abnormal findings in the respiratory system are paramount to comprehensive respiratory care during transport. Essential skills include auscultating breath sounds, evaluating oxygenation and ventilatory adequacy, and setting up and troubleshooting the ventilator.

Concepts such as tidal volume, minute volume, and anatomic dead space are crucial to understanding respiratory function and monitoring the patient's condition, as are a variety of devices and laboratory studies. ABG values, if available, will reveal the acid–base balance and blood levels of oxygen and CO_2. Pulse oximetry, capnography, and ETCO$_2$ detection offer a continuous, noninvasive means of measuring these gases during transport.

CCTPs must have a comprehensive understanding of airway assessment and management strategies. The use of video laryngoscopy is expanding as technologic advances have reduced the cost and enhanced the effectiveness of these devices. CCTPs should develop expertise in the specific video laryngoscopy device available to them, and consider transitioning to it as a primary instrument for most intubations.

Case Study

Your team is dispatched to a rural hospital 75 miles (121 km) away for a 23-year-old, 154-pound (70-kg) woman in status asthmaticus. She was brought to the emergency department 2 hours ago by local EMS for difficulty breathing. She presented to the emergency department in acute respiratory distress, with audible inspiratory and expiratory wheezes, intercostal and supraclavicular retractions, and tripod positioning. Her initial vital signs included the following: respiratory rate, 32 breaths/min and labored; heart rate, 126 beats/min; blood pressure, 126/84 mm Hg; and SpO_2, 92% on an 8-L nebulizer.

Brush fires in the area have placed the county under an air quality warning. The patient's attack occurred after she had taken her dog for a walk. Her medical history includes asthma, which is controlled with daily use of an Advair inhaler. She has been hospitalized three times for asthma-related conditions prior to this episode. One of these admissions resulted in a stay in the intensive care unit for respiratory failure requiring intubation.

A radiograph of the patient's lungs obtained on her arrival at the emergency department demonstrated hyperinflation. The initial ABG reading while the patient was receiving a nebulizer treatment using 8 L of oxygen was pH 7.52, $PaCO_2$ 27 mm Hg, and PaO_2 88 mm Hg. A subsequent ABG reading 45 minutes later with the patient on a nonrebreathing mask at 15 L/min was pH 7.46, $PaCO_2$ 33 mm Hg, and PaO_2 79 mm Hg. All other chemistry and blood values were within normal limits.

You and your team arrive at the emergency department 4 hours after the patient's arrival. While your partner obtains her paperwork and speaks with the nurse caring for her, you assess the patient. You observe a young woman who is minimally responsive to verbal stimuli. She exhibits poor air exchange with shallow respirations accompanied by severe intercostal and supraclavicular retractions and minimal air exchange on auscultation. Current vital signs include the following: pulse rate, 87 beats/min; respiratory rate, 18 breaths/min, labored and shallow; blood pressure, 112/78 mm Hg; and SpO_2, 86% on a non-rebreathing mask with oxygen administered at 15 L/min. As you are completing your assessment of the patient, the nurse brings you the most recent ABG results drawn with the patient on the nonrebreathing mask, showing pH 7.25, $PaCO_2$ 62 mm Hg, and PaO_2 65 mm Hg.

1. Does this patient meet the criteria for intubation?
2. Which factors should be considered when assessing the patient for a difficult airway?
3. Which medications are used during rapid sequence intubation?

Per your protocol, you and your partner prepare for rapid sequence intubation. Using the LEMONS mnemonic, you determine that the patient should not be a difficult intubation. While your partner provides oxygen to the patient using a bag-mask device attached to 100% oxygen and a 15-L nasal cannula, you prepare the following medications for administration: etomidate, 21 mg for sedation; vecuronium, 0.7 mg as a defasciculating agent prior to paralysis; and succinylcholine, 140 mg for paralysis. Your partner administers the etomidate and succinylcholine while you are ventilating the patient and waiting for muscle relaxation. After 90 seconds, you notice that the patient still does not feel completely relaxed and presents with an intact gag reflex. You follow your protocol and administer a second dose of succinylcholine through another IV line. You are able to intubate the patient without difficulty, and confirm correct tube placement by auscultation, visualization, and use of capnography. The patient is placed on the transport ventilator and prepared for the trip back to your facility. Prior to leaving the hospital, you administer an additional 7 mg of vecuronium and 2 mg of lorazepam for continued paralysis and sedation during transport. Additional treatment includes a continuous albuterol nebulizer at 10 mg/h, 125 mg of methylprednisolone sodium succinate, and a normal saline drip at 150 mL/h.

Once you have the patient loaded in the back of your helicopter, you notice that the patient's

ETCO$_2$ is rising and her SpO$_2$ is dropping. Reassessment of the ET tube indicates that the tube has become dislodged and is now ventilating the stomach. You and partner decide to pull the tube and reattempt intubation. After two unsuccessful attempts, you give your partner a chance; your partner is unable to visualize the vocal cords. Your King LT airway is retrieved and inserted without difficulty. After confirming placement of this airway, you secure the tube with a commercial tube holder, place the patient back on the ventilator, and continue your transport.

You arrive at the receiving hospital approximately 90 minutes later following an uncomplicated trip. A detailed patient report is given to the awaiting staff on your arrival, which includes a list of all the medications given, along with the reason for the insertion of the King LT airway.

1. Was it an acceptable practice to administer a second dose of succinylcholine? What are some possible causes for having to repeat the dose?
2. What is a King LT airway, and why could you insert it without difficulty when the ET tube could not be inserted?
3. Was there ever a point in this patient's care when noninvasive positive-pressure ventilation would be considered appropriate?

Analysis

This patient was a candidate for ET intubation due to her decreased mental status and respiratory failure, as shown by ineffective respirations, minimal air movement, and ABG results. Initially, the patient arrived at the emergency department awake and alert in respiratory distress. The first ABG results showed respiratory alkalosis, a common finding in the early stages of an acute asthma attack. The second blood gas analysis came back with close to normal values, with the exception of oxygenation. This finding should be a warning sign and should prompt you to reassess the patient to determine whether her condition is improving or whether she is getting tired and bears close watching. Do not let the numbers trick you!

Patient history and assessment play an important role in the preparation for intubation. Questions that can be answered by a review of patient history include the presence of congenital anomalies, recent surgery, trauma, infection, or cancer. Pertinent assessment findings include patients with short necks, those who are obese, and those with dental abnormalities such as an overbite. Two assessment tools can be used to guide your decision: the Mallampati method and the 3-3-2 rule.

The Mallampati method ranks the difficulty of intubation (class I is the easiest and class IV is the most difficult) based on how well the oropharyngeal structures can be visualized in a patient who is seated in an upright position with a fully open mouth. A class I airway is one in which all oropharyngeal structures can be visualized. With a class II airway, the glottis is only partially visible. With a class III airway, the glottis cannot be exposed, but the corniculate cartilages can be seen. Finally, the class IV airway prevents the visualization of any oropharyngeal structures.

The 3-3-2 rule refers to three easy anatomic methods of assessing candidates for intubation. For the first 3, have the patient open their mouth as wide as possible. This opening should allow for a minimum of three fingerbreadths (approximately 5 cm); an opening of less than three fingerbreadths may be an indicator of a difficult airway. The second 3 is a measurement of the length of the mandible, from the tip of the chin to the hyoid bone. Again, an optimal measurement is the width of at least three fingers. The final measurement, 2, refers to the distance from the hyoid bone to the thyroid notch. An ideal airway would have a distance of at least two fingerbreadths.

Medications administered during rapid sequence intubation are given to premedicate, sedate, and paralyze the patient. Medications given to premedicate the patient include a smaller dose (also known as a defasciculating dose) of a nondepolarizing neuromuscular blocking agent, such as vecuronium; atropine in the pediatric population, to decrease the bradycardic effects associated with succinylcholine; and a sedative, or induction agent (eg, etomidate), to provide sedation and amnesia.

The succinylcholine dose can be repeated if needed using the same dosing regimen. The most likely reason that the succinylcholine did not work in this patient is an infiltrated intravenous line. Alternatively, because succinylcholine is temperature sensitive, that particular vial of medication might have been exposed to extreme temperatures for a prolonged period of time, which in turn contributed to the ineffectiveness of the medication.

The King LT airway is a supraglottic airway that does not require the direct visualization of the vocal cords during its placement. This device is actually inserted into the esophagus, after which a distal and proximal balloon is inflated and the patient's lungs ventilated through fenestrations located between the two balloons. Even though it is a supraglottic device, the patient can be mechanically ventilated without difficulty.

A trial of noninvasive positive-pressure ventilation might have been attempted after the second ABG results were obtained.

Prep Kit

Ready for Review

- The goal of the CCTP is to ensure the adequacy of ventilation and oxygenation of the critically ill patient during transport. To do so, the CCTP must have a good understanding of respiratory function and assessment.
- An understanding of airway anatomy and physiology, including the structures of the nose, mouth, pharynx, larynx, and trachea, is essential to successful airway management.
- The airway anatomy of pediatric patients is different from the anatomy of adults. The small size of the cricothyroid membrane in children younger than 4 years may make needle and surgical cricothyrotomy difficult or impossible. Children also have significantly higher oxygen consumption rates compared to adults.
- The respiratory system is divided into the conducting zone and the respiratory zone, with the conducting zone further divided into the upper airway and lower airway. The pulmonary circulatory system is a low-pressure system.
- An adult lung contains approximately 300 million alveoli, each of which is in contact with a pulmonary capillary. The interface between an alveolus and a pulmonary capillary is called the alveolar-capillary membrane. For gas exchange to occur, blood flow must be in contact with the alveoli.
- Gas exchange occurs as a result of pressure gradient changes across the alveolar-capillary membrane. Through diffusion, molecules of oxygen move out of the alveoli and into the blood because there are fewer oxygen molecules in the blood, and molecules of CO_2 move out of the blood and into the alveoli because there are fewer CO_2 molecules in the alveoli.
- Ventilation-perfusion mismatch factors—due to inadequate ventilation, perfusion, or both—can affect the diffusion of gases across the alveolar-capillary membrane. The mechanics and dynamics of breathing involve the concepts of elastance, compliance, resistance, and pressure gradients.
- The total lung capacity of a healthy male adult ranges between 5 and 6 L of gas, which can be further divided into different lung volumes and capacities.
- Diseases that result in difficulty moving air out of the lungs are classified as obstructive diseases. They include asthma, chronic obstructive pulmonary disease, cystic fibrosis, and bronchiectasis, and involve an increase in airway resistance.
- Diseases that result in difficulty moving air into the lungs are classified as restrictive diseases. These diseases, which result from loss of chest

Prep Kit Continued

or lung compliance, either individually or together, include occupational lung diseases (the pneumoconioses) and idiopathic pulmonary fibrosis, pneumonia, atelectasis, chest wall deformities and injuries, and the neuromuscular diseases that affect breathing.

- Assessment of a patient's respiratory system includes visually inspecting the patient with a focus on the chest, using auscultation sites to check breath sounds, assessing respiratory patterns and breathing rate, and using palpation to check the status of the lungs, skin, subcutaneous tissues, and chest expansion. Prior to transport, the CCTP needs to review the patient care report carefully, noting any medications, underlying disease, or trauma that might compromise ventilation.

- The functioning of the respiratory system is measured using ABG levels, in which blood is obtained from a superficial artery and then analyzed for pH, $Paco_2$ (partial pressure of CO_2 in arterial blood), Pao_2 (partial pressure of oxygen in arterial blood), HCO_3^- (concentration of bicarbonate ion), base excess, and Spo_2 (oxygen saturation of the hemoglobin molecule).

- Respiratory insufficiency is the inability of the respiratory system to keep up with the metabolic demands of the body; it can lead to respiratory depression. Respiratory failure—either oxygenation failure or ventilatory failure—occurs when the respiratory system is unable to meet the body's metabolic needs.

- Basic airway skills are the starting point in the CCTP's initial assessment and treatment of the patient with a respiratory disorder. They include positioning the nontrauma victim in the recovery position; using the head tilt–chin lift, tongue-jaw lift, or jaw-thrust maneuver; or using airway adjuncts such as an oropharyngeal airway or nasopharyngeal airway.

- Suctioning to remove debris (vomit and blood) and turning the patient onto their side while

using a large-bore suction device can restore airway patency and minimize the potential for aspiration.

- Patients with respiratory disorders should receive some form of supplemental oxygen based on the provider's assessment, regardless of documented Spo_2.

- Oxygen delivery may take many forms, including mouth-to-mouth ventilation, barrier device/resuscitation mask, and bag-mask ventilation.

- Definitive airway management is considered to be the placement of an endotracheal (ET) tube or tracheostomy tube within the trachea.

- In anticipation of a difficult airway, several factors need to be considered, including patient history and patient assessment.

- The 3-3-2 rule should be used as part of the airway assessment. A mouth opening of less than three fingers wide, a mandible length of less than three fingers wide, and a distance from the hyoid bone to the thyroid notch of less than two fingers wide indicate a possibly difficult airway.

- Once the decision to intubate a patient has been made, the CCTP needs to determine how to most effectively accomplish the procedure. The goal is to intubate the patient on the first attempt (first-pass success) without inducing hemodynamic compromise or aspiration.

- Orotracheal intubation can be performed in two ways: direct visualization of the vocal cords by displacement of the tongue with a laryngoscope blade or indirect visualization of the vocal cords using video laryngoscopy.

- Nasotracheal intubation has been used only infrequently since the advent of rapid sequence intubation (RSI); however, it may still be indicated in the prehospital setting if RSI is inadvisable. Thus, providers should maintain competency in this technique.

- A bougie is an ET tube introducer that allows the CCTP to perform laryngoscopy in difficult airways. It provides a tactile sensation as the bougie slides alongside the tracheal rings.

Prep Kit Continued

- Advantages of using the laryngeal mask airway (LMA) include greater ease of insertion and superior oxygenation and ventilation compared with bag-mask ventilation; disadvantages are the risk of aspiration and difficulty with obtaining an adequate seal. Use an LMA if the patient is in a deep coma or cardiac or respiratory arrest, or if ET intubation is not possible. The LMA is contraindicated for use in patients with an intact gag reflex or facial or esophageal trauma, or if an airway obstruction by a foreign body is suspected.
- The King LT airway and the i-gel are supraglottic airways that may be placed blindly; once proper placement is verified, the patient must be kept sedated and paralyzed. This kind of airway is used when ET intubation is not possible, if intubation has failed and the patient is in a deep coma or cardiac or respiratory arrest, or to reduce the risk of gastric distention. Contraindications include an intact gag reflex, an upper airway obstruction or suspected foreign body obstruction, facial or esophageal trauma, known esophageal disease, and possible caustic ingestion.
- When a patient cannot be intubated or ventilated, placement of a surgical airway via needle cricothyrotomy, surgical cricothyrotomy (either open or modified), or RSI is required.
- RSI involves the coadministration of both anesthetic agents and neuromuscular blocking agents to produce a state of unconsciousness and paralysis that allow for tracheal intubation.
- Some pharmacologic agents used in RSI are sedative/induction agents, including benzodiazepines such as lorazepam and diazepam, anesthetic agents such as etomidate and ketamine, opiates such as fentanyl, and atropine for pediatric patients.
- Other pharmacologic agents used in RSI are neuromuscular blocking agents, which are either depolarizing or nondepolarizing. Succinylcholine is the only depolarizing neuromuscular blocking agent used in the United States, but several nondepolarizing neuromuscular blocking agents, including vecuronium, pancuronium, rocuronium, atracurium, and cisatracurium, are also used. The nondepolarizing agents are primarily used as pretreatment agents, as the primary paralytic agent, or more commonly, to maintain postintubation paralysis.

Vital Vocabulary

3-3-2 rule A method used to predict difficult intubation. A mouth opening of less than three fingers wide, a mandible length of less than three fingers wide, and a distance from the hyoid bone to the thyroid notch of less than two fingers wide indicate a possibly difficult airway.

adventitious breath sounds Abnormal breath sounds that are heard in addition to, or in place of, normal sounds.

agonal respirations Slow, shallow, irregular respirations or occasional gasping breaths; result from cerebral anoxia.

alveolar ventilation (V_a) The volume of air that comes into contact with the alveolar-capillary membrane surfaces and participates in the exchange of gases between the lung and blood.

anatomic dead space (V_d) Space in airway structures such as the trachea, bronchi, and bronchioles that does not participate in gas exchange. It is defined physiologically as ventilation without perfusion.

apnea The absence of respiration.

apneustic breathing A condition in which lesions in the respiratory center of the brainstem lead to a breathing pattern characterized by prolonged, gasping inspiration, followed by extremely short, ineffective expiration.

Prep Kit Continued

arterial blood gas (ABG) Analysis of the following characteristics of blood: pH, partial pressure of carbon dioxide (in arterial blood), partial pressure of oxygen (in arterial blood), concentration of bicarbonate ion, base excess (indicating whether the patient is acidotic or alkalotic), and oxygen saturation of the hemoglobin molecule.

barotrauma Injury to the chest or lungs as a result of increased intrathoracic pressure.

Biot (ataxic) respiration Breathing characterized by three patterns: (1) slow and deep, (2) rapid and shallow, and (3) apnea. Causes include meningitis, increased intracranial pressure, and central nervous system dysfunction.

bradypnea A respiratory rate that is slower than normal.

bronchovesicular sounds A combination of the tracheal and vesicular breath sounds, heard in places where airways and alveoli are found, including the upper part of the sternum and between the scapulae.

capnography A method for measuring exhaled CO_2, which in most cases correlates with the CO_2 levels in arterial blood. Two different types of devices can be used—an electronic monitor that displays a waveform and a colorimetric device that should turn yellow during exhalation, indicating proper tube placement.

capnometry A method for measuring exhaled CO_2; it is performed the same way as capnography, but provides a light-emitting diode readout of the patient's exhaled CO_2.

central neurogenic hyperventilation A pattern of very deep, rapid respirations at rates of 40 to 60 breaths/min, caused by a midbrain lesion or dysfunction.

Cheyne-Stokes respiration A cyclic pattern of increased respiratory rate and depth with periods of apnea. Causes include increased intracranial pressure, renal failure, meningitis, drug overdose, or hypoxia secondary to congestive heart failure.

cluster breathing An abnormal respiratory pattern in which a cluster of irregular respirations that vary in depth are followed by a period of apnea at irregular intervals.

compliance A change in volume per unit of pressure; $\Delta V/\Delta P$.

crackles A breath sound produced as fluid-filled alveoli pop open under increasing inspiratory pressure; can be fine or coarse.

difficult airway An airway in which the provider anticipates complications in securing an airway.

elastance The tendency to collapse (as in lung tissue).

eupnea Normal breathing at a rate of 12 to 20 breaths/min in the adult patient.

exhalation A passive process in which gas leaves the lungs.

expiratory reserve volume (ERV) The amount of air that can be expelled from the lungs after a normal exhalation.

face-to-face intubation Intubation in which the provider's face is at the same level as the patient's face; used when the standard position is not possible. In this position, the laryngoscope is held in the provider's right hand and the endotracheal tube in the left.

failed airway An unsuccessful intubation attempt in a patient for whom oxygenation cannot be adequately maintained with bag-mask ventilation; three unsuccessful intubation attempts by an experienced operator but with adequate oxygenation; and failed intubation using one best attempt in the "forced to act" situation.

fraction of inspired oxygen (FIO2) Percentage of inhaled oxygen expressed as a decimal. For example, 40% oxygen = FIO2 of 0.40.

functional residual capacity (FRC) The amount of air remaining in the lungs after normal expiration; the sum of the residual volume and the expiratory reserve volume.

Prep Kit Continued

hyperangulated blade A video laryngoscope blade with a high degree of curvature to get around anatomic structures.

hyperpnea A breath that is deeper than normal; it can lead to low levels of CO_2.

hypopnea A shallow breath; it can lead to increased CO_2 levels and decreased oxygen levels.

hypoxemia An abnormally low oxygen level.

I:E ratio An expression for comparing the length of expiration to the length of inspiration. The normal ratio is 1:2, which means that expiration is twice as long as inspiration. This ratio is not measured in seconds.

inspiration An active process in which gas is taken into the lungs.

inspiratory capacity (IC) The maximum amount of air that can be inspired; the sum of the inspiratory reserve volume and the tidal volume.

inspiratory reserve volume (IRV) The amount of air that can be inhaled after a tidal volume is inhaled.

Kussmaul respiration A fast and deep respiratory pattern without any periods of apnea. The rate and depth are greater than the normal rate expected; breathing is labored, with periods of deep breaths punctuated by sighs.

laryngeal mask airway (LMA) A rescue airway with a basic design similar to an endotracheal tube at the proximal end, in that a standard adapter is present to allow ventilation. The distal end is equipped with an elliptical cuff, which, when inflated, covers the supraglottic area and allows ventilation.

Mallampati classification A system for predicting the relative difficulty of intubation based on the amount of oropharyngeal structures visible in an upright, seated patient who is fully able to open their mouth.

minute volume Total volume of air breathed in and out in 1 minute. It is calculated by multiplying the respiratory rate per minute by the tidal volume.

obstructive diseases Diseases that result in difficulty with moving air out of the lungs, such as asthma, chronic obstructive pulmonary disease, cystic fibrosis, and bronchiectasis.

pleural friction rub The result of an inflammation that causes the pleura to thicken, decreasing the pleural space and allowing the surfaces of the pleura to rub together.

positive end-expiratory pressure (PEEP) The amount of pressure above ambient pressure present in the airway at the end of the respiratory cycle.

pressure gradients Differences in pressure, which allow for movement of gas into and out of the lung.

pulse oximetry Measurement of arterial oxygen saturation and the pulse.

rapid sequence intubation (RSI) The coadministration of both anesthetic agents and neuromuscular blocking agents to produce a state of unconsciousness and paralysis, which in turn allows for tracheal intubation.

residual volume (RV) The amount of air remaining in the lungs after the expiratory reserve volume is exhaled.

resistance The amount of force needed to move a gas or fluid through a single capillary tube.

respiratory depression A low respiratory rate (<2 breaths/min in adults) for a prolonged period of time; also called hypoventilation.

respiratory failure A situation in which the respiratory system fails to meet the body's metabolic needs. If not reversed, it may lead to respiratory or cardiopulmonary arrest.

respiratory insufficiency The inability of the respiratory system to keep up with the metabolic demands of the body.

restrictive diseases Diseases that result in difficulty moving air into the lungs, such as occupational lung diseases, idiopathic pulmonary fibrosis, pneumonia, atelectasis, chest wall deformities and injuries, and neuromuscular diseases that affect breathing.

Prep Kit Continued

rhonchi Rattling vibrations produced as air flows through mucus or around obstruction in the larger airways.

rigid stylet A hyperangulated intubation stylet used to facilitate endotracheal tube passage when using an hyperangulated blade.

Seldinger technique A technique for obtaining vascular or other hollow organ access that uses a hollow-bore needle inserted percutaneously, followed by placement of a soft-tipped guide wire. The needle is removed and a dilator is temporarily placed. The dilator is removed, the desired catheter is placed over the guide wire, and the guide wire is removed. The catheter is then secured.

shunt Perfusion without ventilation.

SpO_2 The noninvasive pulse oximetry measurement of oxyhemoglobin saturation by means of a beam of light applied to a superficial capillary bed such as the digits or ear lobe.

standard geometry blade A device used during indirect (video) laryngoscopy that allows the CCTP to visualize the oral cavity on a monitor.

stridor High-pitched sound representing air moving past fluid or mechanical obstruction within or immediately above the glottic opening.

tachypnea An abnormally fast respiratory rate.

tidal volume (V_t) The volume of air moved into and out of the lungs with each respiratory cycle.

total lung capacity (TLC) The maximal amount of air that can fill the lungs; the sum of tidal volume, inspiratory reserve volume, expiratory reserve volume, and residual volume.

tracheal breath sounds Breath sounds heard by placing the stethoscope diaphragm over the trachea or over the sternum; also called bronchial breath sounds.

ventilation-perfusion ($\dot{V}/\dot{Q}$) mismatch A state of inadequate ventilation, perfusion, or both, in which there is inadequate gas exchange.

vesicular breath sounds Softer, muffled sounds in which the expiratory phase is barely audible.

video laryngoscopy An orotracheal intubation technique that involves indirect visualization of the vocal cords via a video camera at the distal end of a blade that provides a video feed to a screen.

vital capacity (V_c) The maximal amount of air that can be exhaled following a maximal inspiration; the sum of tidal volume, inspiratory reserve volume, and expiratory reserve volume; approximately 80% total lung capacity.

$\dot{V}/\dot{Q}$ ratio The relationship between alveolar ventilation and alveolar capillary perfusion. The normal value is 0.8.

wheezes A high-pitched musical sound caused by airflow through a narrowed or constricted airway.

References

Brenner B, Corbridge T, Kazzi A. Intubation and mechanical ventilation of the asthmatic patient in respiratory failure. *J Allergy Clin Immunol.* 2009;124(suppl 2):S19-S28.

Brown CA, Sakles JC, Mick NW. *The Walls Manual of Emergency Airway Management.* 5th ed. Philadelphia, PA: Lippincott, Williams and Wilkins; 2018.

Butler TJ, Close JB, Close RJ. *Laboratory Exercises for Competency in Respiratory Care.* 3rd ed. Philadelphia, PA: FA Davis; 2013.

Cottrell GP. *Cardiopulmonary Anatomy and Physiology for Respiratory Care Practitioners.* Philadelphia, PA: FA Davis; 2001.

Difficult airway course. Stony Brook University Hospital website. https://www.stonybrookmedicine.edu /patientcare/emergencymedicine/difficult_airway_course. Accessed August 14, 2021.

Gausche-Hill M, Henderson D, Goodrich S, et al. *Pediatric Airway Management for the Prehospital Professional.* Sudbury, MA: Jones & Bartlett Learning; 2004.

Gravenstein J, Jaffe M, Gravenstein N, Paulus D, eds. *Capnography.* 2nd ed. Cambridge, UK: Cambridge University Press; 2011.

Hartjes TM. *Core Curriculum for High Acuity, Progressive, and Critical Care Nursing.* 7th ed. Philadelphia, PA: WB Saunders; 2017.

Heuer A. *Wilkins' Clinical Assessment in Respiratory Care.* 8th ed. St Louis, MO: Mosby Year Book; 2018.

Prep Kit Continued

Hung O, Murphy MF. *Management of the Difficult and Failed Airway.* New York, NY: McGraw-Hill Medical; 2011.

Kacmarek RM, Stoller JK, Heuer A. *Egan's Fundamentals of Respiratory Care.* 10th ed. St. Louis, MO: Mosby Year Book; 2013.

Ma OJ, Mateer JR, Reardon RF, Joing SA. *Ma and Mateer's Emergency Ultrasound.* 4th ed. New York, NY: McGraw-Hill; 2020.

Margolis G. *Airway Management: Paramedic.* Sudbury, MA: Jones & Bartlett Learning; 2004.

Mittal MK. Needle cricothyroidotomy with percutaneous trans-tracheal ventilation. *UpToDate* website. https://www.uptodate.com/contents/needle-cricothyroidotomy-with-percutaneous-transtracheal-ventilation. Updated January 8, 2020. Accessed August 14, 2021.

Paix BR, Griggs WM. Emergency surgical cricothyroidotomy: 24 successful cases leading to a simple "scalpel–finger–tube" method. *Emerg Med Australasia.* 2011. https://doi.org/10.1111/j.1742-6723.2011.01510.x.

Rezaie S. Critical care updates: resuscitation sequence intubation—pH kills (part 3 of 3). REBEL EM website. https://rebelem.com/critical-care-updates-resuscitation-sequence-intubation-ph-kills-part-3-of-3/. Published October 3, 2016. Accessed May 16, 2021.

Sakles JC, Bair CA. Video laryngoscopy. In: Brown CA, Sakles, Mick NW, eds. *The Walls Manual of Emergency Airway Management.* 5th ed. Philadelphia, PA: Wolters Kluwer; 2018:157-174.

Tintinalli JE, Stapczynski JS, Ma OJ, et al., eds. *Tintinalli's Emergency Medicine: A Comprehensive Study Guide.* 9th ed. New York, NY: McGraw-Hill; 2019.

Walls RM, Hockberger RS Gausche-Hill M, et al., eds. *Rosen's Emergency Medicine: Concepts and Clinical Practice.* 9th ed. Philadelphia, PA: Elsevier; 2017.

Weingart S. EMCrit Podcast 131—cricothyrotomy—cut to air: emergency surgical airway. EMCrit website. https://emcrit.org/emcrit/surgical-airway/. Published August 26, 2014. Accessed May 16, 2021.

Weingart S. Podcast 3—laryngoscope as a murder weapon (LAMW) series—ventilatory kills—intubating the patient with severe metabolic acidosis. EMCrit website. https://emcrit.org/emcrit/tube-severe-acidosis/. Published May 22, 2009. Accessed May 16, 2021.

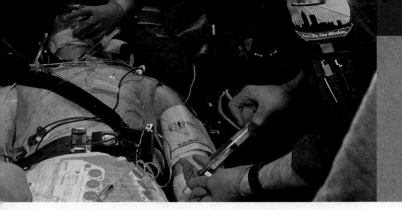

Chapter 7

Ventilation

Michael Schauf, RRT

OBJECTIVES

After completing this chapter, you will be able to:

1. Describe common features and characteristics of mechanical ventilators (p 228).
2. Differentiate between positive-pressure and negative-pressure ventilators (pp 229–230).
3. Differentiate among pressure ventilators, volume ventilators, and flow- and time-cycled ventilators (pp 237–238).
4. Differentiate between invasive and noninvasive ventilation (p 232).
5. Explain the types and uses of nasal cannulas (pp 232–234).
6. Define the various modes of mechanical ventilation (pp 240–241).
7. Define the ventilator parameters of tidal volume, fraction of inspired oxygen, respiratory rate, ratio of the length of inspiratory-to-expiratory (I:E) ratio, mode, and positive end-expiratory pressure (PEEP) (p 244).
8. Explain the use of PEEP (p 245).
9. Differentiate between respiratory distress and respiratory failure (p 248).
10. Describe measures the CCTP may take to ensure proper ventilator function and keep the patient's ventilatory status stable (pp 248–249).
11. Explain the difference between volume-delivered breaths and pressure-delivered breaths (p 249).
12. Describe the use of mechanical ventilation in managing common lung diseases and conditions (p 256).
13. Discuss how the graphics displayed by ventilators aid the clinician (pp 269–271).
14. Troubleshoot problems with mechanical ventilators, including common alarms (pp 271–274).

Introduction

Ventilation may be described most simply as the supply of oxygen delivered into the lungs for adequate gas exchange to take place. Health care providers can provide ventilation manually or with a machine, referred to as **mechanical ventilation**. Mechanical ventilation applies either positive pressure or negative pressure. Positive pressure is most commonly used today and may be applied either invasively (such as through an endotracheal [ET] tube) or noninvasively (with a nasal cannula or full-face mask). The indications for mechanical ventilation include managing the work of breathing, improving the distribution of inhaled gases, protecting the airway, and managing conditions such as apnea and ventilatory or respiratory failure.

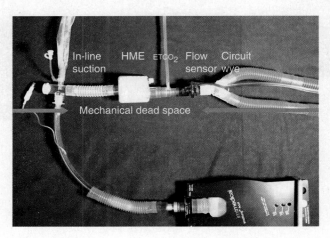

FIGURE 7-1 Example of additional dead space added to the ventilator circuit.

Courtesy of Vent-Pro Training.

Overview of Mechanical Ventilation

A major goal when ventilating a patient is to provide appropriate minute ventilation to meet the patient's metabolic demands. To identify which modality best meets their respiratory needs, the clinician must understand the patient's current lung physiology. Lung function may be assessed through pressure and flow measurements, which provide valuable information such as respiratory volume, resistance, compliance, and work of breathing. Clinicians use this information to evaluate respiratory mechanics and lung function to optimize mechanical ventilatory support.

Review of Common Respiratory Terminology

Dead Space Ventilation

Dead space ventilation, also referred to as wasted ventilation, refers to the volume of gas that moves into and out of the lungs but does not take part in gas exchange. Areas in which dead space ventilation occurs, called anatomic dead space, include the airways in the mouth and nose and the terminal bronchioles. The anatomic dead space for an adult male is approximately one-third of the tidal volume breathed in; the remaining two-thirds of gas inhaled is considered alveolar ventilation. When adding additional pieces, such as in-line suction catheters and heat moisture exchangers, to the ventilator circuit proximal to the wye, you are, in essence, adding dead space (mechanical dead space) to the delivered breath **FIGURE 7-1**. This consideration may be more critical in the neonatal/pediatric population, so using appropriate-size products is essential when caring for these patients.

Alveolar-to-Arterial Oxygen Gradient

The main purpose in calculating an alveolar-to-arterial oxygen (A-a) gradient is to determine the source of hypoxemia. This will help narrow the location of the problem to either inside the lungs or outside the lungs. The A-a gradient is calculated as $P_{AO_2} - P_{aO_2}$ (ie, partial pressure of alveolar oxygen – partial pressure of arterial oxygen), with the component values being determined by an arterial blood gas (ABG) analysis. The alveolar gas equation is used to estimate alveolar oxygen pressure:

$$P_{aO_2} = (P_{atm} - P_{H_2O})\, F_{IO_2} - P_{aCO_2}/RQ$$

where P_{atm} is the atmospheric pressure, P_{H_2O} is the partial pressure of water, F_{IO_2} is the fraction of inspired oxygen, P_{aCO_2} is the partial pressure of carbon dioxide in the alveoli, and RQ is the respiratory quotient. The main variables that affect the alveolar gas equation are the amount of F_{IO_2}, the level of carbon dioxide, and the atmospheric pressure.

A normal A-a gradient equals (Age + 10)/4. Patients with a condition such as pneumonia would typically have an elevated A-a gradient due to the excessive secretions within the lung, which create a physical barrier to gas exchange within the alveoli. This condition would result in ventilation-perfusion ($\dot{V}/\dot{Q}$) mismatch. Hypoxemia with a normal A-a gradient would indicate hypoventilation, in which carbon dioxide overrides alveolar oxygen.

Ventilation-Perfusion Mismatch

When searching for the underlying cause of hypoxemia, it is helpful to understand the $\dot{V}/\dot{Q}$ ratio. In healthy lungs, 4 L of air enters the respiratory tract system while 5 L of blood passes through the pulmonary capillary system. That equates to a $\dot{V}/\dot{Q}$ ratio of 0.8. Any number that is higher or lower than this ratio would be considered a $\dot{V}/\dot{Q}$ mismatch. The goal is to quickly identify the cause of the mismatch and develop a plan to correct the condition.

A ventilation problem is referred to as a shunt. Typical shunt presentations include pneumonia, asthma, chronic obstructive pulmonary disease (COPD) or emphysema, atelectasis, and pulmonary edema. Any condition that prohibits gas from crossing the alveolar-capillary membrane may be considered a shunt.

On the perfusion side of the $\dot{V}/\dot{Q}$ ratio, anything that prohibits normal blood flow through the pulmonary capillary system is considered dead space ventilation. For example, a patient with a pulmonary embolism is experiencing some form of dead space ventilation. A pulmonary embolism may be suspected in the face of hypoxemia with an elevated D-dimer level and confirmed with a computed tomography (CT) pulmonary angiogram.

Minute Volume

Minute volume is measured to determine how many liters of air move into or out of the lungs per minute. It is calculated by multiplying the exhaled tidal volume by the current respiratory rate. The minute volume has a direct correlation to the $Paco_2$ and $ETCO_2$ (end-tidal carbon dioxide) results. Having a higher than normal minute volume will theoretically lower the $Paco_2$ and $ETCO_2$, whereas having a lower than normal minute volume will theoretically increase the $Paco_2$ and $ETCO_2$. A normal minute volume for an adult is anywhere from 5 to 8 L/min, though it can increase with exercise. Methods for calculating minute volume and adjusting the ventilator to meet the patient's needs are discussed later in this chapter.

Features of Mechanical Ventilators

Mechanical ventilation devices range from simple to complex, depending on the needs of the patient and the capabilities of the machine. At one time, the classification and description of ventilators were simple; however, with the increased use of biotechnology, microprocessors, and sophisticated flow-sensing devices in mechanical ventilation, the classification of these devices has become ever more complicated. All ventilators, however, share several common characteristics:

1. **Power source.** All ventilators require an external power source. This source can be electric (AC), battery (DC), or pneumatic (requiring a 50-psi [pounds per square inch] gas source).
2. **Cycling.** This feature refers to which variable terminates the inspiratory phase of a breath. Pressure, volume, time, and flow can terminate a breath, depending on the ventilator.
3. **Breath delivery.** The ventilator can deliver a breath using either negative pressure **FIGURE 7-2** or positive pressure **FIGURE 7-3**. It is important to understand the changes that take place when a positive-pressure system is applied to a system that normally functions as a negative-pressure system.
4. **Parameters.** Mode, tidal volume or inspiratory pressure, respiratory rate, set minute volume, inspiratory-to-expiratory ratio, flow or I time, fraction of inspired oxygen (Fio_2), and positive end-expiratory pressure (PEEP) are all ventilator settings selected by the clinician. Modes and parameters are discussed in detail later in this section.
5. **Ventilator circuit.** An external circuit, which varies depending on the ventilator, is used to connect the ventilator to the patient. Some transport ventilators use a single-limb circuit, some use a dual-limb circuit, and some incorporate the dual-limb circuit into a coaxial circuit.
6. **Alarms.** Varying types of audio and/or visual alarms warn of ventilator malfunction or parameters outside the set alarm limits. They should be set for each individual patient and *never* disabled. Guidelines for alarm settings are discussed later in this chapter. The most important alarms to monitor for volume-targeted breathing are those for the peak inspiratory pressure (PIP) and the plateau pressure. The most important alarm to monitor for pressure-targeted breathing is the low-minute-volume alarm, which will detect a decrease in tidal volume.

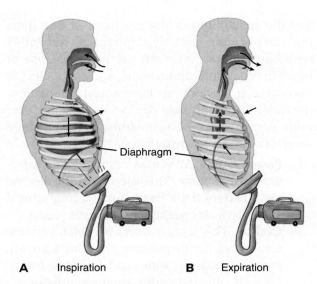

A   Inspiration   **B**   Expiration

FIGURE 7-2 Normal ventilation is negative-pressure ventilation, which is similar to how a vacuum cleaner works. **A.** The diaphragm contracts, expanding the size of the thoracic cavity and creating the negative pressure to help fill the lungs. **B.** When the pressure is released, the diaphragm relaxes and the lungs empty.

© Jones & Bartlett Learning.

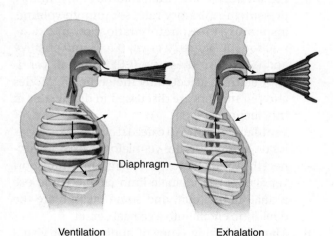

Ventilation   Exhalation

FIGURE 7-3 With positive-pressure ventilation, such as with a bag-mask device, air is pushed into the respiratory tract. This is the opposite of negative-pressure ventilation.

© Jones & Bartlett Learning.

Basic Types of Mechanical Ventilators

Greater use of mechanical ventilation has led to a steadily growing industry to provide these devices. These sophisticated machines may be designed specifically for adult, pediatric, or neonatal patients. Some ventilators safely ventilate only patients up to a certain weight limit, whereas others accommodate patients of all weights. Moreover, these ventilators vary widely in their complexity to accommodate different settings: Some are designed for stationary use, such as in an intensive care unit (ICU) or operating room, and others are portable units for use during transport, whether in the hospital or in the out-of-hospital environment.

Transport ventilators are chosen based on a number of factors. The most important consideration should be the patient population whom the transport team serves. Population characteristics include patient age and weight, patient acuity, type of transport (eg, intrafacility versus interfacility), length of transport, means of transport (ground, rotor aircraft, fixed-wing aircraft), and budget for the equipment and supplies associated with the ventilator.

More sophisticated ventilators may have a flow-sensing device that is attached in close proximity to the patient's airway and transmits information to the ventilator necessary for accurate feedback, allowing the patient to trigger a breath with better synchrony to the ventilator settings. This flow sensor can also provide feedback in the form of pressure, volume, and flow waveforms, allowing providers to adjust the ventilator settings for the specific patient and lungs being ventilated. Pressure/volume and flow/volume loops are available on some of these ventilators, and may be used to visually detect compliance changes, air leaks, and air trapping. Specific training in waveform interpretation is needed to take full advantage of these features.

The transport ventilator's ability to meet a patient's flow demand must be considered prior to use of a specific device. Some transport ventilators are simply unable to meet extremely high flow demands. For example, a patient with severe acute respiratory distress syndrome (ARDS) who is on high levels of PEEP, has a high respiratory rate, and has high pressures may need a transport ventilator that can provide flow ranges from 160 to 240 L/min to effectively oxygenate and ventilate the patient. These higher-flow generators, which are typically turbine driven, are often called blower-driven ventilators. They send gas directly to the output section, and manipulation of a flow control valve enables them to deliver specific ventilator settings. Just as providers should understand the ventilator's ability to meet the patient's needs before connecting the device to the patient, they should also understand the patient's lung condition (if possible) to select the appropriate lung protection strategy.

Transport ventilators can be categorized according to three levels of performance: sophisticated ventilators with features similar to those used in the ICU, midlevel transport ventilators, and simple transport ventilators.

Sophisticated transport ventilators have the following characteristics:

- Turbine/blower driven to reach available flows greater than 150 L/min
- Waveform and loop monitoring available
- Many modes of ventilation available
- Triggering delay less than 100 ms
- Tidal volume control more accurate than with midlevel transport ventilators
- Flow manipulation with rise time (P-ramp) and flow termination in a pressure-delivered breath
- Leak compensation feature
- Measure plateau and auto-PEEP
- Measure static compliance
- Precise F_{IO_2} delivery
- Many alarm settings available
- Allow for hot-swapping of batteries (ie, changing batteries without cutting the power to the unit)

Advantages of sophisticated transport ventilators include the following:

- Deliver consistent ventilator parameters in the presence of dynamic changes in lung mechanics
- Offer performance and modes similar to ICU ventilators
- Provide accurate monitoring and feedback from lung mechanics
- Provide comprehensive alarm settings
- Some are altitude compensated

Disadvantages of sophisticated transport ventilators include the following:

- Extensive training required to master all available functions
- Bias flow during flow triggering may contribute to higher gas consumption (During

high-frequency oscillatory ventilation, bias flow is the continuous "background" flow of gas through the ventilator circuit during expiration. When the ventilator detects a deviation in the set flow, a breath is delivered to the patient.)
- Cost

Midlevel transport ventilators have the following features:

- Pneumatic or piston driven
- Typical available flows of 60 to 100 L/min
- Simple user interface
- Basic scalars available
- Mediocre trigger performance
- Triggering delay greater than 120 ms
- Selective F_{IO_2} delivery
- Lower pressurization performance

Advantages of midlevel transport ventilators include the following:

- Simple user interface
- Basic modes available
- Lower cost

Disadvantages of midlevel transport ventilators include the following:

- Challenging to ventilate patients with poor-compliance and high-resistance lung conditions
- Can create distress in the air-hungry patient receiving noninvasive ventilation

Simple transport ventilators have the following features:

- Pneumatic or compressor driven
- Basic ventilator settings

Advantages of simple transport ventilators include the following:

- Lowest cost
- Ease of use
- Less training required
- Useful during CPR

Disadvantages of simple transport ventilators include the following:

- F_{IO_2} may be fixed
- Poor trigger performance
- Minimal alarms

It is important to know the battery life for each transport ventilator you are managing. According to the American Association for Respiratory Care, transport ventilators should have a minimum of

4 hours of battery life. Many factors affect battery duration, including the patient's pressure or volume, the respiratory rate, the PEEP level, the temperature of the operating environment, and the number of charge cycles the battery has been through. Always check the manufacturer's information on the battery life before operating the ventilator. The ventilator should be plugged into an appropriate external AC power source whenever possible.

Another transport concern is oxygen tank duration. Many variables contribute to oxygen consumption—most importantly, how much FIO_2 the patient requires. The lower the FIO_2, the less oxygen that will be used. The next most important concern is the minute volume the patient requires, which is calculated as respiratory rate $\times$ exhaled tidal volume. Some ventilators use a bias flow throughout the breathing cycle to augment patient triggering, which in turn increases oxygen consumption.

The critical care transport professional (CCTP) is responsible for becoming familiar with the operating characteristics, capabilities, and features of the ventilator being used and to troubleshoot and adapt as necessary. The goal when applying any mechanical ventilation is to maximize the potential benefit and to minimize any potential harm to the patient. Planning each trip on a case-by-case basis will ensure patient safety and comfort.

Noninvasive Ventilation Methods

For years, conventional ventilation required invasive ventilation by placing an artificial airway—chiefly the ET tube or a tracheostomy tube. Because of the hazards and complications associated with ET tubes, however, other interfaces began to emerge. Mouthpieces and masks of varying sizes and styles were attached to conventional ventilators, giving rise to "noninvasive" ventilation. By definition, noninvasive ventilation is any form of mechanical ventilation without an artificial airway. It includes methods such as high-flow nasal cannula (HFNC) therapy, continuous positive airway pressure (CPAP), and bilevel positive airway pressure (BPAP), which deliver a preset pressure or volume to the lungs during a preset or spontaneous breathing pattern.

This chapter focuses primarily on invasive ventilation techniques. Because emergency medical services (EMS) providers are quite familiar with most noninvasive techniques, they are not detailed in this chapter. However, the more advanced noninvasive techniques—HFNC therapy, CPAP, and BPAP—warrant a brief discussion.

In broad terms, each of these techniques has a primary indication. HFNC therapy is most appropriate for patients with purely hypoxemic respiratory failure. CPAP is typically selected to treat hypoxia associated with increased work of breathing. BPAP, commonly referred to by the brand name BiPAP, is extremely effective for patients with hypercarbic respiratory failure.

Nasal Cannula Therapy

When caring for the acutely hypoxic patient, it is common practice to place the patient on supplemental oxygen via a nasal cannula with liter flows ranging from 1 to 6 L/min, often referred to as a low-flow nasal cannula (LFNC). The oxygen percentage that the patient receives with this setup is limited by the patient's minute volume; it is a fixed liter flow of oxygen applied to the variable rate and depth that the patient is breathing on room air (21%). The estimated percentage of FIO_2 a LFNC can deliver at 1 to 6 L/min would be 0.24 to 0.44 FIO_2. If the patient requires more FIO_2, the clinician may try to deliver 35% to 55% oxygen with a simple face mask, 85% to 95% with a nonrebreathing mask, or 100% using an HFNC.

Because of the design of these devices, they cannot create any measurable pressure to provide some level of CPAP, nor do they decrease the work of breathing. Instead, they are designed solely to deliver supplemental oxygen to the patient and do nothing to aid in ventilation.

Furthermore, administering a dry gas such as oxygen can dry out the mucosa within the nasal passages and lungs, potentially causing mucus plugging. Providers should avoid any potential for formation of a mucus plug because it may cause severe hypoxemia due to a $\dot{V}/\dot{Q}$ mismatch. This possibility is especially concerning in a patient with excessive secretions, as occurs in bacterial/viral pneumonia.

The best choice for a more comfortable delivery and precise FIO_2 target might be an HFNC. Initially introduced under the brand name

Vapotherm, these devices can deliver flows of up to 60 L/min of humidified oxygen through a larger-lumen nasal cannula; they reduce both inspiratory resistance and work of breathing by providing flows that exceed the patient's demand. Such a device is designed with an oxygen blender that delivers 0.21 to 1.0 FIO_2 as well as providing heat and humidification through a special cartridge that pulverizes the water molecules to ensure greater patient comfort. The HFNC requires external AC power and a source of oxygen at 50 psi and medical air at 50 psi to be blended to provide a predetermined FIO_2.

Used to treat hypoxic respiratory failure, HFNCs deliver high flow rates that equate to a form of non-invasive ventilation. The high oxygen flows required typically have made HFNC therapy impractical for use during interfacility transports, but prototypes suitable for EMS and critical care transport (CCT) use are in development. The potential need to transport a patient being treated with HFNC therapy makes it important for the CCTP to be familiar with this form of respiratory support.

HFNC therapy uses soft, large-bore nasal prongs (cannulas), humidification and heating mechanisms, and a gas blender. Heating and humidification are accomplished by placing a heater/humidifier similar to those used on mechanical ventilator circuits in line with the HFNC. The delivered gas is a blended mixture of compressed air and oxygen, set from 0.21 to 1.0 FIO_2, that runs through the heater/humidifier, where it is warmed to body temperature and humidified to approximately the same 80% to 90% humidification seen physiologically with air inspired through the mouth and nose. The heating and humidification remedy the major causes of discomfort associated with conventional oxygen therapy: The added moisture can help to liquefy mucus and facilitate expectoration. The high flow washes out nasopharyngeal dead space, improving ventilation and oxygenation. Moreover, some level of PEEP, which is difficult to quantify, results from the high flow. Theoretically, every 10 L/min of gas flow generates PEEP of 1 cm H_2O. This PEEP (or CPAP) effect also decreases the work of breathing and improves oxygenation.

Initiation and titration of HFNC therapy have not yet been studied extensively. Application of this technology typically uses the maximum flow: 40 to 60 L/min for adults, depending on the brand

of equipment used, and up to 8 L/min for infants. FIO_2 should initially be set at 1.0 (100%). The flow can be adjusted for patient comfort and to target respiratory rates between 25 and 30 breaths/min in adults. Before weaning the patient from the flow, FIO_2 should be gradually decreased to at least 0.4 (40%). Once FIO_2 reaches 0.4, the flow can be decreased, typically in increments of 5 L/min, with effects continuously assessed. The temperature of the circuit is usually set to normal body temperature (37°C [98.6°F]) but can be adjusted up or down for comfort. Patients are often more comfortable with a setting lower than body temperature.

Neonatal and pediatric populations have also benefited from the favorable effects of the higher flows delivered by HFNC. Proper fit, flow levels, and oxygen concentration are even more essential in these populations due to their fragility. Much discussion has focused on the optimal flow for these younger patients. The range that is typically considered is 2 to 8 L/min, titrated to decrease the patient's work of breathing and optimize oxygenation status. Recent guidelines for flow selection have included using 1 to 2 L/kg/min as a starting point with a maximum flow rate set.

HFNC therapy can be used as a bridge to support the patient's respiratory status while other therapies and medications are being administered. In the face of respiratory distress, the goal is to prevent respiratory failure while using the least invasive methods. Some common conditions that may benefit from early application of HFNC therapy include bronchiolitis, respiratory syncytial virus, asthma, and postextubation somnolence.

There is some debate over the application of HFNC and how much PEEP it may create, as the PEEP level is difficult to measure when this therapy is applied. Many variables may increase the level of pressure in the lungs, including the applied flow and the use of open- versus closed-mouth breathing. In addition, the patient's size and current lung condition play major roles in how much PEEP the lungs may receive. However, HFNC therapy has been shown to increase **functional residual capacity** and contribute to washing out physiologic dead space.

People normally rebreathe approximately one-third of their exhaled breath. Therefore, a major benefit of the high flows provided by HFNC is to provide continuous fresh gas to the airways, allowing for the presence of more oxygen and less carbon dioxide in the lungs. This action makes this modality a good choice for patients who present with COPD exacerbation or with hypercarbia and hypoxia. Specifically, patients with the following conditions may benefit from HFNC therapy:

- COPD, including emphysema
- Pneumonia
- Coronavirus disease 2019 (COVID-19)
- Asthma exacerbation
- Pulmonary fibrosis
- Cystic fibrosis
- Lung cancer

This approach may also be useful in providing comfort care or preoxygenating patients for rapid sequence intubation.

Thorough planning for the transport of a patient on HFNC therapy is imperative. The high flows required to support this modality present a challenge during transport because the quantity of gas available is limited and, therefore, time sensitive. Some suggested solutions are to carry more oxygen, reduce the flow if tolerated, and/or reduce the FIO_2 if tolerated. Heat and humidification are essential when applying such high concentrations of oxygen at high flows. Several manufacturers offer options to account for this added challenge **FIGURE 7-4**.

If ventilation cannot be maintained in a patient on an HFNC, the gas flow may be increased to meet the patient's demands. However, a patient who is still experiencing respiratory distress may be heading toward respiratory failure, and the decision needs to be made to change modalities. CPAP or BPAP are often viable alternatives. CCTPs should consult with medical control when making this decision.

Another device that is popular in neonatal and pediatric patients is the RAM cannula. This nasal cannula has a 15-mm adapter on the end and can be attached to a ventilator circuit. Considered an interface to deliver noninvasive ventilation, it is often applied in the transport arena and can lead to successful results when used with the appropriate patient population. Using a RAM cannula as an interface with a transport ventilator allows the provider to deliver two levels of pressure with a respiratory rate applied.

While it is possible to transport most HFNC assemblies, doing so can be challenging. The heater/humidifier will require AC power, and the HFNC device requires a level and secure platform to ensure the heater/humidifier remains upright. The high gas flows necessitate large cylinders of both oxygen and compressed air, both connected to a blender that facilitates FIO_2 titration. In most cases, trying to move a HFNC setup is neither practical nor recommended. When impractical, the CCTP will need to choose an equivalent device to provide respiratory support during transport.

Combining a nonrebreathing device with a nasal cannula might be sufficient to match a given HFNC flow and FIO_2, especially when the HFNC settings are not maximized. Pulse oximetry is a necessity for continual monitoring. Not to be overlooked in a patient with HFNC is the PEEP effect. A patient on HFNC at 50 L/min is likely receiving 5 cm H_2O of PEEP from the gas flow. Switching to a nonrebreathing mask might provide the same amount of oxygen, but if the PEEP had served to reduce the work of breathing and improve oxygenation, loss of those benefits might not become evident for 15 to 20 minutes, which would probably coincide with the beginning of the actual transport.

A more suitable replacement for HFNC therapy is CPAP. CPAP or BPAP, when delivered using a transport ventilator, allows providers to adjust the FIO_2 level and enables some degree of PEEP to continue. Disposable CPAP devices can deliver equivalent PEEP but, depending on the manufacturer, may not be able to deliver adequate FIO_2. These units entrain a significant amount of atmospheric air to achieve the gas flows needed, thereby lowering the delivered FIO_2. Adding a nasal cannula under a disposable CPAP mask might provide an adequate level of FIO_2.

Continuous Positive Airway Pressure

Introduced to the medical community in 1971, CPAP found its niche in neonatal ICUs, supporting premature newborns with respiratory distress resulting from underdeveloped lungs. Ten years later, it was tried experimentally in adults with obstructive sleep apnea who, until then, underwent tracheostomies to avoid apnea-related asphyxiation. Today, CPAP is the primary therapy for both premature neonates and people of all ages with obstructive sleep apnea. CPAP indications have also

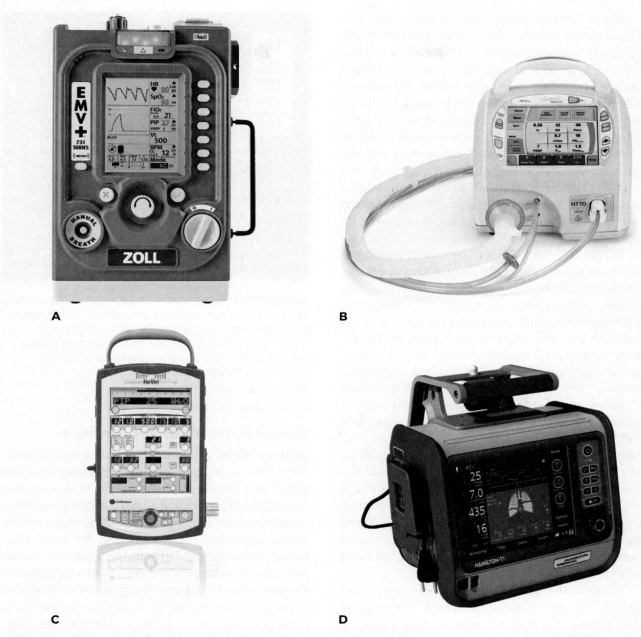

FIGURE 7-4 Examples of mechanical ventilators commonly used in critical care transport. **A.** Zoll 731+ EMV. **B.** Newport (HT70+). **C.** CareFusion. **D.** Hamilton T-1, military version preferred.

expanded to include acute pulmonary edema (APE) plus a wide variety of clinical conditions associated with acute shortness of breath.

The physiologic action of CPAP involves continuous positive pressure applied to the upper airway. The "continuous" aspect of CPAP implies that the pressure remains the same regardless of whether the patient is inspiring or expiring. Airway pressure applied during expiration increases the work of breathing, depending on the pressures used. Higher pressures may interfere with exhalation. Despite the slightly increased work needed to breathe against CPAP during exhalation, the overall effect is a significantly decreased work of breathing owing to its benefits during inspiration and on the airways themselves.

Use of CPAP for APE illustrates a dramatic, immediate, and effective application for CPAP. APE can result from a variety of conditions but is most commonly associated with right-side heart failure resulting from left-side heart failure. In patients with heart failure, significantly elevated pulmonary vascular pressures cause fluid to leak from the pulmonary vessels into the airways. In what is often described as "flash" pulmonary edema, pulmonary vascular fluid quickly fills the terminal airways. CPAP offers multiple benefits for patients with APE, with clinically significant improvement usually seen within the first minute following its application.

For patients with APE, CPAP prevents additional fluid from leaking out of the pulmonary vessels and entering the airways through the creation of a continuous, positive-pressure gradient. Theoretically, CPAP may force fluids congesting the lower airways back into the pulmonary blood vessels. At a minimum, it assists in splinting lower airways open, thereby preventing the collapse of the fluid-filled airways. CPAP also leads to a significant reduction in transpulmonary pressure—the pressure needed inside the chest to draw air into the lungs. In a healthy person, transpulmonary pressures of negative 1 or negative 2 cm H_2O are sufficient to draw air into the lungs. In the presence of significant obstruction caused by fluids, secretions, mucus plugs, or bronchial spasm, however, pressures as high as negative 8 cm H_2O may be needed to inhale. These negative pressures produce retractions in the chest musculature, a telltale clinical finding associated with APE.

In APE, the left ventricle is ejecting blood against a high afterload. Elevated blood pressure, added to a high transpulmonary pressure, is the root cause of the pulmonary edema seen in this condition: The heart simply cannot overcome the resistance it is pushing against. CPAP directly lowers transpulmonary pressures, as seen in **FIGURE 7-5**. The seemingly small decrease in transpulmonary pressure achieved with CPAP is such a powerful force in reducing afterload that patients with APE often improve within seconds following initiation of CPAP. Clinical outcomes are improved through the combined effects of improving oxygenation through oxygen delivered with continuous positive pressure and splinting open terminal airways.

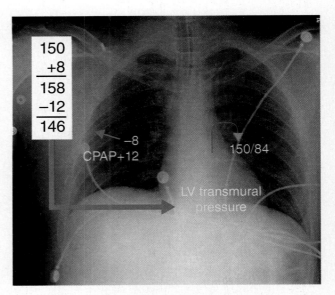

FIGURE 7-5 Transpulmonary pressure in acute pulmonary edema includes systolic blood pressure of 150 (afterload) plus the increased inspiratory force of −8 (normal is −1 to −2). Continuous positive airway pressure quickly reduces both afterload and the work of breathing by lowering the transpulmonary pressure.

Abbreviation: LV, left ventricular

© Jones & Bartlett Learning.

Bilevel Positive Airway Pressure

BPAP, as *bi*level would imply, delivers two different pressures: an inspiratory positive airway pressure (IPAP) and a lower, expiratory positive airway pressure (EPAP). This method allows a higher pressure to be delivered during inspiration, and a lower pressure during expiration, thereby reducing the work of exhaling. The difference between the pressures, a value called pressure support or delta P, is directly related to the patient's tidal volume. The greater the difference in pressures, the higher the patient's tidal volume is likely to be. The ability of BPAP to increase tidal volumes, and thereby lower carbon dioxide levels, is what most differentiates this approach from CPAP. BPAP offers the same support as CPAP, but with the added benefits of further decreasing the work of breathing during exhalation and improving tidal volumes; thus, it clears more carbon dioxide from the patient's respiratory system compared to CPAP. It is a reasonable alternative for patients who are unable to tolerate CPAP, those who require high CPAP pressures, and those whose respiratory failure is primarily related to hypercarbia (high carbon dioxide levels).

The most significant issue with BPAP is apnea induced by higher levels of pressure support than a patient requires. This condition can occur on initial setup or if a patient's respiratory status recovers during transport. All ventilators and machines configured to deliver BPAP monitor respiratory rates and, if they detect apnea, are preset to initiate mechanical ventilation. This level of monitoring and backup support is not available on disposable BPAP units, however. In consequence, providers should remain hypervigilant when using BPAP without respiratory rate monitoring and apnea ventilation capabilities.

BPAP can present a challenge to providers when they are selecting and subsequently adjusting the IPAP and EPAP settings. The IPAP is always set higher than the EPAP; most references suggest an initial IPAP setting of 8 to 10 cm H_2O and EPAP of 3 to 5 cm H_2O. Increasing the IPAP will clear more carbon dioxide, whereas increasing the EPAP will improve oxygenation (in the same way that increasing CPAP pressures improves oxygenation). Patients who are intolerant of high EPAP levels may benefit from an increased IPAP level.

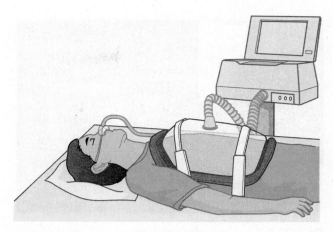

FIGURE 7-6 Biphasic cuirass ventilation.
© Jones & Bartlett Learning.

Negative-Pressure Ventilators

During the polio epidemics of the 1950s, iron lungs were commonly used to ventilate patients experiencing the respiratory effects of this disease. Recall that in normal spontaneous breathing, a breath is initiated by a drop in the transrespiratory pressure gradient. Negative-pressure ventilators operate in the same way. A negative pressure is transmitted by the ventilator to the chest wall, thereby enabling inspiration.

The original iron lung is no longer used, but has instead been replaced by smaller, more convenient devices. The two devices most commonly used as negative-pressure ventilators are the cuirass, or turtle shell, and the poncho type. The cuirass resembles a chest plate of armor and is strapped onto the patient's chest **FIGURE 7-6**. A hose connected to the ventilator sucks on the chest during inspiration. In contrast, the poncho requires a lightweight frame that is fitted onto the patient's chest, with a lightweight airtight jacket placed over the patient's frame. The ventilator hose is then attached to the jacket. Both the cuirass and the poncho require that a tight seal be maintained.

These negative-pressure ventilators are sometimes used in acute care facilities, but are more often used in rehabilitation and long-term care facilities or in the home. They are used chiefly on patients with neuromuscular diseases who still have airway control.

Positive-Pressure Ventilators

Positive-pressure ventilators are more prevalent than negative-pressure ventilators. With these devices, the tidal volume is delivered at pressures greater than ambient pressure; thus, the process is paradoxical to spontaneous breathing.

Several potential hazards are associated with this type of life support. Pulmonary barotrauma is of major concern because it can lead to pneumothorax, subcutaneous emphysema, pneumomediastinum, and pneumoperitoneum. Another major concern while applying positive pressure to the lungs is volutrauma, defined as trauma from excessive lung inflation volumes. Volutrauma is typically a result of overdistending the alveoli. It may occur at minimal tidal volumes due to regional differences in compliance within the lungs. This concern often arises in patients with ARDS because their lung compliance is poor, their airway resistance is high, and heterogeneous lung injury is likely. Positive pressure will overdistend the compliant alveoli, causing volutrauma. Strategies to minimize these complications are discussed later in the chapter. The main consideration is keeping plateau pressures below 30 cm H_2O.

Controversy

Barotrauma, injury due to excessive pressure, is often considered synonymous with *volutrauma*, injury resulting from excessive volume. Both terms remain in use, although barotrauma is more frequently used when referring to injury resulting from overdistention in the lungs.

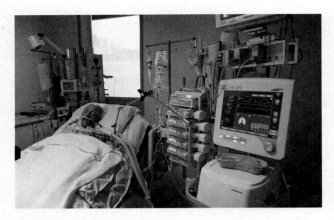

FIGURE 7-7 A critical care ventilator.

© Yon Marsh/Alamy Stock Photo.

Positive-pressure ventilators come in various sizes, power sources, and capabilities, and can be as small and portable as a laptop computer or as large as a desk. Institutions typically select ventilators based on their capabilities and patient needs, as well as their cost and operational factors **FIGURE 7-7**.

Positive-pressure ventilators are often described in terms of which variable the clinician controls to terminate the inspiratory phase of the breath. A pressure ventilator ends the delivery of the tidal volume based on the pressure preselected by the clinician. With a volume ventilator, the breath ends when the predetermined tidal volume is achieved. A flow-cycled ventilator ends inspiration when a predetermined flow rate is achieved, and a time-cycled ventilator ends inspiration after the selected inspiratory time has been achieved. Many of the ventilators in use today allow clinicians to choose which variable terminates the inspiratory cycle, while focusing on patient comfort/synchrony and patient safety. Each of these variables may have a unique benefit to accomplish oxygenation and ventilation but may be accompanied by some limitations. Understanding how each variable works and interacts with patient demand is of utmost importance.

When working with pressure ventilators, remember that the machine terminates inspiration when a preset pressure is reached. Therefore, if the patient is biting down on the ET tube or the patient's airway is obstructed with mucus, the ventilator will still deliver the pressure, but the tidal volume will be significantly decreased. Increased airway resistance and decreased thoracic compliance will also produce this effect. Careful monitoring of breath sounds, oxygen saturation, and ETCO$_2$; visual inspection for adequate chest expansion; and monitoring delivered tidal volume and exhaled minute volume are essential when pressure ventilation is being used. Some ventilators have extensive alarm settings that allow for monitoring minute volume and tidal volumes. When using pressure ventilation, it is strongly suggested that these alarms be used and set to tight ranges to prevent any large deviations from targeted minute volumes.

Volume ventilators deliver a preset volume using varying pressures. The pressure required by the ventilator depends on the size of the tidal volume, flow rate, airway resistance, and lung–chest wall compliance. Because volume ventilators use different pressures, it is important that the CCTP monitor the peak airway pressure. The high-pressure alarm will sound if excessive pressures are being used to deliver the tidal volume. This alarm is set at approximately 10 cm H$_2$O greater than the patient's average peak pressure. Secretions, bronchospasm, and a decrease in thoracic/pulmonary compliance may all result in increased airway pressures. Peak airway pressures may also rise when the patient is asynchronous with the ventilator ("bucking the vent") or is experiencing auto-PEEP. Continuous monitoring and trending of the peak pressure values are extremely important while caring for the patient who is being mechanically ventilated. In any event, an increased PIP requires immediate attention to detect and resolve the issue.

All ventilators, regardless of type, rely on an external circuit that connects the ventilator to the patient. Intrinsic to this circuit is some method for venting the patient's exhaled gas to the environment. On some ventilators, this is accomplished through the exhalation limb of the circuit connected to the ventilator; an internal exhalation valve then regulates exhalation as well as PEEP. Other ventilators use an external exhalation valve.

It is strongly recommended that each circuit be equipped with an in-line heat-moisture exchanger, placed close to the ET tube. This device also acts as a bacterial/viral filter. Note that adding anything proximal to the ET tube will increase dead space to the circuit and may increase Paco$_2$ levels to a slight extent. This possible increase is of particular importance in the neonatal and pediatric populations.

In every case, a closed system must exist between the ventilator and the patient. Any loose connections, cracks, or disconnections will result in ventilator malfunction and can be life threatening. The integrity of the patient–ventilator connection via the circuit, as evidenced by the pressure, should be checked per the manufacturer's procedure and visually inspected throughout transport, and all clinicians operating the ventilator should be familiar with the process of troubleshooting these connections. In the CCT environment, it is imperative that the CCTP read and understand the alarms and troubleshooting guide in the ventilator's operation manual. Each ventilator may display specific codes to identify potential problems and classify their priority level. Some manufacturers' manuals include guidance on potential remedies to correct the alarm. This information should be readily available to the CCTP in the event of an alarm trigger.

A major concern relating to the positive pressure exerted during mechanical ventilation is the effect it has on the patient's hemodynamics. Hypovolemia, high levels of PEEP, and increased **mean airway pressure (MAP)** values may all contribute to hemodynamic compromise. This issue is often overlooked and needs to be monitored closely.

- Positive-pressure ventilation increases intrathoracic pressure, which can result in barotrauma or volutrauma (pneumothorax).
- An increase in intrathoracic pressure can result in reduced venous return to the right side of the heart, leading to a reduction in right ventricular output associated with alveolar inflation that compresses the pulmonary vascular bed.
- The diminished venous return to the right side of the heart leads to poor cardiac output, and possibly hypotension.
- Reduced hepatorenal blood flow may mislead the body into believing it is volume depleted, resulting in changes in hormone levels, such as increased vasopressin and aldosterone activity and decreased levels of atrial natriuretic hormone. All of these changes result in fluid retention.

There is no one-size-fits-all approach to mechanically ventilating patients. Protocols and guidelines offer general guidance, but ultimately a strategy should be developed on a case-by-case basis. The main goal when mechanically ventilating any patient is to support their respiratory needs while focusing on safety and comfort.

Special Populations

Pregnant patients at term have an increased (by approximately 40%) tidal volume and live in a state of compensated respiratory alkalosis. Keep this factor in mind when adjusting ventilator settings.

Calculating Oxygen Cylinder Duration

When oxygen administration is required, how long the available oxygen supply will last is a critical consideration. Although many reliable apps are readily available that you can use on your computer or smartphone, it remains important to learn the following formula to calculate tank duration:

Oxygen tank time (min) = Tank pressure (psi) × Tank conversion factor ÷ Flow rate (L/min)

where the oxygen tank conversion factors are as follows:

D tank = 0.16
E tank = 0.28
G tank = 2.41
H or K tank = 3.14
M tank = 1.56

For example, suppose the patient is on a nonrebreathing mask running at 15 L/min. Your D tank has a 1,600 psi reading on the gauge. To calculate time in minutes until the tank is completely empty, you would perform the following calculation:

1,600 psi × 0.16 ÷ 15 L/min = 17 min

It is recommended that you subtract 500 psi from the tank pressure as a safety factor when using this formula. Thus, in the preceding example, the tank time would more safely be calculated as a little less than 12 minutes: 1,100 psi × 0.16 ÷ 15 L/min = 11.7 min.

Knowing the tank size is crucial. Keep this chart of conversion factors available to calculate oxygen cylinder duration prior to launching the mission. Some ventilators may have an oxygen cylinder duration feature that requires input from the provider.

Ventilator Modes and Parameters

Volume and pressure are often thought of as modes the CCTP can choose when setting up a ventilator. In reality, both volume and pressure are flow targets set to determine when the ventilator should end the inspiratory cycle. Ventilator *modes* describe the *types* of breaths being delivered to the patient—that is, whether the breath is a mandatory or machine breath or a spontaneous breath. Ventilator *parameters* refer to the other settings that may be adjusted and should be monitored continuously by the clinician. The availability of modes, alarms, and other parameters can vary from machine to machine. The basic considerations are discussed in the following sections.

Modes

The various modes of mechanical ventilation may ensure a particular minute ventilation rate and control the work associated with the patient's spontaneous breathing efforts. The result is an alphabet soup of acronyms that can be confusing to the novice ventilator user. You may encounter a situation where you are picking up a patient who is on a ventilator mode with which you are unfamiliar. For every CCTP, it is important to understand what the patient's pulmonary status is and why they were placed on this particular mode. If possible, involve the patient's respiratory therapist in the process of transitioning the patient to your ventilator. Strategies for changing patients to transport ventilators are discussed in detail later in this chapter. Note, however, that not all ventilators

have all modes available. As technology changes at a rapid pace, you will find more transport ventilators able to mirror the more advanced modes commonly available on hospital ICU ventilators. **TABLE 7-1** lists the most common modes of ventilation.

A potentially confusing concept in mechanical ventilation is the mode of ventilation. With more than 170 different names being used for modes, medical professionals have a wide range of choices available. Providers must understand that no one mode fits all situations; all contributing factors must be considered before choosing an appropriate mode. Knowing how the specific lung condition will respond to positive-pressure ventilation is paramount.

The CCTP must be able to safely control the ventilator to increase or decrease oxygenation, adjust ventilation, or liberate the patient from the ventilator. Simply put, a mode can determine whether the delivered breaths are volume or pressure targeted, whether the breaths are mandatory (set) or spontaneous, or a combination of the two, and which situational effects can trigger a change in ventilator response. The main concerns when choosing a mode are ensuring patient safety and comfort (referred to as patient synchrony with the ventilator) and implementing a lung-protective strategy that meets the desired oxygenation and ventilation goals.

TABLE 7-1 Modes of Mechanical Ventilation

Mode	Definition	Indication
Control, or continuous, manual ventilation (CV)	Ventilator delivers a specific set respiratory rate and volume or pressure, controlled by the ventilator. The patient is not allowed any other breaths. (Rarely used mode.)	Used when a specific minute volume is required, such as with a head injury. Can also be used when a patient is fighting, or bucking, the ventilator. The respiratory center is controlled by using a neuromuscular blockade agent and sedation.
Assist/control (AC)	The ventilator guarantees a minimum breath rate or flow. The patient is allowed to breathe over the set rate, but each breath is at the preset tidal volume or preset pressure. Requires properly setting the **sensitivity** (the ventilator control that regulates the amount of negative pressure or flow required by the patient to initiate, or trigger, a breath).	Controls the work of breathing, but allows the patient to set their own respiratory rate. Be aware of the potential for air trapping in the patient with tachypnea.

Mode	Definition	Indication
Synchronized intermittent mandatory ventilation (SIMV)	A set respiratory rate and tidal volume or pressure are delivered and synchronized with each patient-initiated breath. Each patient breath is at the patient-initiated volume. The machine will deliver a preset number of mandatory breaths. All other breaths are spontaneous breaths at the patient's own rate and depth.	Allows the patient to assume some or most of the work of breathing, depending on the mandatory rate. Can also be used as a weaning technique and is often combined with pressure support to overcome airway resistance within the airways, ventilator circuit, and ET tube. The pressure support does not have an inspiratory time attached to it. Careful monitoring of the exhaled volume on the pressure support breath is important; titrate the pressure support for desired volumes.
Pressure control ventilation (PCV)	The machine is set to deliver a preset pressure rather than a preset volume. The PIP or PAP is set and flow is delivered until the set PIP or PAP is reached. Tidal volume may vary significantly with changes in patient pulmonary status.	Used when volume ventilation requires too much pressure, such as in acute respiratory distress syndrome. Commonly used in conjunction with inverse-ratio ventilation (see below). One of the lung-protective strategies. A suggested strategy when fixing a plateau pressure.
Pressure-regulated volume control ventilation (PRVC)	The machine will deliver the desired tidal volume at the least amount of pressure using a decelerating waveform.	Used when both pressure and volume regulation are needed.
Inverse-ratio ventilation	The ventilator is set so that the inspiratory phase is longer than the expiratory phase.	Used to increase oxygenation when the F_{IO_2} is too high (>0.60). Must ensure that all volume is exhaled to prevent breath stacking and hyperinflation. Often used with PCV. The patient should be sedated or paralyzed.
Pressure support	A clinician-selected amount of positive pressure augments a spontaneous breath. There is no set inspiratory time in a pressure support breath.	Used to augment a spontaneous breath. The pressure overcomes the superimposed resistance of the airway and ventilator circuit and improves lung compliance. The patient must be able to initiate a breath.
Continuous positive airway pressure (CPAP)	The baseline pressure for spontaneous breathing is raised above the ambient pressure, increasing both oxygenation and the mean airway pressure.	Improves oxygenation during spontaneous breathing by increasing functional residual capacity. May also increase lung compliance.
Bilevel positive airway pressure (BPAP)	CPAP with the ability to sense inspiration and deliver additional positive pressure. An inspiratory and expiratory pressure is set. A respiratory rate may be added on some ventilators.	Improves oxygenation and ventilation with spontaneous breathing.
Airway pressure release ventilation (APRV)	Uses an inverse I:E ratio strategy. Allows the patient to breathe throughout the respiratory cycle.	Used for acute lung injury, acute respiratory distress syndrome, and atelectasis.
Adaptive support ventilation (ASV)	Maintains an operator-set minute volume percentage and automatically determines an optimal tidal volume/respiratory rate combination based on the Otis equation (calculated by the ventilator).	Full or partial support with low PIP and guaranteed minute volume.

Abbreviations: F_{IO_2}, fraction of inspired oxygen; I:E ratio, inspiratory-to-expiratory ratio; PAP, pressure above positive end-expiratory pressure (PEEP); PIP, peak inspiratory pressure

Airway Pressure Release Ventilation

Whether referred to as airway pressure release ventilation (APRV) or a different name, such as BiLevel, BiVent, BiPhasic, DuoPAP, or BPAP, the same basic concept is at work with this strategy: using high levels of CPAP with a brief, intermittent release in pressure while applying an inverse inspiration-to-expiration (I:E) ratio. Used primarily for patients with severe ARDS, this mode has also demonstrated positive results when implemented for patients in the early stages of ARDS. Once ARDS progresses, the vascular permeability increases and the edema fluid that enters the alveoli will wash out the surfactant and cause further lung instability. In the face of this lung instability, homogenous ventilation is difficult to achieve with a conventional mode that has typical inspiratory times less than 1 second. Some alveoli may need more time to open effectively, allowing gas exchange to take place. This is where the benefits of APRV come into play.

The longer inspiratory times with APRV give the damaged or collapsed alveoli the opportunity to participate in the gas exchange process. The patient may also breathe spontaneously throughout the breathing cycle, which is more comfortable for the patient than inverse-ratio ventilation.

Typical ventilator settings for APRV are a high pressure (P-high) that is sufficient to recruit the alveoli and regain any functional residual capacity. Aim for a P-high with a desired plateau pressure of 20 to 30 cm H_2O. Time high (T-high) should be set equal to 90% of one breath cycle, typically 4 to 6 seconds. Pressure low (P-low) should always be set to 0 cm H_2O. If time low (T-low) is set appropriately, there will always be some PEEP remaining at end expiration. The T-low is the most important setting. It should be set at 75% of the peak expiratory flow rate, which is difficult to accurately measure unless you have high-resolution flow graphics and the ability to freeze the trend and measure the expiratory flow to isolate the 75% mark. Typically, the T-low is less than 5 seconds.

APRV settings may appear as follows:

P-high: 25 cm H_2O
P-low: 0 cm H_2O
T-high: 5 s
T-low: 0.4 s
FIO_2 titrate for saturation greater than 92%

If you achieve the optimal P-high setting, then the T-high setting becomes the means of adjusting oxygenation and ventilation. Lengthening the inspiratory time would aid in oxygenation by holding the alveoli open longer and increasing the surface area at the alveolar-capillary membrane. Shortening the inspiratory time would increase the number of releases and, therefore, increase the minute volume. By changing these settings, you can fine-tune the adjustments for ventilation. The patient's spontaneous breaths will also contribute to the minute ventilation. If your ventilator does not have this mode of ventilation, do not attempt to change the mode—a weaning process must occur before any changes are made. Any deviation from this mode should be further discussed with the provider managing the patient and your medical control.

Adaptive Support Ventilation

Adaptive support ventilation (ASV) is a closed-loop controlled mode that receives feedback related to the patient's lung mechanics and makes adjustments to the pressure applied and respiratory rate received by the lungs to optimize the patient's work of breathing. In addition, it adjusts the inspiratory and expiratory times using time constants. This is accomplished with software that relies on the Otis equation, a formula used to calculate the optimal minute ventilation, tidal volume, and rate using the least amount of pressure when the patient is passive, with the respiratory rate being adjusted to meet the minute volume target set by the clinician. The settings on a ventilator providing ASV may look different from the conventional settings. The most important information input by the clinician is the patient's height and sex, which are used to determine the predicted body weight (PBW). For an adult patient, the normal predicted minute volume is calculated as follows:

$$\text{Minute volume} = 0.1 \text{ L/kg of PBW}$$

For example, an adult patient with a PBW of 80 kg and normal lung function would have an 8 L/min volume requirement.

The percentage of minute volume that should be set as a target depends on the patient's current pulmonary ventilation status. If the patient is experiencing respiratory acidosis due to hypercapnia alone, then increasing the percentage of minute volume would be advantageous to lower the $Paco_2$. Also, the percentage of minute volume should be increased with increasing altitude or when adding mechanical dead space in the circuit. These increases are subtle and should be confirmed with the ventilator's manufacturer.

The clinician must also set the limits and alarms designed to protect the lungs. Set the high-pressure limits not to exceed a chosen plateau pressure and tidal volume. Next, set the oxygenation portion of PEEP and Fio_2. There is no tidal volume, respiratory rate, inspiratory time, or I:E ratio to set. The ventilator's software adjusts for those considerations to reach the desired percentage of minute volume and will automatically make changes based on the patient's lung mechanics and the preset limits.

Although ASV might sound like the perfect mode for all patients, it does have limitations. In a patient experiencing metabolic acidosis with a high respiratory drive, it may become a challenge for the ventilator to match the patient's respiratory demand. Likewise, a patient in diabetic keto-acidosis with Kussmaul breathing may be difficult to ventilate using this mode. Because the patient can breathe spontaneously independent of the set parameters, this mode would be considered pressure-limited, volume-targeted, synchronized intermittent mandatory ventilation.

ASV settings may appear as follows:

% minute volume: 115
PEEP: 5 cm H_2O
Fio_2: 0.6 s

Parameters

The clinician must be familiar with the ventilator being used and should be proficient in its use, understand its application to the patient, be able to set appropriate alarm settings, and know how to perform the troubleshooting process. Gaining competence with these machines may require additional specific training in ventilator management. **TABLE 7-2** describes some key ventilator parameters and alarms, though it is not intended to be a comprehensive list. Some ventilators have many more audio/visual alarms that the CCTP must understand prior to transporting a patient on the ventilator. Reading and understanding the ventilator's

operator manual is essential to safely caring for the mechanically ventilated patient.

Note that expiratory time is not a set parameter in most ventilators. Rather, it is a function of the set respiratory rate and inspiratory time, and is "left over" after inspiration is completed. More important to understand is the inspiratory-to-expiratory ratio, more simply known as the I:E ratio, which the provider can set on some ventilators. Recognizing what constitutes the total cycle time helps with understanding the I:E ratio and its effect on the respiratory rate. The total cycle time for the breath to take place (inspiratory and expiratory phases) is calculated by dividing the respiratory rate into 60 seconds. For example, a respiratory rate of 20, divided into 60 seconds, would give a total cycle time for one breath of 3 seconds. In such a case, if the inspiratory time is set at 1 second, the expiratory time is 2 seconds (ie, total cycle time of 3 seconds minus inspiratory phase of 1 second) and the I:E ratio is 1:2.

Any change in the rate or inspiratory time (I time) will affect the I:E ratio and should be a major concern when setting up or making changes on a ventilator. This consideration is extremely important with patients who have an obstructive disease process such as COPD or asthma. These patients require longer expiratory times as a by-product of their lower respiratory rates and shorter inspiratory times. If the expiratory time is not sufficient for the patient, auto-PEEP becomes a worrisome risk.

Some hospital ventilators and transport ventilators do have a specific setting for the I:E ratio. When setting a specific I:E ratio, the inspiratory time fluctuates with any change in the respiratory rate. Notably, too short of an inspiratory time coupled with a small-diameter ET tube in an adult may cause increased turbulent flow, which will increase the PIP. When setting the I:E ratio, be certain to monitor the inspiratory time when respiratory rate changes are made. Inspiratory times of 0.7 to 1.2 seconds in an adult patient are considered an acceptable range to start with, with these values then being titrated as needed.

Positive End-Expiratory Pressure

PEEP occurs at the end of each breath. Instead of allowing a full exhalation back to ambient pressure, exhalation is set to be stopped at a prescribed pressure. The result is an increase in the amount of air in the alveoli, which increases the functional residual

TABLE 7-2 Ventilator Parameters

Parameter	Definition	Setting Range
Tidal volume	Amount of air delivered with each machine breath. Measured in millimeters.	Approximately 6–8 mL/kg of ideal weight; 4–6 mL/kg if poor lung compliance (eg, from acute lung injury or restrictive or obstructive disease) is present. Smaller volumes may be used to prevent alveolar overdistention.
Respiratory rate	Number of breaths delivered in 1 minute. Measured in breaths per minute.	12–14 based on desired mandatory minute ventilation. Confirm minute volume adequacy with arterial blood gas or ETCO$_2$.
Fraction of inspired oxygen	Percentage of inhaled oxygen, expressed as a decimal.	0.21–1.0. Titrated to achieve adequate oxygenation (oxygen saturation, 0.90%). For initial management, an FIO$_2$ of 1.0 (100%) is used and then titrated downward in an attempt to maintain adequate arterial saturation at the lowest FIO$_2$ possible (50% or less) to avoid oxygen toxicity.
Peak flow	Speed at which the tidal volume is delivered. Measured in liters per minute.	Can vary greatly between 35 and >120 L/min.
Inspiratory time	The time set to deliver the desired flow or tidal volume. Measured in seconds.	Can vary between 0.25 and 1.5 s depending on the patient population.
Peak inspiratory pressure	The peak pressure generated during ventilation. May vary with volume ventilation. Measured in cm H$_2$O.	Set this parameter with pressure ventilation. Should be maintained at the lowest value possible to minimize the risk of barotrauma/volutrauma. It is the proximal airway pressure.
Driving pressure	The change in pressure between the plateau pressure and PEEP. Determined by the elastic properties of the respiratory system and the delivered tidal volume. Measured in cm H$_2$O.	Not an actual setting. The goal is to keep the driving pressure at <15 cm H$_2$O.
Inspiratory plateau pressure	The pressure applied in volume ventilation to the small airways and alveoli. Measured by applying an inspiratory pause. Measured in cm H$_2$O.	Plateau pressure should be maintained at <30 cm H$_2$O in patients with poor lung compliance to minimize the risk of volutrauma. Adult patients with normal lungs should be maintained at <20 cm H$_2$O.
Percentage of minute volume	Amount of desired minute volume, set according to normal minute volume equation (Minute volume = 0.1 L/kg predicted body weight for adult). Measured in liters per minute.	100% for normal lung conditions. Increase for hyperventilation. Decrease to encourage spontaneous breaths or liberation from mechanical ventilation.
Low-pressure alarm	Alerts the clinician to a leak in the system or a patient disconnect.	Set 5–10 cm H$_2$O lower than the average cycling (peak) pressure.
High-pressure alarm	Alerts the clinician that the ventilator is using high pressures to deliver the tidal volume.	Set 10 cm H$_2$O higher than the peak inspiratory pressure.
Power failure/low-battery alarm	Alerts the clinician to a ventilator failure due to a loss of power.	Varies from ventilator to ventilator.

Abbreviations: ETCO$_2$, end-tidal carbon dioxide; FIO$_2$, fraction of inspired oxygen; PEEP, positive end-expiratory pressure

---

capacity and improves oxygenation. PEEP also reduces the shunt fraction and may increase lung compliance, as determined by a targeted transpulmonary pressure measured via esophageal manometry. Detrimental effects of PEEP may include decreased venous return, a resultant decrease in cardiac output, increased intracranial pressure, decreased renal and portal blood flow, and increased risk of barotrauma. When PEEP is increased, the MAP increases correspondingly. PEEP is contraindicated in patients with untreated pneumothorax or bronchopleural fistula.

PEEP values are usually determined by the ability to improve the partial pressure of oxygen in arterial blood (Pao_2) and decrease the Fio_2. An important consideration during transport is to maintain PEEP levels even when using a bag-mask device. An external PEEP valve should be attached to the bag with the appropriate PEEP value set. The patient's hemodynamic status, as well as oxygenation, should be carefully monitored when applying and adjusting PEEP.

If high levels of PEEP are present and the patient must be disconnected from the ventilatory circuit, clamping the ET tube may be required to prevent alveolar collapse even for a moment. This step may be necessary in patients with severe ARDS because the inflammation process may make it difficult to re-recruit alveoli that were once open. Special training is necessary to ensure ET tube integrity and patient safety during the disconnection/reconnection procedure. The goal is to maintain the same level of PEEP while the disconnect takes place as swiftly as possible. Keeping the patient sedated to avoid unwarranted spontaneous breathing is suggested, as this strategy may prevent the patient from taking a breath while the ET tube is clamped. Such a breath could trigger negative-pressure pulmonary edema, owing to the increased negative intrathoracic pressure during the patient's spontaneous breath. This skill should be practiced on a mechanically ventilated manikin, if possible. The goal is to clamp the ET tube and change over the circuit in less than 5 seconds.

Inhaled Gases

When managing a mechanically ventilated patient, the CCTP must adjust the ventilator settings to

Clamping an ET Tube

Special care must be taken when the decision to clamp an ET tube has been made. Clamping the ET tube during a ventilator change protects against any viral or bacterial exposure to the environment, but patients receiving high levels of PEEP may need that level of support to be maintained to facilitate their oxygenation and ventilation. Any interruption in the PEEP level may have disastrous results, as it may take a long time to re-recruit the alveoli lost during a disconnect procedure in patients with some lung conditions (eg, ARDS). Additionally, patients may need to be sedated if spontaneous breathing is present. Clamping the airway on an alert, anxious patient on high levels of PEEP is not recommended without adequate sedation.

Materials needed for this procedure include a clamping device (with a smooth clamp surface, if possible), gauze for protecting the integrity of the ET tube **FIGURE 7-8A**, and a second pair of hands to turn the ventilators first off and then on. This procedure should be done as quickly as possible, and a bag-mask device connected to oxygen should be ready to use if necessary. The steps are as follows:

1. Prepare the receiving ventilator with appropriate settings for the transport, and have it on stand-by to deliver a breath with no delay.
2. Have one person shut off the sending facility's ventilator while a different team member simultaneously clamps the ET tube **FIGURE 7-8B**.
3. Remove the circuit, quickly apply the receiving ventilator's circuit, and turn on the ventilator **FIGURE 7-8C**.
4. Once the ventilator is confirmed "on," remove the clamp.

correct any imbalances in the patient's oxygenation/ventilation status based on ABG values or $Etco_2$ and Spo_2 readings. Certain scenarios may warrant using inhaled gases to correct these imbalances. The CCTP should be familiar with the most commonly encountered gases and their indications.

Nitric Oxide

Nitric oxide (or nitrogen monoxide) is seeing increased use during critical care transports. This is due in part to the introduction of portable inhaled nitric oxide (iNO) administration units and the expansion of the patient populations in whom

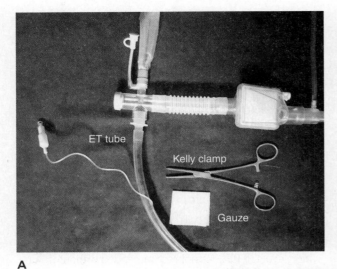

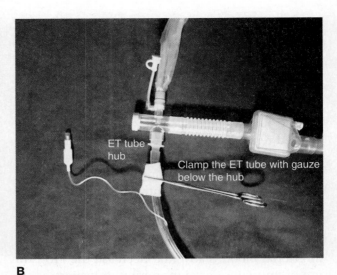

A

B

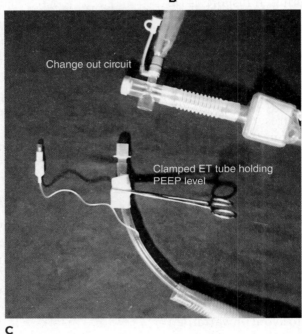

C

FIGURE 7-8 A. Gather the clamp and gauze needed to clamp the endotracheal (ET) tube. **B.** Place the ventilator on standby and then clamp the ET tube. **C.** Disconnect the ventilator circuit and reconnect the patient to the transport ventilator circuit. Unclamp the ET tube and turn on the transport ventilator.

Abbreviation: PEEP, positive end-expiratory pressure

Courtesy of Vent-Pro Training.

iNO has been shown to be effective. Research into use of iNO is ongoing, and many institutions have standing agreements with their institutional review boards to allow compassionate use of iNO in adults with refractory hypoxemia from a wide range of clinical syndromes. Note that nitric oxide (iNO) is not the same as nitrous oxide (N_2O).

When administered as a gas, iNO increases blood flow by promoting vasodilation. This mechanism involves the endothelial blood vessel linings, which receive a signal from the iNO that stimulates smooth muscle to relax. iNO also discourages smooth muscle contraction of the blood vessels. Therefore, when hypoxia results from pulmonary vascular vasoconstriction, iNO can significantly improve flow and oxygenation. However, an overabundance of iNO can contribute to reperfusion injury—for example, if an excess is produced after an ischemic injury.

iNO gas is bled into the inspiratory limb of a ventilator circuit at a dilution measured in parts per million (ppm). Published studies list effective doses ranging from 0.25 to 80 ppm, although the recommended doses may vary by institutional policy and practice. The recommended starting dose for neonates with acute hypoxic respiratory failure is 20 ppm. For adults, the recommended starting dose ranges from 5 ppm to 20 ppm. Doses greater than 20 ppm are not recommended. Effects of iNO vary and are patient specific.

Parameters for titration of iNO need to be defined prior to initiating therapy. Patient assessment modalities, however, vary considerably by institution. Typical measurements that suggest a favorable response to iNO include a 20% improvement in oxygenation and/or a 30% decline in pulmonary vascular resistance. When invasive monitoring is not available, improvements in oxygenation, hemodynamic stability, and less frequent desaturations may be used to gauge the effectiveness of this therapy (or lack thereof).

Abrupt discontinuation of iNO has been associated with a rebound phenomenon, characterized by significant desaturations and hemodynamic instability. Given this risk, CCTPs should calculate the gas volumes and battery lifespan needed and ensure that the needed equipment and supplies will be available to continue iNO administration throughout the entirety of the transport.

iNO gas readily reacts with other gases, including oxygen and water vapor found in ventilator circuit tubing. This oxidative process produces highly corrosive nitrogen dioxide, which poses a significant risk of causing acute lung tissue injury with resultant pulmonary edema. Nitrogen dioxide concentrations are monitored by the commercially available iNO administration device; elevated levels can be remedied by purging the iNO gas system or lowering the iNO bleed rate. Occupational exposure of health care providers to iNO and nitrogen dioxide is a theoretical risk of treatment, but the severity of this risk has yet to be demonstrated in published research.

Methemoglobinemia is another potential complication of iNO therapy. It is caused by oxidation of hemoglobin to methemoglobin, a dyshemoglobin that cannot carry oxygen. In patients receiving iNO therapy, monitoring methemoglobin levels at least daily is important to prevent induction of an iatrogenic hypoxia. Pulse carbon monoxide oximeters capable of measuring methemoglobin are helpful for spot assessment or continual monitoring of methemoglobin levels.

iNO can be a valuable adjunct for CCT of extremely hypoxic patients, to optimize conventional therapies, to continue care started prior to transfer, or as a bridge to more advanced therapies such as extracorporeal membrane oxygenation (ECMO) or high-frequency jet ventilation. The greatest dangers during transport are iatrogenic overdoses of iNO with resultant acute lung injury and pulmonary edema and/or methemoglobinemia. Because abrupt discontinuation of iNO therapy due to gas loss or equipment malfunction can result in catastrophic rebound effects, it is extremely important to have a bag-mask device at the ready that can be used to deliver breaths with the iNO delivery device attached. Use of iNO during transport requires the CCTP to be thoroughly familiar with iNO equipment operation, troubleshooting, and emergency procedures in case of failure. Often a respiratory therapist will accompany the patient and manage the delivery of iNO during the transport.

Epoprostenol

Inhaled epoprostenol is often used in hospitals for treating hypoxemia related to pulmonary hypertension and ARDS. When administered through the ventilator circuit via a specific vibrating mesh device, it produces selective pulmonary vasodilation, which can lead to improvements in the $\dot{V}/\dot{Q}$ mismatch without any systemic hemodynamic compromise. Note that the duration of action for inhaled epoprostenol is 3 to 5 minutes; any interruption in delivering this medication puts the patient at risk for rebound pulmonary hypertension. Precise planning for transporting a patient on epoprostenol is vital, and providers should have enough medication in the event of any unplanned delays.

Heliox

Heliox is a specific blend of helium and oxygen. Combinations of 80% helium and 20% oxygen (80/20) and of 70% helium and 30% oxygen (70/30) are the most commonly encountered mixtures. Because helium is less dense than air, it can contribute to turning turbulent flow into laminar flow and decreasing airway resistance. This therapy is often used to decrease airway resistance in the presence of foreign body obstruction, stridor, and vocal cord dysfunction as a bridge to correcting the underlying issue.

While there is minimal research on its use in asthma or COPD exacerbations, heliox may be used in these scenarios when other interventions have failed. Patients with an intubated asthma exacerbation are sometimes given heliox through a specifically designed ICU mechanical ventilator. These ventilators have a dedicated port to receive this lighter gas and to ensure equivalency of flows and volumes. The evidence base is not currently robust enough to recommend its widespread use in this capacity.

Respiratory Distress and Respiratory Failure

Respiratory distress is a medical emergency that demands immediate treatment. Signs and symptoms include tachypnea, tachycardia, increased anxiety, increased work of breathing, and pallor. Respiratory failure is a medical emergency that may present initially as respiratory distress, but signs and symptoms eventually worsen into cyanosis, hypercapnia, hypoxia, bradycardia, fatigue, shallow breathing, and loss of consciousness. At this point, the pulmonary system fails to meet the body's metabolic demands for oxygenation and ventilation.

There are four classifications of respiratory failure:

- **Type 1 (hypoxemic).** In this type of respiratory failure, the lung loses its ability to deliver adequate amounts of oxygen to the pulmonary vasculature. Typically, the ABG analysis will reveal a Pao_2 of less than 50 mm Hg on room air. Hypoventilation, $\dot{V}/\dot{Q}$ mismatch (low $\dot{V}/\dot{Q}$ ratio), and shunt are common physiologic causes of hypoxemia. Typical origins of a shunt may include atelectasis, pneumonia, cardiogenic pulmonary edema, ARDS, and a lung hemorrhage. Therapies are aimed at recruiting the collapsed alveoli and removing any excess fluid from the lungs.
- **Type 2 (ventilatory).** This type of respiratory failure presents in patients with airflow obstruction, increased work of breathing, poor lung compliance, increased airway resistance, and decreased respiratory drive. If the patient is not chronically retaining carbon dioxide, then a $Paco_2$ of greater than 50 mm Hg is a classic sign of type 2 respiratory failure. Some physiologic reasons for hypercapnia include a decrease in the respiratory rate, a decrease in the tidal or minute volume (drug overdose), or an increase in carbon dioxide production (eg, sepsis, burns, fever). Another consideration for hypercapnia is dead space ventilation, in which blood flow to the alveoli is severely diminished due to pulmonary embolus, hypovolemia, and poor cardiac output.
- **Type 3 (perioperative).** This type of respiratory failure can be a subtype of type 1 and is commonly seen in postoperative patients. The main culprit is atelectasis due to anesthetic effects, accompanying pain, and shallow breathing, which collectively contribute to a decrease in functional residual capacity and airway secretions. The therapy of choice is to reverse the atelectasis.
- **Type 4 (shock).** Hypoperfusion can lead to respiratory distress and failure. The underlying causes may be septic, cardiogenic, or hypovolemic shock. Identifying and treating the underlying cause is the ultimate goal.

Recognizing the underlying type of respiratory failure and its appropriate treatment is essential. The CCTP may benefit from reviewing a recent ABG analysis and correlating the $Paco_2$, Pao_2, and calculated oxygen saturation with the transport monitor's $ETco_2$ and Spo_2 readings. A recent chest radiograph and radiologist report to rule out any abnormalities (eg, a small pneumothorax) that may present an issue on transport, and to confirm ET tube placement, would be helpful.

Ventilator Management

Use of a portable ventilator during patient transport may be necessary in the following situations:

- Impending or actual respiratory failure
- Inadequate respiratory drive or apnea
- Inadequate gas exchange
- To decrease the work of breathing and oxygen cost

Complications of using a portable ventilator include the following possibilities:

- Mechanical failure
- Patient anxiety

- Improper settings
- Increased intrapulmonary pressure
- Cardiovascular compromise
- Gastrointestinal disturbances
- Infection
- Impaired clearance and drying of secretions
- Ventilator unable to meet the patient's flow demand

Most of today's ventilators can match most patients' demands. The most important consideration is to know the capabilities of the equipment and be able to match them to the patient's lung condition. For example, if a patient is on pressure-regulated volume control (PRVC) and your ventilator does not have this mode, find out why the patient is using this mode; based on this information, you can then decide whether you can support the patient's needs with your ventilator. If volume- and pressure-delivered breaths are available with your equipment, you very likely can meet the patient's demands.

During transport of a critically ill patient receiving mechanical ventilation, only necessary adjustments to the ventilator should be made. These adjustments usually focus on maintaining adequate oxygenation, minute ventilation, and patient comfort and safety. If mechanical ventilation is instituted, it is recommended that the guidelines listed in this section be followed after securing a patent airway. In most cases, the CCTP will use the settings already in place, provided the patient's respiratory status is deemed sufficient for the transport. A recent ABG analysis (or venous blood gas analysis, in some institutions) and chest radiograph may be helpful at this time. These guidelines should be considered by the CCTP who is intubating and establishing the patient on the ventilator.

The CCTP may also be called on to transport a patient on an unfamiliar device or mode. For example, a low-stretch lung strategy might call for use of a high-frequency oscillator to ventilate the patient. Although rarely seen today, this strategy may still be employed with a specific patient population. This approach employs a constant MAP to open the lung, similar to the effects of PEEP delivered via a conventional ventilator, and then ventilates the patient at rates of 180 to 900 breaths/min, with small volumes being delivered with each breath. Some transport ventilators use a similar technology. If your equipment consists of a conventional transport ventilator, however, it is helpful to know if the patient can be weaned from the high-frequency oscillator to a conventional ventilator prior to transport. The adult patient should have a MAP of less than 24 cm H_2O before considering any change to conventional ventilation.

Keep in mind that any occult pneumothorax or pneumomediastinum may worsen with the initiation of positive-pressure ventilation. Always perform a pre-use check of the ventilator and circuit per the manufacturer's guidelines before placing the patient on the ventilator. It is recommended to perform this test prior to arrival at the sending facility to troubleshoot any malfunctions.

Adult Ventilation

Suggested guidelines for adult ventilation are as follows:

1. Choose either a volume- or pressure-delivered breath.
2. Choose a target tidal volume of 6–8 mL/kg using the PBW (see Table 7-3).
3. Select an appropriate mode of delivery for the transport, typically assist/control or synchronized intermittent mandatory ventilation.
4. Select an appropriate respiratory rate of 12–14 breaths/min.
5. Select an inspiratory time. Start at 1 second.
6. Start with a PEEP of 5 cm H_2O.
7. Start with an FIO_2 of 6. Titrate for target saturation levels.
8. Set the sensitivity at 3–5 L/min or minus 2 cm H_2O.
9. Set the heat moisture exchange at circuit Y.
10. Set all alarms that involve high pressure, low pressure, minute volume, and apnea.

CCTPs must understand the difference between volume-delivered breaths and pressure-delivered breaths. In volume-delivered breaths, the flow available to the patient is limited to the set (dialed-in) tidal volume and the inspiratory time, although some minor adjustments can be made to increase the flow. In pressure-delivered breaths, the pressure is set and the flow available to the patient is unlimited—at least up to the ventilator's maximum flow capabilities. It follows that pressure control may deliver a more comfortable breath for the air-hungry patient. Because of its decelerating flow pattern, this technique can improve distribution of ventilation in the lungs of patients with acute lung injury. In addition, it is the breath delivery of choice in patients with un-cuffed tracheostomies, in patients with uncuffed ET tubes, and in any patient whose airway cannot be sealed. In such circumstances, the ventilator will continue to pressurize the airway until the I time expires, with the volume breath terminating once the volume is delivered. In contrast, with volume-delivered breaths, the PIP varies depending on lung compliance. In pressure-delivered breaths, the exhaled tidal volume becomes the variable and is also dependent on lung compliance. Many transport ventilators allow the CCTP to manipulate how much flow is delivered at the initiation of the breath (rise time, P-ramp) and when the flow terminates (flow termination, expiratory trigger sensitivity) in a pressure-targeted breath. This allows the CCTP to fine-tune the flow to meet the patient's demand.

It is extremely important to monitor PIP and exhaled minute volume during ventilation. Some ventilators can deliver a pressure breath with a volume target, an approach referred to as dual-control ventilation or PRVC. This mode gives a pressure-delivered breath with a guaranteed minute volume due to the targeted tidal volume.

It has been suggested that using low tidal volume ventilation might reduce volutrauma and should be the standard of care for mechanically ventilated patients with ARDS. Studies have used the 4–8 mL/kg PBW ratios given in **TABLE 7-3** as a strategy; they are based on the following equations:

Males: PBW (kg) = 50 + 2.3 [height (inches) − 60]

Females: PBW (kg) = 45.5 + 2.3 [height (inches) − 60]

This is suggested only as a starting point, because some patients require more tidal volume. As always, the patient's lung condition and disease process should be considered when setting up or making changes on a ventilator.

When transporting a patient who is on a hospital ventilator, it is wise to match their current settings, provided those settings are adequately ventilating and oxygenating the patient. These values can be quickly confirmed using a recent ABG analysis.

TABLE 7-3 Predicted Body Weight and Tidal Volumes

Height (in.)	PBW (kg)	4 mL	5 mL	6 mL	7 mL	8 mL
Females						
4' 0" (48)	17.9	72	90	107	125	143
4' 1" (49)	20.2	81	101	121	141	162
4' 2" (50)	22.5	90	113	135	158	180
4' 3" (51)	24.8	99	124	149	174	198
4' 4" (52)	27.1	108	136	163	190	217
4' 5" (53)	29.4	118	147	176	206	235
4' 6" (54)	31.7	127	159	190	222	254
4' 7" (55)	34	136	170	204	238	272
4' 8" (56)	36.3	145	182	218	254	290
4' 9" (57)	38.6	154	193	232	270	309
4' 10" (58)	40.9	164	205	245	286	327
4' 11" (59)	43.2	173	216	259	302	346

Height (in.)	PBW (kg)	4 mL	5 mL	6 mL	7 mL	8 mL
5' 0" (60)	45.5	182	228	273	319	364
5' 1" (61)	47.8	191	239	287	335	382
5' 2" (62)	50.1	200	251	301	351	401
5' 3" (63)	52.4	210	262	314	367	419
5' 4" (64)	54.7	219	274	328	383	438
5' 5" (65)	57	228	285	342	399	456
5' 6" (66)	59.3	237	297	356	415	474
5' 7" (67)	61.6	246	308	370	431	493
5' 8" (68)	63.9	256	320	383	447	511
5' 9" (69)	66.2	265	331	397	463	530
5' 10" (70)	68.5	274	343	411	480	548
5' 11" (71)	70.8	283	354	425	496	566
6' 0" (72)	73.1	292	366	439	512	585
6' 1" (73)	75.4	302	377	452	528	603
6' 2" (74)	77.7	311	389	466	544	622
6' 3" (75)	80	320	400	480	560	640
6' 4" (76)	82.3	329	412	494	576	658
6' 5" (77)	84.6	338	423	508	592	677
6' 6" (78)	86.9	348	435	521	608	695
6' 7" (79)	89.2	357	446	535	624	714
6' 8" (80)	91.5	366	458	549	641	732
6' 9" (81)	93.8	375	469	563	657	750
6' 10" (82)	96.1	384	481	577	673	769
6' 11" (83)	98.4	394	492	590	689	787
7' 0" (84)	100.7	403	504	604	705	806
Males						
4' 0" (48)	22.4	90	112	134	157	179
4' 1" (49)	24.7	99	124	148	173	198
4' 2" (50)	27	108	135	162	189	216
4' 3" (51)	29.3	117	147	176	205	234
4' 4" (52)	31.6	126	158	190	221	253
4' 5" (53)	33.9	136	170	203	237	271

(Continues)

TABLE 7-3 Predicted Body Weight and Tidal Volumes (continued)

Height (in.)	PBW (kg)	4 mL	5 mL	6 mL	7 mL	8 mL
4' 6" (54)	36.2	145	181	217	253	290
4' 7" (55)	38.5	154	193	231	270	308
4' 8" (56)	40.8	163	204	245	286	326
4' 9" (57)	43.1	172	216	259	302	345
4' 10" (58)	45.4	182	227	272	318	363
4' 11" (59)	47.7	191	239	286	334	382
5' 0" (60)	50	200	250	300	350	400
5' 1" (61)	52.3	209	262	314	366	418
5' 2" (62)	54.6	218	273	328	382	437
5' 3" (63)	56.9	228	285	341	398	455
5' 4" (64)	59.2	237	296	355	414	474
5' 5" (65)	61.5	246	308	369	431	492
5' 6" (66)	63.8	255	319	383	447	510
5' 7" (67)	66.1	264	331	397	463	529
5' 8" (68)	68.4	274	342	410	479	547
5' 9" (69)	70.7	283	354	424	495	566
5' 10" (70)	73	292	365	438	511	584
5' 11" (71)	75.3	301	377	452	527	602
6' 0" (72)	77.6	310	388	466	543	621
6' 1" (73)	79.9	320	400	479	559	639
6' 2" (74)	82.2	329	411	493	575	658
6' 3" (75)	84.5	338	423	507	592	676
6' 4" (76)	86.8	347	434	521	608	694
6' 5" (77)	89.1	356	446	535	624	713
6' 6" (78)	91.4	366	457	548	640	731
6' 7" (79)	93.7	375	469	562	656	750
6' 8" (80)	96	384	480	576	672	768
6' 9" (81)	98.3	393	492	590	688	786
6' 10" (82)	100.6	402	503	604	704	805
6' 11" (83)	102.9	412	515	617	720	823
7' 0" (84)	105.9	421	526	631	736	842

Abbreviation: PBW, predicted body weight

Data from ARDSNet Studies.

Again, before making any major adjustments to the current ventilator settings, it is prudent to consult the respiratory therapist, sending facility physician, or medical control. A quick and easy way to choose transport settings for an adult patient is to choose a target tidal volume of 6 to 8 mL/kg of PBW (4 to 6 mL/kg of PBW for a patient with ARDS) and a respiratory rate of 12 to 16 breaths/min, and to draw an ABG if possible or monitor the ETCO$_2$. Confirm the target tidal volume is not approaching a plateau of less than 30 cm H$_2$O and the I:E ratio is sufficient to allow time for passive exhalation and not contribute to auto-PEEP (which causes air trapping).

The formula to predict minute volume for an adult patient while accounting for volume loss at the alveolar level due to dead space is 100 mL/min/kg of PBW. For example, suppose you need to determine the minute volume for a male patient with a PBW of 75 kg and no known lung history:

$$75 \times 100 \text{ mL} = 7,500 \text{ mL} = 7.5 \text{ L/min}$$

Theoretically, this patient should receive a minute volume of 7.5 L/min. To achieve this goal, you must first determine an adequate target tidal volume. Using the 6 to 8 mL/kg guideline and the PBW of 75 kg, you can start on the low end of 6 mL/kg:

$$6 \text{ mL/kg} \times 75 \text{ kg} = 450 \text{ mL}$$

Thus, the target tidal volume would be 450 mL.

Using the formula "Minute volume = Rate × Tidal volume," plug in the numbers just obtained to determine the respiratory rate:

$$7.5 \text{ L/min} = \text{Rate (breaths/min)} \times 450 \text{ mL}$$

Equation for Adjusting Paco$_2$

Providers can use a simple formula to calculate a target minute volume and Paco$_2$, and thereby improve the accuracy of acid–base adjustment in mechanically ventilated patients:

$$\text{Target minute ventilation} = \frac{\text{Known Paco}_2 \times \text{Known minute volume}}{\text{Target Paco}_2}$$

In this equation, the provider knows the current Paco$_2$ and current minute volume, and wants to calculate the target minute volume and target Paco$_2$. To illustrate this calculation, suppose a patient's status is indicated by the following values:

- Ventilator settings: Assist/control rate, 12 breaths/min; tidal volume, 0.5 L; PEEP, 5 cm H$_2$O; Fio$_2$, 0.6
- ABG values: pH, 7.13; Paco$_2$, 68 mm Hg; Pao$_2$, 100 mm Hg; Hco$_3^-$, 23 mEq/L; O$_2$ saturation, 95%

Suppose further that the provider wishes to arrive at a Paco$_2$ of 40 mm Hg. The provider will use the known values (Paco$_2$, 68 mm Hg; minute volume, 6 L/min) to determine the target minute volume (X) that will produce a Paco$_2$ of 40 mm Hg. Plugging these values into the equation, the provider can calculate the target minute volume:

$$X = 68 \text{ mm Hg} \times 6 \text{ L/min}/40 \text{ mm Hg}$$
$$X = 10.2 \text{ L/min}$$

Provided that this target tidal volume is ideal for this patient (6 to 8 mL of PBW), the provider can then adjust the ventilator settings. Using the tidal volume of 0.5 L and the calculated minute volume of 10.2 L, the provider determines the respiratory rate as follows:

$$10.2 \text{ L/min}/0.5 \text{ L} = 20.4 \text{ breaths/min}$$

The adjusted ventilator settings are as follows: assist/control rate, 20 breaths/min; tidal volume, 0.5 L; and Fio$_2$ 0.6.

This formula does not take into consideration alveolar ventilation and any specific lung physiology. A major concern when adjusting the respiratory rate is the effect on the I:E ratio. Changes should be monitored closely, and providers should also monitor for auto-PEEP.

Three important caveats apply to the end results obtained with the target minute ventilation formula:

- The patient should exhibit a steady metabolic state, where carbon dioxide production is constant. ("Steady" is generally considered 30 minutes of unaltered function.)
- The ratio of dead space to tidal volume needs to remain fixed; thus, any changes to the minute ventilation should be achieved by changing the respiratory rate, not the tidal volume.
- The patient must accept the adjusted minute ventilation without attempting to overbreathe the ventilator.

When respiratory rates are already high and peak pressures allow for upward adjustment of the tidal volume, the actual results will often not correspond to the results calculated with the formula owing to changes in dead space.

To complete the math operation, convert the 7.5 L into milliliters, then divide the minute volume by the tidal volume:

$$7.5 \text{ L} = 7,500 \text{ mL}$$

$$7,500/450 = 16.6 \text{ breaths/min}$$

This calculation results in a tidal volume of 450 mL and a respiratory rate of 16 or 17 breaths/min. A slight adjustment with the inspiratory time or I:E ratio setting may be necessary to allow for more passive exhalation in a patient with an obstructive lung condition.

The mode of delivery also requires considerable attention. The patient will be traveling either by ground or by air during transport, and the environment may change rapidly. For patients who are alert and awake, all of their senses will be stimulated, causing potential stress and anxiety. Gravitational forces and barometric pressure changes may also affect patients' cardiorespiratory status. Some patients may be susceptible to motion sickness. All of these factors need to be considered before placing a patient on the transport ventilator. In addition, if a patient is in the process of weaning off the ventilator, make sure the settings are appropriate for the transport that lies ahead, as active weaning efforts should generally be suspended during transport unless specifically requested.

The respiratory rate should be set and adjusted as necessary for patient demand, and careful monitoring of capnography is necessary throughout the transport. Remember, an increase in the respiratory rate shortens the expiratory time. Check the I:E ratio and adjust the inspiratory time if necessary. The I:E ratio for a healthy lung should be in the range of 1:2 to 1:3 I:E, whereas that for a diseased lung may be 1:3 or greater **TABLE 7-4**.

The inspiratory time can be adjusted slightly to ensure greater patient comfort. Any change in inspiratory time will also affect the I:E ratio, however, so be sure to monitor this ratio. Rarely should you set an inspiratory time of less than 0.7 second for an adult patient, as this might increase turbulent flow within the respiratory tract.

For adults, PEEP should initially be set at 5 cm H_2O to account for physiologic dead space. If more PEEP is needed for oxygenation, it is suggested to make these changes slowly, as PEEP is proportional to MAP. If the patient has a high oxygen requirement

TABLE 7-4 Adjusting I Time Versus Respiratory Rate

Example: Respiratory rate = 10 breaths/min		
Total cycle time	6 s (60 s ÷ 10 breaths = 6 s/breath) I time = 1.0 s E time = 5.0 s I:E ratio = 1:5 (expiratory time divided by inspiratory time)	
	Decreasing I Time	**Decreasing Respiratory Rate**
Respiratory rate	10 breaths/min	6 breaths/min
Total cycle time	6 s	10 s
I time	0.75 s	1.0 s
E time	5.25 s	9.0 s
I:E ratio	1:7	1.9

Abbreviations: E time, expiratory time; I time, inspiratory time; I:E, inspiration-to-expiration ratio

© Jones & Bartlett Learning.

and adjusting PEEP would be of benefit, one strategy suggests raising PEEP to a level at which the CCTP could lower the FIO_2 at the bedside and wait for PEEP to take effect. Then, if the patient becomes hypoxic during transport, the CCTP can consider the option of raising the FIO_2. This strategy depends on what is initially causing the hypoxia. In a patient with severe ARDS, it may take many hours before any positive results from increasing the PEEP appear. Any adjustment in PEEP levels should be discussed with medical control before being applied.

The adult guidelines suggest starting with an FIO_2 of 0.6 and titrating until SpO_2 is greater than 92%. Knowing the patient's baseline oxygen requirement, lung history, age, and PaO_2 are helpful in meeting this goal.

Setting the sensitivity at minus 2 is a safe place to start. With this setting, the patient would need to trigger a breath by inhaling minus 2 cm H_2O of pressure or flow. If the patient has an uncuffed tracheostomy or ET tube and the ventilator is auto-cycling due to a leak from this device, the sensitivity needs to be increased until the auto-cycling stops. Once this is accomplished, the setting can be adjusted to a sensitivity of minus 2 cm H_2O past the leak-related value.

Some ventilators have a leak compensation feature that automatically adjusts the sensitivity for a stable leak. Keep in mind that CCTPs work in a dynamic environment and a leak from an uncuffed tracheostomy or ET tube is rarely stable during patient transport.

As noted earlier, a heat moisture exchanger (HME) is important to use during ventilation because oxygen is a dry gas. The HME is designed to capture the moisture and heat from the patient's exhaled breath and hold it for the next inhaled breath. The CCTP should monitor the integrity of this device throughout the transport, ensuring no mucus or excessive moisture is restricting the flow through it, and in turn causing back pressure and auto-PEEP.

Alarms should be set according to the ventilator manufacturer's guidelines. A suggested starting point is to set the high-pressure limit at 10 cm H_2O above the average PIP. Set the low-pressure alarm at 5 cm H_2O below the average PIP. Set the low-minute-volume alarm at 25% below the resting minute volume. Setting the apnea alarm for 20 seconds is also recommended, but you should check with the manufacturer for the default apnea settings.

Special Considerations: Auto-PEEP and Hyperinflation

Auto-PEEP (intrinsic PEEP) can be described as an incomplete expiration before the next positive-pressure breath is delivered, causing air trapping **FIGURE 7-9**. It is often the culprit when a patient becomes asynchronous with the ventilator and is having trouble triggering a breath. Auto-PEEP can be measured by performing an expiratory hold maneuver on the ventilator, if the ventilator has this capability. Check the ventilator manual to determine its ability to measure auto-PEEP.

Patients who have a high airway resistance are especially susceptible to auto-PEEP when mechanically ventilated. These populations include individuals with asthma or any obstructive disease such as emphysema, as these patients are susceptible to hyperinflation **FIGURE 7-10**.

When auto-PEEP or hyperinflation occurs, it may benefit the patient to administer bronchodilators, chest percussion, suction, and possibly steroids. To decrease the risk of barotrauma/volutrauma, consider lowering the respiratory rate and possibly the inspiratory time, and discuss permissive hypercapnia as an option. Raising the PEEP level to 2 or 3 cm H_2O below the measured auto-PEEP may help with synchrony and lead to decreased work of breathing. This strategy should be discussed with medical control before raising the PEEP level.

Another consideration that may help reduce air trapping is decreasing the airway resistance by shortening the ET tube. The length of the tube is standardized, and is based on its size. Once you verify proper ET tube placement, it is acceptable to shorten the ET tube (thereby removing dead space) in a patient with obstructive or restrictive disease.

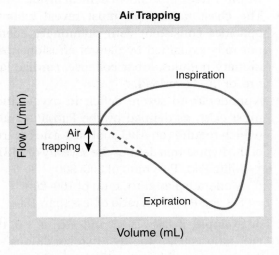

FIGURE 7-9 Auto-PEEP (positive end-expiratory pressure) occurs when an incomplete expiration causes air to become trapped in the lungs.

© Jones & Bartlett Learning.

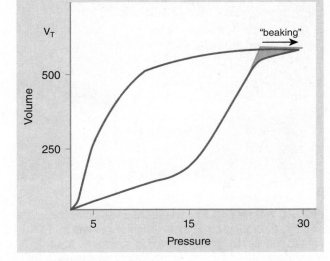

FIGURE 7-10 Hyperinflation.

© Jones & Bartlett Learning.

Management of Lung Diseases and Conditions

Knowing the patient's lung condition is imperative to ensure proper use of ventilation. Many strategies may be employed to ventilate patients with different lung processes. For example, a patient with severe ARDS might require high levels of PEEP and pressure due to the inflammatory process, whereas a patient with severe emphysema might require a lower respiratory rate and a shorter inspiratory time to allow for more expiratory time, along with limiting the tidal volume **FIGURE 7-11**.

The following sections suggest strategies to oxygenate and ventilate patients with some common lung diseases. Note that each patient should be thoroughly evaluated on a case-by-case basis to develop a strategy for ventilator settings. No single mode or setting will fit every lung condition. Instead, providers must interpret the feedback from the ventilator's monitored values, graphics, scales, and loops (if available) and make adjustments to ensure patient safety and maintain patient synchrony with the ventilator. When setting up the ventilator, it is wise to discuss the settings with the sending facility's physician, the respiratory therapist, and your medical control.

Acute Respiratory Distress Syndrome

ARDS is characterized by diffuse damage at the alveolar-capillary membrane, resulting in hypoxemia that is not attributed to cardiogenic pulmonary edema. This cascade of events includes neutrophil activation, cytokine storm, deficiencies in surfactant, and increased permeability of the alveolar-capillary membrane, ultimately resulting in alveolar collapse. As the process continues, some patients with ARDS develop fibrosis, contributing to worsening lung compliance and added dead space ventilation, which may then lead to pulmonary hypertension.

The Berlin definition for ARDS includes the following criteria:

- Respiratory symptoms must have begun within 1 week of a known clinical insult.
- The chest radiograph must reveal bilateral opacities consistent with pulmonary edema not fully explained by pleural effusions, pulmonary nodules, lobar collapse, cardiac failure, or fluid overload.
- A moderate to severe deficit in oxygenation must exist, as defined by the $Pao_2:Fio_2$ ratio (which requires an ABG analysis). The severity of the hypoxemia defines the severity of ARDS:
  - Mild: $Pao_2:Fio_2$ ratio of 200–300
  - Moderate: $Pao_2:Fio_2$ ratio of 100–200
  - Severe: $Pao_2:Fio_2$ ratio of less than 100

For example, if Pao_2 is 88 and Fio_2 is 1.0, the $Pao_2:Fio_2$ ratio is 88. If the first two conditions are met, the patient would be classified as having severe ARDS.

Typically, patients presenting with pulmonary contusions, pneumonia, inhalation of toxic gases,

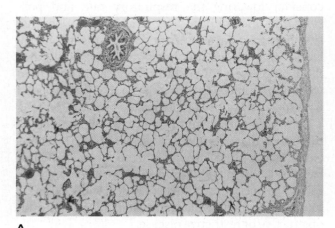

A

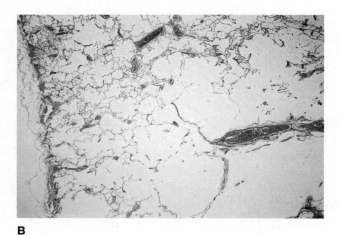

B

FIGURE 7-11 Healthy lung tissue **(A)** and lung tissue affected by emphysema **(B)**. In terms of ventilation, a patient with severe emphysema might require a lower respiratory rate and a shorter inspiratory time to allow for more expiratory time, along with limiting the tidal volume.

© Biophoto Associates/Science Source.

near drowning, and aspiration of gastric contents are susceptible to primary ARDS. Patients who present with sepsis, multiple traumas, pancreatitis, drug overdose, and transfusion of blood products may experience a secondary presentation of ARDS.

Many different strategies may be used to manage the respiratory status of the patient with ARDS. The main goal in treating this patient population is to establish adequate gas exchange while diminishing the negative effects of positive-pressure ventilation. When lung-protective ventilation is the main goal, the strategy may focus on a low tidal volume (4 to 6 mL/kg of PBW), a high level of PEEP, and an increased respiratory rate while maintaining a plateau pressure at less than 30 cm H_2O. The ARDS Network developed a specific protocol for managing the patient with a Pao_2:Fio_2 ratio less than 300 **FIGURE 7-12**.

As yet, no clinical evidence has been published that confirms whether setting a volume target or a pressure target produces better outcomes. If a patient with ARDS is being transported on a mechanical ventilator, it is, as always, best to match the patient's current settings on the hospital ventilator, provided the oxygenation and ventilation goals are met. The CCTP must be aware of the transport ventilator's capabilities, as a patient on high levels of PEEP and high minute volume requirements is best matched with a transport ventilator that can deliver high flow rates, such as a turbine-driven ventilator.

Another ventilation strategy for the patient with ARDS is to focus on an inverse I:E ratio, also known as inverse-ratio ventilation. This is achieved by adjusting the inspiratory time to be longer than the expiratory time **FIGURE 7-13**. The goal with this approach is to increase oxygenation by increasing the MAP. The MAP, which is measured at the opening of the airway, is an average over the complete respiratory cycle. The main factors contributing to the MAP are the inspiratory pressure, PEEP, and length of time spent in each phase of the breathing cycle. The target scheme is a pressure-delivered breath, and the PEEP and inspiratory time are set to achieve the desired goal. Because the inverse-ratio strategy can be extremely uncomfortable, patients receiving this therapy are often given neuromuscular blocking agents (NMBAs).

The more current form of the inverse-ratio strategy is APRV. As discussed previously, this modality has many other names, but is best described as a high level of CPAP with intermittent drops in pressure.

Recruitment maneuvers may also be implemented to improve oxygenation and minimize the risk of atelectrauma in patients with ARDS. Often a CPAP of 40 to 50 cm H_2O for 30 to 40 seconds is applied to the lungs in an attempt to stabilize the collapsed lung areas. This strategy may produce a short-term improvement in oxygenation, but the benefit does not appear to last long.

Recently, esophageal manometry has been implemented in the ICU setting to measure transpulmonary pressures (pressure at the airway opening, minus the pressure in the pleural space) for patients with ARDS. Because the PIP is a poor indicator of lung stress, transpulmonary pressures are often useful to determine the true distending pressures applied to the lungs. This information is extremely valuable for making essential adjustments to the ventilator to prevent atelectrauma and overdistention of the lungs. In this case, the patient will have an esophageal balloon catheter placed in a specific location to monitor transpulmonary pressures.

Another maneuver used in the hospital setting is prone positioning of the patient, often simply called proning, for a specific time. Shifting the gravitational forces may reduce atelectasis, redistribute lung densities, increase lung elastance, minimize alveolar shunting, and improve the $\dot{V}/\dot{Q}$ ratio. Proning the patient is labor intensive. It is associated with significant risk and is not commonly done in transit. It would be advantageous to coordinate the timing to have the patient transported during the supine portion of the prone positioning cycle.

Selective pulmonary vasodilators are often used for patients with ARDS who have developed refractory hypoxemia. Inhaled nitric oxide and inhaled epoprostenol are sometimes administered during transport, and the CCTP should be familiar with the devices employed to deliver these gases. Specifically trained personnel should accompany these transports, and a respiratory therapist will commonly assist with the patient's care.

Administration of NMBAs is considered when providing mechanical ventilation of the patient with ARDS and tachypnea, because the high respiratory rate may cause auto-PEEP. NMBA administration is a short-term solution, however; the goal is to withdraw the NMBA as soon as possible.

Inclusion Criteria: Acute Onset of:

1. $Pao_2/Fio_2 \leq 300$ (corrected for altitude)
2. Bilateral infiltrates consistent with pulmonary edema
3. No clinical evidence of left atrial hypertension

Part I: Ventilator Setup and Adjustment

1. Calculate predicted body weight (PBW).
   Males: 50 + 2.3(height in inches − 60)
   Females: 50 + 2.3(height in inches − 60)
2. Select ventilator mode.
3. Set ventilator to achieve initial tidal volume (V_T) = 8 mL/kg PBW.
4. Reduce V_T by 1 mL/kg at intervals ≤ 2 hours until V_T = 6 mL/kg PBW.
5. Set initial rate to approximate baseline minute ventilation (not > 35 beats/min).
6. Adjust V_T and respiratory rate (RR) to achieve pH and plateau pressure (Pplat) goals, as follows:

Oxygenation Goal: Pao_2 of 55–80 mm Hg or Spo_2 of 88%–95%
Use a minimum positive end-expiratory pressure (PEEP) of 5 cm H_2O. Consider use of incremental Fio_2/PEEP combinations such as shown below (not required) to achieve goal.

Lower PEEP/higher Fio_2

Fio_2	0.3	0.4	0.4	0.5	0.5	0.6	0.7	0.7
PEEP	5	5	8	8	10	10	10	12

Fio_2	0.7	0.8	0.9	0.9	0.9	1.0
PEEP	14	14	14	16	18	18–24

Higher PEEP/lower Fio_2

Fio_2	0.3	0.3	0.3	0.3	0.3	0.4	0.4	0.5
PEEP	5	8	10	12	14	14	16	16

Fio_2	0.5	0.5–0.8	0.8	0.9	1.0	1.0
PEEP	18	20	22	22	22	24

Pplat Goal: ≤ 30 cm H_2O
Check Pplat (0.5-second inspiratory pause) at least every 4 hours and after each change in PEEP or V_T.
If Pplat > 30 cm H_2O: Decrease V_T by 1-mL/kg steps (minimum = 4 mL/kg).
If Pplat < 25 cm H_2O and V_T < 6 mL/kg: Increase V_T by 1 mL/kg until Pplat > 25 cm H_2O or V_T = 6 mL/kg.
If Pplat < 30 cm H_2O and breath stacking or dyssynchrony occurs: May increase V_T in 1-mL/kg increments to 7 or 8 mL/kg if Pplat remains < 30 cm H_2O.

pH Goal: 7.30–7.45
Acidosis (pH + 7.30) management:

- **If pH 7.15–7.30:** Increase RR until pH > 7.30 or $Paco_2$ < 25 mm Hg (maximum set RR = 35 breaths/min).
- **If pH + 7.15:** Increase RR to 35 breaths/min.
  - If pH remains < 7.15, V_T may be increased in 1-mL/kg steps until pH > 7.15 (Pplat target of 30 may be exceeded).
  - May give sodium bicarbonate.

Alkalosis (pH = 7.45) management: Decrease ventilatory rate, if possible.

I:E Ratio Goal: Recommend that duration of inspiration be less than duration of expiration.

Part II: Weaning

A. Conduct a spontaneous breathing trial daily when:

1. $Fio_2 \leq 0.40$ and PEEP ≤ 8 cm H_2O *or* $Fio_2 < 0.50$ and PEEP < 5 cm H_2O.
2. PEEP and Fio_2 are the same or lower than values of previous day.
3. Patient has acceptable spontaneous breathing efforts. (May decrease ventilatory rate by 50% for 5 minutes to detect effort.)
4. Systolic blood pressure ≥ 90 mm Hg without vasopressor support.
5. No neuromuscular blocking agents or blockade.

B. Spontaneous breathing trial:
If all above criteria are met and subject has been in the study for at least 12 hours, initiate a trial of *up to* 120 minutes of spontaneous breathing with $Fio_2 < 0.5$ and PEEP < 5 cm H_2O:

1. Place on T-piece, tracheostomy collar, or continuous positive airway pressure (CPAP) ≤ 5 cm H_2O with pressure support < 5 cm H_2O.
2. Assess for tolerance as below for up to 2 hours.
   a. Spo_2 ≥ 90% and/or Pao_2 ≥ 60 mm Hg
   b. Spontaneous V_T ≥ 4 mL/kg PBW
   c. RR ≤ 35 breaths/min
   d. pH ≥ 7.3
   e. No respiratory distress (distress = 2 or more)
      - Heart rate > 120% of baseline
      - Marked accessory muscle use
      - Abdominal paradox
      - Diaphoresis
      - Marked dyspnea
3. If tolerated for at least 30 minutes, consider extubation.
4. If not tolerated, resume pre-weaning settings.

Definition of *unassisted breathing*
(different from the spontaneous breathing criteria, as pressure support is not allowed)

1. Extubated with face mask, nasal prong oxygen, or room air, *or*
2. T-tube breathing, *or*
3. Tracheostomy mask breathing, *or*
4. CPAP ≤ 5 cm H_2O without pressure support or intermittent mandatory ventilation assistance.

FIGURE 7-12 ARDS Network protocol for managing a patient with a Pao_2:Fio_2 ratio less than 300.
Abbreviations: ARDS, acute respiratory distress syndrome; Fio_2, fraction of inspired oxygen; $Paco_2$, partial pressure of carbon dioxide, arterial; Pao_2, partial pressure of oxygen, arterial; Spo_2, oxygen saturation as measured by pulse oximeter

From NIH NHLBI ARDS Clinical Network: Mechanical Ventilation Protocol Summary. ARDSnet website. http://www.ardsnet.org/files/ventilator_protocol_2008-07.pdf. Accessed December 8, 2021.

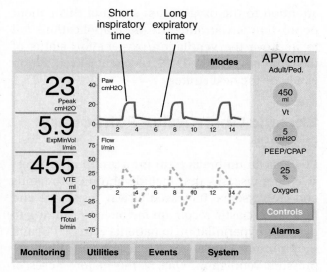

A

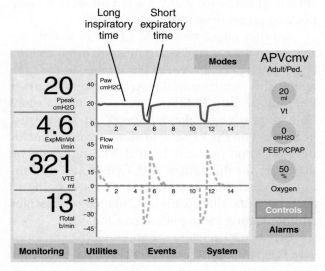

B

FIGURE 7-13 Inverse inspiratory-to-expiratory (I:E) ratio.
A. Conventional ventilation. **B.** Airway pressure release
ventilation.

Courtesy of Vent-Pro Training.

Another consideration is fluid management. It becomes a delicate balancing act in patients with ARDS to provide enough fluid to adequately perfuse the organs while not adding unnecessary fluid to the lungs, which may increase compression atelectasis and hinder gas exchange.

ECMO is on the rise as a rescue therapy and is often used during transports when patients need a higher level of care. This intervention requires specialty teams to accompany the transport team, including a perfusionist or specifically trained RN to manage the ECMO device and a clinician to treat the patient. Implementing ECMO is considered when the patient's Pao_2:Fio_2 ratio is less than 50 and plateau pressures are greater than 32 cm H_2O. The most common form of ECMO support consists of removing the blood from the vena cava (superior or inferior) and infusing it into the right atrium, a practice referred to as veno-venous access.

COVID-19

Most experts agree that patients with COVID-19 who are receiving care in the ICU should be treated similarly to patients who have ARDS if their condition matches the Berlin definition. As with any critically ill patient, treatment decisions for these patients should be made on a case-by-case basis.

Observations and detailed discussions of this patient population have revealed different patterns in their ventilatory response to hypoxemia. Interestingly, some patients present with normal compliant lungs, yet still experience hypoxemia. The assumption is the lungs are being adequately ventilated but the perfusion at the alveolar-capillary membrane is diminished. It is believed that this particular virus can invoke microthrombi in the pulmonary vessels, causing a $\dot{V}/\dot{Q}$ mismatch and high rates of coagulation anomalies throughout the body. Because of this potential diffusion deficiency and good lung compliance, extremely high levels of PEEP have been avoided in patients with COVID-19. PEEP levels typically range from 10 to 14 cm H_2O in these patients, although the ARDS Network's protocol allows PEEP levels as high as 24 cm H_2O in severe cases at an Fio_2 of 1.0. The goal is to keep plateau pressures at less than 30 cm H_2O and driving pressures at less than 15 cm H_2O, if possible, to reduce further lung injury.

Common complications of COVID-19 include elevated liver enzymes, acute kidney injury, and cardiac injury presenting as a late-onset complication. Some patients may develop atypical coagulation profiles leading to thrombosis. The most prominent finding in critically ill patients with COVID-19 is acute hypoxemic respiratory failure. Rarely do these patients present in a hypercapnic state. For most patients with COVID-19, providing supplemental oxygen early in the progression of the infection is paramount. The options available are listed here:

- **Low-flow oxygen.** Typically, a nasal cannula administering 4 to 6 L/min is used to administer low-flow oxygen.
- **Oxypendant.** This nasal cannula incorporates a larger luminal diameter and an oxygen reservoir that is designed to deliver a higher oxygen concentration in each breath, similar to a nonrebreathing mask reservoir.
- **Simple face mask.** A simple face mask may deliver higher F_{IO_2}, ranging from 0.3 to 0.6, with flows up to 10 L/min.
- **Nonrebreathing mask.** A nonrebreathing mask delivers F_{IO_2} of approximately 0.85 to 0.95.
- **HFNC.** This device may deliver flows up to 60 L/min, with F_{IO_2} ranging from 0.21 to 1.0, and the ability to heat and humidify the blended gas.
- **Noninvasive ventilation.** The preferred noninvasive approach uses a full-face mask and either CPAP or BPAP.
- **Self-proning.** Self-proning has been encouraged in this patient population to better ventilate the dorsal lung regions and potentially improve $\dot{V}/\dot{Q}$ matching.

The World Health Organization suggests a targeted SpO_2 of greater than 90% for maintenance oxygen. Hyperoxia should be avoided. Because the transport arena is a dynamic environment, close attention to the oxygenation status of this patient population is warranted. If these applications fail to improve the ventilation/oxygenation status of the patient with COVID-19, mechanical ventilation would be the next strategy.

Chronic Obstructive Pulmonary Disease

COPD is an umbrella term for a group of progressive lung diseases that include chronic bronchitis and emphysema. Increased airway resistance and decreased elastic recoil are factors contributing to dynamic hyperinflation in patients with COPD, and they present challenges when applying positive-pressure ventilation. One of the major causes of COPD is tobacco smoking. If possible, obtain a smoking history from any patient about to receive positive-pressure ventilation.

Another characteristic of COPD is airflow restriction, which may lead to further complications if too much pressure/volume is applied at too high a rate. This patient population is susceptible to air trapping or auto-PEEP and typically needs more time for passive exhalation. Special attention must be focused on the I:E ratio to allow enough time for the exhalation phase. A 1:4 or 1:5 I:E ratio may be necessary for the patient with COPD. Accomplishing this goal becomes particularly challenging in such patients, due to the abundance of variables within the lung mechanics to consider.

Before transporting a patient with COPD, ensure the patient has received all of the medications that are prescribed and due before transport. Medications commonly used to treat these lung diseases include long- and short-acting bronchodilators (beta-2 and anticholinergic), corticosteroids, and antibiotics. The goal is to maximize the lung's ability to oxygenate and ventilate with the least amount of airflow restriction. The patient should be suctioned prior to transport if rhonchi are present.

Noninvasive positive-pressure ventilation (NIPPV) plays an important role for patients with COPD exacerbation and has been widely accepted as the first strategy for treating such patients who present with respiratory distress. Early application of this modality may avoid the need for intubation, and consequently the negative ramifications of mechanical ventilation. Prior to placing a patient on NIPPV, it would be beneficial to obtain a recent chest

Controversies

Research suggests that patients who have, or are suspected of having, COVID-19 may benefit from transport in the prone position. This position has been shown to improve oxygenation and reduce mortality in patients who are awake and undergoing mechanical ventilation when transport time is longer than 15 minutes. Improving oxygenation via this simple technique may help avoid the need to intubate these patients, which is a higher-risk intervention.

A limiting factor in using the prone position is patient tolerance, as patients may find the position uncomfortable, particularly given a long transport. If this position is used, providers should try to make the patient more comfortable by padding the stretcher with pillows and blankets.

Research into this intervention is limited. Providers should follow local protocols when considering transport of a patient in the prone position.

radiograph, ABG analysis, and some history of oxygen requirements. Placing any patient on positive-pressure ventilation carries an inherent risk of barotrauma, volutrauma, and hemodynamic compromise. Because the patient with COPD may already have damaged alveoli due to the nature of the disease process, applying judicious amounts of pressure/volume is essential.

Typical starting pressures for NIPPV using a full-face mask may be a PIP of 10 cm H_2O and a CPAP of 5 cm H_2O, followed by assessment for patient compliance, breath sounds, work of breathing, and oxygenation and ventilation status. Titration of inspiratory pressures assists in achieving the intended exhaled tidal volumes, which may be necessary to reach the target goals for ventilation. The CPAP setting can be adjusted to increase the surface area at the alveolar-capillary membrane, and FIO_2 can be increased to improve oxygenation.

It is important to fully understand how your transport ventilator delivers the pressure-delivered breath. For example, if the ventilator delivers a PIP and your settings are an IPAP of 10 cm H_2O and an EPAP of 5 cm H_2O, and if your strategy is to increase the EPAP to 8 cm H_2O to aid in oxygenation, the change in pressure (delta P) decreases from 5 cm H_2O to 2 cm H_2O, as the PIP will remain the same. This outcome is of great concern because the tidal volume may be drastically reduced, causing increased work of breathing, anxiety, and elevated $Paco_2$ levels in the patient due to the decreased minute volume. However, if your transport ventilator uses PAP for a pressure-delivered breath, and you make the same adjustment from an IPAP of 10 cm H_2O and an EPAP of 5 cm H_2O (which is a PIP of 15 cm H_2O) to an IPAP of 10 cm H_2O and an EPAP of 8 cm H_2O (which is a PIP of 18 cm H_2O), then the change in pressure is unaffected.

Of particular concern is the patient with bullous emphysema—a condition in which the air-filled space in the lung is greater than 1 cm in diameter, and which results from alveolar destruction in the lung parenchyma. The main causes of bullous emphysema are tobacco smoking and alpha-1 antitrypsin deficiency, an inherited genetic condition. Although diagnosing someone with bullous emphysema on a physical exam is impossible, gathering a history and CT scan, chest radiograph, and ABG analysis can be important in formulating a strategy for transporting such a patient **FIGURE 7-14.**

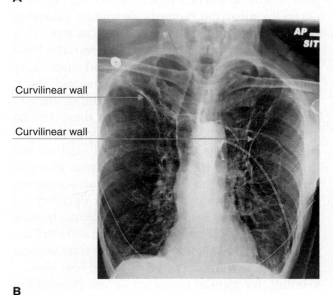

Hyperinflated lungs

Barrel chest

Smaller heart size

Flattened diaphragms

A

Curvilinear wall

Curvilinear wall

B

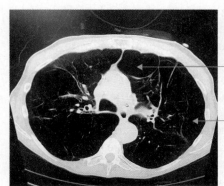

Bullae emphysema

Emphysematous space

Emphysematous space

C

FIGURE 7-14 A. Typical chest radiograph. **B.** Chest radiograph of a patient with bullous emphysema. **C.** Computed tomography scan of a patient with bullous emphysema.

Courtesy of Vent-Pro Training.

Administering positive-pressure ventilation to the patient with end-stage COPD or emphysema may lead to disastrous results, including a pneumothorax. Such patients are often on home oxygen via nasal cannula or an oxypendant. They might do well on a nonrebreathing mask, HFNC, or even a minimal level of CPAP. Treat each case individually to ensure patient safety at all times.

Ventilator settings for this patient population are challenging. If the patient's hospital ventilator settings are acceptable for the transport, then try to match them on your own ventilator. Recognize, however, that the ventilation provided with the transport ventilator will not feel exactly the same as that provided by the hospital ventilator. Some adjustments or a mode change may be necessary to meet the patient's demands. Choosing the right flow target is a great place to start. In a volume-targeted breath, the flow delivered is fixed and is set by the desired volume and inspiratory time. If the tidal volume target has already been set, the only way to increase flow to the air-hungry patient is to lower the inspiratory time. For an air-hungry patient, you might consider setting a pressure target, as the ventilator will deliver the flow in a decelerating pattern and provide as much flow as the machine is rated for. Some ventilators also allow for manipulation of that decelerating flow in the initial inspiratory phase by decreasing the rise time or P-ramp setting, which will send the desired pressure slightly faster. A low tidal volume strategy (6 to 8 mL/kg of PBW) is the best choice, keeping the plateau pressures at less than 30 cm H_2O. If auto-PEEP is present, confirm the settings are appropriate for the patient and aim for an I:E ratio of 1:4 or 1:5, if possible. This may be accomplished by reducing the respiratory rate and decreasing the inspiratory time.

Three factors contribute to dynamic hyperinflation: (1) the I:E ratio, (2) the minute volume (tidal volume × respiratory rate), and (3) the expiratory time constant, a dynamic measurement that is the product of compliance and resistance. If auto-PEEP is accurately measured, a suggested strategy is to set external PEEP at 75% less than auto-PEEP to avoid any increased hyperinflation or hemodynamic compromise. Some ventilators may allow for auto-PEEP measurement by applying an expiratory hold maneuver and then calculating actual PEEP in the circuit minus the set PEEP. Other

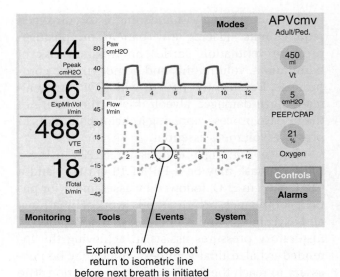

Expiratory flow does not return to isometric line before next breath is initiated

FIGURE 7-15 Some ventilators provide an estimate of auto-PEEP along with flow graphics.

Courtesy of Vent-Pro Training.

ventilators will give an estimate of auto-PEEP along with flow graphics, which can visually alert the CCTP to auto-PEEP; that is, the CCTP can observe the expiratory flow tracing and ensure it returns to the isometric line before the next breath is delivered **FIGURE 7-15**.

Initial ventilator settings for a patient with COPD who is in respiratory failure might appear as follows:

- Pressure or volume target
- Assist/control mode
- Tidal volume: 6 mL/kg of PBW, ensuring plateau pressures less than 30 cm H_2O
- Respiratory rate: 10–12 breaths/min, aiming for an I:E ratio of 1:4 to 1:5
- Inspiratory time: 0.8–1.0 s, aiming for an I:E ratio of 1:4 to 1:5
- PEEP: 5 cm H_2O
- F_{IO_2}: titrate for desired saturation

Some sedation may be necessary, and aiming to keep the patient in a fluid-neutral state is important.

Example ABG values for a patient with COPD might be pH, 7.35; $Paco_2$, 75 mm Hg; Pao_2, 98 mm Hg; serum bicarbonate (HcO_3), 49 mEq/L; base excess, 18.7; calculated oxygen saturation (calc sat) 94%; patient on F_{IO_2} at 1.0. It is important to know the patient's baseline condition before "chasing numbers." For a patient with these ABG values, you would treat the pH, not the hypercapnia, as many patients with COPD have chronic hypercarbia. Decreasing the F_{IO_2} would be indicated.

Pneumonia

Pneumonia is most commonly triggered by a bacterial infection in the lungs, which sets off the invasion of fibrinous exudate and leukocytes, impeding the lung's ability to oxygenate and ventilate effectively. However, it may also be triggered by a viral or fungal infection. In severe cases of pneumonia, the patient may develop ARDS. Empiric antibiotics should be started based on regional guidelines. Ensure blood and, if possible, sputum cultures are sent prior to initiating antibiotic therapy when possible.

If you are transporting a patient with pneumonia on NIPPV, it is important to consider using a heated-wire circuit. This device provides warmed humidification to minimize the risk of drying of secretions that then leads to a mucus plug. Be mindful of these secretions, and perform deep suction whenever possible prior to beginning the transport. Chest physiotherapy and postural drainage are other options to consider for loosening the secretions. The dynamic environment that the transport arena presents may loosen up secretions unexpectedly, and monitoring the PIP can provide a good indicator of airway resistance. The same ventilator strategy used for patients with ARDS may be implemented in this patient population, though they may require more F_{IO_2} to reach the target saturation levels due to the shunting effect that excessive secretions precipitate.

Pulmonary Fibrosis

Pulmonary fibrosis is a respiratory condition that causes scarring of the lung tissue. This incurable disease is thought to have a genetic component, but in most cases its cause is unknown; therefore, the condition is referred to as idiopathic pulmonary fibrosis. Treatment is aimed at slowing the process and improving the patient's quality of life. Patients with idiopathic pulmonary fibrosis receive oxygen when their saturation level falls below 88%. Medications such as pirfenidone and nintedanib may be prescribed to slow the scarring process. Pulmonary rehabilitation is essential to teach patients how to better live with this condition. Because prognoses are poor and life expectancy from the time of diagnoses ranges from 2 to 5 years, lung transplant is a strong consideration. Mechanical ventilation and ECMO may be considered as a bridge to transplant.

You may be tasked with transporting a patient with idiopathic pulmonary fibrosis. Discussion of the strategy for such a transport should involve all parties. Some lung transplant centers may cancel the transplant procedure if the patient is receiving mechanical ventilation. Often supporting the patient with a nonrebreathing mask or HFNC will suffice. Consider using NIPPV at a comfortable level of CPAP and high levels of F_{IO_2} if necessary. Because of the scarring of the lung tissue, adding high levels of PEEP typically will not increase oxygenation.

Asthma

Asthma is a common lung disorder that causes shortness of breath due to inflammation of the airways and increased mucus production. When a patient presents with an asthma exacerbation, rapid assessment and treatment should be the priority, as patients experiencing status asthmaticus need immediate attention to support their ventilation and ultimately oxygenation. It is imperative to recognize the difference between respiratory distress and respiratory failure (explained earlier in the chapter).

Another potential strategy for reducing the increased airway resistance is to administer heliox, as this therapy will help to decrease the work of breathing. A small number of patients may show signs of improvement with intramuscular administration of epinephrine or terbutaline.

A trial of NIPPV can be considered, but if the patient's condition is not improving or is worsening, then intubation and mechanical ventilation would be the next step. Because airway resistance is of great concern with this patient population, choosing an ET tube with the largest appropriate diameter would be prudent due to the potential for auto-PEEP. Ventilator settings should account for the time needed for passive exhalation, meaning the I:E ratio should be near 1:4 or 1:5. A pressure-delivered breath is often used in these scenarios because it limits the pressure delivered; it should be targeted at less than 30 cm H_2O. The mode of choice is often assist control until the patient's respiratory status becomes more stable. Tidal volumes can be on the low side (6 mL/kg or less of PBW) until the patient's lungs respond to medical therapy.

Some patients may need to be heavily sedated or paralyzed to slow their respiratory rate and prevent auto-PEEP. This intervention, termed permissive hypercapnia, is not a goal per se, but rather an end result of preventing volutrauma, barotrauma, and air trapping. It is not uncommon to allow for higher-than-normal $Paco_2$ and $etco_2$ values during the initial stages of caring for a newly intubated patient with asthma exacerbation. Constant monitoring of exhaled tidal volume and minute volume is essential when such patients are receiving pressure-delivered breaths. If you choose a volume target, always monitor and trend the PIP values.

Heart Failure

Acute pulmonary edema (APE) can occur in heart failure patients. When assessing a patient for APE, the initial step to identify whether this condition involves a pump-filling problem (diastolic malfunction) or a pump-contractility problem (systolic malfunction).

When transporting a patient with APE, the goal may be to support oxygenation and ventilation. On auscultation, it is common to hear crackles on end inspiration along with scattered rhonchi, and pulmonary edema may be evident on the chest radiograph or thoracic ultrasonography. If the patient appears dyspneic, NIPPV in the form of CPAP is the first-line strategy to support the patient's respiratory status in addition to standard pharmacologic treatment. Starting at a CPAP of 5 cm H_2O and titrating the pressure up to meet the patient's respiratory demand is a sound initial strategy. Many patients do well with CPAP but may require more assistance if they appear air hungry. Switching to BPAP is another option to help decrease the work of breathing. Typical BPAP settings start with an IPAP of 10 cm H_2O and an EPAP of 5 cm H_2O, which are then titrated upward to obtain the desired results. Using a full-face mask would be beneficial to provide more accurate pressures, but the CCTP needs to be acutely aware of the risk of aspiration. Increasing the gradient between IPAP and EPAP should increase the minute volume and potentially decrease the work of breathing; increasing the EPAP should help with oxygenation.

If intubation is inevitable, using a low tidal volume (6 to 8 mL/kg of PBW) is the best initial strategy. The choice between a volume or pressure target may be determined by how the patient's lungs respond to mechanical ventilation while monitoring for volutrauma and barotrauma. The goal should be to keep the plateau pressures at less than 30 cm H_2O. Initially, use of assist/control mode may benefit the patient until ABG values are stable. Maintain a cautious attitude when applying PEEP. In a patient with low end-diastolic volume, increasing PEEP levels may negatively affect preload. One benefit from PEEP may be improved left ventricular function, as a result of decreasing the left ventricular afterload.

Another benefit of PEEP in the patient with APE is that this therapy moves extravascular lung fluid from the alveoli back into the pulmonary vasculature. Start with a PEEP of 5 cm H_2O; then, if more PEEP is to be applied, do so in small increments of pressure, allowing sufficient time to achieve the desired results while monitoring the patient's hemodynamics and ventilatory status. Adjusting the respiratory rate to achieve a target $Paco_2$ of 35 to 45 mm Hg is common practice.

When weaning from the ventilator is considered for a patient, including the patient with APE, it may be useful to switch the mode to synchronized intermittent mandatory ventilation. In this mode, a set rate and target volume/pressure are established, and the patient can breathe spontaneously between the set rate. A minimum of 5 cm H_2O of pressure support might be added to address any airway resistance within the circuit. Pressure support may then be increased to target a specific exhaled tidal volume if needed.

Patient Monitoring

The CCTP's goal is to deliver the same level of ongoing care and treatment during transport as would be provided in an inpatient critical care unit. All patients with significant respiratory concerns should be continuously monitored with pulse oximetry and continuous waveform capnography.

Nasal capnography is readily available for spontaneously breathing patients and can also be used to monitor the effects of noninvasive ventilation. Make sure you have performed a pre-use check, including a circuit check, on the ventilator prior to placing a patient on this device.

During transport, it is crucial to monitor the values measured for the patient and displayed on the ventilator. Some of these values are summarized here.

Peak Inspiratory Pressure

Record a baseline PIP and monitor this value regularly. If PIP rises, it may indicate compliance/resistance changes or obstruction in the circuit. This finding could also indicate a patient who is asynchronous with the ventilator settings. Corrective action may include assessing the patient's lung sounds, applying suction, or giving bronchodilators if indicated. Inspect the circuit components for malfunctions, including the ET tube and HME. The patient biting on the ET tube, a kinked ET tube, and a closed suction catheter that is not fully withdrawn are common problems and need to be addressed immediately. Always reassess the ventilator settings for patient demand.

Respiratory Rate

Record a baseline respiratory rate and monitor this value regularly, watching for tachypnea. If the patient's respiratory rate increases rapidly, first check the circuit for leaks; such an event could cause the ventilator to autocycle or trigger an unwanted breath. Adjusting the sensitivity should correct this problem if the leak cannot be fixed. If the patient appears air hungry, consider changing the mode, adjusting the volume delivered, increasing the respiratory rate, adjusting the inspiratory time to match the patient's need, and switching to a pressure-delivered breath, which offers the ability to adjust the flow to the patient through rise-time adjustments and flow termination.

Exhaled Tidal Volume

Record a baseline exhaled tidal volume and monitor this value closely. If extreme fluctuations are noted (in the range of 50 to 100 mL), first check the components of the circuit (HME, closed suction catheter, ETCO$_2$ adapter, and ET tube cuff) for leaks. It may be helpful to measure for auto-PEEP by performing an expiratory hold maneuver. If you cannot obtain an exhaled tidal volume measurement, you may instead assess the patient's breathing pattern and breath sounds. If fluctuations in exhaled tidal volume are observed, suction and administer bronchodilator therapy as necessary. Adjusting the ventilator settings may prove beneficial as well.

I:E Ratio

Monitor the I:E ratio, remembering that a ratio of 1:2 or 1:3 is normal for a healthy lung. Patients with obstructive or restrictive lung diseases might need a longer expiratory time, indicated by a 1:4 or 1:5 I:E ratio.

Documentation

Charting of the ventilator settings and monitored values should include the following elements:

- **Settings**
  - Volume or pressure breath
  - Mode
  - Respiratory rate
  - Inspiratory time
  - Tidal volume or pressure
  - PEEP
  - FIO_2
  - Sensitivity
- **Values**
  - PIP
  - Exhaled tidal volume
  - Respiratory rate
  - I:E ratio
  - Minute volume
  - ETCO$_2$
  - Pulse oximetry (SpO$_2$)

This information is valuable when troubleshooting ventilation-related problems during transport. The frequency of the charting is up to the CCTP. It is recommended to record values at least every 30 minutes or after making any changes to the ventilator settings.

Quick Reference: Ventilator Settings for Adult Patients

I. Selection of pressure or volume ventilation

  A. Choose mode

    1. Assist/control (A/C)

    2. Synchronized intermittent mandatory ventilation (SIMV)

    3. Pressure-regulated volume control (PRVC)

    4. Pressure support ventilation (PSV)

    5. Continuous positive airway pressure (CPAP)

    6. Adaptive support ventilation (ASV)

  B. Choose a target tidal volume: 6–8 mL/kg predicted body weight

  C. Choose a respiratory rate: 12–14 breaths/min

  D. Choose a PEEP level: 5 cm H_2O

  E. Choose an inspiratory time: 1 s

  F. I:E ratio: 1:2 to 1:3 (healthy lung)

  G. FIO_2: 0.21–1.0; adjust for saturation >92% to 94%

  H. Sensitivity: 2 L/min (increase for autocycling due to leak)

II. Alarms

  A. High-pressure alarm: 10 cm H_2O above PIP

  B. Low-pressure alarm: 5 cm H_2O below PIP

  C. Low-minute-volume alarm: 25% below baseline minute volume

Always consider the patient's lung condition before placing them on a ventilator. Suctioning and bronchodilator therapy may enhance lung compliance or decrease airway resistance. Monitor for high PIP and auto-PEEP, and adjust the ventilator accordingly.

Quick Reference: Ventilator Settings for Pediatric Patients

I. Selection of pressure or volume ventilation

  A. Choose mode

    1. Assist/control (A/C)

    2. Synchronized intermittent mandatory ventilation (SIMV)

    3. Pressure-regulated volume control (PRVC)

    4. Pressure support ventilation (PSV)

    5. Continuous positive airway pressure (CPAP)

    6. Adaptive support ventilation (ASV)

  B. Choose a target tidal volume: 6–8 mL/kg predicted body weight

  C. Choose a respiratory rate: 15–20 breaths/min

  D. Choose a PEEP level: 5 cm H_2O

  E. Choose an inspiratory time: 0.5–1 s

  F. I:E ratio: 1:2 to 1:3 (healthy lung)

  G. FIO_2: 0.21–1.0; adjust for saturation >92% to 94%

  H. Sensitivity: 2 L/min (increase for autocycling due to leak)

II. Alarms

  A. High-pressure alarm: 10 cm H_2O above PIP

  B. Low-pressure alarm: 5 cm H_2O below PIP

  C. Low-minute-volume alarm: 25% below baseline minute volume

Always consider the patient's lung condition before placing them on a ventilator. Suctioning and bronchodilator therapy may enhance lung compliance. Monitor for high PIP and auto-PEEP, and adjust the ventilator accordingly.

Ongoing Care

The transport team is responsible for ensuring that proper ventilator function and the patient's ventilatory status are maintained during the transport. This can be accomplished by ensuring the following tasks are completed:

- Maintain a stable and patent airway.
- Verify and document the ventilator settings and monitored values before, during, and after arrival.
- Ensure a proper power supply and oxygen are available during the transport.
- Assess and document breath sounds before, during (if possible), and after transport.

- Continuously monitor SpO_2 and ETCO$_2$.
- Have a bag-mask device available at the head of bed if there is any doubt about the ventilator's functioning.

SKILL DRILL 7-1 summarizes the steps for using a portable ventilator, which are described here:

1. Attach the ventilator circuit **STEP 1**.
2. Initiate power **STEP 2**.
3. Select the ventilator rate, inspiratory rate, flow rate, and oxygen concentrations **STEP 3**.
4. Make mode selections: CPAP and PEEP, IMV/SIMV, and assist/control **STEP 4**.

Skill Drill 7-1 Using a Portable Ventilator

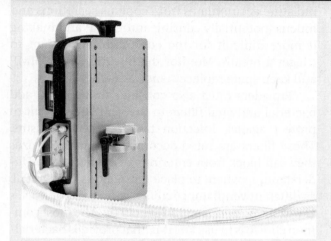

Step 1

Attach the ventilator circuit.

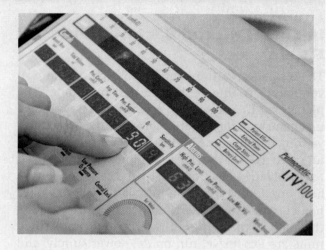

Step 2

Initiate power.

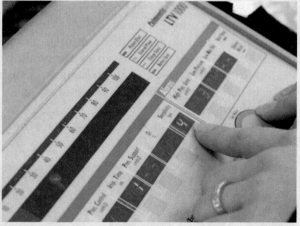

Step 3

Select the ventilator rate, inspiratory rate, flow rate, and oxygen concentrations.

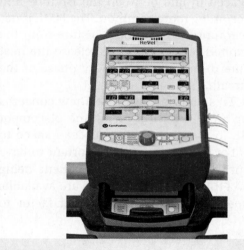

Step 4

Make mode selections: CPAP and PEEP, IMV/ SIMV, and assist/control.

Step 1: The ReVel ventilator image is © 2014 CareFusion Corporation. Used with permission; **Steps 2 & 3:** © Jones & Bartlett Learning; **Step 4:** The ReVel ventilator image is © 2014 CareFusion Corporation. Used with permission.

Flight Considerations

Not all ventilators are able to compensate for changes in altitude in their delivery of tidal volumes. Some studies have shown a 10% increase in tidal volumes at the cabin pressures experienced at 8,000 feet of altitude, a relationship explained by Boyle's law (discussed in Chapter 4, *Aircraft Fundamentals and Flight Physiology*). Boyle's law should also be considered when transporting a patient who has potential for any gas to become trapped in a body cavity, such as happens with pneumothorax. Air in the body cavities can expand as much as 25% at higher altitudes. In such a case, the CCTP should discuss with the pilots whether it is possible to fly at an altitude that would maintain a sea-level cabin pressure to reduce the negative effects on the patient.

In-Line HME and Bacterial/Viral Filters

The air delivered to patients requiring mechanical ventilation should be heated and humidified. By placing an ET tube in the trachea, the physiologic mechanism of the superior airway is bypassed, preventing it from contributing heat or moisture to the lungs. In the ICU, heated humidifiers are often used to supply the delivered breath at a set temperature and humidification. The ventilator circuits have heated wires to prevent temperature drops along the path to the lungs. These heated, humidified units are expensive, run on AC power supply, and require a steady flow of sterile water. To circumvent these factors in the out-of-hospital setting, use of an HME placed in-line between the ET tube and circuit is becoming more common. The HME is designed to capture the heat and moisture from the patient's expired breath and then release the heat and moisture during the inspiratory phase of the delivered breath.

The CCTP should be aware of a few concerns when using an in-line HME. First, the placement of the HME in the circuit will add dead space to the circuit. For this reason, it is important to have the appropriate-size HME for the patient being transported **FIGURE 7-16**. Three sizes are available: neonatal, pediatric, and adult. Another factor to

consider is the resistive load associated with the HME for the critically ill patient. This added resistance to the circuit will be minimal unless excessive moisture accumulates from copious secretions and mucus, potentially causing auto-PEEP and making it more difficult for the compromised patient to trigger a breath. Monitor the integrity of the HME and keep spare replacements available.

Providers must also consider the need to add bacterial and viral filters to the ventilator circuit to protect against infection by airborne organisms. These filters are rated according the particle sizes they can block from entering the environment. Understanding where to place these filters is essential, as different ventilator circuits have exhalation valves at various positions within the circuit. The most common choice is to use an HME that provides bacterial/viral protection, placed close to the patient, as guided by the product's specifications for dead space, resistive load, and particle size filtration.

In-Line Suction Catheters

In-line suction catheters allow providers to suction the patient without opening the circuit and exposing the environment to airborne organisms or losing PEEP **FIGURE 7-17**. Because the transport environment is dynamic, the patient's secretions may become mobilized during transport. The CCTP must closely monitor the patient through auscultation of

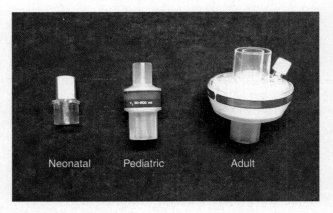

FIGURE 7-16 Example of additional dead space added to the ventilator circuit through placement of an HME.

Courtesy of Vent-Pro Training.

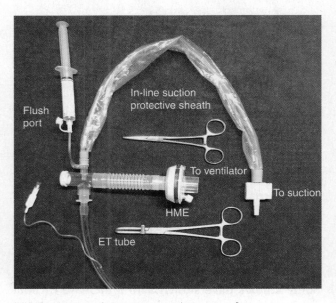

FIGURE 7-17 In-line suction catheter.

Courtesy of Vent-Pro Training.

Transport Management

- HMEs and bacterial/viral filters are beneficial until they are filled with secretions, causing increased airway resistance. Always carry spare filters.

- When using in-line suction, ensure the catheter is withdrawn to its original position and is not partially inserted into the ET tube.

- Always maximize the patient's lung condition before beginning the transport—for example, by suctioning the patient's lungs, administering medications prior to departure, evacuating unwanted air from the stomach, and positioning the patient to optimize lung compliance.

- Calculate oxygen consumption for worst-case scenarios, with the patient requiring an FIO_2 of 1.0.

- Be cautious when adjusting the minute volume and oxygenation based on $ETCO_2$ and pulse oximetry. Knowing the patient's baseline ventilation and oxygenation requirements and current lung physiology is essential when caring for a patient on mechanical ventilation.

- When formulating a strategy for ventilator settings based on an ABG analysis, consider the pH value before manipulating the minute ventilation to correct any hypercarbic or hypocarbic condition.

- Before making any adjustments on the ventilator, consider the expected results and what those adjustments might collaterally affect, and then closely watch the monitored values from the ventilator.

- All ventilators need some time to deliver the target settings. A few breaths may be needed to adjust for lung compliance and airway resistance. Remain calm and inform the patient of this condition.

the lungs and watch for increased PIP in a volume target and decreased exhaled tidal volume in a pressure target.

Use the appropriate-size catheter, as a catheter that is too small may not be able to remove thick secretions and a catheter that is too large may not fit or may get stuck in the ET tube. Many models contain a port where a flush syringe of normal saline can be connected to remove any remaining secretions in the catheter. Flushing the syringe is recommended because the secretions remaining in the catheter may dry out and clog the catheter, rendering it useless for the next attempt.

When suction is completed, confirm that all of the catheter has been removed from the ET tube. Pulling the catheter beyond the gasket may cause

the protective plastic shield to inflate, adding more dead space to the circuit. The suction catheter should be changed out if this occurs.

When checking for leaks in the circuit, the flush port is a common culprit.

Basic Ventilator Waveform Analysis

Many ventilators display various waveforms in the form of scalars and loops that provide a great point-of-care tool. These graphics offer visual information regarding patient–ventilator asynchrony in regard to time, flow, volume, or pressure. Some transport ventilators are capable of displaying waveforms through a graphics package that incorporates sensors and signal processors **FIGURE 7-18**.

On a scalar graphic, three components are plotted against time: the pressure time scalar, flow time scalar, and volume time scalar. When observing these waveforms, note that time is typically plotted on the horizontal x-axis, and pressure, flow, and volume are typically plotted on the vertical y-axis.

Loops are a two-dimensional graphic display containing two scalar values. The first display might be a pressure-volume loop, and the second might

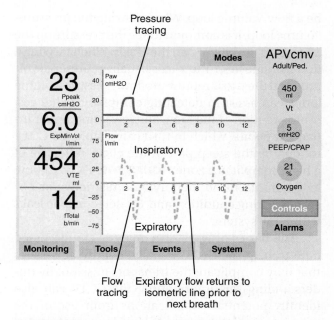

FIGURE 7-18 Some transport ventilators display waveforms through a graphics package that incorporates sensors and signal processors.

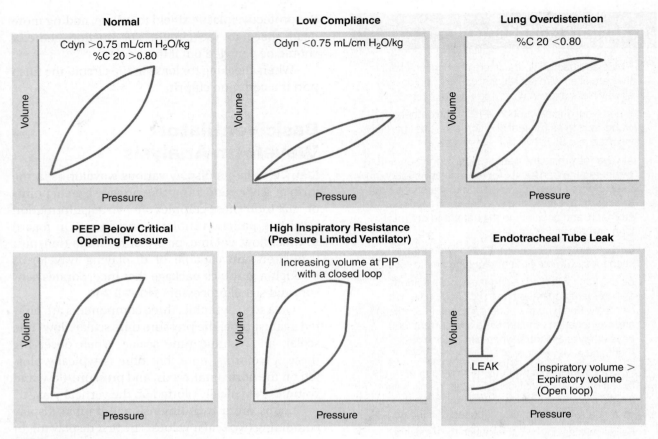

FIGURE 7-19 Pressure-volume loops.

Courtesy of Vent-Pro Training.

be a flow-volume loop. When viewing the pressure-volume loop, it is common to see the pressure on the *x*-axis and the volume on the *y*-axis. When viewing a flow-volume loop, the *x*-axis usually represents volume and the *y*-axis represents flow. Pressure-volume loops can assist in detecting compliance changes, overdistention of the lung, and lower and upper inflection points, which in turn can enable the CCTP to identify the steep part of the curve reflective of a high-compliance zone **FIGURE 7-19**. Flow-volume loops are useful in identifying a restrictive or obstructive lung condition and for detecting air leaks within the system.

The basics of waveform analysis are discussed here to help the CCTP visually identify any issues that may complicate the transport mission. By understanding this information, the CCTP can also identify potential complications from use of the hospital ventilator in the ICU. It is recommended that CCTPs become familiar with all the options available if the transport monitor is equipped with graphic monitoring, so as to optimize the

monitoring capabilities while caring for a mechanically ventilated patient during transport.

The most important scalars to monitor are the flow time scalar and the pressure time scalar. Valuable information can be obtained by observing how the flow time scalar reacts during each breath. The inspiratory flow tracing appears above the isometric line, displaying the positive flow, while the expiratory flow tracing appears below the isometric line, displaying the negative flow. Observing this flow scale can give the CCTP visual clues needed to detect air trapping or auto-PEEP. If the expiratory flow tracing does not return to the isometric line (baseline) before the next breath is initiated, then the CCTP should suspect air trapping and undertake further investigation to correct this situation (see Figure 7-15). The patient's lung history is always the first place to start the investigation.

As always, it is prudent to check the patient, first looking for specific reasons for air trapping, including tachypnea, anxiety, pain, bronchospasm, excessive secretions, and improper ventilator mode and

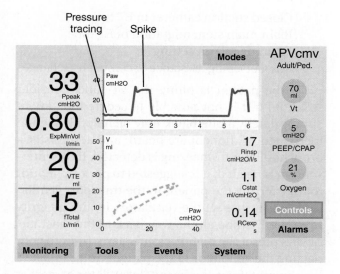

FIGURE 7-20 An initial spike at the peak inspiratory pressure may indicate too much flow is being delivered, causing a turbulent flow situation.

Courtesy of Vent-Pro Training.

settings. The pressure time scalar can be studied to detect the breath going in too fast by observing the slope of the breath in the initial milliseconds. An initial spike at the PIP may indicate too much flow is being delivered, causing a turbulent flow situation **FIGURE 7-20**. This setting may be fine-tuned by slightly increasing the inspiratory time in a volume-targeted breath or increasing the rise time or P-ramp in a pressure-targeted breath.

Troubleshooting and Diagnosing Ventilator Problems

Troubleshooting ventilator function is not as difficult as it might seem. First, it is imperative that the CCT team carry a bag-mask device for every patient on a ventilator. If any doubts about ventilator function arise, use the bag-mask device to ensure the patient's safety. A good rule of thumb when troubleshooting equipment is to start at the patient and work methodically toward the equipment or power source.

Patient Not Tolerating the Change From the Hospital Ventilator to the Transport Ventilator

This problem is a frequent occurrence in the alert and awake patient. The two ventilators may deliver the flow in different patterns, which may feel uncomfortable to the patient. To avoid this problem, match the settings of the hospital ventilator as closely as possible, provided they are oxygenating and ventilating the patient with the lowest amount of risk to the patient's lungs.

The most common settings to match are pressure or volume target, mode, tidal volume or pressure, respiratory rate, PEEP, and F_{IO_2}. A frequently overlooked setting is the patient's inspiratory time or I:E ratio, which plays a major role in what the patient feels upon transfer. It may be difficult to find these settings on the ventilator without going deep into the settings menu. If you are unsure of the inspiratory time or I:E ratio, consult the respiratory therapist who is caring for the patient.

Prior to switching to the transport ventilator, describe the process to the patient and explain that the transport ventilator may feel different. Always assure the patient you will adjust the ventilator to make them comfortable. When you first connect the ventilator to the patient, the time it takes to reach the set volume or set pressure will vary. The machine needs to determine which pressures to apply to the patient's lungs to deliver the target volumes. Making these adjustments may take five to six breaths in some cases. The patient may experience some anxiety during this brief period, but coaching the patient may help relieve any discomfort.

If the patient appears air hungry, then adjustments may be necessary. In a volume-targeted breath, the flow may be set too low for the patient's demand. An obvious adjustment is to increase the target tidal volume, although this strategy has some limitations. The target tidal volume should be 6 to 8 mL/kg of PBW, and PIP should be limited to less than 30 cm H_2O, if possible. The next adjustment in a volume-targeted breath might be to decrease the inspiratory time to increase the fixed flow. Small increments of 0.1 second are recommended while monitoring the patient's response and PIP levels, as decreasing the inspiratory time may cause the pressure to rise.

Another strategy to increase flow to the air-hungry patient would be to change to a pressure-targeted breath. This method typically uses a decelerating flow pattern that reaches the desired pressure quickly. If you are switching from a volume target to a pressure target, note the PIP on the target volume: Do not exceed this pressure. It is important to know how the ventilator delivers the pressure. Most of today's ventilators use a pressure above PEEP (PAP). Therefore, if your PIP in volume-targeted ventilation is 20 cm H_2O and the PEEP is 5 cm H_2O, you would set the PAP at 15 cm H_2O. (PAP plus PEEP equals PIP.) If your ventilator does not set the pressure above PEEP, then you would match the set pressure with the PIP. Often the matched pressure will deliver a larger tidal volume in pressure-delivered breaths. The main concern is to monitor the exhaled tidal volume and titrate the pressure to meet your target tidal volume.

Alarms

When attempting to diagnose and correct a pressure alarm, start by using the DOPE mnemonic:

- **Displacement.** Check for ET tube displacement.
- **Obstruction.** Check the ET tube for any obstruction.
- **Pneumothorax.** Obtain a chest radiograph, observe chest excursion, auscultate the lung fields, and obtain a chest ultrasound.
- **Equipment failure**

High-Pressure Alarm

The high-pressure alarm may be the most important alarm to monitor and trend while caring for the patient on a mechanical ventilator. Typical suggested settings for this alarm, or limit, are 10 cm H_2O above the resting PIP. The high-pressure alarm is designed to prevent the ventilator from delivering pressures that are unfavorable to the specific lungs being ventilated. It is rare to set an alarm above 50 cm H_2O, but this may be necessary when lung compliance is severely diminished.

Following are some of the more common triggers of this alarm:

- Patient biting the ET tube
- Mucus plug
- Pneumothorax
- Bronchospasm
- Excessive secretions
- Patient coughing
- Patient bucking the ventilator
- Air trapping or auto-PEEP
- Circuit kinked
- HME clogged

- Closed suction catheter in ET tube
- Right main stem migration of ET tube
- Improper alarm setting
- Any worsening resistance or compliance changes

If the patient is biting the ET tube, consider sedation. If it is not possible to sedate the patient appropriately, a bite block may be helpful. Suction the patient if rhonchi are heard, and administer a bronchodilator if wheezing is detected. If this intervention is needed, it is suggested to perform it prior to transferring the patient to the transport ventilator. Visually inspect the ventilator circuit's integrity from the ET tube all the way back to the machine. Always preset the high-pressure alarm prior to connecting the ventilator to the patient. You can take a baseline PIP from the hospital ventilator or start at 30 to 35 cm H_2O and titrate accordingly.

Never silence an alarm without evaluating the patient, diagnosing the cause, and remedying the situation.

Low-Pressure Alarm

Most transport ventilators incorporate a low-pressure alarm. The typical setting for this alarm is 5 cm H_2O below the resting PIP. The main reason this alarm activates is a leak in the circuit. Many locations can present with a leak, so it is wise to pressure-check your circuit prior to placing it on the patient. Refer to the ventilator's operator manual for this procedure.

Following are some of the more common triggers for a low-pressure alarm:

- Leak in the ET tube or tracheostomy cuff
- Positional leak in the uncuffed ET or tracheostomy tube
- Open flush port in the closed suction system
- Blown seal in the closed suction catheter
- Cracked HME or removed ETCO$_2$ port cap
- Disconnected flow sensor lines
- Malfunction of the external exhalation valves
- Improvement in the patient's lung compliance

If a leak is detected in the cuff, a decision must be made to either change out the ET or tracheostomy tube or transport the patient with the leak. Both risks and benefits must be considered in regard to changing out the tube, requiring a discussion with medical control. If the team decides to transport the patient with the leak, it might be beneficial to change to a pressure-targeted breath. This method may allow the flow to be manipulated via the rise time or P-ramp to deliver each breath a little more slowly. With a faster flow, the gas will find the path of least resistance and exit through the leak. Always monitor oxygenation and ventilation when a leak is known to be present. Increasing the PEEP slightly may help overcome the leak.

It is rare for the low-pressure alarm to activate because of increased compliance or decreased resistance, but it can happen. This condition may occur following suction or because of the positive effects of a bronchodilator, which would be administered if auscultation reveals wheezing.

Low-Minute-Volume Alarm

The low-minute-volume alarm is typically set at 25% less than the resting minute volume. It essentially monitors the exhaled tidal volume and the respiratory rate. When the alarm is activated, the challenge is detecting which value is causing the alarm. Is it the low tidal volume, the low respiratory rate, or both?

Following are some of the more common triggers for a low minute volume alarm:

- Decrease in the patient's respiratory rate
- Decrease in the patient's expired tidal volume
- Leak in the system

If the transport ventilator is delivering a volume-targeted breath, then the baseline minute volume is set by that volume and the respiratory rate. If you set the low-minute-volume alarm at 25% below that minute volume, the alarm will activate only if there is a leak in the system.

This alarm becomes extremely important when you are delivering a pressure-targeted breath. In this situation, the exhaled tidal volume varies with lung compliance and resistance, and any decrease in exhaled volume will affect the low-minute-volume alarm. In a pressure-delivered breath, this alarm should be set to detect any changes in lung volumes.

The low-minute-volume alarm is also extremely important when caring for a patient on straight pressure support ventilation. In this mode, there is no set respiratory rate or set tidal volume. Instead, there is just a pressure that acts as a "boost" breath to help the patient breathe. The tidal volumes and rate can vary greatly in this mode.

Apnea Backup Ventilation

The apnea backup alarm is designed to deliver a breath when a specific time interval is reached to detect a patient breath. If the ventilator does not detect a patient trigger to breathe, the ventilator will automatically deliver a preset or user-set breath. It is imperative to know how the apnea backup alarm delivers a breath and at what time interval it should be set. Typically, the default time interval is 20 seconds. The type of breath that is delivered may vary from machine to machine. Do not set up a patient on a ventilator without ensuring the apnea backup alarm is set properly for that patient.

Following are common triggers for an apnea alarm:

- Ventilator not detecting a time-set breath by the patient
- Sensitivity setting too high, not allowing the patient to trigger a breath
- Patient stopped breathing spontaneously

Low-Battery Alarm

Like oxygen cylinder duration, battery duration is an important factor when planning for a transport. Many variables can affect battery life, including the battery's age, the air temperature, hours of use, the ventilator settings, and the F_{IO_2} settings. Refer to the operations manual for recommendations for, and limitations of, the ventilator's battery.

This is a high-priority alarm. Best practice is to plug the ventilator into its primary power source whenever possible, rather than relying on battery power.

High/Low-Frequency Alarm

This alarm is set to trigger when the patient's respiratory rate exceeds or falls below the set levels. The provider determines the alarm settings based on the patient's overall condition.

Following are common triggers for the high/low-frequency alarm:

- Apnea
- Agitation, anxiety, or pain
- Tachypnea
- Metabolic acidosis
- Kussmaul breathing

Consider the mode the patient is currently on. It may be necessary to adjust the default settings around the patient's baseline respiratory rate. The target tidal volume, inspiratory time, and PEEP may require adjustment.

Disconnection Alarm (Disconnect Sensor)

If this alarm triggers, inspect the circuit integrity while looking for any disconnection and leaks within the entire circuit. This inspection should be accomplished within 5 seconds. Start with the pressure at the ET tube cuff, as low pressure could trigger a disconnection alarm. Other alarms that will subsequently be triggered are the low-minute-volume alarm and the low-pressure alarm.

Oxygen Supply Failed Alarm (Low O₂ Pressure, Low O₂ Supply)

This alarm is triggered when the ventilator does not detect a specific pressure at the oxygen inlet port. Typically, transport ventilators are connected to a 50-psi source of oxygen. When the pressure drops below 35 psi, an alarm will sound, alerting the user to this extremely dangerous situation.

The most common reason that this alarm activates is failure to properly calculate oxygen consumption for the mission. Other reasons including the following problems:

- Oxygen tank valve off
- Oxygen hose not fully connected
- Oxygen tank <200 psi

Names for this alarm may vary among ventilators, so learn your specific ventilator's verbiage.

High-PEEP Alarm

This alarm activates when the PEEP level exceeds the preset PEEP level. Most ventilators have a default setting and allow adjustments to the value.

The most common trigger for this alarm is patient air trapping (auto-PEEP). Diagnosing the root cause of this auto-PEEP can be quite a challenge. First, consider the patient's lung condition. Typically, patients with an obstructive lung disease are susceptible to air trapping. Confirm that the ventilator mode, flow target, and settings are the optimal choices for this patient. Optimize the lungs'

function prior to transport by performing suction and administering bronchodilators, if necessary.

Another cause of air trapping may be an in-line filter or HME in which excessive secretions are restricting airflow within the circuit. In such a case, immediately replace these filters with new filters.

It is also common for patients who have been liberated from sedation to become anxious during the transfer from hospital ventilator to transport ventilator. If the patient becomes tachypneic, the I:E ratio changes drastically. Depending on the ventilator mode, this response can create auto-PEEP. You may need to discuss other options to diminish the risk of high PEEP levels.

Low-PEEP Alarm

This alarm detects a PEEP level that has fallen below the preset PEEP. Most ventilators have a default setting that may be adjusted by the user.

The most common reason this alarm activates is a disconnect in the circuit or a faulty exhalation valve that is unable to maintain the set PEEP level. Performing another circuit pressure test should help detect any defect within the circuit.

A less common, but often overlooked cause is an air-hungry patient who is sucking air through the circuit beyond the flow delivered, causing the low-PEEP alarm to activate. It may be necessary to adjust the ventilator settings to accommodate this flow demand. Some patients do well with a pressure-targeted breath and appropriate targeted tidal volumes. Check the sensitivity setting and adjust it to allow the patient to trigger a breath with less effort.

Troubleshooting and Diagnosing the Complicated Problem

When transporting the critically ill patient, a few considerations should be prerequisites before launching the mission. First, the CCTP must have a thorough understanding of the transport ventilator's operation. The CCTP should demonstrate proficiency in its use and application to patients with various disease processes on a regular basis through hands-on experience in a ventilator laboratory. The pre-use ventilator and circuit check should always be performed prior to patient application to ensure ventilator and circuit integrity. This is where many malfunctions occur.

Second, the CCTP must be familiar with the ventilator's specifications and ability to meet the specific patient's respiratory demands. Not all transport ventilators can deliver the same flow rates to meet the targets set by the CCTP.

Third, the CCTP must account for the patient's current lung condition and how that condition might change during transport. Consider the length of transport, altitude, temperature, gravitational forces, and vibration when planning the mission. Discussing a strategy for any unforeseen problems ahead of time is a good idea.

Finally, the CCTP must calculate the anticipated oxygen consumption and verify there is enough oxygen on board to meet this demand.

Patient Appears Dyssynchronous With the Ventilator

The patient's level of pain and anxiety must be addressed before attempting to adjust the ventilator settings. Clear the airways of secretions and auscultate lung fields for any bronchospasm; administer bronchodilators, if needed, prior to beginning the transfer if possible. It is important to correct this conflict with the breathing pattern because it will increase the patient's work of breathing, increase the oxygen demand, and complicate any intracranial pressure concerns.

As discussed previously, if you are transferring the patient from the hospital ventilator to the transport ventilator, try to match the current settings, provided the oxygenation and ventilation status meet your target goals, with the monitored values within normal limits. If possible, explain to the patient that the transition to the transport ventilator will feel different and that you may make some adjustments to make them comfortable. A common complaint is patients feeling as if they are not getting enough air. This perception is often related to setting a volume-targeted breath with a fixed flow, which may be less than the hospital ventilator's flow.

Missed Triggering

When setting up the ventilator, pay close attention to the sensitivity setting. If this setting is too high (not sensitive enough), some patients may have difficulty triggering a breath. The patient population of greatest concern includes patients with myasthenia gravis, Guillain-Barré syndrome, paralyzed diaphragm, or any disorder that weakens the patient's ability to create a negative flow or pressure to trigger the ventilator. If the sensitivity level is set too low (overly sensitive), this may contribute to autotriggering or autocycling. In this situation, a stimulus other than the patient's effort triggers the ventilator to deliver a breath. Some common causes of these ominous breaths are excessive secretions in the lungs or circuit, cardiac oscillations, and abrupt motion in transit. An incorrect sensitivity setting may cause asynchrony between the patient and the ventilator. If possible, obtain the sensitivity setting from the hospital ventilator.

Another missed triggering scenario may stem from an uncuffed tracheostomy or ET tube, or even a cuff, that fails to hold pressure. As a result, the patient cannot create enough flow or pressure to signal the ventilator to trigger a breath. If the leak cannot be corrected during transport, then adjusting the sensitivity may help with patient–ventilator synchrony. If a leak in the system is causing autotriggering, one solution is to slowly increase the sensitivity (in flow sensing) to overcome the leak. Watch carefully to determine when the autotriggering stops, and then add another 2 or 3 L/min of flow to the sensitivity. If the autotriggering stops at 6 L/min and you add 2 L/min, the total sensitivity setting would be 8 L/min and the patient could theoretically trigger a breath with a minus 2 L/min inhalation.

A patient who is asynchronous with the ventilator is typically tachypneic and at risk for auto-PEEP. This can be confirmed if your equipment allows for an expiratory hold or displays an estimate of auto-PEEP; alternatively, you can visually detect auto-PEEP on a flow scalar tracing (see Figure 7-15). Another reason to suspect auto-PEEP is an increase in PIP and large discrepancies of more than 75 to 100 mL of exhaled tidal volume.

Double Triggering

Double triggering is loosely defined as two ventilator-delivered breaths with one patient inspiratory effort. It is most commonly attributed to a mismatch in the set inspiratory time on the ventilator and the patient's neural inspiratory times. Such a mismatch usually reflects a short inspiratory time in a fixed-flow, volume-targeted ventilation mode. Although it may be difficult to match the patient's neural inspiratory time, it may be beneficial to slowly increase the I time on the ventilator and observe the patient's response. Always monitor the I:E ratio when making adjustments to the I time or respiratory rate, and consider the patient's lung condition and the potential for causing auto-PEEP. Another suggested strategy is to switch to a pressure-targeted breath, as the flow will vary depending on patient demand, and possibly to increase the pressure to meet target exhaled tidal volumes.

Transporting the Patient With a Tracheostomy

As a CCTP, you may be dispatched to transport a patient with a tracheostomy. Patients may have tracheostomies for many reasons, including the following:

- Congenital anomalies of the airway
- Laryngectomy
- Tumors
- Tracheomalacia
- Subglottic stenosis
- Vocal cord paralysis
- Upper airway burns
- Obstructive sleep apnea
- Diaphragm dysfunction
- COPD-related reduction of dead space
- Severe facial or neck trauma
- Neuromuscular disease with paralysis
- Spinal cord injury
- Failure to wean from the ventilator
- Anaphylaxis

It is important to be familiar with your agency's specific guidelines for caring for this patient population. The biggest challenge is identifying the type of tracheostomy tube in place **FIGURE 7-21A**. If the patient is breathing spontaneously and not ventilator dependent, the tracheostomy tube in place is unlikely to connect well to a bag-mask device in the event of an emergency. Your first priority is ensuring you have a way to manually ventilate the patient, should the need arise.

The next concern is determining the amount of oxygen and humidification the patient will require during the transport. For the nonventilated patient,

specific devices are available that can deliver oxygen and some form of heat and humidification during transport. When preparing for the transport, confirm the portable device will meet the patient's needs and match their F_{IO_2} requirements. Assessing the patient's breath sounds and having the ability to perform deep suctioning of the lungs are extremely important as well. The latter skill needs to be mastered to effectively care for a patient with a tracheostomy. Excessive secretions are common in this patient population, and without humidification and frequent suctioning, mucus plugging is an unwelcome risk. When a tracheostomy is in place, the body's natural heat and humidification system is also bypassed.

Some patients with a tracheostomy may use a speaking valve that allows them to talk **FIGURE 7-21B**. This one-way valve is placed on the end of the inner cannula to allow air into the lungs during inhalation; it closes on exhalation, allowing air to exit past the vocal cords so the patient can speak. If the patient has a cuffed tracheostomy tube, it is imperative to deflate the cuff before placing the speaking valve. Devices often used to provide low-flow oxygen to the patient with a tracheostomy include the tracheostomy collar, a T-piece with in-line suction, and a T-HME with oxygen port.

Gather as much information about the patient's tracheostomy tube as possible. When was the tube placed? Why was the tube placed? Did any complications occur during the procedure? Was it a surgical or percutaneous procedure? Are there any barriers to endotracheal intubation? What size is the tracheostomy tube?

When transporting a patient with a tracheostomy on a ventilator, many issues must be considered before transferring the patient to the transport ventilator. The first concern is the transport ventilator's ability to match the patient's current ventilatory support. The conventional settings applied in the ICU are not always the same as the those used in the long-term acute care setting. If the patient is currently on a home care ventilator, it may be beneficial to leave them on that ventilator if possible. The major benefit of this strategy is that the patient is familiar with this ventilator, so they will feel a difference in the flow delivered with the transport ventilator. The disadvantage of this plan is the CCTP may not be familiar with the home ventilator and

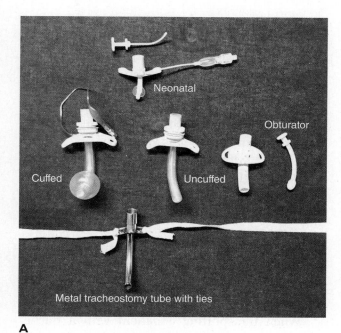

A

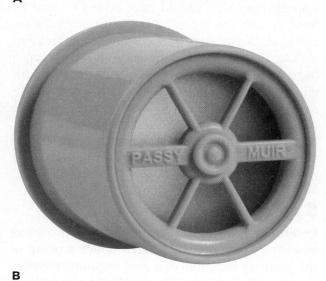

B

FIGURE 7-21 A. Tracheostomy tubes. **B.** Speaking valve.

A: Courtesy of Vent-Pro Training; B: Image courtesy of Passy-Muir, Inc. Irvine, CA.

may have difficulty troubleshooting any potential issues that arise.

When setting up the transport ventilator, the obvious settings to focus on are the mode, respiratory rate, target tidal volume, PEEP, and FIO₂. Often-overlooked settings include the flow targets of a pressure or a volume. Other settings of great importance are the inspiratory time and the sensitivity setting to trigger a breath. This is where the patient

will feel a difference in ventilators and why it is so important to try to match these settings. When fine-tuning the flow, note whether the two ventilators can adjust the rise time (P-ramp) and flow termination (expiratory trigger sensitivity). These features determine how the flow is initially delivered and when it terminates. Discussing these and any other concerns with the respiratory therapist would be extremely helpful to assure the patient's safety and comfort needs before transport. Note that some ventilator rehabilitation facilities may use tidal volumes of 20 mL/kg of PBW during the weaning process. In these cases, a discussion with medical control is advised.

An uncuffed tracheostomy tube or defective cuff can definitely present challenges to the CCTP. When positive pressure is applied to an uncuffed tracheostomy tube, the gas supplied to the lungs will follow the path of least resistance. Therefore, a leak caused by the uncuffed tracheostomy creates a major challenge in delivering the desired volume or pressure to the lungs. This leak may have a positional component, such that any movement of the tracheostomy tube or the patient's neck alters the size of the leak.

If it is not advisable to change out the tracheostomy tube for a cuffed version, then some alternative strategies may be helpful. Some transport ventilators provide a leak-compensation feature that can detect a stable leak and make adjustments to compensate for it. As discussed previously, a leak may create autocycling, a condition in which the ventilator delivers unwanted breaths because the leak is triggering the machine to send a breath. The sensitivity setting can be adjusted to prevent autocycling. Another strategy for dealing with a leak in the system is to perform a trial of pressure-targeted breaths. Most machines allow for manipulation of the flow delivered in a pressure target, and titrating the time the flow is delivered and terminated may prove helpful.

It is mandatory that certain items be transported with the patient. A spare tracheostomy tube and securing device of the same size should be readily available at the head of the bed in case of an emergency. If possible, a spare inner cannulas should be available as well. Appropriate-size suction catheters should be provided for deep suctioning, along with a bag-mask device. An in-line suction catheter is recommended for deep suctioning, as it eliminates the need to disconnect the circuit. Specific-size in-line catheters are available to accommodate the shorter distance needed to suction the patient with a tracheostomy. Saline flush should be used to clean the catheter after suctioning.

It is important to secure the ventilator circuit to minimize any movement that might jostle the tracheostomy tube, potentially causing a cough reflex from the patient. Devices are available that can minimize the movement of the circuit, such as flex tube adapters. Although they can make it difficult to pass a suction catheter and will add some minimal dead space to the circuit, they are still commonly used within the ventilator circuit.

Tracheostomy tube displacement is uncommon but can be fatal. The first concern is recognizing the displaced tube. Because of the dynamic nature of the transport arena, the CCTP must always ensure the tracheostomy tube is secured. If the tube becomes dislodged, an immediate assessment of the patient's respiratory status is key in deciding whether to reinsert the tube or to implement a trial of decannulation. If the patient is breathing spontaneously and needs supplemental oxygen, a nonrebreathing mask may be placed over the stoma. If the tube needs to be reinserted, it is important to evaluate the condition of the patient's stoma. If the patient has received a percutaneous tracheostomy within 14 days of an accidental decannulation, it may be necessary to orotracheally intubate the patient due to the smaller stoma size associated with this procedure. Additional concerns arise with a more recently placed (within 1 week) surgical tracheostomy tube, as the tracheal stoma is not suitably formed and may present complications during reinsertion.

Having a worst-case scenario plan in place is advisable when transporting any patient. Patients with a tracheostomy are no exception, even though they have a definitive airway in place. Replacing a dislodged tracheostomy tube presents many challenges, which may be minimized with some diligent pretransport planning. Placing the tube in a false tract/passage occurs when the tube is inadvertently inserted through the cutaneous stoma but not through the tracheal lumen. A properly placed tracheostomy tube is a clear passage through both the cutaneous stoma and the tracheal lumen. When a false passage is formed and positive pressure is applied, the patient will be in respiratory distress and signs of subcutaneous emphysema will develop. Once this condition is recognized, the tube should be removed immediately and ventilation achieved through alternative means.

The following factors increase the risk for dislodgement of the tracheostomy tube:

- Morbid obesity
- Edema of the neck
- Excessive coughing
- Improper fit of the tracheostomy tube
- Patient anxiety and pulling at the tube
- Ventilator circuit tension
- Loose tracheostomy tube ties

When transporting a patient with a tracheostomy, the CCTP should have access to (and be familiar with the use of) a tracheostomy tube securing device, a spare tracheostomy tube, an inner canula, an obturator, a bougie/Cook catheter, a bag-valve device, and all equipment necessary for endotracheal intubation. More advanced equipment would include a stoma dilator and a portable bronchoscope. Although the likelihood of tracheostomy tube dislodgement may be minimal, training for and awareness of such an event must not be overlooked.

Summary

Determining the need for and means of providing ventilatory support requires an understanding of the patient's lung function and respiratory needs. You must be familiar with any device you will use during patient transport. Gaining competence with each device may require special training and consultation with specialists, including respiratory therapists and other clinicians working with the patient at the sending facility. Before using any complicated and potentially unfamiliar device, review the guidelines provided in the device's operating manual and consult other providers, including medical control.

Concepts such as tidal volume, minute volume, and anatomic dead space are crucial to understanding respiratory function and monitoring the patient's condition, as are a variety of devices and laboratory studies. ABG analysis, if available, will reveal the acid–base balance and blood levels of oxygen and CO_2. Pulse oximetry, capnography, and $ETCO_2$ detection offer a continuous, noninvasive means of measuring these gases during transport.

Transport of the critically ill patient who is receiving ventilation must be planned carefully to ensure patient safety. First, the CCTP should be familiar with the capabilities of the ventilator and should always have a bag-mask device on hand in case of malfunction. Prepare for the transport by confirming the presence of an adequate power and oxygen supply.

Second, the CCTP should know why the patient is being ventilated and what the settings are prior to transport. Obtain baseline assessment parameters for the patient and the ventilator before beginning the transport. Continue to monitor ventilator performance and patient response during the transport. Always have continuous pulse oximetry and waveform capnography in place.

Last, the CCTP should repeat these assessments upon arrival at the destination facility. Verify and document airway patency, respiratory assessment, and parameters at the time of transfer. When these guidelines are followed, the transport should be a safe one for the CCTP and the patient.

Case Study

Your team is dispatched to a rural hospital to transport a patient to a higher level of care. The receiving hospital is 135 miles (214 km) from the sending facility. Incoming weather conditions rule out transport by rotor aircraft, so your team will be transporting the patient by ground. The estimated time for the transport is 2 hours and 10 minutes. The patient is in the ICU and being mechanically ventilated.

On arrival to the ICU, your partner begins to obtain pertinent information regarding the patient's condition while you assess the patient. The patient is a 59-year-old man who weighs 216 pounds (98 kg) and is 73 inches (185 cm) tall. He came to the emergency department (ED) 3 days ago because he was having difficulty breathing and feeling lethargic. The patient has diabetes mellitus type 1 and an extensive smoking history (50 pack-years) but quit 1 year ago. The patient was quickly placed on a nonrebreathing mask; his oxygen saturation readings are in the mid-80s with a good waveform. Vital signs are heart rate, 89 beats/min, normal sinus rhythm; respiratory rate, 28 breaths/min, labored; blood pressure, 139/85 mm Hg, 103 mean; SpO_2, 84%; and temperature, 100.1°F (38.3°C).

The patient was moved to a negative-pressure room and placed on airborne precautions. A nasopharyngeal swab was sent to the lab and subsequently came back with a positive result for COVID-19. The patient was placed on an oxypendant nasal cannula reservoir device at 8 L/min and was encouraged to self-prone for increased $\dot{V}/\dot{Q}$ matching. Unfortunately, the patient was unable to tolerate proning.

The next strategy to aid in this hypoxic situation was HFNC therapy at 60 L/min and FIO_2 of 1.0. An ABG was drawn 1 hour after implementation of HFNC therapy, and a chest radiograph was taken. The ABG revealed pH, 7.21; $PaCO_2$, 51 mm Hg; PaO_2, 81 mm Hg; HcO_3, 30 mEq/L; and calculated saturation, 84%. The chest radiograph revealed bilateral patchy infiltrates with a ground-glass appearance.

Because of the patient's worsening respiratory status, the ED team placed him on a BPAP trial for 1 hour with a starting pressure of 15 cm H_2O of IPAP and 8 cm H_2O of EPAP with a full-face mask. The patient was unable to tolerate the BPAP despite multiple adjustments to improve comfort. Another ABG analysis showed no improvement in oxygenation, so the ED team prepared to intubate the patient because his condition was heading toward respiratory failure.

The patient was intubated with direct laryngoscopy on the first attempt using rapid sequence intubation. A #7 ET tube was placed in the trachea and anchored at 26 cm at the lip. Confirmation of its correct placement was made with capnography and a good waveform present with an $ETCO_2$ reading of 47 mm Hg. Another chest radiograph is pending. Mechanical ventilation was initiated with the following settings: assist/control rate, 14 breaths/min; tidal volume, 700 mL; PEEP, 5 cm H_2O; FIO_2, 1.0. The monitored values on the ventilator read as follows: PIP, 38 cm H_2O; plateau pressure, 34; total respiratory rate, 25 breaths/min; exhaled tidal volume, 600–760 mL, fluctuating; PEEP 5 cm H_2O; minute volume, 14.9 L/min. Breath sounds are diminished on the left side of the patient's chest and clear on the right side, with asymmetric chest excursion.

1. Was the patient managed appropriately on admission in the ED?
2. Do the initial impression, interventions, and lab values lead you to a diagnosis and treatment plan?
3. Was the ET tube size and depth appropriate for this patient?
4. Are the ventilator settings appropriate for this patient?
5. Do the monitored values raise any concerns?

The chest radiograph revealed a right main stem intubation, so the ET tube was withdrawn 5 cm and resecured at 22 cm at the lip. The PIP decreased to 27 cm H_2O, breath sounds were equal, and good chest excursion was present. The patient was given fentanyl 50 mcg and propofol infusion of 20 mcg/kg/min and admitted to the ICU.

You arrive at bedside. During your initial assessment, you note the patient's vital signs are heart rate, 118 beats/min; respiratory rate 23 breaths/min; blood pressure 129/68 mm Hg, 88 mean; and SpO_2, 84%. The patient is currently on a dexmedetomidine drip at 0.2 mcg/kg/h for sedation. The patient has also received dexamethasone and remdesivir since being admitted to the ICU. Breath sounds are equal but diminished throughout. Good chest excursion is noted. The hospital ventilator settings are assist/control rate, 18 breaths/min; tidal volume, 650 mL; PEEP, 8 cm H_2O; and FIO_2, 1.0. Monitored values are PIP, 35 cm H_2O; plateau pressure, 31; total respiratory rate, 25 breaths/min; exhaled tidal volume, 655 mL; PEEP, 8 cm H_2O; and minute volume, 16 L/min. A chest radiograph performed 3 hours ago reveals worsening bilateral pulmonary infiltrates. An ABG sample obtained 6 hours ago reveals pH,

7.31; $PaCO_2$, 29 mm Hg; PaO_2, 67 mm Hg; HCO_3^-, 21 mEq/L; and calculated saturation, 86%.

6. Is the sedation dose adequate for this patient?
7. Are the ventilator settings appropriate for this patient?
8. Is there a specific strategy this patient qualifies for?
9. Is there another mode of ventilation that might better oxygenate this patient?

Based on the Berlin definition of ARDS, this patient has severe ARDS:

- Onset within 1 week of a known insult or of new or worsening respiratory symptoms
- Imaging: Bilateral opacities not fully explained by effusions, lobar or lung collapse, or nodules
- Origin of edema: Respiratory failure not fully explained by heart failure or fluid overload
- PaO_2:FIO_2 ratio of 67 (PaO_2 from the most recent ABG analysis is 67 on an FIO_2 of 1.0.)

At this point, you and your partner decide to call medical control to discuss a strategy for transporting this patient because of the refractory hypoxia. Based on the ABG results and the clinical diagnosis of ARDS with an underlying COVID-19 condition, the recommended strategy is to follow the ARDS Network's protocol. The first adjustment to consider is the target tidal volume and the measured plateau pressure. The patient is 73 inches (185 cm) tall and male, so the PBW is calculated as 176 pounds (80 kg). Following the ARDS Network's protocol, you could try using the 6 mL/kg of PBW for a tidal volume of 480 mL, titrating it lower if needed. Another strategy to address the hypoxia condition is to raise the PEEP to inflate the alveoli for better oxygenation. This increase in PEEP should be done in small increments and monitored for the desired results.

After consulting with medical control, the hospital's ED physician, and the respiratory therapist, it was decided to make some changes to the ventilator settings. The adjusted settings are assist/control rate, 18 breaths/min; tidal volume, 480 mL; PEEP, 12 cm H_2O; and FIO_2, 1.0. The dexmedetomidine dosage was increased because the patient was overbreathing at the ventilator's set rate. The monitored values from the new settings are

PIP, 30 cm H_2O; plateau, 27; total respiratory rate, 19 breaths/min; exhaled tidal volume, 469 mL; PEEP, 12 cm H_2O; and minute volume, 9.1 L/min. An ABG was drawn an hour after the changes were made and the following results obtained: pH, 7.29; $Paco_2$, 55 mm Hg; Pao_2, 121 mm Hg; HCO_3^-, 22 mEq/L; and calculated saturation, 91%.

A major goal in any patient who is being mechanically ventilated is to keep plateau pressures at less than 30 cm H_2O. Another goal is to keep driving pressures (plateau – PEEP) at less than 15 cm H_2O. In this case, the driving pressure is 15 cm H_2O (plateau 27 – PEEP 12 = 15).

To be on the safe side during transport, lowering the tidal volume to 450 mL might be beneficial as part of the lung-protective strategy.

Another consideration is oxygen consumption. The patient is on an Fio_2 of 1.0 with a set minute volume of 9 L/min that can change with spontaneous patient breaths. Some ventilators may calculate oxygen consumption along with the bias flow provided on exhalation.

Another potential strategy for ventilating this particular patient would be APRV. Transport ventilator manufacturers are adding this mode to the menu to match the hospital ventilator modes and help transport patients with complicated respiratory conditions.

Analysis

The patient was managed appropriately on admission to the ED. Attempting to correct the hypoxic presentation and respiratory distress with supplemental oxygen, HFNC therapy, and non-invasive ventilation was an appropriate first-line strategy to address the respiratory issues. Self-proning was attempted but not tolerated well by the patient. The ED team decided to intubate the patient and begin mechanical ventilation before respiratory failure became apparent. The initial diagnosis leaned toward COVID-19 pneumonia with ARDS.

The ET tube may have been small for someone this size, adding some airway resistance, and was inadvertently placed too deeply initially. The initial ventilator settings were aggressive and were based on the patient's actual weight, not the PBW. The plateau pressure was high, at 34 cm H_2O, and the tidal volume should have been corrected prior to the ICU admission. The feedback from the ventilator following the patient's initial intubation contains valuable information that should give the clinician an indication of how the lungs are responding to the positive-pressure breaths delivered by the ventilator.

This patient did not appear to be adequately sedated, as the total breath rate was initially 25 breaths/min. The driving pressure was 29 cm H_2O initially, almost double the target driving pressure of 15 cm H_2O. The other major concern was the lack of PEEP in the presence of hypoxia on an Fio_2 of 1.0. The ARDS Network's protocol could have been instituted earlier in the course of this patient's treatment. The backup plan would have been to use APRV mode to recruit more alveoli if possible. The next option might have been ECMO.

Prep Kit

Ready for Review

- Mechanical ventilation entails the use of a machine to provide ventilatory support. Indications for mechanical ventilation include managing the work of breathing, improving distribution of inhaled gases, protecting the airway, and managing conditions such as apnea and ventilatory or respiratory failure.

- The CCTP must understand common respiratory terminology, including dead

Prep Kit Continued

space ventilation, alveolar-to-arterial oxygen (A-a) gradient, ventilation-perfusion ($\dot{V}/\dot{Q}$) mismatch, and minute volume.

- All ventilators have several characteristics in common, including the use of a power source, cycling, breath delivery, parameters, circuitry and interface, and alarms. Not all ventilators have the same parameters available for adjustment, nor do all ventilators have the same range of features. Specifically, not all transport ventilators compensate for altitude changes.

- Normal ventilation is negative-pressure ventilation. Negative pressure pulls the diaphragm down, causing the lungs to fill. When the pressure is released, the diaphragm relaxes and the lungs empty.

- In positive-pressure ventilation, air is pushed into the respiratory tract. Positive-pressure ventilators are often described in terms of which variable terminates the inspiratory phase of the breath, such as pressure ventilators, volume ventilators, flow-cycled ventilators, and time-cycled ventilators.

- It is important to understand the changes that occur when a positive-pressure system is applied to a negative-pressure system.

- Conventional ventilation requires invasive ventilation by placing an artificial airway, chiefly the endotracheal tube.

- Noninvasive ventilation is any form of mechanical ventilation without an artificial airway, but includes other devices such as continuous positive airway pressure and bilevel positive airway pressure, which use nasal or full-face masks to deliver a certain pressure to the lungs during spontaneous breathing.

- When caring for the acutely hypoxic patient, it is common practice to place the patient on supplemental oxygen via a nasal cannula with liter flows ranging from 1 to 6 L/min, referred to as a low-flow nasal cannula. A high-flow nasal cannula enables more comfortable delivery and a more precise fraction of inspired oxygen (FIO_2) target. The high flows required to support this modality present a challenge during transport, requiring careful pretransport planning by the CCTP.

- Volume and pressure are flow targets that are set for the ventilator to end the inspiratory cycle.

- Ventilator modes describe which types of breaths are being delivered to the patient— that is, whether the breath is a mandatory or machine breath or a spontaneous breath. Ventilator parameters refer to the other settings that may be adjusted and should be monitored continuously by the clinician.
  - Modes include control (or continuous) manual ventilation, assist/control ventilation, synchronized intermittent mandatory ventilation, pressure control ventilation, pressure-regulated volume control ventilation, inverse-ratio ventilation, pressure support, continuous positive airway pressure, bilevel positive airway pressure, airway pressure release ventilation, and adaptive support ventilation.
  - Parameters include tidal volume, respiratory rate, fraction of inspired oxygen, peak flow, inspiratory time, peak inspiratory pressure, driving pressure, inspiratory plateau pressure, percentage of minute volume, low-pressure alarm, high-pressure alarm, and low-battery alarm.

- Positive end-expiratory pressure (PEEP) occurs at the end of a mandatory machine breath. Instead of exhaling back to ambient pressure, the ventilator stops the exhalation at a prescribed pressure, which results in an increase in the air in the alveoli, thereby increasing the functional residual capacity, facilitating gas exchange, and improving oxygenation. PEEP may also improve lung compliance when the clinician finds the optimal ventilator setting for the patient's particular lung disease.

- Inhaled gases with which the CCTP must be familiar include nitric oxide, epoprostenol, and heliox.

Prep Kit Continued

- The CCTP must recognize and guard against the progression from respiratory distress to respiratory failure. Respiratory distress is a medical emergency that demands immediate treatment. Signs and symptoms include tachypnea, tachycardia, increased anxiety, increased work of breathing, and pallor. Respiratory failure is a medical emergency that may present initially as respiratory distress, but signs and symptoms worsen into cyanosis, hypercapnia, hypoxia, bradycardia, fatigue, shallow breathing, and loss of consciousness.
- During patient transport, few ventilator changes generally need to be made, except for adjustments of F_{IO_2} to accommodate changes in oxygenation. The CCTP is responsible for ensuring proper ventilator function and keeping the patient's ventilatory status stable.
- The CCTP must understand the difference between volume-delivered breaths and pressure-delivered breaths. In volume-delivered breaths, the flow available to the patient is limited to the set (dialed-in) tidal volume and the inspiratory time, although some minor adjustments can be made to increase the flow. In pressure-delivered breaths, the pressure is set and the flow available to the patient is unlimited—at least up to the ventilator's maximum flow capabilities.
- The approaches to mechanical ventilation vary by the lung disease or condition being treated. Common conditions for which mechanical ventilation may be used include acute respiratory distress syndrome, chronic obstructive pulmonary disease, pneumonia, pulmonary fibrosis, asthma, and congestive heart failure.
- The CCTP's goal is to transport the patient from one place to another in the safest manner possible while doing no harm. During transport, it is crucial to monitor the patient's measured values on the ventilator, including peak inspiratory pressure, respiratory rate, exhaled tidal volume, and I:E ratio.
- Heat moisture exchangers and bacterial/viral filters will help ensure the patient's airway remains warm and humidified during transport, but can become dangerous to the patient if allowed to fill with secretions. The CCTP must understand how these devices work and how to keep them working properly.
- Ventilators in the ICU display various waveforms in the form of scalars and loops; these displays represent a great point-of-care tool for the clinician who has the formal education to interpret the information.
- The CCTP should be able to troubleshoot ventilator function, and a bag-mask device should accompany every patient who is transported while on a ventilator.

Vital Vocabulary

anatomic dead space Space in airway structures such as the trachea, bronchi, and bronchioles that does not participate in gas exchange. It is defined physiologically as ventilation without perfusion.

arterial blood gas (ABG) Analysis of the following characteristics of blood: pH, partial pressure of carbon dioxide (in arterial blood), partial pressure of oxygen (in arterial blood), concentration of bicarbonate ion, base excess (indicating whether the patient is acidotic or alkalotic), and oxygen saturation of the hemoglobin molecule.

auto-PEEP The nonintended increase in end alveolar pressure due to air trapping.

barotrauma Injury to the chest or lungs as a result of increased intrathoracic pressure.

bilevel positive airway pressure (BPAP) The use of inspiratory positive airway pressure and expiratory positive airway pressure to raise the breathing baseline above the ambient pressure.

Prep Kit Continued

The pressure gradient enhances ventilation, and the reduced expiratory pressure makes exhalation easier and increases patient tolerance.

continuous positive airway pressure (CPAP) A means of raising the breathing baseline above the ambient pressure. The increased pressure across the entire breathing cycle increases the mean airway pressure, stents the airway, and increases the functional residual capacity, thereby improving oxygenation.

flow-cycled ventilator A positive-pressure ventilator that ends inspiration when a predetermined flow rate is achieved.

flow rate The speed of the gas at which the tidal volume is delivered.

fraction of inspired oxygen (F_{IO_2}) Percentage of inhaled oxygen expressed as a decimal. For example, 40% oxygen = F_{IO_2} of 0.40.

functional residual capacity The amount of air remaining in the lungs after normal expiration; the sum of the residual volume and the expiratory reserve volume.

high-flow nasal cannula (HFNC) therapy A form of noninvasive ventilation used to treat hypoxic respiratory failure by delivering up to 100% humidified and heated oxygen at a flow rate of up to 60 L/min.

hypoxemia An abnormally low oxygen level.

I time The time frame for the delivery of the tidal volume.

inspiratory-to-expiratory (I:E) ratio An expression for comparing the length of expiration to the length of inspiration. The normal ratio is 1:2, which means that expiration is twice as long as inspiration.

inspiration An active process in which gas is taken into the lungs.

invasive ventilation Application of mechanical ventilation through an artificial airway such as a tracheostomy or endotracheal tube.

mean airway pressure (MAP) The amount of positive pressure in the airway, averaged over the inspiratory and expiratory phases of the breathing cycle.

mechanical ventilation The application of a device that provides varying degrees of ventilatory support.

minute volume Total volume of air breathed in and out in 1 minute. It is calculated by multiplying the respiratory rate per minute by the tidal volume.

mode The particular way in which a spontaneous or mechanical breath is delivered.

negative-pressure ventilators Mechanical ventilators that operate using pressure that is less than the ambient (atmospheric) pressure.

noninvasive ventilation Application of mechanical ventilation through a mask, mouthpiece, or other interfaces other than an artificial airway.

peak airway pressure The amount of positive pressure generated by the ventilator to deliver the tidal volume.

peak inspiratory pressure (PIP) The greatest volume of air delivered to the lungs during inhalation.

plateau pressure The average pressure applied to airways and alveoli at the end of inspiration during positive-pressure mechanical ventilation.

positive end-expiratory pressure (PEEP) The amount of pressure above the ambient pressure present in the airway at the end of the respiratory cycle.

positive-pressure ventilators Mechanical ventilators that operate using pressure that is greater than the ambient pressure.

pressure ventilator A type of positive-pressure ventilator that ends the delivery of the tidal volume based on a predetermined pressure; therefore, the volume may vary.

pulse oximetry Measurement of arterial oxygen saturation (Spo_2) and the pulse.

respiratory failure A situation in which the respiratory system fails to meet the body's metabolic needs. If not reversed, it may lead to respiratory or cardiopulmonary arrest.

Prep Kit Continued

sensitivity Ventilator control that regulates the amount of negative pressure required by the patient to initiate, or trigger, a breath.

shunt Perfusion without ventilation.

tidal volume The volume of air moved into and out of the lungs with each respiratory cycle.

time-cycled ventilator A type of positive-pressure ventilator in which the ventilator ends inspiration after a selected inspiratory time has been achieved.

ventilation-perfusion ($\dot{V}/\dot{Q}$) mismatch A state of inadequate ventilation, perfusion, or both, in which there is inadequate gas exchange.

volume ventilator A type of positive-pressure ventilator in which the breath ends when the predetermined tidal volume is achieved.

volutrauma Trauma caused by excessive lung inflation volumes.

References

Brown CA, Sakles JC, Mick NW. *The Walls Manual of Emergency Airway Management*. 5th ed. Philadelphia, PA: Lippincott, Williams and Wilkins; 2017.

Butler TJ, Close JB, Close RJ. *Laboratory Exercises for Competency in Respiratory Care*. 3rd ed. Philadelphia, PA: FA Davis; 2013.

Cottrell GP. *Cardiopulmonary Anatomy and Physiology for Respiratory Care Practitioners*. Philadelphia, PA: FA Davis; 2001.

Gausche-Hill M, Henderson D, Goodrich S, et al. *Pediatric Airway Management for the Prehospital Professional*. Sudbury, MA: Jones and Bartlett; 2004.

Hartjes TM. *Core Curriculum for High Acuity, Progressive, and Critical Care Nursing*. 7th ed. Philadelphia, PA: WB Saunders; 2017.

Heuer A. *Wilkins' Clinical Assessment in Respiratory Care*. 8th ed. St Louis, MO: Mosby Year Book; 2018.

Hung OR, Murphy MF. *Management of the Difficult and Failed Airway*. 3rd ed. New York, NY: McGraw-Hill Medical; 2017.

Kacmarek RM, Stoller JK, Heuer A. *Egan's Fundamentals of Respiratory Care*. 11th ed. St. Louis, MO: Mosby Year Book; 2016.

Margolis G. *Airway Management: Paramedic*. Sudbury, MA: Jones and Bartlett; 2004.

Şan I, Yildirim Ç, Bekgöz B, Gemcioğlu E. Transport of awake hypoxemic probably COVID 19 patients in the prone position. *Am J Emerg Med*. 2021;46:420-423.

Wexler HR, Lok P. A simple formula for adjusting arterial carbon dioxide tension. *Canad Anaesth Soc J*. 1981;28(4):370-372.

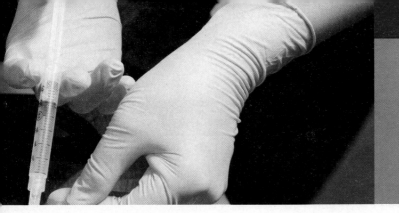

Critical Care Pharmacology

Zlatan Coralic, PharmD, BCPS

Mike McEvoy, PhD, NRP, RN, CCRN

OBJECTIVES

After completing this chapter, you will be able to:

1. Identify reliable resources of medication and pharmacology information (pp 287–288).
2. Outline the principles of medication administration for critical care transport professionals, including patient and medication selection, predicted and desired responses, absorption and elimination principles, side effects or adverse medication reactions, and transport and monitoring considerations (pp 288–289).
3. Discuss the significance of medication pharmacokinetics and pharmacodynamics in the critical care transport setting (pp 289–291).
4. Review principles of medication management, including storage of drugs and maintaining the security of controlled substances (pp 295–296).
5. Discuss the different types and classes of medication used in the critical care arena (pp 296–348).
6. Understand the sequence for medication infusion (p 348).
7. Know how to infuse medication with an infusion pump during transport and through changes in altitude (pp 348–349).

Introduction

Pharmacology is the study of preparation, uses, and actions of medications. Modern health care and modern society are heavily dependent on medications for the management of illness and the alleviation of symptoms. Likewise, medications play an essential role in prehospital and critical care of patients. Critical care transport professionals (CCTPs) need a deep understanding of critical aspects of pharmacology to provide optimal patient care without causing further patient injury or death. Although this chapter includes a brief review of important basics, it assumes a general understanding of the subject of pharmacology. Many specific medications and medication groups are discussed. This list, however, is not comprehensive. As new medications and approaches to treatment of various conditions emerge, it is essential to balance this new information with proven treatment strategies. CCTPs should follow their local regulations, policies, and protocols and consult reliable, current sources when administering any medication.

Pharmacology and Medication Information

CCTPs should stay abreast of newly approved medications and current pharmaceutical research. Up-to-date, reliable medication information may

TABLE 8-1 Sources of Drug Information	
Source	**Description**
Lexicomp, Micromedex, Epocrates	Internet-based drug information databases tailored to pharmacists, physicians, dentists, and nurses. Available to subscribers via desktop or mobile applications. Ideal for rapid retrieval of information from personal/company mobile smartphones.
Individual drug package inserts	Printed documents included in the packaging provided by the drug's manufacturer; generally the same information submitted and approved by the FDA. Drug package inserts will usually provide only FDA-approved uses without mention of off-label indications. Package inserts tend to be bulky and formatted in small print, making them difficult to read during patient transport.
Prescriber's Digital Reference (PDR)	A compilation of prescribing information from drug package inserts. This information is freely available via the *PDR* website or mobile app. As with individual package inserts, information may be limited. The *PDR* was formerly called the *Physicians' Desk Reference*.

Abbreviation: FDA, Food and Drug Administration

© Jones & Bartlett Learning.

be obtained from a variety of sources, many of which are available in both print and electronic formats **TABLE 8-1**. Medication-related reference materials are published by educational institutions, industry organizations, and independent publishing companies. Formats range from simple listings of medications and doses to complex compilations that include an exhaustive list of interactions, overdose/toxicity treatments, pharmacokinetics, and administration guidelines.

The Internet is a readily accessible source of medication information. Take some time to familiarize yourself with reputable and reliable Internet resources, particularly those that are geared toward professional prescribers and health care providers. Mobile applications, such as Epocrates, are also available for smartphones, tablets, and notebook computers. Regardless of the format used, you must perform careful research to determine the source's accuracy and ensure reliable information is obtained for clinical practice.

A Practical Approach to Medication Administration

The optimal medication for a particular patient may or may not be immediately available during patient transport. Notably, CCTPs do not routinely carry many specialized medications, such as antidotes, thrombolytics, and antibiotics, as part of their supplies. The expense of medications, storage concerns, and infrequent use of certain drugs

also limit the number of drugs carried in the critical care transport (CCT) arena. A sending facility and a transport program's sponsoring hospital pharmacy are potential resources when a certain medication is needed emergently but is not carried by the transport team. Before leaving a sending facility, transport crews should obtain a sufficient quantity of any needed medication to cover the anticipated transport time, plus an additional amount to provide a safe margin against unanticipated delays. If a desired medication is unavailable, the transport team must decide if there is an acceptable alternative.

The scope of practice and monitoring capabilities of the transport team must also be considered when selecting a medication. For example, many vasoactive medications are best administered with continuous hemodynamic monitoring and require infusion pumps to ensure controlled delivery and precise dosing. The transport team must be adequately trained and equipped to recognize and effectively manage anticipated side effects or adverse reactions associated with a particular medication. Teams who do not perform adequate monitoring or are unable to properly administer a medication place their patients at grave risk.

Other considerations include the patient's clinical status. If immediate, life-saving interventions are required, it would be best to postpone the administration of scheduled routine medication until the threat has been resolved. Additionally, significant safety or operational priorities related to an aircraft or ambulance may outweigh concerns related to routine medication administration.

CCTPs must consider factors specific to each medication before its administration—specifically, the drug's indications, contraindications, pharmacodynamics, pharmacokinetics, and potential adverse effects. An indication is the specific reason a drug may be used. Indications are based on the US Food and Drug Administration's (FDA) approval of the medication, which specifies the conditions that the medication is officially authorized to treat. However, some medications are used "off-label" when research supports their use in an indication but the drug's manufacturer has not sought FDA approval for that specific purpose.

Pharmacokinetics

Pharmacokinetics is the study of the action of medications within the body, with particular emphasis on the time required for absorption, distribution, metabolism (biotransformation), and elimination.

Absorption

Absorption of a medication occurs either immediately or shortly after its administration. The route of administration affects how quickly and how much of the dose is absorbed. CCTPs generally use intravenous (IV), intraosseous (IO), intramuscular (IM), subcutaneous, oral, inhaled (nebulized), transdermal, nasal, and sometimes rectal routes for medication administration. Routes of administration rarely used by CCTPs include ocular, intra-arterial, otic, epidural, and vaginal administration of drugs.

The route of administration affects a medication's bioavailability, meaning the amount of an administered medication (fraction or percentage) that reaches the patient's systemic circulation without any alteration. IV medications have 100% bioavailability. By comparison, the bioavailability of medications administered orally ranges from 0% to 100%, depending on the substance. Oral digoxin, for example, has a bioavailability of 60% to 80%. Epinephrine and naloxone, in contrast, have close to 0% bioavailability when given orally. Differences in bioavailability illustrate how a dose of a particular medication may be safe when given orally, yet toxic or lethal when given intravenously. For example, significant differences in bioavailability

between oral and IV doses are observed for many drug classes (eg, opioids, beta blockers).

The nasal, sublingual, and rectal routes provide safe, alternative access for some medications when IV access cannot be established. The bioavailability of medications administered by these routes and other non-IV routes depends on numerous factors, including perfusion, skin temperature, membrane pH, and surface area, along with the type of medication, lipophilicity, and its method of preparation.

Distribution

Once absorption has occurred, medication distribution within the body may vary. Blood is the primary distribution vehicle. Substances will become distributed within the body based on the molecule's size, ionization, binding to tissues or plasma proteins, lipid or water solubility, and target tissue penetration. Placental and blood–brain barriers may restrict distribution of certain substances into fetal and brain tissue, respectively. Highly lipid-soluble medications tend to cross these barriers readily, whereas other medications may cross only minimally or not at all. The first-pass effect (also called first-pass metabolism) occurs when the concentration of an oral medication is reduced as it passes through the liver before it enters systemic circulation. The first-pass effect is an important determinant of a drug's bioavailability.

The kidneys and urinary system are the main routes of elimination. Patients with acute or chronic renal disease require careful consideration when medications are administered, because their impaired renal function can result in slower elimination that leads to a potentially toxic buildup of certain agents within the body. Other routes of elimination include the lungs (usually for highly volatile substances or gases), sweat, saliva, stool, and breast milk.

Biotransformation

The liver is the primary site for biotransformation, but many body tissues and cells have the ability to support this process as well. Four possible events occur during biotransformation of a medication:

- An active drug may be changed into an inactive metabolite; this new substance causes no new effects and is ultimately eliminated.

- An active drug may be changed into an active metabolite that causes continued or new clinical effects. For example, morphine is transformed into morphine-3 and morphine-6 glucuronide, centrally active metabolites.
- An active medication may be changed into a reactive metabolite that has a greater potential for action/toxicity than its parent substance. For example, acetaminophen is biotransformed into the highly active metabolite N-acetyl-p-benzoquinone imine.
- A poorly active substance may be changed into an active, potentially toxic substance. For example, codeine is metabolized into morphine through biotransformation.

Active (and reactive) metabolites can complicate the clinical situation and require special consideration when selecting certain medications for use. The presence of active (and reactive) metabolites becomes particularly important when considering the medication's half-life or monitoring a medication plasma levels.

Enzyme systems in the liver perform biotransformation. The cytochrome P450 system, which is present in the liver and in other tissues, is the main pathway responsible for biotransformation of many medications and chemicals. Genetic polymorphism can affect the cytochrome P450 system. The liver enzymes can also be inhibited or induced by concomitant medications. Commonly used agents such as nicotine, grapefruit juice, and broccoli have a significant impact on the functioning of the cytochrome P450 system; thus, intake of these substances may be prohibited when patients are taking certain drugs. The list of medications that either promote or inhibit the action of liver enzymes is extensive.

Elimination

Drugs are primarily eliminated from the body via the urinary route (kidneys) or the fecal route. Patients with acute or chronic renal disease require careful consideration when medications are dosed and given. Impaired renal function can result in slower drug and metabolite elimination, which may amplify the drug's effects and lead to toxicity. To a lesser extent, drugs may also be eliminated via the lungs (usually for highly volatile substances or gases), sweat, saliva, and breast milk.

Drug elimination follows one of two possible patterns. If a substance follows zero-order elimination, a fixed amount of substance is eliminated over a time period, regardless of the amount of substance present in the plasma. Ethanol, for example, follows zero-order elimination. Regardless of how much ethanol is present, only a relatively fixed amount is excreted each hour. However, most medications follow first-order elimination. In this pattern, the amount of substance eliminated over a period of time is proportional to the plasma concentration. Medication half-lives reflect first-order kinetics. A medication steady state occurs when the rate of administration of a medication equals the rate of its elimination—a balance that is desirable with antibiotics and anticoagulants.

Factors affecting both biotransformation and elimination include perfusion, liver and kidney status, metabolism, and the manner and extent of absorption. Biotransformation and elimination are also influenced by chronic exposure to a particular medication or chemical.

Pharmacodynamics

Pharmacodynamics is the branch of pharmacology dealing with a drug's mechanism of action and its effects. It encompasses the various factors that may alter the intended response and any associated adverse events.

Theories of Drug Action

Medications are chemicals that are administered to cure or treat a disease, symptom, condition, or other anomaly. When these chemicals act upon the body to achieve a particular goal, four basic mechanisms may come into play:

- A medication may bind with a receptor site on a particular cell to either promote or inhibit a specific activity of that cell.
- A medication may affect a physical property of a cell, which in turn alters the functioning of that cell.
- A medication may combine directly with other chemicals within the body to alter or limit the effects of this chemical or allow it to be removed.
- A medication may alter a metabolic pathway to achieve the desired result.

Medications that bind to a receptor site are the most widely used, particularly in the prehospital setting. Receptor sites are specialized proteins on a cell that receive chemical mediator messages triggering a particular response. For example, when acetylcholine attaches to receptor sites in the heart, it causes the heart rate to slow. Cellular responses can vary widely, depending on the chemical mediator and the target cells. Generally, a molecule (medication) will have one of two effects when it attaches to a receptor site: (1) It may stimulate the receptor site (ie, act as an agonist) or (2) it may block the receptor site from further stimulation (ie, act as an antagonist). Some medications act as agonist-antagonists. In trying to bind to its receptor, the drug molecule competes with the endogenous or exogenous chemical mediators. For a medication to work effectively, it must have a higher affinity for the receptor than other mediators have. In addition, more than one medication may compete to bind to the same receptor.

The number of available receptors is inconsistent and can be affected by the actual number of sites present, the number already occupied by another chemical mediator, and the number occupied by another medication. Prolonged binding to receptor sites may result in upregulation or downregulation of available receptor sites and the need for dose adjustments to achieve a desired response.

Drug-Response Relationship

When a medication is administered, the onset of action is defined as the amount of time it takes for the concentration of the medication at the target tissue to reach the minimum effective level. The CCTP needs to know how long the medication can be expected to remain above that minimum level and, therefore, exert the intended action (ie, the duration of action). The termination of action is the amount of time after the concentration level falls below the minimum level to the point at which it is considered eliminated from the body.

The therapeutic index is the ratio of a drug's lethal dose for 50% of the population (LD_{50}) to its effective dose for 50% of the population (ED_{50}). In other words, the therapeutic index gives an indication of a medication's margin of safety. The plasma profile also provides information about the medication's biologic half-life ($T\frac{1}{2}$)—that is, the time it takes the body to eliminate half of the amount of the drug present. Despite the name, a medication is not eliminated in two "half-lives." During the second half-life period, only half of what remained after the first half-life is eliminated. After three half-lives, approximately one-eighth of the medication still remains in the body.

In many instances, the duration of action of a medication is unrelated to its half-life. Aspirin, for example, has a half-life of 15 minutes, yet produces antiplatelet effects that last for 7 days. Typically, a medication has no effect after five to seven half-lives.

Factors Affecting Drug Responses

A number of patient characteristics can affect the action of a drug. Consequently, patients differ with respect to how they react to medications. Age, sex, weight, heredity, and clinical conditions can all influence medication choice, medication response, required dose, and elimination characteristics.

Age

Patients of different ages may have vastly different responses to the same drug. Older adults, for example, tend to be much more sensitive to the effects of drugs and often require smaller doses than younger patients do. Many older patients exhibit declining renal function and decreased muscle mass, both of which interfere with estimating creatinine clearance and predicting optimal dosing. Body fat content and fluid status can also influence dose response. Changes in or a reduction of certain neurotransmitters can further complicate medication dosing in older adults.

A patient's metabolism may vary significantly at different ages throughout the lifespan. Pediatric patients, for example, generally have an increased metabolic rate compared with adult and older adult patients, often requiring increases in the dosing amount or the frequency of administration. The issue of concern is not solely a matter of dose, however: Some drugs have altogether different effects in different age groups.

For example, sedative-hypnotic agents tend to exhibit a more profound or prolonged effect in older patients. Paradoxical excitement, rather than sedation, is also possible when older adult patients receive certain medications. Barbiturates, for example, act as sedatives in most adults, but may produce excitement or agitation in older patients. Pediatric patients frequently experience paradoxical drug reactions in which sedative agents cause hyperactivity and agitation, further complicating the clinical situation. Diphenhydramine, chloral hydrate, and certain benzodiazepines are frequently the cause of paradoxical medication reactions in children.

Special Populations

Older adult patients require lower doses of medications because of generally diminished renal and liver function. Additionally, extra doses of medications that have a high first-pass metabolism rate through the liver may be necessary to achieve the optimal serum levels in these patients. Consult a specific, reliable reference for each medication that is being given. Online databases usually describe adult, pediatric, and geriatric considerations for each medication.

Weight

Many drug doses are generally intended for adult patients weighing 154 pounds (70 kg). However, the actual drug concentration may be quite different if the same dose is administered to a 106-pound (48-kg) person or a 300-pound (136-kg) person. To account for such differences, body weight must be taken into consideration during dose selection. Specifically, dosages should be calculated in terms of milligrams or micrograms per kilogram of the patient's body weight (mg/kg or µg/kg, respectively).

Depending on the drug's pharmacokinetics and pharmacodynamics, the doses may be based on total (or actual) body weight, ideal body weight, or adjusted body weight. For example, ketamine should be administered according to a patient's ideal body weight, whereas lidocaine should be administered according to a patient's actual body weight. Ideal body weight is calculated as follows:

- Males (kg): 50 ± (2.3 times patient's height in inches over 5 feet)
- Females (kg): 45.5 ± (2.3 times patient's height in inches over 5 feet)

Research is limited on many other weight-based medication dosages; in general, critical care medications are administered and titrated based on effect.

Sex

General differences in body mass between males and females affect their reactions to medications. Some medications can have varying effects in the different sexes. Females, for example, have increased responses to beta blockers compared to males. They also require lower doses of antipsychotic drugs to control symptoms and experience greater analgesic effects from opioid medications compared to males.

Because many medications can carry reproductive risks, a patient's pregnancy status should always be assessed prior to any medication administration. A good empirical rule is to assume that any woman of childbearing age is pregnant until proven otherwise. You should also use caution when giving medications to breastfeeding women, as many medications are excreted in breast milk.

Environment

The environmental milieu can influence a medication's reaction because of the psychological and physiologic stresses imposed on the patient. In addition, a particular reaction to an environmental factor, such as seasonal allergies, can alter response to a medication. As many medications are sensitive to temperature and light, extra care should be taken to ensure all medications are stored under the proper conditions once they leave the pharmacy.

Time of Administration

When administering oral medications, the timing may influence absorption. Medications may be absorbed differently based on a recent meal. Some medications are inactivated by certain foods, whereas others require a full stomach to ensure optimal absorption. Timing is also important to ensure medications are not stacked if administered before the next dosing time. For example, if repeat opioid doses are given too frequently, they may cause respiratory depression. Thus, CCTPs must be careful to administer all drugs as instructed. They should keep an accurate medication administration record and clearly communicate the medication status with all health care providers involved in the patient's care, especially during transfers and handoffs.

Condition of the Patient

The patient's overall health also affects the response to many drugs. In patients with renal dysfunction, for example, medications may not be excreted efficiently, and the concentration of a drug may reach toxic levels, possibly requiring urgent dialysis for removal. Liver and kidney failure significantly alter the metabolism and elimination of many medications. *Consult a reliable medication reference or seek medical direction before administering medications to patients with significant liver or kidney dysfunction.*

If the patient is in shock or being resuscitated, it may take an extended time for medications to circulate and have an effect. In a situation such as profound anaphylaxis, it may be necessary to administer medications intravenously that are normally administered intramuscularly or subcutaneously.

Be aware that medications may not be effective in hypothermic patients. IV medications are often withheld if a patient's core temperature has fallen below 80°F (30°C) and are given at greater intervals when hypothermic patients have a core temperature above 80°F (30°C). Chapter 19, *Environmental Emergencies*, provides a more detailed discussion of medication administration for the treatment of hypothermia.

Genetic Factors

A patient's genetic makeup may influence a drug's pharmacokinetics and pharmacodynamics. For example, glucose-6-phosphate dehydrogenase (G6PD) deficiency is a common genetic disorder affecting hundreds of millions of people worldwide. The administration of oxidant medications (eg, antimalarial agents), sulfonamides, nitrofurantoin, or phenazopyridine may cause a potentially life-threatening hemolytic anemia. Other genetic disorders, such as primary pulmonary hypertension and sickle cell disease, raise specific concerns related to pharmacology and hemodynamics. Medications with vasoconstrictor properties will adversely affect lung perfusion in patients with pulmonary hypertension. Any medication that causes hypoxia, vasospasm, or dehydration can precipitate or worsen a sickle cell disease crisis.

Pregnancy

Medication administration in pregnant patients carries special risks. Many medications will pass from the pregnant woman's bloodstream into the placenta and may affect the fetus. During pregnancy, patients also experience altered respiration, hemodilution, and altered hemodynamic parameters. Some evidence suggests that catecholamines, such as norepinephrine and epinephrine, have an adverse impact on placental perfusion, although use of these medications is generally limited to extreme situations, such as profound shock or cardiac arrest. Ephedrine, because of its beta-2 and alpha-1 properties, is the preferred vasopressor for maternal shock.

Psychological Factors

For CCTPs, it is crucial to consider psychological factors when administering medications for analgesia and sedation. Patient positioning, temperature regulation, and proactive communication can optimize the effects of analgesia or sedative medications, possibly decreasing the overall amount of each medication required. Occasionally, patients with severe agitation or delirium may require excessive amounts of sedatives to achieve the desired effect. In such cases, the risk of oversedation should always be assessed and mitigation interventions anticipated. Finally, CCTPs should remember that in some instances medications may cause paradoxical reactions; for example, benzodiazepines may cause agitation in older adults.

Predictable Responses

Clinical research generally identifies the dose-response effects that are expected for a particular drug. In addition, during clinical research and through postmarketing surveillance after a medication is used in the broader population, other unexpected and unwanted drug responses (ie, side effects) may be discovered. All medications have side effects, which may be either beneficial or undesirable.

CCTPs need to be able to weigh the risks associated with the use of a medication. If the patient's condition will improve more as a result of the medication's desired effects than its side effects, administering the medication is probably warranted. Conversely, if the risks from side effects outweigh the benefits from drug treatment, it is best to withhold the drug. This concept is known as the risk-benefit ratio. The risk-benefit ratio is evaluated separately for each patient and each intervention.

Sometimes a side effect that is insignificant for one group of patients may have life-threatening implications for others. For example, if a medication causes hypotension as a side effect, its use should be avoided in patients with shock. A medication that prolongs the QT interval may be well tolerated by most patients, but could cause deadly arrhythmias in patients with preexisting cardiac disease. The risks associated with medication side effects should not be underestimated in high-risk or critically ill patients.

Iatrogenic Responses

An iatrogenic response is an adverse condition inadvertently induced in a patient as a result of treatment. The term *iatrogenic* comes from ancient Greek, meaning "brought forth by the healer." For example, a urinary tract infection may develop after the insertion of an indwelling catheter. In pharmacology, a hemorrhagic stroke caused by administration of a thrombolytic or an extrapyramidal reaction due to chlorpromazine is an example of an iatrogenic response.

Unpredictable Responses

Adverse drug events during treatment are common. While some are avoidable, many are not. The most common unpredictable response encountered in the prehospital setting is an allergic reaction. An allergic reaction occurs when the patient has a hypersensitivity to a medication or one of the ingredients used in its particular form or preparation. Such reactions are unpredictable and may range from an isolated rash to a dangerous systemic immune response, or anaphylaxis. They should be anticipated with any drug. Severe reaction to one penicillin-based antibiotic, for example, may indicate the person has a greater chance of cross-reacting to another penicillin-based antibiotic. An allergy to bananas or avocados is highly suggestive of a latex allergy. Numerous other allergy patterns have been identified among foods, environmental allergens, and medications. When possible, CCTPs should always evaluate a patient's allergies prior to administering any medication.

In rare cases, the patient may experience a completely unique response to a medication. This idiosyncratic reaction is unrelated to the pharmacologic action of a medication or the dose administered. For example, in extremely rare cases, patients have developed Stevens-Johnson syndrome after exposure to ibuprofen.

Patients who take a particular medication for an extended period can build up tolerance to it. In these cases, the patient will often require higher-than-normal doses to achieve the desired response. Patients may also develop a tolerance to one medication as a result of prolonged administration of another, a condition known as cross-tolerance. This phenomenon is often seen in patients who take different opioids. For example, a patient taking higher doses of oxycodone may need higher doses of intravenous morphine to control acute pain.

Tachyphylaxis is a condition in which the patient rapidly becomes tolerant to a medication. With tachyphylaxis, increasingly higher doses of a medication are required to achieve the desired effects. This phenomenon most commonly occurs with prolonged treatment with nitroglycerin.

Keep in mind that toxic thresholds may remain unchanged even when tolerance develops. With prolonged administration of a medication, a patient may also become drug dependent. In this case, the person will have significant symptoms if they stop using the medication.

Frequent dosing of a medication over a relatively short time may lead to a cumulative effect, possibly resulting in supratherapeutic or nontherapeutic effects.

Many patients take multiple medications at one time. It is possible for the effects of one medication to alter the patient's response to another medication, a phenomenon known as a drug interaction. For example, a woman on birth control taking rifampin (an antibiotic) may inadvertently become pregnant, as rifampin causes the liver to metabolize the contraceptive at an increased rate. Another example is the administration of epinephrine to a patient taking a monoamine oxidase inhibitor (MAOI). The interaction between these medications can lead to a hypertensive crisis because MAOIs block the breakdown of catecholamines.

If the interaction between two medications causes one drug to enhance the effect of the other, the outcome is known as potentiation. For example, acetaminophen and alcohol, both of which may be hepatotoxic, may interact. When patients with chronic alcohol use disorders ingest acetaminophen, it may precipitate liver toxicity even when taken at therapeutic doses, a phenomenon referred to as alcohol-acetaminophen syndrome. Some potentiation effects are known and can be exploited to achieve a desired effect; in other cases, potentiation may occur unexpectedly. A summation effect occurs when a patient receives two drugs that have the same effect, thus doubling the overall effect. When the patient receives two drugs that produce a response greater than their sum, the result is known as synergism.

A direct biochemical interaction that takes place between two drugs resulting in diminished efficacy is referred to as interference. Inhibition is the opposite of potentiation, with one medication limiting the effects of another.

Avoiding Medication Errors

Medication errors are the most common errors in medicine. While most produce no harm, others can have devastating effects on the patient, their families, and the health care provider. Medication errors may occur at any point during the medication use process, including the selection, administration, and monitoring phases. As part of ensuring the "rights" of medication administration **TABLE 8-2**, CCTPs must evaluate medication decisions made by the sending facility. It is essential that CCTPs confirm the accuracy of any medication infusion they are continuing during transport. Proper labeling of transport medications and infusions is essential for CCTPs when accepting a patient or turning over patient care. Additionally, line incompatibility should be considered for any patient receiving multiple IV infusions. Some IV solutions may be incompatible when mixed in the same line or bag; such a combination may result in inactivation or precipitation of medications. CCTPs should never infuse drugs that have visible precipitants or unexpected discoloration.

Labeling all infusions and cross-checking them with active orders during handoff are key responsibilities of the CCTP. All medication infusions should be labeled both at the distal end of the infusion tubing (proximal to the patient) and on the infusion pump. A CCTP who prepares an infusion should label the bag with, at a minimum, the drug name and concentration, the time and date of preparation, and their initials.

Medication Management
Medication Storage

Some medications may be sensitive to extremes in temperature, exposure to direct sunlight, or excessive humidity. Exposure to such conditions may result in drug inactivation or precipitation. As such, the storage of drugs is a key issue for ensuring safe medication administration during transport.

Each manufacturer provides guidance on the proper medication storage conditions. This information can be found on the drug's package insert or in other drug references. In general, medications should be kept out of direct sunlight and stored at room temperature, as defined in the *United States Pharmacopeia* (ie, 59°F–86°F [15°C–30°C]). During transport, CCTPs and vehicles may be exposed to temperature extremes. It is essential that medications remain within the required temperature ranges. Certain IV medications (eg, diltiazem, lorazepam, succinylcholine) require refrigeration. These medications are stable at room temperature for a limited time and expire quickly. CCTPs should expect transport medications to have different shelf lives, with some remaining stable for years and others expiring in a much shorter time.

Transport vehicles require special consideration in terms of medication storage. CCTPs should monitor the temperature of transport vehicles when they are exposed to extremes of heat or cold. Medications may need to be removed while the vehicle is parked. Smaller electronic devices are now available that can record the temperature of a vehicle and identify periods of deviation from safe medication storage temperatures.

CCTPs should be conscious of these general guidelines, use their best judgment, and ensure medications are stored in areas that are not

TABLE 8-2 Rights of Medication Administration
Right patient
Right medication and indication
Right dose
Right route
Right time
Right education
Right to refuse
Right response and evaluation
Right documentation

© Jones & Bartlett Learning.

routinely or constantly exposed to extreme environments. Every department should have a written policy or procedure for all medication, fluid, and diluent storage and handling. In addition, CCTPs should perform monthly audits to identify soon-to-expire medications and restock as appropriate. Finally, it is best practice to double-check the expiration date prior to any drug administration.

Security of Controlled Medications

Most drugs used in the prehospital setting are prescription medications, and many are controlled substances. State and federal governments heavily regulate the acquisition, storage, transport, usage, and disposal of controlled medications. State pharmacy boards and the US Drug Enforcement Administration have specific regulations that CCTPs must follow in these situations. Minimum requirements for the storage of controlled substances include housing them in an inconspicuous, securely locked, substantially constructed cabinet. Cabinets constructed of materials that are fragile or allow visualization, such as those with glass or plastic fronts, are inappropriate.

A disposition record must be maintained for all controlled substances, and thorough documentation must be completed for any use of a controlled substance, including the disposal of any leftover waste medication not administered during patient care. Any expired controlled substances must be returned to the agency or departmental officer in charge of maintenance and dispersal of controlled substances and must also be documented in the disposition record(s).

Every agency must have a written protocol and procedure for the use, storage, disposition, and documentation of controlled substances.

Specific Medications Used in Critical Care Transport

Common medications used by CCTPs are highlighted in this section. CCTPs will encounter additional medications in clinical practice and should develop a strategy for safe administration of any drug that may be needed. Conversely, not every medication or medication class described here may be relevant to providers who perform only CCT of specialty populations (eg, high-risk obstetric or neonatal populations).

Vasopressors

Vasopressor medications induce arterial vasoconstriction, which in turn elevates mean arterial blood pressure. Their mechanism of action usually involves stimulation of the adrenergic receptors involved in vasoconstriction. Some vasopressors may also exhibit inotropic activity (increasing myocardial contractility). Vasopressors are generally indicated for patients in distributive shock states following correction of any fluid volume deficits. Significant side effects of these medications include tissue necrosis from extravasation and ischemia related to vasoconstriction effects (eg, limb ischemia). **TABLE 8-3** profiles selected vasopressors.

Phenylephrine

Phenylephrine is an alpha-1 agonist. This medication binds to and stimulates the alpha-1 receptors, resulting in systemic arterial vasoconstriction. As with any vasopressor, caution must be exercised when this drug is administered to patients with coronary artery disease because it may precipitate or worsen myocardial ischemia. Further, phenylephrine should be avoided in patients with bradycardia because it may further decrease the heart rate (through baroreflex bradycardia due to increased systemic vascular resistance). Phenylephrine is typically given as an infusion at a rate of 40 to 60 µg/min. It may be necessary to rapidly titrate the dose or give a bolus dose to achieve the desired blood pressure response. Phenylephrine is best used in situations where the patient has a loss of vasomotor tone, without simultaneous impairment of myocardial contractility.

Norepinephrine

Norepinephrine is a beta-1 and alpha-1 agonist. It is most commonly used for blood pressure control in patients who are in cardiogenic or septic shock. Norepinephrine is a first-line vasopressor in patients with septic shock who remain hypotensive after an adequate fluid challenge. It is most commonly dosed in units of µg/min; however, certain hospitals may use µg/kg/min, especially in pediatric patients. Norepinephrine's side effects represent

TABLE 8-3 Vasopressors

Medication	Uses	Mechanism of Action	Route of Administration	Side Effects	Special Considerations
Phenylephrine	Hypotension, shock; decongestant (OTC nasal spray)	Pure alpha adrenergic agonist	IV, IO	Peripheral vasoconstriction, hypertension, ischemia, reflex bradycardia, low cardiac output, anxiety, restlessness	Continuous hemodynamic and cardiac monitoring is essential. Administer via central venous access whenever possible; peripheral administration may cause tissue necrosis with extravasation. Vasopressors may worsen myocardial performance in compromised patients.
Norepinephrine	Hypotension, cardiogenic or septic shock (first-line pressor in adult patients with septic shock)	Stimulates beta-1 and alpha-1 receptors; increases myocardial contractility and heart rate in addition to systemic vasoconstriction; alpha (vasoconstriction) effects are greater than beta (inotropic and chronotropic) effects	IV, IO	Peripheral vasoconstriction, hypertension, ischemia, tachycardia, anxiety, restlessness	Continuous hemodynamic and cardiac monitoring is essential. Administer via central venous access whenever possible; peripheral administration may cause tissue necrosis with extravasation.

(Continues)

TABLE 8-3 Vasopressors (continued)

Medication	Uses	Mechanism of Action	Route of Administration	Side Effects	Special Considerations
Epinephrine	Anaphylaxis, hypotension, severe asthma unresponsive to inhaled beta agonists, cardiac arrest, bradycardia unresponsive to atropine or pacing, shock unresponsive to adequate fluid volume replacement, low cardiac output	Stimulation of alpha-1, beta-1, and beta-2 adrenergic receptors, resulting in bronchial smooth muscle relaxation, cardiac inotropy (increased contractility), and chronotropy (increased rate)	Nebulized, subcutaneous, IM, IV, IO, endotracheal tube	Arrhythmias (tachycardias, ventricular ectopy, fibrillation), hypertension, increased myocardial oxygen consumption, vasoconstriction, ischemia, hyperglycemia, nausea, vomiting, anxiety, tremors, nervousness, restlessness	Continuous hemodynamic and cardiac monitoring is essential. Administer via central venous access whenever possible; peripheral administration may cause tissue necrosis with extravasation. Errors with this agent's use are common, requiring careful dosing and administration, especially in pediatric patients.
Vasopressin	Treatment of hypotension refractory to fluids and catecholamines	Direct systemic vasoconstriction with no inotropic or chronotropic effects through V₁ receptor agonism (non–alpha- or beta-mediated mechanism); additionally decreases urine output and acts as an antidiuretic hormone	IV, IO	Hypertension, reflex bradycardia, peripheral vasoconstriction, ischemia, decreased urine output	Continuous hemodynamic and cardiac monitoring is essential. Administer via central venous access whenever possible; peripheral administration may cause tissue necrosis with extravasation.
Methylene blue	Treatment of drug or chemically induced methemoglobinemia, refractory vasoplegia syndrome following cardiac surgery	Speeds conversion of methemoglobin to hemoglobin; may restore vascular tone by direct inhibition of nitric oxides	IV, IO	Arrhythmias, hypertension, blue skin staining, blue-green fecal discoloration, blue-green urine discoloration, diaphoresis, local ischemia with extravasation	Continuous hemodynamic and cardiac monitoring is essential. Administer via central venous access whenever possible; peripheral administration may cause tissue necrosis with extravasation.

"Push-dose pressors": epinephrine or phenylephrine	Emergent treatment of severe hypotension, typically during volume resuscitation or while vasopressor infusions are being prepared	See information for epinephrine or phenylephrine	IV, IO	See information for epinephrine or phenylephrine	An arterial line should be in place whenever push-dose pressors are employed owing to significantly increased risks of inducing significant hypertension. Errors are common when admixing; use commercially available products if available.
Angiotensin II	Septic or distributive shock	Renin-angiotensin-aldosterone system hormone causing vasoconstriction and aldosterone release, increasing blood pressure	IV (central)	Thrombosis, tachycardia, ischemia, delirium	This vasoactive agent has a unique mechanism of action and is relatively new and costly. It poses considerable risk of thrombosis; all patients must receive prophylactic anticoagulation prior to beginning therapy.

Abbreviations: cAMP, cyclic adenosine monophosphate; DI, diabetes insipidus; IM, intramuscular; IO, intraosseous; IV, intravenous; OTC, over-the-counter; ROSC, return of spontaneous circulation; SVT, supraventricular tachycardia

a continuation of its mechanism of action; they include arrhythmias, tachycardia, hypertension, and decreased peripheral blood flow. The onset is rapid and the half-life is only 2.5 minutes. As such, infusion interruptions may result in rapid effects on the patient's blood pressure. Norepinephrine infusion ceiling doses are usually in the range of 20 to 40 μg/min; however, in practice larger doses have been reported.

Epinephrine

Epinephrine is an alpha/beta agonist that stimulates alpha-1, beta-1, and beta-2 adrenergic receptors, which in turn leads to relaxation of bronchial smooth muscle, inotropic and chronotropic cardiac stimulation, and dilation of skeletal muscle vasculature. Low doses cause beta$_2$ vascular receptor stimulation, resulting in vasodilation; in contrast, higher doses constrict skeletal and vascular smooth muscles. When given intravenously, epinephrine's effects are nearly immediate and last for less than 5 minutes.

Infusions of epinephrine for relief of bronchospastic respiratory distress, anaphylaxis, bradycardia, and cardiogenic shock are generally initiated at 0.05 μg/kg/min and titrated every 3 to 5 minutes in increments of 0.02 μg/kg/min, up to a maximum of 1 μg/kg/min. Usual doses range from 0.05 to 0.5 μg/kg/min.

Epinephrine is a potent vasoconstrictor and should be infused through a central access line as soon as one is available. Its adverse effects include tachycardia, anxiety, restlessness, arrhythmias, limb ischemia, diaphoresis, hyperglycemia, and tremor.

Vasopressin

Vasopressin is a naturally occurring antidiuretic hormone that is typically used in critical care to treat refractory distributive (vasodilatory) shock. This agent is frequently used as a second-line pressor in patients with septic shock who remain hypotensive despite adequate fluids and norepinephrine. Vasopressin exhibits direct vasoconstrictor activity without inotropic or chronotropic effects. It stimulates V_1 receptors and increases systemic vascular resistance and mean arterial blood pressure. Dose ranges for vasopressin infusions vary by indication, but typically range between 0.01 unit/min and 0.1 unit/min; dosing in patients with sepsis is usually 0.04 unit/min. Effects of vasopressin are seen in less than 15 minutes and last for less than 15 to 20 minutes when the infusion is discontinued or decreased.

Adverse reactions to vasopressin may include bradycardia, decreased cardiac output, hyponatremia, and tissue and organ ischemia.

Methylene Blue

Methylene blue is an antidote used for treatment of methemoglobinemia. In critical care settings, it is also employed as a treatment for vasopressor-refractory hypotension. In patients with vasoplegia, methylene blue acts as an inhibitor of nitric oxide and blocks the formation of cyclic guanosine monophosphate; both of these effects reduce vasorelaxation.

Dosing strategies for methylene blue vary and are supported primarily by observational studies rather than prospective clinical trials. For cardioplegia associated with cardiac surgery, the methylene blue IV dose is 1.5 to 2 mg/kg given over 20 to 60 minutes. Improvement is usually observed within 1 to 2 hours. Some clinicians follow the loading dose with an infusion of 0.5 to 1 mg/kg/h for several hours.

Methylene blue is a vesicant, and any extravasation should be treated aggressively. Infusions should be administered through a central line **FIGURE 8-1**. When high doses are given in infants and in patients with G6PD deficiency, methemoglobinemia may occur. Adverse effects include urine discoloration (blue-green color), dysgeusia, limb pain, and interference with pulse oximetry readings.

Push-Dose Pressors

Originating in anesthesia, the use of push-dose pressors has become increasingly prevalent over the past decade. Patients may be given small aliquots of appropriately diluted pressors to treat hypotension that is refractory to fluids. These agents are now used in critical care, emergency medicine, and emergency medical services systems. The two medications most often employed as push-dose pressors are dilute concentrations of epinephrine and phenylephrine.

Indications for push-dose pressors include situations where profound hypotension fails to

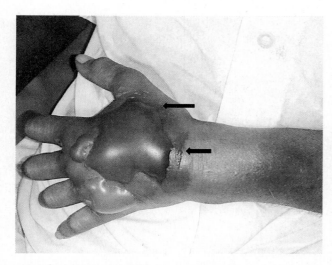

FIGURE 8-1 Extravasation is the leaking of an intravenously administered medication into the surrounding tissues.

Vinod KV, Shravan R, Shrivarthan R, Radhakrishna P, Dutta TK. Acute compartment syndrome of hand resulting from radiographic contrast iohexol extravasation. *J Pharmacol Pharmacother.* 2016;7:44-47, published by Medknow Publications and Media Pvt.

respond to fluid boluses or where vasopressors either are not yet infusing or are not immediately producing an increase in blood pressure. Patients who require such treatment may include those with propofol-induced hypotension, peri- or post-intubation hypotension, hypotension induced by tachyarrhythmias, or profound vasoplegia.

Push-dose epinephrine is usually prepared by adding 0.1 mg of epinephrine to 9 mL of normal saline, with the resulting concentration being 10 µg/mL. Given the onset of action of approximately 1 minute, push-dose pressor doses of 0.5 to 2 mL (5 to 20 µg) would be appropriate to administer every 1 to 5 minutes. Blood pressure, heart rate, and contractility should all increase with the administration of epinephrine.

Unlike epinephrine, phenylephrine has no beta effects and will provide only vasoconstriction with some increase in coronary perfusion. Prepared by either adding 10 mg of phenylephrine to a 100-mL bag of normal saline or adding 10 mg of phenylephrine to a 250-mL bag of saline (the latter is a typical infusion concentration), the resulting concentrations are 100 µg/mL or 40 µg/mL, respectively. With an onset of action of approximately 1 minute, doses consisting of 0.5 to 1 mL of the 100 µg/mL solution (50 to 100 µg) or 1 to 2 mL of the 40 µg/mL solution (40 to 80 µg) would be appropriate to administer every 1 to 5 minutes.

Close patient monitoring is imperative for safety when using push-dose pressors. Ideally, an arterial line should be in place. If not, the patient's blood pressure should be measured at 1-minute intervals. Be careful when preparing push-dose pressors, especially during stressful clinical situations (eg, patients in extremis), as dilution and dosing errors are easy to make and can have devastating consequences. Commercially available products should be considered whenever available.

Angiotensin II

Angiotensin II is a relatively new medication used for blood pressure support in patients with distributive shock. Its mechanism of action differs from the other vasopressors. This agent acts on the renin-angiotensin-aldosterone system, causing vasoconstriction and water retention, both of which increase systemic blood pressure. The usual starting dose is 10 to 20 ng/kg/min, which may be titrated every 5 minutes in increments of 15 ng/kg/min. Once the blood pressure has normalized, angiotensin II can be down-titrated using the same parameters. Maximum doses are usually 80 ng/kg/min during the first 3 hours of treatment and 40 ng/kg/min during maintenance.

During clinical trials, angiotensin II was associated with increased risk of thrombosis, both arterial and venous. To guard against these effects, any patient receiving angiotensin II should be on concomitant venous thromboembolism prophylaxis (eg, heparin, enoxaparin). Due to the significant risk of thrombosis, and its significantly higher cost compared to other vasopressors (ie, $1,800 per vial), few institutions have this drug on their formulary. However, CCTPs may still encounter patients on active infusions of angiotensin II.

Inotropes

Medications may have positive or negative inotropic effects, meaning that they either increase or decrease the force of myocardial contractility, respectively. Inotropic medications increase myocardial contractility and are generally indicated for patients in cardiogenic shock states. Their mechanisms of action vary. Selection typically depends on the diagnosis and provider preference. **TABLE 8-4** profiles selected inotropes.

TABLE 8-4 Inotropes

Medication	Uses	Mechanism of Action	Route of Administration	Side Effects	Special Considerations
Dopamine	Adjunct treatment for cardiogenic shock, hypotension refractory to fluid resuscitation, symptomatic bradycardias unresponsive to atropine or pacing, low cardiac output syndrome	Adrenergic agonist acting on alpha, beta, and dopaminergic receptors to increase contractility and heart rate	IV, IO	Hypertension, tachycardia, increased myocardial oxygen consumption, peripheral vasoconstriction, ischemia, anxiety, nervousness, restlessness	Continuous hemodynamic and cardiac monitoring is essential. Administer via central venous access whenever possible; peripheral administration may cause tissue necrosis with extravasation. Dopamine impairs renal, gastrointestinal, and hepatic perfusion, and impairs respiratory, immune, and endocrine function.
Dobutamine	Short-term management of depressed cardiac output in patients with heart failure, management of sepsis-induced myocardial dysfunction	Stimulates myocardial beta receptors to increase heart rate and contractility; stimulates beta-1, beta-2, and alpha receptors in vasculature; the greater beta effects result in vasodilation	IV, IO	Arrhythmias (dobutamine leads to more tachycardia than dopamine), hypotension, ischemia	Continuous hemodynamic and cardiac monitoring is essential. Administer via central venous access whenever possible; peripheral administration may cause tissue necrosis with extravasation.
Milrinone	Short-term treatment for acutely decompensated heart failure; typically used in patients unresponsive to dobutamine or patients intolerant of dobutamine-induced tachyarrhythmias	Selective phosphodiesterase inhibitor with inotropic and vasodilatory effects; minimal to no chronotropic activity	IV infusion (loading infusion may be given initially)	Hypotension, arrhythmias, headache	Continuous hemodynamic and cardiac monitoring is essential. When initiated without a loading dose, significant effects will be seen in 30 minutes and peak in 2–3 hours. Increased pressor requirements after 24 hours of therapy may signal the need for milrinone weaning.

Abbreviations: AV, atrioventricular; IO, intraosseous; IV, intravenous

Dopamine

Dopamine is an inotrope and is classified as an adrenergic agonist. In its natural endogenous form, it is a precursor to both norepinephrine and epinephrine. The original research that resulted in its popularity in cardiovascular conditions theorized that dopamine had positive inotropic effects by stimulating beta-1 receptors. Additionally, dopamine appeared to stimulate alpha-1 receptors at a higher dose, leading to peripheral vasoconstriction. Dopamine also affects dopaminergic receptors, which are found in the central nervous system (CNS) as well as in the pulmonary arteries and atria of the heart. Stimulation of these receptors increases myocardial contractility and cardiac output.

The wide range of effects found with dopamine allowed for a variety of uses, and clinicians became comfortable with dopamine as a first-line vasopressor in fluid-refractory hypotension. Fear of the ischemic effects of norepinephrine inspired further confidence in the use of dopamine, as clinicians believed its vasopressor and inotropic effects occurred without the renal and gastrointestinal loss of perfusion often seen with other pressors.

Low-dose dopamine, administered at 0.3 to 5 µg/kg/min, was often used and thought to optimize renal perfusion and preserve renal function; this regimen was believed to have minimal effects on cardiac output. More recent studies have challenged the renal and splanchnic (gastrointestinal) protective effects of dopamine and suggested that, in fact, it may do more harm than good in these indications. Significant evidence suggests that dopamine may promote ischemia in the renal medulla, and it may even increase the risk of acute renal failure (ARF) in critically ill patients. The benefits of dopamine in preventing, reversing, or limiting the progression of ARF cannot be substantiated. Norepinephrine, in contrast, has been demonstrated to protect renal blood flow and improve diuresis in patients with shock who have been adequately fluid resuscitated.

Dopamine also creates significant impairment of respiratory function by depressing the carotid body, leading to an impaired response to hypoxemia and hypercapnia. Coupled with regional ventilation-perfusion mismatch, the hypoxemia resulting from dopamine infusions poses significant risks to patients who are not mechanically ventilated or who are weaning from mechanical ventilation. Finally, dopamine significantly depresses endocrine and immunologic function and causes major disturbances in anterior pituitary function. The use of this medication has now fallen out of favor, especially with recent evidence showing norepinephrine to be a superior agent, especially in patients with sepsis.

When used for hemodynamic support, dopamine infusions are titrated from 1 to 20 µg/kg/min in increments of 1 µg/kg/min every 5 to 10 minutes. The drug's onset of action in adults is 5 minutes, but a steady state of action is not seen for 20 minutes. In children, it may take 1 hour to achieve a steady-state effect. The duration of action of dopamine in adults is 10 minutes.

Dopamine is a vesicant and should be infused into a central line whenever possible. Extravasation should be treated aggressively.

Dobutamine

Dobutamine is an inotrope and is classified as an adrenergic agonist. It is commonly used to treat cardiac decompensation secondary to heart failure. Dobutamine stimulates beta-1 receptors to increase myocardial contractility and heart rate. Its effects on the vasculature (beta-2 effects) also result in vasodilation. The vasodilatory and inotropic effects of dobutamine make it an ideal heart failure drug but limit its utility in patients with hypotension. This agent also results in greater tachycardia than other pressors do, owing to the baroceptor stimulation that occurs secondary to its vasodilatory properties.

As a treatment for heart failure, an infusion of dobutamine is started at 5 µg/kg/min and can be increased every 10 minutes in increments of 2.5 µg/kg/min to a maximum dose of 20 µg/kg/min. Some references suggest starting at lower doses (0.5 to 1 µg/kg/min) to minimize adverse effects such as tachyarrhythmias. Onset of action occurs within 1 to 10 minutes, with peak effects observed in 10 to 20 minutes. The duration of action is short, with the drug having a half-life of only 2 minutes.

Dobutamine does not pose the same risks of tissue damage with extravasation associated with other inotropes and pressors. It may be infused into a peripheral IV line. Patients with home infusions will often have dobutamine running through central IV catheters.

Milrinone

Milrinone is a phosphodiaterase-3 enzyme inhibitor that is used as an inotropic agent for patients in cardiogenic shock or advanced stages of heart failure. Milrinone improves inotropy and results in vasodilation with little effect on heart rate. Typically, this agent is used in patients with heart failure who fail to respond to dobutamine. It may be employed for symptom relief in patients with end-stage heart failure who cannot be discharged from the hospital and are not candidates for heart transplantation or cardiac assist devices. Milrinone also produces a favorable lowering of pulmonary artery pressures and may be used in patients with postoperative pulmonary hypertension.

Milrinone infusions are initiated at 0.125 to 0.75 µg/kg/min. Previously, a loading dose of 50 µg/kg administered over 10 minutes was recommended; however, the relatively high incidence of hypotension associated with loading doses has discouraged this practice. While this practice is uncommon, some heart failure specialists may administer milrinone infusions at rates as high as 1.5 µg/kg/min. The onset of action for milrinone is 5 to 15 minutes, and it has a half-life of 2.3 to 2.4 hours. In patients with renal failure, the half-life may be as long as 20 hours.

Major side effects of milrinone include hypotension and arrhythmias (usually ventricular). Hypotension typically responds well to low-dose vasopressors. In patients with new acute decompensated heart failure, recovery over the first 3 to 5 days of milrinone infusion is often associated with increased pressor requirements. Weaning off milrinone will usually decrease the pressor requirements; indeed, with recovery of cardiac function, patients may be completely weaned off milrinone.

Vasodilators and Antihypertensives

Vasodilator medications induce vasodilation, cause preload and/or afterload reduction, and thereby lower mean arterial blood pressure. The mechanism of action for vasodilators is induced relaxation of the smooth muscle in blood vessel walls. Selection of vasodilators depends on the indication for use, patient response, and cost. Hypotension is the most common, and most dangerous, side effect associated with vasodilators. **TABLE 8-5** profiles selected vasodilators.

Sodium Nitroprusside

Sodium nitroprusside is a potent arterial and venous vasodilator. Its vasodilating effects result from its breakdown to nitric oxide, which acts directly on vascular smooth muscle. Nitroprusside is used to treat acute hypertension and acute decompensated heart failure; its therapeutic effects are seen within 2 minutes. The reduction in total peripheral resistance and venous return produced by this medication decreases both preload and afterload; hence, in patients with severe heart failure, nitroprusside can act to increase cardiac output.

Initial dosing is started at 0.25 to 0.5 µg/kg/min and titrated in increments of 0.5 to 1 µg/kg/min every 3 to 5 minutes. The usual dose range is 0.25 to 3 µg/kg/min to a maximum of 10 µg/kg/min. Some references recommend a maximum rate of 3 to 5 µg/kg/min to avoid cyanide toxicity; such metabolic toxicity occurs when nitroprusside combines with hemoglobin, producing cyanide and cyanmethemoglobin. Normally, cyanide detoxification occurs via conversion of cyanide to thiocyanate, which is then excreted in the urine. However, this process has limited capacity and can become overwhelmed with large cyanide exposures. Nitroprusside's hypotensive effects have a short duration, lasting only 1 to 10 minutes. Common adverse effects with this agent include hypotension, reflex tachyarrhythmias, cyanide toxicity, and methemoglobinemia.

Nitroprusside is relatively unstable. Prepared solutions should be wrapped with aluminum foil to protect them from light, which accelerates their decomposition. Mixtures normally have a clear to brown color; decomposition results in a color change to orange, dark brown, or blue. Blue discoloration indicates almost complete decomposition.

Nitroglycerin

Nitroglycerin is an antianginal agent and vasodilator with primarily venous effects. Its primary action is through the relaxation of vascular smooth muscle. Dilation of post-capillary vessels, including large veins, promotes peripheral pooling of blood, decreasing venous return to the heart and thereby reducing preload. Nitroglycerin also reduces peripheral vascular resistance, thereby reducing afterload. In combination, these effects reduce the heart's workload. In addition, nitroglycerin produces dilation of the coronary vessels themselves,

TABLE 8-5 Vasodilators and Antihypertensives

Medication	Uses	Mechanism of Action	Route of Administration	Side Effects	Special Considerations
Sodium nitroprusside	Hypertensive crisis management, acute decompensated heart failure	Direct action on arterial and venous smooth muscles; increases cardiac output by lowering afterload	IV or IO infusion	Hypotension, flushing, tachycardia, methemoglobinemia, metabolic acidosis (secondary to cyanide toxicity), hyperreflexia (secondary to thiocyanate toxicity), headache, light-headedness, dizziness, syncope	Thiocyanate and cyanide toxicity are possible, especially with prolonged or high-dose infusions. Continuous blood pressure monitoring with an arterial line is mandatory. Monitor vital signs, acid–base status, and thiocyanate levels during prolonged treatment. Protect the prepared solution from light. The solution should be clear to brown in color; near-complete decomposition in light results in blue discoloration.
Nitroglycerin	Treatment or prevention of angina, acute decompensated heart failure, vasopressor extravasation injury	Forms a nitric oxide free radical that acts directly on vascular smooth muscle to produce vasodilation; effects are greater on venous than arterial vessels	Sublingual, transdermal, IV, IO	Hypotension, flushing, tachycardia, headache, light-headedness, dizziness, syncope	Monitor vital signs during infusion. Because adsorption occurs with soft plastics, nonpolyvinyl chloride tubing should be used.
Hydralazine	Hypertension, heart failure with intolerance to ACEIs or ARBs, postoperative hypertension, hypertensive emergencies during pregnancy	Causes direct dilation of arterial wall smooth muscle	Oral, IM, IV, IO	Tachycardia, hypotension, rebound hypertension, flushing, nausea, vomiting, edema	Monitor blood pressure and heart rate before and after administration. Onset of action with IV administration is 5–20 minutes and lasts for 1–4 hours, although hypotension may last longer. Expect an increased heart rate.

(Continues)

TABLE 8-5 Vasodilators and Antihypertensives (continued)

Medication	Uses	Mechanism of Action	Route of Administration	Side Effects	Special Considerations
Clevidipine	Hypertension	Calcium channel blocker with potent arterial-vasodilating activity	IV or IO infusion only	Atrial fibrillation, fever, nausea, headache, insomnia	Formulated in an oil-water lipid emulsion; change the tubing every 12 hours. Continuously monitor blood pressure during infusion. Vials and tubing resemble those for propofol, requiring caution during simultaneous infusion (both are milky-white liquids).
Nicardipine	Hypertension, hypertension during acute ischemic stroke	Calcium channel blocker with direct action on arterial and coronary vascular smooth muscle; vasodilates and increases myocardial oxygen delivery in vasospastic angina	IV, IO	Hypotension, flushing, headache, dizziness, edema (dose related), palpitations, tachycardia, bradycardia	Continuously monitor blood pressure and heart rate during infusion. Closely monitor infusion site; administer via central line if possible; change peripheral IV sites every 12 hours.

Abbreviations: ACEI, angiotensin-converting enzyme inhibitor; ARB, angiotensin II receptor blocker; IM, intramuscular; IO, intraosseous; IV, intravenous

© Jones & Bartlett Learning.

theoretically increasing the supply of oxygenated blood to the myocardium.

Therapeutic doses of nitroglycerin will reduce systolic, diastolic, and mean arterial blood pressure. Effective coronary perfusion pressure is usually maintained, but can be compromised if blood pressure falls excessively, or if the increased heart rate leads to decreased diastolic filling time.

Nitroglycerin infusions, which are typically used to manage ischemic chest pain, are initiated at 10 µg/min and titrated every 3 to 5 minutes in increments of 5 to 10 µg/min. Although the maximum dosing is usually listed as 400 µg/min, most patients are unable to tolerate doses greater than 200 µg/min because of headaches. Other side effects include hypotension, tachycardia, flushing, and nausea. When this medication is used for treatment of acute pulmonary edema, more rapid titration is warranted to doses as high as 100 µg/min to achieve sufficient preload reduction. Prolonged infusions (24 to 48 hours) of nitroglycerin may result in tachyphylaxis.

Because nitroglycerin is absorbed by soft plastic, including polyvinyl chloride–based containers, infusions must be prepared in glass bottles, EXCEL containers, or PAB containers. The drug's manufacturers recommend use of IV tubing sets intended specifically for nitroglycerin.

Hydralazine

Hydralazine is a direct arterial vasodilator that acts on the smooth muscle of the arterioles, yet has little effect on venous vessels. This agent is typically used in hypertensive emergencies and is administered as an IV dose of 10 to 20 mg every 4 to 6 hours. The most common adverse effect with this medication is tachycardia, a phenomenon that leads many clinicians to alternate dosing of hydralazine with a beta blocker such as labetalol.

Clevidipine

Clevidipine is a calcium channel blocker that reduces mean arterial blood pressure by decreasing systemic vascular resistance. It does not reduce cardiac filling pressure (preload), so it is unlikely to lead to myocardial ischemia and decreased cardiac output. This potent antihypertensive agent is used for short-term treatment of hypertension in patients who are unable to take oral medications.

Clevidipine infusions are prepared in a lipid-based, oil-in-water emulsion and should be refrigerated. Bottles of this medication remain stable at room temperature for 2 months when unopened; once opened, however, they are stable for only 12 hours. Bottles and tubing should be changed every 12 hours, as the lipid base increases the risk of bacterial growth.

Clevidipine infusions are started at 1 to 2 mg/h and titrated by doubling the dose every 90 seconds. As blood pressure approaches the target goal, titration increments should be reduced by 1 to 2 mg/h every 3 to 5 minutes. Clevidipine's onset of action is 2 to 4 minutes after the infusion begins, and its duration of action is 5 to 15 minutes.

Because the emulsion contains soybean, egg yolk phospholipids, and glycerin, patients with a history of allergies to soy products or eggs should not receive clevidipine. Adverse effects may include tachycardia, atrial fibrillation, fever, and nausea.

Nicardipine

Nicardipine is a calcium channel blocker used for short-term treatment of hypertension in patients who are unable to take oral medications. Its effects are more selective for vascular smooth muscle than for cardiac muscle. When given intravenously, nicardipine produces significant decreases in systemic vascular resistance, leading to a resultant decrease in blood pressure.

Nicardipine infusions are extremely irritating to peripheral veins, owing to the drug's low pH, and should be administered in a central line or large peripheral vessel. If central access is not available, rotating the peripheral venous administration site every 12 hours may minimize venous irritation.

Nicardipine infusions are initiated at 5 mg/h and titrated every 15 minutes in increments of 2.5 mg/h. If rapid control of blood pressure is desired, titration every 5 minutes is recommended. The maximum recommended dosing is 15 mg/h. The manufacturer recommends that the infusion rate be lowered to 3 mg/h once blood pressure control is achieved, although this dosing may be insufficient to maintain control in many patients.

Other than peripheral access site pain and irritation, side effects of IV nicardipine occur relatively infrequently, but include tachycardia, flushing, pedal edema, and headache. Use of this medication in combination with fentanyl has been reported to exacerbate hypotension.

Sedatives, Anesthetics, Analgesics, Antipsychotics, and Anticonvulsants

Sedatives, anesthetics, analgesics, and anticonvulsants all act on the nervous system, typically to depress nervous system activity. Sedatives, which include anxiolytics and hypnotics, act as CNS depressants or relaxants. Anesthesia is a state of unconsciousness induced with anesthetics, whereas analgesia is relief of pain. Anticonvulsants act to stop seizure activity. **TABLE 8-6** profiles selected sedatives, anesthetics, analgesics, and anticonvulsants.

Many medications classified as sedatives, anesthetics, analgesics, or anticonvulsants cross classifications and, depending on the dose and indication, may be considered members of multiple classes. Their mechanisms of action vary widely. While their side effects also vary widely, the most significant and potentially dangerous adverse effect of any CNS depressant is unrecognized respiratory depression. Identification of respiratory depression via continuous monitoring of pulse oximetry, which has long been a standard of care for all critical patients, is significantly delayed; hence, this modality is woefully inadequate as a respiratory depression monitor. Waveform capnography is the standard of care for monitoring when administering anesthetics and sedatives; indeed, it is the only well-validated tool for promptly recognizing respiratory depression. Capnography provides a measure of certainty when administering analgesia and when using anticonvulsants in an actively seizing patient.

Midazolam

Midazolam is a medication often chosen for procedural sedation because of its relatively fast onset (1 to 5 minutes when given intravenously). When used for rapid sequence intubation (RSI), it is usually administered as an adjunct to other sedative-hypnotic agents, rather than as the sole induction agent. Midazolam has a potent amnesic effect, inhibiting the patient's ability to recall the procedure. Because this agent can be stored for a prolonged period at room temperature, it is a popular medication during CCT.

Midazolam is also used for sedation in CCT patients and to terminate status epilepticus seizures. It can be administered orally, intravenously/intraosseously by bolus or continuous infusion, intramuscularly, intranasally, or buccally (off-label). Intranasal administration is likely to cause a burning sensation due to the drug's low pH (adjusted pH is 3). Minimizing the volume administered by using a 5 mg/mL concentration reduces irritation, as does the use of a commercial atomizer device such as the MAD Mucosal Atomizer. The maximum recommended volume is 1 mL per nare.

Midazolam dosing is titrated to effect and can vary by indication. Initial IM dosing in adults for sedation is typically 5 mg. IV midazolam is initially given slowly over at least 2 minutes (to avoid profound hypotension) at doses of 0.5 to 2 mg, repeated every 2 to 3 minutes to a usual dose of 2.5 to 5 mg. Continuous infusions of midazolam are usually prepared by adding 100 mg to 100 mL of normal saline (NS) or dextrose 5% in water (D_5W); the infusion is started at 1 to 2 mg/h for adults, and then titrated upward in increments of 2 mg/h. Often, an analgesic infusion such as fentanyl or morphine is used in combination with midazolam, which potentiates the effects of both medications.

The recommended dosing for status epilepticus is 0.2 mg/kg IV, up to a maximum of 10 mg. If given intramuscularly, a single 10-mg dose is recommended in adults. Close cardiorespiratory monitoring is needed when giving larger midazolam doses.

Midazolam is believed to produce its effects by altering the neurotransmitter gamma-aminobutyric acid (GABA). Thus, midazolam acts as a CNS depressant, though it also has hypnotic and anterograde amnesic properties. Patient recovery time depends on both the dose and the duration of administration.

Diazepam

Diazepam is a moderately long-acting benzodiazepine with similar indications as midazolam. Diazepam is also marketed in a gel designed for rectal administration by caregivers in the community to treat status epilepticus seizures. Rectal gel dosing is 0.5 mg/kg for children age 2 to 5 years, 0.3 mg/kg for children age 6 to 11 years, and 0.2 mg/kg for children 12 years and older. Of note, IV diazepam solution (5 mg/mL) is sometimes used for rectal administration in hospital settings. Although

TABLE 8-6 Sedatives, Anesthetics, Analgesics, and Anticonvulsants

Medication	Uses	Mechanism of Action	Route of Administration	Side Effects	Special Considerations
Sedatives					
Midazolam	Sedation, anxiety, amnesia (during procedures), for induction of general anesthesia, seizures	Enhances the action of the inhibitory neurotransmitter GABA	Oral, IV, IO, IM, intranasal, buccal	Respiratory depression, hypotension, drowsiness, nausea, vomiting	Due to its low pH of 3, burning is likely to occur with intranasal administration. Higher concentrations (ie, 5 mg/mL) are preferred to reduce the total intranasal volume needed. Monitor respiratory status using capnography as well as blood pressure during administration.
Diazepam	Anxiety, acute alcohol withdrawal, muscle spasm, seizures, sedation	Enhances the action of the inhibitory neurotransmitter GABA	Oral, IV, IO, IM, rectal	Hypotension, drowsiness, respiratory depression, localized phlebitis, pain at injection site	Diazepam is a vesicant; avoid extravasation. Monitor respiratory status using capnography as well as blood pressure during administration.
Lorazepam	Anxiety, amnesia, agitation, premedication to general anesthesia, alcohol withdrawal syndrome, seizures, chemotherapy-associated nausea and vomiting	Enhances the action of the inhibitory neurotransmitter GABA	Oral, SL, IV, IO, IM	Hypotension, sedation, respiratory depression	Unopened vials require refrigeration (contact the manufacturer for room-temperature storage information). The injectable solution requires dilution. Its thickness also makes it difficult to withdraw from vial; use larger-gauge needles. Contains propylene glycol or benzyl alcohol; long-term or high-dose infusions may lead to toxicity. Monitor respiratory status using capnography as well as blood pressure during administration.

(Continues)

TABLE 8-6 Sedatives, Anesthetics, Analgesics, and Anticonvulsants (continued)

Medication	Uses	Mechanism of Action	Route of Administration	Side Effects	Special Considerations
Phenobarbital	Seizures, sedation, alcohol and sedative-hypnotic withdrawal, status epilepticus	Depresses the sensory cortex, which slows cerebral metabolism and decreases cerebral oxygen consumption	Oral, IM, IV, IO	Bradycardia, hypotension, syncope, profound CNS depression, respiratory depression	Monitor heart rate, blood pressure, oxygen saturation, and capnography continuously during administration.
Dexmedetomidine	ICU sedation of mechanically ventilated patients, procedural sedation of nonintubated patients	Agonist of alpha-2 adrenergic receptors; exhibits both sedative and anesthetic properties	IV	Sedation, hypotension, bradycardia (risk related to loading doses or higher maintenance doses), agitation/delirium (responds well to benzodiazepines), inhibits salivation	Patients are usually readily aroused with stimulation. Dexmedetomidine is not appropriate for patients who are paralyzed. Monitor heart rate and blood pressure continuously during administration. Use narcotics and benzodiazepines cautiously and in reduced doses; dexmedetomidine enhances their effects.
Anesthetics					
Propofol	Induction of anesthesia, procedural sedation, refractory status epilepticus	Causes global CNS depression through likely agonism of GABA-1 receptors	IV, IO	Hypotension, injection-site burning/pain, apnea, arrhythmias, hypertriglyceridemia with high-dose, long-term infusion (more than 2 days), oversedation, propofol-related infusion syndrome	Monitor heart rate, blood pressure, oxygen saturation, and capnography continuously during administration. Lidocaine may be used to reduce injection-site pain. Requires aseptic handling; the lipid emulsion encourages bacterial growth. Change tubing every 12 hours.

Drug	Indication	Description	Route	Side Effects	Monitoring
Etomidate	Induction of anesthesia, procedural sedation	Ultra-short-acting benzylimidazole general anesthetic	IV, IO	Pain at injection site, nausea and vomiting on emergence from anesthetic effects, myoclonus (up to 33% of patients), transient skeletal movements, uncontrolled eye movements, hiccups, apnea, impaired cortisol synthesis	Monitor heart rate, blood pressure, oxygen saturation, and capnography continuously during administration. Monitor the infusion site carefully; etomidate is very irritating.
Ketamine	Induction and maintenance of general anesthesia, analgesia, procedural sedation, refractory status epilepticus	Produces a cataleptic-like state (dissociation) most likely by NMDA receptor antagonism	IV, IO, IM, oral	Hypertension and increased heart rate (transient); may cause auditory/visual hallucinations, restlessness, vivid dreams, irrational behavior on emergence; tonic-clonic movements resembling seizure	Laryngeal reflexes and respiratory drive usually remain intact during ketamine administration. Bronchodilation occurs. Monitor heart rate, blood pressure, oxygen saturation, and capnography continuously during administration. Laryngospasm is an extremely rare but dangerous side effect.
Antipsychotics					
Haloperidol	Behavioral disorders, delirium, tranquilization of agitated/aggressive/violent patients	Blocks postsynaptic dopaminergic D_2 receptors; first-generation (typical) antipsychotic	Oral, IM, IV, IO (IV is common but unapproved)	QT prolongation (especially at high IV doses), excessive sedation, hypotension, bradycardia, neuroleptic malignant syndrome, and extrapyramidal symptoms	Avoid large doses. Monitor blood pressure and cardiac rhythm. Baseline 12-lead ECG recommended to follow QTc.

(Continues)

TABLE 8-6 Sedatives, Anesthetics, Analgesics, and Anticonvulsants (continued)

Medication	Uses	Mechanism of Action	Route of Administration	Side Effects	Special Considerations
Olanzapine	Treatment of schizophrenia-associated acute agitation, delirium, psychosis or acute agitation, PTSD, Tourette syndrome	Combined antagonism of dopamine and serotonin receptor sites; atypical antipsychotic	IM, oral (ODT available)	Orthostatic hypotension, drowsiness, Parkinson-like syndrome, extrapyramidal syndrome, weight gain (with regular use)	Patients should be monitored closely for excessive sedation.
Quetiapine	Delirium in the critically ill patient, generalized anxiety disorder, bipolar disorder, schizophrenia	Believed to be a combination of dopamine and serotonin receptor antagonism; atypical antipsychotic	Oral	Drowsiness, dry mouth (xerostomia), orthostatic hypotension	Lack of parenteral formulation may be challenging in noncooperative patients.
Analgesics					
Fentanyl	Pain management, adjunct to anesthesia	Binds with opioid receptors in the CNS, preventing painful impulse transmission	Oral, transdermal, IM, IV, IO, intranasal	Respiratory depression, apnea, hypotension, bradycardia, palpitations, flushing, nausea, vomiting, constipation, disorientation, urinary retention	Monitor heart rate, blood pressure, oxygen saturation, and capnography continuously during administration.
Sufentanil	Pain management, adjunct to anesthesia, surgical and postoperative analgesia	Binds with opioid receptors in the CNS, preventing painful impulse transmission	IV, IO, SL	Respiratory depression, apnea, hypotension, bradycardia, palpitations, flushing, nausea	Considerably more potent and shorter acting than fentanyl. Monitor heart rate, blood pressure, oxygen saturation, and capnography continuously during administration.

Morphine	Pain management	Binds with opioid receptors in the CNS, preventing painful impulse transmission	Oral, subcutaneous, IM, IV, IO, intranasal	Respiratory depression, apnea, hypotension, bradycardia, palpitations, flushing, nausea and vomiting (usually related to speed of administration), urinary retention, constipation	Monitor heart rate, blood pressure, oxygen saturation, and capnography continuously during administration. Use with caution in patients with renal dysfunction (may accumulate).
Hydromorphone	Pain management	Binds with opioid receptors in the CNS, preventing painful impulse transmission; produces generalized CNS depression	Oral, subcutaneous, IM, IV, IO, PR	Respiratory depression, apnea, hypotension, bradycardia, palpitations, flushing, nausea, vomiting, abnormal dreams, cognitive dysfunction	Often used in patients who are allergic to or who fail to respond to morphine. Use with caution because of its potency. Monitor heart rate, blood pressure, oxygen saturation, and capnography continuously during administration.
Nalbuphine	Pain management, opioid-induced pruritus (itching)	Agonist and partial antagonist; binds with opioid receptors in the CNS	Subcutaneous, IM, IV, IO	Excessive sedation, respiratory depression, dizziness, nausea, vomiting	Often used for opioid-induced pruritus, especially with epidural opioid infusions. Blood pressure and respiratory monitoring are recommended when nalbuphine is used for analgesia.
Acetaminophen	Temporary relief of minor aches and pains (mild to moderate pain), antipyretic, treatment of moderate to severe pain when combined with an opioid	Believed to activate serotonergic inhibitory pathways; works peripherally to block pain impulses; antipyresis results from inhibition of heat-regulating hypothalamic centers	Oral, PR, IV, IO	Most significant side effect is liver toxicity; maximum daily dose for healthy adults is 4 g; limit to less than 2 g/day for patients with liver disease or EtOH abuse history	Often combined with opioids for treatment of severe pain. Use caution with total daily dose when giving combination products and acetaminophen.

(continues)

TABLE 8-6 Sedatives, Anesthetics, Analgesics, and Anticonvulsants (continued)

Medication	Uses	Mechanism of Action	Route of Administration	Side Effects	Special Considerations
Ketorolac	Short-term (less than 5 days) management of moderate to severe pain, treatment of migraine in adults	Inhibits COX-1 and COX-2 enzymes, decreasing formation of prostaglandin precursors; exhibits antipyretic, analgesic, and anti-inflammatory properties	Oral, IM, IV, IO	Abdominal discomfort, gastritis, headache, renal insufficiency	Use with caution in patients with preexisting renal dysfunction. Ketorolac inhibits platelet function and is contraindicated in patients at high risk of bleeding. Administer IV doses slowly (over more than 15 s).
Anticonvulsants					
Levetiracetam	Seizures, status epilepticus, seizure prophylaxis in patients with subarachnoid hemorrhage	Unknown; believed to have multiple central pharmacologic effects, including calcium channel and facilitation of GABA inhibitory transmission	Oral, IV, IO	Behavioral problems and vomiting in children and adolescents, weakness, CNS depression	Administer IV doses over 15 min or at a rate of 2–5 mg/kg per min.
Phenytoin	Seizures, status epilepticus, prevention of early (within 1 week) seizures following traumatic brain injury	Decreases cellular sodium levels in the motor cortex of the CNS; increases effective refractory period in neural cells; also has antiarrhythmic activity	Oral, IV, IO	Hypotension, CNS depression, nausea, cardiac arrhythmias, venous irritation, skin rash	IV phenytoin should not be infused any faster than 50 mg/min in adults. Slow the infusion rate if hypotension occurs. Monitor IV sites closely for signs of infiltration; phenytoin is a vesicant.
Fosphenytoin	Seizures, status epilepticus	Stabilizes neuronal membranes and influx/efflux of sodium across cell membranes	IM, IV, IO	Hypotension, CNS depression, cardiac arrhythmias, venous irritation; transient and dose-related pruritus, tinnitus, and somnolence	IV fosphenytoin is considered safer for administration than phenytoin. Monitor IV sites closely for signs of infiltration. Continuous respiratory, blood pressure, and ECG monitoring are recommended during loading doses and for 10–20 min after infusion.

Drug	Indications	Mechanism	Route	Side Effects	Monitoring
Valproic acid	Seizures, status epilepticus, bipolar disorder	Increases GABA availability	Oral, IV, IO	Headache, drowsiness, gastrointestinal distress, dose-related thrombocytopenia, tremor, weakness, visual disturbances	Monitor liver function, platelets, prothrombin time/partial thromboplastin time, and serum ammonia levels during therapy.
Pentobarbital	Sedation, status epilepticus refractory to first-line anticonvulsants, barbiturate coma in severe brain injury with elevated intracranial pressure	Depresses the sensory cortex, which slows cerebral metabolism and decreases cerebral oxygen consumption	IM, IV, IO	Bradycardia, hypotension, syncope, profound CNS depression, respiratory depression, nausea, vomiting	Monitor heart rate, blood pressure, oxygen saturation, and capnography continuously during administration.

Abbreviations: CNS, central nervous system; COX-1, cyclooxygenase 1; COX-2, cyclooxygenase 2; ECG, electrocardiogram; EtOH, ethyl alcohol; GABA, gamma-aminobutyric acid; ICU, intensive care unit; IM, intramuscular; IO, intraosseous; IV, intravenous; NMDA, N-methyl-D-aspartate; ODT, oral disintegrating tablets; PR, rectal; PTSD, posttraumatic stress disorder; SL, sublingual

diazepam has been used for procedural sedation in adults, its use for this indication has fallen out of favor due to its longer half-life (and its active metabolite).

Diazepam is incompatible with many other drugs. For this reason, it should never be mixed with other solutions or medications.

Lorazepam

Lorazepam remains the preferred benzodiazepine for emergency treatment of status epilepticus. Unfortunately, its physical and chemical properties pose obstacles to field use. Lorazepam requires refrigeration for its storage, although it may remain stable at room temperature for shorter periods, depending on the manufacturer. Injectable lorazepam is a very thick liquid, making it difficult to draw into a syringe, especially if using a smaller-gauge needle. Finally, propylene glycol is typically used to preserve injectable lorazepam; when the drug is administered as a continuous infusion at higher doses, this preservative can result in toxicity. Collectively, these physical and chemical properties explain why midazolam tends to be the benzodiazepine most often carried by field units.

Lorazepam is an anxiolytic and is commonly used to treat acute alcohol withdrawal. In addition, it is often used as an adjunct antiemetic for anticipatory chemotherapy-induced nausea and vomiting.

Flumazenil is a benzodiazepine reversal agent that competitively inhibits benzodiazepine receptor site activity. This medication is rarely used, especially in patients on long-term benzodiazepines, as it may precipitate seizures (highlighted by a black box FDA warning on its label). Many experts recommend symptomatic management of suspected benzodiazepine overdose (ie, assisted ventilation and supportive treatment of hypotension) rather than administering a reversal agent.

Phenobarbital

Phenobarbital is a long-acting barbiturate used in critical care for treatment of status epilepticus, seizures, and alcohol withdrawal. For treatment of status epilepticus, 20 mg/kg of IV phenobarbital is administered initially at 50 to 100 mg/min. A second dose of 5 to 10 mg/kg can be given 10 minutes after completing the initial loading dose if needed. Phenobarbital results in significant sedation and respiratory depression, and hypotension often occurs during the IV loading dose administration. For treatment of status epilepticus, this agent is usually considered only after other first-line therapies (eg, fosphenytoin, levetiracetam) have failed.

Dexmedetomidine

Dexmedetomidine is a selective alpha-2 adrenergic receptor agonist with analgesic and anxiolytic properties. It is used for sedation in mechanically ventilated patients, as a premedication for induction of anesthesia, for procedural sedation, for relief of pain, and to reduce opioid doses following surgery or trauma. Dexmedetomidine may cause hypotension (24% to 56% of patients) and bradycardia (5% to 42%), though these effects tend to be dose and duration dependent.

Loading doses are occasionally used in adult patients, beginning with an infusion of 0.5 to 1 µg/kg/h for 10 minutes; however, such doses are more likely to cause adverse cardiovascular effects (eg, hypertension, hypotension, bradycardia). Most patients are started on maintenance infusion of 0.2 to 0.7 µg/kg/h. Titration is done in increments of 0.1 µg/kg/h. Dexmedetomidine's onset of action varies between 5 and 10 minutes.

There has been considerable discussion regarding the maximum doses and duration of therapy with dexmedetomidine. Doses as high as 2.5 µg/kg/h have been used, although many reference sources note that doses greater than 1.5 µg/kg/h do not offer additional clinical benefits. In practice, the authors typically use doses of up to 2 µg/kg/h. The manufacturer recommends that the duration of dexmedetomidine infusion not exceed 24 hours, although several clinical trials have shown that dexmedetomidine has safety and efficacy comparable to that for lorazepam and midazolam with infusions of up to 5 days.

There is potential for medication errors when administering dexmedetomidine because recommended doses are expressed in micrograms per kilogram per hour (µg/kg/h), an administration unit quite different from that of other sedatives and analgesics used in the ICU.

Hypotension associated with dexmedetomidine can be lessened by eliminating the loading dose and titrating the dose upward no more often than every 30 minutes. Pressors may be needed to manage the hypotension. Bradycardia, especially when it occurs early in the administration of dexmedetomidine, can be treated with atropine. Later in the course of treatment, symptomatic bradycardia may require discontinuation of dexmedetomidine and may take several hours to resolve because of the drug's prolonged clearance time. Patients sedated with dexmedetomidine at sedative doses are usually arousable and alert when stimulated.

Dosing of dexmedetomidine is very individualized and should be titrated to the desired effects. Weaning should be accomplished by downward titration so that the patient becomes more alert slowly. Acute agitation is best managed with small doses of intravenous benzodiazepines such as midazolam. Patients receiving infusions of dexmedetomidine should receive smaller initial doses of sedatives and narcotics, as these agents' effects tend to be increased in the presence of the dexmedetomidine.

Propofol

Propofol is a general anesthetic. In addition to its use in the operating room for induction and maintenance of anesthesia, this agent is employed as a sedative in mechanically ventilated patients. It provides both anesthetic and amnesic effects that begin, on average, 30 seconds following bolus administration (range, 9 to 51 seconds), with these effects then lasting from 3 to 10 minutes depending on dosing. This very short duration of action is one of the primary advantages of propofol over other sedatives, as it allows for rapid awakening and assessment of the patient.

For sedation in the mechanically ventilated critical care patient, usual propofol doses range from 5 to 50 μg/kg/min to a maximum of 100 μg/kg/min at some institutions. Titration upward and downward is usually done every 5 minutes in increments of 5 to 10 μg/kg/min. When higher doses are required, an additional infusion of a narcotic analgesic may significantly lower the propofol requirements. Bolus dosing, when permitted and necessary for acute agitation, is usually given in 25- to 50-mg increments in a typical adult.

Propofol is formulated in a 1% fat emulsion (10 mg/mL). The lipid base increases the potential for microorganism growth in the solution. Tubing should be changed at 12-hour intervals to lessen this risk, and propofol should not be infused with blood or plasma. Propofol may cause pain on injection into peripheral vessels. Injection-site pain can be lessened by using larger veins of the upper arm or antecubital fossa or by pretreatment with 1 mL of a 1% lidocaine solution.

Close and careful cardiopulmonary monitoring is necessary when using propofol. The most significant cardiac effect of propofol is hypotension, which can be more pronounced in patients who are hypovolemic. Hypotension is also dose related and occurs more frequently with bolus dosing and in patients who are receiving other sedatives or narcotics. Dosing should be titrated to individual effect, with continuous monitoring of the level of sedation. Abrupt discontinuation can result in rapid awakening and acute agitation; to avoid this outcome, the infusion should be titrated to allow for slow awakening. Propofol effects may be more pronounced in patients who are frail or elderly.

Propofol is generally intended for short-term use (less than 48 hours). Both prolonged and high-dose infusions have been associated with **propofol-related infusion syndrome (PRIS)**, a constellation of symptoms including arrhythmias (bradycardia), metabolic acidosis, hyperkalemia, rhabdomyolysis or creatine phosphokinase elevations, and progressive renal and cardiac failure. Mortality from PRIS is high, with estimates of 33% to 66%. When propofol is used for more than 48 hours, especially at doses exceeding 50 μg/kg/min, serum triglyceride levels should be monitored every 3 to 7 days.

Etomidate

Etomidate is an ultra-short-acting general anesthetic used for procedural sedation, induction of general anesthesia, and intubation. Its ultra-short duration of action and favorable side-effect profile make it a popular choice for rapid sequence and emergent intubations. Compared to other induction agents, etomidate results in considerably lower incidence of hypotension. This medication depresses the reticular activating system by stimulating GABA receptors. It decreases oxygen consumption and cerebral blood flow, which may be useful in patients with increased intracranial pressure (ICP).

Administered intravenously at a dose of 0.3 mg/kg (range, 0.2 to 0.6 mg/kg) over 30 to 60 seconds, etomidate reaches its peak effect in 1 minute and provides dose-dependent anesthesia for approximately 4 to 10 minutes. This agent is highly irritating and should not be administered in smaller blood vessels. Pretreatment with lidocaine may be considered.

Other than an allergy to etomidate, there are no absolute contraindications to this medication's use in RSI. Etomidate has been associated with a high incidence of uncomfortable myoclonic muscle movements, an effect that is most apparent when this agent is used as monotherapy for procedural sedation. During RSI, myoclonus is masked by rapid administration of paralytics. Some studies had suggested etomidate was associated with adrenal suppression, leading some to reconsider its use in critically ill patients. More recent data suggest that a single etomidate dose blocks the stress-induced rise in adrenal cortisol production for 6 to 8 hours and potentially up to 24 hours in debilitated or older adult patients, but this effect has not been associated with increased mortality. In patients receiving repeated doses of etomidate who are under severe stress, corticosteroid replacement may be indicated.

Ketamine

Ketamine, a phencyclidine (PCP) derivative, is a general anesthetic that is increasingly being used on an off-label basis in the prehospital arena to provide procedural sedation and analgesia. Ketamine's pharmacodynamics make it particularly attractive for critical care and emergency situations. This agent has a rapid onset of action, produces a dose-dependent profound anesthetic or dissociative state, results in bronchodilation, causes little to no respiratory depression or loss of gag reflex, and tends to increase (rather than lower) blood pressure. In addition to its utility for analgesia and procedural sedation of entrapped patients, ketamine has recently shown promise in rapid sedation of patients exhibiting signs and symptoms of excited delirium syndrome (ExDS). Anesthesia providers may use ketamine in concert with propofol, which at low doses may also allow sedation without intubation. The mixture of ketamine and propofol, nicknamed "ketofol," is commonly prepared in a syringe or given sequentially. See Chapter 25, *Bariatric, Psychiatric, and Special Situations*, for further discussion of ExDS.

Induction of general anesthesia is achieved with 1 to 4.5 mg/kg of ketamine when given intravenously or with 6.5 to 13 mg/kg when given intramuscularly. For procedural sedation (pacing, extrication, cardioversion, ExDS, fracture management), 0.2 to 0.8 mg/kg is the recommended IV or IO dose, or 2 to 4 mg/kg intramuscularly. IV or IO doses should be administered over at least 60 seconds, as rapid administration tends to be associated with respiratory depression, apnea, and unusually high spikes in blood pressure. Some references suggest administration of IV ketamine over 2 to 3 minutes. Laryngospasm is a rare adverse reaction that has been reported with use of this medication.

Anesthetic doses of ketamine given intravenously take effect within 30 seconds and last for 5 to 10 minutes, with full recovery occurring within 1 to 2 hours. IM administration takes effect in 3 to 4 minutes, with the action lasting 12 to 25 minutes and full recovery occurring in 3 to 4 hours. Despite the significant anesthetic effect, ketamine leaves the patient with near-normal pharyngeal and laryngeal reflexes and normal to slightly enhanced skeletal muscle tone, though it sometimes results in transient respiratory depression or episodic apnea. Enhanced skeletal muscle tone in some patients may appear as tonic-clonic movements and be mistaken for seizures. In reality, these movements do not imply an emergence from anesthesia or a need for additional medications. Nystagmus is a common finding in patients dissociated with ketamine.

Ketamine elevates heart rate and blood pressure starting shortly after injection, but these vital signs typically return to preadministration values within 15 minutes. Systolic and diastolic blood pressure may increase as well. Ketamine also results in bronchodilation, increased cerebral blood flow and metabolism, and increased salivary secretions. Anesthesia providers may premedicate patients with atropine (0.4 to 0.6 mg given intravenously 30 to 60 minutes before induction) to reduce salivary secretions.

Emergence from a ketamine-induced anesthetic state may result in tachycardia, a rise in blood pressure, nystagmus, and attempts at swallowing. Return to consciousness is usually gradual.

When other sedatives or narcotics are coadministered, lower doses of ketamine are needed to achieve the desired effects, and the risk of apnea increases. These risks are particularly concerning for patients who fail to receive sufficient analgesia from multiple doses of narcotics prior to escalating to ketamine.

For analgesia, ketamine doses of 0.1 to 0.3 mg/kg IV are commonly recommended. Intranasal dosing for acute pain management using 0.5 to 1 mg/kg of ketamine, repeated if necessary using 0.25 to 0.5 mg/kg after 10 to 15 minutes, can be used when IV access is not available.

Ketamine's label carries a warning about emergence reactions, which appear as the patient emerges from the effects of ketamine sedation. Such emergence reactions, which occur in approximately 12% of patients, comprise psychological manifestations that vary from pleasant dreamlike states, to vivid images and hallucinations, to delirium. They may be associated with confusion, excitement, or irrational behavior, and usually last for only a few hours. Rarely, emergence reactions may recur up to 24 hours later. There is a markedly lower incidence of emergence reactions in patients younger than 15 years and in those older than 65 years. Administration of a benzodiazepine, such as midazolam, diazepam, or lorazepam, in conjunction with ketamine also reduces emergence reactions. Acute emergence reactions should be treated with benzodiazepines.

Clinicians experienced in the use of ketamine for procedural sedation suggest that emergence reactions may be directly influenced by the environment. Informing the patient ahead of time about the expected side effects and ensuring a calm, quiet environment may decrease patient agitation and unpleasant side effects. As ketamine may transiently precipitate symptoms resembling schizophrenia (psychosis), it should be used with caution in patients with schizophrenia. It is not recommended for routine use.

Haloperidol

Haloperidol is an antipsychotic medication that is used in the treatment of delirium and agitation in the critical care setting. Administration of this agent via the IV route is common practice, but is considered an off-label route. For critical care patients with delirium and severe agitation (or escalating agitation that is expected to become severe), haloperidol is administered intravenously at doses ranging from 0.5 to 10 mg, with doubling of the initial dose every 15 to 30 minutes until the patient is calm, and then 25% of the bolus dose being administered every 6 hours as maintenance. Some literature suggests maximum doses greater than 40 mg/d offer no added clinical benefits. In practice, many clinicians find that patients who fail to become calm with several doses of haloperidol do respond to a benzodiazepine.

Haloperidol can be given intramuscularly when IV access is not available. In such cases, this agent is often combined with a benzodiazepine such as lorazepam and sometimes with an antihistamine such as diphenhydramine. The combined effects of these therapies are usually significantly sedating. Additionally, diphenhydramine or benztropine may be used as a prophylactic anticholinergic agent to ameliorate extrapyramidal symptoms when coadministered with haloperidol.

Intravenous haloperidol can result in hypotension. QTc prolongation may occur, especially when given IV. Numerous studies in critically ill patients who were given IV haloperidol have demonstrated that, while QTc prolongation does occur, it is rarely associated with ventricular arrhythmias in patients without preexisting cardiac channel disorders.

Olanzapine

Olanzapine is an atypical antipsychotic used to treat delirium and severe agitation in the critical care environment. While available in a short-acting intramuscular injectable form, the preferred form for administration in the CCT environment is an oral disintegrating tablet; this tablet dissolves rapidly in saliva and can be easily swallowed with or without liquids.

The usual IM adult dose of olanzapine is 5 to 10 mg. A repeat dose may be given 2 hours later, if needed, and a third dose given 4 hours after the second, if needed. The maximum daily adult dose is 30 mg. Parenteral olanzapine and benzodiazepines should not be given together, as their coadministration has been linked with increased mortality.

Quetiapine

Quetiapine is an atypical antipsychotic that is used off-label to treat delirium, confusion, and insomnia in patients in the ICU. Initial dosing is 25 to 50 mg given orally two or three times daily. The dose can be adjusted upward daily to a maximum of 400 mg/d.

Compared to other antipsychotics, many intensivists find quetiapine to be the most efficacious agent for ICU delirium. Unfortunately, quetiapine is available in oral form only, limiting its use in uncooperative patients.

Fentanyl

Fentanyl is a potent, synthetic opioid analgesic with a rapid onset and short duration of action. This agent is 70 to 100 times more potent than morphine; that is, 10 mg of morphine is equivalent to 100 to 150 μg of fentanyl. Fentanyl is an analgesic that is also used for procedural sedation in intubated critical care patients. Prehospital providers often administer fentanyl intranasally as an analgesic or for procedural sedation.

Typical adult dosing of fentanyl for analgesia or sedation includes a dose of 50 to 100 μg administered intravenously over 1 to 3 minutes, followed by an infusion starting at 25 μg/h. Incremental dose changes are typically made in steps of 8 to 10 μg/h, implemented every 5 minutes. Alternatively, weight-based dosing of 0.7 to 10 μg/kg/h can be used. Usual infusion dose ranges for adults vary between 25 and 125 μg/h, up to a maximum of 200 μg/h, although some studies report employing doses of as high as 700 μg/h. When fentanyl is given at a dose of 0.5 to 2 μg/kg, the patient will experience analgesia within about 90 seconds, with an effective duration lasting approximately 30 minutes.

Rapid administration of fentanyl and single IV doses exceeding 150 μg in adults have (rarely) been associated with rigid chest wall syndrome. This chest wall rigidity interferes with ventilation and necessitates immediate treatment with naloxone or a short-acting neuromuscular-blocking agent; either option will facilitate adequate ventilation. The occurrence of chest wall rigidity does not appear to be a contraindication to later use of fentanyl or other opioids.

Fentanyl has minimal cardiovascular effects, although bradycardia, tachycardia, and arrhythmias have been reported with its use. Hypotension is also possible, especially when sympathetic stimulation from pain is artificially producing an increased blood pressure in the patient. Consequently, it is common for patients' hemodynamic, CNS, and respiratory status to decline when painful stimulation is suddenly eliminated by opioid medications.

Sufentanil

Sufentanil is similar to fentanyl, with significant analgesic effects and minimal cardiovascular effects. Sufentanil, however, is 10 times more potent than fentanyl; that is, 100 μg of fentanyl is equivalent to 10 μg of sufentanil. Sufentanil also has a shorter half-life than fentanyl, which makes it an ideal choice for use in surgical settings. CCTPs may encounter patients receiving sufentanil in postoperative ICU settings.

Sufentanil bolus and infusion doses are based on the anticipated duration of surgery. Doses range from 1 to 8 μg/kg prior to surgery, followed by maintenance doses up to 1.5 μg/kg/h.

As is true for other opioid agonists, patients with compromised respiratory systems should not receive sufentanil unless their airway and ventilations can be supported. The adverse reactions observed with this agent are similar to those seen with fentanyl, including chest wall rigidity, cardiac arrhythmias, and respiratory depression.

Morphine

Morphine is an opioid receptor agonist that acts directly on the CNS to produce analgesia. It is used as an analgesic in the critical care environment.

Usual doses of morphine vary widely, depending on the patient. Notably, IV doses are two to three times more potent than the same doses taken orally. Morphine should be diluted and bolus doses administered over 3 to 5 minutes to reduce side effects of nausea and vomiting, hypotension, and respiratory depression. An initial loading dose of 5 to 10 mg of morphine can be given over 3 to 5 minutes. Infusions are typically mixed as a concentration of 1 mg/mL and initiated in adults at 2 mg/h. Upward titration can be done hourly in increments of 2 mg/h. Additional bolus doses of 2 to 5 mg can be given as needed until the patient is comfortable. Due to the longer half-life and safer opioid infusion alternatives, morphine infusions are most commonly used during palliative care in hospital settings. However, morphine is also used during patient-controlled analgesia infusions.

Patients frequently report flushing or an itchy feeling when they receive morphine, which is sometimes mistaken for an allergic reaction. The actual cause is morphine-induced histamine release, which leads to vasodilation and rather bothersome incidence of pruritus. Treatment options for these side effects are limited. Typically, antihistamines are used to manage the itching, although their use often results in additional sedative effects. Low doses of IV nalbuphine may be used to relieve opioid-induced pruritus. Low-dose and continuous low-dose infusions of naloxone have also been shown to produce positive results, but are less effective than antihistamines and may reverse the opioid effect and precipitate withdrawal. Another option for patients with significant histamine-related effects from morphine is a change to fentanyl, whose use results in considerably less, if any, histamine release.

Hydromorphone

Hydromorphone is an opioid analgesic used in the management of moderate to severe pain. It is used when the patient does not obtain relief from morphine or fentanyl.

Dosing of hydromorphone to achieve relief from pain varies widely among patients. The IV doses are two to four times more potent than equal doses taken orally. Compared to the effects achieved with IV morphine, 1 mg of hydromorphone is equivalent to 7 mg of morphine.

Usual adult dosing of hydromorphone is 0.4 to 0.8 mg given intravenously over 3 to 5 minutes, repeated every 2 to 6 hours as needed. Rarely, hydromorphone infusion may be required, starting at 0.5 mg/h and titrated upward every hour in increments of 0.3 mg/h. Like morphine, hydromorphone is often used in patient-controlled analgesia infusions.

Nalbuphine

Nalbuphine is an opioid agonist-antagonist that is typically given at a dose of 10 mg (IV, IM, or subcutaneous) every 3 to 6 hours. While not commonly used as an analgesic in critical care, its agonist-antagonist properties make nalbuphine useful in relieving opioid-induced pruritus. This off-label use is dosed intravenously at 2.5 to 5 mg IV, repeated as needed.

Acetaminophen

Acetaminophen is an analgesic and antipyretic. It is commonly used and available as an over-the-counter product in oral and rectal forms.

Intravenous acetaminophen was approved by the FDA in 2010.

The actual mechanism of action of acetaminophen is poorly understood. This medication remains a common cause of drug-induced liver failure in the United States. Maximum daily doses of acetaminophen should not exceed 4 g in healthy adults, and patients with hepatic insufficiency and those who consume more than three alcoholic drinks daily are susceptible to liver damage at daily intake exceeding 2 g. The CCTP should be aware that combination pain medications may contain acetaminophen.

Adult oral acetaminophen doses range from 325 to 650 mg every 4 to 6 hours. Pills or tablets can be crushed and administered through a feeding tube. The maximum single oral dose is 1,000 mg. Adult rectal doses also range from 325 to 650 mg every 4 to 6 hours.

The cost of IV acetaminophen has led most hospital formulary committees to restrict its use to patients who are unable to receive enteral or rectal doses. When given intravenously, dosing is similar to oral doses.

Ketorolac

Ketorolac is a nonsteroidal anti-inflammatory drug (NSAID) used for pain management. The natural reaction to injury or infection in the body is to promote inflammation in the areas involved, in an effort to build up the body's defenses against the invader and to rebuild cell populations. This inflammation-promotion activity is carried out by prostaglandins, which also play a role in fever and platelet activity. Prostaglandins are created by an enzyme found in the cells called cyclooxygenase (COX). NSAIDs such as ketorolac work by blocking the COX enzymes, thereby decreasing the body's load of inflammation-causing prostaglandins.

In the critical care setting, ketorolac is most often administered intravenously. The usual IV dose for adults is 15 to 30 mg given every 6 hours. In critically ill patients, patients older than 65 years, and patients with renal insufficiency, the IV dose is often reduced or not given at all. IV doses should be administered over a minimum of 15 seconds.

Ketorolac should not be used for more than 5 days, regardless of the route of administration. Multiple concerns have arisen related to this agent's adverse effects. Ketorolac inhibits platelet function, which increases the risk of gastrointestinal bleeding, surgical bleeding, and bleeding from all other causes. It also carries an increased risk of thrombotic cardiovascular events, including stroke and myocardial infarction, as do many other NSAIDs; this risk is both dose and duration dependent. Ketorolac may compromise renal function, especially in patients with volume depletion. In addition, this drug should not be used in patients in labor.

Levetiracetam

Levetiracetam is an anticonvulsant. Following immediate treatment with a short-acting benzodiazepine, this agent may be considered for treatment of status epilepticus. A recent large multicenter trial found that levetiracetam, fosphenytoin, and valproate were similarly efficacious in treatment of established status epilepticus.

For status epilepticus, levetiracetam is given intravenously, with the recommended adult dose range being 1,000 to 4,500 mg, infused at a rate of 2 to 5 mg/kg/min. Pediatric dosing is 20 to 60 mg/kg. Levetiracetam may also be used to prevent seizures following significant brain injury. Dosing for seizure prophylaxis in adults is 1,000 mg given intravenously every 12 hours; for children, it is 15 to 25 mg/kg every 12 hours.

Phenytoin

Phenytoin is an anticonvulsant medication. In the critical care setting, it is used after short-acting benzodiazepines for treatment of status epilepticus. The initial IV dosing is 20 mg/kg, infused at a rate no faster than 50 mg/min. An additional dose of 5 to 10 mg/kg can be administered, if needed, 10 minutes after completion of the initial loading dose.

Phenytoin should not be given to patients with cardiac arrhythmias, including atrioventricular (AV) blocks and bradycardia. This agent can itself cause cardiac arrhythmias, including ventricular fibrillation and AV conduction abnormalities, and can lead to significant hypotension. Often, hypotension is related to the speed of administration. Even with slow administration, however, pressors may be required to counteract the negative cardiac effects.

Of note, phenytoin is compatible with only saline; it will precipitate if mixed with dextrose or other IV solutions. It may also cause significant tissue necrosis if extravasated. Extravasation of IV phenytoin causes "purple glove syndrome," which has required limb amputation in severe situations.

When possible, phenytoin should be administered through a central line. It should not be administered through smaller peripheral veins of the hands or feet. This agent cannot be given as an intramuscular injection.

Oral phenytoin loading is much safer than administration of IV phenytoin and should be contemplated for conscious, stable, low-risk patients. Oral loading will take approximately 6 hours to reach a therapeutic plasma level. Dosing should be considered carefully when patients who are already taking phenytoin present following a seizure with a subtherapeutic plasma phenytoin level.

Fosphenytoin

Fosphenytoin is a precursor to phenytoin; when metabolized, it yields phenytoin. This agent is designed to be modified by the body (biotransformed) into phenytoin, which makes it a **prodrug** of phenytoin. Because it transforms into phenytoin, the dose is documented as milligrams of phenytoin equivalents (PE). For status epilepticus, the IV dose of fosphenytoin is 20 mg PE/kg, administered at rates of up to 150 mg PE/min. If needed, a second dose of 5 mg PE/kg can be administered 10 minutes after completion of the initial loading dose.

Fosphenytoin is compatible with saline, dextrose, and lactated Ringer solutions and can be administered as an intramuscular injection. Dose volumes of up to 20 mL per injection site have been reported.

Valproic Acid

Valproic acid is an anticonvulsant that is used to treat benzodiazepine-resistant status epilepticus. IV dosing for adults is 20 to 40 mg/kg administered at a rate of 3 to 6 mg/kg/min (typically, over a minimum of 5 minutes). If needed, a second dose of 20 mg/kg can be administered 10 minutes after completing the loading infusion. In studies where more rapid infusion rates were used, they seemed to be well tolerated. The loading doses may be followed by a continuous infusion of 1 to 4 mg/kg/h for 24 hours. Liver enzymes and serum ammonia levels should be monitored during treatment with valproic acid. In addition, valproic acid may prolong bleeding times.

Seizures are not the only indication for valproic acid. Indeed, this drug is prescribed for a wide range of other conditions, including migraine headaches, bipolar disorder, neuropathic pain syndromes, diabetic neuropathy, postherpetic neuralgia, and borderline personality disorder.

Pentobarbital

Pentobarbital is a short-acting hypnotic barbiturate and an anticonvulsant. Prior to the advent of many newer sedatives with more favorable side-effect profiles, it was used as a sedative for acutely agitated patients. Today, pentobarbital is more commonly employed to induce a barbiturate coma in severely brain-injured patients with elevated ICP as well as to treat refractory status epilepticus. Patients should be intubated prior to administration of this treatment for status epilepticus or traumatic brain injury, as IV pentobarbital can induce significant respiratory depression as well as laryngospasm. Hypotension requiring pressor support is also commonly seen with the high doses needed to induce a pentobarbital coma. The onset of action with IV pentobarbital typically occurs within 1 minute of its administration.

When pentobarbital is used to treat refractory status epilepticus, the loading dose is 5 to 15 mg/kg administered intravenously at a rate no greater than 50 mg/min. This loading dose can be repeated once and is followed by an infusion of 0.5 to 5 mg/kg/h, titrated to electroencephalogram monitoring. Breakthrough seizures are treated with additional boluses of 5 mg/kg and increases in the continuous infusion of 0.5 to 1 mg/kg/h at 12-hour intervals.

As with most barbiturate medications, quick cessation of pentobarbital's use should be avoided, as it can lead to dangerous withdrawal symptoms—most notably, a return of status epilepticus. Additional withdrawal symptoms may include restlessness, insomnia, nausea, vomiting, diarrhea, diaphoresis, tachycardia, hyperthermia, hallucinations, delirium, and death.

Neuromuscular-Blocking Agents

Neuromuscular-blocking agents (NMBAs) block transmission of neuromuscular signals, resulting in skeletal muscle paralysis. The most common indication in the critical care setting for NMBAs is facilitation of endotracheal intubation. Because NMBAs induce paralysis of respiratory muscles, continuous waveform capnography must be used whenever administering any NMBA. **TABLE 8-7** profiles selected NMBAs.

Long-term chemical paralysis of the patient has serious implications for CCTPs and other health care providers who will care for the patient. Muscle weakness and neuropathies can persist long after the patient has been weaned off paralytic medications. These conditions can impair ventilator weaning, prolong ICU admissions, and further compromise patient recovery. It is essential that patients receive paralytics only for the shortest duration and in the lowest possible dose.

Intensive care providers can use a train-of-four (TOF) measurement, post-tetanic count, or double-burst stimulation to assess for the correct level of neuromuscular blockade in patients receiving NMBAs. Special instruction is required so that CCTPs can perform or interpret these tests. Proper use of NMBAs can help prevent excessive dosing of paralytic medications, which will minimize the risk and severity of long-term complications.

TOF and other paralytic monitoring do not reflect the underlying level of sedation and analgesia in chemically paralyzed patients. For this reason, it is imperative that CCTPs and other health care providers carefully evaluate the level of sedation and analgesia in any patient who is chemically paralyzed. In many patients, but especially those with unstable hemodynamics, assessment of sedation and analgesia using vital signs is unreliable. Conversely, it is common for hypertension and tachycardia to be incorrectly treated with vasoactive medications when the underlying cause is actually undersedation or pain. Unfortunately, inadequate sedation and analgesia in chemically paralyzed patients is commonplace in intensive care and CCT settings. CCTPs must take careful steps to avoid undertreating agitation and pain in any patient whom they transport, especially if the patient is paralyzed. Awareness during paralysis has been linked with poor patient outcomes and posttraumatic stress disorder.

Succinylcholine

Succinylcholine is the only **depolarizing paralytic** agent in widespread use. Depolarizing paralytics

TABLE 8-7 Neuromuscular-Blocking Agents

Medication	Uses	Mechanism of Action	Route of Administration	Side Effects	Special Considerations
Succinylcholine	Fast-acting depolarizing NMBA, facilitation of tracheal intubation	Similar to acetylcholine: depolarizes motor endplates at myoneural junction, leading to sustained flaccid paralysis	IV, IO, IM	Hypertension, hypotension, bradycardia, tachycardia, excessive salivation, muscle fasciculations, hyperkalemia, increased intraocular pressure, malignant hyperthermia, apnea	Monitor ECG, blood pressure, pulse oximetry, waveform capnography, temperature, and neuromuscular function (with a peripheral nerve stimulator) during treatment. Monitor serum potassium prior to and during treatment.
Pancuronium	Long-acting NMBA, to facilitate tracheal intubation, skeletal muscle relaxant during surgery or mechanical ventilation	Blocks acetylcholine from binding to motor endplate receptors (nondepolarizing), inhibiting depolarization	IV, IO	Vagolytic (more than 90% of patients have HR increase of more than 10 beats/min); use cautiously in patients who cannot tolerate increased HR. Clearance prolonged in patients with renal and liver failure.	Monitor ECG, blood pressure, pulse oximetry, waveform capnography, temperature, and neuromuscular function (with a peripheral nerve stimulator) during treatment.
Vecuronium	Intermediate-acting NMBA, to facilitate tracheal intubation, skeletal muscle relaxant during surgery or mechanical ventilation	Blocks acetylcholine from binding to motor endplate receptors (nondepolarizing), inhibiting depolarization	IV, IO	Is not vagolytic (like pancuronium); lower doses needed in patients with renal and hepatic insufficiency (30% is renally excreted, 50% excreted in feces)	Monitor ECG, blood pressure, pulse oximetry, waveform capnography, temperature, and neuromuscular function (with a peripheral nerve stimulator) during treatment.
Rocuronium	Intermediate-acting NMBA, to facilitate tracheal intubation, skeletal muscle relaxant during surgery or mechanical ventilation	Blocks acetylcholine from binding to motor endplate receptors (nondepolarizing), inhibiting depolarization	IV, IO	Very rapid onset of action (less than 2 minutes)	Monitor ECG, blood pressure, pulse oximetry, waveform capnography, temperature, and neuromuscular function (with a peripheral nerve stimulator) during treatment.

Atracurium	Intermediate-acting NMBA, to facilitate tracheal intubation, skeletal muscle relaxant during surgery or mechanical ventilation	IV, IO	Minimal cardiovascular adverse effects but is associated with histamine release at higher doses (flushing, hives, pruritus, wheezing); potential for CNS excitation, especially with higher doses	Monitor ECG, blood pressure, pulse oximetry, waveform capnography, temperature, and neuromuscular function (with a peripheral nerve stimulator) during treatment.
Cisatracurium	Intermediate-acting NMBA, to facilitate tracheal intubation, skeletal muscle relaxant during surgery or mechanical ventilation	IV, IO	Fewer cardiovascular effects; less tendency than atracurium for histamine release	Monitor ECG, blood pressure, pulse oximetry, waveform capnography, temperature, and neuromuscular function (with a peripheral nerve stimulator) during treatment.

Abbreviations: CNS, central nervous system; ECG, electrocardiogram; HR, heart rate; IM, intramuscular; IO, intraosseous; IV, intravenous; NMBA, neuromuscular-blocking agent

© Jones & Bartlett Learning.

Train-of-Four

Train-of-four (TOF) stimulation delivers an electrical impulse to a relevant nerve, allowing a trained observer to assess the level of muscle contraction and thereby estimate NMBA effects. The TOF monitor is a peripheral nerve stimulator capable of delivering a 0- to 80-mA current to the ulnar, facial, or (least commonly) posterior tibial nerve. With the two electrodes properly placed on the skin, pressing the TOF button sends four serial 0.2-ms pulses, spaced 500 ms apart. The number of twitches observed corresponds to the percentage of muscle receptors under NMBA blockade. No twitches suggests 100% of receptors are blocked; one twitch corresponds to 90% blocked; two twitches, 80% blocked; three twitches, 75% blocked; and four twitches, 0% to 75% blocked. Ulnar stimulation causes twitching of the thumb **FIGURE 8-2**, facial stimulation results in twitching of the eyebrow, and posterior tibial stimulation causes plantar flexion of the great (large) toe.

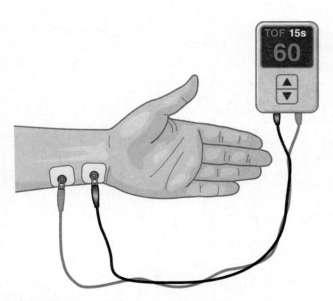

FIGURE 8-2 Train-of-four stimulation of the ulnar nerve causes twitching of the thumb.

© Jones & Bartlett Learning.

act as agonists at nicotinic receptors, mimicking the activity of acetylcholine. Acetylcholine (ACh) is the neurotransmitter that bridges the synapse at the neuromuscular junction. An influx of calcium in the nerves stimulates the release of ACh, which moves across the synapse and binds with the nicotinic receptors on the muscle cells. When ACh makes that connection, depolarization of the muscle takes place and the intended movement or action occurs. Paralytic medications are grouped into one of two categories depending on how they interact with ACh and the nicotinic receptors: *depolarizing* or *nondepolarizing*. Succinylcholine stimulates muscle depolarization but then remains bound to the receptor, thereby preventing it from repolarizing and being triggered again.

In addition to exhibiting activity at nicotinic receptors, succinylcholine stimulates cardiac muscarinic receptors, leading to bradycardia, especially in children. At a dose of 1 to 1.5 mg/kg, patients will experience muscle relaxation in approximately 30 seconds, with total paralysis occurring in about 45 seconds. This rapid onset time, coupled with its duration of action of 4 to 6 minutes, makes succinylcholine an ideal paralytic agent for medication-assisted airway management.

Succinylcholine may increase serum potassium levels, which can cause significant problems in the presence of chronic or acute conditions in which potassium levels may already be elevated. Acute injuries such as crush injuries and spinal cord injuries should be treated with alternative medications, if available. Patients with chronic conditions associated with hyperkalemia, such as renal failure, should also receive an alternative medication.

Succinylcholine can cause a transient increase in ICP. Although the increased ICP from laryngoscopy is of greater concern, this medication-induced ICP must be considered and accounted for in cases of closed head injury.

The most common side effect of succinylcholine is muscle fasciculations, a twitching activity seen as muscles depolarize. Although the twitching may not appear overly dramatic, care should be taken to ensure the patient does not experience injury or inadvertently dislodge IV lines. Some RSI protocols include a reduced dose of a nondepolarizing muscle relaxer that is administered prior to succinylcholine to reduce these fasciculations.

Succinylcholine can cause malignant hyperthermia and, therefore, is contraindicated in patients who have a personal or family history of this condition. (See Chapter 21, *Toxicologic Emergencies*.) Also, providers should expect succinylcholine to have a much longer than normal duration of action when it is administered to any patient who has been exposed to acetylcholinesterase inhibitors, including those found in chemical nerve agents and pesticides. This extended activity is the result of inhibition of acetylcholinesterase, the enzyme that breaks down ACh. A nondepolarizing muscle relaxer may be preferred in these situations. Malignant hyperthermia is discussed in greater depth in Chapter 21, *Toxicologic Emergencies*.

Pancuronium

Pancuronium is a nondepolarizing neuromuscular-blocking agent. A nondepolarizing agent works by competitively antagonizing ACh at the postsynaptic receptors. As a consequence, ACh is unable to cause stimulation at these sites, and muscle depolarization cannot occur. Overall, the major drawback in using nondepolarizing medications is that they tend to have a slower onset of action and longer duration compared to succinylcholine.

Pancuronium is administered as an IV bolus of 0.06 to 0.1 mg/kg, followed by a continuous infusion of 0.8 to 1.7 µg/kg/min (0.048 to 0.102 mg/kg/h). The onset of effect with pancuronium is rapid, occurring within 3 to 5 minutes from administration. While the duration of effect is dose dependent, a typical loading dose will last for about 60 minutes in adults.

Pancuronium must be refrigerated, but is stable at room temperature for as long as 6 months. It can be administered in an undiluted form by rapid IV injection. Its elimination half-life is doubled in patients with renal or hepatic impairment.

Vecuronium

Vecuronium is a nondepolarizing neuromuscular-blocking agent. Initial IV dosing for intubation purposes is 0.08 to 0.1 mg/kg. To maintain paralysis in a critical care setting, a continuous infusion of 0.8 to 1.7 µg/kg/min (0.048 to 0.102 mg/kg/h) is recommended, along with monitoring the depth of neuromuscular blockade every 1 to 2 hours. Usual maintenance infusion doses range from 0.8 to 1.2 µg/kg/min (0.048 to 0.072 mg/kg/h).

Following bolus administration, good intubating conditions occur within 2.5 to 3 minutes. The paralysis lasts for 25 to 40 minutes, with complete recovery occurring approximately 45 to 65 minutes after the initial bolus dose is given.

Vecuronium is manufactured as a powder and must be reconstituted with a compatible diluent prior to use. Vials of powder can be stored at room temperature.

Rocuronium

Rocuronium has the fastest onset time of all the nondepolarizing paralytics, taking effect at 60 to 90 seconds after its administration. It is generally administered at a dose of 0.6 to 1.2 mg/kg, and lasts for as long as 45 minutes with that dose. A higher initial dose (1 mg/kg) permits the shorter onset time needed in RSI procedures. Subsequent maintenance doses can be reduced to 0.5 mg/kg. For maintenance of paralysis, a continuous infusion of 8 to 12 µg/kg/min (0.48 to 0.72 mg/kg/h) is recommended, accompanied by regular monitoring of the depth of neuromuscular blockade.

Rocuronium can be administered in an undiluted form by rapid IV injection. It should be refrigerated when stored. If kept at room temperature, however, it is stable for 60 days.

Atracurium

Atracurium is a nondepolarizing neuromuscular-blocking agent. Initial IV dosing for intubation purposes is 0.4 to 0.5 mg/kg. To maintain paralysis in a critical care setting, a continuous infusion of 4 to 20 µg/kg/min (0.24 to 1.2 mg/kg/h) is recommended, along with monitoring the depth of neuromuscular blockade every 1 to 2 hours. The onset of action of atracurium is dose dependent but, for intubation, typically takes 2 to 3 minutes. Recovery begins 20 to 35 minutes following the initial bolus dose.

Atracurium can be administered in an undiluted form by rapid IV injection. Vials must be refrigerated.

Cisatracurium

Cisatracurium is a nondepolarizing neuromuscular-blocking agent. Initial IV dosing for intubation purposes is 0.15 to 0.2 mg/kg. To maintain paralysis in a critical care setting, a continuous infusion of 1 to 3 µg/kg/min (0.06 to 0.18 mg/kg/h) is recommended, along with monitoring the depth of neuromuscular blockade every 1 to 2 hours. Usual doses range from 0.5 to 10 µg/kg/min (0.03 to 0.6 mg/kg/h). The onset of action of cisatracurium given for intubation is typically 2 to 3 minutes. Recovery begins 35 to 45 minutes following the initial bolus dose.

Cisatracurium can be administered in an undiluted form as a bolus injection over 5 to 10 seconds. Vials must be refrigerated. At room temperature, they remain stable for 21 days.

Histamine Antagonists and Proton Pump Inhibitors

Stress ulcer prophylaxis is undertaken in critically ill patients with associated risk factors such as coagulopathy, severe sepsis, or mechanical ventilation for more than 48 hours. Histamine antagonists and proton pump inhibitors (PPIs) **TABLE 8-8** are used to reduce the effects of gastric acids on the walls of the stomach and intestines. Once these risk factors are resolved, the stress ulcer prophylaxis should be discontinued.

Acids and enzymes are produced in the stomach by cells in the stomach lining, including the gastric parietal cells. Stimulation of these cells can occur when the histamine$_2$ (H$_2$) receptors on the cells are stimulated. The medications used to reduce acid production do so by antagonizing the H$_2$ receptors. These medications are particularly useful because they are very selective for the H$_2$ receptors, have no effect on histamine$_1$ (H$_1$) receptors, and have no anticholinergic effects. At the same time, H$_2$ blockers potentiate the effects of H$_1$ (common antihistamine) medications, which are used to treat allergic reactions and related symptoms. This additive effect is beneficial when treating anaphylaxis and other significant allergic reactions.

Some guidelines recommend the use of PPIs rather than H$_2$ antagonists for stress ulcer prophylaxis. PPIs suppress gastric acid secretion by inhibiting the hydrogen/potassium adenosine triphosphatase enzyme system (H$^+$/K$^+$ ATPase), also referred to as the gastric proton pump. The greater efficacy of PPIs relative to H$_2$ blockers has made these drugs among the most widely sold agents in the world. Studies comparing the efficacy of PPIs and H$_2$ antagonists in patients with active gastrointestinal bleeding have demonstrated consistent and significant reduction in rebleeding with PPIs versus H$_2$ antagonists.

Famotidine

Famotidine is the preferred H$_2$ antagonist in many intensive care units. Unlike cimetidine, it has no significant hemodynamic effects, nor does it alter hepatic drug metabolism. This favorable safety profile, combined with its profound inhibitory effect on gastric acid secretion and its dosing schedule, have made this H$_2$ antagonist exceedingly popular for use as an agent for stress ulcer prophylaxis. For adult patients who are unable to take oral medications or for whom famotidine cannot be given through a gastric tube, the recommended dose is 20 mg IV every 12 hours.

Cimetidine

Cimetidine is an H$_2$ antagonist. While it was used in the past, H$_2$ antagonists with safer profiles and fewer drug interactions have become more popular.

Esomeprazole

Esomeprazole is a PPI commonly used for stress ulcer prophylaxis in critically ill patients. It is administered intravenously at doses of 20 to 40 mg once daily. Aside from headache, dizziness, and some occasional gastrointestinal symptoms such as flatulence, abdominal pain, diarrhea, and nausea, esomeprazole is well tolerated.

Pantoprazole

Pantoprazole is a PPI most commonly used in the critical care setting to prevent rebleeding in patients with peptic ulcer bleeds. This therapy typically consists of an IV loading dose of 80 mg, followed by a continuous infusion of 8 mg/h for 72 hours. However, recent evidence suggests that intermittent administration via a bolus (eg, 40 mg IV twice daily) is as efficacious as continuous infusion therapy. As with other PPIs, side effects of pantoprazole include headache and gastrointestinal symptoms.

Antiemetic/Gastrointestinal Medications

The general classification of antiemetic medications—that is, those medications intended to treat nausea and vomiting—encompasses several more specific categories. **TABLE 8-9** profiles selected antiemetic and other gastrointestinal medications.

Antihistamines and Anticholinergics

Nausea and vomiting are typically triggered in the medulla but can also be triggered by the vestibular system. The vestibular system contains a high

TABLE 8-8 Histamine Antagonists and Proton Pump Inhibitors

Medication	Uses	Mechanism of Action	Route of Administration	Side Effects	Special Considerations
H₂ Blocker Medications					
Famotidine	Gastric acid reduction in patients with ulcers, reflux, or excessive gastric secretions; adjunct to H_1 blockers in patients with allergic or anaphylactic reactions	Inhibition of H_2 receptors, in gastric parietal cells (which release gastric acids)	Oral, IV, IO	Agitation and vomiting in pediatric patients; confusion, delirium, vomiting, headache, dizziness, diarrhea, constipation	IV doses should be given over at least 2 min. Dose reduction is needed in patients with renal insufficiency.
Cimetidine	Gastric acid reduction in patients with ulcers, reflux, or excessive gastric secretions; adjunct to H_1 blockers in patients with allergic or anaphylactic reactions	Inhibition of H_2 receptors, in cells that release gastric acids	Oral	Headache, dizziness, diarrhea, confusion, delirium	Dosing adjustment is needed in patients with renal insufficiency. Significant drug interactions exist.
Proton Pump Inhibitors					
Esomeprazole	Gastric acid reduction in patients with ulcers, reflux, or excessive gastric secretions; reduction of postprocedure risk for ulcer rebleeding	Suppresses gastric acid secretion by inhibiting hydrogen/potassium ATPase enzyme (proton pump) on gastric parietal cells	Oral, IV, IO	Headache, dizziness, flatulence, diarrhea, abdominal pain, nausea, constipation	Administer IV doses over more than 3 min.
Pantoprazole	Gastric acid reduction in patients with ulcers, reflux, or excessive gastric secretions; reduction of postprocedure risk for rebleeding	Suppresses gastric acid secretion by inhibiting hydrogen/potassium ATPase enzyme (proton pump) on gastric parietal cells	Oral, IV, IO	Headache, dizziness, edema, diarrhea, abdominal pain	Administer IV doses over at least 2 min.

Abbreviations: ATPase, adenosine triphosphatase; H_1, histamine₁; H_2, histamine₂; IM, intramuscular; IO, intraosseous; IV, intravenous

TABLE 8-9 Antiemetic/Gastrointestinal Medications

Medication	Uses	Mechanism of Action	Route of Administration	Side Effects	Special Considerations
Dopamine Antagonists					
Promethazine	Prevention and control of nausea and vomiting, treatment of motion sickness, procedural sedation	Blocks dopamine receptors in the cerebral medulla; has some antihistamine properties that also suppress nausea and vomiting	Oral, PR, IV, IO, IM	Hypotension, hypertension, bradycardia, tachycardia, sedation, akathisia (intense feeling of restlessness and anxiety), extrapyramidal symptoms, neuroleptic malignant syndrome, seizures, delirium, disorientation	Monitor for CNS effects. Be cautious with IV administration: Promethazine is a vesicant and can cause serious tissue injury, including gangrene, and has resulted in limb amputations.
Prochlorperazine	Management of severe nausea and vomiting, termination of migraines	Blocks dopamine receptors in the cerebral medulla; believed to also depress the reticular activating system	Oral, PR, IV, IO, IM	Hypotension, hypertension, bradycardia, tachycardia, sedation, akathisia, extrapyramidal symptoms, neuroleptic malignant syndrome, seizures, delirium, disorientation	Administer IV doses slowly, not exceeding 5 mg/min.
Metoclopramide	Gastroparesis, prevention of nausea and vomiting; GERD	Blocks dopamine receptors in the cerebral medulla; at higher doses, also blocks serotonin receptors in the CNS chemoreceptor trigger zone	Oral, IM, IV, IO	Hypotension, hypertension, bradycardia, tachycardia, sedation, akathisia, extrapyramidal symptoms, neuroleptic malignant syndrome	While the manufacturer advises administration of doses 10 mg or less over 1 to 2 min, rapid administration may cause akathisia.

Other

Ondansetron	Prevention of nausea and vomiting	Selectively blocks serotonin receptors both peripherally (vagal nerve terminals) and centrally (chemoreceptor trigger zone)	Oral, IM, IV, IO, ODT	Headache, drowsiness, fatigue, dizziness, constipation; dose-dependent QT prolongation	Theoretically, works best before vomiting starts. Administer IV doses over at least 30 s, preferably over 2 to 5 min.
Octreotide	Gastroesophageal variceal hemorrhage, certain tumors, chemotherapy-associated diarrhea	Mimics endogenous somatostatin: decreases intestinal fluid secretion, gastrointestinal motility, and portal blood flow	Subcutaneous, IM, IV	Vary by dose and route of administration	Potential for QT prolongation, which may be enhanced with vasoconstrictors. Consider obtaining a baseline 12-lead ECG to monitor QT. May also be used for treatment of oral sulfonylurea overdose.
Droperidol	Prevention and treatment of nausea and vomiting from surgical or diagnostic procedures	Blocks dopamine stimulation in the chemoreceptor trigger zone	IM, IV, IO	Dose-dependent QT prolongation, dizziness, drowsiness, extrapyramidal symptoms, restlessness	Obtaining a baseline 12-lead ECG is recommended to follow QT intervals. Cardiac monitoring is recommended.

Abbreviations: CNS, central nervous system; ECG, electrocardiogram; GERD, gastroesophageal reflux disease; IM, intramuscular; IO, intraosseous; IV, intravenous; ODT, orally disintegrating tablet; PR, per rectum

concentration of both histamine and ACh. Certain antihistamine medications can inhibit the activity of the histamine in the vestibular system, thereby suppressing the stimulation of the medulla. The same suppression effect can be accomplished by blocking the ACh receptors. Meclizine and dimenhydrinate are examples of antihistamines used as antiemetics; scopolamine is an anticholinergic used to treat nausea and vomiting. Both drug classes are associated with similar adverse reactions—sedation, visual acuity changes, and, most notably, the potential worsening of narrow-angle glaucoma.

Dopamine Antagonists

The vomiting center of the medulla can be triggered by the neurochemical transmitter dopamine when it activates the D_2 dopamine receptor. Medications that antagonize D_2 receptors, therefore, may be useful in reducing nausea and vomiting. Unfortunately, these medications all have major side effects—notably, considerable sedation, orthostatic hypotension, and extrapyramidal effects.

Promethazine

Promethazine is a phenothiazine-type antiemetic that belongs to the dopamine antagonist category. This agent is typically administered intravenously or intramuscularly at a dose of 12.5 to 25 mg, with even smaller doses being given in frail patients or older adults. Intravenous administration of promethazine has been associated with severe reactions, including tissue necrosis and need for amputation. If possible, the IV route of promethazine should be avoided. Promethazine should also be avoided in children; it is contraindicated in patients younger than 2 years.

Prochlorperazine

Prochlorperazine also blocks dopamine at the D_2 receptor in the medulla. The dose is 2.5 to 10 mg every 3 to 4 hours when given intravenously. This medication may cause extrapyramidal symptoms (eg, Parkinson-like syndromes, dystonia, akathisia).

It is imperative that prochlorperazine be administered slowly or by infusion, as rapid injection may cause orthostatic hypotension. Prochlorperazine, like promethazine, has the potential to lower the seizure threshold and may increase the likelihood of seizures in patients already predisposed to them. Use caution when administering these medications in older adults and other at-risk patients. Prochlorperazine is contraindicated in children younger than 2 years of age.

Metoclopramide

Metoclopramide has similar action on the D_2 receptors as prochlorperazine and promethazine do, but has the added benefit of increasing gastrointestinal motility. This is accomplished by enhancing ACh's effects on receptors in the upper gastrointestinal tract. Metoclopramide can cause drowsiness, dizziness, akathisia, and dystonic reactions, similar to other phenothiazine antiemetics.

Metoclopramide is usually given at a dose of 5 to 10 mg IV or IM. Many providers administer diphenhydramine with metoclopramide as prophylaxis against dystonic reactions. Rapid IV infusion can cause a profound dysphoria. The action of metoclopramide begins within 1 to 3 minutes and persists for 1 to 2 hours.

Ondansetron

Ondansetron is an antiemetic belonging to the selective 5-HT$_3$ receptor antagonist class. This class of antiemetics works by selectively blocking serotonin, both peripherally on the vagal nerve terminals and centrally in the chemoreceptor trigger zone. These drugs have gained popularity owing to their safer adverse-effect profile. The side effects most commonly associated with 5-HT$_3$ receptor antagonists include headache, fatigue, and general malaise.

Ondansetron is used for prevention of postoperative nausea and vomiting via the IV, IM, or oral route. It comes in an oral disintegrating tablet form that readily dissolves with even small amounts of saliva or a sip of water. For chemotherapy-induced nausea and vomiting, 8 mg or larger doses may be used, although single IV doses exceeding 16 mg create a significant risk of QT prolongation with. IV doses should be administered over at least 30 seconds and preferably over 2 to 5 minutes. Larger doses are safest if infused over at least 15 minutes.

Ondansetron is most effective when used to prevent vomiting. Its effectiveness is considerably lessened once a patient has vomited, although it may help to prevent further vomiting episodes.

Octreotide

Octreotide is an antidiarrheal, somatostatin analog used off-label in critical care for patients with bleeding esophageal varices. Somatostatin is a naturally occurring peptide chain that decreases intestinal fluid secretion, slows gastrointestinal motility, and reduces portal blood flow through vascular smooth muscle vasoconstriction. Unfortunately, the half-life of both naturally occurring and synthetic somatostatin is limited to minutes. Octreotide is a synthetic peptide with actions analogous to somatostatin, but a longer, more clinically useful duration of action.

Octreotide is given as a loading IV dose of 25 to 100 µg over at least 3 minutes (the usual bolus dose is 50 µg), followed by an IV infusion of 25 to 50 µg/h for 2 to 5 days. If bleeding is not controlled, the bolus dose may be repeated in the first hour.

Adverse reactions to octreotide vary by dosage. With IV dosing, sinus bradycardia, chest pain, pruritus (itching), and gastrointestinal distress have been reported.

Octreotide is also used subcutaneously or intramuscularly to treat dumping syndrome (often associated with gastric bypass surgery or esophagectomy), acromegaly, a variety of tumors and malignancies, and other gastrointestinal conditions, in addition to its primary use in critical care as a vasoconstrictor in patients with bleeding esophageal varices. Another use of octreotide is for the treatment of hypoglycemia following an overdose of oral sulfonylurea (a hypoglycemic agent for control of type 2 diabetes).

Droperidol

Droperidol is a dopamine-blocking agent that is used in critical care as an antiemetic. Intravenous administration of this drug is used for both treatment and prevention of nausea and vomiting in adults, with doses ranging from 0.625 mg to 1.25 mg given every 6 hours. Such doses should be administered slowly, over 2 to 5 minutes.

Droperidol has QT-prolonging effects and is contraindicated in patients with prolonged QTc intervals (greater than 440 ms in males or greater than 450 ms in females). While considerable debate exists about the clinical significance of droperidol-induced QTc prolongation, the drug has a reasonable safety record with the low doses used to treat nausea and vomiting. Most reported adverse events with droperidol occurred at doses of 2.5 mg and higher—doses that had previously been used for sedation, agitation, and induction of general anesthesia.

Pulmonary Medications

Paramedics are familiar with bronchodilators such as albuterol and anticholinergics such as ipratropium, both of which are used to manage reactive airways. The pulmonary medications listed in this section are typically systemic drugs used in management of life-threating pulmonary conditions such as pulmonary arterial hypertension, refractory hypoxemia, and ductal issues in neonates. **TABLE 8-10** profiles selected medications for pulmonary indications.

Epoprostenol

Epoprostenol is a vasodilator, prostacyclin and prostaglandin, and inhibitor of platelet aggregation used to treat pulmonary arterial hypertension, also known as primary pulmonary hypertension, as well as severe hypoxemia and acute right heart dysfunction. In adults, it has usually been delivered by intravenous infusion; in pediatric patients, it may also be nebulized. In recent years, data showing equal or better efficacy for inhaled epoprostenol compared to inhaled nitric oxide in adults have led to increased use of continuously nebulized epoprostenol in the adult population.

Dosing of IV epoprostenol is initiated at 2 ng/kg/min and increased in increments of 1 to 2 ng/kg/min at intervals of 10 to 15 minutes until the response plateaus or dose-limiting side effects occur. There is no specified maximum dose, but usual doses range from 25 to 40 ng/kg/min, with doses as high as 195 ng/kg/min reported in children. Increased doses should be expected with chronic use; indeed, such doses are usually needed more frequently the first few months after starting the drug. Dose increases should be made in increments of 1 to 2 ng/kg/min. Conversely, when significant symptoms require dose reduction, decreases are made in increments of 2 ng/kg/min.

Continuously nebulized epoprostenol is initiated at 20 to 50 ng/kg/min and titrated upward in increments of 10 ng/kg/min. When this medication is delivered through a ventilator circuit, the

TABLE 8-10 Pulmonary Medications

Medication	Uses	Mechanism of Action	Route of Administration	Side Effects	Special Considerations
Epoprostenol	Treatment of pulmonary arterial hypertension	Direct vasodilation of pulmonary and systemic arterial vascular beds; inhibits platelet aggregation	Continuous jet nebulizer, IV	Flushing, headaches, nausea, vomiting, hypotension, tachycardia	Must be infused through a central line; temporary peripheral infusion is permitted while central access is obtained. Requires special tubing. Do not interrupt the infusion. Avoid bolus injections. Carefully monitor blood pressure.
Alprostadil	Temporary maintenance of patent ductus arteriosus in neonates with ductal-dependent congenital heart lesions until surgical repair, pulmonary hypertension in children with congenital heart defects and left-to-right shunts	Prostaglandin, which causes direct relaxation of ductus arteriosus and vascular smooth muscle	IV	Apnea, flushing, fever, bradycardia, tachycardia, hypotension, hypertension	Anticipate more than a 10% chance of apnea. Carefully monitor respirations.
Aerosolized epinephrine	Treatment of bronchospasm associated with bronchial asthma, croup, stridor	Alpha and beta bronchial tree smooth muscle stimulation (promotes relaxation)	Nebulized	Tachycardia, hypertension	Monitor heart rate and respiratory status.

Abbreviations: IO, intraosseous; IV, intravenous

ventilator tidal volume may require adjustment due to the increased flow. In addition, the vent filter may need to be changed as often as every 2 hours if a glycine buffer diluent is used with this medication.

Epoprostenol can cause nausea, vomiting, headache, jaw pain, hypotension, and flushing of the skin. Abrupt withdrawal due to sudden interruption in medication delivery can result in rebound hypoxemia and pulmonary hypertension. This risk is of significant concern, as the half-life of epoprostenol is only 6 minutes. Loss of IV access or failure of nebulization equipment should be considered an emergency in patients who are receiving this medication. Whenever transporting patients from home, a backup supply of medications and equipment should be requested and brought to the receiving hospital.

Alprostadil

Alprostadil is a prostaglandin and vasodilator used to maintain the patency of the ductus arteriosus in neonates with ductal-dependent congenital heart disease until surgery can be performed. It has also been used in postoperative heart transplant patients to facilitate weaning from cardiopulmonary bypass in the presence of severe pulmonary hypertension.

For neonates, alprostadil continuous infusion is initiated at 0.05 µg/kg/min, using a large vein or an umbilical artery catheter placed at the ductal opening. The dose is then titrated in increments of 0.05 to 0.1 µg/kg/min until a therapeutic response is achieved (evidenced by increased pH, systemic blood pressure, or increased Po_2—typically seen within 30 minutes). At that point, the dose should be reduced to the lowest effective amount. It is often possible to reduce doses by as much as 50% without losing the therapeutic effect. Usual dose ranges are 0.01 to 0.4 µg/kg/min, with the maximum dose being 0.4 µg/kg/min.

One of the more common side effects of alprostadil is apnea, which may occur in 10% to 12% of infants with congenital heart defects, especially in those weighing less than 4 pounds (2 kg) at birth. Apnea usually occurs in the first hour of alprostadil infusion. Fever, flushing, hypotension, and bradycardia have also been reported and are considered dose-dependent side effects. If apnea occurs, the infusion should be discontinued and cautiously restarted at a lower dose.

Aerosolized Epinephrine

Aerosolized epinephrine, or racemic epinephrine, is an alpha and beta agonist. It works by stimulating the alpha adrenergic receptors in the airway, which leads to resultant tightening of the mucosa (mucosal vasoconstriction) and decreased fluid in the airway (subglottic edema), and by stimulating the beta adrenergic receptors, which causes relaxation of the bronchial smooth muscle. Racemic epinephrine is typically used for relief of respiratory distress due to stridor, bronchiolitis, laryngeal edema, and upper airway obstruction. It has also been effective in treating post-extubation edema and croup.

Racemic epinephrine is given by small-volume nebulizer, using 0.5 mL of a 2.25% solution added to 3 mL of normal saline, repeated every 15 minutes to 4 hours as needed. Effects should be evident within 1 minute.

The manufacturer recommends that racemic epinephrine be refrigerated, although it is stable when stored at room temperature. Potential side effects with its use include tremor and tachycardia.

Antiarrhythmics

Antiarrhythmic medications comprise a general, broad-based group of drugs, with subcategories being distinguished based on the medications' mechanisms of action according to the **Vaughan-Williams classification scheme**. This scheme organizes drugs that affect heart rhythms into classes I through IV **TABLE 8-11**. With the advent of newer medications with several simultaneous mechanisms of action (eg, amiodarone), however, the Vaughan-Williams classification system has been found to have significant limitations.

Class I Antiarrhythmic Medications

Class I antiarrhythmic medications work by blocking sodium channels. In doing so, the medication reduces the phase 0 slope and the peak of the action potential. Class I drugs are further divided into subclasses IA, IB, and IC based on their strength and degree of phase 0 reduction. Class IA is considered moderate in effect, class IB is weak, and class IC produces a strong reduction. The general principle behind sodium-channel blockade is reduction of the rate and magnitude of depolarization by decreasing conduction velocity in non-nodal tissue.

TABLE 8-11 Antiarrhythmics

Medication	Uses	Mechanism of Action	Route of Administration	Side Effects	Special Considerations
Class I Antiarrhythmic Medications					
Procainamide	Treatment of various atrial or ventricular arrhythmias (different class I agents are appropriate for different types of arrhythmias)	Blocks fast sodium channels; inhibits depolarization of neuronal cells; decreases myocardial conduction velocity and automaticity	IV	Hypotension, nausea, vomiting, unwanted conduction disturbances	Monitor ECG, blood pressure, and renal function.
Lidocaine	Treatment of ventricular arrhythmias (different class I agents are appropriate for different types of arrhythmias)	Blocks fast sodium channels; inhibits depolarization of neuronal cells; decreases myocardial conduction velocity and automaticity	IV	Hypotension, nausea, vomiting, seizures, altered mental status	Monitor ECG and CNS status. As with amiodarone, considered a first-line agent in patients with ventricular fibrillation or pulseless ventricular tachycardia.
Flecainide	Treatment/prevention of atrial fibrillation/flutter, PSVT, and ventricular arrhythmias	Slows conduction in cardiac tissue by altering ion transport across cell membranes	PO	Dizziness, visual disturbances, dyspnea	Monitor ECG and blood pressure during administration. Proarrhythmic effects including ventricular fibrillation and tachycardia have been reported with use in patients with atrial fibrillation.
Class II Antiarrhythmic Medications					
Labetalol	Treatment of mild to severe hypertension	Competitively blocks beta receptors in heart, blood vessels; also blocks alpha-1 receptors; may affect other beta receptors at higher doses	Oral, IV	Hypotension, bradycardia, conduction abnormalities, dizziness, hypoglycemia	A loss of beta selectivity occurs following high doses or overdose. May exacerbate bronchospasm in patients with reactive airway disease.

Metoprolol	Treatment of hypertension, rate control in atrial fibrillation, tremors, certain psychological disorders, migraines	Selectively inhibits beta-1 receptors; little to no effect on beta-2 receptors at doses <100 mg/d in adults	Oral, IV	Hypotension, bradycardia, conduction abnormalities, dizziness	Avoid use in patients with cocaine toxicity due to theoretical risk of unopposed alpha stimulation. A loss of beta selectivity occurs following high doses or overdose.
Esmolol	Treatment of SVT and control of ventricular rate in atrial fibrillation/flutter; treatment of tachycardia and hypertension	Competitively blocks beta-1 receptors; little to no effect on beta-2 receptors except at high doses	IV	Hypotension, bradycardia, infusion-site reactions	Use cautiously in heart block greater than first degree. Usually given as an infusion, with an optional bolus prior to start of therapy.
Sotalol	Treatment of life-threatening ventricular arrhythmias; maintenance of sinus rhythm in patients with symptomatic atrial fibrillation/flutter	Both beta blocking and cardiac action potential duration-prolonging effects	Oral, IV	Bradycardia, chest pain, palpitations, fatigue; dose-related proarrhythmias such as torsades de pointes	Contraindicated if baseline QTc >450 ms, serum potassium <4 mEq/L, or creatinine clearance <40 mL/min. Monitor QTc during therapy.

Class III Antiarrhythmic Medications

| Amiodarone | Management of life-threatening ventricular arrhythmias, atrial fibrillation in critically ill patients or patients with heart failure, SVT, maintenance of sinus rhythm after conversion of atrial fibrillation | Inhibits alpha and beta stimulation; blocks sodium, potassium, and calcium channels; decreases AV conduction and sinus node function | Oral, IV, IO | QT-interval prolongation, infusion rate–related hypotension, bradycardia, other conduction abnormalities, flushing, edema, hypothyroidism, pulmonary toxicity | Monitor ECG and blood pressure during administration. Central line administration is preferred to decrease the incidence of phlebitis. Long-term effects can be significant, including pulmonary toxicity, hypothyroidism, corneal deposits with visual changes, and abnormal liver function tests. Like lidocaine, considered a first-line agent in patients with ventricular fibrillation or pulseless ventricular tachycardia. |

(Continues)

TABLE 8-11 Antiarrhythmics (continued)

Medication	Uses	Mechanism of Action	Route of Administration	Side Effects	Special Considerations
Class IV Antiarrhythmic Medications					
Verapamil	SVT; oral administration is used for hypertension	Blocks slow calcium channels, especially in the SA and AV nodes; inhibits calcium influx into cells in arterial walls, decreasing systemic vascular resistance	Oral, IV, IO	Hypotension, bradycardia, conduction disturbances, edema, flushing	Monitor blood pressure and ECG during administration. Verapamil is a nondihydropyridine calcium channel blocker and should be used cautiously in patients with heart failure.
Diltiazem	Rate control of narrow-complex tachycardias; vasopressor medications induce vasoconstriction, which in turn elevates mean arterial blood pressure, SVT, and atrial fibrillation; oral administration is used for hypertension	Blocks slow calcium channels, especially in the SA and AV nodes; inhibits calcium influx into cells in arterial walls, decreasing systemic vascular resistance	Oral, IV, IO	Hypotension, bradycardia, conduction disturbances, edema, flushing	Monitor blood pressure and ECG during administration. Diltiazem is a nondihydropyridine calcium channel blocker and should be used cautiously in patients with heart failure.

Abbreviations: AV, atrioventricular; CNS, central nervous system; ECG, electrocardiogram; IO, intraosseous; IV, intravenous; PSVT, paroxysmal supraventricular tachycardia; QTc, corrected QT; SA, sinoatrial; SVT, supraventricular tachycardia

Recall that nodal tissue generates the initial electrical impulse, whereas non-nodal tissue receives stimulation from nodal tissues or neighboring cells to initiate depolarization.

Class IA Medications

Class IA medications have been found to increase the effective refractory period (ERP)—that is, the interval within the cardiac cycle during which cardiac cells (and muscles) are chemically unable to reenergize. During this time, additional action by cardiac tissues is impossible. By increasing the ERP, the medication decreases the cells' ability to recharge and depolarize as quickly, thereby interrupting reentry mechanisms.

The class IA medications are quinidine, procainamide, and disopyramide. Some significant drawbacks are noted with this class, particularly pertaining to their effects on patients with preexisting infarction or structural heart disease. They also tend to trigger significant adverse reactions, including lupus-like syndromes (inflammation of the heart tissue including the valves and pericardium); such reactions occur in as many as 30% of long-term procainamide users, for example. Oral procainamide is not available in the United States.

Of all the class IA medications, procainamide is the most commonly encountered in the acute setting. Given as an infusion, its typical dose is 20 to 50 mg/min, with a maximum dose of 17 mg/kg. When administering procainamide, the CCTP must be mindful of the clinical endpoints for this therapy: a 50% widening of the QRS complex, suppression of the arrhythmia, or hypotension. Along with the lupus-like syndromes, patients may experience side effects such as widening of the PR and QT intervals, AV blocks, seizures, and CNS depression, which may deteriorate into seizures.

Class IB Medications

Class IB medications carry out their functions by decreasing the ERP and the action potential duration (APD)—that is, the length of the action potential cycle. When the ERP and the APD are decreased, automaticity of the cardiac cells is diminished, which reduces their tendency to depolarize in a disorganized fashion. Class IB medications are indicated for ventricular fibrillation, ventricular tachycardia, and ventricular irritability.

Lidocaine is the prototypical class IB medication. It has a greater impact on ventricular cells with longer action potentials than on atrial cells with shorter action potentials. Given at an initial dose of 1 to 1.5 mg/kg and a repeat dose of 0.5 to 0.75 mg/kg, lidocaine remains a treatment option for patients experiencing cardiac arrhythmias originating in the ventricles.

Lidocaine achieves its peak effect in about 5 minutes but has a highly variable duration of action. Caution should be exercised so as not to exceed the maximum dose of 3 mg/kg.

Class IC Medications

Class IC medications work by suppressing the phase 0 repolarization. These medications differ from class IA and class IB medications in that they have virtually no effect on the action potential. By suppressing repolarization, conductivity is reduced through the heart. Class IC medications are used for life-threatening arrhythmias originating in the ventricles. Interestingly, medications in this class can be proarrhythmic as well. Some studies have indicated a propensity for ST-segment elevation with the use of these medications.

Flecainide is a prototypical class IC medication. This oral medication is not routinely used in CCT.

Class II Antiarrhythmic Medications/ Beta Adrenergic Blocking Agents

Class II antiarrhythmics comprise the beta blocking medications. The cardiovascular system is influenced by the sympathetic nervous system, particularly by epinephrine and norepinephrine (**sympathomimetics**) binding to the adrenergic beta-1 and beta-2 receptors. Beta blocking medications work to antagonize the beta receptors by competitively binding to these sites to inhibit stimulation. Earlier beta blocking medications were considered nonselective because they indiscriminately blocked both beta-1 and beta-2 receptors. More recent versions are relatively selective for beta-1 receptors, although some beta-2 binding occurs, particularly with higher doses. These sympathetic nervous system–blocking medications (ie, sympatholytics) have several uses, including the treatment of arrhythmias, hypertension, and heart failure. If the medication causes an excessive blockade, however, the patient may experience bradycardia, heart failure, hypotension, and AV blocks. Especially with the use of nonselective beta blocking medications, bronchoconstriction and hypoglycemia may occur. Propranolol is a commonly used nonselective beta blocking medication.

Labetalol

Labetalol is a medication with both alpha-1 and beta blocking (antagonist) properties. It can be given orally or intravenously for the management of chronic or emergent hypertension, respectively. Health care providers should avoid administering beta blockers, including labetalol, when a patient has a high-degree (greater than first-degree) heart block or sick sinus syndrome. Heart failure, cardiogenic shock, asthma, and obstructive airway disease are other situations in which labetalol should be avoided.

The initial IV dose of labetalol for hypertensive emergency in adults is 10 to 20 mg given over 1 to 2 minutes, followed by subsequent doses of 20 to 80 mg every 10 minutes until the target blood pressure is reached. The manufacturer recommends a cumulative maximum dose of 300 mg, but in practice this maximum dose is sometimes exceeded with careful monitoring. Labetalol can also be administered as a continuous IV infusion of 1 to 2 mg/min. Its effects become evident less than 5 minutes following an IV dose and last up to 4 hours.

Metoprolol

Metoprolol is a selective beta-1 blocking drug that decreases the automaticity of the heart tissue, thereby decreasing cardiac output and systemic blood pressure. For acute rate control, this agent is usually given intravenously at a dose of 5 mg every 2 to 5 minutes for up to three doses. Metoprolol should not be administered to patients with significant heart failure (ejection fraction less than 45%), bradycardia, or cardiogenic shock.

Esmolol

Esmolol is an antihypertensive, beta-1 selective blocker and class II antiarrhythmic. It is used for control of hypertension or tachycardia. Esmolol has an advantage over other antihypertensive and rate control agents in terms of its quick action and very short half-life. Effects are seen within 2 to 10 minutes of starting an infusion of the drug; use of a loading dose can shorten this interval. The duration of action is 10 to 30 minutes following discontinuation of esmolol. With high doses or extended-duration infusions, the duration of action may be longer.

Esmolol infusions are initiated at 50 µg/kg/min and titrated upward in increments of 50 µg/kg/min every 4 minutes to a maximum of 200 µg/kg/min. Some patients with hypertension require higher doses (250 to 300 µg/kg/min). The safety of doses exceeding 300 µg/kg/min has not been studied. At rates greater than 200 µg/kg/min, minimal additional effects on rate control are seen. When immediate control of rate or blood pressure is needed, a bolus of 1 mg/kg can be administered over 1 minute; alternatively, for more gradual lowering, a 0.5-mg/kg bolus can be administered over 1 minute. Both boluses are then followed by an infusion administered at a rate of 50 µg/kg/min.

Esmolol is a vesicant. Thus, although it can be administered through a peripheral IV line, caution should be used to avoid extravasation. Potential side effects include bradycardia, hypotension, heart failure, dizziness, and bronchospasm.

Sotalol

Sotalol is a nonselective beta blocker and class II/III antiarrhythmic. It is indicated for documented sustained ventricular rhythms such as ventricular tachycardia that are judged to be life-threatening as well as for the maintenance of normal sinus rhythm in patients with symptomatic atrial fibrillation or atrial flutter. Sotalol can cause life-threatening ventricular tachycardia associated with significant prolongation of the QT interval (torsades de pointes). Because of this risk, as well as the drug's very high cost, many US hospitals have chosen not to place IV sotalol on their formularies. Consequently, there is very limited clinical experience with IV sotalol.

When administered intravenously over 5 minutes for ongoing hemodynamically stable ventricular tachycardia, the effects of sotalol are usually seen in 5 to 10 minutes. Recommended dosing is 1.5 mg/kg or 100 mg as a one-time dose.

Class III Antiarrhythmic Medications

The third class of antiarrhythmic medications in the Vaughan-Williams classification is composed of the potassium channel blocker medications. Potassium channels open immediately after cardiac cell depolarization and enable repolarization. Potassium channel–blocking medications block these potassium channels, thereby delaying the phase 3 repolarization of the cardiac cells. In turn, both the duration of the action potential and the effective refractory period increase. Because these medications increase the refractory period, the patient's electrocardiogram (ECG) tends to show a prolonged QT interval. This effect makes potassium channel–blocking medications particularly useful for treating reentry tachycardias and arrhythmias occurring as a result of cellular depolarization due to excessive excitability.

Amiodarone is the most commonly used class III antiarrhythmic medication, even though it also has properties that are consistent with other categories. Like some of the other antiarrhythmic medications, the class III medications can be proarrhythmic as well. Amiodarone can precipitate torsades de pointes, AV blocks, and bradycardia; consequently, it is contraindicated in the presence of bradycardia or AV blocks. Numerous dosing patterns are used for different indications. The onset of action varies, and peak effects may not occur for days or weeks. Because amiodarone carries a high risk for many adverse events and has a variable half-life of 15 to 142 days, careful patient-specific risk-benefit assessment is important before initiating long-term therapy.

Class IV Antiarrhythmic Medications/ Calcium Channel–Blocker Medications

The class IV antiarrhythmic medications consist of the calcium channel blockers. Calcium channel–blocking medications bind to the l-type calcium channels in cardiac and vascular smooth muscle cells. These calcium channels play a primary role in cardiac nodal automaticity and phase 0 of the action potential. In other words, the l-type calcium channels influence the impulse-generating and depolarizing activities of the sinoatrial and AV nodes. By blocking the calcium channels, class IV medications cause vasodilation and negative inotropic, negative chronotropic, and negative dromotropic (decreased electrical conduction velocity) effects. Although calcium channel–blocking medications decrease the automaticity of aberrant pacemaker sites, their greatest influence comes through their ability to decrease the conduction velocity through the AV node. This action makes class IV antiarrhythmic medications useful for treating tachyarrhythmias originating in the atria.

Currently, only two nondihydropyridine calcium channel–blocking medications are used for treating arrhythmias: verapamil and diltiazem. Neither medication should be given to patients who have preexisting bradycardias, Wolff-Parkinson-White syndrome, or heart failure. Additionally, patients taking a beta blocking medication may experience a potentiation effect.

Anticoagulants and Thrombolytics

Anticoagulant medications are used to prevent the formation of blood clots; thrombolytics are used to dissolve existing clots.

The goal of anticoagulation therapy is to prevent thrombosis and thromboembolic events. Critically ill patients represent one of the groups at highest risk for development of thromboembolisms, which often lead to pulmonary emboli. The onerous monitoring requirements and bleeding complications associated with anticoagulant use have led to continued development of newer anticoagulants that directly target the enzyme activity of thrombin and factor Xa. While newer agents have more specific action than the conventional heparins and vitamin K antagonists, their reversal has proved to be challenging.

Thrombolytics are indicated to dissolve clots formed in intravenous catheters and vessels such as the coronary, cerebral, and pulmonary arteries. **TABLE 8-12** profiles selected anticoagulants and thrombolytics.

Heparin

Heparin is an anticoagulant used for acute coronary syndromes, for venous thromboembolism, and in any situation where systemic anticoagulation is desired. Many concentrations of this drug are available, and it can be injected subcutaneously, instilled in a central venous or dialysis catheter to maintain patency, or delivered as a continuous infusion to provide systemic anticoagulation. Heparin inactivates thrombin (as well as several coagulation factors and plasmin) and prevents the conversion of fibrinogen to fibrin. Thus, while heparin is an anticoagulant, it is not a thrombolytic; heparin may prevent the growth of existing thrombi, but will not reduce their size or dissolve them.

TABLE 8-12 Anticoagulants and Thrombolytics

Medication	Uses	Mechanism of Action	Route of Administration	Side Effects	Special Considerations
Heparin	Anticoagulation, prophylaxis and treatment of thromboembolic disorders, adjunct to fibrinolysis in STEMI, DVT, and PE prophylaxis and treatment in critically ill patients	Impairs blood fibrin formation by inactivating thrombin as well as other coagulation factors	Subcutaneous, IV	Thrombocytopenia, bleeding	Monitor aPTT during administration of heparin infusions and following IV bolus injections. Adjust doses following local nomograms.
Alteplase	Treatment of acute ischemic stroke, PE, STEMI, frostbite, peripheral arterial occlusions, prosthetic heart valvular thrombus, retinal artery/vein occlusions; also used to restore intravascular catheter function when clotted	Initiates local fibrinolysis (clot lysis) by binding to clot fibrin, converting plasminogen to plasmin	IV	Potentially life-threatening bleeding, hypotension, reperfusion arrhythmias in coronary thrombolysis	Monitor vital signs and ECG during administration. Perform invasive procedures cautiously due to increased risk of bleeding. Carefully monitor IV sites and hemoglobin to assess for bleeding. Follow local protocols and guideline-driven monitoring protocols.
Tenecteplase	Lysis of intracoronary thrombi in STEMI, acute ischemic stroke	Tenecteplase is essentially alteplase with three mutations, making it more fibrin specific and providing a longer duration of action	IV	Potentially life-threatening bleeding, hypotension, fever, reperfusion arrhythmias in coronary thrombolysis	Perform invasive procedures cautiously due to increased risk of bleeding. Carefully monitor IV sites and hemoglobin to assess for bleeding.

Abciximab	Prevention of platelet aggregation in patients undergoing or awaiting PCI	Impairs platelet aggregation by binding to platelet receptors	IV	Potentially life-threatening bleeding, hypotension, chest pain, back pain, antibody development (especially with repeat dosing)	Intended for coadministration with aspirin and heparin infusion to maintain a therapeutic bleeding time measured by ACT. May be administered directly through the catheter during PCI. Monitor coagulation parameters, hemoglobin and platelets, and signs and symptoms of bleeding (especially the sheath insertion site)
Eptifibatide	Treatment of patients with ACS, including those undergoing PCI and those managed medically	Blocks platelet receptors, inhibiting platelet aggregation and preventing thrombosis	IV	Potentially life-threatening bleeding, hypotension, local site reactions	Monitor coagulation parameters, hemoglobin and platelets, and signs and symptoms of bleeding (especially the sheath insertion site).
Tirofiban	Adjunct treatment of NSTEMI/UA patients; prevention of platelet aggregation in patients undergoing or awaiting PCI	Impairs platelet aggregation in a dose- and concentration-dependent manner	IV	Potentially life-threatening bleeding	Monitor coagulation parameters, hemoglobin and platelets, signs and symptoms of bleeding (especially the sheath insertion site).

Abbreviations: ACS, acute coronary syndrome; ACT, activated clotting time; aPTT, activated partial thromboplastin time; DVT, deep venous thrombosis; ECG, electrocardiogram; IV, intravenous; NSTEMI, non–ST-segment elevation myocardial infarction; PCI, percutaneous coronary intervention; PE, pulmonary embolism; STEMI, ST-segment elevation myocardial infarction; UA, unstable angina

Continuous heparin infusion dosing varies by indication. Generally, a loading dose is administered, followed by a continuous, weight-based infusion. Dosing is adjusted to activated partial thromboplastin time (aPTT) levels, which are drawn at 4- to 6-hour intervals, and adjusted to a target of 1.5 to 2 times the upper limit of control (usually 50 to 70 seconds). As an adjunct to fibrinolytics in patients with ST-segment elevation myocardial infarction (STEMI), a heparin bolus of 60 units/kg (maximum 4,000 units) is recommended, followed by a 12 units/kg/h infusion (maximum 1,000 units/h). Heparin dosing and monitoring are most often institution specific and care should be taken to follow local protocols.

Effects of IV heparin are seen immediately, and the medication's duration of action is approximately 20 minutes. Bleeding is the most significant adverse event associated with heparin administration, and patients should be closely monitored for this complication during transport. Most bleeding can be controlled by direct pressure. If serious hemorrhage occurs, heparin should be immediately discontinued and a reversal agent (ie, protamine) considered.

Alteplase

Alteplase is a thrombolytic agent used to treat acute ischemic stroke, acute massive pulmonary embolism, STEMI, acute peripheral artery occlusions, and central catheter clearance. Alteplase triggers local fibrinolysis by binding to the fibrin in a clot (thrombus) and converting plasminogen to plasmin. It begins working immediately once a bolus or infusion is started and continues to exhibit fibrinolytic action for as long as 1 hour after its administration is stopped.

Dosing strategies vary by patient weight and indication, but usually include a loading dose followed by an infusion lasting from 30 minutes to 2 hours. For certain indications, other anticoagulants may be administered simultaneously. However, an important exception is treatment of acute ischemic stroke, as patients should not receive any anticoagulants or antiplatelets for at least 24 hours after treatment.

In patients with STEMI, coronary thrombolysis may result in reperfusion arrhythmias such as accelerated idioventricular rhythms. Bleeding is a risk in all patients and is dose related. Certain conditions increase the risk of bleeding, requiring careful consideration of inclusion/exclusion criteria before administering alteplase. Total alteplase doses should not exceed 90 mg in patients with acute ischemic stroke or 100 mg in patients with acute myocardial infarction or PE. Doses of 150 mg or more are associated with a significantly greater risk of intracranial hemorrhage compared to doses of 100 mg or less. Overall, the bleeding risk with appropriate alteplase therapy is low. If serious hemorrhage occurs, the infusion of alteplase and any other anticoagulants (such as heparin) should be discontinued.

Tenecteplase

Tenecteplase is another thrombolytic agent used in the management of STEMI. Acute ischemic stroke practice guidelines from major medical organizations have recommended alteplase rather than tenecteplase for this indication; however, recent data have shown benefits from tenecteplase in patients with large-vessel occlusion strokes. Additionally, this agent may be associated with better perfusion and potentially fewer bleeding complications.

Tenecteplase promotes fibrinolysis by binding to fibrin and converting plasminogen to plasmin. This medication is essentially alteplase with three mutations that make it more fibrin specific and give it a longer duration of action. The longer half-life (20 to 24 minutes) allows for rapid bolus dosing over 5 seconds, rather than an hour-long infusion as with alteplase.

For STEMI, the total dose of tenecteplase should not exceed 50 mg and is weight based. This agent is administered as a single bolus dose over 5 seconds. Effects are seen immediately and last for 90 to 130 minutes. Adverse effects may include reperfusion arrhythmias and bleeding.

Abciximab

Abciximab is an antiplatelet agent in the glycoprotein IIb/IIIa inhibitor family. It is used during and after percutaneous coronary intervention (PCI) for STEMI and following some carotid stent procedures. It works by blocking the platelet IIb/IIIa receptors, thereby reversibly blocking platelet aggregation and preventing thrombosis.

Abciximab is administered by IV infusion, with a bolus of 0.25 mg/kg given 10 to 60 minutes prior to PCI, followed by an infusion of 0.125 μg/kg/min (maximum 10 μg/min) for 12 hours. In patients with unstable angina and non–ST-segment elevation myocardial infarction (NSTEMI), the infusion may be continued for 18 to 24 hours after PCI. Abciximab is intended for coadministration with aspirin and a continuous heparin infusion.

The most significant adverse effect associated with abciximab is bleeding, which can occur at any site. The precise level of risk depends on multiple variables, including patient susceptibility and concurrent use of other anticoagulating agents. Minor bleeding can be controlled with direct pressure; major bleeding may require discontinuation of abciximab. Consultation with medical control is necessary when discontinuation is contemplated, as a careful risk-benefit assessment is necessary.

Eptifibatide

Eptifibatide is an antiplatelet agent in the glycoprotein IIb/IIIa inhibitor family. It is used for treatment of acute coronary syndrome (ACS) as well as during and after percutaneous coronary intervention. It works by binding to platelet IIb/IIIa receptors, thereby inhibiting platelet aggregation.

Eptifibatide is administered by IV infusion. In patients with ACS, a bolus of 180 μg/kg (maximum 22.6 mg) is administered as soon as possible after diagnosis; the bolus is followed by an infusion of 2 μg/kg/min (maximum 15 mg/h), which is continued until hospital discharge, PCI, or cardiac bypass surgery. In patients undergoing bypass surgery, eptifibatide is discontinued 2 to 4 hours prior to surgery. In patients with PCI, a second bolus is administered 10 minutes after the first, and the infusion is continued for 24 hours post PCI.

The most significant adverse effect associated with eptifibatide is bleeding, which most often occurs at catheter sites. Patients who weigh less than 154 pounds (70 kg) may be at greater risk for bleeding. Minor bleeding can be controlled with direct pressure; major bleeding may require discontinuation of eptifibatide. Consultation with medical control is necessary when discontinuation is contemplated, as a careful risk-benefit assessment is necessary.

Tirofiban

Tirofiban is an antiplatelet agent in the glycoprotein IIb/IIIa inhibitor family. It is used for treatment of ACS as well as during and after PCI. This agent works by binding to platelet IIb/IIIa receptors, thereby inhibiting platelet aggregation. When tirofiban is used as recommended, more than 90% platelet inhibition may be seen within 10 minutes of initiating the infusion, with levels returning to baseline within 4 to 8 hours after discontinuation of the medication.

Tirofiban is administered by IV infusion. A loading dose of 25 μg/kg is administered over 5 minutes or less, followed by a maintenance infusion of 0.15 μg/kg/min, which is continued for 18 to 48 hours depending on the indication. Tirofiban is intended to be used in combination with other anticoagulants and antiplatelet agents.

The most common complication of tirofiban is bleeding. Profound thrombocytopenia (reduced platelet counts) has been reported with its use; if this adverse effect is confirmed, it requires discontinuation of the tirofiban and any concurrent heparin infusion. Consultation with medical control is necessary when discontinuation is contemplated, as a careful risk-benefit assessment is necessary.

Miscellaneous Medications

TABLE 8-13 profiles some other medications that CCTPs are likely to use on a routine basis when caring for patients.

Insulin

Insulin infusions are used for control of hyperglycemia in patients with diabetic ketoacidosis (DKA). In 2001, insulin infusions became popular across the spectrum of critical care after a study suggested that glycemic control conferred a significant mortality benefit. Since then, it has become abundantly evident that hyperglycemia in critically ill patients is associated with an increase in infection and death. Currently, for most critically ill patients, the American Diabetic Association recommends initiating insulin in patients with a blood glucose of 180 mg/dL or higher, with a goal of maintaining blood glucose between 140 and 180 mg/dL. Likewise, protocols and monitoring need to be designed to avoid

TABLE 8-13 Other Medications Used in the Critical Care Transport Setting

Medication	Uses	Mechanism of Action	Route of Administration	Side Effects	Special Considerations
Insulin, regular	Treatment of diabetic ketoacidosis, hyperglycemia during critical illness, hyperkalemia	Regulates metabolism of carbohydrates, protein, and fats; promotes intracellular movement of potassium	Subcutaneous, IV	Hypoglycemia, hypokalemia, hypertrophy at subcutaneous injection sites	For critically ill patients on insulin infusions, monitor blood glucose at a minimum hourly during transport. Arterial or venous whole-blood sampling is recommended for patients in shock, with significant edema, or on vasopressors.
Furosemide	Management of edema associated with heart failure, hepatic or renal disease, acute pulmonary edema, treatment of hypertension	Inhibits reabsorption of sodium and chloride in the ascending loop of Henle and distal renal tubules	Oral, IM, IV, IO	Hypovolemia, electrolyte abnormalities, dizziness, hearing impairment (potentially permanent with rapid IV administration of high doses)	Monitor blood pressure, serum electrolytes (particularly potassium), renal function, and fluid volume status.
Bumetanide	Management of edema secondary to heart failure, hepatic disease, or renal disease	Inhibits reabsorption of sodium and chloride in the ascending loop of Henle and proximal renal tubules; does not act on distal tubules	Oral, IM, IV, IO	Hypovolemia, electrolyte abnormalities, dizziness	Monitor blood pressure, serum electrolytes (particularly potassium), renal function, and fluid volume status.

Abbreviations: IM, intramuscular; IO, intraosseous; IV, intravenous

© Jones & Bartlett Learning.

hypoglycemia (blood glucose ≤70 mg/dL), which is associated with increased mortality—a risk that increases significantly with even brief episodes of severe hypoglycemia (blood glucose ≤40 mg/dL).

Insulin infusions are usually prepared by adding 100 units of regular insulin (U-100 Humulin-R or Novolin-R) to 100 mL of normal saline. If initiating an infusion in a patient whose blood sugar has triggered the need for glycemic control (ie, blood glucose ≥180 mg/dL), the starting dose is usually 1 to 2 units/h. Incremental dose changes are made hourly according to local protocol or in 0.5 to 1 unit/h steps. The dose needed to maintain a blood glucose level within the target range varies by patient.

For treatment of DKA in adults, fluids are usually the first-line therapy. Once the serum potassium is verified, insulin infusions with or without boluses, depending on institution-specific protocols, are initiated. Of note, in patients with serum potassium less than 3.3 mEq/L, insulin is usually held until potassium is repleted and its level is greater than 3.3 mEq/L. Patients may need continuous potassium repletion while receiving IV insulin. The insulin infusion is usually initiated at 0.1 unit/kg/h, with a goal of reducing the blood glucose by 50 to 75 mg/dL in the first hour. If this outcome is not achieved, the insulin dose should be increased per institutional protocols (eg, doubled each hour until the blood glucose falls by 50 to 75 mg/dL/h). When the serum glucose reaches 250 mg/dL, the insulin dose is usually decreased and dextrose-containing IV fluids are infused to maintain blood glucose between 150 and 250 mg/dL until any acidosis is resolved.

Like nitroglycerin, insulin is absorbed by the plastics used in intravenous tubing. Tubing should be primed with 20 to 25 mL (run through the tubing and wasted) to minimize insulin infusion losses to IV tubing lines.

In any patient receiving an insulin infusion, blood glucose should be checked at least hourly and more often with any titration. When hypoglycemia occurs, the infusion should be stopped and the patient's blood glucose checked every 15 minutes. Most protocols suggest restarting insulin infusions that have been held for hypoglycemia at 50% of the previous dose. When hypoglycemia is significant or symptomatic, oral or intravenous dextrose should be administered.

> ### Medication Safety Note
>
> One medication safety issue with insulin is how doses are ordered and charted. The abbreviation "u" should never be used in place of "units" because it may be misinterpreted as a number. Also, a decimal point should always be preceded by a zero in values less than 1 (eg, 0.5 unit, not .5 u). Finally, never follow a decimal point with a zero (eg, 5 units, not 5.0 u). These rules are especially important when charting is handwritten.

Furosemide

Furosemide is a loop diuretic. It inhibits reabsorption of sodium and chloride ions in the proximal and distal renal tubules and loop of Henle, resulting in excretion of sodium, potassium, and excess water into the urine. This agent is used to treat edema associated with heart failure and hepatic or renal disease; it is also administered as an adjunct treatment for oliguria (low urine output) in patients with severe renal impairment.

In the CCT setting, furosemide may be administered as a continuous infusion at rates of 10 to 40 mg/h. When the patient's urine output is less than 1 mL/kg/h, the dose is usually doubled to a maximum of 80 to 160 mg/h. High doses increase the risk of ototoxicity, which can also occur as a result of too-rapid injection of bolus doses (more than 4 mg/min).

The onset of action for IV furosemide is 5 minutes, and its duration of action when given by this route is 2 hours. When furosemide is given orally, its duration of action is 6 hours—hence, the brand name Lasix, which implies the drug lasts 6 hours.

Bumetanide

Bumetanide is a loop diuretic that is significantly more potent than furosemide; in fact, 1 mg of bumetanide is equivalent to 40 mg of furosemide. Bumetanide is often used when patients fail to respond to furosemide.

Like furosemide, bumetanide can be given as a continuous infusion, usually administered at 0.5 to 2 mg/h. The onset of action of IV bumetanide is 2 to 3 minutes, with peak effects usually observed in 15 to 30 minutes. The duration of action is 2 to

3 hours. Boluses of bumetanide should be administered over 1 to 2 minutes.

Medication Infusion Technique

The standard of care for medication infusion during CCT mandates use of infusion pumps for any continuously running infusion. When patients are being transported by aircraft, CCTPs should recognize that actual delivery rates for fluids not infused via pumps will be affected by changes in altitude. Specifically, when altitude increases, IV drip rates will increase; conversely, when altitude decreases, IV drip rates will decrease. Flow rates should not be affected at 1,500 feet to 2,000 feet.

A two-tone alarm from the infusion system indicates that either the infusion is complete or the battery is low. Four quick beeps and a corresponding red light alarm on the screen signal a more serious problem. Silence the alarm and press the *Alarm Channel* key if needed to access alarm information, then press *Start/Stop* to restart fluids.

The sequence for medication infusion is presented in **SKILL DRILL 8-1** and described here:

1. To set up a medication infusion system, press the *On/Off* key for 1 second, and then prime the tubing system **STEP 1**.
2. Pull the white slide clamp on the cassette to the out position, and insert the cassette into the appropriate channel **STEP 2**.
3. After placing the tubing collar into the recessed area, select the appropriate channel by pressing *ABC* on the soft pad that corresponds to the pump **STEP 3**.
4. Set the rate and volume on the system, and press the *Accept* button **STEP 4**.
5. Press *Select* to advance the volume infused; press *Clear* to zero the amount infused **STEP 5**.
6. Press the *Standard Display* key, and then press *Start/Stop* to initiate the infusion **STEP 6**.

Administration of fluids through a dial-a-flow device is not considered reliable and should be switched to an IV infusion pump.

Skill Drill 8-1 Administering Medication With an Infusion Pump

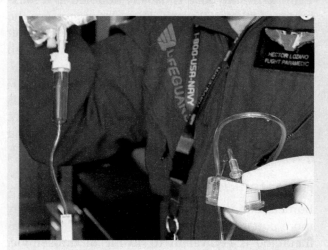

Step 1

Pull the white slide clamp on the cassette to the out position. Insert the cassette into the appropriate channel.

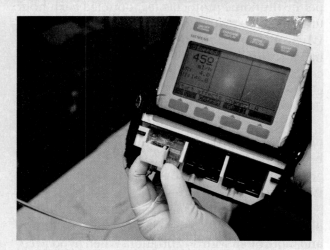

Step 2

Press the *On/Off* key for 1 second, and then prime the tubing system.

Skill Drill 8-1 Administering Medication With an Infusion Pump (continued)

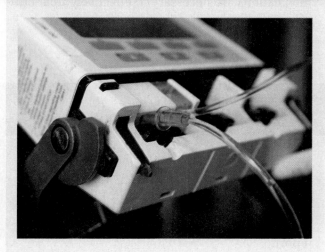

Step 3

Place the tubing collar into the recessed area. Select the appropriate channel by pressing *ABC* on the soft pad that corresponds to the pump.

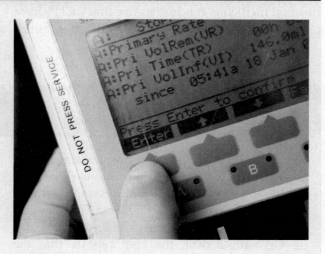

Step 4

Set the rate and press *Accept*. Adjust the volume and press *Accept*.

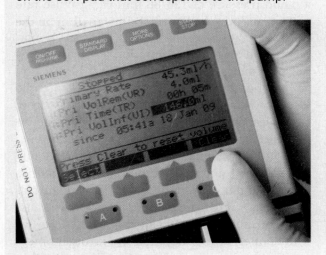

Step 5

Press *Select* to advance the volume infused. Press *Clear* to zero the amount infused.

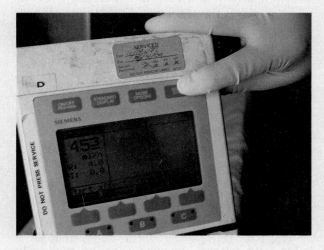

Step 6

Press the *Standard Display* key. Press *Start/Stop* to initiate the infusion.

Summary

Numerous medications are used in critical care medicine, and many of them pose greater risk of harm than the medications used in standard prehospital medicine. It is imperative that CCTPs have an understanding of both the medications used during their transports and the medications they may encounter at sending facilities. Any continuous infusion must be delivered using an infusion pump. Continued review and refamiliarization with medications are necessary to effectively treat critical care patients.

Case Study

You are called to a regional hospital emergency department for a male patient who is experiencing an active STEMI and requires cardiac intervention and emergent air transfer to a tertiary care facility. Transport time by air will be 45 minutes.

On your arrival, the staff reports that the 55-year-old, 269-pound (122-kg) man presented to the emergency department (ED) with chest pain with a rating of 7/10 and mild shortness of breath. He has had chest pain on and off for the past few days and awoke this morning with the current symptoms. His 12-lead ECG revealed an active STEMI.

The patient's medical history and report per the referring registered nurse includes hypertension, coronary artery disease, and hyperlipidemia. This patient's prescription medications include metoprolol, clopidogrel, and aspirin.

In the ED, the patient was placed on the monitor and given oxygen at 2 L/min via nasal cannula to achieve an oxygen saturation of 95%. An 18-gauge angiocatheter was placed in his left forearm, and a 20-gauge angiocatheter was placed in his right hand. Blood samples were obtained. Both IV lines provided 0.9% saline at to-keep-open rates. The patient received three nitroglycerin tablets sublingually, producing total relief of his chest discomfort, and a drip of 10 µg/min was initiated with a concentration of 100 mg/250 mL running at 3 mL/h. Aspirin 325 mg was also given. Serial ECGs revealed ST elevation in the V_3 and V_4 leads, indicative of an anterior infarct. Positive cardiac markers confirmed the ECG findings. A heparin drip of 1,000 units/h was initiated using a concentration of 25,000 units/250 mL running at 10 mL/h. A bolus of 30.5 mg of abciximab was given, and a drip using 9 mg/250 mL was initiated at 10 µg/min, or 16.7 mL/h. The patient also received 5 mg of metoprolol via IV push. His pain is currently a 4/10. His temperature is reported as 98.6°F (37°C). The referring nurse has no further report.

Your assessment reveals the patient is alert and oriented and consents to transfer. He reports chest pain at 4/10, but his shortness of breath feels resolved. Current vital signs at this facility are a blood pressure of 126/86 mm Hg, a pulse rate of 84 beats/min, and normal sinus rhythm on the ECG; respirations of 16 breaths/min and nonlabored; and an oxygen saturation as measured by pulse oximetry (SpO_2) of 96% with 2 L/min oxygen via nasal cannula. The patient feels afebrile to touch. An examination of the patient's head, ears, eyes, nose, and throat reveals equal reactive pupils at 5 mm, a midline trachea, no jugular vein distention, and no audible carotid bruits on auscultation. His chest is symmetric with equal rise and fall, and breath sounds are clear with auscultation. His S_1 and S_2 heart tones are normal on auscultation, and no rubs or gallops are noted. He has a moderately obese abdomen and no organomegaly or pulsatile masses. His extremities are within normal limits, with no trauma, deformity, or other abnormality noted. Pulse quality is normal on palpation. All IV lines are infusing well, and no local redness or swelling is noted. The nitroglycerin is infusing in the right IV line, and the heparin and abciximab are infusing in the left IV line.

You duplicate the flow rates and transfer his IV lines to your pumps. The ECG, blood pressure cuff, and SpO_2 sensors are transferred to your monitors. Oxygen is transferred to your portable cylinder. The patient is transferred to your cot and secured, and IV lines are transferred to the cot. You discharge the patient from the ED, obtain all records, and move to your helicopter. You place the patient in the aircraft, and all oxygen and power needs are transferred to on-board systems. You lift off and transport is begun.

En route, you note no changes in the patient's hemodynamic status, as vital signs remain within the previously described range. The patient continues to report chest pain at 4/10 but has no shortness of breath. He denies having any nausea. Medical control and standing protocols are initiated. You arrive within the 90-minute door-to-balloon time standard at the tertiary care facility, and the patient is moved directly to the catheterization lab and transferred to the facility's staff without incident. You give your report and all paperwork to the charge nurse and retreat to complete your paperwork and prepare your equipment for the next call.

1. Are the medication doses correct?
2. Are any compatibility issues identified?
3. Which further adjustments can be made to current medications to benefit this patient?

Analysis

The case study represents one of the most common scenarios a CCTP will face: The medication dosing is *not* correct. Although all the concentrations are within standards, the dosing for nitroglycerin is not correct. The patient is receiving 20 µg/min with this concentration versus the intended 10 µg/min.

The administration of heparin and abciximab also warrants scrutiny. Although abciximab is not reported as having incompatibility issues when infused via the same IV line in this case, the manufacturer recommends that it be run in a separate IV line. This could be accomplished by placing the nitroglycerin and heparin into the same IV line.

This patient's condition may be better treated by increasing his nitroglycerin dose incrementally and monitoring his responses.

This patient has had, and is receiving, multiple anticoagulant medications. He must be monitored for any bruising or bleeding. If bleeding is suspected, the CCTP should stop the infusions and immediately consult with medical control or follow established protocols. No prescreening information for anticoagulation was readily offered. It is always good practice to ask for this information because it may uncover a contraindication to medication use. Speed is essential in transporting time-sensitive patients, but moving too quickly without paying attention to details is just as detrimental to the patient as moving too slowly.

A standard treatment for STEMI does exist, but treatments and medications vary from region to region because of local preferences, drug availability and cost, and referral patterns related to facilities. CCTPs must be familiar with the protocols used in their region and the common treatment modalities.

The identification of a wrong medication dose is of paramount importance. Although all health care providers strive to provide accurate care, errors can and do occur. The CCTP must ensure a mistake is not repeated. Some of the most common errors involve mistaken concentrations, which result in dosing errors. This risk is increased when IV drips are hand-mixed by the practitioner. The CCTP must ensure concentrations are correct and match the dosing required. All medications administered using IV drips should be checked for flow rate and dosing accuracy. The CCTP must be well versed in many pharmacologic interventions. It is always recommended to consult up-to-date pocket guides or charts to ensure accuracy as well given the large number of medications the CCTP may encounter.

Another issue that the CCTP must consider is compatibility. Although many medications are compatible with each other, many are not. Again, the CCTP is responsible for double-checking all co-infusing medications for compatibility. Adjustments may be required to obtain compatibility in medications administered.

An understanding of pharmacology is a challenging part of CCTP practice. The responsibilities of the CCTP can be as simple as administering an oral medication or as complex as calculating doses, admixing medications, and administering simultaneous infusions. CCTPs are responsible for both maintaining their knowledge of current and emerging pharmacology and performing due diligence in practice.

Prep Kit

Ready for Review

- Pharmacology is defined as the study of the preparation, properties, uses, and actions of medications.
- Current and reliable medication information may be obtained from a variety of print and electronic reference sources.
- Many factors must be considered when selecting the most appropriate medication for a particular condition, including medication availability, the transport team's scope of practice, monitoring capabilities, the patient's clinical status, and medication-specific factors.
- The optimal medication for a particular situation may not be immediately available during patient transport. For example, specialized medications such as antidotes, thrombolytics, and antibiotics are not routinely carried by CCT organizations.
- Pharmacokinetics is the study of the metabolism and action of medications within the body, with particular emphasis on the time required for absorption, distribution in the body, metabolism (biotransformation), and mechanism of excretion.
- The route of administration affects how quickly and how much of an administered dose is absorbed into the patient's body. CCTPs generally use intravenous, intramuscular, subcutaneous, intraosseous, oral, sublingual, transdermal, nasal, and sometimes rectal routes for medication administration.
- The route of medication administration may affect bioavailability—the amount of an administered medication that reaches the patient's systemic circulation without any alteration.
- A medication or other foreign substance in the body undergoes elimination, biotransformation, or both. The kidneys and urinary system are often the primary routes of elimination.
- Biotransformation may lead to any of four outcomes: (1) an active drug may be changed into an inactive metabolite and eliminated;

(2) an active drug may be changed into an active metabolite that causes continued or new clinical effects; (3) an active medication may be changed into a reactive metabolite that has a greater potential for action than its parent substance; and (4) an otherwise inactive substance may change into an active, potentially toxic substance.

- Medications work in one of four ways: (1) by binding with a receptor site on a particular cell to either promote or inhibit a specific activity of that cell; (2) by affecting the physical properties of a cell and, thereby, its functioning; (3) by combining directly with other chemicals within the body to either alter or limit the effects of a chemical or allow it to be removed; and (4) by altering a metabolic pathway.
- In downregulation, as the medication molecules bind to their corresponding receptor sites, the number of receptors decreases. In upregulation, the medication increases the number of receptor sites available for binding.
- The drug-response relationship correlates the amount of medication given with the response it causes.
- The onset of action is defined as how long it takes for the concentration of the medication at the target tissue to reach the minimum effective level.
- The duration of action is defined as how long the medication can be expected to remain above that minimum level to provide the intended action.
- The termination of action is the amount of time after the concentration level falls below the minimum level to the point at which it is eliminated from the body.
- The onset of action, duration of action, and termination of action combine to determine the therapeutic index for a medication, which gives an indication of the medication's margin of safety (defined as the ratio of a drug's lethal

Prep Kit Continued

dose for 50% of the population to its effective dose for 50% of the population).

- Patients of different ages may have vastly different responses to the same drug, owing to age-related factors such as renal function, muscle mass, body water/fat content, and metabolic rate.
- Older adult patients often have slower absorption and elimination times, necessitating modification of the doses of many drugs administered to these patients.
- To correct for differences in weight between patients, drugs are sometimes dosed in milligrams or micrograms per kilogram of the patient's body weight.
- Other factors that may affect the dose-response relationship include the patient's sex, environmental factors (eg, stress), time of the medication's administration, the patient's overall state of health, and genetic factors.
- In pregnant patients, medications may pass from the mother's bloodstream into the placenta and ultimately affect the fetus. Medications may also pass into breast milk in breastfeeding women. When contemplating administration of any medication to a pregnant or a breastfeeding patient, evidence of risk and benefits of that medication should be reviewed.
- Every medication has side effects—that is, reactions that can manifest as undesired signs or symptoms but that are nevertheless expected based on how the medication works.
- The transport team must be adequately trained and equipped to recognize and effectively manage anticipated side effects or adverse reactions associated with a particular medication.
- An iatrogenic response is an adverse condition inadvertently induced in a patient by the treatment given. Some of these responses may be devastating and even potentially lethal.
- The most common unpredictable response encountered in the prehospital setting is an allergic reaction.
- The effects of one medication may alter the response of another medication in sometimes

unexpected ways, resulting in a drug interaction.

- Medication errors are the most common errors in medicine. While many cause little to no harm, others can have serious, even devastating, consequences for the patient, their family, and caregivers involved in the error.
- The critical care transport environment continually exposes personnel and vehicles to temperature extremes; it is essential that medications remain within their required temperature ranges.
- Minimum requirements for the storage of controlled substances include housing them in a securely locked, substantially constructed cabinet with no sign or any other indication that the cabinet is used for the storage of controlled substances.
- Vasopressors include phenylephrine, norepinephrine, epinephrine, vasopressin, and methylene blue; some may be used as push-dose pressors. Vasopressors are typically administered to improve cardiac output.
- Epinephrine (a sympathomimetic agent) increases blood pressure by increasing vascular tone and cardiac stimulation, and supports respiratory function by opening larger airways. It is the drug of choice for treating patients with anaphylaxis.
- In anesthesia practice, providers may draw a syringe of an available diluted vasopressor drip and administer boluses to treat hypotension that is refractory to fluids (ie, push-dose pressors). The two medications most often employed in these combinations are dilute concentrations of epinephrine and phenylephrine.
- Inotropes include dopamine, dobutamine, and milrinone. Dopamine (a sympathomimetic agent) stimulates alpha-1 receptors when given at a higher dose, thereby producing peripheral vasoconstriction. Stimulation of the dopaminergic receptors may also result in increased myocardial contractility and cardiac output, increased renal output, decreased fluid volume, and increased blood pressure.

Prep Kit Continued

- Vasodilators and antihypertensives are used to lower blood pressure; they include sodium nitroprusside, nitroglycerin, hydralazine, clevidipine, and nicardipine.
- The traditional first-line medication for chest pain associated with cardiac ischemia is nitroglycerin. Nitroglycerin may also be used to treat hypertension. Nitroprusside is both an arterial and a venous dilator and is more potent than nitroglycerin; at lower doses, nitroglycerin is only a venous dilating agent.
- Hydralazine is an antihypertensive that is used as an intermittent IV bolus for emergent control of hypertension.
- Benzodiazepines may be used for treatment of anxiety and seizures and to provide sedation. These agents are the initial medications for seizures in prehospital and critical care transport settings.
- Aside from its use in the operating room for induction and maintenance of anesthesia, propofol is used as a sedative in mechanically ventilated patients. It is also commonly used for brief procedures requiring procedural sedation (eg, electric cardioversion).
- Etomidate is an ultra-short-acting general anesthetic used for procedural sedation, induction of general anesthesia, and intubation. Its short duration of action and favorable side-effect profile make it a popular choice for rapid sequence and emergent intubations.
- Ketamine is a general anesthetic that is increasingly being used on an off-label basis in the prehospital arena to provide procedural sedation and analgesia. It has also shown promise in rapid sedation of patients exhibiting signs and symptoms of excited delirium.
- Antipsychotic medications (eg, haloperidol, olanzapine, quetiapine) are often first-line therapies in patients with agitation and psychosis.
- The use of morphine and other opioids is an essential component of patient care during critical care transport. Other analgesic medications used may include ketamine, acetaminophen, and NSAIDs.
- Anticonvulsants are used in patients with seizures, including status epilepticus, as well as in some other indications. They include levetiracetam, phenytoin, fosphenytoin, and valproic acid.
- Long-term chemical paralysis of the patient has serious implications for CCTPs and other health care providers caring for the patient. Intensive care providers can use a train-of-four measurement, post-tetanic count, or double-burst stimulation to assess for the correct level of neuromuscular-blocking agents in patients receiving long-term paralysis, but CCTPs require special training to interpret these tests.
- Paralytic medications are classified into two categories based on how they interact with acetylcholine (ACH) and the nicotinic receptors: depolarizing and nondepolarizing.
- Succinylcholine, the only depolarizing paralytic, stimulates muscle depolarization but then remains bound to the receptor, thereby preventing repolarization.
- Nondepolarizing agents competitively antagonize ACH at the postsynaptic receptors. They include pancuronium, vecuronium, rocuronium, atracurium, and cisatracurium.
- Stress ulcer prophylaxis is undertaken in critically ill patients with associated risk factors such as coagulopathy, severe sepsis, or mechanical ventilation for more than 48 hours. Histamine antagonists and proton pump inhibitors are used to reduce gastric acid secretion.
- Antihistamine medications, which inhibit the activity of histamine in the vestibular system, and medications that block the ACH receptors are often used to treat nausea and vomiting.
- Medications that antagonize the D_2 receptors, such as the phenothiazine-type antiemetics, are used for treatment of nausea and vomiting.

Prep Kit Continued

- The serotonin antagonists exert an antiemetic effect by selectively blocking serotonin receptors in the medulla.
- Octreotide is a synthetic peptide with actions analogous to somatostatin, but a longer, more clinically useful duration of action.
- Epoprostenol is used to treat pulmonary arterial hypertension. Although most commonly given via IV infusion, it may also be nebulized.
- Alprostadil is a vasodilator medication that is used during critical care transport to maintain a patent ductus arteriosus in newborns with certain congenital heart defects.
- Aerosolized epinephrine, which is given by small-volume nebulizer, is typically used for relief of respiratory distress due to stridor, bronchiolitis, laryngeal edema, and upper airway obstruction. It has also been effective in treating postextubation edema and croup.
- The management of cardiac arrhythmias involves several classes of antiarrhythmic medications, many of which are arrhythmogenic.
- Class I antiarrhythmic medications work by blocking sodium channels; they include anticholinergic medications such as quinidine, procainamide, and disopyramide.
- Class II antiarrhythmic medications (beta blockers) work by competitively binding to beta receptor sites to inhibit their stimulation. They are used to treat arrhythmias, hypertension, acute myocardial infarctions, and heart failure.
- Class III antiarrhythmic medications (potassium channel blockers) are particularly useful for treating reentry tachycardias and arrhythmias caused by cellular depolarization as a result of excessive excitability. Their use may produce prolonged QT intervals on the patient's ECG.
- Class IV antiarrhythmic medications (calcium channel blockers) cause vasodilation, negative inotropy, negative chronotropy, and negative dromotropy. Because these medications decrease the conduction velocity through the AV node, they are useful for treating tachyarrhythmias originating in the atria.
- When a patient is taking heparin, the CCTP should review the latest lab values and the partial thromboplastin time prior to transport and monitor the patient closely for bleeding problems.
- Alteplase is a thrombolytic agent used to treat acute ischemic stroke, acute massive pulmonary embolism, ST-segment elevation myocardial infarction (STEMI), and acute peripheral artery occlusions, and to clear clotted central venous catheters. Tenecteplase is an alternative to alteplase in management of STEMI and may be used in the near future for treatment of acute ischemic stroke.
- Glycoprotein IIb/IIIa inhibitors are antiplatelet medications. Abciximab is used during and after percutaneous coronary intervention for STEMI and following some carotid stent procedures; other antiplatelet agents include eptifibatide and tirofiban. All of these agents carry a risk of excessive bleeding.
- For most critically ill patients, interventions to control hyperglycemia should be triggered when the blood glucose level reaches or exceeds 180 mg/dL, with a goal of maintaining this level in the range of 140 to 180 mg/dL. Likewise, protocols and monitoring need to be designed to avoid hypoglycemia (blood glucose ≤70 mg/dL), which is associated with increased mortality.
- Diuretics are widely used by CCTPs for treating patients with fluid volume overload, cerebral edema, hyperkalemia, and rhabdomyolysis. The most commonly administered diuretic is furosemide.
- During air transports, when altitudes increase, IV drip rates will increase; conversely, when altitudes decrease, IV drip rates will decrease.
- Patients should always be placed on infusion pumps to ensure precise medication delivery during critical care transport.

Prep Kit Continued

Vital Vocabulary

absorption   The process by which molecules are taken up into another medium or tissue.

acetylcholine (ACh)   A chemical neurotransmitter of the parasympathetic nervous system.

agonist   A molecule (medication) that binds and activates a receptor, producing a biologic response.

antagonist   A molecule (medication) that blocks a receptor site from being stimulated by an agonist or other chemical mediators.

bioavailability   The amount or percentage of a medication that reaches the systemic circulation without being altered.

biotransformation   The process by which the body alters a medication.

chronotropic   Altering the heart rate.

controlled substances   Drugs whose manufacture, possession, and use are controlled by the government.

cross-tolerance   A form of drug tolerance in which patients who take a particular medication for an extended period can build up a tolerance to other medications in the same class.

cumulative effect   An effect that occurs when several successive doses of a medication are administered or when absorption of a medication occurs faster than its excretion or metabolism.

depolarizing paralytic   A medication that causes neuromuscular blockade by binding and briefly activating receptor sites at the neuromuscular junction, preventing further activation of these sites and causing chemical paralysis.

distribution   The process by which molecules move from the body's systemic circulation to specific organs and tissues.

dromotropic   Influencing the conduction rate within the heart.

drug interaction   The alteration of the action or metabolism of a particular medication when combined with another medication.

duration of action   The amount of time a medication concentration can be expected to remain above the minimum level needed to provide the intended action.

extravasation   An infusion-related complication in which the drug being administered intravenously leaks outside the vein and enters the surrounding tissues; if that substance is a vesicant, it can cause blisters and tissue damage.

first-order elimination   The rate of elimination is proportional to the drug's plasma concentration.

first-pass effect   A process by which the dose of an oral medication is reduced as it passes through the liver (and, for some medications, the gut as well as the liver) before it enters systemic circulation; also called first-pass metabolism.

half-life (T½)   The time period required to eliminate one-half of the plasma concentration. During the second half-life, an additional 25% of the original plasma concentration is eliminated. After three half-lives, one-eighth of the original plasma concentration remains.

histamine   A neurotransmitter that is released by cells in response to injury and in allergic and inflammatory reactions; it causes vasodilation and contraction of smooth muscle tissue.

iatrogenic response   An adverse condition inadvertently induced in a patient by the treatment given.

idiosyncratic reaction   An abnormal (and usually unexplained) reaction by a person to a medication to which most other people do not react.

indication   The reason for using a medication; it may be an official use, approved by the FDA, or an off-label use, for a purpose other than those specifically noted on the medication's label.

inhibition   A condition in which the presence of one medication decreases the effect of another medication.

inotropic   Affecting the force with which cardiac muscle tissue contracts.

Prep Kit Continued

interference A direct biochemical interaction between two drugs.

mechanism of action The way in which a medication produces the intended response.

neuromuscular-blocking agents (NMBAs) Medications that bind to acetylcholine receptors, thereby inhibiting the action of acetylcholine; this effect blocks transmission at the neuromuscular junction and causes paralysis of the muscles.

nicotinic receptors Cholinergic receptors that bind with the neurotransmitter acetylcholine.

nondepolarizing agent A medication designed to cause temporary paralysis by binding in a competitive but nonstimulatory manner to part of the acetylcholine receptor; these medications do not cause fasciculations and have a longer duration of action than succinylcholine does.

onset of action The time needed for the concentration of a medication at the target tissue to reach the minimum effective level.

pharmacodynamics The branch of pharmacology that studies reactions between medications and living structures, including the processes of body responses to pharmacologic, biochemical, physiologic, and therapeutic effects.

pharmacokinetics The study of the metabolism and action of medications, with the particular emphasis on the time required for absorption, duration of action, distribution in the body, and method of excretion.

pharmacology The study of the preparation, properties, uses, and actions of medications.

potentiation The effect of increasing the potency or effectiveness of a drug or other treatment; it may occur when two medications are administered concurrently.

prodrug A medication that, once inside the body, becomes metabolized to a physiologically active form.

propofol-related infusion syndrome (PRIS) A constellation of symptoms, including arrhythmias (bradycardia or tachycardia), metabolic acidosis, hyperkalemia, rhabdomyolysis or creatine phosphokinase elevations, and progressive renal and cardiac failure, associated with use of propofol.

proton pump inhibitors (PPIs) Medications that reduce gastric acid secretion; they are used to treat gastroesophageal reflux disease and peptic ulcers.

receptor sites Specialized proteins on a cell that receive chemical mediator messages.

risk-benefit ratio An evaluation of the therapeutic benefits of a medication versus the risks associated with that medication's side effects.

side effects Reactions that can manifest as signs or symptoms that are not desired but are expected based on how the medication works.

status epilepticus A life-threatening neurologic disorder in which an individual experiences prolonged (more than 5 minutes) seizure or does not recover from such seizures.

steady state A point in drug administration at which the rate of administration (frequency and dose) is equal to the rate of elimination, resulting in a constant plasma medication level.

summation effect The process whereby administration of multiple medications can produce a response that the individual medications alone do not produce.

sympathomimetics Medications that mimic the body's sympathetic nervous system response (fight-or-flight response); include epinephrine and norepinephrine.

synergism An interaction of two or more medications that results in an effect that is greater than the sum of their effects if taken independently.

tachyphylaxis A condition in which the patient rapidly becomes tolerant to a medication.

termination of action The amount of time after the medication's concentration falls below the minimum effective level until the point at which it is eliminated from the body.

therapeutic index The ratio of a drug's lethal dose for 50% (LD_{50}) of the population to its

Prep Kit Continued

effective dose for 50% (ED$_{50}$) of the population; a medication's margin of safety.

tolerance   Physiologic adaptation to the effects of a drug such that increasingly larger doses of the drug are required to achieve the same effect.

vasopressor   A medication that causes constriction of blood vessels, thereby causing blood pressure to rise.

Vaughan-Williams classification scheme   A classification system for antiarrhythmic medications.

vesicant   A substance that causes tissue injury.

zero-order elimination   A process by which medications or chemicals are eliminated from the body at a constant rate, regardless of plasma concentration.

References

American Pharmacists Association. *Drug Information Handbook* (Lexicomp's Drug Reference Handbooks). 25th ed. Hudson, OH: Lexicomp; 2016.

Baglin TP. Heparin-induced thrombocytopenia thrombosis (HIT/T) syndrome: diagnosis and treatment. *J Clin Pathol*. 2001;54:272-274.

Barnet JC, Touchon RC. Short-term control of supraventricular tachycardia with verapamil infusion and calcium pretreatment. *Chest*. 1990;97:1106-1109.

Bersten AD, Handy JM, eds. *Oh's Intensive Care Manual*. 8th ed. New York, NY: Butterworth Heinemann Elsevier; 2018.

Boersma E, Harrington RA, Moliterno DJ, et al. Platelet glycoprotein IIb/IIIa inhibitors in acute coronary syndromes: a meta-analysis of all major randomized clinical trials. *Lancet*. 2002;359(9302):189-198.

Brophy GM, Bell R, Claassen J, et al. Guidelines for the evaluation and management of status epilepticus. *Neurocrit Care*. 2012;17:3-23.

Brown CA III, Sakles JC, Mick NW, eds. *The Walls Manual of Emergency Airway Management*. 5th ed. Philadelphia, PA: Lippincott, Williams and Wilkins; 2017.

Cornelius C. Drug use in the elderly: risk or protection? *Curr Opin Psychiatry*. 2004;17(6):443-447.

Gerber JG, Nies AS. Furosemide-induced vasodilation: importance of the state of hydration and filtration. *Kidney Int*. 1980;18:454-459.

Hamilton RJ, ed. *Tarascon Pocket Pharmacopoeia: 2020 Classic Shirt-Pocket Edition*. 34th ed. Burlington, MA: Jones & Bartlett Learning; 2020.

Harrington L, Leiker C. Dosing of emergency cardiovascular medications in obese patients. *Bariatr Nurs Surg Patient Care*. 2007;2(2):131-139.

Harvey RP, Schocket AL. The effect of H$_1$ and H$_2$ blockade on cutaneous histamine response in man. *J Allergy Clin Immunol*. 1980;65(2):136-139.

Jacobi J, Bircher N, Krinsley J, et al. Guidelines for the use of an insulin infusion for the management of hyperglycemia in critically ill patients. *Crit Care Med*. 2012;40:3251-3276.

Junger WG, Coimbra R, Liu FC, et al. Hypertonic saline resuscitation: a tool to modulate immune function in trauma patients? *Shock*. 1997;8:235-241.

Katzung BG, Vanderah TW, eds. *Basic and Clinical Pharmacology*. 15th ed. New York, NY: McGraw-Hill; 2020.

Kim GH, Hahn DK, Kellner CP, et al. The incidence of heparin-induced thrombocytopenia type II in patients with subarachnoid hemorrhage treated with heparin versus enoxaparin. *J Neurosurg*. 2009;110:50-57.

King C, Henretig FM, eds. *Pediatric Emergency Procedures*. 2nd ed. Philadelphia, PA: Lippincott, Williams and Wilkins; 2008.

Kizior RJ, Hodgson K, eds. *Saunders Nursing Drug Handbook 2020*. St. Louis, MO: Elsevier; 2020.

Lameire N, Vanholder R, Van Biesen W. Loop diuretics for patients with acute renal failure: helpful or harmful? *JAMA*. 2002;288:2599-2601.

Lowson S, Gent JP, Goodchild CS. Anticonvulsant properties of propofol and thiopentone: comparison using two tests in laboratory mice. *Br J Anesth*. 1990;64:59-63.

Mehta RL, Pascual MT, Soroko S, Chertow GM. Diuretics, mortality, and nonrecovery of renal function in acute renal failure. *JAMA*. 2002;288:2547-2553.

Nelson LS, Howland MA, Levin MA, et al., eds. *Goldfrank's Toxicologic Emergencies*. 11th ed. New York, NY: McGraw-Hill; 2019.

O'Donnell CJ, Ridker PM, Hebert PR, Hennekens CH. Antithrombotic therapy for acute myocardial infarction. *J Am Coll Cardiol*. 1995;25:S23-S29.

Olson KR, ed. *Poisoning and Drug Overdose*. 7th ed. New York, NY: Lange/McGraw-Hill; 2017.

Pickkers P, Dormans TPJ, Russel FGM, et al. Direct vascular effects of furosemide in humans. *Circulation*.1997;96:1847-1852.

Powers WJ, Rabinstein AA, Ackerson T, et al. Guidelines for the early management of patients with acute ischemic stroke: 2019 update to the 2018 guidelines for the early management of acute ischemic stroke: a guideline for healthcare professionals from the American Heart Association/American Stroke Association. *Stroke*.

Prep Kit Continued

2019;50(12):e344-e418. https://doi.org/10.1161/STR.0000000000000211.

Selleng K, Warkentin TE, Greinacher A. Heparin-induced thrombocytopenia in intensive care patients. *Crit Care Med*. 2007;35:1165-1176.

Sharma R, Mir S, Rizvi M, Akthar S. Efficacy of magnesium sulphate versus phenytoin in seizure control and prophylaxis in patients of eclampsia and severe pre-eclampsia. *J K Science*. 2008;10:181-185.

Van den Berghe G, Wouters P, Weekers F, et al. Intensive insulin therapy in critically ill patients. *N Engl J Med*. 2001;345:1359-1367.

Wagner LK. Diagnosis and management of preeclampsia. *Am Fam Physician*.2004;70:2317-2324.

Walker M. Status epilepticus: an evidence based guide. *Br Med J*. 2005;331:673-677.

Weingart S. Push-dose pressors for immediate blood pressure control. *Clin Exp Emerg Med*. 2015;2:131-132.

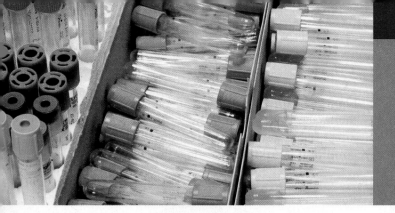

Chapter 9

Laboratory Analysis and Diagnostic Studies

Gregory Peters, MD

Christopher J. Hanowitz, MD

Introduction

Critical care transport professionals (CCTPs), when performing interfacility transports, are often responsible for patients who have undergone a battery of tests and examinations at the referring institution. Laboratory tests (sometimes called labs) can be very useful in determining the seriousness of the patient's condition or in preparing for potential problems while en route. Such tests may include laboratory analyses of the patient's blood, urine, cerebrospinal fluid (CSF), or other body fluids. Similarly, as diagnostic imaging technology continues to advance, the prevalence and relevance of such tests will continue to increase within critical care transport (CCT).

Diagnostic analysis serves many purposes in the CCT environment. A CCTP must know the normal ranges for each lab value, as well as the associated physiologic meaning of each test. These tests are performed to support an evidence-based approach to patient care, in which providers use both well-tested principles and patient-specific knowledge to select and administer treatments. A proper understanding of diagnostic analysis, such as laboratory tests and imaging studies, can be invaluable in preparing for potential incidents, responding to changes in a patient's clinical status en route, and ensuring optimal transfer of care at both the sending and receiving facilities.

Principles of Analysis

Laboratory analysis should run deeper than simply surmising whether the value is outside the normal range for that test. If the normal value range for creatinine is 0.6 to 1.2 mg/dL, for example, then a creatinine value of 4.5 mg/dL for a specific patient is clearly outside the normal range. But what does that actually mean for the patient? The most important point is to understand how this excess level affects the patient now and how it might affect the patient's condition while the transport team is en route to the receiving facility, including the patient's likely response to different interventions or higher risk of experiencing certain medical emergencies. The underlying principles that guide the analysis of all laboratory values must be ever-present in a CCTP's mind.

An appreciation of a lab test's **precision** and **accuracy** is essential to the proper use of that particular lab test. If the lab test is precise, results of performing it repeatedly on the same sample will be similar. For example, if a patient's serum sodium level is measured five times on the same sample, the values may range from 152 to 155 mEq/L. This test exhibits high precision (tightly packed values), but the results would be inaccurate if the patient's true serum sodium level is 140 mEq/L **FIGURE 9-1**. In contrast, if another test of the same patient's serum sodium was performed five times and yielded results of 135 to 145 mEq/L, this test would be fairly accurate but not precise **FIGURE 9-2**. The scientists who design laboratory tests strive for tests that are both precise and accurate, such that repeated measures will yield results that are both consistent and close to the true value.

Laboratory tests also have differing levels of sensitivity and specificity. **Sensitivity** refers to the ability of a test to indicate whether a person does or does not have a certain condition. If a test is

highly sensitive, most of the people with a particular condition would have a positive result. If a test has a low sensitivity, many people with the condition would have a negative result. In other

Precise But Inaccurate Test

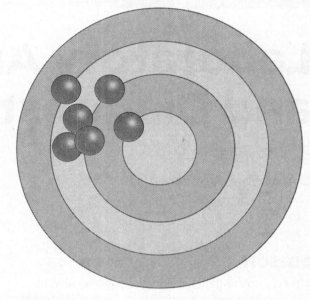

FIGURE 9-1 The sample lab results depicted here are precise (because results cluster together) but inaccurate (because results are out of the normal range [center circle]).

© Jones & Bartlett Learning.

Accurate But Imprecise Test

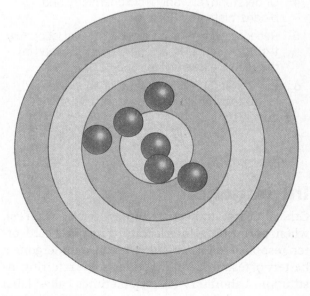

FIGURE 9-2 The sample lab results depicted here are imprecise (because results vary substantially) but accurate.

© Jones & Bartlett Learning.

words, sensitivity is the proportion of people with the target disorder who have a positive test result. Specificity, in contrast, is the proportion of people without the target disorder who have a negative test result FIGURE 9-3.

Let's consider an example that clarifies these concepts. The D-dimer test is a test of hypercoagulability that detects a fragment, D-dimer, from the fibrinolysis process. It is used to help diagnose and monitor diseases and conditions related to inappropriate clotting of the blood. This test provides a good illustration of sensitivity versus specificity. The sensitivity of the D-dimer test for the presence of deep vein thrombosis (DVT) is calculated by dividing the number of patients with a true positive test result by the actual number of patients with the disorder. For example, suppose researchers conduct a study to determine the accuracy of D-dimer tests in diagnosing DVT. If 13 out of the 14 patients included in this study have a true positive test result for DVT, the sensitivity of D-dimer testing would be 93%:

$$13/14 = 0.928, \text{ or } 93\%$$

In other words, the D-dimer test will correctly identify a patient with a DVT 93% of the time; the other 7% of results are false negatives (people with the condition who tested negative).

The specificity of the D-dimer test for the presence of DVT is calculated by dividing the number of patients with a true negative test result by the actual number of patients without the disorder:

$$72/91 = 0.791, \text{ or } 79\%$$

In other words, the D-dimer test will correctly identify a patient without DVT 79% of the time; the other 21% of results are false positives (people without the condition who tested positive).

Therefore, this D-dimer test is more sensitive than specific, meaning that it will be better at ruling out the condition (limiting false negatives) than for definitively diagnosing it (limiting false positives). TABLE 9-1 presents another example depicting the effectiveness of D-dimer testing, this time illustrating values in patients diagnosed with pulmonary embolism.

Providers often combine tests with different sensitivity and specificity profiles to optimize these factors and make decisions about how to use resources more efficiently. For example, highly sensitive tests are typically used as screening tests to limit the number of diagnoses missed initially, and individuals with positive results are then subjected to highly specific tests to confirm the diagnosis in those with the target condition, thereby eliminating the initial false positives. It is also important to have an intention to treat prior to ordering or performing any test, so proper assessment of whether a given test is indicated is fundamental to the interpretation of any result. Unnecessary or misused tests can be difficult to interpret and can lead to faulty decision making.

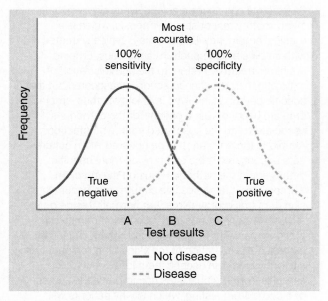

FIGURE 9-3 Graphic representation of the relationship between sensitivity and specificity. **A.** 100% sensitivity. **B.** Most accurate. **C.** 100% specificity.

TABLE 9-1 Results of D-Dimer Measurement Used in the Diagnosis of Pulmonary Embolism		
D-Dimer Test Result	**Pulmonary Embolism**	**No Pulmonary Embolism**
D-Dimer ≥500 µg/L	195	278
D-Dimer <500 µg/L	1	197
Total	**196**	**475**
95% confidence interval	Sensitivity = 99.5%, 97.2–100	Specificity = 41.4%, 37.0–45.9

Reprinted with permission of the American Thoracic Society. Copyright © 2022 American Thoracic Society. All rights reserved. Perrier A, Desmarais S, Goehring C, et al. D-dimer testing for suspected pulmonary embolism in outpatients. *Am J Respir Crit Care Med.* 1997;156(2 Pt 1):492-496. The *American Journal of Respiratory and Critical Care Medicine* is an official journal of the American Thoracic Society.

Certain tests lend themselves to certain levels of analysis. For example, a serologic blood test for the presence or absence of the hepatitis B virus will often show a result as positive or negative, respectively. This is a *qualitative* assessment because the result does not identify the specific level of hepatitis B virus within the blood. If information on the viral load of hepatitis B is desired, a *quantitative* test is performed to indicate the exact amount of the virus within the blood. Sometimes semiquantitative assessments are performed. For example, a urine test looking for blood in the urine may give the result as none, mild, moderate, or severe.

Novices in laboratory analysis can become overly concerned about the notion of normal versus abnormal lab values. One must remember that normal ranges were identified based on findings in healthy people, not the patients being transported by CCTPs. By convention, a normal range is empirically derived and represents values that 95% of *healthy* people would have for the particular test. Thus, for every 100 healthy people tested, 5 will not have results that fall in the normal range, even though their particular level is "normal" for them.

When this idea of normality is applied to patients who have acute conditions, one must be careful not to react too impulsively to spuriously high or low values. Not only is the normal range for a particular lab test subjective in the emergency department (ED) or intensive care unit (ICU) context, but an abnormal result may also be the desired effect of a particular treatment or the body's healthy compensatory response to another condition. Consider the intentional fluid depletion that is implemented with patients who have experienced a traumatic brain injury. Part of the therapy may be to decrease the intravascular volume, which will result in abnormally high serum sodium values. Trying to correct the abnormal serum sodium value would harm the patient in such a case. The message here is simple: Although abnormal lab values cannot be ignored, it is essential to assess them within the context of the patient's entire clinical picture.

With all tests, it is important to keep in mind that errors in specimen collection, identification, labeling, and laboratory analysis may result in erroneous values being reported. In addition, when evaluating laboratory results, it is critical to recognize that different laboratories have different normal ranges for the same tests. In fact, you may find that many of the normal ranges listed in this text differ from the ranges you are accustomed to using in your local practice. Three different labs may very well have three different sets of normal ranges for each test they perform. Thus, you must pay careful attention to the normal values (which are indicated on report forms) when reviewing a particular patient's lab reports and always think critically when interpreting the patient's results.

Specimen Cultures

With a specimen culture, the laboratory technician studies the growth of microorganisms in a biologic sample over a given period of time to learn about suspected infections in the sample's source. Blood, urine, sputum, and other body fluid cultures may all provide information that is used to identify microorganisms and treat specific infections. For example, a sputum culture is obtained when a respiratory infection is suspected. To obtain a sputum sample from a conscious patient, the patient must be well hydrated and able to follow commands to produce sputum from a deep cough. Deep suctioning may be performed to obtain a sputum sample

Bacteremia

Bacteremia can cause a severe systemic inflammatory response called sepsis, which is a medical emergency. Bacteremia is typically treated with empiric broad-spectrum antibiotics. Empiric antibiotic treatment refers to the administration of antibiotic therapy when infection is suspected but the specific pathogen involved is unknown; thus, empiric data are used to treat a patient for the pathogens associated with the suspected source of infection. Antibiotic therapy can then be updated when culture data become available and provide more specific details about the pathogen causing the infection.

Importantly, false-positive cultures can occur when skin flora (microorganisms that normally reside on the skin, such as gram-positive cocci) contaminate the blood sample. This contamination can be caused by inadequate preparation of the skin at the venipuncture site or by breaks in aseptic technique. Taking blood samples from multiple sites can improve the accuracy of blood culture testing, which is why patients will often have two samples in process or completed at the same time.

from an unconscious patient. If the sample is not actually sputum, false results on the laboratory report, based on identification of mixed flora, are likely. Such results are not useful.

Blood culture is a common, important type of culture in which the specimen is a blood sample. Blood cultures can test for the growth of various pathogens, such as aerobic bacteria, anaerobic bacteria, or fungi. The most common indication for collecting blood cultures is concern for **bacteremia**, the presence of bacterial infection in the blood.

Sensitivity testing can be done as well. (Culture and sensitivity testing is sometimes called "C and S.") For bacterial infections, the sensitivity results suggest which antibiotic will most effectively treat the organism causing the infection. A specimen for culture should be obtained before antibiotic therapy is started so that the actions of the antibiotic do not influence the culture result, and so that the proper antibiotic (one to which the microorganism is sensitive) can be selected. Usually, it takes 3 days for a laboratory to complete a culture and sensitivity report; an initial report is generated in approximately 24 hours, but a complete and final report will not be available for 72 hours.

Chemistry Review

Many consider the care of an acute patient to be akin to an advanced experiment in physiology. Physiology is built on the basics of chemistry and cellular biology, the principles of which should be part of the health care provider's educational background. Insightful test interpretation requires a firm grasp of these principles.

Ions

Ions are atoms that have gained or lost electrons. Recall that each electron has a single (-1) negative charge. If electrons are lost, the charge on the atom is less negative; one might also say that the atom is now more positive. The reverse is true if the atom gains electrons. A positively charged ion is referred to as a **cation**; a negatively charged ion is called an **anion**. If one electron is lost from an atom, its charge is $+1$. If two electrons are lost, its charge is $+2$. Conversely, if one electron is gained by an atom, its charge is -1. If two electrons are gained, its charge is -2.

Often ions of opposite charge will join together by forming an **ionic bond**. Sodium chloride (NaCl; table salt) is an example of a molecule whose atoms are joined by an ionic bond. When molecules with ionic bonds interact with water (recall that plasma is 90% water), they often dissociate into their basic ionic forms **FIGURE 9-4**. This is why Na^+ and Cl^- exist as separate ions within plasma, rather than as the compound NaCl. The ionic components of plasma are called electrolytes; they include sodium (Na^+), potassium (K^+), chloride (Cl^-), calcium (Ca^{+2}), and magnesium (Mg^{+2}), among others.

Amounts of ions are expressed in moles or equivalents. A mole is a unit representing 6.02×10^{23} atoms, in much the same way that "a dozen" is used to specify 12 eggs. Equivalents (Eq) are used to measure amounts of charged particles (ie, ions). Essentially, 1 Eq is equal to 1 mole of ionic charges. Given that a single Na^+ atom has one charge, 1 mole of Na^+ atoms has 1 mole of charges (1 Eq). Similarly, calcium (Ca^{+2}) has two charges, so 1 mole of Ca^{+2} has 2 moles of charges (2 Eq). This concept applies only to charged particles; uncharged molecules, such as proteins, are electrically neutral overall.

Osmolarity

Laboratory testing often involves the analysis of certain fluid characteristics. One characteristic of interest to CCTPs is the **osmotic pressure** created by the blood, CSF, or urine sample. Because human

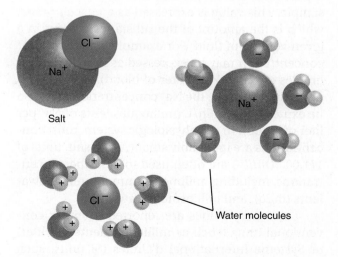

FIGURE 9-4 The ionic bonds of sodium chloride dissociate into their basic ionic forms when they interact with water.

cells have semipermeable membranes, osmosis (the diffusion of water across membranes) is a major mechanism by which fluid moves between the body's different fluid compartments. In the space divided by the semipermeable membrane, the osmotic pressure is created by differences in concentrations of solutes (dissolved substances) found in the solutions on either side of that membrane.

The osmotic pressure generated by the particles in the fluid is called the osmolarity or osmolality, depending on the method of measurement. Physiologic measurement of osmotic pressure in humans yields information on osmolality (though it is often mislabeled as osmolarity). Osmolality measures the amount of dissolved substance in 1 kg of water, where as osmolarity measures the amount of dissolved substance in 1 L of water. Because the volume (liter) of a fluid depends on the temperature of the fluid, osmolality is used in lab tests—the weight (kilogram) of fluid used in this method is independent of temperature. The unit of measurement for osmolality is the osmole (Osm), which is the pressure created by 1 mole of particles in solution.

It is important to note a particular chemical property of osmosis: Osmotic pressure depends only on the number of particles present in the fluid, not on the size of those particles. In other words, a single protein or sugar molecule induces the same osmotic pressure as a single ion of sodium (Na^+).

Ultimately, we want to know the amount of a particular ion or protein that is present in the sample. This value is expressed as a concentration, which is the amount of the substance present in a given volume of fluid. For example, a patient's Na^+ concentration may be expressed as mmol/dL (millimoles of Na^+ per deciliter of blood). Because Na^+ has a single charge, the Na^+ concentration may also be expressed as mEq/L (milliequivalents of Na^+ per liter of blood). In the physiologic system, most concentrations are incredibly small. As a result, units of 1/1,000 (*milli-*) are often used to describe concentrations, including millimoles (mmol), milliequivalents (mEq), and milliosmoles (mOsm).

Laboratory values are reported in either conventional units (such as milliequivalents per liter) or Système International d'Unités (SI units; such as millimoles per liter). Many laboratories use SI values for some tests and conventional units for others, or they might use only conventional units. When reviewing results for a patient, CCTPs need to be sure that the reported units of measure are the same as the units of measure (ie, both conventional or both SI) used to define the normal range.

Each laboratory has its own normal ranges, which usually are printed on the laboratory report along with the patient-specific values. Note that the normal ranges for measurements performed by a certain device may differ from one instrument manufacturer to another. CCTPs should be familiar with the normal ranges for tests often used in the CCT setting, and they should be alert to the normal ranges listed for the tests performed for a specific patient, especially when comparing results from different facilities.

Biochemistry Review

Examining the basic ions and fluid properties provides only part of the story. To ascertain how well an organ (such as the liver) is functioning, it is necessary to look at the levels of various proteins and enzymes in a serum sample. Thousands of different kinds of proteins are found in the human body, and specific laboratory tests examine the amounts of the various types of proteins present in a sample.

Enzymes are critically important proteins that act as catalysts for biochemical reactions. The formation of one biologic substance from another may proceed slowly when just the two substances are present; with the addition of the appropriate enzyme to catalyze the reaction, however, the reaction rate may increase many times. Methods of measuring enzyme levels often rely on this basic catalytic principle. The beginning substrate (material) for the reaction is added to the sample, and the amount of product generated in a given time is measured. By knowing the beginning amount of substrate and the amount of product produced and by assuming normal enzyme function, one can then calculate how much enzyme is present. The function of enzymes is measured in units per liter (U/L), which is the amount of enzyme that catalyzes 1 micromole (μmol) of substrate per minute.

Lab Panels

In laboratory testing, groups of related tests can be performed as a single unit, called a panel (or profile). The single unit comprising these related tests is often named for the common link among those tests. For example, a liver panel consists of a set of tests that examine liver function, whereas a basic electrolyte and metabolite panel may be called a Chem-7 (referring to a chemistry panel of seven tests). In a patient's hospital chart, these panels are written in the form of a matrix.

Serum Chemistry/Metabolic Panels

Examination of the electrolytes and metabolites in the extracellular fluid is one of the most basic and fundamental assessments done in the ED or ICU. Often this testing takes the form of a standard panel—that is, the basic metabolic panel (Chem-7) **FIGURE 9-5**.

Sodium

Sodium (Na^+) is the major extracellular ion; its serum concentration in a healthy person ranges from 136 to 142 mEq/L (mmol/L). In contrast, for intracellular concentrations of Na^+, the normal range is only 3 to 20 mEq/L. Dramatic changes in a patient's serum sodium level are possible, primarily due to changes in extracellular water concentrations. As a patient becomes depleted of free (solute-free) water, the serum sodium concentration increases; that

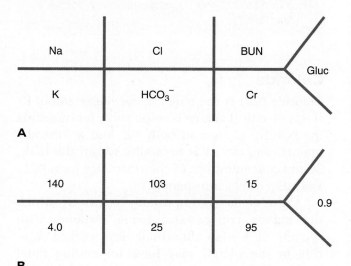

FIGURE 9-5 A. The items measured in a basic metabolic panel, shown in the format in which values are written. **B.** An example of how the values would be written, with each slot representing a particular lab value. These values are for a healthy person.

Abbreviations: BUN, blood urea nitrogen; Cr, creatinine; Gluc, blood glucose level

is, more sodium ions are present per liter of water in the body. The introduction of excess extracellular water (without additional sodium) will, therefore, decrease serum sodium levels by diluting the concentration.

Serum sodium is a convenient marker for a patient's fluid status and one of the key components of the serum osmolality calculation (explained later in this chapter). Unlike with potassium derangements (discussed later), an abnormal sodium level does not manifest as electrocardiographic (ECG) changes. Instead, most signs and symptoms revolve around neurologic sequelae, which stem from changes in osmolality.

Hypernatremia (elevated sodium levels) is not uncommon in the patients seen in the CCT setting. For example, an elevated sodium level may be observed in a patient with a traumatic brain injury as a consequence of treatment at the referring hospital. Hypertonic saline (HTS), mannitol, and diuretics may all be given to such a patient in an effort to reduce cerebral edema. Serum sodium levels in patients with traumatic brain injury, therefore, are often elevated. While no absolute ceiling has been identified, mortality appears to increase when sodium levels exceed 155 mEq/L.

Hyponatremia (an abnormally low level of sodium in the blood) often results from an excess of free water or excessive sodium depletion. It may be seen in patients with endocrine disorders, congestive heart failure, renal failure, or liver disease and in patients undergoing diuretic therapy. Although some debate exists about how rapidly a hyponatremic state should be corrected, slower appears to be better (4 to 6 mEq/L per 24-hour period), to avoid causing subsequent neurologic problems.

Patients with a sodium imbalance (high or low) need to be monitored for intake and output, including oral and IV input. A sodium level of less than 125 mEq/L can result in behavioral changes, confusion, delirium, increased respiratory rate, muscle twitching, increased intracranial pressure, and cardiac abnormalities. Increased sodium levels can cause fluid retention and cardiac abnormalities.

Potassium

Whereas sodium is the major extracellular cation, potassium (K^+) is the major intracellular cation. The extracellular K^+ concentration (as typically measured in blood) is normally 3.5 to 5.0 mEq/L.

Of primary concern is the effect of an elevated K^+ level on cardiac cells, as cardiac arrhythmias tend to occur with hyperkalemia (an abnormally high level of potassium in the blood). If not properly managed, cardiac arrhythmias associated with hyperkalemia pose a high risk of progressing to cardiac arrest and death. Weakness and paralysis are physical findings associated with hyperkalemia. When patients do show ECG changes, the earliest changes, occurring at potassium levels of 5.5 to 6.5 mEq/L, consist of classic peaked T waves and a shortened QT interval. This progresses to lengthening of the PR and QRS intervals, followed by flattened P waves when the potassium level exceeds 7.0 mEq/L. Derangements in other electrolytes (eg, hypocalcemia, hypomagnesemia, and hyponatremia) can exacerbate hyperkalemia. Hyperkalemia can occur in a patient receiving acute care as the result of excessive potassium supplementation, intracellular to extracellular fluid shifts with cellular lysis (seen with crush injuries and tissue necrosis), drug administration (eg, angiotensin-converting enzyme [ACE] inhibitors), metabolic acidosis, and decreased excretion, as might occur in acute renal failure.

CCTPs should be aware that many abnormally high potassium levels seen on lab results are actually erroneous reports. For example, cellular lysis (hemolysis) can cause an elevated potassium level, so if the sample is hemolyzed before its analysis, an incorrect value may be reported. In fact, the most common cause of hyperkalemia diagnosis is lab error, usually involving hemolysis during collection or transportation of the specimen. For this reason, the first consideration when evaluating hyperkalemia is to redraw the specimen, in addition to assessing the patient and checking an ECG for associated changes.

The urgency in correcting hyperkalemia is predicated on the symptoms and cause. Hyperkalemia resulting from massive tissue breakdown (eg, crush injury, tumor lysis syndrome, rhabdomyolysis) can accelerate rapidly and should be treated aggressively. In contrast, chronic hyperkalemia of less than 7.0 mEq/L that is not accompanied by symptoms or ECG changes may not require immediate or aggressive treatment.

Causes of hypokalemia (an abnormally low level of potassium in the blood) include cellular shifts (eg, as the result of insulin administration or hypothermia) and increased excretion of potassium (gastrointestinal [GI] tract or renal losses). Although younger patients may have a higher tolerance for decreased levels of potassium, older patients (especially those taking digitalis preparations) are more likely to have arrhythmias and ECG changes with low K^+ levels.

Low K^+ levels result in muscle pain, hyporeflexia, nausea, vomiting, and orthostatic hypotension. High K^+ levels can cause cardiac abnormalities, particularly atrioventricular and intraventricular blocks. Atrial arrest is likely when the K^+ level reaches 9 mEq/L.

For any patient who has a cardiac history, altered renal function, liver disease, or GI disturbances, or who is receiving insulin, a recent K^+ level should be available for review before transport.

Special Populations

Older patients with decreased potassium levels, especially those taking digitalis preparations, will have cardiac changes. Hyperkalemia can exacerbate digitalis toxicity.

Chloride

Chloride (Cl^-) is the major extracellular anion. Its single electrical charge is responsible for offsetting the positive charges of both Na^+ and K^+, thereby maintaining electrical neutrality within the body. Serum concentrations of chloride range from 96 to 106 mEq/L in healthy people.

Chloride is an important means by which the kidney concentrates urine. Patients with hypochloremia (an abnormally low level of chloride in the blood) may have impending renal dysfunction. Note, however, that patients receiving diuretic therapy may routinely have abnormally low chloride levels. Strangely, patients who experience excess diuresis can also exhibit hyperchloremia (an abnormally high level of chloride in the blood).

In practice, chloride levels mimic sodium levels; that is, when hypernatremia is present, hyperchloremia is often observed as well. Clinically, serum chloride levels help differentiate the various types of metabolic acidosis.

Bicarbonate and Carbon Dioxide

One of the most basic indications of the acid–base status of a patient is the *venous* bicarbonate (HCO_3^-) level. Confusing as it may seem, the carbon dioxide level (CO_2) reported on lab results is not a CO_2 level at all; instead, this test indicates the amount of HCO_3^- in the venous sample. CO_2 and HCO_3^- exist in equilibrium according to the following equation:

$$CO_2 + H_2O \leftrightarrow H_2CO_3 \leftrightarrow H^+ + HCO_3^-$$

Thus, the levels of CO_2 and HCO_3^- in the body are related, although they are actually very different substances.

CO_2 is a gas, so when it is measured, the value should be expressed as a partial pressure. HCO_3^- is an ion; thus, as with the other ions mentioned earlier in this chapter, its measured value is expressed as a concentration. A level below the normal range could indicate metabolic acidosis or respiratory alkalosis, whereas an elevated level could indicate metabolic alkalosis or respiratory acidosis. Therefore, this lab value can be helpful when working to understand the balance between a patient's metabolic and respiratory processes, which produces the current pH of the blood. The normal HCO_3^- value is 21 to 28 mEq/L, and the normal CO_2 value is 22 to 28 mEq/L.

Blood Urea Nitrogen

A product of protein catabolism, urea is related to the amount of protein intake, protein metabolism, and rate of excretion. Urea is considered a useful marker for adequate kidney function because its level in kidney filtrate is often the same as its level in serum. The normal range for blood urea nitrogen (BUN), the test used to measure urea, is 8 to 23 mg/ dL. It is often helpful to interpret BUN values alongside creatinine values, and a BUN to creatinine ratio (BUN:Cr) can sometimes provide helpful indications regarding the cause of acute kidney injury, such as dehydration versus intrarenal disease.

The BUN level tends to increase with age as a consequence of gradually declining renal function; thus, a slightly elevated BUN finding of 28 to 35 mg/dL in older patients is not necessarily a cause for concern. Instead, an elevated BUN level in an older patient should be interpreted in the context of other lab test results and the findings during the patient assessment. Any value of more than 40 mg/dL should be monitored closely.

When patients have high renal output levels, BUN values are a less valid means of assessing kidney health because of the inverse relationship between urine formation and urea reabsorption. Elevated levels of urea occur not only with decreased renal function, but also with consumption of a high-protein diet and in the presence of a high-protein catabolism state (eg, burns, crush injuries).

Occult upper gastrointestinal bleeding may result in an elevated BUN value with a normal creatinine level.

Creatinine

A major storehouse of intramuscular high-energy phosphate, creatine is degraded to creatinine (Cr), a chemical waste product that results from muscle metabolism, at a relatively steady rate by the muscles. Within a particular individual, the rate of Cr production typically varies by only 10% at any particular time. Creatinine is filtered from the blood by the kidneys and, unless reabsorption occurs, is excreted in the urine. Because of its steady rate of production, this by-product of metabolism can be used to assess kidney function: Its clearance by the kidneys is the primary variable that determines its serum concentration under typical conditions. If renal function decreases, serum Cr levels will become elevated (normal range, 0.6 to 1.2 mg/dL).

An abnormal serum Cr level does not pinpoint the exact disease or cause at work, but does indicate some level of decreased renal function. Under certain circumstances, a patient may have an increased Cr level with adequate renal function, such as when the patient has experienced a large amount of muscle damage (owing to protein release from trauma, a process called rhabdomyolysis). Care must be taken when a geriatric patient has a Cr level slightly more than the upper normal value (near 1.5 mg/dL): Owing to the proportionately smaller amount of muscle mass and consequent lower Cr production in older people, a small elevation in the Cr level may reflect greater kidney dysfunction in these individuals than would the same level in a younger patient.

Acute elevation in Cr can sometimes indicate a transient condition from which the patient will fully recover. However, if the cause of the elevated Cr level is not identified and corrected, damage to the kidneys will be permanent. Patients who experience such damage may require dialysis for the rest of their lives or need kidney transplantation.

Creatinine clearance is the most accurate measure of the glomerular filtration rate. The results of a Cr clearance test can be used to determine the most appropriate long-term management of patients with chronic disorders of renal function and to calculate the necessary fluid and electrolyte replacement therapy. Creatinine clearance is calculated by multiplying the concentration of measured urine Cr by the volume of urine during a set time and then dividing this product by the serum concentration of Cr. A single test result does not give a great deal of information, but serial results can be very useful in directing a patient's course of therapy.

Special Populations

Geriatric patients with creatinine levels approaching 1.5 mg/dL warrant careful attention. They may have more kidney dysfunction than might otherwise be suspected, owing to the relatively lower level of creatinine production from the smaller amount of muscle mass present.

Glomerular Filtration Rate

The glomerular filtration rate (GFR) is a measurement of the overall filtration efficiency of all the functioning nephrons. While the exact rate depends on age, sex, and body size, the normal GFR is 90 to 120 mL/min per 1.73 m^2 for both men and women.

Changes in GFR can suggest improvement or decline in kidney function. (But note that GFR declines progressively with age, even in the absence of chronic kidney disease.) Actual measurement of GFR is not possible, however, and its estimation is extremely complex; it is commonly done using blood serum markers in a laboratory analysis. A GFR less than 60 mL/min in any patient suggests renal impairment. Some labs estimate GFRs only when the value is less than 60 mL/min, reporting higher values as simply >60 mL/min.

Glucose

Glucose is the most important carbohydrate in the body, and its quantification is the lab measurement with which CCTPs may be most familiar. Glucose is commonly assessed in the field with a point-of-care testing device, and prehospital care providers often measure the blood glucose level of patients with altered mental status. Concentrations of glucose are normally in the range of 70 to 110 mg/dL (3.9 to 6.1 mmol/L). Maintaining a normal glucose level is an extremely important consideration for CCTPs, because patients may be receiving insulin infusions during transport and may have chronic or acute renal failure, which will affect their blood glucose levels. If a patient is receiving an insulin infusion, a point-of-care glucose test should be done at least hourly, and more often if the patient demonstrates altered mental status or when the CCTP is withholding the infusion for low glucose levels.

Glucose levels that are high (hyperglycemia) or low (hypoglycemia) can lead to coma and death if not properly treated. Hypoglycemia is generally easier to recognize early because of the associated symptoms, such as blurred vision, dizziness, nausea, vomiting, and shakiness. Hypoglycemia can also lead to syncope (loss of consciousness) or seizures, which can result in injuries secondary to falling.

Total Calcium

Calcium is one of the most essential electrolytes found in the body. It is responsible for functions ranging from muscle contraction (including the contraction of cardiac myocytes) to intracellular signal transduction (including the messages sent via neurons). Physiologically, calcium is found in the body in three states: free, chelated, and bound. The largest portion of calcium (47%) is found as a free calcium ion dispersed in the body fluids. Another 43% of calcium in the body is bound to proteins, mostly albumin. Naturally, the amount of calcium bound to proteins depends on the ability of the protein to complex with the calcium ion (Ca^{+2}). Protein binding is a function of the shape of the protein, which in turn is heavily dependent on the surrounding pH. In lower pH states, the amount of calcium bound to proteins decreases, which causes the amount of free calcium to increase. Calcium that is chelated (bound) to other molecules, such as citrate, HCO_3^-, lactate, phosphate, and sulfate, represents only 10% of the calcium in the body.

The sum of all calcium in the body is expressed as the total calcium level (Ca^{+2}_{TOT}). The normal range for Ca^{+2}_{TOT} is 8.5 to 10.2 mg/dL. The Ca^{+2}_{TOT} is increased in elevated parathyroid hormone states, such as hyperparathyroidism and parathyroid-secreting tumors. Low levels of Ca^{+2}_{TOT} are seen with renal insufficiency, hypomagnesemia, and hyperphosphatemia, and in patients who have received a massive blood transfusion or have decreased parathyroid hormone levels.

Ionized Calcium

Only the calcium that is not bound or chelated (ie, free calcium) is physiologically active. In patients whose status is characterized by an altered fraction of bound or chelated calcium, free calcium assessment is warranted. Examples of physiologic states that warrant assessment of ionized calcium include renal failure and nephrotic syndrome (hypoalbuminemia), acid–base derangements (particularly acidosis), and decreases or elevations in chelating compounds (citrate, HCO_3^-, lactate, phosphate, and sulfate). The normal range for ionized calcium is 8.8 to 10.3 mg/dL, which is equivalent to 2.2 to 2.6 mmol/L and 4.4 to 5.2 mEq/L.

Low levels of ionized calcium can result in decreased cardiac output and hypotension and are sometimes associated with arrhythmias. They are also often seen in patients with prolonged cardiac arrest, although calcium administration has not been shown to offer survival benefits to these patients. Use of calcium may be warranted in patients with hyperkalemia, hypocalcemia, or calcium channel blocker overdose. Patients with these conditions are sometimes transported with a magnesium sulfate drip to mitigate the risk of further cardiac arrhythmias or cardiac arrest.

Magnesium

Magnesium (Mg) levels can be affected by disruptions of several body systems, in particular the GI and endocrine systems. The normal serum magnesium level is 1.3 to 2.1 mEq/L. High Mg levels are rarely encountered. When they do occur, generally the causes are renal defects, severe dehydration, overadministration of Mg, untreated diabetic coma, and aspiration of sea water. Low Mg levels are more

commonly seen—for example, in conjunction with GI distress, vomiting and diarrhea, hepatic cirrhosis, and pancreatitis.

Phosphate

Phosphate is an ion in the blood that contains the mineral phosphorus. The blood's phosphate level is primarily regulated by the parathyroid endocrine system and the kidneys. Phosphate plays an important role in bone and dental health.

Normal serum phosphate levels are typically defined as 2.3 to 4.7 mg/dL. Hyperphosphatemia (high phosphate levels) can be caused by hypoparathyroidism and kidney failure, among other diseases, and can lead to calcium disorders and muscle spasms. Hypophosphatemia (low phosphate levels) can be caused by nutritional disorders and hyperparathyroidism, among other diseases, and can lead to altered mental status, seizures, or osteopenia.

Blood Components

FIGURE 9-6 shows a schematic of the abbreviated notation for a complete blood count (CBC) test. This schematic is intended to be used for quick reference to pertinent values. Classically, the CBC

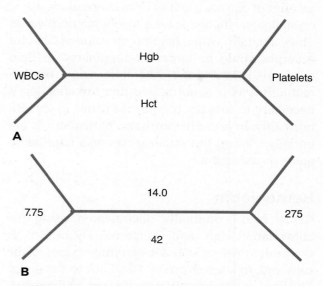

FIGURE 9-6 Complete blood count schematic (abbreviated notation). **A.** The format in which values are written. **B.** An example of values for a healthy person.

Abbreviations: Hct, hematocrit; Hgb, hemoglobin; WBCs, white blood cells test includes counts of red blood cells (RBCs), white blood cells, and platelets, as well as hematocrit and hemoglobin levels. It may also include other values that lie outside the scope of this text, many of which describe various attributes of RBCs that can be used to determine the cause of anemia (an abnormally low RBC count). If one of these values is abnormal, the CCTP would be expected to consult the patient's complete medical record for more information on the patient's condition.

Hematocrit

Hematocrit, commonly documented using the abbreviation Hct, is the percentage of formed elements (ie, cells) in a venous blood sample. A hematocrit value of 45% indicates that 45% of the sample consists of cells or cellular debris, and the other 55% consists of plasma. The normal range for hematocrit is 41% to 50%.

This test's specificity depends on the nature of the relationship between the blood's formed elements and the plasma. With an acutely ill patient, the health care provider is often concerned with a low hematocrit value. A low level of formed elements (which are predominantly RBCs) can indicate decreased capacity of the blood to deliver oxygen to the tissues. A patient who has an excess amount of plasma (such as from overzealous use of crystalloids) will also have a low hematocrit value. Thus, a patient with a hematocrit value of 22%, for example, could be either exsanguinated or fluid overloaded **FIGURE 9-7**. Therefore, when the hematocrit level is abnormal, further investigation is necessary to identify the precise cause of the abnormality. In acute hemorrhage, hematocrit is not initially relevant but rather serves as a baseline to guide resuscitation.

Hemoglobin

Hemoglobin, commonly documented using the abbreviation Hgb (and sometimes Hg or Hb), is the protein responsible for carrying oxygen to the cells and, to a lesser extent, CO_2 back to the lungs. The level of hemoglobin varies by sex, with normal values falling in the range of 135 to 175 g/L (14.0 to 17.5 g/dL) for males and 120 to 160 g/L (12.0 to 16.0 g/dL) for females. Elevated levels are seen in people with hemoconcentration (decreased fluid in the blood, which means that concentrations of other

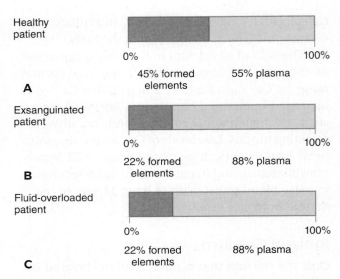

Healthy patient

0%   100%

45% formed elements   55% plasma

A

Exsanguinated patient

0%   100%

22% formed elements   88% plasma

B

Fluid-overloaded patient

0%   100%

22% formed elements   88% plasma

C

FIGURE 9-7 Examples of hematocrit levels and (B and C) potential causes. **A.** Healthy patient. **B.** Exsanguinated patient. **C.** Fluid-overloaded patient.

© Jones & Bartlett Learning.

blood components increase), which can result from dehydration, burns, or excessive vomiting. Of greater concern are low hemoglobin levels, which are typical of most types of anemia (microcytic, normocytic, and macrocytic). Similar to hematocrit, hemoglobin must be interpreted within the context of a patient's hemodynamic stability in the setting of acute hemorrhage; the hemoglobin level may not drop in the setting of hemorrhagic shock until intravascular volume is expanded, either endogenously or exogenously.

Red Blood Cell Count

The red blood cell (RBC) count is the number of erythrocytes (RBCs) per microliter of blood. The normal range for the RBC count is 3.9 to $5.5 \times 10^6/\mu L$. Although the presence of an abnormal number of RBCs does not necessarily equate to the presence of disease, the RBC counts can be elevated with hemoconcentration. Patients with elevated white blood cell counts may have an erroneously high RBC count owing to analysis errors. As would be expected, low RBC counts are seen in all types of anemia.

Along with RBC count, a reticulocyte count may be provided on the CBC report. Reticulocytes are immature RBCs. A high reticulocyte count can indicate that erythropoiesis, the process that produces new RBCs, is actively occurring. The RBC and reticulocyte counts have little clinical utility for the CCTP.

White Blood Cell Count

The white blood cell (WBC) count is a measure of the total number of leukocytes (WBCs) per microliter of blood. An increased number of WBCs, referred to as leukocytosis, can be a healthy response, demonstrating the body's response to a detected threat, such as an infection. An ordinary WBC count does not differentiate among the various types of leukocytes in the sample; a CBC with differential can be performed to provide a detailed summary of the components that contribute to the WBC count (see the following section). The normal range for WBC counts is between 4,500/μL and 11,000/μL.

Low levels of WBCs are seen in patients with certain anemias (eg, aplastic anemia) and vitamin deficiencies, and in patients receiving certain therapies (eg, chemotherapy). Although it might seem counterintuitive, low levels are also seen in sepsis: WBCs are mobilized to fight the infection and are ultimately destroyed at a rate that exceeds their production. Leukocytosis is seen not only with inflammation or infection, but also in certain malignancies (leukemia and lymphoma) and vascular conditions (pulmonary embolism, acute myocardial infarction [AMI], and DVT), with steroid administration, and with the stress of trauma.

White Blood Cell Count Differential

A CBC with differential, also called a WBC differential, is an expanded panel of lab tests that includes counts of specific types of WBCs in the blood, such as neutrophils, lymphocytes, monocytes, eosinophils, and basophils. These values may be expressed as absolute counts, percentages of all WBCs, or both. In a healthy immune response, the nature of the stimulus for the leukocytosis can often be indicated by the differential. For example, a leukocytosis predominated by neutrophils is often associated with bacterial—rather than viral—infection, whereas relatively elevated lymphocyte counts are typically associated with viral infection. Other causes of elevated WBC components beyond infection include hematologic malignancy, autoimmune conditions, medication effects, and other inflammatory conditions. For example, corticosteroid therapy can cause elevated neutrophil counts in the absence of any infection or other potential cause.

Neutropenia is an abnormally low neutrophil count. Neutropenia has various causes, with the most common one being chemotherapy or radiation therapy in patients with cancer. Neutrophils are a key aspect of the immune system's defense against bacterial infection, so bacterial infection in a neutropenic patient is considered a life-threatening emergency. (Neutropenic fever refers to a fever in a patient with neutropenia, which is also considered a medical emergency.)

The WBC differential may also include a band cell count. Band cells (also called immature granulocytes) are precursors to granulocytes, a type of WBC that includes neutrophils. An elevated band cell count (ie, bandemia) is sometimes referred to as a "left shift" associated with granulopoiesis, the process by which new granulocytes are created. It is typically interpreted as a sign of acute inflammatory response, most commonly in the setting of an active infection.

Platelet Count

Maintenance of hemostasis within the body relies on the presence of adequate numbers of functional platelets coupled with sufficient clotting factors. The platelet count, often documented using the abbreviation Plt, is useful in assessing the number of circulating platelets in a patient. The normal range for a whole blood sample is 150 to $350 \times 10^3/\mu L$. Elevated levels of platelets are seen in patients with certain myeloproliferative disorders (diseases in which the bone marrow produces too many RBCs, WBCs, or platelets; examples include polycythemia and chronic myelogenous leukemia), most notably after severe bleeding or following splenectomy. Decreased platelet counts may occur when disease causes decreased production of these cells in the bone marrow. Often thrombocytopenia—an abnormally low level of platelets—is associated with splenomegaly, disseminated intravascular coagulation (DIC), or high levels of circulating platelet antibodies (such as after massive transfusions).

Two thrombocytopenic conditions often seen in critical care patients are heparin-induced thrombocytopenia (HIT) and idiopathic thrombocytopenic purpura (ITP). HIT is an antibody response to a complex formed by platelet factor 4 (PF4) and heparin; it results in platelet activation, leading to significant and sometimes life-threatening thromboses. HIT occurs in 5% of patients exposed to heparin, regardless of the route or dose used, and is treated by rapidly discontinuing all heparin products. ITP is an antibody reaction against platelet antigens and can be difficult to diagnose. In adults, it tends to be a chronic condition, but it may also be present in critically ill patients being treated for other conditions.

Proteins

Total Protein

One of the most basic protein tests, total protein, examines the total quantity of protein in a blood sample. This quantity consists of mostly albumin and immunoglobulins. The normal range for total protein in a serum sample is 6.0 to 8.0 g/dL, and variations are almost always due to fluctuations in serum albumin levels. As a consequence, most clinicians focus on albumin levels. While a commonly performed lab test, total protein has no clinical relevance to the CCTP.

Albumin

By far the most common protein in the body is albumin. Albumin serves many functions: It acts as a transport protein (for free fatty acids, bilirubin, hormones, and drugs), functions as a free-radical scavenger, and serves as the main source (70%) of protein-generated oncotic pressure. This osmotic pressure enables colloids to move from one side of the cell membrane to the other as needed and contributes to the maintenance of adequate intravascular volume. The normal range for albumin is 3.5 to 5.0 g/dL.

A low level of albumin may be due to increased catabolism of the protein (as seen in malnutrition), decreased production, or edema in the spaces between the cells in the tissue. Decreased production is seen in patients who have liver damage or other liver disease. Hypoalbuminemia (an abnormally low level of albumin) from increased interstitial sequestration can occur in high-vascular-permeability states and leads to diseases such as acute respiratory distress syndrome. High levels of albumin generally indicate dehydration; that is, they are not pathologic.

Lactate

Adequate indicators of a patient's end-organ perfusion and oxygenation that can serve as a gold standard for measuring perfusion continue to be sought. One of the best and most readily available standard tests used to assess a patient's end-organ perfusion and oxygenation is the venous lactate level. Once tissue perfusion and oxygen levels in the cells and tissues decrease too much, cells switch to anaerobic metabolism. This mechanism allows the cells to continue to use glucose, albeit less efficiently than if perfusion and oxygenation were adequate. This inefficient metabolic process produces lactic acid as a by-product, which may be measured in the form of serum lactate. Perfusion and oxygenation of the cells and tissues of the body's end organs are considered inadequate if the serum lactate level in the blood is greater than 2 mmol/L (normal range, 0.5 to 1.5 mmol/L).

Lactate levels are a global indicator of perfusion and oxygenation; that is, they do not indicate exactly which tissues are inadequately perfused or oxygenated. Apart from being nonspecific, lactate levels are relatively slow to respond to adequate resuscitation with fluid and oxygen, generally improving only over the course of several hours. Once tissue perfusion and oxygenation return to normal, anaerobic metabolism ceases and lactate is no longer produced. The remaining lactate is then converted into nontoxic metabolic by-products in the liver and kidney and, eventually, to CO_2 and water. Serial lactate measurements can suggest trends in end-organ perfusion, whereas a single lactate value simply provides a snapshot of the current state.

Lactate Dehydrogenase

In the absence of a functioning citric acid cycle, pyruvate (the end product of glycolysis) is metabolized to lactate. (The citric acid cycle is discussed in Chapter 10, *Resuscitation, Shock, and Blood Products.*) The enzyme that catalyzes this reaction is lactate dehydrogenase (LDH). As this enzyme is found in almost all tissues of the body, the LDH level is not sensitive or specific for any disease. The normal range of LDH is 100 to 200 U/L.

The usefulness of the LDH measurement in the clinical setting comes from analysis of LDH's isoenzyme forms (LD_1 to LD_5). Various organs, tissues, and cells differ in terms of the amount of each isoenzyme found within them. For example, LD_1 is found largely in the heart, kidneys, and RBCs. Other tissues, such as skeletal muscle and the liver, contain relatively high amounts of LD_5.

The LDH value was once considered a useful aid in the diagnosis of AMI but has been replaced in routine use by troponin analysis (discussed later in this chapter). LDH can also be helpful in diagnosing *Pneumocystis jirovecii* pneumonia and determining the severity of pancreatitis. In addition, LDH levels are followed in patients with implanted ventricular assist devices, in whom they can provide an early warning of pump thrombosis.

Creatine Kinase

Creatine kinase (CK) is found in muscle, liver, lung, GI, brain, kidney, and spleen tissues. If any of these tissue cells become damaged, CK is released into the vascular space. Most often, CK levels are used to diagnose and monitor response to treatment of rhabdomyolysis. This condition can result from significant exertion (eg, running a marathon), crush or burn injuries, seizures, or prolonged unconsciousness. Though this application is less common today since the advent of troponin analysis, CK has also been used as a less specific marker for myocardial infarction. With myocardial damage, CK levels rise within 4 to 8 hours, peak within 12 to 24 hours, and return to normal within 2 to 4 days. The normal range for the total CK level is 40 to 150 U/L.

The MB fraction of CK, or CK-MB, refers primarily to CK in the heart muscle. The normal range for the CK-MB level is 0 to 7 ng/mL. When this level is less than 10 ng/mL, a myocardial event is unlikely. Results ranging between 10 and 12 ng/mL are not conclusive, and additional workup and serial lab tests are required in such cases. A level of more than 12 ng/mL is indicative of a myocardial event.

Troponin

Troponin is a key protein involved in muscle contraction. This protein has three subunits: T, C, and I. The I subunit has three separate isoforms, one of which is found only in cardiac muscle. Troponin is expressed in the serum *only after* cellular necrosis releases the respective cellular contents. Thus, measurement of the troponin levels offers some advantage over measurement of the CK and LDH levels because CK and LDH are normally present in the serum.

Normal values for the various troponins depend on the method used to do the test, but, in general, the normal ranges are 0 to 0.4 ng/mL for troponin I (often abbreviated cTnI) and 0 to 0.1 ng/mL for troponin T. Elevations in cTnI following myocardial injury are detectable in a serum sample after 4 hours; tests for cTnI are 97% sensitive and 95% specific at 6 hours after an AMI. Peak levels are expressed 8 to 12 hours post injury, but the protein may still be detected 5 to 7 days later. Not only is the cTnI level useful in detecting AMI, but it has also been shown to be predictive of adverse outcomes in patients with severe unstable angina. Newer high-sensitivity cardiac troponin T (hs-cTnT) tests have demonstrated the ability to reliably rule out AMI within even shorter time intervals from the onset of symptoms.

B-Type Natriuretic Peptide

The **B-type natriuretic peptide (BNP)** is released by the ventricles in response to higher filling pressures. The normal value for BNP is less than 167 pg/mL. A high level can be indicative of abnormal ventricular function or heart failure if it is outside the expected range.

Besides evaluating response to heart failure therapies, BNP is used to assess the probability of heart failure in patients presenting with dyspnea. In this application, values greater than 400 pg/mL strongly correlate with heart failure as the cause of dyspnea, whereas values less than 100 pg/mL negatively predict heart failure as a cause of dyspnea. The middle range of 100 to 400 pg/mL has very poor sensitivity and specificity for predicting or excluding heart failure. Additionally, numerous other conditions, such as renal insufficiency, tend to affect BNP values. BNP values are typically most informative when trended over time to assess improvement or exacerbation of heart failure.

Inflammatory Markers

Procalcitonin

Procalcitonin (PCT) is a peptide precursor of calcitonin. Evidence suggests that serum PCT levels rise significantly in the setting of an inflammatory response to a serious bacterial infection such as sepsis. While PCT levels have not yet been integrated into routine evaluation of infection, they are increasingly being used to identify serious bacterial infection in young children and to distinguish bacterial from viral infection when deciding whether to prescribe antibiotics. Reference ranges vary by context, but a typical normal PCT threshold is less than 0.5 µg/L.

C-Reactive Protein

C-reactive protein (CRP) is an acute-phase protein produced by the liver. CRP levels rise quickly in the context of inflammation due to its multiple roles in inflammatory processes. Testing CRP is a useful but nonspecific means to evaluate for the presence of an inflammatory response, including those triggered by infection, autoimmune processes, or tissue damage. Values less than 10 mg/L are typically considered normal.

Erythrocyte Sedimentation Rate

The erythrocyte sedimentation rate (ESR), sometimes abbreviated as "sed rate," is the rate at which RBCs settle at the bottom of a tube containing a blood sample. ESR values rise in the context of an inflammatory response, leading to the use of this test as a marker of the acute-phase reaction, similar to CRP. However, ESR tends to be less specific than CRP due to multiple other factors that can lead to elevated levels. Evidence suggests that ESR threshold values should vary by context, but in general normal is defined as less than 20 mm/h in females and less than 15 mm/h in males, with higher thresholds in older populations.

Liver Function Tests

Although not truly tests of liver function, elevated liver function test (LFT) results suggest liver damage or injury. LFTs measure enzymes that normally appear, to some extent, in liver cells. When the liver is damaged, these enzymes often spill out into the vasculature. LFTs include aspartate aminotransferase, alanine aminotransferase, total bilirubin, direct bilirubin, and alkaline phosphatase.

Aspartate Aminotransferase

Found in large amounts in the liver, the intracellular enzyme aspartate aminotransferase (AST), previously called serum glutamic-oxaloacetic transaminase (SGOT), is also found in skeletal muscle, the brain, RBCs, and the heart. Damage to any of these cells causes them to release their contents, which can then be detected in a blood sample. Low levels of AST are not of serious consequence, considering that the normal range for this enzyme is 10 to 30 U/L. Elevated levels are seen in liver damage, especially with acute conditions such as acute hepatitis or biliary tract obstruction. Chronic liver damage (due to alcoholic cirrhosis, hepatitis, and liver cancer) also produces elevation of the AST level, although the alanine aminotransferase (ALT) level (described in the next section) is affected more dramatically. Acute hepatitis is marked by significant elevations in AST and ALT, whereas AST and ALT may or may not remain elevated in patients with advanced cirrhosis. Elevations in AST may occur in a setting of right heart failure, hypoxia (global or end-organ), or extensive trauma.

Alanine Aminotransferase

Like its counterpart AST, ALT, previously called serum glutamic-pyruvic transaminase (SGPT), is found in large amounts in the liver, kidney, skeletal muscle, and heart. Similar to the findings with AST, the normal range for ALT is 10 to 40 U/L, with low levels considered to be of no consequence. The causes of an elevated ALT level mirror the causes of an elevated AST level, with the exception that the ALT level is higher than the AST level in acute processes and lower than the AST level in chronic processes. The ALT test is considered slightly more specific than the AST test for hepatic injury because fewer organs have ALT than have AST. The ratio of AST to ALT is an important diagnostic tool and is explained further in the calculation section in this chapter.

Although AST and ALT are found in the heart, neither AST nor ALT measurement is valid for diagnosing myocardial infarction. Elevated levels of ALT may be prolonged because this enzyme has a long half-life (between 36 and 60 hours). As a consequence, levels may appear elevated even after resolution of the hepatic dysfunction.

Total Bilirubin

All RBCs are metabolized eventually, with bilirubin being one of the by-products of their breakdown. The initial by-product is unconjugated and, therefore, not water soluble (indirect bilirubin). When bilirubin is conjugated in the liver, it becomes direct bilirubin, which is ultimately excreted in the bile. The normal range for the total bilirubin level is 0.3 to 1.2 mg/dL. The total bilirubin level (direct plus indirect) is often elevated in patients with liver disease; thus, this level is often used as a measure of liver health. Other causes of elevated levels of total bilirubin include biliary tract obstruction and RBC hemolysis.

Direct Bilirubin

In the medical laboratory, bilirubin may be fractionated to determine the respective levels of unconjugated (indirect) and conjugated (direct) bilirubin. Although such tests are sometimes unreliable, the cause of elevated total bilirubin levels may often be derived from the fractionated levels. The indirect bilirubin fraction is typically elevated in conditions characterized by massive hemolysis, such as massive blood transfusions or blood transfusion reactions. If only the direct or indirect bilirubin level is reported, the other value may be obtained by subtracting the reported level from the total bilirubin level. The normal values for direct and indirect bilirubin are 0.1 to 0.3 mg/dL and 0.2 to 0.9 mg/dL, respectively.

Alkaline Phosphatase

Alkaline phosphatase is found in almost all body tissues and is manufactured by the bone, liver, intestine, and placenta. It is essential for proper digestion and absorption of nutrients through the mucous membranes of the GI tract. The measurement of alkaline phosphatase is clinically useful for testing liver function and, in particular, for diagnosing a common bile duct obstruction. The normal range is 30 to 120 U/L.

Elevated LFT values are often described as having either a hepatocellular pattern or a cholestatic pattern. Transaminitis—that is, elevated AST and/ or ALT levels—typically indicates hepatocellular damage, such as from viral or alcoholic hepatitis. In contrast, a cholestatic pattern, indicated by elevated alkaline phosphatase and bilirubin levels, suggests biliary obstruction, such as from gallstones or a mass. Both patterns can be present simultaneously, but relatively greater disturbances in one pattern over the other can suggest the primary etiology.

Amylase

A key enzyme used by the body to metabolize carbohydrates, amylase is produced by the salivary glands and the pancreas. Tissues such as the ovaries, small and large bowels, and skeletal muscle also produce small amounts of amylase. The normal range for amylase is 27 to 131 U/L. Tests for amylase are used to assess for pancreatic insufficiency or damage: Levels of this enzyme are elevated not only with pancreatic disease (such as pancreatitis, pancreatic cancer, and diabetic ketoacidosis), but also with bile duct obstructions and head trauma. A sign of pancreatic insufficiency, low amylase levels are seen in people with cystic fibrosis.

Lipase

The pancreatic enzyme lipase metabolizes lipids. Generally considered more specific than amylase for identifying pancreatic disease, lipase is also produced by the liver, intestine, and stomach. The normal range for lipase is 31 to 186 U/L. In acute pancreatitis, the levels of lipase and amylase are elevated, but the lipase level stays elevated longer. Although measurements of lipase levels have poor sensitivity in terms of identifying chronic pancreatitis and pancreatic cancer, elevated levels are often seen with both diseases. Like amylase levels, lipase levels are often elevated in patients with bile duct obstruction or biliary disease.

Coagulation

Assessment of the coagulation system involves looking at the intrinsic and extrinsic pathways of the coagulation cascade, which are discussed in more detail in Chapter 10, *Resuscitation, Shock, and Blood Products*. The intrinsic pathway (initiated within the body, such as by platelet damage) begins with the activation of factor XII and then factors XI and IX; it ultimately results in the activation of factor X, which initiates the common pathway of coagulation. The extrinsic pathway (initiated outside the body, following tissue injury) begins with tissue factor and factor VII; it also leads to activation of factor X and, in turn, initiates the common pathway of coagulation. Fibrin is eventually produced, resulting in a clot.

Coagulation studies can be used to assess the body's ability to form and prevent clots. This information can be very helpful when abnormal clotting is suspected, in the setting of hemorrhage, or in the preoperative setting. The enzymes involved in coagulation are synthesized in the liver. Some clinicians consider assessments of these enzymes to be the true liver function tests because they are products of the liver, rather than merely being markers of liver cell damage. Many coagulation assessments are functions of time and, therefore, are reported in units of seconds.

Prothrombin Time

A key step in coagulation is the creation of thrombin from prothrombin by prothrombin activator, which is a collection of activated substances. The prothrombin time (PT) is the rate of prothrombin's conversion to thrombin in a blood sample, and it represents the function of the extrinsic pathway. The normal range is 10 to 13 seconds. The PT may be increased in liver disease or with warfarin therapy, and decreased with low levels of vitamin K, in DIC, and after massive transfusions. This measurement is also used to assess for correct therapeutic effect of warfarin.

Activated Partial Thromboplastin Time

The activated partial thromboplastin time (aPTT) indicates the health of the intrinsic and common pathways of the coagulation system. Genetic diseases, such as hemophilia A, hemophilia B, and von Willebrand disease, may cause elevated aPTT levels. The aPTT is often used to assess for DIC, in which the level is often grossly elevated relative to the normal range of 25 to 40 seconds. Heparin therapy also results in elevated aPTT. Some patients being moved by interfacility transport may be receiving heparin therapy or anticoagulant prophylaxis. The aPTT is used to assess for the correct therapeutic effect of heparin.

International Normalized Ratio

Owing to lack of standardization in measuring the PT within different laboratories (especially internationally), a normalizing index has been created based on the international sensitivity index. The normal range for the international normalized ratio (INR) is 0.9 to 1.3. Increased ratios are seen in the same diseases in which PT is increased and in persons receiving anticoagulants.

The typical anticoagulation target for the INR depends on the indication and the type of anticoagulant used. For atrial fibrillation and DVT, and after pulmonary embolus, a usual INR target is 2.0 to 3.0. For mechanical heart valves and some circulatory support devices, a target of 2.5 to 3.5 may be preferred. An INR greater than 5 with bleeding generally requires treatment.

Factor Xa

Factor Xa levels, also known as anti-Xa levels, are most commonly used to inform dosing of anticoagulation therapy. In particular, heparin and low-molecular-weight heparin primarily act by inactivating thrombin and factor Xa, so the factor Xa assay can be used to measure the activity of these medications. By trending factor Xa levels over time, providers can adjust the dosing of anticoagulation therapy to maintain therapeutic levels in the blood, thereby optimizing the benefit (ie, reduce clotting) and limiting the risk (ie, reduce bleeding).

Thromboelastography

Thromboelastography (TEG) is a test used to describe the global viscoelastic properties of a sample of whole blood. It can provide a real-time assessment of clot formation by quantifying the interaction of platelets and the coagulation cascade. TEG typically generates five measures of interest based on the timing of landmark stages in clot formation and degradation, as well as attributes of a waveform. These measures can provide both quantitative and rapid qualitative information.

- **Reaction time (R time).** R time extends from the initiation of the test until the first detection of clot formation. Normal values typically range from 4 to 8 minutes. The R time can be used to assess clotting factor function.
- **Clot formation time (K time).** K time is the duration from initial clot formation (where R time is t = 0) until a standardized level of clot strength is achieved. Normal values typically range from 1 to 4 minutes. The K time can be used to assess fibrinogen and platelet count.
- **Alpha (α) angle.** The α angle is measured between the baseline and the initial slope of the waveform. Normal values typically range from 47° to 74°. The alpha angle can be used in conjunction with the K time to assess fibrinogen and platelet count.
- **Maximum amplitude (MA).** MA is the maximum amplitude of the waveform. Normal values typically range from 55 to 73 mm. MA value can be used to assess platelet function.

- **Lysis time (LY30).** LY30 is the percentage decrease in amplitude 30 minutes after achieving MA. Normal values typically range from 0% to 8%. LY30 can be used to assess fibrinolysis.

Finally, a G value can be calculated to provide an overall assessment of clot strength, which depends on the health of the entire coagulation cascade. Normal values typically range from 5.3-12.4 dynes/cm^2.

Some of the pathologic conditions described by TEG are shown in **FIGURE 9-8**.

D-Dimer

The D-dimer test was introduced earlier as an example of specificity and sensitivity. D-Dimer is a fibrin degradation product that can be detected in the blood and serves as an indicator of fibrinolysis. The D-dimer test is typically used to assess the presence of clotting when a hypercoagulability state is suspected, meaning both clot formation and clot degradation exist, such as in the diagnosis of DVT. A typical reference level is less than 500 ng/mL, but evidence suggests that higher thresholds are appropriate with increasing age. Given the D-dimer test's profile as highly sensitive but less specific, it is often used as an initial screening test for the diagnosis of DVT or pulmonary embolism within relevant decision tools and practice guidelines (eg, Wells criteria, PERC [pulmonary embolism rule out criteria] rule).

Osmolality

The blood contains numerous components that contribute to its tendency to give or extract free water when blood is placed near a semipermeable membrane. As noted in the chemistry review section, this tendency is commonly called osmolarity, although it is measured as osmolality in clinical medicine. Physiologically, the normal range for osmolality is 275 to 295 mOsm/kg. Although this value was used in the past to assess fluid volume status, the most common current application of serum osmolality is to titrate hyperosmolar infusions (such as mannitol) used in patients with elevated intracranial pressure.

Ethanol

Laboratory analysis may have not only patient care implications, but also legal ramifications. For example, ethanol (also called ethyl alcohol [EtOH]) is not a normal physiologic product in the body; therefore, the ethanol value reported on lab tests if the

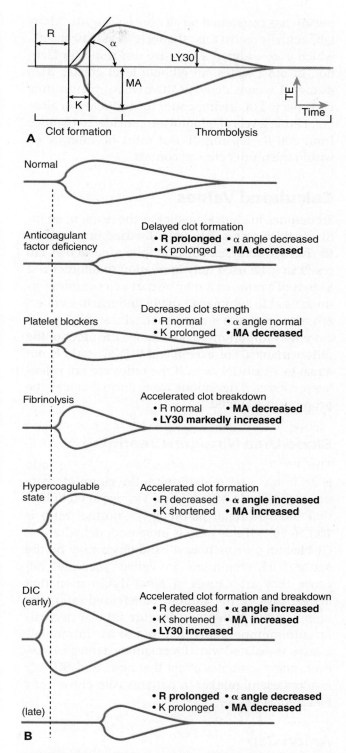

FIGURE 9-8 Visual representation of thromboelastography. **A.** General principle. **B.** Specific pathologic findings. (These images are exaggerated for emphasis.)

Abbreviations: DIC, disseminated intravascular coagulation; K, clot formation time; LY30, lysis time; MA, maximum amplitude; R, reaction time; TE, thromboelastic efficiency

person has consumed no alcohol is 0 mg/dL. Many labs actually report this ethanol level as <10 mg/dL, which is considered a negative test result for alcohol. In most states, an ethanol level greater than 80 mg/dL is considered positive when an individual is suspected of driving under the influence of alcohol. Lethal levels of ethanol are considered to range from 300 to 400 mg/dL but must be interpreted within the proper clinical context.

Calculated Values

Sometimes in clinical medicine, the result of an individual lab test is subsequently used in a formula for further analysis. For example, a particular lab result may be used only in relation to another test as part of a ratio, or it may be part of a complex formula used to summarize many findings in a coherent manner. From a mathematical standpoint, it is extremely important to not change the order of the ratio variables. For example, a BUN:Cr ratio is not equal to a Cr:BUN ratio. If the ratios are not calculated correctly, deviations from normal cannot be properly interpreted.

Blood Urea Nitrogen:Creatinine

The blood urea nitrogen:creatinine (BUN:Cr) ratio is an index used to determine the cause of acute increased levels of BUN and Cr, two metabolites that indicate renal pathology. A normal ratio is 10:1 to 20:1. If this ratio is increased, dehydration, GI bleeding, or increased catabolism may be the cause. Such conditions are called "prerenal" because they are causes of renal dysfunction that are extrinsic to the kidney. A decreased ratio may be present in patients with acute tubular necrosis or autoimmune injury, referred to as "intrarenal" causes associated with direct kidney damage. However, many variables affect this ratio, and BUN:Cr is a less useful marker in patients with chronically elevated values.

Anion Gap

Disturbances in the overall electrical or acid–base balance of the body result from disease and can result in further deterioration in a patient's condition. The primary pathology is usually related to increased production or intake of physiologically active substances, or to respiratory or kidney problems that interfere with their clearance. The major contributors to the overall electrical charge are Na^+, Cl^-, and HCO_3^-. Their relationship, called the anion gap (AG), is portrayed in the following equation:

$$\text{Anion gap} = Na^+ - (Cl^- + HCO_3^-)$$

The normal range for the AG is 8 to 12 mEq/L. An increased AG indicates that unmeasured anions (such as in lactic acid) are present.

One example where the AG can help guide treatment is with states of acidosis such as diabetic ketoacidosis (DKA). As the acidosis progresses, the AG will trend up. As the acidosis is treated and corrected, the AG will trend down. In patients with DKA, when the AG returns to normal levels, it may be interpreted as signaling resolution of the acidotic state.

Blood Gases

A typical arterial blood gas (ABG) panel assesses a patient's acid–base status (pH) based on CO_2 tension ($Paco_2$), HCO_3^-, and base excess (BE). Measures of the patient's oxygen status, oxygen tension (partial pressure of oxygen [Pao_2]), and oxygen saturation (Sao_2) are also provided as part of the ABG panel. There are many reasons for assessing a patient's blood gas parameters, and any patient in the intensive care unit is likely to meet at least one of these criteria.

Venous blood gas (VBG) analysis can be performed as an alternative to the ABG panel, though certain parameters require different reference ranges or are altogether unhelpful when analyzed in venous rather than arterial blood. For simplicity, our discussion of acid–base status focuses on ABG analysis.

Acid–Base Status

The acid–base balance reflects how well the body's respiratory and metabolic systems are functioning. If they are working properly and in harmony, then there is a balance. When they are not, acidosis or alkalosis can occur. Importantly, abnormal values of CO_2 and HCO_3^- can represent primary disturbances or secondary compensatory processes in response to other stimuli; therefore, these values must be interpreted in conjunction with the pH and, of course, within the clinical context.

Hydrogen Ion Concentration

A direct measure of the acid–base status of the patient, hydrogen ion (H^+) concentration, more commonly referred to as pH, quantifies the amount of unbuffered H^+ present. Physiologic pH is related to the amount of CO_2 and the amount of HCO_3^-. An increase in the Pco_2 will result in a smaller fraction component, which translates into a lower pH (acidic). Conversely, an increase in the HCO_3^- will cause a larger fraction component and, therefore, will result in an increased pH (alkaline). The inverse of each of these disturbances will result in the respective opposite effect on the pH. In other words, a decrease in Pco_2 will increase pH, while a decrease in HCO_3^- will decrease pH. Based on the other components of the blood gas panel, the pH derangement (acidosis or alkalosis) can be classified as metabolic or respiratory, respectively.

The normal range for the arterial pH is 7.35 to 7.45; the normal range for the venous pH is slightly lower, 7.31 to 7.41. The body can handle minor variations in pH relatively well. By contrast, once deviations in pH become extreme—for example, 7.0 or less, or 7.6 or more (arterial)—normal physiologic reactions may be drastically affected. With large derangements in serum pH, many proteins and enzymes cease to carry out their normal functions, and vasopressors are inactivated. For example, in patients with severe acidosis, epinephrine is rendered physiologically inactive. Few body systems or enzymes function at extremely low pH levels; a pH of 6.888 is considered to be generally incompatible with survival.

Partial Pressure of CO_2

The natural by-product of cellular respiration, CO_2 is transported back to the lungs by a number of mechanisms. CO_2 exists in the blood as a soluble gas, whose presence is measured as a partial pressure—that is, the partial pressure of CO_2 ($Paco_2$). Because alterations in respiratory function substantially affect the $Paco_2$, this parameter is considered the respiratory component of the blood gas analysis. If the $Paco_2$ is above or below the normal range of 35 to 45 mm Hg, a respiratory derangement is present. Hypercapnia (high $Paco_2$) generally indicates that the patient is experiencing hypoventilation (low minute ventilation), whereas hypocapnia (low $Paco_2$) generally signals the presence of hyperventilation (high minute ventilation). This derangement may be primary (ie, respiratory acidosis or alkalosis) or secondary (ie, compensated metabolic acidosis or alkalosis).

Bicarbonate

In the blood gas panel, whereas $Paco_2$ represents the respiratory component, as noted earlier, HCO_3^- represents the metabolic component. If there is a metabolic aspect to an acidosis- or alkalosis-related condition, a corresponding derangement in HCO_3^- will be seen: The level of this ion will be decreased in metabolic acidosis and increased in metabolic alkalosis. Physiologic alterations in HCO_3^- concentration can also compensate for chronic primary respiratory disturbances.

The normal HCO_3^- level is 22 to 26 mEq/L. The administration of intravenous HCO_3^- to treat metabolic acidosis is controversial.

Base Excess

Base excess (BE) is a measurement of metabolic derangement that is included as part of the ABG panel. Base excess is also known as base deficit (BD) because this value can be either a positive number (excess) or a negative number (deficit). Healthy people do not have an appreciable BE. The BE is measured in units of mEq/L and has a normal range of −2 to +3. If there is an excess amount of acid or a lack of base, the BE is negative. Conversely, if there is an abnormally small amount of acid or an excess amount of base, the BE is positive. Positive values beyond the normal range indicate an excess of HCO_3^- (base), whereas negative values less than the normal range indicate a deficit of HCO_3^-. The more extreme the metabolic derangement, the larger the BE value will be.

Some clinicians use BE value to assess for proper fluid resuscitation. If the amount of fluid present is not adequate to support the body's metabolic activities (as in hypovolemic shock), the patient will experience ineffective energy production, which leads to a concomitant increase in the lactic acid level. The BE value in such a case may be classified as mild (−2 to −6), moderate (−6 to −15), or severe (−15 or greater). If a patient has normal vital signs with a continued high negative BE, a source for the continued shock should be sought.

Oxygenation Status

Partial Pressure of Oxygen

The partial pressure of oxygen (Po_2) measures the amount of oxygen dissolved in the blood. A healthy person has an arterial Po_2 in the range of 80 to 100 mm Hg. Other than in some narrowly defined cases (eg, carbon monoxide poisoning), patients do not benefit from having a Po_2 greater than 100 mm Hg; the most important consideration is simply that the Po_2 remain within the normal range. As the Po_2 falls below 80 mm Hg, the hemoglobin's affinity for oxygen decreases and oxygen is released more readily from the hemoglobin molecule, which results in hypoxia.

Oxygen Saturation

Oxygen saturation measures the percentage of potential oxygen-binding sites on hemoglobin that are currently occupied by oxygen molecules. The oxygen saturation measured transcutaneously (Spo_2), using a saturation monitor and probe, differs from the oxygen saturation calculated from an arterial or venous blood sample (Sao_2) that is reported on a blood gas report, because in the latter case Sao_2 is calculated based on other parts of the blood gas panel. The normal value for measured Sao_2 in a healthy person is greater than 93%. The calculated saturation from the blood gas values can give a falsely elevated saturation when abnormal hemoglobin variants, such as carboxyhemoglobin and methemoglobin, are present in the sample. This consideration is important: Although the Sao_2 value may appear normal, the patient might actually have a poor oxygen distribution because the abnormal hemoglobin variants cannot carry oxygen.

Carboxyhemoglobin

Because carbon monoxide binds very tightly with hemoglobin, the body's ability to transport oxygen can become extremely compromised when too much carbon monoxide is present in the body. Although some carboxyhemoglobin (COHb), a hemoglobin derivative, is always present in the vasculature, normal levels of this compound are thought not to exceed 0.02 (2%). The percentage reported in testing is based on the amount of total hemoglobin.

Assessment of COHb levels is useful in confirming a diagnosis of carbon monoxide poisoning, and it may be used to guide therapy as well. Caution should be used in assessing COHb levels in smokers, as their baseline COHb levels are routinely higher than the levels of nonsmokers. COHb levels are often elevated in critically ill patients for reasons that are poorly understood.

Most blood gas analyses provide a carboxyhemoglobin level as part of a full arterial or venous blood gas report. When carbon monoxide poisoning is suspected, it is not necessary to obtain an arterial blood specimen; venous carboxyhemoglobin levels are closely correlated with arterial values.

Obtaining Blood Samples

Arterial Blood Samples

SKILL DRILL 9-1 shows the steps to obtain an arterial blood sample, which are also described here:

1. Appropriately identify the patient. Explain the procedure. Determine the appropriate arm from which to take the specimen **STEP 1**.
2. Perform an Allen test. First have the patient raise the hand above the level of the heart, and then have the patient make a fist while you simultaneously compress the radial and ulnar arteries **STEP 2**.
3. When the patient's hand turns white or pale, release compression of the ulnar artery and assess circulation. The color should return to baseline in approximately 5 to 7 seconds **STEP 3**.
4. Repeat Steps 2 and 3 while releasing the radial artery. Sluggish return of color may indicate occlusion in one or both of the arteries. Arterial puncture should not be performed on this extremity.
5. Ensure universal precautions.
6. If possible, position the patient's arm with a small towel roll beneath the wrist to slightly extend the wrist (do not overextend) **STEP 4**.
7. Prepare the site per protocol.
8. Palpate the radial artery with your index and middle fingers (do not use your thumb) **STEP 5**.
9. Locate the radial artery and puncture the skin with the bevel of the needle at a 45° angle. The syringe should rapidly fill with bright red blood **STEP 6**. Do not dig or probe with the needle! If you have difficulty, slightly reposition the

needle. If you continue to have difficulty, stop and restart the procedure.

10. Once the appropriate amount of blood has filled the syringe, rapidly remove the needle

and hold pressure on the site for approximately 2 to 5 minutes **STEP 7**.

11. Safely remove the needle and expel any air contained within the syringe **STEP 8**.

Skill Drill 9-1 Obtaining an Arterial Blood Sample

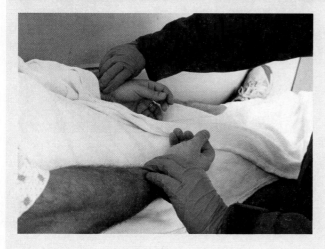

Step 1

Determine the appropriate arm from which to take the specimen.

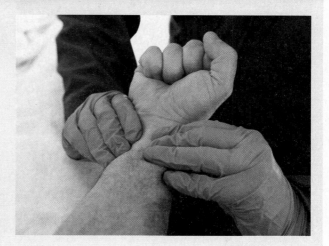

Step 2

Have the patient make a fist. Compress the radial and ulnar arteries.

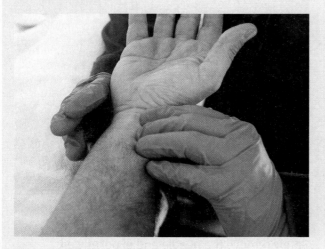

Step 3

When the patient's hand turns white or pale, release compression of the ulnar artery and assess circulation. Repeat for the radial artery. Ensure universal precautions.

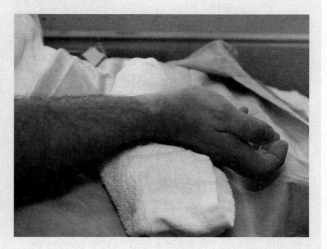

Step 4

Position the patient's arm with a small towel roll beneath the wrist to slightly extend the wrist.

Continues

Skill Drill 9-1 Obtaining an Arterial Blood Sample (continued)

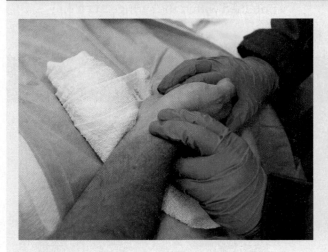

Step 5

Palpate the radial artery with your index and middle fingers.

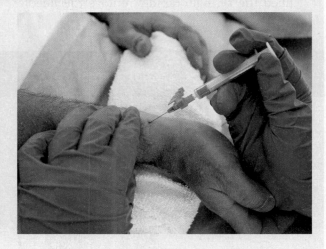

Step 6

Locate the radial artery and puncture the skin with the bevel of the needle at a 45° angle.

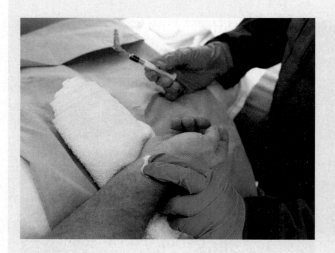

Step 7

Rapidly remove the needle and hold pressure on the site for approximately 2 to 5 minutes.

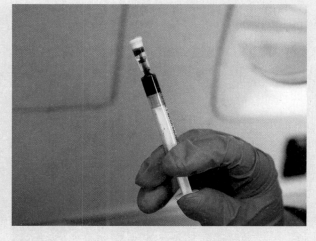

Step 8

Safely remove the needle and expel any air contained within the syringe.

Skill Drill 9-1 Obtaining an Arterial Blood Sample (continued)

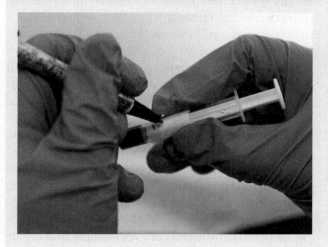

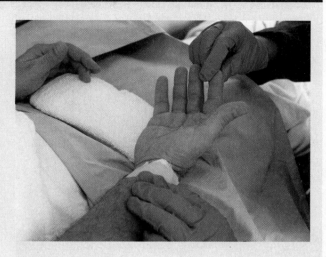

Step 9

Label the syringe with appropriate patient identification.

© Jones & Bartlett Learning.

Step 10

Reassess neurovascular status.

12. Place a rubber stopper on the syringe.
13. Label the syringe with appropriate patient identification **STEP 9**.
14. Immediately perform the test or place the specimen on ice.
15. Reassess the patient's neurovascular status **STEP 10**.

Venous Blood Samples

If the patient has a peripheral IV line and is receiving fluids or medications, if at all possible, the other extremity should be used to obtain a venous blood sample. If the patient has IV lines in both extremities, the one without IV medication or without the medication that is being tested should be used. For example, a finger-stick blood glucose sample should not be obtained in an extremity where an IV infusion containing dextrose is running. The flow of fluid or medication needs to be paused or stopped immediately prior to obtaining the blood sample; otherwise, the sample may become contaminated with infusate. Minimum discard volumes are also recommended when obtaining blood specimens from arterial and central venous lines, as discussed in Chapter 15, *Hemodynamic Monitoring*.

Blood Tube Uses

Blood tubes are selected primarily based on the preservatives or lack of preservatives that they contain. Most laboratories have specific requests regarding tube selection and the number of tubes needed. The desired tube selection is usually communicated by the laboratory **TABLE 9-2** and **FIGURE 9-9**.

Point-of-Care Testing

Traditionally, tests used to make clinical patient care decisions have required the health care provider to send a specimen to a laboratory, where trained personnel run the test and then report its results. Increasingly, however, demands for faster results and miniaturization of laboratory testing instruments have brought testing and reporting to the patient bedside **FIGURE 9-10**. **Point-of-care testing (POCT)** refers to testing done outside of a traditional laboratory, usually near where care is being delivered to a patient, with the results of the testing being used for clinical decision making (ie, changes in patient care). POCT is also called decentralized testing, bedside testing, and ancillary testing.

TABLE 9-2 Blood Tube Uses	
Blood Tube Color	**Use**
Lavender	Complete blood count
Red	Blood banking
Marbled	Serum chemistry tests
Blue	Coagulation studies
Green	Plasma studies
Yellow	Human leukocyte antigen typing
Navy	Trace metals
Gray	Lactate

© Jones & Bartlett Learning.

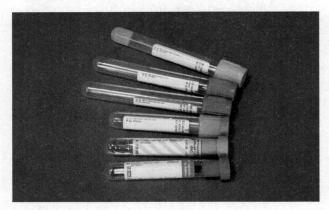

FIGURE 9-9 The colors of blood tube tops relate to their intended use.

© Jones & Bartlett Learning.

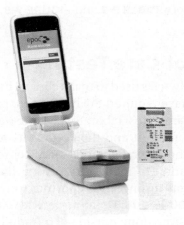

FIGURE 9-10 Point-of-care testing allows testing to be performed outside of a traditional laboratory. The epoc® Blood Analysis System is pictured.

Photo courtesy of Siemens Healthineers. © Siemens Healthcare Diagnostics Inc. 2021.

Regulation of Laboratory and Point-of-Care Testing

Highly publicized cases of deaths attributed to missed cervical cancers from false-negative reads of Pap smears led Congress to pass the Clinical Laboratory Improvement Act (CLIA) in 1988. Today, state and federal regulations cover almost every test performed on specimens from humans, including those done in the home, physician offices, or a CCT unit.

CLIA classifies some laboratory tests as having a low risk for reporting incorrect results. These "waived tests" include tests cleared by the US Food and Drug Administration (FDA) for home use (such as certain blood glucose meters) and other tests approved for a waiver by the FDA using the CLIA criteria. Generally, these tests are very simple and highly accurate, or they pose no reasonable risk of harm if they are performed incorrectly. Health care providers who perform waived tests must have a CLIA certificate authorizing them to do so, and must carefully follow the test manufacturer's instructions.

Nonwaived testing encompasses all other laboratory tests except for provider-performed microscopy. Such tests are divided into moderate or high complexity categories. Providers performing nonwaived testing must have a CLIA laboratory certificate, be inspected, and meet CLIA quality standards, which mandate regular proficiency testing of all test operators.

Implications for Critical Care Transport Professionals

It is critical for CCTPs to be familiar with any POCT equipment they use and to know whether a test they perform is classified as waived, moderate complexity, or high complexity, as this status determines the applicable CLIA or state laboratory requirements. Based on field experience, the FDA may choose to waive tests or revoke previously issued waivers, which can impact the POCT that a CCTP may perform in the field.

In the context of POCT, the term "CLIA exempt" refers to a lab, service, or user that has been licensed or approved by a state where the state laws or regulations are equal to or more stringent than CLIA, and where the state licensure program has been approved by the Centers for Medicare and Medicaid Services (CMS). Washington and New York are two such CLIA-exempt states. CCTPs in CLIA-exempt states must comply with state testing and licensing requirements.

Multiple POCT devices are suitable for use in CCTP units, all of which require various levels of operator training, competency, and credentialing. Each manufacturer offers training to users and assistance with regulatory compliance and policy development.

Urine Lab Values

Urinalysis involves performing various laboratory tests (including some of the same tests performed on blood samples) on a patient's urine **TABLE 9-3**.

TABLE 9-3 Common Urinalysis Values	
Analyte	**Normal Values Reported on a Typical Urinalysis**
Color	Yellow (light/pale to dark/deep amber)
Clarity/turbidity	Clear or cloudy
pH	4.5–8
Specific gravity	1.005–1.025
Glucose	≤130 mg/dL
Ketones	None
Nitrites	Negative
Leukocyte esterase	Negative
Bilirubin	Negative
Urobilirubin	Small amount (0.5–1 mg/dL)
Blood	≤3 RBCs × 10^6/μL
Protein	≤150 mg/dL
RBCs	≤2 RBCs/hpf
WBCs	≤2–5 WBCs/hpf
Squamous epithelial cells	15–20 squamous epithelial cells/hpf
Casts	0–5 hyaline casts/lpf
Crystals	Occasionally
Bacteria	None
Yeast	None

Abbreviations: hpf, high-power field; lpf, low-power field; RBCs, red blood cells; WBCs, white blood cells

© Jones & Bartlett Learning.

Roughly one-fourth of the heart's cardiac output enters the kidneys for filtration, and the urine produced by the kidneys provides a way of investigating the patient's physiologic status. Tests performed on urine may range from simple (such as color) to complex (such as specific gravity). Many drugs can be detected in the urine for hours, days, or weeks after their use. **TABLE 9-4** lists drugs of abuse that can be tested in urine, including how long the drug can be detected in the urine after its use. Urine can also be tested for biomarkers of physiologic processes, such as in pregnancy tests that qualitatively test for the presence of human chorionic gonadotropin (hCG) in the urine.

Color

Color may be the most simplistic laboratory analysis performed. This assessment simply notes the urine color, which is often classified as yellow, pale, clear, and so forth. Urine's color is a function of concentration, with more concentrated urine being darker yellow. Various other particulates in the urine can affect the color as well. If the person's glomeruli or

TABLE 9-4 Drugs of Abuse That Can Be Detected in Urine	
Drug	**Length of Time Detected in Urine**
Alcohol	7–12 hours
Amphetamine	48 hours
Barbiturate	24 hours (short acting); 3 weeks (long acting)
Benzodiazepines	3 days
Cocaine	6–8 hours (metabolites, 2–4 days)
Heroin	36–72 hours
Marijuana	3 days to 4 weeks (depending on dose)
Methadone	3 days
Methaqualone	7 days
Morphine	48–72 hours
Phencyclidine	8 days
Propoxyphene	6–48 hours

© Jones & Bartlett Learning.

renal tubular system is damaged and blood is spilling into the urine, the urine may be reddish. Brown or tea-colored urine often reflects the presence of large amounts of protein in the urine and is a hallmark sign of rhabdomyolysis.

Appearance

Similar to color, urine appearance is a rather coarse assessment. Appearance is categorized as clear (similar to color) or turbid (cloudy or opaque). Turbidity can be indicative of a bladder infection and should be examined further.

Specific Gravity

Specific gravity is a chemical property of a fluid that relates its density to the density of water. Distilled water is arbitrarily given a specific gravity of 1, so fluid that is denser than water has a specific gravity greater than 1. The more concentrated a urine sample is, the denser the sample and the higher its specific gravity will be. Conversely, a low specific gravity indicates a more dilute urine sample. At the simplest level, athletes measure specific gravity to assess their hydration status. Higher-than-normal specific gravity would reflect volume depletion in an otherwise healthy athlete.

The normal range for urine specific gravity is 1.003 to 1.035; in the setting of impaired ability to concentrate urine, the specific gravity may approach 1.001. Numerous factors can affect the kidney's ability to concentrate the urine. For example, if the pituitary gland secretes an abnormally low level of antidiuretic hormone, this condition may lead to diabetes insipidus. This metabolic disorder impairs the ability of the kidney to concentrate the urine (ie, the body reabsorbs free water), so the specific gravity of urine will be very low (ie, there would be copious amounts of dilute urine). Other disorders, such as glomerulonephritis and pyelonephritis, may also impair the kidney's ability to concentrate urine.

pH

The H^+ concentration in the urine can be a useful marker for metabolic acidosis. Unlike serum pH, urine pH has a relatively wide normal range, 4.5 to 8. Patients with acidic urine often have large amounts of unbuffered acid (eg, lactic acid or keto acid). Salt wasting may also occur as the body excretes a positive ion (eg, Na^+) to counteract the negatively charged acid salt of lactate or keto acetate.

Certain renal abnormalities may render the kidneys unable to excrete H^+ in the urine, even in the presence of overwhelming metabolic acidosis. This abnormality is called renal tubule acidosis (RTA). Four types of RTA are distinguished, although the specifics of each type are not included here. Nevertheless, CCTPs should be able to identify the presence of RTA, defined as an arterial pH of less than 7.35 and a urine pH of greater than 6. Generally, the biggest concern is that the kidneys are not able to concentrate urine, which will cause wasting of potassium and magnesium.

Glucose

The presence of glucose in the urine (glycosuria) is almost always indicative of elevated serum glucose levels. In healthy people, the urine does not contain any glucose, so the normal value of this marker is 0. If glucose is present, its amount is graded on a scale of mild to severe, expressed as +1, +2, +3, or +4. The presence of glycosuria may not always signal ineffective insulin production or function (as in diabetes mellitus). For example, in some cases it may result from the administration of a carbohydrate-containing intravenous fluid such as 5% dextrose in water. The specific context for the patient will dictate when a value outside the normal range is pathologic.

Ketone Bodies

Fat catabolism occurs when the available supply of glucose does not suffice to satisfy the tissues' need for energy. If the body does not completely break down fat into CO_2 and water, ketone bodies are produced. The term ketone bodies describes a number (typically three) of organic products: acetoacidic acid, acetone, and beta-hydroxybutyric acid. Acetoacidic acid and beta-hydroxybutyric acid are keto acids that are produced as by-products during a starvation state in which the body is forced to rely on metabolism of lipid stores for energy. For example, diabetic ketoacidosis occurs when inadequate insulin is present and cells are unable to use glucose as a source of energy, forcing the body to engage in lipid metabolism, which yields ketone bodies as a by-product. Although ketone bodies are not normally found in the urine, their presence can help identify inadequately controlled diabetes mellitus. Other causes of ketonuria (ketone bodies in the urine) include alcoholic ketoacidosis and starvation ketosis.

Grading of the level of ketonuria uses the same system as grading of the amount of glucose in urine: +1, +2, +3, or +4.

Protein

Although the body excretes 40 to 80 mg of protein (one-third of which is albumin) in the urine each day, this amount is below the detectable threshold for typical tests; thus, the normal reference value in a qualitative test for protein would be negative (or not detectable). Urinary protein is one of the most important assessments for kidney disease. Detectable levels of urinary protein (proteinuria) can result from either renal causes (such as glomerulonephritis, polycystic kidneys, diabetic nephropathy, toxic nephropathy, nephrosclerosis, and nephritic syndrome) or extrarenal causes (such as preeclampsia, multiple myeloma, urinary tract disease, amyloid disease, systemic lupus erythematosus, heart failure, and constrictive pericarditis).

Blood and Hemoglobin

The presence of blood in the urine is highly suggestive of kidney or urinary tract damage. Recall that blood is not able to cross the glomerular membrane and enter the filtrate. Thus, the presence of hemoglobin in the urine (hemoglobinuria) most often indicates traumatic passage of RBCs through the collecting ducts, urinary bladder, or urinary tract. Urinary hemoglobin may also result from filtering of serum hemoglobin during hemolytic transfusion reactions or certain blood disorders such as hemolytic anemia.

The presence of RBCs in the urine (hematuria) may indicate the presence of glomerular membrane or urinary tract disease. The cause may be an infectious process (commonly a urinary tract infection), neoplasm, ureterolithiasis, or trauma. Note that RBCs detected in a urinalysis performed soon after placement of an indwelling urinary catheter may merely reflect trauma from insertion of the catheter. Myoglobin in the urine (myoglobinuria), caused by rhabdomyolysis, can also cause a positive hemoglobin result. Myoglobinuria, which may indicate a serious threat to the kidneys, can be distinguished from hemoglobinuria by a positive urine hemoglobin result combined with a negative urine RBC result.

Electrolytes

To better understand how the body is eliminating certain electrolytes, a quantitative analysis is performed on the urine. Similar to a basic metabolic panel, this panel analyzes numerous components of the urine. Although their discussion is beyond the scope of this text, urine electrolytes can be useful in clinical management as well, particularly when analyzed alongside serum values.

Diagnostic Imaging

Diagnostic imaging is typically performed by a technologist, and the resulting images are often interpreted by a physician on site or possibly sent off site for interpretation. Typically, copies are included with the patient's charts upon transfer. Note that summaries of findings alone from imaging studies performed at the sending facility are generally insufficient for use at the receiving facility. For example, a typed report describing a femur fracture that requires operative repair will not allow the receiving facility to verify the quality of the images, perform an independent assessment of the findings, and use the data to plan interventions. To undertake an appropriate assessment, the receiving facility must receive a copy of the images, typically stored on a physical disc, unless they can be shared and accessed electronically.

The CCTP should be familiar with these studies and be able to perform basic interpretation for obvious abnormalities, such as long bone fractures, masses, and catheter and tube placements. Contrast dyes can also be used to enhance these imaging modalities, depending on the indication. It is important to have a system for analyzing imaging results and to use that system every time. Think of this process as being akin to the steps of a primary exam: Completing the same steps in the same order will prevent the CCTP from overlooking findings. Extensive interpretation of imaging studies requires significant training and is beyond the scope of this text.

Standard Radiographs

One of the oldest and still frequently used diagnostic imaging modalities is standard or plain radiography. Such images can be obtained rapidly and used for quick diagnostics in patient care.

To create a radiograph, radiation (in the form of x-rays) is projected through the tissue and onto a photographic plate. Different densities of the body cause gradation changes in black and white on the film. Dense objects such as bone or blood appear white on the images, whereas less dense objects such as air appear black. Objects with a medium density such as tissues will appear as shades of gray.

Radiographs can be very useful to examine the integrity of the skeletal system (eg, fractures, dislocations), identify the abnormal presence of air or fluid (eg, hemothorax, pneumoperitoneum), and identify or evaluate foreign bodies (eg, bullet fragments in a gunshot wound, placement of an endotracheal tube or central venous catheter). Radiographs generate two-dimensional images that capture the various densities in the path of the radiation. The lack of a third dimension that would indicate the relative depth of objects, however, makes it difficult to evaluate multiple objects of interest within this axis. Therefore, multiple views can be combined to add greater perspective, such as lateral and anteroposterior (AP) views. Radiography provides the basis for more advanced imaging modalities, such as computed tomography and fluoroscopy (continuous radiography that can provide a radiographic image to guide procedures in real time).

Computed Tomography

Computed tomography (CT), also called computerized axial tomography (CAT) scanning, is an imaging method in which cross-sectional images of the structures in the body plane are reconstructed by a computer program to generate three-dimensional images. Focused beams examine an area of interest and are reconstructed by computer to give a high-resolution view. During this imaging study, the patient lies on a table that moves into and out of the scanner device. (The use of CT may be limited in patients with morbid obesity, because they may not fit into the scanner or may exceed the table's operating limits.) CT scans are typically analyzed by choosing one plane—axial, sagittal, or coronal—and scrolling through a series of two-dimensional slices within that plane to compile a three-dimensional model of the target.

CT scans are commonly used when it is necessary to evaluate different characteristics of tissues, bones, and organs. Because the resulting images are essentially generated using a series of radiographs, low densities (eg, air) are dark and high densities (eg, bone) are white, although various viewing profiles can be used to magnify the contrast between various densities of interest. Unlike conventional radiographs, CT allows differences to be quantified, which can allow for differentiation of tumors from soft tissue, old fractures from new ones, air from fluid, and blood clots from normal blood. The views, or slices, can pick up abnormalities not seen with traditional plain radiography. Interpreting a CT scan can reveal conditions such as aortic dissection, lung injuries, abdominal organ injuries, fractures, pulmonary emboli, pleural effusions, and acute respiratory distress syndrome **FIGURE 9-11**. Interpretation of CT scans is beyond the scope of the CCTP, although it is reasonable to develop a cursory understanding of CT images.

In recent years, CT scanning has undergone major improvements; the newest technologies offer significantly reduced scan times, multiple and finer slice capabilities for greater three-dimensional resolution, and improved overall image quality. CT scans are now a standard diagnostic tool in many disciplines, despite the growing concern about the significantly greater radiation exposure experienced by patients from this imaging modality compared to conventional radiography and the resultant increase in cancer risk. Specifically, a single CT scan can generate radiation exposure equivalent to 5,000 chest radiographs. However, recent advancements in this technology have also resulted in CT protocols that have dramatically reduced the amount of radiation required to generate adequate images, thereby lowering risk.

When transporting a critically ill patient who has had a recent CT scan, the CCTP should attempt to obtain an electronic copy of the scan from the transferring facility to expedite care on arrival at the receiving center. Often scans can be shared between facilities through electronic medical record portals.

CT angiography (CTA) refers to CT imaging that uses intravascular contrast to visualize blood vessels in addition to the surrounding tissues. CTA can be used to diagnose blockages in blood flow

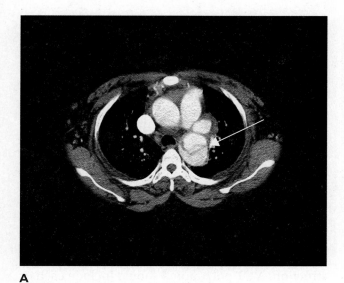

A

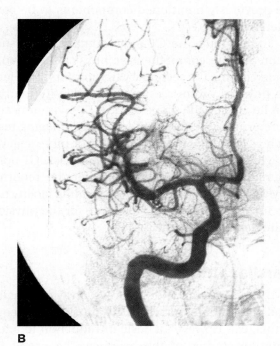

B

FIGURE 9-11 Computed tomography scans. **A.** Acute aortic dissection. **B.** Frontal view of a cerebral angiogram showing recanalization.

A: © Living Art Enterprises, LLC/Science Source; B: © Science History Images/Alamy Stock Photo.

(eg, pulmonary embolism, acute ischemic stroke), stenosis (ie, narrowing of a blood vessel), aneurysm (ie, dilation of the blood vessel wall), or dissection (eg, tear in the blood vessel wall).

Magnetic Resonance Imaging

Magnetic resonance imaging (MRI) is primarily a diagnostic imaging technique; it is most commonly used to visualize the internal structure and function of the body. Most MRI studies are structural, meaning they provide a static three-dimensional image of anatomy. However, functional MRI (fMRI) can also be used to collect physiologic data over time; for example, brain fMRI can be used to track brain activity associated with changes in blood flow across time overlaid on a neuroanatomic image.

MRI provides a much greater contrast between the different soft tissues of the body than a CT scan does. As a result, this technology is especially useful in brain, spinal cord, musculoskeletal, cardiovascular, and oncologic imaging. Another benefit of this imaging modality is that the patient is not exposed to radiation. Even so, despite significant recent advancements in MRI technology that have made MRI faster and more accessible, CT scans remain faster to perform and are more widely used throughout the United States.

MRI uses a large circular magnet and radio waves to align the water molecules in the tissues and generate signals from atoms in the body. An image is obtained based on both this alignment and the speed at which molecules alter or release signals. The strength of the magnetic field requires MRI-compatible patient monitoring, infusion pumps, and special ventilators for intubated patients. When done, such studies are typically used to provide exquisitely detailed images of the brain, spine, skeletal system, heart, abdomen, or pelvis.

MRI may be limited by the patient's size or ability to tolerate an enclosed tunnel like environment for the greater duration of time required to complete MRI studies compared to CT. Certain preexisting ferrous metals in the patient's body may also contraindicate such scans. Many advances have been made in the size and openness of the MRI device, as well as the speed with which it can complete an imaging sequence, allowing for a more tolerable environment.

It is important to adhere to safety guidelines with MRI machines, because the powerful magnet will cause certain metal objects to launch with great force or heat to dangerous temperatures. Keeping your equipment and any other metals you may be wearing away from the control area is essential.

Positron Emission Tomography

Positron emission tomography (PET) is a functional imaging modality used to visualize physiologic changes over time or distinguish various levels of physiologic activity between tissues. The equipment and procedure are similar to those used in CT imaging; indeed, these modalities are often combined as a single procedure (PET-CT imaging).

In PET, radiotracers (ie, radioactive substances) attached to a carrier drug are injected into the patient, or are ingested or inhaled by the patient. Gamma radiation is then emitted, which enables the clinician to detect the radiotracers as they move within the body. The behavior of these tracers reveals processes such as changes in blood flow or differences in metabolic activity. Areas of disease often appear as bright spots on PET scans.

Applications of a PET scan include the following:

- Measuring temporospatial changes in brain activity. For example, this study can help reveal which brain structures are most active when performing a particular task.
- Locating regions of the heart that might be vulnerable to myocardial infarction. This imaging shows myocardial tissue with decreased metabolic activity during a period of increased myocardial stress.
- Identifying metastatic disease in patients with cancer. Tumors are highly metabolically active, so cancerous tissues will absorb a greater amount of radiotracer than surrounding tissues. In turn, they can be easily visualized on PET scans even if they would otherwise be very difficult to identify using other modalities based on tissue density.

Imaging for Polytrauma

The imaging studies commonly used in trauma have already been covered in this section, but a few special considerations for trauma patients are worth noting for CCTPs. The evaluation of polytrauma patients in the acute setting can be associated with numerous challenges—for example, impaired patient participation (secondary to injury and related distraction, therapy, or substance use, among other causes); distraction of providers due to obvious patient injuries; and limitations in the initial trauma survey due to other procedures or immobilization. Although providers are trained to overcome these challenges, imaging studies tend

to provide highly valuable data that can mitigate these challenges and aid in diagnosing occult injury, evaluating surgical candidacy, and planning for surgery. Therefore, thorough imaging of the polytrauma patient and sharing of the original studies (often saved on physical discs) and radiology reports are essential aspects of interfacility transport communication.

In CT polytrauma, also known as a pan-scan, the imaging protocol typically includes CT of the head, cervical spine, chest, and abdomen/pelvis, with the results being combined to generate a continuous image from the top of the head through the pelvis. Additional images (eg, face, spine) can sometimes be generated through image reconstruction. A CT polytrauma should include each of the previously mentioned components to be considered complete.

Importantly, the CT polytrauma is *not* a substitute for the comprehensive physical exam conducted during the secondary trauma survey. In fact, the physical exam is essential to identify injuries that lie outside the scope of the CT polytrauma and to determine the need for additional imaging tests such as imaging of the extremities or more specific imaging tests than those used in the basic CT polytrauma protocol. Moreover, neither the reported physical exam performed at the sending facility nor the imaging studies can substitute for the physical exam performed by the CCTP.

Cardiac Imaging

Cardiac imaging includes a broad array of imaging modalities, many of which lie outside the scope of this text. However, a basic introduction to a few common studies of the heart can be useful for CCTPs. Classic indications for various types of cardiac imaging include concern for structural disease (eg, valvular disease), acute coronary syndrome (eg, blockages in the coronary arteries, regions of hypokinetic or damaged myocardial tissue), or inflammatory conditions (eg, pericarditis, myocarditis, endocarditis).

Echocardiography is the use of ultrasonography to produce dynamic images of the heart (ie, live images of heart activity). Such studies can provide a wealth of information about cardiac function, including left ventricular ejection fraction (a measurement of how much blood is being pumped by the heart with each beat, where normal values typically range from 50% to 75%), valvular disease (ie, problems with heart valves, such as regurgitation or stenosis), wall motion abnormalities (ie, specific regions of the heart that are hypokinetic), presence of effusion (ie, fluid around the heart), and other structural changes (eg, hypertrophy, dilation, or changes in relative size that might indicate abnormal pressures). Transthoracic echocardiography is performed by placing an ultrasonography probe on the skin of the chest, whereas transesophageal echocardiography is performed by using a probe inside the esophagus to obtain higher-quality images for particular diagnostic indications (eg, endocarditis, intracardiac thrombus).

Cardiac MRI is an MRI study of the heart that obtains high-resolution images of the myocardial tissue and surrounding structures. Common indications for cardiac MRI include assessment of the health and composition of the myocardium, such as in patients with myocarditis or cardiac amyloidosis, or assessment of tissue viability following myocardial infarction. It is also used to evaluate valvular disease, cardiac masses, and pericardial disease.

Myocardial perfusion imaging, often referred to as a stress test, is a noninvasive imaging study to assess the perfusion of myocardial tissue via the coronary arteries. Myocardial perfusion imaging is classically performed on patients experiencing angina to evaluate coronary artery disease and resultant myocardial hypoperfusion as a cause of the chest pain. Rather than directly visualizing the blood vessels supplying the heart, myocardial perfusion imaging uses a variety of imaging techniques to detect regions of the heart that are hypoperfused during increased myocardial stress. Clinicians typically induce a state of increased myocardial stress either by having the patient perform physical exercise (ie, a physical or exercise stress test) or by administering a drug that increases myocardial activity and simulates the effects of exercise (ie, a chemical or pharmacologic stress test).

Coronary CTA provides direct visualization of the coronary arteries, typically to aid in the diagnosis of coronary artery disease. In contrast to myocardial perfusion imaging, which provides assessment of the physiologic consequences of coronary artery disease during times of myocardial stress, coronary CT provides anatomic assessment of blockages within the coronary arteries.

Coronary angiography is a minimally invasive imaging study performed using coronary catheterization, a procedure in which a physician inserts a catheter into the vasculature and guides it into the coronary circulation. Coronary angiography is one of several procedures that can be performed during a coronary catheterization procedure. During this study, locally injected contrast dye enables radiographic images of flow through the coronary arteries to evaluate blockages in the vessels. Unlike myocardial perfusion imaging, which evaluates the consequences of coronary artery disease in the form of myocardial hypoperfusion, and coronary CTA, which directly visualizes the coronary arteries, coronary angiography provides direct dynamic imaging of flow through the coronary arteries. This highly sensitive test can both identify the location of blockages and estimate the percentage degree of blockage within coronary vessels, providing very helpful information for interventions performed during the coronary catheterization procedure and for planning future therapy.

Ultrasonography

Ultrasonography is an imaging modality that uses high-frequency sound waves to visualize both static and dynamic anatomic structures. Sound waves are transmitted into the body, and based on the time it takes for them to be reflected back to the probe, an image is constructed. Because the sound waves must be reflected to form an image, they are often referred to as echoes. This principle allows for the real-time visualization of moving elements such as cerebral blood flow with transcranial Doppler studies, or the visualization of moving tendons to assess for tears and other injuries.

While most imaging modalities are largely the domain of radiology, ultrasonography has transcended any one individual medical specialty and is now frequently used by providers at the bedside in the ED, ICU, and various specialty clinics. In some agencies, it is even used in the prehospital setting. The routine use of ultrasonography for bedside procedures has significantly increased its safety margin.

As with MRI, ultrasonography has the advantage of not exposing the patient to ionizing radiation. As such, it is often used for frequent repeat examinations in the point-of-care setting to assess for progression of disease or response to therapy. It has the further advantage of being extremely portable, with some devices consisting of a lightweight ultrasonography probe that can plug into a smartphone or tablet.

One of the most common uses of point-of-care ultrasonography (POCUS) in the ED setting is in the evaluation of trauma. The focused assessment with sonography for trauma (FAST) examination became a standard part of the initial assessment of major trauma in the United States in the 1990s. By obtaining standardized views of the right upper quadrant (perihepatic), left upper quadrant (perisplenic), and retrovesicular space (around the bladder), the operator can assess for the presence of free intraperitoneal fluid. At least one view of the heart, typically the subcostal, is also included to assess for the presence of fluid around the heart causing cardiac tamponade. A highly experienced point-of-care ultrasonographer can detect as little as 100 mL of free fluid; the average user typically will not detect free fluid volumes of less than 500 mL. Any positive findings generally necessitate immediate intervention in the setting of an unstable patient. However, a degree of caution and clinical judgment must be exercised because ultrasonography will not differentiate the type of free fluid, which means ascites will have the same appearance as blood on the images.

POCUS has also seen increased use for thoracic imaging and is sometimes incorporated into trauma assessment, in a protocol known as an eFAST (extended FAST) exam. Since ultrasonography allows for visualization of moving structures, it can be used to assess for the presence of normal lung motion, typically referred to as lung sliding. A lack of normal lung motion, particularly in a trauma patient, may indicate a pneumothorax, though other pathology (eg, consolidations) can also cause the absence of lung sliding.

Ultrasonography is also used to assess for the presence of pleural effusion, both in the setting of trauma (raising concern for hemothorax) and in more routine situations. A further use of ultrasonography in this setting is to assist with drainage of the effusion; it can be used to identify landmarks for the site of the procedure or even to provide direct visualization of needle entry into the pleural space.

Technique

To obtain the cardinal views of the eFAST exam, the operator typically begins with the right upper quadrant view, as this is the most sensitive anatomic location for detecting peritoneal free fluid. All ultrasonography probes have an indicator on one side that corresponds with the indicator on the screen. In this view, the indicator is pointed cephalad, toward the patient's head. Ideally, the operator will have a view displaying the liver, right kidney, and diaphragm. Fluid, if present, will normally collect in the Morison pouch, also termed the hepatorenal space **FIGURE 9-12**. The right upper quadrant view should include the tip of the liver to be considered adequate.

Following interrogation of the right upper quadrant, the left upper quadrant is typically visualized. In this view, the indicator is again pointed cephalad and the view will include the spleen, left kidney, and diaphragm. In this view, fluid will most often collect between the spleen and diaphragm.

Next, the retrovesicular view is obtained. This view has classically been referred to as the pelvic view, but that term is somewhat of a misnomer because the peritoneal space, not the pelvic space, is visualized. The indicator is once again pointed cephalad, with the probe placed midline above the bladder. Fluid will be seen cephalad to the bladder if present. In this view it is important to identify the bladder, which may often be recognized by its smooth edges, because peritoneal free fluid combined with a decompressed bladder may often be interpreted as a false-negative result.

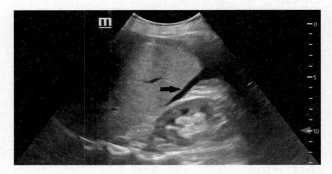

FIGURE 9-12 A right upper quadrant view from a focused assessment with sonography for trauma (FAST) exam demonstrating free fluid in the hepatorenal space. Note that the fluid appears darker than the surrounding tissue. This is because the fluid is less echogenic than the tissue and, therefore, reflects fewer sound waves.

The subcostal view of the heart is obtained next. In this view, the indicator is typically toward the patient's right, with the probe placed beneath the xiphoid process. Of note, when this view is obtained in traditional echocardiography, the indicator is pointed toward the patient's left. This view is used to visualize the heart and allows for assessment of gross pathology. Most importantly, it allows the ultrasonographer to assess for the presence of pericardial effusion.

To complete the eFAST exam, the probe is placed in the midclavicular line of the right and left chest in the second or third intercostal space, with the indicator again cephalad. The interface between the parietal and visceral pleura will have a shimmering appearance, termed "sliding" under normal circumstances. Absence of this finding may indicate a pneumothorax, which in certain clinical settings (eg, high pretest concern for tension pneumothorax) is an indication for decompression.

Applications

Ultrasonography has been used for cardiac imaging, an application called echocardiography, since 1953 **FIGURE 9-13**. In the point-of-care setting, it is used most frequently for applications such as assessing gross left ventricular systolic function, looking for evidence of right heart strain, assessing volume responsiveness, finding significant valvular disease, or assisting during CPR to assess for reversible causes (eg, tamponade) or to look for cardiac standstill. Cardiologists will perform significantly more detailed studies than are typically obtained in the point-of-care setting, including the assessment of blood flow across all valves, which clinically may produce a murmur in an otherwise structurally normal-appearing heart. Sometimes transesophageal echocardiography is also used due to its higher sensitivity (compared to transthoracic echocardiography) for detecting pathology such as valvular vegetations.

The use of ultrasonography during cardiac arrest has gained widespread acceptance in the emergency medicine, critical care, and anesthesia communities over the past several years. One of the initial uses was to distinguish pulseless electric activity (PEA) with electrical mechanical dissociation (EMD) from PEA with true cardiac standstill. Several studies have examined the differences in outcomes for these two conditions; they have typically demonstrated a greater than 25% probability of return of spontaneous circulation in patients with PEA and EMD and a less than 5% probability in patients with PEA and true cardiac standstill. POCUS can be used to help identify reversible causes of cardiac arrest, one of which was previously mentioned in the discussion of the eFAST: pericardial effusion causing tamponade physiology.

POCUS can also be used to assess the chambers of the heart. A dilated right atrium is consistent with pressure overload, which in the setting of cardiac arrest may indicate a massive pulmonary embolism. Underfilled ventricles are consistent with hypovolemia, necessitating aggressive volume resuscitation. Mechanical activity in synch with electrical activity with absent palpable pulses may indicate severe hypotension or vasoplegia requiring the use of additional pressors.

Ultrasonography is used extensively in abdominal imaging. It is considered the standard of care when evaluating the gallbladder for acute cholecystitis because it enables excellent visualization of the gallbladder (including the presence of stones), measurement of the common bile duct, and assessment for point tenderness at the site. Similarly, it

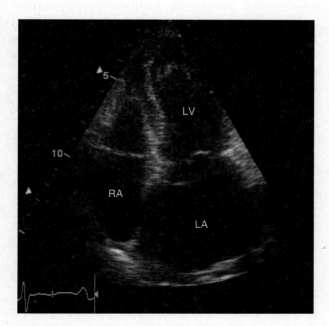

FIGURE 9-13 An echocardiogram. A four-chamber view in systole and diastole shows normal left ventricular systolic function but severely enlarged left atrium.

Abbreviations: LA, left atrium; LV, left ventricle; RA, right atrium provides excellent visualization of the liver and can help providers assess intrahepatic blood flow. It is used in the assessment of appendicitis, particularly in the pediatric population; younger patients tend to be thinner than adults, and the use of radiation is of higher concern in this group. Ultrasonography is also increasingly used for the identification of small bowel obstruction.

Ultrasonography for Identifying Appendicitis

While CT imaging remains the standard of care in the United States for identification of appendicitis and other bowel pathology in the adult population, ultrasonography has become the first-line test in Japan and several other countries.

Ultrasonography is a mainstay in vascular imaging because it enables the assessment of the direction, velocity, and turbulence of blood flow. It is the standard of care for screening and monitoring of abdominal aortic aneurysms and for identifying DVT of both the upper and lower extremities. In this type of study, the probe is used to evaluate the compressibility of the vein; as the operator applies pressure and attempts to collapse the vein, a thrombus will prevent complete compression.

For decades, ultrasonography has been used to evaluate the uterus during pregnancy, partially due to its excellent safety profile compared with other imaging modalities. Both transabdominal and transvaginal imaging are used to assess for the presence of an intrauterine pregnancy early in the course of gestation and further along the course to track development. In the emergent setting, ultrasonography can be used to evaluate for intrauterine pregnancy versus ectopic pregnancy or for ovarian torsion and the presence of ovarian cysts.

As it applies to the genitourinary system, ultrasonography is used in the evaluation of the testicles to identify testicular torsion, epididymitis, and other pathology. It can also help visualize the kidneys and bladder to assess for hydronephrosis and the presence of stones. Doppler ultrasonography allows for the visualization of flow from the ureters into the bladder, the absence of which strongly suggests obstruction.

Ophthalmology was one of the first specialties to adopt the use of ultrasonography and continues to make frequent use of the technology. Since the eyes are superficial fluid-filled structures, they are ideal for imaging with ultrasonography. Ocular ultrasonography is a mainstay in emergency medicine to help identify pathology such as lens subluxation, retinal detachment, and vitreous hemorrhage. It can also be used to identify ocular foreign bodies, just as it is used to find soft-tissue foreign bodies.

One of the most common uses of ultrasonography at the bedside remains its application for procedural guidance. It is routinely used for vascular access procedures ranging from placement of peripheral intravenous catheters to placement of central venous catheters and arterial lines. When used for vascular access, the target vessel is centered on the screen and needle entry is directly visualized. The operator slowly advances the probe to maintain constant visualization of the needle tip as it passes through the soft tissue and enters the targeted structure. Ultrasonography is used to find pockets of intraperitoneal fluid when preparing for paracentesis; as in drainage of pleural effusions, it can be used to visualize and direct needle entry. Frequently, ultrasonography is used to find peripheral nerves, allowing for the injection of local anesthetic and the performance of nerve blocks; this remains one of the most common uses of the modality in anesthesia. Finally, ultrasonography provides excellent visualization of soft tissue, allowing for the identification and drainage of abscesses.

Summary

One of the core goals of CCTPs is to form as complete a clinical picture of the patient as possible. Each patient presents with a unique hemodynamic and ventilatory status, which may be associated with various degrees of end-organ dysfunction. Laboratory analysis allows clinicians to assess or confirm the status of a particular system or organ. A key principle of laboratory interpretation is that no lab result should be analyzed in isolation. Repetition of tests (trending) and confirmation of findings through multiple testing modalities can create a more informed, accurate picture of the patient's condition. If adherence to that principle is maintained throughout the course of the patient's care, clinicians can be confident that their consideration of lab values is of the highest caliber.

The results of a variety of laboratory and point-of-care tests may be used by CCTPs in assessing and treating patients, including tests performed on blood samples, blood gas tests, and urinalysis. In addition, CCTPs must be familiar with the various diagnostic imaging studies and be able to interpret them for obvious abnormalities.

TABLE 9-5 summarizes normal and abnormal lab values.

TABLE 9-5 Normal and Abnormal Lab Values for Adults[a]

Name	Abbreviation	Normal	Critically Low	Critically High
Electrolytes and Other Chemicals				
Sodium (mEq/L)	Na^+	134–142	<125	>145
Potassium (mEq/L)	K^+	3.7–5.1	<3.0	>5.0
Chloride (mEq/L)	Cl^-	98–108	Varies	Varies
Calcium, total (mg/dL)	Ca^{+2}	8.6–10.3	<6.5	>13.5
Calcium, ionized (mmol/L)	Ca^{+2}_I	1.15–1.27	Varies	Varies
Total carbon dioxide (mEq/L)	CO_2	22–30	<15	>40
Phosphate (mEq/L)	PO_4	2.3–4.1	<1.2	>9
Metabolites				
Blood urea nitrogen (mg/dL)	BUN	6–25	<2	>80
Creatinine (mg/dL)	Cr	0.4–1.3	<0.4	>2.8
Lactate/lactic acid (mmol/L)	N/A	Venous: 0.4–2.0 Arterial: 0.5–1.6	Varies	>4.99
Proteins				
Protein, total (g/dL)	N/A	6.5–8.3	Varies	Varies
Albumin (g/dL)	N/A	3.9–5.0	Varies	Varies
Myoglobin (mg/L)	N/A	19–92	Varies	Varies
Troponin I (ng/mL)	cTnI	0–0.4 (negative)	Varies	Varies
Enzymes				
Lactate dehydrogenase (U/L)	LDH	120–300	Varies	Varies
Alanine aminotransferase (U/L)	ALT	5–40	N/A	Varies
Aspartate aminotransferase (U/L)	AST	5–40	N/A	Varies
Alkaline phosphatase (U/L)	ALP	35–110	Varies	Varies
Amylase (U/L)	N/A	27–131	Varies	Varies
Lipase (U/L)	N/A	31–186	Varies	Varies
Creatine kinase (U/L)	CK	40–150	Varies	Varies

(Continues)

TABLE 9-5 Normal and Abnormal Lab Values for Adults[a] (continued)

Name	Abbreviation	Normal	Critically Low	Critically High
Coagulation				
Prothrombin time (s)	PT	10–13	N/A	Varies
Activated partial thromboplastin time (s)	aPTT	25–40	N/A	>60
International normalized ratio	INR	2.0–3.0 (target for therapeutic anticoagulation therapy) Normal range for a patient who is not anticoagulated: 0.8–1.2	Varies	Varies
Serum				
Osmolality (mOsm/kg)	N/A	275–295	<240	>320
Complete Blood Count (CBC)				
Hematocrit (%)	Hct	41–50	<20	>60
Hemoglobin (g/dL)	Hgb	12.0–17.4	<7	>20
Erythrocytes (× 10^6/mL)	RBC	4.0–5.5	Varies	Varies
Leukocytes (/mL)	WBC	4,500–11,000	<2,000	>30,000
Arterial Blood Gases				
Percentage of hydrogen ions	pH	7.35–7.45	<7.2	>7.6
Partial pressure of oxygen (mm Hg)	Pao_2	80–100	<40	N/A
Partial pressure of carbon dioxide (mm Hg)	$Paco_2$	35–45	<20	>77
Bicarbonate (mEq/L)	Hco_3^-	21–28	<10	>40
Base excess (mEq/L)	BE	−2 to +3	<−5	>+5

[a] It is important to know the normal range for the laboratory where the specimen is tested.

Data from Fischbach FT, Fischbach MA, Stout K, eds. *Manual of Laboratory and Diagnostic Tests*. 10th ed. Philadelphia, PA: Lippincott Williams & Wilkins; 2017.

Case Study

You have been dispatched to transport, via helicopter, a 37-year-old man whose pretransport diagnosis is acute renal failure after renal transplantation.

You arrive at a rural hospital at the base of a mountainous region. The physician gives you the following history: The patient and his friend took a day hiking trip into the mountains and got lost. A search-and-rescue team was dispatched after 24 hours. The patient and friend were found 48 hours later. Both were severely dehydrated and confused; they had only a little water to sustain themselves during their ordeal. The patient underwent kidney transplantation approximately 1 year ago. Before today, he has not had any difficulties with the transplant. The patient has missed 2 days of his transplant antirejection drugs. The search-and-rescue team inserted a large-bore IV catheter and provided fluid resuscitation to the patient with 2,000 mL of normal saline before getting him to the local hospital.

The staff gives you the following report: The patient is now alert and oriented with generalized weakness. He has had a total intake of 2,500 mL of normal saline. He has an indwelling urinary catheter in place with 100 mL of urine output since the catheter was placed. His current vital signs are as follows: temperature, 96.0°F (35.6°C); heart rate, 88 beats/min; respirations, 20 breaths/min; and oxygen saturation, 98% with 4 L/min of oxygen per nasal cannula. His blood pressure is 150/90 mm Hg. He has two large-bore IV catheters in place. His current ECG shows a normal sinus rhythm, with a rate of 88 beats/min. There are tall, peaked T waves in the precordial leads V_1 through V_6. His QRS complex is prolonged, measures 130 milliseconds, and shows an incomplete right bundle block pattern.

Lab analysis reveals the following results: sodium, 135 mEq/L; potassium, 7.3 mEq/L; chloride, 100 mEq/L; and total calcium, 8.8 mg/dL. The patient's BUN is 70 mg/dL and his creatinine is 3.0 mg/dL. The physician says that the CBC and glucose levels were normal. He also says that the CK and myoglobin levels were elevated; he does not remember the exact numbers but will send hard copies along on the transport. The physician tells you that the patient is being transported to tertiary care (45 minutes by air) for emergency dialysis and management of his renal failure.

You give the patient 1 g of calcium gluconate IV. You reassess the ECG and notice that the QRS complex is narrower at 90 milliseconds (within normal limits) and the T wave is less peaked. You elect to promptly transport this patient, realizing that he still needs emergency treatment, but the rest of the medications can be given en route. During the transport, you administer 50 mL of 50% glucose in water solution ($D_{50}W$) IV, followed by 10 U of regular insulin IV; sodium bicarbonate, 50 mEq IV; and 5 mg of albuterol in 3 mL of normal saline via nebulizer.

1. What are your priorities in care before this transport?
2. What are your priorities in care during this transport?
3. Which reassessment parameters are important during this transport?

Analysis

In evaluating the situation, you realize that this patient is in acute renal failure with hyperkalemia. You also realize the renal failure could be a result of his severe dehydration, transplant rejection, and/or rhabdomyolysis; however, your transport priority is the hyperkalemia. The markers for emergency treatment of hyperkalemia are profound muscle weakness and marked ECG changes. This patient has generalized weakness and an intraventricular conduction delay along with peaked T waves, and he requires immediate treatment. The most important emergency intervention is the administration of calcium, which directly antagonizes the membrane actions of hyperkalemia. Either calcium chloride or calcium gluconate may be administered. Calcium chloride contains three times as much elemental calcium as calcium gluconate and should be given via a central line placed at the hospital. You elected to give 1 g of calcium gluconate IV. You reassess the ECG and notice that the QRS complex is narrower at 90 milliseconds (within normal limits) and the T wave is less peaked. The effects of calcium are usually seen in 3 to 5 minutes and last approximately 30 to 60 minutes.

While en route, you also want to drive the potassium back into the cells by increasing the availability of insulin; therefore, you administer 10 U of regular insulin IV, followed by 50 mL of $D_{50}W$ IV (the $D_{50}W$ prevents hypoglycemia). These effects are seen within 15 minutes, usually peak in 60 minutes, and can last for several hours.

Another medication that promotes the shift of potassium into the cells is sodium bicarbonate. Raising the systemic pH will also release hydrogen ions from the cells; potassium is then shifted back into the cell to maintain a neutral state. You gave sodium bicarbonate, 50 mEq IV. The effects of this therapy are usually seen within 30 minutes and last a few hours.

Beta-2 adrenergic agonists (such as insulin) also drive potassium back into the cells by increasing the Na^+/K^+ ATPase activity needed for the sodium pump. To accomplish this effect, you elected to give 5 mg of albuterol in 3 mL of normal saline via nebulizer. The onset of action of this therapy is about 30 minutes, and the effects last 2 to 3 hours.

During transport, it is imperative to continuously assess the patient's ABCs. This patient's airway has remained patent, his respiratory rate has been 16 to 20 breaths/min, and oxygen saturation has been 98% with 4 L/min of oxygen. Continuous cardiac monitoring has shown a normal sinus rhythm with a heart rate in the 80s, a normal-appearing T wave, and a normal QRS complex at 90 milliseconds.

You have point-of-care laboratory testing available during transport. You check the patient's blood glucose level and find that it is 130 mg/dL. You are also able to test basic electrolytes en route, and the results are as follows: sodium, 140 mEq/L; potassium, 4.4 mEq/L; chloride, 103 mEq/L; and total CO_2, 23 mEq/L. The patient's extracellular potassium level is now within normal limits.

Last, you assess the patient's strength, because he was previously weak. He has a much stronger upper grip strength, which is equal, and has equal and strong dorsiflexion of his feet. His urine output en route is approximately 200 mL. The patient reports that he generally feels much better.

The patient was admitted directly to the ICU, where you gave a report to the nursing and physician staff. The plan was to restart his antirejection medication and monitor serial lab values to see if the hyperkalemia and kidney function improved. If they did not, emergency dialysis would be performed.

Prep Kit

Ready for Review

- Laboratory tests—including laboratory examinations of the patient's blood, urine, cerebrospinal fluid, or other body fluid—can be very useful in determining the seriousness of a patient's condition or preparing for potential problems en route to the hospital.
- A CCTP must know the normal ranges for each lab value, as well as each test's associated physiologic meaning.
- The value of laboratory analysis is determined by the test's accuracy (a marker of whether the value measured by a test conforms to the true value), precision (a marker of tolerance or variation within multiple measurements), sensitivity (the ability of a certain test to accurately rule out a condition), and specificity (the ability of a certain test to accurately confirm a condition).

- A normal range for a test indicates the values that 95% of healthy individuals would have for the particular test. It may or may not be reflective of the patients who are being transported by CCTPs.
- Although abnormal lab values cannot be ignored, it is essential that they be assessed within the context of the patient's entire clinical picture. Abnormal lab values can arise due to acute or chronic conditions and can be due to primary problems or secondary compensatory processes.
- Errors in specimen collection, identification, and labeling or errors in laboratory analysis procedures may result in erroneous values being reported.
- A culture and sensitivity (C and S) report can be determined for any type of specimen.

Prep Kit Continued

The culture results will reveal what is causing an infection; in bacterial infections, the sensitivity results will indicate which antibiotic will most effectively treat the organism causing the infection.

- The ionic components of plasma that are analyzed in the laboratory are known as electrolytes; they include sodium (Na^+), potassium (K^+), chloride (Cl^-), calcium (Ca^{+2}), and magnesium (Mg^{+2}).

- Fluid characteristics assessed in the laboratory include osmotic pressure, which arises in a space divided by a semipermeable membrane owing to differences in the concentrations of solutes (dissolved substances) found in the solutions on either side of the membrane. Osmotic pressure depends only on the number of particles in the fluid, not on the size of the particles.

- Concentration is the amount of a substance present in a given volume of fluid. In the physiologic system, most concentrations are incredibly small, leading to use of units such as millimoles (mmol), milliequivalents (mEq), and milliosmoles (mOsm) to quantify them.

- Different laboratories may have different normal ranges for the same tests. Laboratory reports should always provide the reference ranges for their tests, which are the proper ones to use for the specific patient.

- Thousands of different kinds of proteins are found in the human body, and specific laboratory tests examine the amounts of the various types of protein present in a sample. For example, tests may assess levels of enzymes, which act as catalysts for biochemical reactions.

- In laboratory testing, groups of related tests can be performed as a single unit, called a panel (or profile).

- The basic metabolic panel examines the electrolytes and metabolites in the extracellular fluid; it is one of the most basic and fundamental assessments done in the emergency department or intensive care unit.

- Serum sodium is a convenient marker for a patient's fluid status and is one of the key components of the serum osmolality calculation. An abnormal sodium level will not manifest as electrocardiographic (ECG) changes.

- Elevated sodium levels are treated with diuretics and restricted fluid intake; the net effect of this treatment is expected to be lower intracerebral pressure. Hyponatremia (an abnormally low level of sodium in the blood) is often encountered in patients with endocrinopathies, congestive heart failure, renal failure, or liver disease and in patients taking diuretics.

- Hyperkalemia (an abnormally high level of potassium in the blood) can lead to cardiac arrhythmias. Potassium levels of 5.5 to 6.5 mEq/L can result in the classic peaked T waves on an ECG, with flattened P waves occurring when the potassium level exceeds 7.0 mEq/L. Hyperkalemia can be an artifact of a hemolyzed sample, or it can reflect a true emergency; therefore, this finding should always be correlated with a clinical exam, an ECG, and often a repeat sample.

- Older patients (especially patients taking digitalis) are more likely to develop arrhythmias and ECG changes with hypokalemia (an abnormally low level of potassium in the blood).

- For any patient with a cardiac history, altered renal function, liver disease, or gastrointestinal disturbances, or any patient receiving insulin, a recent potassium level should be available for review before transport.

- Patients with hypochloremia (an abnormally low level of chloride in the blood) may have impending renal dysfunction. Patients taking diuretics may also have abnormally low chloride levels.

Prep Kit Continued

- Venous HCO_3^- levels below the normal range could indicate metabolic acidosis or respiratory alkalosis, whereas elevated levels could indicate metabolic alkalosis or respiratory acidosis.
- Urea, which is considered a useful marker for adequate kidney function, is measured via the blood urea nitrogen (BUN) test. The BUN level tends to increase with age as a consequence of gradually declining renal function.
- Creatinine levels can be used to assess kidney function, although some patients may have an increased creatinine level with adequate renal function. Geriatric patients with increased creatinine levels may have more kidney damage than might be suspected by testing the creatinine level.
- The glomerular filtration rate (GFR) is a measurement of the overall filtration rate of all the functioning nephrons; changes in GFR can suggest improvement or decline in kidney function.
- The glucose level is commonly assessed in the field with a point-of-care testing device, and prehospital care providers often measure the blood glucose level of patients with altered mental status.
- Total calcium is increased in elevated parathyroid hormone states such as hyperparathyroidism and parathyroid-secreting tumors. It is decreased in renal insufficiency, hypomagnesemia, and hyperphosphatemia; in patients who have undergone a massive blood transfusion; and in patients who have a decreased parathyroid hormone state.
- Low levels of ionized calcium can cause serious arrhythmias and are especially pronounced in prolonged cardiac arrest. Calcium administration may be warranted in patients with hyperkalemia, hypocalcemia, or toxic levels of calcium channel blockers.
- Magnesium levels can be affected by disruptions of several body systems, in particular the gastrointestinal and endocrine systems. High magnesium levels are rarely encountered, but low levels may be seen with gastrointestinal distress, vomiting and diarrhea, hepatic cirrhosis, and pancreatitis.
- A complete blood count (CBC) includes measurements of hematocrit (the percentage of cells in a venous blood sample), hemoglobin (the protein responsible for carrying oxygen to the body's cells and, to a lesser extent, CO_2 back to the lungs), red blood cells (erythrocytes), white blood cells (leukocytes, an integral aspect of inflammatory response), and platelets (useful for assessing coagulation status).
- Protein-based tests include those for total protein and albumin. With albumin, abnormally low levels indicate liver disease, whereas abnormally high levels lead to acute respiratory distress syndrome.
- Lactate levels are a global indicator of poor perfusion and oxygenation; they do not indicate which specific tissues are inadequately perfused or oxygenated.
- Lactate dehydrogenase levels can be helpful in diagnosing *Pneumocystis jirovecii* pneumonia, determining the severity of pancreatitis, and assessing patients with implanted ventricular assist devices as an early warning of pump thrombosis.
- Elevated levels of creatine kinase (CK) are indicative of muscle damage, such as in the context of rhabdomyolysis. The MB fraction of CK (CK-MB) can be used as a more specific marker for the diagnosis of acute myocardial infarction.
- Elevations of cardiac troponin I following myocardial injury are detectable in a serum sample after 4 hours; thus, this protein can be used to assess for acute myocardial infarction. High-sensitivity cardiac troponin T (hs-cTnT) tests can accurately detect myocyte damage even earlier.
- The B-type natriuretic peptide (BNP) is released by the ventricles in response to higher

Prep Kit Continued

filling pressures. Its level can be indicative of abnormal ventricular function or heart failure if outside expected ranges.

- Elevated liver function test results may indicate the presence of liver damage. They measure enzymes that normally appear in liver cells, such as aspartate aminotransferase, alanine aminotransferase, bilirubin, and alkaline phosphatase. Different patterns in these tests can be suggestive of hepatocellular damage versus biliary obstruction.

- Tests of pancreatic function include measurements of amylase (an enzyme used by the body to metabolize carbohydrates) and lipase (more specific than amylase for identifying pancreatic disease).

- Lab tests assessing the coagulation system focus on the prothrombin time (the time from creation of thrombin from prothrombin by the enzyme prothrombin activator), activated partial thromboplastin time (used to assess for various diseases), and the international normalized ratio.

- Thromboelastography is a method used to assess the viscoelastic properties of whole blood that combines multiple measurements of platelet function, the coagulation cascade, and their interaction.

- Ethanol (ethyl alcohol) levels are used to assess blood alcohol concentration in the context of alcohol consumption. Owing to the legal implications of ethanol measurements, precise protocols often govern the technique for obtaining the blood sample and storing and analyzing it.

- An increased BUN:creatinine ratio may indicate dehydration, gastrointestinal bleeding, or increased catabolism. A decreased ratio may be present in patients with acute tubular necrosis or autoimmune injury.

- Disturbances in the overall electrical balance of the serum can indicate disease; the anion gap is a measure of this balance.

- A typical arterial blood gas (ABG) panel assesses a patient's acid–base status and oxygen status.

- The acid–base balance (pH)—which is assessed based on CO_2 tension ($Paco_2$), HCO_3^-, and base excess (BE)—indicates how well the body's respiratory and metabolic systems are functioning. Abnormalities result in acidosis or alkalosis.

- Oxygenation status is measured by assessing the partial pressure of oxygen, as well as arterial (Pao_2) and oxygen saturation (Sao_2) levels.

- Assessment of carboxyhemoglobin levels is useful in confirming a diagnosis of carbon monoxide poisoning, and potentially for guiding therapy as well.

- When possible, initial blood samples should be obtained before administering IV fluids or medications.

- If the patient has an IV line and is receiving fluids or medications, the other extremity should be used for taking a blood sample, if possible. If the patient has lines in both extremities, the one without IV medication or without the medication that is being tested should be used.

- CCTPs must be familiar with any point-of-care testing equipment they use and know whether a test they perform is classified as waived, moderate complexity, or high complexity, because this status determines the applicable regulatory requirements.

- Urinalysis involves performing laboratory tests on a patient's urine that range from simple (eg, color or appearance) to complex (eg, specific gravity). Many drugs of abuse (or their metabolites) can be detected in the urine for a considerable amount of time after the drug's use.

- Other tests performed on urine include pH, glucose, ketone bodies (a prominent finding in diabetic ketoacidosis), protein (one of the most important assessments for kidney diseases),

Prep Kit Continued

and blood and hemoglobin (which are not normally found in urine).

- The CCTP should be familiar with diagnostic imaging studies and be able to perform basic interpretation of their results for obvious abnormalities, such as long bone fractures, masses, and catheter placements.
- Radiographic studies are two-dimensional images that can be useful to examine the integrity of skeletal system, identify the abnormal presence of air or fluid, and identify or evaluate foreign bodies.
- Computed tomography (CT) is a three-dimensional imaging modality in which cross-sectional images of a body plane are reconstructed by a computer. A CT scan can reveal abnormalities not seen with traditional plain radiography. The CCTP should obtain a copy of the scan from the transferring facility to expedite care on arrival at the receiving center.
- Magnetic resonance imaging provides for a much greater contrast of the different soft tissues of the body than a CT scan does, which makes it especially useful in brain, spinal cord, musculoskeletal, cardiovascular, and oncologic imaging. This rapidly evolving technology is becoming faster and more accessible over time.
- Positron emission tomography is a functional imaging modality that uses radiotracers to visualize physiologic changes over time or distinguish various levels of physiologic activity between tissues.
- CT polytrauma, also known as a pan-scan, is an imaging protocol that typically includes CT of the head, cervical spine, chest, and abdomen/pelvis to generate a continuous image from the top of the head through the pelvis. Using the CT polytrauma, additional images can sometimes be generated through image reconstruction.
- Cardiac imaging includes a broad array of imaging modalities designed to assess for structural disease, acute coronary syndrome, or inflammatory conditions.
- Ultrasonography does not expose the patient to any radiation and has the advantage of being a very portable imaging technology that can obtain dynamic images over time to assess organ function and guide procedures.
- One of the most common uses of point-of-care ultrasonography in the emergent setting is in the evaluation of trauma. The focused assessment with sonography for trauma (FAST) examination is a standard assessment component in the context of major trauma.
- Ultrasonography is commonly used at the bedside for procedural guidance.

Vital Vocabulary

accuracy A measure of the likelihood that an average of a set of test values will be similar to the true value.

activated partial thromboplastin time (aPTT) A value that represents the intrinsic coagulation pathway's clotting ability; also known as partial thromboplastin time (PTT).

alanine aminotransferase (ALT) An intracellular enzyme found in large amounts in the liver and in the kidney, skeletal muscle, and heart; formerly known as serum glutamic-pyruvic transaminase (SGPT).

albumin The most common protein in the body; it acts as a transport protein, is a free radical scavenger, and serves as the main source of protein-generated oncotic pressure.

alkaline phosphatase An enzyme that is essential for proper digestion and absorption through the mucous membranes in the gastrointestinal tract; it is clinically useful for testing liver function and for diagnosing a common bile duct obstruction.

amylase A key enzyme used by the body to metabolize carbohydrates; it is produced primarily by the salivary glands and the pancreas.

Prep Kit Continued

anion A negatively charged ion.

anion gap (AG) A summary of the relationship among the three major contributors to the overall electrical charge (Na^+, Cl^-, and HCO_3^-); abnormal AG values may signal disturbances in the overall electrical and acid–base balance of the serum and presence of disease.

arterial blood gas (ABG) panel A collection of lab values used to analyze the following characteristics of blood: pH, partial pressure of CO_2 (in arterial blood), partial pressure of oxygen (in arterial blood), concentration of bicarbonate ion, base excess (indicating whether the patient is acidotic or alkalotic), and oxygen saturation of the hemoglobin molecule.

aspartate aminotransferase (AST) An intracellular enzyme found in large amounts in the liver and in skeletal muscle, the brain, red blood cells, and the heart; formerly known as serum glutamic-oxaloacetic transaminase (SGOT).

bacteremia The presence of bacterial infection in the blood.

base excess (BE) A measure of metabolic derangement that is part of the arterial blood gas panel; also known as base deficit (BD), as the value can be either positive (excess) or negative (deficit).

bicarbonate (HCO_3^-) An ion that is present in the blood; its measurement represents the metabolic component of the arterial blood gas panel.

blood urea nitrogen (BUN) A test used to measure urea, which is a biomarker for adequate kidney function.

blood urea nitrogen:creatinine (BUN:CR) A calculated index used to determine the cause of increased levels of blood urea nitrogen and creatinine.

B-type natriuretic peptide (BNP) A polypeptide whose value is indicative of abnormal ventricular function and congestive heart failure.

carboxyhemoglobin (COHb) A measure of the amount of hemoglobin–carbon monoxide complexes in the blood.

cardiac imaging A broad array of modalities used to assess the cardiac system for structural disease, acute coronary syndrome, inflammatory conditions, and other conditions.

cation A positively charged ion.

CBC with differential An expanded panel of lab tests that includes counts of specific types of white blood cells in the blood, such as neutrophils, lymphocytes, monocytes, eosinophils, and basophils.

computed tomography (CT) An imaging modality in which x-rays are used in a 360° rotation around an object to generate a computed three-dimensional model that can be viewed as multiple slices through a given plane; also called computerized axial tomography (CAT) scan.

concentration The amount of a substance present in a given volume of fluid.

C-reactive protein (CRP) An acute-phase reactant used to identify inflammatory response.

creatine A major storehouse of intramuscular high-energy phosphate.

creatine kinase (CK) An enzyme that cleaves the high-energy phosphate from creatine in muscle tissues and transfers it to adenosine diphosphate to yield adenosine triphosphate; its measurement is used in the assessment for muscle damage.

creatinine (Cr) A chemical waste product of creatine that results from muscle metabolism.

CT polytrauma An imaging protocol that typically includes computed tomography (CT) of the head, cervical spine, chest, and abdomen/pelvis to generate a continuous image from the top of the head through the pelvis; also called a pan-scan.

D-dimer test A test of hypercoagulability that detects a fragment from the fibrinolysis process; the test can be used to help diagnose and monitor

Prep Kit Continued

diseases and conditions related to inappropriate clotting, such as deep venous thrombosis.

direct bilirubin Conjugated bilirubin; the result of bilirubin's conjugation in the liver, which is ultimately excreted in the bile.

enzymes Proteins that act as catalysts for biochemical reactions within the body.

erythrocyte sedimentation rate (ESR) The rate at which red blood cells settle at the bottom of a tube containing a blood sample. This test is used to identify inflammatory response and is generally less specific than testing C-reactive protein.

glycosuria The presence of glucose in the urine.

hematocrit The percentage of formed elements (cells) in a venous blood sample.

hematuria The presence of red blood cells in the urine.

hemoconcentration Decreased fluid in the blood, which means that concentrations of other blood components increase.

hemoglobin The protein responsible for carrying oxygen to the body's cells and, to a lesser extent, carbon dioxide back to the lungs.

hemoglobinuria The presence of hemoglobin in the urine.

hemolysis Destruction of red blood cells, sometimes following massive blood transfusions or blood transfusion reactions.

hyperchloremia An abnormally high level of chloride in the blood.

hyperkalemia An abnormally high level of potassium in the blood.

hypoalbuminemia An abnormally low level of albumin in the blood.

hypochloremia An abnormally low level of chloride in the blood.

hypokalemia An abnormally low level of potassium in the blood.

hyponatremia An abnormally low level of sodium in the blood.

indirect bilirubin A by-product of the metabolism of red blood cells that is unconjugated and, therefore, not water soluble.

international normalized ratio (INR) A comparative rating of a patient's prothrombin time to help standardize the prothrombin time when planning treatment.

ionic bond A type of chemical bond formed between oppositely charged ions.

ionized calcium Calcium that is not bound or chelated; also called free calcium. Its value is useful in assessing for renal failure, nephrotic syndrome, acid–base derangements, and decreases or elevations in chelating compounds.

ketone bodies Organic products of fat catabolism—specifically, acetoacidic acid, acetone, and beta-hydroxybutyric acid.

ketonuria The presence of ketone bodies in the urine.

lactate The form of lactic acid that is physiologically present in the body.

lactate dehydrogenase (LDH) An enzyme that catalyzes the metabolism of pyruvate (the end product of glycolysis) to lactate in the absence of a functioning citric acid cycle.

leukocytosis An abnormally high number of white blood cells.

lipase A pancreatic hormone that metabolizes lipids.

liver function test (LFT) A test for liver damage that measures enzymes that normally appear in liver cells but may spill out into the vasculature with parenchymal damage.

magnetic resonance imaging (MRI) A diagnostic imaging technique that uses a powerful magnet to align water molecules present in body compartments to visualize the internal structure and function of the body; a three-dimensional image is obtained from this alignment and the speed at which molecules alter or release.

neutropenia An abnormally low neutrophil count.

Prep Kit Continued

normal range A range of values encompassing the results that 95% of healthy people would have for the particular test.

osmolality The amount of dissolved substance in 1 kg of water.

osmolarity The amount of dissolved substance in 1 L of water.

osmosis The diffusion of water across membranes.

osmotic pressure The pressure created in a space divided by a semipermeable membrane owing to differences in concentrations of solutes found in the solutions on either side of the membrane.

panel Groups of related tests that are performed as a single unit; also called a profile.

partial pressure of oxygen (Po$_2$) A measurement of the amount of oxygen dissolved in the blood.

platelet count A measurement of the number of platelets in the blood, which is useful for assessing a patient's coagulation status.

point-of-care testing (POCT) Testing done outside of a traditional laboratory, usually near where care is being delivered to a patient, with the results of the testing being used for clinical decision making; also called decentralized testing, bedside testing, and ancillary testing.

positron emission tomography (PET) A functional imaging modality that uses radiotracers to visualize physiologic changes over time or distinguish various levels of physiologic activity between tissues.

precision A measure of how a value is likely to be the same every time a test is performed.

procalcitonin A peptide precursor of calcitonin used to identify serious bacterial infection.

prothrombin time (PT) A value that represents the extrinsic coagulation pathway's clotting ability by taking into account various clotting factors, fibrinogen, the prothrombin ratio, and the international normalized ratio.

radiography basic imaging modality that uses x-ray radiation to generate a two-dimensional image of the internal form of an object.

red blood cell (RBC) count A measure of the total number of erythrocytes in the blood.

renal tubule acidosis (RTA) An inability to excrete H$^+$ in the urine, even in the presence of overwhelming metabolic acidosis.

sensitivity The ability of a certain test to maximize the number of true positives that test positive.

specific gravity The chemical property of a fluid that relates its density to the density of water.

specificity The ability of a certain test to minimize the number of true negatives that test positive.

thrombocytopenia An abnormally low blood platelet count.

thromboelastography (TEG) A method used to assess the viscoelastic properties of whole blood that combines multiple measurements of platelet function, the coagulation cascade, and their interaction to form clots.

total protein The total quantity of protein in a blood sample.

troponin A key protein involved in muscle contraction that is present in the serum only after cellular necrosis releases the cellular contents of cardiac muscle (such as after myocardial infarction).

turbid Cloudy or opaque.

ultrasonography A technique for mapping the echoes produced by high-frequency sound waves transmitted into the body; the denser material reflects waves back to a transducer that produces an image. It is typically used for obstetrics, gynecology, and abdominal diagnostics.

urinalysis Laboratory tests performed on a patient's urine.

white blood cell (WBC) count A measure of the total number of leukocytes in the blood.

Prep Kit Continued

References

Abelow B. *Understanding Acid–Base*. Baltimore, MD: Lippincott Williams & Wilkins; 1998.

Allon M, Shanklin N. Effect of albuterol treatment on subsequent dialytic potassium removal. *Am J Kidney Dis*. 1995; 26(4):607-613.

Clausen T, Everts ME. Regulation of the Na, K-pump in skeletal muscle. *Kidney Int*. 1989;35(1):1-13.

Derr P, Tardiff J, McEvoy M. *Emergency and Critical Care Pocket Guide*. 8th ed. Burlington, MA: Jones & Bartlett Learning; 2013.

Evans KJ, Greenberg A. Hyperkalemia: a review. *J Intens Care Med*. 2005;20(5):272-290.

Fischbach FT, Fischbach MA, Stout K, eds. *Manual of Laboratory and Diagnostic Tests*. 10th ed. Philadelphia, PA: Lippincott Williams & Wilkins; 2021.

Garrett RH, Grisham CM. *Biochemistry*. 6th ed. Clifton Park, NY: Cengage Learning; 2016.

Garth D. Hyperkalemia in emergency medicine. Medscape website. http://emedicine.medscape.com/article/766479-print. Updated August 8, 2019. Accessed May 26, 2021.

Kamel KS, Halperin ML. *Fluid, Electrolyte, and Acid–Base Physiology: A Problem-Based Approach*. 5th ed. Philadelphia, PA: Elsevier; 2016.

Christiansen SL, Iverson C, Flanagin A, et al. Table 17.5.2: selected laboratory tests, with conversion factors. In: *AMA Manual of Style: A Guide for Authors and Editors*.11th ed. New York, NY: Oxford University Press; 2020:798-815.

Kee JL. *Laboratory and Diagnostic Tests with Nursing Implications*. 10th ed. Englewood Cliffs, NJ: Prentice-Hall; 2017.

Marieb E, Hoehn KE. *Human Anatomy and Physiology*.11th ed. New York: Pearson; 2018.

Marino PL. *The ICU Book*. 4th ed. Philadelphia: Lippincott Williams & Wilkins; 2013.

Markovchick V, Pons P, Bakes KA. *Emergency Medicine Secrets*. 5th ed. St. Louis, MO: Elsevier Mosby; 2011.

Masterson W, Hurley C. *Chemistry: Principles and Reactions*. 8th ed. Clifton Park, NY: Cengage Learning; 2016.

Parsons PE, Wiener-Kronish JP, Stapleton RD, Berra L. *Critical Care Secrets*. 6th ed. St. Louis, MO: Elsevier Mosby; 2018.

Skobe C. The basics of specimen collection and handling of urine testing. *LabNotes*. 2004;14:1. http://www.bd.com/vacutainer/labnotes/Volume14number2. Accessed May 26, 2021.

Smith B. Preanalytical errors in the emergency department. *LabNotes*. 2007;17:1. http://www.bd.com/vacutainer/labnotes/volume17number1. Accessed April 20, 2009.

Tintinalli J, Stapczynski JS, Ma OJ, et al. *Trintinalli's Emergency Medicine: A Comprehensive Study Guide*. 9th ed. New York, NY: McGraw-Hill; 2019.

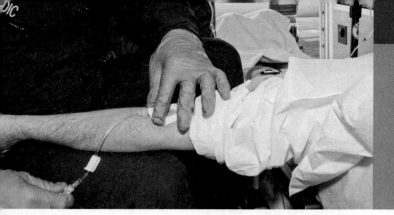

Chapter 10

Resuscitation, Shock, and Blood Products

Amar Deshwar, MD

Sean Kivlehan, MD, MPH

OBJECTIVES

After completing this chapter, you will be able to:

1. Discuss cellular respiration (p 410).

2. Describe oxygen transport and utilization of oxygen by the cell (pp 411–414).

3. Summarize the pathophysiology of shock and its stages: compensatory, decompensatory (progressive), and refractory (irreversible) (pp 414–419).

4. Describe the clinical manifestations associated with the various shock states (pp 414–419).

5. Explain the classification of shock: cardiogenic, hypovolemic, distributive (neurogenic and anaphylactic), and septic (pp 420–432).

6. Identify from a patient presentation which type and stage of shock the patient is experiencing (pp 420–432).

7. Define the following terms: infection, sepsis, sepsis syndrome, systemic inflammatory response syndrome (SIRS), septic shock, and multiple organ dysfunction syndrome (MODS) (pp 419, 430–432).

8. Describe the epidemiology and pathophysiology of shock, sepsis, SIRS, and MODS (pp 432–435).

9. Identify the signs and symptoms that describe the patient in shock, sepsis, SIRS, or MODS (pp 423, 426, 428, 429, 438).

10. Discuss assessment and management of the patient with shock, sepsis, SIRS, and MODS (pp 420–432).

11. List the parameters that should be monitored during the transport of a critical patient experiencing shock, sepsis, SIRS, or MODS (pp 424, 426, 428, 430).

12. Identify the interventions necessary during transport of the critically ill patient experiencing shock, sepsis, SIRS, or MODS (pp 421, 424, 426, 428, 430, 438, 439).

13. Discuss pharmacologic agents used in the treatment of the patient with shock or MODS (pp 427–430).

14. Discuss blood administration, including the ABO blood system, various blood products, and the procedure for administering blood (pp 440–449).

15. Describe the types of adverse transfusion reactions and their etiology (pp 449–451).

16. Summarize management concerns related to blood transfusions (pp 451–452).

Introduction

Shock, sepsis, and multiple organ dysfunction syndrome (MODS) are complex disorders that affect the body in multifaceted dimensions. As unique as each of these conditions is, collectively they share a common denominator—a breakdown in oxygen supply and demand. When oxygen delivery to the cells is compromised, those cells become damaged. A cascade of unfortunate events begins with localized tissue damage and may eventually progress to organ failure and death. Before learning about the pathophysiology of shock, sepsis, and MODS, it is imperative to grasp the basic physiology of how the cell and the microcirculation function. After all, the cell and the microcirculation are the first to experience the insult of inadequate oxygen supply.

Cellular Respiration

All cells require a continuous supply of oxygen, glucose, and other nutrients for normal metabolic function and homeostasis. However, another essential element is also needed for cells to function properly: energy. Energy is required to maintain cellular metabolic processes, much like electricity is needed to power manufacturing plants. The mitochondria within the cell take the nutrients supplied and convert them into energy in the form of adenosine triphosphate (ATP), the primary energy-carrying molecule in the body.

Adenosine triphosphate is manufactured through a complex process known as cellular respiration. Essentially, cellular respiration involves three parts: glycolysis **FIGURE 10-1**, the Krebs cycle **FIGURE 10-2**, and the electron transport chain, otherwise referred to as oxidative phosphorylation. These three components work together in an aerobic environment to produce large amounts of ATP.

The Krebs cycle and the electron transport chain can work only in the presence of oxygen. However, glycolysis—the breakdown of glucose for energy—can occur in an aerobic or anaerobic environment. When there is not enough oxygen for aerobic metabolism of glucose, glycolysis must work alone to produce ATP. This solo attempt to support cellular respiration leads to decreased production of ATP molecules and increased production of lactic acid. As a result, cells are damaged and tissue function is impaired, leading to a cascade of injurious effects.

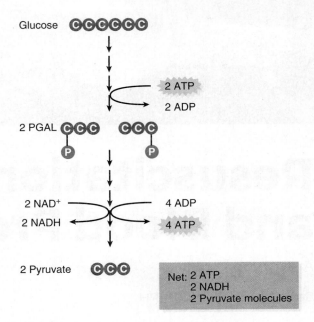

FIGURE 10-1 During glycolysis, glucose is broken down into two molecules of glyceraldehyde-3-phosphate (PGAL), which are converted to pyruvate. The cell nets two adenosine triphosphate (ATP) molecules and two NADH (reduced form of nicotinamide adenine dinucleotide) molecules.
Abbreviation: ADP, adenosine diphosphate

© Jones & Bartlett Learning.

In the ATP molecule, the critical component for energy production is triphosphate. Oxygen molecules connect these phosphate groups to each other within ATP. Under normal conditions, these oxygen molecules have a negative charge and, therefore, repel each other. This property produces the potential energy of ATP. Removing just one of the phosphate groups from this molecule results in conversion of ATP to adenosine diphosphate (ADP) and a release of energy. This conversion from ATP to ADP is crucial for supplying the energy required for biologic functions.

In aerobic metabolism, the ultimate acceptor of electrons is oxygen. The mitochondria use glucose, amino acids, and fatty acids combined with oxygen and ADP to produce ATP, carbon dioxide, water, and heat. The energy is stored as ATP, and the resultant carbon dioxide is eliminated by way of the respiratory tract.

In anaerobic metabolism, an alternative pathway converts glucose to pyruvic acid with the simultaneous production of ATP; however, significantly less ATP results from this process. This process also results in the production of lactate, which is released into the extracellular fluid and

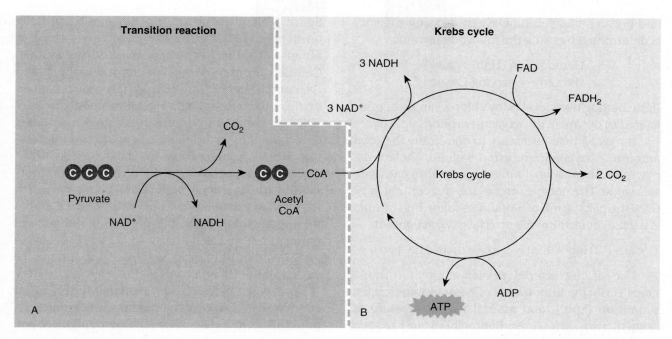

FIGURE 10-2 The Krebs cycle. **A.** Coenzyme A (CoA) is created. **B.** In the mitochondrion, the Krebs cycle liberates two carbon dioxide molecules and produces one adenosine triphosphate (ATP) molecule per pyruvate molecule. Its main products, however, are NADH (a reduced form of nicotinamide adenine dinucleotide) and $FADH_2$ (a reduced form of flavin adenine dinucleotide), which bear high-energy electrons that are transferred to the electron transport system. *Abbreviation*: ADP, adenosine diphosphate

© Jones & Bartlett Learning.

decreases the pH of body fluids. Overall, anaerobic metabolism is less efficient than aerobic metabolism.

Microcirculation and the Cell: Oxygen Transport and Utilization

Understanding the imbalance between oxygen supply and demand is critical to understanding the pathophysiology of shock, sepsis, and MODS. To a large extent, the pathophysiology associated with these disorders can be compared with the mechanisms of injury in trauma. When EMTs and paramedics respond to a vehicular trauma scene, they can identify injuries and correlate the injuries to the impacts the patient endured. Indeed, this activity is part of a good scene size-up. The same principle carries over to understanding the cell and the microcirculation—the nexus between the arterioles and venules, consisting of the capillaries that course between cells of the various organs. These tiny conduits are large enough to allow passage of a single red blood cell (RBC). In cases of shock, sepsis,

and MODS, the "crash site"—that is, the injury and its impact—is hidden deep within the body, at the cellular level.

For cells to function properly, oxygen is required. Oxygen is a key nutrient in maintaining the homeostatic balance within the body. Put another way, the body can maintain homeostasis only when the supply of oxygen is sufficient to meet its cellular demands. To achieve this balance, each of the body's systems must be intact and functioning normally, and the respiratory system must allow oxygen and carbon dioxide exchange across the alveolar-capillary membrane.

Once this transfer occurs, arterial blood transports oxygen to the tissues. Oxygen may be dissolved in plasma (3%) or bound to hemoglobin (97%). Given that the majority of oxygen in the body is bound to hemoglobin, it is important to have an ample supply of hemoglobin. Simple formulas exist to determine the oxygen-carrying capacity of hemoglobin. As a standard, 1 g of hemoglobin carries approximately 1.39 mL of oxygen. (Note: Some texts state that 1 g of hemoglobin carries only 1.34 to 1.36 mL of oxygen, based on the theory that a certain percentage will be bound to methemoglobin, and not to hemoglobin.) Oxygen-carrying capacity is determined by using the following formula:

$$\text{Hemoglobin (Hgb)} \times 1.39 = \text{Oxygen} - \text{Carrying Capacity}$$

If the hemoglobin level is low, blood can be administered to optimize the oxygen-carrying capacity.

It may also be necessary to determine the total amount of oxygen in the arterial blood. The **arterial oxygen content (Cao$_2$)** formula is used to calculate this value. The normal arterial oxygen content is 17 to 20 mL per 100 mL of blood. The following formula is used to determine the arterial oxygen content:

$$\text{Cao}_2 = (\text{Hgb} \times 1.39 \times \text{Spo}_2) + (0.0031 \times \text{Pao}_2)$$

Use of the arterial oxygen content formula helps verify the importance of hemoglobin, oxygen saturation (Spo$_2$), and arterial partial pressure of oxygen (Pao$_2$). However, hemoglobin and oxygen saturation have a greater impact on arterial oxygen content than does Pao$_2$. For this reason, some clinicians use an abbreviated formula for measuring arterial oxygen content:

$$\text{Cao}_2 = \text{Hgb} \times 1.39 \times \text{Spo}_2$$

TABLE 10-1 explains the components of the arterial oxygen content formula.

The cardiovascular system delivers oxygen-rich blood to the tissues. A number of factors can affect this transport process, including blood volume, viscosity, and arterial elasticity. However, the primary determinants of transport effectiveness are blood pressure (BP) and cardiac output.

Systolic blood pressure (SBP) depends primarily on **cardiac output (CO)**, the force and volume of blood ejected from the ventricles during systole. Cardiac output, in turn, depends on heart rate and the components of stroke volume—preload, afterload, and contractility. Diastolic blood pressure (DBP) depends on peripheral resistance, which is determined by arteriolar vasoconstriction. Knowing the BP is necessary to calculate the **mean arterial pressure (MAP)**, which can provide information on how well organs are being perfused. Overall, an adequate cardiac output and a stable BP are essential for proper perfusion and general performance of the body.

The amount of oxygen delivered to the tissues each minute is reflected in the **oxygen delivery (Do$_2$)**. Oxygen delivery is a calculated formula that combines arterial oxygen content with cardiac output. **TABLE 10-2** discusses the components of the formula shown here (CO represents cardiac output, and Cao$_2$ represents arterial oxygen content):

$$\text{Do}_2 = \text{CO} \times \text{Cao}_2$$

If the arterial oxygen content is normal and oxygen delivery is below normal, measures should be taken to enhance the CO. These measures include fluid challenges and administration of an inotropic agent. Once all measures to increase the CO have been attempted, pressor support is used.

When the oxygen-bound hemoglobin reaches the capillaries, the hemoglobin releases the oxygen to the cells in exchange for cellular waste. The amount of oxygen used by the cells and tissues is

TABLE 10-1 Components of the Arterial Oxygen Content Formula

Arterial Oxygen Content Formula: Cao$_2$ = (Hgb × 1.39 × Spo$_2$) + (0.0031 × Pao$_2$)		
Hgb	97% of oxygen bound with Hgb	Hgb × 1.39 = Oxygen-carrying capacity
1.34–1.39 (varies in literature)	Each gram of Hgb is capable of carrying 1.39 mL of oxygen	
Spo$_2$	The amount of oxygen carried on Hgb	Oxygen-carrying capacity × Spo$_2$
0.0031	0.0031 mL O$_2$/100 mL plasma/mm Hg Also known as the solubility coefficient for oxygen	0.0031 × Pao$_2$ = Amount of oxygen dissolved in plasma
Pao$_2$	Partial pressure of oxygen dissolved in plasma (normal is 0.8–1.0 mm Hg)	

Abbreviation: Hgb, hemoglobin

TABLE 10-2 Oxygen Transport and Utilization: Formula Description

Step	Formula Component	Normal Values
Arterial oxygen content (Cao$_2$)		
1. Transfer of oxygen across the alveolar-capillary membrane	$(Hgb \times 1.39 \times SpO_2) + (0.0031 \times PaO_2)$	17–20 mL/100 mL arterial blood
2. Adequate Hgb to carry the oxygen		
Oxygen delivery (Do$_2$)		
3. Adequate cardiac output to deliver the oxygen-rich blood to the tissues	$CO \times CaO_2$	640–1,400 mL/min
Oxygen consumption (V̇o$_2$)		
4. Appropriate release of oxygen from Hgb	$CO \times Hgb \times 13.9 \times (SpO_2 - SvO_2)$	180–280 mL/min
5. Adequate utilization of oxygen by cells	Oxygen extraction ratio (ERo$_2$) $$\frac{\dot{V}o_2}{Do_2}$$	25%

Abbreviations: Hgb, hemoglobin; Pao$_2$, partial pressure of oxygen; Spo$_2$, oxygen saturation; Svo$_2$, venous oxygen saturation

© Jones & Bartlett Learning.

reflected in **oxygen consumption (V̇o$_2$)**. It is calculated as follows:

$$\dot{V}o_2 = CO \times Hgb \times 13.9 \times (SpO_2 - SvO_2)$$

This formula is unique because it subtracts the percentage of oxygen saturation in the venous bed (Svo$_2$) from the oxygen saturation in the arterial bed (Spo$_2$). Mixed venous oxygen saturation (Svo$_2$) is measured much like an arterial blood gas (ABG), except that in measuring the venous saturation, blood is drawn from the distal port of the pulmonary artery (PA) catheter. This value reflects how well the body's tissues are able to extract and use the oxygen attached to hemoglobin. A sample from the distal port of the PA catheter provides a global perspective on how well the tissues are utilizing oxygen. The problem with this test is that some tissues may extract more or less oxygen than others. For example, pulmonary and cardiac tissues extract approximately 40% of the oxygen from hemoglobin. As a result, the Svo$_2$ of venous blood drawn directly from the cardiovascular or pulmonary circulation will normally be approximately 60%. In contrast, the skin typically extracts only approximately 5% of the oxygen from hemoglobin.

Using the tip of the PA catheter to measure Svo$_2$ provides an average of the oxygen extracted from hemoglobin throughout the body. The normal Svo$_2$ level measured in the pulmonary artery is approximately 60% to 80%. When this value is abnormal, there is no way to specify which tissue bed or organ is responsible for the dysfunction. Some specialty catheters allow for direct Svo$_2$ measurements.

Under certain circumstances, oxygen is more readily extracted from hemoglobin or more readily bound to hemoglobin—a property sometimes referred to as hemoglobin's affinity for oxygen. This affinity for oxygen depends on the Pao$_2$, the pH of the blood, the level of carbon dioxide in the blood, the ambient temperature, and the effects of BPG (2,3-biphosphoglycerate—a chemical that binds to deoxygenated hemoglobin, which helps RBCs release oxygen).

The oxyhemoglobin dissociation curve reflects the effects of Pao$_2$ on the oxyhemoglobin saturation of RBCs; this curve is shown in Chapter 6, *Respiratory Emergencies and Airway Management*. Specifically, as the Pao$_2$ decreases, the amount of oxygen bound to hemoglobin in the arterial blood decreases, so that less oxygen is available for utilization by the tissues. A rightward shift of the dissociation curve causes decreased affinity for oxygen by hemoglobin. Conditions that cause a rightward shift include increased carbon dioxide level, BPG level, and temperature as well as decreased pH. A leftward shift of the dissociation curve leads to an increased affinity for oxygen by hemoglobin; in other words, oxygen is more readily bound to hemoglobin, and the body can maintain oxygen saturation with a lower Pao_2. However, release of the bound oxygen to tissues becomes more difficult. The conditions that cause a leftward shift are the opposite of those that cause a rightward shift—namely, decreased carbon dioxide level, BPG level, and temperature and increased pH.

Finally, it is the responsibility of the cells to use the oxygen. The $\dot{V}o_2$ is dependent on the Do_2. The relationship between these two components is reflected in the oxygen extraction ratio (ERo_2), which is defined as follows:

$$ERo_2 = \frac{\dot{V}o_2}{Do_2}$$

Under normal conditions, only 25% of the oxygen delivered to the tissues is extracted. Therefore, the normal Svo_2 when measured in the pulmonary artery is approximately 75%. This allows the body a buffer zone for periods of low oxygen delivery when the cells must extract more oxygen. For example, if the Do_2 drops to 600 mL/min, for $\dot{V}o_2$ to remain within normal limits (180–280 mL/min), the ERo_2 will need to increase 33%. If the $\dot{V}o_2$ drops, cells are forced to work under anaerobic conditions. Mortality rates increase as $\dot{V}o_2$ is compromised. Therefore, treatment is geared toward maximizing $\dot{V}o_2$, which is done partially by maintaining an adequate oxygen supply, providing hemoglobin through administration of blood products, and optimizing cardiac output. If one or more of these components breaks down, the body will suffer a loss of homeostasis.

Shock

Shock is a whole-body response to an inadequate supply of oxygen within cells, tissues, and organs from one or multiple causes. The beginning stages of shock occur at the cellular level. When oxygen supply to the microcirculation is diminished, cells are forced to function in an anaerobic environment, which leads to widespread cellular hypoxia. Shock is a progressive condition that functions on a continuum; however, it is commonly classified into three stages: compensatory, decompensated, and refractory shock.

Compensatory Stage

When the oxygen supply to the microcirculation decreases, as a compensatory mechanism to maintain blood flow to the heart, brain, and adrenal glands, the microcirculatory blood flow to other tissue beds is severely restricted. The initial stage of shock begins as blood flow into the microcirculatory beds decreases to a point that oxygen delivery to the cells falls below the level required to maintain normal aerobic cellular function. Initially, the tissues respond to the restricted oxygen delivery by consuming excess oxygen, thereby increasing oxygen consumption. Eventually, however, the oxygen oversupply is exhausted and cells are unable to extract enough oxygen. The mitochondria cannot function aerobically to produce ATP, secondary to hypoxemia. This anaerobic environment leads to increased lactate and carbon dioxide levels. With ATP production severely reduced, cells are unable to maintain homeostasis and, more specifically, microcirculatory flow to the heart, brain, and adrenal glands.

In the early stages of shock, there are only very subtle clinical signs and symptoms of hypoperfusion, and sometimes no signs at all. Vital signs may change temporarily. For example, the heart rate and respiratory rate may increase, and the MAP may fall somewhat, but the body's compensatory mechanisms are able to return these values to baseline. Research has demonstrated that lactic acidosis begins to increase in the initial stage of shock. Serum lactate elevation is a useful early marker of shock, as it begins to rise before obvious clinical signs materialize. When early signs of shock are recognized, the transport team should increase the frequency of their vital signs checks and monitor the patient closely.

The body uses its own physiologic mechanisms in an attempt to maintain cellular homeostasis. There are three types of compensatory mechanisms, all of which are controlled by the sympathetic nervous system: neural **FIGURE 10-3**, hormonal **FIGURE 10-4**, and chemical **FIGURE 10-5**. The neural mechanism is typically thought of first. It is reflected in the vital signs and physical assessment as an increased heart rate, increased contractility, and vasoconstriction, which help shunt blood to vital organs. In reality, all three compensatory mechanisms—neural, hormonal, and chemical—act simultaneously in an attempt to restore circulating volume and tissue oxygenation. In compensatory shock, the body is still successfully using these mechanisms in an attempt to correct the problem, making it sometimes difficult to

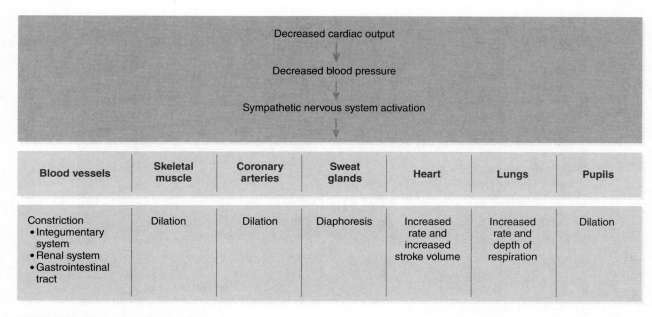

FIGURE 10-3 Neural compensation.

© Jones & Bartlett Learning.

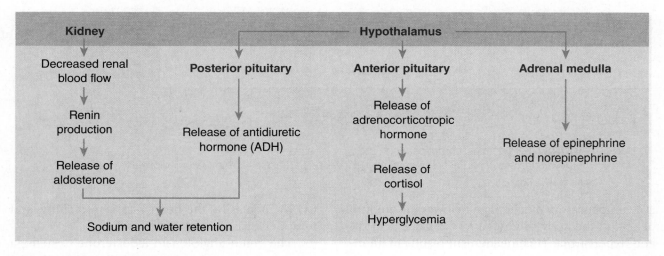

FIGURE 10-4 Hormonal compensation.

© Jones & Bartlett Learning.

recognize the patient in shock. Indeed, signs and symptoms of compensatory shock may be as subtle as mild tachypnea and tachycardia and slightly lower cardiac output.

In compensatory shock, oxygen delivery to the tissues is severely reduced. To compensate for this imbalance, cells try to increase their oxygen consumption by pulling more oxygen from the capillary bed. However, the cells are already working in an oxygen-deprived environment. Trying to work

harder in this anaerobic environment produces more lactic acid and carbon dioxide. Chemoreceptors that are strategically located in the carotid arteries and aortic arch recognize this increase in the carbon dioxide level and relay this information to the brain, which in turn stimulates an increase in the respiratory rate. A patient in compensatory shock may become tachypneic in an attempt to take in more oxygen while concurrently exhaling excess carbon dioxide. Blowing off carbon dioxide

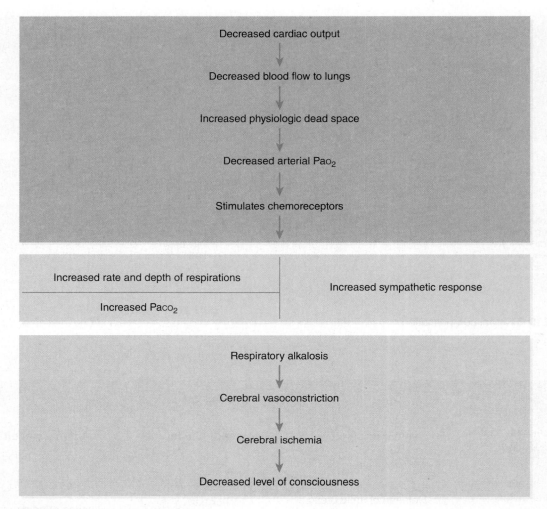

Decreased cardiac output

↓

Decreased blood flow to lungs

↓

Increased physiologic dead space

↓

Decreased arterial Pao₂

↓

Stimulates chemoreceptors

↓

Increased rate and depth of respirations

Increased Paco₂

Increased sympathetic response

Respiratory alkalosis

↓

Cerebral vasoconstriction

↓

Cerebral ischemia

↓

Decreased level of consciousness

FIGURE 10-5 Chemical compensation.
Abbreviations: Pao₂, partial pressure of oxygen; Paco₂, partial pressure of carbon dioxide

is a compensatory mechanism to lower the amount of acid in the body produced by the lactic acidosis and hypercarbia. This mechanism results in an increase in pH.

While the respiratory system is working to balance pH and pull in more oxygen while ridding the cells of waste, the heart and circulatory system are simultaneously attempting to maintain cardiac output. When the stroke volume and MAP begin to fall, baroreceptors in the carotid sinus and aortic arch recognize the change in pressure and send a signal to the vasomotor receptors in the medulla. This activates the autonomic nervous system, which stimulates the sympathetic nervous system and the anterior pituitary to release epinephrine and norepinephrine from the adrenal glands. These hormones work together to increase MAP and CO by increasing the heart rate, contractility, and peripheral vasoconstriction.

The renin-angiotensin-aldosterone system, a hormonal compensatory mechanism, is activated in response to low arterial pressures. Decreased BP stimulates the release of renin, which stimulates first the conversion of angiotensinogen to angiotensin I, and then the conversion of angiotensin I to angiotensin II. Angiotensin II increases arterial BP through four mechanisms: vasoconstriction, stimulation of the thirst receptors in the hypothalamus, stimulation of the release of aldosterone from the adrenal glands, and stimulation of antidiuretic hormone (ADH) secretion from the posterior pituitary gland. Aldosterone increases the circulatory volume by stimulating the reabsorption of sodium and water in the renal tubules.

Low arterial pressures will directly trigger the posterior pituitary gland to release ADH as well. This hormone increases water reabsorption within the kidneys and assists the adrenal hormones in enforcing vasoconstriction to nonvital areas of the body. When vasoconstriction limits the supply of oxygen and blood flow to peripheral areas, shifts in capillary fluid occur. Adequate capillary pressure depends on an adequate perfusion pressure (ie, MAP). When capillary pressure drops, the pressure balance within the capillary bed is lost. As part of the physiology of the capillary pressures, hydrostatic pressure pushes fluid out and osmotic pressure pulls fluid back in. Normally, the hydrostatic pressure at the arterial end of the capillary is higher than the osmotic pressure, causing interstitial fluid to filter through the capillary endothelium into the interstitial space. At the venous end of the capillary, the hydrostatic pressure is lower than the osmotic pressure, causing fluid to diffuse back into the capillary. A loss of the normal pressure balance in the capillaries may lead to edema. Edema results from any disturbance that alters the regulation of fluid transfer in the capillary and interstitial space. Such disturbances can include inflammation (more porous capillaries), decreased colloid osmotic pressure, increased capillary hydrostatic pressure, and lymphatic channel obstruction.

The body's ability to compensate for shock in its early stages often masks what is happening at the cellular level. Compensatory mechanisms can cover up a low circulatory volume, poor stroke volume, and inadequate CO before any noticeable changes in the BP become evident, especially in children and healthy young adults. Even so, other signs—such as tachycardia and tachypnea, which may be subtle—are important indicators of the body's attempt to deal with shock. Laboratory studies are also a useful adjunct to early assessments for shock, as ABGs will show a low pH indicative of acidosis. As mentioned previously, an elevated lactate level in the patient with compensated shock is a concerning finding.

Decompensatory Stage

If its underlying cause remains untreated, shock will progress to an uncompensated state. In this stage, the compensatory mechanisms fail to supply the much-needed oxygen to the cells. Patients with progressive shock exhibit more pronounced signs of shock, including a drop in MAP, altered mental status, and tachycardia. Laboratory analysis continues to show a progression of acidosis, hyperkalemia, and a climbing lactate level.

This clinical picture develops for many reasons **TABLE 10-3**. Hypotension becomes more prominent as the microcirculation loses its ability to autoregulate, leading to increased capillary permeability. Blood starts to pool in the capillary bed, increasing hydrostatic pressure. The marked change in hydrostatic pressure within the microcirculation leads to edema and third spacing, which decreases venous return to the heart—a condition evidenced in a patient in shock by the presence of mottled skin. Hemodynamic effects of this decreased preload

TABLE 10-3 Effects of Shock on the Body	
Organ or System Affected	**Progressive Result of Ischemia**
Heart	Arrhythmias Cardiac failure
Lungs	Pulmonary hypertension Pulmonary edema Acute respiratory distress syndrome
Brain	Ischemia or infarction
Kidney	Decreased urine output Acute tubular necrosis Renal failure
Gastrointestinal	Stress ulcer Ischemic bowel with release of toxins
Pancreas	Ischemia Myocardial depressant factor released
Liver	Hypoglycemia Toxicity
Hematologic and immune	Initial leukocytosis followed by leukopenia Systemic inflammatory response Disseminated intravascular coagulation
Adrenal glands	Adrenal insufficiency, leading to hypotension, and hypoglycemia

© Jones & Bartlett Learning.

are reflected in the BP as hypotension and through other direct and indirect preload assessments. For further discussion, see Chapter 15, *Hemodynamic Monitoring*.

Altered blood flow to the capillary bed, particularly when combined with the inflammation that occurs in sepsis, can cause damage to endothelial cell walls, triggering activation of the intrinsic clotting cascade and development of microemboli. These microclots can form in the tissues and organs, where they inhibit cellular respiration and cause cell damage. The body uses up its clotting factors and fibrinogen faster than the liver can produce them; simultaneously, fibrinolysis occurs in an attempt to reopen the microcirculation. The imbalance between coagulation and fibrinolysis leads to disseminated intravascular coagulation (DIC), a complex coagulopathy that can emerge in critically ill patients for a variety of reasons and cause both bleeding *and* thrombosis FIGURE 10-6. Finally, the movement of RBCs through the microclots damages the cells and can lead to hemolysis—that is, destruction of the RBCs. Rupture of these cells results in the release of hemoglobin and RBC remnants into the bloodstream; in addition, the decrease in the number of RBCs leads to anemia.

Hypotension is also a by-product of increased anaerobic metabolism. Anaerobic metabolism produces a more acidic environment that leads to rupture of the lysosomes, which then spill their contents into the cellular cytoplasm, leading to an even more acidic environment. As the sodium-potassium pump begins to fail, sodium ions accumulate within the cell, eventually drawing fluid into the cell through osmosis. This influx causes cellular swelling and ultimately destruction of the cellular membrane. It is an important consideration in patient management, because a number of devastating effects, such as cardiac arrhythmias, can follow.

As cellular damage becomes more pronounced, cells start to die and release toxins into the microcirculation. For example, lysosomes, which normally defend cells from invaders, rupture and unleash their digestive enzymes, causing further damage within the microcirculation. Cell mediators attempt to counterattack this release and initiate the inflammatory response. The inflammatory response provoked is not isolated to a specific area, but rather occurs throughout the body.

When various complex compensatory components fail, the ensuing vasodilation, smooth muscle contraction, and increased tissue permeability collectively result in hypotension. Unfortunately, this cascade of events only gets worse as clotting mechanisms respond to cell breakdown. The inflammatory response is further discussed in the section on sepsis later in this chapter. The combination of these multifaceted systemic responses to cell breakdown can lead to the process known as systemic inflammatory response syndrome (SIRS), also discussed in detail later in this chapter.

Patients in the decompensatory stage of shock will present as hypotensive, tachycardic, tachypneic, and oliguric, and frequently demonstrate altered mental status. The presence of progressive shock indicates that the body's compensatory mechanisms have failed; this condition is a life-threatening emergency requiring immediate treatment. Patients still have a chance for recovery from this stage of shock, although mortality is significantly increased.

Refractory Stage

When a patient reaches the refractory stage of shock, the body's compensatory mechanisms have failed and permanent organ dysfunction has occurred. Although no consensus definition exists regarding when a patient is in this stage of shock, refractory shock is clinically marked by the need for high-dose vasopressors—though this point is also the subject of debate. At this stage, the survival and outcomes for patients are generally poor, with a mortality rate of approximately 60%; mortality rises to 80% to 90% when greater than 1 mcg/kg/min of norepinephrine is required to maintain a stable MAP.

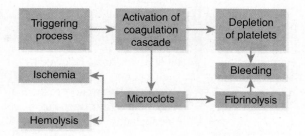

FIGURE 10-6 Development of disseminated intravascular coagulation.

Data from Tintinalli JE, et al. *Tintinalli's Emergency Medicine: A Comprehensive Study Guide*. 7th ed. McGraw Hill; 2020.

A patient in this stage of shock will typically be minimally responsive or unresponsive, severely hypotensive, with cold, cyanotic, and/or mottled skin, and weak and thready to absent peripheral pulses. Urinary output will have progressed from oliguria to anuria.

Multiple Organ Dysfunction Syndrome

Progressive cell death results first in tissue death and eventually in organ failure. When two or more organs stop functioning, the diagnosis of multiple organ dysfunction syndrome (MODS) is made. MODS can be classified as primary or secondary. Primary MODS results from a direct insult such as trauma. Secondary MODS, the more common cause of organ failure, is characterized by a slower, more progressive insult to organs. It frequently results from the sepsis cascade (discussed later in this chapter).

Overall MODS mortality rates range from 44% to 76%. In patients with failure of two to four organs, mortality varies between 10% and 40%, compared to mortality up to 50% with failure of five organs and 100% with failure of seven organs. All organs can be affected in MODS, with some of these changes being amenable to tracking with laboratory values (kidneys and liver), urine output (kidneys), and mental status (brain). A decreased MAP will greatly reduce renal perfusion and function, leading to oliguria. Renal damage is reflected in elevated blood urea nitrogen (BUN) and creatinine levels. Many patients need temporary continuous bedside dialysis to address this renal failure, which greatly increases mortality. Liver damage results in a loss of detoxification ability, decreased clotting capacity, and decreased oncotic protein production. Such damage is diagnosed by markedly increased levels of total bilirubin and liver enzymes, including aspartate aminotransferase and alanine aminotransferase.

As hypotension progresses or hypoxia ensues, there comes a point when the body's compensatory mechanisms can no longer keep the brain adequately perfused and oxygenated. The brain will then experience ischemia, and patients will experience anoxic brain injury with potentially permanent consequences. A broad array of cardiac effects may be seen, including hypotension from decreased cardiac output and arrhythmias from myocyte irritability induced by cellular hypoxia or toxin exposure.

Many inflammatory mediators are released during MODS, which have effects ranging from myocardial depression to vasodilation. These mediators are the focus of ongoing research to better understand and effectively treat MODS.

TABLE 10-4 lists systems and organs commonly affected by hypoperfusion and describes associated signs of dysfunction.

TABLE 10-4 Common Effects of Hypoperfusion

System or Organ	Signs of Dysfunction
Neurologic	Altered level of consciousness Confusion
Pulmonary	Tachypnea Hypoxemia • Pao_2 <70 mm Hg • Spo_2 <90% • Pao_2:Fio_2 ratio <300 Respiratory alkalosis
Cardiovascular	Tachycardia Hypotension Altered hemodynamics • Decreased systemic vascular resistance • Decreased cardiac output • Decreased CVP Arteriovenous shunting • Cellular hypoxia • Lactic acidosis
Renal	Oliguria Anuria Elevated creatinine level
Hepatic	Jaundice Elevated enzyme levels Decreased albumin level Prolonged PT
Hematologic	Decreased platelet count Prolonged PT/activated partial thromboplastin time Decreased protein C level Elevated D-dimer level
Adrenal glands	Hypotension Hypoglycemia

Abbreviations: CVP, central venous pressure; Fio_2, fraction of inspired oxygen; Pao_2, partial pressure of arterial oxygen; PT, prothrombin time; Spo_2, oxygen saturation

Classification of Shock

Shock is traditionally classified by cause. Thus, the three primary classifications of shock are based on the conditions that cause them: cardiogenic, hypovolemic, and distributive. Distributive shock, which is characterized as a relative hypovolemia, can be further broken down into neural and chemical (eg, anaphylactic) causes. More than one type of shock may be present at the same time. For example, many trauma patients present with hypovolemic shock from the injuries they have sustained, but may also have cardiogenic or neurogenic shock.

Cardiogenic Shock

Cardiogenic shock is caused by failure of the heart to pump blood effectively. The definition of cardiogenic shock includes the following elements:

- A sustained SBP of less than 90 mm Hg for greater than 30 minutes

- Hemodynamic criteria including a cardiac index less than 2.2 and pulmonary capillary wedge pressure greater than 15 mm Hg
- Evidence of end-organ damage (altered mental status, urine output less than 30 mL/h, cool extremities, mottled skin)

The diagnosis of cardiogenic shock is made from the combination of clinical presentation, laboratory studies, echocardiography, and electrocardiogram (ECG). If the diagnosis remains uncertain or the presentation is atypical, a PA catheter (Swan-Ganz) can be used to measure central venous pressure (CVP) and pulmonary capillary wedge pressure (PCWP), which will be elevated in left ventricular cardiogenic shock. Measurements from a PA catheter can also assist in differentiating right versus left ventricular heart failure **TABLE 10-5**.

Cardiogenic shock can result from numerous causes, both intrinsic and extrinsic. The most common (intrinsic) cause is left ventricular failure resulting from a large myocardial infarction (MI).

TABLE 10-5 Findings in Cardiogenic Shock

	Left Ventricular Heart Failure	Right Ventricular Heart Failure	Biventricular Heart Failure
Heart rate	Increased	Increased	Increased or decreased
Blood pressure	WNL in the initial stage, then decreases as patient decompensates	WNL in the initial stage, then decreases as patient decompensates	Decreased
Pulse pressure	Narrow	Narrow	Narrow
Central venous pressure/right atrial pressure	WNL	Increased	Increased
Pulmonary capillary wedge pressure	Increased	Decreased	Increased
Cardiac output/cardiac index	Decreased	Decreased	Decreased
Systemic vascular resistance	Increased	Increased	Increased
Svo$_2$	Decreased	Decreased	Decreased
Urinary output	Decreased	Decreased	Decreased
Jugular vein distention	Absent	Present	Present
Heart sounds	S$_3$	Normal	S$_3$ or S$_4$
Edema	Pulmonary	Peripheral	Systemic

Abbreviations: Svo$_2$, venous oxygen saturation; WNL, within normal limits

Other intrinsic causes of cardiogenic shock may include right ventricular failure, valvular disorders, cardiomyopathies, septal defects, papillary muscle rupture, and sustained arrhythmias. These conditions manifest with poor contractility, decreased CO, or impaired ventricular filling. Extrinsic causes of cardiogenic shock include pericardial tamponade, effusion, pulmonary emboli, and tension pneumothorax. Some experts, including those at the American Heart Association, classify extrinsic causes as cardiogenic shock because they lead to impaired filling or emptying of the ventricles, or a combination of the two. Noncoronary causes of cardiogenic shock include myocardial contusion, pericardial tamponade, ventricular rupture, and pulmonary embolus.

Cardiogenic shock occurs in approximately 5% to 12% of patients admitted to the hospital following an MI. Populations at the greatest risk of developing this type of shock are older patients, patients with a history of diabetes mellitus, and patients with a history of MI with an ejection fraction (the portion of the blood ejected from the ventricle during systole) of less than 35%.

Risk stratification of patients in cardiogenic shock formerly was very high, with a mortality rate as high as 80%. Such a high mortality rate led to a very grim prognosis with little chance of survival. In recent years, newer treatment modalities have greatly improved the risk stratification, so that the prognosis for such patients is no longer quite so poor. Recent data suggest that the average mortality rate for cardiogenic shock is now approximately 50%, with the exact rate depending on risk factors and demographics, and patients have an excellent chance for long-term survival. Modern treatment modalities include early percutaneous coronary interventions, early revascularization, hemodynamic management with PA catheters, mechanical support with an intra-aortic balloon pump, and total circulatory support through the use of left-ventricular assist devices, biventricular assist devices, and extracorporeal life support. See Chapter 15, *Hemodynamic Monitoring*, and Chapter 16, *Mechanical Circulatory Support*, for further discussion of these interventions.

Cardiogenic shock occurs when the ventricles are unable to pump blood forward. Because the ventricles cannot contract normally, blood remains trapped in the ventricles. As a result, stroke volume is reduced, ultimately decreasing CO. The five major

determinants of myocardial oxygen consumption are contractility, preload, wall tension, afterload, and heart rate. With inadequate oxygen supply to the periphery, cells must function in anaerobic conditions, enabling the cascade of events leading to SIRS and MODS.

Manifestations of cardiogenic shock vary depending on the underlying cause (Table 10-5). Initially, the patient exhibits signs and symptoms associated with poor CO and low BP. Both right- and left-side heart failure result in hypotension, reflected as a SBP of less than 90 mm Hg for a sustained period or a MAP that is 30 mm Hg below baseline. The decreased stroke volume causes a narrow pulse pressure (less than 25 mm Hg). Patients also demonstrate an altered mental status; cool, pale, diaphoretic skin; and a drop in urine output.

The Meaning of *Pale*

The word "pale," as used in this text, may apply to any patient whose skin presentation suggests reduced blood flow or oxygenation. In general, the mucous membranes inside the inner lower eyelid and the oral mucosa will have a pink coloration in all healthy patients, regardless of their baseline skin color; thus, a white or pale appearance of these areas in any patient suggests reduced blood flow or oxygenation.

Because providers do not necessarily know the patient's normal skin color, they should consider the observations of friends or family members on scene. Simply asking, "Does her skin look like its usual color to you?" or noting when a loved one says, "He's white as a ghost!" may offer useful insight into the person's condition.

The first compensatory mechanism that is likely to be observed is tachycardia. However, the heart cannot sustain or improve CO, and the pulse becomes weak and thready. Heart sounds may be distant, or abnormal heart sounds may appear as S_3 or S_4. Preload is elevated because the heart cannot effectively push the blood forward. This lack of forward movement may cause fluid accumulation in the lungs (acute pulmonary edema), the periphery (jugular vein distention [JVD]), or both, depending on the ventricle(s) affected. Skin becomes cool and clammy as compensatory mechanisms create systemic vasoconstriction. This increases afterload, which in turn increases the pressure that the already struggling myocardium must pump against. If the right ventricle is affected, the right atrial pressure (RAP) and CVP will also be elevated. Cardiogenic shock from right heart failure classically presents with marked JVD and an absence of pulmonary edema.

Analysis of ABGs may reflect hypoxemia with a low Pao_2 level and a corresponding metabolic acidosis with compensatory respiratory alkalosis. Acidosis develops as a result of poor perfusion due to cardiac dysfunction and the heart's inability to pump oxygen-rich blood to the peripheral tissues. Respiratory alkalosis develops as the patient becomes tachypneic and the body attempts to blow off the excess carbon dioxide generated by the increased anaerobic metabolism. Eventually, this compensatory mechanism will fail, in which case the ABGs will reflect metabolic and respiratory acidosis.

Patients with shortness of breath should receive high-flow oxygen therapy, with a goal of maintaining an Spo_2 of more than 92%. One manifestation of cardiogenic shock is pulmonary edema; when it occurs, consider positive-pressure or mechanical ventilation as guided by the patient's clinical presentation and ABG analysis. Supportive therapy is also necessary to eliminate chest pain and reduce anxiety. Arrhythmias are common with cardiogenic shock, so administration of antiarrhythmic agents may be necessary to optimize cardiac function.

Fluid therapy is never wrong when done judiciously **FIGURE 10-7**. Isotonic crystalloids in small 200- to 250-mL (5- to 10-mL/kg) boluses may improve CO. In patients with suspected cardiogenic shock, frequently reassess vital signs, lung sounds, and heart sounds after administering fluid boluses to measure the adequacy of that therapy. Excessive crystalloids may cause new-onset pulmonary edema or worsen existing pulmonary edema.

Inotropic support may be needed to improve contractility, and vasopressors may be necessary for immediate hypotension treatment. The choice of vasopressor for patients with cardiogenic shock is controversial and complicated. Because the use of dopamine has been associated with higher rates of cardiac arrhythmias and mortality, norepinephrine is often the favored first-line therapy in undifferentiated cardiogenic shock. Unfortunately, all vasopressors will increase afterload through

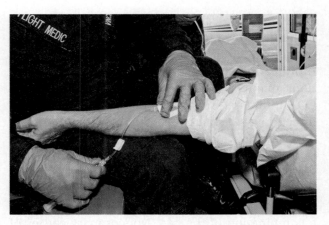

FIGURE 10-7 Administer intravenous fluids judiciously to the critical care patient with cardiogenic shock.
© JHP Travel/Alamy Stock Photo.

vasoconstriction, which in turn will increase cardiac workload and oxygen demand. Dobutamine and milrinone are two alternative options that will improve inotropy without increasing the systemic vascular resistance (SVR). However, these two drugs will cause peripheral vasodilation and should be avoided in the severely hypotensive patient.

Preload and afterload reductions are primary concerns in patients with cardiogenic shock that must be balanced with the need for inotropic and pressor support. Once the BP is stabilized, vasodilators are started. Nitroglycerin and nitroprusside can be used to reduce preload and afterload, respectively; however, these medications must be used in conjunction with close BP monitoring and possibly pressor support. Diuretics such as furosemide (Lasix) or bumetanide (Bumex) are frequently administered as well to reduce volume overload.

Primary management of cardiogenic shock focuses on enhancing CO while decreasing left ventricular workload. If the underlying cause is known, simple procedures to relieve the cause of cardiogenic shock should be implemented first. They may include pericardiocentesis for cardiac tamponade (if protocols allow), along with needle decompression and placement of a chest tube for tension pneumothorax. If the cause is an acute MI (AMI), revascularization should be initiated early (this in-hospital procedure is not performed during transport) and aspirin should be administered. However, clopidogrel (Plavix) and heparin should be administered only in consultation with an interventional cardiologist, as some patients with cardiogenic shock will require coronary artery bypass surgery.

When pharmacologic methods are contraindicated or fail to support the failing heart, both temporary and durable mechanical circulatory-support devices are available for patients in refractory cardiogenic shock. As a whole, the evidence to guide patient and device selection is limited and typically determined by a multidisciplinary team, which will consider multiple patient factors in making this decision. The intra-aortic balloon pump (IABP) is a temporary option for mechanical circulatory support. This large balloon catheter lies in the thoracic aorta and inflates during diastole, displacing blood in the aorta. Balloon inflation forces blood in two directions—back toward the aortic arch and the coronary arteries, and forward through the descending aorta, forcing blood into the peripheral circulation, including the renal and mesenteric arteries. The balloon deflates during systolic contraction, allowing the heart to pump against very low systemic pressures. While this device is still widely used, recent studies have shown no improvement in mortality rates with use of the IABP. See Chapter 6, *Respiratory Emergencies and Airway Management*, and Chapter 7, *Ventilation*, for in-depth discussion of mechanical circulatory support devices.

Other percutaneous options for temporary circulatory support include the Impella, the TandemHeart, and veno-arterial extracorporeal membrane oxygenation. The Impella works as an axial flow pump, with the inflow coming from the left ventricle and the outflow moving through the proximal aorta. This design helps to increase CO and offload the burden placed on the left ventricle. The TandemHeart works as an extracorporeal pump, with the inflow cannula being placed in the left atrium and the outflow cannula in the femoral artery. As both of these devices depend on sufficient left atrial preload, right ventricular failure is a contraindication to use of both the Impella and the TandemHeart. Veno-arterial extracorporeal membrane oxygenation is an increasingly common bridge therapy that can stabilize the patient in cardiogenic shock. A cannula is placed, either centrally or peripherally, in the venous and arterial systems to support the cardiac and respiratory systems via a centrifugal pump and an oxygenator, respectively.

A left ventricular assist device (LVAD) differs from the previously discussed temporary mechanical circulatory support options. In addition to functioning as a bridge therapy to further treatments or a heart transplant, this device can be implanted as a durable option for "destination" therapy, thereby serving as long-term treatment for patients who are waiting on a transplant list or who are not candidates for transplantation. LVADs work by driving a continuous flow from the left ventricular cavity into the ascending aorta. This continuous flow replaces a typical heartbeat on auscultation with a continuous "hum" or machine-like noise, often resulting in a loss of peripheral pulses and rendering the standard noninvasive BP cuffs ineffective in obtaining a BP reading. Instead, the MAP can be calculated by attaching a manual BP cuff to a patient's arm, inflating the pressure to more than 120 mm Hg, and then deflating it while having a Doppler ultrasound probe over the brachial artery and listening for the return of signal. The use of LVADs and other types of assist devices has grown rapidly in recent years, and they appear to be a promising bridge therapy to a heart transplant or recovery.

Hypovolemic Shock

Hypovolemic shock is present when too little blood volume is circulating within the vascular system, resulting in hypotension. Hypovolemia may be present when either internal or external loss of blood or fluids from the intravascular space occurs. Examples of conditions associated with hypovolemia include

---

Signs and Symptoms

Cardiogenic Shock

- Poor CO
- Low BP (SBP of <90 mm Hg or MAP of 30 mm Hg below baseline)
- Altered mental status
- Cool, pale, diaphoretic skin
- Decreased urine output
- Weak and thready pulse
- Distant or abnormal S_3 or S_4 heart sounds
- Fluid accumulation in the lungs or limbs (for example, JVD or pedal edema)
- Tachypnea

Differential Diagnosis

Cardiogenic Shock

- Aortic dissection
- Acute valve rupture
- Chordae tendineae rupture
- Endocarditis
- Myocardial infarction
- Pulmonary hypertension
- Pulmonary embolus
- Pericardial tamponade
- Tension pneumothorax
- Dilated cardiomyopathy
- Restrictive cardiomyopathy
- Acute myocarditis

Transport Management

Cardiogenic Shock

- Perform simple procedures to relieve the cause, including the following:
  - For cardiac tamponade, perform pericardiocentesis if allowed per protocols.
  - For tension pneumothorax, also perform needle decompression and insert a chest tube.
- Provide high-flow oxygen for hypoxia (Spo_2 <92%).
- Eliminate chest pain.
- Reduce anxiety.
- Initiate hemodynamic and cardiac monitoring.
- Provide antiarrhythmic agents if arrhythmias are present.
- Provide judicious fluid therapy.
- Consider administering vasopressors to physician-ordered parameters.
- Consider administering inotropic agents to physician-ordered parameters.
  - Use these medications with caution. Research shows that high doses of inotropic agents lead to a higher incidence of mortality.
- Consider administering diuretics.
- Consider using afterload-reducing agents.
- Monitor urinary output.

fever, vomiting and diarrhea, hemorrhage, burns, and excessive third spacing.

Manifestations of hypovolemic shock are evident early in shock **TABLE 10-6**. The initial stage of hypovolemic shock is characterized by low circulating volume, with minimal signs of hypoperfusion. However, as the body begins to compensate for low venous return, decreased stroke volume, and low CO, patients begin to have tachycardia, hypotension, and signs of poor tissue perfusion, including pallor and delayed capillary refill. Patients become more confused and anxious as oxygen supply to the tissues is compromised and cellular metabolism is altered. Compensatory mechanisms continue to increase the SVR in an attempt to improve hemodynamics. As SVR increases and CO drops, patients exhibit cold and mottled extremities with worsening mental status. Left untreated, the shock will eventually progress to decompensated shock that is refractory to any therapy.

TABLE 10-6 Findings in Hypovolemic Shock

Heart rate	Increased
Blood pressure	Within normal limits in the early stages, then decreases as the patient decompensates
Central venous pressure/renal artery pressure	Decreased
Pulmonary capillary wedge pressure	Decreased
Cardiac output/cardiac index	Decreased
Systemic vascular resistance (SVR)/SVR index (SVRI)	Increased
Svo_2	Decreased
Urinary output	Decreased
Jugular vein distention	Flat
Hematocrit (percentage of whole-blood components versus plasma)	Decreased (with hemorrhage) Increased (with dehydration)

Abbreviation: Svo_2, venous oxygen saturation

The hematocrit value decreases with hemorrhage—but not immediately, as all components of blood are lost equally. A decline in the hematocrit value after blood loss will happen after one to several hours if no fluids are infused in the patient (as interstitial and cellular fluid shifts occur). The hematocrit value decreases faster with exogenous fluid challenges due to hemodilution.

Hypovolemic shock caused by hemorrhage from trauma has been classified by the American College of Surgeons Committee on Trauma into four classes, each of which has its own specific characteristics and treatments **TABLE 10-7**.

Treatment of hypovolemic shock revolves around treating the underlying condition, administering oxygen, and initiating volume replacement. Isotonic crystalloids—that is, normal saline and lactated Ringer solution—are the preferred solutions for fluid resuscitation, and are given in 250- to 500-mL increments to maintain BP in the low normal range. Another option is Plasma-Lyte, an isotonic, buffered intravenous crystalloid solution with a physiochemical composition (140 mmol/L sodium, 5 mmol/L potassium, 1.5 mmol/L magnesium, 98 mmol/L chloride) that more closely

reflects human plasma than either lactated Ringer solution or normal saline. Many trauma surgeons prefer lactated Ringer solution or Plasma-Lyte over normal saline to avoid the development of hyperchloremic acidosis, which can occur in patients with severe hemorrhagic hypovolemia who are given large volumes of normal saline. Whether use of normal saline in this context impacts patient morbidity or mortality remains controversial, however, and all of these solutions will benefit the patient. Alternative solutions for fluid resuscitation, such as hypertonic saline and colloid solutions, have been explored, but have not shown any mortality benefit. For now, replenishment with isotonic fluid consisting of either normal saline, lactated Ringer solution, or Plasma-Lyte is the standard recommendation.

The American College of Surgeons recommends starting blood products in patients with class III hypovolemic shock and beginning a **massive transfusion protocol** for those with class IV hemorrhage. If massive transfusion (more than 10 units of RBCs in 24 hours) is to be initiated, current evidence supports maintaining a 1:1:1 ratio of packed red blood cells (PRBCs), fresh frozen

TABLE 10-7 Estimated Fluid and Blood Loss for a 154-lb (70-kg) Male

	Class I	Class II	Class III	Class IV
Blood loss (mL)	<750	750–1,500	1,500–2,000	>2,000
Blood loss (%)	<15	15–30	30–40	>40
Heart rate (beats/min)	<100	>100	>120	>140
Blood pressure	Within normal limits	Normal	Low	Low
Pulse pressure	Within normal limits	Narrow	Narrow	Very narrow
Capillary refill	Within normal limits	Delayed	Delayed	Absent
Respiratory rate (breaths/min)	14–20	20–30	30–40	>35
Central nervous system/mental status	Slightly anxious	Mildly anxious	Anxious and confused	Confused and lethargic
Skin condition	Cool, normal color	Cool, pale	Cold, pale, moist	Cold, cyanotic
Urine output (mL/h)	>30	20–30	5–15	Minimal or none
Fluid replacement	Crystalloids	Crystalloids	Crystalloids and blood	Crystalloids and blood

Modified from American College of Surgeons Committee on Trauma. *Advanced Trauma Life Support for Doctors: ATLS Student Course Manual.* 9th ed. Chicago, IL: American College of Surgeons; 2012.

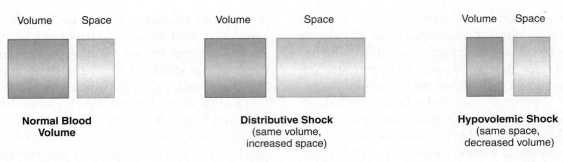

FIGURE 10-8 Conceptual illustration of distributive versus hypovolemic shock.
© Jones & Bartlett Learning.

plasma, and platelets. Of course, any classification system has inherent limitations, so providers must take into account all available clinical information with making decisions about blood product infusion. Some of the confounding factors in this system include patient age (older patients typically have less physiologic reserves), prior use of medications (eg, beta blockers may mask tachycardia), and the time lapse from injury to initiation of treatment.

The next section discusses distributive shock. **FIGURE 10-8** shows a conceptual illustration of distributive versus hypovolemic shock.

Signs and Symptoms

Hypovolemic Shock

- Tachycardia
- Hypotension
- Signs of poor tissue perfusion (pallor and delayed capillary refill)
- Confusion
- Anxiety
- Cold, mottled, and pulseless extremities
- Decreased mentation

Differential Diagnosis

Hypovolemic Shock

- Fever
- Dehydration
- Hemorrhage
- Burns
- Excessive third spacing

Transport Management

Hypovolemic Shock

- Treat the underlying condition.
- Administer oxygen.
- Maintain the airway and ensure optimal ventilation.
- Initiate volume replacement (normal saline, lactated Ringer solution, or Plasma-Lyte in 250- to 500-mL increments).
- Administer blood products early if hemorrhage is suspected.

Distributive Shock

Distributive shock is a catch-all term used to describe several types of shock involving loss of vasomotor tone or increased vascular permeability; it includes neurogenic, anaphylactic, and septic shock. The human body has approximately 60,000 miles of blood vessels and 5 to 6 L of blood. Maintaining homeostasis requires constant regulation of vessel diameter and flow through capillary beds. When a disruption occurs in the vascular compartment causing widespread vasodilation and relative hypovolemia, distributive shock is present.

Neurogenic Shock

Neurogenic shock is a form of distributive shock caused by loss of sympathetic tone, which results in substantial peripheral vasodilation, bradycardia, and altered thermoregulation. Normally, the sympathetic nervous system maintains a baseline level of vasoconstriction within blood vessels, or "tone." Trauma to the brain or spinal cord at the cervical or high thoracic level can disrupt this tone, as the bulk of the sympathetic ganglia reside in the sympathetic trunk running parallel to the thoracic vertebrae.

Neurogenic shock is not limited to trauma, however. Many pharmacologic agents, such as general and spinal anesthetics, opiates, and barbiturates; insulin shock; various toxins; and extreme parasympathetic stimulation may trigger the onset of neurogenic shock. It is important to differentiate neurogenic shock from spinal shock, which is a different entity. Spinal shock is a temporary loss of spinal function following trauma, which recovers after a variable amount of time; it is thought to represent a concussion injury to components of the spinal cord.

Neurogenic shock is characterized by relative hypovolemia as the result of vasodilation. In essence, the amount of fluid in the vasculature remains constant, but the container size is increased. As a result, there are significant drops in the SVR and BP. The signs and symptoms associated with neurogenic shock, however, can be very different from those found in hypovolemic shock **TABLE 10-8**. One profound difference is the presence of bradycardia in the face of hypotension; it is caused by the combination of loss of sympathetic tone and baroreceptor response. Nevertheless, neurogenic shock is a diagnosis of exclusion in the emergent setting, and all hypotensive trauma patients should initially be assumed to be bleeding.

Treatment for neurogenic shock focuses on immediate correction of hypotension. The MAP should be maintained between 85 and 90 mm Hg for the first 7 days following injury if the cause of the neurogenic shock is incomplete spinal cord injury with potential for some recovery of function. Aggressive fluid therapy with isotonic crystalloids should be started, and a transition should be made to inotropes and vasopressors if needed.

Dopamine, norepinephrine (Levophed), and phenylephrine (Neo-Synephrine) are the vasopressor agents that are most commonly used in neurogenic shock. Norepinephrine and phenylephrine raise the BP by directly stimulating alpha adrenergic receptors in the smooth muscle of blood vessels,

TABLE 10-8 Hemodynamic Findings in Distributive Shock Compared With Hypovolemic Shock			
	Hemodynamic Findings in Distributive Shock		
	Neurogenic Shock	**Anaphylactic Shock**	**Comparison With Hypovolemic Shock**
Heart rate	Decreased	Increased	Increased
Blood pressure	Decreased	Decreased	Within normal limits in the initial stage, then decreases as the patient decompensates
Pulse pressure	Normal	Narrow	Narrow
Central venous pressure/ renal artery pressure	Decreased	Decreased	Decreased
Pulmonary capillary wedge pressure	Decreased	Decreased	Decreased
Cardiac output/cardiac index	Decreased	Decreased	Decreased
Systemic vascular resistance (SVR)/SVR index (SVRI)	Decreased	Decreased	Increased
Svo$_2$	Decreased	Decreased	Decreased
Urinary output	Decreased	Decreased	Decreased
Skin	Normal color, warm, dry	Flushed, warm to hot, pruritus, hives	Cool, pale, moist

Abbreviation: Svo$_2$, venous oxygen saturation

causing vasoconstriction. Dopamine, when given in moderate doses, stimulates beta-1 adrenergic receptors, increasing the force of contraction and, therefore, increasing CO. Higher dopamine doses stimulate alpha adrenergic receptors, mimicking the effects of norepinephrine.

Controlling the heart rate is also important in patients with neurogenic shock. Loss of sympathetic tone may result in profound bradycardia. Methods for increasing the heart rate include pacemaker therapy and administration of atropine. Atropine works by blocking acetylcholine (muscarinic) receptors, creating a temporary increase in heart rate.

Transport considerations for patients with neurogenic shock center on ensuring a patent airway, adequate ventilation, and oxygenation: Depending on the level of involvement, the patient may

Signs and Symptoms

Neurogenic Shock
- Relative hypovolemia as the result of vasodilation
- Bradycardia
- Significant drop in BP
- Normal pulse pressure
- Decreased CVP/RAP
- Decreased PCWP
- Decreased CO/cardiac index
- Significant drop in the SVR/SVRI
- Decreased Svo_2
- Decreased urinary output
- Normal color, warm, dry skin

Differential Diagnosis

Neurogenic Shock
- Spinal shock
- Hypovolemic shock
- Trauma to the brain or spinal cord
- Pharmacologic agents such as general and spinal anesthetics, opiates, and barbiturates
- Insulin shock
- Toxins
- Extreme parasympathetic stimulation

Transport Management

Neurogenic Shock
- Correct hypotension immediately.
- Maintain a MAP of 85 to 90 mm Hg for the first 7 days following injury.
- Consider administering vasopressors (dopamine, norepinephrine, phenylephrine). Administer inotropic agents and vasopressors if traditional fluid resuscitation is insufficient to maintain the MAP.
- Initiate fluid therapy with isotonic crystalloids.
- Maintain the heart rate (increase heart rate via pacemaker therapy or atropine administration).

be unable to breathe without assistance or may have impaired ventilatory capabilities. Care also includes cardiac monitoring, administration of IV fluids and vasopressor medications as ordered, and maintenance of spinal motion restriction. The patient also requires placement of an indwelling urinary catheter.

Anaphylactic Shock

Anaphylactic shock is a severe, life-threatening allergic reaction producing systemic vasodilation in response to histamine release. The list of possible antigens in humans is extensive, including diagnostic agents, foods, bites, stings, chemical agents, and several classes of medications, such as antibiotics, immunologic agents, anesthetics, anti-inflammatory agents, narcotics, and hormones.

Two types of anaphylactic shock are distinguished: true and anaphylactoid. **True anaphylaxis** occurs when the allergen binds to immunoglobulin E (IgE) on the cell membranes of basophils and mast cells, stimulating the release of histamine from the cell. In contrast, an **anaphylactoid reaction** is a non–IgE-mediated response that causes the rupture of mast cells and basophils, which then release histamine and other defense mediators. Non–IgE-mediated responses can result in the same reactions as true shock without prior exposure to the antigen. Either reaction can be massive and can happen in minutes after exposure. Alternatively, the response may be delayed for hours or even days—a condition called a delayed hypersensitivity response.

Histamine, a cell mediator, is responsible for the widespread vasodilation and resultant relative hypovolemia, increased capillary membrane permeability, and smooth muscle constriction associated with anaphylactic shock. Increased capillary membrane permeability leads to oropharyngeal and laryngeal edema, and smooth muscle constriction contributes to bronchoconstriction; together, these effects can produce rapid life-threatening airway compromise.

Rapid treatment is necessary to limit the effects of anaphylaxis. Notably, standard oxygen therapy may not be enough to ensure adequate oxygenation. Some patients may need to be intubated, and some may require an emergency cricothyrotomy or tracheostomy to maintain an adequate airway.

Treatment focuses on removing the allergen that caused the severe reaction, including discontinuing the medication causing the reaction or simply removing a stinger after a bee sting. Drug therapy for anaphylaxis focuses on supporting the cardiovascular system and preventing further mediator release. Epinephrine is the drug of choice for anaphylactic shock because it acts as a physiologic antagonist to the leukotrienes and other cell mediators released in anaphylaxis. Epinephrine increases BP through stimulation of alpha-1 receptors, which leads to vasoconstriction. It also has bronchodilation effects owing to its activation of the beta-2 receptors. The initial dose of epinephrine is 0.3 to 0.5 mg (0.3 to 0.5 mL) of a 1 mg in 1 mL solution intramuscularly, given every 5 to 10 minutes as needed. If hypotension persists, initiating an epinephrine drip may be necessary. Epinephrine may not work effectively in patients taking beta blockers; in these cases, glucagon may be given IV at 5 to 15 µg/min. Glucagon mitigates anaphylaxis by increasing the heart rate and contractility via non–beta-receptor-mediated pathways.

Owing to the increased "container size" associated with anaphylactic shock, fluid therapy needs to be started early to maintain a MAP of greater than 65 mm Hg (or a SBP of greater than 90 mm Hg). Normal saline should be administered to sustain adequate preload volumes. Further vasopressor agents may be started if crystalloid therapy and epinephrine prove inadequate in maintaining CO.

Some other pharmacologic agents are also commonly given as treatments for anaphylactic shock; however, clinical data demonstrating their benefits are lacking, so they should be considered second-line agents, with epinephrine being the treatment of choice. Antihistamines such as diphenhydramine (Benadryl) are used to block histamine release from the H_1 receptors on smooth muscles, gland cells, and some nerve endings. The dose of diphenhydramine is 1 to 2 mg/kg IV, repeated every 4 to 8 hours, not to exceed 50 mg. Ranitidine (Zantac), an H_2 blocker, is sometimes used to treat severe allergic reactions because of its effects on the heart, along with its ability to decrease stimulation of acid secretion within the stomach. Bronchodilators are administered to relieve the shortness of breath associated with anaphylaxis. Albuterol is a beta-2 selective bronchodilator that works as a physiologic antagonist toward leukotrienes and other inflammatory mediators, thereby relaxing smooth muscle. Corticosteroids are often given to stabilize the capillary membrane, offsetting the inflammatory response in an effort to prevent a delayed reaction; however, this effect has never been proven.

While anaphylactic reactions following a biphasic course were previously believed to be highly common, newer studies have found that only 4% to 4.5% of such reactions are actually biphasic. The timing of the biphasic reaction has been shown to occur across a relatively wide range, between 1 and 72 hours after the initial reaction. While corticosteroids are often given to patients with anaphylaxis, there is no consensus on whether their administration has a role in preventing the biphasic reaction.

Signs and Symptoms

Anaphylactic Shock
- Increased heart rate
- Decreased BP
- Narrow pulse pressure
- Decreased CVP/RAP
- Decreased PCWP
- Decreased CO/cardiac index
- Decreased SVR/SVRI
- Decreased Svo_2
- Decreased urinary output
- Flushed skin that is warm to hot, with pruritus and hives
- Bronchoconstriction
- Laryngeal edema
- Angioedema
- Airway compromise

Other Forms of Distributive Shock

Additional forms of distributive shock include endocrine causes such as addisonian crisis from mineralocorticoid deficiency, myxedema crisis from hypothyroidism, and thyrotoxicosis such as in thyroid storm. These conditions are covered in Chapter 18, *Endocrine Emergencies*. The most common cause of distributive shock is sepsis, which is a progressive disease that typically results from an infection.

Sepsis

Sepsis is life-threatening organ dysfunction caused by a dysregulated host response to infection. It is part of a spectrum of disease culminating in septic shock, whose distinct classifications and treatment approaches have been outlined by a joint task force sponsored by the European Society of Intensive Care Medicine and the Society of Critical Care Medicine. Initially released in 1991, sepsis definitions and guidelines have been updated several times, most recently in 2016. This section describes the continuum of the disease and then provides a detailed discussion of the pathophysiology, assessment, and management of sepsis.

Types of Sepsis

Systemic inflammatory response syndrome (SIRS) is a widespread inflammatory process with both infectious and noninfectious causes. Acute respiratory distress syndrome (ARDS), burns, pancreatitis, intestinal endotoxins, and major trauma are the most commonly identified triggers for the development of SIRS when no microorganism is involved.

Four variables—temperature, heart rate, respiratory rate, and white blood cell (WBC) count—are used to identify SIRS **TABLE 10-9**. In the past, sepsis was defined as the presence of two or more markers

TABLE 10-9 Systemic Inflammatory Response Syndrome Criteria[a]

Criteria	Marker
Temperature	>38°C (100.4°F) <36°C (96.8°F)
Respiratory rate	>20 breaths/min Pao_2 <32 mm Hg
Pulse rate	>90 beats/min
White blood cell (WBC) count	>12,000/μL <4,000/μL >10% immature band forms

[a]Criteria from the American College of Chest Physicians, 1992.

Data from Levy MM, et al. 2001 SCCM/ESICM/ACCP/ATS/SIS International Sepsis Definitions Conference. *Intens Care Med.* 2003;29(4):530-538.

of sepsis in the setting of a suspected infection. However, the 2016 revision acknowledged that SIRS criteria can be met in noninfected people or not met in infected people, and the presence of these markers is often simply reflective of the body's normal response to infection.

The current diagnosis of sepsis includes the presence of organ dysfunction in the setting of infection. Organ dysfunction is defined by an increase in the Sequential [Sepsis-related] Organ Failure Assessment (SOFA) score of 2 points or more, which is associated with an in-hospital mortality greater than 10% **TABLE 10-10**. Recognizing that the SOFA score variables are rarely obtained outside of the intensive care unit (ICU), the 2016 guidelines introduced the quick SOFA (qSOFA) score to rapidly identify a patient with sepsis at the bedside. In this setting, sepsis is diagnosed if two of the following three signs are present: respiratory rate of 22 breaths/min or greater, altered mentation, or SBP of 100 mm Hg or less. Subsequent studies have challenged the qSOFA's utility as a screening tool, however, demonstrating that this score has reduced sensitivity in detecting sepsis in comparison to the SIRS criteria, with the highest sensitivity found with the use of the National Early Warning Score (NEWS) **TABLE 10-11**. The NEWS is a scoring system derived from six physiologic parameters: respiratory rate, oxygen saturation, SBP, pulse rate, level of consciousness or new confusion, and temperature.

Septic shock is defined as fluid-unresponsive hypotension requiring a vasopressor to maintain a MAP of 65 mm Hg or greater and a serum lactate

TABLE 10-10 Sequential [Sepsis-Related] Organ Failure Assessment (SOFA) Score

System	Score				
	0	1	2	3	4
Respiration Pao$_2$/Fio$_2$, mm Hg (kPa)	≥400 (53.3)	≤400 (53.3)	<300 (40)	>200 (26.7) with respiratory support	<100 (13.3) with respiratory support
Coagulation Platelets, × 10^3/μL	≥150	<150	<100	<50	<20
Liver Bilirubin, mg/dL (μmol/L)	<1.2 (20)	1.2–1.9 (20–32)	2.0–5.9 (33–101)	6.0–11.9 (102–204)	>12.0 (204)
Cardiovascular	MAP ≥70 mm Hg	MAP <70 mm Hg	Dopamine <5 or dobutamine (any dose)	Dopamine 5.1–15 or epinephrine ≤0.1 or norepinephrine ≤0.1[a]	Dopamine > 15 or epinephrine >0.1 or norepinephrine >0.1[a]
Central nervous system Glasgow Coma Scale score[b]	15	13–14	10–12	6–9	<6
Renal Creatinine, mg/dL (μmol/L) Urine output, mL/d	<1.2 (110)	1.2–1.9 (110–170)	2.0–3.4 (171–299)	3.5–4.9 (300–440) <500	>5.0 (440) <200

Abbreviations: Fio$_2$, fraction of inspired oxygen; MAP, mean arterial pressure; Pao$_2$, partial pressure of oxygen

[a]Catecholamine doses are given as μg/kg/min for at least 1 hour.

[b]Glasgow Coma Scale scores range from 3 to 15; higher scores indicate better neurologic function.

Data from Vincent JL, Moreno R, Takala J, et al; Working Group on Sepsis-Related Problems of the European Society of Intensive Care Medicine. The SOFA (Sepsis-related Organ Failure Assessment) score to describe organ dysfunction/failure. *Intens Care Med*. 1996;22(7):707-710.

TABLE 10-11 National Early Warning Score (NEWS)

Score Value	3	2	1	0	1	2	3
Respiratory rate (breaths/min)	≤8		9–11	12–20		21–24	≥25
Spo$_2$ saturation (%)	≤91	92–93	94–95	≥96			
Added o$_2$		Yes		No			
Systolic blood pressure (mm Hg)	≤90	91–100	101–110	111–219			≥220
Heart rate (beats/min)	≤40		41–50	51–90	91–110	111–130	≥131
Level of consciousness[a]				A			V, P, or U
Temperature (°C)	≤35		35.1–36	36.1–38	38.1–39	≥39	

[a]Letters taken from AVPU: Awake and alert, responsive to Verbal stimuli, responsive to Pain, Unresponsive.

Data from Smith GB, Prytherch DR, Meredith P, et al. The ability of the National Early Warning Score (NEWS) to discriminate patients at risk of early cardiac arrest, unanticipated intensive care unit admission, and death. CORE website. https://core.ac.uk/reader/74204518?utm_source=linkout. Accessed July 14, 2021.

level greater than 2 mmol/L (>18 mg/dL) in the absence of hypovolemia. These patients are critically ill and have a mortality rate exceeding 40%.

Epidemiology

Determining the exact number of sepsis cases per year is difficult, as definitions have varied over the years. Nevertheless, all reports agree on one point: The incidence of sepsis-related infections is increasing. An estimated 1.7 million cases of sepsis occur each year in the United States, according to the Centers for Disease Control and Prevention. As this trend continues, CCTPs will likely encounter more cases of sepsis.

Although sepsis affects all populations and age groups, the majority of cases occur in people older than 65 years. This condition is most prevalent in nonwhite males between the ages of 57 and 70 years. A number of coexisting medical conditions have been closely associated with sepsis, including diabetes, hypertension, congestive heart failure, chronic obstructive pulmonary disease (COPD), cirrhosis, human immunodeficiency virus (HIV) infection, cancer, and pregnancy.

The mortality rate for sepsis is roughly 20%, but it increases significantly as the severity of sepsis increases. Septic shock has a reported mortality rate of more than 40% and is a leading cause of death in ICUs.

Despite the development of sophisticated technologies and advancements in medical therapies, sepsis remains a challenge to the medical community. Mortality rates have been decreasing, though, likely due to aggressive management of this condition. Health care professionals must be aware of the many risk factors associated with sepsis to keep mortality rates low. The conditions that place people at greatest risk for developing sepsis are listed in **TABLE 10-12**. Prolonged hospitalization is also a risk factor for sepsis for any person. The longer a patient remains in the ICU (especially) or the hospital, the greater the risk for sepsis becomes. Invasive procedures, comorbidities, and use of immunosuppressants increase this risk even further.

Pathophysiology

To understand the pathophysiology of sepsis, it is necessary to review some basic anatomy and physiology of the immune system. The immune response is typically classified into innate and adaptive arms.

The **innate immune system** is the first line of defense, including what is commonly referred to as the inflammatory response. It represents a generalized, fast-acting response to antigen recognition and is accomplished through the actions of neutrophils, macrophages, natural killer (NK) cells, and complement.

The **adaptive immune system** employs lymphocytes, antibodies, and memory cells; it offers a more

TABLE 10-12 Risk Factors for Sepsis	
Patients with a compromised immune system	Extremes of age: infants and older patients Patients with cancer Transplant recipients Patients with HIV/AIDS Patients with immunosuppressed systems Patients with alcoholism Pregnancy
Chronic and coexisting diseases	Diabetes Chronic obstructive pulmonary disease Cirrhosis Heart failure Renal failure
Infections and exposures	Meningitis Community-acquired pneumonia Cellulitis Urinary tract infections Organisms with antimicrobial resistance
Patients who are critically ill	Increased use of invasive catheters and prosthetic devices Postoperative abdominal surgery

Abbreviations: AIDS, acquired immunodeficiency syndrome; HIV, human immunodeficiency virus

© Jones & Bartlett Learning.

precise response to specific antigens, but requires time to mobilize its defense if the pathogen is unknown. This aspect of the immune response is called "adaptive" because it creates a targeted response to an invading pathogen based on its exposed antigenic signatures. Memory cells remember specific antigens with which they have previously come in contact, so when an antigen tries to invade again, the adaptive immune system can mount a faster response to it.

Taken together, the innate and adaptive immune systems provide a robust immune response that protects the human body from disease. However, prolonged and extensive activation of this system is responsible for many of the problems that arise in patients with sepsis.

Pathogens

The microorganisms that activate the immune system are referred to as pathogens. Sepsis can occur as a result of infection at any body site, including the lungs, abdomen, skin, soft tissue, urinary tract, bloodstream, and central nervous system. Bacteria are the pathogens most commonly associated with the development of sepsis, although fungi, viruses, and parasites can cause this condition as well. Each pathogen has identifiers on it called antigens that can elicit an immune response within the body. A pathogen is recognized in the body when its antigen binds to special cells within the immune system known as antigen-presenting cells (APC); they include B cells, dendritic cells, and macrophages. An APC will engulf, digest, and finally "present" the antigen on its own surface, where T cells can encounter and develop a targeted immune response to the antigen.

This powerful response system must be prevented from attacking the normal body structures and, therefore, must be capable of classifying antigens as "self" or "nonself." Problems with this system can lead to various autoimmune conditions, with its overreaction being responsible for allergies and anaphylaxis.

In addition to the infectious agents just described, the human body is colonized by symbiotic bacterial flora, which assist in digestion and several other functions. The immune system keeps the flora in balance; disruptions of this balance can lead to overgrowth and undergrowth, both of which have negative consequences such as gastrointestinal (GI) upset and yeast infections.

Infectious agents may produce endotoxins and exotoxins that alter the living cells and ultimately destroy them. This action is the primary way that bacteria affect the immune system stimulus response and cause cell death. Endotoxins are lipopolysaccharides that coat the outer surface of gram-negative bacteria and elicit strong immune responses in humans while providing a layer of protection for the bacterium. The bacterial cell can also secrete endotoxins and release them en masse when cell death occurs. Exotoxins are proteins secreted by some bacteria that can directly cause significant damage to host cells while also triggering an immune response.

Gram-negative and gram-positive bacteria are the two types of organisms most commonly responsible for sepsis. A large study of infection among ICU patients showed that positive isolates consisted of 62% gram negative, 47% gram positive, and

17% fungal organisms (with some patients growing multiple organisms). Approximately one-third of patients with sepsis will have negative cultures.

Infection

Infection is the invasion of normally sterile tissue by a pathogen, and bacteremia is the presence of viable bacteria in the bloodstream. The body's first lines of defense against pathogens are its natural barriers—for example, the skin, mucous membranes, and GI tract. Typically, when an infection develops, it is because a pathogen was able to penetrate these natural barriers. Normally, these barriers mitigate infection by inhibiting the entry of nonself pathogens into the body and by keeping a careful watch over self antigens.

Isolated infections are confined to a small area, with the invading organisms being destroyed by immune cells within that location. Components of the innate system recognize foreign antigens through the pattern recognition receptors that activate them and similar cells in the area, initiating the inflammatory process. Characteristic changes in the microcirculation (arterioles, capillaries, and venules) occur near the site of injury secondary to inflammation:

- Blood vessels dilate, increasing blood flow to the area.
- Vascular permeability increases, facilitating an influx of fluid and plasma cells (exudate) into the area.
- Certain WBCs (neutrophils) adhere to the inner walls of vessels and then migrate through the vessel walls to the site of injury. While destroying the pathogen, these phagocytic cells cause the release of lytic enzymes, which are potent enough to damage healthy cells near the area of injury.

Numerous chemical mediators, called cytokines, are released from injured cells (the endothelium of the microcirculation) in response to tissue insult. Some of these cytokines include interleukins, tumor necrosis factor (TNF), histamine, prostaglandins, and bradykinins. These chemicals cause vasodilation, smooth muscle contraction, increased tissue permeability, and pain **TABLE 10-13**. Inflammation is an important process because it helps contain the injury, allowing phagocytes and the complement system to clean up the area.

TABLE 10-13 The Body's Response to Inflammatory Chemical Mediators

Inflammatory Chemical Mediator Action	Body Response
Vasodilation	Redness and heat production
Smooth muscle contraction	Difficulty breathing
Increased capillary permeability	Edema and swelling
Stimulation of pain receptors	Pain

© Jones & Bartlett Learning.

Cytokine communicators also send out distress signals informing the body of the injury. These signals attract neutrophils to the site of infection. There, these WBCs move through the endothelial wall to the site of injury, where they begin their phagocytic role.

Vasodilation and increased capillary permeability also activate the clotting pathways. Tissue factor is released, leading to the production of thrombin, a pro-inflammatory substance that initiates fibrin clot formation in the microvasculature. Fibrin is the final product of the coagulation cascade and is responsible for preventing the spread of infection by building a fibrin clot barrier wall.

Systemic Infection

Systemic infections activate a widespread inflammatory response throughout the body, completely overwhelming and theoretically confusing the immune system **FIGURE 10-9**. SIRS, sepsis, and septic shock are part of a dynamic hypermetabolic, hyperinflammatory response to an infection that leads to a loss of control of the immune response. Left unchecked, the vasodilation and permeability that are initially helpful in fighting an infection may progress to distributive shock.

Sepsis disrupts normal inflammatory modulators. This is an area of intense research, and many mediators that participate in this process have already been identified. Interleukins, TNF, and other cytokines whose release leads to fever, edema, and tissue hypoperfusion are produced rapidly after

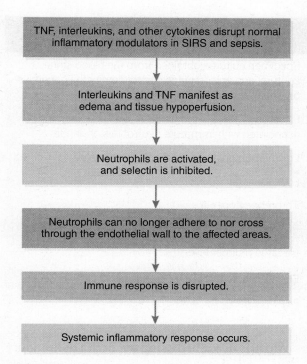

FIGURE 10-9 Summary of the process leading to a systemic inflammatory response.
Abbreviations: SIRS, systemic inflammatory response syndrome; TNF, tumor necrosis factor

© Jones & Bartlett Learning.

insult or injury, and they continue to proliferate as the inflammatory process continues. These chemical mediators lead to activation of neutrophils while simultaneously inhibiting selectin, the protein that adheres neutrophils to the endothelium, allowing these WBCs to move into tissue to fight infection.

The inflammatory process, in association with the complement cascade, damages the endothelium, causing small clots to form in the capillaries. These microemboli can lead to DIC, as described earlier (see Figure 10-6). The progression of DIC is difficult to control and has been the focus of significant research looking for therapeutic modalities.

In summary, microvascular disruption and injury are responsible for hypoperfusion and the shunting of oxygen, resulting in decreased oxygen delivery to the tissues. The profound imbalance between oxygen delivery and consumption causes hypoxia within the cell and tissue. This complex cascade of events is the primary cause of sepsis and its progression to organ dysfunction and failure.

Assessment

Distributive shock caused by sepsis differs from other shock states in that it has two phases. Phase 1 is the hyperdynamic state, commonly referred to as warm shock. Phase 2 is the hypodynamic state, commonly referred to as cold shock. A high-CO state, which may last for hours or days, characterizes the hyperdynamic (warm) phase. This phase may progress to hypodynamic (cold) shock when the patient's condition deteriorates rapidly and a sudden drop in CO occurs. The prognosis is much better for patients in hyperdynamic shock than for those in hypodynamic shock.

To recognize sepsis while it is still in its early stages, the provider must maintain a high index of suspicion for this disorder. A thorough patient history correlated with the patient presentation can ensure early identification and allow for rapid interventions to break the progression of the sepsis process. Do not withhold treatment while searching for the source: In many cases, an infectious cause is never identified. Specimen cultures are obtained from the blood, urine, sputum, and any drainage site to assist in identifying the causative organism. If the pathogen is bacterial, the WBC count is typically elevated and testing will identify immature neutrophils or bands. Once the pathogen is identified, more direct antimicrobial therapy can be initiated.

Many health care providers associate infection with fever. Although fever is certainly one clinical sign of infection, it may not be present in geriatric, newborn, and infant populations; patients with chronic renal failure; and patients receiving steroids or other anti-inflammatory drugs. Hypothermia is present in about 10% of patients with sepsis and is associated with a poor prognosis.

The cardiovascular and respiratory organs are the hardest hit in sepsis and septic shock. The cardiovascular changes seen in sepsis result from its inflammatory process. The massive vasodilation significantly lowers the SVR, so the heart increases CO. Cardiac output is extremely elevated in sepsis states. To produce this high-output state, the heart rate becomes tachycardic, and the stroke volume increases. Initially, normal to low-normal BP is maintained. Skin color and mucous membranes appear normal because of the vasodilation with associated high CO. However, the skin typically feels warm to the touch as the result of fever.

Once hypotension ensues, the patient is considered to be in septic shock. Because septic shock is refractory to fluid challenges, vasoactive agents must be initiated. This pathway is also the means by which progression from hyperdynamic shock to hypodynamic shock occurs. Hypodynamic shock gets its name from the low-CO state observed in these patients. Patients are unable to compensate for the relative hypovolemia in this phase, and their condition deteriorates rapidly, as evidenced by low BP, decreased pulse pressure, and low CO. Skin color and temperature change as blood is shunted to critical organs. The patient becomes cold and clammy, with pallor or cyanosis. In patients with DIC, petechiae may appear, and blood may ooze from mucous membranes, including the nose and mouth, and from any place where invasive procedures were necessary, including IV sites, indwelling urinary catheters, and chest tubes. Diagnostic patterns at this stage can include low hemoglobin and hematocrit reflecting anemia and low platelets and fibrinogen if DIC is occurring. A rising lactate level is perhaps the most ominous sign and can be used as a marker of disease severity.

The respiratory system also manifests changes. In hyperdynamic septic shock, the respiratory rate increases along with the depth of respiration, leading to respiratory alkalosis. As shock progresses, pulmonary edema and ARDS can develop. While pulmonary edema generally results from aggressive fluid resuscitation as well as cardiac pump insufficiency, ARDS—a complication of SIRS—evolves through an intricate process related to unchecked inflammation and alveolar membrane leakiness.

Mechanical ventilatory support is generally needed in patients with sepsis states associated with ARDS and should follow the ARDSNET protocol. A lung-protective strategy should be initiated, with low tidal volumes at 6 mL/kg, while keeping end-inspiratory plateau pressures lower than 30 cm H_2O. End-inspiratory plateau pressures should also be monitored closely. Mild **hypercapnia** can be permitted in patients with sepsis plus ARDS to allow for low tidal volumes and pressures. Ideally, the FIO_2 should be titrated to less than 60%. Therapy goals should be an SpO_2 of greater than 92%. (Treatment of ARDS is discussed in Chapter 6, *Respiratory Emergencies and Airway Management*.)

TABLE 10-14 Lab Abnormalities in Sepsis
Specimen cultures obtained from the blood, urine, sputum, and any drainage site to identify the causative organism
Elevated WBC count (if the pathogen is bacterial) associated with immature neutrophils or bands
Low hemoglobin level and hematocrit value
Low fibrinogen levels
Thrombocytopenia
Prolonged prothrombin time
Elevated D-dimer level
Elevated lactate level (>4 mmol/L)

© Jones & Bartlett Learning.

ARDS is described using the Berlin definition:

- Acute onset of respiratory failure within 1 week of a known clinical insult
- Diffuse bilateral infiltrates evident on chest radiography, not fully explained by effusion, lobar/lung collapse, or nodules
- Respiratory failure not fully explained by cardiac failure or fluid overload
- Hypoxemia, defined on a minimum positive end-expiratory pressure (PEEP) of 5 cm H_2O or greater, as PaO_2/FIO_2 of 300 or less for mild ARDS, PaO_2/FIO_2 of 200 or less for moderate ARDS, and PaO_2/FIO_2 of 100 or less for severe ARDS

TABLE 10-14 lists lab abnormalities seen in patients with sepsis.

Management

Early recognition and early management of sepsis are vital for a positive patient outcome. The primary goal of sepsis treatment is to maintain organ perfusion while enhancing tissue oxygenation. Achieving this goal requires balancing preload, afterload, and contractility to achieve an optimal level of homeostasis. The most current recommendations from the Surviving Sepsis Campaign are outlined in the Hour-1 bundle:

- Measure lactate level. (Remeasure lactate level if the initial level is elevated to >2 mmol/L.)

- Obtain blood cultures before administering antibiotics.
- Administer broad-spectrum antibiotics.
- Begin rapid administration of 30 mL/kg crystalloid for hypotension or lactate ≥4 mmol/L.
- Apply vasopressors if the patient remains hypotensive during or after fluid resuscitation, to maintain a MAP of 65 mm Hg or higher.

While all of the bundle elements may not be completed within the first hour, it is ideal for all of them to have begun within this time frame.

Fluid Resuscitation

The determinants of CO are preload, afterload, heart rate, and contractility. Initial resuscitation includes volume expansion to optimize preload. Isotonic crystalloids should be given in an initial fluid challenge as a 30 mL/kg (2,000 to 3,000 mL of fluid) bolus. The goal is to achieve a MAP of greater than 65 mm Hg. If the patient shows signs of fluid overload, intubation or administration of diuretics may be necessary. There is no evidence that the use of colloids produces any significant improvement in outcomes when compared with the use of crystalloids. Consider the infusion of PRBCs if the hemoglobin level drops below 7.0 g/dL.

Lactate trending can be a useful guide when assessing treatment response. Point-of-care lactate meters have become increasingly available either as stand-alone devices or as part of a blood gas panel. Recent evidence has shown that usual, aggressive care for patients with sepsis is equivalent to the protocolized goal-directed therapy proposed in 2001. Central venous catheters are no longer routinely recommended unless they are specifically indicated by the need to administer vasoactive medications or the need for additional access. Research has shown that using central venous oxygenation to guide treatment response is no better than lactate trending, and the latter approach is far less invasive. Use of CVP as a treatment parameter has become increasingly controversial and is no longer recommended as the sole value to guide fluid resuscitation. However, arterial lines are still recommended whenever vasoactive medications will be infused.

Vasopressor and Inotropic Support

Fluid therapy is not always sufficient to maintain BP in patients with sepsis. If the 30 mL/kg fluid challenge proves inadequate to maintain BP, vasopressors should be started. Detailed profiles of the vasoactive agents used for this purpose—norepinephrine, dopamine, phenylephrine, vasopressin, epinephrine, dobutamine, nitroglycerin, and angiotensin II—are presented in Chapter 8, *Critical Care Pharmacology*.

Norepinephrine is the vasopressor of choice in hypotensive patients with sepsis. This sympathomimetic agent acts directly on alpha adrenergic receptors in the smooth muscle of blood vessels to rapidly increase BP, while also stimulating beta adrenergic receptors that work to increase CO by enhancing contractility. Norepinephrine produces a minimal increase in the heart rate as compared with dopamine; hence, it has emerged as the first-line treatment for sepsis. Norepinephrine is typically started at 2 µg/min and titrated to a desired MAP of greater than 65 mm Hg. In some cases, the initial dose may be as high as 10 µg/min until the BP stabilizes, and max doses vary locally, often ranging from 20 to 40 µg/min.

Dopamine is no longer recommended for routine use in septic shock, as it has been shown to increase arrhythmias and mortality as compared to norepinephrine. Further, there is no evidence that use of low-dose dopamine stimulates renal output, so it is not used for this purpose.

Vasopressin or epinephrine may be administered as a secondary pressor if the patient's hypotension proves refractory to norepinephrine. Vasopressin works as a vasoconstrictor but has no inotropic or chronotropic effects. Therefore, CO may decrease when it is administered, resulting in a decreased blood supply to the spleen. Vasopressin is used in lower doses when complementing another pressor, beginning at 0.01 unit/min and being titrated up to 0.04 unit/min.

Epinephrine is a nonselective adrenergic activator, meaning it stimulates alpha-1, beta-1, and beta-2 receptors. It increases MAP by increasing the cardiac index, stroke volume, SVR, and heart rate.

Other vasopressors such as phenylephrine and dopamine may also be used in sepsis, but only in carefully selected populations or as last-resort efforts. Phenylephrine has pure alpha adrenergic properties that increase BP significantly without affecting the heart rate. However, the vasoconstriction it produces within the visceral tissue and mesentery may increase lactic acidosis, exacerbating the hypoxic state associated with sepsis. Dopamine can cause increased arrhythmias but may be helpful in patients with bradycardia.

Dobutamine is an inotropic agent that has proved very beneficial in treating cardiac depression associated with sepsis. This inotropic agent increases cardiac contractility through its selective beta-1 adrenergic properties. Dobutamine is especially useful when given in conjunction with norepinephrine. An IV infusion typically starts at 2 µg/kg/min and may be titrated to as high as 20 µg/kg/min. When titrating dobutamine, it is important to monitor MAP, Svo_2, and the CO or cardiac index to establish whether the treatment is adequate.

Infection Control

Cultures of all potential infection sources (eg, blood, urine, sputum, wounds) should be obtained as soon as possible and ideally before any antibiotic administration; however, inability to obtain cultures should not delay antibiotic treatment. In addition to cultures, viral test panels should be obtained. The goal of initial therapy with broad-spectrum antibiotics is to cover all likely possible infectious agents. When cultures identify specific microorganisms, antibiotic therapy can be narrowed to be more specific to the pathogen. Administer antibiotics within the first hour of suspecting sepsis to minimize mortality, because every hour of delay in antibiotic administration increases mortality.

Infection control also requires therapy to remove potential infection sources, such as special interventions for wound debridement, abscess drainage, or device removal. Identifying and removing the potential source of infection is key to treating and lowering mortality in sepsis.

Immune-Specific Therapy
Corticosteroids

In sepsis, corticosteroid production drops and a relative adrenocortical insufficiency can develop. Nevertheless, studies on steroid administration have demonstrated mixed outcomes on mortality, and there is currently no consensus opinion on how they should be used. The 2016 Surviving Sepsis guidelines recommend their use in septic shock only when hypotension is refractory to fluid challenges and vasopressors. A recent Cochrane review also concluded that glucocorticoid steroids appear

to improve patient-centered outcomes, such as reducing total days in the ICU. When used in the treatment of septic shock, intravenous hydrocortisone should be given at 200 mg/d.

Signs and Symptoms

Sepsis

- Distributive shock (beginning with hyperdynamic [warm] shock, progressing to hypodynamic [cold] shock)
- Infection, either confirmed or highly suspicious
- Fever may or may not be present
- Hypothermia may be present in later stages
- Cardiovascular changes
- Significantly lowered SVR
- Tachycardia
- Normal to low-normal BP initially; hypotension once in septic shock
- Normal skin color, normal mucous membrane color, but warm skin initially
- Cold, clammy skin with pallor or cyanosis when sepsis is more progressed
- Petechiae
- Blood oozing from mucous membranes and procedure sites
- Decreased pulse pressure
- Increased respiratory rate
- Increased respiratory depth
- Respiratory alkalosis
- ARDS

Postresuscitation Management

Once a patient's condition is stabilized, ongoing management must be active. Fluid resuscitation and vasopressors should be continued to maintain a goal urine output and lactate clearance.

Specifically, following a cardiac arrest, a 12-lead ECG should be performed immediately to evaluate for new evidence of ischemia or ST-segment elevation myocardial infarction and to determine if the patient requires the cardiac catheterization laboratory. It is currently recommended that targeted temperature management be initiated for all comatose patients following cardiac arrest, regardless of whether the initial cardiac rhythm is

Transport Management

Sepsis

- Maintain the following:
  - MAP greater than 65 mm Hg or SBP greater than 90 mm Hg
  - Urine output greater than 0.5 mL/kg/h
  - SpO_2 greater than 92% with administration of supplemental oxygen as needed
- Provide fluid resuscitation (30 mL/kg isotonic crystalloid bolus to stabilize filling pressures).
- Administer vasoactive agents if isotonic fluid bolus is inadequate to maintain BP.
- Monitor D-dimer level.
- Provide mechanical ventilatory support if the patient has ARDS.
  - Maintain low tidal volumes at 6 mL/kg.
  - Provide high PEEP at ranges of 5 to 14 cm H_2O. Increase the PEEP as the need arises to maintain oxygen saturation.
  - Make FIO_2 adjustments for oxygen saturation as needed.
  - Maintain PaO_2 between 55 and 80 mm Hg or SpO_2 between 88% and 95%.
  - Keep end-inspiratory plateau pressures lower than 30 cm H_2O.
  - Monitor $PaCO_2$ closely.
  - Sedation, if needed, must be monitored closely.
- Initiate broad-spectrum antibiotic therapy as ordered.
- Remove potential sources of infection: wound debridement, abscess drainage, and device removal.
- Consider administration of a corticosteroid or recombinant human APCs.

TABLE 10-15 Shock Resuscitation

Common Initial Treatment

- Oxygen
- IV access
- Monitoring

Cardiogenic Shock

- ECG for signs of STEMI
- Aspirin
- Nitroglycerin unless hypotensive
- Inotropic support (dobutamine)
- Consider diuresis for volume overload
- Emergent echocardiogram for structural issue
- Catheter lab for STEMI
- Obstructive shock evaluation:
  - Tension pneumothorax: needle decompression and chest tube
  - Pericardial tamponade: pericardiocentesis

Hypovolemic Shock

- Identify and control bleeding
- Large-bore IV access
- IV fluid bolus and blood transfusion
- Operating room

Distributive Shock (Neurogenic, Anaphylactic, Septic)

- Volume resuscitation with crystalloids
- Vasopressor support
- Evidence of anaphylaxis:
  - Epinephrine IM and gtt as needed
  - Airway control
  - H_1 and H_2 blockers
  - Steroids
- Evidence of sepsis:
  - Broad-spectrum antibiotics
  - Ongoing evaluation with lactate
  - Source control

Postresuscitation Management

- ECG to evaluate for STEMI
- Crystalloid bolus and vasopressors to maintain MAP >65 mm Hg
- Consider targeted temperature management in hospital

Abbreviations: ECG, electrocardiogram; H_1 and H_2, histamine; IV, intravenous; MAP, mean arterial pressure; STEMI, ST-segment elevation myocardial infarction

© Jones & Bartlett Learning.

deemed shockable or nonshockable. This principle was formerly known as therapeutic hypothermia; however, there is ongoing debate over whether the neurologic benefits observed in studies of this treatment are attributable to the mild hypothermia or simply to the avoidance of fever. Cooling the patient's body to a core temperature between 32°C and 36°C (89.6°F to 96.8°F) is advised, with specific temperature targets varying based on institution protocols and depending on patient characteristics. Protocols related to postresuscitation care are generally closely tied to American Heart Association (AHA) guidelines **TABLE 10-15**. CCTPs should always refer to both their local protocols and current AHA guidelines.

Blood Administration

Blood administration can be part of the management of shock, as discussed in the previous section. The decision to give a transfusion to a patient during a critical care transport is more complex than the administration of blood in the hospital setting. The urgency of the transfusion, the out-of-hospital time, the availability of the blood products, **type-and-crossmatch** information, and the appropriate transport and care of the blood product must be considered. A risk-benefit analysis of the "right treatment for the right patient at the right time" must be conducted as well.

Blood administration may be required to restore circulating blood volume, improve the blood's oxygen-carrying ability, or correct specific coagulation components. Blood products for transfusion can take the form of whole blood, RBCs, WBCs, platelets, cryoprecipitate, or other blood products. It is currently less common to transfuse whole blood owing to the expense, uncommon availability, and possibility of volume overload during its administration. Conditions for which blood administration may be considered include hemorrhagic blood loss as a result of trauma, internal hemorrhage, perioperative and postoperative complications, specific disease entities such as leukemia or other cancers, anemia due to illness, and coagulation disorders.

Many CCT programs carry type O blood for field pickups or will take matched blood with the patient from outlying hospitals; however, the availability of blood products in rural health care settings can be a critical issue when blood administration is contemplated. Rural hospitals may have a limited supply of banked blood products, especially of certain blood types and specific blood products required by a critically ill patient. Such limitations alter the desired treatment of the patient.

Time becomes a factor in the transport decisions surrounding a critically ill or injured patient. Awaiting the availability of certain blood products may lengthen the time to definitive care at a tertiary care center; it may be more important to transport the patient urgently than to perform the transfusion. In particular, the out-of-hospital time for the patient must be taken into account. For example, if it would take 15 minutes to obtain the needed blood products but the total transport time would be 20 minutes, it would likely be prudent to transport the patient and forgo the transfusion until the patient reaches the receiving facility. If the patient can tolerate the transport without the en route transfusion, the decision to defer blood administration until arrival at the receiving hospital may be in the patient's best interest.

Blood administration can result in undesirable complications such as transfusion reactions. Complications of this nature are best handled in the controlled environment of a hospital setting and may be difficult to address adequately during transport. Management of transfusion reactions is covered later in this section.

The transfusion of blood or blood products is considered to be a form of human tissue transplantation. For this reason, some states regulate who may initiate blood transfusions. Many state or institutional blood bank regulations require two licensed personnel to check blood and ensure a proper match of the blood unit to the patient. Each unit is treated as a new transfusion, rather than as a continuation of the previous unit.

Care of the blood products must be considered if the transfusion is not initiated before transport. The specific container and ice provided by the sending facility's blood bank must be used to ensure that the quality of the blood product is maintained. The blood products must remain cold throughout transport. For this reason, bags of ice are placed in an insulated icebox with ice beneath and on top of the blood products when transporting whole blood, PRBCs, or platelets. Care must be taken to prevent the ice from melting, including steps such as placing the icebox in a cool area and away from direct sunlight during transport.

The blood bank thaws fresh-frozen plasma and cryoprecipitate under specific guidelines. After thawing, fresh-frozen plasma must be transfused within a 24-hour period and cryoprecipitate must be transfused within a 6-hour period. Blood products are best stored in a refrigerator specially designed to store blood, which includes strict temperature regulations and consistently monitored temperature-recording systems, along with required alarm systems in case the refrigerator fails to maintain the temperature settings.

The extensive requirements for proper storage of banked blood products allow for little tolerance of deviations when blood administration occurs outside the hospital setting. Consequently, an inability to adhere to the stringent care, storage, and temperature monitoring of blood products during transport will result in refusal and waste of transferred blood products by the receiving facility's blood bank. If the patient may need blood products during transport, but it is not certain whether they will be administered, the decision to transport the blood should be made with caution. Most likely, the receiving facility's blood bank will destroy unused blood products from another blood bank. In fact, policies in many institutions forbid the acceptance of transferred blood products from outside blood banks. The possible wasting of a scarce resource, such as blood products, may be important in the decision to transport blood products that may not be absolutely necessary for a patient during transport.

Another key consideration is that blood transfusion requires a skilled health care provider with knowledge and experience in blood product administrations. Therefore, the expertise of the CCTP, medical direction, and prevailing medical protocol may further influence the decision to transfuse blood products during transport.

Once the decision to administer blood products has been made, the steps to provide for proper blood administration must be followed. These include appropriate typing and crossmatching through laboratory analysis. An exception to the required crossmatching of the patient before transfusion may be made during emergency resuscitation for hemorrhagic shock, when type O, Rh-negative blood (the universal donor type) may be administered owing to the urgent need for blood replacement and the critical delay associated with typing and crossmatching the patient before transfusion. In such a case, requirements for the transfusion procedure include appropriate IV access, blood tubing administration sets, priming of the tubing with normal saline, validation of the blood product's match with the specific patient before administration, and continued supervision by a skilled health care provider **FIGURE 10-10**.

When preparing for a potential large-volume resuscitation, the CCTP must understand the fundamental factors that impact flow rate through a cylinder, as defined by Poiseuille's law:

$$Q = \frac{\pi P r^4}{8 \eta l}$$

According to this principle, the flow (Q) of a fluid through a tube is directly proportional to the fourth

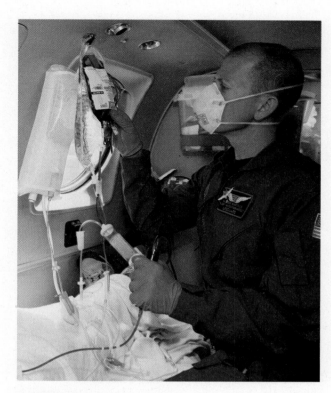

FIGURE 10-10 Proper procedures for blood administration include appropriate IV access, appropriate blood tubing administration sets, validation of the blood product's match with the specific patient before administration, and continued supervision by a skilled health care provider.

© Jones & Bartlett Learning.

power of the radius (r) of the tube and the pressure (P) being applied, and is inversely proportional to the length (l) of the tube and the viscosity (η) of the fluid. Practically speaking, a larger, shorter IV line under pressure will maximize flow rate. When measuring the length of the system, remember that it includes any IV extension tubing that is attached to the infusion set. IV connection tubing is used almost ubiquitously for its convenience and for the advantages it provides against blood loss and exposure, infection, and air embolism. If the objective is large-volume transfusion, however, providers should avoid a needleless IV connector, which can negate the improved flow intended by placing a larger-gauge IV access point. If necessary, use multiple large-bore (14- or 16-gauge) catheters to administer multiple units of blood simultaneously.

Pressure bags or rapid infusion devices can also be used to enhance the flow of the transfusion under emergent resuscitation conditions. In addition to higher flow rates, rapid infusion devices

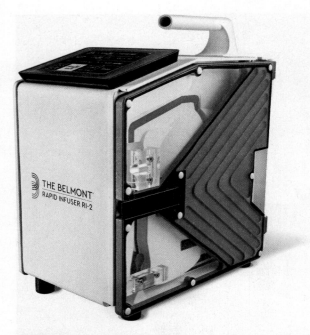

FIGURE 10-11 A rapid infusion device can enhance fluid flow and quickly warm fluids to help prevent hypothermia.

© The Belmont® Rapid Infuser RI-2. Reproduced with permission from Belmont Medical Technologies.

can rapidly warm refrigerated fluids to physiologic temperatures before their infusion **FIGURE 10-11**. This warming helps to avoid hypothermia—one of the three components of the lethal triad of trauma (hypothermia, acidosis, coagulopathy) that has been shown to contribute to worsening coagulopathy, cardiovascular function, and hepatocellular function. If neither a pressure bag nor a rapid infusion device is available in the field, manually squeezing the bag of fluid can significantly improve the flow rate in comparison to gravity alone.

ABO System

Blood contains a variety of antigens, with more than 400 RBC antigens having been identified to date. These antigens influence the compatibility of blood between people. Three types of blood antigens are generally considered important in the setting of blood transfusion—namely, the ABO blood group, Rh factor, and the human leukocyte antigen blood group. The type and crossmatch process focuses on identifying these antigen group characteristics through laboratory testing and ensuring compatibility of blood donor–recipient ABO grouping. Incompatibility at this step may cause the most severe type of transfusion reaction, known as acute hemolysis.

The ABO method of blood typing identifies two antigens on a RBC, known as A and B. If a person has only an A antigen identified, that person is type A. A person who has only a B antigen identified is type B. If both A and B antigens are present, the person is type AB. When neither an A nor B antigen is present, the blood type is O. The most common blood types in the United States are A and O, with 85% of the population having one of these two blood types. Type O is the most common blood type. Type B is found in 10% of the US population, whereas only 5% of the population has type AB blood.

A blood transfusion reaction may occur when a patient possesses antigens to a blood type and receives that blood type. Human error resulting in the misidentification of crossmatch samples or recipients is the most common cause of **ABO-incompatible transfusion reactions**. These reactions have caused an average of two deaths per year over the past decade in the United States. Patients with A antigens in their blood also have anti-B antibodies in their plasma; similarly, patients with B antigens in their blood also have anti-A antibodies in their plasma. Transfusion reactions may occur if patients receive a blood type for which they have antibodies.

People who have type AB blood do not have antibodies and are known as **universal recipients**. They can receive blood types A, B, AB, and O without the threat of an ABO reaction. People who have type O blood are considered **universal donors** because their blood can be transfused into patients with types A, B, and AB blood. However, people with type O blood have antibodies to blood types A and B and, therefore, can receive only type O blood.

Patients should receive transfusions of their own blood type to minimize possible transfusion reactions. In an emergency situation in which the time necessary for crossmatching of blood cannot be taken, type O, Rh-negative blood or plasma can be transfused until crossmatched blood becomes available.

Rh factors are antigens found on the cell membrane of RBCs. These antigens are present in approximately 85% of the US population, who are known as "Rh positive." People lacking the Rh antigen are termed "Rh negative." There are no natural Rh antibodies. Instead, an Rh-negative person may develop an Rh antibody if exposed to Rh-positive blood. This first exposure to Rh-positive blood allows a person to become sensitized. A second

Rh-positive exposure could result in a fatal hemolytic reaction. This type of reaction may occur during a transfusion or pregnancy.

Human leukocyte antigen (HLA) is present on the surfaces of the cell membranes of circulating platelets, WBCs, and most tissue cells. Patients receiving platelets from multiple donors may experience febrile transfusion reactions from the infusion of HLAs. The ensuing antigen-antibody reaction destroys the platelets, reducing the benefits derived from the transfusion. HLA-matched platelet transfusions dramatically diminish this antigen-antibody reaction and are optimal for patients receiving multiple transfusions.

Blood Products

Blood component therapy has become common in the United States, with nearly 21 million of these transfusions taking place each year. Many of these transfusions occur in surgical and obstetric patients. Such transfusions provide benefits including increased tissue oxygenation, decreased blood loss, and improved clinical outcomes. The risks and costs of transfusions must always be considered, however. Transfusion reactions and the risk of transmission of multiple infectious diseases must be factored into any decision to transfuse blood products.

Blood Components and Derivatives

Blood transfusions became possible in the early 1900s after discovery of the A, B, O, and AB blood types. The first blood bank was founded in the United States in 1937. During World War II, the use of whole blood and plasma was widespread. Subsequently, the introduction of plastic blood storage containers and apheresis instruments allowed for the use of blood components as therapy. By the 1970s, blood component therapy had gained acceptance and its use surpassed the use of whole blood. Recently, however, whole blood has been regaining its popularity as a treatment for patients in hemorrhagic shock.

Whole Blood

Whole blood contains all blood components, including RBCs, WBCs, platelets, plasma, and electrolytes. The usual volume is approximately 450 to 500 mL/U. Transfusion of whole blood is indicated only in cases of acute massive blood loss,

Controversies

Retrospective study of soldiers with combat injuries in the Middle East who required large volumes of blood transfusion demonstrated improved survival when they were given plasma in a roughly equal ratio to red blood cells. Since then, civilian trauma studies have demonstrated that in patients who required activation of massive transfusion protocols, outcomes were improved when these patients received a more balanced resuscitation of RBCs, plasma, and platelets in a 1:1:1 ratio. This balanced resuscitation approach is seen as an approximation of whole blood and has prompted protocol shifts in the US military and a small number of civilian trauma centers to recommend whole blood as the preferred prehospital fluid for the resuscitation of patients with hemorrhagic shock.

Proponents of whole-blood resuscitation point to the fact that 1 unit of whole blood is more concentrated than the equivalent component products, which contain additive solutions; therefore, patients may require fewer transfusions and be exposed to fewer foreign donor antigens. Moreover, proponents for whole blood use argue that transfusing 1 unit of whole blood is easier than keeping track of a 1:1:1 ratio in the midst of a massive transfusion. Thus far, however, meta-analysis comparing whole blood to balanced resuscitation of components has not demonstrated a difference in outcomes, and blood component therapy remains the most common transfusion option.

where its effects of blood volume expansion and increased oxygen-carrying capacity are urgently needed. Whole-blood transfusions should be considered only in patients who have lost at least 25% of their total blood volume. Whenever possible, loss of blood should be treated with options other than whole blood, such as blood components, crystalloids, or colloid solutions. Administration of whole blood may cause fluid volume overload in patients with cardiac compromise.

Whole blood is stored at a temperature between 34°F and 43°F (1°C and 6°C). The expiration date depends on the anticoagulant preservative, but most commonly a citrate phosphate-dextrose solution is used that can allow for refrigerated storage up to 21 days. If not treated with a preservative solution, whole blood will begin to degrade after 24 hours of storage. This cell breakdown causes elevated potassium levels, the formation of microaggregates, damaged platelets and granulocytes, and decreased clotting factors.

Whole-blood transfusions must be ABO matched with the recipient because of the presence of antibodies. Hemoglobin levels should rise 1 g/dL per infusion of each unit of whole blood. Administer whole-blood transfusions as rapidly as possible while maintaining hemodynamic stability. Whole blood may be administered through an IV catheter as small as 20 gauge, with normal saline solution, and within a 4-hour period. The patient must be closely monitored during the infusion for possible fluid volume overload and transfusion reactions.

Packed Red Blood Cells

Packed red blood cells (PRBCs) retain all of the characteristics of whole blood, with the exception of the extraction of approximately 250 mL of platelet-rich plasma from each unit of whole blood. This constitutes the removal of nearly 90% of the fluid around the RBCs. An anticoagulant preservative is then added that can allow RBCs to last for up to 42 days. Each unit of PRBCs retains the same concentration of RBCs as a unit of whole blood and is approximately 250 mL in volume.

PRBCs are indicated for the restoration and maintenance of blood's oxygen-carrying ability. Anemia and blood loss are possible indications for PRBC administration. A patient's hemoglobin level is expected to rise 1 g/dL per unit of administered PRBCs.

Nearly 70% of the leukocytes are removed from each unit of PRBCs, which reduces the risk for febrile, nonhemolytic reactions. Proper ABO compatibility and Rh factor matching are required before administration of these blood products.

Special Populations

Pediatric patients have proportionately higher blood and plasma volumes compared to adults. Transfusion of PRBCs is calculated by weight. Children younger than 4 months are initially given 10 mL/kg of PRBCs, whereas children 4 months of age or older can be transfused with 10 to 20 mL/kg depending on their lab values and clinical condition. Increased attention to volume overload during blood product administration is particularly important in the pediatric population.

Washed blood products are RBC or platelet products in which the small amount of noncellular fluid has been replaced, typically with saline. This process removes all of the plasma proteins—for example, antibodies, cytokines, electrolytes, and preservative solution. The removal of the plasma proteins can decrease the risk of severe allergic reactions. In pediatric patients, the removal of potassium in particular reduces the risk of hyperkalemia.

In **leuko-reduced blood products**, the WBCs and platelet fragments have been filtered from donated blood products. While in some countries this filtering is done universally, in the United States leuko-reduction of donated blood is performed in approximately 95% of platelets and only 75% of RBCs. The use of leuko-reduced blood products can reduce the risk of febrile nonhemolytic transfusion reactions in patients with a history of prior reactions or chronic transfusions, and the risk of HLA alloimmunization in patients awaiting organ transplantation.

In **irradiated blood products**, lymphocyte DNA has been exposed to radiation, which damages the DNA and thereby limits its ability to replicate. The resulting blood products are given to severely immunocompromised patients, in an effort to avoid the rare but often fatal condition of transfusion-associated graft-versus-host disease (ta-GVHD). This disease is estimated to occur in less than 1% of at-risk populations. Such populations include but are not limited to patients with congenital immunodeficiency syndromes, acute leukemia, or lymphoma; patients who have received organ transplants; and oncology patients undergoing chemotherapy. While they likely reduce this risk as well, leuko-reduced blood products are not considered to be an effective protective mechanism against the development of ta-GVHD.

Platelets

Platelets are blood components that are manufactured in the bone marrow; they consist of cytoplasmic fragments containing enzymes necessary for normal clotting response. In the United States, nearly 7,000 units of platelets are transfused daily. These products can be frozen and kept for up to 2 years, but are most commonly stored at room temperature and kept under constant agitation to prevent aggregation and clumping, resulting in a shelf life of 5 days. Indications for platelet transfusions include patients who are bleeding because of thrombocytopenia or, in rare cases, the presence of abnormally functioning platelets. Patients experiencing low platelet counts (less than 5,000 to 10,000 cells/μL) may benefit from platelet transfusions on a prophylactic basis. Platelet therapy may also be considered before surgery or extensive invasive procedures in those patients with platelet levels of less than 50,000 cells/μL. Patients who are receiving chemotherapy, have disseminated intravascular coagulation, or need massive transfusions may be candidates for platelet therapy as well.

ABO-identical platelets are ideal whenever available, with Rh-negative platelets matched to Rh-negative patients as frequently as possible for transfusion. If a patient must receive multiple transfusions of platelets, single-donor platelets should be administered.

Each bag of platelet concentrate contains 5.5×10^{10} of platelets in 50 to 70 mL of plasma. A single unit raises the platelet count by 5,000 cells/μL. The calculation for dosing of platelet therapy is based on 6 to 10 U and 1 U/10 kg of body weight.

Administration of platelets requires a filtered component IV drip set with normal saline solution. Premedication of the patient before transfusion may include antihistamines or acetaminophen to reduce or prevent chills, fever, and allergic reactions.

Fresh-Frozen Plasma

Fresh-frozen plasma (FFP) consists of uncoagulated plasma that has been separated from the RBCs. This plasma is primarily composed of water, proteins, salts, and metabolites, and is rich in clotting factors. As the name implies, FFP is kept frozen, so it must be thawed before use; after thawing, it can be kept refrigerated for up to 24 hours. Indications for the administration of FFP may include blood loss, coagulation deficiencies, warfarin reversal, and thrombotic thrombocytopenic purpura.

Transfusions of FFP must be ABO compatible; Rh matching is not required. Blood administration sets and normal saline solution are required for rapid infusion. Because the citric acid preservative in FFP may bind with calcium during transfusion and can lead to hypocalcemia, close patient monitoring for hypocalcemia is required during transfusion. FFP must be infused within 24 hours of being thawed.

Cryoprecipitate

Cryoprecipitate is a frozen blood product created from the plasma of a donor. It contains factor VIII, fibrinogen, von Willebrand factor, and factor XIII; it follows that indications for administering cryoprecipitate include hemophilia A, fibrinogen deficiency, von Willebrand disease, and factor XIII deficiency. Cryoprecipitate is useful in treating patients with clotting disorders, because it replaces fibrinogen. It is typically given to patients with fibrinogen levels of less than 50 to 60 mg/dL. Each bag contains 80 to 100 U of factor VIII. A patient may need as much as 10 U of cryoprecipitate to restore the fibrinogen level to 100 mg/dL.

Administration of cryoprecipitate does not require compatibility testing, but ABO compatibility is preferred. An Rh match is not necessary.

A blood administration set can be used for infusion, and cryoprecipitate should be administered as rapidly as tolerated. Cryoprecipitate must be administered within 6 hours of thawing. Whole-blood donor requirements and the preparation of cryoprecipitate are the same as those for platelets and FFP.

Albumin

Albumin is prepared by the fractionation of pooled plasma. This product is available as a 5% or 25% solution and is used for volume replacement in patients with conditions such as burns, trauma, surgery, or infections. However, large studies have failed to find a comparative benefit when using albumin instead of crystalloid fluids; consequently, its use remains controversial. The 25% solution will expand to five times its volume in extravascular water and move into the vascular space. Thus, it is important that patients receiving 25% albumin have adequate extravascular water and the compensatory abilities to handle this blood volume expansion.

ABO and Rh compatibility are not a consideration with albumin products. The manufacturer-provided tubing should be used for albumin administration, and the infusion rate should be set in accordance with the patient's condition and response. Patients with cardiac and pulmonary disease must be monitored closely during albumin administration because of the risk of heart failure from volume overload.

Plasma Protein Fractions

Plasma protein fraction contains 83% albumin and 17% globulins. This blood product is available in a 5% preparation and is indicated for volume expansion in patients with hypovolemia and hypoproteinemia. Clinical indications for its administration include shock and burns. Plasma protein fraction is available in 250-mL containers and can be stored for 5 years at 35.6°F to 50°F (2°C to 10°C).

Synthetic Blood Substitutes

The quest for synthetic substitutes for blood transfusions continues to move forward despite several setbacks and disappointments. The most studied product thus far has been the Hb-based oxygen carrier, Hemopure (HBOC-211), which is made from purified bovine hemoglobin. Clinical trials of HBOC-211 have raised concerns about patient tolerance of the volume associated with its infusion, as well as increased methemoglobin levels. Several other products have been developed or are in active trials, but none of these agents is FDA approved for clinical use in the United States. Under compassionate use authorization, HBOC-211 can be used at some centers for patients with critical anemia who are unable to receive blood products.

Tranexamic Acid

Tranexamic acid is a synthetic antifibrinolytic agent that has several uses in medicine, most notably for patients undergoing elective surgery and for trauma patients with hypovolemic shock. It works by inhibiting plasminogen activation, thereby preventing fibrin clot breakdown and promoting clotting. A large European study demonstrated a mortality reduction in trauma patients receiving tranexamic acid when compared to placebo, particularly when those patients received tranexamic acid early, within 3 hours of injury onset. Further, there was no increase in the number of adverse events such as pulmonary embolism or stroke. EMS systems are beginning to adopt this new therapy, and CCTPs may encounter patients who have received tranexamic acid before transport.

For trauma patients, tranexamic acid is dosed as a 1-g bolus given over 10 minutes, followed by infusion of 1 g over 8 hours. Aside from its use in trauma indications, tranexamic acid has been demonstrated to have benefits in controlling bleeding from epistaxis, hemoptysis, and postpartum hemorrhage.

In contrast, a recent randomized controlled trial of tranexamic acid in patients with an acute GI bleed showed no improvement in outcomes, and its use is not recommended in this group.

Anticoagulants

For many years, warfarin (Coumadin) and heparin were the mainstays of anticoagulation; however, since the first direct-acting oral anticoagulant (DOAC) was approved in 2010, use of DOACs has become increasingly prevalent in daily practice. These medications are generally administered for thromboembolic prophylaxis in patients with atrial fibrillation or a mechanical heart valve, as well as in postsurgical patients or patients confined to bed. They are used therapeutically to treat deep vein thrombosis, pulmonary embolism, and other thromboembolic diseases.

Warfarin works by inhibiting the vitamin K–dependent clotting factors (II, VII, IX, and X) and requires frequent checks of the patient's international normalized ratio to maintain the goal therapeutic level. A variety of medications, such as certain antibiotics, can increase or decrease its effectiveness.

Heparin can be used in its natural, unfractionated form, or as a fractionated low-molecular-weight version (Enoxaparin or Lovenox). Both types are injectable medications that work by indirectly inhibiting factor Xa.

DOACs work by directly inhibiting either thrombin itself (dabigatran [Pradaxa]) or factor Xa (rivaroxaban [Xarelto], apixaban [Eliquis]). While these medications offer significant advantages over warfarin, such as higher dosing reliability and fewer lab checks, their effects can be more challenging to reverse. Warfarin and heparin have well-established reversal protocols that can be implemented in the setting of a traumatic bleeding event. A four-factor prothrombin complex concentrate (PCC) containing high dosages of factors II, VII, IX, and X (Kcentra) is FDA approved for the emergent reversal of warfarin, and protamine can be used to bind to unfractionated heparin to inactivate it. For patients on dabigatran who require emergent reversal, the monoclonal antibody idarucizumab (Praxbind) can be administered to inactivate its anticoagulant effects. If idarucizumab is not available, dialysis is another option to remove dabigatran from the patient's system. For patients taking rivaroxaban or apixaban, andexanet alfa (Andexxa) can be used to reverse life-threatening bleeds. Andexanet alfa is a compound that binds directly to factor Xa inhibitors to inactivate them; however, a randomized controlled trial has not been conducted to determine its superiority to four-factor PCC. Further, andexanet alfa is significantly more expensive than four-factor PCC. Thus, both techniques of Xa inhibitor reversal are in use currently, depending on facility resources.

Procedure

The procedure for administering blood is discussed in this section.

Indications

Indications for administering blood include the following:

- Significant hypovolemia as the result of acute blood loss
- Symptomatic anemia
- Decreasing hemoglobin level
- Decreasing hematocrit value
- Increase oxygen-carrying ability
- Decreased clotting factors
- Presurgical care in selected cases

Equipment/Materials

Upon receiving a physician's orders to administer blood, the CCTP needs to prepare the following equipment and materials:

- Physician's orders
- Blood product, typed and crossmatched (in some cases may be cryoprecipitate, platelets, or plasma)
- Dedicated venous access line (18-gauge or larger needle)
- Filtered administration set
- Thermometer

Complications

Potential complications of administering blood include the following:

- Anaphylaxis
- Hemolytic reaction
- DIC
- Transfusion reaction
- Infection

Signs of complications include the following:

- Body temperature of 2°F (1°C) or more above the baseline temperature
- Hives, itching, or skin symptoms
- Swelling, soreness, or hematoma at the venous site
- Flank pain
- Tachycardia
- Respiratory distress (wheezing and dyspnea)
- Hypotension
- Bleeding from widely varied sites or previously clotted wounds
- Blood in the urine
- Anaphylaxis
- Nausea and vomiting

Steps

SKILL DRILL 10-1 shows the steps for administering blood products. These steps are also described here:

1. Prepare the patient by following these steps:
   a. Confirm the order or protocol **STEP 1**.
   b. Check the patient for the following "rights": right patient, right blood product, and right type. Have a second provider confirm steps a and b with you **STEP 2**.
   c. Assess the patient's baseline vital signs and temperature **STEP 3**.
   d. Ensure suitable venous access (usually requires 18-gauge or larger needle) **STEP 4**. At this point, patient preparation is complete and the transfusion procedure begins.
2. Check the blood for the following "rights": right patient, right blood product, and right type. Also check the blood's expiration date.
3. Assess the patient for the possibility of a transfusion reaction, and consider the prophylactic administration of ibuprofen or acetaminophen and diphenhydramine.
4. Maintain the temperature of the blood product.
5. Flush the tubing with normal saline **STEP 5**.
6. Connect the blood to the tubing **STEP 6**.
7. Saturate the administration filter with the blood.
8. Piggyback into the IV line of normal saline **STEP 7**.
9. Start the transfusion slowly **STEP 8**.
10. Monitor every 5 minutes for adverse reactions.

Skill Drill 10-1 Administering Blood Products

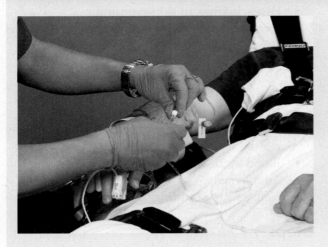

Step 1

Confirm the order or protocol.

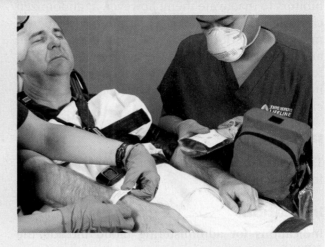

Step 2

Check the patient for the following: right patient, right blood product, and right type. Have a second provider confirm steps 1 and 2 with you.

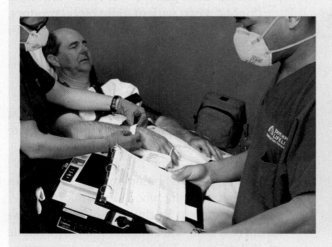

Step 3

Assess the patient's baseline vital signs and temperature.

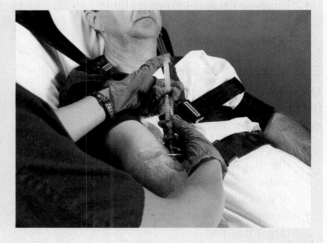

Step 4

Ensure suitable venous access. Check the blood for the following: right patient, right blood product, right type, and expiration date. Assess the patient for the possibility of a transfusion reaction, and consider prophylactic administration of medications. Maintain the temperature of the blood product.

Skill Drill 10-1 Administering Blood Products (continued)

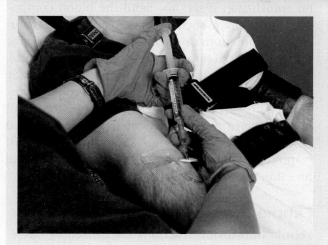

Step 5

Flush the tubing with normal saline. Cover the administration filter with blood.

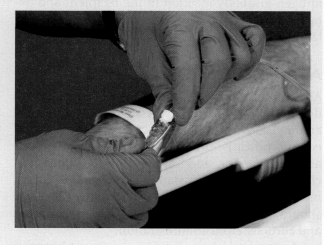

Step 6

Connect the blood to the tubing.

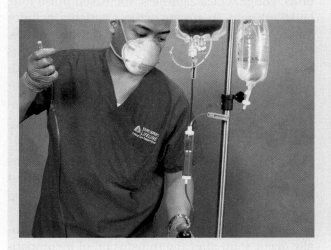

Step 7

Piggyback into the IV line of normal saline.

© Jones & Bartlett Learning.

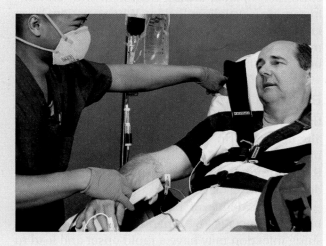

Step 8

Start the transfusion slowly. Monitor for adverse reactions.

It is important to follow these transfusion precautions:

- Do not mix blood with 5% dextrose in water (causes hemolysis).
- Do not mix blood with lactated Ringer solution (causes clotting).

- Do not mix blood with medications (may react).
- Have a second venous access available.

Transfusion Reactions

Transfusion reactions are of great concern and play a significant role in the decision to administer blood products. These reactions can be as mild as chills or as catastrophic as death. Reactions can include both endogenous reactions caused by an antigen-antibody reaction in the recipient and exogenous reactions caused by external factors related to the transfused blood.

Allergic Reactions

Allergic reactions are caused by allergens in the donated blood and are evidenced by symptoms of anaphylaxis, including chills, facial and laryngeal edema, pruritus, urticaria, and wheezing, as well as fever, nausea, and vomiting. Management includes the use of antihistamines and careful patient monitoring and assessment. Additionally, providers should consider the indications for epinephrine and corticosteroid administration.

Isolated reactions such as urticaria or hives may occur during transfusion without additional signs or symptoms of anaphylaxis and without further sequelae. The transfusion does not need to be discontinued in such a case; treatment with an antihistamine is usually sufficient. When a patient has a known history of this type of allergic reaction, premedicate the patient with an antihistamine before beginning the transfusion.

Bacterial Contamination

Bacterial contamination of blood components usually occurs during one of the following phases of blood administration: during phlebotomy, during the component preparation or processing, or during thawing of the blood components.

The incidence of bacterial contamination of blood products is low. When it does occur, the ensuing infection may have a rapid onset and lead to death. Platelets present a particularly high risk of infection. Report all cases of suspected bacterial contamination of blood products to the local department of public health.

Bacterial contamination usually results from endotoxins produced by organisms capable of surviving the cold, such as *Pseudomonas*, *Staphylococcus*, and *Yersinia enterocolitica*. Presenting symptoms may occur rapidly or within 30 minutes after transfusion and include chills, fever, vomiting, abdominal cramping, bloody diarrhea, hemoglobinuria, shock, renal failure, and DIC. It is essential to rapidly recognize sepsis caused by blood products contaminated by bacteria. Stop the transfusion immediately upon the onset of symptoms. Keep the IV line open, and implement the protocol for transfusion reactions. Send the blood component unit, any associated fluids, and the transfusion equipment to the blood bank immediately for thorough inspection, Gram staining, and culture. Draw blood cultures from the patient as soon as possible to identify the presence of aerobic or anaerobic organisms. Consider the administration of broad-spectrum antibiotics, corticosteroids, and vasopressors; treatment for shock; fluid support; respiratory ventilation; and maintenance of renal function in the management of these patients.

Febrile Transfusion Reactions

Febrile transfusion reactions are caused by bacterial lipopolysaccharides or antileukocyte recipient antibodies directed against donor WBCs. Patients may experience temperatures as high as 104°F (40°C), chills, headache, facial flushing, palpitations, cough, chest tightness, increased pulse rate, and flank pain. Treatment of these patients includes administration of antipyretics and antihistamines. Consider modifications if future blood transfusions are anticipated in these patients, including the administration of frozen RBCs and the use of leukocyte filters as modifiers.

Hemolytic Transfusion Reactions

Hemolytic transfusion reactions may be caused by ABO or Rh incompatibility, intradonor incompatibility, improper crossmatching, or improper blood storage.

Immediate hemolytic transfusion reactions usually occur soon after the transfusion of incompatible RBCs. The RBCs are quickly destroyed, resulting in the release of hemoglobin and cell remnants into the bloodstream. This process leads to the onset of hemoglobinuria and abnormal bleeding from open sites, accompanied by hypotension. The reaction time varies between 1 hour and 2 hours, with the onset of symptoms occurring within minutes after the blood transfusion begins. Symptoms include chest pain, facial flushing, shortness of breath, chills, fever, hypotension, flank pain, hemoglobinuria, oliguria, bloody oozing at the infusion site, burning along the vein receiving the blood, shock, signs of renal failure, and DIC. These reactions are relatively rare, representing only 0.41% of all reported adverse effects to transfusion.

Treatment of immediate hemolytic transfusion reactions focuses on prevention and supportive management. If a hemolytic transfusion reaction is suspected, immediately stop the transfusion. The use of diuretics to augment renal diuresis in an effort to prevent renal failure is recommended. The patient must be closely monitored for the risk factors related to DIC and hypotension is required. Hypotension is managed with fluid resuscitation and vasoactive agents. Consider the use of blood component therapy, including FFP, cryoprecipitate, and platelets, in patients with bleeding complications or significant coagulation abnormalities.

Human error is the cause of most cases of immediate hemolytic transfusion reactions; therefore, these reactions are considered preventable. The extensive policies and procedures necessary to ensure proper patient identification, sample collection and labeling, unit identification, patient testing, handling, and correct transfusion must be strictly enforced.

Delayed hemolytic transfusion reactions most often occur in patients who have been sensitized through a previous transfusion, pregnancy, or transplant and who possess an antibody undetectable by standard pretransfusion testing. In cases of delayed hemolytic transfusion reactions caused by secondary response, the onset of symptoms does not occur until 1 to 30 days after transfusion. The production of antibodies sufficient to generate the signs and symptoms of delayed hemolytic transfusion reactions occurs during this time period. Clinical signs and symptoms usually consist of mild fever, chills, and moderate jaundice. Generally, the reaction is mild; severe cases and death are rare. Treatment focuses on the prevention and treatment of severe complications should they arise. Support of renal function includes IV fluids to maintain adequate fluid status.

Plasma Protein Incompatibility

Plasma protein incompatibility results from immunoglobulin A incompatibility. Clinical presentations include abdominal pain, diarrhea, shortness of breath, chills, fever, flushing, and hypotension. Management of this form of incompatibility includes oxygen administration, fluids, epinephrine, and corticosteroids as indicated.

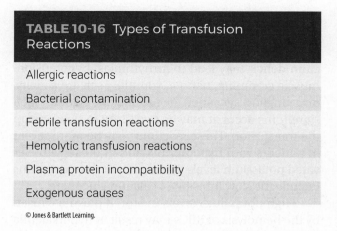

TABLE 10-16 Types of Transfusion Reactions
Allergic reactions
Bacterial contamination
Febrile transfusion reactions
Hemolytic transfusion reactions
Plasma protein incompatibility
Exogenous causes

© Jones & Bartlett Learning.

Other Causes

Other exogenous transfusion reactions include bleeding tendencies, circulatory overload, hypocalcemia, hypothermia, and potassium intoxication **TABLE 10-16**. Bleeding tendencies may be caused by low platelet counts in banked blood, which then cause thrombocytopenia in patients who receive these products. Clinical presentations include abnormal bleeding and oozing from breaks in the skin or gums, abnormal bruising, and petechiae. Management involves the consideration of transfusion of platelets, FFP, or cryoprecipitate as needed.

Blood Transfusion Management Considerations

Transfusion-associated circulatory overload (TACO) is a potential complication during blood administration. As noted earlier, administering whole blood has the possible disadvantage of infusing an increased total volume of blood product, which may be poorly tolerated by certain patients. Caution should be exercised with the administration of whole blood in patients with cardiac and pulmonary disease, who are at higher risk for experiencing congestive heart failure. The use of PRBCs in lieu of whole blood administration is recommended in this patient group. The use of diuretics should be considered if circulatory overload is suspected.

Transfusion-related acute lung injury (TRALI) is another recognized complication of blood administration. In this condition, neutrophil activation in the lung parenchyma leads to an ARDS-like presentation.

Hypocalcemia may result from citrate toxicity during blood transfusions when blood products containing citrate are infused too quickly and bind to calcium. The ensuing depletion of circulating calcium results in calcium deficiency in the patient. This calcium deficit may lead to arrhythmias, hypotension, muscle cramping, nausea, vomiting, seizure activity, or a tingling sensation in the fingers. Should such symptoms occur, it may be necessary to slow or stop the transfusion. These reactions may be more severe in patients with hypothermia and in those with elevated potassium levels. Management considerations include the slow infusion of calcium gluconate.

High potassium levels in stored plasma caused by the hemolysis of RBCs may result in hyperkalemia during blood administration. Clinical manifestations of this electrolyte imbalance may include diarrhea, intestinal colic, flaccidity, muscle twitching, oliguria, signs of renal failure, bradycardia, ECG changes with visible tall peaked T waves, and cardiac arrest. Treat the patient for hyperkalemia according to standard protocols. See Chapter 17, *Gastrointestinal and Genitourinary Emergencies*, for further discussion of hyperkalemia treatment.

The induction of hypothermia is possible when large amounts of cold blood products are infused too rapidly. Hypothermia symptoms may include chills, shivering, hypotension, arrhythmias, bradycardia, or cardiac arrest if the body temperature falls below 86°F (30°C). Treatment considerations may include stopping the transfusion, warming the patient, obtaining a diagnostic 12-lead ECG, and warming the blood if the transfusion is resumed.

The risk-benefit analysis of blood administration must be approached with caution. Blood transfusion can be a life-saving intervention, but the many complications and adverse reactions that are possible with administration of blood products require the thoughtful care of highly skilled providers and vigilance in the health care setting.

Flight Considerations

In the transport environment, a patient in shock or with sepsis or MODS will most likely be in a very labile state, requiring diligence by CCTPs in monitoring and adjusting therapy to maintain adequate oxygenation and hemodynamic status. It is important to pay close attention and ensure that all infusions are dosed properly and are compatible. Ventilator transfers and settings must also be managed carefully because oxygen desaturation may occur easily. In addition, movement and agitation can have a negative effect on these patients.

Transport of patients with sepsis over long distances by fixed-wing transport is an infrequent event. However, when it does occur, altitude and cabin pressure require ventilator adjustments to compensate for the pressures at altitude.

Summary

In the transport environment, a patient with sepsis will often be critically ill, and the therapeutic regimen will include use of multiple support devices and treatments. The referring facility may have exhausted its ability to care for the patient. CCTPs must be well versed in the many aspects of the management of shock, sepsis, SIRS, and MODS. Multiple therapies may be needed concurrently in the care of patients in critical condition because of these disorders.

Case Study

You are called to a regional hospital ICU for emergency ground transfer of a male patient to a tertiary facility. Three days earlier, the patient fell, sustained splenic trauma, and underwent emergency repair of a splenic tear. Transport time by ground will be 1 hour.

Upon your arrival, the staff reports that 3 days ago EMS providers brought the patient, a 35-year-old, 170-pound (77-kg) man who fell from a scaffold, to the emergency department. He has no medical history, smokes half a pack of cigarettes per day, and is an occasional drinker. He was diagnosed with a splenic tear and underwent surgical repair. He was admitted to the ICU after surgery, has had worsening hemodynamic status, and is being referred to a tertiary facility for ongoing care. During his stay, the patient received PRBCs, normal saline, and FFP for surgery and stabilization. A PA catheter was inserted, and norepinephrine was initiated to maintain hemodynamic status. He was given cefazolin (Ancef) as surgical prophylaxis. He continues to need a ventilator as well.

This patient is currently mildly responsive, with a Glasgow Coma Scale score of 7T ("T" indicates that the patient is intubated). He is intubated with a 9.0 endotracheal tube and ventilated with synchronized intermittent mandatory ventilation. The tidal volume is 700 mL, the rate is 10 breaths/min, F_{IO_2} is 50%, and PEEP is 5 cm H_2O. Occasional suctioning is required. Two peripheral lines are in place, with normal saline running at 100 mL/h. Norepinephrine is infusing at 6 μg/min. The patient is receiving enteral nutrition via a nasally inserted duodenal tube. His PA catheter reveals lowered PCWP, decreased SVR, and increased CO. An available chest radiograph reveals bilateral diffuse infiltrates. Current monitoring reveals the following: heart rate, 133 beats/min; BP, 84/43 mm Hg; temperature, 102°F (38.9°C); MAP, 55 mm Hg; CVP, 3 mm Hg; PA pressure, 20/10 mm Hg; PCWP, 7 mm Hg; SpO_2, 89%; and end-tidal carbon dioxide, 35 mm Hg. Current lab values are as follows: hemoglobin, 11.0 g/dL; hematocrit, 33.1%; WBC count, 24, 100/μL; platelet count, 51×10^3/μL; BUN, 61 mg/dL; creatinine, 2.1 mg/dL; Na^+, 146 mEq/L; K^+, 4.8 mEq/L; Cl^-, 111 mEq/L; glucose, 225 mg/dL; pH, 7.29; PcO_2, 52 mm Hg; PaO_2, 47 mm Hg; and Hco_3^-, 14 mEq/L. Urine output has been scant, at less than 50 mL/h.

Your assessment confirms the preceding information. The patient feels febrile to the touch. The examination reveals equal and reactive pupils at 5 mm. The enteral feeding tube is placed nasally and secured. The endotracheal tube is secured at 23 cm at the lip line. The trachea is midline. Other portions of the head, eye, ear, nose, and throat exam have normal findings. The chest has equal rise and fall with ventilations. A PA catheter is placed in the right side and is secure. Lung sounds reveal bilateral, diffuse, light crackles. The abdomen reveals a splenic surgical incision that is intact and dressed; no exudate is noted. An indwelling urinary catheter is noted with a pelvic exam. The lower extremities are cool and pale. Pedal pulses can be detected by Doppler ultrasonography only. Faint radial pulses are noted. Capillary refill is delayed.

You transfer the patient's IV lines to your pumps, then transfer the ECG and hemodynamic lines and calibrate them to your monitors. You move the patient to your litter and duplicate his ventilator settings on your portable ventilator, increasing the F_{IO_2} to 80%. You discharge the patient from the ICU, obtain all records, and move to your mobile ICU. The patient is placed in the mobile ICU, all oxygen and power needs are transferred to onboard systems, and transport is begun.

En route, no change in the patient's hemodynamic status is noted, and the patient continues to be hypoxic, with an oxygen saturation of 89%. You contact medical control, and standing protocols are initiated.

Immediate attention is given to increasing the oxygenation and perfusion. Norepinephrine is increased to 10 μg/min, and epinephrine is considered as another pressor agent to increase the BP and SVR. The ventilator F_{IO_2} is increased to 100% and PEEP to 10 cm H_2O. Only slight improvements of oxygenation (90%) and hemodynamics (BP, 88/46 mm Hg) are noted. Hydrocortisone is also considered. Further discussions are held to maintain current patient status, and further therapy will ensue on admission to the tertiary facility. No further changes are noted during the transport course, and the patient is delivered to the tertiary facility ICU without further incident.

1. What is your differential diagnosis?
2. Which other treatment may be beneficial to this patient?
3. Is this an appropriate transfer based on the patient's condition?

Analysis

This patient is most likely experiencing sepsis and SIRS. MODS should be considered a possible diagnosis because of the patient's respiratory failure and renal insufficiency. The infection could have occurred secondary to the surgical exploration, or it might be the result of the mechanical ventilation (pneumonia) or perhaps an invasive line or catheter (intravascular or urinary).

Treatments en route to the receiving facility may include the following:

- Further increasing ventilator support by increasing FIO_2, minute volume, and PEEP. Tidal volume should not be increased.
- Administering chemical paralytics to facilitate ventilation. Sedatives must be used with paralytics, and the hypotensive effects may require increased pressor doses.
- Performing adequate fluid resuscitation *before* increasing any vasopressor doses; 4 to 6 L may be required. Blood products would be considered if the hematocrit value is less than 21%.
- Adding an infusion of another vasopressor agent, such as epinephrine or vasopressin, *after* adequate fluid resuscitation.
- Instituting dobutamine therapy, which may enhance tissue oxygen delivery, only *after* adequate fluids and vasopressor support.

This is an appropriate transfer because the patient will benefit from further treatment at a tertiary facility, such as the following:

- Further ventilator support
- Studies and determination of appropriate antibiotic therapy
- Possible surgical consult and intervention
- Anticoagulation and inflammatory therapies

Sepsis and MODS present complex challenges to CCTPs. Despite recent advances in the critical care arena, these conditions continue to have high mortality and morbidity rates. New therapies are helpful, but early detection and intervention remain the cornerstones of positive outcomes. Identification of risk factors and subtle changes in the patient's condition are required to identify early onset of these disorders and to initiate aggressive therapy to reverse the process and obtain a favorable outcome. Although CCTPs are limited in terms of the therapeutic options they may implement to reverse the process, such care still serves a vital role in supporting these extremely ill patients. Transport staff members have sufficient resources to address these patients' challenges and must remain vigilant in providing support for failing organ systems, restoring intravascular volume, and ensuring adequate oxygenation to meet the body's metabolic demands.

Prep Kit

Ready for Review

- All cells require energy, a continuous supply of oxygen, and nutrients. From those nutrients, mitochondria manufacture energy in the form of adenosine triphosphate (ATP), in a process called cellular respiration.
- Cellular respiration has three parts: glycolysis, the Krebs cycle, and the electron transport chain (oxidative phosphorylation). Unlike the other two parts of cellular respiration, which require oxygen, glycolysis can occur in an anaerobic environment as well as the usual aerobic environment. Nevertheless, such a solo attempt to support cellular respiration reduces the amount of ATP produced and increases lactic acid production, which can result in cell damage, impaired tissue function, and a cascade of injurious effects.
- To get oxygen to the body's cells, the respiratory system must allow oxygen and carbon dioxide exchange across the alveolar-capillary membrane. Once this transfer occurs, arterial blood transports oxygen to the tissues; in this blood, the oxygen is either dissolved in plasma (3%) or bound to hemoglobin (97%).
- Various factors can affect the delivery of oxygen-rich blood to the tissues, including blood volume, viscosity, and arterial elasticity. However, the primary determinants of

Prep Kit Continued

adequate transport are BP (it must be stable) and cardiac output (it must be adequate).

- Under normal conditions, the cells extract only 25% of the oxygen delivered to the tissues of the body. This allows the body a buffer zone for periods of low oxygen delivery, during which the cells must extract more oxygen.
- Shock is a progressive, whole-body response to an inadequate supply of oxygen within cells, tissues, and organs, from one or multiple causes. It is commonly organized into stages, and the mortality rate increases with progression through these stages:
  - In the compensatory stage of shock, neural, hormonal, and chemical mechanisms attempt to compensate for the severely reduced delivery of oxygen. In effect, they cover up for low circulatory volumes, poor stroke volume, and falling cardiac output, especially in children and healthy young adults. Common signs and symptoms may be as subtle as mild tachypnea and tachycardia. Mean arterial pressure (MAP) may decrease 10 to 15 mm Hg from baseline, and cardiac output may drop slightly.
  - In the decompensatory stage, multifaceted systemic responses to cell breakdown affect nearly every organ of the body. Compensatory mechanisms begin to fail, such that patients demonstrate more pronounced signs of shock, including altered mental status, tachycardia, and a drop in MAP from baseline. Laboratory analysis shows a progression of acidosis, hyperkalemia, and climbing lactate levels. This life-threatening emergency requires immediate treatment.
  - In the refractory stage, compensatory mechanisms have failed. The patient is unresponsive to verbal stimuli, BP is inadequate, the heart rate is increased, the respiratory rate is increased, and respirations are shallow. The skin is cold, cyanotic, and/or mottled, and peripheral pulses are weak and thready to absent. Urinary output decreases

and bowel sounds are absent. Anaerobic metabolism progresses to permanent organ dysfunction, and treatment can no longer reverse the mass effects. Multiple organ failure ensues and the risk of mortality is at its highest.

- Management of shock focuses on maximizing oxygen consumption by maintaining an adequate oxygen supply, providing hemoglobin through administration of blood products, and optimizing cardiac output. If a breakdown in one or more of these components occurs, a loss of homeostasis will occur.
- Multiple organ dysfunction syndrome (MODS) is diagnosed when two or more organs stop functioning. The organs affected early in MODS are the brain, kidneys, liver, adrenal glands, and heart. Sepsis is the leading cause of MODS.
- Shock traditionally is classified by cause. More than one type of shock may be present at the same time.
- Cardiogenic shock results when the ventricles are unable to pump blood forward, ultimately decreasing cardiac output. Manifestations vary depending on the underlying cause, but common signs and symptoms are low BP; altered mental status; cool, pale, diaphoretic skin; decreased urine output; weak and thready pulses; distant or abnormal S_3 or S_4 heart sounds; fluid accumulation in the lungs or limbs; and tachypnea. Management focuses on enhancing cardiac output while decreasing the left ventricular workload.
- In hypovolemic shock, too little circulating blood volume is present within the vascular system, which results in hypotension. Manifestations include tachycardia; hypotension; signs of poor tissue perfusion; altered mental status; and cold, mottled, and pulseless extremities. Management revolves around treating the underlying condition, administering oxygen, and initiating volume replacement.
- Distributive shock encompasses several types of shock involving loss of vasomotor tone or increased vascular permeability—namely,

Prep Kit Continued

neurogenic shock, anaphylactic shock, and septic shock.

- Neurogenic shock results from conditions that impede the sympathetic nervous system's ability to control the constriction and dilation of vessel walls, such as trauma to the brain or spinal cord. The signs and symptoms associated with neurogenic shock can be very different from those found in hypovolemic shock; most profound is the presence of bradycardia in the face of hypotension. It is vital to piece together all possible causes of hypotension to determine the best treatment, which generally focuses on maintaining MAP at greater than 85 mm Hg.

- Anaphylactic shock is a severe, life-threatening allergic reaction producing systemic vasodilation in response to histamine release. The reaction can be massive, and it can occur minutes after exposure, or hours or days later. Manifestations include bronchoconstriction, laryngeal edema, and angioedema resulting in airway compromise, which requires rapid treatment to limit its effects. Standard oxygen therapy may not be enough to maintain adequate oxygenation; patients may require intubation, an emergency cricothyrotomy, or tracheostomy to maintain an adequate airway.

- Sepsis is a life-threatening organ dysfunction caused by a dysregulated host response to infection. Septic shock is a subset of sepsis in which particularly profound circulatory, cellular, and metabolic abnormalities are associated with a greater risk of mortality than is noted with sepsis alone.

- Septic shock is a progressive disease that typically stems from an infection. It usually starts as a localized infection and then develops into a widespread inflammatory process, referred to as systemic inflammatory response syndrome (SIRS). When hypotension develops, septic shock is diagnosed.

- Infection is the leading cause of SIRS and septic shock. However, any shock state can trigger SIRS and lead to sepsis, and ultimately to multiple organ failure. The minimum criteria for early recognition of SIRS relate to temperature, heart rate, respiratory rate, and WBC count.

- The prevalence of sepsis-related infections is increasing. Such infections, which affect all populations and age groups, are especially associated with diabetes, hypertension, congestive heart failure, chronic obstructive pulmonary disease, cirrhosis, HIV infection, cancer, and pregnancy. Prolonged hospitalization is a risk factor, as are invasive procedures, comorbidities, and use of immunosuppressants. The mortality rate for sepsis increases with its severity.

- Bacteria are the pathogens most commonly associated with the development of sepsis, although fungi, viruses, and parasites can also cause this condition. Infection can occur at any body site, including the lungs, abdomen, skin, and urinary tract; it can also be a primary bloodstream infection. Gram-negative and gram-positive bacteria are the two types of organisms most commonly responsible for sepsis.

- Sepsis is part of a dynamic hypermetabolic, hyperinflammatory response to an infection that leads to a loss of control of the immune response. Left unchecked, the vasodilation and permeability that are initially helpful in fighting an infection may progress to distributive shock.

- Microvascular disruption and injury are responsible for hypoperfusion and the shunting of oxygen, which result in decreased oxygen delivery to the tissues. The profound imbalance between oxygen delivery and consumption causes hypoxia within the cells and tissues. This complex cascade of events is a primary cause of sepsis and its progression to organ dysfunction and failure.

- The first priority in recognizing sepsis is to maintain a high index of suspicion for the two phases of distributive shock: hyperdynamic (warm shock) and hypodynamic (cold shock). High cardiac output lasting hours or days

Prep Kit Continued

characterizes the hyperdynamic phase. It can progress to the hypodynamic phase, which features a rapid deterioration of the patient's condition accompanied by a sudden drop in cardiac output. Other manifestations of sepsis may include fever, hypothermia (in later stages), tachycardia, normal-to-low BP progressing to hypotension, normal skin progressing to cold and clammy skin with pallor or cyanosis, petechiae and blood oozing from mucous membranes and procedure sites, decreased pulse pressure, increased respiratory rate and depth, respiratory alkalosis, and acute respiratory distress syndrome.

- Management of sepsis aims to maintain organ perfusion while enhancing tissue oxygenation. It requires balancing preload, afterload, and contractility to achieve the targeted criteria for an optimal level of homeostasis.

- Fluid resuscitation is a key component of sepsis treatment, but it is not always sufficient to maintain BP. When it proves inadequate, vasopressors and inotropic agents may be administered in an effort to interrupt the septic cascade. Infection control and immune-specific therapy are other components of the multipronged sepsis treatment algorithm.

- Blood administration is sometimes performed to manage shock and should be considered when patients have hemorrhagic blood loss as a result of trauma, internal hemorrhage, perioperative and postoperative complications, specific disease entities, anemia due to illness, or coagulation disorders.

- The decision to give a transfusion during transport is complex. Factors to consider include the urgency of the transfusion, the amount of time out of the hospital, the availability of blood products, type and crossmatch information, and appropriate transport and care of the blood product.

- Steps for proper blood administration include appropriate typing and crossmatching, obtaining appropriate IV access, securing the appropriate blood tubing administration sets, priming the tubing with normal saline, validating the blood product's match with the specific patient before administration, and continued supervision by a skilled health care provider.

- In an emergency situation in which there is not enough time for crossmatching, type O, Rh-negative (universal donor type) blood or plasma can be transfused until crossmatched blood becomes available.

- Blood contains a variety of antigens that influence the blood's compatibility in various persons. Three types of blood antigens are the ABO blood group, Rh factor, and the HLA blood group; they are all considered during the crossmatching process.

- A person with only an A antigen is type A; a person with only a B antigen is type B. If both A and B antigens are identified, the person is type AB. When neither A nor B antigens are identified, the person's blood type is O.

- People with type AB blood are universal recipients; they can receive blood types A, B, AB, and O without the threat of an ABO reaction. People with type O blood are universal donors; their blood can be transfused into patients with type A, B, and AB blood.

- Rh factors are antigens found on the cell membrane of RBCs. An Rh-negative person may develop an Rh antibody if exposed to Rh-positive blood. A second Rh-positive exposure could then result in a fatal hemolytic reaction.

- Human leukocyte antigens (HLAs) are present on the cell membrane surfaces of circulating platelets, WBCs, and most tissue cells. Patients receiving platelets from multiple donors may experience febrile transfusion reactions due to an HLA reaction. This type of reaction destroys the platelets, reducing the benefits obtained from the transfusion.

- Blood can be administered in many different forms: whole blood, packed red blood cells

Prep Kit Continued

(PRBCs), platelets, fresh-frozen plasma (FFP), cryoprecipitate, albumin, plasma protein fractions, and synthetic blood substitutes. Specific groups of immunocompromised patients may require blood products that have been irradiated, leuko-reduced, or washed prior to transfusion.

- Whole blood contains all blood components (RBCs, WBCs, platelets, plasma, and electrolytes). Transfusion with whole blood is indicated only in acute massive blood loss for blood volume expansion and increased oxygen-carrying capacity. This type of transfusion has some significant disadvantages, including fluid volume overload in patients with cardiac compromise and degradation of the stored whole blood after 24 hours of storage.

- PRBCs retain all of the characteristics of whole blood, with the exception of the extraction of approximately 250 mL of platelet-rich plasma from each unit of whole blood. Anemia and blood loss are possible indications for PRBC administration.

- Platelet therapy may be considered for patients with extremely low platelet levels, those who are bleeding due to thrombocytopenia, and those with abnormally functioning platelets. If a patient must receive multiple transfusions of platelets, the platelets should come from a single donor.

- FFP is uncoagulated plasma that has been separated from the RBCs. Indications for its administration include blood loss, coagulation deficiencies, warfarin reversal, and thrombotic thrombocytopenia purpura. Patients must be closely monitored for hypocalcemia during FFP transfusions.

- Cryoprecipitate is a frozen blood product created from the plasma of a donor. It contains factor VIII, fibrinogen, von Willebrand factor, and factor XIII, and is useful in treating patients with clotting disorders. Administration of cryoprecipitate does not require compatibility testing.

- Albumin is prepared by the fractionation of pooled plasma. It can be used for volume replacement in patients with conditions such as burns, trauma, surgery, or infections. Patients with cardiac and pulmonary disease must be monitored closely during albumin administration.

- Plasma protein fraction contains 83% albumin and 17% globulins. It is indicated for volume expansion in patients with hypovolemia and hypoproteinemia. Clinical indications for the administration of plasma protein fraction may include shock and burns.

- Other types of blood products include synthetic blood substitutes, which have proved disappointing in clinical use to date; tranexamic acid, a synthetic antifibrinolytic agent that may be used in trauma patients with hypovolemic shock; and direct-acting oral anticoagulants.

- When performing blood administration, it is important to follow transfusion precautions:
  - Do not mix blood with 5% dextrose in water (causes hemolysis).
  - Do not mix blood with lactated Ringer solution (causes clotting).
  - Do not mix blood with medications (may react).
  - Have a second venous access line available.

- Blood administration can result in transfusion reactions, which can be as mild as chills or as catastrophic as death. Signs of such a reaction include body temperature that is 2°F (1°C) or more above the baseline temperature; hives, itching, or skin symptoms; swelling, soreness, or hematoma at the venous site; flank pain; tachycardia; respiratory distress (wheezing and dyspnea); hypotension; bleeding from widely varied sites or previously clotted wounds; blood in the urine; anaphylaxis; and nausea and vomiting.

- The main types of transfusion reactions include allergic reactions, bacterial contamination, febrile transfusion reactions, hemolytic transfusion reactions, and plasma protein incompatibility.

Prep Kit Continued

- Allergic reactions caused by allergens in the donated blood may produce symptoms of anaphylaxis (ie, chills, facial and laryngeal edema, pruritus, urticaria, and wheezing) as well as fever, nausea, and vomiting. Management includes the use of antihistamines, careful patient monitoring and assessment, and possibly epinephrine and corticosteroid administration.
- Bacterial contamination of blood components usually occurs during phlebotomy, component preparation or processing, or thawing of the blood components. Presenting symptoms may occur within 30 minutes after the transfusion begins and include chills, fever, vomiting, abdominal cramping, bloody diarrhea, hemoglobinuria, shock, renal failure, and DIC. It is essential to rapidly recognize these symptoms, stop the transfusion immediately, and implement the protocol for transfusion reactions.
- In febrile transfusion reactions, symptoms include a temperature as high as 104°F (40°C), chills, headache, facial flushing, palpitations, cough, chest tightness, increased pulse rate, and flank pain. Treatment includes the administration of antipyretics and antihistamines.
- Hemolytic transfusion reactions are caused by ABO or Rh incompatibility, intradonor incompatibility, improper crossmatching, or improper blood storage.
- Immediate hemolytic transfusion reactions may occur during the transfusion or within the first 24 hours after transfusion. Such reactions destroy RBCs, such that hemoglobin and cell remnants are released into the bloodstream. Symptoms include chest pain, facial flushing, shortness of breath, chills, fever, hypotension, flank pain, hemoglobinuria, oliguria, bloody oozing at the infusion site, burning along the vein receiving the blood, shock, signs of renal failure, and DIC. Treatment of immediate hemolytic transfusion reactions focuses on prevention and supportive management.
- Delayed hemolytic transfusion reactions occur 1 to 30 days after transfusion. Signs and symptoms are usually mild, including mild fever, chills, and moderate jaundice. Treatment focuses on the prevention and treatment of severe complications should they arise.
- Plasma protein incompatibility is caused by immunoglobulin A incompatibility. Clinical presentations include abdominal pain, diarrhea, shortness of breath, chills, fever, flushing, and hypotension. Management includes oxygen administration, fluids, epinephrine, and corticosteroids as indicated.
- Hypocalcemia may occur when blood products containing citrate are infused too quickly and bind to calcium, causing calcium deficiency and leading to arrhythmias, hypotension, muscle cramping, nausea, vomiting, seizure activity, or a tingling sensation in the fingers. Slowing or stopping the transfusion may be indicated. Management considerations include the slow infusion of calcium gluconate.
- High potassium levels in stored plasma may result in potassium intoxication during blood administration. Clinical manifestations may include diarrhea, intestinal colic, flaccidity, muscle twitching, oliguria, signs of renal failure, bradycardia, ECG changes with visible tall peaked T waves, and cardiac arrest.
- Hypothermia may result from a rapid infusion of large amounts of cold blood products. Symptoms may include chills, shivering, hypotension, arrhythmias, bradycardia, or cardiac arrest. Treatment may include stopping the transfusion, warming the patient, obtaining a diagnostic 12-lead ECG, and warming the blood if the transfusion is resumed.
- Patients with sepsis are rarely transported over long distances by fixed-wing transport; when they are, altitude and cabin pressure require ventilator adjustments to compensate for the pressures at altitude.

Prep Kit Continued

Vital Vocabulary

ABO-incompatible transfusion reactions Transfusion reactions in which the patient possesses antigens to a blood type and receives that blood type.

adaptive immune system The secondary mechanism that protects the host by reacting with and eliminating specific antigens, but that requires more time than the innate immune system to mobilize its defenses against unknown pathogens.

aerobic metabolism A form of energy production in which mitochondria use glucose, amino acids, and fatty acids combined with oxygen and ADP to produce ATP, carbon dioxide, water, and heat.

albumin A blood product containing this specific protein found in the blood, which is prepared by the fractionation of pooled plasma; used for volume replacement in certain conditions.

anaerobic metabolism A less efficient form of energy production in which an alternative pathway converts glucose to pyruvic acid with the simultaneous production of ATP; it also results in the production of lactate.

anaphylactic shock A severe hypersensitivity reaction that involves bronchoconstriction and cardiovascular collapse.

anaphylactoid reaction A non–IgE-mediated response that causes the rupture of mast cells and basophils, which then release histamine and other defense mediators.

antigens Substances that can create an immune response in the body.

arterial oxygen content (Cao_2) The total amount of oxygen in the arterial blood.

bacteremia The presence of viable bacteria in the bloodstream.

cardiac index A hemodynamic value that adjusts a patient's cardiac output to take into account the total body surface area.

cardiac output (CO) The amount of blood pumped by the heart per minute, calculated by multiplying the stroke volume by the heart rate per minute.

cardiogenic shock A condition caused by loss of 40% or more of the functioning myocardium; the heart is no longer able to circulate sufficient blood to maintain adequate oxygen delivery.

cryoprecipitate A blood product created from plasma and in which clotting factors, especially factor VIII, are concentrated; it is used to treat patients with coagulation disorders.

cytokines Chemical messengers that enhance cell growth, promote cell activation, direct cellular traffic, stimulate macrophage function, and destroy antigens. Interleukins are a type of cytokine.

delayed hemolytic transfusion reactions Transfusion reactions that do not occur until 3 to 30 days after transfusion.

disseminated intravascular coagulation (DIC) A complex condition arising from different causes that activate coagulation mechanisms, resulting in obstructed blood flow as a result of microclots as well as fibrinolysis, while the body attempts to reopen the microcirculation. Bleeding, thrombosis, and, potentially, organ dysfunction result.

distributive shock A condition characterized by widespread dilation of the resistance vessels, the capacitance vessels, or both.

ejection fraction The portion of the blood ejected from the ventricle during systole.

endotoxins Lipopolysaccharides that coat the outer surface of gram-negative bacteria and elicit strong immune responses in humans while providing a layer of protection for the bacterium; they can also be secreted from the cell and are released en masse when cell death occurs.

exotoxins Proteins that are secreted by some bacteria and can directly cause significant damage to host cells while also triggering an immune response.

Prep Kit Continued

fresh-frozen plasma (FFP) A blood product in which uncoagulated plasma has been separated from the red blood cells; it is primarily composed of water, proteins, salts, metabolites, and clotting factors.

hemolysis The destruction of red blood cells, which results in the release of hemoglobin and cell remnants into the bloodstream.

hemolytic transfusion reactions Transfusion reactions caused by ABO or Rh incompatibility, intradonor incompatibility, improper cross-matching, or improper blood storage.

human leukocyte antigen (HLA) An antigen present on the cell membrane surfaces of circulating platelets, white blood cells, and most tissue cells.

hypercapnia Greater than normal amounts of carbon dioxide in the blood.

hyperdynamic state The first stage of distributive shock, which is characterized primarily by high cardiac output and low peripheral vascular resistance; also known as warm shock.

hypodynamic state The second stage of distributive shock, which is characterized primarily by a subnormal temperature, a low white blood cell count, profound hypotension and hypoperfusion, and a sudden drop in cardiac output; also known as cold shock.

hypovolemic shock A condition in which the circulating blood volume is inadequate for delivering sufficient oxygen and nutrients to the body.

immediate hemolytic transfusion reactions Transfusion reactions that usually occur soon (between 1 and 2 hours) after the transfusion of incompatible red blood cells.

infection The invasion of normally sterile tissue by a pathogen.

innate immune system The primary nonspecific antigen and immunogen defense mechanism that protects the host by eliminating microbes and other antigens in an effort to prevent infection and allergic reactions.

irradiated blood products Blood products in which lymphocyte DNA has been exposed to radiation to damage it, and thereby limit the cells' ability to replicate and cause the rare but often fatal condition of transfusion-associated graft-versus-host disease.

leuko-reduced blood products Blood products in which the white blood cells and platelet fragments have been filtered from donated blood products.

leukotrienes A class of biologically active compounds that occur naturally in leukocytes and that produce allergic and inflammatory reactions.

massive transfusion protocol The rapid administration of large amounts of blood products in fixed ratios (usually 1:1:1) for the management of hemorrhagic shock.

mean arterial pressure (MAP) The average (or mean) pressure against the arterial wall during a cardiac cycle.

microcirculation Circulation that occurs in the microvasculature, the body's smallest vessels (arterioles, capillaries, and venules).

multiple organ dysfunction syndrome (MODS) Altered organ function in acutely ill patients, which is diagnosed when two or more organs stop functioning.

neurogenic shock Circulatory failure caused by paralysis of the nerves that control the size of the blood vessels, leading to widespread dilation; it is seen in spinal cord injuries.

neutrophils A type of leukocyte (white blood cell); these numerous phagocytic microphages usually are the first of the mobile phagocytic cells to arrive at the site of injury or infection.

oxygen consumption ($\dot{V}o_2$) The amount of oxygen used by the cells and tissues.

oxygen delivery (Do_2) The amount of oxygen delivered to the tissues each minute.

oxygen extraction ratio (ERo_2) The relationship between oxygen consumption and oxygen

Prep Kit Continued

delivery; a measure of the cells' ability to use oxygen.

packed red blood cells (PRBCs) A blood product that retains all of the characteristics of whole blood, with the exception of the extraction of approximately 250 mL of platelet-rich plasma from each unit of whole blood.

pathogens Microorganisms that activate the immune system and cause disease; they include viruses, parasites, fungi, and bacteria.

plasma protein fraction A blood product that contains 83% albumin and 17% globulins.

primary MODS Multiple organ dysfunction syndrome that results from a direct insult such as trauma.

refractory stage The stage of shock characterized by persistently low mean arterial blood pressure despite vasopressor therapy and adequate fluid resuscitation.

Rh factors Antigens found on the cell membrane of red blood cells.

secondary MODS Multiple organ dysfunction syndrome that presents a slower, more progressive insult to organs and frequently results from the sepsis cascade.

sepsis A condition of life-threatening organ dysfunction caused by a dysregulated host response to infection.

septic shock A subset of sepsis in which particularly profound circulatory, cellular, and metabolic abnormalities are associated with a greater risk of mortality than occurs with sepsis alone.

systemic inflammatory response syndrome (SIRS) A widespread inflammatory process associated with infectious and noninfectious causes, without end-organ damage.

transfusion reactions Reactions resulting from an endogenous or exogenous factor related to transfused blood.

true anaphylaxis An anaphylactic reaction that occurs when the allergen binds to immunoglobulin E on the cell membranes of basophils and when mast cells stimulate the release of histamine from the cell.

tumor necrosis factor (TNF) A protein mediator that is released primarily by macrophages and T lymphocytes, and that helps regulate the immune response.

type-and-crossmatch The test to determine compatibility between patient serum and donor red blood cells prior to transfusion.

universal donors Persons who have type O blood.

universal recipients Persons who have type AB blood.

washed blood products Red blood cell or platelet products in which the small amount of noncellular fluid has been replaced, typically with saline.

References

Acute Respiratory Distress Syndrome Network. Ventilation with lower tidal volumes as compared with traditional tidal volumes for acute lung injury and the acute respiratory distress syndrome. *N Engl J Med.* 2000;342(18):1301-1308.

American College of Surgeons Committee on Trauma. *Advanced Trauma Life Support for Doctors: ATLS Student Course Manual.* 10th ed. Chicago, IL: American College of Surgeons; 2018.

American Red Cross. Blood needs and blood supply. https://www.redcrossblood.org/donate-blood/how-to-donate/how-blood-donations-help/blood-needs-blood-supply.html. Accessed March 28, 2021.

Annane D, Siami S, Jaber S, et al; for the CRISTAL Investigators. Effects of fluid resuscitation with colloids vs crystalloids on mortality in critically ill patients presenting with hypovolemic shock: The CRISTAL randomized trial. *JAMA.* 2013;310(17):1809-1817.

ARDS Definition Task Force; Ranieri VM, Rubenfeld GD, Thompson BT, et al. Acute respiratory distress syndrome. *JAMA.* 2012;307(23):2526-2533.

Assinger A, Schrottmaier WC, Salzmann M, Rayes J. Platelets in sepsis: an update on experimental models and clinical data. *Frontiers Immunol.* 2019;10:1687.

Ausset S, Glassberg E, Nadler R, et al. Tranexamic acid as part of remote damage-control resuscitation in the prehospital

Prep Kit Continued

setting: a critical appraisal of the medical literature and available alternatives. *J Trauma Acute Care Surg.* 2015;78(6 suppl 1):S70-S75.

Bassi E, Park M, Pontes Azevedo LC. Therapeutic strategies for high-dose vasopressor-dependent shock. *Crit Care Res Pract.* 2013. doi:10.1155/2013/654708.

Bellumkonda L, Gul B, Masri SC. Evolving concepts in diagnosis and management of cardiogenic shock. *Am J Cardiol.* 2018;122(6):1104-1110.

Boldt J. Use of albumin: an update. *Br J Anaesth.* 2010;104(3):276-284.

Bonanno FG. Clinical pathology of the shock syndromes. *J Emerg Trauma Shock.* 2011;4(2):233.

Centers for Disease Control and Prevention. Sepsis: clinical information. https://www.cdc.gov/sepsis/clinicaltools/index.html. Reviewed December 7, 2020. Accessed March 28, 2021.

Christiaans SC, Wagener BM, Esmon CT, Pittet JF. Protein C and acute inflammation: a clinical and biological perspective. *Am J Physiol-Lung Cell Molec Physiol.* 2013;305(7):L455-L466.

Cohen J, Vincent J-L, Adhikari NKJ, et al. Sepsis: a roadmap for future research. *Lancet Infect Dis.* 2015;15(5):581-614.

CRASH-2 Trial Collaborators. Effects of tranexamic acid on death, vascular occlusive events, and blood transfusion in trauma patients with significant haemorrhage (CRASH-2): a randomised, placebo-controlled trial. *Lancet.* 2010;376:23-32.

De Backer D, Biston P, Devriendt J, et al; for the SOAP II Investigators. Comparison of dopamine and norepinephrine in the treatment of shock. *N Engl J Med.* 2010;362:779-789.

Epstein L, Dantes R, Magill S, et al. Varying estimates of sepsis mortality using death certificates and administrative codes—United States, 1999–2014. *MMWR.* 2016;65(13):342-345.

Finfer S, Bellomo R, Boyce N, et al; for the SAFE Study Investigators. A comparison of albumin and saline for fluid resuscitation in the intensive care unit. *N Engl J Med.* 2004;350(22):2247-2256.

Gourd NM, Nikitas N. Multiple organ dysfunction syndrome. *J Intens Care Med.* 2020;35(12):1564-1575.

Holcomb JB, Tilley BC, Baraniuk S, et al; for the PROPPR Study Group. Transfusion of plasma, platelets, and red blood cells in a 1:1:1 vs a 1:1:2 ratio and mortality in patients with severe trauma: the PROPPR randomized clinical trial. *JAMA.* 2015;313(5):471-482.

Jahr JS, Guin NR, Lowery DR, et al. Blood substitutes and oxygen therapeutics: a review. *Anesth Analg.* 2021;132(1):119-129.

Kalil A. Septic shock. http://emedicine.medscape.com/article/168402-overview. Updated October 7, 2020. Accessed March 28, 2021.

Kim F, Nichol G, Maynard C, et al. Effect of prehospital induction of mild hypothermia on survival and neurological status among adults with cardiac arrest: a randomized clinical trial. *JAMA.* November 17, 2013. [Epub ahead of print]. doi:10.1001/jama.2013.282173. PubMed: 24240712.

Levy MM, Evans LE, Rhodes A. The surviving sepsis campaign bundle: 2018 update. *Intens Care Med.* 2018;44(6):925-928.

Lilly CM. The ProCESS trial: a new era of sepsis management. *N Engl J Med.* 2014;370(18):1750-1751.

Liumbruno G, Bennardello F, Lattanzio A, et al. Recommendations for the transfusion of plasma and platelets. *Blood Transfus.* 2009;7(2):132-150.

Mandawat A, Rao SV. Percutaneous mechanical circulatory support devices in cardiogenic shock. *Circulation Cardiovasc Interv.* 2017;10(5):e004337. doi:10.1161/CIRCINTERVENTIONS.116.004337.

Mayr FB, Yende S, Angus DC. Epidemiology of severe sepsis. *Virulence.* 2014;5(1):4-11.

Nandhabalan P, Ioannou N, Meadows C, Wyncoll D. Refractory septic shock: our pragmatic approach. *Crit Care.* 2018;22(1):1-5.

National Heart, Lung, and Blood Institute (NHLBI) ARDSNet. NIH NHLBI ARDS Clinical Network mechanical ventilation protocol summary. http://ardsnet.org/files/ventilator_protocol_2008-07.pdf. Accessed March 28, 2021.

Pourmand A, Robinson C, Syed W, Mazer-Amirshahi M. Biphasic anaphylaxis: a review of the literature and implications for emergency management. *Am J Emerg Med.* 2018;36(8):1480-1485.

Rhee C, Dantes R, Epstein L, et al. Incidence and trends of sepsis in US hospitals using clinical vs claims data, 2009–2014. *JAMA.* 2017;318(13):1241-1249.

Rhodes A, Evans LE, Alhazzani W, et al. Surviving Sepsis campaign: international guidelines for management of sepsis and septic shock: 2016. *Intens Care Med.* 2017;43(3):304-377.

Rivers E, Nguyen B, Havstad S, et al. Early goal-directed therapy in the treatment of severe sepsis and septic shock. *N Engl J Med.* 2001;345(19):1368-1377.

Roberts I, Blackhall K, Alderson P, Bunn F, Schierhout G. Human albumin solution for resuscitation and volume expansion in critically ill patients: review. *Cochrane Library.* 2011;11. Cochrane Collaboration; John Wiley & Sons.

Shaz BH, Hillyer CD, Reyes Gil M, eds. *Transfusion Medicine and Hemostasis: Clinical and Laboratory Aspects.* 3rd ed. Elsevier Science; 2019.

Simpson SQ. SIRS in the time of Sepsis-3. *Chest.* 2018;153(1):34-38.

Singer M, Deutschman CS, Seymour CW, et al. The Third International Consensus Definitions for Sepsis and Septic Shock (Sepsis-3). *JAMA.* 2016;315(8):801-808. doi:10.1001/jama.2016.0287.

Prep Kit Continued

Storch EK, Rogerson B, Eder AF. Trend in ABO incompatible RBC transfusion related fatalities reported to the FDA, 2000–2019. *Transfusion*. 2020;60(12):2867-2875.

Thiele H, Zeymer U, Neumann F-J, et al; for the IABP-SHOCK II Trial Investigators. Intraaortic balloon support for myocardial infarction with cardiogenic shock. *N Engl J Med*. 2012;367(14);1287-1296.

Unverzagt S, Buerke M, de Waha A, et al. Intra-aortic balloon pump counterpulsation (IABP) for myocardial infarction complicated by cardiogenic shock: review. *Cochrane Library*. 2015;3. Cochrane Collaboration; John Wiley & Sons.

Unverzagt S, Wachsmuth L, Hirsch K, et al. Inotropic agents and vasodilator strategies for acute myocardial infarction complicated by cardiogenic shock or low cardiac output syndrome: review. *Cochrane Library*. 2014;1. Cochrane Collaboration; John Wiley & Sons.

Usman OA, Usman AA, Ward MA. Comparison of SIRS, qSOFA, and NEWS for the early identification of sepsis in the emergency department. *Am J Emerg Med*. 2019;37(8):1490-1497.

Van Diepen S, Katz JN, Albert NM, et al. Contemporary management of cardiogenic shock: a scientific statement from the American Heart Association. *Circulation*. 2017;136(16):e232-e268.

Volbeda M, Wetterslev J, Gluud C, Zijlstra JG, van der Horst ICC, Keus F. Glucocorticosteroids for sepsis: systematic review with meta-analysis and trial sequential analysis. *Intens Care Med*. 2015;41(7):1220-1234.

Wang J-W, Li J-P, Song Y-l, et al. Hypertonic saline in the traumatic hypovolemic shock: meta-analysis. *J Surg Res*. 2014;191(2):448-454.

Weinberg JA, Farber SH, Kalamchi LD, et al. Mean arterial pressure maintenance following spinal cord injury: Does meeting the target matter? *J Trauma Acute Care Surg*. 2021;90(1):97-106.

Wiersinga WJ, Seymour CW, eds. *Handbook of Sepsis*. Vol. 8. Springer International Publishing; 2018.

Yasuyuki K, Ito T, Nakahara M, Yamaguchi K, Yasuda T. Sepsis-induced myocardial dysfunction: pathophysiology and management. *J Intens Care*. 2016;4(1):1-10.

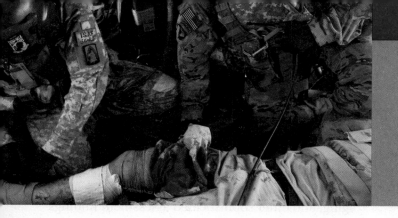

Chapter 11

Trauma

Christopher McLaughlin, MD, MBA

OBJECTIVES

After completing this chapter, you will be able to:

1. Understand the critical care transport professional's impact on preventing trauma deaths by performing proper prehospital care and transporting patients to the appropriate trauma center (p 466).
2. Explain the significance of trauma management for morbidity and mortality (pp 466–467).
3. Understand Newton's first, second, and third laws of motion, and explain how they relate to patterns of injury (p 467).
4. Discuss the types of trauma (pp 467–468).
5. Describe the various trauma scoring systems, including the Glasgow Coma Scale, the trauma score, the revised trauma score, the Abbreviated Injury Scale, the Injury Severity Score, and the trauma injury severity score, and explain how they are used (pp 468–472).
6. Discuss the classifications of trauma centers defined by the American College of Surgeons' Committee on Trauma, including Level I, II, III, and IV trauma centers (pp 472–473).
7. Understand how to assess a patient in a hospital setting prior to initiating interfacility transport (pp 473–474).
8. Describe the elements of the hypothermia–acidosis–coagulopathy triad, including how to manage them (pp 474–475).
9. Understand how and when diagnostic imaging, including standard radiographs, computed tomography, ultrasonography, transthoracic echocardiography, transesophageal echocardiography, magnetic resonance imaging, and intra-abdominal pressure monitoring, are used and their implications (pp 475–480).
10. Explain how to recognize, assess, and manage the most common thoracic trauma injuries, including pneumothorax (open, simple, and tension), hemothorax, flail chest, pericardial tamponade, aortic dissection, myocardial contusion, diaphragmatic rupture, tracheobronchial disruption, pulmonary contusion, esophageal perforation, and traumatic asphyxia (pp 481–504).
11. Explain how to insert and manage a chest tube, including pigtail catheters (pp 488–495).
12. Describe how to recognize, assess, and manage ear, eye, neck, and tracheal trauma injuries (pp 505–511).
13. Identify the signs and symptoms of abdominal and pelvic injuries, including both hollow and solid organ injuries, and describe how to manage them (pp 511–514).
14. Understand the indications for and use of resuscitative endovascular balloon occlusion of the aorta (REBOA) (pp 514–516).
15. Identify the most commonly encountered types of fractures, and describe how to manage them (pp 520–524).
16. Explain how to recognize, monitor, and manage compartment syndrome, rhabdomyolysis, and crush syndrome (pp 524–527).
17. Discuss specific trauma considerations for special populations (pp 527–528).

Introduction

Trauma poses a significant threat to life. Since emergency medical services (EMS) began to evolve in the 1960s, more emphasis has been placed on rapidly identifying injuries and transporting patients to an appropriate trauma center for definitive care. The severity of the injuries in a traumatic incident may range from minor to life threatening. All trauma patients need a trauma assessment to determine if they have serious injuries. Most local community hospitals should be able to manage and treat patients with minor injuries.

The ability of the critical care transport professional (CCTP) to provide appropriate care for trauma patients en route to the trauma center can help decrease the incidence of morbidity and mortality related to their injuries. The emphasis on identifying life-threatening illnesses and injuries as soon as possible and transporting the patient to an appropriate facility has certainly improved patient outcomes. Unfortunately, trauma remains the leading cause of death in persons younger than 45 years. According to the Centers for Disease Control and Prevention, traumatic injuries accounted for more than 170,000 deaths in the United States in 2019. Many preventable trauma deaths occur in the prehospital environment, further highlighting the importance of proper prehospital care.

Renewed emphasis on education has helped to focus prehospital care providers' priorities at the scene of a trauma incident. These priorities include scene safety, rapid motion restriction/stabilization, and transport.

Scenarios Involving Trauma Patients

CCTPs may encounter trauma patients in two very different situations. The first scenario is the scene call, in which CCTPs usually back up field basic life support (BLS) and/or advanced life support (ALS) providers. In these cases, the CCTP will be working in more austere and less controlled conditions with less sophisticated assessment tools than are available in an interfacility transport. During a scene call, the CCTP may be asked to provide care that is outside the scope of the standard field responder, such as rapid sequence intubation (RSI), or to provide a speedy transport of the patient to a facility for immediate surgery or blood transfusion, such as by rotor-wing aircraft.

In the second scenario, the CCTP is involved in transferring critical patients, usually from smaller facilities to trauma centers. In this situation, the CCTP will be able to review laboratory results, imaging, and other sophisticated assessment findings prior to beginning the transport. The CCTP may also be able to enlist the assistance of the transferring physician or other house staff to help with stabilization efforts prior to transport. These steps may include securing difficult airways, inserting chest tubes, and hanging blood or other treatments that may be better performed in the referring hospital than in a moving transport vehicle. Diplomatically enlisting this aid and advocating for the patient are other jobs of the CCTP in this situation.

In both types of calls, the time it takes to stabilize the patient's condition for transport must be balanced against the need to transport an unstable patient immediately for definitive care that cannot be provided in the field. A top priority of the CCTP is to determine the treatment that needs to be provided before transport versus what can be done en route.

Morbidity and Mortality

Managers and practitioners in trauma systems in the United States spend considerable time and effort in researching ways to decrease morbidity and mortality rates. The terms *morbidity* and *mortality* are often used synonymously with *disability* and *death*, because these outcomes are ultimately what advanced trauma systems are working to prevent. Morbidity refers to nonfatal injury and disability, whereas mortality refers to deaths caused by injury and disease. Reducing their incidences is an area of concern for all trauma systems in the United States, because trauma is the leading cause of death in the pediatric population and a leading cause of death overall. One-half of all deaths of children result from trauma, and this cause accounts for more than 14,000 deaths annually.

Prevention and quality trauma care are two major factors that contribute to decreasing morbidity and mortality rates. High-quality prevention programs keep the trauma system and its patients from the effect of life-threatening and life-altering injuries related to trauma. This role is especially significant because a vast majority of trauma deaths are related to motor vehicle crashes (MVCs). Such crashes are often caused by factors such as alcohol, excessive speed, lack of physical restraints, and poor judgment. Most of these factors can be easily addressed with an established and efficiently functioning prevention program.

An alarming statistic related to MVCs is the number of people who survive the crash but sustain a debilitating injury that leaves them incapacitated. Many of these injuries involve the head and the spinal cord. To prevent these kinds of negative outcomes, the CCTP must realize the importance of avoiding secondary injury caused by improper handling of the patient. Patients with long-term debilitating injuries will spend the rest of their lives dependent on others for basic everyday needs and may require advanced nursing care, resulting in a huge cost to society and to the patients and their families, both financially and emotionally.

Overview of Trauma
Newton's Laws of Motion

By far one of the foremost scientific intellects of all time, Sir Isaac Newton discovered three laws of motion. These laws factor into the mechanism of injury for trauma patients, which in turn affects the care that EMS responders provide to these patients. We review them here.

Newton's First Law

Newton's first law of motion deals with force and velocity, both of which play key roles in MVCs. Essentially, Newton says, "A body in motion remains in motion in a straight line unless acted upon by an outside force." The CCTP must understand this concept to predict patterns of injuries. For example, suppose a vehicle traveling at 50 mph hits a tree head on and comes to an abrupt stop. The chain of events during the collision includes the vehicle striking the tree, the patient's chest striking the steering wheel, and the patient's internal organs striking the rib cage. During this sequence, the exchange of energy within the body causes many different types of damage. A solid understanding of Newton's first law of motion better prepares the CCTP to deliver the appropriate standard of care to patients with traumatic injuries.

Newton's Second Law

Newton's second law of motion refers to an object's behavior when an outside force is applied. According to this law, acceleration depends on two variables—the mass of the object and the force upon the object. In essence, if force is increased, so is acceleration. If mass is increased, the acceleration is decreased. Essentially, an object accelerates in the direction in which it is pushed. If you push the object twice as hard, it accelerates twice as much. Conversely, if the mass of an object increases, the acceleration must decrease proportionally if force is to remain constant as F (force) $= m$ (mass) $\times a$ (acceleration).

Newton's Third Law

Newton's third law of motion is most commonly paraphrased as "To every action, there is an equal and opposite reaction." In other words, if a motor vehicle strikes a wall at 70 mph, the wall pushes back at 70 mph. A solid understanding of the third law is of particular importance to the CCTP when evaluating the mechanism of injury and understanding the predictability of injuries. For example, the CCTP would have a higher index of suspicion of a chest injury if the patient is a passenger in a motor vehicle that was traveling at 70 mph when it hit a tree head on than if the vehicle had been traveling at 5 mph.

Types of Trauma

Traumatic injuries are generally classified into one of two categories: blunt or penetrating. Patients may have injuries that fit into both classifications at the same time. For example, an individual who is stabbed in the back (penetrating injury) and then falls down a flight of steps (blunt injury) could experience both types of injuries. Blunt injuries result from an energy exchange between an object and the body, without intrusion through the skin **FIGURE 11-1**. Examples include rapid forward decelerations (crashes), rapid vertical decelerations (falls), and energy transferred from blunt instruments such as a stick or bat. Penetrating injuries refer to injuries caused by external forces in which the skin is penetrated by an object. Examples include projectiles, such as bullets, knives, and fragments from explosions and falls upon fixed objects.

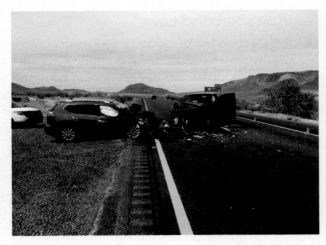

FIGURE 11-1 A front-end collision should prompt the CCTP to suspect potential head, neck, and chest injuries.

© Uncredited/AP/Shutterstock.

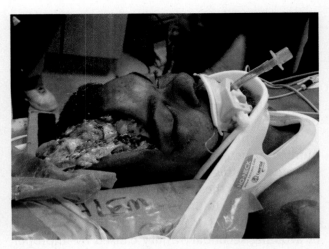

FIGURE 11-2 An overwhelming injury can cause a CCTP to focus on the visual horror, while missing more serious emergencies such as severe internal blood loss.

© E.M. Singletary, MD. Used with permission.

Deceleration injuries are caused by a sudden stop of the body's forward motion. These blunt injuries can result from falls, MVCs, or abuse such as shaken baby syndrome. Common injuries involve shearing, avulsing, or rupturing of body organs, fascia, nerves, and other soft tissue. Often these types of injuries are not visible to the CCTP, so a thorough understanding of the types of mechanisms of injury and effective assessment skills is imperative.

Forces that disrupt or damage the tissues of the body cause external force injuries. These injuries can result from gunshot wounds, stabbings, and projectiles. The severity of the injury depends on the anatomic area involved, the mass, and, most importantly, the velocity of the foreign object that enters the body. The kinetic energy (KE) of an object is the energy associated with that object in motion. It reflects the relationship between the weight (mass) of the object and the velocity at which it is traveling, and is expressed mathematically as follows (m = mass, v = velocity):

$$KE = \frac{1}{2}mv^2$$

External force injuries require the CCTP to use excellent patient assessment skills to prioritize the patient's injuries and the treatments for them. When doing so, the CCTP must be careful not to develop tunnel vision. Tunnel vision occurs when people devote all of their attention to what is immediately in front of them, ignoring their peripheral vision. For example, the CCTP with tunnel vision might focus on

a visible injury, which may or may not be life threatening, yet ignore other injuries to the patient that may well be life threatening **FIGURE 11-2**. Maintaining a calm, professional demeanor and using a systematic approach will allow the CCTP to maintain a high index of suspicion and keen attention to detail.

Trauma Scoring Systems

Several trauma scoring systems are used in the critical care transport environment to provide assessment information and as indicators of patient survivability. Trauma scoring systems are an important tool for regional trauma centers, which use them in conjunction with their quality assurance programs.

Glasgow Coma Scale

The Glasgow Coma Scale (GCS) is a validated tool that is widely used by health care professionals to assess the neurologic status of a wide variety of patients. This scoring system is used to determine a patient's level of consciousness by measuring and assigning point values, or scores, for three basic indicators of neurologic function: eye opening, verbal response, and motor response. The highest score is 15; the lowest score is 3. The lower the score, the more severe the extent of brain injury. **TABLE 11-1** shows how the numerical values are determined.

The GCS score is an important tool when caring for trauma patients and can be used for numerous

TABLE 11-1 Glasgow Coma Scale

Eye Opening		Best Verbal Response		Best Motor Response	
Spontaneous	4	Oriented conversation	5	Obeys commands	6
In response to sound	3	Confused conversation	4	Localizes to pressure	5
In response to pressure	2	Words	3	Withdraws from pressure	4
No response	1	Sounds	2	Abnormal flexion	3
		None	1	Extension	2
				No response	1

a Some systems assign a "Not testable" (NT) score for any element that cannot be tested. Eye opening cannot be tested in a patient whose eyes are closed due to a local factor, such as swelling; verbal response cannot be tested in a patient who has a preexisting factor interfering with communication, such as mutism; and motor response cannot be tested in a patient who has preexisting paralysis or other limiting factor.

Scoring:

13–15 may indicate mild dysfunction, although 15 is the score a person without neurologic impairment would receive.

9–12 may indicate moderate dysfunction.

8 or less is indicative of severe dysfunction.

© Jones & Bartlett Learning.

other types of patients. Many medical emergencies, such as drug overdoses, metabolic disorders, and neurologic emergencies, will benefit from frequent patient evaluation using the GCS. Ongoing assessments assist CCTPs in rapidly identifying treatable conditions.

Patients who present with a GCS score of less than 8 warrant immediate consideration for intubation or further advanced airway intervention, as they likely have significant neurologic impairment. While not without its critics, the GCS score is one of the most frequently used means of objectively assessing the central nervous system when invasive monitoring devices are not available. Even in an intubated patient, the GCS score provides useful information; the CCTP merely needs to note when a patient's inability to verbalize may be impaired by a device in their airway, rather than a decrease in neurologic function. Always give detailed explanations of abnormal GCS findings in the narrative section of your patient care record.

In many situations, successful management of the unresponsive patient with a head injury depends on ongoing examinations. Neurologic changes can occur in a matter of minutes, which may necessitate obtaining a GCS score as often as every 5 minutes. Ongoing GCS assessment scores must always be compared to the baseline score. It is important to look for changes that signal deterioration, as well as any improvements. Any changes must be reported to the receiving facility.

Special Populations

It is just as important to obtain an accurate neurologic exam in children as it is in adults, although doing so may be more difficult with pediatric patients. Depending on the age of the child, modifications may be necessary to accurately identify any neurologic deficits. These modifications are made based on the child's age and stage of pediatric development.

Just as in adults, a poor GCS score in a pediatric patient usually indicates the patient requires some type of immediate intervention, such as airway control or aggressive resuscitation. Chapter 24, *Pediatric Emergencies*, discusses the pediatric GCS score and its application in the management of pediatric patients.

Trauma Score

The trauma score is a predictor of the likelihood of patient survival. The score ranges from 1 to 16, with 16 being the best possible score, and takes into account the GCS score, respiratory rate, respiratory expansion, systolic blood pressure, and capillary refill. The trauma score, however, does not accurately predict survivability in patients with severe head injuries. Therefore, the revised trauma score (discussed next) has replaced the trauma score as a means of assessment.

Special Populations

The pediatric trauma score takes into account the child's weight, systolic blood pressure, airway status, central nervous system status, the presence of an open wound, and the presence of musculoskeletal trauma. Chapter 24, *Pediatric Emergencies*, discusses the pediatric trauma score and its application in the management of pediatric patients.

Revised Trauma Score

The numeric scoring of trauma patients as a means of determining the severity of their injuries is common practice. Several different trauma scoring systems have been developed, with the most commonly used system being the **revised trauma score**.

The revised trauma score measures three physiologic parameters: respiratory rate, systolic blood pressure, and GCS score **TABLE 11-2**. Total scores range from 0 to 13, with more seriously injured patients receiving lower scores. The score can also be weighted; the result then ranges from 1.0 to 7.8408. When the scores are weighted, the GCS score is given more weight to account for a patient's compensatory mechanisms that could prevent vital signs from accurately reflecting the patient's condition.

The weighted score is not practical for use in clinical care but is a helpful research tool when studying mortality among trauma patients. Much time and effort are spent researching ways to decrease morbidity and mortality in trauma patients, and extensive research has shown that low revised trauma scores are correlated with high mortality rates **FIGURE 11-3**. This relationship simply reinforces the effectiveness of the various trauma scores.

TABLE 11-2 Components of the Revised Trauma Score	
Revised Trauma Score	**Components**
4	GCS score: 13–15 Systolic blood pressure: >89 mm Hg Respiratory rate: 10–29 breaths/min
3	GCS score: 9–12 Systolic blood pressure: 76–89 mm Hg Respiratory rate: >29 breaths/min
2	GCS score: 6–8 Systolic blood pressure: 50–75 mm Hg Respiratory rate: 6–9 breaths/min
1	GCS score: 4–5 Systolic blood pressure: 1–49 mm Hg Respiratory rate: 1–5 breaths/min
0	GCS score: 3 Systolic blood pressure: 0 mm Hg Respiratory rate: 0 breaths/min

Abbreviation: GCS, Glasgow Coma Scale

© Jones & Bartlett Learning.

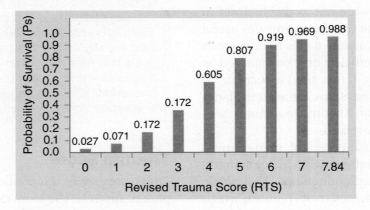

FIGURE 11-3 Survival probability by revised trauma score.

Modified from Survival Probability by Revised Trauma Score. © Trauma.org.

The revised trauma score does not readily identify the small percentage of severely injured trauma patients whose vital signs, because of compensatory mechanisms, do not accurately represent their conditions. For example, a patient with severe trauma who is in compensated shock may not present with abnormal vital signs (eg, low systolic blood pressure and increased respiratory rate) because the body is compensating for the blood loss. The body's ability to compensate for this blood loss may last for only a brief period. When the patient begins to decompensate, the vital signs will begin to deteriorate. Importantly, aggressive resuscitation should begin *before* the patient's vital signs deteriorate. Regardless of the revised trauma score calculated at a particular moment, the CCTP needs to be prepared for each trauma patient's condition to deteriorate with time, once the body becomes unable to compensate for the injury. For patients with a revised trauma score of less than 11, the American College of Surgeons recommends transfer to a Level I or II trauma center. *A high index of suspicion for potential decompensation should be maintained in all trauma patients.*

Abbreviated Injury Scale

Developed in 1969, the Abbreviated Injury Scale (AIS) is an anatomic scoring system that is designed to provide a reasonably accurate means of ranking the severity of injury. This scale categorizes injuries into six body regions—head, neck, thorax, abdomen, spine, and extremities—and assigns an individual score to each injury. Injuries are ranked on a scale of 1 to 6 in the AIS system:

- Minor injury: 1
- Moderate injury: 2
- Serious injury: 3
- Severe injury: 4
- Critical condition: 5
- Unsurvivable: 6

Areas that are not injured are typically given a score of 0 or not recorded. The AIS allows for the determination of the severity of an individual injury but does not take into account multisystem injuries. Such scores are typically calculated for research purposes and in conjunction with trauma center outcome reporting. The AIS scoring system is not used in the clinical setting but is important for identifying injury patterns.

Injury Severity Score

The Injury Severity Score (ISS) is an anatomic scoring system that provides a single overall score for patients with multiple injuries. It quantifies multisystem injuries through the use of AIS scores. The ISS is determined by adding the squares of the three highest AIS scores. The ISS is a number between 0 and 75, with 1 being an isolated minor injury and 75 being severe multisystem injury. Any ISS body region that is assigned an AIS score of 6 (nonsurvivable) equates to an ISS of 75. **TABLE 11-3** shows an example of the ISS calculation.

TABLE 11-3 Sample ISS Calculation			
ISS Region	**Injury**	**AIS**	**Square of the Top Three AIS Scores**
Head and neck	No injury	0	
Face	Unstable facial fracture	4	16
Chest	Flail chest	5	25
Abdomen	Liver laceration	4	16
Extremity	No injury	0	
External	Abrasion to right upper quadrant of abdomen	3	
Totals		16	57

Abbreviations: AIS, Abbreviated Injury Score; ISS, Injury Severity Score

As with AIS scores, trauma registry personnel often use the ISS for data collection and research purposes. Generally, an ISS greater than 15 is associated with major trauma requiring care at a Level I facility. Once data such as ISS scores are collected, some variances can occur with this scoring system. For example, any error made in AIS scoring will increase the likelihood of errors with the ISS.

Trauma Injury Severity Score

The trauma injury severity score (TRISS) is another scoring system that calculates the survival probability of the critically ill or injured patient. This scoring system uses the results of the ISS and the revised trauma score along with the patient's age, so it incorporates the patient's physiologic and anatomic indicators. This score is rarely used in the transport setting.

It is important for CCTPs to use their triage skills in the field when determining where to transport a patient. Ultimately, the various trauma scoring systems are not as useful as expert triage skills, because a full description of the patient injuries is not known.

Trauma Systems
Levels of Trauma Care

The CCTP is often called to incident scenes and outlying facilities to transport critically injured trauma patients to more definitive care. For this reason, it is important to be familiar with how the American College of Surgeons' Committee on Trauma (ACS-COT) classifies echelons of trauma care. Trauma centers are classified into Levels I through IV, with Level I having the most resources, followed by Levels II, III, and IV, respectively.

A Level I facility is a comprehensive resource center that serves as the major referral hospital in a mature trauma system. Level I facilities must be capable of providing every aspect of trauma care from prevention through rehabilitation; therefore, the facility must have adequate personnel and resources to support that care. Because of the extensive requirements, most Level I facilities are large, university-based teaching hospitals that serve larger cities or heavily populated areas. These centers have subspecialty care, such as neurosurgery, orthopedic

surgery, and intensive care units, readily available, in addition to dedicated surgery department access.

Level II centers are expected to provide definitive care during the initial trauma hospitalization, regardless of injury severity. These facilities are usually academic institutions or public/private community facilities located in less densely populated areas and may not have all the subspecialties of a Level I facility. Because of its location and resource limitations, the Level II trauma center may not be able to provide the same comprehensive care as a Level I trauma center.

Level III facilities typically serve communities that do not have access to Level I or II facilities. These facilities provide assessment, resuscitation, stabilization, and transfer when necessary. Level III facilities must have transfer agreements with a Level I or II trauma center and must have protocols in place to transfer patients whose needs exceed the facility's resources.

Level IV facilities are typically found in remote, outlying areas where no higher level of care is available. They provide advanced trauma life support (ATLS) prior to transfer. Such a facility may be a clinic or urgent care facility, and may or may not be staffed with a physician.

A mature and inclusive trauma system will leave no facility without a direct link to a Level I or II facility. All facilities, no matter the level, are expected to provide the same high quality of initial stabilization regardless of the trauma center's level.

Trauma centers can be either adult trauma centers or pediatric trauma centers, but are not necessarily both. Pediatric trauma centers are not as common as adult trauma centers. When transporting a pediatric trauma patient, you must be certain to transport the patient to the closest appropriate facility—a pediatric trauma center, if that is the closest option.

Since 1987, the ACS-COT has provided a consultation and verification program through which hospitals can be evaluated to see if they are meeting ACS-COT criteria. In addition, it provides consultation on developing and evolving trauma systems to states, regions, counties, and cities.

Classification of Trauma Patients

Trauma centers often have multiple tiers of trauma activations. The ACS-COT provides minimum criteria for Level I (full trauma team) activation. When one or more of the following criteria are present in the trauma patient, the full trauma team should be available and ready to provide ALS:

- Confirmed blood pressure less than 90 mm Hg at any time in adults and age-specific hypotension in children
- Gunshot wounds to the neck, chest, or abdomen or extremities proximal to the elbow/knee
- Glasgow Coma Scale score less than 9, with a mechanism of injury attributed to trauma
- Patients transferred from other hospitals who are receiving blood to maintain vital signs
- Patients requiring advanced airways who are transferred from the scene
- Patients who have respiratory compromise or are in need of an emergent airway
  - Includes intubated patients who are transferred from another facility with ongoing respiratory compromise
  - Does not include patients intubated at another facility who are now stable from a respiratory standpoint
- Emergency physician's discretion

The ACS-COT has also developed criteria to consider transfer of a trauma patient from a Level III facility to a Level I or II facility. These criteria, which are listed in **TABLE 11-4**, represent some of the more common reasons for trauma patient transfer. The CCTP should be familiar with the presentation and management of these conditions.

Interfacility Transport Trauma Management

Paramedics are already well versed in prehospital management of trauma. Interfacility management of trauma patients will often involve patients who are severely injured and in need of close assessment and continued monitoring. Some of these patients may undergo damage-control surgery prior to transfer. This treatment involves surgical correction of life-threatening injuries and initiation of resuscitation, followed by transfer to a critical care unit or tertiary hospital for longer-term stabilization and monitoring. Definitive surgery, in contrast, is performed after the patient's life-threatening injuries

TABLE 11-4 Criteria for Consideration of Transfer From Level III Centers to Level I or II Centers

1. Carotid or vertebral artery injury
2. Torn thoracic aorta or great vessel
3. Cardiac rupture
4. Bilateral pulmonary contusion with PaO_2:FIO_2 ratio <200
5. Major abdominal vascular injury
6. Grade IV or V liver injuries requiring transfusion of more than 6 units of red blood cells in 6 hours
7. Unstable pelvic fracture requiring transfusion of more than 6 units of red blood cells in 6 hours
8. Fracture or dislocation with loss of distal pulses
9. Penetrating injuries or open fracture of the skull
10. Glasgow Coma Scale of less than 14 or lateralizing
11. Spinal fracture or spinal cord deficit
12. Complex pelvis/acetabulum fractures
13. More than two unilateral rib fractures or bilateral rib fractures with pulmonary contusion (if no critical care consultation is available at the referring facility)
14. Significant torso injury with advanced comorbid disease (such as coronary artery disease, chronic obstructive pulmonary disease)

Abbreviations: FIO_2, fraction of inspired oxygen; PaO_2, partial pressure of arterial oxygen

have been stabilized. For patients who meet certain criteria, injuries may be managed without surgery. Regardless of the approach taken, management after the patient's initial arrival at a hospital should follow ATLS guidelines.

Just as in the prehospital setting, the ABCs are addressed first during an interfacility transport call. On arrival at the facility, the CCTP should ensure the ABCs have been assessed and managed before initiating transfer. In addition, the CCTP should assess the placement of the endotracheal tube (if present), presence of breath sounds, and capnography waveform. If any doubt exists about the endotracheal tube's proper placement, transport should not be initiated until the airway status is stabilized. Cardiovascular status should be assessed, including the patency of all vascular access devices and the total volume of fluids infused since the patient presented at the receiving facility. A thorough neurologic exam, including GCS score, should be performed and documented. Although this effort might seem to duplicate earlier care, it is imperative to assess the patient from head to toe for external injuries prior to initiating transfer and in collaboration with the initial trauma team if possible. Previously unseen injuries can prove fatal during interfacility transport if they are not discovered and addressed prior to departure. Repeated head-to-toe assessments will decrease the possibility of missed injuries, which occur more often in patients with multisystem trauma.

Elicit as much medical history as possible from the patient or hospital staff. Consider whether the patient might have drug or alcohol intoxication; as many as one-third of all trauma patients are drug or alcohol dependent. The CCTP must also be prepared to detect and treat complications on initial evaluation and treatment, including fluid overload, transfusion reactions, contrast-induced renal issues, abdominal compartment syndrome, bleeding, and shock.

The Hypothermia–Acidosis–Coagulopathy Triad

The lethal triad of hypothermia, acidosis, and coagulopathy is often described in the trauma literature as the cornerstone of understanding proper resuscitation of the bleeding trauma patient. Each element of the lethal triad exacerbates the effect of the other two, and can accelerate patient decompensation without timely intervention.

Hypothermia

Hypothermia, defined as a core body temperature less than 35°C (95°F), is commonly encountered in trauma patients. In fact, studies have shown that the incidence of hypothermia in trauma patients can be as high as 50%. Moreover, hypothermia in trauma is associated with higher mortality rates.

Hypothermia can generally be attributed to either the environment or the treatment provided. Extended time in the field during an extrication process can contribute to hypothermia in trauma patients. Even on a warm day, loss of blood and thermoregulation in trauma can result in this condition. Additionally, a major component of ATLS is complete exposure and assessment, which often means removing clothing and blankets that could cover up injuries. Hypothermia can also be induced or exacerbated by the CCTP by exposing the patient for an exam, failing to increase the ambient temperature in patient care areas, and infusing fluids. Administration of nonwarmed infusions requires the body to warm up the fluid internally, resulting in further decreases in core temperature, energy expenditure, and further stress to thermoregulation mechanisms.

The CCTP must diligently prevent hypothermia and work to reverse it if it does occur before and during transport. Limit exposure of the patient as much as possible. Increase the ambient temperature by using warm blankets and raising the temperature in the patient compartment of the transport vehicle. This increase in temperature may be needed even on a warm day. Use of warmed fluids may be helpful, although fluids stored in a warmer have not been shown to maintain significant warmth when infused. To administer truly warm fluids, it is necessary to use a device that actively warms fluids while they are infusing. Warmed and humidified oxygen may be beneficial as well. For critically injured patients, esophageal temperature probes can provide continuous monitoring of core body temperature during their transfer. The CCTP should also be cognizant of the multiple other side effects of hypothermia, such as reduced drug clearance **TABLE 11-5**.

Acidosis

Hypothermia can directly lead to acidosis, as can administration of large volumes of acidic crystalloid solutions during resuscitation efforts. Normal saline, which has a pH of 5.5 and a very high level of chloride, can worsen underlying acidosis. The acidotic pH and tendency to induce a hyperchloremic metabolic acidosis, in addition to the existing lactic acidosis, make large volumes of normal saline a potentially harmful resuscitation fluid. Lactated Ringer solution, with a pH of 6.5, is an imperfect alternative because of the lactate content and incompatibility with other fluids, medications, and blood products. More recently, Plasma-Lyte A and Plasma-Lyte 148 have made their way into critical care as balanced-pH, multiple-electrolyte fluids of

TABLE 11-5 Effects of Hypothermia on Trauma Patients

Impaired Cardiorespiratory Function

Cardiac depression
Myocardial ischemia
Arrhythmias
Peripheral vasoconstriction
Impaired tissue oxygen delivery
Elevated oxygen consumption during rewarming
Blunted response to catecholamines
Increased blood viscosity
Metabolic acidosis

Bleeding Diathesis

Decreased kinetics of coagulation factors
Reduced platelet function

Reduced Clearance of Drugs

Decreased hepatic blood flow
Decreased hepatic metabolism
Decreased renal blood flow

Increased Risk of Infection

Decreased white blood cell number and function
Impaired cellular immune response
Wound infection
• Thermoregulatory vasoconstriction
• Decreased subcutaneous oxygen tension
• Impaired oxidative killing by neutrophils
• Decreased collagen deposition
Pneumonia
Sepsis

Insulin Resistance With Hyperglycemia

Reproduced from Smith CE. *Prevention and Treatment of Hypothermia in Trauma Patients. Trauma Care International* ITACCS. http://www.itaccs.com/traumacare/archive/04_01_Spring_2004/prevention.pdf. Accessed April 23, 2009.

choice for large-volume crystalloid resuscitation. The patient's respiratory status, such as acidosis from hypoventilation, should be taken into consideration as well.

Coagulopathy

Coagulopathy, which is seen in 25% of severely injured patients, can be precipitated by hypothermia and acidosis, or by acute blood loss. Dilutional coagulopathy occurs when providers resuscitate a bleeding trauma patient with fluid or blood products that do not contain the same clotting factors lost in the whole blood. Aggressively managing hemorrhage, including early replacement of both clotting factors and packed blood cells, is important to reverse or prevent progressive coagulopathy. New trauma recommendations call for a 1:1:1 ratio of plasma, platelets, and packed red blood cells for replacement, especially in the context of massive transfusion protocols, while minimizing crystalloid infusions. The CCTP should be familiar with the different types of blood products and the goals of administration for each type.

Diagnostic Imaging for Trauma

Obtaining and understanding imaging studies related to trauma is an integral component of the trauma care paradigm for the CCTP. The use of diagnostic imaging helps direct further care for the trauma patient. Diagnostic imaging also confirms the previous care that has been delivered, such as endotracheal tube placement and invasive catheters.

Many exciting advances and new procedures have been introduced in regard to diagnostic imaging. This section briefly covers the developments related to CCTPs' practice in trauma care.

Standard Radiographs

Standard radiographs, such as a chest radiograph, are part of the initial assessment of the patient with multisystem trauma. They can provide information on endotracheal tube depth, fractures, and chest injuries. Examples of normal and abnormal cervical spine radiographs are shown in **FIGURE 11-4** and **FIGURE 11-5**.

Typical interpretation of radiographs involves the following elements:

• Structure and landmark verification
• Proper size and placement of anatomic structure or devices
• Symmetry of structures
• Foreign object identification

Computed Tomography

Computed tomography (CT) is another imaging study that is essential in diagnosing traumatic injury. For trauma patients, it is typically used for

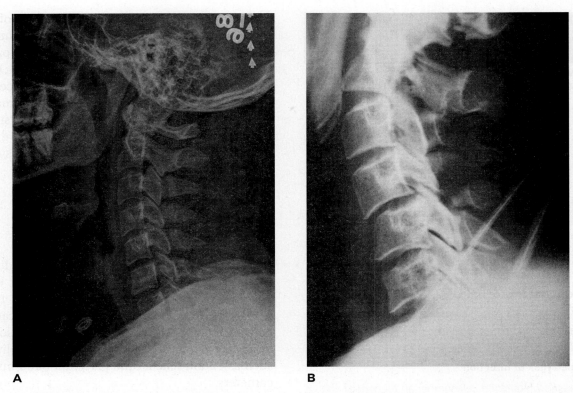

FIGURE 11-4 A. Normal cervical radiograph. **B.** Abnormal cervical radiograph.

A. Courtesy of Andrew N. Pollak, MD, FAAOS; **B.** © Dr. P. Marazzi/Science Source.

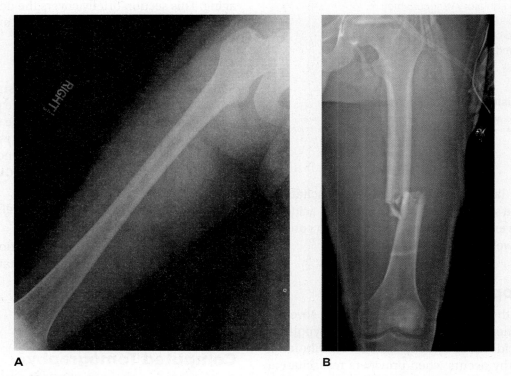

FIGURE 11-5 A. Normal long bone radiograph. **B.** Abnormal long bone radiograph (transverse femur fracture in an adult with shortening and marginal comminution).

Courtesy of Andrew N. Pollak, MD, FAAOS.

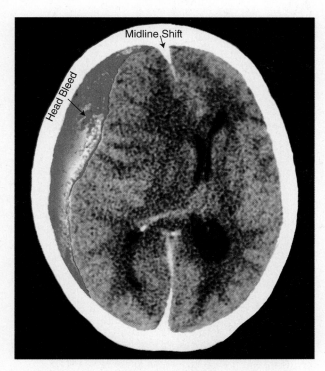

FIGURE 11-6 A computed tomography scan showing a head bleed with a midline shift.

© Zephyr/Science Source.

head injury identification (**FIGURE 11-6**), identification of bleeding, and complex fractures. Typical studies will scan the head, cervical spine, thoracic and lumbar spines, chest, and abdominal-pelvic regions. Interpretation of CT images is similar to that for plain radiographs because the images depict the contrast between different structures.

Ultrasonography

Focused assessment with sonography for trauma (FAST) is an ultrasonographic examination directed at identifying the presence of pericardial or intraperitoneal free fluids. It was first described in the early 1970s and has since been adopted by a multitude of practitioners who perform point-of-care ultrasonography in the trauma setting. Recent studies have validated the use of the FAST examination as noninferior to more invasive methods of clinical investigation such as **diagnostic peritoneal lavage (DPL)** or CT scan. For the FAST examination to be effective, approximately 150 to 200 mL of free fluid must be present. Notably, negative imaging, especially in early assessments, does not necessarily rule out evolving injuries.

The role of ultrasonography in *blunt* abdominal trauma has been well studied. Excellent evidence supports the use of the FAST examination as the initial diagnostic modality for the evaluation of peritoneal free fluid in these patients. In the context of blunt abdominal trauma, practitioners accept the accuracy rate for ultrasonography as being nearly equivalent to that of DPL or CT. The adoption of the noninvasive FAST examination serves as an important diagnostic tool in determining which patients will require **exploratory laparotomy**—that is, open surgical exploration of the abdomen to look for a source of unexplained acute blood loss.

The evidence is less clear for the use of ultrasonography in the setting of *penetrating* thoracoabdominal trauma. The current literature demonstrates that ultrasonography is an excellent screening tool for penetrating pleural and cardiac injuries and has a high sensitivity for detecting injuries requiring acute intervention. For abdominal injuries, however, the sensitivity for detection of injury is low; thus, the utility of ultrasonography as a screening tool is limited in patients with such injuries. Most cases of penetrating thoracoabdominal trauma will require operative exploration, diminishing the value of imaging during the initial assessment.

The FAST examination is performed by imaging the pericardial space and three distinct areas of the abdomen. Several different cardiac views can be used while evaluating for an **anechoic** (an area free from echo; black on ultrasonogram) stripe between the heart and the pericardium. The abdominal area that is the most sensitive for the detection of free fluid—and is imaged first—is the hepatorenal space or Morison pouch. This region of the right upper quadrant is the interface between the liver and the right kidney. Free fluid will appear as an anechoic stripe between the organs in imaging of the hepatorenal space. The second area imaged is the left upper quadrant or splenorenal space; on imaging of this area, free fluid may be observed either under the diaphragm (superior to the spleen) or between the spleen and the left kidney. The third area of the abdomen imaged is the pelvis. Free fluid will accumulate here dependently in the rectouterine space (pouch of Douglas) in women or in the vesicorectal space in men. The FAST examination can be repeated if concern for evolving injury or ongoing bleeding exists.

Studies have also shown that the extended FAST (e-FAST) exam can reliably identify thoracic injuries such as pneumothorax and hemothorax. In the supine patient, the anterior chest wall is evaluated for contact between the pleural layers, shown by the lung sliding against the pleura. When this contact is confirmed, it excludes the possibility of air or fluid in the pleural space. The lung bases are evaluated for free fluid when evaluating for hemothorax. When present, anechoic free fluid will be visualized just above the diaphragm.

The FAST examination does have some limitations. First, it does not evaluate directly for solid-organ injury, but rather looks for the bleeding that occurs and accumulates as a result of injury to such an organ. Second, it does not evaluate the retroperitoneal space, so injuries to organs such as the pancreas or aorta may go undetected. Finally, the FAST examination evaluates for the presence of fluid, but does not identify the specific type of fluid. As a consequence, it may be impossible to differentiate blood from pericardial effusion, pleural effusion, or ascites. The presence of free fluid must always be assessed within the clinical context of the patient.

The FAST approach has been adopted by some transport services as well as for use in the prehospital setting, using smaller and more portable equipment **FIGURE 11-7**. It has shown much promise in the early identification of thoracoabdominal bleeding and may assist in transport decisions when varying levels of trauma care are available. Training standards for performing this procedure vary, but at a minimum usually require specific credentialing and substantial experience.

See Chapter 9, *Laboratory Analysis and Diagnostic Studies*, for further discussion of ultrasonography.

Transthoracic Echocardiography and Transesophageal Echocardiography

Critical care clinicians sometimes use other focused exam algorithms such as HEARTscan, FATE, FEEL, FEAR, and BLEEP, all of which are intended to rapidly determine pathology in critically ill or injured patients using transthoracic echocardiography (TTE). Additionally, transesophageal echocardiography (TEE), which involves inserting a probe

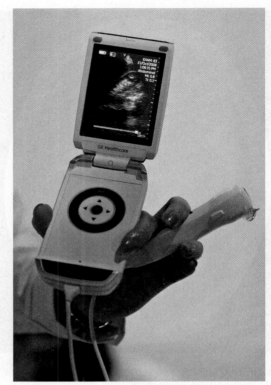

A

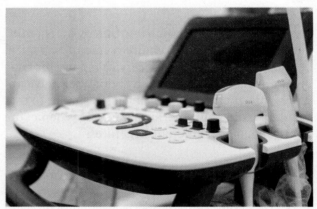

B

FIGURE 11-7 A. A handheld ultrasonography unit. **B.** A portable ultrasonography unit.

A. © Bloomberg/Getty Images; **B.** © Borkin Vadim/Shutterstock.

into the esophagus, has revolutionized intraoperative cardiac monitoring. TEE is widely employed in cardiothoracic and vascular surgery cases to provide real-time evaluation of cardiac function and fluid volume status during surgery. As esophageal probe technology becomes more miniaturized, intensive care unit (ICU) clinicians, including critical care nurses, are beginning to use TEE for longer-term evaluation, assessment, and monitoring of patients' hemodynamics.

Magnetic Resonance Imaging

The contrast differences illuminated by magnetic resonance imaging (MRI) are sometimes used to identify abnormalities in trauma patients **FIGURE 11-8**. Nevertheless, MRI is typically of limited use in trauma patients because these devices are not always readily available and it takes considerable time to obtain the images—time that critically injured patients may not have.

Intra-abdominal Pressure Monitoring

Intra-abdominal pressure (IAP) is the static pressure inside the abdominal compartment. Normally, IAP is approximately 0 to 5 mm Hg, with variations caused by respirations. Nonpathologic increases in IAP can occur with obesity. Recent studies of IAP in critically ill medical and surgical patients have found elevated pressures to be relatively common. The deleterious effects of intra-abdominal hypertension (IAH) can lead to abdominal compartment syndrome (ACS) and death if left untreated. ACS is thought to play a significant role in end-organ damage and multisystem organ failure during critical illness.

IAP can be measured with a variety of commercial devices or with user-assembled equipment. The current reference standard uses a transducer connected to an indwelling urinary drainage catheter located within the bladder. IAP is expressed in millimeters of mercury (mm Hg); it is measured at end expiration with the patient supine and the pressure transducer placed at the iliac crest at the midaxillary line. The recommended technique uses a pressure transducer connected by tubing at or near the aspiration port of the urinary catheter drainage tubing. To measure IAP, follow these steps:

1. Clamp the tubing distal to the connection.
2. Instill 50 mL or less of sterile room-temperature saline through the pressure measurement system into the bladder.
3. Record the measured pressure after a 30- to 60-second stabilization period **FIGURE 11-9**.

IAH is defined as a sustained IAP of greater than or equal to 12 mm Hg. It has multiple causes, not all of which are associated with trauma or surgical procedures to the abdomen.

ACS is defined as a sustained IAP of greater than 20 mm Hg with new-onset single- or multiple-organ system failure. ACS is classified into three types:

- *Primary:* Results from surgical interventions or injuries to the abdominal-pelvic region—for

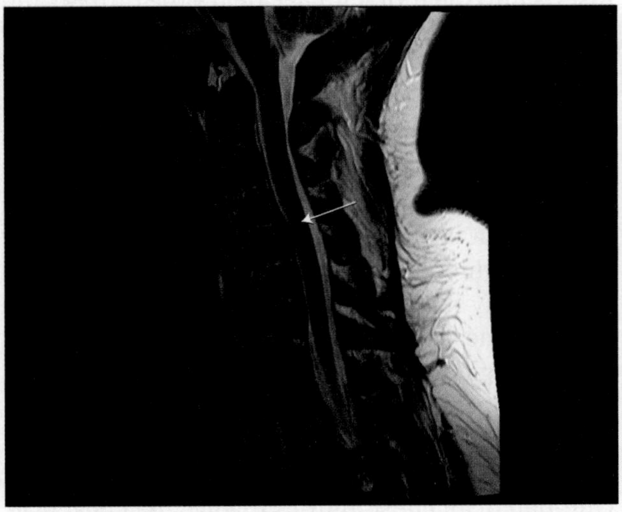

FIGURE 11-8 Magnetic resonance image showing C4-C5 bulge with pressure on the spinal cord (arrow).

Courtesy of Andrew N. Pollak, MD, FAAOS.

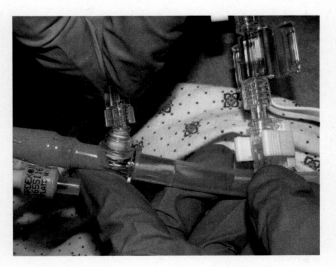

FIGURE 11-9 The CCTP may be asked to obtain intra-abdominal pressure measurements during transport.

© Jones & Bartlett Learning.

example, in conjunction with damage-control exploratory laparotomy, massive retroperitoneal hematomas, liver transplantation, and failed nonoperative management of injury or disease.

- *Secondary:* Develops as a result of conditions outside the abdomen, such as sepsis, burns, and capillary leakage resulting from massive fluid resuscitation.
- *Recurrent:* Recurrence of ACS following initially successful surgical or medical treatment of primary or secondary ACS.

Although definitive treatment for acute ACS is surgical decompression (often with the abdomen left open until swelling is decreased), prevention through careful monitoring and targeted medical management is highly encouraged. Interventions to reduce the risk of IAH and to prevent IAH from progressing to ACS include neuromuscular blockade, drainage of free fluid in the abdominal cavity (**paracentesis**), decompression of the gastrointestinal tract using gastric tubes, prokinetic drugs (to stimulate intestinal motility), and close attention to prevention of fluid volume overload.

The CCTP may observe IAP monitoring equipment being used in the ICU or emergency department (ED) setting and may be asked to obtain IAP measurements during transport. Familiarity with the equipment used for this purpose is necessary to accurately obtain measurements.

Transport Considerations

Given the need to provide rapid care to the trauma patient, not all indicated studies may have been performed at the point in time when the CCTP encounters such a patient. Nevertheless, the CCTP should have and maintain some proficiency in interpreting imaging for obvious abnormalities. Reviewing imaging that has been performed can limit liability, confirm suspicions about the diagnosis, and document accurate placement of tubes and lines or performance of procedures. Various methods of training are available to the CCTP, and most services provide internal training sessions as well.

Even with advances in technology and the electronic transmission of imaging, the CCTP should always ask for and ensure that all copies of the imaging studies are present in the patient care record or have been uploaded to a portal accessible to the receiving facility. Some data storage devices may be as small as a disk or thumb drive, so be careful not to misplace or lose them.

Thoracic Trauma

Thoracic trauma accounts for approximately one-third of trauma-related deaths in the United States. Of all trauma deaths, one in four (25%) is directly associated with thoracic injuries. Falls and motor vehicle accidents are the leading causes of chest trauma, but these mechanisms can also cause underlying lung injury that does not become obvious until days after an accident. Given these statistics, it is imperative for the CCTP to have a thorough understanding of the complex anatomy and physiology of the thoracic cavity. Note that only 15% to 20% of these potentially catastrophic injuries require open chest surgery; the majority can be managed with relatively simple interventions within the scope of the CCTP.

The thorax is essentially a bony cage consisting of 12 pairs of ribs that join anteriorly with the sternum and posteriorly with the thoracic spine **FIGURE 11-10**. The chest consists of two thoracic cavities, each containing one lung. The mediastinum, which contains the heart, superior and inferior venae cavae, aorta, bronchi, trachea, and esophagus, is located between the two cavities. The diaphragm inserts into the thoracic cage below the fifth rib and separates the chest and abdominal cavities.

The primary function of the thorax is to facilitate adequate oxygenation and circulation. Thus, injuries to the chest must be promptly found and managed to avoid compromise to this critical function. Injuries to the thoracic region can result from either blunt or penetrating injuries, and the CCTP must conduct a thorough assessment to avoid missing any such life-threatening injuries.

The chest is normally a closed compartment with a single inlet and outlet through the trachea. The changes in pressure necessary for ventilation depend on the ribs, diaphragm, and pleural membrane all being intact and working properly. One-half of all chest injuries involve the chest wall. Recent research has emphasized the importance of this anatomic relationship and the critical nature of normal intrathoracic pressures for adequate circulation and ventilation. Especially when the patient

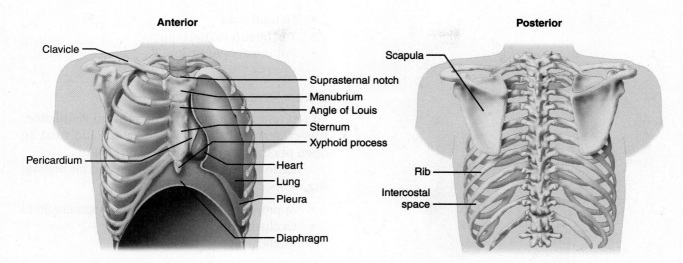

FIGURE 11-10 The thorax, anterior and posterior views.
© Jones & Bartlett Learning.

has hypotension, excessive intrathoracic pressure can interfere with adequate venous return or preload. Therefore, care must be taken in trauma patients to ensure adequate positive-pressure ventilations without allowing intrathoracic pressure to rise too high.

Maintaining this balance may become a challenge during flight. Atmospheric pressure declines as the aircraft goes higher, allowing gas volume to expand in a closed space. This gas expansion may make a small tension pneumothorax larger. In addition, less gas will be needed to ventilate a patient using a gas-powered ventilator.

Pneumothorax

A pneumothorax, which can be either open or closed **FIGURE 11-11**, is reported to be present in 15% to 50% of chest injuries. An open pneumothorax (also known as a communicating pneumothorax) is commonly called a sucking chest wound **FIGURE 11-12**, even though it does not always make a sucking noise. A tension pneumothorax occurs when a defect in the chest wall allows air to enter the thoracic space, disrupting the normal adherence between the pleura (think of the suction between a wet glass and the countertop), but not escape, which causes the lung to collapse **FIGURE 11-13**. This condition often results from a penetrating injury to the outer chest, such as a stab wound, but it can also occur internally from a sharp broken rib end.

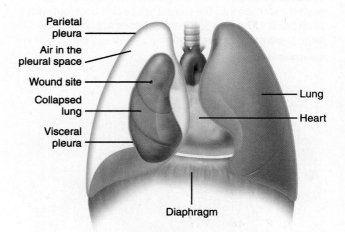

FIGURE 11-11 A pneumothorax occurs when air leaks into the space between the pleural surfaces from an opening in the chest or the surface of the lung. The lung collapses as air fills the pleural space.
© Jones & Bartlett Learning.

These types of injuries cause air to be drawn into the thoracic cavity with each breath. The air enters the space in the pleural cavity, increasing the pleural pressure and causing the lung to collapse due to its relative lower pressure. As the lung collapses, it does not oxygenate the blood, resulting in hypoxia and shortness of breath. A collapse as small as 10% can be life threatening if the patient has other comorbidities; additionally, a pneumothorax this small may be difficult to appreciate by auscultation.

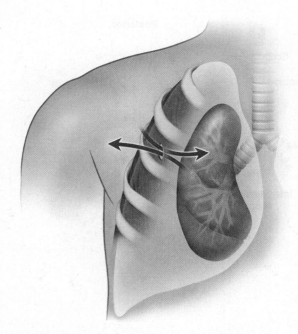

FIGURE 11-12 With a sucking chest wound, air passes from the outside into the pleural space and back out with each breath. The size of the defect does not need to be large to compromise ventilation.

© Jones & Bartlett Learning.

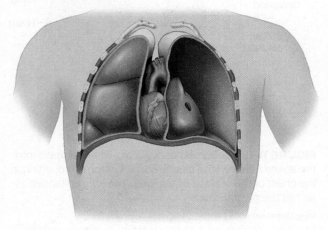

FIGURE 11-13 In a tension pneumothorax, air accumulates in the pleural space, eventually causing compression of the heart and great vessels.

© Jones & Bartlett Learning.

The differential diagnosis for respiratory distress in chest trauma includes the following conditions:

- Simple pneumothorax
- Tension pneumothorax
- Flail chest

- Hemothorax
- Tracheobronchial injury
- Pulmonary contusion

Open Pneumothorax

To promote adequate oxygenation and ventilation, it is critical that the CCTP recognize and treat an open pneumothorax as soon as possible.

The following equipment is needed for managing an open pneumothorax:

- Appropriate personal protective equipment (PPE)
- Occlusive dressing
- Medical tape

Indications for this treatment include emergency relief of dyspnea secondary to open pneumothorax. Contraindications include tension pneumothorax.

Sealing a sucking chest wound may induce a tension pneumothorax if air can enter the thoracic cavity but not escape. This condition can occur if air enters the pleural cavity from the lung side of the wound and builds up, or if the seal is incomplete. If this happens, the CCTP should "burp" the dressing by releasing an edge and allowing the pressure to equilibrate. Many techniques of sealing sucking chest wounds attempt to address these issues, but pressure buildup or an ineffective seal may still occur. Once a seal is applied, constant surveillance is necessary to guard against either possibility. Assisted ventilation and/or needle decompression may be necessary. Of note, debate exists regarding the most appropriate means of achieving an occlusive seal over an open chest wound. Regardless of the method employed, the objective is to achieve an occlusive seal and prevent or relieve subsequent pressure buildup.

SKILL DRILL 11-1 illustrates the clinical procedure for managing an open pneumothorax, which is described here:

1. Maintain an open airway and administer appropriate oxygen therapy **STEP 1**.
2. Immediately cover the chest wound **STEP 2**. This can be initially accomplished by the use of a gloved hand. However, to reduce the risk of a tension pneumothorax, apply an occlusive dressing, taped down on three or four sides **STEP 3**. Adequate overlap on the open edge is required to create a good seal. Many commercial devices are available for this purpose.

Skill Drill 11-1 Managing an Open Pneumothorax

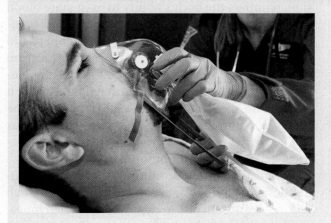

Step 1

Maintain an open airway and administer appropriate oxygen therapy.

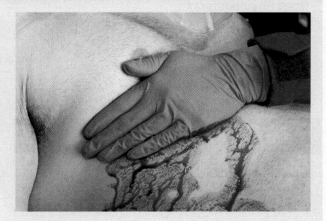

Step 2

Immediately close the chest wound, initially with a gloved hand.

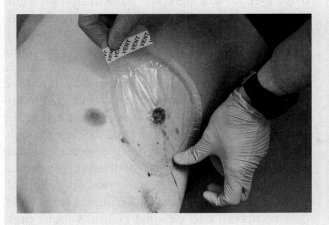

Step 3

Apply an occlusive dressing, preferably during patient exhalation, that is taped down on three or four sides.

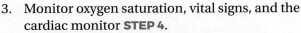

All images © Jones & Bartlett Learning.

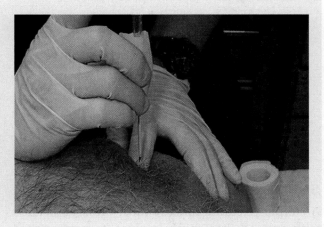

Step 4

Monitor oxygen saturation, vital signs, and the cardiac monitor. Watch for development of a tension pneumothorax or an inadequate seal, and stay alert to the need for needle decompression or assisted ventilation.

3. Monitor oxygen saturation, vital signs, and the cardiac monitor **STEP 4**.
4. Watch for development of a tension pneumothorax or an inadequate seal, and stay alert to the need for needle decompression or assisted ventilation.
5. Transport the patient to an appropriate facility.

Possible complications include converting an open pneumothorax to a tension pneumothorax. The CCTP should watch for increasing difficulty in breathing, elevated peak inspiratory pressures (PIPs), increased work of breathing, restlessness, and agitation. Late signs may include tracheal tugging, tracheal deviation, and jugular venous distention (JVD).

Simple Pneumothorax

A simple pneumothorax is most often associated with a closed chest injury, such as from a fractured rib being driven inward into the lung or a collapsed lung that results from a medical cause—a condition often called a spontaneous pneumothorax. Loss of the negative pressure holding the two layers of the pleura together allows the lung to collapse like an empty balloon. The term "simple pneumothorax" actually refers to any pneumothorax that is not a tension pneumothorax; thus, it may be used to refer to an open or closed pneumothorax as long as there is no buildup of pressure in the pleural cavity outside the lung.

Tension Pneumothorax

A tension pneumothorax is a life-threatening injury that results from a continual influx of air into the pleural space. It may occur secondary to a closed simple pneumothorax or after sealing an open pneumothorax, which increases intrathoracic pressure, hampers the body's ability to oxygenate blood or eliminate carbon dioxide from blood, and eventually collapses the affected lung. The collapse in the lung causes the mediastinum to shift away from the injured side, resulting in ventilatory and circulatory compromise from the collapsed lung. The great vessels and the heart become deformed under the pressure. Failure to treat a tension pneumothorax will cause the patient to progress to pulseless electrical activity and cardiopulmonary arrest.

Clinical signs and symptoms of a tension pneumothorax include dyspnea, anxiety, JVD (although this may be absent due to hypovolemia), tachypnea, and tracheal deviation (a late sign not often observed in the prehospital setting). Tracheal tugging during inspiration—a much more subtle sign—is observed much earlier in the process; the CCTP should actively look for this sign. The most important signs, however, are increasing dyspnea, decreasing ventilatory compliance with assisted ventilations, and increasing PIPs or peak airway pressures, depending on the settings if the patient is receiving ventilation. Auscultation of lung sounds will reveal diminished or absent breath sounds (which are difficult to appreciate in an aircraft and at noisy scenes) on the affected side if the pneumothorax is large enough. Pulsus paradoxus (a pulse that disappears on inspiration and that also can be associated with a drop in systolic blood pressure), electrical alternans (alternating between a large QRS complex and a small QRS complex), and elevated central venous pressure (CVP) may be present as well. In a patient with tension pneumothorax, PIP will increase despite the patient having an open airway.

Management of tension pneumothorax is performed by immediate needle decompression. The following equipment is needed to perform this procedure:

- Appropriate PPE, including sterile gloves
- 14-gauge or larger intravenous (IV) catheter (minimum 3.25 inches [8 cm] in length)
- 10-mL syringe with 1 to 2 mL of sterile saline in it, which enables the CCTP to see bubbling air escaping (it is too difficult to hear in many cases)
- 2% chlorhexidine

- Flutter valve (Heimlich or nonlubricated condom or glove finger) optional
- Sterile dressings

Indications for this treatment include emergency relief of tension pneumothorax. Contraindications include patients without signs of a tension pneumothorax.

SKILL DRILL 11-2 demonstrates the clinical procedure for managing a tension pneumothorax, which is described here:

1. Assess the patient to ensure that the presentation matches that of a tension pneumothorax **STEP 1**.

Skill Drill 11-2 Needle Decompression (Thoracentesis) of a Tension Pneumothorax

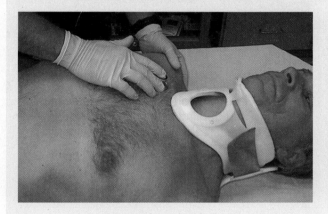

Step 1

Assess the patient.

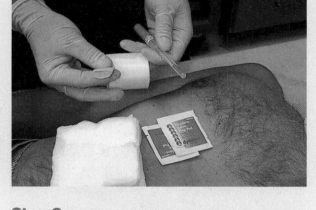

Step 2

Prepare and assemble all necessary equipment.

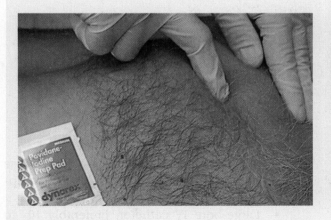

Step 3

Locate the appropriate site. The midclavicular line between the second and third ribs is shown here, but the space between the fifth and sixth ribs at the anterior axillary line may also be used.

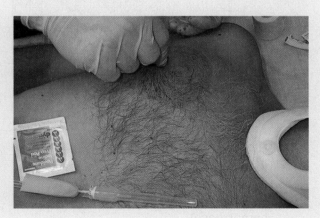

Step 4

Cleanse the appropriate area using an aseptic technique.

Continues

Skill Drill 11-2 Needle Decompression (Thoracentesis) of a Tension Pneumothorax (continued)

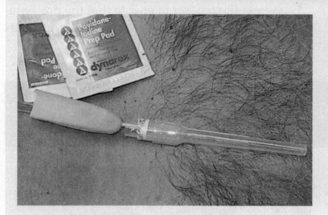

Step 5

Insert the needle at a 90° angle to the skin and chest wall.

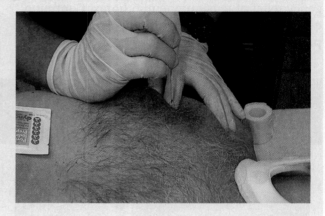

Step 6

Remove the needle and listen for the release of air or look for bubbling in the syringe. Properly dispose of the needle in a sharps container.

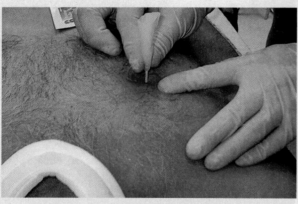

Step 7

Secure the catheter in place. Monitor the patient closely for recurrence of the tension pneumothorax.

All images © Jones & Bartlett Learning.

- Difficult ventilation despite an open airway (decreasing compliance or increasing PIP or peak airway pressure)
- JVD (may not be present with associated hemorrhage)
- Absent or decreased breath sounds on the affected side
- Hyperresonance to percussion on the affected side
- Tracheal deviation away from the affected side (a late sign that is not always present)
- Electrical alternans and pulsus paradoxus
- Elevated CVP
- Signs of impending cardiovascular collapse

2. Prepare and assemble the necessary equipment **STEP 2**.
   - Large-bore IV catheter, preferably 10- to 14-gauge and at least 3.25 inches (8 cm) long on a syringe filled with 1 to 2 mL of sterile saline
   - Alcohol or 2% chlorhexidine
   - Adhesive tape

3. Select the appropriate site **STEP 3**: The placement shown is midclavicular, second

intercostal space, above the third rib. Alternatively, you may use the anterior axillary line, above the fifth or sixth rib **FIGURE 11-14**. Go over the rib to avoid the neurovascular bundle under each rib.

4. Select the largest available needle. Optional: Attach the needle to a syringe with a few milliliters of saline so the bubbles are visible.
5. Cleanse the site with an appropriate aseptic technique **STEP 4**.
6. Insert the needle at a 90° angle over the rib **STEP 5**.
7. Remove the needle and listen for a rush of air or look for bubbles in the syringe **STEP 6**.
8. Advance the catheter over the needle and secure it in place **STEP 7**.
9. Dispose of the needle in a sharps container.
10. Closely monitor vital signs, oxygen saturation, and lung compliance.
11. Be prepared to repeat decompression if necessary.

Complications of needle decompression may include improper placement, which could lead to injury to the intercostal vessels and significant hemorrhage. Also, passing the needle into the chest may injure the lung parenchyma.

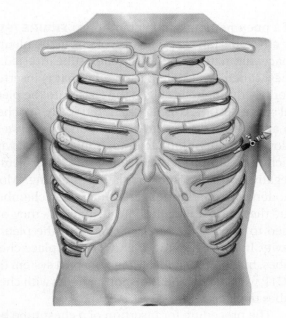

FIGURE 11-14 Correct placement for needle decompression if placing between the fifth and sixth ribs at the anterior axillary line. The positions of nerves, arteries, and veins are shown in relation to the ribs.

© Jones & Bartlett Learning.

Signs and Symptoms

Tension Pneumothorax

- Dyspnea
- Anxiety
- JVD
- Tachypnea
- Tracheal deviation
- Tracheal tugging during inspiration
- Decreasing ventilatory compliance to bagging
- Increasing PIP or peak airway pressure, if the patient is on a ventilator
- Diminished or absent breath sounds on the affected side, if the pneumothorax is large enough
- Pulsus paradoxus
- Electrical alternans
- Elevated CVP

Transport Management

Tension Pneumothorax

- Perform immediate needle decompression.
- Consider inserting a chest tube if your protocol allows.
- Maintain the chest tube on suction during transport.

Hemothorax

Blood in the pleural space is called a hemothorax **FIGURE 11-15**. Each of the body's thoracic cavities can accommodate the accumulation of as much as

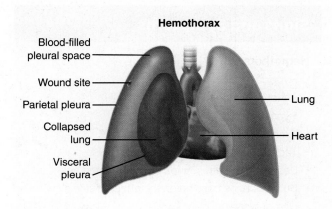

FIGURE 11-15 A hemothorax is a collection of blood in the pleural space produced by bleeding within the chest.

© Jones & Bartlett Learning.

3,000 mL of blood. A massive hemothorax occurs when at least 1,500 mL of blood collects in a thoracic cavity. The obvious threat from a hemothorax is hypovolemic shock, although the presence of a large amount of blood in the pleural cavity can also interfere with lung function. Hemothorax can be caused by blunt trauma, but is more commonly the result of penetrating trauma. A torn intercostal artery can bleed at a rate of 50 mL/min. Medical causes include a tumor eroding through great vessels.

Clinical signs and symptoms of a hemothorax include hypoxia, agitation, hypotension, tachycardia, tachypnea, decreased breath sounds on the affected side, dullness to percussion on the affected side, hemoptysis, and worsening shock. A patient with a hemothorax rarely presents with JVD or tracheal deviation.

Management of a hemothorax is supportive and includes the following interventions:

1. Maintain an open airway and apply appropriate oxygen therapy.
2. Immediately transport if in the field.
3. Initiate IV fluids to maintain peripheral perfusion; however, raising blood pressure above 90 mm Hg systolic or 65 mm Hg mean arterial pressure (MAP) may increase blood loss, dislodge a clot, or restart bleeding.
4. Be alert for development of a tension pneumothorax.

Management: Chest Tube Insertion

Patients with a pneumothorax, tension pneumothorax, hemothorax, hemopneumothorax (combination

Signs and Symptoms

Hemothorax

- Hypoxia
- Agitation
- Hypotension
- Tachycardia
- Tachypnea
- Decreased breath sounds on the affected side
- Dullness to percussion on the affected side
- Hemoptysis
- Worsening shock
- Falling CVP

Transport Management

Hemothorax

- Maintain an open airway; apply appropriate oxygen therapy.
- Immediately transport if in the field.
- Initiate IV fluids.
- Be alert for the development of a tension pneumothorax.
- Consider inserting a chest tube or pigtail catheter if your protocol allows.
- Maintain the chest drain on suction during transport.

Controversies

Use of fluids in patients with uncontrolled internal bleeding is controversial. Although raising the blood pressure may increase blood loss or dislodge a clot, an adequate blood pressure of 90 mm Hg systolic or a MAP of 65 mm Hg must be maintained to perfuse the heart and brain. The ideal fluid for use is one that carries oxygen, such as blood.

of a pneumothorax and hemothorax) **FIGURE 11-16**, or empyema (an accumulation of pus in the pleural space) ultimately may need a chest tube inserted. A chest tube is a flexible plastic tube that is inserted sterilely through the side of the chest into the pleural space **FIGURE 11-17**. It was traditionally attached to an underwater seal to create a one-way system allowing for air or fluid to drain from the chest with each exhalation, reestablishing the interpleural negative pressure and reinflating the lung. Most modern systems no longer use a water chamber, but they have the same effect—namely, they are used to remove air, fluid, or pus from the pleural cavity. In some systems, the CCTP may place chest tubes, but in every critical care transport system the CCTP will care for and transport patients with chest tubes in place.

The procedure for insertion of a chest tube begins with collecting the needed equipment (often packaged as a "tray"):

- Appropriate PPE, including sterile gloves
- Scalpel

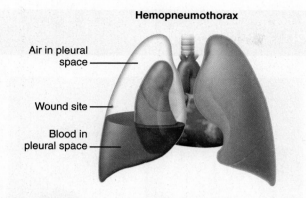

Hemopneumothorax

Air in pleural space

Wound site

Blood in pleural space

FIGURE 11-16 In a hemopneumothorax, both blood and air are present.

© Jones & Bartlett Learning.

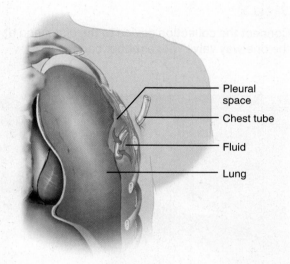

Pleural space

Chest tube

Fluid

Lung

FIGURE 11-17 A chest tube is inserted through the side of the chest into the pleural space.

© Jones & Bartlett Learning.

- Sterile chest tube: 28- to 36-French
- Kelly clamps (curved and straight)
- Sterile occlusive dressing
- Suturing material (typically a 0-silk or other large, nonabsorbable suture)
- 2% chlorhexidine
- A local anesthetic if the patient is awake
- A fluid collection device with a one-way valve that allows air, fluid, or pus to flow out of the chest; if not available, an indwelling catheter bag with a one-way valve may be used
- Tape
- Mechanical suction device (not always used)

Indications for insertion of a chest tube include the following:

- Pneumothorax
- Hemopneumothorax
- Empyema

Numerous complications are possible:

- Recurrent pneumothoraces
- Accidental removal
- Broken collection chamber
- Parenchymal injury
- Subcutaneous emphysema
- Laceration of intercostal vessels
- Creation of a hemothorax or bleeding
- Misplacement below the diaphragm
- Infection

SKILL DRILL 11-3 shows the clinical procedure for inserting a chest tube, which is described here:

1. Select the appropriate site: midaxillary over the fifth rib **STEP 1**.
2. Connect the collection device or the indwelling catheter bag to the distal end of the one-way valve with a rubber band **STEP 2**. Ensure the arrow on the valve is facing away from the patient.
3. Cleanse the site with an appropriate aseptic technique **STEP 3**.
4. Anesthetize the area, including the pleura and periosteum, over the fifth rib **STEP 4**, if the patient is conscious and time permits.
5. Mark the tube for the desired length of insertion.
6. Clamp the distal end of the tube with a large clamp (such as a Kelly clamp) and the proximal end of the tube with a curved clamp.
7. Make a transverse incision over the fifth rib in the midaxillary line **STEP 5**. If the patient has fractured ribs, use the anterior axillary line (between the midaxillary line and the nipple line).
8. Tunnel over the fifth rib with a large curved clamp, push through the pleura, spread the clamp, and replace the clamp with a finger. In a hemothorax, sudden evacuation of some blood is not uncommon. Ensure there are no palpable structures within the pleural cavity, such as pleural adhesions, that may prevent proper chest tube placement **STEP 6**.
9. Grasp the clamp attached to the end of the chest tube and advance it through the space

Skill Drill 11-3 Chest Tube Insertion

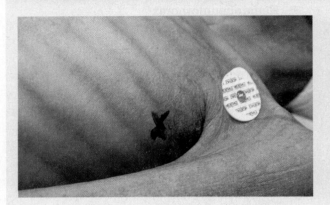

Step 1

Select the appropriate site.

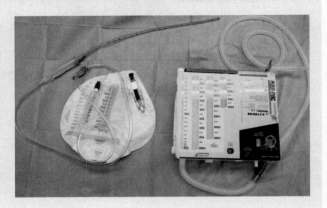

Step 2

Connect the collection device to the distal end of the one-way valve with a rubber band.

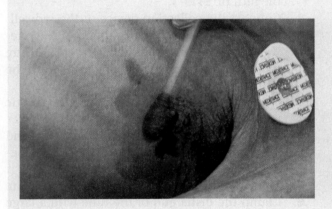

Step 3

Cleanse the site with an appropriate aseptic technique.

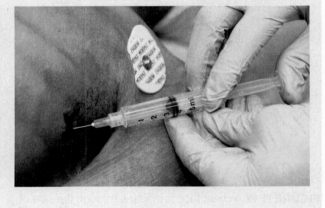

Step 4

Anesthetize the area, including the pleura and periosteum, over the fifth rib.

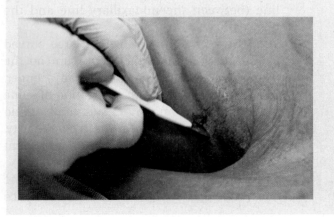

Step 5

Mark the tube for the desired length of insertion. Clamp the distal end of the tube with a large clamp and the proximal end of the tube with a curved clamp. Make a transverse incision over the fifth rib at the midaxillary line. If the patient has fractured ribs, use the anterior axillary line (between the midaxillary line and the nipple line).

Skill Drill 11-3 Chest Tube Insertion (continued)

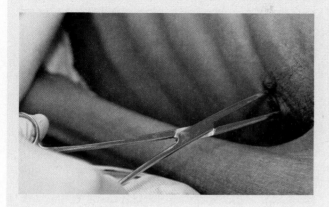

Step 6

Tunnel over the fifth rib with a large curved clamp, push through the pleura, spread the clamp, and replace the clamp with a finger.

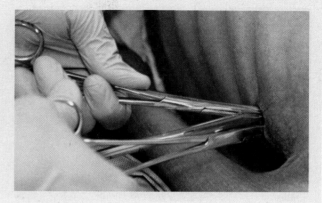

Step 7

Grasp the clamp attached to the end of the chest tube and advance it through the space created by the first clamp.

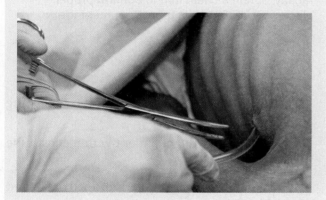

Step 8

Remove the clamps and advance the tube to the predetermined mark indicated on the tube, at least 5 cm past the most proximal hole, directed posteriorly and superiorly.

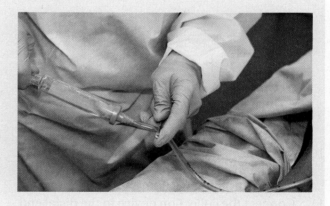

Step 9

Connect the collection device with the one-way valve.

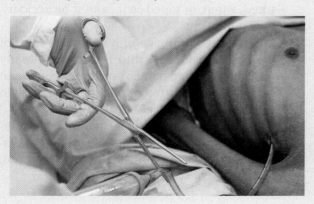

Step 10

Remove the distal clamp.

Continues

Skill Drill 11-3 Chest Tube Insertion (continued)

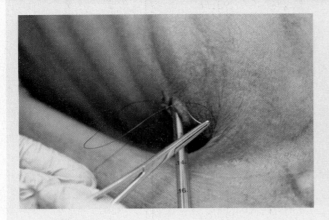

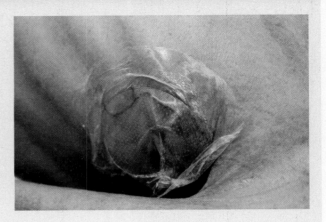

Step 11

Suture the tube in place and close the wound according to local protocols.

All images © Jones & Bartlett Learning.

Step 12

Cover the insertion site with an occlusive dressing. Upon arrival at the receiving facility, obtain a chest film to confirm proper placement of the chest tube. Document the procedure.

created by the first clamp, directing it posteriorly and superiorly toward the patient's head **STEP 7**.

10. Remove the clamps and advance the tube to at least 2 inches (5 cm) beyond the last hole, typically to around the 10- to 14-cm mark **STEP 8**.

11. Connect the collection device to the distal end of the chest tube **STEP 9**.

12. Remove the distal clamp **STEP 10**.

13. Suture the tube in place and close the wound according to local protocols **STEP 11**.

14. Note the depth of the tube at the skin (marked on the tube) and mark it with a felt-tip pen if possible.

15. Cover the insertion site with an occlusive dressing and reinforce all connections with tape **STEP 12**.

16. On arrival at the receiving facility, obtain a chest radiograph to confirm proper placement of the chest tube.

17. Document the procedure, including the size of the chest tube inserted, the amount of return of air/fluid after insertion of the tube, and any

changes in the patient's condition (including oxygen saturation).

When transporting a patient with a chest tube in place:

- Make sure all connections are taped or banded with wire to prevent accidental separation.
- Ensure that the dressing over the insertion site is securely taped and occlusive. Use a felt-tip marker to mark the depth of the tube; if there are markings, note the depth of the tube on the transfer chart. Make sure the tube is sutured, wired, or taped so it cannot be accidentally pulled out.
- Maintain the drainage unit below the level of the chest at all times during transport. Many units include bed hangers so that the unit can be hung on the stretcher. If there is water in the unit, keep it upright at all times.
- If the tube is attached to a suction device, determine whether the patient can tolerate discontinuing the vacuum for transport; if not, attach the chest tube to portable suction.

- Keep the tubing coiled to prevent kinks or dependent loops.
- Access and document bubbling in the water seal (does not have to be continuous), any output in the collection chamber, and its type (eg, frank blood).
- Do not clamp tubes for transport, as this is likely to cause a tension pneumothorax.
- Continuous bubbling may be a sign of tracheobronchial laceration. Large amounts of frankly bloody drainage need to be balanced by transfusion.

Pigtail Catheter

Pigtail catheters are small-bore (6- to 12-French) tubes inserted using a sterile Seldinger (catheter-over-wire) technique, often under ultrasonographic guidance. They are less painful for patients, produce less scarring, and do not require tissue dissection or skin closure on removal. Overall, there is less risk for complications with these devices than with the larger-bore versions. Recent studies comparing the effectiveness of pigtail versus larger conventional chest drainage tubes show no significant differences in resolution of pneumothoraces, hemothoraces, empyemas, or effusions. Pigtail catheters are managed in much the same way as chest tubes. In the future, it is possible that insertion of pigtail catheters will be included in some CCTPs' scope of practice.

The procedure for inserting a pigtail catheter begins with collecting the needed equipment (often packaged as a "tray"):

- Appropriate PPE, including sterile gloves
- Ultrasonography unit
- Scalpel
- Pigtail catheter: 6 to 12 French
- Sterile occlusive dressing
- Suturing material
- 2% chlorhexidine
- A local anesthetic if the patient is awake
- A fluid collection device with a one-way valve that allows air, fluid, or pus to flow out of the chest; if not available, an indwelling catheter bag with a one-way valve may be used
- Tape

SKILL DRILL 11-4 shows the clinical procedure for inserting a pigtail catheter, which is described here:

1. Select the appropriate site. Ultrasonographic guidance has been shown to reduce complications and misplacement **STEP 1**.
2. Connect the collection device to the distal end of the one-way valve with a rubber band or set up a chest tube drainage system.
3. Cleanse the site with an appropriate aseptic technique.
4. Anesthetize the area, including the pleura and periosteum, over the fifth rib **STEP 2**.
5. Measure the pigtail catheter against the chest to determine the insertion distance. Keep in mind that pigtail catheters can be withdrawn but cannot be further inserted following completion of the procedure.
6. Draw a few milliliters of sterile water into the finder needle so you can visualize aspiration of air during insertion. Insert the needle over the superior aspect of the rib while aspirating the syringe. Once in the pleural space, the syringe plunger will provide a way to aspirate bubbles in a pneumothorax and pleural fluid or blood in an effusion or hemothorax.
7. Disconnect the syringe from the needle and pass the guide wire in far enough to clear the needle **STEP 3**. Inserting the wire too far will make it difficult to direct the pigtail catheter superiorly.
8. Remove the needle over the wire and make a small incision adjacent to the guide wire (as when inserting a central line) to accommodate the dilator and catheter. Pass the dilator over the wire into the pleural space **STEP 4**. You should feel the dilator "pop" once you are in the correct location. Ensure there are no kinks by verifying that the guide wire moves easily in and out of the dilator.
9. Pass the pigtail and trocar over the wire, ensuring you advance them sufficiently to locate all holes in the pleural space.
10. Remove the trocar and guide wire. Suture the pigtail catheter in place and connect it to the drainage device **STEP 5**.
11. Cover the insertion site with an occlusive dressing. On arrival at the receiving facility, obtain a chest film to confirm proper placement of the pigtail catheter. Document the procedure.

Skill Drill 11-4 Pigtail Catheter Insertion

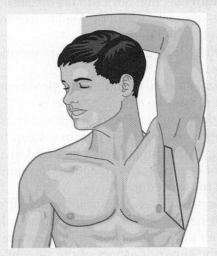

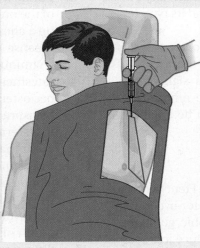

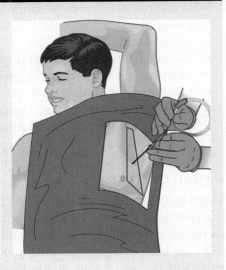

Step 1

Select the appropriate site. Connect the collection device to the distal end of the one-way valve with a rubber band or set up a chest tube drainage system.

Step 2

Anesthetize the area, including the pleura and periosteum, over the fifth rib.

Step 3

Disconnect the syringe from the needle and pass the guide wire in far enough to clear the needle.

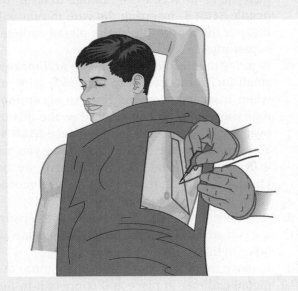

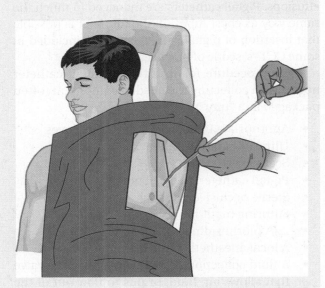

Step 4

Remove the needle over the wire and make a small incision adjacent to the guide wire.

Step 5

Pass the dilator over the wire into the pleural space. You should feel the dilator "pop" once you are in the correct location. Verify that the guide wire moves easily in and out of the dilator. Remove the trocar and guide wire. Suture the pigtail catheter in place and connect it to the drainage device.

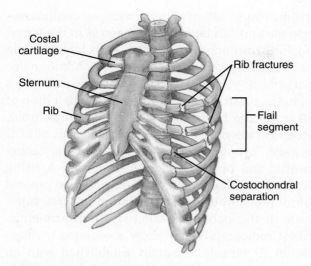

FIGURE 11-18 In flail chest injuries, two or more adjacent ribs are fractured in two or more places. A flail segment may move paradoxically when the patient breathes, although this sign is usually present only in very young children, older adults, or other patients with underdeveloped pectoral and latissimus muscles.

© Jones & Bartlett Learning.

Flail Chest

A fracture in two or more places of two or more adjacent ribs is known as a flail chest or a flail segment **FIGURE 11-18**. This condition is relatively common in trauma patients. In one study, flail chest was found to be present in as many as one-third of serious chest injuries. Many of these injuries escape detection for as long as 6 hours following hospital admission.

A flail segment may appear to move paradoxically relative to the chest wall, but actually is stationary while the rest of the chest moves around it. This movement may be more obvious in unconscious patients who are no longer "splinting." Often, bruises to the underlying tissue may cause a pulmonary or myocardial contusion and represent the most dangerous sequelae of a flail chest. Flail segments are generally caused by blunt trauma, such as striking a steering wheel in an MVC. A central flail involves the sternum.

Clinical signs and symptoms of a flail chest are dyspnea, severe pain, decreased breath sounds on the affected side, tenderness, and crepitus to palpation, with possible bruising over the area. Signs and symptoms are often difficult to assess as a result of the patient's efforts to splint the area and ease the

pain that occurs with respiration. The pain associated with flail segments may mask abdominal tenderness. When this condition is present, the CCTP must maintain a high clinical suspicion for underlying injury.

Flail segments pose a threat to the patient's ability to breathe, increase the risk for developing a hemothorax or pneumothorax, and require immediate treatment. Definitive treatment for flail chest with significant symptoms involves pain control and positive-pressure ventilation.

Management of a flail chest is as follows:

1. Maintain an open airway and apply appropriate oxygen therapy. Analgesia is a major determinant of a patient's ability to ventilate unassisted, and proper pain control should be initiated and maintained.
2. Assist ventilation with a trial of noninvasive ventilation (continuous positive airway pressure or bilevel positive airway pressure), and be prepared to intubate.
3. Immediately transport the patient if the call involves a field transport.
4. Monitor the patient's oxygen saturation, vital signs, and cardiac monitor. Be alert for development of tension pneumothorax, hemothorax (shock), or respiratory failure secondary to a pulmonary contusion.
5. The gold-standard treatment for flail chest is positive-pressure ventilation (also known as internal fixation) with a sedated patient who has been adequately treated for pain. It may be possible to manage some patients conservatively with pain medications and noninvasive ventilation alone.

Attempts to splint (also called external fixation) or wrap the chest have been shown to be ineffective, and this practice has been abandoned.

Signs and Symptoms

Flail Chest

- Dyspnea
- Severe pain
- Decreased breath sounds on the affected side
- Tenderness
- Crepitus to palpation
- Bruising over the area

Pericardial Tamponade

Pericardial tamponade is a life-threatening condition that may require immediate treatment. This condition is reported in 2% of penetrating injuries to the chest and upper abdomen. It is more common in stab wounds to the heart (occurring in as many as 80% of such cases) than in gunshot wounds.

The pericardium normally contains a small amount of fluid that cushions and lubricates the heart as it expands and contracts. When an abundance of blood or fluid accumulates in the pericardial sac, it compresses the ventricles of the heart, which in turn compromises cardiac filling and output. Abnormal amounts of fluid may result from any of the following conditions:

- Pericarditis caused by infection and inflammation
- Trauma
- Surgery or other invasive procedures performed on the heart (ie, pacemaker insertion, ablation)
- Cancer
- Myocardial infarction and congestive heart failure
- Renal failure

The classic clinical signs and symptoms of a pericardial tamponade are summarized as the **Beck triad**: narrowing pulse pressure, JVD, and muffled heart tones. However, Beck triad is present in only 10% to 40% of patients with pericardial tamponade and can be difficult to assess in the transport environment. In patients with hypovolemia or hemorrhage, there may be no JVD. Additionally, patients may present with a paradoxical pulse (loss of radial pulse on inspiration, often with a drop of 10 to 15 mm Hg in the systolic pressure as well), electrical alternans, progressive decreases of ECG voltage, hypotension, cyanosis, dyspnea, tachycardia, and pulseless electrical activity. A rising CVP greater than 15 cm H_2O may also be present (until precipitous decompensation occurs), especially if the patient is otherwise normovolemic. Chest radiographs may show a widened mediastinum. Diagnosis is usually established with an ultrasonographic (FAST) exam, using a portable ultrasonography unit.

Most often, prehospital management of pericardial tamponade is only supportive, and administering a fluid bolus may prevent decompensation. On some occasions, with proper training and certification, the CCTP may be called upon to perform or assist in an emergency **pericardiocentesis FIGURE 11-19**. The equipment needed for this procedure includes:

- Appropriate PPE, including sterile gloves, gown, and mask
- Cardiac monitor and defibrillator
- Pericardiocentesis kit (Mansfield catheter)

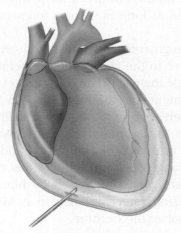

Pericardiocentesis

FIGURE 11-19 Pericardiocentesis in pericardial tamponade.

© Jones & Bartlett Learning.

- 50-mL Luer-lock syringes
- Sterile tubes for specimen collection
- 2% chlorhexidine
- Appropriate medications (cardiac, sedating, and numbing)
- Pigtail catheter
- Drapes
- 16- to 18-gauge by 5.5-inch (14-cm) spinal needle
- Three-way stopcock
- Sterile alligator clip
- Scalpel
- Assorted needles and syringes
- Preferably, the availability of ultrasonographic imaging

Indications for pericardiocentesis include the following conditions:

- Chest trauma with patient in extremis, such as those with pulseless electrical activity
- FAST exam showing pericardial blood with clinical signs

Contraindications include:

- No demonstrable pericardial effusion
- Severe thrombocytopenia or noncorrectable coagulopathy
- Skin or soft-tissue infection at the proposed needle site (except in a critical patient)

Pericardiocentesis is associated with several potential complications:

- Malignant ventricular arrhythmias, including cardiac arrest
- Puncture of the ventricles or atria (most commonly the right ventricle)
- Laceration of the coronary arteries and lung
- Pericardial tamponade from a myocardial laceration
- Air embolism
- Acute pulmonary edema
- Puncture of the liver or stomach
- Infection

SKILL DRILL 11-5 illustrates the clinical procedure for pericardiocentesis, which is described here:

1. Prepare the equipment and obtain baseline vital signs, including pulse oximetry findings.
2. Place the patient into a supine position with the head of the stretcher elevated to a 20° to 30° angle as tolerated.
3. Premedicate per your protocol or online medical control.
4. Don a mask, gown, hair cover, and sterile gloves.
5. Cleanse the site with an appropriate aseptic technique and drape the area **STEP 1**.
6. Identify the needle entry site directly below the xiphoid—approximately 0.4 inch (1 cm) left of midline **STEP 2**.
7. Infiltrate the area with 1% lidocaine into the skin and deeper tissues, if the patient is conscious **STEP 3**.
8. Insert the needle-on-syringe, with 2 to 3 mL of sterile saline in it, at the identified entry site, at a 30° angle directed toward the left shoulder or directly cephalad **STEP 4**.
9. Gently aspirate while inserting the needle **STEP 5**. Some resistance may be felt as the needle enters the pericardial sac. *If the needle is advanced too far, the myocardium will become irritated. The needle may vibrate with the pulse. Pull back the needle slightly until you can aspirate fluid.*
10. If blood is withdrawn and placed in an open container, it should not clot if it comes from the pericardial sac. Place the sample into the collection container and transport it with the patient.
11. Administer medications per your protocol or online medical control.
12. Monitor for postprocedural complications.
13. Monitor vital signs and for JVD at 15-minute intervals for 1 hour, and then every hour for 4 hours.
14. The entire procedure should occur under ultrasonographic guidance, when possible, to visualize entry into the pericardium and prevent cardiac injury.
15. In some cases, a catheter or drain may be placed, with the stopcock being opened for periodic drainage as needed.

Pericardial Window

CCTPs should be familiar with the anatomic landmarks of a pericardial window (an in-hospital surgical procedure) and postprocedural monitoring.

Skill Drill 11-5 Pericardiocentesis

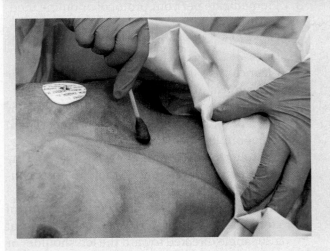

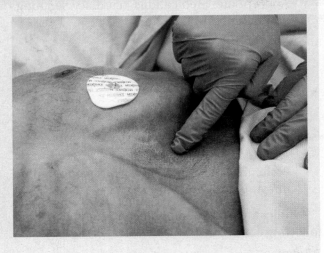

Step 1

Prepare the equipment and obtain baseline vital signs, including pulse oximetry findings. Place the patient into a supine position with the head of the stretcher elevated to a 20° to 30° angle as tolerated. Premedicate per your protocol or online medical control. Don a mask, gown, hair cover, and sterile gloves. Cleanse the site with an appropriate aseptic technique and drape the area.

Step 2

Identify the needle entry site directly below the xiphoid.

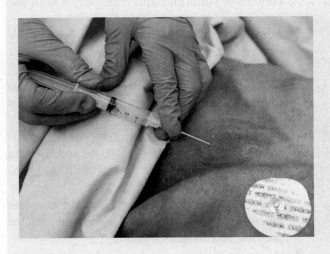

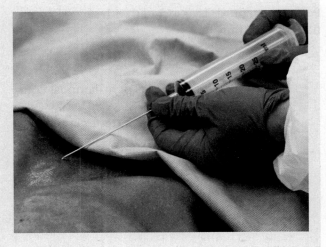

Step 3

Infiltrate the area with 1% lidocaine into the skin and deeper tissues.

Step 4

Insert the needle-on-syringe at the identified entry site, at a 30° angle directed toward the left shoulder or directly cephalad.

Skill Drill 11-5 Pericardiocentesis (continued)

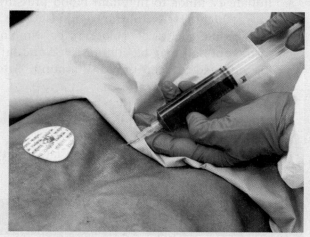

All images © Jones & Bartlett Learning.

Step 5

Gently aspirate while inserting the needle. *If the needle is advanced too far, the myocardium will become irritated. Pull the needle back slightly until you can aspirate fluid.* Place the blood sample into the collection container and transport it with the patient. Administer medications per your protocol or online medical control. Monitor for postprocedure complications. Monitor vital signs and for JVD at 15-minute intervals for 1 hour, and then every hour for 4 hours.

Signs and Symptoms

Pericardial Tamponade
- Beck triad: narrowing pulse pressure, JVD, and muffled heart tones
- Paradoxical pulse
- Electrical alternans
- Progressive decreases of ECG voltage
- Hypotension
- Cyanosis
- Dyspnea
- Tachycardia
- Pulseless electrical activity
- Increasing CVP (greater than 15 cm H_2O)
- Widened mediastinum on chest radiograph

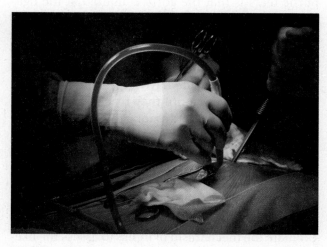

FIGURE 11-20 A large pericardial window. Sutures ensure that all the layers stay in place.

© miralex/iStock/Getty Images Plus/Getty Images.

Transport Management

Pericardial Tamponade
- Provide supportive care.
- Administer a fluid bolus.
- If necessary, perform an emergency pericardiocentesis or pericardial window.

A pericardial window is performed by incising the skin just inferior to the xiphoid process, in the midline, and dissecting down to the anterior and inferior surface of the pericardium **FIGURE 11-20**. Once identified, the pericardium is incised and fluid is allowed to drain. Typically, a small section, approximately 1 × 1 inch (2.5 × 2.5 cm), is removed to prevent reaccumulation of fluid and tamponade recurrence. Sudden decompensation can occur if cardiac preload is not adequate during the initial phases of this procedure. The pericardial window procedure concludes with placement of a drain through the dissection tract into the pericardium. For the CCTP, it is important to note the quality and color of drainage and the drain output on initial contact with the patient and to monitor for post-procedural complications, such as arrhythmia or recurrence of tamponade.

Aortic Dissection/Transection

Traumatic aortic rupture is the most common cause of immediate death in MVCs. The body's entire blood volume passes through the aorta; therefore, it is easy to understand how death could occur immediately when the aorta is torn. Most people with aortic rupture die within minutes, often prior to the arrival of the CCTP. Those who do survive require emergent surgical intervention as soon as possible.

The most widely accepted etiology of traumatic aortic tears is that the aorta is injured at the ligamentum arteriosum, the remnant of the fetal ductus arteriosus, as a result of decelerating injuries and shear force. Tears in the ascending aorta are almost uniformly immediately fatal, but patients with tears on the descending side have approximately a 15% chance of surviving until they reach the operating room. The mortality rate among those patients who make it to the hospital is 30%. Some trauma centers are now using endovascular stenting with some success to treat patients with aortic rupture.

Diagnosis of traumatic aortic tears is very difficult in the prehospital setting and may even be missed in the hospital. The CCTP should closely evaluate the mechanism of injury to assess the likelihood of an aortic injury. A pulse deficit or blood pressure difference from one arm to the other, usually greater than 15 to 20 mm Hg, may be noted if the dissection is at the top of the arch of the aorta (ie, beyond the left subclavian artery). Level of consciousness may be decreased due to decreased carotid pressure. Other signs include hypertension of the upper extremities; decrease of pulse amplitude in the lower extremities; chest pain; chest wall bruising; widened mediastinum on chest radiograph with blurring of the aortic knob; and fractures of the first and second ribs.

Definitive diagnosis is made with CT and TEE. Potential aortic tears are managed as follows:

1. Maintain an open airway and apply appropriate oxygen therapy.
2. Assist ventilation and be prepared to intubate.
3. Initiate IV fluids to maintain blood pressure *only* at 90 mm Hg systolic or 65 mm Hg MAP.
4. Medications such as beta blockers (eg, esmolol or metoprolol) may be administered and fluids withheld to keep the MAP around 65 to 70 mm Hg.
5. Initiate transport immediately.
6. Monitor oxygen saturation, vital signs, and the cardiac monitor.
7. Transport the patient to an appropriate facility with early advance notification.

Signs and Symptoms

Traumatic Aortic Rupture

- Pulse deficit or blood pressure difference from one arm to the other
- Hypotension
- Decreased level of consciousness
- Hypertension of the upper extremities
- Decreased pulse amplitude in the lower extremities
- Decreased blood pressure
- Chest pain
- Chest wall bruising
- Widened mediastinum on chest radiograph with blurring of the aortic knob
- Fractures of the first and second ribs

Transport Management

Traumatic Aortic Rupture

- Maintain an open airway; apply appropriate oxygen therapy.
- Assist ventilation; be prepared to intubate.
- Initiate IV fluids.
- Administer beta blockers (eg, esmolol or metoprolol) and withhold fluids to keep the MAP at 65 to 70 mm Hg (90 mm Hg systolic blood pressure).
- Begin immediate transport.
- Monitor oxygen saturation, vital signs, and the cardiac monitor.
- Transport to an appropriate facility with early advance notification.

Myocardial Contusion

A contusion, or bruise, results from damage to small blood vessels, causing localized bleeding and direct trauma to cells. A contusion to the myocardium primarily results from blunt trauma to the anterior chest wall. MVCs are an obvious mechanism of injury, but other blunt trauma to the anterior part of the chest (eg, gunshot to a bulletproof vest, baseballs) may also cause this condition. Myocardial contusions have been reported even in low-speed (20 to 35 mph) MVCs, without external chest wall bruising. Estimates of this injury's frequency vary widely, ranging from 16% to 76% of all blunt chest trauma cases.

The amount of damage to myocardial cells also varies widely in these injuries. Areas downstream of injured blood vessels may no longer be perfused, resulting in damage similar to that caused by a myocardial infarction resulting from atherosclerotic coronary artery disease. In turn, the most common signs and symptoms are similar to those associated with acute myocardial infarction: chest pain, palpitations, and arrhythmias. Arrhythmias may develop as late as 12 to 72 hours after injury. Irregular rhythms to watch for include premature ventricular complexes, ventricular tachycardia, and ventricular fibrillation. The appearance of premature ventricular contractions should prompt high suspicion for an evolving cardiac injury. ST-segment elevations may be evident on the 12-lead ECG, particularly in the right-side (V_4R) leads. Bundle branch blocks, especially on the right (anterior) side of the heart, and atrioventricular blocks may develop if the intraventricular septum is involved. The wider the QRS in a bundle branch block, the more the ventricles are out of phase, reducing the ejection fraction and compromising cardiac output. Other signs include cardiac murmur, pericardial friction rub, and persistent tachycardia. If the injury is large enough, cardiogenic shock may result from the myocardium's reduced contractibility.

Lab tests for myocardial contusion may be performed in the field with a point-of-care device but are more likely to be performed in the hospital. They include measurements of troponin I and troponin T. These proteins are very specific to cardiac injury and are elevated in the presence of myocardial injury. The creatine kinase MB–fraction test is not used to assess for this condition.

Current recommendations for the management of myocardial contusion are mostly supportive. Treatment modalities include assessment of cardiac function (typically with echocardiography), oxygen administration if indicated, resuscitation without fluid overload, and continuous ECG monitoring for the development of arrhythmias.

Signs and Symptoms

Myocardial Contusion

- Chest pain
- Palpitations
- Arrhythmias: premature ventricular complexes, ventricular tachycardia, and ventricular fibrillation
- ST-segment elevation on the 12-lead ECG, particularly the V_4R leads
- Bundle branch blocks, especially on the right side
- Atrioventricular blocks
- Cardiac murmur
- Pericardial friction rub
- Persistent tachycardia without other cause
- Cardiogenic shock

Transport Management

Myocardial Contusion

- Administer appropriate oxygen therapy.
- Provide pharmacologic treatment of arrhythmias.
- Watch closely for development of hemopericardium, leading to pericardial tamponade, myocardial rupture, or ventricular aneurysm.

Diaphragmatic Rupture

Either blunt or penetrating trauma may lead to rupture of the diaphragm. Penetration inferior to the nipple line or scapula may lacerate the diaphragm. These lacerations are usually small and not an immediate problem, but will require eventual surgical repair. A larger problem is blunt compression of the abdomen that causes a large rupture and herniation of abdominal organs into the thoracic cavity. This displacement impinges on lung function and decreases venous return, such that both ventilatory function and cardiac output are reduced.

Signs and symptoms of diaphragmatic rupture include chest and/or abdominal pain, acute respiratory distress, decreased breath sounds, and abdominal sounds in the chest cavity. Patients may also have subcutaneous emphysema or obvious penetration in the thoracic region.

Management of diaphragmatic rupture includes supporting ventilation and oxygenation. Nasogastric or orogastric decompression of the stomach may temporarily assist in reducing the volume of abdominal organs in the thoracic cavity. Surgical repair is the definitive treatment for these patients, and transport should not be delayed to perform additional prehospital procedures.

Signs and Symptoms
Diaphragmatic Rupture • Chest or abdominal pain • Acute respiratory distress • Decreased breath sounds • Abdominal sounds in the chest cavity • Subcutaneous emphysema • Obvious penetration in the chest or abdomen

Transport Management
Diaphragmatic Rupture • Assist ventilation. • Administer appropriate oxygen therapy. • Insert a nasogastric or orogastric tube to decompress the stomach if advised by medical control.

Tracheobronchial Disruption

Tracheobronchial injuries are rare, but often life threatening. They occur in less than 3% of blunt and penetrating (the more common cause) chest injuries, but may have a fatality rate as high as 30%. Most tracheobronchial injuries occur within 1.5 inches (4 cm) of the carina, although they can occur anywhere along the tracheobronchial tree. The leakage of air may cause a tension pneumothorax or tension pneumomediastinum, which will act like a cardiac tamponade. Signs and symptoms include severe respiratory distress, hypoxia, tachycardia, subcutaneous emphysema (especially in the neck), hemoptysis, JVD, and tracheal deviation.

An apparent tension pneumothorax that does not improve after needle thoracostomy or one associated with continuous flow of air from the needle or chest tube is probably a tracheobronchial tear. Management includes judicious use of ventilatory support. If positive-pressure ventilation makes the patient worse and no relief is obtained from needle decompression, then oxygen supplementation alone may be necessary.

Signs and Symptoms
Tracheobronchial Disruption • Severe respiratory distress • Hypoxia • Tachycardia • Subcutaneous emphysema, especially in the neck • Hemoptysis • JVD • Tracheal deviation • Continuous air leak after chest tube placement

Transport Management
Tracheobronchial Disruption • Administer appropriate oxygen therapy. • Provide positive-pressure ventilation, unless it worsens the patient's condition. • Perform needle decompression, if necessary. • Insert a chest tube or pigtail catheter, if necessary and if protocols allow. Patients may need more than one in rare cases of very proximal bronchial injury.

Pulmonary Contusion

Tearing and lacerations to the lung tissue can cause bleeding and leakage of plasma into the alveoli and the interstitial spaces around them **FIGURE 11-21**. This damage occurs when the lung hits the inside

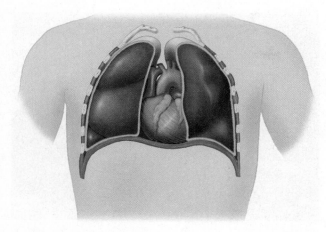

FIGURE 11-21 Pulmonary contusion.

© Jones & Bartlett Learning.

of the chest wall (such as in blunt chest injury) or as a result of shearing force causing stretching and tearing of capillaries and alveoli. Pressure waves from explosions may also stretch and tear lung tissue. With this injury, blood in and around the alveoli interferes with gas exchange and leads to severe hypoxemia. The bleeding may begin soon after the impact, but more often develops over hours; the patient's deterioration may occur over a period of 24 hours or longer. Uninjured parts of the lung undergo gradual thickening of the alveolar capillary membranes as the inflammatory process evolves. Close monitoring is necessary for at least 48 hours after injury, as the inflammatory response of the lung to trauma can cause fluid shifts that compromise the ability to exchange gases across capillary membranes.

Patients with flail chest or similar significant mechanisms of injury may be assumed to have a developing pulmonary contusion. Signs and symptoms may initially be absent, but over time the trauma patient's condition will deteriorate; at that point, the CCTP may be called to transfer the patient to a medical center that has more sophisticated technology. The primary sign of this deterioration is increasing hypoxia. Although definitive chest radiographs will show an opacity in the area of chest wall damage, a clear chest radiograph does not rule out a pulmonary contusion. Worsening oxygenation and increased difficulty ventilating over time with a pertinent mechanism of injury are sufficient to make this diagnosis.

Treatment is to support ventilation with mechanical ventilation—traditionally done with pressure-control ventilation and a positive end-expiratory pressure of 10 to 15 cm H_2O. Today, however, more patients are being successfully supported with noninvasive ventilation. In either case, and especially in patients with rib fractures or flail chest, adequate analgesia is imperative. Fluid restriction may be helpful as well, but volume resuscitation in difficult-to-ventilate patients has become controversial unless physiologic parameters suggest volume resuscitation would be beneficial. In the field, resuscitation fluids should be given as needed for systolic pressure support.

Signs and Symptoms

Pulmonary Contusion

- Initially absent (no signs and symptoms)
- Increasing hypoxia over hours to days
- Opacity in the area of chest wall damage on chest radiograph
- Worsening oxygenation and increased difficulty ventilating over time as fluid accumulates in the lungs secondary to inflammation

Transport Management

Pulmonary Contusion

- Provide ventilatory support: either (1) pressure-control or another pressure-limited mode of ventilation with positive end-expiratory pressure of 10 to 15 cm H_2O or (2) noninvasive ventilation.
- Provide adequate analgesia.

Esophageal Perforation

Esophageal perforations are most often caused by penetrating injuries, such as projectiles, or caustic ingestion. They can also result from a medical cause, such as cancer or gastroesophageal reflux disease erosions. Excessive vomiting may cause a Mallory-Weiss tear.

Signs and symptoms of esophageal perforation include pain, fever, dysphagia, subcutaneous air in the neck and neck stiffness, and pleuritic-type pain. Free mediastinal air or widening may be found on imaging studies. The air introduced into the mediastinum may produce a crunching sound on auscultation.

Treatment is supportive of the ABCs. Nasogastric tube insertion is usually contraindicated.

Traumatic Asphyxia

Traumatic asphyxia describes a severe, sudden crushing injury to the chest and abdomen, such as occurs when a patient is caught between a truck and a loading dock or when a vehicle falls off a jack. This injury forces blood backward out of the right side of the heart, engorging the veins of the chest, neck, and head. The deoxygenated blood makes the chest, neck, and head look blue or purple, as in extreme cyanosis, giving rise to the name "asphyxia" **FIGURE 11-22**. Traumatic asphyxia is not a form of asphyxia, nor is it by itself fatal, despite its undeserved reputation for high mortality. Associated injuries, if present, are far more serious—for example, brain hemorrhage, possible cardiac rupture, eye injuries, flail chest, ruptured diaphragm, and pulmonary or myocardial contusions. If the patient survives the initial injury, the dramatic purple color will fade after several weeks.

Specific assessment findings, besides the mechanism of injury and the purple discoloration,

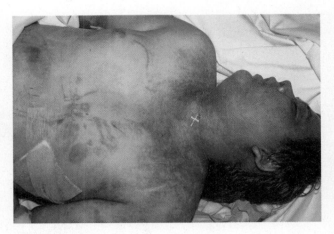

FIGURE 11-22 Traumatic asphyxia.
© Charles Stewart, MD, EMDM, MPH.

include JVD, conjunctival or scleral petechiae, and a sharp line of demarcation with normal skin color below it. Treatment is primarily supportive, including treatment for the associated injuries. If the patient is found entrapped, IV lines and a treatment plan to deal with sudden hypotension and possible release of myoglobin and potassium are necessary when the patient is freed. (The patient may have crush syndrome, depending on how long the individual was entrapped.)

Facial Trauma

Facial trauma can be life threatening and has many implications for patients both socially and in terms of self-image. Such trauma can be distracting for providers as well. Facial injuries are of special significance because the patient experiences an immediate life threat as a result of airway compromise and the loss of sensory inputs through sight and hearing. CCTPs must also be aware of their own emotional response and reactions to these injuries.

Ear Injuries

Ear injuries are generally not considered an area of concern for CCTPs because they are not life threatening and do not involve technology for transport. Ear injuries may be present in patients who have other more serious injuries, but they usually do not need much attention on either a scene call or an interfacility transport. A punctured eardrum, however, may cause vertigo and nausea, which the CCTP may need to control with medication. The patient should be protected from aircraft noise.

External Ear Injury

External ear injuries are considered a local injury with no acute systemic implications. The long-term possibility of infection or deformity (cauliflower ear) is not usually life threatening. Standard soft-tissue injury care applies **FIGURE 11-23**.

Blood or fluid coming from the auditory canal indicates a more serious injury. A halo test for cerebrospinal fluid mixed with blood, indicating basilar skull fracture, is easily done with a piece of filter paper or a gauze pad. Do not pack the ear canal; rather, use a loose dressing. Chapter 12, *Neurologic Emergencies*, covers neurologic emergencies in depth.

Ruptured Tympanic Membrane

A ruptured tympanic membrane may be the result of overpressure injury, such as occurs with an explosion or a direct blow to the ear. Rupture may also result from failure to equalize middle ear pressure during scuba diving. In the absence of infection, most of these injuries will heal spontaneously and are not life threatening, but their presence should raise the suspicion for other, much more serious

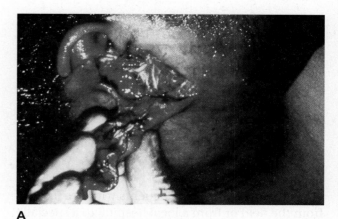

A

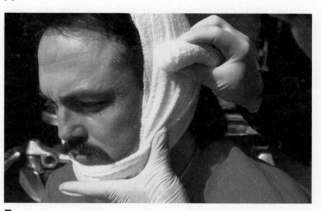

B

FIGURE 11-23 A. A major laceration of the ear. **B.** Place a soft, sterile pad behind the ear, between it and the scalp. Then wrap a roller gauze bandage (eg, Kling or Kerlex) around the head to include the entire ear.

A. © American Academy of Orthopaedic Surgeons; **B.** © Jones & Bartlett Learning.

overpressure injuries. Principal signs and symptoms are pain and vertigo, possibly accompanied by vomiting. Sometimes blood may be visible in the ear canal. Treatment includes an external dressing to reduce the chance of infection (do not pack the ear canal), and possibly use of an antiemetic. This injury is a relative contraindication to aircraft transport of the patient.

Signs and Symptoms

Ruptured Tympanic Membrane
- Pain
- Vertigo
- Vomiting
- Blood visible in the ear canal

Eye Injuries

The CCTP may transport patients with eye injuries from the field or from a local hospital to a specialty center with ophthalmologic services. Eye injuries, although often dramatic, are not life threatening. Although vision loss is serious, there is usually little for the CCTP to do other than protect the eye from further injury and transport the patient to the ophthalmology service.

The major exception to this rule is chemical burns to the eye **FIGURE 11-24**—a case in which transport can actually interfere with appropriate care. Adequate washing is essential and should be performed with (preferably) sterile saline or dextrose solution for at least 10 minutes prior to transport for acid burns and at least twice as long for alkali burns. Lavage should then continue en route if possible, though such care may be difficult to administer in an aircraft. Use of topical anesthesia such as tetracaine (TetraVisc) or proparacaine (Alcaine) is necessary for flushing to be effective. The CCTP must be alert to the possibility of other more serious injuries that may have been overlooked and should always be treated first. Many techniques may be used when irrigating the eyes; the Morgan Lens is one.

Eyelid Lacerations

Soft-tissue injuries to the eye and surrounding structures include lacerations and swelling. Direct pressure, applied in a manner so as not to push on the globe (pressure directly on the globe may cause vagal stimulation), will usually stop any bleeding. Application of cold may reduce swelling. The CCTP should have concern for concomitant eye injuries when an eyelid laceration is observed.

Conjunctival and Corneal Injuries

The most common conjunctival and corneal injuries are abrasions and foreign bodies. More serious

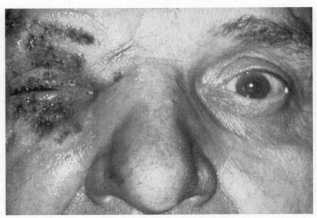

A

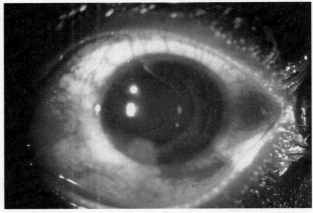

B

FIGURE 11-24 A. Chemical burns typically occur when an acid or alkali is splashed into the eye. **B.** A chemical burn from lye, an alkaline solution.

© American Academy of Orthopaedic Surgeons.

injuries involve shrapnel from high-speed equipment such as drills and saws. These types of injuries often involve objects impaled in the eye. If possible, the eye and the object should be prevented from movement for transport. A cup or shield is generally used for this purpose **FIGURE 11-25**. The unaffected eye may need to be patched to prevent sympathetic movement, although this practice has fallen out of favor, as little evidence supports any benefit to the patient. Removal of most objects will need to be visualized with a slit lamp or ocular loupe under local anesthetic.

Hyphema

A hyphema is a collection of blood in the anterior chamber of the eye **FIGURE 11-26**. It may result from blunt trauma to the eye or a medical cause. A

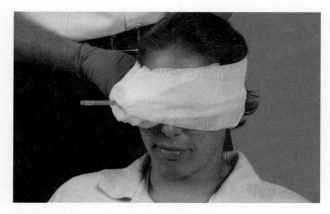

FIGURE 11-25 An impaled object is secured with a protective barrier and a bulky dressing.

© Jones & Bartlett Learning.

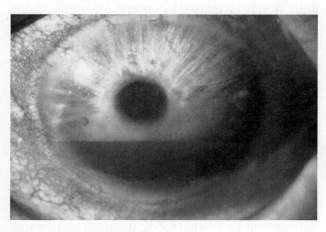

FIGURE 11-26 A hyphema.

© American Academy of Orthopaedic Surgeons.

hyphema may also be a marker of damage to other structures of the eye and, therefore, requires a full ophthalmologic examination. One concern that arises with this condition is blood clotting in the canal connecting the anterior chamber of the eye to the posterior chamber, causing an acute rise in intraocular pressure. The patient will complain of reduced vision directly proportional to the size of the hyphema. Often the blood is visible unaided, but shining a penlight obliquely at the globe may help to visualize the blood, which will pool with gravity.

Grading of hyphemas is based on four categories:

- Grade 1: Layered blood occupying less than one-third of the anterior chamber
- Grade 2: Blood filling one-third to one-half of the anterior chamber
- Grade 3: Layered blood filling one-half to less than the total anterior chamber
- Grade 4: Total clotted blood, often called a blackball or 8-ball hyphema

If there are no other contraindications, transport should occur with the patient sitting as upright as possible and with eye patches applied per protocols or local medical direction. Pain should be managed with acetaminophen; medications with antiplatelet effects (eg, aspirin) should be avoided. An anxiolytic may facilitate transport.

Signs and Symptoms

Hyphema

- Patient complaint of reduced vision (directly proportional to the size of the hyphema)
- Pool of blood in the eye; may be visualized either directly or by shining a penlight obliquely at the globe

Transport Management

Hyphema

- Patch both eyes (controversial).
- Transport the patient sitting as upright as possible.
- Administer analgesics; avoid antiplatelet agents.
- Administer an anxiolytic if necessary to facilitate transport.

Ocular Globe Rupture

Rupture of the globe with ensuing leak of the vitreous humor may be the result of penetration with a foreign body or blunt trauma. Signs of an open globe include penetrating lid injury, bullous conjunctival hemorrhage, blood in the anterior chamber (hyphema), peaked or deformed pupil, lens dislocation, vitreous hemorrhage, and decreased visual acuity. Management for transport includes protecting the affected eye with a rigid eye shield or cup, rather than a soft patch. Antiemetics and pain medication should be given for transport. Sometimes antitussives are also used to prevent any increase in intraocular pressure as the result of coughing.

Signs and Symptoms

Ocular Globe Rupture

- Penetrating lid injury
- Bullous conjunctival hemorrhage
- Blood in the anterior chamber (hyphema)
- Peaked or deformed pupil
- Lens dislocation
- Vitreous hemorrhage
- Decreased visual acuity

Transport Management

Ocular Globe Rupture

- Protect the affected eye with a rigid eye shield or cup.
- Administer antiemetics and pain medication.
- If necessary, administer an antitussive to prevent increased intraocular pressure as the result of coughing.

Ocular Avulsion

Enucleation of the eyeball from the eye socket is possible from a trauma **FIGURE 11-27**. Multiple facial fractures may increase the chance of this injury. The globe may actually be hanging from the optic nerve. Despite the dramatic presentation, loss of vision is not inevitable. Proper care includes protecting the

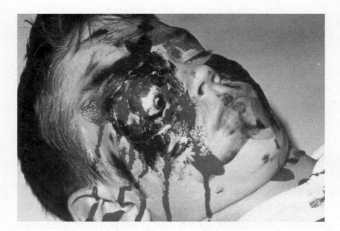

FIGURE 11-27 Ocular avulsion.
© American Academy of Orthopaedic Surgeons.

eye from further trauma in transit by using a protective cup or other rigid protective device with moistened gauze padding.

Transport Management

Ocular Avulsion

- Protect the eye from further trauma with a protective cup or other rigid protective device with moistened gauze padding.

Traumatic Retinal Detachment

Retinal detachment refers to separation of the inner layers of the retina from the pigmented epithelium. It may be caused by several other conditions besides trauma, including diabetic retinopathy and sickle cell disease.

Initially, the patient complains of the sensation of flashing light, often accompanied by a shower of floaters and vision loss. The vision loss may be described as filmy, cloudy, irregular, curtain like, or wavy. Patients may also complain of black spots, especially in the center of the visual field, or spiderweb-like vision.

When retinal detachment is suspected, it is imperative to avoid pressure to the globe. A rigid metal eye shield, rather than a soft patch, should be used to protect the eye. Although some types of retinal detachment are treated medically, most require surgery within 24 hours. In the past, retinal detachment uniformly led to blindness. Today, however, rapid diagnosis and surgery may be truly sight saving.

Signs and Symptoms

Traumatic Retinal Detachment

- Sensation of flashing light, often accompanied by a shower of floaters and vision loss
- Black spots, especially in the center of the visual field
- Spiderweb-like vision

Transport Management

Traumatic Retinal Detachment

- Avoid pressure to the globe.
- Protect the eye with a rigid metal eye shield.

Mandibular Fracture and Dislocation

The mandible is the only movable bone in the skull and makes up the lower third of the face. Because of its U shape, single blows to this bone can cause multiple fractures anywhere around its length. The mandible can also become anteriorly dislocated, causing the mouth to be locked in an open position. Signs of fracture include crepitus, trismus, swelling, and patient complaints that the jaw does not feel right or close normally (malocclusion).

Treatment is usually not necessary on a scene call, but transfers to rehabilitation facilities or tertiary centers may involve a patient with a jaw wired shut in maxillomandibular fixation. Provision must be made for inserting an emergency airway during such transfers. This may involve having wire cutters available to open the jaw, using nasotracheal intubation skills and equipment, and being prepared to obtain emergency surgical access.

Signs and Symptoms

Mandibular Fracture or Dislocation

- Crepitus
- Trismus
- Swelling
- Patient complains the jaw does not feel right or close normally (malocclusion)

Transport Management

Mandibular Fracture or Dislocation

- If the patient's jaw is wired shut, have wire cutters available to open the jaw in case an emergency airway is needed.
- Have nasotracheal intubation skills and equipment available.
- Be prepared to make emergency surgical access.

Dental Avulsion

Avulsed teeth have a good chance of successful re-implantation if replaced within 1 hour. Until that time, the tooth or teeth must be handled carefully.

The American Dental Association has developed the following guidelines for managing dental avulsion:

- Never place an avulsed tooth in anything that can dry or crush the outside of the tooth.
- Do not handle the tooth roughly. Do not rinse it off or rub, scrape, or disinfect the outside of the tooth.
- Place the tooth in a soft transport device, preferably in Hank's solution (a pH-balanced, isotonic, glucose/calcium/magnesium solution). Do not use tap water. Some recommendations suggest whole milk as a second-best solution to Hank's solution. A third choice is saline, but only for less than 1 hour.

Neck Injuries

The critical structures running through the neck are relatively unprotected and, therefore, are susceptible to many types of injuries. In addition to damage to critical airway and vascular structures, the possibility of an unstable cervical spine and spinal cord injury must be considered in a trauma patient. For scene calls, use of selective spinal motion restriction criteria has become standard practice. If a patient has a cervical collar in place at the sending facility and the sending physician has not cleared the cervical spine, the cervical collar should be kept in place. The CCTP can achieve an acceptable degree of additional spinal motion restriction by properly securing the patient to the transport stretcher. Use of rigid backboards and spinal motion restriction devices for prolonged periods (ie, several hours), as is common with CCT, is fraught with potential complications.

Always consider patients with neck injuries as potentially having a "difficult airway." Deterioration of the patient's airway in the back of a transport vehicle with limited space and personnel can be disastrous; thus, airway insertion should be completed prior to transport whenever there is a high index of suspicion that an artificial airway will be needed. Special airway considerations in the presence of neck injuries include bleeding into the airway field, expanding hematomas, and tracheal disruption.

The CCTP should immediately attempt to achieve hemorrhage control in any patient with signs of a major vascular, airway, or digestive tract injury. In case of an air leak or expanding hematoma, the CCTP should also attempt to achieve definitive airway control. Following these attempts, the patient should be taken directly to the operating room for surgical exploration.

For the purposes of assessment and management, the neck is typically divided into three zones, each with unique hemorrhage control and surgical limitations **FIGURE 11-28**:

- Zone 1—the most inferior—is defined by the clavicle and sternal notch inferiorly and the horizontal plane dissecting the cricoid cartilage superiorly. Structures in zone 1 include the proximal common carotid arteries; the vertebral and subclavian arteries; the subclavian, innominate, and jugular veins; the trachea; the recurrent laryngeal and vagus nerves; the esophagus; and the thoracic duct.
- Zone 2 is defined by the cricoid cartilage inferiorly and the angle of the mandible superiorly. It includes the carotid arteries, jugular and vertebral veins, pharynx, larynx, proximal trachea, recurrent laryngeal and vagus nerves, and spinal cord.
- Zone 3 is defined by the angle of the mandible inferiorly and the base of the skull superiorly. It includes the extracranial carotid and vertebral arteries, the jugular veins, the spinal cord, cranial nerves IX through XII, and the sympathetic trunk.

Zones 1 and 3 have a higher incidence of vascular injury with penetrating trauma because vessels in these zones are fixed to other structures. There is significant incidence of esophageal injury with penetrating zone 1 injuries; because these injuries are often asymptomatic, they can be missed, often with devastating consequences. Nearly all zone 1 and zone 3 injuries and any asymptomatic zone 2 injuries can usually be evaluated with CT angiography (CTA) or other dedicated vascular imaging. If an injury in any zone requires surgical repair, the patient should be taken to the operating room without delay. Patients with symptomatic zone 2 injuries should go directly to surgery upon arrival at the hospital.

For neck trauma resulting in hoarseness accompanied by skin lacerations, ecchymosis, tenderness, subcutaneous emphysema, or stridor, an immediate otolaryngology consult is recommended. Indeed, this consultation may be the reason for the patient's transport to a larger hospital. Humidified oxygen, inhaled corticosteroids, and nebulized epinephrine may be ordered for patients with these types of neck injuries. If concern for airway compromise exists, a secure airway should be established before initiating transport.

The thyroid is located mainly in zone 1 of the neck, inferior to the cricoid cartilage, with some extension of the superior poles into zone 2. The thyroid is very vascular, and direct trauma to the front of the neck that affects this endocrine gland can cause hematomas of sufficient size to impinge on the airway. If surgical airway management is required, the entry location may need to be inferior to the usual site and inferior to the thyroid gland. Scattered reports of thyrotoxicosis, or thyroid storm, after thyroid trauma have been noted. The treatment is the same as that of thyroid storm due to other causes. See Chapter 18, *Endocrine Emergencies*, for more information.

Neck wounds may need to be dressed with occlusive dressings. If the wound affects the lower neck or clavicular area, vascular access in the lower extremity should be considered as the result of compromised drainage from the arms.

Laryngotracheal Injuries

Laryngotracheal injuries account for fewer than 1% of all traumatic injuries. Most occur in the area of the cervical trachea, and direct blunt trauma is the most common cause. Examples include contact with a steering wheel to the extended throat, hanging, strangulation, and "clothesline" injury during sports such as mountain biking or snowmobiling.

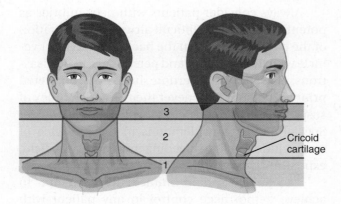

FIGURE 11-28 Neck zones.
© Jones & Bartlett Learning.

Penetrating laryngotracheal injuries represent 10% of all penetrating neck injuries.

Bubbling from a neck wound and subcutaneous air, along with dysphonia, dyspnea, stridor, visible wounds, and swelling, are all signs of laryngotracheal injury. These injuries can appear stable for a time, only to be followed by rapid and catastrophic deterioration.

The most severe cases involve laryngotracheal disruptions. It is vital that paralytics and muscle relaxants not be used in patients with such injuries, because the only support for the trachea may be the surrounding musculature. If the patient is paralyzed, the trachea may retract into the chest, making it impossible to ventilate the patient. If the trachea is visible through the neck wall, the endotracheal tube should simply be passed through the neck into the trachea.

Signs and Symptoms

Laryngotracheal Injury
- Bubbling from a neck wound
- Subcutaneous air
- Dysphonia
- Dyspnea
- Stridor
- Visible wounds
- Swelling

Transport Management

Laryngotracheal Injury
- Airway management with careful endotracheal intubation
- Occlusive dressing for open neck wounds, especially if bubbling is present
- Spinal precautions
- Transport to a trauma center

Vascular Neck Injuries

Injury to the carotid, subclavian, and vertebral arteries and external and internal jugular veins can produce rapid exsanguination, hematoma formation, or embolization of air. One-fourth of all penetrating neck trauma cases involve vascular neck injuries. Mortality may be as high as one-half of these patients. If there is concern for an expanding hematoma from an injured vessel in the neck, securing the airway as soon as possible is crucial to patient survival. If delays occur, the airway may become unsalvageable without surgical intervention.

Many of the complications of vascular neck injuries do not appear until days to weeks after the trauma and involve thromboemboli causing neurologic problems. Because of the possibility of venous air embolism, direct pressure with an occlusive dressing should be applied to open vascular neck injuries while the patient is kept in the Trendelenburg position. Keep in mind that the Trendelenburg position may lead to respiratory compromise and that ventilatory assistance may be needed.

Accidental or improper removal of a central venous line or catheter can also readily lead to significant air embolism. Should a central catheter become dislodged during transport, the CCTP should act quickly to apply pressure with an occlusive dressing. Maintain a high index of suspicion when symptoms appear in a patient who recently had a central catheter discontinued prior to transport. When removing a central catheter, the patient should be placed in a Trendelenburg position prior to discontinuing the line.

Transport Management

Vascular Neck Injury
- Secure the airway early.
- Apply direct pressure to the injury with an occlusive dressing.
- Keep the patient in the Trendelenburg position.

Abdominal Trauma

Traumatic injuries to the abdomen are some of the most difficult injuries for the CCTP to recognize. Whether providing care at a trauma scene or transferring a critical patient from the ED to a trauma center, it is important to document an accurate history and physical exam for later comparison. At the sending facility, it is usually worthwhile to interview the crew who brought the patient from the field.

Knowing the extrication time, scene details, and trends in patient condition is important in caring for trauma patients. With interfacility critical care transport calls, always try to review all studies that have been done, including lab tests, radiography, ultrasonography (FAST exam), and CT imaging, as well as any procedures that have been performed.

Considerations in Blunt Versus Penetrating Abdominal Trauma

As with other injuries, abdominal trauma can be classified into two categories: blunt and penetrating.

Blunt abdominal trauma occurs when an external force is placed on the abdominal cavity, such as during a fall, MVC, or motorcycle crash. One of the most commonly missed culprits in blunt abdominal trauma is the seat belt, which can act as a force vector of injury. Approximately 40% of lumbar spine fractures in MVCs are associated with intra-abdominal injury, as the seat belt causes the spine to flex/extend and compresses intra-abdominal contents. Use of seat belts has significantly decreased the incidence of morbidity and mortality related to MVCs, but these restraining devices continue to cause less noticeable abdominal injuries.

Penetrating abdominal trauma can involve many different objects, such as knives, guns, tree limbs, or metal rods. Such injuries will be very difficult for the CCTP to assess because detailed information on the object involved is often not available (eg, the size of the knife, the length of the blade, and whether it had a jagged or straight edge). In many instances, even if this information is available, it will still be very difficult to rapidly identify which structures inside the abdominal cavity were injured without the assistance of diagnostic imaging studies. Penetrating injuries usually require operative exploration to assess the extent of injury, and transport should not be delayed to perform additional imaging.

Challenges in Diagnosing Abdominal Trauma

The abdominal cavity is an extremely large space that houses many different vital organs. In many instances, the patient may experience either blunt or penetrating trauma to the abdominal cavity, yet signs or symptoms of injury may remain very subtle until shock becomes obvious. Because of the size of the abdominal cavity, a significant amount of blood can collect within this area and go unnoticed. Unlike other vital organs in the body, those in the abdominal cavity have very little protection, which makes them that much more susceptible to injury.

The following organs, structures, and vessels are located within the abdomen, and, if injured, can cause potential harm to the patient:

- Spleen
- Liver
- Kidneys
- Aorta
- Urinary bladder
- Gallbladder
- Small and large intestines
- Pancreas
- Stomach

Blunt or penetrating trauma to many of these organs can cause a life-threatening hemorrhage and serious organ damage. It is important for the CCTP to focus attention on the mechanism of injury, instead of becoming unduly distracted by the outward signs of trauma found on assessment. Injuries to any of the previously listed organs may not readily present with outward signs and symptoms—a fact that makes it that much more important for the CCTP to perform a detailed assessment and a thorough ongoing assessment during the transport, looking for subtle changes that might indicate a progressing condition. If a significant abdominal injury is suspected or confirmed, the most important treatment that the CCTP can provide is rapid transport to the trauma center for definitive care.

Once the CCTP recognizes the need for immediate transport to the trauma center, their job is to stabilize and maintain the patient's hemodynamic status as efficiently as possible until arrival at the trauma center. This task will be difficult and may require the administration of a crystalloid solution, blood products, or even vasoactive medications in more severe cases. Grey Turner sign **FIGURE 11-29** and Cullen sign **FIGURE 11-30** are indications of internal abdominal bleeding.

Assessment

When beginning the physical assessment of the patient with abdominal trauma, the CCTP should try to ascertain as many details about the events leading up to the injury as possible. Gathering more

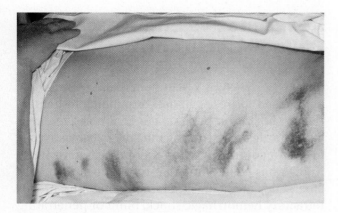

FIGURE 11-29 Grey Turner sign.

"Images of Memorable Cases - 50 years at the bedside" by Herbert L. Fred, MD and Hendrik A. van Dijk.

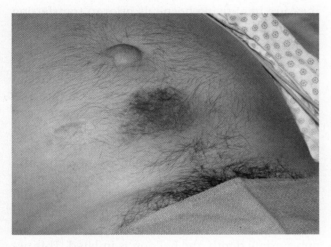

FIGURE 11-30 Cullen sign.

"Images of Memorable Cases - 50 years at the bedside" by Herbert L. Fred, MD and Hendrik A. van Dijk.

information will make diagnosing and treating the problem that much quicker and oftentimes simpler. The initial physical exam to rapidly identify blood loss is the most important task. When performing this exam, remember to always inspect, auscultate, and palpate—in that order. The primary assessment needs to be completed at the bedside, before beginning transport, as it will be very difficult to obtain an accurate assessment in the back of a moving helicopter or ambulance. This assessment must be repeated frequently during the transport, with the CCTP being ready to provide immediate interventions if necessary. In particular, the CCTP will need to monitor the patient's level of consciousness, heart rate, and blood pressure, watching for changes that would indicate a progressively worsening condition. Additionally, changes in the abdominal exam

should be documented. Special note should be made if the abdomen becomes tense or if pain increases with palpation or becomes worse when palpation is removed from the abdomen.

Patients who experience massive amounts of blood loss may compensate initially but will eventually begin to present with signs of shock. Signs and symptoms for which the CCTP should be wary include the following:

- Altered mental status
- Tachycardia
- Absence of palpable pulses
- Skin that is paler than baseline, moist, and mottled
- Poor peripheral perfusion
- Hypotension

Although the assessment should not be limited to these symptoms, they are some of the most common warning signals of hypovolemic shock.

Management

Regardless of the findings obtained during the initial assessment, all patients suspected of having abdominal injuries should be transported with appropriate supplemental oxygen and fluid administration. A minimum of two IV lines (as with most CCT patients) should be established, and central lines may need to be considered. Placing CVP and arterial pressure lines is a very good idea because noninvasive blood pressure monitoring performed in transit can yield inaccurate results, especially in patients with hypotension. However, permissive hypotension should also be considered, especially if an aneurysm of a great vessel is suspected. The patient's blood pressure should be maintained at 80 to 90 mm Hg systolic or 60 to 65 mm Hg MAP.

Boluses of crystalloids should be given in 250-mL to 500-mL amounts titrated to blood pressure, MAP, or CVP until blood is available. Patients with more severe abdominal injuries may need aggressive airway management and blood administration; most transport programs carry packed red blood cells (O negative) for such emergency situations. Some EMS units carry whole blood, which is preferred to packed red blood cells. To prevent hemodilution, protocols should allow the administration of human blood if a large volume of fluids is deemed necessary. Research into many new fluids with oxygen-carrying capacity continues, and many of these products are expected to eventually reach the market.

Except in cases of suspected urethral injury, all patients with serious abdominal trauma should, in addition to the vascular access, have an indwelling urinary catheter placed prior to transport. Completing this step prior to transport will help the CCTP evaluate shock by quantifying the amount of urine output. In addition, the presence of frank blood in the urinary catheter indicates renal system damage. Patients should be kept warm, and open abdominal wounds should be covered first with a sterile dressing and then with an occlusive dressing to prevent evaporative cooling.

Signs and Symptoms

Abdominal Injury

- Altered mental status
- Tachycardia
- Absence of palpable pulses
- Tense or rigid abdomen
- Skin that is paler than baseline, moist, and mottled
- Poor peripheral perfusion
- Hypotension

Transport Management

Abdominal Injury

- Administer appropriate oxygen therapy, fluids, or blood.
- Establish large-bore vascular access; consider placement of a central line.
- Keep the patient's blood pressure at 80 to 90 mm Hg systolic or 60 to 65 mm Hg MAP.
- Administer boluses of crystalloids in 250- to 500-mL amounts titrated to blood pressure, MAP, or CVP.
- If necessary, secure the airway.
- If necessary, administer blood products.
- Except in cases of suspected urethral injury, insert an indwelling catheter prior to transport.
- Keep the patient warm (prevent hypothermia/hyperthermia).
- Cover open abdominal wounds first with a sterile dressing and then with an occlusive dressing to prevent evaporative cooling.

Resuscitative Endovascular Balloon Occlusion of the Aorta

Resuscitative endovascular balloon occlusion of the aorta (REBOA) is a treatment that is increasingly being used for resuscitation of patients in hemorrhagic shock who have sustained a massive blood loss. First described during the Korean War as a technique for controlling intra-abdominal hemorrhage, REBOA has gained traction in trauma surgery and emergency medicine as a temporizing measure for refractory hemorrhagic shock, blunt or penetrating abdominal trauma, pelvic fractures with significant hemorrhage, and ruptured abdominal aortic aneurysms. It may also be applied as a temporizing measure in outlying hospitals prior to transferring a trauma patient to a higher-level trauma center. Importantly, REBOA has not yet been proved safe for aeromedical transfer, and ongoing research is examining the effects of altitude on the occlusion balloon. Consultation with both the sending and the receiving facilities is paramount for ensuring patient safety in the event of interfacility transfer with a REBOA in place.

The REBOA procedure involves insertion of a small balloon catheter through a femoral artery into the proximal aorta **FIGURE 11-31**. The insertion depth depends on the goal of treatment and the anatomic location of bleeding. Once inserted to the appropriate depth, the balloon is inflated. This occludes the aorta, preventing additional bleeding below the level of the balloon and increasing cardiac afterload above the level of the balloon.

As part of the REBOA approach, the aorta is divided into three zones **FIGURE 11-32**:

- Zone 1 spans from the origin of the left subclavian artery to the celiac trunk.
- Zone 2 extends from the celiac trunk to the lowest renal artery.
- Zone 3 extends from the lowest renal artery to the bifurcation of the femoral arteries.

Indications for zone 1 placement include temporary control of severe intra-abdominal hemorrhage, severe retroperitoneal hemorrhage, and traumatic arrest with suspected infradiaphragmatic injury as the source of hemorrhage. Indications for zone 3 placement include patients with severe pelvic, junctional (groin/perineum), or proximal lower extremity hemorrhage that cannot be controlled by other methods. Zone 2, the smallest area of the

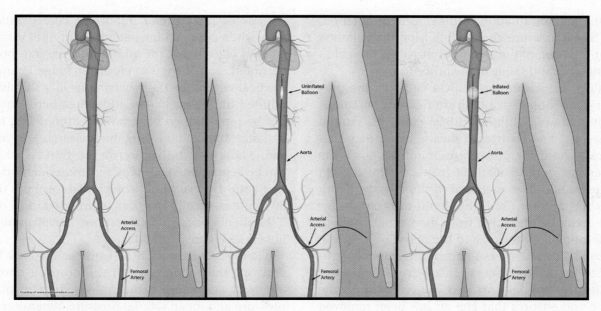

FIGURE 11-31 Resuscitative endovascular balloon occlusion of the aorta (REBOA). **A.** Central arterial tree. **B.** REBOA catheter placed in zone 1. **C.** REBOA catheter with balloon inflated.

Courtesy of Prytime Medical Devices, Inc. www.prytimemedical.com.

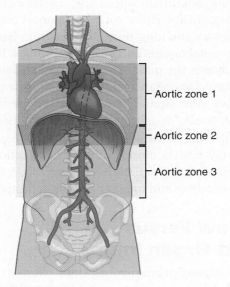

FIGURE 11-32 Aortic zones.

Data from Stannard A, Eliason JL, Rasmussen TE. Resuscitative endovascular balloon occlusion of the aorta (REBOA) as an adjunct for hemorrhagic shock. *J Trauma.* 2011;71(6):1871. doi:10.1097/ta.0b013e31823fe90c.

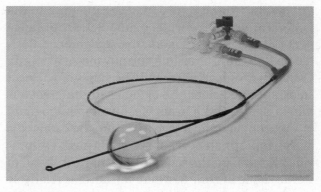

FIGURE 11-33 A catheter designed for resuscitative endovascular balloon occlusion of the aorta.

Courtesy of Prytime Medical Devices, Inc. www.prytimemedical.com.

aorta, is typically used intraoperatively only in selected vascular or aortic procedures.

While placement of a REBOA catheter is not currently within the CCTP's scope of practice, familiarity with the placement procedure is important in understanding the function and maintenance of the device. These catheters should be placed in a sterile environment. As shown in **FIGURE 11-33**, the REBOA catheter has a flexible, transducing tip for pressure monitoring, a balloon with radio-opaque markers at either side, and markings to measure the insertion depth over the length of the tubing. The REBOA catheter also features two sets of bold markings that indicate the average insertion depth for zone 1 (45 to 49 cm) and zone 3 (26 to 29 cm). There are two ports: one for the balloon (clear; marked BAL) and one for arterial access (red; marked ART). Finally, at the most proximal end of each catheter is a paper tab that has spaces to record the insertion depth, balloon inflation volume, time of inflation, and blood pressure change following the balloon's inflation. Each of these measurements is critical to the stability and safety of the procedure.

Prior to placing the REBOA catheter, the provider must obtain femoral arterial access. Unlike traditional arterial lines, REBOA catheters require at least a 7-French arterial sheath, larger than that typically used for pressure monitoring. Once the 7-French arterial sheath is in place, the REBOA catheter should be prepared. If the average depth markings are not used, the depth of insertion for zone 1 can be measured from the sternal notch to the femoral access site, and the depth of insertion for zone 3 can be measured from the xiphoid process to the femoral access site. Next, the provider flushes the arterial port and catheter with sterile saline and ensures that any air has been removed from the balloon by gently inflating it with about 2 to 3 mL of sterile saline and then withdrawing the fluid immediately. The orange peel-away sheath is used to extend the flexible distal tip of the REBOA catheter just before inserting it through the 7-French arterial line. To place the REBOA catheter into the femoral artery, the provider manipulates the orange peel-away catheter to guide the straightened flexible tip into the arterial line and advance it to 15 cm. Catheter advancement should be smooth. The next steps are to advance the catheter to the predetermined depth, and if available, obtain a radiograph or ultrasonographic image to ensure the catheter is at the appropriate level. Once confirmed, the provider can inflate the balloon starting with 2 mL of sterile saline in zone 3, where the aorta is relatively smaller, or 8 mL of sterile saline in zone 1, where the aorta is wider.

After initial inflation of the balloon, an arterial blood pressure tracing should be obtained. Additional sterile saline should be slowly infused into the balloon until a sudden increase in the blood pressure tracing is observed. This sudden increase indicates occlusion of the aorta. Distal pulses should not be palpable in the lower extremities. The provider can then secure the femoral arterial catheter and REBOA catheter in place with sutures and dressings. Finally, imaging should be performed to confirm correct placement and balloon inflation. The insertion depth, time of balloon inflation, amount of saline in the balloon, and blood pressure change should be recorded.

For CCTPs, several important considerations arise when approaching patients with REBOA catheters in place. First, the arterial line tracing should be noted, and if the waveform or range changes, medical control or the receiving facility should be notified immediately. The REBOA catheter should not be repositioned or removed without first fully deflating the balloon. Ongoing research is investigating how long the balloon on the REBOA catheter can be kept inflated. General recommendations are that zone 1 should not be occluded for more than 60 minutes, ideally less than 30 minutes, and zone 3 should not be occluded for more than 90 minutes, ideally less than 60 minutes.

Removal of the REBOA catheter involves first deflating the balloon, which will drop the cardiac afterload and cause a precipitous drop in blood pressure and mean arterial pressure. Whenever the REBOA catheter is manipulated, providers should be prepared to treat a sudden decrease in the patient's blood pressure, and the balloon should be deflated slowly.

While potentially lifesaving, aortic occlusion poses significant risks, such as femoral artery or aortic injury and long-term damage from ischemia to abdominal organs and lower extremities. REBOA use indicates the patient is in imminent danger of cardiovascular collapse and death, so transport to definitive care should not be delayed under any circumstances. As more experience is gained with use of REBOA, its indications and practice will undoubtedly evolve, along with the implications for transport by CCTPs. Clearly, use of REBOA creates a time-sensitive and urgent need for definitive care.

Hollow Versus Solid-Organ Injury

Hollow organs primarily leak their contents when injured, whereas solid organs bleed. Treatment of injury to either type of organ should be oriented toward treating shock and expeditious transport.

Solid organs include the liver (in the upper right quadrant), the spleen (in the upper left quadrant), and the pancreas and kidneys (in the retroperitoneal space). Solid-organ injuries are increasingly being managed nonoperatively with observation or in an interventional radiology suite, where imaging can be used to identify the injured vessel(s) and catheter-deployed treatments provided. Management with interventional radiology is a common option. The primary concern with any solid-organ injury is hemorrhage resulting in hypovolemic shock.

The hollow organs consist of the digestive tract including the stomach (in the upper left quadrant), the small and large intestines (throughout all quadrants), and the gallbladder (under the liver in the upper right quadrant). Additionally, hollow organs in the midline include the urinary bladder and ureters, the uterus, and the great vessels of the descending (abdominal) aorta and the inferior vena cava. The primary concern with hollow-organ injury is peritonitis resulting in distributive shock.

Spleen

The spleen is a bean-shaped organ in the left upper quadrant that serves as a site for maturation of white blood cells and filtration of senescent (old) red blood cells. This organ gets a direct vascular supply from the aorta, and its drainage goes directly to the inferior vena cava. Approximately 5% of circulating blood filters through the spleen every minute. Given this volume, injury to the spleen can produce massive hemorrhage very quickly.

The spleen is the most commonly injured organ in the abdominal cavity. It can even be injured by what seems to be minor trauma. Young adults and patients with sickle cell disease or mononucleosis are at particular risk of such injuries, as a result of their spleens being relatively larger.

Located in the upper left quadrant of the abdomen, the spleen is partially protected by the lower rib cage, but lacks a strong exterior capsule. Injuries that do not disrupt the structure of this organ will likely produce only minimal bleeding. In contrast, more significant bleeding may occur if the exterior capsule is damaged.

The presence of normal vital signs does not rule out an injury to the spleen. The patient may simply complain of pain on the primary assessment, with symptoms of shock developing later. In some cases, symptoms may arise as late as 2 to 3 weeks after the original injury. This understanding is especially important in patients who have a history of splenic trauma but present with sudden decompensation. Delayed splenic rupture can occur when splenic injury is managed nonoperatively but the splenic capsule weakens and eventually ruptures.

A helpful tool for recognizing a splenic injury through referred pain is the **Kehr sign**. This sign presents as pain in the shoulder as a result of the presence of blood or other irritants along the diaphragm and superior peritoneum. Pain in the left shoulder is considered a classic symptom of a ruptured spleen, but may also result from any free blood irritating the diaphragm. The same phenomenon also occurs on the right side with irritation to the liver or gallbladder.

Failure to recognize, understand, and treat the signs and symptoms of hypovolemic shock related to internal hemorrhage will rapidly lead to the patient's death. Nevertheless, many spleen injuries can be managed through bed rest and careful observation, because this organ sometimes heals over time and invasive interventions are not always needed. Embolization of the spleen is another increasingly common nonoperative management technique and may be employed in circumstances where surgery needs to be avoided but the patient has signs and symptoms of ongoing hypovolemia.

Signs and Symptoms

Spleen Injury
- Pain in the area of the spleen
- Kehr sign: pain in the shoulder despite no evident injury to the shoulder

Transport Management

Spleen Injury
- Provide oxygen and monitor ABCs as indicated.
- Treat the patient for signs and symptoms of hypovolemic shock.

Liver

The largest organ in the abdominal cavity, the liver is also the most vascular organ and receives 25% of the total cardiac output. The liver has a little more protection than the spleen does, because it is surrounded by many different structures of the thorax, including ligaments that stabilize the organ to the diaphragm and abdominal wall, reducing the risk of impact. However, the ligament in front of the liver (ligamentum teres) can injure the liver in the case of a sudden deceleration. Additionally, the liver's close proximity to the lower rib cage makes it susceptible to injury after a rib fracture occurs. Liver injuries will cause pain in the right upper quadrant, along with pain in the right shoulder as blood accumulates around the diaphragm.

In the past, the majority of liver injuries were surgically repaired. Studies have since shown that many less severe liver injuries can tolerate 1 or 2 days of observation before making a decision to surgically repair them. In most instances, simple observation is the only intervention needed, because the liver heals over time and invasive interventions are not always necessary. Angioembolization, an interventional radiology technique, is also growing in popularity as a hemorrhage control method, as long as the bleed is confined to one side of the liver. However, in severe liver injuries, surgery may be the only means to prevent exsanguination.

Stomach

Damage to the stomach from trauma is rare. Blunt trauma to this organ most commonly occurs during MVCs when a full stomach is caught against the steering wheel. The stomach can also be damaged in penetrating injuries. In trauma patients who are intubated, placing a nasogastric or orogastric tube can help decompress the stomach.

Large and Small Intestines

The intestines are hollow organs that occupy much of the space within the abdominal cavity. Penetrating trauma is the most common cause of injury to the intestines because they lie very close to the surface of the abdomen. When objects such as knives or bullets penetrate the abdominal wall, injury to the intestines is likely.

Although penetrating trauma is the most common source of injury to these organs, blunt trauma to the abdominal wall—especially from a seat belt—can also damage the small bowel. The lap portion of the seat belt lies along the lower quadrants of the abdominal cavity. The patient with such an injury would likely present with an ecchymotic area across the lower portion of the abdomen (seat belt sign), which should prompt an assessment for internal injuries **FIGURE 11-34**.

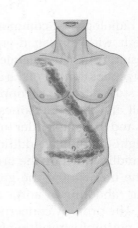

FIGURE 11-34 Seat belt sign.
© Jones & Bartlett Learning.

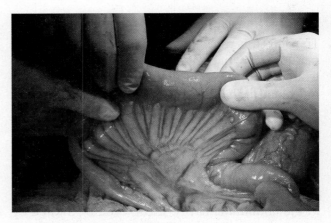

FIGURE 11-35 Bowel mesentery.
© Kaushik_Ghosh/iStock/Getty Images Plus/Getty Images.

Injuries to the wall of the small or large intestine can cause digestive material to leak out of the lumen, leading to both peritonitis and pain. The bowel mesentery is the fatty sheet containing the blood vessels that supply the bowel wall **FIGURE 11-35**. It is often a source of hemorrhage in blunt and penetrating trauma patients; injury to the mesentery usually requires surgical repair. Approximately 80% of gunshot wounds to the abdomen and 30% of stab wounds penetrate the small or large bowel. Because the jejunum and ileum are anchored to the abdominal wall via the ligament of Trietz, the mesentery and its vasculature often are torn with such injuries, causing hemorrhage.

A lack of visible injury should not be used as a rationale for ruling out internal injury. Instead, CCTPs must rely on their assessment skills to detect abnormalities. In some cases, the presence of pain with palpation to the abdomen might be the only indicator of injury. In addition to the pain with palpation, other indicators, such as guarding, abdominal distention, rebound tenderness, and vomiting, may be present.

The large intestine or colon is the organ most frequently injured by penetrating trauma. Such an injury was found in 96% of penetrating trauma cases in one study, with gunshots accounting for more than 90% of the injuries. Ruptures of the colon or rectum are particularly susceptible to sepsis and peritonitis.

Signs and Symptoms

Intestinal Injury

- Ecchymotic area across the lower portion of the abdomen (seat belt sign)
- Presence of pain with palpation to the abdomen
- Guarding
- Abdominal distention
- Rebound tenderness
- Vomiting

Transport Management

Intestinal Injury

- Maintain a high index of suspicion for occult injury.
- Establish large-bore IV access.
- Consider other injuries, such as chest, neck, and lumbar spine injuries.
- Provide rapid transport.

Duodenum

The duodenum deserves special note because it is a retroperitoneal organ and, therefore, is well protected. If ruptured, because of its retroperitoneal location, it may not produce symptoms. Nevertheless, because of its close proximity to the stomach, liver, pancreas, gallbladder, bile ducts, aorta, and inferior vena cava, the duodenum is never the only organ injured. An injury to the duodenum should be suspected with high-velocity blunt trauma to the midabdomen, such as when a child is thrown off a bicycle and the abdomen strikes the handlebars.

Vascular Injuries

Unfortunately, injuries that occur to the vessels of the abdomen are usually life threatening. The abdominal aorta is a large vessel that carries blood away from the heart, supplies all the abdominal organs, and continues its distribution of blood and oxygen to the toes. Severe blunt trauma may disrupt these vessels, although the most common cause of vascular injury is, once again, penetrating trauma. In instances of blunt trauma, the shearing force at impact causes the vessels to break away from their branches, allowing blood to flow freely into the abdominal cavity. The following major blood vessels in the abdomen can be injured in trauma events:

- Aorta
- Inferior vena cava
- Left or right renal artery
- Superior or inferior mesenteric artery
- Left or right iliac artery

Bleeding from an injury to any of the major abdominal vessels may occur rapidly, and signs of shock may not be noticed as blood accumulates in the abdomen. Aggressive treatment of patients with such injuries is required but may not prove very helpful, because arterial injuries will cause exsanguination unless immediate surgery is available. Therefore, rapid transport to a hospital capable of immediate surgery may be the best possible treatment. The abdominal cavity is also home to several large veins whose rupture will cause the body to lose large amounts of blood, albeit not at the rapid pace of an arterial rupture. Bleeding into the abdominal cavity may slowly occur without obvious signs or symptoms.

The treatment of vascular injuries is similar to the treatment of the other abdominal injuries. Airway patency is the key concern, because patients who are experiencing massive blood loss are likely to demonstrate an altered mental status. Immediate steps should be taken to perform endotracheal intubation to secure the patient's airway if necessary. The CCTP should focus on treating the hypovolemic shock and transporting the patient to a center capable of trauma surgery. REBOA may be indicated depending on the level of injury, availability of femoral arterial access, and provider training. In the initial treatment of such a patient, aggressive fluid resuscitation is necessary to maintain a systolic blood pressure of at least 80 mm Hg but not higher than

90 mm Hg, with progression toward blood products as soon as possible.

If the patient survives the transport, the surgical team needs to intervene as soon as possible and attempt to surgically repair the disturbed vessel. Even if the patient survives to surgery, several serious complications can occur afterward—for example, disseminated intravascular coagulation (DIC), continued bleeding, and thrombosis formation. All are life threatening, and will be treated as such by the team caring for the patient.

Signs and Symptoms

Abdominal Vascular Injury
- Potentially none
- Altered mental status
- Hypovolemic shock

Transport Management

Abdominal Vascular Injury
- Maintain airway patency; ensure adequate ventilation.
- Administer judicious fluid resuscitation; ensure adequate tissue perfusion.
- Transport the patient immediately to a center capable of trauma or vascular surgery.

Pelvic Trauma
Pelvic Fracture

Pelvic fractures typically result from trauma due to MVCs (approximately 60% to 70% of all cases), pedestrian–versus–motor vehicle incidents (12% to 18%), motorcycle crashes (5% to 10%), and falls (up to 10%). Because of the significant force involved, the presence of a pelvic fracture should alert the CCTP to the potential for other injuries in the abdomen and pelvis. In one study, mortality from blunt pelvic fractures was as high as 50%. Most of the threat to life from these injuries comes from internal hemorrhage from the associated vasculature within the pelvis.

The pelvis is made of three paired bones—the ilium, the ischium, and the pubis—that are collectively called the innominate bones. The innominate bones are connected posteriorly by the sacrum and coccyx. Their very rich blood supply comes from the left and right iliac arteries. The veins in the pelvis lack valves and adhere to the pelvic wall. Because these blood vessels have thin walls, they are easily torn, and fractures to the pelvis can result in catastrophic hemorrhage.

The pelvis also houses the reproductive organs and the urinary bladder. When full, the bladder can rise above the pelvic rim and rupture as part of a seat belt injury. The uterus, ovaries, and fallopian tubes are well protected in the nonpregnant patient. Injuries to these organs are usually found after the patient is transported to the trauma center, when the patient is assessed using CT.

Subjective assessment of potential pelvic fracture includes a good history of the mechanism of injury, location, and radiation of pain, as well as an assessment of the presence of hematuria and the possibility of pregnancy. Objective examination includes observing for the rotation or uneven height of the iliac crests and uneven length of the legs. Palpation of the posterior aspect of the pelvic ring should not elicit tenderness. Gentle lateral compression posteriorly and inward compression medially at the iliac crests should not result in pain, crepitus, or movement. This test should be done one time, carefully, and stopped and not repeated if any instability is felt.

Management of pelvic injury depends on the type of fracture. Field treatment consists of splinting and treatment for shock. Soft-tissue damage to the genitalia can be managed like any other soft-tissue injury. Packaging for transport of suspected or confirmed pelvic fracture entails immobilization of the pelvis with a pelvic binder **FIGURE 11-36**. The patient should be moved on a scoop stretcher or backboard to minimize pelvic movement.

Open-Book Fractures

Open-book fractures, a subset of pelvic fractures, account for approximately 15% of pelvic fractures and involve the loss of stability of the pelvic ring. They result from anterior-posterior compression forces that separate the pelvis at the symphysis pubis. The greatest danger with this injury is from hemorrhage. Reduction of these fractures decreases the bleeding.

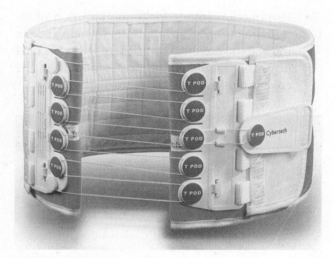

FIGURE 11-36 A pelvic binder.

Courtesy of Pyng Medical Corp.

Assessment and treatment of an open-book fracture are the same as for any pelvic fracture, and patients should be transported on a well-padded backboard or scoop. Pelvic binders or even pneumatic antishock garments have also been used successfully to manage these injuries during transport.

Signs and Symptoms

Pelvic or Open-Book Fracture

- Rotation or uneven height of the iliac crests
- Uneven length of the legs
- Tenderness upon palpation of the posterior aspect of the pelvic ring
- Pain, crepitus, or movement upon gentle lateral compression posteriorly and inward medial compression

Transport Management

Pelvic or Open-Book Fracture

- Splint the fracture by restricting movement and stabilizing the pelvis.
- Treat the patient for signs and symptoms of shock.
- Manage any soft-tissue damage to the genitalia.
- Package the patient for transport using motion restriction measures on a scoop stretcher or similar transfer device; alternatively, use a pelvic binder.

Extremity Trauma
Musculoskeletal Injuries

Musculoskeletal injuries are rarely life threatening. They include fractures, sprains, strains, dislocations, muscular contusions, and compartment and crush syndromes. Often dramatic, they may suggest the amount of energy transferred to the body and the likelihood of additional injury. However, the CCTP must not let the dramatic picture presented by these fractures distract from a proper primary and secondary assessment.

Initial motion restriction on the scene can be accomplished by using a backboard as a whole-body splint to decrease on-scene time for patients who have experienced multiple trauma. During interfacility transports, there is usually time to make sure individual fractures are properly splinted. In both cases, adequate pain control should be used. All musculoskeletal injuries should be assessed for the six Ps—pain, pallor, pulselessness, paresthesia, paralysis, and pressure—before and after any manipulation. These findings should be documented on the patient's chart, and pulse locations should be marked with a felt-tip or skin marker on the patient to speed rechecking during transport.

Fractures

A **fracture** is a break in the continuity of a bone. It may be either open or closed. With any fracture, the CCTP's priorities are prevention of further injury due to movement and pain assessment and management. The CCTP should use appropriate analgesic medications as permitted by the system's protocols to reduce the patient's pain and upset.

In a closed fracture, the skin over the bone remains intact, reducing the risk of infection. However, closed fractures can be as dangerous as open fractures due to bleeding into the surrounding tissues. Depending on the anatomic area where a closed fracture occurs, a large amount of blood could be lost before enough pressure is achieved internally to tamponade the bleeding. For example, a closed fracture of one femur could easily result in the loss of 1 L of blood, whereas bilateral femur fractures could result in the loss of 2 L of blood **TABLE 11-6**. Multiple fractures of trauma patients can cause massive internal hemorrhage and even death, despite no external bleeding being noted.

TABLE 11-6 Estimated Blood Loss by Fracture Type

Estimated Potential Blood Loss (mL)	Fracture Type
125 each	Rib
250–500	Radius or ulna
500–750	Humerus
500–1,000	Tibia or fibula
1,000–2,000	Femur
1,000 to massive	Pelvis

© Jones & Bartlett Learning.

In an open fracture, the skin over the bone is broken, introducing the additional risk of infection, which could lead to sepsis and increases the risk of mortality. Open fractures typically result from high-energy injuries, so they have the potential for more blood loss and concomitant injuries than closed fractures do.

Clinical signs and symptoms of fractures include pain, swelling, deformity, rigidity, limb shortening, ecchymosis, guarding, and crepitus. The patient could have either one of these signs and symptoms or a combination of them.

Management of isolated fractures is as follows:

- Maintain an open airway and apply appropriate oxygen therapy.
- Assess pulses and motor and sensory function distal to the fracture site.
- Control bleeding with direct pressure and pressure dressings; if that is not effective, use a tourniquet. Apply a sterile dressing to any exposed bone or tissue.
- Initiate IV fluids to maintain peripheral perfusion.
- Consider administering analgesic medication titrated to the patient's pain level prior to manipulating the fracture if the patient is hemodynamically stable.
- Splint the fracture site in a normal anatomic position with an appropriate splint while maintaining circulation.
- Reassess pulses and motor and sensory function distal to the fracture site after application or manipulation of a splint.
- Monitor oxygen saturation, vital signs, and the cardiac monitor.

- Use traction splints for immobilization of femur fractures, if appropriate, to help reduce muscle spasms and control hemorrhage. Local protocols should guide the assessment of the risks versus the benefits of traction splinting.

Signs and Symptoms

Extremity Fractures

- Pain
- Swelling
- Deformity
- Rigidity
- Shortening
- Ecchymosis
- Guarding
- Crepitus

Differential Diagnosis

Extremity Fractures

- Fracture
- Sprain
- Contusion
- Compartment syndrome

Transport Management

Extremity Fractures

- Maintain an open airway; apply appropriate oxygen therapy.
- Assess pulses and motor and sensory function distal to the fracture site.
- Control bleeding with direct pressure and pressure dressings; if that is not effective, apply a tourniquet.
- Apply a sterile dressing to any exposed bone or tissue.
- Initiate IV fluids.
- Consider administering analgesic medication.
- Splint the extremity in its normal anatomic position with an appropriate splint while maintaining circulation.
- Reassess pulses and motor and sensory function distal to the fracture site after application or manipulation of the splint.
- Monitor oxygen saturation, vital signs, and the cardiac monitor.

Femur Fracture

The femur is the largest bone in the body and is surrounded by some of the body's most powerful muscles. When the femur is broken, the muscles contract, causing sharp bone ends to override each other, damaging soft tissue and increasing the rate of blood loss. More importantly, the slack muscle can provide a large space for the collection of blood. Generally, femur fractures lead to a loss of at least 1 L of blood from circulation.

The traction splint was theorized to pull the slack muscles taut again, tamponading the bleeding. When first invented during the Crimean War in the 1850s, this intervention reduced mortality from femur fractures secondary to gunshot wounds from 80% to 20%. Nevertheless, a number of contraindications and dangers arise with use of traction splints. The contraindications include hip and pelvic fractures, knee injury, and ankle damage. The dangers include damage or worsening damage to the neurovascular bundle of the thigh; this includes the sciatic and femoral nerves and the vasculature of the area. Local protocols should include a risk-versus-benefit assessment when traction splinting is being considered.

Spinal Injury

Patients being transported from one facility to another who have not definitively had their spines cleared should be transported with motion restriction in place. The CCTP should apply an appropriately fitted cervical collar and firmly secure the patient to the transport stretcher. It is not necessary to place patients with motion restriction in a recumbent position, but care should be taken to keep the spine in line and minimize flexion or extension. Advance planning for airway management and prevention of aspiration, especially in small aircraft, must be undertaken prior to transport.

Thoracic Fracture

Thoracic fractures can lead to a loss of innervation of the intercostal muscles, which then contributes to respiratory insufficiency. Sympathetic nervous control arises from the thoracic and high lumbar spinal cord. Although it is rare, a condition called spinal shock can affect the thoracic area or higher. In this type of shock, hypotension is accompanied by bradycardia, instead of tachycardia. Pulse pressure will be normal or widened, instead of narrowed as in hypovolemia. The area above the fracture will be pale and cool, but the area below it will be warm. Treatment should consist of fluids and vasopressors to maintain the patient's MAP in the range of 80 to 90 mm Hg.

Lumbar Spine Fracture

The lumbar vertebrae are the largest vertebrae. Because they are not supported—as the thoracic vertebrae are—by the ribs, they are susceptible to injury. Jackknifing, such as over a seat belt, is frequently the mechanism of injury in lumbar spine fracture and is associated with intra-abdominal injury in as many as 40% of these fractures. Motion restriction for transport is the appropriate treatment.

Rib Fracture

Single rib fractures are rarely life threatening. They may cause pneumothorax, and torn intercostal arteries can lead to significant blood loss or hemothorax. Multiple rib fractures will negatively impact respiratory excursion, even without a flail segment.

The goal of treatment for rib fractures is analgesia to improve inspiration. The CCTP should provide sufficient pain medication so that the patient is less inclined to self-splint, which can interfere with respiration. In rare cases, multiple rib fractures may require ventilatory assistance; however, adequate analgesia should be achieved prior to airway intervention.

Extremity Fracture

Casting

With fractures of the extremities in trauma patients, casts made of fiberglass or plaster are applied by an orthopaedic surgeon after acute swelling has gone down. Casting usually takes place at least 24 hours after the injury occurs. Swelling under a cast can cause compartment syndrome.

Any patient with a cast who is transported by a CCTP should be evaluated for neurovascular function distal to the cast prior to transport and periodically during transport. It is recommended that the location where pulses are found be marked on the skin and documented in the patient care record.

Reduction/Realignment

Typically, reduction and realignment of a fractured extremity is not a priority of care in the critical patient—instead, resuscitation of cardiovascular status must always take priority. Usually, reductions are done by an orthopaedic surgeon as part of the resuscitation team or soon thereafter. Realignment becomes a priority if the neurovascular function distal to the injury is compromised. This is accomplished by applying gentle traction in the anatomic direction of the bone distal to the fracture while stabilizing the bone proximal to the break. The bone is then brought into alignment or to a position in which the maximal pulse is felt, and is splinted in that direction.

External Fixation

External fixation of fractures has become more common, especially in critically ill patients. Placed by an orthopaedic surgeon, external fixation uses external rods held to the bone with plates and screws. The apparatus is placed surgically. The external joints are then adjusted over time as needed by the orthopaedist. Occasionally, CCTPs will transport patients with this device in place. Adequate padding and comfortable positioning are required for such transports.

Internal Fixation

Internal fixation is the placement of rods with plates and screws in the operating room to hold fractures in place for healing. The rods may be removed later, or they may be left in place permanently. Occasionally, the rods work themselves out of position and may need surgical revision. Generally, this equipment is not of concern during transport.

Compartment Syndrome

In compartment syndrome, bleeding or swelling occurs within the nonstretchable fascia that surrounds different muscle groups and divides each extremity into compartments. Because the compartments can accommodate only a small amount of bleeding or swelling, this condition increases the pressure within the compartment, which eventually compresses arteries and veins, prevents adequate perfusion of the muscle, and causes pain. Although the anatomic locations where compartment syndrome most commonly occurs are the lower legs and the forearms, this condition can develop in any extremity and the buttocks. In one study, 69% of compartment syndrome cases were associated with fracture (one-half of the fractures were to the tibia), but burns, external compression from splints or bandages, and crushing injury were also noted to lead to this complication. In the same study, 31% of patients with compartment syndrome had soft-tissue injuries without a fracture. Compartment syndrome usually develops over a period of hours, so frequent assessments are imperative.

Clinical signs and symptoms of this condition initially present as pain out of proportion to the evident injury, sometimes described as burning and paresthesia over the compartment site. Additional signs include tension of a muscle when not in use, loss of distal sensation or pulses, and extreme pain on extension or voluntary movement. The presence of pulses or Doppler blood flow does not rule out compartment syndrome, as pulselessness is typically the last symptom to appear. The signs are commonly referred to as the six Ps—pain, pallor, pulselessness, paresthesia, paralysis, and pressure. Sometimes a seventh P is added, **poikilothermia**, or a coldness of the affected extremity relative to the contralateral side.

Management of compartment syndrome is as follows:

1. Maintain an open airway and apply oxygen therapy as necessary.
2. Assess pulses, motor, and sensory function.
3. Elevate the extremity above the heart.
4. Place ice packs over the extremity.
5. Initiate IV fluids to maintain peripheral perfusion.
6. Consider loosening any constrictive splint material and/or clothing.
7. Administer pain medication.
8. Monitor carefully for signs of, and be prepared to treat, rhabdomyolysis, hyperkalemia, and myoglobinuria.

For interfacility transport, several methods may be used to monitor actual compartment pressures invasively. In a noncontracting muscle, the normal mean interstitial tissue pressure is close to 0 mm Hg. If this pressure becomes elevated to 30 mm Hg or more, small vessels in the tissue can become compressed, resulting in reduced blood flow, ischemia, and pain. Pay close attention to both compartment pressure and diastolic blood pressure **FIGURE 11-37**. It is considered an emergency if the diastolic blood pressure drops to less than 30 mm Hg over the compartment pressure. When compartment pressure exceeds diastolic pressure, the blood flow in the extremity stops.

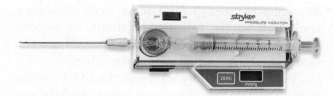

FIGURE 11-37 Compartment pressure monitoring device.
Courtesy of Stryker.

Untreated compartment syndrome–mediated ischemia of the muscles and nerves will lead to eventual irreversible damage and death of the tissues within the compartment. Definitive treatment involves fasciotomy—that is, cutting the fascia and opening the compartment to release the pressure. This procedure is typically performed in the operating room under general anesthesia. The compartment is then left open until bleeding is controlled and swelling is resolved.

Signs and Symptoms

Compartment Syndrome

- Pain
- Pallor
- Pulselessness
- Paresthesia
- Paralysis
- Pressure
- Poikilothermia (affected extremities may be colder on the affected side)

Transport Management

Compartment Syndrome

- Maintain an open airway; apply oxygen therapy as necessary.
- Assess pulses and motor and sensory function frequently.
- Elevate the extremity above the heart.
- Place ice packs over the extremity.
- Initiate IV fluids to maintain peripheral perfusion.
- Consider loosening any constrictive splint material and/or clothing.
- Administer pain medication.
- Monitor carefully for signs of, and be prepared to treat, rhabdomyolysis, hyperkalemia, and myoglobinuria.

Rhabdomyolysis and Crush Syndrome

Rhabdomyolysis is damage to the sarcolemma (muscle membrane) from any cause. This damage allows an influx of calcium and sodium, followed by water, into the cells. When these cells then rupture, they release myoglobin, aspartate transaminase, lactate, creatine kinase, potassium, uric acid, and phosphorus into the surrounding tissues. These substances are then absorbed into the circulation. The membrane damage also results in extracellular hypocalcemia and hyperkalemia; hyperkalemia leads to cardiac arrhythmias. The release of myoglobin combined with hypovolemia and acidosis leads to the blockage of renal tubules, causing acute renal failure.

Rhabdomyolysis has multiple etiologies, both traumatic and medically induced. The leading causes are exercise, alcohol, drugs, infections, trauma, compression, and seizures. This condition may also stem from metabolic myopathies, drugs and toxins (including cocaine and hallucinogens such as phencyclidine hydrochloride [PCP] and 3,4-methylenedioxymethamphetamine [MDMA]), infections, electrolyte abnormalities (including hypokalemia, hypophosphatemia, and both hypernatremia and hyponatremia), electrical current injuries, hypoxia (including carbon monoxide poisoning and sickle cell crisis), hyperthermia (including heat stroke, neuroleptic malignant syndrome, and malignant hyperthermia), and idiopathic causes.

Assessment

Assessment must start with a high index of suspicion, given the many causes of rhabdomyolysis. Any patient who lies in one position without being able to move for several hours is at risk. Physical examination may reveal motor weakness, obvious evidence of trauma or compression, and sensory loss. All of these symptoms may be accompanied by evidence of dehydration and dark or brown urine. The urine on a dipstick will show blood, with only a few red blood cells apparent on microscopic urine analysis, and a blood test will reveal significant creatine kinase levels of five times normal or higher. The upper normal level of creatine kinase is 150 U/L, but several hundred thousand units per liter may be present in rhabdomyolysis.

Electrolyte analysis will demonstrate the presence of hyperkalemia (potassium level greater than 5.5 mEq/L), with the expected ECG changes of tall, pointed T waves with a narrow base that widens as the potassium level increases, and then a flattening P wave. Hypocalcemia may also be present; it is defined as a calcium level lower than 8.2 mg/dL (2.05 mmol/L) or, in the case of ionized calcium, a concentration of less than 4.6 mg/dL (less than 1.15 mmol/L). In addition, a prolonged QT interval may be evident on ECG.

Management

When a CCTP is called to a scene that involves prolonged (longer than 2 hours) entrapment of a large muscle area of the patient, it is imperative that evaluation and treatment be started prior to the release of the entrapped patient. Crush syndrome is known as the smiling death—a sobriquet attributable to the pattern of extricated patients being happy and smiling until the released potassium reaches their heart, at which point sudden death ensues. Immediately prior to rescue, 2 L or more of saline (not potassium-containing lactated Ringer solution) should be infused and 1 mEq/kg of sodium bicarbonate given. It has been theorized—and now demonstrated in at least one published case report—that application of a tourniquet to the proximal, unentrapped portion of a pinned extremity (or extremities) delays release of hyperkalemic and acidotic blood back into circulation for the duration of time that the tourniquet is in place. Such a practice may allow for stabilization of other injuries; the tourniquet can then be released in the more controlled in-hospital setting or operating room.

The entrapped patient should be placed on a heart monitor when released. If the patient develops signs suggestive of an elevated potassium level, then calcium gluconate should be given as often as every 5 minutes as a slow IV push. Once an indwelling urinary catheter is placed, fluids should be given to maintain output of 300 mL/h. Bicarbonate should be given to keep urine pH at or greater than 7.65. This can be done by adding 3 ampules of bicarbonate to 1 L of 5% dextrose in water to maintain an isotonic solution. Mannitol is the diuretic of choice: It is both an osmotic diuretic, reducing swelling of the damaged muscle, and an intravascular volume expander. Mannitol also dilates and flushes the renal tubules. As a free radical scavenger,

this agent reduces direct damage from these ions. Loop diuretics (eg, furosemide) should be avoided in patients with suspected rhabdomyolysis or crush syndrome, because they acidify the urine.

During interfacility transfers, the CCTP should follow the patient's electrolyte levels carefully and use them to guide therapeutic interventions. This includes an electrolyte analysis completed immediately prior to transfer and, if available, use of bedside electrolyte monitoring during transport, such as with an i-STAT device **FIGURE 11-38**.

Signs and Symptoms

Rhabdomyolysis

- Motor weakness
- Obvious evidence of trauma or compression
- Sensory loss
- Dehydration
- Dark or brown urine
- Blood with only a few red blood cells on microscopic urine analysis
- Significant elevations of creatine kinase (5 times normal or higher)
- Hyperkalemia (>5.5 mEq/L), plus ECG changes of tall, pointed T waves with a narrow base that widens as potassium increases, and then a flattening P wave
- Hypocalcemia (<8.2 mg/dL [<2.05 mmol/L] or <4.6 mg/dL [<1.15 mmol/L ionized]), plus a prolonged QT interval on ECG

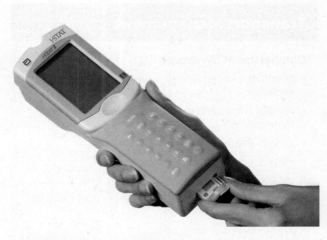

FIGURE 11-38 An i-STAT bedside electrolyte monitoring device for use during transport.

Courtesy of Abbott Laboratories.

Transport Management

Rhabdomyolysis

- Administer 2 L (or more) of saline.
- Administer 1 mEq/kg of sodium bicarbonate.
- Place the patient on a heart monitor.
- If signs of elevated potassium develop, give calcium as often as every 5 minutes as a slow IV push. Discontinue if severe bradycardia develops.
- Insert an indwelling urinary catheter, and give enough fluids to maintain output of 300 mL/h.
- Give enough bicarbonate to keep urine pH equal to or greater than 7.65, by adding 3 ampules per 1 L of D_5W (5% dextrose in water) given.
- Administer mannitol if the patient is producing urine.
- During interfacility transfers, monitor electrolytes.

Pulseless Extremity

Although a traumatized pulseless extremity may be repositioned successfully to reestablish circulation, this maneuver carries inherent dangers. Such repositioning should be done with manual traction in anatomic alignment with the long bone. Traction should reduce—not cause—pain if it is done in the correct anatomic direction. If the injury involves a dislocation rather than a fracture, analgesia and benzodiazepines may help relax the muscles to facilitate the repositioning. Position the extremity to maximize the strength of the pulse and splint it in this position. Mark the skin where pulses are obtained to make reassessment faster.

Trauma to Special Populations

Geriatric trauma and trauma to pregnant patients are covered here. Pediatric trauma is covered in Chapter 24, *Pediatric Emergencies*.

Geriatric Trauma

Some 54 million Americans (16.5%) were older than 65 years in 2019, a number expected to increase to 98 million by 2060. Geriatric refers to patients age 65 years and older; regarding trauma, mortality rates start to climb after the age of 30 years. The incidence of complicating comorbid conditions also increases after age 30 years. These coexisting medical conditions may cause lesser traumas to have a higher mortality due to increased physiologic stress.

Although patients older than 65 years account for only 11% of pedestrian incidents, they make up 25% of the fatalities in such incidents. A driver older than 65 years is five times more likely to be fatally injured in an MVC than a younger driver is. In another example of the greater vulnerability of older adults, the 1-year mortality rate for hip fractures in the over-65 population is 20% and the 2-year rate is 33%. One in five burn center admissions is a patient older than 65 years (approximately 1,500 people per year), and these older patients have a fatality rate seven times that of younger patients.

Some special considerations are necessary when dealing with geriatric patients who have experienced trauma. For example, assessment of the airway needs to include the presence of dentures or other dental devices that may have become dislodged. Removing dentures may make intubation easier, but without having them in place, achieving a satisfactory mask seal becomes more difficult. Broken teeth are at an increased risk of becoming a foreign body obstruction in older patients.

Kyphosis in geriatric patients can cause problems in terms of both motion restriction and airway management. Extra padding to fill the void under the patient's head and additional personnel to assist with motion restriction may be necessary. Geriatric patients also have reduced subcutaneous fat, so extra padding should be used between any applied splints and the skin.

Because of a reduced cough reflex and an increased risk of aspiration, additional attention to suctioning may be necessary in older adults. Their nasal tissues are more fragile and, if the patient is on anticoagulants, the risk of bleeding may render the use of both basic and advanced nasal airways problematic. Respiratory assessment must take into account reduced vital capacity and decreased ability for chest excursion, even prior to injury. Reduced tidal volume and lower minute volume can lead to a significant reduction in oxygen and carbon dioxide exchange as a baseline. Progressive hypoxia can result from even minor chest injury. Increased PIP may be necessary as a result of chest wall stiffness. Older patients are often more dependent on diaphragmatic excursion, and any restriction of the abdomen may interfere with this respiratory movement.

In addition, assessment for shock and perfusion may be difficult in older adults. Capillary refill may be normally delayed in these patients. Furthermore, cardiovascular assessment of the geriatric patient may be complicated by the ongoing use of medications such as beta blockers or other antihypertensive agents. These medications may interfere with compensatory mechanisms of shock, keeping the heart rate artificially low in the face of hypovolemia. Likewise, patients with pacemakers may be unable to compensate by raising their heart rate. Preexisting hypertension means that decompensated shock may present as what appears to be a normal blood pressure to the observer. A slow or absent vasoactive response means that the patient is more dependent on preload for maintaining an adequate circulation.

Fluid resuscitation remains the mainstay of traumatic shock resuscitation in older patients. Nevertheless, caution must be exercised to prevent fluid overload owing to the inability of the older person's cardiovascular system to adjust to rapid changes in fluid volumes.

Slow responses to questions or a lack of orientation to a location or date may not be a sign of head trauma in the geriatric patient, but rather part of the patient's baseline. Therefore, if the patient is conscious, history taking may require more patience when waiting for answers. The use of open-ended questions is recommended. If a family member is available, obtaining a sense of the geriatric patient's baseline mental status can assist in identifying changes or deficits.

Trauma During Pregnancy

Abdominal Injuries to Pregnant Patients

Injuries to pregnant patients are complicated by the multiple physiologic changes experienced by the pregnant woman and the fact that the CCTP is responsible for two lives. The primary cause of fetal demise in a mother who experiences trauma is maternal shock and death. Therefore, the best treatment for the fetus is to resuscitate the mother. Trauma occurs in 7% of pregnancies and is the leading cause of nonobstetric death in pregnancy, accounting for 7% of all maternal deaths and 80%

of fetal deaths. The most common cause of trauma during pregnancy is MVCs, followed by assault. Approximately 8% of women between ages 15 and 40 years who present to trauma centers do not even know they are pregnant. Chapter 22, *Obstetric and Gynecologic Emergencies*, describes the physiologic changes in pregnancy in more detail.

Some of the changes associated with pregnancy can mimic shock. For example, in the first trimester, the woman's systolic blood pressure drops about 5 mm Hg and diastolic blood pressure drops 15 mm Hg. The pregnant patient's heart rate also increases as much as 20 beats/min. Other changes may hide shock as well. Blood volume increases by about 50% in midpregnancy, and a relative anemia results from hemodilution. Consequently, the pregnant trauma patient may lose as much as 40% of her blood volume before the signs of shock become obvious. Because of the increased levels of coagulation factors and fibrinogen associated with pregnancy, the risk of deep vein thrombosis, pulmonary embolus, and DIC increases, especially in patients with multisystem trauma. Because of the increase in blood flow to the uterus to more than 0.5 L/min during pregnancy, along with venous congestion of the pelvic vessels, the risk of massive blood loss is considerably increased with trauma to the bony pelvis of a pregnant patient.

Any pregnant patient who sustains a pelvic injury or fracture is at very high risk for a bladder and/or uterine injury. At term, the uterus/placenta is perfused with approximately 600 to 800 mL of blood *per minute*. There should be a high rate of suspicion for these injuries, because these patients may exsanguinate rapidly.

Abruptio Placentae

In pregnant women who experience blunt trauma, as many as 70% of fetal deaths are the result of abruptio placentae. Sudden deformation of the uterine wall can shear the placenta from the site of implantation, without any external signs of this injury. Signs of abruption include vaginal bleeding (seen in only 37% of cases), abdominal cramping, and symptoms of maternal hypovolemia. The most important sign is fetal distress. Ultrasonograms are less than 50% accurate in finding an abruption. Women with an abruption are at an extremely high risk for DIC as a result of release of thromboplastin from the placenta.

Management

Fetal resuscitation focuses on maternal resuscitation, and maternal resuscitation starts with the ABCs. Given a higher risk of aspiration and the increase in gastric acidity in pregnant patients, isolating and monitoring the airway is of vital importance. Because of their increased oxygen consumption and reduced reserve, all pregnant patients should have their oxygenation maximally optimized. Hypoxia alone can cause a 30% reduction in uterine blood flow. Increased tidal volume and respiratory alkalosis as a baseline must be taken into account when using ventilators and end-tidal carbon dioxide ($ETCO_2$) monitoring. The target for $ETCO_2$ should be 30 mm Hg, rather than the usual 40 mm Hg. Early IV access with judicious fluid resuscitation should be initiated before signs of shock appear. Beyond 20 weeks' gestation, the patient should be tilted left laterally to at least a 15° angle to prevent inferior vena cava compression. CVP is helpful in guiding fluid administration, but remember that

Signs and Symptoms

Abruptio Placentae
- Vaginal bleeding
- Abdominal pain
- Back pain
- Uterine tenderness
- Signs of shock
- Lack of fetal heart sounds

Differential Diagnosis

Abruptio Placentae
- Ectopic pregnancy
- Placenta previa
- Preterm labor
- Spontaneous abortion

Transport Management

Abruptio Placentae
- If the patient is beyond 20 weeks' gestation, tilt her laterally to the left, to at least a 15° angle, to prevent vena cava compression.
- Provide bleeding control.
- Maintain the patient's airway; provide appropriate oxygen therapy.
- Initiate early IV access and implement judicious fluid resuscitation (eg, with lactated Ringer solution).
- Provide rapid transport.

CVP normally trends down to as low as 3 mm Hg as pregnancy progresses.

Flight Considerations

The principles presented in this chapter apply to both ground and air critical care transport. Given the critical nature of their injuries, however, patients with severe trauma are more likely to be transported by air, especially in situations in which ground transport time could take considerably longer than air.

Summary

Caring for patients with traumatic injuries requires the CCTP to have a solid understanding of the trauma system used in the United States. Knowledge and application of commonly used trauma scoring systems are essential parts of the CCTP's scope of practice. The CCTP must apply this knowledge and the appropriate assessment skills to assess, triage, and treat patients with traumatic injuries, and to transport them to the most appropriate facility. It is imperative that the CCTP be competent in clinical skills, understand why certain injuries occur, and have knowledge of which emergency procedures need to be performed to decrease morbidity and mortality. By mastering these skills, the CCTP becomes an integral part of the overall trauma care and management process, which in turn maximizes the patient's acute care, rehabilitation, and recovery.

Case Study

You are working the day shift with a nurse-medic–staffed helicopter. You have been dispatched to a scene. You receive a report from your communications center stating that you are going to a farm site where an older man has been kicked by a bull. The patient is currently alert and his vital signs are stable, as reported by the paramedics on the scene. The closest Level I trauma center from the scene is a 30-minute flight.

Upon landing, you and your partner approach the scene, which is in the pasture of a beef cattle farm. You survey the scene to ensure your safety. You receive a report from the local paramedics. The patient, a 68-year-old man, was assisting in feeding cattle when one of the bulls attacked him, first striking him in the chest with his head (horns removed) and then kicking him in the chest. The medic states that the patient is complaining of shortness of breath and severe chest pain, but otherwise he is alert and oriented and his vital signs remain stable.

Your assessment reveals a well-developed man who appears to be extremely short of breath. He is wearing a nonrebreathing mask and is receiving oxygen at 15 L/min; his oxygen saturation is 90%. In looking at his chest wall, you see a significant defect on the left side of the chest, with paradoxical chest wall motion. The patient is alert and oriented, with a GCS score of 15. The ground medics report that his breaths are becoming progressively shorter. The patient has two large-bore IV lines in place and has already received 1,000 mL of normal saline. His vital signs include a blood pressure of 110/70 mm Hg, a pulse rate of 118 beats/min, a respiratory rate of 32 breaths/min, and an oxygen saturation of 90%.

You and your partner discuss the patient's need for pain medication. You administer 2 μg/kg of IV fentanyl. The patient's heart rate slows down to approximately 100 beats/min, but his respiratory status does not improve. You and your partner discuss managing this patient's airway/ventilator status and elect to intubate the patient orally before leaving the scene. Using your local protocol, you administer etomidate, 0.3 mg/kg IV, and succinylcholine, 2.0 mg/kg IV. The intubation

is performed without difficulty. After intubation, you hear bilateral breath sounds but crackles in the left base. You apply capnography and monitor the patient's $ETCO_2$. His initial reading after intubation was 60 mm Hg, so you increase the ventilator minute volume. You finish packaging the patient and begin transport.

In flight, you administer long-term paralytics and additional sedation agents, and continue to treat the patient's pain. His vital signs remain stable, with a blood pressure of 98/70 mm Hg, a pulse rate of 90 beats/min, and ventilations at 16 breaths/min with 97% saturation. His $ETCO_2$ reading is 40 mm Hg, which shows that he is adequately ventilated. You and your partner discuss IV flow rates and elect to keep both IV lines open. The patient is admitted to the Level I trauma center and a report is given to the attending staff.

1. Why did you elect to intubate this person when the standard of care for flail chest is to keep the patient off mechanical ventilation if it all possible?
2. Why did you decide to continue the patient's fluids in fight?

Analysis

In cases of flail chest, the patient's pain is treated aggressively. With the pain under control, many times the patient is then able to ventilate adequately on their own. In this patient, two issues needed to be considered. First, the patient was dyspneic and was not breathing adequately, as shown by his poor oxygen saturation despite appropriate oxygen therapy. Even after his pain was treated and his heart rate slowed down, his oxygen saturation was borderline at best. Second, the patient faced the prospect of a 30-minute flight, and the chance that his condition would continue to deteriorate seemed high. In the treatment of flail chest, mechanical ventilation should be reserved for patients who have persistent respiratory insufficiency or failure, after adequate pain control. This patient met that standard; therefore, intubation is appropriate, and rapid sequence intubation should be performed. Follow the local protocol for appropriate medication use. In this patient, it is imperative that you continue to treat his pain after administering long-term paralytics and sedation. Patient monitoring after intubation must include continuous waveform capnography; a capnography reading is an excellent indicator of respiratory rate and adequate ventilation in flight.

Many services now carry continuous positive airway pressure devices on the helicopter. This patient would have been a candidate for continuous positive airway pressure in flight, thereby avoiding mechanical ventilation. The CCTP would have to be astute in ongoing pulmonary assessment to realize when the patient's condition is failing and would need to provide mechanical ventilation if necessary.

When chest trauma is significant enough to break multiple ribs, there is a higher associated risk of underlying parenchymal injury to the lung. Aggressive fluid resuscitation only worsens the interstitial fluid leak, which leads to ventilation-perfusion mismatch and, in turn, worsening pulmonary contusion. This patient had already received 1,000 mL of fluid, which probably worsened his lung condition.

The patient's mean arterial pressure (MAP) should be maintained at or above 65 mm Hg. His current reading is approximately 79 mm Hg, which is adequate for end-organ perfusion. This patient's IV fluids should be slowed. If his blood pressure dictates, titrate the patient's fluids according to his MAP.

Prep Kit

Ready for Review

- A paradigm shift in the care of critically injured trauma patients has resulted in an emphasis on rapidly identifying and treating those patients who need immediate transport to an appropriate trauma center.
- The ability of the CCTP to rapidly identify life-threatening injuries while recognizing the need for transport to a trauma center can help decrease the incidence of morbidity and mortality related to these traumatic injuries.
- CCTPs may encounter trauma patients during a scene call, when they are called to back up field BLS or ALS providers. In these cases, the CCTP will be working in more austere and less controlled conditions with less sophisticated assessment tools than are available in an interfacility transport.
- CCTPs may also aid in transferring critical patients with trauma, usually from smaller facilities to higher-level trauma centers. In this situation, the CCTP may have access to the

results of any assessment findings identified prior to transport and may be able to enlist the aid of the sending physician or other house staff to help with stabilization efforts prior to transport.
- The balance of treatment before transport versus what can be done en route should always be a top priority in the CCTP's decision-making process.
- Trauma is the leading cause of death in children and adults younger than 45 years in the United States.
- Many people survive an MVC, only to sustain a debilitating injury that leaves them incapacitated. Providers must appreciate the importance of avoiding secondary injury caused by improper handling of these patients.
- Understanding Newton's first law of motion—"A body in motion remains in motion in a straight line unless acted upon by an outside force"—enables the CCTP to predict

Prep Kit Continued

patterns of injuries in trauma incidents and deliver the appropriate standard of care.

- Traumatic injuries are generally classified into one of two categories: blunt or penetrating.
- Blunt injuries result from energy exchange between an object and the body, without intrusion through the skin—for example, rapid forward decelerations (crashes), rapid vertical decelerations (falls), and energy transferred from blunt instruments (assault).
- Penetrating injuries refer to injuries caused by external forces in which the tissue is penetrated by an object—for example, injuries caused by projectiles such as bullets, knives, fragments from explosions, and falls upon fixed objects.
- Deceleration injuries are caused by a sudden stop of the body's forward motion. Because they may not be visible to the CCTP, an excellent understanding of the types of mechanisms of injury and effective assessment skills are imperative for detecting them.
- External force injuries occur when forces violate the tissues of the body. Their severity depends on the anatomic area involved as well as the mass, size, and the velocity of the foreign object that enters the body.
- The CCTP must not develop tunnel vision; that is, the CCTP must not focus on a visible injury, which may or may not be life threatening, while paying little or no attention to other, genuinely life-threatening injuries.
- Maintaining a calm, professional demeanor and using a systematic approach allows the CCTP to maintain a high index of suspicion and attention to detail.
- Trauma scoring systems are used in the CCT environment to provide assessment information, to report quality outcomes, and as indicators of patient survivability.
- The Glasgow Coma Scale (GCS) is a neurologic assessment tool that assigns a numerical value to the patient's condition based on three body functions: best eye-opening response, best verbal response, and best motor response.

- The GCS should be used regardless of the cause of central nervous system alteration. It is predominantly applied and the score reported during the care of critically ill and injured patients when their current level of consciousness is pertinent to their acuity level.
- Patients who present with GCS scores of less than 8 typically require intubation or another form of advanced airway intervention.
- The trauma score takes into account the GCS score, respiratory rate, respiratory expansion, systolic blood pressure, and capillary refill rate. This score, which ranges from 1 to 16 (the best possible score), reflects the likelihood of patient survival.
- The revised trauma score measures three physiologic parameters: respiratory rate, systolic blood pressure, and GCS score. The total score ranges from 0 (the most severely debilitated patient) to 13 or, when a weighted system is used, from 1.0 to 7.8408.
- The revised trauma score is considered flawed because it measures the body's physiologic response to the injury and fails to identify a small percentage of severely injured trauma patients.
- The Abbreviated Injury Scale (AIS) is an anatomic scoring system that provides a reasonably accurate means of ranking the severity of an injury by categorizing injuries into six body regions. Scores for each region range from 1 (minor injury) to 6 (unsurvivable), but do not take into account multisystem injuries.
- The Injury Severity Score (ISS) is an anatomic scoring system that provides an overall score for patients with multiple injuries. Scores range from 1 (minor injury) to 75 (high mortality).
- A patient with an ISS of greater than 15 is frequently considered to have major trauma and requires immediate attention and, in most cases, transfer to a Level I facility.
- The trauma injury severity score is used to determine the survival probability of the

critically ill and/or injured patient. It takes into account the ISS, the revised trauma score, and the patient's age, which collectively summarize the patient's physiologic and anatomic indicators.

- Trauma centers are classified into Levels I through IV. Level I centers (regional centers that provide every aspect of trauma care) have the most resources, followed by Level II centers (facilities that provide initial definitive care), Level III centers (facilities that provide assessment, resuscitation, emergency medical care, and stabilization, and then transfer patients to higher-level centers), and Level IV centers (clinics that provide ATLS prior to patient transfer).

- Patients with severe trauma (Level I patients) are more likely to be transported by air, especially in situations in which ground transport time could take longer than air transport.

- Interfacility care for trauma patients will often involve patients who are very ill and in need of close assessment and continued monitoring. Management after these patients' arrival at a hospital should follow ATLS guidelines.

- As in the prehospital setting, immediate attention during interfacility transport is directed at the ABCs. It is also imperative to assess the patient from head to toe for external injuries.

- The CCTP must be prepared to detect and treat complications of the initial evaluation and treatment, including fluid overload, transfusion reactions, contrast-induced renal issues, abdominal compartment syndrome, bleeding, and shock.

- Hypothermia, acidosis, and coagulopathy are the lethal triad of trauma. Every effort should be made to avoid these pathologies in caring for trauma patients.

- The incidence of hypothermia in trauma patients can be as high as 50%, and mortality rates can approach 100%. Treatment should focus on prevention or reduction of hypothermia in these patients.

- Hypothermia can lead to acidosis, as can administration of large volumes of acidic crystalloid solutions like normal saline, which has a pH of 5.5 and a very high level of chloride.

- Coagulopathy can be precipitated not only by hypothermia and acidosis, but also by acute blood loss. Aggressively managing hemorrhage and ensuring early replacement of clotting factors through transfusion of blood products are important interventions to reverse or prevent progressive coagulopathy.

- Obtaining and understanding imaging studies related to trauma is an integral component of the trauma care paradigm for the CCTP.

- Standard radiographs are part of the initial assessment of the patient with multisystem trauma; they can provide confirmation of endotracheal tube placement, lead to identification of fractures, and suggest the need for further intervention prior to initiation of transport.

- In trauma patients, computed tomography scanning is typically used to identify head injury, bleeding, and complex fractures. Typical studies will scan the head, chest, and abdominal-pelvic regions.

- Focused assessment with sonography for trauma (FAST) ultrasonography is used to identify the presence of free intraperitoneal or pericardial fluids, and has replaced diagnostic peritoneal lavage and laparotomy for this indication.

- Critical care clinicians may also use focused-exam imaging modalities such as transthoracic and transesophageal echocardiography.

- Magnetic resonance imaging provides much better resolution that can help identify abnormalities in trauma patients, but requires substantial amounts of time to obtain. It is infrequently used in the initial care for trauma patients.

Prep Kit Continued

- Intra-abdominal pressure (IAP) is the static pressure inside the abdominal compartment. Deleterious effects of intra-abdominal hypertension (IAH) can lead to abdominal compartment syndrome (ACS) and death if untreated. Definitive treatment is surgical decompression, but many interventions can be implemented to help prevent IAH and ACS. The CCTP may be asked to obtain IAP measurements during transport.
- When transporting trauma patients, CCTPs should always ask for and ensure that all copies of any imaging studies are included as part of the patient care record.
- Approximately 25% of all trauma deaths are directly associated with thoracic injuries.
- The primary function of the thorax is to support adequate oxygenation and circulation. Therefore, injuries to the chest must be found and managed promptly.
- Care must be taken in trauma patients to ensure adequate positive-pressure ventilations without allowing intrathoracic pressure to rise too high; this may become an issue during flight.
- Pneumothorax injuries cause air to be drawn into the thoracic cavity with each breath. A collapse as small as 10% can be life threatening if the patient has other comorbid issues.
- Sealing a sucking chest wound can cause a tension pneumothorax if air is still able to enter the pleural cavity from the lung side of the wound and builds up, or if the seal is ineffective. Monitoring the airway and breathing in these patients is critical.
- A simple pneumothorax is most often associated with a closed chest injury, such as from a fractured rib being driven inward into the lung or from a medical cause that leads to collapse of the lung.
- A tension pneumothorax is a life-threatening injury that results from a continual influx of air into the pleural space. It may occur secondary to a closed simple pneumothorax or after sealing an open pneumothorax.
- Management of a tension pneumothorax consists of immediate needle decompression.
- Hemothorax can be caused by blunt or penetrating trauma, as well as a tumor eroding through the great vessels. It may potentially lead to hypovolemic shock or, if a large amount of blood accumulates in the pleural cavity, respiratory distress.
- Patients with a pneumothorax, hemothorax, hemopneumothorax, or empyema ultimately may need a chest tube inserted. In addition, CCTPs routinely care for and transport patients with chest tubes in place.
- Because of the potential for massive hemorrhage from thoracic trauma, the CCTP must be familiar with the administration of blood and blood products.
- Recent studies comparing the effectiveness of pigtail versus larger conventional chest drainage tubes show no significant differences in resolution of pneumothoraces, hemothoraces, empyemas, and effusions.
- A flail chest (flail segment) consists of a fracture in two or more places to two or more adjacent ribs. Bruises to the underlying tissue causing a pulmonary or myocardial contusion are the most dangerous sequelae of a flail chest.
- Flail segments pose a threat to the patient's ability to breathe, increase the risk for developing a hemothorax or pneumothorax, and require immediate treatment.
- The gold-standard treatment for flail chest is mechanical ventilation with a sedate, paralyzed patient who has been adequately treated for pain. Some patients may be managed conservatively with pain medications and oxygen supplementation alone.
- Pericardial tamponade is a life-threatening condition that requires immediate treatment. It occurs in 2% of penetrating injuries to

Prep Kit Continued

the chest and upper abdomen, and is more common in stab wounds to the heart than in gunshot wounds.

- Most often, prehospital management of pericardial tamponade is only supportive; sometimes, however, the CCTP may need to perform or assist in an emergency pericardiocentesis.
- A pericardial window procedure involves removing a section of the pericardium to create a window, allowing fluid that has accumulated in the pericardium to drain, and leaving a drain in place. Monitoring drain output and frequent cardiovascular assessments can prevent recurrence of cardiac tamponade.
- Traumatic aortic rupture is the most common cause of immediate death in MVCs.
- Tears in the ascending aorta are almost uniformly immediately fatal, but patients with tears on the descending side have a 15% chance of making it to the operating room. Even so, there is a 30% mortality rate among those patients who do survive until arrival at the hospital.
- The ligamentum arteriosum is the most common cause of aortic dissection in trauma patients.
- Myocardial contusion (bruise to the myocardium) is primarily the result of blunt trauma to the anterior chest wall, such as trauma that occurs during MVCs or with other blows to the front of the chest (eg, gunshot to a bulletproof vest).
- With myocardial contusion, damage to small blood vessels may cause local bleeding and direct trauma to cells. Because the areas downstream from the damaged vessels are no longer perfused, the damage may resemble that associated with myocardial infarction.
- If blunt compression of the abdomen occurs (eg, from blunt or penetrating trauma), it may cause diaphragmatic rupture and herniation of abdominal organs into the thoracic cavity. This impairs lung expansion and decreases venous

return, resulting in decreased ventilatory and cardiac output.

- Tracheobronchial injuries are rare, but often life threatening. The leakage of air that occurs with such damage may cause a tension pneumothorax or tension pneumomediastinum, which will act like a cardiac tamponade.
- Management of tracheobronchial disruption includes judicious use of ventilatory support.
- Lacerations and bruising of the lung tissue (pulmonary contusion) can cause bleeding and leakage of plasma into the alveoli and interstitial space. This damage interferes with gas exchange and can lead to severe hypoxemia.
- Patients with pulmonary contusion may be managed with noninvasive, continuous positive airway pressure, adequate analgesia, and resuscitation fluids as needed.
- Esophageal perforations are most often caused by penetrating injuries, such as from projectiles, or by caustic ingestion, but can also be caused by an underlying medical issue, such as cancer, gastroesophageal reflux disease erosions, or excessive vomiting.
- Traumatic asphyxia—a severe sudden crushing injury to the chest and abdomen—is not a form of asphyxia, nor is it by itself fatal. Associated injuries, if present, tend to be far more serious.
- Facial trauma can be life threatening as a result of airway compromise and the threat to the patient's ability to get sensory information through sight and hearing; it also has many social and self-image implications for the patient and can be distracting for caregivers.
- A punctured eardrum may cause vertigo and nausea, which the CCTP may need to control with medication. The patient should be protected from aircraft noise.
- Blood or fluid coming from the auditory canal indicates a more serious injury and should be assessed with the halo test.

Prep Kit Continued

- A ruptured tympanic membrane is not life threatening, but should raise the suspicion for other, much more serious overpressure injuries.
- Eye injuries, although often dramatic, are not life threatening. Care typically consists of protecting the eye from further injury and transporting the patient to the ophthalmology service.
- In patients who have chemical burns to the eye, adequate washing is essential and should be performed for at least 10 minutes prior to transport for acid burns and at least 20 minutes for alkali burns.
- If an object is impaled in the eye, both the eye and the object should be prevented from movement, if possible, during transport.
- Hyphema—a collection of blood in the anterior chamber of the eye—may be a marker of damage to other structures of the eye and requires a full ophthalmologic examination.
- Rupture of the ocular globe with leak of vitreous humor may be the result of penetration by a foreign body or blunt trauma.
- Despite the dramatic presentation of enucleation of the eyeball from the eye socket, loss of vision is not inevitable with such an injury. Proper care includes protecting the eye from further trauma in transit by using a protective cup or other rigid protective device with gauze padding.
- Retinal detachment—that is, separation of the inner layers of the retina from the pigmented epithelium—may be caused by trauma, diabetic retinopathy, and sickle cell disease. With rapid diagnosis and surgery, blindness may sometimes be avoided in such cases.
- Treatment is usually not necessary on a scene call for mandibular fracture or dislocation, but provision must be made for inserting an emergency airway during the transfer of any patient whose jaw is wired shut.
- Avulsed teeth have a good chance of successful reimplantation if replaced within 1 hour.
- The critical airway and vascular structures running through the neck are relatively unprotected during trauma events. In addition, the possibility of unstable cervical spine and cord injury must always be considered.
- Securing the airway with endotracheal intubation should be considered prior to transporting any patient with a neck injury. Deterioration of the patient's airway in the back of a transport vehicle with limited space and few personnel available to manage this condition can be disastrous.
- Most laryngotracheal injuries occur in the area of the cervical trachea and are often caused by direct blunt trauma. These injuries can appear stable for a time, only to then be followed by rapid and catastrophic deterioration.
- In case of laryngotracheal disruptions, paralytics and muscle relaxants are absolutely contraindicated.
- Direct trauma to the front of the neck (including the thyroid gland) can cause hematomas of sufficient size to impinge on the airway. Thyrotoxicosis (thyroid storm) has a 20% to 30% mortality rate and has been rarely seen following thyroid trauma.
- Injury to the carotid, subclavian, and vertebral arteries, and to the external and internal jugular veins, can produce rapid exsanguination, hematoma formation, or embolization of air, usually resulting in mortality.
- Widespread use of seat belts has significantly decreased the incidence of morbidity and mortality related to MVCs, but these devices can cause less obvious abdominal injuries.
- Penetrating injuries may be very difficult for the CCTP to assess because detailed information about the penetrating object is often not available. Even when this information can be obtained, it is difficult to rapidly identify which structures inside the abdominal cavity

Prep Kit Continued

were injured without the assistance of imaging studies.

■ If the patient has experienced blunt or penetrating trauma to the abdominal cavity, signs or symptoms of injury may be very difficult to identify until shock becomes obvious. Because of the size of the abdominal cavity, a significant amount of blood can collect within this space and go unnoticed.

■ With abdominal injuries, it is important for the CCTP to focus attention on the mechanism of injury, instead of the outward signs of trauma found on assessment.

■ If a significant abdominal injury is suspected or confirmed, the most definitive treatment that the CCTP can provide is rapid transport to the trauma center, while stabilizing and maintaining the patient's hemodynamic status as effectively as possible, so that surgical intervention can be performed if needed.

■ In case of abdominal injury, performing a physical exam to rapidly identify the presence of blood loss is the most important task for the CCTP.

■ The primary assessment of a patient with abdominal injury should be completed before beginning transport, and repeated frequently during transport, watching for changes that require immediate intervention.

■ All patients suspected of having abdominal injuries should be transported on appropriate oxygen therapy with fluid administration. More severe cases may need aggressive airway management and blood administration.

■ Resuscitative endovascular balloon occlusion of the aorta (REBOA) has recently gained traction in trauma surgery and emergency medicine as a temporizing measure for refractory hemorrhagic shock, blunt or penetrating abdominal trauma, pelvic fractures with significant hemorrhage, and ruptured abdominal aortic aneurysms.

■ Before a REBOA catheter can be placed, femoral arterial access must be obtained. Continuous

arterial waveform monitoring should be used to monitor blood pressure and ensure correct placement of the REBOA catheter.

■ Indications for zone 1 placement of a REBOA catheter include temporary control of severe intra-abdominal hemorrhage, severe retroperitoneal hemorrhage, and traumatic arrest with suspected infradiaphragmatic injury as the source of hemorrhage.

■ Indications for zone 3 placement of a REBOA catheter include severe pelvic, junctional (groin/perineum), or proximal lower extremity hemorrhage that cannot be controlled by other methods.

■ The insertion depth, time of balloon inflation, amount of saline in the balloon, and blood pressure change should be recorded after insertion of the REBOA catheter.

■ Ongoing research is examining the safety of REBOA catheters in transport.

■ The primary concern with hollow-organ injury is the potential for peritonitis and shock to develop.

■ The spleen is the most commonly injured organ in the abdominal cavity. Young adults and patients with sickle cell disease are at particular risk for spleen injury.

■ Failure to recognize, understand, and treat the signs and symptoms of hypovolemic shock related to internal hemorrhage will rapidly lead to the patient's death.

■ The falciform ligament in front of the liver can slice the liver in a sudden deceleration. The liver's close proximity to the lower rib cage also makes it susceptible to injury after a rib fracture occurs.

■ Although penetrating trauma is the most common source of injury to the intestines, blunt trauma to the abdominal wall—often caused by a seat belt—can also damage the small bowel.

■ Approximately 80% of gunshot wounds to the abdomen and 30% of stab wounds lacerate the jejunum and ileum.

Prep Kit Continued

- Injuries that occur to the vessels of the abdomen are usually life threatening. Although severe blunt trauma may disrupt these vessels, the most common cause of vascular injury is penetrating trauma.
- Rapid transport of patients with an injury to any of the major abdominal vessels to a hospital capable of immediate surgery is the best possible treatment.
- The presence of a pelvic fracture should alert the CCTP to the possible existence of other injuries, given the force that must be exerted to cause pelvic fracture; the potential for (possibly fatal) internal hemorrhage is high in such cases.
- Subjective assessment for pelvic fracture includes identification of the mechanism of injury, location and radiation of pain, presence of hematuria, and possibility of pregnancy. Objective examination should include observing for the rotation or uneven height of the iliac crests and uneven length of the legs, palpating the posterior aspect of the pelvic ring, and exerting gentle lateral compression posteriorly and inward medial compression once.
- Musculoskeletal injuries, although often dramatic, may distract the CCTP from more serious injuries. Nevertheless, their presence may be an indicator of the amount of energy transferred to the body and suggest the likelihood of additional injury.
- All musculoskeletal injuries should be assessed for the six Ps—pain, pallor, pulselessness, paresthesia, paralysis, and pressure—before and after any manipulation.
- Regardless of whether a fracture is open or closed, the CCTP must prioritize prevention of further injury as a result of movement, along with pain assessment and management.
- Closed fractures can be as dangerous as open fractures because of their potential to cause internal bleeding into the tissues involved.
- In an open fracture, the skin over the bone is broken, adding the potential danger of infection, which could lead to sepsis and death.
- Femur fractures can lead to a loss of at least 1 L of blood from circulation.
- Patients being transported from one facility to another who have not definitively had their spines cleared should be transported with motion restriction in place. The CCTP should apply an appropriately fitted cervical collar and firmly secure the patient to the transport stretcher.
- Planning for airway management and prevention of aspiration (especially in small aircraft) must be undertaken prior to transport of any patient with a spinal injury.
- Thoracic fractures can lead to a loss of innervation of the intercostal muscles, which then leads to respiratory insufficiency. Spinal shock, in which hypotension is accompanied by bradycardia instead of tachycardia, can affect the thoracic area or higher.
- Any patient with a cast who is transported by a CCTP should be evaluated for neurovascular function distal to the cast both prior to transport and periodically during transport. It is recommended that the locations where pulses are found be marked on the skin and documented in the patient care record.
- External fixation of fractures using external rods held to the bone with plates and screws has become common. Adequate padding and comfortable positioning are required when transporting patients with these devices.
- Swelling under a cast can cause compartment syndrome. The most common anatomic locations for compartment syndrome are the forearms and legs, but this condition can develop in any extremity and the buttocks.
- If the diastolic blood pressure drops below 30 mm Hg over the compartment pressure, it is considered an emergency. When the compartment pressure exceeds the diastolic pressure, the blood flow in the extremity stops.
- Rhabdomyolysis, which is characterized by hyperkalemia, hypocalcemia, and myoglobinuria,

Prep Kit Continued

initiates a cascade of events that ultimately results in cardiac arrhythmias and acute renal failure. The leading causes of rhabdomyolysis are exercise, alcohol, drugs, infections, trauma, compression, and seizures.

- When a CCTP is called to a scene involving a patient with prolonged entrapment of a large muscle area, it is imperative to start evaluation and treatment (IV fluids and sodium bicarbonate) prior to the release of the entrapped patient to avoid the mortality associated with crush syndrome.

- Although a traumatized, pulseless extremity may be repositioned successfully to reestablish circulation, doing so carries some risks. If attempted, repositioning should be done with manual traction in anatomic alignment with the long bone.

- Considerations when treating geriatric patients with trauma include several aging-related issues: presence of dentures or other dental devices, kyphosis, reduced cough reflex and increased risk of aspiration, fragility of the nasal tissues, increased risk for bleeding and use of antiplatelet or anticoagulant medications, reduced vital capacity and decreased ability for chest excursion, chest wall stiffness, difficulty of assessing for shock and perfusion, preexisting cardiovascular abnormalities or use of cardiovascular medications, tendency toward fluid overload, slower mental processing, and difficulties in thermoregulation.

- The primary cause of fetal demise in the pregnant patient who experiences trauma is maternal shock and death. Therefore, the best treatment for the fetus is to resuscitate the mother.

- Some of the normal changes in pregnancy can mimic shock, which makes it difficult to diagnose true shock in a pregnant trauma patient.

- The risk of massive blood loss is considerably increased with trauma to the bony pelvis of a pregnant patient. Any pregnant patient who sustains a pelvic injury most certainly has a bladder and/or uterine injury.

- Fetal resuscitation centers on maternal resuscitation, and maternal resuscitation starts with the ABCs.

Vital Vocabulary

Abbreviated Injury Scale (AIS) A trauma scoring system that ranks injury severity by assigning an individual injury score of 1 to 6 to six body regions, with 1 being a minor injury and 6 being an injury with a high mortality rate; does not account for multisystem injuries.

abdominal compartment syndrome (ACS) A condition that can result from intra-abdominal hypertension, including decreased end-organ perfusion with evidence of failure; if untreated, it can lead to death.

anechoic Free from echo.

Beck triad The combination of a narrowed pulse pressure, muffled heart tones, and jugular venous distention associated with cardiac tamponade; usually resulting from penetrating chest trauma.

crush syndrome The combination of shock and renal failure after a crush injury; it may lead to the death of an entrapped person after the patient is freed from the entrapment.

diagnostic peritoneal lavage (DPL) A surgical procedure to assess for bleeding or intestinal perforation in the abdomen. Classically, a liter of crystalloid is infused into the abdomen and then drawn out to examine for the presence of blood or intestinal contents.

empyema An accumulation of pus in the pleural space.

exploratory laparotomy Surgical exploration of the abdomen.

flail chest A fracture in two or more places to two or more adjacent ribs.

Prep Kit Continued

focused assessment with sonography for trauma (FAST) An ultrasonographic examination directed at identifying the presence of free intraperitoneal or pericardial fluids, performed by transducing four distinct areas of the abdomen.

fracture A break in the continuity of a bone.

Glasgow Coma Scale (GCS) An evaluation tool used to determine level of consciousness, which evaluates and assigns point values (scores) for eye opening, verbal response, and motor response, which are then totaled; effective in helping predict patient outcomes.

hemothorax An accumulation of blood in the pleural space.

hyphema A collection of blood in the anterior chamber of the eye.

Injury Severity Score (ISS) A trauma scoring system that adds the squares of the three highest abbreviated injury scale scores to create a score between 1 and 75 that accounts for multiple injuries, with 1 being a minor injury and 75 being an injury with a high mortality rate.

intra-abdominal hypertension (IAH) Sustained increased abdominal pressure of more than 12 mm Hg.

intra-abdominal pressure (IAP) The static pressure inside the abdominal compartment; normally 5 mm Hg, with variations caused by respirations.

Kehr sign Left shoulder pain that may indicate a ruptured spleen. (Right shoulder pain may indicate trauma to the liver.) This referred pain stems from diaphragm irritation by intra-abdominal bleeding.

morbidity The number of nonfatally injured or disabled people. Usually expressed as a rate, meaning the number of nonfatal injuries in a certain population in a given time period divided by the size of the population.

mortality Deaths caused by injury and disease. Usually expressed as a rate, meaning the number of deaths in a certain population in a given time period divided by the size of the population.

open pneumothorax A communicating chest wound, in which air enters the pleural space from the environment; also called a sucking chest wound.

paracentesis A procedure used to drain free fluid from the abdominal cavity.

pericardial tamponade Impairment of diastolic filling of the right ventricle as a result of significant amounts of fluid in the pericardial sac surrounding the heart, leading to a decrease in the cardiac output.

pericardiocentesis A procedure in which a needle or angiocatheter is introduced into the pericardial sac to relieve cardiac tamponade.

pneumothorax An accumulation of gas or fluid in the pleural space that causes the lung to become detached from the chest wall.

poikilothermia Inability to regulate temperature in an extremity due to lack of perfusion, which may result in abnormally cold extremities.

resuscitative endovascular balloon occlusion of the aorta (REBOA) A surgical procedure in which arterial access is gained through a femoral approach, a balloon catheter is floated into the aorta, and the balloon is inflated to occlude flow; a temporizing measure for refractory hemorrhagic shock, blunt or penetrating abdominal trauma, pelvic fractures with significant hemorrhage, and ruptured abdominal aortic aneurysms, and possibly for outlying hospitals prior to transfer of a trauma patient to a higher-level trauma center.

retinal detachment Separation of the inner layers of the retina from the pigmented epithelium.

revised trauma score A trauma scoring system that rates injury severity by comparing the Glasgow Coma Scale score, the systolic blood pressure, and the respiratory rate and assigning a score ranging from 0 to 13 based on these

Prep Kit Continued

three values; in some cases the parameters are weighted, resulting in a score ranging from 1.0 to 7.8408.

rhabdomyolysis Damage to the sarcolemma (muscle membrane) from any cause, leading to a release of potassium and myoglobin.

tension pneumothorax A pneumothorax in which an intact chest wall allows air that has entered the thoracic space to progressively accumulate, resulting in catastrophic collapse of pulmonary and cardiac structures in the chest.

thyrotoxicosis An excess of thyroid hormones resulting in a hypermetabolic crisis, including tachycardia greater than 140 beats/min; hyperthermia (sometimes greater than 103.9°F [39.9°C]); coma with agitation, nausea, vomiting, diarrhea, and unexplained jaundice; and pulmonary edema; marked by an elevated thyroxine level. Also called thyroid storm.

tracheal deviation A late sign of a tension pneumothorax in which the trachea is tugged to one side of the neck, usually opposite the side of the pneumothorax.

tracheal tugging Downward traction of the trachea toward the thoracic cavity during inspiration.

trauma injury severity score (TRISS) A scoring system that uses the results of the Injury Severity Score, the revised trauma score, and the patient's age to calculate the survivability rate; rarely used in the transport setting.

trauma score A score ranging from 1 to 16 that takes into account the Glasgow Coma Scale score, respiratory rate, respiratory expansion, systolic blood pressure, and capillary refill, and relates to the likelihood of patient survival; not accurate for patients with severe head injuries.

traumatic asphyxia A condition resulting from severe, sudden crushing injury to the chest and abdomen, which forces blood backward out of the right side of the heart; engorges the veins of the chest, neck, and head; and gives the chest, neck, and head an extremely cyanotic appearance.

References

American Geriatrics Society, National Association of Emergency Medical Technicians. *Geriatric Education for Emergency Medical Services*. 2nd ed. Burlington, MA: Jones & Bartlett Learning; 2015.

Aspesi M, Gamberoni C, Severgnini P, et al. The abdominal compartment syndrome: clinical relevance. *Minerva Anesth*. 2002;68(4):138-146.

Ball CG, Kirkpatrick AW, McBeth P. The secondary abdominal compartment syndrome: not just another post-traumatic complication. *Can J Surg*. 2008;51(5):399-405.

Balogh Z, McKinley BA, Cocanour CS, et al. Supranormal trauma resuscitation causes more cases of abdominal compartment syndrome. *Arch Surg*. 2003;138(6):637-643.

Bernstein MP, Mirvis SE, Shanmuganathan K. Chance-type fractures of the thoracolumbar spine: imaging analysis in 53 patients. *AJR Am J Roentgenol*. 2006;187(4):859-868. doi: 10.2214/AJR.05.0145. PMID: 16985126.

Brenner M, Bulger EM, Perina DG, et al. Joint statement from the American College of Surgeons Committee on Trauma (ACS COT) and the American College of Emergency Physicians (ACEP) regarding the clinical use of resuscitative endovascular balloon occlusion of the aorta (REBOA). *Trauma Surg Acute Care Open*. 2018;3(1). doi: 10.1136/tsaco-2017-000154.

Busti A, Hinston J. Chest tube thoracostomy. *Evidence-Based Med Consult*. https://www.ebmconsult.com/articles/chest-tube-placement-thoracostomy-procedure. Updated September 2015. Accessed April 9, 2021.

Campion EM, Fox CJ. Prehospital hemorrhage control and REBOA. *Curr Trauma Rep*. 2019;5(3):129-136.

Centers for Disease Control and Prevention, National Center for Health Statistics. Accidents and unintentional injury. https://www.cdc.gov/nchs/fastats/accidental-injury.htm. Reviewed March 1, 2021. Accessed April 8, 2021.

Centers for Disease Control and Prevention, National Center for Injury Prevention and Control. Ten leading causes of death by age group, United States—2018. https://www.cdc.gov/injury/wisqars/pdf/leading_causes_of_death_by_age_group_2018-508.pdf. Accessed April 8, 2021.

Cheatham ML, Malbrain ML, Kirkpatrick A, et al. Results from the International Conference of Experts on Intra-abdominal Hypertension and Abdominal Compartment Syndrome, II: recommendations. *Intens Care Med*. 2007;33(6):951-962.

Clemency BM, Tanski CT, Rosenberg M, May PR, Consiglio JD, Lindstrom HA. Sufficient catheter length for pneumothorax needle decompression: a meta-analysis. *Prehosp Disaster Med*. 2015;30:249-253.

Prep Kit Continued

Committee on Trauma, American College of Surgeons. *Resources for Optimal Care of the Injured Patient*. American College of Surgeons website. https://www.facs.org/-/media/files/quality-programs/trauma/vrc-resources/resources-for-optimal-care.ashx. Published 2014. Accessed April 9, 2021.

De Backer D, Cortes DO. Characteristics of fluids used for intravascular volume replacement. *Best Pract Res Clin Anaesthesiol*. 2012;26(4):441-451.

Edgecombe L, Sigmon DF, Galuska MA, Angus LD. Thoracic trauma. *StatPearls* [Internet]. https://www.ncbi.nlm.nih.gov/books/NBK534843/. Updated June 1, 2020. Accessed April 9, 2021.

Gabbe BJ, Cameron PA, Finch CF. Is the revised trauma score still useful? *ANZ J Surg*. 2003;73(11):944-948.

Gallagher J. Intra-abdominal hypertension. *AACN Adv Crit Care*. 2010;21(2):205-217.

Gentilello LM, Jurkovich GJ, Stark MS, et al. Is hypothermia in the victim of major trauma protective or harmful? A randomized, prospective study. *Ann Surg*. 1997;226(4):439-449.

Helm M, Lampl L, Hauke J, Bock KH. Accidental hypothermia in trauma patients: is it relevant to preclinical emergency treatment? *Anaesthetist*. 1995;44:101-107.

Holcomb JB, Tilley BC, Baraniuk S, et al. Transfusion of plasma, platelets, and red blood cells in a 1:1:1 vs a 1:1:2 ratio and mortality in patients with severe trauma: the PROPPR randomized clinical trial. *JAMA*. 2015;313(5):471-482.

Hughes CW. Use of an intra-aortic balloon catheter tamponade for controlling intra-abdominal hemorrhage in man. *Surgery*. 1954;36:65-68.

Kashuk JL, Moore EE, Millikan JS, Moore JB. Major abdominal vascular trauma: a unified approach. *J Trauma*. 1982;22(8):672-679.

Kauvar DS, Lefering R, Wade CE. Impact of hemorrhage on trauma outcome: an overview of epidemiology, clinical presentations, and therapeutic considerations. *J Trauma*. 2006;60(suppl 6):S3-S11.

Kirkpatrick AD, Roberts DJ, De Waele J, et al. Intra-abdominal hypertension and the abdominal compartment syndrome: updated consensus definitions and clinical practice guidelines from the World Society of the Abdominal Compartment Syndrome. *Intens Care Med*. 2013;39(7):1190-1206.

Martin SR, Kilgo PD, Miller PR, et al. Injury-associated hypothermia: an analysis of the 2004 National Trauma Data Bank. *Shock*. 2005;24(2):114-118.

Martinelli T, Thony F, Decléty P, et al. Intra-aortic balloon occlusion to salvage patients with life-threatening hemorrhagic shocks from pelvic fractures. *J Trauma*. 2010;68:942-948.

Marx JA, Hockberger RS, Walls RM. *Rosen's Emergency Medicine: Concepts and Clinical Practice*. 8th ed. St Louis, MO: Mosby; 2013.

McNelis J, Soffer S, Marini CP, et al. Abdominal compartment syndrome in the surgical intensive care unit. *Am Surg*. 2002;68(1):18-23.

Moffatt SE. Hypothermia in trauma. *Emerg Med J*. 2013;30(12):989-996.

Petrella F, Radice D, Colombo N, Mariolo AV, Diotti C, de Marini F. Pericardial-peritoneal window for malignant pericardial effusion. *Shanghai Chest*. 2018;2:1-6.

PHTLS Committee, National Association of Emergency Medical Technicians. *Prehospital Trauma Life Support*. 9th ed. Burlington, MA: Jones & Bartlett Learning; 2020.

Prytime Medical Devices. *The ER-REBOA Catheter Quick Reference Guide*. Boerne, TX. http://prytimemedical.com/wp-content/uploads/2017/08/ER-REBOA-Catheter-Quick-Reference-Guide-wall-poster.pdf. Accessed December 20, 2020.

Sasser SM, Hunt RC, Sullivent EE, et al. Guidelines for field triage of injured patients: recommendations of the national expert panel on field triage. *MMWR Recomm Rep*. 2012;61(RR-1):1-20.

Shiroff AM, Gale SC, Martin ND, et al. Penetrating neck trauma: a review of management strategies and discussion of the "no zone" approach. *Am Surg*. 2013;79(1):23-29.

Singer KE, Morris MC, Blakeman C, et al. Can resuscitative endovascular balloon occlusion of the aorta fly? Assessing aortic balloon performance for aeromedical evacuation. *J Surg Res*. 2020;254:390-397.

Sperry JL, Moore EE, Coimbra R, et al. Western Trauma Association critical decisions in trauma: penetrating neck trauma. *J Trauma Acute Care Surg*. 2013;75:936-940.

Stannard A, Eliason JL, Rasmussen TE. Resuscitative endovascular balloon occlusion of the aorta (REBOA) as an adjunct for hemorrhagic shock. *J Trauma*. 2011;71:1869-1872.

Trauma in pregnancy: a unique challenge. Mayo Clinic website. https://www.mayoclinic.org/medical-professionals/trauma/news/trauma-in-pregnancy-a-unique-challenge/mac-20431356. Published October 6, 2017. Accessed April 9, 2021.

Wang HE, Callaway CW, Peitzman AB, et al. Admission hypothermia and outcome after major trauma. *Crit Care Med*. 2005;33(6):1296-1301.

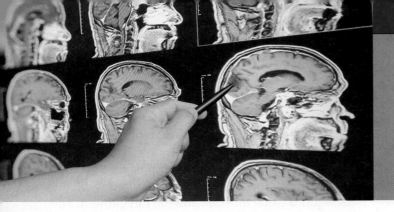

Chapter 12

Neurologic Emergencies

Heidi Hutchison, MD

OBJECTIVES

After completing this chapter, you will be able to:

1. Describe the major anatomic structures of the nervous system and their physiology (pp 544–561).

2. Describe how to perform a neurologic assessment, including the following specific assessments: Mini-Mental State Examination; assessment of speech abnormalities, cranial nerves, eyes, motor function, and sensory function; reflex testing; and evaluation of meningeal irritation (pp 561–575).

3. Discuss the pathophysiology of traumatic brain injury, including primary and secondary brain injuries (pp 579–581).

4. Explain the significance of cerebral perfusion pressure and mean arterial pressure (p 580).

5. Discuss the pathophysiology of specific neurologic injuries, including scalp injuries, skull fractures, facial fractures, epidural hematoma, subdural hematoma, and diffuse axonal injury (pp 581–589).

6. Define intracranial pressure (ICP) (p 590).

7. Explain the pathophysiology of increased ICP (pp 592–593).

8. Discuss clinical manifestations of increased ICP (p 593).

9. Discuss the concept of ICP monitoring, including indications, contraindications, complications, methods, and procedures (pp 593–601).

10. Describe the elements of multimodality monitoring (pp 601–603).

11. Discuss management of ICP during transport (p 606).

12. Discuss the pathophysiology of brain herniation (p 606).

13. Describe spinal cord injuries, including primary and secondary spinal cord injuries, complete and incomplete spinal cord injuries, and spinal and neurogenic shock (pp 607–609).

14. Explain the assessment, management, and complications of spinal cord injuries (pp 609–613).

15. Discuss types of stroke, including their assessment and management, and the use of fibrinolytic therapy (pp 613–616).

16. Describe the pathophysiology and management of intracerebral hemorrhage (p 618).

17. Describe the pathophysiology and management of subarachnoid hemorrhage (pp 618–619).

18. Describe the pathophysiology and management of Guillain-Barré syndrome (pp 619–620).

19. Discuss seizures and epilepsy, including their transport management (p 620).

20. Discuss transport considerations for patients with neurologic injuries—prior to transport, on scene, and during interhospital transport (pp 621–622).

21. Discuss considerations for managing neurologic emergencies in flight (p 622).

Introduction

Critical care patients with neurologic complications present a variety of assessment and management challenges during transport for the critical care transport professional (CCTP). The CCTP will find that an understanding of the underlying principles of neurologic structure, function, and dysfunction provides a sound basis for these patients' care. Patients with neurologic illness and injury require skilled care that includes a thorough history and physical examination as well as a variety of specialized interventions. An in-depth understanding of the various types of neurologic injuries, their pathophysiology, and current (evidence-based) management trends is fundamental to ensuring the best possible patient outcomes.

Anatomy and Physiology

The human nervous system is a truly remarkable arrangement of fibers running throughout the body that allows the body to interact with and adapt to differing environments by regulating the activities of virtually every other body system. An intimate understanding of the anatomy and physiology of the nervous system is essential to the delivery of competent medical care—and especially assessment—by the CCTP. This section reviews the structures and functions of the components of the nervous system that are most pertinent to the CCTP's care.

Nervous System Organization

The nervous system is perhaps the most diverse and highly organized organ system in the human body. Its various components are classified in terms of either their location or their function.

When classifying the parts in terms of their location, the nervous system is divided into the central nervous system (CNS), which consists of the brain and spinal cord, and the peripheral nervous system (PNS), which consists of the spinal and cranial nerves (CN). The parts of the PNS are also differentiated on the basis of which information is transmitted via the fibers. Most activities mediated by the nervous system occur as a result of sensory stimulation sensed by special receptors, such as visual, auditory, or tactile receptors. Afferent pathways (ascending pathways) carry sensory impulses toward the CNS. Efferent pathways (descending pathways) carry impulses away from the CNS to effector organs, such as muscles (smooth and skeletal) or glands **FIGURE 12-1**.

Physiologically, the nervous system consists of voluntary and involuntary divisions. The voluntary (somatic) nervous system is composed of nervous system fibers that connect the structures of the CNS with skeletal muscles and the integument. The involuntary (autonomic) nervous system is divided into sympathetic and parasympathetic branches, both of which are composed of nervous system fibers that connect the structures of the CNS with smooth muscle, cardiac muscle, and glands. Using these fibers, the involuntary nervous system regulates the body's internal environment by controlling specific organ systems. For example, the sympathetic nervous system is responsible for sweating, pupil dilation, ejaculation, and temperature regulation, as well as the shunting of blood from the periphery to the core—the flight-or-fight response.

Central Nervous System

The CNS consists of the brain and the spinal cord, both of which are encased in and protected by bone. The brain, located within the cranial cavity, is the largest component of the CNS. It contains billions of neurons that serve a variety of vital functions.

Cranial Anatomy and Physiology

The brain is a very delicate, gelatinous-like substance that requires the protection afforded by the skull. Although the skull primarily serves a protective function, excessive forces can cause a fracture to the adult skull and force bone fragments into vulnerable brain tissue.

The skull, or cranium, consists of the neurocranium (brain box) and the viscerocranium (the 14 bones that make up the facial skeleton). The neurocranium is the part of the skull that encloses the brain and provides a protective vault for this vital organ **FIGURE 12-2**. It has a domelike roof—the calvaria (skullcap)—and a cranial base. The neurocranium includes eight bones: the frontal bone, paired parietal bones, paired temporal bones, an occipital bone, a sphenoid bone, and an ethmoid bone.

When the skull is observed from the inside, the superior surfaces form a smooth inner wall. In contrast, the basilar skull contains many ridges and folds with sharp edges that normally provide structure for the support of many parts of the

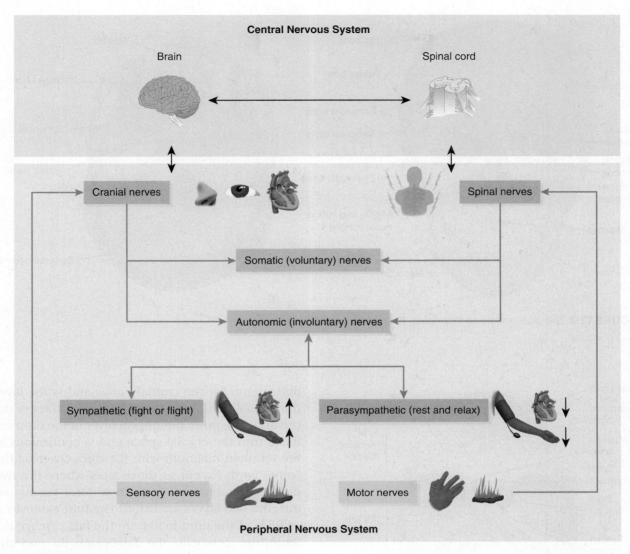

FIGURE 12-1 Organization of the nervous system.

© Jones & Bartlett Learning.

brain **FIGURE 12-3**. When the head comes into contact with significant forces, the brain may shift over this base and become lacerated or contused by the sharp edges. This mechanism is a culprit in many of the brain injuries encountered by the CCTP.

The base of the skull also contains openings, or foramina, that allow cranial nerves and blood vessels to enter and exit the cranial cavity. These openings also weaken the area, leaving it susceptible to fracture.

Meningeal Anatomy and Physiology

The entire CNS is enclosed by a set of three membranes collectively known as the meninges

Special Populations

Children have extremely pliable skull bones and often have not healed their suture lines or closed their fontanelle before the age of 8 years. Excessive forces can cause a fracture in the adult skull, but in a child they are more likely to result in brain injury without skull fracture.

FIGURE 12-4. The cranial meninges (internal to the neurocranium) protect the brain and form the supporting framework for arteries, veins, and venous sinuses. The cranial meninges consist of three layers:

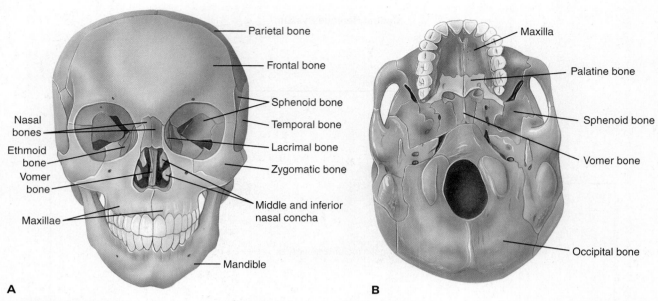

A

B

FIGURE 12-2 The skull and its components. **A.** Anterior view. **B.** Interior view.

© Jones & Bartlett Learning.

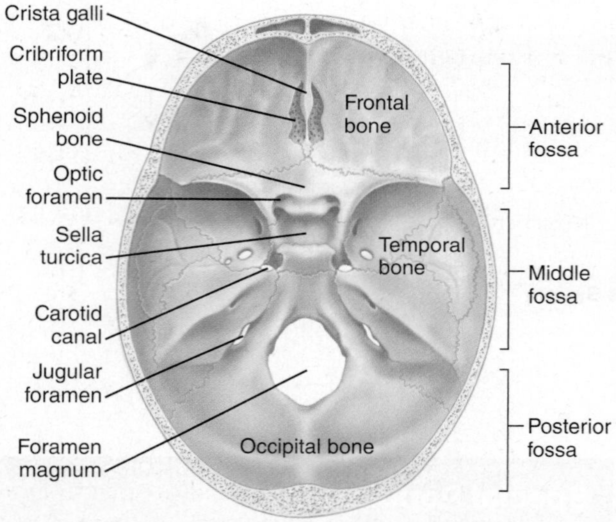

FIGURE 12-3 The floor of the cranial vault and its anatomy.

© Jones & Bartlett Learning.

(1) the **dura mater**, an external thick, dense fibrous membrane; (2) the **arachnoid mater**, an intermediate, delicate membrane; and (3) the **pia mater**, an internal delicate, vascular membrane.

The dura mater, which adheres to the internal surface of the cranium, is actually a two-layered membrane. The outer layer comprises the periosteum for the cranial bones and is the layer that actually connects to the internal surface of the calvaria. The inner meningeal layer of the dura extends into the cranial space and is continuous at the foramen magnum with the dura covering the spinal cord. Except at those sites where the two dural layers separate to form a dural venous sinus, the two layers are fused. The four extensions or folds of the dura mater are the falx cerebri, the tentorium cerebelli, the falx cerebelli, and the diaphragma sellae.

The **falx cerebri** is a double fold of dura mater that divides the cerebrum into right and left hemispheres by descending vertically into the longitudinal fissure that extends from the frontal lobe to the occipital lobe. This structure is observed to *shift* on computed tomography (CT) scan during times of increased intracranial pressure due to swelling or bleeding. It extends posteriorly by becoming continuous with the tentorium cerebelli.

The falx cerebri attaches to the **tentorium cerebelli** in the midline and holds it up, giving this extension a tent like appearance. The tentorium cerebelli separates the occipital lobes of the cerebrum from the cerebellum and brainstem. This fold of the dura mater divides the brain into an upper compartment (supratentorial) and a lower compartment (infratentorial). The tentorium cerebelli

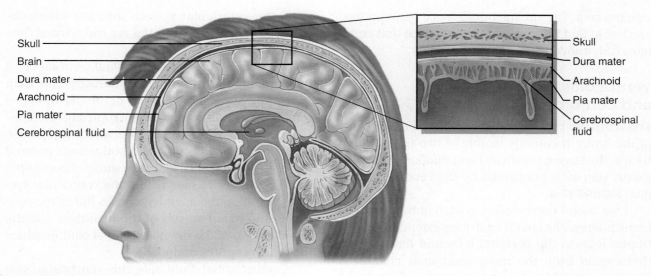

FIGURE 12-4 The meninges.

© Jones & Bartlett Learning.

is noted for its role in brain swelling or bleeding; it is the location where the **uncus** (the medially curved anterior part of the hippocampal gyrus) of the temporal lobe slips off of the tentorium and compresses cranial nerve (CN) III, which lies underneath the dural structure. This process causes a unilateral fixed and dilated pupil, characteristic of uncal herniation.

The **falx cerebelli** forms the division between the two lateral lobes of the cerebellum. The final extension of the dura mater, the **diaphragma sellae**, forms a roof over the sella turcica, which contains the pituitary gland.

Further dural separations form the **dural venous sinuses**, which are endothelial cell–lined spaces between the periosteal and meningeal layers of the dura mater. Large veins from the surface of the brain empty into these sinuses, and all blood from the brain ultimately drains through them into the internal jugular veins. These dural sinuses contain arachnoid granulations—tufted prolongations of the arachnoid mater that protrude through the meningeal layer of the dura into the venous sinuses and transfer cerebrospinal fluid (CSF) to the venous system.

The arachnoid mater is an extremely thin and delicate layer that loosely encloses the brain. It is in close contact with the meningeal layer of the dura mater owing to the pressure of the circulating CSF beneath the arachnoid layer. Web like arachnoid trabeculae (small protrusions of connective tissue)

pass between the arachnoid and the pia, connecting the two layers and forming the subarachnoid space, which contains CSF and a variety of cerebral arteries and veins. Although it is commonly stated that the brain *floats* in CSF, the brain is actually suspended in the CSF-filled subarachnoid space by the arachnoid trabeculae. In essence, the meninges and CSF form a fluid-filled cushion that protects the brain and spinal cord.

The pia mater is a vascular membrane that adheres to the surface of the brain and follows its contours. It is rich in small blood vessels that supply a large volume of arterial blood to cerebral tissues. In fact, at the point where the cerebral arteries penetrate the cerebral cortex, the pia follows them for a short distance, forming a pial coat and creating a periarterial space. Tufts or folds of the pia mater in the lateral, third, and fourth ventricles form a portion of the choroid plexus, which is responsible for the production of CSF.

Three meningeal spaces are associated with the cranial meninges. The **extradural space** (also known as the epidural space) is normally not an actual space but only a potential one between the cranial bones and the periosteal layer of the dura. It becomes a real space only when blood from torn vessels pushes the periosteum from the cranium and accumulates there. Likewise, the dura-arachnoid junction, also called the **subdural space**, is normally only a potential space but may develop into a real one after a blow to the head causes bleeding into the area. The subarachnoid space between the arachnoid and the pia is an actual space that contains CSF, trabeculae, arteries, and veins.

Ventricular System and Cerebrospinal Fluid

The ventricular system is the central CSF-filled core of the brain. It consists mainly of two lateral ventricles (the largest ventricles) and midline third and fourth ventricles connected by the cerebral aqueduct **FIGURE 12-5**.

One lateral ventricle lies in each of the cerebral hemispheres. The lateral ventricles extend from the frontal lobe to the occipital lobe and have horns that extend from the main ventricular chamber. They are named for the respective area of the cerebrum in which they are contained. These ventricles are important structures when **intracranial pressure (ICP)** monitoring, CSF drainage, or placement of a CSF shunt becomes necessary.

The **foramen of Monro** connects the two lateral ventricles with the third ventricle, a central cavity. Situated directly above the midbrain, the third ventricle lies between the structures of the thalamus in the diencephalon.

The **cerebral aqueduct**, the narrowest portion of the ventricular system, provides communication with the fourth ventricle, which lies between the brainstem and the cerebellum. Because of its small size, it is vulnerable to obstruction. At the base of the fourth ventricle, two openings, the **foramen of Luschka** and the **foramen of Magendie**, open the ventricular system into the subarachnoid space and are essential for the normal flow of CSF.

The **choroid plexus** of the lateral ventricles and the third and fourth ventricles produces more than 70% (approximately 500 mL/d) of the CSF by active transport and diffusion. Microscopically, the choroid plexus has the appearance of a delicate sponge, consisting of a collection of blood vessels covered by a thin coating of cells. These surfaces constantly secrete CSF. Other sites within the ventricular system, including the ependymal cells lining the ventricles and blood vessels of the meninges and the blood vessels of the brain and spinal cord, produce the remaining 30% of the CSF.

Cerebrospinal fluid fills the ventricular system and surrounds the brain and spinal cord in the subarachnoid space. It provides some measure of protection for the CNS by acting as a *shock absorber* in minor acceleration and deceleration incidents; it also participates in the removal of waste products from cerebral tissue. CSF is normally clear, colorless, and odorless. The total volume of CSF is approximately 150 mL, of which only 23 mL is found in the ventricles; the remaining 127 mL fills the subarachnoid space surrounding the brain and spinal cord. Under normal conditions, CSF contains very few cells and is low in proteins, glucose, potassium ions, and calcium ions relative to plasma **TABLE 12-1**. In contrast, it is high in magnesium, sodium, and chloride ions as compared to plasma.

Cerebrospinal fluid also has a slightly lower osmolality (289 mOsm/L) compared with serum (290 to 300 mOsm/L). This osmotic gradient is responsible for the transport of small molecules, metabolic products, and drugs from the surrounding brain tissue into the CSF. Likewise, administration of hypertonic solutions promotes diffusion in the opposite direction, removing CSF from the brain and spinal cord.

No feedback mechanisms exist for the regulation of the rate or volume of CSF production. That is, the choroid plexus continues to produce CSF even if the ventricles and subarachnoid spaces are filled and the pressure is high. Consequently, any obstruction to the normal flow of CSF, either in the ventricular system or at the level of the arachnoid granulations, may produce high CSF pressure and lead to brain damage.

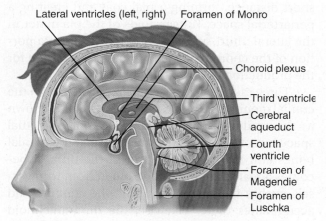

Lateral ventricles (left, right)   Foramen of Monro
Choroid plexus
Third ventricle
Cerebral aqueduct
Fourth ventricle
Foramen of Magendie
Foramen of Luschka

FIGURE 12-5 The ventricles of the brain and the cerebral aqueduct.

© Jones & Bartlett Learning.

TABLE 12-1 Composition of Cerebrospinal Fluid

Property (Substance)	Value (Normal Range)
pH	7.35–7.45
Specific gravity	1.007
Glucose	70–110 mg/dL
Protein	5–8 g/dL
Pressure	7–20 cm (lumbar puncture) 3–15 mm Hg (brain ventricle)
Potassium	3.5–5.0 mEq/L
Sodium	136–142 mEq/L
Chloride	96–106 mEq/L
Calcium	4.60–5.08 mg/dL
Magnesium	1.3–2.1 mEq/L
Carbon dioxide	22–28 mEq/L

© Jones & Bartlett Learning.

Once the CSF is formed in the ventricles, it flows within the closed system. Fluid formed in the two lateral ventricles passes into the third ventricle by way of the two foramina of Monro. The fluid then flows through the cerebral aqueduct into the fourth ventricle. CSF exits the fourth ventricle by taking one of two paths. In the first path, it exits medially through the foramen of Magendie, where it is then directed to the subarachnoid space of the spinal cord. In the second path, CSF exits the fourth ventricle laterally through the two foramina of Luschka, where it is directed to the subarachnoid space surrounding the brain.

On entering the subarachnoid space, CSF moves over the surface of the spinal cord and brain, then ultimately leaves the subarachnoid space and enters the dural venous sinuses via the arachnoid villi. The arachnoid villi are highly permeable one-way valves that allow CSF to exit easily from the subarachnoid space into the venous sinuses, but do not allow blood to enter the subarachnoid space. Blockage of CSF's movement into the dural venous sinuses leads to a condition known as communicating hydrocephalus. If CSF cannot leave the ventricular system, the condition is called noncommunicating hydrocephalus.

Anatomy and Physiology of the Brain

The brain gives humans the ability to reason, function intellectually, express personality and mood, and interact with their environment. This organ weighs approximately 3 pounds (1 kg), a meager 2% of body weight, yet consumes 20% of the total cardiac output. The three major areas of the brain are the cerebrum, the brainstem, and the cerebellum.

Cerebrum

The cerebrum is, by mass, the largest part of the brain, accounting for 80% of its weight. It consists of two cerebral hemispheres that are incompletely separated by the longitudinal cerebral fissure. Both hemispheres are connected at the base of the longitudinal cerebral fissure by the **corpus callosum**, a large tract of transverse fibers that provides a communication link between the two cerebral hemispheres. The hemispheres are further separated from the underlying brainstem and cerebellum by the transverse cerebral fissure. Both the longitudinal and transverse cerebral fissures contain meninges and thick folds of dura: specifically, the falx cerebri and the tentorium cerebelli.

The surface of the cerebrum is characterized by numerous convolutions called **gyri**. The gyri functionally increase the cortical surface area. Grooves between adjacent gyri are called **sulci**, and the deepest grooves are referred to as **fissures**.

The **cerebral cortex** is the outermost layer of the cerebrum. This layer is 2 to 5 mm thick and contains billions of unmyelinated cell bodies of dendrites and neurons, which are often referred to as gray matter. Underneath the cerebral cortex are the white matter (myelinated) tracts, which communicate impulses from the cerebral cortex to other areas of the brain. Three types of fibers are found in the white matter; they are named for the role they play in communicating information:

- *Commissural* (transverse) fibers are tracts that communicate between corresponding parts of the two hemispheres. The corpus callosum is the largest of these fiber tracts.
- *Projection* fibers communicate between the cerebral cortex and lower portions of the brain and spinal cord.
- *Association* fibers allow communication between various regions of the same hemisphere.

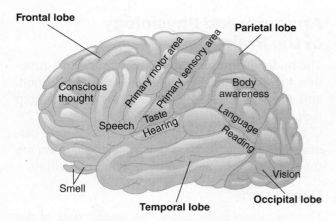

FIGURE 12-6 The lobes of the cerebrum.

© Jones & Bartlett Learning.

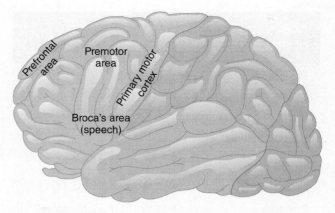

FIGURE 12-7 The frontal lobe of the cerebrum is divided into specific areas based on function.

© Jones & Bartlett Learning.

The **cerebral hemispheres** are divided into four paired lobes, based on the divisions demarcated by the fissures: the frontal lobes, the parietal lobes, the temporal lobes, and the occipital lobe **FIGURE 12-6**. In everyday speech, and indeed throughout this chapter, the paired lobes are referred to in the singular form; for example, *the frontal lobe* can be understood to mean the structure comprising both lobes. Another area found deeper inside the cerebrum, the so-called limbic lobe, is also classified as a lobe, although it is technically part of the temporal lobe.

Frontal Lobe

The largest of the four lobes of the cerebral hemispheres is the **frontal lobe**, which accounts for approximately one-third of the total cortical tissue. The frontal lobe lies underneath the frontal bone of the skull; it is separated posteriorly from the parietal lobe by the central fissure and inferiorly from the temporal lobe by the lateral fissure. It is further divided into different areas based on the functions for which those regions are responsible **FIGURE 12-7**.

The **prefrontal area** of the frontal lobe is responsible for a variety of higher functions. This area controls thought, concentration, depth perception, abstract thinking, memory, and autonomic nervous system responses to emotional changes, with help from the thalamus and hypothalamus.

The **premotor area** lies adjacent to the motor area. These areas are connected by cranial nerves III, IV, VI, IX, X, and XII, allowing for coordination of certain movements. For example, stimulation of the lateral portion results in gross generalized movements, such as turning of the eyes and head, turning of the trunk with the head, and coordinated eye movements.

The **motor area** contains pyramidal cells that control voluntary motor function on the opposite side of the body. Body parts that require a great deal of dexterity, such as the thumb and tongue, are allotted a larger motor area than are body parts that do not require much dexterity, such as the shoulder and trunk.

The **Broca area**, located at the inferior frontal gyrus, is an associative area that participates in the formulation of words. Any damage to this area, from either primary injury (direct trauma) or secondary injury (ischemia), results in expressive or nonfluent aphasia.

Parietal Lobe

The **parietal lobe** is situated directly posterior to the frontal lobe and lateral to the central fissure. This lobe is largely responsible for sensory functions, including the integration of sensory information; awareness of body parts; interpretation of touch, pressure, and pain; and recognition of object size, shape, and texture. The parietal lobe consists of a sensory strip that lies adjacent to the motor strip of the frontal lobe. Sensory areas for certain parts of the body are located close to the motor areas for the same body part. Fibers going to the sensory strip carry input associated with cutaneous and deep sensibility sensations, as well as cutaneous sensations of touch, pressure, position, and vibration. Input from the thalamus also reaches the sensory strip.

Associative areas of the parietal lobe interpret sensory input in terms of size, shape, texture, and weight. They enable individuals to localize sensations and define them in terms of pressure, temperature, or vibration. Interpretive aspects of the parietal lobe's response to stimuli include awareness of body parts, orientation in space, and recognition of environmental spatial relationships.

Occipital Lobe

Occupying the most posterior portion of the cerebrum, the occipital lobe is separated from the cerebellum by the tentorium cerebelli. This area of the brain is the primary receptive area for vision, specifically the interpretation of visual stimuli. The primary visual cortex receives impulses from projections of the optic tract; these impulses are then referred to the visual associative areas for interpretation and integration. A person who sustains an injury to the visual associative areas will be able to see objects but will not be able to recognize or identify them (a condition known as visual agnosia).

Temporal Lobe

Located beneath the temporal bone of the cranium, the temporal lobe lies in the lateral portion of the cerebrum. It is separated from the frontal and parietal lobes by the lateral fissure. The primary functions of this region relate to hearing, speech, behavior, and memory.

Within the temporal lobe, the primary auditory receptive areas receive sound impulses and assist in determining the sound's source and interpreting its meaning. The auditory associative area is part of the superior temporal gyrus and is known as the Wernicke area. Usually the largest part of the dominant hemisphere, it is responsible for comprehension of both written and spoken words. If the Wernicke area becomes damaged, a person may hear sounds, but they will be meaningless (a condition known as receptive aphasia).

In the superior portion of the temporal lobe, at the junction of the frontal, parietal, and temporal lobes, lies the interpretative area. This area is responsible for integrating the auditory, visual, and somatic associative areas to form complex thoughts and memory. It plays a significant role, along with the frontal lobe, in cerebration.

Limbic Lobe

The limbic lobe (also called the rhinencephalon) is, strictly speaking, an anatomic part of the temporal

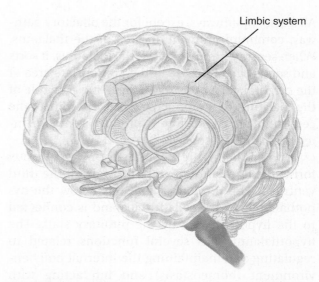

FIGURE 12-8 The limbic system is the seat of emotions, instincts, and other functions.
© Jones & Bartlett Learning.

lobe, although its function is sometimes discussed separately from the temporal lobe. This area forms the border of the lateral ventricles and contains the hippocampus, uncus, primary olfactory cortex, and amygdaloid nucleus. Functions of the limbic lobe include self-preservation, primitive behavior, moods, the visceral processes associated with emotion, short-term memory, and the interpretation of smell **FIGURE 12-8**.

Diencephalon

The diencephalon is a major division of the cerebrum, which itself is divided into four regions: the thalamus, the hypothalamus, the subthalamus, and the epithalamus. The lowest structure of the cerebrum, the diencephalon actually lies on top of the brainstem surrounding the third ventricle. Also found in this region are the pituitary gland and the internal capsule.

The thalamus, the largest portion of the diencephalon, consists of a pair of egg-shaped masses of gray matter that form the lateral walls of the third ventricle and are connected to the midbrain. This structure acts as a relay station for motor and sensory activity; basic neuronal activity, such as the processing of brain activity; and memory, thought, emotion, and complex behavior. The relay role performed by the thalamus is a complex function coordinated with the parietal lobe of the cerebrum.

All sensory pathways, except for the olfactory pathway, communicate with an area of the thalamus. When sensory impulses reach the thalamus, it sorts and sends each impulse to the appropriate area of the cerebral cortex for final processing. The role of the thalamus in motor activity is to coordinate the cerebrum and cerebellum to produce a smooth, integrated motor response.

Located below the thalamus, the **hypothalamus** forms the floor and the anterior walls of the third ventricle. The pituitary gland lies below the hypothalamus in the sella turcica and is connected to the hypothalamus by the pituitary stalk. The hypothalamus has several functions related to regulating and maintaining the internal body environment (homeostasis) and interacting with the limbic system to generate physical responses to emotions (implementation of behavioral patterns). The hypothalamus exerts its influence through the endocrine system and neuronal pathways **TABLE 12-2**.

The **epithalamus** is located in the **dorsal** portion of the diencephalon and contains the pineal gland, which is thought to play a role in physical growth and sexual development. The **subthalamus**, which is located below the thalamus, is closely related to the basal ganglia in terms of its function.

Basal Ganglia

The **basal ganglia** comprise several masses of nuclei located deep within the cerebral hemispheres. These structures are primarily associated with fine motor function, particularly of the hands and lower extremities. They provide a pathway between, and assist in processing information from, the cerebral motor cortex and the thalamus. Much of the basal ganglia's function is conducted through the extrapyramidal (involuntary) pathways.

Internal Capsule

As radiation and projection fibers coming from various parts of the cerebral cortex converge at the brainstem, they form the corona radiata. At the point where the fibers enter the thalamus-hypothalamus region, they are collectively called the **internal capsule**. Thus, the capsule is a massive bundle of efferent and afferent fibers connecting the various subdivisions of the brain and spinal cord.

TABLE 12-2 Functions of the Hypothalamus

Function	Mechanism
Temperature regulation	Temperature of blood flowing through the hypothalamus is monitored. Impulses are sent to the sweat glands, peripheral vessels, and muscles (shivering).
Regulation of food intake	The hunger center produces the sensation of hunger when stimulated. The satiety center decreases the desire for food when the stomach is full or blood glucose is high.
Regulation of water intake	The hypothalamus monitors serum osmotic pressure; it triggers the release of antidiuretic hormone when osmotic pressure is high and inhibits this hormone's release when osmotic pressure is low.
Control of pituitary gland secretion	Releasing or inhibiting factors are sent from the hypothalamus to the pituitary gland.
Control of behavioral responses	The hypothalamus mediates visible physical expressions in response to emotions, such as blushing, dryness of mouth, and clammy hands.
Control of the autonomic nervous system	Stimulation responses of the anterior region of the hypothalamus elicit the parasympathetic system response. The posterior region of the hypothalamus mediates the sympathetic system response.

© Jones & Bartlett Learning.

Brainstem

The brainstem acts as a bridge between the cerebral hemispheres and the spinal cord; it is the only structure connecting the cerebellum with the cerebral cortex. All motor and sensory fibers, both those ascending to the cerebral hemispheres and those descending to the spinal cord, travel through the brainstem. The brainstem consists of three parts: the midbrain, the pons, and the medulla oblongata.

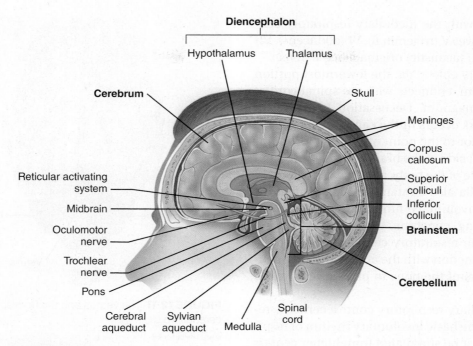

FIGURE 12-9 The midbrain.

© Jones & Bartlett Learning.

The **midbrain** is a small area extending between the diencephalon, the pons, and the third ventricle **FIGURE 12-9**. Several important structures are found in the midbrain, including the cerebral aqueduct (Sylvian, which connects the third and fourth ventricles), the superior colliculi (which controls visual reflexes and the center for upward gaze) and inferior colliculi (auditory system), cranial nerves III (oculomotor) and IV (trochlear), and the reticular activating system (RAS).

The midbrain's major function is to relay stimuli involved in voluntary motor movement of the body. The tectospinal and rubrospinal tracts of the extrapyramidal (involuntary) motor system are also found in this region: The **tectospinal tract** controls reflex motor movements in response to visual and auditory stimuli, whereas the **rubrospinal tract** controls the tone of flexor muscles. The **Edinger-Westphal nucleus** is located in the midbrain and is responsible for mediating the autonomic reflex centers that govern pupillary accommodation to light.

Located between the midbrain and the medulla oblongata, the **pons FIGURE 12-10** relays information to and from the brain and spinal cord along fiber tracts. Motor tracts for motor movement descend through the pons, and sensory tracts necessary for touch, pressure, proprioception, pain, and

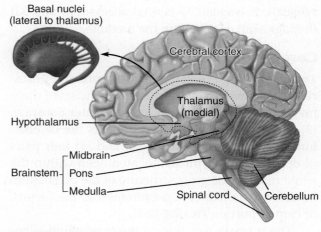

FIGURE 12-10 The pons.

© Jones & Bartlett Learning.

temperature ascend through the pons. The **ventral** surface of the pons contains fibers that connect to the cerebellum, which allows for efficient and smooth transmission of information from the cerebellum to the cerebral cortex. Two respiratory control centers are found in the pons: the apneustic center, which is responsible for stimulating and producing sustained respirations, and the pneumotaxic center, which antagonizes the apneustic center, clinically inhibiting inspiration. Both centers of control communicate with the medullary respiratory center. Cranial nerves V (trigeminal), VI (abducens), VII (facial), and VIII (acoustic) originate in the pons.

The **medulla oblongata**, the lowermost portion of the brainstem, connects with the spinal cord at the foramen magnum. Decussation (crossing) of the motor fibers occurs in the caudal aspect of the medulla. Inferior to the point of decussation, stimuli from the left side of the brain control movement on the right side of the body, and vice versa.

The medulla also contains groups of neurons that control involuntary functions such as swallowing, vomiting, coughing, vasoconstriction, and respiration. The respiratory center of the medulla works in conjunction with the apneustic and pneumotaxic centers of the pons to produce controlled respirations.

The medullary respiratory control center is responsible for the basic involuntary rhythm of respiration, but must be stimulated from higher centers to maintain a life-sustaining respiratory pattern. The reticular formation also has its beginnings in the medulla, with cranial nerves IX (glossopharyngeal), X (vagus), XI (spinal accessory), and XII (hypoglossal) exiting from the medulla.

Cerebellum

The cerebellum is located just superior and posterior to the medulla oblongata and consists of three major parts: (1) the cortex, or gray outer covering; (2) the white matter, which connects the cerebellum to other parts of the CNS; and (3) four pairs of deep cerebellar nuclei, located deep within the white matter. The gross structure of the cerebellum includes two distinct hemispheres and the vermis, or central portion **FIGURE 12-11**.

The primary function of the cerebellum is coordination of voluntary movement. The vermis is responsible for trunk control. The three lobes of the hemispheres are responsible for upper and lower extremity control, including control of antigravity muscles, proprioception, tactile impulses, motor tone facilitation, volitional breaks in movement, synergy of movement, and equilibrium. Input is received from sensory pathways of the spinal cord, the brainstem, and the cerebrum; output is transmitted through the descending motor pathways. Cerebellar influences work through continual excitatory and inhibiting stimuli, resulting in smooth motor movements instead of rapid, erratic movements.

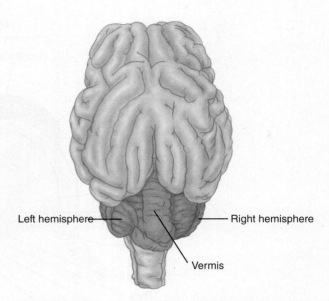

FIGURE 12-11 The vermis and the hemispheres of the cerebellum.

© Jones & Bartlett Learning.

Reticular Formation

The **reticular formation (RF)** comprises a set of neurons that extends from the upper level of the spinal cord, through the medulla, pons, and midbrain, and into the thalamus and cerebral cortex. Composed of both motor and sensory tracts, the RF is closely tied to functions of the basal ganglia, thalamus, cerebellum, and cerebral cortex. This bundle of neural fibers has many excitatory and some inhibitory capabilities, and can enhance, suppress, or modify impulse transmission. The main role of the descending RF is to provide a balance between the excitatory and inhibitory stimuli so as to maintain normal muscle tone, which supports the body against gravity. Also located in the RF are centers for blood pressure (BP), respiration, and heart rate function. The ascending RF is essential for arousal, attention, and perceptual association.

Reticular Activating System

The **reticular activating system (RAS)** is a diffuse system—not an actual anatomic structure—that extends from the lower brainstem to the cerebral cortex. Input from multiple sensory pathways is received in the RAS, and signals are transmitted to various areas of the cerebral cortex, providing multiple opportunities for stimulation of the RAS.

The lower portion of the RAS, which is rooted in the brainstem, assists with control of sleep-wakefulness cycles and consciousness; the upper portion, which is in the thalamus, facilitates focusing attention on a specific task. When the upper portion of the RAS sustains damage, the person enters a vegetative state, exhibiting sleep-wake cycles and other brainstem functions but no upper levels of cerebration.

Cerebral Circulation

The brain makes huge demands on the other body systems: 15% to 20% of total cardiac output and 40% of the oxygen in the available blood are required to meet normal cerebral metabolic needs. The predominant metabolic process that occurs in the brain is the oxidation of glucose to provide energy. Therefore, the overall goal of cerebral circulation is to provide enough blood to supply oxygen, glucose, and nutrients for this process.

The total amount of blood received by the brain is distributed carefully among those areas with high metabolic demands. Carbon dioxide serves as the primary regulator for blood flow in the CNS. A potent vasodilator, its presence causes more blood to flow to certain areas of the brain. The brain is supplied blood by two pairs of arteries: the two vertebral arteries and the two internal carotid arteries **FIGURE 12-12**.

Circle of Willis

The circle of Willis is a collection of arteries located at the base of the skull that is divided into anterior and posterior circulation branches **FIGURE 12-13**. Its physiologic significance derives from the fact that this structure may be able to compensate for reduced blood flow from any one of the major contributors to cerebral circulation. Some individuals, however, may have hypoplastic or missing communicating vessels, which may inhibit this compensatory mechanism.

The circle of Willis is fed by the internal carotid and basilar arteries. The three cerebral arteries (anterior, middle, and posterior) supplying each hemisphere are connected by communicating arteries to form a complete circle. **TABLE 12-3** lists the areas of the brain supplied by the cerebral arteries.

Vertebral Arteries

The vertebral arteries, or posterior circulation, arise from the subclavian arteries and enter the skull through the foramen magnum, ventrolateral to the spinal cord. At the level of the pons, the two vertebral arteries join to form the basilar artery. The basilar artery then divides at the level of the midbrain to form paired posterior cerebral arteries. The vertebral arteries and their branches predominantly

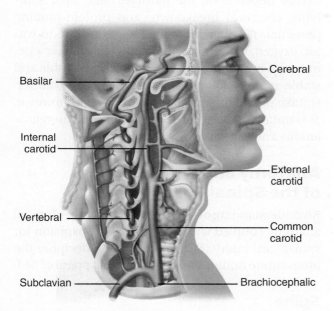

FIGURE 12-12 Blood supply to the brain via arteries.
© Jones & Bartlett Learning.

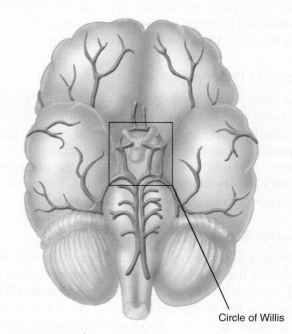

FIGURE 12-13 The circle of Willis.
© Jones & Bartlett Learning.

TABLE 12-3 Major Cerebral Arteries	
Cerebral Artery Origin	**Structures Supplied**
Anterior	Basal ganglia, corpus callosum, medial surface of cerebral hemispheres, and superior surface of frontal and parietal lobes
Middle	Frontal lobe, parietal lobe, and cortical surface of temporal lobe
Posterior	Occipital lobes and the medial and lateral aspects of the temporal lobe

© Jones & Bartlett Learning.

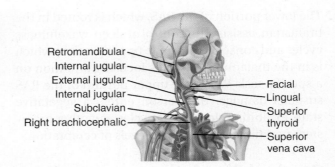

FIGURE 12-14 The veins of the neck.

© Jones & Bartlett Learning.

supply blood to the cerebellum, brainstem, and spinal cord, as well as to some parts of the cerebrum. The basilar artery continues upward into the posterior portion of the circle of Willis and into the two posterior cerebral arteries.

Internal Carotid Arteries

The internal carotid arteries anteriorly supply a proportionately greater amount of blood flow. They originate from the common carotid arteries and enter the cranium through the base of the skull. At the base of the brain, the internal carotid arteries connect to the circle of Willis and then branch into the anterior and middle cerebral arteries, which provide the majority of the anterior circulation.

Venous Drainage

The superficial and deep veins of the brain enter the dural venous sinuses, which subsequently drain into the internal jugular veins. Cerebral veins on the superolateral surfaces of the brain drain into the superior sagittal sinus. Cerebral veins on the postero-inferior aspect drain into the straight, transverse, and superior petrosal sinuses **FIGURE 12-14**.

Blood–Brain Barrier

Several protective mechanisms act together to maintain the delicate balance of the brain's internal environment. Particularly noteworthy in this respect is the blood–brain barrier, the network of endothelial cells and astrocytes (neuroglia) that envelops the fragile cerebral capillaries. The blood–brain barrier is found throughout the brain except in small areas of the fourth ventricle, hypothalamus, and pineal gland, where chemoreceptors and osmoreceptors sample the circulating plasma. This barrier regulates the transport of nutrients, ions, water, drugs, and waste products through the process of selective permeability.

From a functional standpoint, the blood–brain barrier features tight junctions between adjacent capillary endothelial cells; in contrast, the capillaries found elsewhere in the body have pores between adjacent endothelial cells. Some molecules are easily transported through the endothelial cells in the blood–brain barrier, whereas this barrier blocks other toxic or harmful compounds so as to protect the fragile neurons.

Passage of substances across the blood–brain barrier depends on the particles' size, lipid solubility, chemical breakdown, and protein-binding potential. This barrier is readily permeable to water, oxygen, carbon dioxide, and glucose. Likewise, most drugs or compounds that are lipid soluble and stable at a physiologic pH rapidly cross the barrier. Uptake of sodium and potassium is slow, however, as is uptake of dyes and other organic and inorganic anions and cations.

Anatomy and Physiology of the Spinal Cord

An understanding of the form and function of spinal anatomy coupled with a high level of suspicion for spinal cord injury (SCI) is required to decipher the often subtle findings associated with a possible SCI.

Spine

The spine usually consists of 33 irregular bones (vertebrae) that articulate to form the vertebral

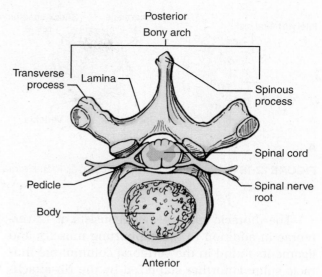

FIGURE 12-16 The human vertebra.

© Jones & Bartlett Learning.

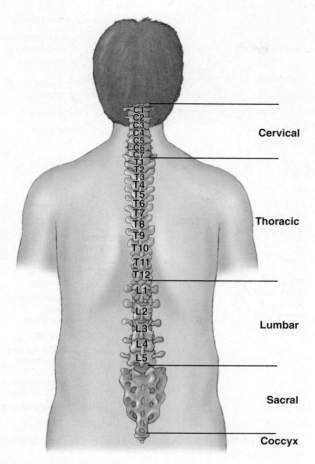

FIGURE 12-15 The sections of the vertebral column, with the letter/number of each vertebra labeled.

© Jones & Bartlett Learning.

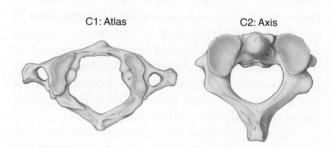

FIGURE 12-17 Superior view of the structure of the atlas and axis.

© Jones & Bartlett Learning.

column, which is the major structural component of the axial skeleton **FIGURE 12-15**. Some patients may have 32 or 34 vertebrae. These skeletal components are stabilized by both ligaments and muscles. Together these components support and protect neural elements while allowing for fluid movement and erect stature.

Vertebrae are identified according to their location as cervical, thoracic, lumbar, sacral, or coccyx. Each vertebra is unique in appearance, but collectively they share basic structural characteristics. The **vertebral body**, or anterior weight-bearing structure, is made of bone that provides support and stability. Shared components of most vertebrae include the body, lamina, pedicles, and spinous processes **FIGURE 12-16**.

The inferior border of each pedicle contains a notch forming the **intervertebral foramen**. This space in the middle of the vertebra allows for the exit of a peripheral nerve root and spinal vein as well as the entrance of a spinal artery on both sides at each vertebral junction.

The transverse spinous processes constitute the junction of each pedicle and the lamina on each side of a vertebra. They project laterally and posteriorly and form points of attachments for muscles and ligaments. The posterior spinous process is formed by the fusion of the posterior lamina and serves as an attachment site for muscles and ligaments.

The cervical spine includes the first seven bones of the vertebral column and its supporting structures. In addition to protecting the cervical spinal cord, the cervical spine supports the weight of the head and permits a high degree of mobility in multiple planes. The atlas (C1) and axis (C2) are uniquely suited to allow for rotational movement of the skull **FIGURE 12-17**.

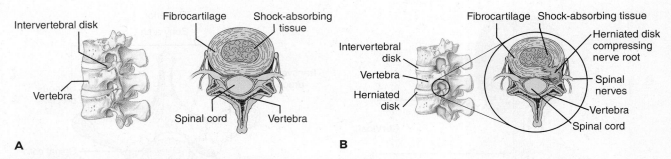

FIGURE 12-18 A. Normal, uninjured vertebral disk. **B.** Herniated disk.

© Jones & Bartlett Learning.

The thoracic spine usually consists of 12 vertebrae in addition to the supporting muscles and ligaments found in the vertebral column; the thoracic spine is further stabilized by the rib attachments. The spinous processes in this section of the spine are slightly larger, reflecting their role as attachment points for the muscles that hold the upper body erect and assist with the movement of the thoracic cavity during respiration. In patients with more than five lumbar vertebrae, there will be fewer than 12 thoracic vertebrae. Although this may seem insignificant, for the purposes of radiographic interpretation, thoracic and lumbar bodies are usually counted together rather than separately.

The lumbar spine, which includes the five largest bones in the vertebral column, is integral in carrying a large portion of the upper body weight. It is especially susceptible to injury because of this weight-bearing capacity.

The sacrum is composed of five fused vertebrae that form the posterior plate of the pelvis. The coccyx is made up of three to five small fused vertebrae. Coccyx injuries, although often extremely painful, are typically clinically insignificant.

Each vertebra is separated and cushioned by intervertebral disks that limit bone wear and act as shock absorbers. As the body ages, these disks lose water content and become thinner, causing the height loss associated with aging. Stress on the vertebral column may cause a disk to herniate into the spinal canal, resulting in a spinal cord or nerve root injury **FIGURE 12-18**.

Although the vertebrae must be able to stabilize the spinal cord, the muscles, tendons, and ligaments that connect the vertebrae do allow the vertebral column a degree of flexion and extension. The vertebral column can sustain normal flexion and extension of 60% to 70% without stressing the spinal cord. Flexion or extension beyond those

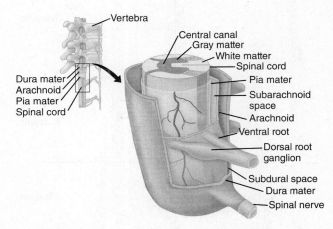

FIGURE 12-19 The spinal cord and its layers. The meninges enclose the brain and spinal cord.

© Jones & Bartlett Learning.

limits may damage structural ligaments and allow excess vertebral movement that could expose the spinal cord to injury.

Spinal Cord

The spinal cord transmits nerve impulses between the brain and the rest of the body. Located at the base of the brain, it represents the continuation of the CNS. This bundle of nerve fibers leaves the skull through a large opening at its base called the foramen magnum. The large size of the foramen magnum relative to other foramina makes it a common location for brain herniation.

The spinal cord extends from the base of the skull to L2; here it separates into the cauda equina, a collection of individual nerve roots. Thirty-one pairs of spinal nerves arise from the different segments of the spinal cord; each pair is named according to its corresponding segment.

A cross section of the spinal cord **FIGURE 12-19** reveals a butterfly-shaped central core of gray matter that is composed of neural cell bodies and

TABLE 12-4 Major Spinal Tracts

Spinal Tract	Function
Anterior	
Anterior spinothalamic tracts (ascending)	Carry sensation of crude touch and pressure sensation to the brain
Lateral spinothalamic tracts (ascending)	Carry pain and temperature information
Spinocerebellar tracts (ascending)	Coordinate impulses necessary for muscular movements by carrying impulses from muscles in the legs and trunk to the cerebellum
Corticospinal tracts (descending)	Voluntary motor commands
Reticulospinal tracts (descending)	Muscle tone and sweat gland activity
Rubrospinal tracts (descending)	Muscle tone
Posterior	
Fasciculus gracilis and cuneatus	**Proprioception**, vibration, light touch, deep pressure, **two-point discrimination**, and **stereognosis**

© Jones & Bartlett Learning.

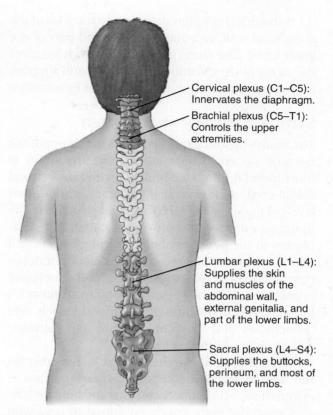

FIGURE 12-20 Nerve roots converge in plexuses, allowing them to function as a group.

© Jones & Bartlett Learning.

Image labels:
Cervical plexus (C1–C5): Innervates the diaphragm.
Brachial plexus (C5–T1): Controls the upper extremities.
Lumbar plexus (L1–L4): Supplies the skin and muscles of the abdominal wall, external genitalia, and part of the lower limbs.
Sacral plexus (L4–S4): Supplies the buttocks, perineum, and most of the lower limbs.

synapses. This gray matter is divided into posterior (dorsal) horns, which carry sensory input, and anterior (ventral) horns, which innervate the motor nerve of that segment. Surrounding the gray matter on each side are three columns of peripheral white matter composed of myelinated ascending and descending fiber pathways. Messages are relayed to and from the brain through these spinal tracts.

The brainstem connects the spinal cord to the remainder of the brain. All but two of the 12 cranial nerves exit from the brainstem. Specific groups of nerves are named based on their source of origin and point of termination. Ascending tracts carry information to the brain, and descending tracts carry information to the rest of the body **TABLE 12-4**.

Peripheral Nervous System

Spinal Nerves

The 31 pairs of spinal nerves emerge from each side of the spinal cord and are named for the vertebral region and level from which they arise. The eight cervical roots perform different functions in the scalp, neck, shoulders, and arms. The 12 thoracic nerve roots have varying functions: The upper thoracic nerves supply muscles of the chest that help in breathing and coughing, whereas the lower thoracic nerves provide abdominal muscle control and are part of the sympathetic nervous system. The five lumbar nerve roots supply hip flexors and leg muscles, as well as provide sensation to the anterior legs. The five sacral nerves provide for bowel and bladder control, sexual function, and sensation in the posterior legs and rectum. The coccyx has a single nerve root.

Nerve roots occasionally converge in a cluster called a **plexus** that permits peripheral nerve roots to rejoin and function as a group **FIGURE 12-20**. For example, the cervical plexus includes C1 through C5; the phrenic nerve (C3 through C5) arises from this plexus and innervates the diaphragm. The brachial plexus (C5 through T1) joins nerves controlling the upper extremities; the main nerves arising from this plexus are the axillary, median, musculocutaneous, radial, and ulnar nerves. The lumbar plexus

(L1 through L4) supplies the skin and muscles of the abdominal wall, external genitalia, and part of the lower limbs. The sacral plexus (L4 through S4) gives rise to the pudendal and sciatic nerves and supplies the buttocks, perineum, and most of the lower limbs.

Sympathetic Nervous System

The brain's hypothalamus controls the sympathetic nervous system. Information from the brain is transmitted through the brainstem and the cervical spinal cord, then exits at the thoracic and lumbar levels of the spine to reach the target structures. The thoracolumbar system provides sympathetic stimulation to the periphery largely through alpha and beta receptors. Alpha receptor stimulation induces contraction of smooth muscles in blood vessels and bronchioles. Beta receptors respond to stimulation by relaxing smooth muscles in blood vessels and bronchioles, and have chronotropic and inotropic effects on myocardial cells.

An SCI at or above the level of T6 may disrupt the flow of sympathetic communication. Loss of sympathetic stimulation can disrupt homeostasis and leave the body poorly equipped to deal with changes in its environment. Stimulation of sympathetic nerves without parasympathetic input can cause sympathetic overdrive, resulting in autonomic dysreflexia.

Parasympathetic Nervous System

The parasympathetic nervous system includes fibers arising from the brainstem and upper spinal cord that carry signals to organs of the abdomen, heart, lungs, and the skin above the waist. The vagus nerve (or 10th cranial nerve) travels from its origins outside of the medulla to the heart via the carotid arteries; thus, vagal tone remains intact following a spine injury. When the sympathetic nerves are stimulated and produce autonomic dysreflexia, the parasympathetic nerves attempt to control the rapidly increasing BP by slowing the heart rate. Parasympathetic nerves that supply the reproductive organs, pelvis, and legs begin at the sacral level (S2 through S4). The parasympathetic nervous system is also responsible for stimulating salivary gland secretions and peristalsis, micturition (urination), and sexual arousal (erection). Disruption of the lower parasympathetic nerves in the sacrum results in the loss of bowel/bladder tone and sexual function.

Axonal Transport

The intracellular transport of protein and organelle materials is essential for all mammalian cells, especially the neurons. Most neuron cell bodies have dendrites on one end and an axon on the opposite end. Because most neuronal proteins are synthesized in the cell body, mechanisms are required to direct their transport along the axon or along the dendrite. Additionally, the distance over which materials have to be moved in the nervous system far exceeds the distances in other cell types; the length of a human motor neuron can span more than 1 m. Finally, even within an individual axon, materials being transported must be targeted to specific compartments.

The feature of neurons that supports the delivery of cellular components to the appropriate site of action is a long-range microtubule-based transport system. This system is composed of two key elements: molecular motors, which drive the transport of cellular components, and microtubules, which direct cellular components to the correct site. The type of molecular motor present determines the direction of transport, either away from the cell body and toward the synapse or toward the cell body.

Axonal transport is commonly divided into fast and slow axonal transport based on the speed of the bulk cargo movement. Cellular components such as vesicles and mitochondria move at fast axonal transport speeds, whereas cytoskeleton components move at slow axonal transport speeds.

When transport of materials becomes disrupted, disease can result. Indeed, axonal and cell body accumulations of organelles and other proteins are hallmark pathologies for many human neurodegenerative diseases, such as Alzheimer and related diseases, Parkinson disease, and amyotrophic lateral sclerosis.

Local anesthetics are medications that cause reversible local anesthesia and loss of nociception (pain sensation). They can also be used on specific nerve pathways (nerve block) to produce analgesia and paralysis. Local anesthetics belong to one of two drug classes, aminoamide or aminoester local anesthetics, which differ in terms of the chemical linkage (amide linkage or ester linkage) between the lipophilic part and the intermediate chain of the molecule. Local anesthetics act mainly by inhibiting sodium influx through sodium-specific ion channels in the neuronal cell membrane. When this occurs, an action potential cannot be generated and signal conduction is inhibited.

Neurologic Examination

Critical patients with neurologic complications present a variety of examination and management challenges during care and transport. Examination of the patient with neurologic dysfunction is the essential starting point for the entire patient care process.

Some specific neurologic tests may or may not be performed in the critical care transport environment. With interfacility transports, many of these tests will have been done as part of the initial assessment at the hospital. In some cases, the CCTP may perform these tests if the initial assessment was shortened by time pressure or if the CCTP has time during transport, but some may not be possible to carry out in cramped quarters. Which evaluations are performed depends on the patient's condition; if they are needed, the CCTP will perform them as appropriate. Regardless of whether the CCTP actually performs all possible exams, transport team members must know how to interpret these findings and alter their care based on the results.

Mental and Emotional Status

The mental/emotional component of the neurologic examination assesses the patient's ability to understand and interact with the environment. Specific areas tested in this component include level of consciousness; general behavior; and thought processes, including memory, attention and concentration, abstract thought, and judgment. Not every component of the examination will be relevant in all critical care situations and, therefore, may not be tested. Nevertheless, the CCTP should understand how all components are integrated and how they influence decision making for patient care.

Assessment of the level of consciousness (LOC) is an extremely important component of the neurologic examination. The CCTP should assess the LOC of all patients, considering each patient's ability to perform elements of the assessment and modifying assessment techniques as necessary. For example, intubated patients who are otherwise awake and aware may gesture or write answers to questions instead of verbalizing them.

TABLE 12-5 AVPU Scale
Awake: eyes open spontaneously
Verbal: arouses to stimulation by voice
Painful: purposeful movement to a painful stimulus such as a pectoral pinch
Unresponsive: not responsive to any stimuli

© Jones & Bartlett Learning.

Arousal and awareness are the most important qualitative markers in assessing LOC. They should be evaluated and documented repeatedly. *Arousal,* or the absence thereof, is the most basic measure of cognitive function. The evaluation of arousal is essentially an assessment of the patient's RAS and its connection with the thalamus and the cerebral cortex. Arousal may be described using either the AVPU scale **TABLE 12-5** or the Glasgow Coma Scale (GCS).

In most critical care settings, where time for gathering data may be limited, the GCS is commonly used to document and trend a patient's level of arousal. This scale evaluates three parameters: eye opening, verbalization, and movement. The best response for each category is recorded. A minimum score of 3 indicates a completely unresponsive patient, whereas a score of 15 indicates the patient is awake and alert. Generally, a GCS score of 7 or less indicates a coma. The GCS is discussed in greater detail in Chapter 11, *Trauma.*

Awareness denotes the content of consciousness, which is a higher-level function than arousal. It is described by terms such as disoriented, lethargic, or obtunded **TABLE 12-6**. In evaluating the patient's awareness, the CCTP should assess orientation to person, place, and time **TABLE 12-7**.

Providers assess awareness by asking the patient to provide appropriate answers to a variety of questions. Findings may be documented as alert and oriented (A&O $\times$ 3, A&O 2/3, or A&O 1/3) or as awake, alert, and oriented (AAO $\times$ 3). The three aspects of awareness, or orientation, disappear in the order of time, then place, then person (self), as the patient becomes more disoriented. Changes in the patient's answers that indicate increasing confusion and disorientation may, therefore, be an early sign of neurologic dysfunction.

Simple observation is the primary tool used to assess the patient's behavior. General behavior is best

TABLE 12-6 Terms Used to Describe a Patient's Awareness

Confusion: inability to think rapidly and clearly

Disorientation: confusion in reference to time, followed by place, and then self

Lethargy: limited spontaneous movement or speech; easy arousal with normal speech or touch; may not be oriented to person, place, or time

Obtundation: mild to moderate reduction in arousal with limited responses to the environment; falls asleep unless stimulated verbally or tactilely; answers questions with minimal response

Stupor: a condition of deep sleep or unresponsiveness from which the person may be aroused or caused to open eyes only by vigorous and repeated stimulation; response is often grabbing at or withdrawal from stimulus

Coma: no verbal response to the external environment or to any stimuli; noxious stimuli such as deep pain may or may not yield motor movement

> **Light coma:** associated with purposeful movement on stimulation
>
> **Coma:** associated with nonpurposeful movement only on stimulation
>
> **Deep coma:** associated with unresponsiveness or no response to any stimulus

Data from McCance K, Huether S. *Pathophysiology: The Biologic Basis for Disease in Adults and Children.* 7th ed. St. Louis, MO: Elsevier Mosby; 2014.

TABLE 12-7 Questions Pertaining to Patient Orientation

Category	Sample Questions	Order of Loss
Time	What day is it? What is the date? What is the month, the year? What is the season? What is the time of day?	
Place	What is the name of the place we are in? Which type of vehicle are we in? What is the name of the town or city?	
Person	What is your name? What is your job? Where do you live?	

© Jones & Bartlett Learning.

assessed by observing gestures, facial expressions, mood, affect, and posture. During this component of the examination, family members or close friends may be able to help establish whether the patient's responses are normal or abnormal. A variety of neurologic pathologies—including pain, hypoxia, anxiety, and expanding intracranial lesions—may initially manifest through changes in general behavior.

Most critical care patients will not be able to undergo lengthy tests to assess their cognitive functioning. The Mini-Mental State Examination **TABLE 12-8** provides a simple, easily applied test of higher cognitive functions. It consists of a series of questions that test orientation, registration, attention and calculation, recall, and language. The highest possible score is 30 points; a score of less than 24 indicates cognitive dysfunction.

Speech Function

Abnormalities of speech may need to be considered early on in the neurologic examination, because they may interfere with the CCTP's ability to accurately assess other, higher-level functions. Abnormalities of speech can reflect dysfunction in any component or process of communication. They include the following:

- Deafness: Profound hearing loss or complete inability to hear
- Aphasia: Any loss or impairment of language function (expressive or receptive) as a result of brain damage
- Dysphonia: Difficulty producing intelligible speech caused by physical impairment at the level of the larynx
- Dysarthria: Difficulty articulating words caused by neurologic impairment affecting the vocal apparatus

Aphasia is generally the focus of the CCTP's assessment of speech function because it is more commonly associated with an acute process. Sounds are recognized as language in the Wernicke area, which is connected to the concept area, where the meaning of the words becomes understood. The concept area is connected to the Broca area, where speech output is generated. The Wernicke area is also directly connected to the Broca area via the arcuate fasciculus. Because the arcuate fasciculus connects the speech comprehension area (Wernicke area) to the speech production area (Broca

TABLE 12-8 Mini-Mental State Examination Components

Parameter	Task	Possible Points[a]
Orientation	Assign 1 point for correct answers to each of the following questions:	
	• What is the time? Date? Day of the week? Month? Year?	5
	• What is the name of this country? State? County? Town? Hospital?	5
Registration	Name three objects arbitrarily. Assign 1 point for each object the patient repeats, in the correct order that you named them, on the first attempt. Encourage the patient, even with prompting, to repeat all three, so you can test recall later.	3
Attention and calculation	Ask the patient to subtract 7 from 100, and then 7 from the result, and so forth through five iterations. Assign 1 point for each correct calculation.	5
Recall	Ask the patient to state the three objects listed during the registration test, assigning 1 point for each object recalled.	3
Language	Indicate two objects (a pencil and a watch). Assign 1 point for each object correctly named.	2
	Assign 1 point if the patient correctly repeats the following phrase: "No ifs, ands, or buts."	1
	Have the patient perform a three-stage task. Assign 1 point for each stage the patient performs successfully. For example, you could state, "With the index finger of your right hand, touch the tip of your nose and then your left ear."	3
	On a blank piece of paper, write, "Close your eyes" and ask the patient to obey what is written. Assign 1 point if the patient closes their eyes.	1
	Ask the patient to write a sentence. Assign 1 point if the sentence makes sense and contains a subject and a verb.	1
	Ask the patient to draw two pentagons. (You can explain that a pentagon has five sides.) A portion of the two pentagons should intersect. For example:	1
	Assign 1 point if the patient's drawing matches the description.	
Total		**30**

[a]Scores of less than 24 indicate cognitive dysfunction. Speech must be intact for the test to be valid.

area), damage to this area impairs the patient's ability to repeat words and phrases. These areas are found in the dominant hemisphere of each person's brain (left dominant is most common). It is important to realize that patients who are aphasic, or unable to speak normally, may still be hearing and understanding everything being said around them.

Assessment of Cranial Nerves

Assessment of the cranial nerves, which are located between the midbrain and the pons, provides invaluable information on pressure changes within the cranium and its effects on the brainstem in particular. Many of the cranial nerve tests require patient participation, so they may not be feasible in some critically ill or injured patients. Cranial nerve dysfunction may result from several pathologies, including lesions to the nerve; lesions in the nucleus, the communicating pathways to and from the cortex, the diencephalon, the cerebellum, or other parts of the brainstem; or generalized problems involving the nerve or muscle.

Knowledge of all cranial nerves (ie, the areas that they serve, the expected response to testing, and indications of abnormal response) is necessary to complete a thorough neurologic examination. Nevertheless, certain nerves are more commonly tested in patients who are critically ill or injured—namely, the optic (CN II), oculomotor (CN III), trochlear (CN IV), trigeminal (CN V), abducens (CN VI), facial (CN VII), acoustic (CN VIII), glossopharyngeal (CN IX), vagus (CN X), and hypoglossal (CN XII) nerves. **TABLE 12-9** provides an overview of the cranial nerves, their functions, and methods of testing.

Owing to the nature of the environment in which the CCTP works, most patients encountered

TABLE 12-9 Cranial Nerves

Cranial Nerve Number	Cranial Nerve Name	Function	Test
I	Olfactory	Sense of smell	Patient smells aromatic substance (coffee or soap but not ammonia or other irritants)
II	Optic	Vision	Visual acuity test—the Snellen chart Optic disk—fundoscopy Fields—confrontation
III	Oculomotor	Medial and upward/downward movement of the eye Constriction of the pupil Elevation of eyelids Consensual light response Accommodation and convergence	Extraocular movements, pupillary size and equality, and symmetry of response to a light shined in the eyes
IV	Trochlear	Moves eyes upward and downward	Tested with cranial nerves III and VI
V	Trigeminal	Sensation for face, scalp, cornea, and nasal and oral cavities Movement of jaw	Prick the patient's face with a pin and touch the face lightly with a piece of cotton Patient clenches their teeth together
VI	Abducens	Moves eyes laterally	Tested with cranial nerves III and IV
VII	Facial	Controls facial expression and taste for interior two-thirds of tongue	Direct the patient to smile, whistle, bare the teeth, and pucker lips Also, the patient should close their eyes and wrinkle the forehead
VIII	Acoustic	Hearing and equilibrium	Caloric test in unconscious patients Doll's eyes test
IX	Glossopharyngeal	Voluntary muscles for swallowing and phonation Secretory and salivary glands Carotid reflex	Test for palatal elevation, swallowing and gag reflexes,[a] and glottal and palatal sounds
X	Vagus	Voluntary muscles for phonation and swallowing Involuntary activity of visceral muscles of the heart, lungs, and digestive tract Carotid reflex	Test for palatal elevation, swallowing and gag reflexes,[a] and glottal and palatal sounds
XI	Spinal accessory	Shrugging of shoulders and turning of head	Ability to shrug shoulders and turn head against resistance
XIII	Hypoglossal	Movement of tongue and taste for posterior third of the tongue	Ability to protrude tongue and push tongue against cheek

[a]Ten percent of the normal population lacks a gag reflex.

TABLE 12-10 Cranial Nerves and Their Exam Results

Cranial Nerve Group	Specific Test	Significance
III, IV, VI	Extraocular movements	Dysconjugate gaze indicates compression or injury of nerve; eyes are unable to turn together in the same direction
V, VII, IX, X, XII	Swallowing	Potential for aspiration
III, VI, VIII	Oculocephalic reflex (doll's eyes)	Brainstem dysfunction
III, VI, VIII	Oculovestibular reflex (caloric test)	Brainstem dysfunction
IX, X	Gag reflex	Loss of protective reflex caused by brainstem dysfunction or nerve injury
V, VII	Corneal reflex	Loss of protective reflex caused by brainstem compression or nerve injury

Data from Kinney MR, Brooks-Brunn JA, Molter N, et al. *AACN Clinical Reference for Critical Care Nursing*. St Louis, MO: Mosby; 1999.

will be critically ill or injured. Consequently, it may be necessary to perform rapid exams that test the function of the most important cranial nerves simultaneously. **TABLE 12-10** outlines such nerve groups and their exam results.

Olfactory Nerve

The CCTP should assess cranial nerve I, which is responsible for olfaction, in patients in whom head trauma has occurred, when pathology at the base of the skull is suspected, and in patients who exhibit an altered mental status. Use familiar odors such as coffee, vanilla, soap, and lemon oil to conduct the exam. *Never* use irritant substances such as ammonia or vinegar as olfactory stimulants.

One interesting phenomenon that is occasionally observed is Foster Kennedy syndrome, which involves the olfactory nerve and is caused by a tumor or abscess at the base of the frontal lobe. Signs and symptoms of this syndrome include ipsilateral blindness and anosmia, ipsilateral atrophy of the olfactory and optic nerves, and contralateral papilledema.

Optic Nerve

The optic nerve (CN II) arises from cells in the retina and then passes into the orbit, where it is enclosed in meningeal sheaths. After the fibers have passed through the optic chiasm, this nerve's name changes to the optic tract. The fibers from the nasal half of the retina decussate (intersect to form an "X") within the optic chiasm; those from the lateral (temporal) half do not.

Evaluate each eye individually to assess the optic nerve. The tests should include evaluation of visual acuity, visual fields, and the fundi (via fundoscopy). **TABLE 12-11** describes the assessment parameters.

To formally evaluate visual acuity, use a Snellen chart **FIGURE 12-21** to check each eye individually. With the patient at a distance of 20 feet (6 m) from the chart, ask them to read the line with the smallest letters they can decipher. The number beside each line on the chart is the distance at which a person with normal vision can read the letters. This number is the denominator when recording the vision.

As an alternative to the Snellen chart, the Rosenbaum Pocket Vision Screener **FIGURE 12-22** can be used at a more practical distance of 14 inches (36 cm) versus 20 feet (6 m). Calculate the ratio in the same manner as is done with the Snellen chart.

Examination of the visual fields provides invaluable information that can often enable the CCTP to determine the location of a lesion on the visual pathway. A normal visual field extends 60° to the nasal side, 100° on the temporal side, and 130° vertically. The confrontation test is used to evaluate the visual fields. In this test, the CCTP faces the patient at a distance of 2 feet (0.5 m), and then asks the patient to cover one eye lightly and look at the CCTP's eye directly opposite. The CCTP should then present a stimulus in each of the four quadrants—upper and lower nasal and upper and lower temporal—of the visual field. Acceptable stimuli include finger movement, rapid finger counting, and hand comparison. The CCTP should assess for the presence of a *scotoma*, or spot, which is an abnormal deficit

TABLE 12-11 Assessment Parameters of the Eye

Structure	Normal	Abnormal	Interpretation of Abnormal Findings
Optic disk	Round or slightly oval in shape Yellow-red color Clearly defined margins	Papilledema: swelling of the disk, including disappearance of the optic cup	Increased intracranial pressure, usually within 24–48 h
		Papillitis: inflammation of the optic nerve	Multiple sclerosis, idiopathic
		Optic atrophy: decreased visual acuity and a change in color of the optic disk to light pink, white, or gray	Primary: optic nerve compression, optic nerve ischemia Secondary: following papilledema
Optic cup	Slightly on the nasal side of the center of the optic disk Diameter is normally <50% of the disk	Cup may appear deep	Chronic (or idiopathic) glaucoma
Blood vessels	Arteries are lightly colored and are two-thirds the diameter of veins	Arterial narrowing and vessel irregularity	Hypertensive retinopathy
	Veins are burgundy colored and may pulsate near the disk	Tortuous vessels	Hypertensive retinopathy
Retinal background	Pigmented background: normal in people with dark skin; if striped, it is called *tigroid* Pale: clear is normal in people with fair skin	Red lesions • Dot hemorrhages: microaneurysms seen adjacent to blood vessels	Diabetic retinopathy
		• Blot hemorrhages: bleeds in the deep retinal layer from microaneurysms	Hypertensive retinopathy
		• Flame hemorrhages: superficial bleed, shaped by nerve fibers into a fan that points toward the disk	Subarachnoid hemorrhage
		• Subhyaloid hemorrhages: irregular superficial hemorrhages usually with a flat top	Diabetes and hypertension
		White/yellow lesions • Hard exudates: yellow, sharply edged lesions that may form a ring around the macula	Diabetes, systemic lupus erythematosus, acquired immunodeficiency syndrome
		• Cotton wool spots: white fluffy spots caused by retinal infarcts	Hypertension

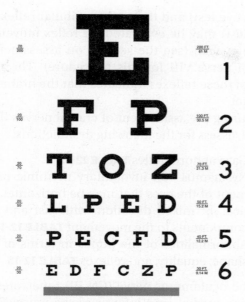

FIGURE 12-21 The Snellen chart.

© Germán Ariel Berra/Shutterstock.

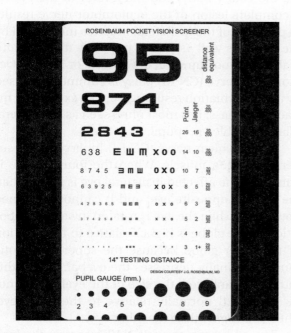

FIGURE 12-22 The Rosenbaum Pocket Vision Screener (eye chart).

© Hopkins Medical Products (www.hopkinsmedicalproducts.com). Used with permission.

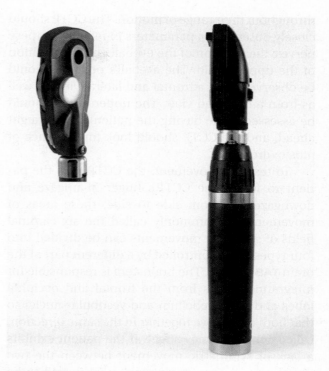

FIGURE 12-23 An ophthalmoscope.

Main photo: © Cameron Swinton/Shutterstock.

of the visual field surrounded by normal vision. The *blind spot*, which is normal, represents the location of the optic disk within the visual field, because the optic disk does not have the rods, cones, or ganglion cells necessary for vision.

The **fundus** of each eye includes the optic disk, macula, and blood vessels on the back wall of the internal eyeball; it should be examined using the ophthalmoscope **FIGURE 12-23**. During the examination, the patient should look at a distant object, and the CCTP should attempt to observe the optic disk, the blood vessels, and the retinal background. With the ophthalmoscope dial set on zero, locate the pupillary red reflex (the point at which the retinal reflex is seen glowing pink in the pupil) from a distance of about 2 or 3 feet (0.5 or 1 m). Slowly approach the patient's eye as if viewing the eye through a keyhole. At the same time, dial the plus or minus lenses, as needed, on the ophthalmoscope to focus on the patient's retina. The **optic disk** is located by directing the ophthalmoscope toward the nasal side of the patient's retina. The most prominent structure visible, it represents the termination of the optic nerve.

Ocular, Trochlear, Trigeminal, and Abducens Nerves

The oculomotor, trochlear, and abducens nerves (CN III, IV, and VI, respectively) are usually examined as a group because they act together in producing eye movement and controlling ocular muscles to ensure that the eyes remain parallel throughout their range of motion. The CCTP should closely observe two parameters in relation to these nerves: the position of the eyeball and the position of the upper eyelid. The eyeball's position should be observed from a frontal and lateral view as well as from a cephalad view. The upper eyelid should be assessed while having the patient look straight ahead, and the CCTP should look for evidence of ptosis (drooping).

To test eye movement, the CCTP asks the patient to follow the CCTP's finger in upgaze and downgaze and from side to side; these areas of movement are commonly called the six cardinal fields of gaze. Eye movements can be divided into four types, each controlled by a different part of the brain **TABLE 12-12**. The brainstem is responsible for integrating inputs from the frontal and occipital lobes and the cerebellum and vestibular nuclei so that both eyes move together in the same direction, called conjugate movement. If the patient exhibits a lack of symmetric movement between the two visual axes, dysconjugate movement is said to be present. Diplopia, or double vision, may occur if the patient is unable to move the eyeball in one particular direction.

In conducting a neurologic examination on an unconscious patient, the oculocephalic reflex (doll's eye test) and the oculovestibular reflex (caloric test) may be evaluated for reflex movement of the eyeball (see the section on assessment of cranial nerve VIII for this procedure). The presence of these reflexes indicates that the brainstem is intact.

During the assessment of cranial nerves III, IV, and VI, assess for the following dysfunctions:

- Gaze abnormalities **TABLE 12-13**
- Nystagmus—an involuntary rhythmic movement of the eyes that may be horizontal, vertical, or mixed direction, with fast and slow components to the movement **TABLE 12-14**
- Abnormalities of the pupils in terms of size, shape, equality, and reflexes **TABLE 12-15**

The oculomotor nerve (CN III) innervates the superior, medial, and inferior rectus muscles; the inferior oblique muscle; the constrictor of the pupil; the ciliary body; and the levator of the eyelid. A complete lesion of the oculomotor nerve results in paralysis of the ipsilateral muscles innervated by the nerve as well as ptosis, pupillary dilation, and inability to look upward, downward, or inward. Oculomotor nerve (CN III) palsy is commonly caused by uncal herniation resulting from an expanding intracranial mass; it is most often seen as a unilateral dilated, or "blown," pupil.

The trochlear nerve (CN IV) innervates the superior oblique muscle. When the fourth nerve is damaged, the affected ipsilateral eye is higher than the normal opposite eye, and it cannot be turned downward when the eye is rotated inward. The position of the globe is higher relative to the position of the other globe because the superior oblique muscle normally depresses the eyeball. When this muscle is paralyzed, the size of the eyeball will not be depressed normally relative to the other eye. Thus, it is *higher* than the other eye.

The abducens nerve (CN VI) controls the ipsilateral lateral rectus muscle, which makes the eye look outward (laterally). Defects in abduction (from a lesion of the sixth cranial nerve, for example) give the patient a *cross-eyed* appearance. The normal eye is oriented straight ahead; by comparison, the affected eye is rotated slightly inward (medially) owing to the unopposed action of the medial rectus muscle on that side.

The trigeminal nerve (CN V) has both motor and sensory functions. In sensory testing, its

TABLE 12-12 Eye Movements		
Type of Eye Movement	**Definition**	**Site of Control**
Saccadic (command)	Rapid movement from one point of fixation to another	Frontal lobe
Pursuit	Slow eye movement used to maintain fixation on a moving object	Occipital lobe
Vestibular-positional	Eye movements that compensate for movement of the head/neck to maintain fixation	Cerebellar vestibular nuclei
Convergence	Movements that maintain fixation as an object is brought close to the face	Midbrain

© Jones & Bartlett Learning.

TABLE 12-13 Gaze Abnormalities

Type of Gaze	Description	Causes
Normal gaze	Eye movements are smooth and conjugate	N/A
Horizontal gaze	Deviation of both eyes toward the same side	Destructive hemispheric lesion: both eyes deviate *toward* the side of the lesion Irritative hemispheric lesion (eg, hemorrhage): both eyes deviate *away* from the side of irritation, but later the conjugate gaze becomes paralyzed
Vertical gaze	Deviation of both eyes upward	Upper brainstem lesion
Medial-longitudinal fasciculus	Dysconjugate gaze	Lesion between the pons and the midbrain
Skewed deviation	One eye looks downward and the other looks upward	Lesion in the pons on the same side as the eye that is directed downward
Roving-eye movements	Spontaneous, slow, random deviation	Seen in comatose patients with intact brainstem oculomotor function
Ocular bobbing	Episodic, intermittent, usually conjugate, downward, brisk eye movement followed by a return to the resting position by a "bobbing action"	Severe destructive lower pontine lesions

© Jones & Bartlett Learning.

TABLE 12-14 Nystagmus Types

Type of Nystagmus	Description	Cause(s)
Retraction nystagmus	Irregular jerks of the eyes backward into the orbit, initiated by an upward gaze	Midbrain tegmental damage
Convergence nystagmus	Slow, spontaneous, drifting, ocular divergence with a final quick, convergent jerk	Midbrain lesion
See-saw nystagmus	A rapid, pendular, dysconjugate see-saw movement accompanied by severe visual field deficits and loss of visual acuity	Lesion around optic chiasm
Downbeat nystagmus	Irregular jerks initiated by a downward gaze	Lower medullary lesion
Optokinetic nystagmus	A test in which a striped drum is spun in front of the eyes, normally evoking nystagmus in the opposite direction of the spin	Present in most patients
Vestibular nystagmus	Mixed nystagmus that can be horizontal, rotational, or both	Vestibular disease
Toxic nystagmus	Nystagmus occurring while the head is in a specific position, caused by certain drugs or alcohol	Induced by treatment with certain drugs, such as phenytoin, barbiturates, and bromides; also caused by alcohol ingestion

© Jones & Bartlett Learning.

TABLE 12-15 Pupillary Exam Results

Size	2–6 mm (average, 3.5 mm)
Shape	Round
	Patients who have had previous cataract surgery may have the shape of a keyhole
Equality	Diameters are equal
	Be aware of anisocoria, a nonpathologic unequal pupil found in 15% of the population

© Jones & Bartlett Learning.

innervation includes the face up to the vertex of the scalp, but spares the angle of the mandible. The sensation from the oral and nasal cavities is transmitted through the trigeminal nerve, although these areas are not usually included in the routine neurologic examination.

Pain and temperature should be tested in the three divisions of the fifth cranial nerve: ophthalmic, maxillary, and mandibular. The ophthalmic division innervates the scalp as far back as the vertex of the skull, forehead, cornea, conjunctiva, and skin of the side and tip of the nose. Corneal sensation is tested by gently touching the corneas with a cotton tip or tissue paper while the patient looks in the other direction. This maneuver exercises the afferent limb of the corneal reflex. The normal response is a rapid, partial, or complete blinking movement of the eyelid elicited by the efferent limb of the corneal reflex via the facial nerve.

The second trigeminal division, the maxillary nerve, conducts stimuli from the skin of the cheek, far lateral aspect of the nose, upper teeth, and jaw. The third division, the mandibular nerve, carries sensory and motor impulses. Tests of the sensory distribution address the skin of the lower jaw, pinna of the ear, lower teeth and gums, and the side of the tongue.

The motor fibers supply the muscles of mastication: the temporal, masseter, and pterygoid muscles. The temporal and masseter muscles are examined by having the patient close the jaw together while the CCTP palpates these muscles. The *jaw-jerk reflex* is elicited by a gentle tap on the chin, with resultant closure of the jaw by the masticatory muscles and is considered an abnormal finding.

Facial Nerve

The facial nerve (CN VII) is a complex nerve with motor, sensory, and parasympathetic fibers. Its motor portion innervates the muscles of facial expression and is tested by instructing the patient to wrinkle the forehead, close the eyelids tightly, smile or grimace to show the teeth, and whistle. Two types of facial motor weakness are possible: one with involvement of the upper motor neuron (corticonuclear/corticobulbar pathways), and the other with involvement of the lower motor neurons (*peripheral* seventh nerve palsy). *Central* (upper) motor facial palsy is characterized by the inability to retract the corner of the mouth, whereas forehead function and eyelid closure remain largely unaffected. Lesions in the facial nucleus or the nerve proper will cause paralysis of one-half of the entire face, with inability to wrinkle the forehead or to close the eyelids and lips on the affected side.

The sensory portions of the seventh nerve originate from the taste buds in the anterior two-thirds of the tongue and from the posterior wall of the external ear canal. Although this test is rarely performed in the field, taste is examined using sugar, salt, or quinine solutions. The patient is instructed to protrude the tongue; then the test substance is applied with a cotton-tipped applicator on one side of the tongue. The patient must identify the test substance before drawing the tongue back into the mouth. The facial nerve also carries parasympathetic fibers to the maxillary and lacrimal glands.

Vestibulocochlear Nerve

The eighth cranial nerve is made up of two divisions: (1) the cochlear division, which affects the sense of hearing, and (2) the vestibular division, which affects the sense of balance.

The vestibular division of the acoustic nerve is assessed by using rotational and caloric stimuli to produce changes in the endolymph current in the semicircular canals. Both types of stimuli are also used to determine the brainstem function of unconscious patients. Typically, patients with vestibular dysfunction complain of vertigo, nausea and vomiting, and difficulty with balance, especially with movement of the head.

The **caloric test**, or Bárány test, is commonly used to assess vestibular function; it should not be performed on any patient with a ruptured tympanic membrane. This assessment involves raising and lowering of the temperature in the external auditory canal, which induces convection currents in the endolymph of the semicircular canals and stimulates the vestibular nerve endings. With the patient lying down and the head elevated 30° such that the lateral semicircular canal is vertical, instill cool water (86°F [30°C]), usually about 250 mL, into one ear over 40 seconds. If the patient is conscious, direct them to look forward while the water is being instilled. Repeat this step in the other ear with warm water (111°F [44°C]). Then observe the direction of nystagmus. **TABLE 12-16** identifies the normal and abnormal responses to the caloric test.

The doll's eye test, or oculocephalic reflex test, is performed on the unconscious patient by rapidly rotating the head from side to side and observing the eye movement **FIGURE 12-24**. This procedure

TABLE 12-16 Caloric Test Responses	
Conscious patient	Cold: nystagmus away from stimulated ear
	Warm: nystagmus toward stimulated ear
	Remember the mnemonic COWS (cold–opposite/warm–same)
Unconscious patient	Cold: nystagmus toward stimulated ear
	Warm: nystagmus away from stimulated ear

© Jones & Bartlett Learning.

is contraindicated if neck or cervical spine injury is suspected. If the reflex is intact or doll's eyes are present (indicating adequate brainstem function between CN III, VI, and VIII), the eyes will deviate opposite the movement of the head. The absence of doll's eyes occurs when the eyes move in the same direction of the head as it is turned; this abnormal response indicates severe brainstem dysfunction.

Glossopharyngeal and Vagus Nerves

The glossopharyngeal and vagus nerves (CN IX and X, respectively) are usually tested together owing to their co-innervation of the pharynx. The glossopharyngeal nerve supplies sensory components to the pharynx, tonsils, soft palate, and posterior third of the tongue. It also supplies motor fibers to the muscle that elevates the pharynx. The vagus nerve is responsible for sensation to the pharynx and larynx; motor function of the soft palate, pharynx, and larynx; innervation of the thoracic and abdominal visceral organs; and sensory input from the heart, lungs, and digestive tract.

To test these nerves **FIGURE 12-25**, direct the patient to open their mouth and say, "Ah." Note the upward movement of the soft palate and any deviation of the uvula. As part of this assessment, you may stimulate the gag reflex (using a tongue depressor or cotton swab), which is also mediated by cranial nerves IX and X. Note that 10% of the population does not have a gag reflex.

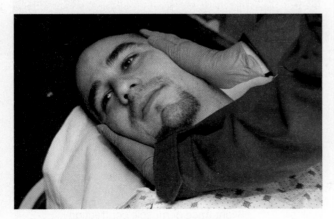

FIGURE 12-24 The doll's eye test, also known as the oculocephalic reflex test.

© Jones & Bartlett Learning.

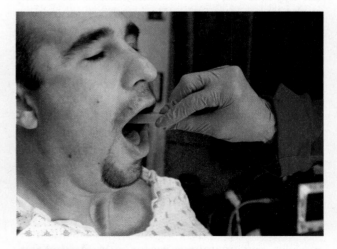

FIGURE 12-25 The test for cranial nerve IX, the glossopharyngeal nerve, evaluates palatal elevation, swallowing and gag reflexes, and glottal and palatal sounds.

© Jones & Bartlett Learning.

Spinal Accessory Nerve

The spinal accessory nerve (CN XI) is tested in two segments. First, the CCTP palpates the trapezius muscle and evaluates its strength while the patient shrugs their shoulders against resistance. Second, the patient turns their head to one side and pushes their chin against the examiner's hand; the CCTP should then palpate the sternocleidomastoid for tone and strength. This test should not be performed on patients with a suspected injury to the base of the skull or the upper neck.

Hypoglossal Nerve

The hypoglossal nerve (CN XII) innervates the musculature of the tongue. To test this nerve, the CCTP observes the tongue for fasciculations and atrophy, tests for muscle strength by having the patient push the tongue against the inside wall of the cheek, and checks for tongue protrusion. Tongue protrusion is straight when the two hypoglossal nerves are working together; when only one branch is working, however, the tongue will deviate toward the injured side. Neck trauma, tumor, or brainstem lesions usually cause unilateral weakness. In contrast, bilateral weakness typically results from degenerative neurologic diseases.

Assessment of Motor Function

The motor examination includes a consideration of muscle tone and strength. This exam proceeds from the upper limbs, to the neck and trunk, and finally to the lower extremities. During this examination, the CCTP should compare the symmetry of each side of the body.

The assessment of motor function evaluates how both the voluntary and involuntary motor pathways are functioning. The voluntary motor pathway is a descending pathway that originates in the precentral gyrus of the frontal lobe and ends at all levels of the spinal cord (suprasegmental level). The descending neuron synapses with motor neurons of the spinal cord (segmental level), and final motor output is achieved at the muscle level (myoneural junction). Voluntary muscle control involves the orchestrated effort of the skeletal structures, muscles, and involuntary motor pathways that control posture, balance, and reflexive activities.

To assess the patient's voluntary motor pathway, the CCTP should palpate the muscles through the normal range of motion. Abnormalities are characterized as follows:

- Spasticity or undue resistance of the muscles owing to passive lengthening because of injury to the corticospinal system
- Rigidity or a more constant state of resistance that involves the extrapyramidal motor system
- Flaccidity or a decreased muscle tone (hypotonia)

To assess muscle strength, the CCTP puts the patient's muscles of the major joints through their normal range of motion. Strength should also be assessed against gravity and finally against resistance. Muscle strength is rated using a scale of 0 to 5 **TABLE 12-17**. To record the data from this exam, the CCTP should draw a stick figure and place values at various points along the figure to indicate the assessed motor response.

Assessment of Sensory Function

Evaluation of the sensory system seeks to determine the patient's ability to perceive various types of sensations with the eyes closed. Sensation arises from specialized receptors in the body that are designed to recognize and transmit stimuli to the CNS (usually the cerebrum or brainstem), where processing takes place and an appropriate response can be initiated. To reach these sites, the sensory impulses travel along specialized tracts in the nervous system.

TABLE 12-17 Muscle Strength Grading Scale	
Grade	**Description**
5	Normal; full strength against resistance
4	Active movement; minimal weakness against resistance
3	Active movement; barely able to overcome gravity and does not overcome active resistance
2	Active movement; does not overcome gravity
1	Slight trace of muscle contraction
0	No muscle contraction

© Jones & Bartlett Learning.

Sensory examination assesses the integrity of both the receptors and the tracts of conduction. It is not useful for all patients, however, as altered levels of consciousness or preexisting conditions may interfere with the conduct of a proper examination or may produce abnormalities unrelated to the present illness or injury. The CCTP should be comfortable using a dermatome chart **FIGURE 12-26** to locate sensory areas supplied by a single spinal nerve and should be especially familiar with certain key dermatomes, such as C4, C7, T2, T10, L5, S1, and S5.

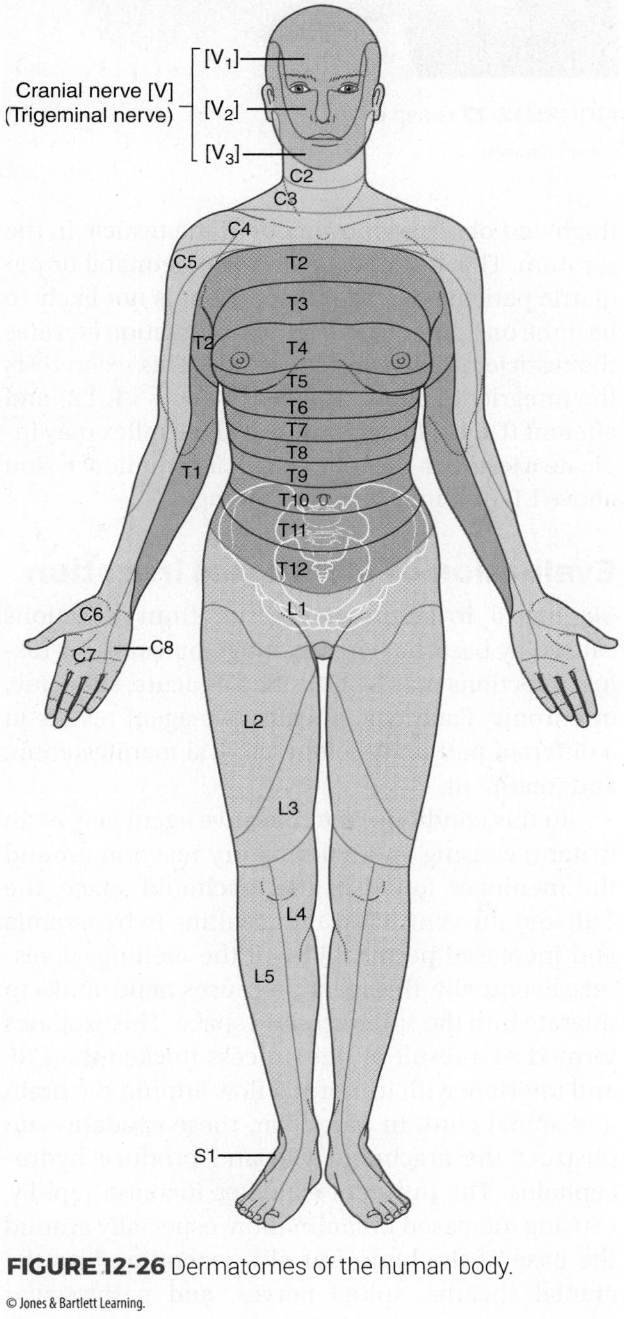

As part of a detailed assessment of sensory function, the CCTP should examine and document the patient's perception of pain, temperature, and touch. These methods of testing compare symmetric areas on both sides of the body and evaluate distal and proximal areas of the arms and legs for pain, temperature, and touch sensation. The stimuli should be scattered to sample most dermatomes and major peripheral nerves. During this assessment, the patient's eyes should remain closed.

To test the patient's perception of pain, ask the patient to close their eyes, then randomly apply both sharp (using a disposable pin) and blunt stimuli, and note the patient's response. Always begin in areas of known altered sensation and move toward areas of normal sensation to find the edges.

Assess touch using a fine wisp of cotton or an alcohol pad. Instruct the patient to close their eyes during the exam, and then stroke their skin with the cotton or alcohol pad symmetrically on alternating sides of the body. This test measures anesthesia or hyperesthesia.

Reflex Testing

Examination of deep tendon reflexes gives information about the integrity of the spinal nerves and may indicate brainstem or spinal cord lesions. A tendon reflex results from the stimulation of a stretch-sensitive afferent nerve from a neuromuscular spindle, which, via a single synapse, stimulates a motor (efferent) nerve, leading to a muscle contraction. Tendon reflexes are increased in upper motor neuron lesions and decreased in lower motor neuron lesions **TABLE 12-18**. The following scale should be used to grade reflexes:

- 0 = absent
- 1+ = reduced or hypoactive
- 2+ = normal
- 3+ = increased or hyperactive
- 4+ = clonus

Pathologic Reflexes

The following list includes the most common pathologic reflexes, all of which indicate pyramidal tract disease. The Babinski reflex (Babinski sign) is perhaps the most important of the pathologic reflexes.

FIGURE 12-26 Dermatomes of the human body.

© Jones & Bartlett Learning.

TABLE 12-18 Reflex Locations

Reflex	Nerve	Root
Biceps	Musculocutaneous	C5, C6
Brachioradialis	Radial	C5, C6
Triceps	Radial	C7
Finger	Median and ulnar	C8
Knee	Femoral	L3-L4
Ankle	Tibial	S1-S2

© Jones & Bartlett Learning.

- **Plantar reflex.** The provider rapidly strokes the lateral aspect of the sole of the foot with a blunt object, such as the back of a pen, from the heel to the ball of the foot. A normal plantar response will lead to toe flexion and is considered a negative test. An extensor (or up-going toe) response is the Babinski sign, a positive (abnormal) test result. Note that infants will usually demonstrate an extensor response as a primitive reflex.
- **Oppenheim sign.** The provider strokes the anterior medial tibial muscle. An extensor response is a positive finding.
- **Gordon sign.** The provider firmly squeezes the gastrocnemius muscle. An extensor response is a positive finding.
- **Hoffmann sign.** The provider flicks the distal phalanx of the index or middle finger. A sudden clawing of the fingers and thumb is a positive finding.

Grasp Reflex

To test the grasp reflex, the CCTP asks the patient to grasp the CCTP's index finger. The CCTP then asks the patient to let go of the finger as they pull their hand away from the patient. A normal response is present if the patient is able to let go. An abnormal response consists of the involuntary flexion of the fingers, causing an uncontrollable grasp of the CCTP's hand **FIGURE 12-27**. Such a positive grasp reflex indicates a frontal lobe lesion.

Superficial Reflexes

To assess the cremasteric reflex in men, the CCTP strokes downward on the inner aspect of the upper

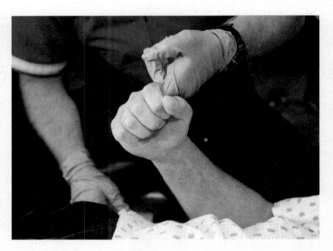

FIGURE 12-27 Grasp reflex.

© Jones & Bartlett Learning.

thigh and observes movement of the testicle in the scrotum. This test may be done on neonatal or pediatric patients during transport but is not likely to be done on adults. Cremasteric contraction elevates the testicle on the stimulated side. This exam tests the integrity of afferent (femoral nerve L1, L2) and efferent (L1, L2) fibers. Absence of the reflex may indicate a lesion in the reflex arc or a pyramidal lesion above L1, or it may be nonpathologic.

Evaluation of Meningeal Irritation

Meningeal irritation may result from infections caused by bacteria, viruses, fungi, parasites, or toxins. Infections may be classified as acute, subacute, or chronic. Each type of causative agent results in a different pathophysiology, clinical manifestation, and treatment.

In this condition, the causative agent acts as an irritant, causing an inflammatory reaction around the meninges found in the arachnoid space, the CSF, and the ventricles, and resulting in hyperemia and increased permeability of the meningeal vessels. Eventually, this reaction causes neutrophils to migrate into the subarachnoid space. The exudates formed as a result of this process thicken the CSF and interfere with its normal flow around the brain and spinal cord. In particular, these exudates can obstruct the arachnoid villi and produce hydrocephalus. The purulent exudates increase rapidly, causing increased inflammation, especially around the base of the brain but also extending into the cranial sheaths, spinal nerves, and perivascular spaces of the brain's cortex. The meningeal cells become edematous. Over time, the combination of purulent exudates and cell edema results in increased ICP.

The clinical manifestations of meningeal irritation can be grouped into meningeal, infectious, and neurologic signs. The meningeal signs include generalized throbbing headache progressing in severity, progressive photophobia, nuchal rigidity, Kernig sign, and Brudzinski sign **FIGURE 12-28**.

To test for nuchal rigidity, while the patient is lying flat, the CCTP places their hand behind the patient's head and gently flexes the head forward until the chin touches the chest, if possible. Marked

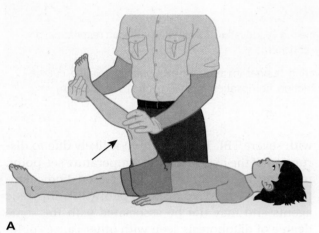
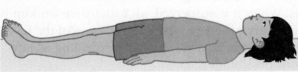
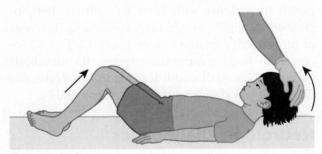

FIGURE 12-28 A. Kernig sign. Meningeal irritation results in the inability to straighten the leg with the hips flexed. **B.** Brudzinski sign. Meningeal irritation results in an involuntary flexion of the knees when the head is flexed toward the chest.

© Jones & Bartlett Learning.

resistance to head movement in any direction is suggestive of meningeal irritation. This test should not be performed if cervical spine injury is suspected.

Lhermitte Phenomenon

In the Lhermitte phenomenon, forward flexion of the neck produces an electric shock feeling, usually running down the back. The presence of this sensation indicates cervical pathology.

Vital Signs

As part of the neurologic examination, the CCTP should obtain vital signs. The centers for control of vital functions are found within the brainstem **TABLE 12-19 FIGURE 12-29**. Thus, any changes in vital signs, which may be subtle, can provide invaluable information concerning the critical care patient's overall neurologic status. Such changes may include those related to breathing **TABLE 12-20** or cardiac function **TABLE 12-21**.

Blood Pressure

The effect on BP most often seen as a result of neurologic injury is hypertension (an increase in BP), especially in the case of rising ICP. As cerebral perfusion decreases, ICP increases; in response, the body attempts to maintain adequate perfusion by increasing BP. Hypertension is commonly seen in conjunction with bradycardia and an abnormal respiratory pattern—a trio of symptoms collectively known as the Cushing triad.

Cerebral injury rarely causes hypotension except in the last stages of injury. The CCTP should, however, take all steps necessary to ensure that the patient does not become hypotensive (systolic blood pressure [SBP] less than 90 mm Hg): Even one episode can be associated with high mortality owing to its detrimental effects on cerebral perfusion.

Pulse pressure is also a valuable tool in the evaluation of neurologic injury. The CCTP may observe widening of the pulse pressure (to greater than 40 mm Hg) in the presence of increasing ICP (discussed later).

Body Temperature

Monitor the patient's body temperature closely for changes. Alterations in body temperature, either hypothermia or hyperthermia, are possible in the

TABLE 12-19 Control Center Location and Function

System	Location	Function
Cardiovascular System		
Cardiac center	Medulla	Regulates rate and force of contraction
Vasomotor center	Medulla	Regulates blood pressure
Respiratory System		
Dorsal respiratory group	Medulla	Initiates inspiration; sets the basic rhythm of respiration
Ventral respiratory group	Medulla	Almost inactive except when increased ventilatory effort is needed
Apneustic center	Pons	Exact function is unclear; sends signals to the dorsal respiratory group to prevent apnea (especially in injury)
Pneumotaxic center	Pons	Modifies inspiration rate
Temperature Regulation		
Anterior hypothalamus (response to heat)	Hypothalamus	Activates cutaneous vasodilation, sweating, increased respiration, anorexia, apathy, and inertia
Posterior hypothalamus (response to cold)	Hypothalamus	Activates shivering, hunger, increased catecholamine release, cutaneous vasoconstriction, horripilation (bristling of hairs on the skin)

© Jones & Bartlett Learning.

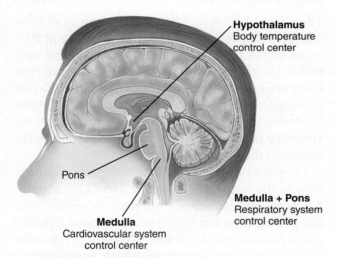

Hypothalamus
Body temperature control center

Pons

Medulla + Pons
Respiratory system control center

Medulla
Cardiovascular system control center

FIGURE 12-29 The locations of the respiratory system, the cardiovascular system, and body temperature control centers in the brain.

© Jones & Bartlett Learning.

presence of neurologic injury, especially if the hypothalamus is involved.

Neurogenic fever (NF), or fever in a patient with traumatic brain injury (TBI) not associated with an infection, was once thought to be relatively uncommon; more recent data, however, suggest that it may occur in as many as one-third of all patients with severe TBI. This condition is likely due to disruption of the hypothalamic temperature set-point, resulting in an abnormally increased body temperature. NF tends to respond poorly to antipyretic agents and may not be associated with the same degree of diaphoresis seen with other causes of fever. When it is suspected, an exhaustive workup is necessary to rule out infectious causes of the fever, as the diagnosis is made by first excluding all infectious possibilities.

Nutritional supplementation should be adjusted in patients with fever to address their increased catabolic demands, particularly in cases of prolonged, sustained fever. Every 1.8°F (1°C) increase in body temperature raises the metabolic rate by 13%, and this additional stress on a critically ill patient can significantly increase morbidity.

Neurologic Diagnostics

This section discusses the neurologic diagnostic tools with which the CCTP should be familiar.

Computed tomography (CT) scanning provides a mathematically reconstructed cross-sectional view of the body, including the brain, and is performed on almost every patient with abnormal neurologic findings. The image is obtained by passing

TABLE 12-20 Breathing Patterns

Breathing Pattern	Location of Injury
Normal	Response to external stressor—not associated with central nervous system dysfunction
Posthyperventilation apnea	Associated with diffuse bilateral metabolic or structural disease of the cerebrum
Cheyne-Stokes respirations	Bilateral dysfunction of deep cerebrum, diencephalonic structures (thalamus and/or hypothalamus), or basal ganglia
Central neurogenic hyperventilation	Dysfunction of midbrain or upper pons
Apneustic breathing	Respiratory control mechanisms located at the pontine level
Cluster breathing	Dysfunction of lower pontine and upper medullary areas
Ataxic (Biot) breathing	Dysfunction of medullary control centers
Agonal gasps	Failing medullary control centers

Data from McCance K, Huether S. *Pathophysiology: The Biologic Basis for Disease in Adults and Children*. St Louis, MO: Mosby; 2002.

TABLE 12-21 Cardiovascular Variances

Cardiovascular Variance	Probable Causes
Bradycardia	Increasing ICP
	SCI involving the sympathetic pathways
Tachycardia	Shock
	The end stage of a neurologic injury
Arrhythmias	Increasing ICP
	Other intracranial pathologic conditions

Abbreviations: ICP, intracranial pressure; SCI, spinal cord injury

© Jones & Bartlett Learning.

intersecting x-ray beams through the area of interest and measuring the density of substances through which the x-ray beams pass. As the density of a substance increases, its image appears more white. As the density of a substance decreases, its image appears more black. In a normal CT scan of the head, bone appears white, blood appears off-white, brain tissue appears shaded gray, CSF appears off-black, and air appears black.

A CT scan can be performed with or without the use of an intravenous (IV) contrast medium. Noncontrast CT is typically undertaken to examine the intracranial area for evidence of intracranial hemorrhage, cerebral edema, or displacement of structures. Computed tomography angiography (CTA) adds the injection of an IV contrast agent into the patient moments before CT scanning. This variant allows for enhancement of vascular areas and better detection of vascular lesions. Patients receiving contrast should be monitored during infusion of the dye and for 10 to 20 minutes after the infusion for evidence of anaphylactic reaction. Patients should also be monitored for evidence of acute tubular necrosis.

The role of CTA has expanded recently, with this technology being used to diagnose large-vessel occlusion (LVO) that may be amenable to neurointerventional procedures. Several large randomized controlled trials—most notably, the MRClean and EXTEND-IA studies—have demonstrated the benefits of neurointerventional treatment with cerebral angiography after IV administration of tissue plasminogen activator (tPA). As a result of these recent advances, most stroke imaging protocols now include a brain CTA after IV administration of tPA based on a negative noncontrast CT. CCTPs will likely be increasingly called upon to transfer patients who have experienced stroke from a primary stroke center to a comprehensive stroke center for neurovascular procedures when CTA demonstrates the patient has a clot amenable to treatment with this regimen.

Magnetic resonance imaging (MRI) produces images with greater detail than does CT and has become the standard diagnostic study for many conditions. A non–iodine-containing contrast medium is usually administered as an IV infusion before performing the procedure. The patient is then placed in a large magnetic field and radiofrequency waves that cause resonance of protons are introduced. A computer uses this resonance to create an image of internal structures and tissues.

Cerebral angiography allows for visualization of the lumens of vessels to provide information about those vessels' patency, size, irregularities, or occlusion. It is typically used in the diagnosis and treatment of cerebral aneurysm, arteriovenous malformation (AVM), and carotid artery disease. In this procedure, a catheter is inserted into the patient's femoral artery, threaded through the aorta, and enters into the origin of cerebral circulation. Once the catheter is in place, a radiopaque contrast medium is injected, facilitating visualization of circulation with the use of serial radiologic imaging. Neurointerventional treatments administered through the catheter can include embolization, clot lysis, and placement and removal of stents or coils. Potential complications associated with this procedure include contrast medium hypersensitivity and renal dysfunction.

Transcranial Doppler (TCD) ultrasonography allows monitoring of cerebral blood flow velocity through thinner areas of the skull; specifically, temporal bone (transtemporal), the eye (transorbital), and the foramen magnum (transoccipital). Blood flow velocities can be measured in the anterior, middle, or posterior cerebral arteries and the vertebral and basilar arteries depending on the angle of the Doppler ultrasound probe. This imaging procedure is commonly used in patients following rupture of an intracranial aneurysm to assess for vasospasm, a problem commonly observed following rupture of a cerebral vessel. It can also be performed to identify intracranial lesions following a stroke and to detect cerebral blood flow changes associated with increased ICP.

Electroencephalography (EEG) involves the recording of electrical impulses generated by the brain to localize abnormal electrical activity. This technology is commonly used as a bedside test in patients with suspected seizure activity, cerebral infarct, metabolic encephalopathies, altered consciousness, infectious disease, and some types of head injuries, and to confirm brain death. Continuous EEG monitoring is often employed in critical care units for patients with known or suspected seizure activity or those at high risk of deterioration.

With this technology, electrodes placed on the patient's head allow electrical impulses to be transferred to a recording unit. Five types of waves are most commonly seen: delta, theta, alpha, beta, and gamma.

- *Delta bands* are normally observed in adults during sleep, and are also normal in infants.

Pathologic causes of these waveforms include various types of lesions (including subcortical, diffuse, and deep midline lesions), as well as metabolic encephalopathy and hydrocephalus.

- *Theta bands* are normally associated with young children, drowsy older children, and drowsy adults, and are sometimes seen during meditation. Pathologic causes are similar to those for delta bands (focal subcortical lesions, deep midline disorders, metabolic encephalopathy, and some kinds of hydrocephalus).
- *Alpha bands* are normal when relaxing or closing the eyes, but are also associated with coma.
- *Beta bands* are normal when a person is active, working, or anxious. They may also appear following use of benzodiazepines.
- *Gamma bands* are normal and are associated with performing cognitive motor functions.

An EEG finding of intermittent slowing with triphasic wave morphology is associated with metabolic encephalopathy. Continuous generalized slowing in the delta or theta range indicates the presence of anoxic damage. Other abnormal EEG findings that are suggestive of a poor prognosis include the combination of alpha waves that do not change with stimulation and a coma state (alpha coma), occasional generalized bursts of activity with intermittent inactivity (burst suppression), generalized spikes at fixed intervals of 1 to 2 Hz, and no activity (electrocerebral silence).

Lumbar puncture is typically performed by entering the subarachnoid space in the lumbar region of the vertebral column with a needle to obtain diagnostic information or to provide a therapeutic intervention. CSF samples can be taken and evaluated for the presence of subarachnoid blood (subarachnoid hemorrhage) or infection, or sent for laboratory analysis (refer to Table 12-1 on CSF composition). The most common complication of this procedure is headache.

Laboratory Assessment

Laboratory studies, other than routine blood studies, biopsy, and CSF analysis, have not traditionally been used in the diagnosis and management of neurologic emergencies. For most patients, a complete blood count (CBC), basic chemistry panel, coagulation study, and cardiac biomarkers should be obtained.

The CBC serves as a baseline study and may reveal a cause of stroke, such as polycythemia or thrombocytosis, or provide evidence of a concurrent illness, such as anemia. The chemistry panel also serves as a baseline study and may reveal the origin of coma, such as hypoglycemia, or provide evidence of concurrent illness, such as renal insufficiency. Coagulation studies may reveal coagulopathy and are useful when the administration of fibrinolytics or anticoagulants is being considered. Cardiac biomarkers are important because of the association of cerebral vascular disease and coronary artery disease. Finally, a toxicology screening may be useful in selected patients in whom a harmful drug or chemical is the suspected cause of an altered level of consciousness, other abnormal neurologic finding, or vital sign anomalies, such as tachycardia or hypertension. See Chapter 21, *Toxicologic Emergencies*, for more information.

Traumatic Brain Injury

Although the rigid cranial vault protects it, the brain may be damaged when high forces impact the skull. Current understanding of the pathophysiology of TBI emphasizes the importance, or role, of two types of injury. Primary (direct) injury occurs as a result of traumatic forces that cause physical or functional disruption of brain tissue. Secondary (indirect) processes occur after injury and cause brain dysfunction or cellular damage (eg, hypoxia and ischemia). Secondary injuries (ie, physiologic derangements) occur rather frequently in the period following primary injury, but often cannot be recorded by standard monitoring equipment. Failure to identify the presence of these injuries may lead to a poor outcome.

Primary Brain Injury

The head is only one part of a collision in an accident; the brain is the other component involved. Primary brain injury can result from two mechanisms: contact phenomena injuries and acceleration-deceleration injuries.

Contact phenomena injuries occur as the direct result of trauma to the head; they include all local effects such as scalp laceration, skull fracture, hematoma, and intracerebral hemorrhage. For years, clinicians believed that contact phenomena injuries were the major factors causing damage in TBI. Subsequent research, however, has shown

that the brain itself is often damaged by abrupt changes in velocity, which may cause strains, compression, tension, and shearing injuries to cerebral tissue. Sudden changes in velocity (acceleration-deceleration) cause the brain to move across its bony interior, resulting in damage. When the head is subjected to translational force, the head's center of gravity moves along a linear path; when it is subjected to rotational force, the head moves around its center of gravity. Rotational injuries result when forces cause the brain to twist within the cranial cavity, resulting in stretching or tearing of neurons in the white matter as well as tearing of the blood vessels that secure the brain to the skull.

Areas of the brain associated with rough portions of the skull (ie, the frontal and temporal lobes) have higher incidences of injury compared with areas with smoother surfaces, such as the occipital lobe. The term contrecoup injury is used to describe a situation in which an impact occurs on one side of the head, causing the brain to move within the cranial vault and forcibly contact the opposite side of the skull, resulting in damage on that side of the brain. This phenomenon is also referred to as transitional injury, because forces can be transferred to the opposite side of the brain **FIGURE 12-30**.

Most of the current literature cites work by Ommaya and his centripetal theory as the best model to explain the lesions observed after head injury. Ommaya's research simulated acceleration-deceleration injuries and found that certain types of brain injuries can be reproduced without any contact force acting on the head. Additionally, his research showed that the higher the magnitude of the injuring forces, the

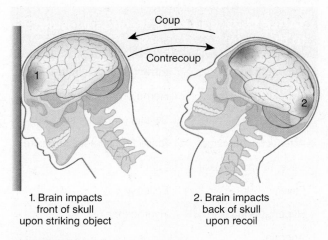

1. Brain impacts front of skull upon striking object

2. Brain impacts back of skull upon recoil

FIGURE 12-30 Contrecoup injury.

deeper the functional and structural damage that occurred to brain structures. As forces increase, the brainstem eventually becomes involved. Even without direct involvement of the brainstem, however, interruption of afferent nerve impulses may be sufficient to produce prolonged loss of consciousness.

Secondary Brain Injury

Secondary brain injury involves the more delayed mechanisms of brain damage. These physiologic derangements, if left uncorrected, will adversely affect brain function integrity. Secondary brain injuries may be classified as insults of either systemic or intracranial origin **TABLE 12-22**.

The pathophysiology of secondary brain injury is well understood. After a brain injury occurs, the normal protective mechanisms may no longer maintain blood flow in the face of falling perfusion pressure, or they may not increase blood flow during hypoxemia. As a consequence, ischemic or hypoxic damage is more likely to occur **FIGURE 12-31**.

Mechanically injured neurons are more susceptible to the effects of hypoxemia and cerebral hypoperfusion. They are also vulnerable to damage by the high concentrations of neurotransmitters (eg, glutamate and aspartate) and toxic metabolites that accumulate in the extracellular environment in the wake of TBI.

Neuronal swelling, edema, and cerebral hyperemia from carbon dioxide retention combine to raise the ICP and lower the **cerebral perfusion pressure (CPP)**. This relationship can be expressed mathematically as **mean arterial pressure (MAP)** minus ICP equals CPP:

$$MAP - ICP = CPP$$

where

$$MAP = DBP + \tfrac{1}{3}(SBP - DBP)$$

As an example, suppose a patient has a BP of 190/100 mm Hg. The calculation of MAP would be

$$MAP = 100 + \tfrac{1}{3}(190 - 100)$$
$$= 100 + \tfrac{1}{3}(90)$$
$$= 100 + 30$$
$$= 130$$

CPP is the primary determinant of blood flow to injured brain tissue when the injury has impaired the ability of the cerebral circulation to autoregulate in response to fluctuations in systemic BP **FIGURE 12-32**. The situation is exacerbated if the ICP is further raised by the presence of a space-occupying lesion or by swelling, or if the CPP is further reduced by extracranial blood loss. The resulting positive feedback loop rapidly causes irreversible clinical deterioration if cerebral perfusion and oxygenation are not quickly improved.

TABLE 12-22 Causes of Secondary Insult to the Brain	
Systemic Origin	**Intracranial Origin**
Hypoxia	Hematoma
Hypercarbia	Swelling, vasospasm
Arterial hypotension	Raised intracranial pressure
Severe hypocarbia	Infection
Fever	Epilepsy
Hyponatremia	Hydrocephalus
Anemia	

© Jones & Bartlett Learning.

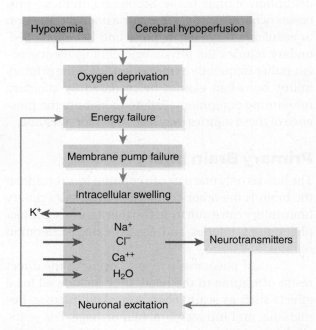

FIGURE 12-31 Pathophysiology of secondary brain injury.

Data from McCance K, Huether S. *Pathophysiology: The Biologic Basis for Disease in Adults and Children*. St. Louis, MO: Mosby; 2002.

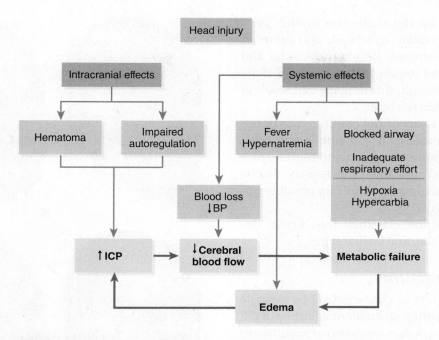

FIGURE 12-32 Cerebral perfusion pressure acts as the primary determinant of blood flow to injured brain tissue.
Abbreviations: BP, blood pressure; ICP, intracranial pressure

Data from McCance K, Huether S. *Pathophysiology: The Biologic Basis for Disease in Adults and Children*. 7th ed. St. Louis, MO: Elsevier Mosby; 2014.

Normal ranges for CPP, MAP, ICP, and end-tidal carbon dioxide (ETCO₂) in adults are as follows:

- CPP: 70 to 90 mm Hg; should not go below 70 mm Hg
- MAP: 70 to 110 mm Hg
- ICP: 5 to 15 cm H_2O
- ETCO₂: 35 to 45 mm Hg

Specific Neurologic Injuries
Scalp Injuries

Injury to the scalp is oftentimes the first indication that a patient has a brain injury. The forces involved in the primary injury determine the type and extent of scalp injury that may be visible. Common injuries to the scalp include abrasions, contusions, lacerations, and avulsions. Like facial injuries, scalp injuries tend to bleed profusely because of the highly vascular nature of the scalp.

Abrasions involve the top layer of the scalp, which may be rubbed away, as evidenced by minor bleeding. Treatment usually focuses on controlling bleeding and cleaning and dressing the area. It is important to remember that some scalp injuries can occur simultaneously secondary to the mechanism of injury.

When examining an abrasion, the CCTP may also note an underlying contusion. Contusions are scalp bruises with possible accumulation of blood in the subcutaneous layer. Definitive control of bleeding is often best achieved by stapling or suturing significant scalp lacerations. It is also important to rule out more significant (deeper) injuries.

Lacerations can be more serious. In these injuries, the scalp is violently torn, leaving a jagged opening that may extend through multiple layers of tissue and even down to the skull itself. Bleeding may be profuse, and deeper injury to the brain tissue or skull is very likely.

Avulsions result from forceful, partial, or complete tearing away or separation of the scalp tissue, which appears as a flap. The primary concerns with this type of injury are the underlying integrity of the skull and the risk of infection resulting from introduction of contaminants. Treatment should focus on evaluation of the skull for fractures and a thorough cleaning of the tissue under the avulsion.

Skull Fractures

Skull fractures result from a direct, and often high-force, blow to the cranium; they are present in more than 50% of patients with a severe TBI. Any of the bones that make up the skull—the frontal, parietal, temporal, occipital, sphenoid, and ethmoid bones—may be fractured. Between the skull and the dura, large blood vessels can be damaged; if the impact is severe enough, this damage can result in hemorrhaging within the brain.

Although not a part of the cranium, the bones of the face—the maxillary, zygomatic, nasal, lacrimal, and palatine bones; vomer; mandible; and part of the ethmoid and sphenoid bones—may also be fractured. Such fractures may indicate possible underlying brain injury.

Skull fractures are classified into linear, depressed, comminuted, and basilar types.

Linear Skull Fractures

A linear skull fracture is characterized by a single fracture line and is often an incidental finding of CT. This kind of fracture occurs when two or more bones of the skull separate at the suture line. Hematomas, soft-tissue swelling, and point tenderness are usually present over the site of impact **FIGURE 12-33A**. A simple closed linear fracture rarely requires any surgical intervention.

Stellate fractures of the skull (and other bones) are also possible. A linear stellate fracture comprises multiple linear fractures radiating from the site of impact. These fractures have the potential to do damage depending on the number and depth of the fracture(s). In contrast, a diastatic stellate fracture involves the separation of an epiphysis when it is the center site of impact. Diastatic stellate fractures are prevalent in abused children. Thus, the presence of a diastatic fracture to a long bone in a child should arouse suspicion of possible head trauma or shaken baby syndrome.

Depressed Skull Fractures

In a depressed skull fracture, a portion of the skull is depressed, and the scalp and/or dura may or may not be torn **FIGURE 12-33B**. This type of fracture may produce soft-tissue swelling over the site of the trauma; a bony step-off may be palpated as well. Depressed skull fractures may be classified as open or closed, indicating the presence, or lack thereof, of a breach in the dura mater in conjunction with the fracture. An open depressed skull fracture **FIGURE 12-33C** is the more serious of the two injuries.

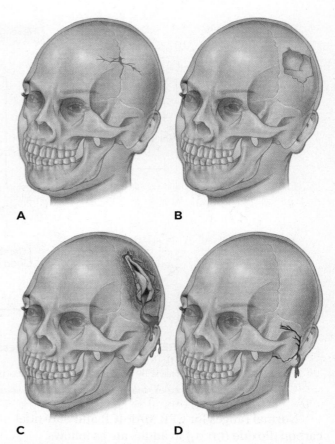

FIGURE 12-33 Types of skull fractures. **A.** Linear. **B.** Depressed. **C.** Open. **D.** Basilar.
© Jones & Bartlett Learning.

Three types of depressed skull fractures are distinguished: true, flat, and ping-pong ball fracture. In a true fracture (the most common type), the fracture has contact with the cranial vault. A flat fracture features a depressed segment without any connection with the cranial vault and is the least common type. A ping-pong ball fracture is a pediatric greenstick fracture of the skull. Although these distinctions may be of importance in the hospital setting, during the prehospital phase of the transport, the most important considerations are to identify the existence of a depressed skull fracture, to classify it as open or closed, and to treat it appropriately.

Comminuted Skull Fractures

A fracture in which the skull is splintered or shattered into many pieces is referred to as a comminuted fracture. These pieces may then act as projectiles and cause direct injury to the meningeal layers or the brain tissue itself. A great deal of blunt force is required to cause this type of skull fracture.

Basilar Skull Fractures

A basilar skull fracture involves fractures along the base of the skull **FIGURE 12-33D**. This area is punctuated by multiple foramina that accommodate the spinal cord, nerves, and blood vessels. Because of the many hollow or open spaces within the skull (eg, the sinuses, eye orbits, nasal cavities, external auditory canals, middle and inner ears), the skull is weaker here and susceptible to basilar fractures. Basilar fractures usually result from a blow to the parietal, temporal, or occipital regions of the skull, with the temporal area being the most commonly affected.

Tearing of the dura mater during a basilar skull fracture may also occur, resulting in a wound between the brain and the external environment. This condition may present with leakage of CSF, which may be combined with blood through the dural tear either into the nasal cavity or via the external auditory canal **FIGURE 12-34**. Openings in the dura mater also provide a conduit for infectious agents to enter the meninges or brain tissue. The halo test for leaking CSF is accomplished by collecting escaping fluid from the nose, mouth, or ears, onto a gauze pad. The appearance of a "target" or "halo" symbol consisting of a dark red circle surrounded by a lighter yellow one is considered a positive halo sign **FIGURE 12-35**. The CCTP must exercise caution when using the halo test as the sole diagnostic evaluation of a CSF leak, because other fluids such as lacrimal fluid, nasal fluid, or saliva may cause a similar response.

Other clinical signs may be evident depending on the location of the injury. Fractures involving the auditory canal and lower lateral areas of the skull may result in the migration of blood to the mastoid region, posterior and slightly inferior to the ear, resulting in discoloration referred to as retroauricular ecchymosis or Battle sign **FIGURE 12-36**. Similarly, orbital fractures and hemorrhaging into the surrounding tissue are known as periorbital ecchymosis or raccoon eyes **FIGURE 12-37**. Raccoon eyes and Battle sign may take several hours to develop and become evident after the injury; thus, these signs are not often seen by emergency paramedics during initial evaluation of a head-injured patient

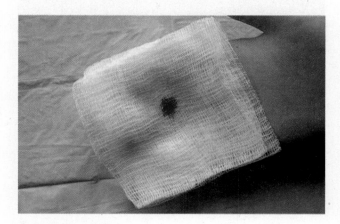

FIGURE 12-35 Halo sign.
© American Academy of Orthopaedic Surgeons.

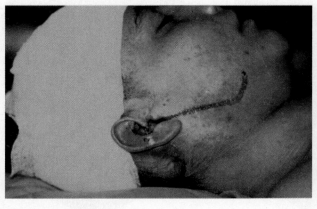

FIGURE 12-34 Blood leaking from the external auditory canal after a head injury may contain cerebrospinal fluid and suggests a basilar skull fracture.
© American Academy of Orthopaedic Surgeons.

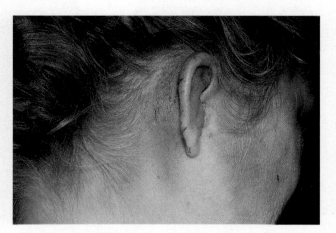

FIGURE 12-36 Battle sign consists of ecchymosis behind the ear or over the mastoid process.
© American Academy of Orthopaedic Surgeons.

at the scene of initial trauma but may be seen by the CCTP during transport and/or subsequent treatment of the patient.

Facial Fractures

As many as 60% of patients with significant facial injuries sustain trauma to other organ systems, including the brain. Unfortunately, many facial injuries have very grotesque presentations accompanied by copious bleeding—characteristics that may potentially distract the CCTP from other, more

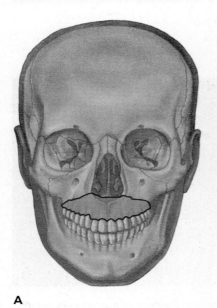

FIGURE 12-37 Raccoon eyes are characterized by ecchymosis under or around the eyes.

serious injuries. Fractures of the facial bones are usually very painful and require massive amounts of analgesia to maintain patient comfort. This is especially true with mandible fractures, which can cause life-threatening airway compromise if the patient is in the supine position. Because of the instability of the mandible, the tongue no longer has support and can become lodged in the back of the airway, obstructing this passageway.

Airway control is the first assessment priority in patients with facial injuries. After securing the airway, the CCTP can assess for the presence of facial fractures by grasping the hard palate and rocking it back and forth. The CCTP should also check for malocclusion and dental trauma, test extraocular muscles to rule out orbital fractures, and look for facial elongation ("monkey face") and periorbital ecchymosis.

Some of the most serious facial injuries are maxillary fractures, which result from high-energy forces to the face. These fractures are classified using the Le Fort criteria **FIGURE 12-38**.

- *Le Fort I* is a transverse fracture separating the hard palate from its bony frame. This fracture exhibits slight instability to the maxilla with no associated displacement.
- *Le Fort II* is a fracture involving the central maxilla and palate; it has a pyramidal appearance (the fractured portion is shaped like a

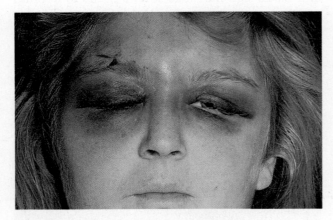

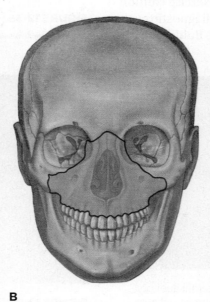

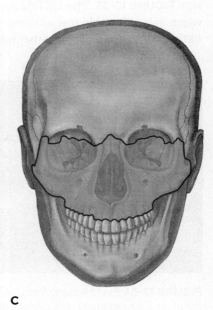

A   **B**   **C**

FIGURE 12-38 Le Fort fractures. **A.** Le Fort I. **B.** Le Fort II. **C.** Le Fort III.

pyramid). This fracture extends through both maxilla and the nasal bones.

- *Le Fort III* is effectively a craniofacial disruption, with fractures extending from the frontozygomatic sutures, orbits, and nasoethmoidal regions. This fracture is unstable and is associated with oral and nasal patency problems. It can leave the patient with a "monkey face" appearance, resulting from the protrusion of the face secondary to its instability.
- *Le Fort IV* is essentially a Le Fort III fracture with a concurrent frontal bone fracture.

Le Fort III fractures usually result in leakage of CSF.

Brain Injuries

Injuries to the brain can be either focal or diffuse. Focal lesions are those large enough to be observed directly. In contrast, diffuse injuries are not associated with gross localized and visible lesions, but include concussions and diffuse axonal injuries **TABLE 12-23**.

Focal Injuries

Contusions and Lacerations

A cerebral contusion is a bruising of the brain tissue. Patients with isolated cerebral contusions may exhibit altered mental status, but rarely develop coma. Contusions commonly occur with rapid deceleration injuries and typically appear on the tips of the frontal and temporal lobes, where the skull

TABLE 12-23 Brain Injury Types	
Focal	**Diffuse**
Contusion Hematoma Epidural Subdural	Axonal injury
Intracerebral	Hypoxia/ischemia
Swelling	Diffuse vascular
Infarct	Fat embolism
Pressure necrosis	Subarachnoid
Abscess	Meningitis

© Jones & Bartlett Learning.

base has an irregular shape. Contusions appearing on the same side of the impact are known as coup injuries, whereas injuries on the side opposite the impact are known as contrecoup injuries (see Figure 12-30).

Treatment for patients with cerebral contusions is largely supportive; no surgical intervention is usually needed. The patient should be monitored for evidence of increasing ICP resulting from hematoma or edema formation; if either of these conditions occurs, it should be treated aggressively.

Special Populations

Indirect and hemorrhagic brain injuries are much more common in older adults. The brain tends to atrophy with aging, so older patients can tolerate more swelling before herniation occurs, making it easier to tear the bridging veins.

Lacerations that result in penetration of the cranium may cause tearing of the cortical surface of the brain. A major difference between a contusion and a laceration is that the pia mater and arachnoid mater are torn over a laceration but remain intact over a contusion. Treatment for cerebral lacerations is identical to that for cerebral contusions, with the CCTP monitoring for signs of increasing ICP.

Epidural Hematomas

An accumulation of blood between the inner periosteum and the dura mater is known as an **epidural hematoma (EDH)**, also called an extradural hematoma. Most EDHs are arterial in origin, occurring when a blow strikes the temporal region and causes concomitant disruption of the middle meningeal artery. Blood may accumulate quickly in the potential space as the high arterial pressure gradually strips the dura away from the inner surface of the skull, forming an oval-shaped mass that exerts pressure on the underlying brain tissue **FIGURE 12-39**. An EDH can be caused by venous bleeding but is limited by the space between the dura and the skull. As the hematoma enlarges, however, the temporal lobe may be displaced and squeeze over the tentorium.

The patient with an EDH may present with a history of a brief period of unconsciousness, followed by a lucid period lasting for minutes to several hours. The lucid period ends with a rapid deterioration of consciousness from drowsiness, to lethargy, and then to coma as a mass effect and herniation develop. If tentorial herniation (herniation of the tentorium of the cerebellum) occurs, the third cranial nerve may become compressed, causing an ipsilateral fixed and dilated pupil **FIGURE 12-40**. Tentorial herniation may also occur on the opposite side, causing either contralateral or bilateral blown pupils (Kernohan notch phenomenon). As ICP continues to rise, the patient may develop bradycardia, Cheyne-Stokes respiratory patterns that progress to brainstem patterns, and brain distortion. Other clinical manifestations may include headache, seizures, hemiparesis or hemiplegia, decorticate or decerebrate posturing **FIGURE 12-41**, respiratory distress, and death. The most common presentation includes vomiting, seizures, unilateral hyperreflexia with a positive Babinski sign, and elevated CSF pressure.

Large hematomas produce a mass effect (ie, act as a space-occupying lesion) and increased ICP. If herniation occurs or will likely occur, the hematoma should be evacuated with a craniotomy. The torn vessel will also be repaired during the craniotomy.

The bleeding with EDH can sometimes be so severe that, in some cases, the brain is actually displaced (midline shift) within the skull. Some medications, such as osmotic diuretics (mannitol), can be given in the early stages of midline shift to slow the progression of this condition until surgical intervention can be obtained.

Mannitol is an osmotic diuretic used to reduce the increased ICP resulting from an increased volume of CSF. It is also used to reduce intraocular pressure. In the case of brain hemorrhage, increases in CSF result from inflammation of brain tissue caused by blood or damage to the subarachnoid villa, which impedes reabsorption of CSF. Mannitol is also useful for patients with cerebral edema not related to a brain bleed. It has little effect in reducing the volume of blood that accumulates owing to the hemorrhage, however. The dosage for adults and children older than 12 years is 1.5 to 2 g/kg in a 15%, 20%, or 25% IV solution given over 30 to 60 minutes via an infusion pump.

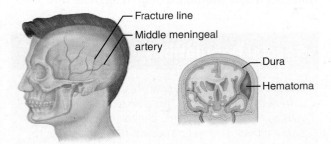

FIGURE 12-39 An epidural hematoma, caused by a blow to the temporal region of the head and concomitant disruption of the middle meningeal artery, with the accumulation of blood between the inner periosteum and the dura mater.

© Jones & Bartlett Learning.

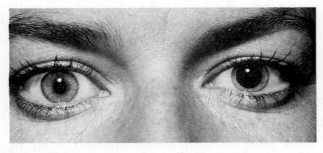

FIGURE 12-40 Ipsilateral fixed and dilated pupil.

© American Academy of Orthopaedic Surgeons.

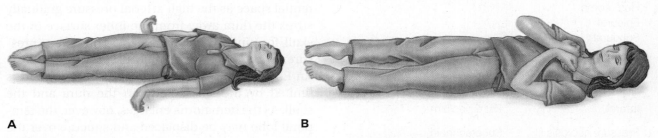

A   B

FIGURE 12-41 Posturing indicates significant intracranial pressure. **A.** Decerebrate (extensor) posturing. **B.** Decorticate (flexor) posturing. (Think of the arms being pulled to the core of the body.)

© Jones & Bartlett Learning.

Hypertonic saline may also be administered to reduce ICP. Given either by bolus or by continuous infusion, hypertonic saline likely reduces ICP through osmotic effects. Concentrations and volumes administered vary significantly, with concentrations ranging from 1.5% to 23.5% and volumes from 10 to 30 mL/kg.

Brainstem herniation is a primary concern with EDH. It occurs when the expanding blood pushes the brain down the foramen magnum, causing a shearing-type force on the brain. Once this takes place, death is imminent, because this condition is irreversible.

Signs and Symptoms

Epidural Hematoma

- Brief period of unconsciousness, followed by a lucid period lasting for minutes to several hours
- Following the lucid period, rapid deterioration of consciousness (drowsiness to lethargy to coma)
- Ipsilateral fixed and dilated pupil
- Contralateral or bilateral blown pupils (Kernohan notch phenomenon)
- Headache
- Bradycardia
- Cheyne-Stokes respiratory pattern, progressing to brainstem breathing patterns
- Possible seizures
- Hemiparesis
- Hemiplegia
- Decorticate or decerebrate posturing
- Respiratory distress
- Vomiting
- Seizures
- Unilateral hyperreflexia with a positive Babinski sign
- Elevated CSF pressure
- Elevated ICP with brain distortion
- Death

Transport Management

Epidural Hematoma

- Provide rapid transport.
- Consider administering an osmotic diuretic (mannitol).

Subdural Hematomas

High-energy impacts may also result in bleeding that accumulates between the dura and arachnoid mater, known as a **subdural hematoma (SDH)**. SDHs are six times more common than EDHs and have a higher mortality rate. Most SDHs result from a disruption of the bridging veins located over the crest of the brain and their subsequent bleeding. SDHs are categorized based on the time that elapses between the initial injury and the appearance of signs and symptoms as well as the appearance of the blood and fluid composition **FIGURE 12-42**.

Acute SDH—that is, SDH in which signs and symptoms appear within 24 hours of the injury—is commonly seen with acceleration-deceleration injuries. With this type of injury, clotted blood may be visible on CT as crescent-shaped collections of blood with high attenuation usually along the cranium. Patients usually present with a gradual or sometimes rapid deterioration in level of consciousness, pupillary changes, and hemiparesis or hemiplegia.

In subacute SDH, signs and symptoms appear between 2 days and 2 weeks after the initial injury because the blood accumulates more slowly. This type of hematoma consists of a mixture of clotted and fluid blood; on CT, it may appear as areas that are isodense, hypodense, or of mixed density depending on the age of the lesion **FIGURE 12-43**. Patients with subacute SDH present with gradual mental status and/or personality changes as well as many of the symptoms for the acute hematoma that evolve as the lesion expands.

Chronic SDH manifests as clinical signs and symptoms more than 2 weeks after the injury. This type of hematoma is composed of fluid only.

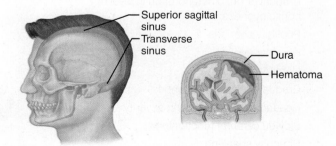

FIGURE 12-42 A subdural hematoma, in which venous bleeding occurs beneath the dura mater but outside the brain.

© Jones & Bartlett Learning.

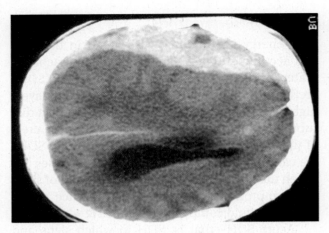

FIGURE 12-43 Computed tomographic scan of an acute subdural hematoma.

© Living Art Enterprises/Science Source.

Because the lesion expands very slowly, the patient may experience headache (progressing in severity), slowed cerebral functioning, confusion, drowsiness, and possibly seizures.

Treatment of SDHs depends on the size of the hematoma and the patient's symptoms, and ranges from watchful waiting to surgical intervention. Small SDHs may be observed and allowed to reabsorb without surgery. SDHs accompanied by signs and symptoms of increasing ICP usually require surgical intervention to evacuate the expanding mass and stop the bleeding. A newer, less invasive technology, known as the Subdural Evacuating Port System (SEPS), can be inserted at the bedside

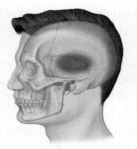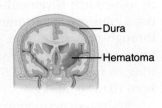

Dura

Hematoma

FIGURE 12-44 An intracerebral hemorrhage is a result of direct bleeding into the brain parenchyma.

© Jones & Bartlett Learning.

through a 5-mm burr hole under local anesthesia to drain chronic and subacute SDHs. The SEPS allows for evacuation of SDHs using a closed system, often avoiding the need for surgical intervention.

Transport Management

Subdural Hematoma
- Provide supportive care.

Other Types of Brain Hemorrhage

An **intracerebral hemorrhage** results from direct bleeding into the brain parenchyma and can be observed in as many as 15% of patients with brain injuries **FIGURE 12-44**. Many of these hemorrhages occur in the same areas as cerebral contusions, making it appear that the rough internal areas of the cranium are often to blame for these injuries. Intracerebral hemorrhages act as space-occupying lesions, producing headaches, deteriorating levels of consciousness, hemiplegia on the contralateral side, and a dilated ipsilateral pupil. They are discussed in more detail later in this chapter.

Patients may also develop a **delayed traumatic intracranial hemorrhage (DTICH)** within the first 3 to 10 days following an injury to the occipital-parietal region via a coup-contrecoup mechanism. Serial CT scans should be performed within the first 72 hours after injury if DTICH is suspected, as part of the effort to decrease the mortality and morbidity that result from such bleeding.

The presentation of a patient with a **subarachnoid hemorrhage (SAH)** depends on the size of the hemorrhage and the coexisting injuries.

Signs and Symptoms

Subdural Hematoma
- Gradual or rapid deterioration in level of consciousness
- Pupillary changes
- Hemiparesis
- Hemiplegia
- Gradual personality changes
- Headache (progressing in severity)
- Slowed cerebral functioning
- Difficulty speaking
- Confusion
- Drowsiness
- Possible seizures

With this type of injury, bleeding occurs between the arachnoid mater and the dura mater of the brain, resulting in the patient reporting the "worst headache in my life." Patients with SAH are also more likely to have hypoxia, hypotension, and increased ICP, all of which contribute to secondary brain injury. Signs and symptoms include altered mental status, coma, paralysis, slurred speech, mood changes, and seizures, and appear to be due to increased ICP and meningeal irritation. SAH is discussed in more detail later in this chapter.

Diffuse Injuries

Concussion, also known as mild TBI, is a traumatically induced physiologic disruption of brain function that occurs without structural damage. This injury is manifested by at least one of the following signs and symptoms:

- Any loss of consciousness
- Any loss of memory for events immediately before (retrograde) or events immediately after (anterograde) the event that precipitated the injury
- Any alteration in mental status at the time of the injury (eg, feeling dazed, disoriented, irritable, drowsy, giddy, or confused)
- Focal neurologic deficits in which the patient is not unconscious for longer than 30 minutes; after 30 minutes, the patient has a GCS score of 13 to 15

Deep areas of the brain may also be involved in a TBI; such injuries are referred to as diffuse axonal injury (DAI). The mechanism for DAI is usually very rapid acceleration-deceleration forces. In these injuries, shearing forces damage the integrity of the axon at the node of Ranvier, which consequently alters the axoplasmic flow (the flow in the cytoplasm of the axon). Areas especially susceptible to this type of injury, because they contain a significant amount of white matter, include the corpus callosum, the brainstem, and sometimes the cerebellum.

Diffuse axonal injury accounts for approximately 50% of all primary brain injuries and 35% of TBI-related deaths. It is characterized by microscopic findings of wide and asymmetric axonal swelling, which appear within hours of the injury and may persist for much longer, and by focal hemorrhagic lesions. The resulting injury is graded based on pathologic findings:

- **DAI grade 1.** Histologic evidence of axonal damage in the white matter of the cerebral hemispheres, corpus callosum, brainstem, and, less commonly, cerebellum
- **DAI grade 2.** In addition to evidence of axonal injury, lesions in the corpus callosum
- **DAI grade 3.** In addition to the findings seen in grades 1 and 2, lesions in the dorsolateral quadrant of the rostral brainstem

The clinical presentation of DAI includes a sequence of events beginning with immediate unconsciousness (termed *coma* in this context), leading to a longer period of confusion and associated posttraumatic amnesia, and followed by a protracted recovery time. DAI can be clinically classified as mild, moderate, or severe based on the patient's signs and symptoms.

- **Mild DAI.** Coma lasts from 6 to 24 hours, with the patient beginning to obey commands by 24 hours. Death is rare with mild DAI, but cognitive and neurologic deficits are common.
- **Moderate DAI.** Coma lasts longer than 24 hours, but prominent signs of brainstem damage are absent. Patients who survive usually have an incomplete recovery.
- **Severe DAI.** Coma is protracted and associated with prominent signs of brainstem damage (eg, decortication, decerebration, abnormal respiratory pattern). Patients usually die or experience severe disability.

Treatment for all types of DAI is supportive.

Signs and Symptoms

Diffuse Axonal Injury
- Sequence of events:
  - Immediate unconsciousness
  - Longer period of confusion and posttraumatic amnesia
  - Protracted recovery time
- Mild DAI: Coma lasts from 6 to 24 hours, with the patient beginning to obey commands by 24 hours
- Moderate DAI: Coma lasts longer than 24 hours, but prominent signs of brainstem damage are absent
- Severe DAI: Coma is protracted and associated with prominent signs of brainstem damage (decortication, decerebration, and abnormal respiratory pattern)

Intracranial Pressure
Physiology

In adults, the normal ICP is 5 to 15 mm Hg. ICP is not a static state, but rather may be influenced by multiple factors. A recording of ICP will show two forms of pressure fluctuations: (1) a rise with cardiac systole, owing to the distention of the intracranial arteriolar tree that follows it, and (2) a slower change in pressure with respiration, with ICP falling with each inspiration and rising with each expiration. Straining and compression of the neck veins can also cause a sudden, considerable rise in pressure.

The Monro-Kellie doctrine describes the cranium as a rigid box that is filled with a nearly incompressible brain and whose total volume tends to remain constant. This doctrine assumes that the cranium volume includes three compartments: (1) the brain and medulla spinalis, along with the meninges; (2) the blood vessels and blood; and (3) the CSF space. Expansion of any of these three volumes occurs at the expense of the other two elements; intracranial bleeding, cerebral edema, mass formation, or inability to regulate the production and removal of CSF may precipitate such an event.

CSF is secreted constantly within the brain. After circulating, it is absorbed at a rate equal to the rate at which it is produced. CSF circulation is a slow process, with only 500 to 700 mL being circulated each day. At any given time, the cranium contains approximately 75 mL of CSF. Excesses of CSF can be displaced through the foramen magnum into the spinal theca, a sac between C1 and C2. This process may help in cases of cribriform plate damage if the channel for drainage becomes blocked. The spinal dural sheath can accept a quantity of CSF because it does not adhere closely to the canal and is surrounded by a layer of loose areola tissue and a plexus of epidural veins. In addition, during periods of increased ICP, blood flow through venous emissaries increases.

Intracranial circulation of blood is approximately 1,000 L/d, delivered at a pressure of 100 mm Hg. At any given time, the cranium contains approximately 750 mL of blood. Obstruction to venous outflow leads to an increase in the volume of intracranial blood, resulting in increased ICP. As the ICP increases, the cerebral venous pressure increases in parallel so that it remains 2 to 5 mm higher than the ICP, a differential that prevents the collapse of the venous system.

Increased ICP can result from changes in CSF, edema, expansible masses, and changes in vessel size. The ability of the skull contents to compensate for the increased pressure depends on the location and rate of expansion of the lesion and the brain tissue compliance—that is, the volume-buffering capacity of the system. (Brain tissue compliance is defined as the change in brain volume resulting from a change in pressure.)

Cerebral Blood Flow

The brain accounts for only 2% of total body weight, yet its blood flow represents 15% of the resting cardiac output and it uses 20% of the total amount of oxygen consumed by the body. Every 24 hours, the brain requires 1,000 L of blood in addition to its normal diet of 71 L of oxygen and 100 g of glucose. The cerebral blood flow (CBF) remains constant over a wide range of arterial pressures between 60 mm Hg and 150 mm Hg. With a rise to more than 150 mm Hg, however, blood flow increases. CBF ceases when MAP drops to 20 mm Hg, except in the chronically hypertensive patient, in whom this autoregulation limit appears to be reset. The exact nature of this autoregulation is not known; we know only that many factors, including direct reaction of the cerebral arterial smooth muscle to stretching, various by-products of metabolism, and direct control by nerves surrounding vessels, seem to have a role.

In patients with a normal cerebrovascular system and BP, even moderate alterations of Pco_2 (partial pressure of carbon dioxide) are capable of markedly altering CBF. Within the Pco_2 range of 30 to 60 mm Hg, there is a 2.5% change in CBF as the Pco_2 changes by 1 mm Hg. With a pressure of less than 20 mm Hg or more than 80 mm Hg, there is no further change. As the body ages and with the development of arteriosclerosis, there is a marked decrease in Pco_2 influence on CBF.

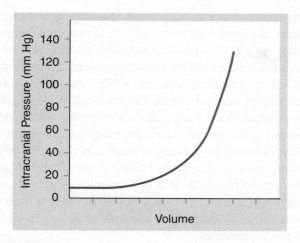

FIGURE 12-45 An intracranial pressure curve.

© Jones & Bartlett Learning.

The effect of P_{O_2} (partial pressure of oxygen) changes is not as obvious as the effect of changes involving carbon dioxide. Moderate variations of oxygen pressure above or below the normal level do not affect CBF. Increased P_{O_2} causes vasoconstriction of nonischemic areas of the brain as well as a reduction in CBF. In contrast, in the ischemic areas of the brain, increasing the P_{O_2} has no effect. Cerebral vasodilation begins with a P_{O_2} of 50 mm Hg, resulting in increasing CBF. By the time the P_{O_2} falls to 30 mm Hg, CBF may have already tripled.

ICP influences the CBF through the CPP, which is the difference between MAP and ICP. An increase in ICP leads to a fall in the CPP. Every effort should be made to maintain the CPP at 70 mm Hg or more during treatment of increased ICP **FIGURE 12-45**.

For the CCTP, the following key points related to CBF are crucial:

- A number of physiologic factors may affect or change CBF. For example, increases in CBF as a result of hypoxia or hypercapnia (increased levels of carbon dioxide in the blood) will cause an increase in ICP once the normal compensating mechanisms have been exhausted.
- Poor airway and ventilatory control contributes to hypoxia, hypercapnia, and hypotension, and will further damage the already critically ill brain.

Cerebral Perfusion Pressure

Cerebral perfusion pressure is responsible for the movement of blood through the brain and is the result of the difference between MAP and ICP (CPP = MAP − ICP). This relationship represents the pressure gradient driving CBF, and hence oxygen and metabolite delivery. The uninjured brain is capable of autoregulating its blood flow to provide a consistent flow of blood, regardless of BP, by altering the resistance of cerebral blood vessels.

After head trauma, however, these homeostatic mechanisms are often lost. As a consequence, a patient with TBI may have increased cerebral vascular resistance, making the brain more susceptible to changes in BP. Those areas of the brain that are ischemic or at risk for ischemia are critically dependent on an adequate CBF and, therefore, CPP.

For the CCTP, the following key points related to CPP are crucial:

- Maintenance of CPP reduces mortality in severe head injury.
- CPP should be maintained between 70 and 90 mm Hg to reduce the risk of poor outcomes for patients with increased ICP.
- Systemic hypotension (SBP less than 90 mm Hg) is associated with a poor prognosis.
- Maintenance of an adequate CPP is the cornerstone of modern brain injury therapy.

After brain injury, and especially in the patient who has sustained multisystem trauma, CBF may be dangerously low, bordering on ischemia. To prevent further neuronal death (secondary brain injury), the flow of well-oxygenated blood must be restored as soon as possible. The optimal level of CPP has not yet been determined, but the CPP target lies within the range of 70 to 90 mm Hg. When CPP is maintained above 70 mm Hg in the absence of cerebral ischemia through the aggressive administration of fluids and pressors, there is a significantly increased risk of acute respiratory distress syndrome.

CPP may be maintained by either raising MAP or lowering ICP. In practice, ICP is usually controlled so that it remains within normal limits (less than 20 mm Hg), and MAP is raised therapeutically to a level greater than 90 mm Hg. Although it is unknown whether ICP control is necessary, given that outcomes from severe TBI related to ICP seem to rely more on its role in determining CPP, it is clear that ICP plays a role in herniation. Current data support initiating treatment when ICP exceeds 20 mm Hg.

Substantial evidence indicates that early hypotension (SBP of less than 90 mm Hg) is associated with increased morbidity and mortality following severe brain injury. Even patients with one episode of hypotension during their intensive care unit (ICU) stay have a significantly poorer prognosis. To ensure that patients remain normovolemic, the CCTP must be vigilant in controlling other sites of hemorrhage while providing adequate oxygenation.

Many patients with TBI, because of the extent of their injuries, will require intensive neurologic monitoring. As previously discussed, CCTPs should perform serial neurologic examinations, especially for patients with TBI. They may also be required to maintain (but not place) invasive neurologic monitoring devices. Each device must be maintained in accordance with the manufacturer's requirements, and each CCTP is responsible for becoming familiar with all aspects of each device prior to using it on a patient. Because of the often subtle, yet devastating effects created by rising ICP, invasive monitoring can be a valuable tool that gives a more detailed picture of the patient's overall neurologic condition.

Pathophysiology of Increased ICP

The brain is encapsulated within the skull and surrounded by CSF generated in the choroid plexus and reassimilated by the subarachnoid villa to balance ICP between 5 and 15 cm H_2O. Because the skull is essentially an immovable structure, any change diminishing its volume will create an increase in ICP. The most common causes of increased ICP are cerebral hemorrhage, tumors, hydrocephalus, and trauma.

Variations in CSF volume result from many causes, including overproduction of CSF, decreased absorption of CSF, and obstructions in cerebral circulation. All of these conditions lead to an increased volume of CSF within the cranial vault and, therefore, to increased pressure on brain tissue.

Brain tissue is the most difficult component within the cranial vault to manipulate without surgical intervention. The parenchyma can respond to increases in ICP, changes in CSF or blood volume, and changes in vessel size (which affect the volumes carried). Minimal volume changes incite the tissue to react with partial collapse of the cisterns, ventricles, and vascular system, which leads to decreased production and increased absorption of CSF.

Increased ICP is defined as a sustained elevation in pressure to more than 20 cm H_2O. During compensation, the ICP rises and plateaus, at which time the increased level of CSF absorption keeps pace with the increase in volume. Intermittent expansion causes only a transient rise in ICP at first. When a sufficient amount of CSF has been absorbed to accommodate the volume, ICP returns to normal. Once compensatory mechanisms are no longer effective, however, pressure increases rapidly, followed by shifting of the brain tissue toward open spaces in the skull. This shift, which results in decreased blood flow to the medulla, is accompanied by dilation of small arteries in the pia mater and some slowing of venous flow, followed by pulsatile venous flow.

The following compensatory mechanisms help maintain ICP:

- Shunting of CSF into the spinal subarachnoid space
- Increased CSF absorption
- Decreased CSF production
- Shunting of venous blood out of the skull

When ICP rises to the level of the arterial pressure, a cascade of events known as Cushing triad begins. Cushing triad comprises progressively increasing SBP, progressively decreasing diastolic blood pressure (DBP; widening pulse pressure), and bradycardia. It is a sign of increased ICP, which occurs as the result of Cushing reflex (a vasopressor response). Vasoconstriction occurs as the body attempts to shift fluid volumes in the cranium, thereby reducing ICP. If ICP continues to rise, brain displacement accelerates, putting pressure on the medulla oblongata by pushing it into the foramen magnum, and in turn resulting in disturbances in breathing, heart rate, and BP. The Cushing triad—hypertension, bradycardia, and respiratory irregularities—is a late sign and often indicates that severe and even irreversible injury has occurred within the cranial cavity. Its identification is important because it suggests severe ischemia in the brain. Possible causes include cerebral hemorrhage, a brain tumor, or brain herniation, which can be fatal.

If ICP increases to the level of systemic arterial pressure, cerebral circulation will be terminated. This situation can be reversed only if arterial pressure rises sufficiently higher than ICP, which restores CBF. If this effort fails, brain death occurs.

The cause of the rise in ICP and the rate at which it occurs are also important. Many patients with benign intracranial temperature (ICT) or obstructive hydrocephalus may show few or no ill effects despite their increased ICP, because the brain is normal and autoregulation is intact. Conversely, cerebral blood flow may be compromised even when ICP is relatively low if parenchymal lesions—such as tumors, hematomas, and contusions—cause the brain to shift and disrupt autoregulation. In acute hydrocephalus, a rapid deterioration occurs because there is no time for compensation.

Disruption of brain function secondary to ICP may include the following conditions:

- Reduction in CBF.
- Transtentorial or foramen magnum herniation resulting in selective compression and ischemia of the brainstem.
- Transtentorial herniation with brainstem compression that leads to clinical deterioration even with adequate CBF. A temporal mass may cause uncal herniation without raised ICP. Similarly, a frontal mass can cause axial distortion and impair brainstem perfusion.

Clinical Manifestations of Increased ICP

The clinical features of increased ICP result from the presence of Cushing triad and are indicated by arterial hypertension, bradycardia, and respiratory changes. It has traditionally been thought that the hypertension and bradycardia result from ischemia or pressure on the brainstem. More recently, some sources have suggested that cerebral ischemia might eliminate supratentorial inhibition of brainstem vasopressor centers and that bradycardia occurs independently of the rise in BP.

Respiratory changes depend on the level of brainstem involved. Midbrain involvement results in Cheyne-Stokes respirations. When both the midbrain and the pons are involved, sustained hyperventilation occurs. With upper medulla involvement, rapid and shallow respirations are followed by ataxic breathing in the final stages.

Increased ICP also has pulmonary effects. Pulmonary edema seems to reflect increased sympathetic activity caused by the effects of increased ICP on the hypothalamus, medulla, or cervical spinal cord. This is a direct result of the disruption of the pulmonary capillary integrity and increased left arterial pressures.

ICP Monitoring

The primary goal of ICP monitoring is to improve the ability to maintain adequate CPP and oxygenation. Intracranial hypertension (sustained ICP of 15 mm Hg or greater) results when the brain's protective mechanisms to shunt CSF to the subarachnoid space or to vasoconstrict cerebral arterioles fail to maintain the ICP at less than 15 mm Hg. Intracranial hypertension compromises the relationship between systemic BP and the resistance that must be overcome to accomplish cerebral perfusion. When CPP falls below 50 mm Hg, secondary brain ischemia, herniation, and ultimately brain death occur. ICP monitoring allows for early detection of intracranial hypertension and subsequent aggressive management of the underlying pathology.

Key points in monitoring ICP are as follows:

- The baseline requirements are oxygen saturation (Spo_2), electrocardiography (ECG), MAP, $ETCO_2$, central venous pressure, and urine output.
- ICP and BP monitoring are the only way to reliably determine CPP and assess cerebral hypoperfusion in patients with severe brain injury.
- Multimodality monitoring, including jugular venous oxygen saturation (Sjo_2), brain tissue oxygen tension ($P_{br}o_2$), and TCD ultrasonography, should be used when ICP and CPP cannot be maintained by standard methods.

ICP monitoring is a complex task that requires knowledge and understanding of the technical components of fluid-filled monitoring systems, the pathophysiology of the CNS, and the interaction between these systems. Personnel performing the setup, data collection, or maintenance procedures should be appropriately trained and credentialed and should be competent in the following areas:

- The technical setup and operation of the pressure monitoring system
- CNS physiology and pathophysiology
- ICP waveform analysis
- Appropriate response to adverse reactions
- Application of universal precautions

Problems associated with ICP monitoring include its cost, the risk of infection, and the risk of hemorrhage. Effective, ongoing ICP monitoring requires a team effort.

Indications for ICP Monitoring

The primary reason for ICP monitoring is a critical injury or illness involving components of the skull, specifically the brain. In addition, ICP monitoring undoubtedly helps in the management of conditions in which prolonged intracranial hypertension is expected. It is difficult to determine a numerical value for ICP clinically, and direct ICP measurement and monitoring is a helpful tool for selecting the most appropriate therapy and accurately studying the effectiveness of that treatment. ICP monitoring should be employed in all salvageable patients with severe TBI who have a GCS score of less than 8 but greater than 3 after resuscitation and an abnormal CT scan (eg, hematomas, contusions, swelling, herniation, or compressed basal cisterns).

ICP monitoring is also indicated for patients with severe TBI with a normal CT scan if two or more of the following conditions are noted at admission:

- Age older than 40 years
- Unilateral or bilateral motor posturing
- SBP of less 90 mm Hg

When clinical monitoring is not possible, such as during hyperventilation therapy and high-dose barbiturate therapy, ICP monitoring may prove helpful. Preoperative monitoring, for example, assists in assessment of **normal-pressure hydrocephalus (NPH)** before a shunting procedure takes place. ICP monitoring can provide an additional assessment in the event of suspected brain death because brain perfusion effectively ceases once ICP exceeds DBP.

Other indications for ICP monitoring are debated. Generally, though, the following specific indications may warrant this kind of monitoring:

- Severe TBI
- Intracranial hemorrhage
- Cerebral edema
- Prior craniotomy
- Space-occupying lesions, such as epidural and subdural hematomas, tumors, abscesses, or aneurysms that occlude the CSF pathway
- Patients with Reye syndrome who develop coma, posturing, and abnormal responses to noxious stimuli
- Encephalopathy from lead ingestion, hypertensive crisis, or hepatic failure
- Meningitis/encephalitis resulting in malabsorption of CSF

- GCS score of less than 8 or a positive CT (ie, evidence of a brain hemorrhage or evidence of a condition that will lead to a brain hemorrhage)

Contraindications to ICP Monitoring

The relative contraindications for ICP monitoring are as follows:

- CNS infection
- Coagulation defects
- Coagulopathy
- Scalp infection
- Severe midline shift resulting in ventricular displacement
- Cerebral edema resulting in ventricular collapse

Complications of ICP Monitoring

In general, complications related to ICP monitoring are rare. The greatest concern is ventriculitis (meningitis), although it has not been demonstrated in prospective studies of clinically significant intracranial infections following ICP measurement. Bacterial colonization does occur (5% of cases are ventricular/subarachnoid, and 15% are parenchymal), however, and its incidence increases markedly after five consecutive days of monitoring. Irrigation of ICP devices to restore patency of the ventriculostomy catheter using either an isotonic sodium chloride solution or antibiotic solution significantly increases the risk of colonization. Definitive treatment entails removal of the ICP monitoring bolt.

The risk of hematoma formation associated with ICP monitors varies. Parenchymal catheters have a higher incidence of hematoma than do other monitoring methods. Malfunction of the devices does occur, and readings of more than 50 mm Hg may be inaccurate, with higher rates of obstruction and loss of signal.

Complications of ICP monitoring can be summarized as follows:

- Intracranial infection
- Intracerebral hemorrhage
- Air leakage into the ventricle or subarachnoid space
- CSF leakage
- Over-drainage of CSF, leading to ventricular collapse and herniation
- Occlusion of the catheter with brain tissue or blood

- Inappropriate therapy because of erroneous ICP readings owing to dampened waveforms, electromechanical failure, or operator error (ie, inappropriate leveling)

ICP Monitoring Methods

ICP can be monitored using either noninvasive or invasive techniques. Noninvasive ICP monitoring simply involves assessing for clinical deterioration in the patient's neurologic status. Signs such as bradycardia, increased BP, and pupillary dilation are reliable signs of rising ICP. Invasive methods, by comparison, provide a quantitative measure of pressure, and some allow for CSF drainage. Although several invasive devices are available **FIGURE 12-46**, the most commonly used are the intraventricular catheter (IVC) and the subarachnoid screw. ICP monitoring devices are placed in the hospital setting—never during transport. It is more common to transport a patient to a facility to have an ICP device inserted than to transport a patient with the device already in place.

Intraventricular Catheters

Intraventricular monitoring is considered the gold standard of ICP monitoring techniques, especially in patients with ventriculomegaly (an enlarged ventricle of the brain). An additional advantage of this method is that it is both diagnostic and therapeutic, with the potential for draining CSF. Insertion of a ventricular catheter is technically difficult and has an associated risk of infection (20%, increasing with

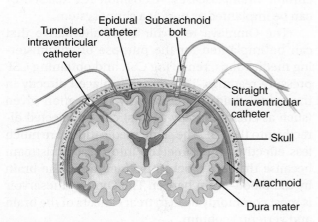

FIGURE 12-46 Invasive methods for intracranial pressure detection and cerebrospinal fluid drainage.

© Jones & Bartlett Learning.

the duration of placement) as well as hemorrhage (2%, and even greater in patients with coagulopathy disorders).

Advantages of an IVC are as follows:

- Allows for drainage of CSF to lower ICP
- Allows CSF cultures to be obtained
- Provides increased accuracy in ICP monitoring
- Is accurate and reliable

Risks associated with use of an IVC include the following problems:

- Infection
- Injury to the brain
- Clot formation
- Hemorrhage
- Collapsed ventricle
- Technically difficult (or impossible) placement, especially when ventricular compression is present as a result of trauma or cerebral edema

Placement of a ventricular catheter requires the insertion of a soft catheter through a burr hole into the lateral ventricle. As noted earlier, the catheter allows for both monitoring of ICP and therapeutic drainage of CSF to reduce ICP. IVCs connect to a transducer set, which is never pressurized. Complications associated with the IVC include infection and hemorrhage. The device must also be carefully leveled at the foramen of Monro (halfway between the outer canthus of the eye and the tragus of the ear). Any fluid drained must be monitored for amount, color, and clarity at hourly intervals. The CCTP should avoid manipulating the catheter, and should recalibrate it only if given approval by medical direction and if properly trained in operation of the device in use.

Intraparenchymal Devices

Intraparenchymal devices are inserted directly into the brain parenchyma through a small burr hole and utilize a thin cable with a fiberoptic or electronic transducer at the tip of a thin cable. They carry less risk of infection or hemorrhage (less than 1%) compared to IVCs, but do not allow for CSF drainage. Moreover, their accuracy has a tendency to "drift" over time, as these devices' transducers cannot be recalibrated after insertion (although several reliability studies have found only small variations in their accuracy). Their complex design also increases the risk of failure. The most widely used intraparenchymal catheter is the Camino fiberoptic system.

Epidural Catheters

Another ICP monitoring device, the epidural catheter, rests against the dura mater just beneath the skull. It offers two advantages: a decreased rate of infection compared to the IVC and a lower risk that its placement will injure the brain. However, this device is also less accurate than the IVC, and it cannot be used to drain CSF. Measurements from epidural catheters are often inaccurate, as the dura tends to dampen pressure transmitted to the epidural space. Nevertheless, these catheters are often utilized in coagulopathic patients owing to their considerably lower risk of hemorrhage (4%) versus intraventricular devices.

Subarachnoid Screws and Bolts

The subarachnoid screw (or bolt) uses a fluid-filled screw placed adjacent to the dura through a burr hole. A subdural bolt is inserted beneath the dura mater and above the pia mater; a subarachnoid bolt is placed beneath the arachnoid mater and above the pia mater. Placement of either type of device punctures the dura, allowing CSF drainage, although the screw often becomes clogged. Screws or bolts allow ICP monitoring, although their measurements are less accurate than those provided by the more direct ventriculostomy drain.

The most commonly used subarachnoid devices are the Richmond screw, the Becker bolt, the Philly bolt, the Leeds screw, and the Landy screw. The Richmond screw and Becker bolt are used extradurally.

Oftentimes a fiberoptic monitor is inserted through the subarachnoid bolt. Fiberoptic monitoring devices have a pressure sensor at the tip and do not require leveling or zeroing. The fiberoptic cable is fragile, however, and can break if twisted, stretched, or bent.

An alternative to fiberoptic monitoring is to use a fluid-filled catheter connected to an arterial pressure monitoring system. The CCTP should avoid manipulating this catheter, and should recalibrate it only if given approval by medical direction and if properly trained to operate the device in use.

Advantages of subarachnoid screws and bolts include the following:

- Not as invasive as an IVC or epidural catheter
- Lower rate of infection
- Less injury to the brain
- Easier to place

Disadvantages of these devices include the following:

- Less accurate monitoring
- Cannot drain CSF
- Risk of bleeding and brain injury
- Higher rate of infection than with an epidural catheter
- Requires a closed, intact skull
- Tendency to become clogged with debris, rendering readings unreliable

Other ICP Monitoring Devices

A fiberoptic transducer-tipped probe is a catheter with a pressure-sensing device that is placed into the subdural space, brain parenchyma, or ventricle. This non–fluid-filled continuous intact system offers the advantages of a good waveform, reliable and accurate pressure readings, and lack of air bubble formation within the catheter. Disadvantages include the inability to access the ICP unless an IVC setup is used and the inability to zero the unit once it is in place.

Mechanically coupled surface monitoring devices include cardio-search pneumatic sensors that are used subdurally or extradurally. Electronic devices (the Camino and Galtesh designs) are fully implantable systems and are valuable in the small group of patients who require long-term ICP monitoring for brain tumors, hydrocephalus, or other chronic brain diseases. A Cosmon ICP telesensor can be implanted as part of a shunt system.

The Ommaya reservoir is an alternative that can be implanted for the purpose of administering medications, removing CSF, and obtaining CSF pressure readings. This device is placed directly in the spinal fluid; therefore, any medication given (such as chemotherapy agents) can be injected directly into the CSF. The same medications are much less effective when injected into the bloodstream because they are blocked from entering the brain by the blood–brain barrier. The Ommaya reservoir is most commonly used to treat cancers of the brain and vertebral column.

Alternatively, a fluid-filled catheter that is placed in the subdural space and connected to an arterial pressure monitoring system is a cost-effective solution that adequately serves the purpose of ICP monitoring. The ICP waveform obtained through this system resembles a dampened arterial BP waveform and is considered normal when the pressure is between 0 and 15 mm Hg. In addition, a stopcock within the system allows for therapeutic drainage of CSF and for sampling for infection surveillance.

The Ladd device uses a fiberoptic system to detect distortions in ICP. It can be used in the subdura, on an extradural basis, and even extracutaneously.

ICP Waveform Analysis

While obtaining an average ICP over time is certainly useful for monitoring a patient's neurologic status, interpretation of the waveform itself provides the clinician with real-time information about brain compliance. This information, in turn, may provide clues about impending deterioration and allow for earlier targeted interventions.

The ICP waveform is typically 1 to 4 mm Hg in amplitude and corresponds to the arterial pulse, reflecting the pressure interaction of the vascular system with the CSF system. A normal ICP waveform contains three peaks: P1, P2, and P3. P1, the "percussion wave," is the result of the pressure from arterial pulsation being transmitted into the CSF. In a normal ICP waveform, P1 is the largest-amplitude component. P2, the "tidal wave," represents pressure reflected back from parenchyma. In a normal waveform, P2 has a smaller amplitude than P1. However, as brain compliance decreases, pressure is transmitted through parenchyma less easily, increasing P2. A waveform with P2 greater than P1 reflects decreased intracranial compliance. P3, the "dicrotic wave," reflects the pressure transmitted through the venous system from aortic valve closure. The end of P2 and the beginning of P3 correspond with the dicrotic notch on an arterial pulse waveform **FIGURE 12-47**.

Respirations cause an expected small change in the baseline reading, which may be thought of as an additional larger waveform. Normal ICP baseline variations range from 2 to 10 mm Hg and are caused by changes in venous pressure associated with respiratory-induced intrathoracic pressure changes. Increased ICP causes decreased respiratory variations and thus decreases the amplitude of this waveform.

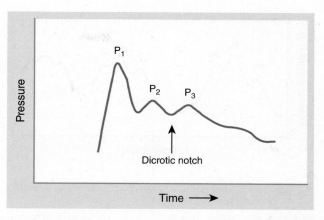

FIGURE 12-47 An intracranial pressure pulse waveform: P1, percussive wave; P2, tidal wave; and P3, dicrotic wave.
© Jones & Bartlett Learning.

The CCTP should be familiar with the classic pathologic ICP waveform changes. As ICP increases, the respiratory variation decreases and, conversely, the ICP waveform increases in amplitude. As ICP increases further, P2 amplitude increases more than P1 and P3 and eventually becomes the predominant wave in the waveform **FIGURE 12-48A**. There may also be a "rounding off" effect of the waveform, with loss of distinct peaks.

Lundberg A waves are sharp increases in ICP of 50 to 100 mm Hg that last 5 to 10 minutes before decreasing again. These waves are associated with cerebral ischemia and impending herniation **FIGURE 12-48B**. Lundberg B waves are rhythmic, short-duration (lasting 1 to 2 minutes) ICP elevations of up to 30 to 50 mm Hg that represent ongoing cerebral injury and a gradual increase in baseline ICP **FIGURE 12-48C**.

Some of these pathologic changes may occur before the average ICP becomes significantly elevated. Thus, paying close attention to the ICP waveform may facilitate more proactive management of the underlying pathology.

Performing ICP Monitoring

Before performing any procedure, including ICP monitoring, the appropriate equipment should be available and the patient should be prepared for the procedure. It is necessary to ensure the procedure is done in a controlled environment with adequate support staff. Every effort must be made to anticipate difficulties, and providers must have a thorough understanding of troubleshooting techniques.

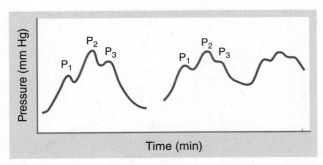

A

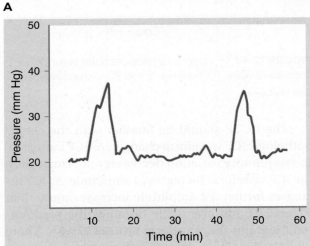

B

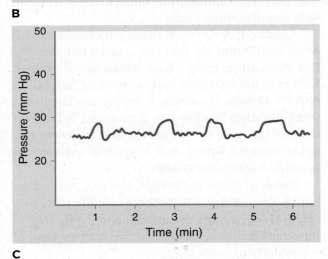

C

FIGURE 12-48 Pathologic intracranial pressure waveform changes. **A.** P2 greater than P1 and P3, followed by rounding off of the waveforms. **B.** Lundberg A waves. **C.** Lundberg B waves.

© Jones & Bartlett Learning.

Equipment

The equipment necessary for ICP monitoring includes the following items:

- External drainage system with a mounting card

- Pressure transducer with 48-inch (122-cm) pressure tubing
- Sterile 0.9% sodium chloride (NaCl) with a sterile 20-mL syringe
- Pressure monitoring cable
- IV tubing
- Manual resuscitator, mask, and 100% oxygen source
- Cardiopulmonary monitor
- Body substance isolation–compliant attire

Procedure

SKILL DRILL 12-1 shows the procedure for monitoring ICP with the Cordis EDS device **FIGURE 12-49**, one of the devices most commonly used for this purpose. The procedure is also described here:

1. Assemble the Cordis EDS as instructed per the package insert and per the mounting card diagrammatic instructions, using 0.9% NaCl to flush the system. Place the 48-inch (122-cm) tubing, with connected pressure transducer, on the plastic mounting card **STEP 1**.
2. Avoid tension or kinking of the pressure monitoring cable.
3. Place the patient in semi-Fowler position and position the zero reference point at the outer canthus of the eye **STEP 2**.
4. Obtain the ICP waveform on the cardiopulmonary monitor. Turn the stopcock nearest the patient so that the ICP waveform is visualized **STEP 3**.
5. Zero the transducer at the distal stopcock **STEP 4**.
6. Record the ICP on the printer, and mark and post the strip. Calculate and record the CPP on the strip **STEP 5**.
7. For continuous drainage, turn the stopcock nearest the patient so that drainage resumes and pressure monitoring is discontinued. *Note:* It is recommended that pressure monitoring and CSF drainage not be done simultaneously **STEP 6**.
8. Maintain a clean and intact dressing. If the dressing is soiled or contaminated, change it using a sterile technique.

Precautions

To minimize the risk of an infectious agent entering the CNS during ICP monitoring, an aseptic technique must be used at all times when assembling,

Skill Drill 12-1 Performing ICP Monitoring

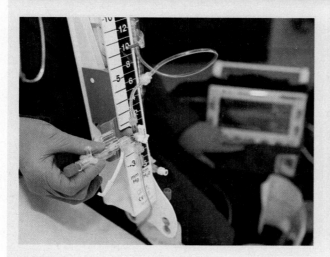

Step 1

Assemble the device as instructed per the package insert and per the mounting card, using 0.9% NaCl to flush the system. Place the 48-inch (122-cm) tubing, with connected pressure transducer, on the plastic mounting card. Avoid tension or kinking of the cable.

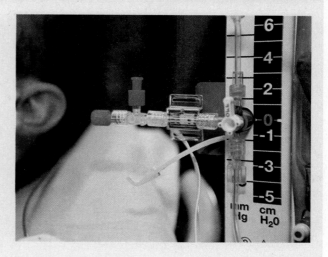

Step 2

Place the patient in semi-Fowler position and position the zero reference point at the outer canthus of the eye.

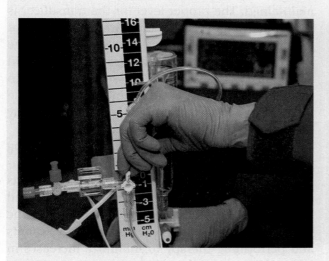

Step 3

Obtain the ICP waveform on the cardiopulmonary monitor. Turn the stopcock nearest the patient so that the ICP waveform is visualized.

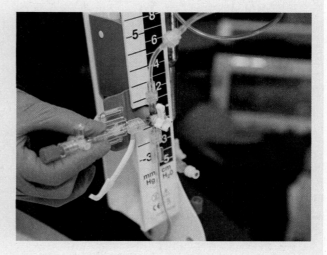

Step 4

Zero the transducer at the distal stopcock.

Continues

Skill Drill 12-1 Performing ICP Monitoring (continued)

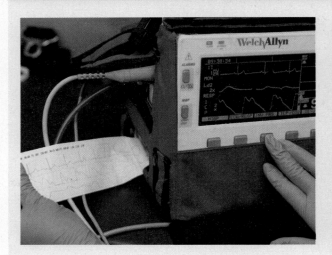

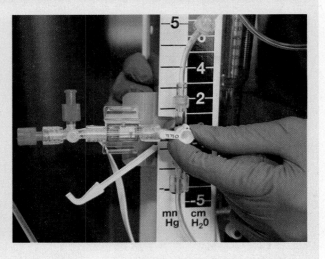

Step 5

Record the ICP on the printer, and mark and post the strip. Calculate and record the CPP on the strip.

© Jones & Bartlett Learning.

Step 6

For continuous drainage, turn the stopcock nearest the patient so that drainage resumes and pressure monitoring is discontinued. Maintain a clean and intact dressing.

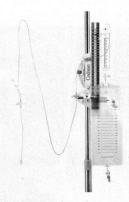

FIGURE 12-49 The Cordis EDS.

Used with permission of Codman, A Johnson & Johnson Company.

manipulating, or accessing the fluid-filled monitoring system. Tight connections must be maintained, and the system must remain free of air to ensure maximal accuracy. Never use a flush device for ICP monitoring. Use only sterile 0.9% NaCl to fill the pressure tubing; do not use a heparinized solution.

To ensure optimal accuracy of the ICP readings, proper leveling and zeroing of the system must be maintained. The proper level for the transducer is at the foramen of Monro, measured at the level of the outer canthus of the eye or, alternatively, at the spine for lumbar drainage. ICP transducers should be capable of measuring a pressure range of 0 to 100 mm Hg, with an accuracy of 2 mm Hg in the range of 0 to 20 mm Hg and at least 10% accuracy for the rest of the measurable range.

Utmost care must be taken when positioning and turning the patient to avoid accidental decannulation or disconnection of the tubing. Patients are maintained at a 30° to 45° angle, head-up, and neutral position when necessary to minimize the ICP. Use extreme caution when positioning patients and performing therapy to minimize increases in ICP and associated degradations in CPP.

Avoid flexion and hyperextension of the patient's neck and use of the Trendelenburg position, all of which may increase ICP. The system's alarm for high ICP must be maintained in the on position at all times.

Use care when manipulating the drainage system to avoid getting the filter wet. The drainage cylinder should remain in an upright position at all times. If the filter becomes wet and drainage slows or stops, some time may be required for the filter to dry out sufficiently before adequate drainage is reestablished.

Simultaneous drainage and pressure monitoring are not recommended. To ensure precise pressure measurements, perform pressure monitoring only when the stopcock to the drainage system is closed.

Only a small amount of CSF (not to exceed 3 mL) should be drained at one time. Rapid cerebral decompression from CSF over-drainage may result in herniation; such excessive drainage may occur if the system is inadvertently left open or if the patient's ICP is maintained at a higher level than the reference point on the system (as per physician order). The height of the drainage cylinder determines the rapidity with which CSF will drain. The physician's order for drainage must include a pressure reading in either mm Hg or cm H_2O and the height (as marked on the mounting card) at which the drainage cylinder must be maintained. The zero reference point for ICP monitoring always remains the outer canthus of the eye (or for lumbar drainage, the spine).

Adverse Reactions and Interventions

Some patients may experience adverse reactions to ICP monitoring. These reactions and the appropriate interventions to mitigate them are discussed here.

First, if blood is visualized in the pressure tubing (from intracranial hemorrhage), notify the physician.

If a good waveform or accurate ICP cannot be obtained (ie, a dampened waveform appears), flushing the fluid-filled monitoring system (with sterile 0.9% NaCl) may be attempted. First check all connections for tightness. Never flush the system while it is open to the patient. Close the stopcock to the patient, and then attempt to flush the monitoring system. Resume pressure monitoring by reopening the system to the patient. If a poor waveform persists, troubleshoot the system as you would any other device, including debubbling, releveling and zeroing, and changing the electrical cable. If all of these maneuvers fail to correct the poor waveform, notify the physician. The catheter may be occluded with blood or tissue, requiring physician intervention.

An acutely low ICP may indicate acute decompression due to leakage or over-drainage of CSF. Never attempt to tamponade or block leakage from the site around an ICP monitoring device. In this situation, notify the physician immediately.

In the event of acute decompensation (ie, sustained ICP $\geq$15 mm Hg), hyperventilation may be beneficial. Notify the physician.

Notify the physician immediately if the patient shows signs of decompensation, including altered level of consciousness, restlessness, agitation, lethargy, confusion, motor weakness, seizures, alteration in breathing pattern, increases in BP, bradycardia, vomiting, decortication/decerebration, or coma.

Post-Procedure Care and Documentation

Once ICP monitoring is established, do the following:

1. Ensure that all connections are tight and that the drainage system is positioned at the precise height for drainage according to the physician's order before leaving the bedside.
2. Relevel and zero the system every 4 hours and as needed.
3. Change the transducer pressure tubing according to local policy (usually every 72 to 96 hours).
4. Post a strip of the ICP in the patient's chart at least once per shift, although ICP will most likely be measured much more frequently. Each posted strip should also have documentation of the corresponding CPP.

Multimodality Monitoring

Although maintaining CPP is important, CPP is only one parameter affecting the delivery of oxygen to the neurons. Ultimately, the CBF and oxygen content of the blood are the prime parameters of concern. Although CPP provides a pressure gradient governing CBF, flow is subsequently affected by the resistance of the cerebral vessels. Neuronal demand for oxygen is governed by the metabolic rate of the neurons; that is, neurons with high activity levels require greater amounts of oxygen than do quiescent neurons. Globally, this principle is described as the **cerebral metabolic rate for oxygen ($CMRo_2$)**:

$$CMRo_2 = CBF \times OEF \times Spo_2$$

The oxygen extraction fraction (OEF) indicates how much oxygen is extracted as it passes by and is, therefore, available to support brain functions. It can be measured by the Fick principle based on measurements of the arterial and venous oxygen content. The Fick principle is used to determine cardiac output; it states that the amount of oxygen uptake of blood as it passes through the lungs is equal to the oxygen concentration difference between mixed venous and arterial blood.

In essence, monitoring only the ICP and CPP provides little information about the overall state of the injured brain and no information about oxygen delivery and usage. Multimodality monitoring involves using a combination of jugular venous bulb oximetry, brain tissue oxygen tension, and transcranial Doppler ultrasonography, thereby providing for a greater understanding of cerebral circulation and oxygen consumption.

In jugular venous bulb oximetry, a sampling catheter is placed in the internal jugular vein, directed upward, so that its tip rests in the jugular venous bulb at the base of the brain. Blood samples drawn from this location measure the mixed venous oxygen saturation (Svo$_2$) of blood leaving the brain, which is normally in the range of 50% to 75%. The Svo$_2$ may fall when there is an imbalance between oxygen consumption and delivery, when CBF decreases, when oxygen use increases, or when cerebrovascular resistance (CVR) increases. Vascular spasm and elevation of CVR are very common after brain injury and are significantly worsened by hyperventilation. Use jugular venous bulb oximetry whenever the patient has experienced prolonged hyperventilation.

Brain tissue oxygen tension (P$_{br}$o$_2$) monitoring is accomplished by inserting a commercial probe (capable of measuring temperature and oxygenation) into the brain tissue through a bolt. The placement technique is similar to that for ICP monitoring devices and can be done simultaneously with ICP monitoring placement. Brain tissue oxygenation monitoring is more sensitive to focal disruptions of blood flow to particular areas of the brain (depending on catheter placement). Compared to jugular venous bulb oximetry, which detects only global ischemic insults, brain tissue oxygen tension appears to be more accurate and may be more practical for continuous monitoring.

Transcranial Doppler ultrasonography is a noninvasive method of assessing the state of the intracranial circulation. The velocity of flow can be measured in the middle, anterior, and posterior cerebral arteries; the ophthalmic artery; or the internal carotid artery. Doppler ultrasonographic waveform analysis can give further information about the state of blood flow, such as flow acceleration and pulsatility index:

(Systolic velocity – Diastolic velocity) / Mean velocity

Vasospasm is common after head injury and can be an important cause of neurologic deterioration. This condition usually occurs in the presence of traumatic subarachnoid hemorrhage. Because it leads to an increase in flow velocity, TCD can be useful for monitoring at-risk patients for signs of vasospasm. TCD is indicated for patients whose intracranial hypertension and CPP cannot be maintained by standard therapy.

All of these monitoring technologies assess oxygen delivery to and extraction by the brain; none measures cerebral activity directly. A full EEG is too complex for continuous use in the ICU, but the cerebral function monitor (CFM) and the cerebral function analysis monitor (CFAM) can both provide summed, averaged, and (in CFAM's case) analyzed outputs of the general state of brain activity. A CFM records a single-channel EEG from two electrodes placed on either side of the head; a third electrode acts as a ground. The CFM is used to assess brain wave activity, indicate the effects of medication administration, and identify seizure activity. It is particularly useful in evaluating the effects of sedation and paralytics.

Patients with severe TBI are intubated to protect their airway and facilitate maximal oxygenation. Standard monitoring for these patients is required, including Spo$_2$, ECG, MAP, and urine output. When ETCO$_2$ cannot be continuously monitored, these patients also require frequent determination of arterial blood gases, which can be achieved by placement of an intra-arterial catheter. Patients are maintained euvolemic (normal fluid volume status), and central venous pressure measurements are used to guide their therapy. Central venous pressure measurement is covered in Chapter 15, *Hemodynamic Monitoring*.

Normocapnia (normal carbon dioxide tension) is vital for maintenance of ICP, and patients' ETCO$_2$ levels should be continuously measured using waveform capnography. These measurements represent the baseline monitoring requirements for patients with TBI. Patients receiving pressors to maintain MAP and/or CPP would also benefit from an arterial line for continuous monitoring of drug effects.

The role of multimodal monitoring devices remains under investigation but addresses a long-standing need in neurocritical care to obtain information about cerebral blood flow and metabolism in the brain. Treatment thresholds have been published for Sjo_2 (less than 50%) and for $P_{br}o_2$ (less than 15 mm Hg), which are currently the only monitoring systems that have yielded sufficient outcome data in patients with TBI.

Treatment Options for Increased ICP

The best treatment for increased ICP is obviously the removal of the causative lesion, such as a tumor, hydrocephalus, or hematoma. Postoperative increased ICP has become less common with more widespread use of the microscope and special techniques to avoid brain retraction. A patient whose basal meningioma (a tumor near the base of the meninges) has been completely removed usually has a smooth postoperative period. By contrast, a convexity or even falx meningioma (a tumor near the falx cerebri of the meninges) may be easily removed, but the postoperative period may prove difficult. In such a case, problems may arise because of impairment of venous drainage, from either intraoperative injury to veins or postoperative diuretic therapy (a practice in some centers).

Debate persists about whether increased ICP is the cause or the result of brain damage. Not all midline shifts seen in CT scans indicate increased ICP; they may simply mean that ICP was high during the shift. A midline shift takes longer to reverse even after ICP returns to normal. In any event, increased ICP tends to be a temporary phenomenon that lasts for a short time unless the patient experiences a fresh secondary injury due to a clot, hypoxia, or an electrolyte disturbance.

First-Line Versus Second-Line Management

Treatment of increased ICP aims at preventing the secondary events. Clinical and ICP monitoring definitely help in this regard. First-line management consists of general measures geared toward making the

patient comfortable, along with effective handling of the ABCs of trauma management. Careful attention to nutrition and electrolytes, bladder and bowel functions, and appropriate treatment of infections should be instituted promptly. Adequate analgesia is often forgotten, but is a must even in unconscious patients.

Second-line management of increased ICP focuses on inducing cerebral vasoconstriction. Osmotherapy consisting of mannitol, hypertonic saline, glycerol, urea, or furosemide may be implemented. Anesthetic agents, including barbiturates, gamma-hydroxybutyrate, and etomidate, and paralytic agents, may also be administered. During transport, preventing hypoxia and hypercarbia, ensuring adequate analgesia, and preventing increased anxiety with reassurance and anxiolytics can all help to avert additional increases in ICP.

Surgical decompression remains controversial. This procedure is performed to counteract increased ICP, which is assumed to be present when neurologic deterioration occurs or when monitoring reveals that ICP is higher than 25 cm H_2O.

Controversies

A small group of surgeons initiate second-line management measures in patients in whom ICP is expected to rise without waiting for that increase to actually occur. Many other physicians believe that institution of measures to reduce ICP invariably compromises CBF; they prefer to wait for the rise in ICP before initiating second-line measures.

There is also debate about the appropriate second-line management of increased ICP. Some prefer hyperosmolar therapy; others prefer measures to induce cerebral vasoconstriction, thereby reducing both CBF and ICP. Finally, some providers believe it prudent to initiate both treatments.

Specific Therapeutic Options

Transport treatment is aimed at reducing ICP and providing rapid transport of the patient to a neurologic facility for definitive treatment. Ways to manage increased ICP during transport include the following measures:

1. Maintain elevation of the head of the stretcher at a 30° to 45° angle and maintain alignment of the patient's head and neck in a neutral position.

2. Consider intubation and mechanical ventilation. For patients with intracranial hemorrhage, increase the minute volume to maintain a carbon dioxide level of 30 to 35 mm Hg.

3. Consider administering an osmotic diuretic. Osmotic diuretics are low-molecular-weight substances that produce a rapid loss of sodium and water by inhibiting their reabsorption in the kidney tubules and the loop of Henle. They also increase the osmolality of plasma, increasing the diffusion of CSF. Osmotic diuretics are used to reduce intracerebral pressure created by excess CSF. Mannitol is the most commonly used osmotic diuretic, but glycerol is also used for this purpose.

4. Consider administering dexamethasone or methylprednisolone sodium succinate, both of which are corticosteroids, to control inflammation and swelling of brain tissue.

5. Maintain SBP at less than 150 mm Hg. Avoid hypotension, which can be equally deleterious.

6. If a surgical drain (bolt) has been installed, drain the CSF if ICP is greater than 20 cm H_2O.

7. Patients with an intracranial hemorrhage and those who have been taking warfarin (Coumadin), such as patients with atrial fibrillation, should have either plasma or platelets administered en route.

Hyperventilation

As a temporizing measure, hyperventilation is recommended to control elevations in ICP. Hyperventilation aims at keeping the Pco_2 between 30 and 35 mm Hg, so that CBF falls and capillary blood volume is reduced, thereby reducing the ICP. Although this intervention is widely used, the reduction of CBF carries a significant risk of inducing cerebral ischemia, especially during the first day following injury, when CBF has been demonstrated to approach one-half the normal value. Prophylactic hyperventilation is not recommended. Hyperventilation should also be avoided in the first 24 hours following injury when CBF is often critically reduced.

Some experts have claimed that a Pco_2 of less than 20 mm Hg results in ischemia, although no experimental proof has definitively shown such a relationship. The present trend is to maintain ventilation with Pco_2 in the range of 30 to 35 mm Hg and with Po_2 in the range of 120 to 140 mm Hg to prevent hypoxia; this is the standard of care for head injuries. When clinical deterioration such as pupillary dilation or widened pulse pressure is observed, hyperventilation may be instituted (preferably by increasing the minute volume) until the ICP decreases. Whenever hyperventilation is implemented, cerebral oxygen delivery should be continuously assessed using jugular venous oxygen saturation or brain tissue oxygen tension measurement.

While the current standard of care recommends maintaining Pco_2 in the range of 30 to 35 mm Hg for prophylactic hyperventilation, some experts continue to recommend a range of 25 to 35 mm Hg in the setting of documented or suspected herniation. There is no evidence suggesting this lower limit offers greater benefit or causes harm.

Hyperosmolar Therapy

Hyperosmolar therapy using mannitol also carries the risk of further reducing perfusion to the brain. Mannitol is effective at reducing ICP, but only if it is used properly. Note that this agent is *not* inert and harmless.

Several theories have been advanced concerning the mechanism by which mannitol reduces ICP:

- Mannitol increases cardiac output, which leads to better CPP and cerebral oxygenation.
- Mannitol decreases CSF production.
- Mannitol's diuretic effect may occur mainly around the lesion, where the blood–brain barrier integrity is impaired, so that the drug has no significant effect on the normal brain. For this reason, intra-axial lesions respond better to mannitol than do extra-axial lesions.
- Mannitol may withdraw water across the ependyma of the ventricles in a manner analogous to that associated with ventricular drainage.
- Mannitol may cause cerebral vasoconstriction, with the resultant changes in CBV being responsible for reduction in ICP.

Mannitol is usually given as a 20% solution in bolus doses, as opposed to a continuous infusion. Boluses of 0.25 to 0.5 g/kg given over 10 to 20 minutes may be used and repeated depending on the patient's response.

Mannitol's effect on ICP reaches its maximum 30 minutes after infusion and lasts for a variable period, ranging from 90 minutes to 6 hours or more. The correct dose is the smallest one that will have sufficient effect on ICP. When repeated doses are required, the baseline serum osmolality gradually increases. If this level exceeds 330 mOsm/L, mannitol therapy should cease; there is no role for dehydration in such a case. Further infusions of mannitol will be ineffective in this scenario and are likely to induce renal failure.

Hypertonic saline has been shown to be equal, if not superior, to mannitol in reducing ICP. Although protocols vary, 5% sodium chloride (NaCl) is the concentration most commonly used. Hypertonic saline can be administered in boluses of 100 mL for acute situations, but is more commonly administered as a continuous infusion at rates of 30 to 150 mL/h, adjusted to maintain serum sodium at less than 160 mEq/L.

Diuretics such as furosemide, given either alone or in conjunction with mannitol, can accelerate mannitol's excretion and reduce the baseline serum osmolality prior to the next dose. It is speculated that furosemide complements mannitol and also increases the output. Furosemide may be given before mannitol, so that it reduces circulatory overload.

Special Populations

Children are much more sensitive to fluid shifts than adults. Be very careful when administering fluids to children.

Barbiturates

Barbiturates can lower ICP when other measures fail, but they have no prophylactic value. Barbiturates and hypnotic drugs such as propofol and etomidate act by reducing the $CMRo_2$ and, concomitantly, reducing CBF. (They also decrease brain metabolism and energy demand, which facilitates healing.) The consequent reduction in CBV leads to a parallel fall in ICP.

Among the barbiturates, phenobarbital is most widely used for this purpose. A loading dose of 10 mg/kg over 30 minutes and a subsequent infusion at 1 to 3 mg/kg/h is a widely used regimen. Close monitoring of ICP and hemodynamic instability should accompany any barbiturate therapy.

Corticosteroids

High-dose corticosteroid therapy (eg, methylprednisone, dexamethasone) is used to lower ICP.

Corticosteroids restore cell-wall integrity and help in recovery by reducing edema.

Surgery

Decompressive craniotomies, such as subtemporal decompression, are not recommended to relieve increased ICP. Herniation of the brain through a defect may cause further injury, further edema, and further increased ICP in some patients who undergo this procedure. In occasional cases, when every other measure has failed, a decompression craniotomy may be justified. This action would need to be substantiated by clear evidence of neurologic deterioration and a CT scan that shows an intracranial lesion.

Hyperbaric Oxygen and Hypothermia

Hyperbaric oxygen and hypothermia are experimental techniques (used especially frequently in Japan) to induce cerebral vasoconstriction and reduce CBV and ICP. Considerable evidence supports the use of mild to moderate hypothermia (89.6°F to 93.2°F [32°C to 34°C]) as a treatment for increased ICP, especially when target temperatures are maintained for longer than 48 hours. Cooling reduces the cerebral metabolic rate, leading to a reduction in CBF, ICP, and glutamate release. Fever increases the cerebral metabolic rate and $CMRo_2$ and occurs commonly in brain-injured patients, especially after intracranial hemorrhage. Therefore, temperature monitoring and control are vital to patient outcomes.

Hyperbaric oxygen therapy (HBOT) has been shown to be neuroprotective in multiple neurologic disorders, but its efficacy in the management of TBI remains controversial. The complementary, synergistic actions of HBOT include improved tissue oxygenation and cellular metabolism as well as anti-apoptotic and anti-inflammatory mechanisms.

Signs and Symptoms

Increased Intracranial Pressure
- Cushing triad: widening pulse pressure, bradycardia, and abnormal respiratory patterns
- Hypertension (increased BP)
- Increased respiratory rate
- Pulmonary edema

Transport Management

Increased Intracranial Pressure

- Intubate and mechanically ventilate the patient. Do not hyperventilate the patient unless acute deterioration occurs.
- Consider administering an osmotic diuretic (mannitol).
- Consider administering dexamethasone or methylprednisolone sodium succinate to control inflammation and swelling.
- Control BP to maintain systolic pressures at less than 150 mm Hg.
- If a surgical drain (bolt) has been installed, drain the CSF if the ICP is greater than 20 cm H_2O.
- For patients who have sustained a hemorrhage and who have been taking anticoagulants, administer reversal agents in an attempt to limit the size and extent of the bleed.

Brain Herniation

Brain herniation is a condition in which a portion of the brain is displaced because of increased ICP, resulting in progressive damage to brain tissue that may include life-threatening damage to the brainstem. This condition is commonly the result of brain swelling (cerebral edema) from a head injury, but it may also result from hemorrhagic stroke or space-occupying lesions, such as primary brain tumor, metastatic brain tumor, or other lesions within the brain. Brain herniation may also occur with bacterial meningitis.

The most common type of brain herniation occurs when a portion of the temporal lobe is displaced through the tentorium (uncal herniation), resulting in compression of cranial nerve III, the midbrain, and the posterior cerebral artery. Uncal herniation typically leads to coma and respiratory arrest.

Another critical type of brain herniation occurs when part of the cerebellum is displaced through the foramen magnum (tonsillar herniation). This compresses the brainstem, resulting in destruction of the respiratory center, apnea, decreased perfusion to the rest of the brain, and death. Because this herniation involves the brainstem and spinal cord, the patient will likely be in a coma, present with decerebrate or decorticate posturing, have ipsilateral pupil dilation, and have difficulty maintaining respirations, heart rate and rhythm, and BP. These patients need immediate surgery to install a drain to remove blood and fluids to alleviate the excess pressure. From a transport point of view, management includes the following measures:

1. Intubate the patient and place them on a mechanical ventilator. Hyperventilate the patient to maintain carbon dioxide levels of 25 to 35 mm Hg.
2. Administer mannitol or an equivalent osmotic diuretic.
3. Consider administering corticosteroids such as dexamethasone, especially in the case of a brain tumor.
4. Provide rapid transport to a neurosurgical facility.

Other areas of the brain may sustain herniation, although such injuries occur with less frequency than either uncal herniation or foramen magnum herniation.

Signs and Symptoms

Brain Herniation

- Tachycardia (inability to control heart rate and rhythm)
- Decreased BP (inability to control BP)
- Decreased respiratory rate (inability to control respirations—irregular breathing)
- Abnormal posturing (decorticate/decerebrate)
- A worsening (progressive) LOC (GCS score of 5 or less)
- Pupil changes (dilation of one or both pupils or failure of pupils to constrict with light)

Transport Management

Brain Herniation

- Intubate the patient and place them on a mechanical ventilator, hyperventilating to maintain carbon dioxide levels of 25 to 35 mm Hg.
- Administer mannitol or an equivalent osmotic diuretic.
- Consider administering corticosteroids such as dexamethasone, especially in the case of a brain tumor.
- Provide rapid transport to a neurosurgical facility.

Spinal Cord Injuries

CCTPs may be called on to provide appropriate transportation of patients with SCIs. Suspicion for these injuries may be high as a result of the mechanism of injury, or SCIs may be identified at the transferring facility through imaging studies. These injuries may be either isolated or associated with other injuries, and their presence can complicate management priorities. Rapid and safe transportation of the patient with an SCI to a facility that can provide definitive care is the optimal outcome.

Mechanism of Injury

Acute injuries of the spine are classified according to the mechanism, location, and stability of the injury. Vertebral fractures often occur with or without associated SCI. Simply put, the spine is composed of three anatomic columns. As first described by Francis Denis, MD, the spine is divided longitudinally into the anterior, middle, and posterior columns. The anterior column includes the anterior longitudinal ligament, the anterior half of the vertebral body, and the anterior half of the intravertebral disk. The middle column is composed of the posterior half of the vertebral body, the posterior half of the intravertebral disk, and the posterior longitudinal ligament. Finally, the posterior column consists of all other structures posterior to the posterior longitudinal ligament, including the pedicles, lamina, spinous process, interspinous ligaments, and ligamentum flavum. Disruption of two of three of these columns is, by definition, an unstable injury.

Generally, the types of forces or mechanisms that affect the vertebral column include flexion/extension, vertical compression/longitudinal distraction, rotational, and combined mechanisms.

Flexion-Extension Injuries

Flexion-extension injuries are typically the result of rapid deceleration or a direct blow to the occiput. They most often involve the cervical region; the spinal cord may be injured as a result by compression in the canal. Hyperextension of the head and neck can result in fractures, ligamentous injury, and SCIs of variable stability. The C5-C6 level is most susceptible to this injury from a mechanical standpoint.

Vertical Compression

Vertical compression forces are transmitted through vertebral bodies and directed either inferiorly through the skull or superiorly through the pelvis or feet. They typically result from a direct blow to the crown (parietal region) of the skull or rapid deceleration from a fall through the feet, legs, and pelvis. Compression forces can cause herniation of disks, subsequent compression of the spinal cord and nerve roots, and fragmentation of vertebral bodies into the canal. Forces transmitted through the vertebral body may cause fractures, ultimately shattering the vertebral body and producing a "burst" or compression fracture, either with or without associated SCI. In falls, most injuries involve the thoracolumbar junction; the lower cervical spine is often involved, with axial loads being placed on the vertebral column **FIGURE 12-50**.

Rotation With Flexion

A rotation-flexion injury often occurs in the thoracolumbar interface. These injury patterns can involve stable or unstable fractures and dislocations.

Primary Versus Secondary Spinal Cord Injury

Primary SCI

Primary spinal cord injury is a result of the initial trauma. Penetrating trauma may either lead to

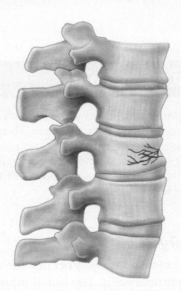

FIGURE 12-50 A compression fracture of the vertebra.
© Jones & Bartlett Learning.

transection of neural elements or cause concussive injury to the spinal cord (as in gunshot wounds); the outcomes may be either complete or incomplete injuries. Blunt trauma may displace ligaments and bone fragments, resulting in compression of points of the spinal cord or an incomplete dislocation of the vertebral body. Hypoperfusion and ischemia may also result from this type of injury to the spinal vasculature. Necrosis from prolonged ischemia leads to permanent loss of function.

Spinal cord contusions may be caused by fracture, dislocation, or direct trauma. These injuries are associated with edema, tissue damage, and vascular leakage. Hemorrhagic disruption may cause temporary or permanent loss of function despite normal radiographs.

Cord laceration usually occurs when a projectile or bone enters the spinal canal. Such an injury is likely to result in hemorrhage into the cord tissue, swelling, and disruption of some portion of the cord and its associated communication pathways.

Special Populations

Osteoporosis in older adult patients contributes to a high rate of spinal injury, which may occur even with minimal trauma (eg, ground level falls or falls from a seated position). The CCTP should maintain a high index of suspicion for spinal injury in this population, paying special attention to possible C1-C2 injuries that include dens fractures and transverse ligament disruption.

Special Populations

Patients with a history of ankylosing spondylitis or diffuse idiopathic skeletal hyperostosis warrant extra care and attention. These conditions put patients at increased risk of spinal fractures. Even nondisplaced fractures in this population can be unstable and lead to potential SCI.

Secondary SCI

Secondary spinal cord injury occurs due to progression of the primary SCI. The initial injury can trigger a cascade of inflammatory responses that may result in further deterioration. These effects can be exacerbated by exposing neural elements to further hypoperfusion, hypoxemia, hypoglycemia, and hypothermia. Although some SCIs may be unavoidable, the prehospital provider should minimize the risk of further (secondary) injury by providing stabilization—that is, through spinal motion restriction and neutral alignment. In addition, minimizing heat loss and maintaining oxygenation and perfusion are key elements in the care of a patient with a possible SCI.

Complete Versus Incomplete SCI

As noted earlier, SCIs may be classified as complete or incomplete. The degree of SCI is best determined 24 hours after the initial injury; the initial dysfunction may be temporary, and there may be some potential for recovery.

Complete SCI

Complete spinal cord injury involves complete disruption of all tracts of the spinal cord, with no sensory and motor function more than three segments below the level of injury. When the injury affects the patient's cervical spine, quadriplegia can result. Injury to the thoracic spine can result in paraplegia.

Incomplete SCI

In an incomplete spinal cord injury, the patient retains some degree of cord-mediated function more than three segments below the level of injury. Several types of incomplete SCI syndromes have been identified.

Anterior cord syndrome results from the displacement of bony fragments into the anterior portion of the spinal cord, often as the result of flexion injuries or fractures. The anterior spinal artery provides blood to the anterior two-thirds of the spinal cord; disruption of this flow presents as an anterior cord syndrome. Typical physical findings include motor paralysis below the level of the insult, with loss of pain and temperature sensation, but preservation of proprioception.

In central cord syndrome, hyperextension injuries to the cervical area present with hemorrhage or edema to the central cervical segments. This type of damage is rarely associated with fractures or bone disruption; more often, it occurs in conjunction with tears to the anterior longitudinal ligament.

Central cord syndrome is frequently seen in older patients, who may already have a significant degree of cervical spondylosis and stenosis as the result of arthritic changes. A brief episode of hyperextension can exert pressure on the spinal cord within the relatively diminished spinal canal. Within the central cord, motor (efferent) fibers are distributed in a unique fashion, with more cervical and thoracic motor and sensory tracts being found there than in the periphery of the cord. The patient with central cord syndrome will present with greater loss of function in the upper extremities than in the lower extremities, with variable loss of sensation to pain and temperature (sacral sparing). The patient may also have some bowel and bladder dysfunction. The prognosis for central cord syndrome is typically good; many patients regain all motor function or have only some residual weakness in the hands.

Brown-Séquard syndrome occurs when penetrating trauma is accompanied by hemisection of the cord and complete damage to all spinal tracts on the involved side. Injury to the corticospinal motor tracts causes motor loss on the same side as the injury, but below the lesion. Damage to the dorsal column causes loss of sensation to light touch, proprioception, and vibration on the same side as the injury (below it). Disruption of the spinothalamic tracts causes loss of sensation to pain and temperature on the opposite side of the injury, below the lesion.

Posterior cord syndrome is associated with extension injuries. This relatively rare syndrome produces dysfunction of the dorsal columns, presenting as decreased sensation to light touch, proprioception, and vibration, while most other motor and sensory functions remain intact. Recovery of function is less likely than with central cord syndrome, but the overall prognosis remains good with therapy and rehabilitation.

Spinal and Neurogenic Shock

Spinal shock is a temporary local neurologic condition that occurs immediately after spinal trauma and involves impaired function of reflex arcs at and below the level of the injury. Patients may present with variable degrees of acute spinal injury, potentially with flaccid paralysis, flaccid sphincters, and absent reflexes. Sensory function below the level of injury will be impaired. Spinal shock usually subsides within 24 to 72 hours, when the spinal cord–mediated reflex arc below the level of injury resumes function. Patients who regain functionality of this arc, yet still have absence of distal motor or sensory function below the level of injury, have a complete cord injury and are unlikely to regain neurologic function. Those with some motor and sensory function below the level of injury are considered to have incomplete injury.

Neurogenic shock results from the temporary loss of sympathetic tone at and below the level of injury; the resultant unchecked parasympathetic stimulation then leads to cardiovascular consequences. The marked hemodynamic and systemic effects typically manifest as the triad of hypotension, bradycardia, and warm, flushed skin. Hypotension occurs as the result of absent or impaired peripheral vascular tone with the loss of alpha receptor stimulation; blood pools in the enlarged vascular space, causing relative hypovolemia and making the patient extremely sensitive to sudden position changes; and cardiac preload decreases, resulting in decreased stroke volume and cardiac output. Bradycardia is the product of the unopposed vagal response: The adrenal gland loses its sympathetic stimulation and does not produce epinephrine or norepinephrine to compensate for the loss of vascular tone. Warm, flushed skin is a result of peripheral vasodilation. Central hypothermia and absence of sweating are also seen because of the loss of sympathetic stimulation and thermoregulation. The classic presentation of neurogenic shock is a hypotensive, bradycardic patient whose skin is warm, flushed, and dry below the level of the spinal lesion.

Transport Management

Evaluate patients for decubitus ulcers, and document any findings in the medical chart. Consideration during packaging should include appropriate positioning to avoid putting pressure on areas at risk for tissue breakdown. Pay particular attention to the coccyx, occiput, and heels.

Assessment of SCI

A patient with an SCI should have a thorough assessment by the CCTP before transport. During this initial assessment, the CCTP should perform a comprehensive neurologic exam. This assessment will provide a baseline with which to compare future assessments when looking for acute changes. SCIs may be severe enough to threaten patients' lives and often leave patients with significant disability.

As part of the initial assessment prior to transport, the CCTP should take the time to perform a physical examination of the patient before packaging. For patients with SCI, it may be particularly important to focus on the following aspects of patient assessment.

When appropriate, visually inspect the neck. Look for obvious deformities and assess crepitus or the presence of pain while maintaining appropriate spinal motion restriction.

Evaluate the patient's airway before transportation. If the patient is not already intubated, perform a thorough and complete assessment of the airway. Consider the likelihood of respiratory failure and the need for definitive airway management during transportation. Patients with high SCI (above C3 through C5) may have an altered ability to breathe and ventilate during transport. They may also tire from the work of breathing as the result of muscular weakness from the SCI or owing to an inability to clear secretions. Managing the airway in a patient with cervical fracture or SCI can be difficult in the best of circumstances. If judged to be appropriate, intubate the patient at the referral facility under controlled circumstances and with appropriate support, if available, depending on that facility's resources (eg, anesthesia, surgeon, emergency medicine).

If appropriate and not previously done, assess the patient's back for tenderness and deformity. Palpate the spine for tenderness and deformity (such as step-offs). Assess for strength in the upper and lower extremities and the presence of sensation, including comparison of both sides.

Ongoing patient assessment, particularly of the patient's pulse, motor, and sensory function, is extremely important, because increased swelling can contribute to progressive deterioration of the patient's neurologic status. On arrival at the receiving facility, it will be important to provide an accurate and up-to-date patient report to the accepting medical staff.

Management of SCI

A patient with an SCI should be treated as having a true neurologic emergency, and the CCTP should

Controversies

When spine clearance cannot be done clinically, CT scans of the cervical spine should be performed. Plain radiographs of the cervical spine can be used with pediatric patients but have poor sensitivity in adults. Sometimes, however, a transferring hospital cannot perform a rapid CT scan while awaiting arrival of the CCTP team, such as when a CT scan would delay the transport. It is also prudent to limit CT exposure when possible to decrease a younger person's risk of cancer later in life; with younger patients, radiographs are still frequently used to minimize this risk. It is also prudent to avoid exposing women of childbearing age to excess radiation when possible.

The CCTP should always confirm whether spine clearance has been done, and obtain specific details from the transferring personnel. Appropriate documentation of this clearance should be evident in the medical record before transport begins.

In general, patients with identified or highly suspected cervical or thoracolumbar injury should not be cleared and should be transported with appropriate spinal motion restriction (ie, supine on the stretcher, with a properly fitted cervical collar and sufficiently secured shoulder and torso straps to limit gross motion). In most cases, patients with neurologic deficits despite the absence of identified radiologic abnormalities should be assumed to have injury and should be transported with appropriate spinal motion restriction in place. An isolated cervical spine injury may be initially managed with an appropriately fitted collar in place. Thoracolumbar fractures should be managed with lower spinal motion restriction during transport. If in doubt, implement full spinal motion restriction precautions.

Unless contraindicated based on their specific injury, patients should be transported with the head of the stretcher elevated at least to a 30° angle to minimize the risk of aspiration.

make every effort to rapidly assess, treat, and transport the patient to the closest appropriate facility while maintaining appropriate spinal motion restriction. These patients should be transported in a way that minimizes jostling and movement to prevent further SCI. Immediate identification and aggressive management of hypotension and hypoxia will also help to prevent anoxic injury to the spinal cord.

Special Populations

Children younger than 10 years have heads that are proportionally larger than their bodies—an anatomic factor that frequently leads to spinal injuries from the occiput to C3. In contrast, children older than 10 years have injury patterns similar to those of adults. Because the head is proportionally larger in younger children, it is important to appropriately immobilize these pediatric patients in a neutral position. This may require padding under the shoulders and back to maintain a neutral alignment in relation to the head.

Signs and Symptoms

Spinal Cord Injury

- May have flaccid paralysis below the level of injury
- May have loss of sensation to pain, temperature, and proprioception below the level of injury; loss may be unilateral
- May have disproportionate upper extremity motor impairment compared with lower extremities
- Bradycardia
- Hypotension
- Hypothermia
- Priapism in males

Transport Management

Spinal Cord Injury

- Identify and correct life-threatening problems (ABCs).
- Maintain spinal stabilization and neutral alignment of the vertebral column.
- In patients with multiple injuries, provide appropriate volume resuscitation with IV fluids and blood component therapy as appropriate.
- Rapidly identify and treat hypotension and hypoxia.
- Maintain normothermia.
- In patients with an isolated SCI, support BP after adequate resuscitation with vasoactive medications such as phenylephrine, norepinephrine, or dopamine.
- Patients may require atropine, transcutaneous pacing, or transvenous pacing for bradycardia.
- Provide rapid, safe transportation to a definitive care facility.

Management Priorities

Priorities of management include rapid identification and correction of life-threatening problems. Appropriately secure and manage the airway, especially in patients with higher-level cervical fractures. Use mechanical ventilation or bag-mask ventilation to support breathing in patients who are intubated or have tracheotomies. End-tidal capnography and pulse oximetry are mandatory for assessing and monitoring respiratory status. Careful assessment, including pulse oximetry, of breathing in nonintubated patients is important when monitoring for progressive respiratory failure.

Frequent monitoring of BP by noninvasive means or by an arterial line during transport will alert providers to hypotension. Appropriate large-bore IV access (minimum of two IV sites) or appropriate central venous access should be in place prior to transport, as should bladder catheterization.

Adequate volume resuscitation with appropriate IV fluids and blood component therapy is necessary for patients with multiple injuries. These patients should be suspected to be experiencing hemorrhage and hemorrhagic shock unless these conditions were ruled out at the transferring facility. Patients with identified isolated neurogenic shock should be treated with volume resuscitation and vasoactive medications.

Patients with SCI may have a loss of thermoregulation from vasodilation and require monitoring of temperature and treatment to maintain normothermia, including warm IV fluids, blankets, and increased temperature in the transporting vehicle. Because bradycardia sometimes results from SCI, the use of atropine, transcutaneous pacers, and transvenous pacemakers may be warranted in patients with high-level cervical lesions (C1 through C5).

Pharmacotherapy

Patients with SCI may require various pharmacologic interventions during transport. Pain associated with fractures or other injuries will require judicious use of opioids. IV opiates can be useful in the management of pain associated with transportation, movement, and the injury itself. Fentanyl, a short-acting synthetic opiate, has less of an effect on BP and may be used as first-line therapy for these patients to control pain and to reduce the risk of hypotension. Midazolam (Versed) or lorazepam (Ativan) may be used for sedation after appropriate pain control has been established and other correctable causes of agitation such as hypoxia have been excluded. The risk of secondary injury as the result of movements from acute agitation must be balanced with potential airway and ventilatory compromise as well as the value of conducting a reliable neurologic exam.

The use of corticosteroids in the acute phase of SCI is no longer recommended.

As noted earlier, patients with SCI may also have neurogenic shock. This condition requires vasoactive medications to support BP (eg, phenylephrine) once adequate resuscitation has occurred. Patients in neurogenic shock may also have bradycardia; in such a case, atropine is required on an urgent basis to support the heart rate and BP.

Controversies

Recent outcomes data on use of corticosteroids immediately following initial SCI and during interfacility transfer have failed to show significant improvements and, in fact, have suggested rates of important complications are increased with this therapy. As a consequence, most spine surgeons have abandoned the practice of administering corticosteroids to patients with SCI.

Complications of SCI

The complications of SCI are consistently implicated in the high morbidity and mortality and the high financial cost associated with this type of injury. Acute-phase complications of SCI include the potential for aspiration or respiratory arrest, especially with high cervical injuries. Lower cervical lesions may preserve the diaphragm, but the loss of intercostal muscles will ultimately impair coughing and deep breathing, predisposing the patient to atelectasis and pneumonia. To prevent these complications, transport patients with the head of the stretcher elevated at least to a 30° angle as appropriate based on any underlying vertebral column instability.

Deep vein thrombosis and pulmonary embolism are late complications that may result from immobility and can become potentially life threatening. Consider applying sequential compression devices to the lower legs for prolonged transports to reduce the risk of deep vein thrombosis subsequent to pulmonary embolism.

Pressure ulcers from immobility are also problematic in conjunction with SCI. Proper padding and positioning are important during the transfer phase.

To reduce the occurrence of urinary tract infections in patients with SCI, avoid the use of Foley catheters. When these catheters are necessary, use appropriate sterile technique during their placement, securing the device to the patient's leg and keeping the Foley bag in a dependent location to prevent backflow of urine into the bladder.

Autonomic dysreflexia is typically a late complication of SCI but may occur acutely. It commonly occurs with injuries above T6 and results from the loss of coordinated autonomic responses. In this condition, an irritation, pain, or stimulus affects the nervous system below the SCI. The affected area sends signals to the brain, but they are unable to reach the brain. The body responds with a reflex action that constricts the blood vessels and increases BP. If left uncontrolled, this cascade can cause a stroke, seizure, and even death. Patients present clinically with evidence of a massive, uninhibited, uncompensated cardiovascular response as the result of noxious stimulation of the sympathetic nervous system below the level of injury. Unabated sympathetic nervous system stimulation results in vasoconstriction and hypertension (SBP sometimes exceeds 200 mm Hg). This leads to compensatory parasympathetic stimulation and causes bradycardia and vasodilation above the level of the lesion, whereas vessels below the SCI remain constricted. The selective vasodilation results in flushed, diaphoretic skin and nasopharyngeal vessel congestion. Other symptoms include headache, nausea, and anxiety.

Common precipitators of autonomic dysreflexia include bladder distention, bowel impaction, bladder infection, pressure ulceration, fractures, and constrictive clothing. Indwelling catheters should be evaluated for obstruction or kinking and flushed to ensure their patency. In patients without an indwelling catheter, draining the bladder acutely with a temporary catheter should be considered to rule out distention as a cause. Identify irritating foci and treat them appropriately, such as removing light clothing, resolving bowel/bladder problems, or treating a decubitus ulcer.

If the source of autonomic dysreflexia cannot be found or minimized to an effective extent, it may be necessary to reduce the patient's BP with vasodilators. Agents to consider are ones with a rapid action and a short duration (eg, nitrates, nitropaste, hydralizine, labetolol). A trial of beta blockers may also help to reduce cardiovascular response. If autonomic dysreflexia is left untreated, the patient may experience seizures, intracranial hemorrhage, and even death.

Signs and Symptoms

Autonomic Dysreflexia

- Hypertension
- Headache
- Nasal congestion
- Anxiety
- Nausea
- Blurred vision
- Bradycardia common, but tachycardia may also occur
- Diaphoresis and flushing above SCI
- Piloerection above SCI

Transport Management

Autonomic Dysreflexia

- Monitor BP frequently.
- Search for, identify, and correct inciting stimuli (ie, reposition the patient and check the bladder and bowels for irritation or obstruction).
- If the source cannot be found or minimized, reduce the BP with a beta blocker or vasodilators.

Stroke
Mechanism of Injury

Stroke, also referred to as cerebrovascular accident, occurs when a disruption of blood flow to the brain results in a neurologic deficit persisting for more than 24 hours. When deficits completely resolve within 24 hours, the event is referred to as a transient ischemic attack (TIA). Perfusion to oxygen-sensitive brain tissue may be interrupted when a blood vessel is occluded or when the structural integrity of a blood vessel is compromised, allowing blood to escape into the brain tissue or into the subarachnoid space. Care must be initiated quickly to restore proper blood flow and reduce loss of normal neurologic function.

Types of Stroke

A hemorrhagic stroke occurs when there is bleeding in the intraparenchymal space (intracerebral hemorrhage) or subarachnoid space (subarachnoid hemorrhage), causing direct or secondary damage to cerebral tissue. This type of stroke is less common and produces worse outcomes as compared to ischemic strokes.

An ischemic stroke occurs when cerebral blood flow is decreased, usually because of an occlusion of a blood vessel. The occlusion can be due to either a thrombus or an embolus. Hypoperfusion secondary to hypotension can also cause an ischemic stroke. An estimated 87% of all strokes are ischemic strokes.

A thrombotic stroke is largely the result of an accumulation of atherosclerotic plaques inside cerebral blood vessels, especially at bifurcations, which narrow the lumen of the vessel and hinder blood flow. Rupture of a local plaque can lead to localized clotting, which then significantly diminishes or completely stops blood flow distal to the occlusion.

In an embolic stroke, an embolus from the heart or lower circulation travels and lodges in a smaller cerebral vessel, resulting in loss of blood supply. Only 30% of ischemic strokes are thought to be caused by an embolus. Myocardial complications, such as atrial fibrillation, valvular heart disease, myocardial infarction, ventricular aneurysm, and cardiomyopathy, are known risk factors for embolus formation.

A focal ischemic stroke occurs when an area of marginally perfused tissue, the ischemic penumbra, surrounds a core of ischemic cells. As blood flow continues to dwindle, the ischemic cells become injured and finally die. The result is infarction and irreversible loss of brain tissue, which eventually softens and becomes necrotic. The size of the stroke depends on the size and location of the occluded vessel and the availability of collateral blood flow.

In a global ischemic stroke, severe hypotension or cardiac arrest produces a transient drop in blood flow to all areas of the brain. The areas of the brain affected first, known as the watershed areas, consist of the cortical territories between the anterior cerebral artery, the middle cerebral artery, and the posterior cerebral artery.

Assessment of Stroke

The hallmark of stroke is the sudden onset of focal neurologic signs that often occur in combination, corresponding to the anatomic area of ischemia or infarction. The CCTP can use abbreviated prehospital stroke assessment tools to identify patients suffering from stroke. Examples include the Cincinnati Prehospital Stroke Scale **TABLE 12-24** and the Los Angeles Prehospital Stroke Screen **TABLE 12-25**. There are multiple acceptable prehospital stroke assessment tools and little evidence to show strong superiority of one over the others. Choice of a prehospital stroke assessment tool varies by region and system. Although useful in the hospital setting, the National Institutes of Health's stroke scale is not

TABLE 12-24 Cincinnati Prehospital Stroke Scale[a]

Assessment	Normal	Abnormal
Facial Droop. Ask the patient to smile and show the teeth.	Both sides of the face move equally well.	One side of the face does not move as well as the other.
Arm Drift. Ask the patient to close the eyes and hold the arms out with palms up for 10 seconds.	Both arms move the same, or both arms do not move.	One arm does not move, or one arm drifts down compared with the other.
Abnormal Speech. Ask the patient to say, "The sky is blue in Cincinnati" or "You can't teach an old dog new tricks."	The patient uses the correct words with no slurring.	The patient slurs words, uses inappropriate words, or is unable to speak.

[a]Interpretation: If any assessment criterion is abnormal, the probability of a stroke is 72%.

© Jones & Bartlett Learning.

TABLE 12-25 Los Angeles Prehospital Stroke Screen[a]

Criteria	Yes	Unknown	No
1. Age >45 years	☐	☐	☐
2. History of seizures or epilepsy absent	☐	☐	☐
3. Symptoms <24 hours	☐	☐	☐
4. At baseline, patient is not wheelchair bound or bedridden	☐	☐	☐
5. Blood glucose between 60 and 400 mg/dL	☐	☐	☐
6. Obvious asymmetry (right versus left) in any of the following three exam categories (must be unilateral):	**Equal**	**Right Weak**	**Left Weak**
Facial smile/grimace	☐	☐ Droop	☐ Droop
Grip	☐	☐ Weak grip ☐ No grip	☐ Weak grip ☐ No grip
Arm strength	☐	☐ Drifts down ☐ Falls rapidly	☐ Drifts down ☐ Falls rapidly

[a]Interpretation: If criteria 1 through 6 are marked yes, the probability of a stroke is 97%.

© Jones & Bartlett Learning.

practical for evaluating patients during transport because it is very involved; nonetheless, the CCTP should become familiar with this scale's values because they indicate the severity of illness.

In addition to focal neurologic signs and stroke tools, noncontrast CT scanning is important to help determine whether the patient's symptoms are being caused by an occlusion or bleeding or whether any hemorrhagic conversion (a secondary hemorrhage at the site of an ischemic stroke lesion) is present. These findings have significant implications for decision making about treatment.

Early in the evaluation, the CCTP should consider possible "stroke mimics." These conditions can cause symptoms clinically similar to stroke, but actually involve a different pathologic process that may benefit from other interventions. A stroke mimic of particular importance to the CCTP is hypoglycemia. All patients with suspected stroke should be assessed for hypoglycemia early in their assessment and treated as indicated. Other possible stroke mimics include seizure, migraine, hyponatremia, and other metabolic derangements, all of which may be considered in the hospital setting.

Complications of Stroke

In addition to neurologic deficits corresponding to the anatomic areas of infarction, other complications from strokes are possible. Cerebral edema sufficient to produce clinical deterioration occurs in 10% to 20% of patients with ischemic stroke and can result in intracranial hypertension. In this case, the edema results from a loss of normal metabolic function of cells and peaks at 3 to 5 days. Intracranial hypertension may, in turn, cause significant complications, as discussed earlier in this chapter. Hemorrhagic conversion can also occur. In addition, patients who have had a stroke may exhibit seizure activity due to damaged neurons.

Management of Stroke

Once stroke is suspected, the CCTP should determine the time of symptom onset or "last known well" time, as this information is key to hospital care providers' determination of the most appropriate therapy. The "last known well time" is either the time of symptom onset, if known, or the last time the patient was known to be at their baseline.

In general, during evaluation and transport, the CCTP should support the patient's cardiopulmonary function, provide continuous monitoring of neurologic function, and maintain normal blood glucose levels. Patients with stroke are at increased risk for respiratory compromise from aspiration, upper airway obstruction, and hypoventilation. Frequent reassessment of airway and respiratory function is necessary because hypoxemia will worsen ischemic brain injury, contributing to a worse outcome. Patients with suspected stroke should not routinely be given supplemental oxygen unless they are hypoxic.

Hemodynamic status is also vital information in stroke patients. BP targets vary depending on the clinical situation. In patients with known ischemic stroke, simple measures may be taken to improve CPP, such as positioning the patient supine and allowing permissive hypertension. Many systems' parameters allow BPs up to 220/120 mm Hg in patients not being treated with fibrinolytic therapy in an effort to maintain adequate CPP. Local protocols may vary regarding the exact vital sign parameters.

After evaluation in the hospital setting, clinicians will determine whether the patient would benefit from a reperfusion therapy such as fibrinolytic therapy or mechanical thrombectomy. This decision depends on the patient's last known well time, type of symptoms, and comorbidities.

Fibrinolytic Therapy

In some cases, the CCTP may provide transport for patients who have experienced a stroke and have received or are actively receiving fibrinolytic therapy. If a stroke patient's symptoms are disabling, a CT scan shows no hemorrhage, the symptom onset is within 4.5 hours, and the patient does not have any contraindications, fibrinolytic therapy may be administered to restore circulation to ischemic brain tissue. Studies have shown that in appropriate patient populations, earlier fibrinolytic therapy produces better neurologic outcomes, underscoring the importance of timely evaluation and treatment of these patients. Fibrinolytic therapy may also be available in certain circumstances when the time of symptom onset is unknown, such as in cases of "wake-up" stroke after a cerebral perfusion scan has been completed in the hospital setting and shows the patient would benefit from the therapy.

The only fibrinolytic agent currently used for the treatment of ischemic stroke is tPA, also referred to as alteplase. A thrombolytic agent, tPA binds to fibrin on a clot surface and converts plasminogen to plasmin, which degrades the clot. It is typically given as an initial bolus, followed by an infusion over an hour. Therefore, the CCTP may provide transport to a patient actively receiving tPA and should be aware of possible complications of this treatment.

Before therapy is initiated, inclusion and exclusion criteria for IV fibrinolytic therapy should be reviewed to decrease the risk of complications. Refer to the American Heart Association's website for the most up-to-date list of inclusion and exclusion criteria. Exclusion criteria generally include the following concerns:

- History of intracranial neoplasm, AVM, or aneurysm
- Bleeding concerns, in the form of either current bleeding or a bleeding disorder
- History of recent stroke
- Recent noncompressible vascular puncture
- Major surgery or trauma in the past 3 months
- SBP of greater than 180 mm Hg
- Pregnancy and up to 1 month postpartum

Possible complications of tPA therapy include intracranial hemorrhage, orolingual angioedema, acute hypotension, and systemic bleeding. When transporting a patient who has received or is receiving tPA, the patient's hemodynamic status should be closely managed, with a BP goal of less than 180/105 mm Hg; risk of hemorrhage increases with higher BP levels. The patient should be continuously monitored for any neurologic deterioration, which would be concerning for possible intracranial hemorrhage. Sudden mental status change, neurologic deterioration, sudden vital sign changes, or severe headache may be signs of intracranial hemorrhage in this setting.

If intracranial hemorrhage is suspected, the tPA infusion should be stopped immediately and the base hospital should be contacted for further orders. The BP goal may be lowered. The patient should be closely monitored for mental status deterioration and need for airway interventions. In the hospital setting, a patient would be taken for an immediate repeat CT scan to evaluate for hemorrhage. If such a bleed is found, reversal of thrombolytic and anticoagulation therapy would be initiated with cryoprecipitate, tranexamic acid, and possibly other medications or blood products, depending on the clinical situation. Reversal of anticoagulation therapy is discussed further in Chapter 10, *Resuscitation, Shock, and Blood Products*.

Endovascular Interventions

Rapid technological advances in recent years have made endovascular interventions for reperfusion therapy increasingly valuable. IV tPA is less effective for strokes caused by proximal or large-vessel occlusions, and the subset of patients with these kinds of strokes can benefit significantly from endovascular interventions. As technology rapidly evolves in this field, the window of time for these patients to receive endovascular interventions will continue to expand.

Intra-arterial thrombolysis uses an endovascular approach to administer local tPA at the site of the occlusion. It may be combined with a mechanical intervention. One study found improved clinical outcomes with this intervention at 90 days post treatment, but more recent studies have not shown any significant clinical benefit compared to standard treatment. The current American Heart Association/American Stroke Association guidelines state that intra-arterial thrombolysis may be considered in a subset of patients who have contraindications to IV fibrinolysis.

Controversies

The standard of care for LVO strokes has been to administer IV tPA to these patients prior to transfer to the neurointerventional radiology suite. However, since the promising results of several landmark studies from 2014 to 2015 (MR. CLEAN, ESCAPE, EXTEND IA, SWIFT-PRIME, and REVASCAT) were published, hospitals have begun using acute endovascular therapy for these patients. More recently, studies have brought the role of tPA into question, demonstrating a reperfusion rate of only 7% to 15% when this medication is used to treat LVO strokes. Further, a 2020 study published in the *New England Journal of Medicine* found that endovascular therapy alone was noninferior to tPA plus endovascular therapy.

Additional studies are ongoing at large comprehensive stroke centers, but early data support a shift in the treatment of LVO stroke, with patients receiving rapid transfer for endovascular interventions without IV tPA.

Mechanical thrombectomy is an endovascular surgical intervention that has been shown to have a significantly positive effect on neurologic outcomes compared to fibrinolytic therapy alone in stroke patients with an LVO. In this procedure, arterial catheterization is performed and a device is used to retrieve the clot, with the aim of restoring circulation to the affected area of cerebral tissue. In general, patients with an LVO stroke who are within 24 hours of symptom onset may be considered for mechanical thrombectomy. As with fibrinolytic therapy, the benefit of mechanical thrombectomy depends heavily on time from symptom onset: It should be done as expeditiously as possible for maximum benefit. Factors such as the exact vessel affected, time since symptom onset, and severity of symptoms may affect the level of benefit. These procedures are typically performed at endovascular-capable comprehensive stroke centers.

Signs and Symptoms

Left Hemisphere Ischemic Stroke

- Right hemiparesis
- Right-side sensory loss
- Right visual field deficit
- Poor right conjugate gaze
- Dysarthria
- Aphasia
- Difficulty in reading, writing, or calculating

Right Hemisphere Ischemic Stroke

- Left hemiparesis
- Left-side sensory loss
- Left visual field deficit
- Poor left conjugate gaze
- Dysarthria
- Extinction of left-side stimuli
- Neglect of the left visual space
- Spatial disorientation

Brainstem/Cerebellum/Posterior Hemisphere Ischemic Stroke

- Motor or sensory loss in all four limbs
- Crossed signs
- Limb or gait ataxia
- Dysarthria
- Dysconjugate gaze
- Nystagmus
- Amnesia
- Bilateral visual field deficits

Small Subcortical Hemisphere or Brainstem (Pure Motor) Ischemic Stroke

- Weakness of the face and limbs on one side of the body without abnormalities of higher brain function, sensation, or vision

Small Subcortical Hemisphere or Brainstem (Pure Sensory) Ischemic Stroke

- Decreased sensation of the face and limbs on one side of the body without abnormalities of higher brain function, motor function, or vision

Adapted from Adams HP, Brott TA, Crowell RM, et al. Guidelines for the management of patients with acute ischemic stroke: a statement for healthcare professionals from a special writing group of the Stroke Council, American Heart Association. *Circulation.* 1994;90(3):1588.

Transport Management

Stroke

- Determine the time of symptom onset.
- Support the patient's cardiopulmonary function.
- Provide continuous monitoring of neurologic function.
- Maintain normal blood glucose levels.
- Reassess airway and respiratory function frequently.
- Maintain oxygen saturation greater than 94%.

Stroke Systems of Care

Given the prevalence of stroke and the time-sensitive nature of effective interventions, organized and coordinated stroke systems of care are extremely important. Regions should have a plan in place that addresses the following needs:

- Strategy for minimizing stroke morbidity and mortality using public education
- Dispatch instructions and triage strategies
- EMS protocols and training
- Coordination between primary stroke centers, comprehensive stroke centers, and rehabilitation centers
- Continuous quality improvement

Further, the regional plan should define criteria for activating the stroke system and for selecting the appropriate transport destination.

The rapid advancements in endovascular interventions have prompted stroke systems to continually evolve. As mentioned, criteria for stroke system activation change frequently due to the ever-expanding time window during which patients may benefit from time-sensitive interventions. It is vital that prehospital and CCT agencies stay current with these changes.

Controversies

Given the significant benefit of endovascular interventions for patients with LVO strokes, the medical community continues to debate how transport destinations should be determined for stroke patients from the field. Historically, given the time-dependent nature of tPA, nearly all stroke patients have been brought to the nearest tPA-capable facility, which is usually not a comprehensive stroke center. At that facility, if imaging reveals the presence of an LVO, the patient may be transported to an endovascular center if indicated. Clearly, this system delays time to mechanical thrombectomy for some patients. Systems must improve early access to mechanical thrombectomy while avoiding delay of tPA therapy for patients who need it or overtriaging patients to comprehensive stroke centers. Many systems are piloting programs to address this problem, such as implementation of mobile stroke units or field triage directly to comprehensive stroke centers for certain patients. This is an emerging area of research in the EMS community and a consensus on best practice does not yet exist.

Intracerebral Hemorrhage

Intracerebral hemorrhage is bleeding directly into the cerebral tissue that causes cerebral tissue destruction, cerebral edema, and increased ICP. The most common cause of spontaneous intracerebral hemorrhage is hypertension-induced vessel rupture. Other causes include anticoagulation or fibrinolytic therapy, coagulation disorders, drug abuse, and hemorrhage into cerebral infarcts or brain tumors.

Symptoms of intracerebral hemorrhage may begin as local neurologic dysfunction related to the area of the brain in which a vessel has ruptured. The patient may also report the presence of a severe headache, nausea, and vomiting. As ICP continues to rise, however, the patient will oftentimes become unconscious (a key finding that helps differentiate this condition from ischemic stroke) and may require ventilatory support. The time it takes for deterioration to progress is related to the amount and speed of bleeding.

The CCTP should provide adequate attention to the management of cardiopulmonary function. If intubation is necessary, the CCTP should perform it as soon as the patient's level of consciousness becomes inadequate for airway control or vomiting begins to endanger airway patency. If intracerebral hemorrhage has been confirmed before transport, orders may be given to reduce BP to decrease ongoing bleeding. An overly aggressive reduction in BP, however, may compromise cerebral perfusion pressure, especially in the patient with an elevated ICP.

Patients on anticoagulation therapy, such as those taking warfarin, will likely need to be given reversal agents. Reversal agents may be in progress during transport. Reversal of anticoagulation is discussed further in Chapter 10, *Resuscitation, Shock, and Blood Products.*

Subarachnoid Hemorrhage

Subarachnoid hemorrhage is bleeding into the subarachnoid space; this bleeding is usually arterial in nature. Most subarachnoid hemorrhages are caused by rupture of a cerebral aneurysm or AVM. Other causes include hypertensive intracerebral hemorrhages that progress to subarachnoid hemorrhage and bleeding from a cerebral tumor. This chapter focuses on the two most frequent causes of subarachnoid hemorrhage.

An **aneurysm** is an outpouching of the wall of a blood vessel that results from weakening of the vessel's wall. Although most aneurysms are congenital, others can be attributed to trauma or infection, or are idiopathic in nature. As an individual with a congenital cerebral aneurysm matures, BP rises and places stress on the wall of the weakened vessel. Eventually, the vessel balloons, which may lead to compression of adjacent brain tissue and focal neurologic dysfunction. If the aneurysm ruptures, arterial blood is sent into the subarachnoid space at high pressure. As blood fills the space, ICP rises and cerebral perfusion pressure falls.

An **arteriovenous malformation (AVM)** is a tangled mass of arterial and venous blood vessels that shunt blood directly from thickly walled arteries to thinly walled veins without the benefit of pressure being reduced by an intervening capillary bed. One or more cerebral arteries, known as feeders, provide blood to an AVM. These feeders enlarge over time, increase the volume of blood shunted through the malformation, and increase the overall mass effect on adjacent brain tissue. Eventually, veins may no longer be able to accommodate the high mean pressure; they may then rupture, causing blood to fill the subarachnoid space. As this happens, ICP rises and cerebral perfusion pressure falls.

Like patients with intracerebral hemorrhage, patients on anticoagulation therapy for subarachnoid hemorrhage will likely need to be given reversal agents, which may be in progress during transport. Reversal of anticoagulation is discussed further in Chapter 10, *Resuscitation, Shock, and Blood Products.*

Assessment of Subarachnoid Hemorrhage

The patient with a subarachnoid hemorrhage characteristically has an abrupt onset of pain, oftentimes described as "the worst headache I have ever had." A loss of consciousness, nausea, vomiting, focal neurologic deficits, photophobia, and nuchal rigidity may accompany the headache. As ICP increases, the patient may become comatose or die.

Management of Subarachnoid Hemorrhage

When caring for a patient with a subarachnoid hemorrhage, the CCTP must focus on maintaining cardiopulmonary function. This frequently involves airway management and ventilatory support as the patient's level of consciousness and vomiting endanger the airway. The CCTP may also take steps to prevent an unnecessary rise in ICP, such as limiting head movement and elevating the head during transport. Common complications of subarachnoid hemorrhage include rebleeding (ie, a second subarachnoid hemorrhage in an unsecured aneurysm), cerebral vasospasm, hyponatremia, and hydrocephalus.

Signs and Symptoms

Subarachnoid Hemorrhage
- Onset of pain
- Worst headache of the patient's life
- Loss of consciousness
- Nausea
- Vomiting
- Focal neurologic deficits
- Photophobia
- Nuchal rigidity

Transport Management

Subarachnoid Hemorrhage
- Take measures to maintain the patient's cardiopulmonary function.
- Manage the patient's airway.
- Provide ventilatory support if necessary.
- Limit movement of the patient's head; elevate the head during transport.

Acute Guillain-Barré Syndrome

Guillain-Barré syndrome (GBS) comprises a group of immune-mediated polyneuropathies, all of which share a common constellation of features often provoked by an infection. The overall worldwide incidence of GBS is 1 to 2 per 100,000 people, with the incidence increasing by 20% for every 10 years of life. This syndrome is more common in males.

The primary clinical presentation of GBS is a progressive, usually symmetric muscle weakness that varies from mild to complete paralysis. Patients often present for medical care several days to a week after the onset of symptoms. Typically, the weakness begins in the legs, but in 10% of patients it may begin in the upper extremities or face.

Patients with known or suspected acute GBS may be transported to referral centers and may exhibit significant or complete paralysis of all four extremities, respiratory, and facial muscles. Ventilator support is required in as many as 30%

of all patients with GBS and is highly likely to be required in patients with acute GBS. Autonomic nervous system dysfunction is also common in patients with acute GBS, who may demonstrate wide swings in BP, significant tachycardia, and hemodynamic changes requiring ICU-level monitoring and treatment. Pain, primarily in the back and extremities, is present in 66% of patients with this condition.

Initial diagnosis of GBS is based on clinical presentation, including progressive, mostly bilateral (symmetric) muscle weakness with depressed or absent deep tendon reflexes. Confirmatory diagnosis of GBS can be made if CSF and neurophysiology studies show a typical pattern of abnormalities.

Treatment, especially during transport, is largely supportive. Close observation of respiratory effort in nonintubated patients with GBS is imperative, as deterioration can occur rapidly. Tachycardias rarely require treatment. Pressors may be needed for hypotension once any fluid volume deficits are corrected. Beta blockers or other antihypertensives may be needed for significant hypertension (sustained MAP >125 mm Hg), although careful consideration should be given to identifying potential causes of autonomic dysreflexia such as pain, acute urinary retention, or hypoxemia. These patients may also have significant pain, requiring narcotic analgesia.

Seizures and Epilepsy

When a nerve cell is stimulated, its action is transmitted to other cells by excitatory neurotransmitters and balanced by inhibitory neurotransmitters that slow communications. Overactivity by excitatory transmitters or underactivity by inhibitory transmitters can result in a seizure.

Seizure activity can be caused by many different factors, such as fever, glucose imbalance, electrolyte imbalances, head injuries and hemorrhagic strokes, and toxins. Epilepsy, for example, is a disorder featuring recurrent seizures caused by abnormal discharges in the brain cells; it is often idiopathic. Although monitoring of nonmotor seizures may be the only care needed, tonic-clonic and focal seizures that may compromise the airway require immediate action.

Care for patients with seizure should initially center on maintaining the airway, protecting the patient, and providing oxygen. Do not attempt to restrain a patient who is actively seizing. Instead, establish an IV line and monitor the patient's cardiac status. Also, check the patient's blood glucose level, and administer glucose if indicated. Check the patient's temperature to ensure that fever is not an issue. Body temperature can be lowered by administering normal saline, giving acetaminophen, and cooling down the patient without causing shivering.

If the patient is actively seizing, administer an anticonvulsant. The drugs most commonly given during transport for this purpose are lorazepam, diazepam, midazolam, and levetiracetam. Patients with a history of epilepsy are often taking phenytoin or levetiracetam, both of which can be given intravenously. In the prehospital arena, and for initial management of seizures in an emergency or critical care setting, midazolam has shown superiority to other agents and is considered the first-line drug of choice. Midazolam can be administered intranasally, intravenously, intramuscularly, or through an oral or rectal tube.

Transport Management

Seizures

- Manage the patient's airway.
- Maintain oxygen saturation greater than 92%.
- Do not attempt to restrain the patient if the patient is actively seizing.
- Establish an IV line.
- Monitor the patient's cardiac status.
- Check the patient's blood glucose level and administer glucose if indicated.
- Check the patient's temperature.
- To lower the patient's body temperature, administer normal saline, give acetaminophen, and cool the patient without causing shivering.
- If the patient is actively seizing, administer an anticonvulsant (eg, lorazepam, diazepam, midazolam, levetiracetam).
- If the patient has epilepsy, give levetiracetam, phenytoin, fosphenytoin sodium, carbamazine, or phenobarbital.

Transport Considerations

Prior to Transport

Before considering transport of a patient with a neurologic emergency, it is imperative to consider potential complications that the patient may experience. To this end, it is advisable to ensure that all diagnostic tests and surgical procedures have been completed when at all possible before transport.

Although patient-related risk factors are difficult to identify, equipment-related complications (which occur in as many as one-third of transports) may be controlled more easily. During critical care transport, the following types of equipment may be present and may require troubleshooting:

- Cardiac monitor, to monitor cardiac status: Check for sufficient batteries, charging, a general check, and waveform capnography.
- Ventilator with waveform capnography, to monitor and control ventilation: Check for sufficient oxygen and gas supply, ventilator tubing, oxygen and circuit connections, and capnography hookup.
- Infusion pumps, to administer medications: See the manufacturer's troubleshooting chart.
- ICP monitoring, to measure and control ICP: Check for sterility, keep the fluid level, and refer to the manufacturer's troubleshooting manual.
- Cerebral function monitor, to assess sedation, monitor brain wave activity, predict and monitor seizure activity, and monitor the onset and effectiveness of paralytics: See the manufacturer's troubleshooting chart.

Most interfacility transports do not involve ICP monitoring or CFM monitoring. When such monitoring is used, patients are usually placed on a ventilator, cardiac monitor, and medications administered by IV pump.

Scene and Interhospital Transport Considerations

Apart from intracranial hemorrhage, the major early risks to the patient with head injury are hypoxia and hypertension. The ABCs are always the first priority. Urgent attention to the ABCs will help reduce cerebral hypoxia and hypoperfusion. Normoxia and normocarbia should be achieved as soon as practically possible.

The patient with a severe closed head injury should be presumed to have an elevated ICP, and factors that may further increase ICP should be avoided. Some critical care transport systems advocate the use of ear and eye protection for such patients to prevent spikes in ICP caused by outside stimuli from aircraft or sirens (mostly applicable in patients with seizure). Overperfusion, hypertension, inadequate sedation, hyperpyrexia, and inappropriate anesthetic agents can increase ICP as well. Likewise, intubation and endotracheal suction cause sharp, albeit transitory, spikes in ICP. In patients with a reduced volume reserve (hypovolemic), however, these stimuli may initiate a prolonged increase in ICP. Pressure waves may be avoided by providing fluid resuscitation adequate to maintain CPP. Any sedation should be administered at a level that is sufficient to prevent coughing or gagging during transport.

Minimum requirements for monitoring patients during transport are continuous ECG, pulse oximetry, and intermittent measurements of BP, respiratory rate, and pulse rate. In specific patients, capnometry, continuous BP reading, and further monitoring (eg, monitoring of ICP and cardiac output and filling pressures) may be beneficial. Unfortunately, many of the complications reported during transport are caused by equipment malfunction. Given this reality, the CCTP must be familiar with all equipment and monitoring devices in use to ensure optimal patient outcomes and avoid complications from equipment misuse or malfunction.

Of particular importance is the possibility of measuring the major ventilation parameters, such as tidal volume or minute ventilation. Although many transport ventilators do not display the actual tidal volumes delivered, judicious use of $ETCO_2$ monitoring will allow the CCTP to observe the effects of mechanical ventilation on the patient during transport and to make appropriate adjustments. One way to reduce inadvertent ventilation problems is to use the best possible monitoring equipment, particularly equipment that focuses on tidal or minute ventilation. Bearing in mind the limitations of many portable ventilators, consider the use of sophisticated transport carts equipped with a standard ICU ventilator and the necessary gas supply. Such carts can be hooked to the patient's bed and moved fairly easily. Monitoring devices and infusion pumps can be integrated into the cart and powered with its battery. Such equipment is being increasingly used during interhospital transports.

Flight Considerations

Most fixed-wing aircraft used for medical transport have the ability to pressurize the cabin as the altitude increases and to depressurize the cabin as the altitude decreases. These aircraft have a chart indicating cabin pressure as a function of altitude. Ideally, the cabin pressure should closely match the original ground pressure. Thus, when feasible, the pilot should fly at altitudes where cabin pressure can be maintained as near to the original departure pressure as possible.

If this synchronization of pressures cannot be achieved in flight, adjustments must be made. If the patient is intubated, the endotracheal cuff pressure should be decreased with altitude to prevent damage to the trachea, and then reinflated during descent to prevent leakage. While recent research suggests that altitude-induced changes in cuff pressures may be clinically inconsequential, the CCTP should be equipped to monitor cuff pressures during transport and adjust them as needed. Adjust the pressure inside indwelling catheters and colostomy bags to prevent breakage. If the patient has a drain and the ICP is monitored, maintain the ICP at less than 20 cm H_2O by draining off excess fluids. If the patient does not have a drain, monitor for any changes in status. If the patient shows changes in the respiratory rate or pattern, or develops any changes in cardiac function (ie, arrhythmias or significant changes in heart rate), these signs may indicate herniation. In such a case, the aircraft must immediately descend to an altitude at which the condition can be managed.

When targeting ventilation to specific ETCO$_2$ parameters, remember that high altitudes require lower ETCO$_2$ values to achieve the same results seen at sea level.

Summary

Management of neurologic emergencies requires an in-depth understanding of brain, spinal, and cranial nerve anatomy and physiology. In addition, the CCTP must be familiar with the complexity of severe TBI, recognize the early signs and symptoms of TBI, and understand how early intervention can influence these patients' outcomes.

The CCTP should make every effort to preserve cerebral perfusion and oxygenation as the primary goal in the initial care for patients with neurologic emergencies. Current guidelines call for careful monitoring of oxygenation and preventing hypoxia by keeping Pao$_2$ (partial pressure of arterial oxygen) above 60 mm Hg and/or oxygen saturation greater than 90% at all times. In patients who exhibit signs and symptoms of cerebral herniation during field management or transport, initial management consists of hyperventilation. Mannitol may be helpful in treating increased ICP and cerebral herniation, but should be used judiciously given its other physiologic effects. The use of analgesia, sedation, and neuromuscular blockade is critical during transport to minimize the risks associated with increased ICP and to maximize safety in the transport setting. The CCTP should also be mindful of the potential for hypoglycemia in patients with neurologic emergencies, because this condition may mimic TBI or stroke; thus, hypoglycemia should be considered in all patients with an altered LOC until ruled out by applicable diagnostic and laboratory confirmations.

To a large extent, the treatment of neurologic emergencies depends on the ability to distinguish between primary and secondary injuries. A key aspect of managing secondary injuries is managing the effects of the injury—namely, CPP and ICP.

A CCTP who is involved in the transport of patients with neurologic emergencies should be mindful of the complexities associated with these conditions. If possible, most diagnostic tests and treatments should be performed prior to transport. Although a number of patient-related risk factors can be identified in any neurologic transport, the rate of equipment-related adverse events in transport is substantially higher with these types of injuries. This requires careful attention to the personnel, equipment, and monitoring in use at any given time.

Case Study

You and your critical care transport team are requested at the three-bed emergency department (ED) of a small community hospital to transfer a 60-year-old woman who was brought in moments ago by local EMS complaining of a severe headache.

As part of your history taking, you interview the patient's husband, who is present at her bedside. He reports that his wife just buried her mother yesterday and has been under a lot of stress dealing with her mother's affairs. He states that she has been complaining of a headache for the past few days, but it has become worse, increasing in severity.

When the patient's husband arrived home after work, he found his wife lying on the couch. He dimmed the lights, put a cool washcloth on her forehead, and gave her two aspirins. He went into the kitchen to start preparing dinner when he heard her vomiting. Upon entering the room, he saw that his wife was projectile vomiting and called 9-1-1.

During your interview with the patient, she confirms what her husband reported and adds that she has been having blurred vision today as well. She attributed the headache and nausea to stress over her mother's death. While you are obtaining information on her past medical conditions, the patient reports that she has a history of high BP and has not been taking her medication for the past week, trying to save money to pay for her mother's funeral. She denies having any other medical problems or taking any other medications.

Your initial physical exam of the patient reveals a normal GCS score of 15. She is able to follow complex commands and move all extremities. She has no decreased level of consciousness and has equal strength bilaterally in all extremities, and all of her cranial nerves are intact. Her BP is 192/110 mm Hg, consistent with the ED staff's measurements. The patient is on a cardiac monitor, which reveals a heart rate of 95 beats/min, with normal sinus rhythm. Her respiratory rate is 18 breaths/min, and her lungs are clear to

auscultation in all lung fields. Oral temperature is 99.6°F (37.6°C). The patient rates her headache as a 10 on a scale of 0 to 10, with 10 being the worst pain in her life.

The patient is prepared for transport. The ED staff has placed an IV line in the patient's right antecubital vein, infusing normal saline at a keep-the-vein-open rate. The patient is placed on the stretcher with the head of the bed elevated at 45° angle. You and your team load the patient into your critical care ambulance and initiate seizure precautions during the transport.

During transport to the referral center, the patient has a tonic-clonic seizure. You administer 2 mg of lorazepam IV and no further seizures occur.

1. What is going on with this patient?
2. Why is the head of the bed elevated at a 45° angle?
3. Why are seizure precautions initiated, and what does the seizure precaution entail for the ambulance crew?
4. What are some possible complications that could occur during the transport of this patient and how would the critical care transport team handle them?

At the referral center, an emergency CT scan of the patient's head is ordered. It reveals a small, right subarachnoid hemorrhage with bleeding into the suprasellar cistern, indicating a grade 2 subarachnoid hemorrhage. (In 1968, Drs. Hunt and Hess developed a grading scale for the classification of cerebral aneurysm. The grading scale ranges from grade 1, an asymptomatic or minor headache, to grade 5, a deep coma.) Neurosurgery is consulted and a cerebral angiogram is ordered. The cerebral angiogram reveals a 4-mm, berry-shaped, right middle cerebral aneurysm located at a bifurcation.

The patient is admitted to the neurosurgery ICU and scheduled for surgery the next morning. A clipping of the right middle cerebral artery is performed without complication. An IVC is placed to monitor the patient's ICP. The surgeon's postoperative order states to maintain a SBP of 140 mm Hg or lower, to perform hourly neurologic exams, and to maintain an ICP of less than 15 mm Hg and a CPP of greater than 80 mm Hg. The patient remains on the ventilator until the following morning, when a postoperative CT scan is performed. The scan reveals no complications and no recurrence of bleeding. She is extubated that day and discharged home 6 days later without further complications.

5. What are some of the common reasons why an individual might have a cerebral aneurysm?

6. List the three major postoperative complications that may occur following a cerebral aneurysm.

Analysis

This patient has a cerebral aneurysm. Elevating the head of the bed will help reduce her increased ICP.

Seizure precautions include the following measures: avoiding the use of lights and siren; keeping lights dimmed in the ambulance compartment; padding the side rails of the patient's stretcher; verifying that airway equipment is readily available, such as oxygen delivery systems, nasal and oral airways, bag-mask device, suction, catheters, and suction equipment; and being prepared to administer diazepam or lorazepam.

Possible complications in this patient include increased ICP, hypertension, respiratory depression and failure, and brain herniation. The CCTP should not treat her hypertension during the transfer unless directed to do so by the receiving facility or neurosurgeon. The hypertension state is intended to provide increased cerebral perfusion to any potentially vasospastic areas. In general,

patients should be maintained in a normotensive state with a SBP of 110 to 160 mm Hg. Keeping the head of the bed elevated and avoiding overstimulation of the patient will help reduce her ICP.

Patients with respiratory depression and failure may require rapid sequence intubation. Patients with potential increased ICP should be premedicated with a short-acting opioid such as fentanyl, usually 3 mcg/kg IV. A sedative should always be used unless the patient is deeply comatose.

Nondepolarizing neuromuscular blockers such as rocuronium or vecuronium, unlike succinylcholine, do not cause fasciculations. Etomidate may be used as an alternative induction agent. This hypnotic agent will not increase ICP, but it is contraindicated in patients younger than 10 years. If etomidate is used, lidocaine is theoretically unnecessary.

The patient's $Paco_2$ level should be maintained between 36 and 42 mm Hg. Hyperventilation should be avoided unless the patient shows signs of herniation.

Causes of cerebral aneurysms include neoplastic disease, atherosclerosis, brain trauma, infection, and congenital defects. Clip ligation—a surgical procedure that blocks the aneurysm from the circulation by placement of a clip—is usually performed to repair cerebral aneurysms.

Potential postoperative complications of clip ligation of a cerebral aneurysm include recurrence of bleeding (especially in the first 24 hours), cerebral vasospasm, and electrolyte disturbances, such as hypernatremia. Vasospasm will decrease blood flow to the brain and cause the death of nerve cells, so medication may be administered to prevent it. The patient may also be given medications to address other potential complications.

Prep Kit

Ready for Review

- A majority of patients with neurologic emergencies who require transport will have traumatic brain injury (TBI).
- The nervous system can be divided into the CNS, which consists of the brain and spinal cord, and the PNS, which consists of the spinal and cranial nerves.
- Afferent pathways (ascending pathways) carry sensory impulses toward the CNS; efferent pathways (descending pathways) carry motor impulses away from the CNS to effector organs, such as muscles (smooth and skeletal) or glands.
- The voluntary (somatic) nervous system is composed of nervous system fibers that connect the structures of the CNS with skeletal muscles and the integument; the involuntary (autonomic) nervous system is divided into the sympathetic and parasympathetic branches.
- The brain is a very delicate organ that requires the protection afforded by the skull. Although the skull is primarily a protective structure, excessive forces can cause a fracture to the adult skull and force bone fragments into the vulnerable brain tissue.
- Openings at the base of the skull (foramina) allow cranial nerves and blood vessels to enter and exit the cranial cavity. These openings also weaken the area, leaving it susceptible to fracture.
- The cranial meninges consist of three layers: the dura mater (a two-layer structure adherent to the internal surface of the cranium), the arachnoid mater (a thin layer loosely enclosing the brain), and the pia mater (a vascular membrane that adheres to the surface of the brain and follows its contours).
- The lateral ventricles extend from the frontal lobe to the occipital lobe of the brain. These structures are important when ICP monitoring, cerebrospinal fluid (CSF) drainage, or placement of a CSF shunt is undertaken.
- Cerebrospinal fluid fills the ventricular system and surrounds the brain and spinal cord in the subarachnoid space. It protects the CNS by acting as a shock absorber in case of minor acceleration and deceleration and by helping to remove waste products from cerebral tissue.
- Any obstruction to the normal flow of CSF may produce high CSF pressure and lead to brain damage.
- The cerebrum consists of two cerebral hemispheres, which are divided into four paired lobes: the frontal, parietal, temporal, and occipital lobes.
- The brainstem acts as a bridge between the cerebral hemispheres and the spinal cord; all motor and sensory fibers travel through this structure. The brainstem consists of three parts: the midbrain, the pons, and the medulla oblongata.
- The cerebellum, which coordinates voluntary movement, consists of three major parts: the cortex, the white matter, and four pairs of deep cerebellar nuclei.
- The reticular formation, which is composed of both motor and sensory tracts, includes centers for BP, respiration, and heart rate function.
- The overall goal of cerebral circulation is to provide enough blood to supply oxygen, glucose, and nutrients so that oxidation of glucose can take place.
- The blood–brain barrier regulates the transport of nutrients, ions, water, drugs, and waste products to and from the brain through the process of selective permeability.
- The spine usually consists of 33 irregular bones (vertebrae) that articulate to form the vertebral column; ligaments and muscles stabilize these skeletal components.
- Flexion of the vertebral column beyond the range of 60% to 70% may damage structural ligaments and allow excess vertebral movement that could expose the spinal cord to injury.

Prep Kit Continued

- The spinal cord transmits nerve impulses between the brain and the rest of the body. The 31 pairs of spinal nerves emerge from each side of the spinal cord and are named for the vertebral region and level from which they arise.
- The sympathetic nervous system is controlled by the brain's hypothalamus. A SCI at or above the level of T6 may disrupt the flow of sympathetic communication.
- When the sympathetic nerves are stimulated and produce autonomic dysreflexia, the parasympathetic nerves attempt to control the rapidly increasing BP by slowing the heart rate.
- The intracellular transport of protein and organelle materials is essential for all mammalian cells, especially neurons; when it becomes disrupted, disease can result.
- The foundation of neurologic care is a thorough serial assessment, which not only allows the CCTP to track patient trends but also may allow the CCTP to identify which parts of the system are damaged.
- In some cases, the CCTP may assess cranial nerves, motor function, and sensory function; perform reflex testing; and evaluate meningeal irritation if the initial assessment was done quickly or if there is time for these assessments during transport.
- The mental and emotional component of the neurologic examination assesses the patient's ability to understand and interact with the environment by addressing the level of consciousness; general behavior; and thought processes, including memory, attention and concentration, abstract thought, and judgment.
- Awareness and arousal are the fundamental constituents of consciousness and should be evaluated and documented repeatedly.
- Arousal is assessed initially by the AVPU scale. The Glasgow Coma Scale is then commonly used to document and trend the patient's level of arousal over time.
- When evaluating the patient's awareness, the CCTP should assess the patient's orientation to time, place, and person.
- A variety of neurologic pathologies—including pain, hypoxia, anxiety, and expanding intracranial lesions—may initially manifest themselves through changes in general behavior.
- The Mini-Mental State Examination is a simple, easily applied test of higher cognitive functions that consists of a series of questions testing orientation, registration, attention and calculation, recall, and language.
- Abnormalities of speech can reflect dysfunction in any component or process of communication. For example, aphasia encompasses any loss or impairment of language function as a result of brain damage.
- Certain nerves are more commonly tested in patients who are critically ill or injured: optic (CN II), oculomotor (CN III), trochlear (CN IV), trigeminal (CN V), abducens (CN VI), facial (CN VII), acoustic (CN VIII), glossopharyngeal (CN IX), vagus (CN X), and hypoglossal (CN XII).
- Cranial nerve I, which is responsible for olfaction, should be assessed in patients with head trauma, when pathology at the base of the skull is suspected, and in patients who exhibit an altered mental status.
- Each eye should be evaluated individually to assess the optic nerve. These tests should include evaluation of visual acuity, visual fields, pupillary response, and the fundi.
- The CCTP should closely observe two parameters to assess the oculomotor, trochlear, and abducens nerves: the position of the eyeball and the position of the upper eyelid.
- To test the motor portion of the facial nerve, the CCTP should instruct the patient to wrinkle the forehead, close the eyelids tightly, smile or grimace to show the teeth, and whistle.
- Rotational and caloric stimuli are used to assess the vestibular division of the acoustic nerve. The CCTP performs this evaluation

Prep Kit Continued

to determine the brainstem function of unconscious patients.

- To test the glossopharyngeal and vagus nerves, the CCTP should direct the patient to open their mouth and say, "Ah," then should stimulate the gag reflex with the tongue blade.
- To assess the hypoglossal nerve, the CCTP observes the tongue for fasciculations and atrophy, tests for muscle strength by having the patient push the tongue against the inside wall of the cheek, and checks for deviation with tongue protrusion.
- The motor examination focuses on muscle tone and strength, as the CCTP puts the muscles through the normal range of motion.
- As part of the assessment of sensory function, the CCTP should examine and document pain, temperature, and touch.
- The most common pathologic reflexes, all of which indicate pyramidal tract disease, include the plantar response, Babinski sign (the most important), Oppenheim sign, Gordon sign, and Hoffmann sign.
- Signs of meningeal irritation include generalized throbbing headache progressing in severity, progressive photophobia, and nuchal rigidity.
- The presence of the Lhermitte phenomenon, in which forward flexion of the neck produces an electric shock feeling, indicates cervical pathology.
- The centers for control of vital functions are found within the brainstem, so changes in vital signs can signal changes in the patient's overall neurologic status.
- The CCTP should repeatedly check the following physiologic variables: BP, heart rate and rhythm, respiratory rate, pulse oximetry, end-tidal carbon dioxide, central venous pressure, temperature, and ICP.
- Hypertension is the effect on BP most often seen as a result of neurologic injury, especially in case of increased ICP.
- Alterations in body temperature—hypothermia or hyperthermia—are possible in the

presence of neurologic injury, especially if the hypothalamus is damaged.

- Neurologic diagnostics with which the CCTP should be familiar include computed tomography, computed tomography angiography, magnetic resonance imaging, cerebral angiography, transcranial Doppler ultrasonography, electroencephalography, and lumbar puncture.
- Laboratory studies, other than routine blood studies, biopsy, and CSF analysis, are not routinely used in the diagnosis and management of neurologic emergencies.
- Two types of TBI are distinguished: primary (direct) injury, in which traumatic forces cause physical or functional disruption of brain tissue; and secondary (indirect) processes, which occur after the initial injury and lead to brain dysfunction or cellular damage (eg, hypoxia and ischemia).
- Primary brain injury can occur as a result of two mechanisms: contact phenomena injuries (direct trauma to the head) and acceleration-deceleration injuries (sudden changes in velocity).
- Secondary injury involves more delayed mechanisms of brain damage; if left uncorrected, it will adversely affect brain function integrity.
- Cerebral perfusion pressure (CPP) is the primary determinant of blood flow to injured brain tissue when an injury has impaired the ability of the cerebral circulation to autoregulate in response to fluctuations in systemic BP.
- Common injuries to the scalp include abrasions, contusions, lacerations, and avulsions. Treatment usually focuses on controlling bleeding, cleaning and dressing the area, and, in case of avulsions, evaluating for fractures.
- Skull fractures result from a direct, and often high-force, blow to the cranium; they are present in more than 50% of patients with a severe TBI.

Prep Kit Continued

- To perform the halo test for leaking CSF, collect escaping fluid from the nose, mouth, or ears onto a gauze pad. The appearance of a target or halo symbol, consisting of a dark red circle surrounded by a lighter yellow one, is considered a positive halo sign. This sign should be interpreted with caution, as it has poor sensitivity and specificity.
- Raccoon eyes (periorbital ecchymosis) and Battle sign (retroauricular ecchymosis) may not appear until several hours after a head injury.
- Fractures of the bones of the face may indicate possible underlying brain injury.
- Many facial injuries have very grotesque presentations accompanied by copious bleeding and may potentially distract the CCTP from other, more serious injuries.
- Mandible fractures can cause life-threatening airway compromise if the patient is in the supine position.
- Airway control is the first assessment priority for patients with facial injuries. After securing the airway, the CCTP can assess for the presence of facial fractures by grasping the hard palate and rocking it back and forth. The CCTP should also check for malocclusion and dental trauma, test extraocular muscles to rule out orbital fractures, and look for facial elongation and periorbital ecchymosis.
- Injuries to the brain can be either focal (lesions large enough to be observed directly) or diffuse (eg, concussions and diffuse axonal injuries).
- Treatment for patients with cerebral contusions and lacerations is largely supportive. It includes monitoring for—and aggressively treating—evidence of rising ICP resulting from hematoma formation.
- An epidural hematoma is an accumulation of blood between the inner periosteum and the dura mater as the result of an injury. The patient with an EDH may present with a history of a brief period of unconsciousness, followed by a lucid period lasting for minutes to several hours, which ends with a rapid deterioration of

consciousness from drowsiness, to lethargy, and to coma as a mass effect and herniation develop.
- Mannitol is an osmotic diuretic that can reduce both the increased ICP resulting from an increase in CSF volume and intraocular pressure. It does not reduce the volume of blood that accumulates in the case of an EDH.
- High-energy impacts may result in a subdural hematoma—bleeding that accumulates between the dura mater and arachnoid mater. These injuries are six times more common than EDHs and have a higher mortality rate.
- Intracerebral hemorrhages often occur in the same areas as cerebral contusions. They produce headaches, deteriorating levels of consciousness, hemiplegia on the contralateral side, and dilated ipsilateral pupils.
- Signs and symptoms of mild TBI include loss of consciousness, loss of memory for events immediately before or after the event that precipitated the injury, altered mental status, and focal neurologic deficits.
- The clinical presentation of diffuse axonal injury includes a sequence of events beginning with immediate unconsciousness, leading to a longer period of confusion and associated posttraumatic amnesia, and followed by a protracted recovery time. Treatment for this condition is supportive.
- In adults, the normal ICP is 5 to 15 mm Hg. Increased ICP may be precipitated by intracranial bleeding, cerebral edema, mass formation, or inability to regulate the production and removal of CSF.
- Many physiologic factors may alter cerebral blood flow (CBF). Increases in CBF resulting from hypoxia or hypercapnia (increased levels of carbon dioxide in blood), for example, will cause an increase in ICP once the normal compensating mechanisms have been exhausted.
- Poor airway and ventilatory control contribute to hypoxia, hypercapnia, and hypotension, and will further damage the already critically ill brain.

Prep Kit Continued

- CPP is responsible for the movement of blood through the brain. The homeostatic mechanisms that manage CPP are often lost after head trauma, such that the patient with TBI may have increased cerebral vascular resistance; this phenomenon renders the brain more susceptible to changes in BP.
- CPP should be maintained between 70 and 90 mm Hg—by using fluids and pressors if necessary—to reduce the risk of poor outcomes for patients with increased ICP.
- Increased ICP is a sustained elevation in pressure above 20 mm Hg. The most common causes of increased ICP are cerebral bleeding, tumors, hydrocephalus, and trauma.
- Cushing triad is the combination of progressively increasing SBP (widening pulse pressure), abnormal respirations, and bradycardia.
- Respiratory changes noted with increased ICP include Cheyne-Stokes respirations (with midbrain involvement), sustained hyperventilation (with midbrain and pons involvement), and rapid and shallow respirations followed by ataxic breathing (with upper medulla involvement).
- Increased ICP produces pulmonary edema owing to the increased sympathetic activity resulting from the effects of this increased pressure on the hypothalamus, medulla, or cervical spinal cord.
- The primary goals of ICP monitoring are identification of ICP trends and evaluation of therapeutic interventions to minimize ischemia in the brain-injured patient.
- Contraindications to ICP monitoring include CNS infection, coagulation defects, anticoagulant therapy, scalp infection, severe midline shift resulting in ventricular displacement, and cerebral edema resulting in ventricular collapse.
- Potential complications of ICP monitoring include intracranial infection, intracerebral hemorrhage, air leakage into the ventricle or subarachnoid space, CSF leakage, over-drainage of CSF (leading to ventricular collapse and herniation), occlusion of the catheter with brain tissue or blood, and inappropriate therapy because of erroneous ICP readings.
- Noninvasive ICP monitoring involves assessment for clinical deterioration in neurologic status, evidenced by signs such as bradycardia, increased BP, and pupillary dilation.
- Intraventricular monitoring is one of the most popular techniques for invasive ICP monitoring. It is also therapeutic, as it provides the ability to drain CSF; the CCTP must monitor any fluid drained for amount, color, and clarity at hourly intervals.
- A subarachnoid screw (bolt) may be used to monitor ICP, although its accuracy is less than that of the more direct ventriculostomy drain.
- Interpretation of the ICP waveform provides the CCTP with real-time information that may provide clues about the patient's impending deterioration and allows for earlier targeted interventions.
- To minimize the risk that an infectious agent will enter the CNS during ICP monitoring, aseptic technique must be used at all times when assembling, manipulating, or accessing the fluid-filled monitoring system.
- To ensure optimal accuracy of ICP readings, proper leveling and zeroing of the ICP monitoring system must be maintained.
- Avoid flexion and hyperextension of the neck and positioning the patient in a Trendelenburg position when conducting ICP monitoring. Simultaneous drainage and pressure monitoring are not recommended.
- Notify the physician immediately if a patient with increased ICP shows signs of decompensation—altered LOC, restlessness, agitation, lethargy, confusion, motor weakness, seizures, alteration in breathing pattern, increases in BP, bradycardia, vomiting, decortication/decerebration, or coma.

Prep Kit Continued

- Patients with TBI should be intubated to protect the airway and allow maximal oxygenation. Standard monitoring for all such patients is required, including oxygen saturation, ECG, mean arterial pressure, and urine output.
- Normocapnia (normal carbon dioxide tension) is vital for maintaining ICP, and neurologic patients' ETCO$_2$ levels should be continuously measured using a capnometer.
- To perform brain tissue oxygen tension monitoring, a commercial probe (capable of measuring temperature and oxygenation) is placed into the brain tissue through a bolt. This type of monitoring is relatively sensitive for monitoring focal disruption of blood flow to particular areas of the brain.
- The best treatment for increased ICP is the removal of the causative lesion (eg, tumor, hydrocephalus, or hematoma). In the field, treatment aims at preventing the secondary events associated with increased ICP, by reducing ICP and providing rapid transport of the patient to a neurologic facility for definitive treatment.
- First-line management of increased ICP consists of general measures aimed at making the patient comfortable (including adequate analgesia), along with effective handling of the ABCs of trauma management.
- Second-line management of increased ICP involves induced cerebral vasoconstriction, which may take the form of hyperventilation, hyperbaric oxygen, or hypothermia. Osmotherapy consisting of mannitol, glycerol, urea, or furosemide may also be implemented.
- Anesthetic agents, including barbiturates, gamma-hydroxybutyrate, and etomidate, and paralytic agents may also be used in patients with increased ICP.
- Hyperventilation aims at keeping the PCO$_2$ between 30 and 35 mm Hg, so that CBF falls and CBV is reduced, thereby reducing ICP. Prophylactic hyperventilation is not recommended.
- Hyperbaric oxygen and hypothermia are experimental techniques to induce cerebral vasoconstriction and reduce CBV and ICP.
- Brain herniation is a condition in which a portion of the brain is displaced because of increased ICP, resulting in progressive harm to brain tissue that may include life-threatening damage to the brainstem. Transport management includes intubation, mechanical ventilation, administration of an osmotic diuretic (eg, mannitol) and possibly corticosteroids, and rapid transport.
- Acute injuries of the spine are classified according to the associated mechanism, location, and stability of the injury.
- Stable vertebral fractures do not involve the posterior column; therefore, they pose less risk to the spinal cord. Unstable injuries involve the posterior column of the spinal cord and carry a higher risk of complicating SCI and progression of injury without appropriate treatment.
- Flexion injuries result from forward movement of the head, typically as the result of rapid deceleration (eg, in a car crash), or from a direct blow to the occiput. Rotation-flexion injuries, which often result from high acceleration forces, can produce a stable dislocation in the cervical spine. Hyperextension of the head and neck can result in fractures and ligamentous injuries of variable stability.
- Vertical compression injuries typically result from a direct blow to the crown (parietal region) of the skull or rapid deceleration from a fall through the feet, legs, and pelvis. In these injuries, forces transmitted through the vertebral body ultimately shatter the vertebral body and produce a "burst" or compression fracture with or without associated SCI; patients may also develop herniation of disks, subsequent compression of the spinal cord and nerve roots, and fragmentation into the canal.
- Primary SCI—injury that occurs at the moment of impact—can involve either

Prep Kit Continued

penetrating or blunt trauma. Penetrating trauma typically results in transection of nonregenerative neural elements and complete injuries; blunt trauma may displace ligaments and bone fragments, resulting in compression of points of the spinal cord or an incomplete dislocation of the vertebral body. Spinal cord concussion, spinal cord contusion, and cord laceration are all types of primary SCI.

- Secondary SCI occurs when multiple factors permit a progression of the primary SCI and result in further deterioration. Exposing neural elements to further hypoxemia, hypoglycemia, and hypothermia can exacerbate these effects.
- The CCTP should minimize the chance of secondary SCI through stabilization (ie, spinal motion restriction and neutral alignment). Minimizing heat loss and maintaining oxygenation and perfusion are other key elements in the care of a patient with a possible SCI.
- The degree of SCI—that is, complete versus incomplete—is best determined 24 hours after the initial injury; the initial dysfunction may be temporary, and there may be some potential for recovery.
- Spinal shock is a temporary local neurologic condition that occurs immediately after spinal trauma and involves reflex arc dysfunction; neurogenic shock results from the temporary loss of autonomic function, which controls cardiovascular function, at the level of injury.
- A patient with SCI should be treated as having a true neurologic emergency, and the CCTP should make every effort to rapidly assess, treat, and transport the patient to the closest appropriate facility while maintaining in-line stabilization of the vertebral column.
- Short-acting, reversible sedatives are recommended for the acute, agitated patient after a correctable cause of the agitation (eg, hypoxia) has been excluded.

- Acute-phase complications of SCI include the potential for aspiration or respiratory arrest, especially in patients with high cervical injuries.
- Autonomic dysreflexia is evidenced by hypertension, headache, blurred vision, anxiety, cool clammy skin, and sweating above the injured site. Treatment consists of identifying and treating the cause (ie, repositioning the patient and checking the bladder and bowels for irritation or obstructions) and reducing the BP with a beta blocker.
- Stroke occurs when blood flow to the brain is disrupted, resulting in a neurologic deficit persisting for more than 24 hours. When deficits completely resolve within 24 hours, the event is referred to as a transient ischemic attack.
- Types of stroke include ischemic (caused by occlusion of a blood vessel by a thrombus or embolus), thrombotic (caused by accumulation of atherosclerotic plaques inside cerebral blood vessels that block blood flow), embolic (occurring when an embolus lodges in a smaller cerebral vessel), focal ischemic (caused by ongoing reduction of blood flow to already ischemic cells), and global ischemic (caused by severe hypotension or cardiac arrest that produces a transient drop in blood flow to all areas of the brain).
- The hallmark of stroke is the sudden onset of focal neurologic signs that oftentimes occur in combination.
- The CCTP can use abbreviated prehospital tools to identify patients suffering from stroke, such as the Cincinnati Prehospital Stroke Scale and the Los Angeles Prehospital Stroke Screen.
- Once stroke is suspected, the CCTP should determine the time of symptom onset or the last known well time.
- The CCTP should support the stroke patient's cardiopulmonary function, provide continuous monitoring of neurologic function, and maintain normal blood glucose levels.
- Frequent reassessment of airway and respiratory function is needed to avoid

Prep Kit Continued

hypoxemia in patients with stroke; supplemental oxygen may be given to hypoxemic patients.

- If a stroke patient's symptoms do not resolve, a CT scan shows no hemorrhage, and the symptom onset occurred within the last 4.5 hours, fibrinolytic therapy may be used to restore circulation to ischemic brain tissue. Providers must understand the role of tissue plasminogen activator, a thrombolytic agent, for patients who have experienced a stroke.
- Endovascular interventions are now the gold-standard reperfusion therapy for strokes caused by large-vessel occlusion.
- Given the prevalence of stroke and the time-sensitive nature of the most effective interventions, organized and coordinated stroke systems of care can improve patient outcomes.
- Intracerebral hemorrhage is bleeding directly into the cerebral tissue. The most common cause of spontaneous intracerebral hemorrhage is hypertension-induced vessel rupture. Symptoms include local neurologic dysfunction, severe headache, nausea, and vomiting. As the ICP continues to rise, the patient may lose consciousness and require ventilatory support. Intubation may be necessary, and orders may be given to reduce BP to decrease ongoing bleeding.
- The patient with a subarachnoid hemorrhage (typically caused by either an aneurysm or an arteriovenous malformation) characteristically has an abrupt onset of pain, sometimes accompanied by loss of consciousness, nausea, vomiting, focal neurologic deficits, photophobia, and nuchal rigidity. As the ICP increases, the patient may become comatose or die.
- Care for the patient with a subarachnoid hemorrhage includes measures to maintain

cardiopulmonary function, manage the airway, provide ventilatory support (if necessary), and limit movement of the patient's head.

- Guillain-Barré syndrome (GBS) comprises a group of immune-mediated polyneuropathies, all of which share a common constellation of features often provoked by an infection.
- Fever, glucose imbalance, electrolyte imbalances, head injuries, hemorrhagic strokes, and toxins can cause seizure activity.
- Epilepsy is a disorder characterized by recurrent seizures caused by abnormal discharges in the brain cells.
- Care for patients with seizure focuses on the ABCs and administration of an anticonvulsant, if the patient is actively seizing.
- Minimum requirements for monitoring patients with neurologic emergencies during transport are continuous ECG, pulse oximetry, and the intermittent measurement of BP, respiratory rate, and pulse rate.
- Other pieces of equipment that should be available—and working properly—to monitor the patient with neurologic emergency during transport include a cardiac monitor, a ventilator with waveform capnography, infusion pumps, an ICP monitor, and a cerebral function monitor.
- Apart from intracranial hemorrhage, the major early risks to the patient with head injury are hypoxia and hypotension. For this reason, management of the ABCs is always the first priority.
- The biggest challenge when transporting patients by aircraft is dealing with pressure variations and oxygen availability at increasing altitudes. Oxygen content in pressurized cabin air is less than that at normal ground level, so the CCTP must be prepared to administer supplemental oxygen to nonintubated patients.

Prep Kit Continued

Vital Vocabulary

afferent pathways Ascending pathways that carry sensory impulses toward the central nervous system.

aneurysm A weakened portion of the wall of an artery where the blood creates a localized dilation or bulge; it can involve the intact wall or be classified as dissecting, in which case the artery wall ruptures and blood pools between the inner and outer artery wall.

anterior cord syndrome Displacement of bony fragments into the anterior portion of the spinal cord, often as the result of flexion injuries or fractures, that disrupts blood flow in the anterior spinal artery.

aphasia Any loss or impairment of language function as a result of brain damage.

arachnoid mater The middle layer of the meninges, which contains blood vessels that give it the appearance of a spider web.

arteriovenous malformation (AVM) A cluster of abnormally formed blood vessels that have a higher rate of bleeding than average vessels.

autonomic dysreflexia A potentially life-threatening complication of spinal cord injury that results from the loss of parasympathetic stimulation. It is characterized by a massive, uninhibited, uncompensated cardiovascular response as the result of some stimulation of the sympathetic nervous system below the level of injury. Also called autonomic hyperreflexia.

axonal transport The movement of organelles and proteins along a nerve cell axon into and out of the cell body.

basal ganglia Masses of nuclei located deep in the cerebral hemispheres that play a major role in fine motor function.

basilar skull fracture A fracture along the base of the skull.

Battle sign Migration of blood to the mastoid region, posterior and slightly inferior to the ear, resulting in discoloration; also called retroauricular ecchymosis.

blood–brain barrier A network of endothelial cells and astrocytes (neuroglia) in the brain that regulates the transport of nutrients, ions, water, drugs, and waste products to and from the brain through the process of selective permeability.

brain herniation Displacement of a portion of the brain from its correct location within the cranial cavity to a different location.

brain tissue compliance The change in brain volume resulting from a change in pressure.

brain tissue oxygen tension ($P_{br}O_2$) A method of monitoring temperature and oxygenation via placement of a commercial probe into the brain tissue through a bolt; it can be done simultaneously with ICP monitoring placement.

Broca area Part of the frontal lobe that is located at the inferior frontal gyrus and that participates in the formulation of words.

Brown-Séquard syndrome Loss of function as a result of penetrating trauma accompanied by hemisection of the spinal cord and complete damage to all spinal tracts on the involved side; it is characterized by loss of motor function and sensation of light touch, proprioception, and vibration on the ipsilateral side and loss of temperature and pain sense on the contralateral side.

caloric test A method for assessing vestibular function that involves the raising and lowering of the temperature in the external auditory canal; also called Bárány test.

cauda equina The collection of individual nerve roots into which the spinal cord separates at the L2 vertebra.

central cord syndrome A syndrome in which cavities form in the central portions of the spinal cord, usually in the cervical area; it may be due to a tumor, a genetic mutation, or trauma. The

Prep Kit Continued

syndrome presents along with hemorrhage or edema to the central cervical segments.

cerebral angiography A procedure that uses imaging and a contrast material or dye to view and find abnormalities in the blood vessels in the brain.

cerebral aqueduct The narrowest portion of the brain's ventricular system; it provides communication with the fourth ventricle, which lies between the brainstem and the cerebellum.

cerebral blood flow (CBF) The amount of blood flow the brain requires to maintain homeostasis. In a 24-hour period, the brain requires 1,000 L of blood to obtain 71 L of oxygen and 100 g of glucose.

cerebral cortex The outermost layer of the cerebrum.

cerebral function analysis monitor (CFAM) A device that can provide summed, averaged, and analyzed outputs of the general state of brain activity.

cerebral function monitor (CFM) A device that can provide summed and averaged outputs, but not analysis, of the general state of brain activity.

cerebral hemispheres The name for each half of the brain (right or left); each of these areas contains one of the paired lobes (occipital, parietal, temporal, and frontal).

cerebral metabolic rate for oxygen ($CMRo_2$) A measurement used to determine neuronal demand for oxygen. Neurons with high activity rates require greater amounts of oxygen.

cerebral perfusion pressure (CPP) The pressure gradient across the brain; it provides an estimate of perfusion adequacy: CPP = MAP − ICP.

choroid plexus A cluster of nerve roots at the lateral and the third and fourth ventricles of the brain that produce cerebrospinal fluid.

circle of Willis A system of arteries located at the base of the skull that (in most people) is able to compensate for reduced blood flow from any one of the major contributors to cerebral circulation.

comminuted fracture A type of skull fracture in which the skull is splintered or shattered into many pieces.

complete spinal cord injury A complete disruption of all tracts of the spinal cord, with permanent loss of all cord-mediated functions below the level of transaction.

computed tomography (CT) A type of scan that provides a mathematically reconstructed view of multiple cross-sections of the body, including the brain; it should be performed on almost every patient with abnormal neurologic findings.

computed tomography angiography (CTA) A form of imaging that includes the injection of an IV contrast agent into the patient moments before CT scanning and results in improved imaging of arterial structures.

conjugate movement Movement of both eyes together in the same direction.

contact phenomena injuries Injuries that occur as the direct result of trauma to the head, including local effects such as scalp laceration, skull fracture, hematoma, and intracerebral hemorrhage.

contrecoup injury A situation in which an impact occurs on one side of the head, causing the brain to move within the cranial vault and forcibly contact the opposite side of the skull, resulting in damage on that side of the brain; also called transitional injury.

corpus callosum A large tract of transverse fibers that provides a communication link between the two cerebral hemispheres.

cranial nerves (CN) The 12 nerves arising directly from the brain that govern many of the senses and the functions of muscles in the eyes, face, and pharynx.

Cushing triad A cascade of events provoked when intracranial pressure rises to the level of the arterial pressure, vasoconstriction occurs in an effort to shift fluid volumes in the cranium, and the ensuing brain displacement puts pressure

Prep Kit Continued

on the medulla oblongata by pushing it into the foramen magnum, resulting in disturbances in breathing, heart rate, and blood pressure.

delayed traumatic intracranial hemorrhage (DTICH) Hemorrhage that occurs within the first 3 to 10 days following an injury to the occipital-parietal region via a coup-contrecoup mechanism.

depressed skull fracture A type of skull fracture in which a portion of the skull is depressed; the scalp and dura may or may not be torn.

diaphragma sellae An extension of the dura mater that forms a roof over the sella turcica, which contains the pituitary gland.

diastatic stellate fracture A fracture involving injury to a bone with separation of an epiphysis; it is prevalent in abused children.

diencephalon Portion of the cerebrum consisting of the thalamus, the hypothalamus, the subthalamus, and the epithalamus.

diffuse axonal injury (DAI) A deep-brain injury in which shearing forces damage the integrity of the axon at the node of Ranvier, which consequently alters the axoplasmic flow.

diplopia Double vision.

doll's eye test An oculocephalic reflex test that is performed on the unconscious patient by rapidly rotating the head from side to side and observing the eye movement.

dorsal Toward the back surface of an object; posterior.

dura mater The outer membrane of the meninges.

dural venous sinuses Endothelial-lined spaces between the periosteal and meningeal layers of the dura mater.

dysarthria Difficulty articulating words caused by neurologic impairment affecting the vocal apparatus.

dysconjugate movement Lack of symmetric movement between the two visual axes.

dysphonia Difficulty producing intelligible speech caused by physical impairment at the level of the larynx.

Edinger-Westphal nucleus Part of the midbrain that is responsible for mediating the autonomic reflex centers for pupillary accommodation to light.

efferent pathways Descending pathways that carry motor impulses away from the central nervous system.

electroencephalography (EEG) A procedure that records the electrical activity of the brain by measuring brain waves.

embolic stroke A condition in which a blood clot, known as an embolus, forms in one part of the body and travels through the bloodstream to the brain or neck.

epidural hematoma (EDH) An accumulation of blood between the inner periosteum and the dura mater; also called extradural hematoma.

epithalamus An area of the cerebrum that is located in the dorsal portion of the diencephalon and contains the pineal gland.

extinction A test of sensation discrimination in which the CCTP simultaneously touches opposite, corresponding areas of the patient's body and asks the patient where the touch is felt; it is intended to identify sensory inattention.

extradural space A potential space between the cranial bones and the periosteal layer of the dura that becomes a real space only when blood from torn vessels pushes the periosteum from the cranium and accumulates; also called epidural space.

falx cerebelli A fold of dura mater that forms the division between the two lateral lobes of the cerebellum.

falx cerebri A double fold of dura mater that divides the cerebrum into right and left hemispheres by descending vertically into the longitudinal fissure that extends from the frontal lobe to the occipital lobe.

Prep Kit Continued

Fick principle A method of indirectly determining cardiac output, in which the amount of oxygen uptake of blood as it passes through the lungs is equal to the oxygen concentration difference between mixed venous and arterial blood.

fissures Deep grooves between adjacent gyri of the brain.

flat fracture The least common type of depressed skull fracture, in which the depressed segment does not have any connection with the cranial vault.

flexion-extension injury A spinal cord injury that results from forward movement of the head, typically as the result of rapid deceleration, or from a direct blow to the occiput.

focal ischemic stroke A condition in which an area of marginally perfused tissue, the ischemic penumbra, surrounds a core of ischemic cells; the cells will eventually die without medical intervention.

foramen magnum The opening at the base of the skull through which the bundle of nerve fibers constituting the spinal cord exits.

foramen of Luschka An opening at the lateral portion of the base of the fourth ventricle that leads to the subarachnoid space and is essential for the normal flow of cerebrospinal fluid; part of the brain's ventricular system.

foramen of Magendie An opening at the medial portion of the base of the fourth ventricle that leads to the subarachnoid space and is essential for the normal flow of cerebrospinal fluid; part of the brain's ventricular system.

foramen of Monro An opening in the skull that connects the two lateral ventricles with the third ventricle, a central cavity; part of the brain's ventricular system.

Foster Kennedy syndrome A tumor or abscess at the base of the frontal lobe that affects the olfactory nerve.

frontal lobe The largest of the four lobes of the brain; it lies underneath the frontal bone of the skull and is separated posteriorly from the parietal lobe by the central fissure and inferiorly from the temporal lobe by the lateral fissure. The frontal lobe is responsible for a variety of cognitive and motor functions.

fundus The optic disk, macula, and blood vessels on the back wall of the internal eyeball.

global ischemic stroke A condition in which severe hypotension or cardiac arrest produces a transient drop in blood flow to all areas of the brain.

gyri Convolutions on the surface of the cerebrum that functionally increase the cortical surface area.

halo test A test for leaking CSF that is accomplished by collecting and assessing fluid that drains from the nose, mouth, or ears; a dark red circle of fluid surrounded by a lighter yellow one is a positive halo sign.

hemorrhagic conversion The condition in which, after the brain tissue surrounding the stroke has died, renewed blood flow to the region (eg, triggered by medication) is no longer held in place by the tissue, resulting in hemorrhage.

hemorrhagic stroke A condition in which bleeding in the intraparenchymal space or subarachnoid space causes direct or secondary damage to cerebral tissue.

hypothalamus An area of the cerebrum located below the thalamus that forms the floor and the anterior walls of the third ventricle. It is responsible for the maintenance of homeostasis and the implementation of behavioral patterns.

incomplete spinal cord injury A disruption of the tracts of the spinal cord in which the patient retains some degree of cord-mediated function.

internal capsule A massive bundle of efferent and afferent fibers connecting the various subdivisions of the brain and spinal cord.

intervertebral foramen A space in the middle of the vertebra that allows the exit of a peripheral nerve root and spinal vein as well as the entrance

Prep Kit Continued

of a spinal artery on both sides at each vertebral junction.

intracerebral hemorrhage Direct bleeding into the brain parenchyma.

intracranial pressure (ICP) The pressure exerted by brain tissue, intracranial vascular contents, and cerebrospinal fluid in the closed, nondistensible cranial cavity.

intracranial temperature (ICT) Core brain temperature or homeostatic mean gradient temperature of 101.1°F (38.4°C).

involuntary (autonomic) nervous system The sympathetic and parasympathetic branches of the nervous system, whose fibers connect the structures of the CNS with smooth muscle, cardiac muscle, and glands.

ischemic stroke A condition in which an artery to the brain becomes blocked by a thrombus, embolus, trauma, or vasospasm (often due to drugs).

jugular venous bulb oximetry A technique in which a sampling catheter is placed in the internal jugular vein and directed upward so that its tip rests in the jugular venous bulb at the base of the brain; samples of blood can then be drawn to measure mixed venous oxygen saturation (Svo_2).

Le Fort criteria A categorization of facial fractures involving the maxilla in which the fractures are differentiated based on the location of fracture lines and the extent of mobility of facial structures on physical examination.

Lhermitte phenomenon A condition in which forward flexion of the neck produces an electric shock feeling, usually running down the back.

limbic lobe Part of the temporal lobe that is the seat of emotions and instincts; also called the rhinencephalon.

linear skull fracture A type of skull fracture characterized by a single fracture line.

linear stellate fracture A fracture with multiple linear fractures radiating from the site of impact.

lumbar puncture A procedure in which a needle is inserted first into the lumbar portion of the back and then into the subarachnoid space to obtain spinal fluid for testing or to administer drugs.

magnetic resonance imaging (MRI) A noninvasive procedure that obtains computer images of internal organs and the body through the use of radiofrequency pulses and a magnetic field.

mean arterial pressure (MAP) The mean between the systolic and diastolic blood pressures (SBP and DBP): MAP = DBP + (SBP − DBP).

medulla oblongata The lowermost portion of the brainstem.

midbrain A small area of the brainstem extending between the diencephalon, the pons, and the third ventricle.

mild TBI Concussion; a traumatically induced physiologic disruption of brain function that occurs without structural damage.

Mini-Mental State Examination A simple, easily applied test of higher cognitive functions.

mixed venous oxygen saturation (Svo_2) A measurement of the oxygenation of blood leaving the brain, which is normally in the range of 50% to 75%.

Monro-Kellie doctrine A theory developed by two Scottish anatomists, who stated that the central nervous system is enclosed in a rigid compartment along with cerebrospinal fluid, whose total volume tends to remain constant; an increase in any component—whether brain, blood, or CSF—will cause an increase in pressure and decrease the volume of one of the other elements.

motor area Part of the frontal lobe containing pyramidal cells that control voluntary motor function on the opposite side of the body.

neurocranium The part of the skull that encloses and protects the brain.

neurogenic shock A temporary loss of autonomic function, which controls cardiovascular function, at the level of a spinal cord injury; it is

Prep Kit Continued

characterized by marked hemodynamic and systemic effects.

normal-pressure hydrocephalus (NPH) An accumulation of CSF that causes the ventricles of the brain to enlarge. The enlarged ventricles of a patient with this condition may not cause increased intracranial pressure.

nuchal rigidity Marked resistance to head movement in any direction that is suggestive of meningeal irritation.

occipital lobe The lobe of the brain that occupies the most posterior portion of the cerebrum; it is the primary receptive area for vision, specifically the interpretation of visual stimuli.

optic disk The most prominent structure visible in the eye; it represents the termination of the optic nerve.

oxygen extraction fraction (OEF) The fraction of oxygen extracted from the blood as it passes by to maintain normal oxygen delivery and, consequently, normal brain functions.

parietal lobe The lobe of the brain situated directly posterior to the frontal lobe on the other side of the central fissure; it is largely responsible for sensory functions.

pia mater The innermost layer of the meninges, which rests directly on the brain or spinal cord.

ping-pong ball fracture A pediatric greenstick fracture of the skull.

plexus A cluster of nerve roots that permits peripheral nerve roots to function as a group.

pons Part of the brainstem located between the midbrain and the medulla oblongata; it relays information to and from the brain and spinal cord along fiber tracts.

posterior cord syndrome Extension injury that produces dysfunction of the dorsal columns, presenting as decreased sensation to light touch, proprioception, and vibration.

prefrontal area Part of the frontal lobe that provides control of thought, concentration, depth and ability to think abstractly, memory, and autonomic nervous system response, concomitant to emotional change.

premotor area Part of the frontal lobe that is adjacent to the motor area and helps coordinate certain movements.

primary spinal cord injury Spinal cord injury that occurs at the moment of impact.

proprioception The ability to perceive the position and movement of one's own body or limbs.

ptosis Drooping of an eyelid.

raccoon eyes Orbital fractures and hemorrhage into the surrounding tissue; also called periorbital ecchymosis.

reticular activating system (RAS) A diffuse system that extends from the lower brainstem to the cerebral cortex; it controls the sleep-wakefulness cycle, consciousness, the ability to direct attention to a specific task, and the perception of sensory input that might alter behavior.

reticular formation (RF) A set of neurons that extends from the upper level of the spinal cord; through the medulla, pons, and midbrain; and into the thalamus and cerebral cortex. It has both excitatory and some inhibitory capabilities, and can enhance, suppress, or modify impulse transmission.

rotation-flexion injury A spinal cord injury to C1-C2, the only area of the spine that allows for significant rotation, in which rotation with abrupt flexion produces a stable dislocation in the cervical spine. In the thoracolumbar spine, rotation-flexion forces typically cause fracture rather than dislocation.

rotational force An injury-producing force in which the head moves around its center of gravity.

rubrospinal tract Part of the midbrain that controls the tone of flexor muscles.

secondary spinal cord injury Spinal cord injury in which multiple factors permit a progression of the primary spinal cord injury; the ensuing cascade of inflammatory responses may result in further deterioration.

Prep Kit Continued

spinal shock The temporary local neurologic condition that occurs immediately after spinal trauma; it is characterized by swelling and edema of the spinal cord and can lead to a physiologic transection, mechanically disrupting all nerve conduction distal to the injury.

stereognosis The ability to sense an object's form through touch.

stroke A disruption of blood flow to the brain that results in a neurologic deficit persisting for more than 24 hours.

subarachnoid hemorrhage (SAH) Bleeding between the arachnoid mater and the dura mater.

subdural hematoma (SDH) Bleeding that accumulates between the dura mater and the arachnoid mater.

subdural space The dura-arachnoid junction; this potential space may develop into a real one if a blow to the head causes a loss of blood into the cranial meninges.

subthalamus An area of the cerebrum that is located below the thalamus and is closely related to the basal ganglia in function.

sulci Grooves between adjacent gyri.

tectospinal tract Part of the midbrain that controls reflex motor movements in response to visual and auditory stimuli.

temporal lobe The lobe of the brain that is located beneath the temporal bone of the cranium; its primary functions relate to hearing, speech, behavior, and memory.

tentorium cerebelli A fold of the dura mater that separates the occipital lobes of the cerebrum from the cerebellum and brainstem, thereby dividing the brain into upper and lower compartments.

thalamus The largest portion of the diencephalons. It acts as a relay station for motor and sensory activity; basic neuronal activity; and memory, thought, emotion, and complex behavior.

thrombotic stroke A condition that occurs when the blood supply to part of the brain is disrupted by a thrombus, or blood clot.

transcranial Doppler (TCD) ultrasonography A noninvasive method of assessing the state of intracranial perfusion and monitoring of cerebral blood flow velocity through thinner areas of the skull. It is used in patients following rupture of an intracranial aneurysm to assess for vasospasm, to identify intracranial lesions following a stroke, and to detect cerebral blood flow changes associated with increased ICP.

transient ischemic attack (TIA) A temporary disruption in the blood flow to the brain that lasts less than 24 hours and has temporary side effects.

translational force An injury-producing force in which the head's center of gravity moves along a linear path.

true fracture The most common type of closed skull fracture, in which the depressed segment has contact with the cranial vault.

two-point discrimination A test of sensation discrimination that measures the shortest distance at which the sides of two separate points of a compass or calipers can be distinguished from each other.

uncal herniation The most common type of brain herniation, in which a portion of the temporal lobe is displaced, resulting in compression of cranial nerve III, the midbrain, and the posterior cerebral artery.

uncus The medially curved anterior part of the hippocampal gyrus.

ventral Toward the abdomen; anterior.

vertebral body The anterior weight-bearing structure within the spine.

vertical compression Forces transmitted through vertebral bodies and directed either inferiorly through the skull or superiorly through the pelvis or feet (eg, from a direct blow to the parietal region of the skull or rapid deceleration from a fall through the feet, legs, and pelvis).

viscerocranium The bones making up the facial skeleton.

Prep Kit Continued

voluntary (somatic) nervous system The nervous system fibers that connect the structures of the CNS with skeletal muscles and the integument.

Wernicke area Part of the temporal lobe that is responsible for comprehension of both written and spoken words.

References

Adeoye O, Nyström KV, Yavagal DR, et al. Recommendations for the establishment of stroke systems of care: a 2019 update; a policy statement from the American Stroke Association. *Stroke*. 2019;50:e187-e210. doi: 10.1161/STR.0000000000000173.

Berkhemer OA, Fransen PS, Beumer D, et al. A randomized trial of intraarterial treatment for acute ischemic stroke. *N Engl J Med*. 2015;372(1):11-20.

Blei AT, Olafsson S, Webster S, et al. Complications of intracranial pressure monitoring in fulminant hepatic failure. *Lancet*. 1993;341(8838):157-158.

Brain Trauma Foundation, American Association of Neurological Surgeons, Congress of Neurological Surgeons, et al. Guidelines for the management of severe traumatic brain injury. *J Neurotrauma*. 2007;24(suppl 1):S59.

Campbell BCV, Mitchell PJ, Kleinig TJ, et al. Endovascular therapy for ischemic stroke with perfusion-imaging selection. *N Engl J Med*. 2015;372:1009-1018.

Fuller G. *Neurological Examination Made Easy*. 5th ed. Edinburgh, UK: Churchill Livingstone; 2013.

Goyal M, Menon BK, van Zwam WH, et al. Endovascular thrombectomy after large-vessel ischaemic stroke: a meta-analysis of individual patient data from five randomised trials. *Lancet*. 2016;387(10029):1723-1731.

Kinney MR, Brooks-Brunn JA, Molter N, et al. *AACN Clinical Reference for Critical Care Nursing*. St. Louis, MO: Mosby; 1999.

Kirkness CJ, Mitchel PH, Burr RL, et al. Intracranial pressure waveform analysis: clinical and research complications. *J Neurosci Nurs*. 2000;32(5):271-277.

Le Roux P. Intracranial pressure monitoring and management. In: Laskowitz D, Grant G, eds. *Translational Research in Traumatic Brain Injury*. Boca Raton, FL: CRC Press/Taylor and Francis Group; 2016.

Lynn-McHale Weigand DJ, ed. *AACN Procedure Manual for Critical Care*. 6th ed. St. Louis, MO: Elsevier; 2013.

McCance K, Huether S. *Pathophysiology: The Biologic Basis for Disease in Adults and Children*. 7th ed. St. Louis, MO: Elsevier Mosby; 2014.

McTaggart RA, Holodinsky JK, Ospel JM, et al. Leaving no large vessel occlusion stroke behind: reorganizing stroke systems of care to improve timely access to endovascular therapy. *Stroke*. 2020;51:1951-1960.

Mortazavi MM, Romeo AK, Deep A, et al. Hypertonic saline for treating raised intracranial pressure: literature review with meta-analysis. *J Neurosurg*. 2012;116(1):210-221.

Nag DS, Sahu S, Swain A, Kant S. Intracranial pressure monitoring: gold standard and recent innovations. *World J Clin Cases*. 2019;7(13):1535-1553.

Powers WJ, Rabinstein AA, Ackerson T, et al. Guidelines for the early management of patients with acute ischemic stroke: 2019 update to the 2018 guidelines for the early management of acute ischemic stroke: a guideline for healthcare professionals from the American Heart Association/American Stroke Association. *Stroke*. 2019;50(12):e344-e418. doi: 10.1161/STR.0000000000000211. [Published correction appears in *Stroke*. 2019;50(12):e440-e441.]

Rabinstein AA. Principles of neurointensive care. In: Daroff RB, Fenichel GM, Jankovic J, Mazziotta JC, eds. *Bradley's Neurology in Clinical Practice*. 6th ed. Philadelphia, PA: Saunders Elsevier; 2012.

Raboel PH, Bartek J Jr, Andresen M, Bellander BM, Romner B. Intracranial pressure monitoring: invasive versus non-invasive methods—a review. *Crit Care Res Pract*. 2012. doi: 10.1155/2012/950393.

Thompson HJ, Pinto-Martin J, Bullock MR. Neurogenic fever after traumatic brain injury: an epidemiological study. *J Neurol Neurosurg Psychiatry*. 2003;74:614-619.

Yang P, Zhang Y, Zhang L, et al. Endovascular thrombectomy with or without intravenous alteplase in acute stroke. *N Engl J Med*. 2020;382(21):1981-1993.

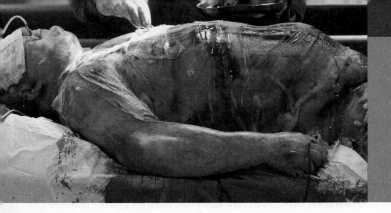

Chapter 13

Burns

Jeremy Lacocque, DO

OBJECTIVES

After completing this chapter, you will be able to:

1. Describe the layers and functions of the skin (pp 642–643).
2. List the major causes of burn injury (p 644).
3. Describe the anatomy of a burn (pp 644–645).
4. Explain the process of the body's systemic inflammatory response to a burn (p 645).
5. Explain the factors that determine the classification of burn injury, including body surface area and burn depth (p 646).
6. Describe the classifications of burn injuries, including superficial burns, partial-thickness burns, deep partial-thickness burns, full-thickness burns, subdermal burns, as well as major burns, moderate burns, and minor burns (p 645).
7. Identify the methods for calculating the total body surface area burned, including the rule of nines and the Lund-Browder chart (p 648).
8. Describe criteria for referral of patients to a burn center (pp 648–649).
9. Discuss assessment considerations for a burn patient's airway, breathing, and circulation (pp 649–652).
10. List situations in which the critical care transport professional (CCTP) should suspect an inhalation injury (pp 652–654).
11. Discuss the roles of edema and compartment syndrome in relation to a burn injury (pp 659–660).
12. Describe the process of stopping a burn, including irrigation, cooling, decontamination, and special considerations (p 652).
13. Discuss management of a burn patient's airway, breathing, and circulation (pp 652–655).
14. Explain various fluid resuscitation formulas, including the American Burn Association's *Advanced Life Support Course* 2018 guidelines and the Parkland formula (pp 654–655).
15. Describe the parameters for adjusting the fluid infusion rate (pp 654–655).
16. Describe how to manage and dress burn wounds (pp 655–656).
17. Discuss pain management of burn patients (p 657).
18. Discuss special situations relating to burn injuries, such as hypothermia, the need for gastric decompression, renal failure, and rhabdomyolysis (pp 657–658).
19. Discuss management of specific burns, including ocular burns, facial burns, ear burns, circumferential burns, hand and foot burns, genitalia burns, pediatric burns, electrical burns, and chemical burns (pp 658–665).
20. List the types of burns that may suggest potential child maltreatment (p 662).
21. Discuss toxic epidermal necrolysis and Stevens-Johnson syndrome, including the similarity between their management and the management of patients with severe burns (pp 665–666).

Introduction

According to the American Burn Association (ABA), approximately 1 million burn injuries occur each year in the United States, resulting in approximately 486,000 emergency department (ED) visits, 40,000 hospitalizations, and 3,275 fire- and burn-related deaths. The highest incidence of burns occurs (1) in the first few years of life and (2) between 20 and 29 years of age. Serious burns occur most often in males (71%), with the majority of these burns resulting from flame. Of patients who seek medical attention for burns, 85% utilize emergency medical services (EMS), suggesting that while burns account for a very small percentage of EMS responses, the majority of critically burned patients will be seen by field EMS providers.

Approximately 30,000 patients are admitted to specialized burn centers or burn units each year, with the majority of these patients requiring transfer to receive this specialized care. Burn centers are large facilities that admit more than 100 patients per year, whereas burn units are specialized facilities that have fewer than 100 admissions per year. In 2020, there were 132 burn centers in the United States, with an average of 200 admissions per facility per year. The average size of a burn injury that requires admission is 14% of total body surface area (TBSA). Approximately 4% of patients admitted to burn centers do not survive.

The principles of acute burn management taught in paramedic and nursing courses are the foundation for caring for these patients. However, the first 24 hours of care after a burn are crucial. Factors such as unrecognized injuries from associated trauma, complications of treatment such as fluid overload, and comorbidities such as diabetes or chronic obstructive pulmonary disease (COPD) may complicate care, and the condition of a patient who initially appears to be stable may worsen acutely. Given that complications of burns may develop during the transport of the patient to a burn facility, the critical care transport professional (CCTP) must ensure that adequate resuscitation and stabilization continue during transport. Knowledge of common complications and the timing of treatments are important for safe and effective transport to specialty care centers.

Anatomy and Function of the Skin

The skin is the largest organ of the body, and its function is as vital to survival as that of any other organ. A basic understanding of skin anatomy and function will help the CCTP understand burn treatment and potential complications. The skin is a multilayered structure, in which the epidermis and the dermis represent the principal components **FIGURE 13-1**. The epidermis and dermis are divided into additional levels that have specific functions.

The Epidermis

The epidermis generally consists of four layers (thin skin), except on the palms, fingertips, and soles of the feet, where it has five layers (thick skin). Each layer has a different composition. The layers of the epidermis, in order from deep to superficial, are the stratum basale, which is attached to the underlying dermis; the stratum spinosum (prickly layer); the stratum granulosum; the stratum lucidum (thick skin only); and most superficially, the stratum corneum.

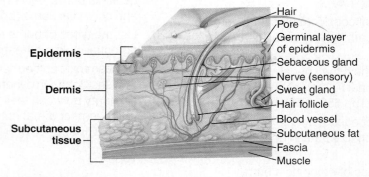

FIGURE 13-1 The skin has two principal layers: the epidermis and the dermis.

The epidermis contains pigment cells known as melanocytes, immune cells known as Langerhans cells, and a network of capillaries found in its lower layers. While the epidermis does contain some receptors for touch, the nerve receptors that transmit pain are actually located in the deeper dermis layer. The outer layer of the epidermis, the stratum corneum, provides a barrier to prevent water loss from deeper structures, and is constantly losing cells as a result of sloughing. It takes approximately 2 to 3 weeks for a cell to make its way from the lowest layer of the epidermis to become a keratinocyte and eventually be sloughed off. Because the epidermis serves as the first barrier to injury and infection, it is injured more often than other layers and is constantly repairing itself.

The Dermis

The **dermis** lies beneath the epidermis and is a dynamic layer of thick connective tissue that, like the epidermis, is in a state of constant turnover. The cell types found here are fibroblasts, macrophages, white blood cells, and the occasional mast cell. The dermis is also richly supplied with nerve fibers, blood vessels, and lymphatic vessels. The major portions of the hair follicles and the oil and sweat glands are also found in the dermis.

The dermis is divided into two layers: the papillary and reticular layers. The thin, superficial papillary layer is composed of connective tissue, which forms the anchoring system for the epidermis. It is also heavily invested with blood vessels and has the highest blood flow of all the dermal layers, which is important for temperature regulation. These blood vessels are found in nipple-like projections called dermal papillae that indent the overlying epidermis. The dermal papillae also house free nerve endings (pain receptors) and touch receptors.

The reticular layer accounts for 80% of the dermis. Its dense, irregular connective tissue is responsible for the durability of the skin and anchors skin appendages. Interlocking collagen fibers run through the reticular layer in various planes, usually parallel to the skin. Regions between these bundles form **lines of cleavage** in the skin **FIGURE 13-2**. These lines run longitudinally in the skin of the head and limbs and in a circular pattern around the neck and trunk. Understanding these anatomic features is important when considering where to make incisions for escharotomies and fasciotomies, because incisions made parallel to these lines cause the skin to gape less and heal more readily than incisions made across cleavage lines.

Collagen fibers give the skin both strength and resiliency against injury. Collagen also helps maintain hydration of the skin—an important concern after a major burn. Another concern is the adverse effect that burns have on the elastin fibers, which provide the stretch–recoil properties of the skin.

Deep in the dermis lies the hypodermis, which is composed of subcutaneous fat, connective tissue, sweat glands, muscle, and bone.

The Process of Healing

Proteins that are produced in the dermis, such as collagen and fibronectin, support the continuously reproducing epidermis and play a major role in wound healing. Multiple cell types are contained in the dermis when it is undamaged, but many more are attracted to the area when it is wounded.

Fibroblasts produce proteins such as collagen, fibronectin, and other substances responsible for skin repair. Macrophages are normally present in the tissues, but increase in number after an injury. They release chemical messages that help attract

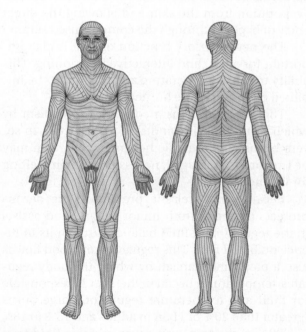

FIGURE 13-2 The skin's lines of cleavage. Incisions made parallel to these lines heal more easily than incisions made perpendicular to these lines.

© Jones & Bartlett Learning.

other cells to the wound site and orchestrate organized healing. Endothelial cells build capillaries and restore blood flow after an injury. Collectively, the fibroblasts, macrophages, platelets, and endothelial cells play a vital role in the wound healing process of the skin. Unfortunately, the inflammatory response that is responsible for burn healing may also create multiple complications, as discussed later in this chapter.

Functions of the Skin

The skin has multiple functions, including protective, immunologic, thermoregulation, maintenance of fluid and electrolyte balance, metabolic, neurosensory, and social functions. All of these capabilities are essential for the body's normal functioning, and any or all of them can be impaired in a burn injury. The degree of dysfunction is determined by the extent and depth of the burn.

The epidermis serves as a barrier that protects the body from desiccation (drying out) and maintains fluid balance by preventing excess loss of fluid through evaporation. An intact epidermis is also relatively effective at preventing the entry of toxins and bacteria. Burn injuries result in damage to the epidermis, increasing the risk of fluid loss through evaporation from the skin and allowing the direct entry of bacteria through the compromised skin.

The neurosensory function of skin is also important for social and interactive functioning. This ability to sense temperature and touch may be impaired or absent in the burned patient.

The skin maintains a complex mechanism by which wound healing and skin repair occur. In severe burns, this intrinsic healing mechanism may be irreparably damaged, necessitating skin grafting for wound closure.

Because of its elastic properties, the dermis protects the body from minor trauma and assists in the regulation of fluid balance through its influence on blood flow. This regulation of blood flow is also a major mechanism by which the body regulates temperature. Because the skin is responsible for fluid and temperature regulation, large burns (greater than 20% of TBSA in adults and 15% to 18% of TBSA in children) can cause massive fluid loss, shock, and hypothermia, even on a hot day.

Damaged skin is also more susceptible to pressure injuries such as pressure sores. Finally, the skin is

a sensory organ, so burns can cause intense pain and jeopardize the patient's ability to recognize touch.

Physiology of Burns
Causes of Burns

Burns can occur from a variety of mechanisms: flame/flash, scald (eg, water or grease), contact, electrical, chemical inhalation, radiation, or any thermal source. In addition, some medical conditions such as Stevens-Johnson syndrome and toxic epidermal necrolysis (TEN) syndrome cause burnlike injuries and are treated similarly to thermal burns. Regardless of the mechanism of injury, all burns share common features—the destruction of skin and an impairment of its ability to perform its functions.

The agent, temperature, and duration of exposure determine the size and depth of a burn. A thermal burn created by exposure to a heat source having a temperature greater than 113°F (45°C) can cause cell damage and denaturing of cellular proteins; the latter phenomenon eventually causes cell death. At temperatures of 120°F (48.9°C), an exposure for 5 minutes is enough to cause a full-thickness burn, and at temperatures greater than 159°F (70.6°C), it takes only 1 second to create a full-thickness burn in a healthy adult. These temperatures and times may vary when children and older adults are affected.

Anatomy of a Burn

The most heavily damaged area of a burn is referred to as the zone of coagulation; it is the area of skin that came into direct contact with the source of heat. In the zone of coagulation, the tissue is destroyed and clotting results in impairment of circulation to the surrounding tissues.

The surrounding areas of injury are referred to as the zone of stasis and the zone of erythema. The zone of stasis is characterized by injured tissue and stagnant blood flow resulting in ischemic tissues. It may appear red and hyperemic (filled with an increased amount of blood) initially, but within 24 hours after injury, blood flow will cease in the area and ischemia results. By the third day after the injury, the zone of stasis becomes white because of avascular necrosis.

The area surrounding the zone of stasis is the outermost area known as the zone of erythema owing to its increased blood flow. This area has sustained minimal damage and will recover from the injury.

Systemic Inflammatory Response of the Burned Patient

Although inflammation is necessary for the normal healing process to occur, excessive inflammation results in undesirable effects on other tissues and organs. Burns of greater than 20% of TBSA trigger a systemic inflammatory response, in which cells in the body migrate to the areas of injury to effect repairs. A blood-rich environment is necessary for these cells to function properly.

In larger areas of injury, the vascular endothelium becomes "leaky," allowing the "repairing" cells to make their way from the vasculature into the wound. When this process occurs at noninjured sites in the body, undesirable results may occur, including the following:

- Proteins may leak into subcutaneous tissues at uninjured sites, or the pressure at which proteins and fluids are exuded into the lungs may be lowered, making pulmonary edema more likely.
- The mediators can suppress the immune system.

- The leaky endothelial cells of the intestinal vasculature may allow bacteria normally found in the bowel to flow into the bloodstream (a process known as translocation), causing sepsis, even in the absence of a burn wound infection.
- Cardiac output may be impaired. Although the mechanism is unclear, myocardial contractility is suppressed after a significant burn injury.

Regardless of the cause, the inflammatory response from a burn injury, although necessary to promote burn healing, may result in untoward effects.

Classification of Burn Injuries

The severity of a burn depends on (1) the extent, depth, and location of the burn injury; (2) the age of the patient; (3) the etiologic agents involved; (4) the presence of inhalation injury; and (5) any coexisting injuries or preexisting illnesses.

Two classification systems for the depth of burns exist. The system describing first- through fourth-degree burns is widely known and used, but is less predictive of the need for surgical intervention than the simple partial- or full-thickness descriptions **TABLE 13-1**. Both systems are discussed here.

TABLE 13-1 Classification of Burns

Depth	Color and Vascularity	Surface Appearance and Pain	Swelling, Healing, and Scarring
Superficial (first degree)	Erythematous, pink and red	No blisters Dry and tender	Slight edema Heals easily without scarring
Superficial to partial thickness (second degree)	Erythematous, bright pink/red, mottled Blanches with brisk capillary refill	Intact blisters, moist when removed Weeping wounds and extremely painful	Moderate edema Easily heals but with skin discoloration
Deep to partial thickness (second degree)	Red, waxy-white Blanches with slow capillary refill	Broken blisters, wet Sensitive to pressure, but not to light touch	Marked edema Heals slowly with hypertrophic scars
Full thickness (third degree)	White, black to red/tan No blanching, vessels thrombosed Poor distal circulation	Dry, leathery Hairs pull out easily Anesthetic	Skin grafting required Scarring likely after healing
Subdermal (fourth degree)	Charred	Obvious subcutaneous tissue involvement Anesthetic	Skin grafting and/or flap required Scarring after healing

Burn Extent and Depth

A superficial burn, or first-degree burn, involves only the epidermis and is usually the result of ultraviolet light exposure (sunburn), very minor scald injury, or flash burn. The skin is hyperemic but not blistered with such a burn, and healing occurs without scarring in approximately 7 days.

A partial-thickness burn, or second-degree burn, is classified as superficial or deep. In a superficial partial-thickness burn (superficial second-degree burn), the epidermis and part of the dermis are involved, but the deeper layers of the dermis are spared, including the sweat glands, sebaceous glands, and hair follicles. These burns are typically caused by hot liquids or minimal contact with flame. Blisters form, and the injured skin is red and painful to touch. These burns do not typically require skin grafting unless they are extensive and occur on areas of the body with thin skin such as the face, hands, genitals, and feet. Superficial partial-thickness burns will heal in 14 to 21 days, and the extent of scarring depends on the extent of the burn. A deep partial-thickness burn (deep second-degree burn) is most often the result of steam, oil, or flames, and involves the deeper layers of the dermis. These burns may be difficult to distinguish from full-thickness burns. The skin is blistered but not charred and is painful to touch. Healing takes 21 days or more and may require surgical grafts. Scarring may be moderate and depends on the extent and location of the burn.

A full-thickness burn, or third-degree burn, involves the entire thickness of the dermis down to the subcutaneous fat. All epidermal and dermal structures, including nerve endings in the burned area, are destroyed, resulting in a pale, painless, leathery charred area of skin. Full-thickness burns will not heal spontaneously, and surgical skin grafting is necessary. These burns result in significant scarring.

A subdermal burn, or fourth-degree burn, involves the deep structures of muscle and bone, larger blood vessels, and nerves. These injuries are severe and life threatening. Like full-thickness burns, they will not heal spontaneously and require surgical intervention.

Superficial, partial-thickness, full-thickness, and subdermal burns are shown in **FIGURE 13-3**.

Burn Size

As stated previously, the depth of the burn is only one factor determining its severity; the size of the burn also informs this determination. Numerous methods are available to estimate the body surface area (BSA) involved in a burn. Regardless of the method used, accuracy improves with experience in applying that method.

The rule of nines is the most commonly used formula. It is based on the fact that large regions of the adult body can be divided into areas that represent roughly 9% of the total body surface area (TBSA), or multiples of 9% **FIGURE 13-4**. For infants and children, an amended rule is used that adjusts the rule of nines to account for the relatively large head and small lower extremities.

Special Populations

Fetal mortality is closely linked to maternal mortality when considering burn patients. Generally speaking, a pregnant patient with burns greater than 60% TBSA has a high rate of fetal mortality.

For patients with scattered irregular burns or small burns, the patient's hand may be used to estimate the burn area. In children and adults, the patient's hand represents 1% of the patient's TBSA.

Studies have shown that the Lund-Browder chart **FIGURE 13-5** is actually more accurate than the rule of nines for calculating the BSA burned. Consequently, it is the preferred method for estimating burn size in most burn centers. However, this chart is difficult to memorize, so the rule of nines remains the most commonly used method in the prehospital environment.

Burn Severity

The ABA classifies burns into three categories: major, moderate, and minor.

Major Burn Injury

Major burn injuries include the following:

- Burns involving 25% or more of TBSA in adults
- Burns involving 20% or more of TBSA in children younger than 10 years and adults older than 40 years

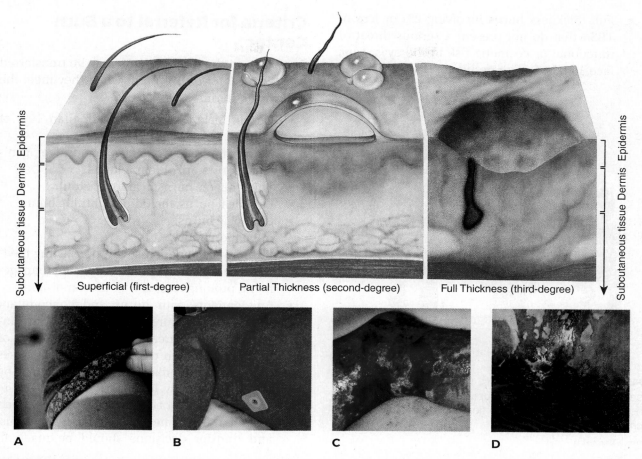

FIGURE 13-3 Classification of burns. **A.** Superficial (first-degree) burns involve only the epidermis. **B.** Partial-thickness (second-degree) burns involve some of the dermis but do not destroy the entire thickness of the skin. The skin is mottled, white to red, and often blistered. **C.** Full-thickness (third-degree) burns extend through all layers of the skin and may involve subcutaneous tissue and muscle. The skin is dry, leathery, and often white or charred. **D.** Subdermal (fourth-degree) burns involve deep structures such as muscle, bone, large blood vessels, and nerves.

© Jones & Bartlett Learning; **A:** © ITisha/Shutterstock; **B:** © E. M. Singletary, MD. Used with permission; **C:** © Mark C. Ide; **D:** © Charles Stewart, MD, EMDM, MPH.

- Full-thickness burns involving 10% or more of TBSA
- All burns involving the face, eyes, ears, hands, feet, or perineum that may result in functional or cosmetic impairment
- High-voltage electrical burns
- Burns complicated by inhalation injury or major trauma
- Burns sustained by high-risk or debilitated patients

Moderate Burn Injury

Moderate burn injuries include the following (note that this list excludes high-voltage injuries):

- Burns of 15% to 25% of TBSA in adults with less than 10% full-thickness injury

- Burns involving 10% to 20% of TBSA in children younger than 10 years and adults older than 40 years with less than 10% full-thickness injury
- Full-thickness burns involving 10% of TBSA or less in any patient younger than 50 years that do not present a threat to functional or cosmetic impairment of the eyes, ears, face, hands, feet, or perineum

Minor Burn Injury

Minor burn injuries include the following:

- Partial-thickness burns involving less than 15% of TBSA in adults
- Burns involving 10% of TBSA in children younger than 20 years and adults older than 50 years

- Full-thickness burns involving 2% or less of TBSA that do not present a serious threat of functional or cosmetic risk to the eyes, ears, face, hands, feet, or perineum

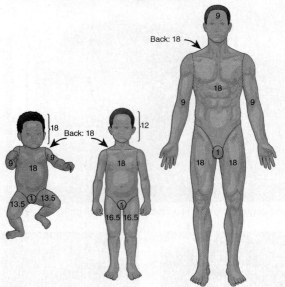

FIGURE 13-4 The rule of nines. The body is divided into sections, each representing approximately 9% of the total body surface area. The proportions differ for infants, children, and adults.

© Jones & Bartlett Learning.

Criteria for Referral to a Burn Center

According to the ABA, patients may be transferred to a burn center or burn unit when they meet the following criteria:

- Partial-thickness burns greater than 10% of TBSA.
- Burns that involve the face, hands, feet, genitalia, perineum, or major joints.
- Third-degree burns in any age group.
- Electrical burns, including lightning injury.
- Chemical burns.
- Inhalation injury.
- Burn injury in patients with preexisting medical disorders that could complicate management, prolong recovery, or affect mortality.
- Any patients with burns and concomitant trauma (eg, fractures) for whom the burn injury poses the greatest risk of morbidity or mortality. In such cases, if the trauma poses the greater immediate risk, the patient may be stabilized initially in a trauma center before being transferred to a burn center. Physician judgment will be necessary in such situations, and transfer decisions should be made in

Region	%
Head	
Neck	
Ant. trunk	
Post. trunk	
Right arm	
Left arm	
Buttocks	
Genitalia	
Right leg	
Left leg	
Total burn	

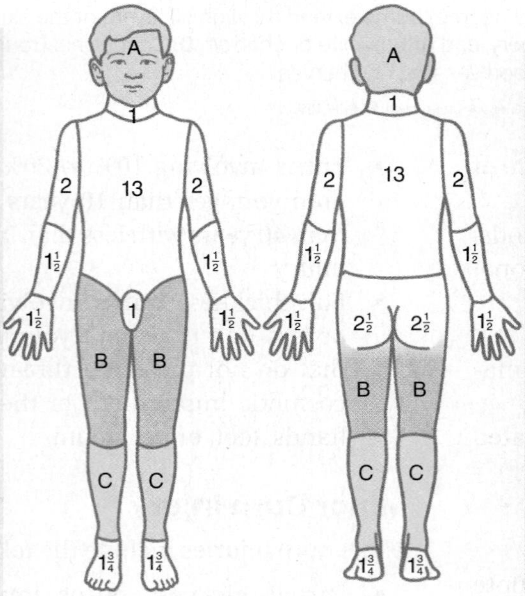

Relative percentages of body surface area affected by growth

Age (years)	A ($\frac{1}{2}$ of head)	B ($\frac{1}{2}$ of one thigh)	C ($\frac{1}{2}$ of one leg)
0	$9\frac{1}{2}$	$2\frac{3}{4}$	$2\frac{1}{2}$
1	$8\frac{1}{2}$	$3\frac{1}{4}$	$2\frac{1}{2}$
5	$6\frac{1}{2}$	4	$2\frac{3}{4}$
10	$5\frac{1}{2}$	$4\frac{1}{4}$	3
15	$4\frac{1}{2}$	$4\frac{1}{2}$	$3\frac{1}{4}$
Adult	$3\frac{1}{2}$	$4\frac{3}{4}$	3

FIGURE 13-5 The Lund-Browder chart.

Data from Lund CC, Browder NC. The estimation of areas of burns. *Surg Gynecol Obstet.* 1944;79:352-358.

concert with the regional medical control plan and triage protocols.

- Burned children in hospitals without qualified personnel or equipment for the care of children.
- Burn injury in patients who will require special social, emotional, or rehabilitative interventions.

Patients who meet these criteria or have a major burn injury should be transferred to a specialized burn center to ensure appropriate acute care, rehabilitation, and long-term care. Patients who meet the criteria for moderate burn injury should be hospitalized and consideration given to transferring care to a specialized burn center. Patients with minor burn injuries can usually be managed as outpatients.

Assessment

The CCTP should assess burn patients much as they would any other patient. Nevertheless, particular complications and findings associated with burns must be detected and the appropriate corrective actions taken to ensure the optimal outcome for the patient **FIGURE 13-6**.

A complete initial assessment and focused history and physical exam should be performed on patients with burns, always using caution whenever a cervical spine injury is suspected. Keep in mind that explosions may produce cervical spine injuries that may not be as obvious as the visible multiple burns. The CCTP should not rely on the history and examinations conducted by others because their level of training may not be equivalent to that of the CCTP. In addition, the patient's condition may have changed since the last physical exam.

As always during interfacility transfers, the CCTP should perform an initial evaluation of the patient for life-threatening conditions and then obtain a history from the patient and/or family members and a report from the nursing staff. To avoid an excessive delay in initiating the transfer, the CCTP should review the chart for the most relevant information. The CCTP can then fill in the remaining details by asking the patient, staff, or family. A focused history and physical exam of the patient should be

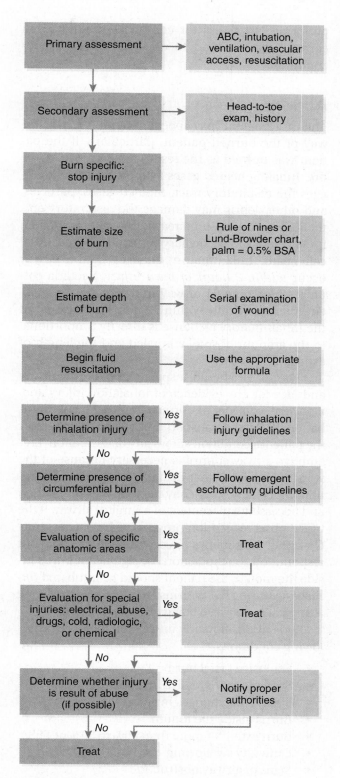

FIGURE 13-6 Algorithm for initial assessment of a burn injury.

Abbreviations: ABC, airway, breathing, and circulation; BSA, body surface area

© Jones & Bartlett Learning.

performed to assess for complications that need corrective action and to document the patient's condition.

Airway

The CCTP should pay special attention to the airway of the burned patient, particularly if the patient was burned as the result of a confined-space fire. Inhaling heated gases from combustion damages the respiratory tract. Inhaled gases, particles, and other debris may damage the respiratory epithelium, resulting in increased mucus production, impairment of mucociliary function, and eventual cell death. Inflammatory changes in the airway occur *within 2 hours of burn injury*. Bacteria colonize the damaged airway and infection is present microscopically within 72 hours. The extent of the inflammatory response is directly proportional to the amount of smoke inhaled and the length of exposure.

The CCTP should inspect the patient's airway and face for any evidence of inhalation injury and, if present, consider performing rapid sequence intubation (RSI) if the transport time will be prolonged or the patient's condition shows any deterioration. Preemptive airway control is necessary because of the worsening edema that occurs after fluid resuscitation, which may potentially cause airway obstruction and necessitate placement of a surgical airway. If the CCTP observes stridor, progressive hoarseness, any change in the patient's voice, wheezing that does not respond to bronchodilators, or significant burns inside the mouth, the patient should be intubated *immediately using RSI*, with instruments for performing a surgical airway also being readily accessible.

Indications for early intubation include the following conditions:

- Extensive facial burns
- Stridor or progressive hoarseness
- Significant changes in voice
- Burns inside the mouth
- Burn extent of more than 40% to 50% of TBSA
- Difficulty swallowing
- Signs of airway obstruction
- Use of accessory muscles
- Respiratory fatigue
- Poor oxygenation or poor ventilation
- Inability to handle secretions (need for frequent nasotracheal suctioning)

- Significant edema or risk for significant edema
- Mental status inadequate for airway protection

Singed nasal hairs alone are *not* an indication for intubation.

The CCTP should reevaluate the patient's airway frequently to assess for potential compromise due to edema. In addition, the airway should be secured in patients with an altered mental status or a Glasgow Coma Scale score of 8 or less after a major burn or any injury. If the patient is to be intubated for an elevated carboxyhemoglobin level, water should be used to fill the endotracheal tube cuff in preparation for hyperbaric therapy. However, it is often difficult for the CCTP to predict which patients will need hyperbaric oxygen, and an air-filled cuff can always be changed to water prior to initiating hyperbaric treatment.

If RSI is not within the scope of practice for CCTPs in your jurisdiction, note that attempted intubation in the setting of an inhalation injury is likely to result in worsened edema and potentially a failed airway. In this situation, the CCTP must perform a risk-benefit assessment of airway management without RSI. Consider delaying the transfer of the patient until someone skilled in airway management and capable of RSI can manage the airway.

Breathing

During the initial assessment, the CCTP should assess the patient's breathing rate and depth along with the breath sounds (also known as lung sounds). Even though noncardiogenic pulmonary edema may develop as a result of inhalation injury or fluid overload from aggressive fluid replacement, needed fluids should never be withheld. Start appropriate oxygen therapy immediately in the patient with major burns. Although COPD often raises concerns regarding oxygen therapy, high-flow oxygen should never be withheld from a hypoxic patient, and the CCTP should be prepared to assist with ventilation if needed.

Examination of the patient's chest should include a search for full-thickness circumferential burns, which may significantly impair ventilation by limiting expansion of the chest. A field escharotomy, a procedure in which an incision is made through the edematous burned skin to restore mobility to the chest or circulation to an extremity, is rarely, if ever, needed. Although it takes time for tissues to desiccate (dry out) and a constrictive eschar (the leathery covering of a burn injury) to develop, the CCTP will encounter burn patients at varying times after injury and an escharotomy may sometimes be necessary. For example, the CCTP may need to perform chest wall escharotomies in extreme cases with extended transport times. Emergent chest wall escharotomy may be performed (if the CCTP's scope of practice allows) to facilitate adequate movement of the chest wall.

If available, the CCTP should review the arterial blood gas levels as part of breathing assessment, paying particular attention to the oxygenation and carboxyhemoglobin levels. Treat wheezing with bronchodilators, as is standard practice. Another therapy to consider is delivery of humidified oxygen for inhalation injuries (in the absence of wheezing) using a nebulizer with normal saline only and no bronchodilators.

Burn patients may have experienced significant trauma from explosions or motor vehicle crashes (MVCs) resulting in fires. In such situations, it is easy to overlook conditions such as a pneumothorax or hemothorax while treating the obvious burn. Repeated patient examinations should be aimed at identifying these conditions.

Patients with carbon monoxide poisoning may present with symptoms of hypoxia, but without cyanosis. The classical teaching is that patients present with cherry red skin, although this condition may not be identified until postmortem. The CCTP should be aware of the limitations of pulse oximetry in the patient with carbon monoxide poisoning; it may not provide an accurate depiction of the patient's oxygenation status. Carbon monoxide poisoning is covered in Chapter 21, *Toxicologic Emergencies*.

Cyanide poisoning should be considered if the assessment of the burn patient reveals intense air hunger, metabolic acidosis, or sudden cardiovascular collapse and the patient has been the victim of a confined-space fire. Begin appropriate therapy such as hydroxocobalamin.

Circulation

Burn patients may have impaired cardiac output. This decreased cardiac output may stem from a variety of causes, including high levels of circulating inflammatory mediators, carbon monoxide poisoning, or cyanide poisoning. Assessment of the burned patient should include an evaluation of cardiac output, capillary refill, jugular vein distention, breath sounds, pulse rate, and blood pressure. Burn patients who have been victims of other trauma such as MVCs or explosions may have myocardial contusions, cardiac tamponade, or abdominal or solid-organ injuries.

Assessment of the patient's circulation should include evaluation of the extremities and digits for circumferential burns that have impaired circulation. Edema in the arms and legs may also impair circulation. Circumferential deep partial-thickness burns cause impairment of circulation because of their tough, leathery nature. Impaired circulation may result in an absence of pulses, delayed capillary refill, or mottling and discoloration of the extremity. Early identification of circulatory impairment in the extremities is crucial to preventing tissue necrosis and amputation. The CCTP should perform escharotomy on patients with circumferential burns and a lack of distal circulation if the local scope of practice allows.

In the arms and legs, edema may develop deep in compartments created by the tough nonelastic fascia surrounding and separating the muscles. This edema can compress the blood vessels and nerves, which impairs blood flow and sensation and results in compartment syndrome. The symptoms of compartment syndrome are collectively known as the five Ps: pain, pallor, paralysis, paresthesias, and pulselessness. The affected extremities may also be cold (poikilothermia, sometimes called the sixth P). Providers should be mindful that many of these signs are late findings in compartment syndrome. Pain, considered the hallmark of this condition, is an early sign. It is typically out of proportion to the injury or physical findings and may occur on passive stretching of the compartment. Nevertheless, compartment syndrome may be difficult to detect on this basis in burn patients, because burns are expected to be painful. To treat compartment syndrome, patients undergo fasciotomy, a surgical incision of the tough and fibrous fasciae that separate the compartments to relieve the pressure. Fasciotomies are typically not performed by prehospital providers and should be carried out only by properly trained personnel.

The assessment of a patient's circulation should also include determining the adequacy of fluid resuscitation. Fluid resuscitation in burn patients should be guided by formulas such as the ABA and Parkland formulas (discussed later in the chapter); however, in patients with significant comorbid conditions such as congestive heart failure or renal failure, the assessment of the patient's fluid status may play a greater role in guiding fluid replacement. Pulse rate, oxygen saturation, and breath sounds must all be considered in determining the patient's fluid balance. In patients with adequate renal function, the CCTP should monitor urine output closely to ensure an output of at least 50 mL/h (0.5 to 1.0 per kilogram of body weight per hour) for the adult. Pulse rate is not a good indicator of the adequacy of fluid resuscitation, as it may remain elevated because of pain and the release of catecholamines associated with burns. If myoglobinuria (an accumulation of myoglobin in the renal tubules) develops, give additional fluids to reach a urine output of at least 100 mL/h. Myoglobinuria should be suspected if the urine becomes dark, brown, or bloody.

Signs and Symptoms

Compartment Syndrome
- The five Ps: pain, pallor, paralysis, paresthesias, and pulselessness
- Possibly cold-affected extremities (poikilothermia)

Transport Management

Compartment Syndrome
- Keep the involved extremity elevated.
- Monitor pulses, sensation, and motor function.
- Do not place anything on the extremity that is compressive, such as splints or bandages.
- Monitor for increased pain (pain out of proportion is the hallmark of this syndrome).
- Provide supportive care (ie, maintain body temperature, analgesics, IV fluids, and appropriate oxygen).

Signs and Symptoms

Myoglobinuria
- Dark, brown, or bloody urine

Transport Management

Myoglobinuria
- Administer additional fluids so that urine output is at least 100 mL/h.

Management

The CCTP's management of burns includes many different areas of focus. **FIGURE 13-7** shows an algorithm for the management of a burn patient.

Stopping the Burn

Removing the patient from the source of the burn is an obvious first step. Cooling with irrigation to stop the burning process is appropriate but should last for no longer than 3 to 5 minutes. Studies of burn patients treated by EMS show a tendency toward overcooling, such that 42% of patients arrive at the hospital in a hypothermic state. Irrigation of a thermal burn older than 30 minutes provides little to no benefit. Copious irrigation is indicated for chemical burns but may also be beneficial if molten metals, synthetic materials, or tar adhere to the skin. Irrigation dissipates heat, so it should be continued until the burning has stopped and the material is cool **FIGURE 13-8**. In addition, cold inhibits lactate production and acidosis, thereby promoting catecholamine function and cardiovascular homeostasis in the wound.

All of the patient's clothing and jewelry should be removed because they may trap chemicals. Wet clothing may contribute to heat loss and cause hypothermia. After cooling or decontamination, keep the patient warm and place the patient in clean, dry linens prior to transport.

Airway and Breathing

Managing the burn patient's airway is a difficult challenge. Inhalation injury, cervical spine injury, circumferential chest burns, and poisoning from noxious fumes are all challenging scenarios. The CCTP must assess the patient for the possibility of inhalation injury and manage the airway with endotracheal intubation if stridor, progressive hoarseness, or any other evidence of airway compromise is present. Because inhalation injuries result in airway edema, the CCTP should anticipate a difficult airway and be prepared to perform a surgical airway

Immediate Care
• Stop the burning.
• Address the ABCs.
• Take cervical spine precautions.

Emergency Management
• Airway and breathing
  – Administer 100% oxygen.
  – Keep suction and a bag-mask device available
    to support ventilation.
  – Intubate early if an inhalation injury is
    suspected; assess for the following:
    • Injury in an enclosed space
    • Carbonaceous sputum
    • Soot in the mouth
    • Singed nasal hairs
    • Facial burns
    • Stridor, inability to clear secretions
    • Dyspnea, cough
    • Hypoxia
    • Voice changes, hoarse voice
    • Circumferential neck burns
  – Insert a nasogastric tube for intubated patients and
    those with greater than 20% body surface area burned.
• Circulation
  – Insert two large-bore IV catheters.
  – Determine fluid resuscitation requirements based on
    weight in kilograms and surface area burned and start
    fluids immediately; titrate to urine output.
  – Lactated Ringer solution is the preferred fluid but
    normal saline is an acceptable alternative.
  – Insert a Foley catheter.
• Wound care
  – Remove clothing and debris.
  – Cover burns with clean and dry sterile gauze or sheets.

Obtain Patient History
• How was the victim burned?
• Related injuries
• Medical and surgical history
• Current medications
• Allergies
• Drug, alcohol, and tobacco use

Consult Burn Center
• Pediatric fluid resuscitation
• Circumferential neck, chest, or extremity injury
• Dark pink or dark urine not clearing with IV fluids
• Decreased urine output not responding to IV fluids

FIGURE 13-7 Algorithm for the management of a burn injury.

Abbreviations: ABC, airway, breathing, and circulation; IV, intravenous

© Jones & Bartlett Learning.

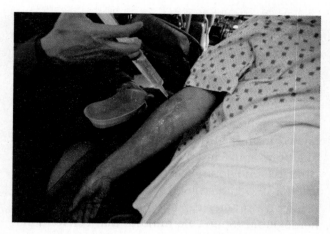

FIGURE 13-8 Management of burn injuries includes irrigation.

© Jones & Bartlett Learning.

(slowly). If the patient is hemodynamically unstable, the CCTP must judge whether sedation is appropriate or whether the risk of profound hypotension is too great to sedate the patient. Many RSI protocols incorporate drugs such as ketamine that increase, rather than lower, blood pressure.

Although succinylcholine is the drug of choice in RSI, it is contraindicated in patients with burn injuries greater than 72 hours old and in patients with known rhabdomyolysis secondary to their burn injuries because it may cause an extremely dangerous rise in potassium level. In these situations, a nondepolarizing agent such as vecuronium or rocuronium should be used instead. Because of the extended time of paralysis when these agents are administered, the CCTP should also carefully weigh the risk of being unable to intubate the patient against the benefits of intubation. Most often the benefits of intubation outweigh the risks associated with paralytic-assisted intubation with a nondepolarizing agent. The CCTP should also consider sedation-only assisted intubation (with a medication such as etomidate) or awake intubation as an alternative in a patient in whom the administration of succinylcholine is contraindicated.

Airway management in the burn patient can be difficult, if not impossible. Not only can airway edema make intubation difficult, but it can also preclude the introduction of airway devices selected for use with failed intubation. Most of these devices rely on the ability to ventilate the patient through an intact glottic opening, which may not be present in the burn patient with inhalation injury. For

intervention should endotracheal intubation fail. For patients who require endotracheal intubation, RSI should be performed per local protocol.

If the patient becomes apneic, develops significant respiratory depression, or experiences a drop in oxygen saturation or significantly elevated end-tidal carbon dioxide ($ETCO_2$) level at any point, the CCTP has no choice except to ventilate the patient

all these reasons, it is imperative that the CCTP be prepared to surgically manage the airway if orotracheal intubation fails.

Carbon monoxide poisoning, asphyxiation, and cyanide poisoning are major concerns in burn patients; indeed, most early fatalities are a result of carbon monoxide poisoning. Poisoning may be suspected from historical information such as report of a burn injury in an enclosed space. An elevated carboxyhemoglobin level may be diagnosed via an arterial or venous blood gas determination or by using an oximeter capable of measuring carboxyhemoglobin (Spco). Be mindful that conventional pulse oximetry cannot distinguish between carboxyhemoglobin and oxyhemoglobin, leading to significant inaccuracies in estimating oxygen saturation in the setting of elevated carboxyhemoglobin levels. Chapter 21, *Toxicologic Emergencies*, covers the treatment of carbon monoxide poisoning and cyanide poisoning.

Cyanide can be produced from the burning of any substance that contains carbon and nitrogen. Good supportive care in the absence of an antidote can save many cyanide poisoning victims. The treatment for cyanide poisoning is described in detail in Chapter 21, *Toxicologic Emergencies*.

If any of these conditions is suspected, the CCTP should treat the patient with 100% oxygen via nonrebreathing mask. In most burn patients, oxygen, preferably humidified, should be administered immediately.

Signs and Symptoms

Inhalation Injury

- Facial burns
- Stridor or progressive hoarseness
- Carbon deposits and acute inflammatory changes in the oropharynx
- Carbonaceous (black) sputum
- History of impaired mentation and/or confinement in a burning environment
- Explosion with burns to head and torso
- Circumferential neck burns
- Carboxyhemoglobin level greater than 10% if the patient is involved in a confined-space fire
- Soot around the nose and mouth
- Increased mucus production
- Impairment of mucociliary function

Transport Management

Inhalation Injury

- Consider performing early endotracheal intubation using RSI, especially if the transport time is prolonged; if the patient has stridor, progressive hoarseness, or any change in their voice; or for any deterioration in the patient's condition.
- Be prepared to perform surgical intervention should intubation fail.
- Consider administering humidified oxygen (in the absence of wheezing) using a nebulizer with normal saline only and no bronchodilators.

Circulation

In the past, the essentials of circulatory management included early, aggressive, sustained fluid management. This practice is no longer recommended. Judicious fluid management can avoid many of the complications resulting from hypervolemia, primarily those related to hemodilution and hypervolemia. Burns can result in large intravascular fluid losses as a result of the loss of the body's protection against desiccation and evaporation. In addition, circulating inflammatory mediators cause fluid from capillaries to leak into the interstitial space (ie, neither in the vasculature nor in the cell). The inflammatory process at the site of injury results in plasma "weeping" into the burned area. The larger the surface area involved, the greater the fluid loss.

Deep second-degree or larger burns can cause hypotension, so fluid resuscitation should begin within 60 minutes following such an injury. If possible, obtain IV access through unburned skin; however, access through burned skin is acceptable if necessary. Given the delays associated with obtaining access and the lack of early benefit from this intervention, the ABA no longer recommends the administration of prehospital fluids for burn patients whose transport times are less than 60 minutes.

Numerous formulas have been developed to determine the appropriate fluid resuscitation for the first 24 hours after a burn. The most commonly used is the ABA's *Advanced Life Support Course* 2018 guidelines, which recommend resuscitation during the first 24 hours following burn injury with lactated Ringer solution of 2 mL/kg per percentage of TBSA (partial- and full-thickness burns) for adults and 3 mL/kg for children age 14 years or younger and who weigh less than 88 pounds (40 kg). Half of the fluid should be administered over the first 8 hours, 25% should be given over the second 8 hours, and the remaining 25% should be infused over the third 8-hour period.

Urine output is used to monitor fluid status, with goals of 0.5 mL/kg/h output in adults, 1 mL/kg/h output in children weighing less than 88 pounds (40 kg), and 1 to 2 mL/kg/h in neonates. Lactated Ringer solution infusion rates should be increased or decreased by one-third if the urine output declines or increases by more than one-third of these target outputs for more than 2 consecutive hours. The urine output should also serve to guide the subsequent fluid replacement rates beyond the initial 24 hours after injury. If the patient's urine is dark brown or red, indicating it contains hemochromogens, titrate the fluids to maintain a urine output of 1.0 to 2.0 mL/kg/h in adults and 2 mL/kg/h in children, until the pigments have cleared and the urine is straw colored.

Controversies

As mentioned previously, the ABA no longer recommends IV fluids in the prehospital environment if transport times are less than 60 minutes. When arrival time at an ED is expected to exceed 60 minutes from the time of burn injury, administer lactated Ringer solution at 500 mL/h for patients age 14 years and older, 250 mL/h for patients ages 6 to 13 years, and 125 mL/h for children age 5 years or younger.

Traditionally, the most commonly used fluid resuscitation method relied on the Parkland formula, which recommends resuscitation with lactated Ringer solution (normal saline is an acceptable substitute) of 4 mL/kg per percentage of BSA burned; half of this amount should be given over the first 8 hours (from the time of injury), one-fourth of the total amount should be given over the second 8 hours, and one-fourth of the total amount should be given over the third 8 hours. All calculations are determined from the time of the injury, so fluid boluses may be necessary to correct deficits in fluid resuscitation because of either a delay in presentation or under-resuscitation. It may also be necessary to administer fluids more aggressively if the patient is in shock and has unstable vital signs. The goal for

all fluid replacement is to maintain a urine output of 0.5 to 1.0 mL/kg/h.

The formulas used to calculate a burn patient's fluid requirements should serve only as a guide. Monitoring the patient's overall perfusion status, mental status, urine output, and breath sounds is essential. If the patient is too aggressively hydrated, pulmonary or cerebral edema may result. If the patient is not adequately resuscitated, inadequate perfusion of the kidneys or mesentery may worsen organ system damage.

Burn centers often want to participate in the calculation of fluid requirements for children. Ideally, the CCTP should know the preference of the receiving facility or contact it prior to transport to discuss fluid resuscitation strategies. When assuming responsibility for a patient, the CCTP should check all fluids and infusion rates to confirm that they are appropriate, inventory the fluids given already, and reconcile urine output since injury. It is a good idea for the CCTP to empty the indwelling urinary catheter bag when assuming care of any patient to allow for accurate measurement of urine output during transport **FIGURE 13-9**.

Wound Management and Dressings

Wound management is critical, especially when burn injury compromises the skin's ability to act as a barrier to infection and a regulator of the body's temperature. Proper dressings help reduce infection, decrease pain, and prevent heat loss.

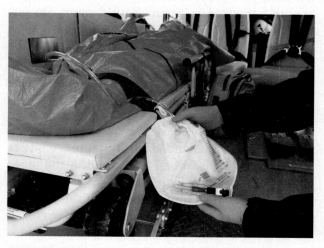

FIGURE 13-9 Empty the indwelling urinary catheter bag when you assume care of any patient to allow for accurate measurement of urine output during transport.

© Jones & Bartlett Learning.

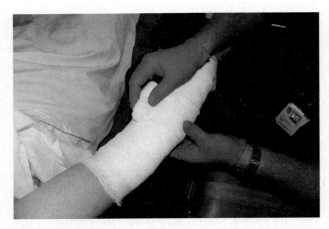

FIGURE 13-10 Dress wounds with dry, clean dressings. Do not use wet dressings.

© Jones & Bartlett Learning.

After cooling, irrigating, and decontaminating, the wounds should be dried and dressed with *dry*, clean dressings **FIGURE 13-10**. A common mistake when caring for burn patients is using wet dressings, which contribute to heat loss and are ineffective barriers to infection. Bulky dressings may be used to pad pressure points and sensitive areas. No ointments or creams are necessary, but if wounds are already dressed with ointments or creams, they may be left in place. All wounds should be examined to confirm that the BSA and the fluid resuscitation calculation are accurate.

Wounds must generally be debrided to remove dead skin, which can serve as a source for infection and prevent healthy tissue from repairing the burned area. Wound debridement consists of removing any dead or nonviable tissue from the wound. The debridement of most wounds will be performed at the receiving burn unit. As a general rule, the CCTP should not perform this intervention except in the setting of chemical exposure and blisters formed by chemical agents.

The treatment of blisters is somewhat controversial. On the one hand, exposing a broken blister can result in local wound infection; on the other hand, fluid confined by necrotic skin can result in a closed-space infection. As a general rule, blisters are left intact unless they are caused by a chemical burn. Blisters from chemical burns should be broken during decontamination because they may trap the causative agent and worsen the extent of injury.

Patients with tar and asphalt burns can present a challenge to providers. When tar that is heated to

form a liquid comes in contact with skin, heat transfer occurs, causing a burn injury. Asphalt cements become a liquid at lower temperatures (275°F to 300°F [135°C to 148.9°C]) compared with tar, which requires a higher temperature to remain in a liquid state (450°F to 500°F [232.2°C to 260°C]). Therefore, more serious burns occur with tar than with asphalt. As tar and asphalt cool, they solidify and adhere to hair; there is little direct bonding between these substances and skin. The tar or asphalt should be bathed with water until hardened and cool. After the material is cooled, the patient may be transported to the burn center.

If an attempt to remove the tar or asphalt is made prior to transfer to the burn unit, several ointments and solvents may assist in this process. Tar must be removed because it will serve as an occlusive dressing and cause infection. Naphthalene, hexane, and other carbon solvents may be useful for removing asphalts, whereas coal tars respond only to aromatic hydrocarbons (benzene, toluene, or naphthalene). Unfortunately, these solvents can be absorbed, producing toxic side effects; therefore, a specific type called long-chain aliphatic hydrocarbons (hexanes or pentanes) should be used, or removal of coal tars may need to be delayed until the patient reaches the burn center. Sunflower oil, butter, baby oil, and commercial surface-active agents such as polysorbate 80 have been shown to be highly effective and inexpensive means of tar and asphalt removal.

Wound Infections and Treatment

Wound infections do not occur during the first few hours after a burn; consequently, antibiotic

---

Transport Management

Burn Wounds

- Dry and dress wounds with dry, clean dressings.
- Use bulky dressings to pad pressure points and sensitive areas.
- Do not use ointments or creams. However, if wounds are already dressed with ointments or creams, leave them in place.
- Examine all wounds to confirm that the BSA and the fluid resuscitation calculation are accurate.

prophylaxis by the CCTP is not warranted. Early antibiotic administration without proven infection may select for resistant bacteria, which makes fighting future infections difficult.

Topical antibiotic preparations are generally used to dress wounds. Agents such as bacitracin or a combination preparation of neomycin sulfate and polymyxin B sulfate (Neosporin) are generally used on the face and areas of thin skin, whereas silver sulfadiazine (Silvadene) is commonly used on other parts of the body. Silvadene should never be used on the face, because it can cause skin discoloration.

The exception to the rule about early wound infection is tetanus; its potential for development should be considered in patients without sufficient immunization against this disease. Patients at highest risk for tetanus are immigrants from developing countries and patients who have not had a booster in the previous 5 years. Patients who have not had a tetanus booster in 5 years require 0.5 mL of diphtheria and tetanus toxoids intramuscularly. Patients who have not had the primary series of three immunizations will require tetanus immunoglobulin in addition to starting the primary immunization series.

Pain Control

Burns can be excruciatingly painful, and pain control in the burn patient must be taken seriously. An opioid such as morphine sulfate, in doses of 4 to 8 mg IV (0.1 mg/kg), is the agent of choice in patients who are not allergic, and may be repeated until adequate pain control is achieved. Alternatively, agents such as fentanyl (Sublimaze) or hydromorphone (Dilaudid) may be used. Some burn specialists prefer use of fentanyl over morphine on the theoretical basis that the histamine release seen with morphine administration may promote increased capillary leak, leading to greater edema.

Morphine sulfate may also be used for children. An initial dose of 0.1 mg/kg up to a maximum of 5 mg per dose should be given. Fentanyl is dosed at 1 µg/kg.

Pain should be assessed and treated every 10 minutes until the patient is comfortable. Burn victims may require large doses of opioids for adequate pain control; if patients say they are in pain, treat their pain. Titration of opioids should be based on the patient's perception of pain, with additional doses withheld in cases of altered level of consciousness, respiratory depression, or hypotension. The patient should be reassessed often and treated as needed. Individual requirements for opioids are different, and the CCTP should ensure that the patient is neither undermedicated nor overmedicated.

CCTPs should also be careful not to confuse sedation and analgesia. Sedatives such as lorazepam (Ativan) do not have analgesic properties, and patients who are receiving ventilation will likely require sedation in addition to analgesia. The CCTP should monitor the patient's condition closely to prevent oversedation. Oxygenation does not equal ventilation, and patients who are oversedated will experience increased partial pressure of carbon dioxide long before any drop in the partial pressure of oxygen becomes apparent. Therefore, clinical assessment of the patient's ventilatory status or ETCO$_2$ level must be used as the gauge to assess for oversedation.

All medications for burn patients should be given intravenously—never intramuscularly, unless special circumstances exist. Long transports may require large quantities of medications, and the CCTP should make sure enough medication is available for sedation and pain control during transport. Burns are particularly distressing injuries, and almost any burn patient the CCTP encounters would likely benefit from administration of anxiolytics. Use of anxiolytics also facilitates pain management, often lowering the doses of opioids needed.

Other Issues

Hypothermia

Every effort should be made to maintain a normal body temperature in the patient. The patient's temperature should be measured prior to transport. Removal of wet clothing, dressings, and linens is essential. Dry sheets and blankets are preferred to cover and warm the patient.

Gastric Decompression

Patients with greater than 20% BSA burned are susceptible to ileus (loss of intestinal motility) because of the systemic inflammatory response that occurs with large burns. The administration of opioid pain medications decreases gastric and intestinal motility, which in turn increases the likelihood of an ileus developing. An ileus can cause abdominal distention, discomfort, and vomiting. To avoid these problems, nasogastric tubes should be placed in these patients. Decompression of the stomach with low intermittent suction will reduce distention, discomfort, and vomiting. Any patient who is endotracheally intubated should also have an orogastric tube in place to evacuate the stomach and prevent regurgitation.

Signs and Symptoms

Ileus
- Abdominal distention
- Discomfort
- Vomiting

Transport Management

Ileus
- Perform gastric decompression.
- Use nasogastric tubes.
- Place an orogastric tube in patients who have been intubated.

Special Situations

Burn centers provide care and expertise for many different types of injuries. A basic knowledge of these special situations is important to prevent further injury and provide appropriate treatment during transport.

Renal Failure and Rhabdomyolysis

Despite adequate fluid resuscitation of burn patients, their urine output may not be adequate. Given that urine output is a highly reliable indicator of adequate fluid resuscitation, patients with inadequate urine output can be extremely challenging for any health care provider. Inadequate urine output may occur for any of several reasons. Severe shock may have caused kidney damage, or the patient may have preexisting renal failure. The patient may also have renal dysfunction as a result of the mobilization of muscle proteins impairing

filtration, a condition known as **rhabdomyolysis**. Rhabdomyolysis occurs most often with crush injuries, electrical burns, or large full-thickness burns. Treatment of rhabdomyolysis is discussed in more depth in Chapter 11, *Trauma*.

Ocular Burns

Every burned patient should have a thorough eye exam. Corneal abrasions and corneal burns may occur from many mechanisms. Friction burns from auto airbags, blast injuries, thermal burns, and chemical burns are common sources of injury.

In awake and alert patients, eye injuries are rarely overlooked because the patient complains of pain or visual changes. If the patient is sedated, is unconscious, or has distracting injuries, however, clinical suspicion must remain high to avoid missing injuries. Because facial edema may develop quickly, early intervention is important. After the eyelids swell, it may be difficult to open the patient's eyes for an exam or treatment **FIGURE 13-11**.

Corneal injuries can be very painful and should be treated with appropriate opioids. Instillation of topical anesthetics such as tetracaine may alleviate the pain from corneal injuries and aid in irrigation, although topical anesthetic drops should not be used repeatedly.

In case of chemical burns of the eyes, the eyes should be irrigated with copious amounts of water for at least 20 minutes or until the conjunctival sac pH has returned to 7. Irrigation of the eyes can be difficult if attempted manually. Morgan lenses—contact lenses with tubing connected to IV fluids—should be placed to facilitate irrigation. Lactated

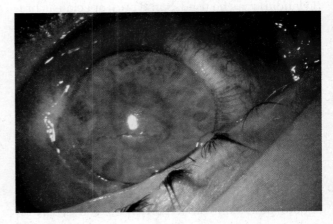

FIGURE 13-11 Examine the burn patient's eyes early; facial edema may develop quickly and make assessment difficult.
© Western Ophthalmic Hospital/Science Source.

Ringer solution is better tolerated as an irrigation fluid than is normal saline, but either is acceptable. Topical anesthetics should be instilled prior to placement of the Morgan lenses.

Injuries to the eyes caused by an airbag should also be irrigated. Airbags may cause friction burns because the bag deploys faster than the eye can react and close to prevent the injury. In addition, the propellant that inflates the bag can release heat or chemicals that can burn the eyes.

For the critically burned patient with nonchemical burns to the eyes, application of topical ophthalmic preparations (if patient care demands allow for this treatment) will suffice as a short-term remedy until the patient can receive a more definitive examination and treatment at the receiving facility.

Transport Management

Ocular Burns
- Treat corneal injuries with appropriate opioids.
- Chemical burns of the eyes: Irrigate with copious amounts of water for at least 20 minutes or until the pH of the conjunctival sac has returned to 7.
- Nonchemical burns to the eyes: Apply a topical ophthalmic preparation.

Facial Burns

Facial burns require special attention owing to the risk of ocular and airway injuries. Significant facial burns are especially suggestive of accompanying airway injury. Rapid and repeated airway evaluation is crucial, and early intubation should be considered for any airway injury.

The face develops edema quickly. Therefore, an early eye exam is important. To help reduce facial edema, the head of the stretcher should be elevated at a 30° angle if spinal injury is not suspected.

Transport Management

Facial Burns
- If no spinal injury is suspected, elevate the head of the stretcher at a 30° angle to reduce facial edema.

Ear Burns

The ears are also prone to significant swelling when they are burned. The ear canal and eardrum should be examined before edema develops. Discuss this issue with the transporting or receiving physician prior to departure. Prevent additional trauma by avoiding pressure dressings; likewise, do not use a pillow to cushion the ear. Only large, dry, bulky dressings are required.

Transport Management

Ear Burns
- Use large, bulky dressings.
- Avoid pressure dressings.
- Do not use a pillow.

Circumferential Burns and Compartment Syndrome

Burns that encircle the chest, an extremity, or the penis present a difficult challenge. Chest burns can cause respiratory impairment if the development of eschar limits chest excursion. Edema in the extremities and penis may result in vascular compromise. These injuries may require an escharotomy to restore mobility to the chest or circulation to an extremity **FIGURE 13-12**. Again, most burn specialists discourage the use of field escharotomy unless absolutely and immediately necessary to preserve life or limb.

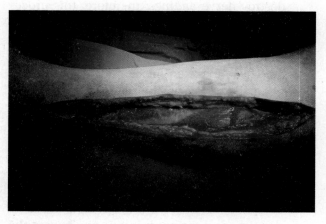

FIGURE 13-12 An escharotomy, in which an incision is made to restore circulation in the context of a circumferential extremity burn.

© Pthawatc/Shutterstock.

The following equipment is needed to perform an escharotomy:

- Scalpel
- Pain medication
- Sedation
- Sterile dressing
- 4-inch × 4-inch (10-cm × 10-cm) gauze pads

An escharotomy may be necessary in the following circumstances:

- Circumferential burns
- Full-thickness burns
- Compartment syndrome (requires fasciotomy)
- Thermal burns
- High-voltage electrical burns
- Tissue pressure measurements greater than 35 mm Hg (obtained by placing a needle into the compartment in question, usually done by an orthopaedist)

Complications of an escharotomy may include these conditions:

- Bleeding
- Infection
- Nerve damage
- Limited range of motion due to improper technique

SKILL DRILL 13-1 shows the steps for performing an emergency escharotomy, which are described here:

1. Prepare the equipment.
2. Administer sedation and pain medications. Burns that cause such injuries are deep and destroy nerve endings; therefore, this procedure can be performed without anesthesia.
3. Maintain an aseptic technique **STEP 1**.
4. Determine a well-defined incision pattern. For the chest, make an incision along both anterior axillary lines or, alternatively, transversely. For an extremity, make an incision parallel to the bone. A single incision may be sufficient for an extremity. The incision should be of sufficient depth for an obvious release in pressure on the skin and for fat to bulge through the incision. For the penis, a single dorsal incision is adequate (the dorsum of the penis is the anterior surface if the penis is pointing toward the feet). Hand escharotomies are performed with incisions in the medial and lateral surfaces of each finger and of the palm.
5. Incise the derma of the burned tissue **STEP 2**. Built-up pressure should cause the tissue to open even more.
6. Prepare to manage bleeding **STEP 3**.
7. Apply a sterile dressing over the incision.

The most qualified person should perform the procedure; however, situations may arise that make escharotomy necessary on an emergent basis to save life or limb. An escharotomy should be performed only after discussion with the receiving burn center or transport service medical direction (if the local scope of practice allows the CCTP to carry out this procedure).

Signs and Symptoms

Circulation Problems Due to Circumferential Burns

- Absence of pulses
- Delayed capillary refill
- Mottling and discoloration of an extremity

Transport Management

Circulation Problems Due to Circumferential Burns

- Escharotomy, if allowed per protocol

Controversies

The necessity of prehospital escharotomies is a subject of debate. Many believe that the efficacy of field escharotomies is limited, as revealed by a risk-benefit analysis. With field escharotomies, there is the potential for blood loss, severe hypotension, contamination of the wound, and damage to the nerves. Because of the amount of time it takes for an eschar to form, the likelihood that an escharotomy will be needed in the field is low. However, the CCTP must also consider the potential benefit of performing an escharotomy if the interfacility transport will require an extended length of time. When performed in a facility as opposed to the field, the benefit may outweigh the risk of the procedure.

Skill Drill 13-1 Performing an Emergency Escharotomy*

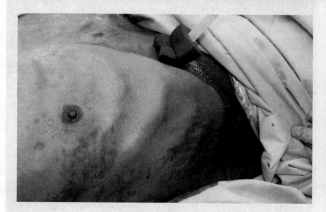

Step 1

Prepare your equipment. Administer sedation and pain medications. Maintain an aseptic technique. Determine a well-defined incision pattern.

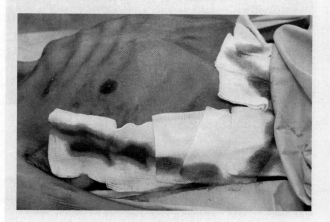

Step 2

Incise the derma of the burned tissue.

Step 3

Prepare to manage bleeding. Apply a sterile dressing.

*Note: The procedure was performed on a cadaver and does not show the burned tissue associated with this injury.

© Jones & Bartlett Learning.

Hand and Foot Burns

Burns on the hands and feet can cause significant disability and require specialized care. Circulation is the main concern with these injuries, because edema may impair blood flow to the periphery of the extremity, causing extensive damage. Simple interventions such as elevating the injured extremity above the heart and avoiding constricting dressings are important. Loose, dry dressings that allow easy assessment of the patient's circulation may be used during transport; however, no dressing is required. Do not apply creams or ointments. Likewise, do not apply ice packs because they may cause frostbite.

Transport Management

Hand and Foot Burns

- Elevate the injured extremity above the heart.
- Avoid constricting dressings; use loose, dry dressings or no dressing.
- Do not apply creams or ointments.
- Do not apply ice packs.

Genitalia Burns

Burns on the genitalia and perineum should not distract health care providers from life-threatening injuries. However, certain aspects of the treatment of patients with such injuries require prompt attention. An indwelling urinary catheter should be placed immediately before edema develops. The penis should be examined for circumferential burns and monitored for impaired circulation. A dorsal escharotomy of the penis may be necessary, albeit as a highly unlikely event.

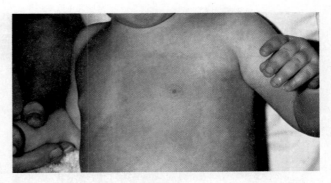

FIGURE 13-13 An accidental burn.

© Dr. P. Marazzi/Science Source.

Transport Management

Genitalia Burns

- Immediately place an indwelling urinary catheter.
- If a penis has a circumferential burn, monitor for impaired circulation.

Pediatric Burns and Child Abuse

Children present special challenges when burned because their physiology and composition differ from those of adults. Children have relatively more surface area per kilogram, which necessitates close attention to their fluid resuscitation. Infants also have relatively less glycogen stores than adults, making them susceptible to hypoglycemia if deprived of oral intake for several hours. The CCTP should consider adding glucose to resuscitation fluids in such young patients; however, this treatment should be guided by local burn center preference. Other strategies include frequently checking glucose levels and correcting any hypoglycemia as it occurs, rather than administering glucose-containing fluids. The blood glucose level should be maintained between 60 and 120 mg/dL.

Approximately 25% of all childhood burns result from child abuse; consequently, the CCTP caring for a child should consider this possibility. When children with burns receive care more than 24 hours after the incident, suspect maltreatment. Accidental burns in children most often result from scalding and more commonly occur in the "spill area"—the area of the face and chest that is exposed when children pull a container of hot liquid onto themselves **FIGURE 13-13**. Burns to other areas with well-demarcated edges and in a stocking-glove distribution should raise the suspicion of abuse **FIGURE 13-14**. The CCTP should report any suspicion of child maltreatment to child protection authorities and the receiving facility.

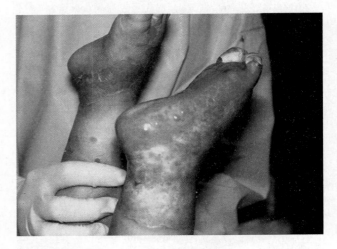

FIGURE 13-14 Stocking-glove distribution.

Courtesy of Ronald Dieckmann, MD.

Transport Management

Pediatric Burns

- Consult with a local burn center regarding adding glucose to resuscitation fluids.
- Check blood glucose levels frequently.
- Correct hypoglycemia.

Electrical Burns

Injuries from electricity may result from alternating current or direct current. Alternating current is found in homes and businesses and is the most common source of electrical injury. Direct current is found in motor vehicle electric systems and some lighting systems, and may be found in some industries. Lightning is also direct current.

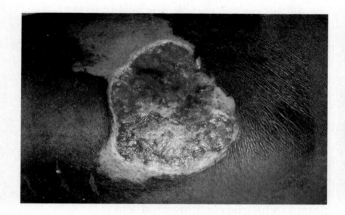

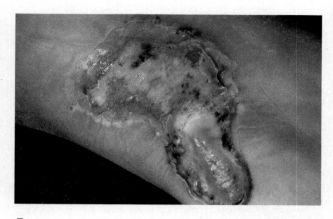

A **B**

FIGURE 13-15 A. An electrical burn entry wound on the shoulder of a patient. **B.** An electrical burn exit wound on the foot of a patient.

© Charles Stewart, MD, EMDM, MPH.

Electricity releases heat as it travels through or across the body, causing extensive tissue damage. All tissues have a different resistance to current flow, with the nervous system being the least resistant. Bone is the most resistant, but all tissues are susceptible to damage. Electricity may enter and exit the body at any point. The hands are the most common point of entry **FIGURE 13-15A**, and the feet are the most common point of exit **FIGURE 13-15B**. The path that electricity follows between entrance and exit is erratic and unpredictable. Severe charring frequently occurs at the point of entry and may be the only obvious injury. Damage to deeper structures may not be evident if the superficial structure such as the skin is uninjured.

Early evaluation of the extent of electrical injury is difficult. Some common patterns of injury do occur, however. Damage to the cardiac conduction system may present as cardiac arrest, and high voltages may lead to respiratory arrest by paralyzing the diaphragm. Alternating current typically causes ventricular fibrillation and is the most common cause of death. Direct current typically causes asystole. Cardiac arrest in the electrocuted patient is treated with the standard advanced cardiac life support protocol. Other arrhythmias may develop at any time after injury, necessitating continuous cardiac monitoring for the first 24 hours. Notably, a normal electrocardiogram or rhythm soon after the event does not rule out injury.

Skin burns sometimes occur without deeper structures being damaged in electrical injury.

Clothing may ignite without an electrical current entering the body. These injuries are treated as other cutaneous burns.

Because the electrical current can travel deep into the skin, structures such as muscle, bone, tendon, blood vessels, and nerves may be severely damaged, despite little evidence appearing on the skin. Massive muscle damage and cell death will release muscle proteins into the bloodstream. In addition, compartment syndrome may develop in the extremities as a result of deep burns; progressive pain, paresthesias, and decreased circulation are clues to this injury. Consult with the transferring and receiving physicians about fasciotomy before transport.

Electric current may also cause violent muscle contractions that break bones or cause joints to dislocate. Spinal motion restriction should be employed and suspected fractures immobilized prior to transport. Care should be taken to protect open fractures from additional contamination.

Lightning injuries are a common source of burns. Patients with lightning injuries may experience any of the injuries already mentioned. In addition, they may experience extensive superficial cutaneous burns in a fern or reticular pattern as electricity passes across the skin **FIGURE 13-16**. The eardrum may rupture as a result of the pressure wave created by the rapid heating of the surrounding air, and the patient may have displacement to the lens of the eye from the pressure gradient produced.

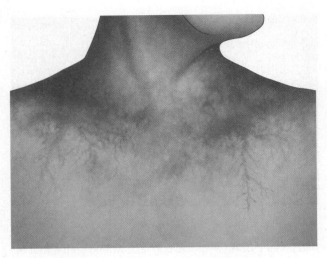

FIGURE 13-16 Fern pattern as a result of a lightning injury.

© Jones & Bartlett Learning.

Transport Management

Electrical Burns
- Treat the same as other cutaneous burns.

Chemical Burns

Common household, industrial, and farm products can be toxic and cause significant burns. The active ingredients responsible for injury are usually acids, alkalis, and a few other organic compounds. The extent of damage depends on the type of agent, its relative strength, and the duration of contact.

Cutaneous burns are not the only risk from chemical exposure; some chemicals may be absorbed systemically, causing organ damage or failure. Such injuries may not become apparent until 6 to 24 hours after exposure. Patients with relatively minor-appearing injuries may require transport for observation at a center for specialized care.

When chemical burns are suspected, it is crucial to decontaminate the patient quickly and thoroughly. Because chemicals can settle in clothing, shoes, linens, and jewelry, the patient should be completely disrobed and then irrigated with copious amounts of water. Attempts to neutralize one chemical with another can produce an exothermic reaction (producing heat) and worsen the burn; therefore, this should not be attempted. After decontamination, the patient should be placed on clean, dry linens. Management of chemical wounds is generally the same as for thermal injuries, with the exception of applying calcium gluconate gel to hydrofluoric acid burns (discussed in the next subsection).

Acid Burns

Acids are found in chemical products such as drain openers, drain cleaners, bathroom cleaners, swimming pool products, and rust removers. They are also found in hair care products such as hair relaxers. Acids are used extensively in industry for production of other compounds and are found in potent industrial cleaning products.

Duration of contact is the main determinant of damage from acids. The initial treatment consists of rapid, copious irrigation with water. Acids tend to cause burns that are more self-limiting than the burns caused by alkalis. When acids come in contact with skin, their damage takes the form of coagulation necrosis. The coagulum, or scar, limits the penetration of the acid, thereby limiting the damage done. This results in a burn with well-demarcated edges and often in a pattern that suggests liquid spilling.

Some acids such as hydrofluoric acid also have other mechanisms of injury and require special attention. Hydrofluoric acid is used in microelectronics, petroleum processing, glass and metal etching, wheel cleaners, rust removal, and many other applications. It is capable of inflicting progressive injury despite irrigation. After this chemical penetrates the skin, fluoride ions are released and cause nerve damage and severe pain. Calcium binds to fluoride and reduces its damage. Therefore, topical calcium gluconate gel should be applied immediately after irrigation. Commercial preparations of calcium gluconate gels are available, but mixing calcium gluconate with a water-based, water-soluble lubricant (such as K-Y Jelly) will suffice if these products are not available. This mixture can be squirted into an exam glove and applied directly to the patient's hand. Intradermal injection of calcium gluconate and intra-arterial calcium gluconate may also be used to alleviate pain.

Oxalic acid is not as toxic as hydrofluoric acid but may also require calcium gluconate therapy. Calcium *chloride* should not be administered intradermally or intra-arterially.

Alkali Burns

Alkalis are found in many household and industrial products and are capable of producing significant burns. Oven cleaners, drain cleaners, lime, lye, and cement are all commonly encountered alkali substances. These agents, when combined with fat, produce soap; thus, they are able to penetrate deeply and rapidly into the tissues. Alkali exposures continue to burn for extended periods of time and require irrigation for more than 20 minutes. Because there is no coagulum to restrict the penetration of alkalis into the tissues, burns caused by these chemicals typically have poorly defined edges and diffuse spreading of the injury. Special care must be taken during decontamination to avoid unnecessary heat loss.

Dry lime is a commonly used agricultural product. When combined with water, it may also generate an exothermic reaction and cause burns.

With alkali burns, all dry powders should be brushed away to reduce the amount of chemical present before irrigation is performed with flowing water. Fast-flowing water will help dissipate heat, but the higher pressure may cause or worsen tissue damage. When using water under pressure, avoid self-contamination from splashing.

Because of the deep penetration of alkalis, systemic toxicity is also a significant concern with these burns. Care of systemic complications is supportive.

Hydrocarbon Burns

Hydrocarbons such as petroleum fuels may cause burns after immersion or prolonged contact with these chemicals. They can also cause significant systemic toxicity if absorbed. Treatment is supportive, including copious irrigation and observation.

Hydrocarbons (including most petroleum products such as gasoline) can cause myocardial depression leading to hypotension and cardiovascular collapse. Halogenated hydrocarbons (chlorofluorocarbons, including Freon and those found in many solvents like oven cleaner), such as those used in propellants, are known to cause central nervous system depression or excitability. In particular, the halogenated hydrocarbons may potentially create a fatal arrhythmia.

Stevens-Johnson Syndrome and Toxic Epidermal Necrolysis Syndrome

Stevens-Johnson syndrome and toxic epidermal necrolysis syndrome are severe mucocutaneous reactions that typically result from certain medications, environmental allergies, infections, and unknown toxins. The medication phenytoin (Dilantin), among others, is well known for causing this reaction. Other medications often implicated include allopurinol, sulfonamides, and certain nonsteroidal anti-inflammatory drugs (NSAIDs). More rarely, other medications such as acetaminophen can be associated with this reaction.

Stevens-Johnson syndrome and toxic epidermal necrolysis are both immune-mediated illnesses that cause sloughing of the skin, mucous membranes, and the cells lining the respiratory system. Both can also present respiratory and wound care challenges that are as difficult to manage as severe burns of other types **FIGURE 13-17**. They are considered to be on the same continuum, with Stevens-Johnson syndrome being the milder of the two. The spectrum of illness from Stevens-Johnson syndrome to toxic epidermal necrolysis is as follows:

- In Stevens-Johnson syndrome, epidermal detachment involves less than 10% of the total body skin area. In more than 90% of patients, mucous membranes are involved. Mortality is approximately 10%.
- In Stevens-Johnson syndrome–toxic epidermal necrolysis, overlap is defined by an epidermal detachment between 10% and 30%.

Transport Management

Chemical Burns

- Decontaminate patients quickly and thoroughly.
- Copiously irrigate the burn until the burning has stopped or the material is cool.
- The length of the irrigation process should be guided by the pH of the wound assessed in the base of the wound.
- If you are unable to measure pH, continue copious irrigation for at least 20 minutes.
- After decontamination, place the patient on clean, dry linens.
- Break blisters.
- Remove all clothing and jewelry.
- Do not attempt to neutralize one chemical with another.
- For burns from hydrofluoric acid, apply topical calcium gluconate gel immediately after irrigation.

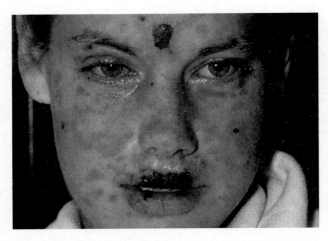

FIGURE 13-17 Patients with toxic epidermal necrolysis or Stevens-Johnson syndrome can present treatment challenges that are similar to those associated with patients with severe burns.

© Dr. P. Marazzi/Science Source.

- Toxic epidermal necrolysis is defined by an epidermal detachment of greater than 30%. Its mortality often approaches 30%.

Patients with toxic epidermal necrolysis are frequently treated in burn centers because their wounds are analogous to burn injuries. Treatment is primarily supportive, in addition to the skin care.

Summary

Mastering the care of burn patients is a continuous process. Research is ongoing to discover optimal wound management and resuscitation techniques. Additional training is available from various sources, and most burn centers and units offer educational programs that can be an invaluable resource to local providers.

Case Study

You are dispatched to a rural community hospital for an interfacility transport of a 45-year-old woman who is experiencing dyspnea and pain after being burned in a house explosion secondary to a natural gas leak.

As you enter the treatment room to begin your assessment, you find a woman with multiple partial- and full-thickness burns to her arms, chest, abdomen, and face. She is experiencing severe dyspnea and crying out in pain, having just arrived via EMS. She is conscious, confused, and difficult to understand because of the hoarseness of her voice. You continue your assessment, while your partner sets up equipment for RSI. The patient is complaining of severe pain throughout the burned areas of her body.

Her vital signs include a blood pressure of 118/80 mm Hg; respiratory rate of 38 breaths/min and labored with audible stridor despite three albuterol nebulizer treatments by EMS providers; and a pulse rate of 140 beats/min. You note burns in the mouth; soot around the nose and mouth; partial-thickness burns to the chest, abdomen, and arms; and full-thickness burns to the face. You estimate the patient's partial- and full-thickness burns to be approximately 30% of her TBSA.

Your partner advises you that she is ready to begin RSI. You use an established IV line to administer 2 mg/kg of ketamine and 2 mg/kg of succinylcholine. You insert the laryngoscope, but you are unable to visualize the vocal cords or pass the endotracheal tube because of pronounced edema. You direct your partner to ventilate the patient using a bag-mask device and 100% oxygen while you prepare the surgical airway kit. You are successful in securing a surgical airway. On confirmation of placement using waveform capnography and bilateral breath sounds, you make a note that breath sounds are slightly decreased on the patient's right side as compared to her left side. You quickly cover all burns with dry, sterile dressings and prepare for transport by placing the patient onto your equipment and rapidly performing a hot load (with the engine running and rotors turning) for transport to the closest burn center.

In flight, the patient's vital signs remain stable; you administer 0.1 mg/kg of vecuronium and 1 µg/kg of fentanyl, and you start administering lactated Ringer solution at 100 mL/h. Approximately 2 minutes from the burn center, your partner, who is ventilating the patient, reports that she is meeting resistance. You assess breath sounds and do not hear anything on the right side, although you are uncertain of this finding because of the amount of noise in the helicopter. End-tidal carbon dioxide has remained at 35 mm Hg with a normal waveform. Because of the burns and swelling, you are unable to determine whether jugular vein distention or tracheal deviation is present. You confirm that the surgical airway has not moved and then decide to do a needle decompression, which your partner reports makes ventilating much easier.

On arrival at the burn center, you do a hot off-load of the patient and transport the patient to the trauma bay, where you give a report to the trauma team. You and your partner clean your equipment and get the aircraft back in service.

Once you return to base, you complete your report for the medical record and discover that you miscalculated the initial IV fluid rate according to the Parkland formula. You notify the nursing staff at the burn unit of the error and complete a protocol deviation form. Finally, you notify the referring EMS agency of the outcome.

1. What should the IV fluid rate have been?
2. What is the rationale for the resistance met during ventilation that led to a needle decompression?
3. According to the American Burn Association, which classification of burns did the patient in the case present?

Analysis

Although the Advanced Burn Life Support fluid resuscitation formula is slowly replacing the Parkland formula, many protocols continue to utilize the Parkland formula. The Parkland formula recommends resuscitation with lactated Ringer solution of 4 mL/kg per percentage of BSA burned. In this case, the initial fluid rate should have been 750 mL/h.

Burn patients may experience significant trauma from explosions or motor vehicle crashes resulting in fires. With the presence of such trauma, the possibility exists that you might overlook conditions such as a pneumothorax or hemothorax while treating the obvious burns. Careful repeated examinations should focus on identifying these conditions. Physical assessment is important in such cases, because monitoring devices such as capnography and pulse oximetry may not display appreciable changes until the patient has significantly decompensated.

This patient met several criteria for major burn injuries, including partial-thickness burns involving more than 25% of BSA in an adult, burns involving the face, and burns complicated by inhalation injury or major trauma.

Caring for patients with burn injuries requires the CCTP to deploy aggressive critical thinking, assessment, and intervention skills. The CCTP must use an organized, rapid approach to assess, prioritize, and treat both the burns and any secondary injuries found. Because of the early fluid losses associated with burn injuries, aggressive and sustained fluid management is essential. Determining the severity and extent of burns is important to arrange for transportation to the most appropriate treatment facility.

Prep Kit

Ready for Review

- The initial 24 hours of care after a burn are crucial. The CCTP must have an understanding of the common complications of burns that can develop during the transport of the patient to a burn facility.

- The skin, which is composed of the epidermis and the dermis, is the largest organ of the body and is vital to survival.
- The layers of the epidermis contain pigment cells, immune cells, and capillaries in the lower

layers. The epidermis is the first barrier to injury and infection; it is constantly repairing itself, because it is injured more often than the other layers. Its outer layer provides a barrier to prevent water loss from deeper structures.

- The dermis lies beneath the epidermis and contains fibroblasts, macrophages, white blood cells, nerve cells, lymphatic vessels, blood vessels, portions of the hair follicles, and oil and sweat glands.

- Proteins such as collagen and fibronectin, which are produced in the dermis, support the continuously reproducing epidermis and play a major role in wound healing, along with fibroblasts, macrophages, platelets, and endothelial cells. The inflammatory response, which is important in the burn healing process, is also responsible for multiple complications of injuries.

- The skin has multiple functions, including protection from infection, maintaining fluid and electrolyte balance, thermoregulation, and neurosensory functioning, which is important for social interaction.

- Burns occur from a variety of mechanisms, including flame/flash, scald (eg, water, grease), contact, electrical, chemical inhalation, radiation, and any type of thermal source. The agent, temperature, and duration of exposure determine the size and depth of a burn.

- The zone of coagulation is the most heavily damaged area of a burn and is the area of skin that came into direct contact with the source of heat.

- The zone of stasis encompasses the injured tissue in a burn and may appear red and hyperemic (filled with an increased amount of blood) initially. Within 24 hours after the injury, it has a stagnant blood flow resulting in ischemic tissues, which by the third day become white because they are avascular and necrotic.

- The zone of erythema, which has increased blood flow, is the outermost area surrounding the zone of stasis; it has minimal damage and will recover.

- Burns affecting more than 20% of the total body surface area (TBSA) result in a systemic inflammatory response, which can result in undesirable effects on other tissues and organs, including pulmonary edema, suppression of the immune system, sepsis, and impaired cardiac output.

- The severity of a burn depends on the extent, depth, and location of the burn; the age of the patient; the etiologic agents involved; the presence of inhalation injury; and coexisting injuries or preexisting illnesses.

- The classification of burns includes four categories:
  - Superficial (first-degree) burns, which involve only the epidermis
  - Partial-thickness (second-degree) burns, which involve some of the dermis but not the entire thickness of the skin
  - Full-thickness (third-degree) burns, which involve all layers of the skin and perhaps some subcutaneous tissue and muscle
  - Subdermal (fourth-degree) burns, which involve deep structures such as muscle, bone, large blood vessels, and nerves

- Burn size also influences burn severity. A common approach to determining severity is the rule of nines, which is the method most commonly used in the prehospital environment. The Lund-Browder chart is more accurate than the rule of nines, but is rarely used by prehospital providers.

- The American Burn Association (ABA) classifies burns into three major categories: major, moderate, and minor. Patients who meet the ABA criteria or have a major burn injury should be transferred to a specialized burn center to ensure appropriate acute care, rehabilitation, and long-term care.

- Assessment for burn patients should be similar to assessment for any other patient, with attention paid to each organ system, but especially to the patient's airway, breathing rate and depth, and cardiac output.

- Burn management includes removing the patient from the source of the burn, cooling, and irrigation.
- Airway management for a burn patient can present difficult challenges because of airway edema resulting from inhalation injuries. The patient must be assessed for the possibility of inhalation injury and the airway managed with endotracheal intubation if stridor, progressive hoarseness, or any other evidence of airway compromise is present.
- Judicious fluid management is important, because burns can result in large intravascular fluid losses due to the loss of the body's protection against desiccation and evaporation. Formulas to calculate fluid resuscitation for the first 24 hours after a burn include the ABA's *Advanced Life Support Course* 2018 guidelines (the most commonly used) and the Parkland formula.
- Burn wounds should be dressed with clean, dry dressings (never wet dressings), and blisters should be left intact. In general, the CCTP should not perform wound debridement.
- Antibiotic prophylaxis by the CCTP is not warranted in patients with burns, although deficiencies in tetanus coverage should be remedied.
- Burn victims may require large doses of opioids for adequate pain control, and pain should be assessed and treated every 10 minutes until the patient is comfortable.
- Other issues of burn management include maintaining a normal body temperature to prevent hypothermia and performing gastric decompression if necessary.
- Despite adequate fluid resuscitation of a burn patient, inadequate urine output may occur as a result of severe shock resulting in kidney damage, preexisting renal failure, or rhabdomyolysis.
- Ocular burns can occur from many different sources, including friction burns from auto airbags, blast injury, thermal burns, and chemical burns. A burn patient's eyes need to be examined early, because edema can develop quickly and make subsequent assessment difficult.
- Treat corneal injuries with appropriate opioids, chemical burns of the eye with irrigation, and nonchemical eye burns with a topical ophthalmic preparation.
- Ocular and airway injuries are the major concerns that arise with facial burns. Airway evaluation is important in such cases, given that early intubation may be necessary.
- Ear burns are susceptible to increased swelling, and an exam should be done before edema develops.
- Circumferential burns (burns that encircle the chest, an extremity, or the penis) and the resultant compartment syndrome present difficult challenges for the CCTP. These injuries may require an escharotomy to restore mobility to the chest or circulation to an extremity.
- Hand and foot burns can cause significant disability. They are treated by elevating the injured extremity above the heart and by using either loose, dry dressings or no dressing.
- Genitalia burns require placement of an indwelling urinary catheter before edema develops. If a penis has a circumferential burn, the CCTP should monitor for impaired circulation.
- Approximately 25% of all childhood burns result from child maltreatment, and the CCTP should consider this possibility when caring for a burned child. Accidental burns in children often result from scalding and frequently occur in the "spill area" (the area of the face and chest that is exposed when children pull a container of hot liquids onto themselves).
- Early evaluation of the extent of injury from an electrical burn is difficult. Damage to the cardiac conduction system may present as cardiac arrest, and high voltages may lead to respiratory arrest by paralyzing the diaphragm.
- Alternating current typically causes ventricular fibrillation and is the most common cause of death, whereas direct current typically causes asystole. Lightning can cause extensive

Prep Kit Continued

superficial burns in a fern pattern as electricity passes across the skin.

- Patients with chemical burns should be decontaminated quickly and thoroughly, irrigating until the burning has stopped and the material is cooled, or for at least 20 minutes. Take care to avoid unnecessary heat loss when performing irrigation.

- Toxic epidermal necrolysis syndrome, the most severe form of skin reaction to certain medications, environmental allergies, or other unknown toxins, and a milder form, Stevens-Johnson syndrome, can present management challenges similar to those presented by severe burn patients.

Vital Vocabulary

compartment syndrome A condition that develops when edema and swelling result in increased pressure within soft tissues, causing circulation to be compromised, possibly resulting in tissue necrosis.

deep partial-thickness burn A burn in which the skin is blistered but not charred and is painful to the touch; it is usually the result of steam, oil, or flames and involves the deeper layers of the dermis.

dermis The layer of skin that lies beneath the epidermis; it is a dynamic layer of thick connective tissue.

epidermis The outer layer of the skin, which generally consists of four layers (thin skin), except on the palms, fingertips, and soles of the feet, which have five layers (thick skin).

eschar The leathery covering of a burn injury, formed after the burned tissues dry out.

escharotomy A surgical incision in an eschar to lessen constriction; sometimes necessary (although rarely performed in a prehospital setting) to prevent edema from building up, impairing capillary filling and causing ischemia.

fasciotomy A surgical incision into an area of fascia—for example, to relieve pressure between two compartments; not usually performed in a prehospital setting.

full-thickness burn A burn that extends through the epidermis and dermis into the subcutaneous tissues beneath, in which skin is pale, painless, leathery, and charred; also called a third-degree burn.

hyperemic An increase in blood flow into a tissue or organ; congested with blood.

ileus Loss of intestinal motility.

lines of cleavage Regions between interlocking collagen fibers that run in various planes, usually parallel to the skin; they run longitudinally in the skin of the head and limbs and in a circular pattern around the neck and trunk, and are used when deciding where to make incisions for escharotomies and fasciotomies.

Lund-Browder chart A detailed version of the rule of nines chart that takes into consideration the changes in body surface area that occur with growth.

major burn According to the American Burn Association classification system, any of the following: (1) partial-thickness burns involving more than 25% of total body surface area (TBSA) in adults or 20% of TBSA in children younger than 10 years and adults older than 40 years; (2) full-thickness burns involving 10% or more of TBSA; (3) burns involving the face, eyes, ears, hands, feet, or perineum that may result in functional or cosmetic impairment; (4) high-voltage electrical injury; (5) burns complicated by inhalation injury or major trauma; and (6) burns sustained by high-risk or debilitated patients.

minor burn According to the American Burn Association classification system, any of the following: (1) partial-thickness burns involving less than 15% of total body surface area (TBSA)

Prep Kit Continued

in adults or 10% of TBSA in children younger than 20 years and adults older than 50 years; and (2) full-thickness burns involving 2% or less of TBSA that do not present a serious threat of functional or cosmetic risk to the eyes, ears, face, hands, feet, or perineum.

moderate burn According to the American Burn Association classification system, any of the following: (1) partial-thickness burns involving 15% to 25% of total body surface area (TBSA) in adults or 10% to 20% of TBSA in children younger than 10 years and adults older than 40 years; and (2) full-thickness burns involving 10% or less of TBSA in patients younger than 50 years that do not present a serious threat to functional or cosmetic impairment of the eyes, ears, face, hands, feet, or perineum.

myoglobinuria The presence of myoglobin, a respiratory pigment of muscle tissue, in the urine.

Parkland formula A formula that recommends giving 4 mL of lactated Ringer solution or normal saline for each kilogram of body weight, multiplied by the percentage of body surface area burned; sometimes used to calculate fluid needs during lengthy transport times.

partial-thickness burn A burn that involves the epidermis and part of the dermis, characterized by pain and blistering; also called a second-degree burn.

rhabdomyolysis The destruction of muscle tissue leading to a release of potassium and myoglobin, which then accumulate in the blood and urine and impair filtration; occurs most often with crush injuries, electrical burns, or large full-thickness burns.

rule of nines A system that assigns percentages to sections of the body, allowing calculation of the amount of skin surface involved in the burn area.

Stevens-Johnson syndrome A milder form of toxic epidermal necrolysis, in which epidermal detachment involves less than 10% of the total body surface area; it causes sloughing of the skin, mucous membranes, and cells lining the respiratory system.

subdermal burn A severe, life-threatening burn involving the deep structures of muscle, bone, larger blood vessels, and nerves; also called a fourth-degree burn.

superficial burn A burn involving only the epidermis, producing very red, painful skin; also called a first-degree burn.

superficial partial-thickness burn A burn involving the epidermis and part of the dermis, but not the deeper layers of the dermis; also called a second-degree burn.

thermal burn A burn caused by heat, contact with hot objects, ignited liquids, steam, or hot liquids.

toxic epidermal necrolysis (TEN) syndrome A severe skin reaction to certain medications, environmental allergies, and other unknown toxins, in which epidermal detachment is greater than 30%.

zone of coagulation The center of a burn, which is usually the deepest and most severely affected area.

zone of erythema The outermost area of a burn, which represents the least severely burned area; usually an area of first-degree burn.

zone of stasis The area found just outside the zone of coagulation, which represents a burned area that is less severely damaged.

References

Advanced Burn Life Support Course: Provider's Manual 2018. Chicago, IL: American Burn Association; 2018.

Blumetti J, Hunt JL, Arnoldo BD, Parks JK, Purdue GF. The Parkland formula under fire: is the criticism justified? *J Burn Care Res*. 2008;29(1):180-186.

Burn center regional map. American Burn Association website. http://ameriburn.org/public-resources/burn-center-regional-map/. Accessed April 12, 2021.

Burn incidence and treatment in the United States: 2016. American Burn Association website. http://www.ameriburn.org/resources_factsheet.php. Accessed April 10, 2021.

Prep Kit Continued

Chung KK, Wolf SE, Cancio LC, et al. Resuscitation of severely burned military casualties: fluid begets more fluid. *J Trauma*. 2009;67(2):231-237.

Dulhunty JM, Boots RJ, Rudd MJ, Muller MJ, Lipman J. Increased fluid resuscitation can lead to adverse outcomes in major-burn injured patients, but low mortality is achievable. *Burns*. 2008;34(8):1090-1097.

Evers LH, Bhavsar D, Mailänder P. The biology of burn injury. *Exp Dermatol*. 2010;19(9):777-783.

Fast facts on US hospitals 2020. American Hospital Association website. www.aha.org/statistics/fast-facts-us-hospitals. Accessed April 12, 2021.

Giardino AP, Alexander R, eds. *Child Maltreatment: A Clinical Guide and Photographic Reference*. 3rd ed. St. Louis, MO: G. W. Medical Publishing; 2005.

Hockberger RS, Walls RM, eds. *Rosen's Emergency Medicine: Concepts and Clinical Practice*. 7th ed. St. Louis, MO: Mosby; 2009.

Klein MB, Hayden D, Elson C, et al. The association between fluid administration and outcome following major burn: a multicenter study. *Ann Surg*. 2007;245(4):622-628.

Ma OJ, Cline DM, Tintinalli JE, Kelen GD, Stapczynski JS. *Emergency Medicine Manual*. 6th ed. New York, NY: McGraw-Hill Medical Publishing Division; 2009.

Orgill DP, Piccolo N. Escharotomy and decompressive therapies in burns. *J Burn Care Res*. 2009;30(5):759-768.

Perel P, Roberts I. Colloids versus crystalloids for fluid resuscitation in critically ill patients. *Cochrane Database Syst Rev*. 2012;6:CD000567.

Rockwell WB, Ehrlich HP. Should burn blister fluid be evacuated? *J Burn Care Rehab*. 1990;11(1):93-95.

Sekula P, Dunant A, Mockenhaupt M, et al. Comprehensive survival analysis of a cohort of patients with Stevens-Johnson syndrome and toxic epidermal necrolysis. *J Invest Dermatol*. 2013;133(5):1197-1204.

Singer AJ, Taira BR, Thode HC Jr, et al. The association between hypothermia, prehospital cooling, and mortality in burn victims. *Acad Emerg Med*. 2010;17(4):456-459.

Sullivan SR, Ahmadi AJ, Singh CN, et al. Elevated orbital pressure: another untoward effect of massive resuscitation after burn injury. *J Trauma*. 2006;60(1):72-76.

Toon MH, Maybauer MO, Greenwood JE, Maybauer DM, Fraser JF. Management of acute smoke inhalation injury. *Crit Care Resusc*. 2010;12(1):53-61.

Weaver MD, Rittenberger JC, Patterson PD, et al. Risk factors for hypothermia in EMS-treated burn patients. *Prehosp Emerg Care*. 2014;18(3):335-341.

Chapter 14

Electrophysiology, Pacemakers, and Defibrillators

Mike McEvoy, PhD, NRP, RN, CCRN

OBJECTIVES

After completing this chapter, you will be able to:

1. Describe the anatomy and physiology of the cardiovascular system (pp 675–681).
2. Describe how to monitor a patient by using electrocardiography (ECG) during a critical care transport (CCT) (p 684).
3. Explain how to correctly place leads from a 12-lead ECG monitor (pp 684–687).
4. Explain how to correctly place additional precordial leads for diagnosing right ventricular and posterior infarctions (p 687).
5. Discuss the step-by-step systematic approach that should be used when interpreting an ECG (pp 688–691).
6. Explain how to determine the heart's electrical axis (p 691).
7. Describe how to identify a bundle branch block on an ECG (pp 695–703).
8. Explain the care for a patient with a bundle branch block during CCT (p 698).
9. Describe how to identify a hemiblock on an ECG (pp 698–700).
10. Explain the care for a patient with a hemiblock during CCT (pp 698–700).
11. Describe the significance of ST-segment and T-wave changes (p 703).
12. Explain how ST-segment and T-wave changes are identified on an ECG (pp 703–704).
13. Identify criteria suggestive of right and left atrial enlargement (pp 704–705).
14. Describe the clinical implications of right and left atrial enlargement (pp 704–705).
15. Identify criteria for determining the presence of left ventricular hypertrophy (LVH), right ventricular hypertrophy (RVH), and the presence of strain (pp 705–707).
16. Describe the clinical significance of LVH, RVH, and the presence of strain (pp 705–707).
17. Describe the ECG changes that indicate the presence of Wolff-Parkinson-White syndrome (pp 707–709).
18. Identify ECG changes that could indicate the presence of pericarditis (p 709).
19. Describe the potential implications of a prolonged QT interval (pp 709–710).
20. Describe how to identify ventricular tachycardia on an ECG, including when it occurs in conjunction with wide complex tachycardia (pp 710–712).
21. Explain the care for a patient with ventricular tachycardia, including when it occurs in

Introduction

Critical care transport professionals (CCTPs) routinely encounter patients with cardiac arrhythmias and need to be familiar with interpretation and monitoring of the 12-lead electrocardiogram (ECG), including the electrophysiology underlying the ECG changes and its implications for the patient. In addition, familiarity with temporary and implanted pacemakers and defibrillators, including transport safety and the ability to troubleshoot problems that may arise with these cardiac devices, is a key skill for CCTPs.

The 12-lead ECG graphically represents electrical activity in cardiac tissue. Cardiac monitoring in the CCT setting typically includes a view of the heart's electrical rhythm in three or more leads and, when indicated, the serial evaluation of 12-lead ECGs. In some cases, additional precordial leads are placed for the diagnosis of right ventricular and posterior infarctions. A key role of the CCT team is to continuously monitor the cardiac rhythm and serial 12-lead ECGs, responding to changes with rapid and appropriate interventions. With that in mind, this chapter provides concise methods and patterns of interpretation to help CCTPs develop a deeper understanding of electrophysiology and of both typical and unusual changes observed in electrical activity as a result of injury or illness.

Traditionally, cardiac arrhythmias have been treated pharmacologically. Unfortunately, cardioactive medications often have side effects that can reduce the patient's quality of life; in some cases, they may be ineffective, even when prescribed appropriately and taken with good compliance. The tremendous evolution of pacing technology has allowed more types of arrhythmias to be treated electrically, with patients often having little to no awareness of the times when electrical therapy is being delivered.

Implanted pacemakers, temporary (transvenous and transcutaneous) pacemakers, wearable defibrillators, and implantable cardioverter-defibrillators (ICDs) vastly broaden the array of therapeutic options for patients with advanced heart failure (HF) and for patients with cardiac arrhythmias. These adjuncts also require care providers, including CCTPs, to have considerable levels of technological expertise in their use. This chapter describes aspects of implantable, temporary, and wearable devices and the electrical therapies that may be important during transport.

Cardiac Anatomy and Physiology
The Heart

Although CCTPs are already familiar with cardiac anatomy and physiology, this section provides a brief review. **FIGURE 14-1** shows the anatomy of the heart.

Myocardial cells require an uninterrupted supply of oxygen and nutrients. Indeed, the cardiac demand for oxygen is particularly unremitting because the heart never stops to rest (without catastrophic consequences). Thus, it is essential that the heart have an absolutely reliable blood supply. Oxygenated blood reaches the heart through the coronary arteries **FIGURE 14-2**, which branch off the aorta at the coronary ostia, just above the leaflets of the aortic valve. The numerous connections (anastomoses) between the arterioles of the various coronary arteries allow for the development of collateral circulation in case of blockage. Unfortunately, the coronary arteries are also vulnerable to narrowing from atherosclerotic heart disease. When the lumen

of one of the arteries becomes so narrowed that blood flow through it is impeded, the symptoms of angina occur.

Heart Sounds

The purpose of listening to heart sounds is to identify the "lub-dub" that indicates the cardiac valves are operating properly. The major heart sounds are the two normal sounds, S_1 and S_2 **FIGURE 14-3**, and the two abnormal sounds, S_3 and S_4 **FIGURE 14-4**.

S_1 occurs near the beginning of ventricular contraction (systole), when the tricuspid and mitral valves close. The closing of these two valves should occur simultaneously as the pressure within the ventricles increases, an action that creates the "lub" sound. Any delay in the closing of these two valves, heard as a split sound, is considered abnormal.

S_2 occurs near the end of ventricular contraction (systole), when the pulmonary and aortic valves close. As the ventricles relax, these valves close because of backward flow in the pulmonary artery and aorta. The two valves can close simultaneously or with a slight delay between them under normal physiologic circumstances; this action creates the "dub" sound.

S_3 is the result of the end of the rapid filling period of the ventricle during the beginning of diastole. An S_3 sound should occur 120 to 170 ms after S_2, if it is heard at all. S_3 is generally heard in children and young adults. When it is heard in older adults,

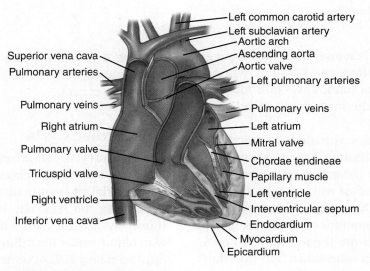

FIGURE 14-1 Anatomy of the heart.
© Jones & Bartlett Learning.

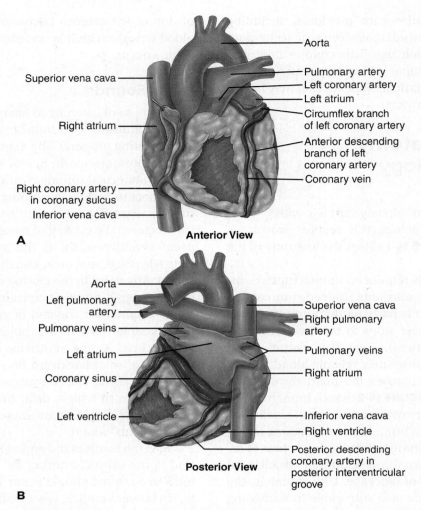

FIGURE 14-2 Coronary arteries. **A.** Anterior view, showing the takeoff point of the left and right main coronary arteries from the aorta. **B.** View from below and behind, showing the coronary sinus.

© Jones & Bartlett Learning.

it often signifies HF. S₃ is sometimes called a gallop, to help differentiate it from the S_4 sound. When S_3 is present, the heartbeat sounds like "dub-lub-dub" (the second sound is the most pronounced, as in the word "Kentucky").

S_4, if heard, coincides with atrial contraction at the end of ventricular diastole. If heard at any other time, it usually means patients have resistance to ventricular filling, as occurs with a weak left ventricle. S_4 is also normally heard in children and young adults. This sound is sometimes called an S_4 gallop, to help differentiate it from the S_3 sound. When S_4 is present, the heartbeat sounds like "lub-dub-dub" (the first sound is more pronounced than the latter two, as in the word "Tennessee").

TABLE 14-1 lists some of the most common heart sounds, where they are heard, and potential associated causes.

The Cardiac Cycle

The cardiac cycle comprises one complete phase of atrial and ventricular relaxation (diastole) followed by one atrial and ventricular contraction (systole).

During the relatively longer relaxation phase (normally 520 ms), the left atrium fills passively with blood, under the influence of venous pressure. Approximately 80% of ventricular filling also occurs during this time as blood flows through the open tricuspid and mitral valves.

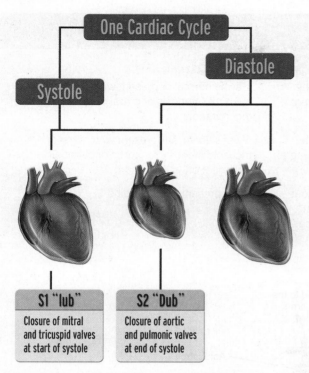

FIGURE 14-3 The normal S_1 and S_2 heart sounds.
© Jones & Bartlett Learning.

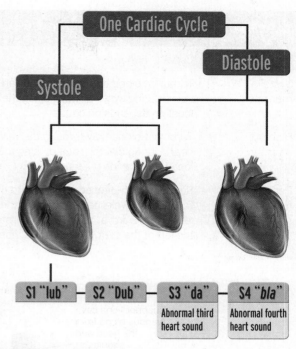

FIGURE 14-4 The abnormal S_3 and S_4 heart sounds.
© Jones & Bartlett Learning.

TABLE 14-1 Heart Sounds		
Heart Sound	**Usual Location**	**Cause**
S_1	Loudest in the mitral area; heard using the diaphragm of the stethoscope	Normal
Split S_1	Between the apex of the heart and the sternum, usually during expiration; heard using the diaphragm	May be normal, nonsynchronous closing of mitral and tricuspid valves or pathologic, such as in a bundle branch block, an atrial septal defect, or pulmonary stenosis
S_2	Loudest in the aortic area; heard using the diaphragm	Normal
Split S_2	Loudest in the pulmonic area, usually on inspiration; heard using the diaphragm	May be normal, nonsynchronous closing of aortic and pulmonic valves or pathologic, such as in hypertension
S_3/ventricular gallop	Heard in early diastole just after the S_2; heard at the apex (left ventricular gallop) or at the left sternal border (right ventricular gallop); loudest on expiration with the patient in the lateral position; heard using the bell of the stethoscope	Always abnormal in older adults; indicates ventricular filling; may be normal in children and young adults or present with diseases such as mitral valve regurgitation, hyperthyroidism, and heart failure
S_4/atrial gallop	Heard late in diastole just before S_1, at the apex or over the suprasternal notch; heard best with the bell	May be normal (children and young adults); indicates increased resistance to ventricular filling after the atrial contraction; often present after a myocardial infarction

(Continues)

Heart Sound	Usual Location	Cause
Systolic murmur	Turbulent blood flow through the valves of the heart, during systole; heard using the diaphragm; location depends on cause	May be normal or present with aortic or pulmonic stenosis or mitral or tricuspid regurgitation
Diastolic murmur	Turbulent blood flow through the valves of the heart, during diastole; heard using the diaphragm; location depends on cause	Always abnormal; present with mitral or tricuspid stenosis, or aortic or pulmonic regurgitation
Pericardial friction rub	Scratchy, high-pitched sound heard throughout the cardiac cycle; best heard with the patient leaning forward, at the third intercostal space to the left of the sternum, using the diaphragm	Often present in pericarditis

TABLE 14-1 Heart Sounds (continued)

© Jones & Bartlett Learning.

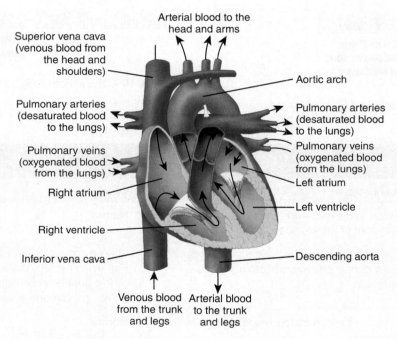

FIGURE 14-5 Blood flow through the heart.

© Jones & Bartlett Learning.

With atrial contraction, the contents of each atrium are squeezed into the respective ventricle to complete ventricular filling (atrial kick). Approximately 70% to 90% of the blood in the atria fills the ventricles by gravity; the remaining 10% to 30% comes from atrial contraction or atrial kick. At the beginning of ventricular contraction, the atrioventricular (AV) valves snap shut, the two ventricles contract (ventricular systole), and the semilunar valves are forced open. Blood squeezed out of the right ventricle moves forward, through the pulmonic valve, and into the pulmonary arteries. Blood from the left ventricle is pushed through the aortic valve and out into the aorta. Systole is usually accomplished in a little more than half the time it takes to fill the ventricles, about 280 ms.

Functionally, the heart is actually two pumps: a right pump and a left pump, separated by a thin wall (the interventricular septum). These pumps are, for purposes of efficiency, housed in one organ and work in parallel **FIGURE 14-5**.

The right side of the heart is a low-pressure, thin-walled pump: It pumps against the relatively low resistance of the pulmonary circulation. The right atrium collects oxygen-poor venous blood from the superior and inferior venae cavae and the coronary sinus and delivers it to the right ventricle, which then pumps the blood into the pulmonary artery for distribution to the alveoli and oxygenation.

After the blood's passage through the alveoli, the pulmonary veins collect the now oxygen-rich blood and return it to the left atrium, which delivers it to the more thickly walled left ventricle. The left side of the heart is a high-pressure pump: It drives blood out of the heart against the relatively high resistance of the systemic arteries.

At any given time, a major proportion of the body's blood flow may be shunted into one of the two circulation systems: the systemic circulation or the pulmonary circulation. If the right side of the pump fails or weakens and cannot squeeze out its contents efficiently, blood will back up behind the right atrium into the systemic veins, which then become engorged and distended. Distention of the external jugular veins signals a back pressure from the right side of the heart throughout the systemic circulation. As pressure increases within the systemic veins, fluid leaks into the surrounding tissues, causing edema. When enough fluid has leaked into the interstitial spaces, edema becomes visible in the subcutaneous tissues (particularly the sacrum and lower extremities); it is less readily visible but equally present in the liver, walls of the intestine, and other internal tissues.

By contrast, if the left side of the pump fails or weakens, blood backs up behind the left atrium into the pulmonary circulation. As pressure builds in the pulmonary veins, fluid is squeezed into the alveoli, producing the characteristic signs and symptoms of pulmonary edema: dyspnea, crackles, and pink, frothy sputum.

The Blood Vessels

FIGURE 14-6 provides a review of the major arteries in the body.

The arterial walls are highly sensitive to stimulation from the autonomic nervous system. In response to such signals, the arterial diameter may change significantly as arteries contract or relax. Baroreceptors sense changes in blood pressure and, in turn, stimulate the autonomic nervous system. Increased blood pressure activates baroreceptors within the parasympathetic nervous system, resulting in a lowered heart rate and decreased myocardial contractility. Decreased blood pressure activates baroreceptors within the sympathetic nervous system, resulting in an increased heart rate and greater myocardial contractility. Blood pressure is influenced not only by the cardiac output and the fluid volume present in the system, but also by the relative constriction or dilation of the arteries.

Chemoreceptors also play a role in autonomic nervous system activation in response to continual monitoring of the partial pressure of oxygen (Po_2) and pH or the partial pressure of carbon dioxide (Pco_2). Chemoreceptors not only stimulate the autonomic nervous system (thereby affecting heart rate and myocardial contractility), but also promote release of dopamine and ultimately cause the respiratory centers in the brainstem to increase or decrease minute ventilation. For example, when the chemoreceptors sense a hypoxia, acidosis, or hypercarbia condition, they trigger sympathetic stimulation, resulting in an increased heart rate and contractility. In contrast, hyperoxia, alkalosis, and hypocarbia lead to parasympathetic stimulation, which produces a decreased heart rate and lessened contractility.

Functioning of the Pump

The following terms are important to understand how the heart functions as a pump:

- *Cardiac output (CO)* is the amount of blood that is pumped out by either ventricle. The left and right ventricles are approximately equal in interior size, so the two ventricles have relatively equivalent outputs. The normal CO for an average adult is 4 to 6 L/min.
- *Stroke volume (SV)* is the amount of blood pumped out by either ventricle in a single contraction (heartbeat). Normally, the SV is 60 to 100 mL, but the healthy heart has considerable spare capacity and can easily increase the SV by at least 50%.
- *Heart rate (HR)* is the number of cardiac contractions (heartbeats) per minute—in other words, the pulse rate. The normal rate for adults is 60 to 100 beats/min.

The volume of blood that either ventricle pumps out per minute equals the volume of blood

Major arteries

Internal carotid
External carotid
Common carotid
Subclavian
Innominate
Axillary
Pulmonary
Ascending aorta

Brachial

Descending aorta

Common iliac
Ulnar
Radial
Palmar arches

Digital

Deep femoral
Superficial femoral

Popliteal

Anterior tibial
Posterior tibial

Peroneal

Dorsalis pedis
Arcuate

Major veins

Internal jugular
External jugular
Innominate
Subclavian
Axillary
Superior vena cava

Pulmonary
Cephalic
Brachial
Antecubital
Inferior vena cava

Common iliac

Volar digital

Great saphenous
Femoral

Popliteal
Anterior tibial

Peroneal
Posterior tibial

Dorsal venous arch

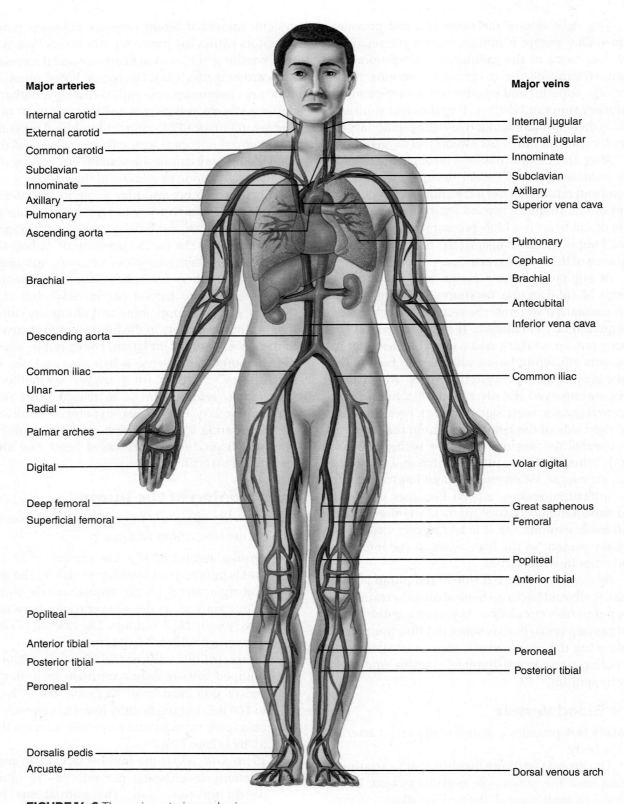

FIGURE 14-6 The major arteries and veins.

© Jones & Bartlett Learning.

it pumps out in a single contraction times the number of contractions per minute:

$$CO = SV \times HR$$

When the body has an increased demand for oxygen, the heart must be able to increase its output several times over. The heart can achieve this feat by increasing SV, increasing HR, or both.

The heart has several ways of increasing SV. One characteristic of cardiac muscle is that, when it is stretched, it contracts with greater force up to a limit, a property called the Frank-Starling mechanism. If an increased volume of blood is returned from the systemic veins to the right side of the heart or from the pulmonary veins to the left side of the heart, the muscle surrounding the cardiac chambers must stretch to accommodate the larger volume. The more the cardiac muscle stretches, the greater the force of its contraction is, the more completely it empties, and, therefore, the greater the SV will be. From the CO equation, it is clear that any increase in SV, with HR held constant, will cause an increase in the overall CO.

The volume of blood returned by the veins to the heart influences preload (the pressure under which a ventricle fills). In situations of increased oxygen demand, the body returns more blood to the heart (preload increases), and CO consequently increases through the Frank-Starling mechanism. In a diseased heart, the same mechanism is used to achieve a normal resting CO (which explains why some diseased hearts become enlarged).

The heart can also vary the degree of contraction of its muscle *without* changing the stretch on the muscle, an ability called contractility. Changes in contractility may be induced by medications that have a positive or negative inotropic effect. The ventricles are never completely emptied of blood, however. The percentage of blood actually ejected, called the ejection fraction, is a reasonable reflection of overall myocardial function. If the heart is more contractile, a larger percentage of the ventricular blood will be ejected, thereby increasing SV and, hence, CO. The nervous system regulates contractility from beat to beat. When the body requires increased CO, nervous signals increase myocardial contractility, thereby augmenting SV.

The heart can also increase its CO, given a constant SV, by increasing HR (the number of contractions per minute). This change is referred to as a positive chronotropic effect.

The Frank-Starling mechanism is an intrinsic property of heart muscle; that is, it is not under nervous system control. By contrast, contractility and changes in HR are regulated by the nervous system.

The Electrical Conduction System of the Heart

Heart muscle can generate its own electrical impulses without nervous system stimulation, a property called automaticity. In addition, the heart is endowed with an electrical conduction system, consisting of specialized conduction tissue that can rapidly propagate electrical impulses to the muscular tissue of the heart. The provider may record these impulses on the ECG; therefore, all CCTPs need to understand the relationship between the activities of the body's electrical conduction system and 12-lead ECG interpretation.

Visualizing the process of impulses traveling in different directions helps to clarify what is happening in the heart. Visualizing the travel of impulses also promotes an understanding of how changes in the structure or function of the heart can alter that travel.

The Dominant Pacemaker: The Sinoatrial Node

Theoretically, any cell within the heart's electrical conduction system can act as a pacemaker. In the normal heart, however, the dominant pacemaker is the sinoatrial (SA) node **FIGURE 14-7**. The SA node receives blood from the right coronary artery (RCA). If the RCA is occluded, as in a myocardial infarction (MI), the SA node may become ischemic. The subsequent death of the conduction cells will prevent the SA node from firing.

The SA node initiates the electrical discharge that passes through the intra-atrial pathways (or intranodal pathways); in physiology, these are sometimes called atrionodal pathways and include the anterior or Bachman bundle, middle bundle, and posterior internodal system. The SA node is the fastest pacemaker in the heart. Electrical impulses generated in this node spread across the two atria through internodal pathways in the atrial wall in approximately 80 ms, causing the atrial tissue to depolarize as they pass. In 85% to 90% of the population,

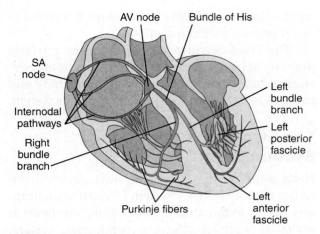

FIGURE 14-7 The electrical conduction system.

© Jones & Bartlett Learning.

the blood supply for the SA node comes from a branch of the RCA; in the remaining 10% to 15% of the population, it comes from a branch of the left circumflex artery. The conduction of the impulse is delayed in the AV node for approximately 120 ms so that the atria can empty into the ventricles.

When the atrial rate becomes very rapid, not all atrial impulses can get through the AV junction. Normally, however, impulses pass through it into the bundle of His and then move rapidly into the right and left bundle branches located on either side of the interventricular septum. Next, they spread into the Purkinje fibers, which comprise thousands of fibrils distributed through the ventricular muscle. It takes approximately 80 ms for an electrical impulse to spread across the ventricles, during which time the ventricles contract simultaneously. The effect on the velocity of conduction is referred to as the dromotropic effect.

Depolarization and Repolarization

As the electrical impulses travel along these pathways, they come in contact with the cardiac cells, which continue the process of generating electrical impulses or depolarization through the properties of automaticity and conductivity. Depolarization, the process by which muscle fibers are stimulated to contract, comes about through changes in the concentration of electrolytes across cell membranes. Myocardial cells, like all cells in the body, are bathed in an electrolyte solution. Chemical pumps inside the cell maintain the concentrations of ions within the cell, in the process creating an electrical

gradient across the cell wall. Consequently, a resting (polarized) cell normally has a net charge of –90 mV with respect to the outside of the cell.

When the myocardial cell receives a stimulus from the conduction system, the permeability of the cell wall changes as specialized channels are opened in such a way that sodium ions (Na^+) rush into the cell, causing the inside of the cell to become more positive. Calcium ions (Ca^{+2}) also enter the cell, albeit more slowly and through a different set of specialized channels, helping maintain the depolarized state of the cell membrane and supplying calcium ions for use in contraction of the cardiac muscle tissue. This reversal of electrical charge (ie, depolarization) starts at one spot in the cell and spreads in a wave along the cell until the cell is completely depolarized. The entire process causes a "wave of depolarization" as the electrical charges pass in all directions from one cell to another. The larger the mass of cardiac muscle, the larger this wave of depolarization will be. As each cell depolarizes, it creates a small electrical vector. In the wave of depolarization, the sum of all these small vectors creates the electrical axis, described later in more detail.

As the cells depolarize and calcium ions enter them, mechanical contraction of the cardiac cells occurs. During diastole, the coronary arteries fill and cardiac circulation occurs. As the cells contract from the base of the heart through the apex, blood is pumped through the pulmonary and systemic circulation.

Following depolarization, each cell must recharge by shifting intracellular electrolytes back into place to ready itself for this continual process. The cell is able to recover from depolarization through a process called repolarization. Repolarization starts with the closing of the sodium and calcium channels, which stops the rapid inflow of these ions. Next, special potassium channels open, allowing a rapid escape of potassium ions (K^+) from the cell. This process helps restore the inside of the cell to its negative charge; the proper electrolyte distribution is then reestablished by pumping sodium ions out of the cell and potassium ions back in. After the potassium channels close, this sodium–potassium pump helps move sodium and potassium ions back to their respective locations. For every three sodium ions that this pump moves out of the cell, it moves two potassium ions into the cell, thereby maintaining the polarity of the cell membrane. To accomplish this task, the sodium–potassium pump moves ions against the natural gradient through a process called active transport, which requires the expenditure of energy.

TABLE 14-2 summarizes the roles of the various electrolytes in cardiac function.

A myocardial cell cannot respond normally to an electrical stimulus from the conduction system unless it is fully polarized. The period when the cell is depolarized or in the process of repolarizing (the **refractory period**) consists of two phases. In the **absolute refractory period**, the heart muscle has been drained of energy and needs to recharge; it will not contract during this period. In the **relative refractory period**, the heart is partially charged, but not strongly enough to create a full contraction.

Secondary Pacemakers

The SA node normally has the most rapid intrinsic rate of firing (60 to 100 times per minute), so it will literally outpace any slower conduction tissue. If it becomes damaged or is suppressed, any component of the conduction system may act as a secondary pacemaker. The further down the conduction system the pacemaker is, the slower its intrinsic rate of firing will be. Thus, the AV junction will spontaneously fire 40 to 60 times per minute, whereas the ventricular Purkinje system, which is further removed from the SA node, will spontaneously fire only 20 to 40 times per minute.

Measuring the Electrical Conduction Activity of the Heart

The electrical conduction events in the heart can be recorded on an ECG as a series of waves and complexes **FIGURE 14-8**. The depolarization of the atria produces the P wave. It is followed by a brief pause as conduction is momentarily slowed through the AV node or AV junction, which can be seen on the ECG as the **PR interval**. Collectively, the electrical impulses that pass through the right and left bundle branches and Purkinje fibers, representing depolarization of the ventricles, are depicted by the **QRS complex**. Repolarization of the atria and ventricles produces the **T wave**; however, the atrial repolarization wave is small and is buried within the QRS complex, so it is not seen on the ECG. The

TABLE 14-2 The Role of Electrolytes in Cardiac Function	
Electrolyte	**Role in Cardiac Function**
Sodium (Na$^+$)	Flows into the cell to initiate depolarization
Potassium (K$^+$)	Flows out of the cell to initiate repolarization • Hypokalemia → increased myocardial irritability • Hyperkalemia → decreased automaticity, conduction, and contractility
Calcium (Ca^{+2})	Has a major role in the depolarization of pacemaker cells (maintains depolarization) and in myocardial contractility (involved in contraction of heart muscle tissue) • Hypocalcemia → decreased contractility and increased myocardial irritability • Hypercalcemia → increased contractility
Magnesium (Mg^{+2})	Stabilizes the cell membrane; acts in concert with potassium, and opposes the actions of calcium • Hypomagnesemia → prolonged conduction • Hypermagnesemia → increased myocardial irritability

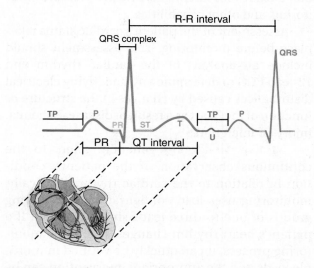

FIGURE 14-8 The electrocardiogram and cardiac events.

larger ventricular T wave follows the QRS complex. The ST segment, which comprises the section of the complex spanning from the end of the QRS complex to the beginning of the T wave, is important in ECG interpretation and represents the period of inactivity between ventricular depolarization and repolarization. Mechanically, it represents the time that the myocardium is maintaining contraction. Finally, a U wave may be present after the T wave. It is unclear exactly what the U wave represents, but its presence can suggest certain conditions discussed later in this chapter.

Any event that changes the structure or function of the cardiac cells typically results in changes in the normal size and shape (morphologic features) of the complexes recorded on the ECG. The strategically placed ECG leads detect this electrical wave of depolarization in the selected positive lead, and the wave is recorded on the ECG as the familiar P-QRS-T waveform.

Cardiac Monitoring: 12-Lead ECG
Monitoring Versus Assessment

Today's cardiac monitors and defibrillators are typically multiparameter devices that can combine continuous 3-lead ECG monitoring, 12-lead electrocardiography, semiautomatic and manual defibrillation, external pacing, capnography, pulse oximetry, blood pressure monitoring, end-tidal carbon dioxide measurements, invasive pressure monitoring, and other capabilities.

Assessment of the patient's cardiac status takes place before monitoring. This assessment should include an analysis of the cardiac rhythm and 12-lead ECG to determine any underlying electrical disturbances caused by changes in the structure or function of the heart as a result of disease, ischemia, injury, or infarction.

Cardiac monitoring generally refers to the continuous observation of the patient's condition in relation to the cardiac rhythm. Typically, monitoring uses lead configurations for viewing groups of one to three leads simultaneously. If a patient's heart rhythm changes during the monitoring process, it can quickly be verified in multiple leads and the appropriate intervention can be initiated.

Lead Placement

The equipment used to record the ECG may vary widely. Lead placement could also vary when using a machine that derives the 12-lead ECG from a 5- to 6-lead system. Several manufacturers currently produce this equipment, and each has its own proprietary lead set and lead configurations. Major problems can result from using different techniques to acquire the "standard" 12-lead ECG. The gold standard for 12-lead ECG interpretation is the ability to perform serial evaluations for comparison; however, it is important to use consistent lead placements to ensure that all providers compare "apples to apples." Therefore, for simplicity and consistency, in this chapter the discussion of 12-lead ECG will use the "standard" lead placements and the views recorded from them.

The terms *lead*, *electrode*, and *cable* are often used interchangeably, which can be misleading; standard terminology should be used to avoid confusion. The electrode is the sensing device that connects directly to the skin; it is usually a self-adhesive pad with some form of conduction media embedded in it to improve the connection of the electrode to the skin, thus improving the quality of the ECG. The lead is the designated position of the electrode (ie, limb and precordial/chest leads); it names the electrode placement, which explains why these two terms are often used synonymously. The cable is the physical wire that connects the electrode to the ECG monitor.

Before connecting the electrodes to the patient's chest, the CCTP should prepare the patient's skin to help improve the quality of the ECG. The skin should be clean and dry, and should be slightly abraded by rubbing with a gauze pad. In addition to drying the skin, the latter step helps remove oils and improves the connection with the electrode. The skin may also be wiped with an alcohol pad to assist in drying the skin and removing oils. In a patient with excessive chest hair (or back hair, when additional nonstandard posterior leads are used), the hair should be clipped with a safety razor before connecting the electrodes. Other unusual conditions affecting the quality of the connection with the electrode to the skin should be corrected as necessary. In patients with extreme diaphoresis, it may be necessary to use topical benzoin or another skin preparation compound to enhance adherence of electrodes to the skin.

The importance of the conduction medium applied to the skin electrode cannot be overemphasized. Because this medium is most often a gel and subject to drying if exposed to air, electrodes applied to the patient should be replaced daily. Additionally, electrodes and pacer/defibrillator pads should remain sealed in their packaging prior to use to prevent drying of the conductive medium, which usually occurs within 24 hours of being exposed to air.

To get an accurate illustration and record the electrical activity of the heart, the leads must be placed so that each provides a unique view **FIGURE 14-9**. The six limb leads (I, II, III, aVR, aVL, and aVF [a, augmented; V, voltage; R, right arm; L, left arm; F, foot]) provide a view of the heart in a vertical plane, also called the frontal plane. In contrast, the six precordial leads (V_1 to V_6), or chest leads, show a horizontal plane. When the leads are placed in the standard locations, each provides a view of a particular region of the heart. For this reason, it is important to place the leads in the proper location each time. The combination of limb leads and precordial leads provides a three-dimensional view of the heart **FIGURE 14-10** and **FIGURE 14-11**. The six limb leads are created using only four electrodes (right arm, left arm, right leg, and left leg); the four electrodes on the body create six actual readings on the ECG.

The average of all electrical impulses generated in the heart can be detected and recorded by the ECG monitor through the combination of leads. These electrical impulses are displayed on the cardiac monitor and can be printed in a standard ECG format.

To better understand the normal waveforms such as P-QRS-T and any additional electrical impulses or changes in the typical presentation, CCTPs should recall that electricity flows from negative toward positive. All ECG leads are considered positive when selected to record the electrical impulse. If the flow of electrical activity proceeds unimpeded toward a positive lead, it will be represented as a positive deflection on the ECG. If the flow of electrical activity flows away from a positive lead, it will be deflected negatively. An electrical impulse that crosses perpendicular to a positive lead is called isoelectric **FIGURE 14-12**.

If the electrical impulse of the heart is deflected by a change in structure or function, it will be less positive, aberrantly conducted, or deflected away from the selected electrode. Because the heart is a three-dimensional organ and the electrical impulses travel through the cardiac tissue in all directions, the leads of the cardiac monitor must be placed in the proper anatomic location to detect these impulses. Traditionally, leads have been categorized as unipolar or bipolar, depending on how they function. The standard limb leads I, II, and III are bipolar leads because they use two leads, a positive and a negative, to measure the electrical

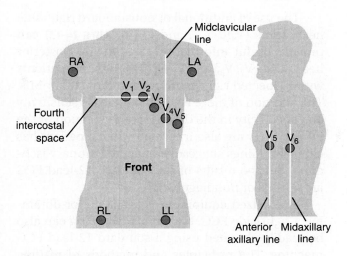

FIGURE 14-9 Limb lead and precordial lead placement.
Abbreviations: LA, left arm; LL, left leg; RA, right arm; RL, right leg

© Jones & Bartlett Learning.

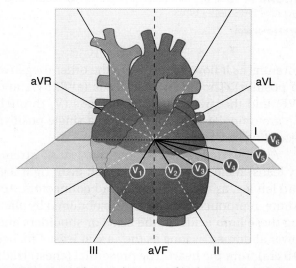

FIGURE 14-10 The combination of limb and precordial leads provides a three-dimensional view of the heart.

© Jones & Bartlett Learning.

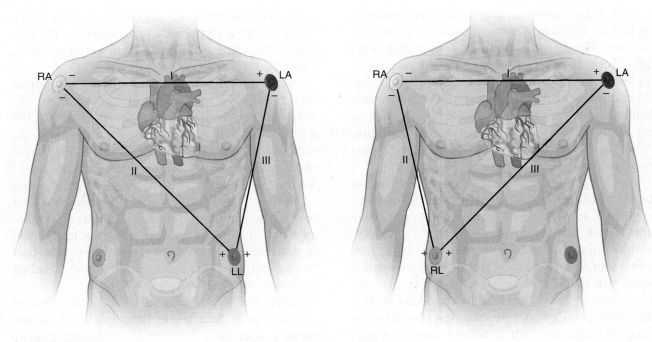

FIGURE 14-11 Each bipolar lead has a positive end and a negative end.

Abbreviations: LA, left arm; LL, left leg; RA, right arm; RL, right leg

Reproduced from *Introduction to 12-Lead ECG: The Art of Interpretation*, courtesy of Tomas B. Garcia, MD.

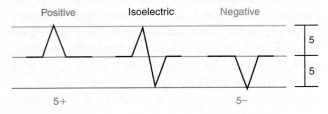

FIGURE 14-12 Representation of positive, isoelectric, and negative QRS deflections.

© Jones & Bartlett Learning.

potential as it flows from one to the other (negative to positive). The augmented leads (aVR, aVL, and aVF) and the precordial (chest) leads (V_1 through V_6) are unipolar because they use a single positive recording electrode.

As shown in Figure 14-9, the limb leads (extremity leads) include the right arm, left arm, right leg, and left leg, as marked on the lead connectors. Accurate, reproducible ECGs can be obtained by placing these limb leads on the arms or shoulders and lower abdomen as long as they are at least 4 inches (10 cm) from the heart. The precordial (chest) leads must be consistently placed in the proper locations:

- V_1 is placed in the fourth intercostal space to the right side (patient's right) of the sternum.

- V_2 is placed in the fourth intercostal space to the left side (patient's left) of the sternum.
- V_3 is placed between V_2 and V_4.
- V_4 is placed in the fifth intercostal space (patient's left) midclavicular line.
- V_5 is placed between V_4 and V_6.
- V_6 is placed in the fifth intercostal space (patient's left) midaxillary line.

The use of additional or nonstandard right-side heart leads (V_4R, V_5R, and V_6R **FIGURE 14-13**) can provide useful information, as can the posterior heart leads V_7, V_8, and V_9 **FIGURE 14-14**, in patients with suspected right ventricular and posterior MIs. The addition of these leads can increase sensitivity and specificity in the detection and location of the infarct. They are also indicated when a patient has clinical findings suggestive of acute coronary ischemia, but the results of the standard 12-lead ECG are normal or nondiagnostic.

Specialized equipment is available for obtaining a right-side ECG, but such a recording can also be readily obtained using a standard 12-lead ECG machine. The principles and methods of reading the additional-lead ECG remain the same as for the 12-lead ECG, except that the leads are "looking" at a different anatomic location. When switching

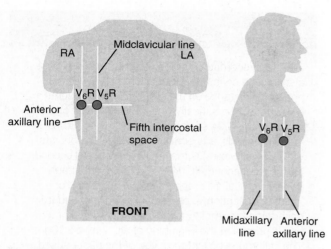

FIGURE 14-13 Placement of right-side leads.

Abbreviations: LA, left arm; RA, right arm

© Jones & Bartlett Learning.

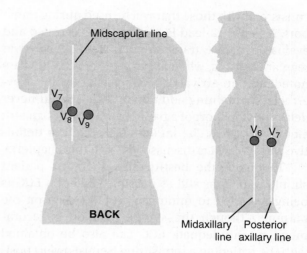

FIGURE 14-14 Placement of posterior leads.

© Jones & Bartlett Learning.

standard 12-lead ECG leads to conform to the non-traditional right-side and posterior leads, the ECG printout should be labeled to represent the leads recorded.

Prior to running an ECG with right-side leads, a standard 12-lead ECG should be completed. Then, the additional leads are attached as follows, using the precordial (chest) leads (in these descriptions, "right" and "left" refer to the patient's right and left sides, respectively):

- V_4R is placed in the right midclavicular line, fifth intercostal space, and connected using the V_3 lead. V_4R has the greatest diagnostic accuracy for RV infarct.
- V_5R is placed in the right anterior axillary line, on a straight line from V_4R, and connected using the V_2 lead.
- V_6R is placed in the right midaxillary line, on a straight line from V_5R, and connected using the V_1 lead.
- V_7 is placed in the left posterior axillary line, on a straight line from V_6, and connected using the V_4 lead.
- V_8 is placed in the left midscapular line, on a straight line from V_7, and connected using the V_5 lead.
- V_9 is placed in the left paraspinal line, on a straight line from V_8, and connected using the V_6 lead.

In the past, the bipolar lead MCL_1 (modified chest lead 1) has been used as a substitute for

cardiac monitoring when using a 3-lead system. Recent research, however, has shown that QRS morphologic features, when recorded simultaneously with V_1 and MCL_1, are different in a significant number of cases (38%). Thus, this recording is not recommended when it is possible to obtain a true V_1 lead. Given the monitoring systems used in the CCT setting, the 12-lead ECG and multiple-lead monitoring should be the standard of care.

Confirmation of Lead Placement

Confirming lead placement might seem like a redundant act, but in the CCT environment, there are innumerable opportunities for leads to become disconnected. As described later in this chapter, because each lead "looks" at a particular anatomic area of the heart, mixing up the leads will cause erroneous ECG readings, which could result in inappropriate therapeutic interventions. Placement should be confirmed before transport and periodically during transport.

Recording the 12-Lead ECG

The acquisition of a 12-lead ECG is a simple procedure that takes only a few minutes. In the CCT setting, it can be assumed that the patient has already had baseline ECG evaluations and that the ECG monitoring system has been connected to the patient before transport. With interfacility transports, CCTPs must ensure that the monitoring system and lead configuration at the initial facility are consistent with those that will be used during transport. A "new" 12-lead ECG should be recorded and evaluated before transport and then repeated at regular intervals, when any changes in the ECG are noted, and on arrival at the receiving facility. Nevertheless, obtaining additional ECGs should never delay the transport of a patient with an **ST-segment elevation myocardial infarction (STEMI)** to definitive care (STEMI is discussed later in this chapter).

To obtain the best-quality ECG, the patient should remain as still as possible while the ECG is being recorded to minimize artifacts seen on the output. Although the supine position is recommended, an adequate ECG can also be obtained with the patient in a semisitting (semi-Fowler) position. (Any patient position other than supine during ECG acquisition should be noted on the ECG tracing.) The patient's condition will dictate the position of evaluation during transport. If all required electrodes for 12-lead ECG monitoring have not been applied to the skin, they should be placed before the patient is moved. The skin should be prepared as previously described to provide adequate contact with the electrodes. Following this preparatory phase, with the leads connected to the corresponding electrodes, the 12-lead ECG can be obtained.

Before obtaining a 12-lead ECG, standardization (ie, calibration) is necessary. With the 12-lead ECG, amplitude and duration are important factors, especially in analyzing ST segments and making other measurements. Depending on the equipment, the calibration or standardization should be set so that 1 mV is 10 mm high and 200 ms wide. Some equipment can be set to half-standard calibration. This calibration is usually done when the complexes are so tall that they overlap each other on the ECG paper when recorded. Another calibration on newer machines is the paper speed, which should be set at the standard 25 mm/s, not 50 mm/s, which may have been set as the speed to help evaluate the morphologic features of ECG complexes in a tachycardic rhythm. Be sure to check your machine's calibration. Most newer 12-lead ECG machines can provide a printout of all 12 leads, along with a rhythm strip in lead II or another designated lead.

Interpretation of the 12-Lead ECG

Acquisition and interpretation of the 12-lead ECG in the CCT setting can pose unique challenges.

ECG Paper

ECGs are recorded on graph paper that moves past a stylus at a constant speed (25 mm/s). Thus, the horizontal distance on the graph paper represents a given period. Specifically, one small (1 mm) box is the equivalent of 0.04 second (1/25th of a second), or 40 milliseconds, and one large box (which consists of five small boxes) is the equivalent of 0.20 second, or 200 milliseconds (0.04 × 5 = 0.20). The graph paper's vertical axis represents the amplitude or "gain" of deflection, expressed in mV. The standard calibration for amplitude is 10 mm/mV. A calibration box is printed at the beginning of all 12-lead ECGs. The calibration box informs you of the paper speed and amplitude. It measures 5 mm wide by 10 mm tall, representing the standard 25-mm/s paper speed and 10-mm/mV gain.

Typically, time is critical, and using ECG calipers, rulers, axis wheels, and straightedges is particularly difficult in a moving vehicle. These challenges call for greater familiarity with the standard practices and principles of 12-lead ECG interpretation and monitoring. This text emphasizes understanding the electrophysiology underlying ECG changes, which affects how they are depicted on the ECG monitor or printout. Some field-expedient methods of interpretation are discussed to help build the base knowledge expected of the CCTP.

Appearance of the 12-Lead ECG

FIGURE 14-15 provides a graphic representation of what the electrical impulses look like when transmitted to the 12-lead ECG. The configuration of

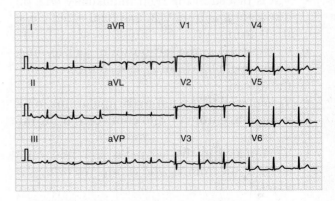

FIGURE 14-15 A normal 12-lead electrocardiogram.

© Jones & Bartlett Learning.

the complexes varies somewhat from lead to lead; therefore, before attempting to identify any abnormalities, CCTPs must know what a typical complex looks like from each lead. In addition, CCTPs must know what a normal 12-lead ECG pattern looks like. If the ECG does not fit this pattern, the CCTP should consider an abnormality to be present.

In the limb leads, the P wave is typically upright in leads I, II, aVL, and aVF. It is frequently biphasic in lead III and is purely negatively deflected in lead aVR. In the precordial leads, the P wave is typically upright in leads V_5 and V_6. Lead V_1 is biphasic, and leads V_2 and V_4 are variable. These are the typical presentations for the P wave, although its appearance can vary from person to person. A change in the P-wave morphology suggests an ectopic atrial focus.

The rules for measuring the PR interval remain unchanged from those used in routine cardiac monitoring. The PR interval is a representation of the time from the start of atrial depolarization to the start of ventricular depolarization and includes the delay in conduction that occurs at the AV junction. The PR interval usually lasts from 120 to 200 ms (0.12 to 0.20 s).

The QRS complex is a representation of ventricular depolarization. The septal fascicle delivers the electrical impulse to the interventricular septum, which is the first part of the ventricles to depolarize. Septal depolarization is not always seen on the ECG, but when it is, a small Q wave may be seen in leads I, aVL, V_5, and V_6. **FIGURE 14-16** provides examples of each precordial lead and demonstrates the concept of R-wave progression.

The T wave will usually be recorded in a positive deflection in the same leads that record a positive deflection of the R wave. In other words, positive T waves are usually found in the same leads that have tall R waves.

As discussed in the lead placement section, each lead provides an enhanced view of a particular region of the heart. The electrical activity picked up by this lead placement is then recorded as complexes from these different perspectives. Understanding that each lead represents a different enhanced view of the heart is the first step in learning to scan the 12-lead ECG by anatomic location **FIGURE 14-17** and **TABLE 14-3**. This skill becomes more relevant as CCTPs begin "localizing" areas of the heart to determine where ischemia, injury, and infarction have occurred. The colors in Table 14-3 will be used to represent these same leads and areas in figures later in this chapter.

It is also useful to know the intrinsic rates of cardiac cells because the CCTP may be able to identify a problem simply by determining the heart rate that is produced **FIGURE 14-18**. The higher the cardiac cell is located in the conduction system in the heart, the faster its "firing rate" will be. The slower pacers found lower in the conduction system will not "normally" fire as long as the higher pacers are functioning properly.

A Systematic Approach to Interpretation of the 12-Lead ECG

A variety of approaches to reading 12-lead ECGs have been recommended by multiple sources.

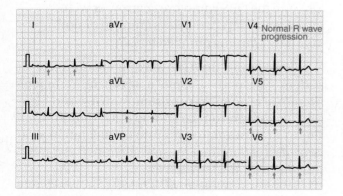

FIGURE 14-16 A small Q wave in leads I, aVL, V_5, and V_6 representing septal depolarization. This electrocardiogram also shows normal R-wave progression.

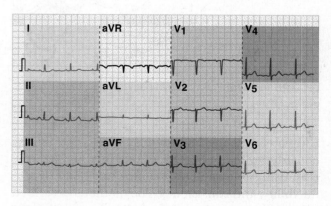

FIGURE 14-17 The relationship between leads and views of the heart.

TABLE 14-3 Leads Listed by the Area of the Heart That They View

Lead	Localized Area
V_1	Septum
V_2	Septum
V_3	Anterior
V_4	Anterior
II	Inferior
III	Inferior
aVF	Inferior
I	Lateral
aVL	Lateral
V_5	Lateral
V_6	Lateral
aVR	None

© Jones & Bartlett Learning.

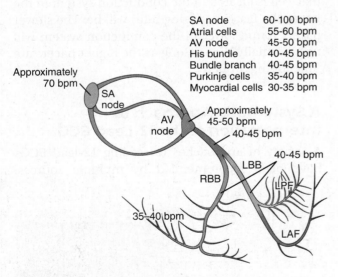

SA node	60-100 bpm
Atrial cells	55-60 bpm
AV node	45-50 bpm
His bundle	40-45 bpm
Bundle branch	40-45 bpm
Purkinje cells	35-40 bpm
Myocardial cells	30-35 bpm

Approximately 70 bpm

SA node

AV node — Approximately 45-50 bpm

40-45 bpm

40-45 bpm

LBB

RBB

LPF

35-40 bpm

LAF

FIGURE 14-18 Intrinsic rates of pacing cells.

© Jones & Bartlett Learning.

Ultimately, the method used is not as important as consistency in application of that method. Repeatedly using one method ensures reliability, reproducibility, and consistency. The methods described here assume a basic understanding of the elements essential to the fundamentals of ECG interpretation and 12-lead ECGs.

The keys to being able to quickly read an ECG are experience and, as stated, consistency. Interpretation of a 12-lead ECG is a skill that must be practiced repeatedly using a standard method of analysis. However, even specialists can reach widely divergent conclusions when examining a routine ECG tracing. The reason this discrepancy is mentioned is to encourage the use of sound methods of interpretation, documentation of findings, and consideration of every piece of patient information.

During the transport of a critically ill patient, the ECG rhythm must be monitored continuously for changes that require intervention. In this setting, however, monitoring should not be mutually exclusive of serial evaluations of the 12-lead ECG. For systematic analysis of the 12-lead ECG, the interpretation of rhythm and arrhythmias is a fundamental building block. In rhythm and arrhythmia interpretation, there are, in general, 10 key elements that must be assessed.

General

1. Is the rhythm fast or slow?
2. Is the rhythm regular or irregular? If irregular, is it regularly irregular or irregularly irregular?

P waves

3. Are there any P waves?
4. Are all the P waves the same?
5. Does each QRS complex have a P wave?
6. Is the PR interval constant?

QRS complexes

7. Are the P waves and QRS complexes associated with one another?
8. Are the QRS complexes narrow or wide?
9. Are the QRS complexes grouped or not?
10. Are there any dropped beats?

Considering the ever-moving environment of patient transport, a rapid assessment technique should be adapted to consistently review and identify changes seen on the 12-lead ECG. The approach shown in **TABLE 14-4** takes into consideration a variety of situations that must be identified and monitored and/or treated right away.

When examining an ECG tracing, CCTPs should document findings as they are discovered to keep an accurate, complete record of changes for serial evaluations. The ECG is a relatively simple test that can provide information about cardiac anatomy,

TABLE 14-4 Rapid 12-Lead ECG Assessment

Verify that aVR is negative (helps to ensure proper lead placement).

Assess rate and rhythm.

Determine the axis (leads I and aVF; also determined by the cardiac monitor's internal diagnostic hardware and printed on the 12-lead ECG).

Identify conduction abnormalities:
- Left bundle branch block
- Hypertrophy
- Aneurysm
- Pericarditis
- Drug or electrolyte imbalance effects
- Early repolarization

Find signs of ischemia, injury, and infarction:
- T-wave inversions
- ST-segment elevation
- Significant Q waves

Identify acute myocardial infarction patterns:
- Anterior
  - ST-segment elevation in V_1, V_2, V_3, and V_4
  - ST-segment depression in II, III, and aVF
- Inferior
  - ST-segment elevation in II, III, and aVF
  - ST-segment depression in V_1, V_2, V_3, or I, and aVL
- Lateral
  - ST-segment elevation in I, aVL, V_5, and V_6
  - ST-segment depression in II, III, and aVF
- Septal
  - ST-segment elevation in I, aVL, V_1, and V_2
- Posterior
  - Tall, wide R waves and ST-segment depression in V_1 and V_2
  - T-wave inversion and ST-segment elevation in alternative posterior leads V_7, V_8, and V_9
- Right ventricular
  - ST-segment elevations in V_4R, V_5R, and V_6R

Consider the patient's clinical picture.

© Jones & Bartlett Learning.

pathology, and pathophysiology as well as effects of treatment.

The 12-lead ECG shows groupings of complexes that are recorded simultaneously by each lead. The rhythm strip, which typically appears at the bottom of the ECG, records for the entire time that the 12-lead ECG is being obtained. For comparison of cardiac electrical events, the series of complexes viewed in lead I is recorded at the same time as the complexes in the other leads. Their appearances are different because of the angle at which the electrical vectors are viewed.

Axis Determination

As previously mentioned, each cell in the heart can produce its own electrical impulse. Each impulse, in turn, varies in intensity and direction. The term *vector* is used to describe these electrical impulses, and the *axis* is the direction of the wave of depolarization as it passes through the heart. The sum of all of the electrical impulses is called the **mean electrical axis**.

As the electrical impulses or vectors travel through the heart toward the larger muscle mass of the left ventricle, the mean electrical axis should progress in a downward and leftward direction. Because the mean electrical axis is the sum of all vectors traveling in different directions, a change in the patient's normal or preexisting axis indicates that a change has occurred in the structure or function of the heart. For example, in a patient with ventricular hypertrophy, the sum of the electrical vectors will shift toward the enlarged ventricle. If an infarction occurs, the area of myocardium affected will not transmit electrical impulses or will transmit them abnormally, causing a shift away from the infarction. If a section of the electrical conduction system is diseased or blocked, the impulses or vectors will shift away from the affected area.

Although the electrical axis is measured and evaluated by the internal diagnostic software of the cardiac monitor and printed on most standard 12-lead ECGs, any health care provider who reads ECGs must know how these determinations are made. This section explains how to determine the direction of the mean electrical axis.

The Hexaxial System

The **hexaxial system** uses a circular diagram divided into 12 equal segments to describe the frontal plane that is created using the limb leads (I, II, III, aVR, aVL, and aVF) **FIGURE 14-19**. As mentioned earlier, the mean electrical axis is the sum of all vectors generated in the wave of depolarization. To isolate the direction of the axis, two leads are required. To illustrate how this combination of leads is used, the hexaxial circle is divided into four quadrants moving clockwise from 0° to +90°, +90° to 180°, 180° to −90°, and −90° to 0°. A wave of depolarization directed into one of these quadrants will give the general direction of the mean electrical axis.

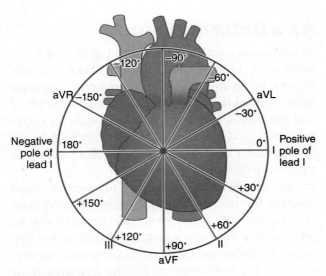

FIGURE 14-19 The hexaxial system.

© Jones & Bartlett Learning.

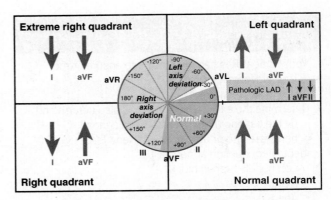

FIGURE 14-20 Electrocardiographic axis presentation of left axis deviation (LAD) and right axis deviation (RAD).

© Jones & Bartlett Learning.

The QRS complex is a representation of the depolarization of both ventricles. The sum of all the vectors generated creates the mean QRS vector in a direction downward and to the patient's left. The mean QRS vector is used to determine the mean electrical axis.

The first lead examined to determine the direction of the mean QRS vector is lead I. Electrical impulses that flow toward the positive electrode create an upright deflection, whereas an electrical impulse that flows away from the positive electrode has a negative deflection. Lead I is the positive lead located at 0°. As the wave of depolarization travels toward lead I, it is shown as a positive deflection on the ECG. If the QRS complex is negatively deflected in lead I, the wave of depolarization shifts away from the left, which means that it is "deviated" toward the right: a right axis deviation (RAD).

The second lead examined to determine the axis is lead aVF. In aVF, the positive electrode is located on the left leg or lower left abdomen at least 4 inches (10 cm) from the heart. Electrically, this placement is at +90°. If the wave of depolarization is downward, it is moving toward the positive electrode in lead aVF and will be shown as a positive deflection of the QRS on the ECG. If the QRS is positive in leads I and aVF, the mean electrical axis is downward (aVF) and toward the patient's left (lead I). This is the normal axis range **FIGURE 14-20**.

If the QRS complex is deflected positively in lead I, the axis is directed toward the left. A QRS complex that is negatively deflected in lead aVF at the same time that it is positive in lead I indicates that the axis is deflected upward and to the left: a left axis deviation (LAD).

If lead I is deflected negatively, the axis is deviated to the right. If lead aVF is deflected negatively at the same time, the axis is shifted upward and to the right, causing an extreme RAD. Extreme RAD, –90° to 180°, is rare. It occurs when the heart is depolarizing inferiorly to superiorly. Extreme RAD can be seen in ventricular tachycardia (VT), atypical MIs, hyperkalemia, and, occasionally, right ventricular hypertrophy (RVH).

FIGURE 14-21 shows sample ECG waves for practice in determining the quadrant in which the mean electrical axis is located. The mean QRS axis is in a "quadrant" of normal, RAD, extreme RAD, or LAD. Noting a change in the electrical axis during the transport of a critically ill patient alerts CCTPs to search for the cause of the deviation. Once an abnormal axis is determined, other associated abnormalities can be found. Further evaluation can suggest the appropriate intervention. In the CCT environment, noting the change of axis is more important than calculating the degree of axis. Nevertheless, some rapid assessment techniques can be used to help narrow down the degree of axis.

Normal Versus Pathologic Measurements

Before determining the degree of the mean electrical axis, it is important to recognize that the quadrants may overlap to some extent. The methods already discussed provide good approximations of

Remember, use your calipers!

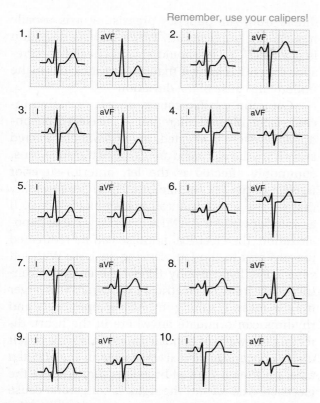

FIGURE 14-21 Sample electrocardiographic waves from which to determine the mean electrical axis.

Reproduced from *Introduction to 12-Lead ECG: The Art of Interpretation*, courtesy of Tomas B. Garcia, MD.

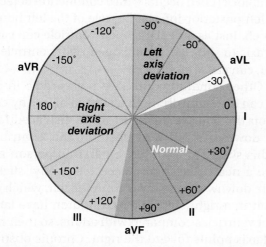

FIGURE 14-22 Pathologic measurements of the hexaxial system.

© Jones & Bartlett Learning.

the axis by isolating the quadrant in which it lies. The true pathologic measurements on the hexaxial system are shown in **FIGURE 14-22**.

The normal ranges for the electrical axis extend from –20° to +100°. The 10° overlap from +90° to

+100° in the right quadrant is not clinically significant. If the axis lies in either of the two right quadrants, the patient has an RAD.

In determining the left axis, it should be noted that normal extends to –20°. The area from –21° to –29° is considered the "physiologic" left axis and is neither pathologic nor normal. The area from –30° to –90° is the true pathologic area of the left quadrant, or LAD. The techniques already discussed should be used to isolate the axis in the left quadrant by determining if the QRS is positive in lead I and negative in lead aVF. If lead II is also negatively deflected, the left axis is between –30° and –90° and indicates the presence of a true pathologic LAD.

Calculation of Axis Direction and Intensity

As shown in Figure 14-19, there are a number of ways to calculate the direction and intensity of the electrical axis. An easy way to make this determination is to use the hexaxial system mentioned earlier. This system uses a circular diagram oriented in the frontal (coronal) plane. The diagram is divided into 12 equal segments around the heart, and each division of the diagram is labeled in degrees. The divisions of the lower half of the diagram are given values ranging from 0° to 180°, and the divisions in the upper half of the diagram have values ranging from 0° to –180°. The limb leads (I, II, III, aVR, aVL, and aVF) are overlaid onto this diagram, with each being oriented to its electrical position on the ECG. Lead I is located at 0°, lead II at +60°, lead aVF at +90°, lead III at +120°, lead aVR at –150°, and lead aVL at –30°. On the hexaxial diagram, each lead has a corresponding lead that is 90° away or perpendicular to the other **FIGURE 14-23**.

To use this system to determine the mean electrical axis, first locate the QRS complex that has the lowest amplitude and is the most isoelectric in one of the limb leads. Then, find the corresponding perpendicular lead. For example, if the most isoelectric QRS complex is in lead II, located at +60°, the corresponding perpendicular lead would be lead aVL, which runs between +150° and –30°. Next, determine whether the QRS is deflected positively or negatively in the perpendicular lead. If it is positive, the mean electrical axis is +150°. If the QRS is negatively deflected, the mean electrical axis is –30°.

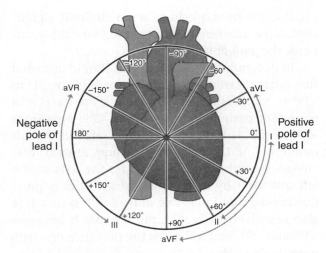

FIGURE 14-23 Perpendicular leads of the hexaxial system.

© Jones & Bartlett Learning.

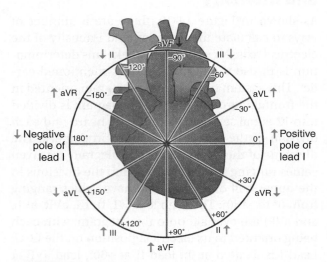

FIGURE 14-24 The hexaxial system with labeled limb leads, degrees, and arrows indicating the QRS deflection.

© Jones & Bartlett Learning.

FIGURE 14-24 shows both ends of each limb lead and their corresponding values. (The arrows show which is positive and which is negative.)

Causes of Axis Deviations

Obtaining a baseline ECG on the cardiac monitor to be used during transport is required before transporting a critically ill patient. A complete assessment of the ECG should be made, noting any abnormalities, including the mean electrical axis. An axis that deviates outside the normal range or differs from the patient's preexisting axis usually has clinical implications. When an axis deviation is detected, CCTPs should always check for corresponding ECG changes that can provide clues to the underlying cause of the deviation.

Common cardiac causes of axis deviation include ischemia and infarction. If the electrical conduction system is affected, the axis will be directed away from the damaged area. One of the areas most commonly affected is the left anterior-superior fascicle of the left bundle branch, an abnormality that results in a left anterior hemiblock (LAH). If an inferior wall MI (IWMI) stops the wave of depolarization, the electrical impulse can be redirected upward and to the left, causing an LAD. With left ventricular hypertrophy (LVH), the enlarged ventricle can draw the electrical axis toward this larger muscle mass, resulting in LAD. Ectopic beats and rhythms can originate anywhere in the heart, directing the wave of depolarization in a right or left direction, causing an axis deviation in the affected area. An RAD is caused by events that redirect the electrical axis toward the right. A congenital cause is **dextrocardia**, which occurs when the heart develops in a right-facing position, creating a mirror image of the normal left-facing heart. Left posterior hemiblock (LPH) occurs with a conduction defect to the left posterior-inferior fascicle of the left bundle branch. Just as an enlarged left ventricle can cause the axis to shift left, an enlarged right ventricle, or RVH, can cause an RAD.

Other conditions that are not cardiac in origin can also contribute to a shift in axis. Any condition that causes the heart to be displaced from the downward leftward position can contribute to this shift. For example, a tall, thin person may have a heart that is displaced (vertically) slightly more downward and away from the left, which can result in a right shift in axis. Children have larger right ventricles compared with adults, so their normal axis points toward the right. Chronic obstructive pulmonary disease (COPD) can lead to RVH, causing an RAD. An LAD can also be caused by mechanical shifts. In patients who are obese or pregnant, the increased intra-abdominal pressure can push up on the diaphragm, displacing the heart into a more horizontal or left position, resulting in an LAD.

TABLE 14-5 summarizes possible causes of various axis deviations.

TABLE 14-5 Possible Causes of Axis Deviation	
Axis Deviation	**Possible Cause**
Right	Right ventricular hypertrophy Left posterior hemiblock Chronic obstructive pulmonary disease Dextrocardia Ectopic beats and rhythms Normal in children
Left	Left anterior hemiblock Left ventricular hemiblock Inferior wall myocardial infarction Ectopic beats and rhythms Obesity Pregnancy

© Jones & Bartlett Learning.

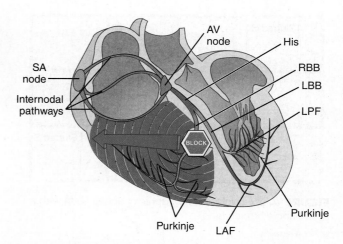

FIGURE 14-25 Right bundle branch (RBB) block.

Abbreviations: AV, atrioventricular; LAF, left anterior fascicle; LBB, left bundle branch; LPF, left posterior fascicle; SA, sinoatrial

© Jones & Bartlett Learning.

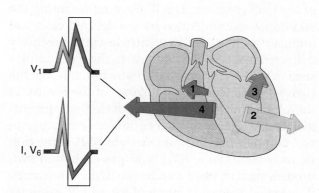

FIGURE 14-26 The effect of a right bundle branch block on the electrocardiogram.

© Jones & Bartlett Learning.

Bundle Branch Blocks and Hemiblocks

When a disruption of the electrical or mechanical response to the wave of depolarization occurs in the heart, bundle branch blocks and hemiblocks may occur. These events may be identified through characteristic changes on the ECG.

Bundle Branch Blocks

A bundle branch block (BBB) is a delay or obstruction along the pathway that electrical impulses travel within the heart.

Right BBB

To recognize a block in electrical conduction through the right bundle branch, think of how the wave of depolarization progresses. The electrical impulses that originate in the atria proceed as normal up to the block, with no change in waveforms or intervals. The impulses then continue down the left bundle branch and its fascicles as usual, but are stopped in the right bundle branch **FIGURE 14-25**.

Diagnosis

When a block occurs, the wave of depolarization must continue through the right ventricle by cell-to-cell conduction. Because cell-to-cell conduction progresses more slowly than conduction through the normal electrical conduction pathway, the representative complex displayed on the ECG will occur late as well, causing a prolonged QRS interval of 120 ms or more. The ECG initially shows the upstroke of the R wave conducted by the left ventricle and its fascicles. Immediately behind this is the delayed right ventricle depolarization resulting in a second R wave called R′ (R prime). The combination of the normally conducted electrical impulse through the left bundle branch and the delayed conduction through the right bundle branch results in the up and down ("rabbit ear") appearance of the QRS complex **FIGURE 14-26**.

The best lead in which to view the changes associated with a right BBB is the precordial lead, V_1,

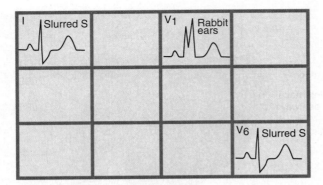

FIGURE 14-27 Electrocardiographic changes seen with a right bundle branch block.

© Jones & Bartlett Learning.

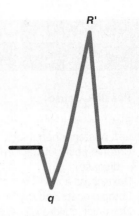

FIGURE 14-28 The qR' wave.

© Jones & Bartlett Learning.

which shows the rsR' complex. Lead V_2 can also show the rsR' complex. The rsR' complex is one in which a second R wave appears in the second half of the QRS complex. The R' wave representing the additional vector created by the delayed electrical impulse through the right ventricle will be positively deflected in lead V_1. In addition to the rsR' complex seen in lead V_1, the delayed conduction through the right ventricle causes a "slurring" of the S wave in the lateral limb lead, lead I, and the left-side precordial lead, V_6. Because other conditions can cause an rsR' complex (eg, incomplete right BBB, some pulmonary conditions, RVH, and pre-excitation syndromes such as Wolff-Parkinson-White syndrome), the slurred S wave is required for an rsR' complex to be diagnostic of a right BBB. **FIGURE 14-27** represents the various leads on an ECG and shows relevant areas for a right BBB diagnosis. (Note: This style of illustration is used repeatedly in this chapter.)

Therefore, the main criteria for the diagnosis of right BBB are as follows:

- QRS prolongation of 120 ms or more
- Slurred S wave in leads I and V_6 (S-wave duration greater than R-wave duration, or S-wave duration greater than 40 ms)
- rsR' pattern in V_1 and V_2, with the R' wave taller than the R wave

A right BBB can occur with disruption of the electrical conduction system, and it can be present in a normal healthy heart.

The QR' Wave

Of the many potential causes of an R' wave in lead V_1, the one that demands the most attention is the Qr' or qR' wave (when their names are written, the larger of the two waves is represented by the upper-case letter) **FIGURE 14-28**.

V_1 is one of the precordial leads that represents the depolarization of the anterior septum (V_2 is the other). A Q wave that occurs in lead V_1 in the presence of a right BBB is evidence of infarction. If this waveform appears during transport of a patient in critical condition, early intervention may prevent ischemia from progressing to infarction.

FIGURE 14-29 provides an example of a right BBB. With practice, by using pattern scanning of the ECG, CCTPs will see the rsR' complex in the precordial leads that represent septal depolarization. Because the rsR' complex alone is not sufficient to make a diagnosis of right BBB, the lateral leads, I and V_6, should also be scanned.

Management

There is no specific treatment required for isolated right BBB. Nevertheless, patients with this condition should have periodic follow-up evaluations.

Left BBB

A left BBB is caused by a disruption of the electrical conduction of the left bundle or both fascicles (the **left anterior fascicle** and the **left posterior fascicle**) of the left bundle. The electrical impulses that originate in the atria proceed as normal, with no change in waveforms or intervals up to the block. The electrical impulses continue to flow unimpeded down the right bundle. With the electrical conduction of the left bundle branch blocked, the wave of depolarization must then proceed by cell-to-cell transmission from right to left **FIGURE 14-30**.

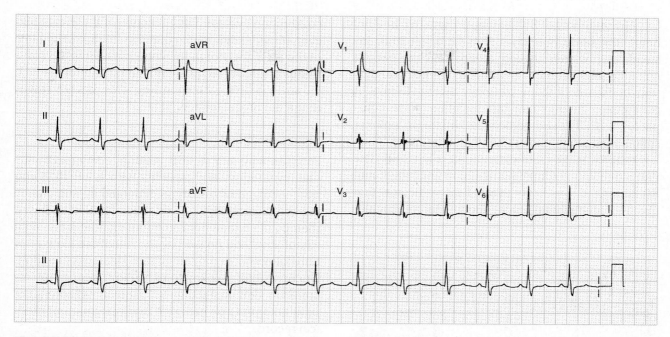

FIGURE 14-29 A 12-lead electrocardiogram showing a right bundle branch block.

Reproduced from *Introduction to 12-Lead ECG: The Art of Interpretation*, courtesy of Tomas B. Garcia, MD.

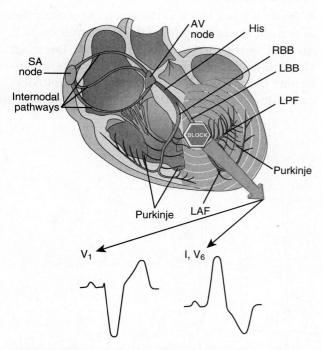

FIGURE 14-30 Left bundle branch (LBB) block.

Abbreviations: AV, atrioventricular; LAF, left anterior fascicle; LPF, left posterior fascicle; RBB, right bundle branch; SA, sinoatrial

© Jones & Bartlett Learning.

Diagnosis

The delay of electrical conduction in the left bundle branch or its fascicles results in a complex that is 120 ms or longer in duration. Because normal ventricular depolarization proceeds down and to the left, the inferior and lateral leads (I, V_5, and V_6) will show the most direct results of the block. With left BBB, the complexes in these leads will not have Q waves, but rather will typically have tall monomorphic R waves. When the conduction of electrical impulses is delayed, the normal sharp rise of the R wave is replaced with a more gradual or bowed, upward appearance. The peak of the R wave is notched, wide, or both. Reciprocal findings are present in the right-side chest leads in the form of wide, deep, monomorphic S waves. Repolarization is also affected in BBBs. In a left BBB, the T waves should be discordant—that is, deflected in the direction opposite to the terminal deflection of the QRS complexes **FIGURE 14-31**.

The main criteria for the diagnosis of a left BBB are as follows:

- QRS complex duration of 120 ms or longer
- V_6 should have a notched R wave with no Q wave
- Wide, deep S waves in lead V_1; may also have a small r wave with a large S wave

Lowercase letters are used to represent small waves, whereas capital letters are used to represent large waves. Therefore, "r wave" represents a small wave, whereas "R wave" represents a large wave.

Although a right BBB can be present in a healthy heart, the same is seldom true for a left BBB. Instead, its presence usually means that the patient has a serious problem within the conduction system or ischemia from coronary artery disease. A pacemaker rhythm can also produce wide complexes, so CCTPs should be watchful for pacemaker spikes with a rhythm that has this appearance.

FIGURE 14-32 is an example of a left BBB. The pattern of wide complexes of 120 ms or longer and discordant T waves in every lead indicates that this is a disturbance that affects the ventricular conduction system. The presence of P waves, however, provides assurance that the rhythm originates in the atria and not in the ventricles. The QRS complexes are deflected positively in the lateral leads (I, V_5, and V_6) with corresponding wide, deep S waves in the reciprocal lead, V_1.

Management

Patients with a left BBB require a thorough cardiac evaluation, and patients with a left BBB and near-syncope or history of syncopal episodes may require a pacemaker. Guidelines for device-based therapy of cardiac rhythm abnormalities have been established and revised by the American College of Cardiology and the American Heart Association. Documentation is key to treatment; hence, any recordings demonstrating left BBB in symptomatic patients should be included in the permanent medical record.

Hemiblocks

A **hemiblock** is a block in the electrical conduction of one of the two fascicles of the left bundle branch. An LAH is the same as a left anterior fascicular block, and an LPH is the same as a left posterior fascicular block. Unlike complete BBBs, hemiblocks cause little to no widening of the QRS complexes

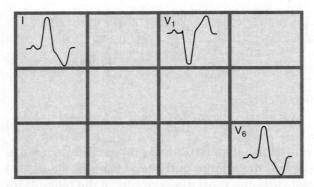

FIGURE 14-31 Electrocardiographic changes seen with a left bundle branch block.

© Jones & Bartlett Learning.

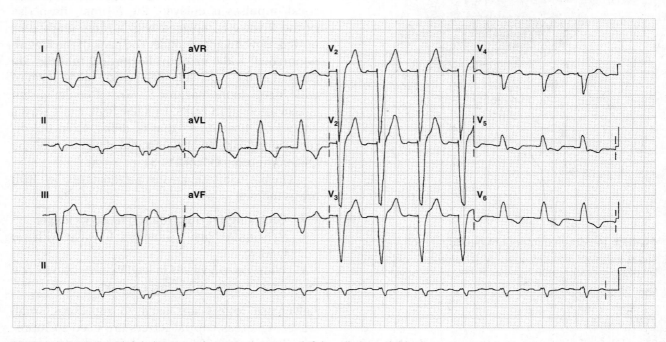

FIGURE 14-32 A 12-lead electrocardiogram showing a left bundle branch block.

Reproduced from *Introduction to 12-Lead ECG: The Art of Interpretation,* courtesy of Tomas B. Garcia, MD.

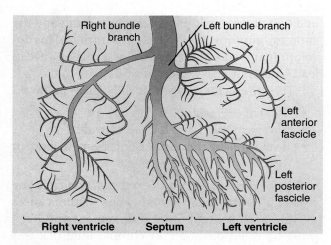

FIGURE 14-33 Ventricular electrical conduction system.

© Jones & Bartlett Learning.

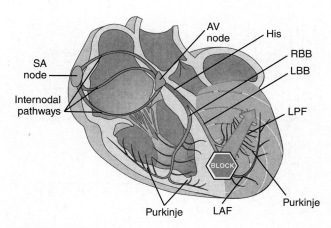

FIGURE 14-34 Left anterior hemiblock.

Abbreviations: AV, atrioventricular; LAF, left anterior fascicle; LBB, left bundle branch; LPF, left posterior fascicle; RBB, right bundle branch; SA, sinoatrial

© Jones & Bartlett Learning.

because the resultant cell-to-cell transmission of the electrical impulses is much less.

Each fascicle branches off of the left bundle branch. The structures of the two fascicles are quite different, however **FIGURE 14-33**. The left anterior fascicle forms a thin bundle of fibers that conducts electrical impulses to the anterior and lateral walls of the left ventricle. In contrast, the left posterior fascicle forms a broad network of fibers that conducts electrical impulses to the inferior and posterior walls of the left ventricle.

The structural differences between these two fascicles clarify why a hemiblock occurs more frequently in the left anterior fascicle. Specifically, it would take a smaller area of ischemia or infarction to impede the electrical conduction to a single strand of fibers than to block the conduction to a broad network of fibers. Even though the blood supply to all areas of the heart varies somewhat from person to person, the left posterior fascicle typically receives blood from branches of the left and right coronary arteries, which means that coronary occlusions would have to occur in both sources of blood supply to have a major effect on the left posterior fascicle.

Left Anterior Hemiblock

An LAH occurs when electrical conduction to the left anterior fascicle is blocked **FIGURE 14-34**.

When conduction to the anterior-superior part of the left ventricle is blocked, depolarization of this area comes from the interventricular septum and retrograde conduction from the inferior and posterior walls. The direction of the wave of depolarization for the blocked area spreads upward and to the left, shifting the electrical axis to the pathologic left, which makes an LAD between −30° and −90° the main criterion for the diagnosis of LAH. Additional findings on the ECG may include a qR complex or a large R wave in lead I. An rS complex also may be found in lead III. These small q and r waves are the result of the interventricular septum depolarizing in an unopposed manner.

The criteria for diagnosing LAH are as follows:

- Left axis deviation within −30° to −90°
- qR complex or large R wave in lead I
- rS complex in lead III (likely to also appear in leads II and aVF)

FIGURE 14-35 is an example of an LAH. The most obvious feature is an LAD. The QRS complex is positively deflected in lead I and negatively deflected in lead aVF. To further isolate this vector to the pathologic range (−30° to −90°), lead II should be examined. Negative deflection, as in this example, confirms the diagnosis of LAD and is presumptive of LAH. Other criteria for LAH are also evident in this example. There is a qR complex in lead I, and there are rS complexes in leads II, III, and aVF. The Q waves that appear in leads I and aVL are insignificant; they are normal and represent the first vector of ventricular depolarization. For a Q wave to be significant and represent an MI, it must be more than one-third the total height of the QRS complex

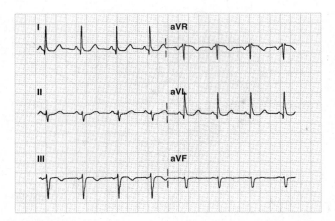

FIGURE 14-35 A 12-lead electrocardiogram showing a left anterior hemiblock.

Reproduced from *Introduction to 12-Lead ECG: The Art of Interpretation*, courtesy of Tomas B. Garcia, MD.

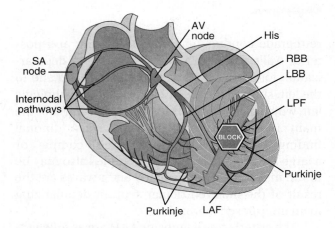

FIGURE 14-36 Left posterior hemiblock.

Abbreviations: AV, atrioventricular; LAF, left anterior fascicle; LBB, left bundle branch; LPF, left posterior fascicle; RBB, right bundle branch; SA, sinoatrial

© Jones & Bartlett Learning.

with which it appears and must also be more than 40 ms in duration.

Left Posterior Hemiblock

An LPH is exceedingly rare because of the dual blood supply to the area and the broad network of fibers that must be blocked to create this condition **FIGURE 14-36**. In addition to being rare, LPH is more difficult to diagnose. When the depolarization of the inferior and posterior portions of the left ventricle is delayed, the resultant wave of depolarization is directed farther inferior and to the right. This rightward deflection results in an RAD. The electrical impulses conducted up to the block are unopposed

and depolarize the interventricular septum and the superior-anterior walls of the left ventricle. This development is shown on the ECG as a small r wave in lead I and a small q wave in lead III.

The criteria for diagnosing LPH are as follows:

- RAD of 190° to 180°
- r wave in lead I and q wave in lead III
- Exclusion of right atrial enlargement and/or RVH

An LPH is a diagnosis of exclusion, which is one reason it is more difficult to diagnose. Other causes of RAD, such as right atrial enlargement and RVH, must be ruled out. Certain chronic lung diseases that cause an overload of the right atrium can be the cause of an RAD. With these additional factors to consider in diagnosing LPH, when an RAD is found, an r wave in lead I and a q wave in lead III should be sought. With no other evidence of right atrial enlargement or RVH, LPH needs to be considered.

FIGURE 14-37 is an example of an LPH. The figure shows an RAD, as well as an s wave in lead I and an insignificant q wave in lead III. There is no evidence of right atrial enlargement.

A pulmonary condition that makes the diagnosis of LPH impossible in many cases is pulmonary embolism. In 15% to 30% of patients with a pulmonary embolism, there is an ECG pattern of $S_1Q_3T_3$ caused by acute right ventricular strain (S_1Q_3 is also a criterion for LPH). This pattern features an s wave in lead I, and a q wave and an inverted T wave in lead III. In this situation, a clinical history suggestive of pulmonary embolism is important information. A thorough history should be obtained, and the reason for transport should be considered.

Bifascicular Blocks

As its name implies, bifascicular block is a condition in which two conduction pathways are blocked at the same time. Such a block includes concurrent findings of right BBB with LAH or LPH.

When right BBB with LAH occurs as a chronic condition, it is considered stable. A new onset of bifascicular block with ischemia, however, is not stable. This presentation will be apparent as a right BBB pattern with a slurred s wave in leads I and V_6 and an up-and-down (rabbit ear) appearance of the RSR′ complex in V_1. The QRS duration will be 120 ms or longer. In addition, with LAH, the typical pattern will include an LAD and rS waves in lead III.

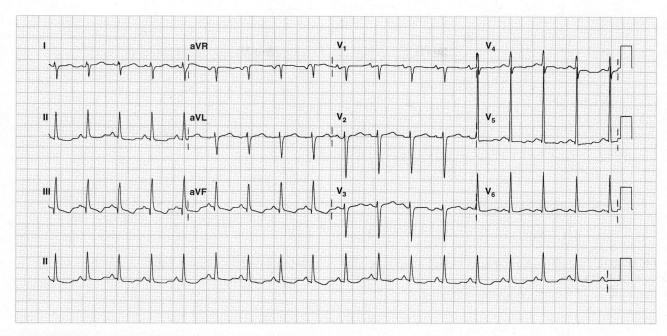

FIGURE 14-37 A 12-lead electrocardiogram showing a left posterior hemiblock.

Reproduced from *Introduction to 12-Lead ECG: The Art of Interpretation*, courtesy of Tomas B. Garcia, MD.

A bifascicular block with a right BBB and an LPH is always considered an unstable rhythm. Owing to the amount of myocardium that must be damaged to cause a true LPH, the defect commonly involves other conduction pathways of the ventricles (right bundle branch). This kind of block often deteriorates into a complete heart block, especially in the presence of an acute MI. Because of the extensive damage it takes to cause an LPH, it does not take much more to progress to a higher degree of block. When a bifascicular block includes a right BBB and an LPH, the typical right BBB pattern with RAD and a small q wave in lead III will be found. **FIGURE 14-38** illustrates two bifascicular block patterns. The right BBB is in black, the LAH is in blue, and the LPH is in green.

FIGURE 14-39 provides an example of a bifascicular block that includes a right BBB with an LAH. To identify it, first scan the ECG for abnormal patterns. In the example, the QRS intervals are 120 ms or more. There is a slurred S wave in leads I and V_6. An RSR′ complex is present in lead V_2. (RSR′ can be found in the septal precordial leads V_1 and/or V_2.) These criteria so far indicate a right BBB. Continue the evaluation, and determine the mean electrical axis. The QRS complex is positively deflected in lead I and negatively deflected in lead aVF,

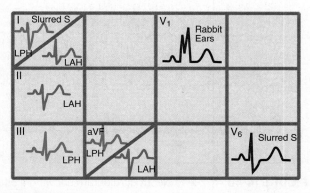

FIGURE 14-38 Electrocardiographic changes seen with a bifascicular block.

© Jones & Bartlett Learning.

indicating LAD. To further isolate the axis, examine lead II. It is negatively deflected, placing the axis between −30° and −90°, the pathologic left axis. This finding provides the additional criterion necessary to determine that an LAH is present.

Bifascicular blocks with a right BBB and an LAH are generally stable unless they occur in the presence of an acute MI. The additional ischemia and tissue death could take out the remaining left posterior fascicle, causing a complete heart block. In a critically ill cardiac patient with an existing bifascicular block consisting of a right BBB and an LAH,

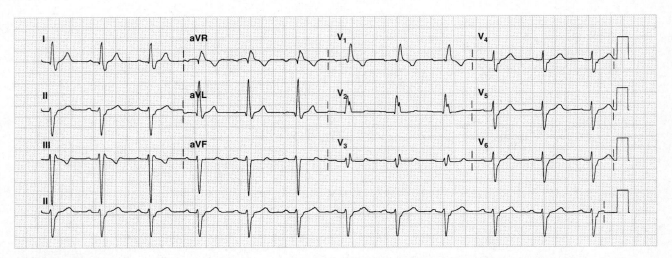

FIGURE 14-39 A 12-lead electrocardiogram showing a bifascicular block with a right bundle branch block and a left anterior hemiblock.

Reproduced from *Introduction to 12-Lead ECG: The Art of Interpretation*, courtesy of Tomas B. Garcia, MD.

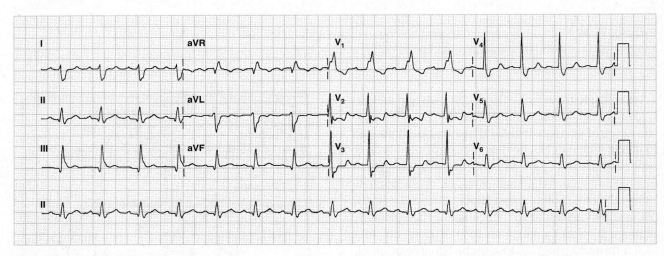

FIGURE 14-40 A 12-lead electrocardiogram showing a bifascicular block with a right bundle branch block and a left posterior hemiblock.

Reproduced from *Introduction to 12-Lead ECG: The Art of Interpretation*, courtesy of Tomas B. Garcia, MD.

signs of ischemia or infarction suggest the need for urgent pacemaker placement, especially in the presence of a second- or third-degree AV block. This procedure will not likely be available in the transport setting, so medical control should be consulted and pads placed for external cardiac pacing. The receiving facility may need to be prepared to place a temporary pacemaker and should be notified of the patient's condition so that a transvenous pacemaker setup is available without delay on arrival. In some cases, depending on the patient's condition and the resources available at the time, a permanent pacer may be implanted immediately.

FIGURE 14-40 provides an example of a bifascicular block with a right BBB and an LPH. To identify it, first scan the ECG for abnormal patterns. Slurred S waves are found in leads I and V_6. There is an RSR′ complex in V_1 consistent with a right BBB. The axis is determined to be in the right quadrant because the rsR is negatively deflected in lead I and positively deflected in lead aVF. To further isolate the axis, find the most isoelectric limb lead with the smallest amplitude. In this example, it is lead aVR. In the hexaxial system, the lead perpendicular (90° away) to aVR is lead III. Assess lead II to determine whether it is positively or negatively deflected. In this case, lead II is positive, placing the mean electrical axis at +120° (RAD). There is also an S wave in lead I and a qS complex in lead III, consistent with an LPH. There are no exclusionary findings to contradict a diagnosis of LPH. Finally, in this example, there is also a first-degree heart block.

This pattern of a right BBB with an LPH is an inherently unstable rhythm owing to the extensive myocardial damage necessary to cause the LPH in the first place. Additional ischemia or even a small infarction could extend the conduction defect to include the anterior fascicle as well.

Trifascicular Blocks

The term trifascicular block is used to describe the combination of a bifascicular block (right BBB with a block in the left anterior fascicle or left posterior fascicle) with a first-degree heart block (prolonged PR interval). Trifascicular block is important to diagnose because it is difficult to tell if the prolonged PR interval seen with the first-degree heart block component is the result of disease in the AV node or is caused by diffuse distal conduction system damage. If the block at the AV node level becomes a complete heart block, the escape rhythm will originate from the bundle of His. This escape rhythm will produce heart rates in the 40s and lead to symptoms of fatigue, near-syncope, or complete syncopal episodes. If diffuse conduction system damage is present, the escape rhythm may be fascicular or ventricular, which may result in heart rates that are life-threateningly low.

The presence of a trifascicular block after an MI implies the presence of extensive cardiac damage. True trifascicular blocks require immediate temporary pacing, followed by the placement of a permanent pacemaker.

Selected ECG Findings

The ECG findings discussed in this section have been selected for review because they can appear alone or coexist with the conditions already discussed. They may help CCTPs identify the many changes in structure and function that occur with chronic conditions or during an acute cardiac event. Ideally, CCTPs will use these findings to help put the pieces of the clinical puzzle together and recognize how they are reflected in the ECG.

Hyperacute T waves

Within the first few minutes of coronary occlusion, the T wave can become tall and narrow because of the ischemia that is present. This peaking is sometimes referred to as a hyperacute T wave. Such a presentation is transient, beginning within minutes to a few hours before the T wave inverts (flips). The first change that might appear with hyperacute T waves is an upward slanting of the ST segment and a subtle enlargement of the T wave that is disproportionate to the QRS complex. The hyperacute T waves are localized to the area of ischemia and infarction and may be associated with depression of the J point and a prolonged QT interval.

Hyperacute T waves differ from those seen in other conditions. In hyperkalemia, for example, the T wave peaking will be tall and narrow and have a "tenting" appearance. These T-wave changes will appear throughout all leads of the ECG. In contrast, hyperacute T waves that occur as a result of ischemia and infarction appear only in leads that view the area of ischemia and infarction.

ST-Segment Elevation

ST-segment elevation is caused by changes that affect ventricular depolarization and repolarization. Non-MI changes can also cause this condition, including left BBB, ventricular rhythms, LVH, pericarditis, and early repolarization.

As the complete ECG picture of infarction evolves, within a few hours the ST segment usually returns to baseline. A persistent ST-segment elevation may indicate the formation of a ventricular aneurysm.

In addition to myocardial injury, ST-segment elevation can be seen in a number of other conditions, such as early repolarization, and is signaled by elevation of the J point. The J point is where the ST segment "takes off" from the QRS complex, and its elevation in the absence of other findings has no pathologic implications. The way to determine the difference between benign elevation of the J point and elevation caused by myocardial injury is to identify the distinctive configuration seen with myocardial disease. In benign J-point elevation, the T wave is clearly distinguished as a separate wave. With myocardial disease, the elevated J point bows upward and merges with the T wave **FIGURE 14-41**.

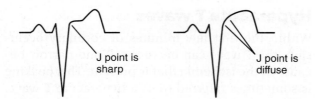

FIGURE 14-41 Sharp and diffuse J points.

© Jones & Bartlett Learning.

Differential Diagnosis

ST-Segment Elevation

- Myocardial disease
- Left BBB
- Ventricular rhythms
- LVH
- Pericarditis
- Early repolarization
- Ventricular aneurysm

Hypertrophy

Hypertrophy is thickening or excessive growth; in this chapter, the term refers to growth of any chamber of the heart. *Hypertrophy* is an increase in muscle mass caused by an increased workload on the heart when it has to pump against resistance; *dilation* is an enlargement of the chamber cavity. These conditions can occur together. The end result is that the heart has a larger mass in the affected area. As discussed in the section on axis determination, the larger the muscle mass, the higher the concentration of electrical impulses or vectors will be.

Left Atrial Enlargement

Left atrial enlargement results in a prolonged electrical conduction time through the left atrium. When normal electrical conduction is initiated by the SA node in the right atrium, the initial impulse is transmitted without delay through this smaller chamber and is recorded on the ECG as the beginning or leading side of the P wave. If the electrical impulse is delayed through an enlarged left atrium, it gives rise to the end or trailing side of the P wave. Overall, the resulting P wave has a notched double-humped appearance.

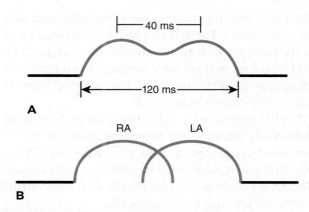

FIGURE 14-42 A. A notched P wave greater than 120 ms in the limb leads shows P mitrale. **B.** The cause of a notched P wave.

Abbreviations: LA, left atrium; RA, right atrium

© Jones & Bartlett Learning.

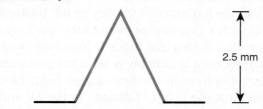

FIGURE 14-43 P pulmonale.

© Jones & Bartlett Learning.

A P wave that is greater in duration than 120 ms in limb leads I and II and has a notched appearance is known as **P mitrale FIGURE 14-42**.

Right Atrial Enlargement

Right atrial enlargement is caused by cardiac and pulmonary conditions affecting the pressures in the right atrium. Causes may include mitral stenosis or regurgitation, COPD, and pulmonary emboli. Right atrial enlargement commonly occurs in conjunction with the pulmonary condition known as **P pulmonale**, which is characterized by tall, peaked P waves in leads II and III that have an amplitude of 2.5 mm (2.5 mV) or more. P waves can be peaked in other conditions, but must be 2.5 mm or higher to make a diagnosis of P pulmonale; if they are less than 2.5 mm, they are not typically associated with right atrial enlargement **FIGURE 14-43**.

When the evidence suggests atrial enlargement but the measurements are not enough to make the diagnosis, some different P-wave patterns might emerge. **Biphasic** P waves in lead V_1 are common. The biphasic P wave indicates nonspecific **intra-atrial conduction delay (IACD)**. Often, biphasic

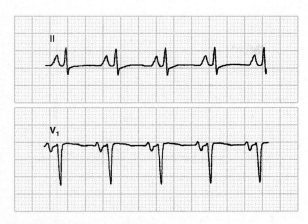

FIGURE 14-44 Biatrial enlargement.

Reproduced from *Introduction to 12-Lead ECG: The Art of Interpretation*, courtesy of Tomas B. Garcia, MD.

P waves seen in IACD are related to atrial enlargement, but the wave is not significant enough to be classified as P mitrale or P pulmonale.

Comparing the P waves in leads V_1 and V_6 can be helpful. When the leading half of the P wave is taller and wider in V_1 than it is in V_6, right atrial enlargement is probable. If the trailing half of the P wave is wider and deeper than the leading upright half is in V_1, left atrial enlargement is probable. If the trailing end of the P wave is wider and deeper than one small block on the ECG (1 mm in height by 40 ms in duration), left atrial enlargement is likely.

Both atria can be enlarged at the same time, a condition referred to as biatrial enlargement. To make the determination of biatrial enlargement, any combination of the aforementioned criteria can be applied. For example, in the inferior leads II, III, and aVF, with lead II being the best view for left atrial enlargement, a notched P wave greater than 120 ms in duration or a tall, peaked P wave of 2.5 mm or more in amplitude is found. Then in lead V_1, there is a biphasic P wave meeting the criteria for right or left atrial enlargement. Any combination of right atrial enlargement and left atrial enlargement equals biatrial enlargement **FIGURE 14-44**.

Left Ventricular Hypertrophy

LVH consists of an enlargement or an increase in the muscle mass of the left ventricle. It represents the end-organ response to the increased pressure or overload seen in hypertension. With increased detection and aggressive treatment of hypertension, there has been a relative decrease in the ECG-observed incidence of LVH. Patients who have

evidence of LVH on the ECG have a higher risk of developing coronary artery disease, making them more susceptible to the sequelae of that disease. People who have LVH are actually more susceptible to increased mortality than people who experience an MI without LVH.

Although a normal axis is the most common finding with LVH, a physiologic LAD is often present. A pathologic left or right axis deviation can occur with LVH, but the hypertrophy is usually not the cause. In general, the increased R-wave amplitude in the leads that look at the left ventricle is the basis for an ECG diagnosis of LVH. The increased amplitude of waves seen on the ECG—in particular, in the precordial leads—is caused by a two-fold process. First, as the left ventricle enlarges, a greater concentration of vectors occurs, increasing the wave of depolarization toward the precordial leads. Second, the increase in muscle mass typically extends anteriorly, bringing the heart physically closer to the electrodes on the chest. This positioning may be the reason for the finding of a normal axis instead of a pathologic axis deviation.

Several ECG criteria are used to diagnose LVH; however, to simplify the discussion, increased R-wave amplitude in the leads overlying the left ventricle and increased S-wave amplitude in the leads overlying the right ventricle are considered here. To assess for LVH, find the deepest S wave in V_1 or V_2, followed by the tallest amplitude of the R wave in V_5 or V_6. If the sum of the deepest S wave and the tallest R wave is 35 mm or more, LVH is likely.

The following criteria are very useful in making a determination of LVH. The more criteria that are present, the greater the likelihood that the patient has LVH.

- Any precordial lead of 45 mm or more
- An R wave in lead aVL of 11 mm or more
- An R wave in lead I of 12 mm or more
- An R wave in lead aVF of 20 mm or more

FIGURE 14-45 demonstrates several criteria for the diagnosis of LVH.

The ECG in **FIGURE 14-46** also demonstrates several criteria for the diagnosis of LVH. First, the S wave is largest in V_1, which is added to the largest R wave found in V_6; the sum is 45 mm or more. Second, the R wave in lead aVL is well beyond the criterion of being 11 mm or more. In lead I, the R wave is clearly 12 mm or more. More than one of the criteria

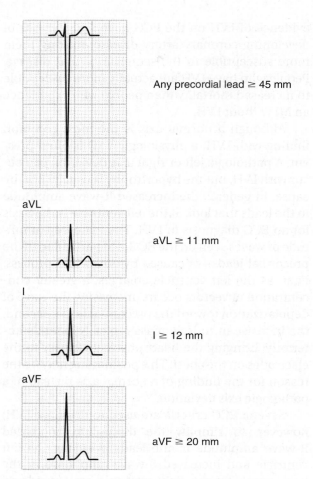

Any precordial lead ≥ 45 mm

aVL ≥ 11 mm

I ≥ 12 mm

aVF ≥ 20 mm

FIGURE 14-45 Examples of criteria for left ventricular hypertrophy.

Reproduced from *Introduction to 12-Lead ECG: The Art of Interpretation*, courtesy of Tomas B. Garcia, MD.

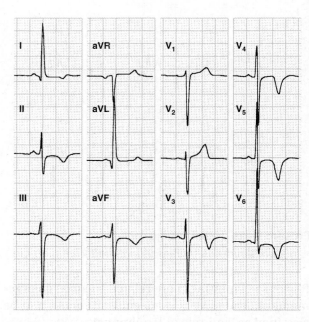

FIGURE 14-46 A 12-lead electrocardiogram showing several criteria for left ventricular hypertrophy.

Reproduced from *Introduction to 12-Lead ECG: The Art of Interpretation*, courtesy of Tomas B. Garcia, MD.

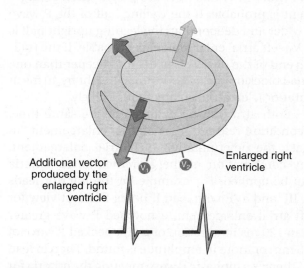

FIGURE 14-47 Right ventricular hypertrophy.

© Jones & Bartlett Learning.

typically are met on the same ECG, and as many as possible should be found when diagnosing LVH.

Right Ventricular Hypertrophy

The right ventricle can also become enlarged. This growth in size is usually caused by right ventricular overload because of a pulmonary disease such as pulmonary hypertension. The ECG is quite different in RVH than in LVH because the electrical vectors are drawn in the anterior and rightward direction with RVH. Therefore, a right shift in axis in leads I and aVF and in precordial leads V_1 and V_2 for increased R-wave deflection would be expected **FIGURE 14-47**.

In RVH, the first finding is often a large R wave in lead V_1 or V_2. This should stand out because during normal conduction, there would be a larger S wave. Owing to the large R waves seen in V_1 or V_2, the normal R-wave progression pattern is altered. The shift

of electrical vectors may also create an S wave in V_6 that is larger than the R wave. The other criterion for RVH is the RAD that lies between 100° and 180°.

Strain Pattern

When severe ventricular hypertrophy occurs, the myocardium can become so thick that the coronary blood supply is reduced. As a result, the subendocardium, or innermost layer of the heart, is likely to become ischemic. When hypertrophy is uncomplicated by ischemia, the changes seen in QRS complexes are used to diagnose ischemia. When subendocardial ischemia is present, changes to the ST segment and T wave also appear as a **strain pattern**.

In LVH, the strain pattern in the right precordial leads, V_1 to V_3, is seen as ST-segment elevation with a concave appearance of the upward slope. The T wave is upright and asymmetric in these leads. The precordial leads V_4 to V_6 show a downward-sloping ST-segment depression with an inverted asymmetric T wave. The key to identifying the strain pattern is to note that it is greatest in the lead with the tallest and deepest QRS pattern.

The ECG in **FIGURE 14-48** shows LVH with strain. First, the criteria are met to make the diagnosis of LVH by adding the S wave in V_2 to the R wave in V_5; this sum is 35 mm or more. The strain pattern is demonstrated by the concave upward sloping of the ST segments in the right precordial leads V_1 and V_2 with asymmetric upright T waves. The right precordial leads V_5 and V_6 show the strain pattern as downward-sloping ST segments with asymmetric inverted T waves.

Strain patterns also occur in RVH. In such a condition, the mean electrical axis is anterior and to the right, causing an RAD. This situation causes an increased R wave in the right precordial leads V_1 and V_2. The associated strain pattern shows a downward-sloping depressed ST segment and inverted asymmetric T waves. If the T wave is biphasic instead of inverted, the leading half will usually be negatively deflected and the trailing half will be positive in RVH.

It is important to distinguish between the strain pattern and the ST-segment and T-wave changes seen in ischemia and infarction. The strain pattern is problematic, but the ST-segment and T-wave changes can be immediately life threatening. The key to distinguishing between these conditions is to look closely at the shapes of the patterns. The ST-segment elevations or depressions in ischemia are usually flat and not sloping; the T waves are usually symmetric and not asymmetric. Another criterion used to define the two entities is the J point. In ischemia or infarction, the J point is sharper or more clearly defined, and the point at which the T wave takes off from the ST segment is seen. In contrast, in LVH with strain, the J point is usually more diffuse and slopes up or down depending on the lead being viewed. The clinical correlation between ECG findings and other patient information is most important in distinguishing between the strain pattern and ischemia/infarction.

Pre-excitation Syndromes

The pre-excitation syndrome that is of most interest in the CCT setting is **Wolff-Parkinson-White (WPW) syndrome**, which is briefly reviewed here. This condition occurs in less than 1% of the population.

WPW syndrome occurs when an accessory pathway, known as the bundle of Kent, allows electrical current to bypass the AV node and enter (or reenter) the ventricles. This accessory pathway does not have the same ability to slowly conduct electrical impulses as does the AV node, which puts people with WPW syndrome at risk for extremely fast heart rates that may result in significant hemodynamic instability. The accessory pathway can occur on the right side, connecting the right atrium to the right ventricle, or on the left side, connecting the left atrium to the left ventricle.

Two hallmarks are seen when premature ventricular depolarization occurs through an accessory pathway. First, the PR interval is shortened to less than 120 ms. Second, the QRS complex is widened

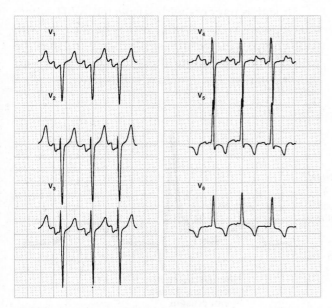

FIGURE 14-48 Precordial leads showing left ventricular hypertrophy with strain.

Reproduced from *Introduction to 12-Lead ECG: The Art of Interpretation*, courtesy of Tomas B. Garcia, MD.

to more than 100 ms. The widening is not the result of a delay in ventricular activation, but rather is attributable to premature activation. Typically in WPW syndrome, most of the ventricular depolarization is activated through the normal conduction pathways. The electrical impulse that passes unobstructed through the bundle of Kent causes early depolarization of a section of the ventricle, resulting in a QRS complex that has a characteristic slurred upstroke called a delta wave **FIGURE 14-49**. The delta wave is not seen in all leads, so every lead should be checked to confirm its presence or absence.

In many people with WPW syndrome, the preexcitation causes few clinical problems. It is well documented, however, that this syndrome can predispose a person to dangerous and even lethal tachyarrhythmias. The two tachyarrhythmias that occur most often in WPW syndrome are paroxysmal supraventricular tachycardia (a supraventricular tachycardia [SVT] that starts and ends abruptly) and atrial fibrillation (AF). In the CCT setting, CCTPs should be aware of the potential for development of wide complex tachycardia, which is difficult to distinguish from VT.

In WPW syndrome, when tachycardia is present, the electrical impulses can travel down the normal conduction pathway, through the AV node, and back up the accessory pathway. This condition, which is called orthodromic AV reciprocating tachycardia (AVRT), usually results in narrow complex tachycardia. The abnormal conduction can progress the other way as well, with the electrical impulse traveling through the accessory pathway and back up through the AV node. This condition, which is called antidromic AVRT, causes wide complex tachycardia. The antidromic tachycardias can be very fast if caused by AF or atrial flutter with one-to-one transmission or conduction of impulses.

Treatment of WPW tachyarrhythmias may require electrical cardioversion if these rhythms are unstable. Electrical cardioversion is considered the safest treatment, as management with drug therapy tends to produce unpredictable results. First-line treatment for stable patients with orthodromic AVRT is vagal maneuvers, followed by intravenous (IV) adenosine, followed by an IV calcium channel blocker such as verapamil or diltiazem.

In consultation with a cardiologist, procainamide may also be administered in stable patients, while watching the patient for hypotension and widening of the QRS. Procainamide blocks the accessory pathway but increases conduction through the AV node. Because of the risk of hypotension with too-rapid IV administration of this agent, slow IV infusion is required. Procainamide given slowly has a prolonged onset of action and may not reach therapeutic levels for 40 to 60 minutes. It may control the AF rate through the accessory pathways, but because of the increased conduction through the AV node, it can also create an extremely fast conventional AF. Thus, in any patient with WPW syndrome and AF who is hemodynamically unstable, cardioversion is the treatment of choice.

In stable patients with suspected AVRT where the diagnosis is not certain, as may be the case with wide complex tachycardias, IV procainamide is the recommended first-line therapy, followed by cardioversion if procainamide is ineffective.

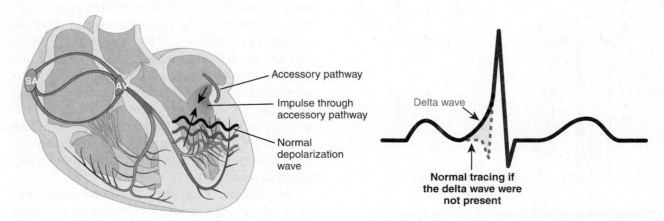

FIGURE 14-49 Impulse propagation through an accessory pathway and formation of the delta wave.

The definitive treatment for WPW syndrome is ablation of the accessory pathway.

Controversies

Although amiodarone is often thought to be safe in patients with AF and WPW syndrome, it is not. In a case series of 12 patients who received amiodarone, 7 experienced ventricular fibrillation. The safest treatment for unstable WPW tachyarrhythmias is cardioversion.

Pericarditis

Pericarditis is an inflammation of the pericardium, the membrane that surrounds the heart. It can be caused by a number of disorders and conditions, such as infection, MI, autoimmune disorders, chest trauma, cancer, and drugs, among others.

Pericarditis may cause ST-segment elevation and T-wave flattening or even inversion. These ECG findings are consistent with evolving MI, and the signs and symptoms of pericarditis can also mimic an MI. Some features on the ECG can be helpful to distinguish these two possibilities. First, the ST-segment and T-wave changes in pericarditis tend to appear throughout all leads of the ECG. In contrast, the same changes seen with ischemia, injury, and infarction tend to occur only in the leads that are viewing the affected area of the heart. Also, in pericarditis, the T wave usually does not invert until the ST segment has returned to baseline; in infarction, inversion of the T wave occurs after ST-segment elevation. Finally, Q waves do not form in pericarditis.

Another finding on an ECG that is consistent with pericarditis is the appearance of low voltage in all leads because of the pericardial effusion that often accompanies pericarditis. ST-segment and T-wave changes can usually still be seen in this situation. Fluid in the pericardial sac can cause **electrical alternans**, a condition in which the electrical axis varies from beat to beat, because the heart is able to move or rotate. Electrical alternans is most easily recognized on the ECG by the varying amplitude of each complex. Other changes often seen with pericarditis include PR depression, notched J points and, in lead aVR, reciprocal ST depression and PR elevation.

Long QT Syndrome

Long QT syndrome (LQTS) is typically a congenital disorder that can be worsened by a variety of factors, including physical exertion, female sex, electrolyte disturbances (hypokalemia and hypomagnesemia), hypothermia, abnormal thyroid function, structural heart disease, bradycardia, medications, and drug abuse/overdose **TABLE 14-6**. LQTS is characterized by a prolonged QT interval on the ECG; under certain conditions, it has a tendency to deteriorate into ventricular tachyarrhythmias, including **torsades de pointes** (often abbreviated TdP; a very rapid rhythm related to VT), which can lead to syncope or sudden cardiac death. The rhythm is often too fast to maintain effective CO, so the patient loses consciousness, usually without warning. LQTS can also be an acquired syndrome, usually as a result of drug therapy.

It is the deterioration of LQTS that poses a management challenge for CCTPs. Carefully evaluating the ECG, reviewing the patient's medications, and obtaining a medical history will provide clues to the diagnosis and alert CCTPs to the possibility of a tachyarrhythmia developing during transport. For example, CCTPs who will be transporting a cardiac patient who has recently started taking an **antiarrhythmic** agent known to increase the QT interval (eg, amiodarone or sotalol) should be prepared to treat any adverse effects from these medications.

As mentioned, LQTS occurs primarily as a congenital defect but can also be caused by a variety

---

TABLE 14-6 Drug Classes That May Worsen Long QT Syndrome

Antianginal
Antiarrhythmic
Antibiotics
Anticancer
Antihistamine
Anti-infectives
Antimalarial
Antinausea
Antipsychotic
Gastrointestinal stimulants
Opiate agonists
Sedatives

of conditions, medications, and drug abuse/overdoses. The measurement of the QT interval depends on the heart rate: The faster the heart rate, the shorter the QT interval will be; the slower the heart rate, the longer the QT interval will be. Thus, the QT interval must be corrected to account for this factor. The corrected QT interval (QTc), as printed on the 12-lead ECG, has already been corrected for heart rate by the cardiac monitor's diagnostic software.

The QT interval is measured from the start of the Q wave to the end of the T wave. Normal values for the QTc range from 350 to 440 ms for men and from 350 to 460 ms for women. During transport, if the patient's QTc reaches 500 ms and the patient's heart rhythm has not deteriorated into a ventricular tachyarrhythmia such as torsades de pointes, preventive medical intervention may be indicated. Such intervention includes correcting electrolyte imbalances, administering beta blockers (such as metoprolol), and being prepared to treat a developing ventricular tachyarrhythmia.

Typically, LQTS remains asymptomatic until the patient becomes physically active or experiences emotional stress (eg, during CCT). Symptoms usually begin in the preteen to teenage years, but can present anywhere from immediately after birth to middle age. The initial clinical sign of sudden loss of consciousness is often misdiagnosed as a vasovagal event or seizure. To make the correct diagnosis, a health care provider should give close attention to a history of loss of consciousness during physical activity.

Long-term treatment for this condition focuses on beta blockers. These medications should be started for women who have QTc-interval prolongation of greater than 460 ms and for men who have a QTc-interval prolongation of greater than 440 ms. Patients who cannot tolerate or do not respond well to the medication may need a pacemaker, an ICD (discussed later in this chapter), or a surgical procedure called a left cervicothoracic stellectomy.

CCTPs should watch for the prolonged QTc and the tachyarrhythmias that may develop as a result of this condition. Hypokalemia and hypomagnesemia make patients more susceptible to torsades de pointes, which can occur either in short bursts of 15 seconds or less or as a longer hemodynamically unstable rhythm. The treatment for torsades de pointes includes correcting the underlying cause, overdrive pacing, and IV administration of 1 to 2 g

of magnesium sulfate. Other therapies for unstable patients may include electrical cardioversion and defibrillation. All treatment should be under direct supervision of a physician or within the standing protocols approved by your agency or jurisdiction.

Transport Management

Long QT Syndrome

Preventive Measures

- Correct the electrolyte imbalance.
- Administer a beta blocker (eg, metoprolol).
- Be prepared to treat a developing ventricular tachyarrhythmia.

Torsades de Pointes

- Consult with a physician or standing protocols.
- Apply basic life support (BLS) and advanced life support (ALS) measures.
- Correct the underlying causes (eg, hypomagnesemia, drug overdose).
- Consider initiating overdrive pacing.
- Consider administering magnesium sulfate.
- Consider initiating electrical cardioversion or defibrillation for patients in unstable condition.

Ventricular and Wide Complex Tachycardia

Wide complex tachycardia in general refers to a cardiac rhythm of more than 100 beats/min with a QRS duration of 120 ms or more. This rhythm can present a diagnostic dilemma for health care providers because it can be of either ventricular or supraventricular origin. Identifying the origin of the arrhythmia can lead to the correct diagnosis and proper therapeutic interventions.

The differential diagnosis for wide complex tachycardia includes the following major categories:

- VT (most common)
- SVT with aberrance
- Pre-excited tachycardias
- Electrographic artifact
- Ventricular paced rhythms

Evaluation of the ECG is critical to make the correct diagnosis of wide complex tachycardia. A variety of diagnostic criteria have been suggested to distinguish the different origins of wide complex tachycardia, and each set of criteria has its own sensitivity and specificity. This section discusses some of the more common methods of making the diagnosis.

Diagnosis

The most useful ECG criterion for establishing the diagnosis of VT is the presence of AV dissociation with more ventricular events than atrial events. This finding practically rules out an SVT origin. An AV dissociation can be implied during wide complex tachycardia by the presence of fusion beats—that is, simultaneous activation of the ventricular myocardium through normal conduction and from an ectopic ventricular focus. In the context of VT, a capture beat or Dressler beat is a narrow QRS complex resulting from an atrial electrical impulse (P wave) that captures the ventricular myocardium through the normal conduction system. A narrow complex beat can also be seen during wide complex tachycardia in a patient with SVT and BBB when a premature ventricular beat originates from or close to the nonconducting bundle branch and fuses with the impulse traveling down the contralateral bundle. This results in a simultaneous ventricular depolarization on both sides of the septum and is demonstrated by a narrow QRS complex.

The QRS duration can also be used to help distinguish between VT and SVT. Studies have shown that nearly 70% of VTs have a QRS duration greater than 140 ms; in contrast, SVTs typically never have a QRS duration greater than 140 ms. To further expand this criterion, in a patient with a right BBB with a QRS duration of greater than 140 ms, VT is the likely diagnosis. In a patient with a left BBB, a QRS duration of greater than 160 ms suggests VT.

The electrical axis seen during wide complex tachycardia is also useful to determine the origin of the arrhythmia. If the axis is 180° to −90° (extreme RAD), the wide complex tachycardia is not likely to be an SVT because this pattern is inconsistent with any type of typical bundle branch or fascicular block. If electrical concordance across the precordium is noted (ie, all QRS complexes point in the same direction in ECG leads V_1 through V_6), the tachycardia is more likely a VT and is rarely consistent with an SVT.

The morphologic features of the QRS complex provide another way to identify the different origins of wide complex tachycardia. The utility of distinguishing VT from SVT in wide complex tachycardia is limited, however, because some measurements are required, making this diagnostic method less accurate and more time consuming when applied in a moving transport vehicle. The following discussion of QRS morphologic features in wide complex tachycardia is provided to help CCTPs better understand the various ECG findings associated with wide complex tachycardia from different origins:

- In a patient with a right BBB, the precordial lead V_1 should be examined. If the left R wave is taller than the R′ wave, or if the QRS complex is biphasic with an Rs or qR pattern, the origin of the wide complex tachycardia is likely VT.
- In a patient with a left BBB, the precordial lead V_1 should also be examined. If the duration of the initial r wave is greater than 30 ms, the time from the beginning of the QRS complex to the nadir of the S wave is greater than 70 ms, and the downstroke of the S wave is notched, the origin is likely to be VT.
- If the QRS complex in precordial lead V_6 has a monophasic QS or biphasic rS wave with an r to S ratio of less than 1 during a right BBB wide complex tachycardia, VT is likely.
- If the intrinsicoid deflection (from the beginning of the QRS complex to the beginning of the downslope of the R wave) in the precordial lead V_6 is greater than 80 ms, VT is the likely origin of the wide complex tachycardia.

Management

The initial management of wide complex tachycardia primarily depends on the patient's hemodynamic status. Patients who have low blood pressure, pulmonary edema, severe chest pain, or other evidence of poor perfusion associated with the wide complex tachycardia should be promptly treated using synchronized cardioversion.

When a patient with wide complex tachycardia remains in hemodynamically stable condition, more time can be spent reviewing information from the history, physical examination, and ECG findings. As mentioned, the majority of cases of wide complex tachycardia involve VT. Making the correct diagnosis, however, is the safest approach to management.

For a patient in hemodynamically stable condition in whom the cause of wide complex tachycardia is uncertain, vagal maneuvers may be diagnostic, if not therapeutic. If the etiology of a stable wide complex tachycardia is uncertain, a trial of adenosine may terminate some SVTs. This medication works by slowing conduction through the AV node, which serves to cut off the tachycardia circuit in most SVTs. It can sometimes terminate atrial tachycardias and, rarely, VT. Because adenosine has a very short half-life, it rarely causes complications in patients with wide complex tachycardia. An exception is the patient with an irregular wide complex tachycardia as a result of AF and pre-excitation over an accessory pathway. In this case, adenosine can block conduction through the AV node, allowing only conduction through the accessory pathway, and may lead to ventricular fibrillation. Beyond adenosine, other drugs used to treat SVT (eg, calcium channel blockers and beta blockers) may result in significant hemodynamic deterioration if the wide complex tachycardia is actually a stable VT. Additional treatments depend on the response to vagal maneuvers and adenosine, and should be based on expert consultation.

While some experts proceed with elective cardioversion for patients with stable wide complex tachycardias unresponsive to initial therapies, procainamide (class IA), is a reasonable alternative but must be used with caution. Notably, it can cause a sudden drop in blood pressure with rapid IV administration and is contraindicated in patients with complete heart block during wide complex tachycardia because it suppresses the nodal or ventricular pacemakers and can result in asystole. As with all drugs, the indications and contraindications of procainamide should be fully understood before administering it to any patient.

Lidocaine (Xylocaine; class IB) is useful for VT of ischemic origin, but does not terminate SVT. In a patient who is conscious and in a hemodynamically stable condition, higher doses of lidocaine can cause confusion, altered mental status, and even seizures.

Following termination of wide complex tachycardia, preventive treatment aimed at maintaining a stable rhythm should be initiated. This treatment will help prevent recurrent episodes, minimize the patient's symptoms, and protect the patient from sudden cardiac death. For CCTPs, interventions are generally limited to pharmacologic treatment with antiarrhythmic drugs, usually a continuation of the drug that terminated the wide complex tachycardia. Additional in-hospital treatments may include the use of an ICD and catheter ablation procedures.

Patients whose rhythm converts to wide complex tachycardia rhythm can pose a diagnostic dilemma, especially for a transport team in transit. At times, only minimal information about the patient's history and clinical and laboratory findings may be known. If wide complex tachycardia develops during transport, a rapid evaluation must be performed and the appropriate treatment must be initiated in a confined environment with relatively limited resources. If the patient is in a hemodynamically unstable condition, wide complex tachycardia should be managed as if it were VT until proven otherwise, and synchronized cardioversion is the initial therapy of choice.

Polymorphic or pulseless VT should be treated as ventricular fibrillation. If it is a witnessed condition that occurs during transport, the patient should already be connected to a cardiac monitor and have a patent IV line. Immediate defibrillation is indicated, and the CCTP should provide cardiopulmonary resuscitation (CPR) if necessary.

Differential Diagnosis

Wide Complex Tachycardia
- VT
- SVT with aberrance
- Pre-excited tachycardias
- Electrographic artifact
- Ventricular paced rhythms

Electrolyte Imbalances and Drug Effects

Electrolytes have an essential role in the proper functioning of cells and are found in both intracellular and extracellular fluids. Important electrolytes are sodium, potassium, calcium, and magnesium. It is the exchange of electrolytes into and out of cells that generates the electrical energy for cellular depolarization and repolarization. As the cells depolarize electrically, they exhibit a mechanical response in the form of contraction; when they repolarize, they relax and expand back to their original states. In the cardiac muscle, this process is repeated continuously over the individual's entire lifetime. Proper levels of the electrolytes are essential to keep the cells functioning correctly. When changes in electrolytes occur, their effects are often seen on the ECG.

Certain drugs affect the electrolyte channels of the cell membranes, changing how the electrolytes flow into and out of the cells. These drugs can alter conduction patterns and, in turn, their representation on the ECG. Cardiac medications can increase the rate and force of contraction or slow and protect the heart from increased demands. Virtually any function of the heart can be altered by design. Other classes of pharmaceuticals that are not cardiac medications may have expected or unexpected cardiac side effects. It is beyond the scope of any text to address the effects of the countless illicit drugs that are available on the street or even online. Rather, the key point is that an endless number of drug effects may alter what is ultimately seen on the ECG. **TABLE 14-7** provides a brief overview of the cardiac effects associated with a few of these drug classes.

This section discusses ECG effects of two of the most clinically important electrolytes, potassium and calcium, because they produce the most recognizable changes on the ECG. In addition, a more in-depth discussion of digoxin toxicity is provided; this drug is one of the most notorious agents causing ECG changes.

Hyperkalemia

Potassium is the primary intracellular ion (the other is phosphate). An elevation of the potassium level is called hyperkalemia. Hyperkalemia is the most dangerous of all electrolyte abnormalities: It can cause death and prevents some drugs used in resuscitation efforts from being effective. On the ECG, hyperkalemia can cause changes in the appearance of all waveforms, indicating that a change has occurred within the cell, and can cause virtually any arrhythmia. Rapid recognition and correction of this electrolyte disturbance is essential to reversing any harmful effects. When hyperkalemia is suspected, a confirmatory potassium level should be obtained.

TABLE 14-7 Common Toxic Drug Effects	
Drug Class	**Possible Toxic Effects**
Class I antiarrhythmics	Lengthened QRS and QTc intervals Possible AV blocks Slowed or completely blocked SA node Arrhythmias
Calcium channel blockers	Blocked AV node primarily, but extent of block varies significantly among different drugs in this class
Beta blockers	Slowed automaticity of the SA node and the Purkinje system Blocked AV node
Amiodarone	Slowed conduction everywhere: the SA node, atrium, AV node, Purkinje system, and ventricles
Phenothiazines and tricyclic antidepressants	Widened QRS and QTc intervals T-wave abnormalities Arrhythmias common in overdoses

Abbreviations: AV, atrioventricular; SA, sinoatrial

Reproduced from *Introduction to 12-Lead ECG: The Art of Interpretation*, courtesy of Tomas B. Garcia, MD.

The main ECG changes found in hyperkalemia are the following:

- T-wave abnormalities (tall and peaked)
- Intraventricular conduction delays
- P-wave abnormalities (missing or decreased amplitude)
- ST-segment changes simulating an injury pattern
- Cardiac arrhythmias (predominantly bradycardias)
- Sinusoidal ECG pattern

On the ECG, T-wave abnormalities are typically the first to appear with hyperkalemia. These changes start to appear when the potassium level exceeds 5.5 mEq/L in patients without renal disease and when it exceeds 6 mEq/L in patients with renal disease. The most common changes are tall, narrow, peaked T waves, but these changes are not seen in every patient with hyperkalemia. A prolonged QT interval may be present. As the potassium level increases, the height of the T wave decreases and

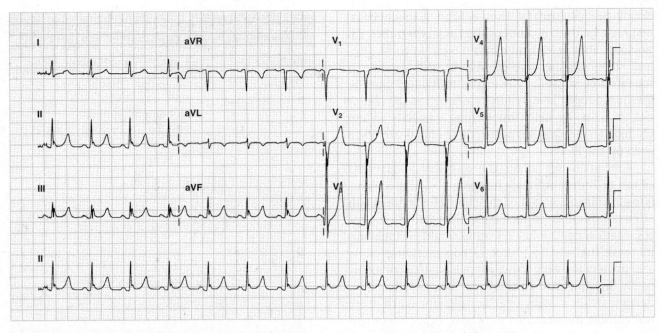

FIGURE 14-50 A 12-lead electrocardiogram showing T-wave changes with acute hyperkalemia.

Reproduced from *Introduction to 12-Lead ECG: The Art of Interpretation*, courtesy of Tomas B. Garcia, MD.

widens; the PR, QRS, and QT intervals also widen; and the amplitude decreases.

The ECG in **FIGURE 14-50** represents acute hyperkalemia. Tall, narrow, peaked T waves are visible in leads V_2 through V_4. Tall T waves also appear in the inferior leads II, III, and aVF. When the T wave is two-thirds the height of the R wave, it is considered pathologic.

A patient who has known hyperkalemia or who has renal failure with suspected hyperkalemia should receive supportive treatment including IV access and cardiac monitoring. In the presence of severe hyperkalemia (potassium level ≥ 6.5 mEq/L in patients without renal failure or ≥ 7 mEq/L in patients with renal failure) with marked ECG changes, calcium should be administered initially for cardioprotection. When central access is available, 1 g calcium chloride should be administered over 5 to 10 minutes; for peripheral administration, 1 to 2 g calcium gluconate over 5 to 10 minutes should be given. Dosing can be repeated in 5 minutes if ECG changes persist. Although calcium has no effect on potassium levels, its cardioprotective effects begin within 1 to 2 minutes and last for 10 to 30 minutes. When ECG changes are not present, or following administration of calcium when ECG changes are present, 10 units of regular insulin should be given

via IV push with 25 g of dextrose over 1 to 3 minutes. If the serum glucose is greater than 250 mg/dL, consider holding the IV dextrose. Additionally, 10 to 20 mg of albuterol should be administered by nebulizer over 10 minutes. Insulin and albuterol serve to shift potassium into the cells. Providers should attempt to facilitate potassium removal by using a binding resin such as sodium polystyrene sulfonate or sodium zirconium cyclosilicate and, if the patient is hypervolemic, 20 to 40 mg of IV furosemide.

Additional medical treatments include sodium bicarbonate: 50 mEq IV over 2 to 5 minutes

Transport Management

Hyperkalemia

- Provide supportive treatment with IV access and cardiac monitoring.
- In the presence of hypotension or marked QRS widening, give IV calcium, insulin together with 50% dextrose, and albuterol.
- Give magnesium sulfate for digoxin toxicity–related cardiac arrhythmias.
- Give additional medical treatments, such as furosemide and binding resins.

or 150 mEq in 1 L of D_5W over 2 to 4 hours, including fluid hydration if the patient is hypovolemic. If severe hyperkalemia does not resolve with medical management, dialysis may be needed.

Hypokalemia

A decrease in the level of potassium is called hypokalemia. Hypokalemia does not cause the dramatic changes on the ECG that are seen with hyperkalemia. Some mild, nonspecific changes are apparent, such as ST-segment depression, slightly decreased amplitude of the T waves, and minimal prolongation of the QRS interval. Probably the most common abnormality in hypokalemia is the presence of a prominent U wave. This U wave (shown in Figure 14-8) is usually small and follows the T wave. Hypokalemia does not typically cause arrhythmias by itself.

Differential diagnoses for U waves include the following:

- Hypokalemia
- Bradycardia
- LVH
- Central nervous system events
- Drug use: digoxin, class I antiarrhythmics, phenothiazines

Treatment for hypokalemia is aimed at decreasing potassium losses, replenishing potassium stores, evaluating for potential toxic effects, and determining the cause to prevent additional losses.

In the transport setting, a few steps can be taken to decrease potassium losses. First, if possible, the use of diuretics should be discontinued. If diuretics are required for severe fluid overload, potassium-sparing diuretics should be used, diarrhea and vomiting should be treated, and H_2 blockers should be administered to decrease loss of potassium through nasogastric suction.

Replacing lost potassium is done by measuring the loss and estimating the replacement. IV potassium is not well tolerated peripherally because it can be highly irritating to veins and must be given only in relatively small doses (ie, 10 mEq/h). Potassium supplementation is best administered through a central line. In an emergency situation, in consultation with medical control, as much as 40 mEq/h can be given.

In evaluating patients for the potential toxic effects of hypokalemia, monitoring for cardiac arrhythmias and prompt treatment are essential. Hypokalemia is one condition in which a more aggressive approach to electrolyte replacement is warranted.

Differential Diagnosis

Hypokalemia

- Bradycardia
- LVH
- Central nervous system events
- Drug use: digoxin, class I antiarrhythmics, phenothiazines

Transport Management

Hypokalemia

- Discontinue diuretics (and any laxatives).
- Use potassium-sparing diuretics if required for severe volume overload.
- Treat diarrhea and vomiting.
- Use H_2 blockers to decrease nasogastric suction losses.
- Measure the potassium loss, estimate the replacement, and administer it through a central line.
- Monitor for cardiac arrhythmias, and treat them promptly if they occur.

Hypercalcemia

Hypercalcemia is a disorder that is most commonly caused by malignancy or primary hyperparathyroidism. Other causes of an elevated calcium level are less common and not typically considered until the most common causes are ruled out. ECG changes are minimal with this electrolyte imbalance, with the most significant change being a shortening of the ST segment, which in turn shortens the QT interval. The ST segment may become so short that there appears to be ST elevation. The PR interval may be prolonged; at higher levels, the QRS interval may lengthen and T waves may become flat or even invert. Because hypercalcemia affects conduction times, a variable degree of heart block may develop. Arrhythmias seldom occur as a result of hypercalcemia.

Treatment of hypercalcemia includes supportive management of the ABCs and increased hydration. Often, treatment also includes a loop diuretic (eg, furosemide) to increase calcium excretion and prevent overload from hydration therapy alone.

Transport Management

Hypercalcemia
- Manage the ABCs.
- Provide hydration.
- Administer a loop diuretic.

Hypocalcemia

Hypocalcemia that occurs acutely can be the result of medication or surgical effects. It is recognized as a significant problem in critically ill patients because of depressed myocardial contractility and resultant hypotension. ECG changes seen include a prolongation of the ST segment that produces an apparent lengthening of the QTc interval. The cardiopulmonary effects of hypocalcemia may include wheezing, stridor, bradycardia, and pulmonary crackles (rales), and an S_3 heart sound may be heard. The prolonged QT interval can lead to ventricular arrhythmias (eg, torsades de pointes).

Treatment during interfacility transfer mainly includes supportive measures, including IV fluids, oxygen, and monitoring of vital signs and the ECG. An infusion with calcium gluconate can be given over a period of 5 to 10 minutes. Administration of magnesium may be considered in patients with a prolonged QTc interval to help prevent torsades de pointes.

Signs and Symptoms

Hypocalcemia
- ECG findings: prolonged ST segment and apparent lengthening of the QTc interval
- Wheezing
- Stridor
- Bradycardia
- Pulmonary crackles (rales)
- S_3 heart sound
- Ventricular arrhythmias (eg, torsades de pointes)
- Tetany (carpopedal spasms), paresthesia

Transport Management

Hypocalcemia
- Initiate IV access.
- Administer oxygen to maintain saturation at greater than 92%.
- Monitor vital signs and the ECG.
- Provide an infusion of calcium gluconate.
- Consider administration of magnesium to help prevent torsades de pointes.

Digoxin Toxicity

Among the countless medications on the market that are specifically designed to alter the function of the heart, the most notorious is digoxin, a digitalis preparation. According to the American Association of Poison Control Centers, observed mortality rates are high with digoxin toxicity. Understanding the actions of digoxin and treating its adverse effects are essential to decreasing the mortality when toxicity occurs.

Digoxin is a cardiac glycoside that produces positive inotropic and negative chronotropic activity in the heart. It is primarily indicated to treat chronic HF and to control the ventricular rate in atrial tachyarrhythmias (such as AF). The inotropic effects are a result of inhibiting the sodium–potassium adenosine triphosphatase pump. This action causes an increase in intracellular calcium and sodium and a decrease in intracellular potassium. The movement of these intracellular electrolytes results in an increased force of myocardial muscle contraction, thereby causing the positive inotropic effect.

Therapeutic concentrations of digoxin (1.0 to 2.0 ng/mL) cause the desired positive inotropic effect and decreased electrical conduction between the SA and AV nodes. Therapeutic levels of digoxin also decrease automaticity and increase the diastolic resting membrane potential.

The margin between toxic and therapeutic doses is small, however, and many factors influence digoxin levels. One of the most common causes of digoxin toxicity is drug–drug interaction(s). In the CCT setting, patients already taking digoxin may be given other medications that result in digoxin toxicity. Any drug interaction or disease state (eg, hypothyroidism or renal impairment) that can interfere with the absorption or elimination of digoxin can cause an increased serum concentration.

Levels of the electrolytes potassium and calcium must be evaluated in conjunction with suspected digoxin toxicity. If the patient is given diuretic therapy, hypokalemia can develop, resulting in increased automaticity. Hyperkalemia exacerbates the digoxin-induced conduction delays. Also, hypercalcemia increases ventricular automaticity and can increase the effects of digoxin.

At toxic levels, the excessive increase of intracellular calcium elevates the resting potential and predisposes the heart to arrhythmias. Almost any arrhythmia can occur in conjunction with digoxin toxicity, and none is specific to this condition. CCTPs need to be alert to any manifestation of increased automaticity in the face of impaired electrical conduction.

The clinical manifestations of acute digoxin intoxication may not appear for several hours. When they do, they typically include gastrointestinal symptoms of nausea, vomiting, or abdominal pain. Neurologic symptoms may include lethargy, confusion, and weakness. Symptoms associated with chronic digoxin intoxication may be difficult to distinguish from those associated with other medical conditions.

The most common ECG changes in the setting of digoxin toxicity include AV, junctional, or ventricular ectopic beats; first-degree AV block; slow ventricular response in AF; and an accelerated AV or junctional rhythm. More severe arrhythmias may also be seen, including severe bradycardia, high-degree heart blocks, and malignant ventricular rhythms. As this list of potential rhythms suggests, there is no signature arrhythmia that points directly to digoxin toxicity. Instead, to diagnose digoxin toxicity, CCTPs should review the patient's medications before transport. In a patient known to be taking digoxin, when an arrhythmia occurs, especially in the presence of other clinical findings, digoxin toxicity should be considered as an underlying cause. In general, any accelerated rhythm with conduction delays should raise the level of suspicion for digoxin toxicity.

Any patient taking digoxin who develops an altered level of consciousness or gastrointestinal symptoms with or without ECG changes needs further evaluation for toxicity. CCTPs typically work with data collected before the transport began, however, and new electrolyte values and drug assays are usually not available en route to the receiving facility. The one value that can be obtained before transport that has some prognostic value and can provide clues to the diagnosis of digoxin toxicity (in the presence of other clinical findings that develop during transport) is the potassium level. In a patient with digoxin toxicity, a potassium level greater than 5.5 mEq/L (normal serum potassium level, 3.5–5.0 mEq/L) with normal renal function is associated with higher mortality. Toxicity can occur in a patient with normal therapeutic levels of digoxin if a drug–drug interaction interferes with absorption or elimination of digoxin or in the presence of increased automaticity and impaired conduction.

If the CCTP suspects digoxin toxicity during transport based on ECG changes along with associated signs and symptoms, the initial concern is to manage the ABCs and stabilize the patient's hemodynamics. Clearing the gastrointestinal tract of very recently ingested digoxin can be beneficial; in the field, this can be accomplished with the administration of activated charcoal. This measure not only helps prevent further absorption of the drug, but also may increase its excretion from the body. Atrioventricular, junctional, or ventricular ectopy; first-degree AV block; slow ventricular response to AF; and accelerated AV or junctional rhythms will typically respond to administration of atropine.

For treatment of severe digoxin toxicity, the standard of care is administration of digoxin-specific antibodies (Fab fragments or digoxin-immune Fab). Fab fragments neutralize free digoxin, decrease potassium levels, and increase renal excretion.

Laboratory tests for electrolyte levels, glomerular filtration rate, creatinine level, and urea level should be obtained as soon as possible. Further treatment includes the administration of insulin and glucose to treat the associated hyperkalemia and to provide the proposed cardioprotective effects. (Insulin may have a cardioprotective effect in digoxin toxicity.) The use of calcium chloride to stabilize the myocardium is controversial. If Fab fragments are used in the treatment of digoxin toxicity, the use of sodium polystyrene sulfonate to treat hyperkalemia is *not* recommended because it will overcorrect the serum potassium level. Fab fragments have also virtually eliminated the need for a pacemaker or cardioversion in patients with digoxin toxicity. Early recognition and aggressive treatment of digoxin toxicity is lifesaving.

Signs and Symptoms

Digoxin Intoxication

- Nausea
- Vomiting
- Anorexia
- Abdominal pain
- Weight loss
- Delirium
- Confusion
- Dizziness
- Disorientation
- Drowsiness
- Headache
- Hallucinations
- Amblyopia (partial or complete loss of vision in one eye)
- Photophobia (painful sensitivity to light)
- Scotoma (area of diminished vision within the visual field)
- Chromatopsia (visual disturbance in which objects appear abnormally colored)
- Xanthopsia (visual yellow discoloration)

Transport Management

Digoxin Intoxication

- Manage the ABCs.
- Stabilize the patient's hemodynamics.
- Administer activated charcoal to clear the gastrointestinal tract in patients who have recently ingested digoxin.
- Administer atropine to address AV, junctional, or ventricular ectopy; first-degree AV block; slow ventricular response to AF; or accelerated AV or junctional rhythms.
- Administer digoxin-specific antibodies (Fab fragments).

Conditions That Mimic Myocardial Infarction

Multiple conditions may mimic the clinical and ECG findings that occur with ischemia, injury, and infarction. The following is a synopsis of these conditions:

- Pericarditis: ST-segment elevation, T-wave inversion (possible)
- Left BBB: ST-segment elevation, QS complexes
- LVH: ST-segment elevation
- Ventricular rhythms: ST-segment elevation, QS complexes
- Early repolarization: ST-segment elevation, tall T waves

Cardiac Disease
Coronary Artery Disease and Angina

Coronary artery disease (CAD) is the most common form of heart disease and is a leading cause of death in US adults. The coronary arteries supply oxygen and nutrients to the myocardium. If one of these blood vessels becomes blocked, the muscle it supplies will be deprived of oxygen (ischemia). If this oxygen supply is not restored quickly, the ischemic area of heart muscle will eventually die (undergo infarction).

Atherosclerosis is of particular concern because it affects the inner lining of the aorta and the cerebral and coronary blood vessels, leading to the narrowing of these vessels and the reduction of blood flow through them. The atherosclerotic process begins, probably in childhood, when small amounts of fatty material are deposited along the inner wall (intima) of arteries, usually at points of turbulent blood flow, such as where the arteries bifurcate or where the arterial wall has been damaged. As the streak of fat enlarges, it becomes a mass of fatty tissue, known as an atheroma, which gradually calcifies and hardens into a plaque. The atheromatous plaque infiltrates the arterial wall and decreases its elasticity. At the same time, the plaque narrows the arterial lumen and interferes with blood flow through the lumen. The narrowed, roughened area of the arterial intima provides a locus for the formation of a fixed blood clot, or thrombus, which may then obstruct the artery altogether (in a coronary artery, such a clot is known as a coronary thrombosis). In addition, calcium may precipitate from the bloodstream into the arterial walls, causing arteriosclerosis, which greatly reduces the elasticity of the arteries.

Risk factors for atherosclerosis and CAD include hypertension, cigarette smoking, diabetes, high serum cholesterol levels, lack of exercise, obesity, family history of heart disease or stroke, and male sex.

Peripheral Vascular Disorders

Although atherosclerosis is rarely the primary cause of medical emergencies, it is a major contributor to other conditions that may become medical emergencies. For example, arterial bruits (turbulence or "swishing" sounds heard with a stethoscope placed over the carotid arteries) signal the presence of atherosclerosis and increased risk of vascular disease. Atherosclerosis can also contribute to claudication, a severe pain in the calf muscle caused by narrowing of the arteries in this muscle and leading to a painful limp. Finally, atherosclerosis may be associated with phlebitis: inflammation, swelling, and pain along the veins that can lead to the formation of blood clots and thrombophlebitis, which is venous inflammation associated with a thrombus (blood clot). If dislodged from their original sites, these thrombi become emboli that could travel to the heart and through its right side, lodging in the pulmonary arterial tree and causing a pulmonary embolism.

An estimated 10% of Americans are affected by significant peripheral vascular disorders annually. The most dangerous complication of these disorders is pulmonary embolism, which causes approximately 100,000 deaths each year. Risk factors for peripheral vascular disorders include age, oral contraceptive use, smoking, recent surgery, recreational IV drug use, trauma, and extended immobilization. Identification of these risk factors has a significant role in the diagnosis of peripheral vascular occlusions. Signs of peripheral vascular occlusion may include pain, flushing, swelling, warmth, and tenderness in the extremity, although these signs are present in only approximately half of all cases. The presence of claudication indicates a significant narrowing of the peripheral arteries associated with peripheral vascular disorders. Arterial bruits are another sign of vascular narrowing that can contribute to ischemia and stroke.

Unfortunately, a CCT team can do little for a patient with peripheral vascular disease. If a blockage or potential embolus is suspected, IV heparin should be administrated initially as a bolus and then as an infusion. If ultrasonography or Doppler imaging is available on the transport vehicle, the CCTP should frequently assess the affected limb. In addition to administering anticoagulant therapy, apply warm compresses to maximize blood flow to the extremity. It is also helpful to keep the leg in the position of comfort and minimize movement.

In the CCT setting, all patients should undergo cardiac monitoring, but any patient who is being transported for a long distance and has a blood clot with the potential to become a pulmonary embolus should be given a baseline ECG before transport and must undergo frequent 12-lead ECG monitoring. ST-segment depression in the limb leads and the precordial leads accompanied by an increase in right axis deviation may indicate a pulmonary embolus. Historically, the McGinn-White sign—that is, an $S_1Q_3T_3$ pattern (ie, a large S wave in lead I, and a Q wave and inverted T wave in lead III)—was considered a classic indicator of right heart strain. This pattern, however, is seen in only 10% of patients with pulmonary emboli. Anterior-inferior T-wave inversion is now considered a better indicator of pulmonary embolus. Of note, these findings are not unique to pulmonary embolism and could suggest any condition leading to right heart strain or hypertrophy. As a diagnostic tool, the ECG is neither specific nor sensitive for pulmonary embolism.

Signs and Symptoms

Peripheral Vascular Disorders

- Pain, flushing, swelling, warmth, and tenderness in the extremity
- Claudication
- Arterial bruits

Transport Management

Peripheral Vascular Disorders (Suspected Blockage or Embolus)

- Give IV heparin or another anticoagulant, initially as a bolus and then as an infusion.
- Monitor the affected limb with ultrasonography or Doppler imaging, if available.
- Maximize blood flow to the extremity by using warm compresses.
- Keep the affected limb in the position of comfort.
- Minimize movement of the affected limb.
- Apply a cardiac monitor, record a baseline ECG before transport, and perform frequent 12-lead ECG monitoring.

Acute Coronary Syndrome

The American Heart Association and the American College of Cardiology have published guidelines for the care of patients with STEMI. In these guidelines, the term **acute coronary syndrome (ACS)** is used to describe conditions that cause an episode of ischemic discomfort (chest pain) as the result of disruption of plaque within a coronary artery.

Plaques occur as the natural evolution of atherosclerosis. The plaques that are susceptible to disruption are usually nonobstructive but have a large amount of macrophages and other inflammatory cells associated with them. After the plaques are disrupted within a coronary artery, these substances promote a chain reaction of platelet activation, adhesion, aggregation, thrombin formation, and, ultimately, thrombus formation. The end product is a complete occlusion of the coronary artery or one of its branches. If there is not enough collateral circulation from branches of adjacent coronary arteries, myocardial necrosis begins within 15 minutes and spreads from the endocardium toward the epicardium.

The term ACS is used to describe any group of clinical symptoms consistent with acute myocardial ischemia. ACS represents a sudden deterioration of the condition of a coronary blood vessel. Acute myocardial ischemia typically presents as chest pain stemming from insufficient blood supply to the heart muscle, which itself is a result of CAD. The life-threatening ACS disorders are responsible for much of the emergency medical care and hospitalization in the United States.

The broad term *acute coronary syndrome* includes unstable angina, MI without ST-segment elevation (NSTEMI), and MI with ST-segment elevation (STEMI). Patients with STEMI have a high probability (greater than 90%) of experiencing coronary thrombus occlusion. In comparison, patients with stable angina have only a 1% probability of having a coronary thrombus. Among those patients with unstable angina or NSTEMI, 35% to 75% may have a coronary thrombus. These percentages are not good predictors for identifying those patients in whom MIs with Q waves eventually develop: Not every STEMI leads to the development of Q waves, and Q waves may develop in NSTEMI.

All patients experiencing a possible cardiac event should have a 12-lead ECG performed. Analysis of the 12-lead ECG enables the health care provider to categorize two groups of patients who have experienced ACS: patients with ST-segment elevation and patients without ST-segment elevation.

Many patients whose ECG displays ST-segment elevation ultimately will have a STEMI. Patients who have ischemic discomfort (chest pain) without an ST-segment elevation are having unstable angina or an NSTEMI that usually leads to a non–Q-wave MI; these conditions are collectively known as UA/NSTEMI (unstable angina/NSTEMI). Patients with non–ST-segment elevation are ultimately diagnosed as either having or not having unstable angina (depending on whether cardiac enzymes or biomarkers indicate evidence of cardiac injury). Patients who experience angina may also have ST-segment depression. Finally, some patients experiencing angina or MI may have no changes indicated by the ECG.

Early recognition of the signs and symptoms of a STEMI is essential to initiate treatment or to ensure the patient is transported to a facility where the appropriate care can be provided. These signs and symptoms (which are discussed later in this chapter in the section on MI) include chest and arm pain, lower jaw pain, shortness of breath, and diaphoresis. Most deaths resulting from STEMI occur within the first 1 to 2 hours after the onset of symptoms and are usually caused by ventricular fibrillation. To avoid this dire outcome, rapid intervention with the most appropriate reperfusion therapy must start as soon as a diagnosis of STEMI has been confirmed.

The CCTP should perform a 12-lead ECG within 10 minutes of contacting a patient with chest discomfort or other signs and symptoms suggestive of STEMI. If this initial ECG is not diagnostic of STEMI but the patient remains symptomatic and there is a high degree of suspicion for STEMI, serial 12-lead ECGs should be performed at 5- to 10-minute intervals while maintaining continuous cardiac (ST-segment) monitoring. Newer 12-lead ECG machines are equipped with multiparameter monitoring capabilities that can assess ST-segment deviation every 30 seconds. In patients with IWMI, right-side chest leads should be evaluated for ST-segment elevation suggestive of right ventricular MI (RVMI). The 12-lead ECG in the CCT setting is central to the therapeutic decision pathway because it provides evidence of ST-segment elevation in patients who will benefit from reperfusion therapy. Preemptive defibrillator pad placement on STEMI patients and NSTEMI patients with significantly increased cardiac enzymes should be considered prior to beginning transport.

In patients with STEMI, the more leads that show ST-segment elevation on a 12-lead ECG, the higher the mortality rate is. In other words, if the occlusion occurred high enough in a coronary artery that it has affected a large area of the heart, multiple patterns of ischemia will appear. Other important predictors of mortality are STEMI occurring in conjunction with a left BBB and in a predominantly anterior location. The classic guidelines for the ECG diagnosis of acute MI require at least 1 to 2 mm (0.1 to 0.2 mV) of ST-segment elevation in at least two contiguous leads. (Each small block measured vertically on the ECG paper equals 1 mm.) More detailed consensus criteria can help suggest different categories of AMI.

When no ST-segment elevation is present or the ECG is normal or shows nonspecific changes, there is no evidence to suggest fibrinolytic therapy will provide any benefit; in fact, in such cases, fibrinolytic therapy has been shown to be harmful. If clinical signs and symptoms continue, the 12-lead ECG should be repeated every 5 to 10 minutes and monitored continuously for any ST-segment changes until serologic testing for cardiac enzymes or biomarkers can be done.

All patients with ACS should receive antithrombin and antiplatelet therapy regardless of the presence or absence of ST-segment elevation. Patients with persistent ST-segment elevation are candidates for prompt reperfusion therapy, either pharmacologic or catheter based, to restore blood flow in the occluded artery. Patients without ST-segment elevation should receive anti-ischemic therapy and be considered for catheter-based therapy when indicated. Medications such as heparin or glycoprotein IIb/IIIa inhibitors can be continued in the field, but revascularization will occur in the hospital.

Another situation that warrants fibrinolytic therapy is marked ST-segment depression in leads V_1 through V_4 with tall R waves in the right precordial leads and upright T waves suggestive of a true posterior wall MI (PWMI). In this case, placement of additional electrodes in the posterior position to form leads V_7, V_8, and V_9 is recommended. Primary percutaneous coronary intervention may be appropriate in patients with true PWMI.

Lethal ventricular arrhythmias may develop in patients with STEMI, so continuous ECG monitoring is mandatory. Because many patients with STEMI are transferred to a higher level of care for therapeutic interventions, CCTPs are in a unique position to be able to monitor them during transport and to respond quickly and appropriately if these events occur. The value of setting alarm parameters on the transport monitor to immediately notify the CCTP of acute changes cannot be overstated.

Most patients diagnosed with ACS are experiencing an MI in progress or severe ischemia, which can quickly become an infarction. The gold-standard treatment is prompt arrival at a facility where the location of the blockage can be identified by cardiac catheterization and subsequently alleviated by percutaneous coronary intervention (PCI) such as stenting or angioplasty. Unfortunately, most hospitals do not have this capability.

The role of the CCT team is to transport the patient from a basic-care hospital to a cardiac hospital as expeditiously as possible without deterioration of the patient's condition en route. Priorities are as follows:

1. Prevent further damage to the heart muscle.
2. Reduce afterload.
3. Prevent a thrombus from getting larger.
4. Reduce myocardial oxygen demand.
5. Maximize oxygen delivery.
6. Reduce or eliminate pain and anxiety.
7. Consider thrombolytic therapy to dissolve the clot(s).

The patient will usually be placed on an anticoagulant heparin drip; in some cases, an IV drip of an antiplatelet medication, such as eptifibatide, may be added to the heparin regimen. These drips must be administered via an infusion pump. The CCTP should monitor the patient en route for signs of serious bleeding. Minor bleeding, especially around the mouth, is common and is not a reason to discontinue or alter the drip rates.

If thrombolytic therapy has not been initiated and is not planned during transport, the CCTP should confer with the transferring provider about administration of 324 mg of aspirin with 180 mg of ticagrelor orally prior to departure. For patients who have previously received or are currently receiving thrombolytics, consider a loading dose of an adenosine diphosphate (ADP) inhibitor such as clopidogrel. Typical ADP inhibitors are administered as oral medications and have been shown to improve PCI outcomes when administered early. The CCTP should also confirm that aspirin administration has occurred or that a contraindication has been clearly documented in the medical record.

Give the patient sufficient oxygen to maintain an oxygen saturation of greater than 92%, but avoid hyperoxia (more than 97% oxygen saturation). Use continuous waveform capnography to monitor patients who require mechanical ventilation, and maintain the carbon dioxide level between 35 and 45 mm Hg.

When transport times will be long or the degree of blockage is severe to the point of being life threatening, administration of a thrombolytic agent may be indicated. Thrombolytics dissolve clots, but their actions are not specific to where these clots might be located. Before administering a thrombolytic, locally determined exclusion criteria need to be met. Such criteria are based on a combination of symptom onset and the estimated delay until PCI can be performed. Examples of thrombolytic exclusion criteria include the following:

- Significant hypertension (eg, systolic blood pressure [SBP] >200 mm Hg and/or diastolic blood pressure [DBP] >110 mm Hg)
- Right versus left SBP difference greater than 15 mm Hg (suggests potential dissection)
- Significant closed head or facial trauma in the previous 3 months
- Stroke in the previous 3 months
- Any history of intracranial hemorrhage
- Recent (2–4 weeks) history of major trauma, surgery, or gastrointestinal/genitourinary bleed
- Pregnant female
- Bleeding disorder, coagulopathy, or anticoagulated state
- Serious systemic disease
- Shock states (eg, hypotension, pulmonary edema)

Reperfusion arrhythmias are commonly seen in patients following thrombolytic therapy or after PCIs such as stent placement or angioplasty. When cardiac tissue becomes ischemic, potassium leaves the intracellular space. With reperfusion, the potassium rapidly returns to the intracellular spaces, resulting in rhythm disturbances. Usually these disturbances are short-lived, but serious rhythm disturbances, including cardiac arrest, have occurred. Patients also should be monitored for signs of bleeding (eg, femoral or retroperitoneal hematomas, rigid

abdomen, hypotension, unexplained tachycardia) and a headache with an altered level of consciousness. If severe bleeding occurs, the CCTP should turn off the heparin drip. Hypotension is managed with fluids or pressors, and the transport may need to be diverted to the closest hospital for stabilization and treatment of the patient, possibly including a blood transfusion.

Transport Management

Acute Coronary Syndrome (Interfacility Transport)

- Control blood pressure.
- Provide analgesia.
- Provide anxiolytics, if indicated.
- Collaborate with the sending provider to assure an ADP inhibitor has been administered, if indicated.
- Assess for and treat pulmonary edema.
- Monitor the heparin (anticoagulant) and/or eptifibatide (antiplatelet) drips.
- Monitor the patient for signs of bleeding and headache with altered level of consciousness.
- Give sufficient oxygen to maintain an oxygen saturation of 92% to 97%.
- If the patient required mechanical ventilation, monitor with continuous waveform capnography, and maintain the carbon dioxide level between 35 and 45 mm Hg.
- Monitor the cardiac rhythm.
- Administer thrombolytics, if indicated.
- If severe bleeding occurs, discontinue any anticoagulant, thrombolytic, or antiplatelet infusions; manage hypotension with fluids or pressors; and consider diversion to the closest hospital for stabilization and further treatment.

Angina Pectoris

The principal symptom of CAD is angina pectoris. Angina occurs when the supply of oxygen to the myocardium is insufficient to meet the demand. As a result, the cardiac muscle becomes ischemic, and a switch to anaerobic metabolism leads to an accumulation of lactic acid and carbon dioxide. A person who experiences angina caused by CAD while at rest, when oxygen needs are minimal, has more severe CAD than a person who experiences angina only with vigorous exercise.

When obtaining the medical history from a patient with chest pain, it is important to distinguish between stable angina and unstable angina. Stable angina follows a recurrent pattern: A person with stable angina experiences pain after a certain, predictable amount of exertion, such as climbing one flight of stairs or walking for three blocks. The pain also has a predictable location, intensity, and duration.

Chronic, stable angina is the result of an atherosclerotic lesion that diminishes the myocardial oxygen supply available during exertion. Patients with this type of angina often take nitroglycerin or some other form of nitrate for relief of anginal pain. In the CCT environment, nitroglycerin should be given intravenously, especially for long transports. IV nitroglycerin is better able to control anginal pain compared to other forms of nitroglycerin. When IV nitroglycerin is given, it is advisable to discontinue all other forms of nitroglycerin. If a patient who is being transported is not taking nitroglycerin and suddenly develops chest pain, a sublingual nitroglycerin tablet or spray may be used initially to reduce the discomfort while delivery of IV nitroglycerin is being established or titrated upward.

Unstable angina is much more serious than stable angina and indicates a greater degree of obstruction of the coronary arteries. In many cases, it is caused by a thrombus or plaque rupture. This condition is characterized by noticeable changes in the frequency, severity, and duration of pain, and often occurs when the patient is not experiencing predictable stress. The patient may report that the anginal attacks have grown more frequent and severe during the past several days or weeks, that they awaken the individual from sleep, or that they occur when the individual is otherwise at rest. Nitroglycerin is often not effective with this type of angina. Such attacks are often warning signs of an impending MI.

Finally, silent ischemia refers to the presence of angina without clinical manifestations, which is detected only when ST-segment elevation is noted on the ECG.

Myocardial Infarction

An MI can occur as a result of the cardiac muscle being deprived of coronary blood flow long enough for myocardial tissue death to ensue. Narrowed vessels (eg, from atherosclerotic disease), coronary artery occlusion (eg, by a thrombus), spasm of a coronary artery, and reduction of overall blood flow (eg, from shock, arrhythmias, or pulmonary embolism) are all potential causes of an MI.

The location and size of an MI depend on which coronary artery is blocked and where along its course the blockage occurred. The majority of infarcts involve the left ventricle. When the anterior, lateral, or septal walls of the left ventricle are infarcted, the source is usually occlusion of the left coronary artery or one of its branches. In most cases, IWMIs are the result of an RCA occlusion. When the ischemic process affects only the inner layer of muscle, the infarct is referred to as a subendocardial MI. By comparison, an infarct that extends through the entire wall of the ventricle is described as a transmural MI. The infarcted tissue is invariably surrounded by a ring of ischemic tissue—an area that is relatively deprived of oxygen but still viable. That ischemic tissue tends to be electrically unstable and is often the source of cardiac arrhythmias.

Acute MI is a leading cause of death in the United States, and more than 800,000 people experience MI each year in this country. Given that more than 70% of sudden cardiac arrests occur outside the hospital, emergency medical services (EMS) providers clearly have a crucial role in recognizing and promptly managing this condition. Patients at risk for sudden cardiac death include those with the following characteristics:

- Prior sudden cardiac arrest
- Prior MI
- HF, class II to IV
- Ejection fraction of less than 40%
- Family history of sudden cardiac arrest
- Prolonged QT interval

Of all deaths from acute MI, 90% are due to arrhythmias, usually ventricular fibrillation, which typically occur during the early hours of the infarct. Arrhythmias can be prevented or treated, so most deaths from acute MI are considered preventable.

Infarct Recognition and Localization

Many cardiac patients are transported from one facility to another where they can receive specialized procedures that are not available at the sending hospital. The physical and emotional stressors of the transport itself can place an additional burden on a patient in already critical condition. CCTPs must always remain acutely aware of the patient's cardiac status and ensure rapid identification of both new findings, including MI, and evolving and changing events.

The diagnosis of an MI relies on three initial components: the history and physical examination, testing for cardiac enzymes, and interpretation of ECG changes associated with an MI. An MI evolves from a normal state to ischemia, injury, and, ultimately, infarction when an event occludes vessels and limits the supply of oxygen-enriched blood reaching the cells. Ischemia and injury are reversible conditions that must be identified and treated to help prevent death of cardiac muscle.

As soon as a chief complaint of a cardiac nature has been noted, start treatment of the patient; obtaining a focused history and performing a physical examination can wait. However, for purposes of discussion, this section proceeds through the history and physical examination.

Cardiac Enzymes

In the past, serum testing for cardiac enzymes was not typically done during transport. Today, however, point-of-care testing devices are increasingly available, and CCTPs should be familiar with these assessment tools. Moreover, such test results are frequently available in the patient's chart and may help put the patient's cardiac status into perspective.

Although the ECG does not directly represent levels of cardiac enzymes that are released as cells are damaged, ECG changes are seen as an aftermath of cell damage because of the change in cell function. When myocardial cells die during an infarction, their internal contents leak into the bloodstream. Troponins T and I are contractile proteins of the myofibril that are specific for detecting myocardial cell injury; although not specific to STEMI/NSTEMI, they are the forms most commonly measured in testing. The levels of these proteins rise during the first 2 to 6 hours after injury, then peak from 12 to 16 hours after the MI. The cardiac troponin I level can remain elevated for 5 to 10 days, and the cardiac troponin T level can stay elevated for 5 to 14 days. Recently, high-sensitivity troponin assays are being used for faster diagnosis of MI.

Creatine kinase (creatine phosphokinase) is an enzyme found in heart (MB fraction) and skeletal (MM fraction) muscle as well as in the brain (BB fraction). The creatine kinase level increases in more than 90% of MIs. Because it is also found in skeletal muscle and the brain, this enzyme can be elevated during trauma and physical exertion, in postoperative patients, in patients with seizures, and in patients with other conditions in which cells are damaged. In an MI, the creatine kinase level begins to rise in 4 to 6 hours, peaks in 24 hours, and returns to normal in 3 to 4 days.

The creatine kinase isoenzyme MB fraction is specific to cardiac muscle. It rises and returns to normal sooner than the total creatine kinase level; that is, the MB fraction rises in 3 to 4 hours and returns to normal in 2 days.

Myoglobin is an oxygen-transport protein. Damage to skeletal or cardiac muscle causes its release into the circulation. After an MI, the myoglobin level rises in the first 2 hours, peaks in 6 to 8 hours, and finally returns to normal in 20 to 36 hours. An increased myoglobin level can also be found in skeletal muscle injury and renal failure, which explains why these values are no longer utilized in evaluation of ACS.

Because levels of several of these markers can be elevated in other medical conditions, they must be used in conjunction with other clinical and laboratory findings when a cardiac event is suspected. Current national and international guidelines for diagnosis of ACS suggest that when the troponin level is available, neither creatine kinase nor myoglobin measurement is useful for diagnosis of ACS.

Blood Supply

Before proceeding further, it is important to review how blood circulates throughout the heart, so as to better understand the ECG changes seen in an MI. The heart is a muscle and, like any muscle, requires an oxygen-enriched blood supply to survive. The blood supply to the heart is delivered through two main coronary arteries and their branches during diastole. Areas that are supplied by more than one source are said to have collateral circulation.

The right and left coronary arteries originate at the base of the aorta just above the aortic valve. The major branches of the right coronary artery are the marginal, posterior (descending) interventricular, and SA nodal branches. The RCA supplies blood to the right atrium, the right ventricle, and portions of the left atrium and left ventricle. The sinus node branch supplies blood to the sinus node, and the AV nodal branch supplies blood to the AV node.

The major branches of the left coronary artery are the anterior interventricular (also known as the left anterior descending) and left circumflex branches. The left coronary artery supplies both ventricles, the interventricular septum, and the left atrium. The left anterior descending artery supplies the right and left bundle branches.

The deoxygenated blood is returned to the venous circulation through the coronary sinus.

By understanding the coronary blood flow and the areas of the heart represented by the ECG, CCTPs can use ECG changes to identify which branch of the blood supply is affected during an MI. Be aware, however, that coronary artery distribution may vary slightly from patient to patient.

Ischemia, Injury, and Infarction

Decreased blood flow to the heart can result from a chronic condition, called coronary vascular disease, or from an acute injury, in which a coronary artery or one of its branches becomes occluded by an embolus. The heart begins in a normal state in which it is receiving an adequate blood supply. Increased oxygen demand caused by an increased workload or a decrease in supply caused by coronary vascular disease or a blocked artery can lead to ischemia, injury, and, ultimately, infarction. Ischemia and injury are reversible, and when evidence of either is present, rapid intervention can often prevent infarction.

When ischemia develops, the tissue becomes more electrically negative compared with the unaffected surrounding tissue. This change causes a pattern of ST-segment depression. The T wave is also inverted (flipped) because of repolarization occurring along abnormal pathways **FIGURE 14-51**.

Other causes of T-wave inversion are also possible, including ventricular hypertrophy with strain, BBB, and cerebral hemorrhage. To help distinguish ischemia from one of the other causes of T-wave inversion, examining the shape of the T wave may be helpful. With myocardial ischemia, the T wave inverts symmetrically. With other causes, the T-wave inversion is often asymmetric or "slurred."

As ischemia continues uninterrupted, injury develops. The injured area does not repolarize

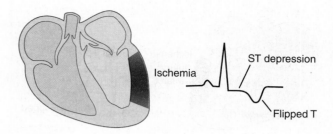

FIGURE 14-51 Ischemia.
© Jones & Bartlett Learning.

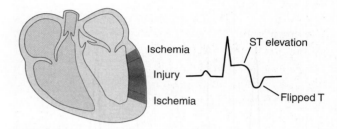

FIGURE 14-52 Ischemia and injury.
© Jones & Bartlett Learning.

completely, causing it to become more electrically positive than the unaffected area surrounding it. This change causes the ST segment to become elevated. The T wave remains inverted because it continues to repolarize through abnormal pathways. As the injury progresses, the elevation of the ST segment can increase **FIGURE 14-52**.

If ischemia and injury continue uninterrupted, infarction can occur. The infarcted tissue no longer generates or transmits electrical impulses, so the area becomes "electrically neutral." Because this tissue can no longer generate or transmit electrical impulses, no direct wave is recorded on the ECG. Electrical impulses are deflected away from the area of infarct and are represented by Q waves. Another way of looking at Q-wave formation is as the result of electrical impulses being generated by the other wall of the ventricle and passing unopposed away from the positive electrode. Because ischemia and injury continue to be present until the infarct process is completed, ST-segment elevation and inverted T waves will still be noted on the ECG **FIGURE 14-53**.

Sometimes small Q waves are seen in the left lateral leads (I, aVL, V_5, and V_6) and occasionally in the inferior leads (especially II and III) in patients with normal hearts. The normal small Q waves occur as

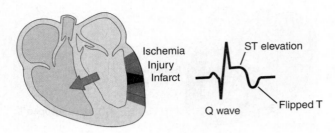

FIGURE 14-53 Ischemia, injury, and infarction.

© Jones & Bartlett Learning.

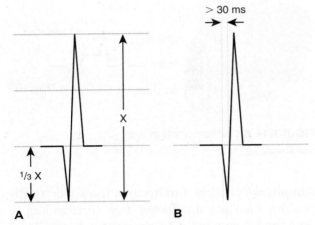

FIGURE 14-54 Q-wave significance. **A.** If the Q wave is more than one-third the total height of the QRS complex, it is a pathologic Q. **B.** If the Q wave is more than 30 ms wide, it is a pathologic Q.

© Jones & Bartlett Learning.

a result of early left-to-right depolarization of the interventricular septum. For Q waves to be significant, indicating pathology, they must be more than one-third the total height of the QRS complex with which they appear and wider than 40 ms in duration **FIGURE 14-54**.

An MI can occur with or without Q waves. Q waves can develop as discussed, especially when larger areas of myocardium are affected. With a smaller infarct, the cell-to-cell conduction of electrical impulses can hide the smaller resulting Q wave. Because ischemia and injury are always present in the setting of MI, ST-segment and T-wave abnormalities will still be present. When a patient has a history, signs and symptoms, and ECG changes suggestive of a cardiac event, a full workup is indicated. In this case, evaluation of cardiac enzymes can be the key to making the correct diagnosis.

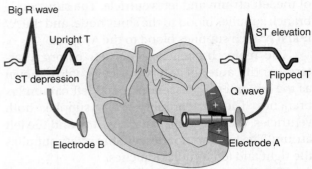

Note: The complexes above are color coded for each of the zones.

FIGURE 14-55 Reciprocal changes.

© Jones & Bartlett Learning.

Generally, STEMIs are associated with a higher incidence of HF and death because of the larger area of heart tissue damaged. NSTEMIs tend to lead to a higher incidence of long-term mortality because of life-threatening arrhythmias that arise from the area of infarction. Quick recognition of ischemia, injury, and infarction, followed by rapid intervention, can reduce the area of infarction and decrease the incidence of subsequent cardiac events that might lead to death.

As mentioned earlier in this section, the infarcted myocardial tissue becomes electrically neutral. As a result, the electrical current will be directed away from the area of infarction. The electrode that lies over the area of infarction will record a deep negative deflection, a Q wave. The electrical current that is directed away from the area of infarction causes **reciprocal changes** in leads located 180° from the site of infarction. Reciprocal leads must be 180° from the lead in question and lie in the same plane. Limb leads and precordial leads cannot be reciprocal, because limb leads lie in the frontal or vertical plane, whereas precordial leads lie in the horizontal plane. The apparent increase in electrical force moving toward the opposite lead will be recorded as tall, positive R waves. This applies not only to Q waves, but also to ST-segment and T-wave changes. For example, a Q wave, an ST-segment elevation, and a T-wave inversion recorded in leads II, III, and aVF will be recorded as a tall R wave, ST-segment depression, and an upright T wave in the reciprocal leads I and aVL **FIGURE 14-55** and **TABLE 14-8**.

TABLE 14-8 Reciprocal Leads and Their Corresponding Locations

Location	Facing Leads	Reciprocal Leads
Anterior	V_3, V_4	None
Inferior	II, III, aVF	I, aVL
Lateral	I, aVL, V_5, V_6	II, III, aVF
Septum	V_1, V_2	None
Posterior	None	V_1, V_2

© Jones & Bartlett Learning.

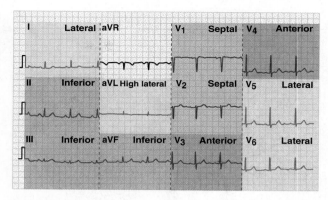

FIGURE 14-56 Correlation between areas of the heart and leads on the electrocardiogram.

© Jones & Bartlett Learning.

Localizing the Infarction

The area of myocardium that infarcts depends on which coronary arteries are occluded and the extent of the collateral blood flow. It is important to localize where an infarction has occurred because the prognostic and therapeutic implications are determined largely by which area of the heart has died. Each of the coronary arteries perfuses more than one area in the heart. Thus, if one coronary artery becomes blocked, more than one region of the heart can become ischemic and develop injury and, ultimately, infarction. ECG findings, therefore, do not always fall neatly into one anatomic area of infarction.

Acute MIs often involve more than one region of the heart. For example, an inferior MI is often an inferoposterior MI, an anterior MI can become anteroseptal or anterolateral, lateral MIs are often posterolateral, and so forth **FIGURE 14-56**. Q waves from old infarctions can be present with findings of a new MI and can obfuscate the process of making the correct diagnosis from the ECG. In the CCT setting, the patient by definition is in serious condition and will likely have evidence of one or more underlying conditions. This makes it even more important to review an "old" ECG from the patient's chart, acquire a new 12-lead ECG before transport, and make serial evaluations along the way. To be sure an ECG change has occurred, CCTPs must know what was there before they came in contact with the patient.

With all this in mind, in general, infarctions can be grouped into several general anatomic categories **TABLE 14-9**.

Acute Anterior Myocardial Infarction

An anterior wall MI seldom occurs alone. It involves the anterior surface of the left ventricle and

TABLE 14-9 Coronary Artery Relationships to Area Perfused

Area of the Heart	Main Arteries That Perfuse the Area
Inferior	RCA (90%), LCx (10%)
Inferior right ventricle	Proximal RCA
Inferoposterior	RCA (90%), LCx (10%)
Isolated right ventricle	LCx
Isolated posterior	RCA (90%), LCx (10%)
Anterior	Left anterior descending
Anteroseptal	Left anterior descending
Anteroseptal-lateral	Proximal left anterior descending
Anterolateral, inferolateral, or posterolateral	LCx

Abbreviations: LCx, left circumflex artery; RCA, right coronary artery

© Jones & Bartlett Learning.

is usually caused by occlusion of the left anterior descending artery **FIGURE 14-57**. Leads V_3 and V_4 are considered the anterior leads **FIGURE 14-58**. In an anterior MI, the normal pattern of R-wave progression may not occur, a situation called poor R-wave progression.

Even without significant Q-wave formation, poor R-wave progression may signify an anterior MI. Poor R-wave progression can also be seen in

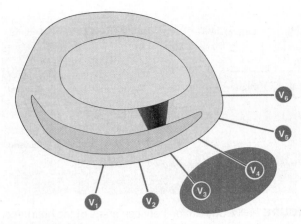

FIGURE 14-57 Anterior wall myocardial infarction.

© Jones & Bartlett Learning.

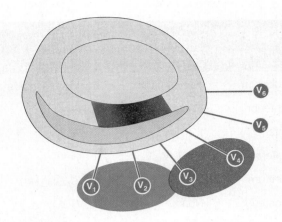

FIGURE 14-59 Anteroseptal myocardial infarction.

© Jones & Bartlett Learning.

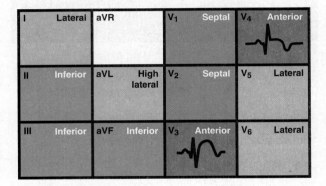

FIGURE 14-58 Anterior leads.

© Jones & Bartlett Learning.

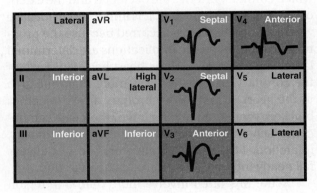

FIGURE 14-60 Anteroseptal leads.

© Jones & Bartlett Learning.

patients with RVH and chronic lung disease and with improper lead placement. By itself, it is not specific for the diagnosis of anterior MI.

Acute Anteroseptal Myocardial Infarction

An anteroseptal MI is common with an occlusion of the left anterior descending artery. As with all anterior MIs, this presentation is often associated with hemodynamic compromise and cardiogenic shock. The leads that offer the best view of this MI pattern are the septal leads V_1 and V_2 and the anterior leads V_3 and V_4 **FIGURE 14-59** and **FIGURE 14-60**.

The ECG in **FIGURE 14-61** represents an acute anteroseptal MI. The anterior and septal leads, V_1 through V_4, show marked elevation and flattening of the ST segment, which is typical of this pattern

of infarction. Further evaluation of the ECG shows some minimal elevation of the ST segment in lead aVL. The left anterior descending artery perfuses all three areas. ST-segment depression is found in the reciprocal leads, II, III, and aVF.

Acute Anteroseptal Myocardial Infarction With Lateral Wall Extension

If the proximal left anterior descending artery is occluded, an acute anteroseptal MI with lateral wall extension may result. Changes can be seen in all precordial leads (specifically, V_5 and V_6 for the lateral extension) and in leads I and aVL. With the loss of electrical impulses in the anterior infarcted tissue, there is not always significant Q-wave formation. Reciprocal changes can be found in leads II, III, and aVF **FIGURE 14-62** and **FIGURE 14-63**.

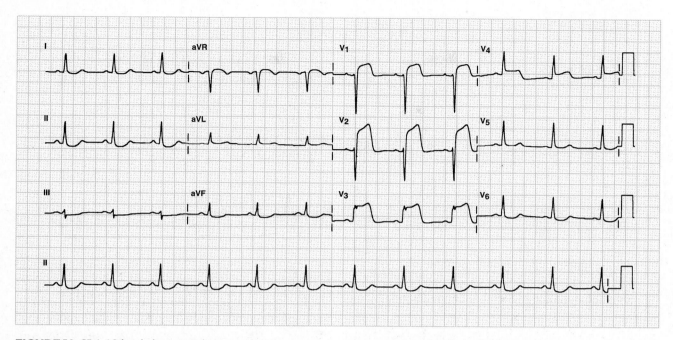

FIGURE 14-61 A 12-lead electrocardiogram showing an acute anteroseptal myocardial infarction.

Reproduced from *Introduction to 12-Lead ECG: The Art of Interpretation*, courtesy of Tomas B. Garcia, MD.

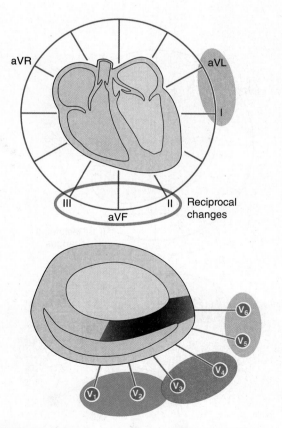

FIGURE 14-62 Acute anteroseptal myocardial infarction with lateral wall extension.

© Jones & Bartlett Learning.

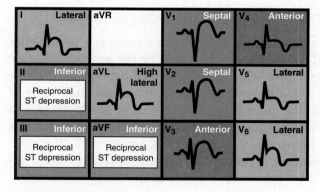

FIGURE 14-63 Electrocardiographic changes seen in an anteroseptal myocardial infarction with lateral wall extension.

© Jones & Bartlett Learning.

The ECG in **FIGURE 14-64** represents an acute anteroseptal MI with lateral wall extension. The ST-segment elevation in leads V_2 through V_6 extends to leads I and aVL. Reciprocal changes are seen in leads III and aVF. In addition to the signs of ischemia and injury, Q waves are forming in leads V_3 to V_6 and in leads I and aVL. In this ECG, the ST segments are very elevated and the T waves are tall and peaked; this phenomenon, often referred to as hyperacute T-wave changes, indicates an early acute MI. The hyperacute T-wave changes occur

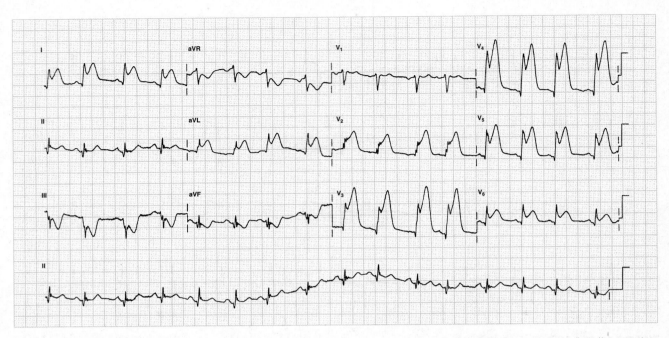

FIGURE 14-64 A 12-lead electrocardiogram showing an acute anteroseptal myocardial infarction with lateral wall extension.

Reproduced from *Introduction to 12-Lead ECG: The Art of Interpretation*, courtesy of Tomas B. Garcia, MD.

only during the first 15 to 30 minutes of an acute MI. When they occur outside the hospital, they are seldom seen because responders usually arrive after the period when these changes are visible. If these changes are found during transport, CCTPs are in a unique position to initiate care, even if it is only to notify the receiving facility to decrease the door-to-treatment time. Early revascularization has a good outcome because the period of ischemia has been relatively short and less permanent damage has been done.

Acute Lateral Wall Myocardial Infarction

An acute lateral wall MI involves the left lateral wall of the heart. It can occur alone or with other patterns of infarction. This type of MI is often the result of occlusion of the left circumflex artery. ECG changes may occur in the lateral leads (I, aVL, V$_5$, and V$_6$), while reciprocal changes may be seen in the inferior leads (II, III, and aVF) **FIGURE 14-65** and **FIGURE 14-66**.

The ECG in **FIGURE 14-67** represents an acute lateral wall MI. There is ST-segment elevation in the lateral leads I and aVL, and reciprocal changes are

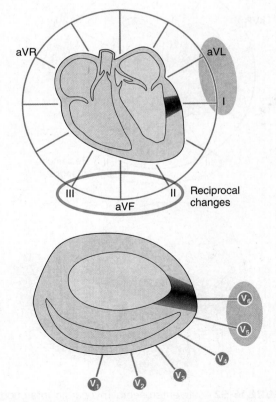

FIGURE 14-65 Lateral wall myocardial infarction.

© Jones & Bartlett Learning.

apparent in the inferior leads II, III, and aVF. Further evaluation shows T-wave inversions in the lateral precordial leads V$_5$ and V$_6$. Because the inverted T waves are symmetric, they are related to the acute lateral wall MI and not associated with LVH with strain. An LVH pattern shows an asymmetric inverted T wave.

Acute Inferior Wall Myocardial Infarction

An IWMI involves the diaphragmatic surface of the heart. It is caused by occlusion of the right coronary

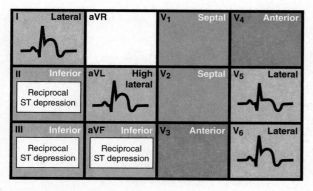

FIGURE 14-66 Electrocardiographic changes seen with lateral wall myocardial infarction.

© Jones & Bartlett Learning.

artery in 90% of patients and by occlusion in its descending branch or the left circumflex artery in 10% of patients. The characteristic ECG changes of infarction can be seen in the inferior leads II, III, and aVF. Reciprocal changes are seen as ST-segment depression in leads I and aVL, unless the high lateral wall is included in the infarction. An IWMI is commonly seen with patterns involving the lateral wall, the posterior wall, and RVMIs. Q waves persist for the lifetime of the patient in most cases, though not necessarily in inferior infarctions. Nearly 50% of inferior infarctions fail to meet the criteria for significant Q waves within 6 months. Small Q waves in the inferior leads may suggest an old inferior infarction. Small inferior Q waves may be present in healthy hearts, so it is important to use the patient's clinical history in decision making **FIGURE 14-68** and **FIGURE 14-69**.

The ECG in **FIGURE 14-70** represents an acute IWMI. Pathologic Q waves appear in leads II and aVF. There are no acute ST-segment or T-wave changes present that would be consistent with an acute infarction. There are also no reciprocal changes found in leads I or aVL. Without signs of acute infarction, pathologic Q waves are considered age indeterminate; without a good patient history, there is no other way to know how old they are.

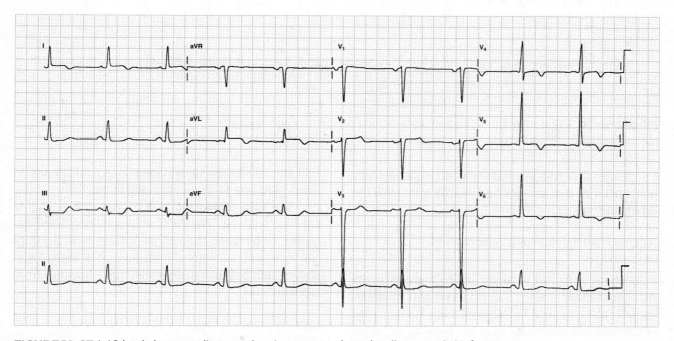

FIGURE 14-67 A 12-lead electrocardiogram showing an acute lateral wall myocardial infarction.

Reproduced from *Introduction to 12-Lead ECG: The Art of Interpretation*, courtesy of Tomas B. Garcia, MD.

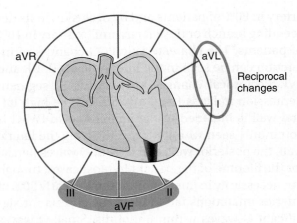

FIGURE 14-68 An inferior wall myocardial infarction.

© Jones & Bartlett Learning.

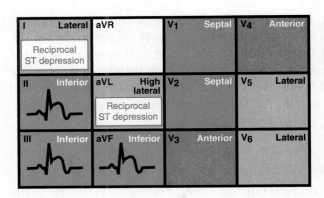

FIGURE 14-69 Electrocardiographic changes seen with inferior wall myocardial infarction.

© Jones & Bartlett Learning.

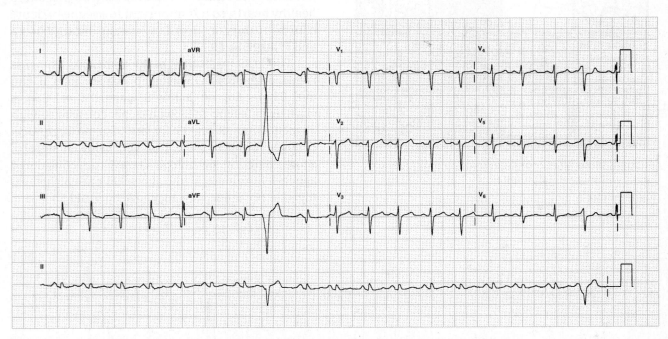

FIGURE 14-70 A 12-lead electrocardiogram showing an acute inferior wall myocardial infarction.

Reproduced from *Introduction to 12-Lead ECG: The Art of Interpretation*, courtesy of Tomas B. Garcia, MD.

There are also two premature ventricular ectopic beats present that are not necessarily related to the other findings.

Acute Inferolateral Myocardial Infarction

ECG changes found in acute inferolateral MIs are seen in inferior leads II, III, and aVF and in lateral leads I, aVL, V_5, and V_6. ST-segment changes may occur and will be found in leads V_2 to V_4 if the infarct extends anteriorly. When anterior extension is present, classic ST-segment and T-wave changes will always be seen in the lateral precordial leads, V_5 and V_6 **FIGURE 14-71** and **FIGURE 14-72**.

The ECG in **FIGURE 14-73** represents an acute inferior wall MI. The ECG shows ST-segment elevation in leads II, III, and aVF. Reciprocal findings are visible as ST-segment depression in leads I and aVL, which helps to distinguish these findings from pericarditis.

Acute Apical Myocardial Infarction

An apical MI is an extension of an inferolateral MI. It covers a large area of the inferior part of the heart

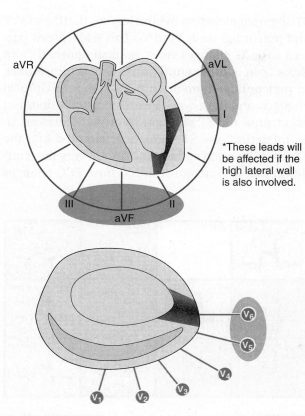

*These leads will be affected if the high lateral wall is also involved.

FIGURE 14-71 Inferolateral leads.

© Jones & Bartlett Learning.

and extends further anteriorly and laterally. The acute apical MI occurs in a patient with RCA dominance. Direct ECG changes can be found in inferior leads II, III, and aVF; lateral leads I and aVL; and precordial leads V_2 through V_6. Because of the diffuse ECG changes, an acute apical MI may be confused with pericarditis **FIGURE 14-74** and **FIGURE 14-75**.

The ECG in **FIGURE 14-76** represents an acute apical MI. Because of the large area affected, the ECG changes are diffuse and can take the form of

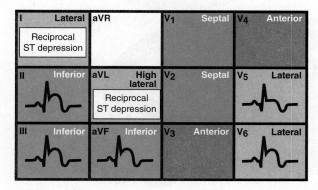

FIGURE 14-72 Electrocardiographic changes seen with acute inferolateral myocardial infarction.

© Jones & Bartlett Learning.

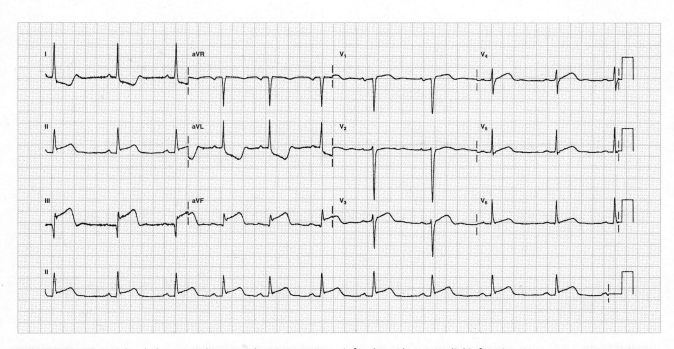

FIGURE 14-73 A 12-lead electrocardiogram showing an acute inferolateral myocardial infarction.

Reproduced from *Introduction to 12-Lead ECG: The Art of Interpretation*, courtesy of Tomas B. Garcia, MD.

ST-segment elevation in limb leads I, II, III, and aVF and precordial leads V_2 to V_6. This widespread pattern of ECG changes must be distinguished from those seen in other conditions such as pericarditis. In pericarditis, there are no Q waves or reciprocal changes, and the T-wave inversion usually does not occur until the ST segment returns to baseline. In an infarction, the ST segment is elevated and the T wave is inverted at the same time. A very rare condition that also demonstrates diffuse ECG changes

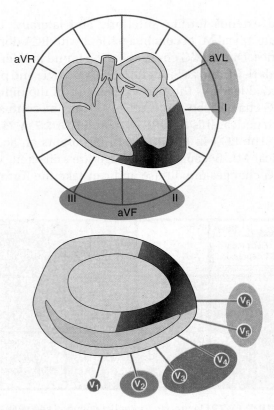

FIGURE 14-74 Acute apical myocardial infarction leads.

© Jones & Bartlett Learning.

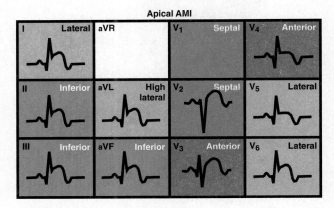

FIGURE 14-75 Electrocardiographic changes seen with an acute apical myocardial infarction.

© Jones & Bartlett Learning.

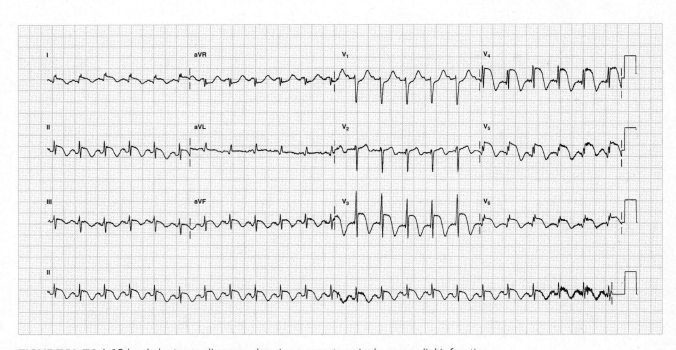

FIGURE 14-76 A 12-lead electrocardiogram showing an acute apical myocardial infarction.

Reproduced from *Introduction to 12-Lead ECG: The Art of Interpretation*, courtesy of Tomas B. Garcia, MD.

is aortic dissection, which occludes the coronary ostea (the origin of the coronary arteries) on the aorta just distal to the aortic valve. This blockage, among other things, causes a global infarction of the heart because it occludes the source of both main coronary arteries.

To rule out some of the more serious differential diagnoses when acute apical MI is suspected, a complete history and clinical evaluations are needed; in addition, radiographic testing, echocardiograms, and more sophisticated tests such as cardiac catheterizations may be necessary. Problematically, no single exam or test is completely reliable for diagnosing acute apical MI.

Acute Right Ventricular Myocardial Infarction

This section predominantly deals with the criteria for identifying RVMI. Further study of RVMI is suggested to obtain a better understanding of its pathophysiology, clinical diagnosis, and management.

RVMI is strongly associated with IWMIs in 30% to 50% of cases **FIGURE 14-77** because both of these

areas are most often perfused by the RCA and its branches. An occlusion of the RCA would likely affect both regions of the heart at the same time. In a small percentage of cases, the left circumflex artery can supply regions of the inferior wall and right ventricle; in these cases, an occlusion in the left circumflex artery could, therefore, cause the same pattern of infarction. RVMIs accompany an additional 10% of anterior wall MIs. Because of the high coexistence of RVMI with IWMI, it is important for CCTPs to maintain a high index of suspicion and check for other criteria.

When RVMI is present, the ST segment is greater in lead III than in lead II **FIGURE 14-78**. Because of the RVMI, the electrical impulse flows unopposed from the interventricular septum and is directed anteriorly, inferiorly, and to the right. Because this impulse flow causes the vector to move toward the lead III electrode, it is recorded with greater amplitude there than in lead II.

With ST-segment elevation in (septal) lead V_1 and (inferior) leads II, III, and aVF, RVMI should be suspected. Because the electrical impulses are not being transmitted through infarcted tissue, they continue to travel unopposed in all other directions. The alteration in the wave of depolarization generally causes ST-segment elevation in V_1 and ST-segment depression in V_2. Depending on the extent of the MI in the involved heart tissue, ST-segment elevation can sometimes extend through V_5 or V_6.

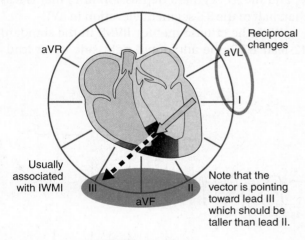

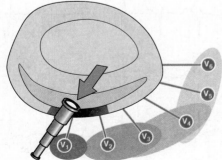

FIGURE 14-77 A right ventricular infarction.

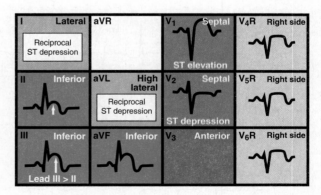

FIGURE 14-78 Electrocardiographic changes seen with a right ventricular infarction. Note the ST-segment elevation in lead V_1. Depending on how much of the RV is affected, this ST-segment elevation can extend up to V_6. In addition, the amount of ST-segment depression has to be less than half of the ST-segment elevation in lead aVF to warrant the diagnosis of RVMI.

As mentioned, ST-segment elevation will occur in V_1, but it will usually be depressed in V_2. This difference arises because MI-related alterations in the electrical impulse will cause the vector to travel more directly toward V_1 and past V_2.

An ST-segment depression in V_2 that is less than half the height of the ST-segment elevation in aVF indicates the infarct is localized to the inferior right ventricular region. An ST-segment depression in V_2 that is more than half the height of the ST-segment elevation in aVF indicates that the infarct is larger and includes the inferior wall, right ventricle, and posterior wall.

The use of nonstandard or additional leads on the right side of the chest is important for localizing an infarction. An ST-segment elevation of 1 mm or more in the right-side chest leads, V_4R to V_6R, is the most specific indication for RVMI. Evidence of IWMI (eg, ST-segment elevation and T-wave inversion in leads II, II, and aVF) combined with 1 mm or more ST-segment elevation in V_4R is considered diagnostic of an inferior RVMI. If right-side chest leads are being obtained, a complete set, including V_4R through V_6R, should allow for a more complete view of the right ventricle. In the presence of IWMI, right ventricular leads should always be recorded as well.

The criteria for diagnosing RVMI are as follows:

- IWMI
- ST-segment elevation greater in lead III than in lead II
- ST-segment elevation in V_1 that could extend through V_5 or V_6
- ST-segment depression in V_2 (unless the ST-segment elevation extends through V_5 or V_6)
- ST-segment depression in V_2 that is not more than half of the ST-segment elevation in aVF
- 1 mm or more of ST-segment elevation in the right-side leads (V_4R to V_6R)

The ECG in **FIGURE 14-79** represents an RVMI. The first notable changes on the standard 12-lead ECG are the classic findings of an IWMI and ST-segment elevation in leads II, III, and aVF, with reciprocal findings of ST-segment depression in leads I and aVL. An RVMI is suspected because of the IWMI; lead III shows an ST-segment elevation greater than that noted in lead II. Additional criteria for RVMI are met with the ST-segment elevation in V_1 and the ST-segment depression in V_2 that is less than half of the ST-segment elevation in aVF.

With the criteria met for RVMI in the standard 12-lead ECG, the additional right-side chest leads

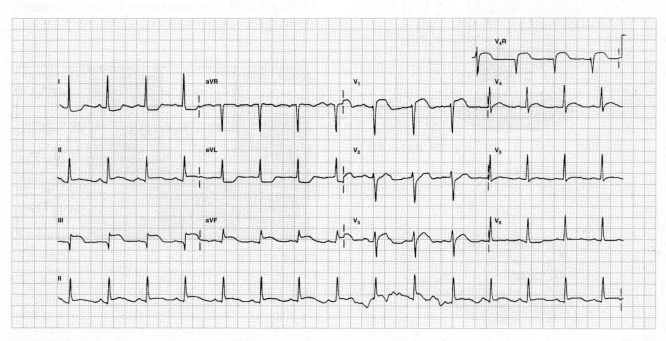

FIGURE 14-79 A 12-lead electrocardiogram showing a right ventricular infarction.

Reproduced from *Introduction to 12-Lead ECG: The Art of Interpretation*, courtesy of Tomas B. Garcia, MD.

V_4R to V_6R should be considered. The ST-segment elevation in lead V_4R completes the diagnostic criteria for RVMI. (Note: The example in Figure 14-79 shows only lead V_4R.)

Acute Posterior Wall Myocardial Infarction

A PWMI is caused by an occlusion of the RCA. The RCA bifurcates into the posterior descending artery and the right posterolateral artery in 80% to 85% of the population; the posterior descending artery comes off of the left circumflex artery in the remaining 15% to 20% of the population. The posterior descending artery, which is sometimes called the posterior interventricular artery, supplies the inferior wall, ventricular septum, and posteromedial papillary muscle. The right posterolateral artery divides into branches that supply the posterior surface of the left ventricle.

On a standard 12-lead ECG, there are no leads that specifically look at the posterior surface of the heart. Thus, when using standard 12-lead ECG technology, the diagnosis of PWMI is made by looking for reciprocal changes in leads V_1 and V_2. These changes include ST-segment depression, upright T waves, and tall R waves. Normally, the QRS complex in lead V_1 has a small R wave and a deep S wave. **FIGURE 14-80** shows the characteristic reciprocal changes of a PWMI as seen in leads V_1 and V_2. The addition of posterior leads can record a direct representation of electrical impulses through the posterior wall.

An R wave with greater amplitude than the corresponding S wave is highly suggestive of a PWMI. In RVH, an R wave greater than the corresponding S wave is also present in lead V_1. The difference is that RVH also requires the presence of an RAD, which is not present in a PWMI.

Because the posterior descending artery branch of the right coronary artery also perfuses regions of the inferior wall, posterior and inferior wall MIs often occur together.

As discussed earlier, nonstandard or additional leads can be used to provide a direct view of the posterior wall of the heart. When there is reciprocal evidence of a PWMI, the CCTP should maintain a high index of suspicion and record the posterior leads (V_7, V_8, and V_9) for comparison. Record a standard 12-lead ECG first. Then add the additional posterior electrodes, attach the precordial leads as described,

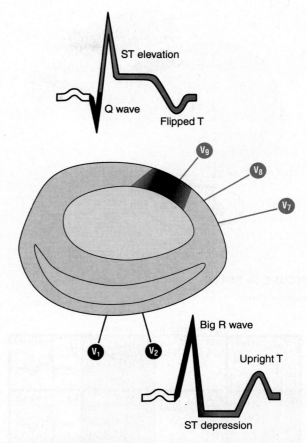

FIGURE 14-80 A posterior wall myocardial infarction.

© Jones & Bartlett Learning.

and record and "label" the posterior leads to avoid confusion. In the posterior leads, the electrical impulses must travel through the larger muscle mass of the back, which increases the electrical resistance. The complexes are typically positive but tend to have a lower amplitude.

FIGURE 14-81 and **FIGURE 14-82** permit comparison of the reciprocal changes of PWMI seen in leads V_1 and V_2 with those in posterior leads V_7, V_8, and V_9.

The ECG in **FIGURE 14-83** represents a PWMI with reciprocal changes seen on a standard 12-lead ECG. This ECG shows tall R waves in leads V_1 and V_2, as well as ST-segment depression with an upright T wave. These changes are all suggestive of a PWMI.

As mentioned, in the majority of the population, the coronary blood supply to the posterior wall is also shared by the inferior wall and right ventricle. In consequence, patterns of infarction with changes associated with the inferoposterior and inferior-right ventricular-posterior areas are often seen.

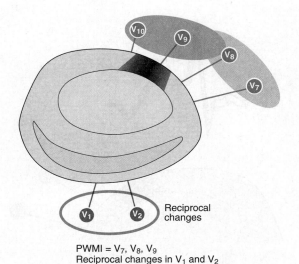

PWMI = V$_7$, V$_8$, V$_9$
Reciprocal changes in V$_1$ and V$_2$

FIGURE 14-81 A posterior wall myocardial infarction.

© Jones & Bartlett Learning.

Posterior Wall MI (PWMI)

I	Lateral	aVR		V$_1$	Septal	V$_7$	Posterior
II	Inferior	aVL	High lateral	V$_2$	Septal	V$_8$	Posterior
III	Inferior	aVF	Inferior	V$_3$	Anterior	V$_9$	Posterior

FIGURE 14-82 Electrocardiographic changes seen with a posterior wall myocardial infarction.

© Jones & Bartlett Learning.

Cardiomyopathy

Cardiomyopathy is a general term for diseases in which the myocardium becomes dilated, enlarged, or stiffened, ultimately progressing to HF, acute MI, or death. One variant, hypertrophic cardiomyopathy, is an autosomal-dominant hereditary disease. The main feature of hypertrophic cardiomyopathy is an excessive thickening of the heart muscle (*hypertrophy* means "to thicken or grow excessively"). In addition, microscopic examination of the heart muscle shows that it is abnormal. Patients may have shortness of breath, chest pain, palpitations, or syncope. Progression of cardiomyopathy is common, even with treatment, and sudden cardiac death can occur. A wide range of medications are used to arrest or delay progression of HF. Many patients require pacemaker and/or defibrillator implantation. Some will be referred for ventricular assist devices or heart transplant.

Heart Failure

Formerly known as congestive heart failure (CHF; also called chronic heart failure), the more contemporary term **heart failure (HF)** refers to a decline in the ability of the heart, for any reason, to pump powerfully enough or fast enough to empty its chambers. Although development of HF is not always a result of acute MI, the basic principles of diagnosis and treatment are similar, whatever the precipitating factors. It was previously believed that congestion and fluid overload were largely responsible for

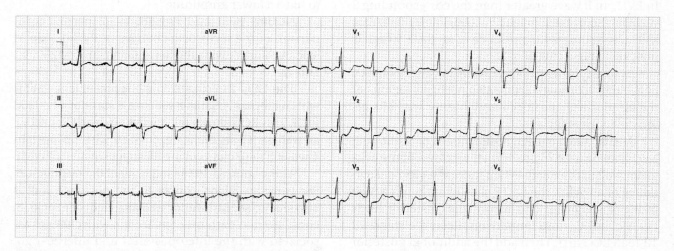

FIGURE 14-83 A 12-lead electrocardiogram showing a posterior wall myocardial infarction.

Reproduced from *Introduction to 12-Lead ECG: The Art of Interpretation*, courtesy of Tomas B. Garcia, MD.

the dyspnea and edema of HF. Newer evidence has demonstrated that a significant number (perhaps as many as half) of patients presenting with acute decompensated HF are actually intravascularly volume depleted rather than fluid overloaded. This factor, coupled with the difficulty in differentiating HF from pulmonary causes of dyspnea and orthopnea, has significantly reduced the role of diuretics as first-line therapy in patients with dyspnea and adventitious lung sounds.

More than 6.2 million people in the United States have HF, and an additional 550,000 cases are diagnosed each year. One-fourth of the patients with HF classified as severe die within 1 year of diagnosis, half of patients die within 5 years of their HF diagnosis, and the remaining 25% die within 10 years. Severe cases are defined as patients with acute pulmonary edema and marked limitations of their physical activity; cases involving cardiogenic shock are life threatening. HF is often described in relationship to preserved or reduced ejection fraction (HFpEF or HFrEF).

HF can have a number of causes, including the following:

- Wall abnormalities (dilated and hypertrophic)
- Valve failure (mitral, tricuspid, aortic, and pulmonic)
- Damage as the result of infarctions
- Conduction abnormalities

In most cases, HF begins with a major infarction involving one or more of the left ventricle walls (septum, anterior, or lateral). Major infarctions can often involve the right side and inferior walls. In any case, the combination of subsequent inadequate coronary artery oxygenation and cardiac damage often leads to conduction path disturbances, particularly AV nodal blocks requiring pacemaker implantation.

Another problem occurs around the areas of a major infarction. The new nerve fibers develop with an increased density that results in hyperinnervation. In turn, this condition can lead to VT and ventricular fibrillation, requiring ICD implantation.

In cases of infarctions involving the septum, synchronization between the ventricles is lost and the ejection fraction is reduced. Patients often require biventricular pacing to restore synchrony.

Left-Side Heart Failure

The left ventricle is most commonly damaged during an acute MI. Likewise, in chronic hypertension, the left ventricle tends to reflect the long-term effects of having to pump against an increased afterload (constricted peripheral arteries). In both cases, the right side of the heart continues to pump relatively normally and to deliver normal volumes of blood to the pulmonary circulation. By comparison, the left side of the heart may no longer be able to adequately pump the blood being delivered from the pulmonary vessels. As a result, blood backs up behind the left ventricle, and the pressure in the left atrium and pulmonary veins increases. As the pulmonary veins become engorged with blood, serum is forced out of the pulmonary capillaries and into the alveoli. This serum mixes with air in the alveoli to produce foam (in pulmonary edema).

When fluid fills the alveoli, oxygenation is impaired. The patient experiences that impairment as shortness of breath (dyspnea), particularly when in a recumbent position. Such orthopnea may occur in conjunction with **paroxysmal nocturnal dyspnea**—that is, severe shortness of breath occurring at night after several hours of recumbency, during which fluid builds up in the lungs; the person is forced to sit up to breathe. Paroxysmal nocturnal dyspnea is caused by left-side HF or the decompensation of COPD. If left ventricular failure is the result of chronic overload (as opposed to acute MI), the patient is likely to give a history of a week or two of paroxysmal nocturnal dyspnea. To compensate for the impairment in oxygenation, the patient's respiratory rate increases (tachypnea); even so, if the patient's condition is advanced enough, hypoxia may become evident. In some patients with pulmonary edema, especially elderly patients, Cheyne-Stokes respirations may be present.

Fluid from the pulmonary vessels also leaks into the interstitial spaces in the lungs, and increasing interstitial pressure causes narrowing of the bronchioles. Air passing through the narrowed bronchioles creates wheezing, whereas air bubbling through the fluid-filled alveoli produces crackles. Furthermore, the patient may cough up edematous fluid in the form of foamy, blood-tinged sputum. As the airways narrow and the lungs grow moist from the accumulation of fluid, the work of breathing increases, which puts an even greater strain on the already floundering heart. Dyspnea and hypoxemia produce a state of panic, which induces the release of epinephrine from the adrenal glands. The heart is pushed to work even harder, and its oxygen demand is increased precisely when fluid in the alveoli is reducing the amount of oxygen available.

To make matters worse, the sympathetic nervous system response produces peripheral vasoconstriction: Peripheral resistance (afterload) increases, and the weakened, hypoxic heart finds itself trying to push blood out into smaller and smaller pipes. Clinically, peripheral vasoconstriction is apparent as pallor and elevated blood pressure. The massive sympathetic discharge also produces sweating of the pale, cold skin.

It is not unusual for a patient with left-side HF to become frantic from air hunger. The patient may pace or thrash about or may even be combative and struggle with health care providers. Furthermore, hypoxemia results in inadequate oxygen supply to the brain, often manifested as confusion or disorientation. If hypoxemia is severe, brady-asystolic cardiac arrest may follow.

Signs and Symptoms of Left-Side Heart Failure

The signs and symptoms of left-side HF include extreme restlessness and agitation, confusion, severe dyspnea and tachypnea, tachycardia, elevated blood pressure, crackles and possibly wheezes, and frothy, pink sputum. Sometimes, it may be difficult to distinguish the wheezing of asthma from that of left-side HF. Capnography waveform analysis is often helpful in differentiating bronchoconstriction from respiratory distress secondary to pulmonary edema.

Management of Left-Side Heart Failure

If a CCT team is transporting a patient with left-side HF, the patient has probably experienced or is having an acute MI.

Pulmonary edema occurs as the result of the reduced ejection fraction and CO of the left ventricle. Because the CO from the right ventricle is normal, pulmonary hydrostatic pressure is increased. This greater pressure causes fluids to cross the alveolar-capillary membranes, filling the alveoli.

The priorities when managing left-side HF are as follows:

1. Decrease pulmonary congestion.
2. Reduce afterload.
3. Normalize myocardial oxygenation.
4. Decrease myocardial oxygen demands.

From a critical care point of view, if the patient is conscious and is able to maintain their airway, application of noninvasive ventilation (such as continuous positive airway pressure [CPAP] or bilevel positive airway pressure [BPAP]) addresses all of these objectives. Noninvasive ventilation provides a positive end-expiratory pressure (PEEP) that opens the terminal bronchi, expands the alveoli, and creates enough pressure to overcome the increased pulmonary hydrostatic pressure, theoretically forcing fluids back into the capillaries and reducing afterload.

If the patient's level of consciousness is such that they cannot maintain the airway, endotracheal intubation is indicated. Once successful intubation has been achieved, apply PEEP using a transport ventilator and manage secretions with endotracheal suctioning. Waveform capnography must be used to monitor ventilation.

Once the airway and ventilation are controlled, the blood pressure must be managed. If the patient has significant fluid overload, consider administering a diuretic to promote increased urine output.

Hypertension should be managed with IV antihypertensive medications. IV nitroglycerin is used to manage cardiac chest pain. This medication is usually started at a rate of 10 mcg/min, with the dose then being increased in 10-mcg increments until the patient obtains pain relief. The ceiling is considered to be a rate of 200 mcg/min, although many patients will experience intolerable headaches at lower doses of nitroglycerin.

Hypotension should be managed with pressors and cautiously with volume repletion. Use of a pressor that also provides inotropic support is likely to be more helpful than administration of a pure pressor agent alone. Although the best choice is currently unclear, dopamine, epinephrine, and norepinephrine are often chosen initially. Hypotensive patients with LV failure are quite likely to be in cardiogenic shock. An ideal IV agent for patients with such HF is dobutamine, as it provides both inotropic support and afterload reduction by vasodilation. Dobutamine is contraindicated in patients with hypotension.

When fluid overload is suspected, IV diuretics can be considered. Furosemide is often the first-line choice. Dosing is variable, but this medication is usually given as 0.5 to 1 mg/kg, not to exceed 80 mg. Continuous infusions of diuretics are also effective for patients with significant volume overload.

With all patients with HF or pulmonary edema, the CCTP should obtain a 12-lead ECG and monitor the patient for arrhythmias.

If there is evidence of an evolving or acute MI, the therapies discussed previously for ACS will also be needed during transport.

Signs and Symptoms

Left-Side Heart Failure
- Extreme restlessness and agitation
- Confusion
- Severe dyspnea and tachypnea
- Tachycardia
- Elevated blood pressure
- Crackles and possibly wheezes
- Frothy, pink sputum

Right-Side Heart Failure

Right-side HF most commonly occurs as a result of left-side HF. As blood backs up from the left side of the heart into the lungs, the right side has to work increasingly harder to pump blood into the engorged pulmonary vessels. Eventually, the right side of the heart cannot keep up with the increased workload, and it, too, fails. Right-side HF may also occur as a result of pulmonary embolism or long-standing COPD, especially chronic bronchitis.

When right-side HF occurs, blood backs up from the right ventricle, increasing pressure in the systemic veins and causing them to become engorged. Distention can be seen in surface veins, such as the external jugular veins. Over time, as the pressure within the systemic veins increases, serum is forced out of the veins and into the surrounding tissues, producing edema. This edema is most evident in dependent parts of the body, such as the legs and feet in an ambulatory patient (pedal edema) or the lower back in a bedridden patient (sacral edema). Edema is also present in parts of the body that are *not* visible; a painful liver that is easily palpable in the right upper quadrant, for example, signals engorgement and swelling (hepatomegaly).

The development of right-side HF can actually improve left-side HF because the failing right side of the heart can no longer pump as much blood

Transport Management

Left-Side Heart Failure
- If the patient is conscious and is able to maintain a patent airway, apply noninvasive ventilation (CPAP or BPAP).
- Intubate the patient if they cannot maintain the airway.
- Use the transport ventilator to apply PEEP to manage pulmonary edema.
- Suction the endotracheal tube, if in place, to manage secretions.
- Use continuous waveform capnography to monitor the patient's response to ventilation.
- Manage the patient's blood pressure (with vasodilators or pressors).
- Consider inotropic therapy for patients with significant HF symptoms.
- Obtain a 12-lead ECG.
- Monitor for arrhythmias.
- Provide analgesia and, if indicated, anxiolytics.
- If acute MI is identified, consider STEMI/ACS interventions (eg, antiplatelet agents, heparin, ADP inhibitors).

into the lungs. The decrease in right-side output amounts to a decrease in preload for the left side of the heart and may lessen pulmonary congestion.

Right-side HF, by itself, is seldom a life-threatening emergency. Usually it develops gradually over days to weeks; likewise, it requires days to weeks to reverse the process, with therapy focusing on slowly ridding the body of excess salt and water. Field treatment of right-side HF, therefore, is simply to make the patient comfortable, which is generally accomplished by placing the patient in the semi-Fowler position. Monitoring is always indicated in any patient with significant cardiac disease. If signs of associated left-side HF are present, treat them as outlined in the previous section.

Signs and Symptoms

Right-Side Heart Failure
- Edema

Transport Management

Right-Side Heart Failure

- Provide supportive care.
- Place the patient in a comfortable position, preferably a semi-Fowler position.
- Treat any signs of associated left-side HF.

Pulmonary Edema

Noninvasive ventilation, which includes CPAP, BPAP, and, in the opinion of some experts, high-flow nasal cannula (HFNC), is the mainstay of treatment for acute pulmonary edema in patients who are able to maintain their airways. Depending on the modality employed, noninvasive ventilation may improve alveolar ventilation and gas exchange, decrease the work of breathing, decrease preload and afterload, and increase lung compliance and functional residual capacity. (Ventilator support is discussed in Chapter 6, *Respiratory Emergencies and Airway Management*, and Chapter 7, *Ventilation*.)

Intubation of patients with acute respiratory distress resulting from asthma, COPD, or pulmonary edema should be seen as a last resort. Noninvasive ventilation leads to fewer complications and greater

Transport Management

Pulmonary Edema

- Use noninvasive ventilation if the patient is able to maintain their own airway.
- Continue any afterload-reducing agents, inotropic agents, or diuretic infusions started prior to transport.
- Place the patient in a position of comfort.

Special Populations

Cardiovascular complications can be exacerbated by pregnancy. It is not uncommon for CCTPs to transport a pregnant patient to a tertiary center for aortic or mitral valve issues, coronary artery disease, thromboembolic events (including pulmonary embolism), or (although rare) aortic dissection.

patient comfort. Transport ventilators should be capable of providing both CPAP and BPAP. Although currently available HFNC units are not designed for transport, if a sufficient gas supply is available, these devices may be utilized in CCT. HFNC units designed for transport are in development.

Cardiac Electrophysiology

Although electrocardiography is routinely used to monitor cardiac rhythms, disturbances may require more sophisticated monitoring and, in some cases, evaluation in an electrophysiology lab. Using equipment and facilities similar to those found in a cardiac catheterization lab, an electrophysiologist is able to evaluate and map the focus of many cardiac rhythm disturbances. The specialty of electrophysiology involves evaluation and management of cardiac rhythm disturbances including VTs, SVTs (including AF), bradycardias, AV blocks, and syncope suspected to be of cardiac origin.

In a hospital setting, an electrophysiologist may conduct an electrophysiology study to assess the electrical activity of the heart by stimulating and recording activity from multiple catheters at several sites in the heart. Such a study records and maps electrical signals from the heart to determine the location of a heart block (AV node versus bundle of His), the origin of tachycardia (supraventricular versus ventricular), and other important considerations, such as the response to specific medications or devices used in treatment of arrhythmias. These clinical data assist in the following:

- Determining whether the patient's symptoms are related to a tachyarrhythmia
- Assessing the risk for lethal tachyarrhythmias
- Developing and testing appropriate therapies based on the induced tachyarrhythmia and its mechanism

An electrophysiologist may also perform catheter ablation of areas where irritable foci originate. This type of ablation uses radiofrequency, cryothermy, microwave, laser, or surgical catheters or procedures to isolate or eliminate sources of rhythm disturbances.

The CCTP's role during transport of a patient who requires electrophysiology studies or procedures is to anticipate the rhythm disturbances that initiated the referral and to address them as necessary during transport.

Patients presenting with symptoms suggestive of cardiac arrhythmias may be fitted with a Holter monitor, a battery-operated wearable device that continuously records ECG data. Holter monitoring is usually done for a minimum of 24 hours and can be continued for several weeks, depending on the indication and frequency of symptoms. In patients with difficult-to-determine rhythms or when long-term monitoring is required, an implantable loop recorder (ILR), also called an implantable loop monitor, may be used **FIGURE 14-84**. Made by pacemaker manufacturers, ILRs are USB-size, bipolar (single)-lead ECG monitoring devices that are implanted subcutaneously, usually in the patient's left parasternal area. The ILR's loop memory is capable of recording and storing 48 to 49 minutes of ECG data. Data recording is either activated by the patient (or a bystander) or automatically triggered by the occurrence of preprogrammed bradyarrhythmia or tachyarrhythmia **FIGURE 14-85**. These data

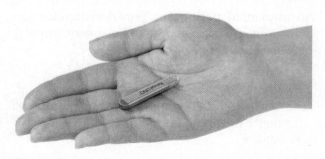

FIGURE 14-84 An implantable loop recorder.

can then be downloaded in a physician's office or transmitted telephonically. Loop recorders have a typical battery life of 3 years.

Therapeutic Options for Patients With Arrhythmias

Pharmacologic, electrical, and surgical therapies for patients with arrhythmias have evolved tremendously over the years, and they continue to advance rapidly. The primary in-hospital arrhythmia therapies are catheter ablation, pharmacologic treatment, and implantable devices, such as pacemakers and ICDs.

Catheter Ablation

Ablation (destruction or isolation) of discrete areas in the heart may reduce or eliminate susceptibility to arrhythmias. Radiofrequency catheter ablation, microwave catheter ablation, cryothermy ablation, laser catheter ablation, and surgical ablation procedures can be highly effective for WPW syndrome and other SVTs, including atrial flutter, atrial tachycardia, AV node reentrant tachycardia **FIGURE 14-86**, and some VTs. Improvements in mapping techniques have made a wider variety of arrhythmias eligible for ablation.

Catheter ablation has completely changed the approach to the long-term care of patients with recurrent SVTs. Electrophysiologists often are able to perform ablation as an outpatient procedure. Ablative therapy is effective 90% to 98% of the time, frequently offers a long-term cure, and has a very low incidence of complications. For many patients with SVT, ablation eliminates the need for long-term

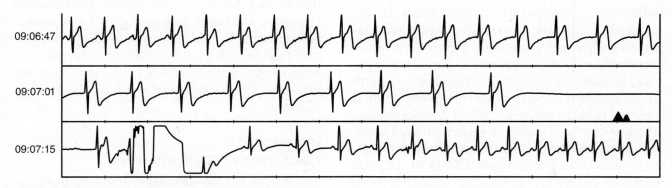

FIGURE 14-85 Data recorded by an implantable loop recorder.
Reproduced from Lombardi F, Calosso E, Mascioli G, et al. Utility of implantable loop recorder (Reveal Plus®) in the diagnosis of unexplained syncope. *EP Europace*. 2005;7(1):19-24. doi: 10.1016/j.eupc.2004.09.003.

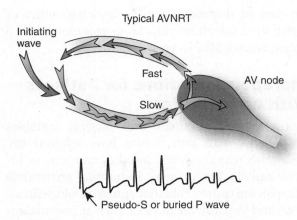

FIGURE 14-86 Atrioventricular (AV) node reentrant tachycardia (AVNRT).

© Jones & Bartlett Learning.

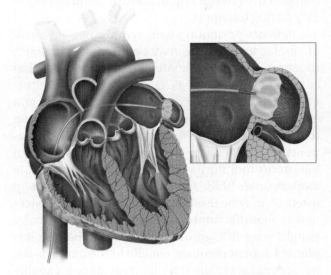

FIGURE 14-87 The Watchman device is percutaneously inserted into the left atrial appendage to permanently close off this portion of the heart.

© ilusmedical/Shutterstock.

medical therapy, which can result in drug-induced adverse events and reduced quality of life. Patients who are poorly compliant with prescribed medications or are reluctant to undergo long-term drug therapy may be candidates for catheter ablation.

Medications may also be used to interfere with electrical conduction or impulse formation at the AV node, accessory pathway, or origin of a focal tachycardia. Examples include digoxin, calcium antagonists, beta blockers, class IA agents (procainamide, disopyramide, quinidine gluconate, quinidine sulfate), class IC agents (propafenone, flecainide), and class III agents (amiodarone, sotalol). Long-term digoxin therapy is contraindicated in patients with WPW syndrome and patients with the capability of rapid **antegrade conduction** over the accessory pathway.

Atrial Ligation

While not a treatment for AF itself, left atrial appendage (LAA) ligation, occlusion, or excision is increasingly being employed as a preventive measure against thromboembolic events such as stroke, especially in patients with contraindications to long-term anticoagulation. In patients with AF, the left atrium is believed to be the primary source of thromboemboli. The LAA can be occluded or excised during cardiac bypass or valve surgery. Percutaneously inserted devices, such as the Watchman **FIGURE 14-87**, may also deployed into the LAA using a transseptal approach (ie, across the atrial septal wall).

Implanted Pacemakers

An implanted pacemaker provides impulse generation in a diseased heart whose own impulses may be characterized as follows:

- Intermittent
- Irregular
- Occurring at an inappropriate rate for the patient's metabolic demand
- Absent

A block can occur at any point within the SA node, AV node, bundle of His, or distal conduction system.

Contemporary pacemakers support heart function in multiple ways. They provide effective and consistent cardiac depolarization, prevent unnecessary pacing by sensing cardiac activity, synchronize right and left heart depolarization, increase the heart rate to match metabolic or physical demands, and store information about events and physiologic changes.

Implantable Cardioverter-Defibrillators

The **implantable cardioverter-defibrillator (ICD)** has been shown to prevent sudden death in patients with

HF and in patients with a history of being resuscitated from sudden cardiac death. Evidence has confirmed that patients receive a greater benefit from ICD therapy than from antiarrhythmic drugs for the treatment of life-threatening ventricular tachyarrhythmias. Studies have also shown that ICDs are as much as 99% effective in terminating life-threatening ventricular tachyarrhythmias. All ICDs currently on the market also have pacing capability.

Wearable Cardioverter-Defibrillators

Patients at risk of sudden arrhythmogenic cardiac death may be prescribed a wearable cardioverter-defibrillator (WCD). These devices are discussed in greater detail later in this chapter.

Pacemakers

The first implantable pacemakers, developed in 1960, were asynchronous; they paced without regard to the heart's intrinsic action. The North American Society of Pacing and Electrophysiology (NASPE)/British Pacing and Electrophysiology Group (BPEG) Generic (NBG) codes appear later in this chapter in Table 14-10, which explains abbreviations related to pacemaker (also called pacer) function.

Single-chamber demand pacemakers appeared in the late 1960s. In 1979, the first dual-chamber pacemaker was introduced. Subsequently, the first single-chamber, rate-responsive pacemaker came into use in 1985. Today, dual-chamber pacemakers are available with a wide variety of programmable functions that allow rate-responsive pacing that mimics the heart's innate ability to respond to exercise and changes in metabolic needs. These devices are also equipped with antitachycardia pacing modes that aim to take rate control away from irritable foci in the atria or ventricles and restore normal rate and rhythm without cardioversion or defibrillation.

In a normally functioning heart, the SA node stimulates depolarization of the ventricles. When the SA node becomes impaired or otherwise dysfunctional, artificial pacing may be needed. The primary indications for pacing are as follows:

- Sinus node dysfunction (SND) with documented symptomatic bradycardia, including frequent sinus pauses that produce symptoms

- Symptomatic chronotropic incompetence (inability to sufficiently increase or lower the heart rate)
- Symptomatic sinus bradycardia resulting from necessary drug therapy
- Reflex syncope
- Third-degree and advanced second-degree AV blocks associated with symptomatic bradycardia, pauses, AF, or after catheter ablation of the AV node
- Cardiac resynchronization in certain patients with HF
- Hypersensitive carotid sinus syndrome
- Overdrive or antitachycardia pacing for atrial or ventricular tachycardias

Pacing Fundamentals

The Pacing Impulse

Electricity is the flow of electrons along a conductive medium. A pacing impulse has current, voltage, and impedance.

- Current is the movement of electrons through an electrical circuit over time, measured in amperes.
- Voltage is the force that causes current to flow, measured in volts. Voltage in a pacing system, referred to as amplitude, reflects the strength or intensity of a pacing pulse.
- Resistance to current, called impedance, is the sum of all factors that resist the flow of current along the conduction pathway, measured in ohms. One ampere is produced by 1 volt, acting through a resistance of 1 ohm.

The main sources of resistance in a pacing circuit are the lead conductor, the electrode, and the concentration of electrically charged ions at the electrode–tissue interface (polarization). Electrode resistance improves pacing efficiency; lead conductor resistance and polarization do not. Reviewing the following definitions and formulas will help CCTPs understand the basic concept of electricity as it pertains to pacing.

Ohm's law is an expression of the relationship between current (I), voltage (V), and resistance (R). Ohm's law states the following:

$$I = \frac{V}{R}$$

Consequently,

$$V = I \times R$$

$$R = \frac{V}{I}$$

With these equations, volts, current, and resistance may be calculated if the other parameters are known. If the voltage drops by half, the current flow does as well. Doubling impedance will also cut the current flow in half. Voltage and impedance are important determinants of battery longevity.

A joule is a measurement of energy:

$$\text{Energy} = \text{Volts} \times \text{Current} \times \text{Time}$$

Energy is expressed in joules or microjoules, as appropriate for the device.

The Pacing Circuit

A pacing system forms an electrical circuit in the patient's body in combination with body tissue and fluid. A pacing circuit consists of a power source, lead, cathode, anode, and body tissue, which form a conduction pathway along which electricity flows.

The pacemaker battery is the power source that generates electrical impulses. The lead conductor wire carries the impulses to the tissue. The cathode is an electrode with a negative charge that delivers the impulse to the myocardium. The impulses return through the anode, an electrode with a positive charge, after stimulating the heart. Body tissue and fluids between the anode and the cathode are also part of the conduction pathway. Passage of the pacemaker's electrical impulse between the cathode and the anode, through cardiac tissue and body fluids, is the event in the pacing circuit that stimulates cardiac depolarization. In a bipolar system, body tissue is part of the circuit only in the sense that it affects impedance at the electrode–tissue interface. In a unipolar system, contact with body tissue is essential to ground the implantable pulse generator (IPG).

During pacing, an electrical impulse begins in the pacemaker battery, travels along the lead to the cathode, stimulates the heart, and then returns through body tissues to the anode to complete the pacing circuit **FIGURE 14-88**.

Pacemaker Components and Functions

Pacemakers stimulate cardiac depolarization, sense intrinsic cardiac activity, respond to metabolic

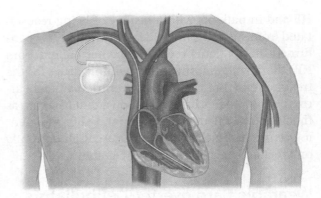

FIGURE 14-88 The pacing circuit. The electrical impulse travels along the lead, stimulates the heart, and returns through body tissues.

© Jones & Bartlett Learning.

needs, and store diagnostic information. All pacemakers can provide fixed-rate pacing, in which the heart is paced at a predetermined rate. Most also provide rate-adaptive (rate-responsive) pacing, increasing and decreasing the pacing rate in response to input from rate sensors. This feature prevents the pacemaker from competing with normal cardiac function. In addition, modern pacemakers collect and store information about the patient's heart and the implanted pacemaker. This information allows clinicians to monitor pacing therapy, optimize programmed settings, and check battery and lead status. A basic pacing system consists of the following components:

- An IPG that contains a power source (ie, the battery that generates the impulse) and sensing, timing, and output circuitry that controls pacemaker operation
- Leads—one or two insulated wires that deliver electrical impulses from the pulse generator to the heart and return electrical signals from the heart to the pulse generator
- Electrodes—conductors at the ends of the leads that deliver impulses to the heart

Most IPGs include a telemetry coil for sending and receiving programming instructions and receiving diagnostic data. Many have sensors that measure indicators of exertion and use the results to change heart rate.

Leads. Lead insulation prevents contact between the conductor wire and body tissue, ensuring that stimulation occurs only at the tip of the electrode.

About 95% of pacing leads are endocardial (transvenous) leads, which are threaded through veins—usually subclavian or cephalic—to the right atrium or ventricle. Their placement involves an introducer (hollow tube) and a stylet (stiff wire). The clinician uses imaging, usually fluoroscopy, to guide insertion and final placement. Epicardial leads, which attach to the external surface of the heart with sutures or another fixation device, account for the other 5% of pacing leads. Because epicardial placement requires a thoracotomy (chest incision), epicardial leads are considered desirable only when endocardial placement is not an option or fails to achieve capture when placed.

A pacing lead may be unipolar or bipolar. A unipolar lead has one conductor wire connecting to a single electrode. The cathode is in contact with the heart, and the IPG housing is the anode. A pacing pulse travels from the IPG to the tip of the electrode (cathode) to stimulate the heart and returns to the IPG housing through chest tissues to complete the pacing circuit. The current flows through a substantial part of the chest and forms a large current loop; the resulting pacing spike is readily visible on an ECG.

A bipolar lead has two conductor wires; both the anode and the cathode are in contact with the heart. The anode—that is, the ring electrode located 0.8 inch to 1.2 inches (2 to 3 cm) above the cathode—has a separate lead connecting it to the IPG. The pacing pulse travels from the IPG to the cathode and then through tissue to the ring electrode. It returns to the IPG by way of the second conductor wire. Because the current loop is small, passing through only a limited area of cardiac tissue, the pacing spike on the ECG is also small.

Electrodes. As mentioned, a cathode is the electrode that is in contact with heart tissue. It is negatively charged when electrical current is flowing. The anode is the electrode that receives the electrical impulse after depolarization of cardiac tissue. It is positively charged when electrical current is flowing.

Small electrodes with a porous surface increase electrode resistance and reduce the effects of polarization. The porosity significantly increases the electrode surface area without increasing the radius and, therefore, reduces the wasteful effects of polarization. The porous surface also promotes tissue ingrowth and improves sensing by providing a larger electrode–tissue contact area.

Steroid Elution. There are two types of transvenous pacemaker leads: passive fixation and active fixation. The active fixation leads require higher stimulation than the passive fixation leads do. Nevertheless, they are preferred for the following reasons:

- Passive fixation leads involve atrial appendage placement, which is difficult in patients who have undergone prior cardiac surgery.
- Active fixation leads allow for more placement areas.
- Active fixation leads reduce the incidence of dislodgement.

To make the active fixation more beneficial, a steroid-eluting lead was developed. In the past, the steroid reservoir in the tip of the lead contained dexamethasone sodium phosphate. The inclusion of the steroid-eluting reservoir in the active fixation lead improved stimulation thresholds and was found to extend the pulse generator's longevity.

Steroid elution reduces inflammation and the growth of fibrous tissue at the electrode site. Both inflammation and fibrosis decrease the electrical excitability of cardiac tissue, requiring increased output to achieve capture. By inhibiting their development, the steroid helps maintain a better electrode–tissue interface.

Steroid-eluting electrodes have a silicone plug that contains a small dose (less than 1 mg) of steroid. Body fluids seep into the electrode and gradually dissolve the steroid, which then flows in the body fluids to the electrode–tissue interface. Initially, the rate of steroid elution is high, but it decreases over time. The steroid typically lasts for several years.

Single-Chamber Versus Dual-Chamber Systems. A single-chamber pacing system uses one lead that may be placed in either the right atrium or the right ventricle **FIGURE 14-89**. A dual-chamber pacing system uses two leads, with one lead placed in each of these chambers **FIGURE 14-90**. The dual-chamber approach compensates for two potential limitations of single-lead systems: the inability to coordinate AV timing (AV synchrony) and the lack of ventricular backup pacing in the absence of AV conduction.

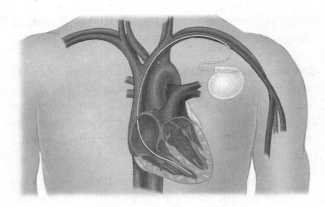

FIGURE 14-89 A single-chamber pacing system.

© Jones & Bartlett Learning.

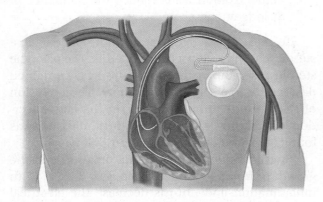

FIGURE 14-90 A dual-chamber pacing system.

© Jones & Bartlett Learning.

NBG Codes

Developed by a joint effort of North American and British electrophysiology groups, NBG codes (NASPE/BPEG Generic codes) provide a succinct way to describe pacemaker functions and capabilities. These terms may be encountered in patient documentation; a general familiarity with them is very helpful in determining appropriate pacemaker function. **TABLE 14-10** lists the codes and their meanings.

The first letter in the NBG code identifies the chamber where the pacing occurs: either the atrium, the ventricle, both, none, or single (which can signify the atrium or ventricle). The second letter in the NBG code identifies the chamber where the pacing is sensed. The options in this category are the same as those in the first category.

The third letter indicates how the pacemaker responds to sensing. Options in this category include triggered, inhibited, dual, and none. The I (inhibited response) setting indicates that the pacemaker is set to fire only under certain conditions. For example, the pacemaker may fire only when the patient's heart rate falls below a certain rate. In other words, when the pacemaker senses an impulse from the patient, it inhibits or does not fire its own impulse. The T (triggered response) setting indicates that the pacemaker, after sensing an impulse from the patient, triggers a pacemaker impulse. The D (dual)

TABLE 14-10 NBG Codes				
I **Chamber Paced**	**II** **Chamber Sensed**	**III** **Response to Sensing**	**IV** **Programmable Functions; Rate Modulation**[a]	**V** **Antitachyarrhythmia Functions**
V: Ventricle	V: Ventricle	T: Triggered	P: Simple programmable[c]	P: Pace
A: Atrium	A: Atrium	I: Inhibited	M: Multiprogrammable[d]	S: Shock
D: Dual (A + V)	D: Dual (A + V)	D: Dual[b]	C: Communicating[e]	D: Dual[f]
O: None	O: None	O: None	R: Rate modulating	O: None
S: Single (A or V)	S: Single (A or V)		O: None	

[a] This sequence is hierarchical; it is assumed that if a pacemaker has rate modulation capabilities (R), it can also communicate (C).
[b] Inhibited and triggered. In single-chamber mode, *triggered* means initiating a pacing pulse immediately after sensing an intrinsic event. In dual-chamber mode, this term means that a sensed atrial event will initiate an atrioventricular (AV) delay.
[c] Rate and/or output.
[d] Rate, output, sensitivity, and so forth.
[e] Can send information to and receive information from the programmer.
[f] Pace and shock available.

© Jones & Bartlett Learning.

setting indicates that the pacemaker can perform in either an inhibited manner or a triggered manner, as needed. The O (no response) setting may be used when a technician wants to ignore sensed beats from the patient and fire the pacemaker regardless of any underlying patient rhythm.

The fourth letter identifies the pacemaker's programmability and rate-modulation capability, which is simply a representation of how much programming can be done externally. Pacemakers may have many external programming options (M) or just a few (P). C (communicating) indicates that the pacemaker can transmit data, such as with telemetry. R (rate modulation) means that the pacemaker can adjust its rate depending on the body's needs.

The fifth letter represents antitachyarrhythmia functions. P (pacing) indicates that a tachyarrhythmia is converted by pacing. S (shock) indicates that a tachyarrhythmia is converted by defibrillation administered by the pacemaker. D (dual) indicates that the pacemaker can pace and administer a shock to address a tachyarrhythmia.

An example of an NBG code is VVI. In a VVI pacemaker, pacing occurs in the ventricle, sensing occurs in the ventricle, and the response setting is inhibited. In day-to-day practice, only the first three letters of the NBG code are typically used.

Types of Pacemakers

Five major categories of cardiac pacemakers are available:

- Transcutaneous
- Implantable
- Transthoracic and epicardial
- Transvenous
- Leadless

Transcutaneous Pacemakers

The most basic pacer is the transcutaneous pacemaker (TCP), which is most commonly used as an initial emergency pacer. With this device, multifunction TCP pads (electrodes) are attached to the patient's chest wall in the anterior-posterior positions. The electrical pacing impulse is transferred to the heart through the skin and thoracic cavity. Although this is the quickest and most convenient method of pacing, it requires the greatest amount of energy and is the least reliable option owing to

the relatively poor quality of the skin-to-pad contact and the thoracic impedance that must be overcome. A TCP is also extremely uncomfortable for most patients and often requires administration of analgesics and/or sedatives to alleviate the muscle discomfort resulting from transthoracic electrical stimulation. Such a device is generally used as a temporary measure until a transvenous pacing wire can be placed. The TCP is useful as an emergency tool both to initiate pacing and in case other pacing modalities fail.

Implantable Pacemakers

Implantable pacemakers consist of a battery-operated pulse generator attached to pacing/sensing leads. An interventional cardiologist or thoracic surgeon implants the lead or leads in the myocardial wall, usually by accessing the subclavian vein and traversing the myocardium until the desired location is reached, which differs depending on the pacer indication. The pulse generator is then surgically implanted in the patient's body, usually in a sac created between the pectoral muscle and the cutaneous layer of the skin. In some cases, when leads cannot be placed conventionally or capture cannot be achieved with traditional leads, the pacemaker electrode(s) are screwed onto the myocardial wall.

Implanted pacers can have a variety of lead configurations. They may be programmed to deliver single-chamber, dual-chamber, atrial, ventricular, biventricular, biatrial, atrial–ventricular, overdrive, antitachycardia, and synchronizing pacing, among other less common modes.

Pacemakers can operate on demand; alternatively, the patient's heart can be fully paced. A demand pacer intervenes when the patient's normal rhythm fails. In this case, the ECG will show the patient's normal rhythm with periodic pacer intervention. In contrast, an ECG for a patient with a fully paced heart will show only the paced rhythm.

Most pacers today are atrial and ventricular, and many include a built-in ICD. Virtually all newer pacemakers are compatible with magnetic resonance imaging (MRI). Biventricular pacers are used in patients with ventricular asynchrony (often seen in cardiomyopathies) to restore right and left ventricular synchrony and improve ejection fraction. Pacer circuitry is less complicated than defibrillator circuitry and requires less power. Statistically, pacer circuits show a lower incidence of failure compared to ICDs. The most common sources of failure are the following:

- Battery failure
- Lead wire failure or detachment

Less common sources of failure are as follows:

- Failure of the pulse-generator circuitry
- Dislodgment from the myocardial wall

Transthoracic and Epicardial Pacemakers

A third class of pacers comprises the transthoracic and epicardial pacers. This type of pacing is done only by interventional cardiologists or cardiac surgeons and involves placing pacing electrodes directly into the heart through the thoracic cavity. Such pacing is limited to the inpatient setting and would be encountered in the CCT environment only if the CCTP were called to transport a patient postoperatively. Epicardial wires are attached to the atria and/or ventricles and brought out through the chest wall. A connector cable is used to attach epicardial wires to the same type of temporary pulse generator used for transvenous pacing.

Transvenous Pacemakers

Transvenous pacemakers are employed as a temporary method of pacing until the problem requiring pacing is resolved or until a permanent pacemaker can be implanted. A transvenous pacing wire is considered more reliable compared to transcutaneous pacing. Because it has direct myocardial contact, the wire is located in the heart itself, and it requires considerably less energy to achieve capture. Additionally, because an external pulse generator is attached directly to the pacing wire, tighter control and more sophisticated settings can be used than with transcutaneous pacing. An interventional cardiologist or other credentialed practitioner places the transvenous lead wires and connects the battery-operated pulse generator externally to the pacing leads **FIGURE 14-91**.

The external pulse generator provides the following controls:

- Pacing rate
- Output
- Sensitivity

The lead wires are externally connected to the pulse generator.

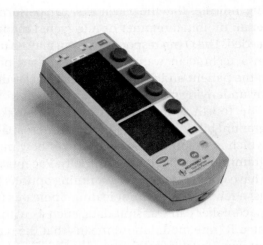

A

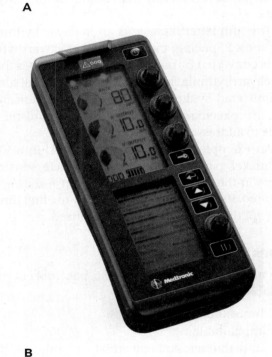

B

FIGURE 14-91 Dual-chamber temporary transvenous pacemakers.

Reproduced with permission of Medtronic.

It is recommended that CCTPs become familiar with the types of transvenous wire(s) and temporary pacemakers used by local hospitals and receive a tutorial on troubleshooting these devices. The difficulty most likely to be encountered during transport is migration of the pacing wire in the heart with subsequent loss of capture or disconnection of lead wires. The CCTP can take specific steps to prevent these and other potential issues that might arise during transport.

Four important pieces of information are needed when transporting a patient with a temporary pacemaker:

1. When and why was the temporary pacemaker wire inserted?
2. What is the underlying rhythm?
3. Is the patient hemodynamically dependent on the pacer?
4. What are the present settings?
   - Milliamperes (mA) (output)
   - Rate
   - Sensitivity
   - Mode

Knowing why a temporary pacemaker was inserted, what the underlying rhythm is, and whether the patient's hemodynamic stability depends on the pacemaker will prepare the CCTP to react aggressively should a loss of capture occur or the pacemaker fail. The duration for which the pacer has been in use may provide a window into any problems that have occurred during that time, but also suggests whether the pacemaker output might need to be increased. Over time, owing to local inflammation and scarring at the site, many temporary pacing wires require a gradual increase in output (mA) to achieve capture. The CCTP should also have some familiarity with the amount of leeway in the present settings for the pacemaker, should adjustments become necessary during transport. For example, a patient who requires 20 mA output to achieve ventricular capture is close to the maximum output available from most temporary pacers. In such a case, there is little margin for increases should a higher output be needed.

After gathering the necessary information about the indications, underlying rhythm, and settings of the pacer, take the following steps during patient packaging:

1. Confirm that the settings provided are the actual settings on the temporary pacemaker. Pay particular attention to the mode, especially with ventricular pacing. It is not uncommon during surgical procedures or insertion of a pacing wire to set an asynchronous or fixed (VOO) mode. For patient safety (to avoid an "R-on-T" event, in which an electrical stimulus is delivered to the ventricle during the repolarization period), the mode should be switched to demand pacing (VVI) as soon as practical.

2. Confirm electrical and mechanical capture. A pulse oximeter waveform is a helpful visual aid that can be compared to the ECG.
3. Place transcutaneous pacing pads on the patient during packaging. Gaining access to the patient to place pads in an emergency situation during transport is fraught with difficulty. Patient safety concerns require the CCTP to be prepared for emergencies.
4. Ensure that transvenous or epicardial pacing wires are looped at their exit sites and securely taped to the patient's body to avoid inadvertent dislodgement should they become ensnared during movement.
5. Tape all connecting wires, cables, and adapters to prevent inadvertent disconnection.
6. Place the temporary pacemaker in a readily accessible location, such as hanging on an IV pole, secured between the patient's legs, or at the head of the stretcher. The CCTP must be able to readily reach the pacer should adjustments be needed.
7. Ensure that there is a fresh battery in the temporary pacemaker and that a spare battery is available for the transport.
8. Ensure that there is a quality ECG tracing on the transport monitor and that the monitoring lead chosen offers the best view of pacing spikes.

In addition to the typical problems that may be encountered with any pacemaker (eg, loss of capture, disconnection, undersensing), one problem frequently encountered in the transport environment is oversensing. Many forms of energy, including vibration, electromagnetic interference, cellular or radio signal interference, on-board inverters, generators, and engine artifact have been

Pacing Spikes

Transport monitors are often configured to eliminate artifactual noise experienced while moving patients and, as a consequence, may not display pacing spikes in patients who are being paced. A quick remedy to this potential loss of information is to print a rhythm strip; most monitors will not only display pacing spikes on the printed strips, but also mark the spikes on the bottom of the ECG.

known to interfere with pacemakers in demand mode. Decreasing the pacemaker's sensitivity is an appropriate action to resolve interference that may be inhibiting necessary pacing.

Leadless Pacemakers

Leadless pacemakers are self-contained pacemakers with pacing/sensing leads implanted as a unit directly into the right ventricle **FIGURE 14-92**. While it is considered in the category of implanted pacemakers, the leadless pacemaker is 90% smaller and is implanted using a transcatheter approach via a femoral vein. There are no chest incisions and no pacemaker

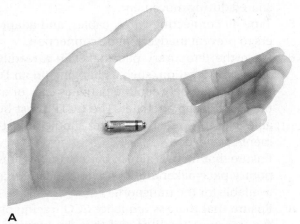

A

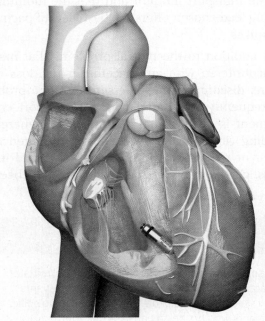

B

FIGURE 14-92 A. Photo of a leadless pacemaker. **B.** Illustration showing placement of a leadless pacemaker in the right ventricle.

pocket in the skin. Leadless pacemakers provide single-chamber ventricular pacing, are MRI compatible, and have a battery life of 5 to 15 years, after which they can be turned off and a new pacemaker implanted. Leadless pacemakers are theoretically retrievable, but, like conventional pacemaker leads, they are likely to become encapsulated in cardiac tissue.

Pacemaker Troubleshooting

Pulse-generator failure is a rare occurrence; its incidence is 0.46%, or 1.3 malfunctions per 1,000 persons annually. By comparison, pacemaker system malfunction occurs occasionally. The primary areas of failure are the following:

- Battery failure
- Problems at the lead electrode–tissue interface
- Coiling or damage to the lead–generator interface
- Insulation failure of the lead wires
- Dislodgement of the lead at the implantation site (very rare)
- Pacemaker programming
- Pacemaker pocket stimulation (muscle tissue in the vicinity of the implanted pacemaker is stimulated by the pacer itself; more common with unipolar pacers than with other types)
- Diaphragmatic stimulation
- Electromagnetic interference (cell phones and other personal electronic devices)

Electromagnetic interference is the collective effect of radiofrequencies and other signals from environmental sources that may be picked up by the pacemaker. This interference may enter a pacemaker by conduction if the patient is in direct contact with the source or by way of radiation if the patient is in an electromagnetic field with the pacemaker lead acting as an antenna. Exposure to electromagnetic interference can affect pacers in various ways, all of which can prevent it from functioning appropriately.

TABLE 14-11 details the four general types of in-hospital solutions available to correct abnormal pacing behavior. These kinds of remedies cannot be applied during transport except with temporary external pulse generators.

During transport, CCTPs must be aware of the signs of pacemaker failure. The cardiac monitor will show failure to capture, and a 12-lead ECG is helpful, but even more important is patient assessment.

TABLE 14-11 Options for Correcting Pacer Malfunction

Solution	Use or Indication
Reprogramming	Correct oversensing, undersensing, and loss of capture As a temporary solution in some cases of an insulation break Adjust the atrioventricular intervals and rate response to optimize pacing therapy
Repositioning the lead	A lead slips out of position and pacing and/or sensing is compromised Muscle, diaphragmatic, or phrenic nerve stimulation occurs Pacing the left side of the heart unintentionally (a lead may traverse the septal wall or innominate vein) Leads are reversed in the implantable pulse generator header block at implant
Replacing the lead or the pacemaker	Lead failure is confirmed The battery is depleted The patient is symptomatic (hemodynamically compromised) as a result of single-chamber pacing The passive fixation lead does not remain in place after attempts to reposition it True circuit malfunction
Observation	Transient problems with the following: • Lead maturation • Changes in drug therapy

© Jones & Bartlett Learning.

First, the CCTP should confirm that the patient's pulse corresponds to the pacer presentation on the ECG. Next, the CCTP should determine whether the patient shows signs of decompensation, such as the following:

- Syncope
- Dizziness
- Palpitations
- Bradycardia
- Heart blocks
- Hypotension
- Tachycardia
- Extracardiac stimulation (sometimes shown by hiccups)

If these conditions exist, alternative treatment should be initiated.

To troubleshoot the device quickly, look for obvious sources of malfunctions, such as cell phones or other personal electronic devices. If the patient is using such a device, it should be shut off and the patient should be reevaluated. If a device in the ambulance has just been turned on and the pacemaker malfunctions, the device should be shut off and the patient should be reevaluated. If these quick fixes do not improve pacemaker performance, begin immediate treatment of the patient. If bradycardia, heart blocks, or syncope exists, apply transcutaneous pacer (multifunction) pads and initiate transcutaneous pacing. Tachycardia as the result of pacemaker runaway (pacemaker-mediated tachycardia) has been largely eliminated; if tachycardia is observed on the ECG, however, confirm it by checking the patient's pulse before considering treatment. Tachycardias that allow for adequate perfusion should be left alone, but tachycardias that result in inadequate perfusion should be treated following advanced cardiac life support (ACLS) protocols.

Identifying the exact cause of pacemaker failure is difficult for CCTPs who do not have training in the use of an external diagnostic device. The easiest cause to diagnose is extracardiac stimulation, which is evidenced by frequent hiccups. The hiccups are caused by pacing electrodes being placed too far into the apex of the ventricle, causing stimulation of the diaphragm.

Unfortunately, CCTPs cannot do much to correct implanted pacemaker malfunction because the device is not accessible to them. Even if the device were accessible, a CCTP would need specific training in the repair of the particular device to initiate reprogramming. Some manufacturers provide a doughnut-type, bar, rectangle, or horseshoe magnet that may be helpful in correcting pacemaker malfunctions **FIGURE 14-93**. Various responses are seen to magnet application, depending on the pacemaker's programming. All pacemakers switch to an asynchronous mode when a magnet is placed near them. DDD pacers switch to DOO; VVI to VOO; and AAI to AOO. The pacer rate depends on its programming and the battery status.

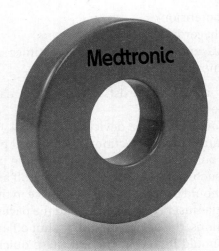

FIGURE 14-93 A pacemaker magnet may help correct malfunction of implanted pacemakers.

Reproduced with permission of Medtronic.

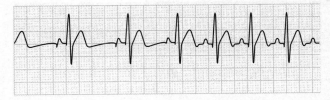

FIGURE 14-94 An electrocardiogram from a patient with an atrial pacer (AAI). Mode: AAI; rate setting: 60.

© Jones & Bartlett Learning.

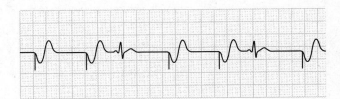

FIGURE 14-95 An electrocardiogram from a patient with a ventricular pacer (VVI). Mode: VVI; rate setting: 60.

© Jones & Bartlett Learning.

Transport Management

Pacemaker Failure

- Shut off the patient's cell phone or other personal electronic device.
- If the pacemaker malfunction occurred after a device in the ambulance was turned on, shut off that device and reevaluate the patient.
- If the malfunction persists and the patient has bradycardia, heart blocks, or syncope, initiate transcutaneous pacing.
- Confirm tachycardia with a pulse reading; treat tachycardias that result in inadequate perfusion per ACLS protocols.

Pacemakers and the ECG

Single-Chamber Systems

The sole electrode in a single-chamber pacemaker system is implanted on the atrium or ventricle. Single-chamber systems require implantation of only one lead, but they do not provide AV synchrony or ventricular backup in the absence of AV conduction.

Pacing in the ventricular pacer (VVI/R) mode and loss of AV synchrony can lead to **pacemaker syndrome**, a variety of symptoms that result from hemodynamic deterioration and cause nonphysiologic timing of atrial and ventricular contractions. This asynchrony can result in a rate that does not respond to physiologic needs. Atrial pacemakers are appropriate only for patients who have proven AV conduction and have regular access to follow-up testing.

Atrial and Ventricular Tracings

FIGURE 14-94 shows an example of atrial pacing. The strip begins with an atrial pacemaker firing at a rate of 60 beats/min. A pacemaker spike precedes the P wave in these complexes. The ventricular rate is 60 beats/min. The paced P waves are conducted through the ventricles via a normal conduction pathway. Starting with the fourth complex, the intrinsic pacemaker begins depolarizing at a rate of 94 to 100 beats/min. There are no pacemaker spikes with these complexes. The pacemaker continues to sense the intrinsic atrial depolarizations. Implications for the CCTP depend on the patient's history (ie, what caused the intrinsic pacemaker to fail in the first place) and hemodynamic status.

FIGURE 14-95 shows an ECG from a patient with a ventricular pacer (VVI). Following the second paced ventricular beat, a capture beat appears and is conducted normally. The pacemaker does not fire during this capture beat because it is sensed as normal depolarization. When another capture beat fails to appear, the ventricular pacemaker senses this and fires, depolarizing the ventricles. It paces two beats, and then another capture beat appears and is conducted. The pacemaker senses when this does not produce a sustained rhythm, and begins firing again at a rate of 60 beats/min. The implication for the CCTP is that this patient's heart is probably failing, but still has the ability to generate electrical impulses periodically. Monitor the patient's hemodynamic status and treat accordingly.

Many implanted pacemakers do not show prominent spikes on the ECG, necessitating that the CCTP check several leads to identify spikes. Many transport monitors require reconfiguration to identify pacemaker spikes. It is a good idea to ask the sending nurse which type of pacer the patient has and what the paced beats looked like on the hospital's ECG monitors.

Dual-Chamber Systems

Dual-chamber pacemaker systems feature two leads, one each in the atrium and the ventricle. This ensures AV synchrony and provides for ventricular depolarization even without AV conduction. This mode of pacing is known as atrial synchronous pacing, atrial tracking, or AV sequential pacing.

As outlined in Table 14-10, DDD and DVI are pacemaker acronyms that refer to dual-chamber pacemaker systems. DDD stands for dual sensed, dual paced, and dual mode (fixed or demand), and DVI stands for dual sensed, ventricular paced, and inhibited (demand) mode. DDD is the most common type of pacemaker in use today. Figures 14-96 through Figure 14-99 show samples of ECG rhythms from dual-demand pacemakers.

FIGURE 14-96 shows a dual-chamber intrinsic atrial pacemaker depolarizing at a rate of approximately 60 beats/min. The pacemaker senses atrial electrical activity and does not need to provide atrial pacing. The atria depolarize but conduction is blocked and does not reach the ventricles. The ventricular mode of the DDD senses no conduction and fires to depolarize the ventricles at a rate of 60 beats/min. Pacemaker spikes precede each ventricular

complex. This patient has a severe conduction problem, as impulses are not reaching the ventricles. For the CCTP, the implications would be to monitor the patient's hemodynamic status and treat accordingly.

FIGURE 14-97 shows a demand dual-mode pacer sensing intrinsic pacemaker depolarizing at a rate of approximately 80 beats/min. The electrical activity is transmitted from the atria to the ventricles without interruption. The underlying rhythm is a regular sinus rhythm at a rate of approximately 78 beats/min. The implication for the CCTP is to always compare ECG findings with the patient's clinical presentation.

FIGURE 14-98 shows a dual-demand mode pacemaker rhythm. On this strip, the demand DDD pacemaker does not sense any intrinsic electrical activity and depolarizes the atria, as indicated by a spike preceding each P wave at a rate of 60 beats/min. With no ventricular activity and the atrial pacing not being transmitted through to the ventricles, the ventricular mode of the DDD fires, depolarizing the ventricles at a rate of 60 beats/min. The implication for the CCTP is that the patient's cardiac electrical activity depends solely on the pacemaker. As always, compare the ECG findings with the clinical findings and treat the patient accordingly.

FIGURE 14-99 shows another demand dual-mode pacemaker rhythm. The underlying rhythm appears to not be producing an atrial intrinsic pacemaker

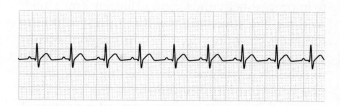

FIGURE 14-97 Mode DDD; lower rate setting, 60; upper rate setting, 120. Atrial and ventricular sensing.

© Jones & Bartlett Learning.

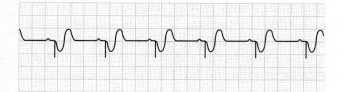

FIGURE 14-96 Mode DDD; lower rate setting, 60; upper rate setting, 120. Atrial sensing and ventricular pacing.

© Jones & Bartlett Learning.

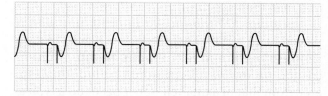

FIGURE 14-98 Mode DDD; lower rate setting, 60; upper rate setting, 120. Atrial and ventricular pacing.

© Jones & Bartlett Learning.

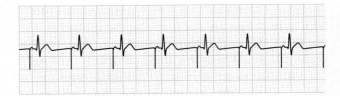

FIGURE 14-99 Mode DDD; lower rate setting, 60; upper rate setting, 120. Atrial pacing and ventricular sensing.

© Jones & Bartlett Learning.

rhythm. The DDD pacer senses this and paces a rhythm at 60 beats/min. Note the pacemaker spike preceding each P wave. The electrical impulse generated by the pacemaker is transmitted through to the ventricles without interruption, allowing the ventricles to depolarize "normally" from above. This indicates that there is no AV block. The ventricular portion of the pacemaker continues to sense the ventricular conduction and does not need to fire. There should be no implications for the CCTP with this rhythm (unless it started after the transport began, which could indicate the patient's condition is deteriorating).

Atriobiventricular Pacing (Cardiac Resynchronization Therapy)

A CCTP may transport a patient with HF to a facility for cardiac resynchronization therapy (CRT) pacemaker insertion. Mortality and morbidity rates are high for patients with HF, but one treatment shown to improve quality and length of life relies on a modified cardiac pacemaker or ICD to resynchronize the heart chambers (ie, CRT). As cardiomyopathy progresses, the right and left ventricles often begin to contract asynchronously, resulting in an unnatural back-and-forth movement of the ventricular septum that further impairs ventricular ejection. A biventricular pacemaker synchronizes ejection of the right and left ventricles of the heart, resulting in more effective ejection. To accomplish this coordination, pacing leads are placed in both ventricles and then their synchronization is optimized.

In a typical biventricular implant, one lead is placed in an atrium and one lead is placed in each ventricle (right and left) **FIGURE 14-100**. A biventricular pacing waveform would be indistinguishable from that of a dual-chamber pacer on a typical monitor lead, because the ventricles are paced simultaneously **FIGURE 14-101**. Analysis by 12-lead ECG and history would lead to a more definitive answer regarding the type of device implanted.

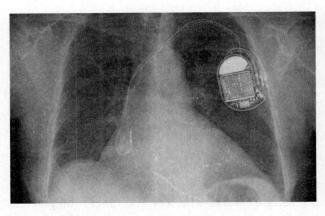

FIGURE 14-100 An implanted atriobiventricular pacing system.

Used with permission of BIOTRONIK.

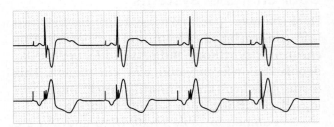

FIGURE 14-101 An example of a 12-lead electrocardiogram with cardiac resynchronization therapy pacing.

© Jones & Bartlett Learning.

Implantable Cardioverter-Defibrillators

ICDs automatically attempt to convert a fibrillating heart to sinus rhythm using a shock from voltage **FIGURE 14-102**. Since their introduction in 1985, the estimated number of ICD implants has increased steadily to more than 200,000 each year. As their numbers rise, so does the frequency of ICD-related issues.

Basic Function

Components

Each patient with an ICD has a custom ICD system consisting of a housing (can) and a variable number of pacing and high-voltage leads. The leads can be placed in the abdominal or pectoral region **FIGURE 14-103A**; the lead is itself often one of the electrodes in the system. Most ICDs have one or two transvenous leads that are used for pacing and shocking. The leads enter the venous system through the subclavian or cephalic vein, for placement into the right ventricle or the superior vena

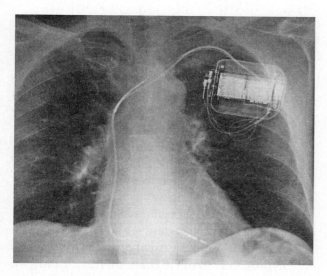

FIGURE 14-102 An implantable cardioverter-defibrillator is attached directly to the heart and continuously monitors heart rhythm, delivering shocks as needed. The electricity from the device is so low that it has no effect on rescuers.

© American Academy of Orthopaedic Surgeons.

cava. Early ICD implants required the pacing leads and high-voltage patches to be placed directly on the epicardial surface **FIGURE 14-103B**. Patients with mechanical heart valves are also limited to epicardial placement.

Sensing and Therapies

An ICD delivers therapy when it determines that the heart is in a tachyarrhythmia, based on the ventricular rate. The ICD counts the number of R-R intervals that are faster than a programmed threshold. When the count reaches the threshold, the device delivers electrical therapy. Because an ICD bases its decision on the ventricular rate alone, atrial arrhythmias and electromagnetic interference can lead to inappropriate shocks.

For ICD purposes, fast heart rhythms are loosely classified into two groups: VT and ventricular fibrillation. An ICD may deliver antitachycardia pacing or cardioversion shocks for episodes of VT. Antitachycardia pacing consists of a series of 6 to 15 pacing pulses with cycle lengths of 70% to 95% of the arrhythmia **FIGURE 14-104A**. In Figure 14-104A, when VT is sensed, antitachycardia pacing begins as indicated by pacemaker spikes (arrow at right). In cardioversion, high-voltage shocks are synchronized to an intrinsic R wave **FIGURE 14-104B**. The device delivers unsynchronized defibrillation shocks for episodes of ventricular fibrillation. In Figure 14-104B, when VT is sensed, a single cardioversion shock is

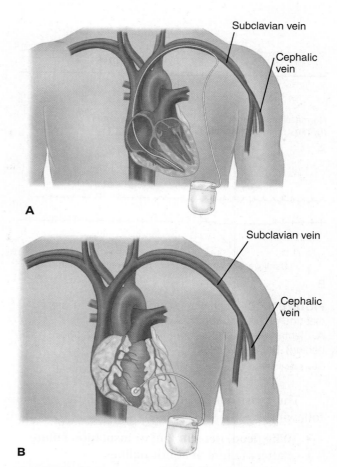

FIGURE 14-103 Typical implantable cardioverter-defibrillator systems. **A.** The ICD enters the heart through the abdominal or pectoral region. **B.** The ICD is placed directly on the epicardial surface.

© Jones & Bartlett Learning.

administered, as indicated by the large spike. The rhythm is converted to a supraventricular rate of approximately 70 beats/min. There appears to be a first-degree AV block with a prolonged PR interval.

ICDs will administer a preprogrammed number of shocks (usually four or five) for each episode of an arrhythmia. Hence, if a patient is in VT, an ICD will stop therapy after the preprogrammed number of shocks, if there is no change in the rhythm. If it detects a different rhythm for which shocks are indicated, it will again deliver its predetermined number of shocks.

Implantable Cardioverter-Defibrillator Troubleshooting

Because an ICD is an implantable device within the patient, it is not accessible to CCTPs. The device must be explanted (in the hospital) to correct the malfunction.

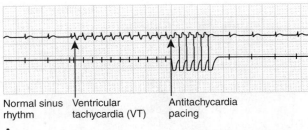

Normal sinus rhythm | Ventricular tachycardia (VT) | Antitachycardia pacing

A

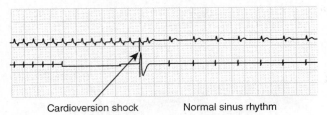

Cardioversion shock | Normal sinus rhythm

B

FIGURE 14-104 Implantable cardioverter-defibrillator electrotherapies for ventricular tachycardia.
A. Electrotherapy for tachycardias (antitachycardia pacing). **B.** Cardioversion.

© Jones & Bartlett Learning.

The most common sources of failure are the following:

- Wire (lead) detachment or insulation failure
- Battery failure or abnormalities
- Pulse-generator failure
- Movement of the wire tip in the ventricle

In addition, dual-chamber ICDs are subject to all of the problems described in the pacemaker section earlier in this chapter. When a magnet is applied over an ICD, most of these devices suspend antitachycardia therapy (ie, rapid pacing and defibrillation) but continue to operate in pacemaker mode.

Information Gathering

If an ICD fires during the care of a patient, everything possible should be done to gather information that will help specialists confirm later whether the therapy was appropriate. After such an event, the patient's electrophysiologist will want to review the transport documentation and data from the ICD. Programming equipment that is unique to the ICD model makes it possible to retrieve detailed information from the device.

Many patients who have been shocked before recognize the symptoms of ventricular arrhythmias and can correctly identify appropriate and inappropriate therapies. A number of historical factors can have a role in ICD malfunction or offer clues about the nature of the problem. Among the most useful are the following:

- *Number of times shocked.* In patients with VT "storms," the device may give more than 100 shocks in a 24-hour period. When a patient has an atrial arrhythmia that conducts rapidly to the ventricle, it is common to deliver repeated unsuccessful therapies. Application of a pacemaker magnet over the ICD will temporarily suspend shocks.
- *Recent medical procedures.* Surgical and medical procedures can damage an ICD system, especially when performed on areas of the body in proximity to the ICD. Diathermy, lithotripsy, MRI, and radiation treatments are among the most common offenders.
- *Recent changes in medical condition or in patient adherence to the medication regimen.* It is not uncommon for patients to stop taking antiarrhythmic drugs if they have been arrhythmia free for several months or years. Likewise, patients withdrawing from benzodiazepines, alcohol, or other substances may experience increased arrhythmias.
- *Activity at the time of shock.* During intense exercise, an ICD may inappropriately shock a sinus tachycardia. Likewise, a patient with an ICD who experiences new-onset AF may receive unwarranted shocks.
- *Proximity to water or an electrical source.* Poorly grounded water pipes can produce trickle electrical currents that the ICD may pick up as a rapid heart rate. Likewise, a nearby source of electromagnetic interference can cause the ICD to discharge inappropriately.

Identifying the Problem

Occasionally, a patient with an ICD will experience multiple inappropriate defibrillator discharges as the result of defibrillator malfunction. This phenomenon is uncomfortable and agitating to the patient, to say the least, and may cause damage to the myocardium if allowed to continue. A magnet can be used to temporarily disable the ICD to prevent further discharges. Manufacturers of ICDs often provide special magnets (usually doughnut shaped) that are placed directly over the pulse generator. The magnet creates a magnetic field that trips a reed switch in the ICD. When the magnet is applied, detection of tachycardia and therapy are discontinued. For most applications, a single magnet is all that is required; however, for patients with obesity or edema, two magnets may be necessary. Before using the magnet, multifunction pads must be placed on the patient and hooked to the monitor; then the ICD can be deactivated.

Some ICD manufacturers make an external interrogation device that will help identify the source of the problem and, in some cases, allow reprogramming of the ICD. CCTPs should receive special training before using such a device.

In a patient with cardiac arrest, external defibrillation can be delivered, but the paddles or pads should not be placed directly over the ICD. CPR can also be performed on a patient with an ICD, with no danger to providers, the patient, or the implanted device. When delivering defibrillation, it is important to use anterior-posterior placement and position the pads away from the ICD.

FIGURE 14-105 and **FIGURE 14-106** illustrate some of the common problems with ICDs. The ICD stores the data for the episode in each case; this information can be retrieved later with the appropriate programming equipment.

In Figure 14-105, the ICD is oversensing the electrical activity that is present. The initial three pacer spikes function as expected, and each generates a QRS complex. However, after that the pacemaker

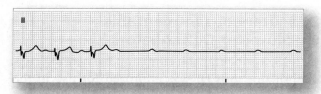

FIGURE 14-105 An electrocardiogram in which the implantable cardioverter-defibrillator is oversensing the P wave.

© Jones & Bartlett Learning.

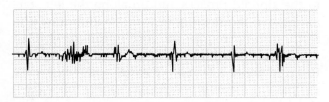

FIGURE 14-106 An example of pacemaker lead malfunction.

© Jones & Bartlett Learning.

inappropriately oversenses the P wave and is suppressed by it. This suppression of the pacemaker leads to the complete heart block seen in the remainder of the rhythm strip, with only P waves present initially. In this case, the CCTP should first check the patient's clinical status. If the patient is unconscious and unresponsive (which would likely be imminent with this ECG), the CCTP should check the patient's pulse and initiate ACLS protocols.

Figure 14-106 shows an example of lead malfunction. Intervals in the range of 120 to 150 ms are usually not physiologic, but more likely indicate electromagnetic interference or a problem with the sensing lead. In this case, there appears to be an irregular rhythm conducting at a rate of 60 to 80 beats/min. The ECG indicates the ventricular pacemaker is sensing at an irregular rate as well (malfunction). There are no clear pacemaker spikes indicating that it is firing appropriately. In this case, the CCTP should monitor the patient for hemodynamic stability and initiate CPR and external pacing as indicated.

Atrial Tachycardia Implantable Cardioverter-Defibrillators

Atrial fibrillation is one of the most common arrhythmias. Significant risks associated with AF include thromboembolism and a resulting increased incidence of stroke. Conventional methods to convert AF have centered on antiarrhythmic medications and external cardioversion. For recurrent arrhythmias, internal cardioversion or antitachycardia pacing with an atrial ICD is the preferred mode of treatment. Advances in lead design and the use of biphasic energy waveforms have made this therapy possible. With a biphasic waveform, lower energy levels may be used to effectively convert AF to a normal sinus rhythm.

Three modes for activating the atrial tachycardia ICD are currently in use. In the patient-activated mode, the patient uses a small, handheld remote device to initiate therapy after the device notifies the patient that AF is present. Alternatively, a physician may activate the device to provide appropriate therapy. A third option is even more commonly used today: The pacemaker or ICD is programmed to automatically deliver therapy after detecting the arrhythmia. All ICDs can act as pacemakers, and their atrial and ventricular leads may be dual purpose.

Wearable Cardioverter-Defibrillators

Short-term use of WCDs has been a treatment option since 2001. Candidates for use of these devices include patients at high risk for sudden cardiac death, such as those with a recent MI, low ejection fraction, new-onset arrhythmias, or survival of a recent or suspected sudden cardiac death episode. A WCD may also be appropriate for patients who require explant of an infected ICD while awaiting resolution of an infectious process. Use of WCDs is increasing, and CCTPs are likely to encounter these devices in their patients.

In the United States, this technology is available in the form of the ZOLL LifeVest WCD. LifeVest consists of a lightweight monitor that is worn around the waist or from a shoulder strap and an electrode belt with a garment worn around the patient's chest **FIGURE 14-107**. The electrodes are dry and nonadhesive. Gel in the therapy pads is released just prior to the device delivering a treatment shock. The device is programmable. The essential performance of the LifeVest WCD is that it detects ventricular fibrillation or ventricular tachycardia, then delivers a defibrillating shock. When it detects a treatable arrhythmia, it begins an alarm sequence that provides a conscious patient with enough time to stop the shock by holding two response buttons. If the patient fails to respond or releases the response buttons, the treatment sequence continues, including continued alarms and voice warnings to bystanders that a shock will be delivered. If the initial shock is ineffective, up to five additional defibrillations may be given. The entire sequence from detection to first shock typically occurs in about 1 minute. Shock energies are biphasic, programmable from 75 to 150 joules, with a default setting of 150 joules.

Patients download the data collected by the WCD via a hotspot in the device charging station to the ZOLL Patient Management Network, thereby allowing health care providers to see ECG recordings, uses, and device-related information. A warning label on the WCD garment advises rescuers to remove the WCD if the patient requires conventional defibrillation, because the WCD may interfere with defibrillation or may be damaged by automated external defibrillators (AEDs) or manual defibrillators. Audible and vibratory alarms include messages on the monitor screen, a gong alarm that tells the patient when to adjust the belt or electrode pads, and a siren alarm that sounds when an arrhythmia has been detected.

Patients prescribed WCDs should wear them continuously except when bathing or showering. The greatest risk to patients is while the WCD is not being worn.

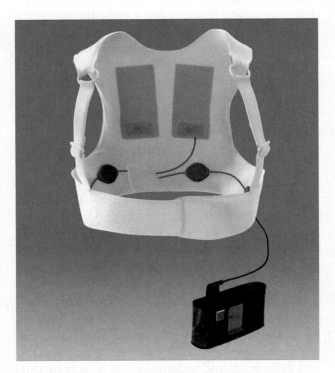

FIGURE 14-107 A wearable cardioverter-defibrillator.

Subcutaneous Implantable Cardioverter-Defibrillators

In 2015, a subcutaneous implantable cardioverter-defibrillator (S-ICD) was approved for use in the United States **FIGURE 14-108**. The S-ICD uses a low-profile ICD called a "can" that is surgically placed in the subcutaneous tissue near the fifth and sixth ribs at the midaxillary line. An electrode/defibrillator lead is then tunneled from the can to the xiphoid process and up along the left sternal border, terminating near the manubrium. The S-ICD does not require any venous leads or wires, so it is associated with less risk of infection compared to a traditional ICD. It has pacing capability in case the patient requires ventricular pacing following a shock, but it is not recommended for patients who have symptomatic bradycardia or arrhythmias that respond to antitachycardia pacing.

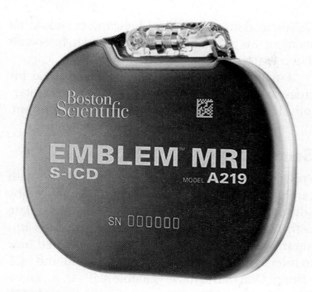

FIGURE 14-108 A subcutaneous implantable cardioverter-defibrillator.

Transport Considerations

When caring for and transporting cardiac patients, CCTPs must recognize that familiarity with temporary and implanted pacemakers and defibrillators is invaluable. Thus, ensuring transport safety and troubleshooting problems that may arise with these cardiac devices are key skills for CCTPs.

Preparation

The management of patients with a pacemaker or ICD begins well in advance of any transport request. CCTPs should receive advance training on any pacemaker or cardioverter-defibrillator device that they might encounter in the field. Pacemakers and defibrillators from a variety of manufacturers may be implanted at different sending facilities, requiring CCTPs to exercise additional scrutiny when picking up or dropping off patients at these facilities. Services transporting critically ill cardiac patients should have a magnet capable of temporarily reprogramming an implanted pacemaker or ICD readily available. It may be necessary to review the instructions for a particular device while en route to a patient transport if the CCTP has not used the relevant equipment recently.

Transport-Related Issues

Any patient with a pacemaker or defibrillator device must have electrical and mechanical pacemaker capture assessed and confirmed. A CCTP may make a potentially lethal error by mistakenly assuming that the electrical capture present on an ECG tracing represents the true mechanical capture. Mechanical capture is demonstrated by palpable pulses (or evidence of myocardial contraction exhibited on a pulse oximeter waveform or ultrasound) with each pacemaker complex on the ECG. Sometimes electrical capture may appear on the ECG without any actual contraction and pumping of the heart, disguising an underlying arrhythmia or cardiac arrest. If it goes unrecognized, lack of mechanical capture may have lethal consequences.

It is not always possible to continue using the same transcutaneous pacemaker or transvenous or transthoracic pulse generator for transport that is being used at the sending facility. Switching from the device used in a sending facility to the device used by the transport team is often a source of anxiety for CCTPs and other providers. Transvenous and transthoracic pacemaker leads are typically compatible with pulse-generator devices from many, if not all, manufacturers. Care must be taken to ensure equipment compatibility and to correctly match rate, output, mode, and sensitivity settings as the devices are switched. CCTPs must carefully check the patient for electrical and mechanical capture, in addition to other clinical indicators, when a change from one pacemaker to another is implemented. If the CCT team does not have a compatible device available, it may be worth considering using the device from the sending facility for the transport and returning it promptly after the transport has been completed, although this may not be possible in many situations. Many transcutaneous pacemakers have adapters that allow for the use of pads from multiple manufacturers. If such adapters are not available, it may be necessary to completely change the transcutaneous pacing pads for the duration of the transport.

CCTPs should also inquire about whether the patient has an ICD. The presence of an ICD may require use of an alternative site (not over the device) for transcutaneous pacing or defibrillation if needed during transport. An improperly functioning ICD has the potential to inappropriately discharge, causing patient discomfort, myocardial damage, and changes on the ECG. Inappropriate shocks are the most common ICD complication. CCTPs may use a pacemaker-type magnet to temporarily suspend cardioversion or defibrillation when an ICD administers continued inappropriate shocks.

A properly functioning ICD may terminate certain potentially lethal arrhythmias without the need for a CCTP to perform any external cardioversion or defibrillation during transport. Even so, it is still essential to have an external cardioverter-defibrillator immediately available. CCTPs may experience a mild sensation if they are in contact with a patient as an ICD discharges, but no serious injuries to bystanders or health care providers have been reported.

Factors in the transport environment may require special consideration for patients with pacemakers or ICDs. Electromagnetic interference is the major cause of pacemaker dysfunction, particularly in older pacemakers that lack adequate internal shielding. Modern chip-based pacemakers are less susceptible to this type of interference. Neither small single-engine airplanes nor larger commercial aircraft pose an increased risk for electromagnetic interference affecting implanted pacemakers or ICDs.

CCTPs should be aware that devices such as headphones and microphones with internal magnets may cause interference in older pacemakers when placed within 1 to 2 inches (2.5 to 5 cm) of the device. The American Heart Association recommends that any type of headphone remain more than 1 inch (3 cm) from the pacemaker to avoid the risk of electromagnetic interference. If patients are provided with headsets or intercom systems during air transport, CCTPs should take care to keep these items safely away from the pacemaker device, which is usually visible as a mass under the patient's skin.

Flight Considerations

Pacemaker malfunction does not usually occur as a result of the flight environment. Some isolated reports have described helicopter vibration affecting pacemaker function; occasionally, rate-responsive pacemakers increase their firing rate as a result of vibration during helicopter transport. Nevertheless, in a study involving helicopter transport of dozens of patients with pacemakers, no pacemaker malfunctions occurred. This sort of issue rarely arises in the fixed-wing environment, although it could occur if the aircraft encounters significant turbulence.

CCTPs working on medical helicopters should be aware of this potential and be prepared to intervene if necessary.

Finally, always remember that as altitude increases, monitoring oxygen saturations to determine if supplemental oxygen is needed is important.

Summary

Providers' ability to diagnose and treat patients with cardiac arrhythmias has been greatly enhanced by advances in technology, and keeping up-to-date with the latest developments on this front is imperative for all CCTPs. This chapter reviewed how to interpret 12-lead ECGs in the context of the CCT setting. One of the most valuable skills that can be learned is the ability to better identify an early MI, relay this information to the receiving facility or treating physician, and decrease the time to treatment. In addition to identifying an MI, acquiring a diagnostic-quality 12-lead ECG in the field, even if the findings are normal, will provide the treating staff with a baseline against which to compare serial ECGs done as part of the follow-up evaluation of the patient.

Over the years, pacemakers and ICDs have evolved through a variety of designs with varying functions and capabilities. Although detailed information about a patient's implanted device is often not readily available to CCTPs, general familiarity with basic concepts will always be helpful in determining whether these devices are functioning properly.

Pacers and ICDs share numerous basic components and functions. Modern devices all sense heart rate and use programmed circuitry to decide whether or how to respond. The exact types of sensing they perform and the therapies they deliver are where the types of devices differ the most.

Knowing the NBG codes is perhaps the single most valuable tool in a CCTP's approach to a patient with a pacemaker. Studying ECGs of real patients with pacers and ICDs will help CCTPs prepare for identifying and managing problems in the transport environment. In any case of suspected or certain malfunction, it will be important to the electrophysiologist that the CCTP obtain ECG recordings, ensure availability of data from the device, and provide detailed written documentation of the incident.

Case Study

Just as you are finishing your lunch, dispatch advises you of an emergency transfer of a critical cardiac patient from Community Hospital to St. Patrick's Hospital. Your crew, which consists of an emergency medical technician (EMT) driver, you, and a fellow paramedic, responds in 12 minutes to the Community Hospital emergency department (ED).

On arrival, you obtain a report from the transferring physician, Dr. Jans, who states that your patient is a 67-year-old, 245.5-lb (111.36-kg) Native American man who arrived in the ED approximately 45 minutes ago complaining of severe substernal chest pain. The patient also had hypertension. The patient's 12-lead ECG revealed no acute ST-segment changes, but bloodwork showed an elevated troponin level, suggesting ACS. His medications in the ED included 324 mg of aspirin; 0.4 mg of nitroglycerin, 2 doses; 3 mg of morphine IV; 300 mg of clopidogrel; and 20 mg of eptifibatide. Currently, the patient is receiving a continuous infusion of nitroglycerin at 20 mcg/min and an eptifibatide infusion at 222 mcg/min. The patient is being transferred to Dr. Webb at St. Patrick's catheterization laboratory for emergency cardiac catheterization.

When you assess the patient, you obtain the following readings: heart rate, 94 beats/min, sinus rhythm; respiratory rate, 18 breaths/min, with clear and equal breath sounds bilaterally; blood pressure, 145/88 mm Hg; temperature, 99.1°F (37.3°C); pulse oximetry reading, 95% on room air; carbon dioxide, 42 mm Hg; heart tones, normal with no rubs, gallops, or murmurs; and peripheral edema, 1+ in the lower extremities.

Further interview of the patient reveals a past medical history of hypertension and hepatitis. At present, he takes no medications and has no allergies. The patient states that the pain started approximately 90 minutes ago and began radiating to his left arm. Initially, he rated the pain as 10 on a 10-point scale; after morphine was given, the score decreased to 2 on a 10-point scale. As your partner secures the patient onto the stretcher, you transfer the infusions to your transport IV pump.

As you review the patient's lab studies, you note the following values of interest:

- Glucose: 98 mg/dL (normal range, 70 to 110 mg/dL)
- Chloride: 110 mmol/L (normal range, 96 to 106 mmol/L)
- Potassium: 4.1 mmol/L (normal range, 3.5 to 5.0 mmol/L)
- Calcium: 8.6 mg/dL (normal range, 8.2 to 10.2 mg/dL)
- Magnesium: 1.7 mEq/L (normal range, 1.3 to 2.1 mEq/L)
- Blood urea nitrogen (BUN): 13 mg/dL (normal range, 8 to 23 mg/dL)
- Creatinine: 1.3 mg/dL (normal range, 0.6 to 1.2 mg/dL)
- BUN/creatinine ratio: 10.0 calculated (normal range, 12.0 to 20.0 calculated)
- Prothrombin time: 14.1 s (normal range, 10 to 13 s)
- Activated partial thromboplastin time: 53.0 s (normal range, 25.0 to 40.0 s)
- Troponin T: 1.6 ng/mL (normal range, 0.0 to 0.1 ng/mL)
- Brain-type natriuretic peptide: 140 pg/mL (normal range, <167 pg/mL)
- Alanine aminotransferase: 392 U/L (normal range, 10 to 40 U/L)
- Aspartate aminotransferase: 110 U/L (normal range, 10 to 30 U/L)

You load the patient into the ambulance and proceed on an emergency basis to St. Patrick's Hospital, which is located approximately 110 miles away. The patient appears to be in a moderate amount of distress; however, he rates his pain as 2 on a 10-point scale. As you reassess the patient, your partner increases the nitroglycerin to 25 mcg/min in an attempt to make the patient more comfortable. The patient acknowledges the improvement: "Thanks, that helps me relax and not hurt quite as bad."

Your partner repeats a 12-lead ECG to compare with the ECG that was done in the ED, and it is unchanged. The remainder of the transport is unremarkable, and you deliver the patient to Dr. Webb and the waiting catheterization laboratory team.

1. If this patient did not have any ECG changes, how were you able to determine that he was experiencing an MI?
2. Why was this patient receiving nitroglycerin? Eptifibatide?
3. What are the side effects of these medications?
4. What are the possible complications that may be experienced en route with this patient?

Analysis

Because of your critical care training, you are able to recognize that this patient was experiencing an NSTEMI based on the given lab values. You know that troponin will increase 3 to 6 hours after infarction and is the most specific cardiac marker.

Nitroglycerin is indicated in MI situations owing to its vasodilatory properties on systemic and large coronary vessels. Systemic venodilation reduces preload, lowering ventricular volume. To a much lesser degree, arterial vasodilation also occurs, reducing afterload. The subsequent decrease in cardiac workload results in increased oxygen and blood supply to ischemic cardiac tissue. The possible side effects of using nitroglycerin for this patient are hypotension, reflex tachycardia, and cardiac arrhythmias.

Eptifibatide is indicated in patients with unstable angina or NSTEMI to reduce the risk of acute ischemic events. This antiplatelet medication selectively blocks the platelet glycoprotein IIb/IIIa receptor. Possible side effects of eptifibatide are uncontrollable bleeding, anemia, and thrombocytopenia.

Owing to the nature of this patient's situation and the different medications that have been administered, careful monitoring en route is essential. Some of the potential problems that might occur en route include hypotension from inadvertent nitrate overdose, cardiogenic shock caused by pump failure, respiratory arrest due to narcotic potentiation, and, ultimately, cardiopulmonary arrest.

That evening, as you are delivering another patient to the ED at St. Patrick's, you see Dr. Webb and ask about the status of the patient whom you brought in earlier. According to the physician, the patient underwent cardiac catheterization that revealed significant narrowing of the left anterior descending artery. Owing to the severity of the narrowing, placing a stent was contraindicated, so the patient underwent an emergency coronary artery bypass graft in which a section of the left internal mammary artery was removed and grafted to the left anterior descending artery. The patient is expected to make a complete recovery and be released in 3 to 5 days.

Prep Kit

Ready for Review

- Oxygenated blood reaches the heart through the coronary arteries, which are vulnerable to blockage and narrowing by plaque formation, a condition called atherosclerosis.
- The major heart sounds are the two normal sounds, S_1 and S_2, and the two abnormal sounds, S_3 and S_4.
  - S_1 (the "lub" sound) occurs near the beginning of ventricular contraction

(systole), when the tricuspid and mitral valves close. Any delay in the closing of these two valves, heard as a split sound, is considered abnormal.
  - S_2 (the "dub" sound) occurs near the end of ventricular contraction (systole), when the pulmonary and aortic valves close. The two valves can close simultaneously or with a slight delay between them under normal physiologic circumstances.

- S_3 ("dub-lub-dub") signals the end of the rapid filling period of the ventricle during the beginning of diastole. In older adults, it often signifies heart failure.
- S_4 ("lub-dub-dub") coincides with atrial contraction at the end of ventricular diastole. If heard at any other time, the patient may have resistance to ventricular filling.

- The cardiac cycle comprises one complete phase of atrial and ventricular relaxation (diastole), followed by one atrial and ventricular contraction (systole).
- During diastole (normally 520 ms), the left atrium fills passively with blood under the influence of venous pressure, and approximately 80% of ventricular filling occurs.
- In systole (normally 280 ms), ventricular filling is completed, the atrioventricular (AV) valves snap shut, the two ventricles contract (ventricular systole), and the semilunar valves are forced open. Blood squeezed out of the right ventricle moves into the pulmonary arteries; blood from the left ventricle is pushed into the aorta.
- If the right side of the heart fails, blood backs up behind the right atrium, evidenced by distention of the external jugular veins, and fluid leaks into the surrounding tissues, causing edema in the subcutaneous and internal tissues.
- If the left side of the heart fails, blood backs up behind the left atrium, and fluid is squeezed into the alveoli, producing pulmonary edema, evidenced by dyspnea, bubbling crackles, and frothy sputum.
- In addition to the output of the heart and the volume of blood present in the system, the relative constriction or dilation of arteries, which is controlled by the autonomic nervous system, influences blood pressure.
- Key parameters associated with the heart's functioning include CO (the amount of blood pumped out by either ventricle), stroke volume (the amount of blood pumped out by either

ventricle in a single contraction), and heart rate (the number of cardiac contractions per minute).
- Changes in the heart's contractility (the degree of contraction of its muscle without changing the stretch on the muscle) may be induced by medications that have a positive or negative inotropic effect.
- The heart can generate its own electrical impulses without stimulation from nerves (automaticity) and has specialized conduction tissue that can rapidly propagate electrical impulses to the muscular tissue of the heart.
- The dominant pacemaker in the heart is the sinoatrial (SA) node; if the right coronary artery is occluded, as in a myocardial infarction (MI), the SA node may become ischemic.
- Depolarization of the heart, the process by which muscle fibers are stimulated to contract, occurs because of an influx of sodium and calcium ions into the myocardial cells. It results in a "wave of depolarization" as the electrical charges pass in all directions from one cell to another.
- Repolarization occurs when the sodium and calcium channels close and potassium channels open; during this process, sodium ions move out of the cell and potassium ions flood back in.
- In the absolute refractory period, the heart muscle has been drained of energy; it will not contract during this period. In the relative refractory period, the heart is partially charged, albeit not strongly enough to create a full contraction.
- The electrical conduction events in the heart can be recorded on an electrocardiogram (ECG) as a series of waves and complexes. Depolarization of the atria produces the P wave; as the electrical impulse slows through the AV node or AV junction, it can be seen on the ECG as the PR interval; depolarization of the ventricles produces the QRS complex;

Prep Kit Continued

repolarization of the atria and ventricles produces T waves.

- A U wave may be present after the T wave, although there is no definitive agreement as to what it represents.
- The 12-lead ECG graphically represents electrical activity in cardiac tissue.
- Today's cardiac monitor-defibrillators typically combine continuous 3-lead ECG monitoring, 12-lead electrocardiography, semiautomatic and manual defibrillation, external pacing, capnography, pulse oximetry, blood pressure monitoring, end-tidal carbon dioxide measurements, invasive pressure monitoring, and other capabilities.
- Assessment of the patient's cardiac status, which takes place before monitoring, should include analysis of the cardiac rhythm and 12-lead ECG to determine any underlying electrical disturbances caused by changes in the heart's structure or function as the result of disease, ischemia, injury, or infarction.
- Cardiac monitoring, the continuous observation of the patient's condition in relation to the cardiac rhythm, typically uses lead configurations that allow for viewing the rhythm simultaneously from one to three leads.
- The gold standard for 12-lead ECG interpretation is the ability to perform serial evaluations for comparison; however, it is important to use consistent lead placements to ensure that all providers compare "apples to apples."
- The electrode is the sensing device that connects directly to the skin; the lead is the designated position of the electrode (ie, limb and precordial leads). The cable is the physical wire that connects the electrode to the ECG monitor.
- The six limb leads (I, II, III, aVR, aVL, and aVF) provide a view of the heart in a coronal or vertical plane (the frontal plane); the six precordial leads (V_1 to V_6), or chest leads,

show a transverse or horizontal plane. The combination of limb leads and precordial leads provides a three-dimensional view of the heart.

- If the flow of electrical activity proceeds unimpeded toward a positive lead, it appears as a positive deflection on the ECG. If the flow of electrical activity moves away from a positive lead, it is deflected negatively. An electrical impulse that crosses perpendicular to a positive lead is called isoelectric.
- If the heart's electrical impulse is deflected by a change in structure or function, it will be less positive, aberrantly conducted, or deflected away from the selected electrode.
- Placement of additional or nonstandard right-side heart leads V_4R, V_5R, and V_6R and posterior heart leads V_7, V_8, and V_9 is indicated in suspected right ventricular and posterior MIs and when a patient has clinical findings suggestive of acute coronary ischemia, but the standard 12-lead ECG is normal or nondiagnostic.
- Before running the ECG with right-side leads, the critical care transport professional (CCTP) should complete the standard 12-lead ECG. Then, using the precordial (chest) leads, the additional leads are attached as follows: V_4R, V_5R, V_6R, V_7, V_8, and V_9.
- The CCTP should confirm placement of leads before transport and several times during transport.
- A "new" 12-lead ECG should be recorded and evaluated before transport and repeated at regular intervals, when any changes in the ECG are noted, and on arrival at the receiving facility.
- The transport of a patient with STEMI to definitive care should not be delayed for the sake of obtaining additional ECGs.
- Placing the patient in a supine position is recommended when obtaining ECGs; however, an adequate ECG can be obtained with the patient in a semisitting (semi-Fowler) position.

Prep Kit Continued

- Before obtaining a 12-lead ECG, the device should be standardized or calibrated at 1 mV = 10 mm high and 200 ms wide.
- In the limb leads, the P wave is typically upright in leads I, II, aVL, and aVF. It is frequently biphasic in lead III, and is purely negatively deflected in lead aVR. A change in the P-wave morphology suggests an ectopic atrial focus.
- In the precordial leads, the P wave is typically upright in leads V_5 and V_6. Lead V_1 is biphasic, and leads V_2 and V_4 are variable.
- The PR interval spans the time from the start of atrial depolarization to the start of ventricular depolarization; it also includes the delay in conduction that occurs at the AV junction. It usually lasts from 120 to 200 ms.
- The QRS complex is a representation of ventricular depolarization. Septal depolarization is not always seen on the ECG; when it is, a small Q wave may be visible in leads I, aVL, V_5, and V_6.
- The keys to being able to quickly read an ECG are experience and consistency. Interpretation of 12-lead ECGs is a skill that must be practiced repeatedly using a standard method of analysis.
- Interpretation of rhythms and arrhythmias is a fundamental building block for ECG analysis.
- The 12-lead ECG shows groupings of complexes that are recorded simultaneously by each lead. The rhythm strip, which typically appears at the bottom of the ECG, records for the entire time the 12-lead ECG is being obtained.
- Each cell in the heart can produce its own electrical impulse (vector), which varies in intensity and direction. The axis is the direction of the wave of depolarization as it passes through the heart.
- The sum of all the electrical impulses is called the mean electrical axis. It should progress in a downward and leftward direction; a change in

the axis indicates that a change has occurred in the structure or function of the heart.
- To calculate the direction and intensity of the electrical axis, the hexaxial system, which relies on a circular diagram oriented in the frontal (coronal) plane, can be used.
- Before transporting a critically ill patient, a baseline ECG should be acquired and analyzed on the cardiac monitor and abnormalities should be noted, including in the mean electrical axis. An axis that deviates outside the normal range or is different from the patient's preexisting axis usually has clinical implications. In such a case, the CCTP should check the ECG for corresponding changes suggestive of the underlying cause of the deviation.
- Cardiac causes of axis deviation include ischemia, infarction, left or right ventricular hypertrophy, ectopic beats and rhythms, dextrocardia, and conduction defect of the left posterior-inferior fascicle of the left bundle branch.
- Other conditions that are not cardiac in origin can contribute to a shift in axis; examples include anatomy (such as tall, thin stature), young age, chronic obstructive pulmonary disease, obesity, and pregnancy.
- A disruption of the electrical impulse in the right and left atria will result in a change in the shape of the P wave.
- An injury to the tricuspid and mitral valves or disruption of the electrical impulse in the AV node can result in lengthening or shortening of the PR interval.
- Injuries in the bundle of His, the left and right bundle branches, the fascicles, and the Purkinje fibers can result in a bundle or fascicular block.
- With a right bundle branch block (BBB), the representative complex displayed on the ECG includes a prolonged QRS interval of 120 ms or more; a slurred S wave in leads I and V_6; and the RSR′ pattern in lead V_1, with the R′ wave being taller than the R wave.

Prep Kit Continued

- No specific treatment is required for an isolated right BBB, but the patient should be seen for periodic follow-up evaluations.
- With a left BBB, the representative complex displayed on the ECG includes a prolonged QRS interval of 120 ms or more; V_6 should have a notched R wave with no Q wave; and wide, deep S waves should be seen in lead V_1 (this lead may also have a small r wave with a large S wave).
- A left BBB usually indicates the presence of a serious cardiac problem within the conduction system or ischemia from coronary artery disease. Patients with this condition require complete cardiac evaluation.
- A hemiblock is a block in the electrical conduction of one of the two fascicle branches of the left bundle branch. It causes little to no widening of the QRS complexes.
- The criteria for diagnosing left anterior hemiblock are left axis deviation within –30° to –90°; a qR complex or large R wave in lead I; and an rS complex in lead III (likely to also appear in leads II and aVF).
- A bifascicular block (ie, two conduction pathways blocked at the same time) is diagnosed by concurrent findings of a right BBB with a left anterior hemiblock or left posterior hemiblock. A new onset of bifascicular block with ischemia is not stable and often deteriorates into a complete heart block, especially in the presence of an acute MI.
- When transporting a critically ill cardiac patient with an existing bifascicular block consisting of a right BBB and left anterior hemiblock, if signs of ischemia or infarction develop, the patient will likely need acute pacemaker placement, especially in the presence of second- or third-degree AV block. The CCTP should contact medical control, prepare the patient for external cardiac pacing, and notify the receiving facility to be urgently prepared for pacemaker placement.
- A trifascicular block is the combination of a bifascicular block (a right BBB with a block in the left anterior or left posterior fascicle) that occurs with a first-degree heart block (prolonged PR interval); its presence after an MI implies extensive cardiac damage. True trifascicular blocks require immediate temporary pacing followed by the placement of a permanent pacemaker.
- Hyperacute T waves that appear as a result of ischemia and infarction appear only in the leads that view the area of ischemia and infarction.
- In addition to being present after an MI, ST-segment elevation is observed with a left BBB, ventricular rhythms, left ventricular hypertrophy, pericarditis, and early repolarization. A persistent ST-segment elevation may indicate the formation of a ventricular aneurysm.
- The combination of hypertrophy and dilation means that the heart has a larger muscle mass in the affected area and the chamber is enlarged. The larger the muscle mass, the higher the concentration of electrical impulses or vectors is.
- Left atrial enlargement produces a P wave with a notched, double-humped appearance.
- The characteristic findings in right atrial enlargement are tall, peaked P waves in the inferior leads II, III, and aVF that have an amplitude of 2.5 mm or more. The tall, peaked P waves are known as P pulmonale.
- Patients with left ventricular hypertrophy (LVH) have a higher risk for coronary artery disease, making them more susceptible to the sequelae of that disease, and exhibit increased mortality relative to patients who experience an MI without LVH. Increased R-wave amplitude in the leads that look at the left ventricle informs the ECG diagnosis of LVH.
- Patients with right ventricular hypertrophy exhibit a right shift in axis in leads I and aVF,

Prep Kit Continued

and precordial leads V_1 and V_2 show increased R-wave deflection.

- When hypertrophy is uncomplicated by ischemia, the changes in QRS complexes are used to make the diagnosis. When subendocardial ischemia is present as well, changes to the ST segment and T wave appear as a strain pattern.

- It is important to distinguish between the strain pattern and the ST-segment and T-wave changes seen in ischemia and infarction, because the ST-segment and T-wave changes can be immediately life threatening.

- In people with Wolff-Parkinson-White syndrome (WPW), the bundle of Kent (accessory pathway) does not have the same ability to slowly conduct electrical impulses as does the pathway through the AV node. This condition puts the person at risk for extremely fast heart rates that may cause hemodynamic instability. On the ECG, WPW is signaled by the presence of a slurred upstroke known as a delta wave.

- The two tachyarrhythmias that occur most often in WPW are paroxysmal supraventricular tachycardia (SVT) and atrial fibrillation. CCTPs should be aware of the potential for a wide complex tachycardia developing that is difficult to distinguish from ventricular tachycardia (VT).

- Treatment of unstable WPW tachyarrhythmias may require electrical cardioversion; management with drug therapy produces unpredictable results.

- Pericarditis (inflammation of the pericardium) may cause ST-segment elevation, T-wave flattening or inversion, and the appearance of low voltage in all leads.

- Long QT syndrome (LQTS) is characterized by a prolonged QT interval on ECG and has a tendency to deteriorate into ventricular tachyarrhythmias, including torsades de pointes, which can lead to syncope and sudden cardiac death. In this condition, the rhythm is

too fast to maintain effective CO, so the patient loses consciousness, often without warning.

- The deterioration of LQTS poses a management challenge for CCTPs. Carefully evaluating the ECG, reviewing the patient's medications, and obtaining a medical history will help provide clues to the diagnosis and alert the CCTP to the possibility of a tachyarrhythmia developing during transport.

- Treatment for torsades de pointes includes correcting the underlying cause, overdrive pacing, and administering magnesium sulfate. Other therapies for patients in unstable condition may include electrical cardioversion and defibrillation.

- Wide complex tachycardia is any cardiac rhythm of more than 100 beats/min with a QRS duration of 120 ms or more. This arrhythmia can be of ventricular or supraventricular origin; identifying its origin can lead to the correct diagnosis and proper therapeutic interventions.

- The most useful ECG criterion in establishing the diagnosis of VT is the presence of AV dissociation with more ventricular events than atrial events.

- In a patient with a right BBB with a QRS duration of greater than 140 ms, VT is the likely diagnosis. In a patient with a left BBB, a QRS duration of greater than 160 ms suggests VT.

- If the electrical axis is in the range of 180° to −90°, the wide complex tachycardia is not likely to be SVT. Electrical concordance across the precordium (all QRS complexes pointing in the same direction in leads V_1 through V_6) is more likely to be VT and is rarely consistent with SVT.

- Patients with wide complex tachycardia who have low blood pressure, pulmonary edema, severe chest pain, or other evidence of poor perfusion should be promptly treated using synchronized cardioversion.

- When a patient with wide complex tachycardia remains in hemodynamically stable condition, more time can be spent reviewing the history, physical examination, and ECG findings, so as to make the correct diagnosis.

- When a patient has wide complex tachycardia of an uncertain cause, yet remains in hemodynamically stable condition, procainamide is the drug of choice because it can terminate SVT and VT. This agent is also useful in patients with a poor ejection fraction.

- Procainamide can be used with caution in a patient with wide complex tachycardia who remains in hemodynamically stable condition. This drug can cause a sudden drop in blood pressure with rapid IV administration and is contraindicated in patients with complete heart block.

- Lidocaine is useful for VT of ischemic origin but does not terminate SVT.

- If SVT is suspected, adenosine is a useful and diagnostic medication. When irregular wide complex tachycardia is the result of atrial fibrillation and pre-excitation over an accessory pathway, however, adenosine may lead to ventricular fibrillation.

- Following termination of wide complex tachycardia, preventive treatment for maintaining a stable rhythm should be initiated, usually in the form of an antiarrhythmic drug (eg, continuation of the drug that terminated the wide complex tachycardia).

- In patients presenting with a wide complex tachycardia rhythm, BLS is the first step in patient management, closely followed by ACLS practices. If the patient is in hemodynamically unstable condition, wide complex tachycardia should be managed as if it were VT until proven otherwise, with synchronized cardioversion being the initial therapy of choice.

- Polymorphic or pulseless VT should be treated as ventricular fibrillation: Give immediate defibrillation, secure the airway, provide CPR, perform endotracheal intubation, support ventilations, and administer an antiarrhythmic medication.

- When changes in electrolytes, especially potassium and calcium, occur, their effects are often seen on the ECG.

- Hyperkalemia, the most dangerous of all electrolyte abnormalities, can cause death and prevent some drugs used in resuscitation efforts from being effective. On the ECG, hyperkalemia can cause changes in the appearance of all waveforms, and it can cause virtually any arrhythmia. Rapid recognition and correction of this electrolyte disturbance is essential.

- Hypokalemia does not cause the dramatic changes on the ECG, but rather is associated with mild, nonspecific changes such as ST-segment depression, a slightly decreased amplitude of the T waves, minimal prolongation of the QRS interval, and the presence of a prominent U wave.

- ECG changes associated with hypercalcemia include a shortened ST segment, a shortened QT interval, a prolonged PR interval, and flattened or inverted T waves. A variable degree of heart block may also develop.

- Hypocalcemia that occurs acutely can be the result of medications or surgical effects. It causes the opposite effects of hypercalcemia.

- There is a higher incidence of adverse effects with use of calcium channel blockers and beta blockers, but the mortality rate is higher in patients who experience digoxin toxicity. The margin between toxic and therapeutic doses of digoxin is small.

- At toxic levels of digoxin, the excessive increase of intracellular calcium associated with this medication elevates the resting potential and predisposes the heart to arrhythmias. The most common ECG changes seen in patients with digoxin toxicity include AV, junctional, or ventricular ectopic beats; first-degree AV block; slow ventricular response in atrial fibrillation; and an accelerated AV or junctional rhythm. More severe arrhythmias may include severe bradycardia, high-degree

Prep Kit Continued

heart blocks, and malignant ventricular rhythms.

- Early recognition and aggressive treatment of digoxin toxicity are lifesaving.
- If one of the coronary arteries becomes blocked, the muscle it supplies will be deprived of oxygen (ischemia). If this oxygen supply is not quickly restored, the ischemic area of heart muscle will eventually die (undergo infarction).
- In atherosclerosis, plaque infiltrates the arterial wall and decreases its elasticity; it also narrows the arterial lumen and interferes with blood flow through the vessel. The narrowed, roughened area of the arterial intima provides a locus for the formation of a fixed blood clot (thrombus) that may obstruct the artery, and calcium may begin to precipitate from the bloodstream into the arterial walls, causing arteriosclerosis.
- Atherosclerosis is rarely the primary cause of medical emergencies but is a major contributor to other conditions that may become medical emergencies.
- Arterial bruits (turbulence or "swishing" sounds heard with a stethoscope placed over the carotid arteries) signal the presence of atherosclerosis and contraindicate the use of carotid sinus massage.
- Other peripheral vascular disorders associated with atherosclerosis include claudication and phlebitis. An example of claudication is a severe pain in the calf muscle caused by narrowing of the arteries in this muscle and leading to a painful limp. Phlebitis is inflammation, swelling, and pain along the veins that can lead to the formation of blood clots and thrombophlebitis, which is venous inflammation associated with a thrombus.
- The most dangerous complication of peripheral vascular disorders is pulmonary embolism, in which a thromboembolus travels to the heart and through its right side, lodging in the pulmonary arterial tree.

- Signs of peripheral vascular occlusion may include pain, flushing, swelling, warmth, and tenderness in the extremity; claudication; and arterial bruits.
- If a blockage or potential embolus is suspected, the CCTP should administer IV heparin or other anticoagulant, monitor the affected limb via ultrasonography or Doppler imaging (if available), and maximize blood flow to the extremity by using warm compresses.
- A patient being transported over a long distance with a blood clot that has the potential to become a pulmonary embolus should have a baseline ECG performed before transport begins and must undergo frequent 12-lead ECG monitoring. ST-segment depression in the limb and precordial leads accompanied by an increase in right axis deviation may indicate a pulmonary embolism. As a diagnostic tool, the ECG is neither specific nor sensitive for pulmonary embolism.
- Acute coronary syndrome (ACS) comprises any group of clinical symptoms consistent with acute myocardial ischemia. Acute myocardial ischemia typically presents as chest pain as the result of insufficient blood supply to the heart muscle because of coronary artery disease.
- ACS includes conditions that cause episodes of ischemic discomfort (chest pain) as the result of disruption of plaque within a coronary artery. These substances promote a chain reaction of platelet activation, adhesion, aggregation, thrombin formation, and, ultimately, thrombus formation, with the end result being complete occlusion of the coronary artery or one of its branches.
- The 12-lead ECG is used to categorize two groups of patients who have experienced ACS: patients with ST-segment elevation MI (STEMI) and patients without STEMI (NSTEMI).
- A 12-lead ECG should be performed within 10 minutes of contacting a patient with chest discomfort or other signs and symptoms suggestive of STEMI. If the findings are

Prep Kit Continued

not conclusive, but the patient remains symptomatic and a high degree of suspicion is present, serial 12-lead ECGs should be performed while maintaining continuous ST-segment monitoring.

- All patients with ACS should receive antithrombin and antiplatelet therapy, regardless of the presence or absence of ST-segment elevation. Patients with STEMI are candidates for prompt reperfusion therapy, either pharmacologic or catheter based, to restore blood flow in the occluded artery; patients with NSTEMI should receive anti-ischemic therapy and be considered for catheter-based therapy.

- Marked ST-segment depression in leads V_1 through V_4, with tall R waves in the right precordial leads and upright T waves, is suggestive of a true posterior wall MI. Placement of additional electrodes in the posterior position to form leads V_7, V_8, and V_9 is recommended to confirm the diagnosis because primary percutaneous coronary intervention may be appropriate in patients with true posterior MI.

- Lethal ventricular arrhythmias may develop in patients with STEMI, so continuous ECG monitoring is required.

- Many patients whose ECG displays ST-segment elevation will ultimately have a STEMI.

- In case of ACS, the role of the CCT team is to transport the patient from a basic-care hospital to a cardiac-specialty hospital with the least possible decline in the patient's condition and to prevent further loss of heart muscle. If transport times will be long or the degree of blockage is severe to the point of being life threatening, administration of tissue plasminogen activators may be required.

- Angina occurs when the supply of oxygen to the myocardium is insufficient to meet the demand. When obtaining a history from a patient with chest pain, it is important to distinguish between stable angina (follows a recurrent pattern) and unstable angina (follows no pattern).

- In the CCT environment, nitroglycerin should be given intravenously to patients with stable angina, especially for long transports.

- Unstable angina is characterized by noticeable changes in the frequency, severity, and duration of pain and often occurs without predictable stress. It is often a warning sign of an impending MI.

- An MI occurs when the cardiac muscle is deprived of coronary blood flow long enough for death of myocardial tissue to occur. Causes include narrowed vessels, coronary artery occlusion, spasm of a coronary artery, and reduction of overall blood flow.

- Acute MI is the leading cause of death in the United States. The majority of infarctions involve the left ventricle.

- The infarcted tissue is invariably surrounded by a ring of ischemic tissue, an area that is relatively deprived of oxygen but still viable. This ischemic tissue is often the source of cardiac arrhythmias.

- The three initial components for the diagnosis of an MI are history and physical examination, testing for cardiac enzymes, and interpretation of ECG changes associated with an MI.

- Biomarkers for MI include troponin I and troponin T, both of which increase after an MI. When troponin assays are available, creatine kinase and myoglobin are no longer considered useful for diagnosis of ACS.

- Increased oxygen demand caused by an increased workload or a decrease in supply caused by coronary artery disease or a blocked artery can lead to ischemia, injury, and, ultimately, infarction. Ischemia and injury may be reversible, and rapid intervention when they occur can often prevent infarction.

- On the ECG, findings associated with ischemia include ST-segment depression and an inverted T wave. With MI, the T wave inverts symmetrically; when other causes (such as

Prep Kit Continued

ventricular hypertrophy with strain and a BBB and cerebral hemorrhage) are to blame, the T-wave inversion is often asymmetric or "slurred."

- If ischemia continues uninterrupted, the injured area does not repolarize completely, leading to an elevated ST segment.

- If ischemia and injury continue uninterrupted, infarction can occur. Because the infarcted tissue no longer generates or transmits electrical impulses, no direct wave is recorded on the ECG. Electrical impulses, which are deflected away from the area of infarct, are represented by Q waves.

- For Q waves to be significant (ie, indicating pathology), they must be more than one-third the total height of the QRS complex with which they appear and wider than 40 ms in duration.

- The prognosis and therapeutic implications for a patient who has had an MI are determined largely by which area of the heart has died.

- Q waves from old infarctions can be present with findings of a new MI and can complicate the process of making the correct diagnosis from the ECG. For this reason, CCTPs should review an "old" ECG from the patient's chart, acquire a new 12-lead ECG before transport, and make serial evaluations along the way.

- In an anterior wall MI, the normal pattern of R-wave progression may not occur, a phenomenon called poor R-wave progression.

- An anteroseptal MI is common with an occlusion of the left anterior descending artery and is often associated with hemodynamic compromise and cardiogenic shock. To identify this pattern of MI, the CCTP should analyze the septal leads V_1 and V_2 and the anterior leads V_3 and V_4.

- In an acute anteroseptal MI with lateral extension, changes can be seen in all precordial leads (specifically, V_5 and V_6 for the lateral extension) and in leads I and aVL; significant Q-wave formation is not always present, but

reciprocal changes can be found in leads II, III, and aVF.

- Hyperacute T-wave changes occur only during the first 15 to 30 minutes of an acute MI. If these changes are found during transport, the CCTP is in a unique position to initiate care, even if it is only early notification of the receiving facility to decrease the door-to-treatment time.

- In an acute lateral wall MI, ECG changes are often seen in lateral leads I, aVL, V_5, and V_6. Reciprocal changes may be seen in inferior leads II, III, and aVF.

- With an inferior wall MI, characteristic ECG changes can be seen in inferior leads II, III, and aVF. Reciprocal changes are seen as ST-segment depression in leads I and aVL unless the high lateral wall is included in the infarction.

- In a patient without signs of acute infarction, pathologic Q waves are considered to have an indeterminate age; that is, without a good patient history, there is no way to tell how old the infarction is.

- In an acute inferolateral MI, ECG changes are seen in inferior leads II, III, and aVF and in lateral leads I, aVL, V_5, and V_6. ST-segment changes will be found in leads V_2 to V_4 if the infarct extends anteriorly, and classic ST-segment and T-wave changes will be evident in lateral precordial leads V_5 and V_6.

- In an acute apical MI, direct ECG changes can be found in inferior leads II, III, and aVF; lateral leads I and aVL; and precordial leads V_2 through V_6. Because of the diffuse ECG changes, this type of MI can be confused with pericarditis.

- Right ventricular infarction is strongly associated with an inferior wall MI, so when it is present, CCTPs should maintain a high index of suspicion and check for other criteria. Right ventricular infarction should be suspected with ST-segment elevation in (septal) lead V_1 and (inferior) leads II, III, and aVF.

Prep Kit Continued

- The diagnosis of a posterior wall MI is made by looking for reciprocal changes in leads V_1 and V_2—specifically, ST-segment depression, upright T waves, and tall R waves.
- When there is reciprocal evidence of a posterior wall MI, CCTPs should maintain a high index of suspicion, and record posterior leads (V_7, V_8, and V_9) for comparison.
- Patients with cardiomyopathy may have shortness of breath, chest pain, palpitations, or syncope; sudden cardiac death is also possible.
- Heart failure occurs when the heart cannot pump powerfully enough or fast enough to empty its chambers; as a result, blood backs up into the systemic circuit, the pulmonary circuit, or both.
- In left-side heart failure, the left side of the heart is no longer able to pump the blood being delivered from the pulmonary vessels. As a consequence, blood backs up behind the left ventricle, the pressure in the left atrium and pulmonary veins increases, and serum is forced out of the pulmonary capillaries and into the alveoli.
- Pulmonary edema occurs as the result of a reduced ejection fraction and CO of the left ventricle, as serum mixes with air in the alveoli.
- The priorities when managing left-side heart failure are to remove the fluid from the lungs, reduce afterload, increase oxygen supply to the heart, and decrease myocardial oxygen demands.
- Right-side heart failure most commonly occurs as a result of left-side heart failure, but may also occur as a result of pulmonary embolism or long-standing chronic obstructive pulmonary disease, especially chronic bronchitis.
- The edema associated with right-side heart failure is most likely to be visible in dependent parts of the body (eg, the feet in a person who is sitting or standing or the lower back in a bedridden patient). It is also present in parts of the body that are not visible, such as the liver.

- Electrophysiology studies are not done during transport, but in the hospital setting they may be performed to assess electrical activity of the heart.
- The primary in-hospital arrhythmia therapies are catheter ablation; atrial ligation; pharmacologic treatment; implantable devices, such as pacemakers and implantable cardioverter-defibrillators (ICDs); and wearable cardioverter-defibrillators.
- The transcutaneous pacemaker is most commonly used as an initial emergency pacer (a temporary measure). It is the quickest and most convenient method of pacing, but also requires the most energy and is the least reliable owing to the quality of the skin-to-pad contact and the thoracic impedance that must be overcome.
- Many patients are transported between medical facilities with transvenous pacemakers accompanied by an external pulse generator. Generally, these transvenous pacers require little attention and are quite reliable; the primary sources of problems are battery failure and lead disconnection at the generator. Voltage (the force that causes current to flow) and impedance (resistance to current) are important determinants of battery longevity in a pacemaker.
- The main sources of resistance in a pacing circuit are the lead conductor, the electrode, and the concentration of electrically charged ions at the electrode–tissue interface. Electrode resistance improves pacing efficiency; lead conductor resistance and polarization do not.
- Passage of the pacemaker's electrical impulse between the cathode and the anode—through cardiac tissue and body fluids—is the event in the pacing circuit that stimulates cardiac depolarization.
- Pacemakers stimulate cardiac depolarization, sense intrinsic cardiac activity, respond to metabolic needs, and store diagnostic information. All pacemakers can provide

Prep Kit Continued

fixed-rate pacing; most also provide rate-adaptive (rate-responsive) pacing, increasing and decreasing the pacing rate in response to input from the rate sensors.

- Endocardial (transvenous) leads are threaded through veins, usually subclavian or cephalic, to the right atrium or ventricle. Epicardial leads are attached to the external surface of the heart with sutures or another fixation device.

- Steroid-eluting electrodes have a silicone plug that contains a small dose of steroid. Its release reduces inflammation and the growth of fibrous tissue at the electrode site.

- Pacemaker system malfunction may occur as a result of battery failure, problems at the lead electrode–tissue interface, coiling or damage to the lead–generator interface, insulation failure of the lead wires, dislodgement of the lead at the implantation site (very rare), pacemaker programming, pocket stimulation, diaphragmatic stimulation, or electromagnetic interference.

- If pacemaker failure occurs during transport, the cardiac monitor will show failure to capture a signal. To confirm the pacing failure, the CCTP should compare a 12-lead ECG with the patient's pulse and assess the patient for signs of decompensation.

- Pacing in the ventricular pacer mode and loss of AV synchrony in a single-chamber pacemaker can lead to pacemaker syndrome, which results from hemodynamic deterioration and causes nonphysiologic timing of atrial and ventricular contractions.

- Atriobiventricular pacemakers, which coordinate the actions of the right and left ventricles of the heart, may be used as a treatment for heart failure to resynchronize the heart's chambers.

- ICDs automatically attempt to convert a fibrillating heart into a sinus rhythm using a shock from voltage. Each patient with an ICD has a custom ICD system consisting of a housing (can) and a variable number of pacing and high-voltage leads.

- Most ICDs are implanted with one or two transvenous leads used for pacing and shocking. The leads enter the venous system through the subclavian or cephalic vein for placement into the right ventricle or the superior vena cava.

- An ICD bases its decision to deliver a shock (to treat tachyarrhythmias) on the ventricular rate alone; thus, atrial arrhythmias and electromagnetic interference can lead to inappropriate shocks.

- If an ICD fires during care of a patient, the provider should gather the following information: the number of times shocked, recent medical procedures, recent changes in medical condition or changes in patient adherence to the medication regimen, presence of a coexisting pacemaker, patient's activity at the time of shock, and proximity to water or an electrical source.

- If a patient with an ICD experiences multiple inappropriate defibrillator discharges as the result of defibrillator malfunction, the ICD can be temporarily disabled by use of a magnet, which will prevent further discharges.

- In case of cardiac arrest, a CCTP can deliver external defibrillation to a patient with an ICD, although the paddles or pads should not be placed directly over this device. Providers can also perform CPR on a patient with an ICD.

- Significant risks associated with atrial fibrillation are thromboembolism and the resulting increased incidence of stroke. Methods to convert atrial fibrillation include antiarrhythmic medications, external cardioversion, and (the preferred method) internal cardioversion and/or antitachycardia pacing with an atrial ICD.

- Candidates for short-term use of wearable cardioverter-defibrillators include patients at high risk for sudden cardiac death and those who require explant of an infected ICD.

Prep Kit Continued

These vest-like devices notify patients of treatable arrhythmias and perform defibrillation automatically if the patient does not respond.

- In 2015, a subcutaneous implantable cardioverter-defibrillator (S-ICD) was approved for use in the United States. This device does not require any venous leads or wires, so it is associated with less risk of infection compared to a traditional ICD.

- CCTPs should expect to transport patients who have or need a pacemaker or ICD, and should be prepared to manage any adverse situations related to either device. They should receive training on any transthoracic or epicardial, transcutaneous, or transvenous pacemaker device that their agencies use, and should be prepared to use a magnet to temporarily reprogram an implanted pacemaker or ICD if their agencies transport critically ill cardiac patients.

- When accepting a patient from a sending hospital for CCT, the CCTP must assess and confirm electrical and mechanical pacemaker capture for any patient with a transthoracic or epicardial, transvenous, transcutaneous, implanted, or leadless pacemaker device.

- Switching from the device used in the sending facility to the device used by the transport team is often a source of anxiety for CCTPs and other providers. If a compatible device is not available to the transport team, it may be worth considering using the device from the sending facility for the transport and returning it promptly after the transport has been completed.

- The presence of an ICD may require use of an alternative site (not over the device) for transcutaneous pacing or defibrillation if either of those measures is needed during transport. It is essential to have an external cardioverter-defibrillator immediately available when transporting a patient with an ICD.

- Electromagnetic interference is the major cause of pacemaker dysfunction, particularly in older-style pacemakers lacking adequate internal shielding; they may be vulnerable to interference from headsets and intercom systems in air transport.

- Rate-adaptive pacemakers appear to be sensitive to helicopter vibrations. CCTPs working on medical helicopters should be aware of this potential and be prepared to intervene if necessary.

Vital Vocabulary

ablation Removal of a pathway or function by electrocautery or radiofrequency.

absolute refractory period The early phase of cardiac repolarization, wherein the heart muscle cannot be stimulated to depolarize.

acute coronary syndrome (ACS) Any group of clinical symptoms consistent with acute myocardial ischemia.

anode The electrode in a pacing circuit that is positively charged when current is flowing.

antegrade conduction Conduction in the normal direction between cardiac structures.

antiarrhythmic A medication used to treat and prevent cardiac rhythm disorders.

arterial bruits Turbulence or "swishing" sounds heard with a stethoscope placed over the carotid arteries that signal the presence of atherosclerosis.

bifascicular block The combination of a right bundle branch block and a block of one of the fascicles of the left bundle, the left anterior or left posterior fascicle.

biphasic A descriptor for a wave with negative and positive components; typically used in conjunction with P and T waves.

Prep Kit Continued

bipolar lead A conduction lead comprising two electrodes attached at specific body sites with different polarity, which is used to examine electrical activity by monitoring changes in the electrical potential between those sites.

bipolar system A closed system consisting of bipolar leads and a module to generate impulses and measure response.

bundle branch block (BBB) A disturbance in electric conduction through the right or left bundle branch from the bundle of His.

cable The physical wire that connects the electrode to the electrocardiography monitor.

cardiac monitoring The continuous observation of the patient's condition in relation to the cardiac rhythm.

cardiomyopathy A general term for diseases in which the myocardium becomes thin, flabby, dilated, or enlarged, ultimately progressing to heart failure, acute myocardial infarction, or death.

cathode The electrode in a pacing circuit that is negatively charged when current is flowing.

chronotropic A medication that affects the rate of contraction of the heart.

claudication A severe pain in a muscle caused by narrowing of the arteries in that muscle and leading to ischemic pain with slight exertion such as that associated with walking.

current The movement of electrons through an electrical circuit over time, measured in amperes.

delta wave The slurring of the upstroke of the first part of the QRS complex that occurs in Wolff-Parkinson-White syndrome.

depolarization The process of discharging resting cardiac muscle fibers by an electrical impulse that causes them to contract.

dextrocardia A congenital cause of right axis deviation, in which the heart develops in a right-facing position, creating a mirror image of the normal left-facing heart.

digoxin A cardiac glycoside that produces positive inotropic and negative chronotropic activity in the heart and is primarily indicated in the treatment of chronic heart failure and to control the ventricular rate in atrial tachyarrhythmias.

discordant A descriptor for T waves that are in the opposite direction from the terminal portion of the QRS complex in bundle branch blocks.

dromotropic Affecting the velocity of conduction.

dual-chamber pacemaker An artificial pacemaker with two leads (one in the atrium and one in the ventricle) so electromechanical synchrony can be achieved.

ejection fraction The percentage of blood actually ejected from the ventricles.

electrical alternans An electrocardiogram pattern in which the QRS vector changes with each heartbeat. This pattern is pathognomonic of cardiac tamponade.

electrode In the context of a 12-lead electrocardiogram, an electrical sensor placed on the chest to record the bioelectrical activity of the heart. In the context of a pacemaker, a conductor in contact with cardiac tissue at the end of a pacing lead; it delivers impulses to that tissue.

electrophysiology The cardiac specialty that involves evaluation and management of rhythm disturbances.

endocardial (transvenous) leads Pacemaker leads guided by angiography and attached to the endocardium.

epicardial leads Pacemaker leads attached to the epicardium (outer surface of the myocardium); placement and troubleshooting of these leads are done in the hospital and require surgery and anesthesia.

heart failure (HF) A decline in the ability of the heart, for any reason, to pump powerfully enough or fast enough to empty its chambers; as a result, blood backs up into the systemic circuit, the pulmonary circuit, or both.

Prep Kit Continued

hemiblock Blocking of one of the fascicles of the left bundle branch, the left anterior or left posterior fascicle.

hexaxial system The system developed to describe the coronal plane that is created by the limb leads (I, II, III, aVR, aVL, and aVF).

hypercalcemia An increased level of calcium in the blood.

hyperkalemia An increased level of potassium in the blood.

hypertrophy An increase in the size of the cells as the result of synthesis of more subcellular components, leading to an increase in tissue and organ size.

hypocalcemia A low level of calcium in the blood.

hypokalemia A low level of potassium in the blood.

impedance Resistance to the flow of current along an electrical pathway, measured in ohms.

implantable cardioverter-defibrillator (ICD) A small, battery-powered electrical impulse generator that is implanted in patients at risk for sudden cardiac death as the result of ventricular fibrillation or pulseless ventricular tachycardia.

implantable pulse generator (IPG) The largest implanted element in a pacemaking system, containing the battery and control circuitry.

inotropic An effect on the contractility of muscle tissue, especially cardiac muscle.

intra-atrial conduction delay (IACD) Delayed conduction within one of the atria, often associated with left or right atrial enlargement.

intra-atrial pathways The anterior or Bachman bundle, middle bundle, and posterior internodal system, through which the electrical impulse passes after the sinoatrial node; represented by the P wave on the electrocardiogram. Also called intranodal pathways.

isoelectric When referring to a wave, the status of the wave as neither positive nor negative.

joule A unit of measurement for energy.

lead In the context of the 12-lead electrocardiogram, the designated position of the electrode, or the name of the electrode placement. In the context of a pacemaker, an insulated wire that carries signals in a pacemaking system between the implantable pulse generator and the heart tissue.

left anterior fascicle The portion of the electrical conduction system responsible for innervating the anterior and superior areas of the left ventricle. It is a single-stranded cord terminating in the Purkinje cells.

left posterior fascicle The portion of the electrical conduction system responsible for innervating the posterior and inferior areas of the left ventricle. It is a widely distributed, fanlike structure terminating in the Purkinje cells.

limb leads The electrocardiography lead electrodes attached to the limbs that form the hexaxial system, dividing the heart along a coronal plane into the anterior and posterior segments.

long QT syndrome (LQTS) A prolonged QT interval on the electrocardiogram that is primarily caused by a congenital disorder. Under certain conditions, it tends to deteriorate into ventricular tachyarrhythmias and can lead to syncope or sudden cardiac death; the patient loses consciousness, often without warning.

mean electrical axis The sum of all electrical impulses.

NBG codes North American Society of Pacing and Electrophysiology/British Pacing and Electrophysiology Group Generic codes; five-letter codes used to categorize pacemakers by their functions and capabilities, developed by a joint effort of North American and British electrophysiology groups.

Ohm's law The principle given by the equation $V = IR$, which states that applied voltage is equal to the current times the resistance of the circuit.

pacemaker syndrome The occurrence of symptoms relating to the loss of atrioventricular

Prep Kit Continued

synchrony in ventricularly paced hearts or symptoms caused by inadequate timing and ventricular contractions in paced hearts.

pacing circuit The conduction pathway along which the pacing impulse flows; formed by a power source, one or two lead–electrode pairs, and body tissue.

pacing impulse The electrical impulse sent to the heart to stimulate the heart to beat.

paroxysmal nocturnal dyspnea Severe shortness of breath occurring at night after several hours of recumbency, during which fluid pools in the lungs; the person is forced to sit up to breathe. It is caused by left-side heart failure or decompensation of chronic obstructive pulmonary disease.

paroxysmal supraventricular tachycardia A supraventricular tachycardia that starts and ends abruptly.

pericarditis An inflammatory process involving the pericardium.

phlebitis Inflammation, swelling, and pain along the veins that can lead to the formation of blood clots and thrombophlebitis (venous inflammation associated with a thrombus).

P mitrale A double-humped, M-shaped P wave that is 120 ms wide or greater, with the tops of the humps 40 ms apart or greater. Found in limb leads I, II, and III, it represents left atrial enlargement.

poor R-wave progression An abnormal R-wave pattern; one of the factors that may signify anterior infarction.

P pulmonale A tall P wave that is 2.5 mm high or greater. Found in leads II and III, it indicates right atrial enlargement.

precordial leads The chest leads in an electrocardiogram.

PR interval The interval of time that occupies the space between the beginning of the P wave and the beginning of the QRS complex.

QRS complex Deflections in the electrocardiogram produced by ventricular depolarization.

reciprocal changes An electrocardiogram pattern in which a lead shows a pattern that is the opposite of the one shown in the lead located 180° from the other; for example, the electrode over the area of infarction records ST-segment elevation, whereas the electrode over the lead that is 180° away records ST-segment depression.

refractory period A short period immediately after depolarization in which the myocytes are not yet repolarized and are unable to fire or conduct an impulse.

relative refractory period The period in the cell-firing cycle during which it is possible but difficult to restimulate the cell to fire another impulse.

repolarization A state in which the cell becomes more negative, moving away from equilibrium with the extracellular fluid; it is an active process.

single-chamber demand pacemaker A pacemaker with the pacing lead placed in only one chamber of the heart, in which the generator stimulus is inhibited by a signal derived from the heart's depolarization, thus minimizing the risk of pacemaker-induced fibrillation.

strain pattern An electrocardiogram pattern that involves ST-segment changes and flipped, asymmetric T waves associated with right or left ventricular hypertrophy.

ST segment The section of the electrocardiogram complex from the end of the QRS complex to the beginning of the T wave, which represents the period of inactivity between ventricular depolarization and repolarization; mechanically, it represents the time that the myocardium is maintaining contraction.

ST-segment elevation myocardial infarction (STEMI) A myocardial infarction that shows ST-segment elevation on the electrocardiogram; patients with STEMI have a high probability of coronary thrombus occlusion.

Prep Kit Continued

thrombus A blood clot.

torsades de pointes An undulating sinusoidal rhythm in which the axis of the QRS complexes changes from positive to negative and back in a haphazard manner.

trifascicular block The combination of bifascicular block (a right bundle branch block with a block in the left anterior fascicle or left posterior fascicle) that occurs with a first-degree heart block (prolonged PR interval).

T wave The upright, flat, or inverted wave following the QRS complex of the electrocardiogram, representing ventricular repolarization.

unipolar lead A lead in which one of the electrodes is placed in the heart and the other lead is placed in an area of zero potential.

unipolar system A type of pacemaker system in which contact between the pacemaker itself and the body tissue forms the ground lead for the implantable pulse generator.

voltage The force that causes current to flow in a circuit, measured in volts; also called *amplitude* in a pacing system.

wide complex tachycardia A cardiac rhythm of greater than 100 beats/min with a QRS duration of 120 ms or greater; it can be of ventricular or supraventricular origin.

Wolff-Parkinson-White (WPW) syndrome A syndrome characterized by short PR intervals, delta waves, nonspecific ST-T wave changes, and paroxysmal episodes of tachycardia caused by the presence of an accessory pathway.

References

Abuzaid A, Fabrizio C, Felpel K, et al. Oxygen therapy in patients with acute myocardial infarction: a systemic review and meta-analysis. *Am J Med.* 2018;131:693.

Amsterdam EA, Wenger NK, Brindis RG, et al. 2014 AHA/ACC guideline for the management of patients with non-ST-elevation acute coronary syndromes: executive summary: a report of the American College of Cardiology/American Heart Association Task Force on Practice Guidelines. *Circulation.* 2014;130:2354.

Ben Salem C, Badreddine A, Fathallah N, Slim R, Hmouda H. Drug-induced hyperkalemia. *Drug Saf.* 2014;37(9):677-692.

Brown DW, Croft JB, Giles WH, Anda RF, Mensah GA. Epidemiology of pacemaker procedures among Medicare enrollees in 1990, 1995, and 2000. *Am J Cardiol.* 2005;95:409-411.

Cevik C, Perez-Verdia A, Nugent K. Implantable cardioverter defibrillators and their role in heart failure progression. *Europace.* 2009;11:710-715.

Chung MK. The role of the wearable cardioverter defibrillator in clinical practice. *Cardiol Clin.* 2014;32:253-270.

Collet JP, Thiele H, Barbato E, et al. 2020 ESC guidelines for the management of acute coronary syndromes in patients presenting without persistent ST-segment elevation. *Eur Heart J.* 2021;42:1289.

De Rotte AA, Van Der Kemp P. Electromagnetic interference in pacemakers in single-engine fixed wing aircraft: a European perspective. *Aviat Space Environ Med.* 2002;73:179-183.

Ellenbogen KA, Kaszala K, eds. *Cardiac Pacing and ICDs.* 7th ed. Malden, MA: Wiley & Sons; 2020.

Ellenbogen KA, Wilkoff BL, Kay N, Lau CP, Auricchio A. *Clinical Cardiac Pacing, Defibrillation and Resynchronization Therapy.* 5th ed. Philadelphia, PA: WB Saunders; 2017.

Epstein AE, DiMarco JP, Ellenbogen KA, et al. 2012 ACCF/AHA/HRS focused update incorporated into the ACCF/AHA/HRS 2008 guidelines for device-based therapy of cardiac rhythm abnormalities: a report of the American College of Cardiology Foundation/American Heart Association Task Force on Practice Guidelines and the Heart Rhythm Society. *J Am Coll Cardiol.* 2013;61:e6-e75.

Essebag V, Halabi AR, Churchill-Smith M, Lutchmedial S. Air medical transport of cardiac patients. *Chest.* 2003;124:1937-1945.

French RS, Tillman JG. Pacemaker function during helicopter transport. *Ann Emerg Med.* 1989;18:305-307.

Fromm RE Jr, Taylor DH, Cronin L, McCallum WBG, Levine RL. The incidence of pacemaker dysfunction during helicopter air medical transport. *Am J Emerg Med.* 1992;19:333-335.

Furman S, Hayes DL, Holmes DR. *A Practice of Cardiac Pacing.* 3rd ed. Mount Kisco, NY: Futura; 1993.

Garcia T. *12-Lead ECG: The Art of Interpretation.* 2nd ed. Burlington, MA: Jones & Bartlett Learning; 2013.

Garcia T, Garcia DJ. *Arrhythmia Recognition: The Art of Interpretation.* 2nd ed. Burlington, MA: Jones & Bartlett Learning; 2019.

Garcia T, Holtz N. *Introduction to 12-Lead ECG: The Art of Interpretation.* Sudbury, MA: Jones & Bartlett; 2003.

Prep Kit Continued

Hayes DL, Asirvatham SJ, Friedman PA. *Cardiac Pacing and Defibrillation: A Clinical Approach*. 3rd ed. Hoboken, NJ: Wiley-Blackwell; 2013.

Heart disease facts. Centers for Disease Control and Prevention website. https://www.cdc.gov/heartdisease/facts.htm. Reviewed September 27, 2021. Accessed November 3, 2021.

Hollander-Rodriguez JC, Calvert JF. Hyperkalemia. *Am Fam Physician*. 2006;73(2):283-290.

Kang GH, Oh JH, Chun WJ, et al. Usefulness of an implantable loop recorder in patients with syncope of an unknown cause. *Yonsei Med J*. 2013;54(3):590-595.

Krahn AD, Klein GJ, Skanes AC, Yee R. Insertable loop recorder use for detection of intermittent arrhythmias. *Pacing Clin Electrophysiol*. 2004;27(5):657-664.

Lacunza-Ruiz FJ, Moya-Mitjans A, Martínez-Alday J, et al. Implantable loop recorder allows an etiologic diagnosis in one-third of patients. *Circ J*. 2013;77(10):2535-2541.

Nikoo MH, Aslani A, Jorat MV. LBBB: state-of-the-art criteria. *Int Cardiovasc Res J*. 2013;7(2):39-40.

O'Gara PT, Kushner FG, Ascheim DD, et al.; American College of Cardiology Foundation/American Heart Association Task Force on Practice Guidelines. 2013 ACCF/AHA guideline for the management of ST-elevation myocardial infarction: a report of the American College of Cardiology Foundation/American Heart Association Task Force on Practice Guidelines. *Circulation*. 2013;127(4):e362-425. doi:10.1161/CIR.0b013e3182742cf6. Erratum in: *Circulation*. 2013;128(25):e481. PMID:23247304.

Opreanu M, Wan C, Singh V, et al. Wearable cardioverter-defibrillator as a bridge to cardiac transplantation: a national database analysis. *J Heart Lung Transplant*. 2015;34:1305-1309.

Otto LA, Aufderheide TP. Evaluation of ST segment elevation criteria for the prehospital electrocardiographic diagnosis of acute myocardial infarction. *Ann Emerg Med*. 1994;23:17-23.

Page RL, Joglar JA, Caldwell MA, et al. 2015 ACC/AHA/HRS guideline for the management of adult patients with supraventricular tachycardia: a report of the American College of Cardiology/American Heart Association Task Force on Clinical Practice Guidelines and the Heart Rhythm Society. *Circulation*. 2016;133:e506. doi:10.1161/CIR.0000000000000310.

Palmer BF, Carrero JJ, Clegg DJ, et al. Clinical management of hyperkalemia. *Mayo Clin Proc*. 2021;96(3):744-762.

Reddy VY, Doshi SK, Kar S, et al. 5-Year outcomes after left atrial appendage closure: from the PREVAIL and PROTECT AF Trials. *J Am Coll Cardiol*. 2017;70:2964.

Ruskin JN, Camm AJ, Zipes DP, Hallstrom AP, McGrory-Usset ME. Implantable cardioverter defibrillator utilization based on discharge diagnoses from Medicare and managed care patients. *J Cardiovasc Electrophysiol*. 2001;13:38-43.

Sperzel J, Burri H, Gras D, et al. State of the art of leadless pacing. *Europace*. 2015;17:1508.

Surawicz B, Childers R, Deal BJ, et al.; American Heart Association Electrocardiography and Arrhythmias Committee, Council on Clinical Cardiology; American College of Cardiology Foundation; Heart Rhythm Society. AHA/ACCF/HRS recommendations for the standardization and interpretation of the electrocardiogram: part III: intraventricular conduction disturbances: a scientific statement from the American Heart Association Electrocardiography and Arrhythmias Committee, Council on Clinical Cardiology; the American College of Cardiology Foundation; and the Heart Rhythm Society. Endorsed by the International Society for Computerized Electrocardiology. *J Am Coll Cardiol*. 2009;53(11):976.

Thygesen K, Alpert JS, Jaffe AS, et al. Fourth universal definition of myocardial infarction (2018). *J Am Coll Cardiol*. 2018;72:2231.

2021 Heart disease and stroke statistics update fact sheet: at-a-glance. American Heart Association website. https://www.heart.org/-/media/PHD-Files-2/Science-News/2/2021-Heart-and-Stroke-Stat-Update/2021_heart_disease_and_stroke_statistics_update_fact_sheet_at_a_glance.pdf. Published 2021. Accessed November 3, 2021.

Virani SS, Alonso A, Aparicio HJ, et al. Heart disease and stroke statistics—2021 update. *Circulation*. 2021;143:e254-e743. doi:10.1161/CIR.0000000000000950.

Chapter 15

Hemodynamic Monitoring

Mike McEvoy, PhD, NRP, RN, CCRN

OBJECTIVES

After completing this chapter, you will be able to:

1. Describe cardiovascular anatomy and physiology, including the phases of the cardiac cycle (pp 784–787).
2. Discuss the principles of and indications for invasive hemodynamic monitoring (p 786).
3. Interpret hemodynamic values (p 788).
4. Discuss the indications, contraindications, and complications for arterial lines (pp 795–796).
5. Discuss indications, contraindications, and complications for central venous lines (pp 804–805).
6. Describe the significance of each pressure reading used in patient care (pp 801, 813).
7. Describe general transport considerations and troubleshooting procedures for common problems with invasive lines and hemodynamic monitoring devices during transport (p 812).
8. Discuss flight considerations related to invasive hemodynamic monitoring (p 828).

Introduction

The fundamental role of critical care, in terms of hemodynamic monitoring, is correction of perfusion deficits. The evolution of intensive care units (ICUs) began some 50 years ago to provide the specialized monitoring, personnel, and sophisticated treatments needed to monitor and correct perfusion deficits resulting from illness and injury. As the level of care across the spectrum of medicine advances, technologies that once required an ICU environment for their application have gradually become safer, more portable, less invasive, and more capable of being used for patient monitoring and treatment on medical–surgical wards, in transport vehicles, in long-term care facilities, and, in some cases, in patients' homes.

Accurate assessment of perfusion, or of the adequacy of the delivery of oxygen and nutrients to the tissues of the body, often eludes clinicians. Conventional physical assessment of vital signs, mentation, skin color, and urine output may provide clues about the presence of poor perfusion, but without the information obtained through more advanced technological monitoring, clinicians may be led to incorrectly believe that a patient has adequate perfusion.

Improved technology and better understanding of perfusion have shifted much of the focus of hemodynamic monitoring from central measurements to assessment of tissue-level circulation or microcirculation. The terminal end of vascular blood distribution consists of capillaries, arterioles, postcapillary venules, and subunits where oxygen is actually delivered to tissues. Measuring this microcirculation or its surrogates has become a primary focus of hemodynamic monitoring.

As monitoring technology evolves, lessons from the past 50 years have taught us that no single measurement on its own provides a complete hemodynamic picture of a critically ill patient. Additionally, critical care interventions must be personalized according to the individual's current needs. This type of responsive, personalized care necessitates use of multiple monitoring devices and dynamic variables sensitive to changes in the patient's condition over time.

Cardiovascular Anatomy and Physiology

A solid understanding of the anatomy and physiology of the pulmonary and cardiovascular systems is important when using and interpreting hemodynamic monitoring equipment and cardiac-assist devices. By way of review, a normal human heart is the approximate size of an individual's clenched fist. It lies in the thoracic cavity beneath the sternum; approximately two-thirds of it is left of the midsternal line.

The **atrioventricular (AV) valves** (mitral and tricuspid) lie between the atria and the ventricles, and the **semilunar valves** (aortic and pulmonic) are the exits from the ventricles **FIGURE 15-1**. The AV valves have **chordae tendineae**, which attach the edge of the valve to the **papillary muscles**, which are themselves attached to the endocardium. The chordae tendineae hold the AV valves in place in

the closed position and prevent them from prolapsing into the atria during systole, or ventricular contraction. In contrast, the semilunar valves do not have chordae tendineae but are attached to the respective vessels at the outer edges. The valve action depends on the valve leaflets (the thin, leaf-like cusps or flaps that compose the valves) being pushed together by the force of the blood trying to flow back into the heart, which keeps them in a closed position, much like a parachute opening. The opening and closing of the semilunar valves is related to the pressure changes that occur in the heart, aorta, and pulmonary artery.

The purpose of each of the cardiac valves is to prevent the backward flow of blood in the heart. If a valve is structurally defective, then a backward flow of blood through the valve is referred to as valvular regurgitation or insufficiency. A valve scarred so severely that its lumen is reduced while in the open position is referred to as stenotic.

The coronary arteries supply the heart muscle with oxygen. The ostia (openings) to the coronary arteries are located at the base of the aorta, just **caudal** to the attachment points of the aortic valve leaflets **FIGURE 15-2**. This anatomy is extremely important because the location means the ostia are obstructed when the aortic valve is in the open position. Therefore, although this is the time that the heart is ejecting blood, almost none of it can get into the coronary arteries. In addition, because

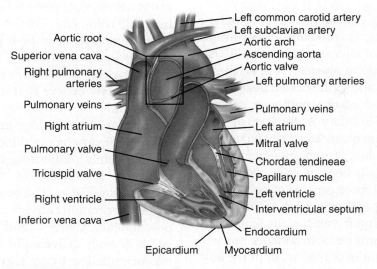

FIGURE 15-1 Anatomy of the heart.
© Jones & Bartlett Learning.

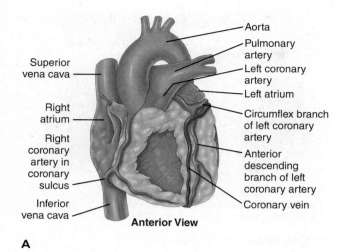

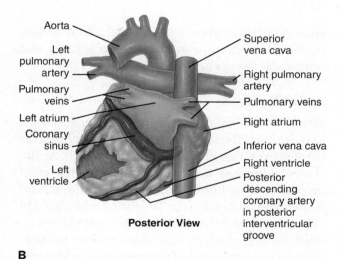

FIGURE 15-2 Coronary arteries. **A.** Anterior view, showing the takeoff points of the left and right main coronary arteries from the aorta. **B.** Posteroinferior view, showing the coronary sinus.

© Jones & Bartlett Learning.

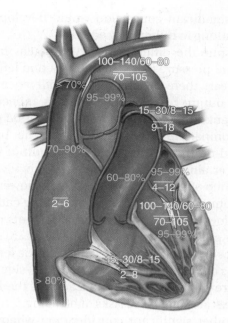

FIGURE 15-3 Pressures (in mm Hg shown in white; mean values are indicated with a bar over the values) and oxygen saturations (shown in yellow) within the circulatory system.

© Jones & Bartlett Learning.

the coronary arteries are embedded in the myocardium, resistance in these blood vessels increases greatly during systole. As a result of these two factors, almost all coronary perfusion occurs during diastole.

Blood returns to the heart through the inferior and superior venae cavae, mixing in the right atrium (RA) before passing through the tricuspid valve into the right ventricle. The tricuspid valve is particularly susceptible to infection from foreign material or organisms introduced into the bloodstream (eg, from intravenous [IV] drug abuse or

line sepsis). From the right ventricle, blood travels via an outflow tract through the pulmonic valve and pulmonary arteries into the lungs. Despite their name (ie, "arteries"), the pulmonary arteries actually carry the most deoxygenated blood found in the body **FIGURE 15-3**. Measurement of oxygen saturations in a pulmonary artery is valuable, when compared to arterial oxygen saturation, in assessing perfusion. Maximally oxygenated blood returns from the lungs to the left atrium (LA) and passes through the mitral valve en route to the left ventricle (LV). From the LV, blood exits an outflow tract leading to the aortic valve and then enters the central circulation.

The anatomy of the myocardium is often incorrectly illustrated. Quite obviously, the heart is a biventricular system with much lower pressures on the right side than on the left side. Perfusing the brain and splanchnic organs necessitates the creation of higher pressures than are needed to deliver blood a few inches from the heart to the lungs. Hence, the LV is a more muscular chamber than the right ventricle, generating significantly higher pressures. Were those same pressures delivered to the lungs, significant congestion would develop, rapidly resulting in pulmonary edema.

Despite the differences in ventricular muscle mass and pressure between the right and left sides of the heart, there is ordinarily little difference in the cardiac output between the two sides. Indeed, any significant difference for a prolonged period would be incompatible with life, because the backup of blood on the side with the lower output would most certainly be fatal. Invasive hemodynamic monitoring often takes advantage of the lower pressures found in the right heart by placing catheters in this low-pressure system. Measurements of cardiac output on the right side of the heart are generally considered equivalent to those on the left side, whereas direct measurements on the left side of the heart are difficult to obtain because of the higher pressures and increased risks of bleeding.

Another significant consideration when using hemodynamic monitoring equipment is coronary perfusion. Most people have two coronary arteries: a right coronary artery (RCA) and a left main coronary artery (LMCA). The LMCA quickly divides into the left anterior descending artery and the circumflex, which together supply most of the LV. The RCA supplies much of the right ventricle and, in most people, also feeds the ventricular septum, including the cardiac conduction system. An assessment of blood pressure (BP) or flow through the coronaries would reveal that the heart receives its blood supply during diastole. Hence, an adequate diastolic BP (DBP) is critical to maintain coronary perfusion. The anatomic positioning of the myocardium in the thoracic cavity, where the right ventricle is the predominant anterior (forward-facing) feature, suggests that chest wall injuries should be monitored for arrhythmias when suspicion of myocardial contusion is present. The role of the RCA in supplying the conduction system also suggests that patients with significant arrhythmias should undergo cardiac catheterization to check the patency of their RCAs.

Cardiac Cycle

The cardiac cycle consists of two main stages: systole, the contraction phase of the heart cycle (ie, the period of work), and diastole, the relaxation phase of the heart cycle (ie, the period of rest). Systole and diastole can be further divided into five

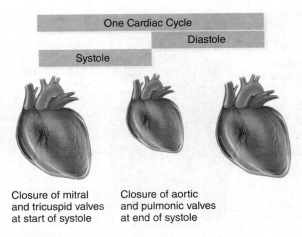

FIGURE 15-4 Systole and diastole.

Closure of mitral and tricuspid valves at start of systole

Closure of aortic and pulmonic valves at end of systole

© Jones & Bartlett Learning.

phases: atrial systole, isovolumetric contraction, ventricular ejection, isovolumetric relaxation, and ventricular filling **FIGURE 15-4**.

Atrial Systole

Atrial systole begins in response to an electrical impulse from the sinoatrial (SA) node, indicated as the P wave on an electrocardiogram (ECG). As the electrical impulse is conducted through the atrial myocardium and internodal pathways, the atrium depolarizes and contracts. The mitral and tricuspid valves are open before atrial systole, with blood already flowing passively from the atria into the ventricles. The contraction of the atria ejects additional blood into the ventricles and accounts for 20% to 30% of the ventricular filling volume (preload). This "atrial kick" raises the ventricular volume and pressure and is important to the effective contraction of the ventricle because of the relationship between the stretching of the myocardium and the force of contraction of the ventricles, known as the Frank–Starling curve or Frank–Starling law (discussed later in this chapter).

Isovolumetric Contraction

During isovolumetric contraction, the electrical impulse from the atria moves through the AV node to the ventricular conduction system, causing the ventricles to depolarize and contract. Immediately after ventricular contraction begins, ventricular pressure rises abruptly, closing the AV valves. The volume of blood in the ventricles just before these valves close is the ventricular preload. Ventricular preload is important to cardiac function because of the relationship between ventricular preload and contractility (Frank–Starling curve).

During isovolumetric contraction, the pressure in the aorta and pulmonary arteries is higher than the pressure in the ventricles and, therefore, the semilunar valves remain closed. The pressure in the ventricles continues to rise during ventricular contraction but, because all of the cardiac valves are closed, no change in ventricular blood volume occurs. (*Isovolumetric* means "same volume.")

Ventricular Systole

Once the pressure in the pulmonary artery is equaled by the pressure in the right ventricle, the pulmonary valve opens and the right ventricle begins to eject blood into the pulmonary artery. The pulmonary valve opens slightly before the aortic valve because the pressure gradient is less for the pulmonary circulation. As the pressure in the LV exceeds the pressure in the aortic root (the section of the base of the aorta that is attached to the heart, including the leaflets of the aortic valve and the openings where the coronary arteries attach), the valve leaflets open and allow the LV to eject the blood into the aorta. During ventricular ejection, the aortic valve leaflets are forced against the wall of the aorta (the open position). No coronary perfusion occurs at this stage because when the aortic valve leaflets are open, they block the coronary arteries.

Isovolumetric Relaxation

Near the end of ventricular ejection, the ventricles begin to relax as the ventricular tissue starts to repolarize. The pressure in the ventricles then drops below the arterial pressure, and the semilunar (aortic and pulmonary) valves close as the blood attempts to flow backward into the heart. During this isovolumetric relaxation phase, the AV valves have not yet opened. Continued ventricular relaxation leads to the decrease in ventricular pressure that will soon allow the AV valves to open as atrial pressure increases.

Ventricular Filling

When the pressure in the ventricles drops below the pressure in the atria, the mitral and tricuspid valves open and ventricular filling begins. Blood flows passively from the atria through the AV valves into the ventricles. When the SA node produces an electrical impulse that initiates atrial systole, the cardiac cycle begins again.

The five phases of the cardiac cycle are summarized in **TABLE 15-1**.

TABLE 15-1 Summary of the Cardiac Cycle

Phase	Events
Atrial systole	The SA node gives impulse. Atrium depolarizes. Atria contract, forcing blood into ventricles. Ventricular volume and pressure are increasing.
Isovolumetric contraction	Impulse travels through the AV node. Ventricles depolarize. Mitral and tricuspid valves close. Ventricular pressure rises abruptly.
Ventricular ejection (systole)	Pressure in the pulmonary artery equals pressure in the right ventricle. Pulmonary valve opens; right ventricle ejects. Pressure in the LV exceeds pressure in the aortic root. Aortic valve opens; LV ejects blood.
Isovolumetric relaxation	Ventricles relax and repolarize. Pressure in ventricles drops to less than arterial pressure. Aortic and pulmonary valves close owing to blood attempting to flow backward.
Ventricular filling (diastole)	Ventricular pressure drops below pressure in the atria. Mitral and tricuspid valves open. Blood flows through the atria and into the ventricles. Cardiac cycle begins again.

Abbreviations: AV, atrioventricular; LV, left ventricle; SA, sinoatrial
© Jones & Bartlett Learning.

Cardiac Output

Cardiac output (CO) is the amount of blood the heart ejects each minute, usually expressed in liters per minute. Normal CO in a healthy adult is in the range of 4 to 8 L/min. Healthy adults can readily increase their CO to more than 20 L/min when needed to meet intense physical demands. The CO is the product of stroke volume (SV) and heart rate (CO = SV × Heart rate). The SV, or amount of blood ejected with each ventricular contraction, is determined by the preload, afterload, and contractility of the heart. Normal SV in adults is 60 to 100 mL. Because SV results from three combined influences, heart rate has a far greater contribution and more immediate effect on CO than does any one component of SV. When confronted with a low CO, the critical care transport professional (CCTP) should investigate the patient's heart rate before evaluating the constituents of SV.

To account for differences in body size, some hemodynamic values are indexed. Indexing divides a hemodynamic parameter by the patient's total body surface area (TBSA), which is stated in terms of meters squared. The TBSA can be derived from a paper-and-pencil chart, but is most commonly calculated by hemodynamic monitoring software after the clinician enters the patient's height and weight values. For example, a cardiac index (CI) (average = 2.5 to 4.2 L/min/m^2) is the patient's CO divided by TBSA:

$$\text{Cardiac Index (CI)} = \frac{\text{CO}}{\text{TBSA}}$$

A CO of 4.5 L/min may be perfectly adequate for a 17-year-old, 100-pound (45-kg) female involved in a multivehicle collision, but not for a 21-year-old, 325-pound (147 kg) male athlete who crashed his motorcycle. The indexing of various hemodynamic parameters is often applied to ventricular work values, SVs, and calculations of oxygen consumption.

The formula most commonly used to calculate TBSA is the Dubois formula:

$$\text{TBSA (m}^2) = \text{height (cm)}^{0.725} \times \text{weight (kg)}^{0.425} \times 0.007184$$

Of particular concern to clinicians is the potential for error if the patient's height or weight is entered incorrectly into the software being used to perform hemodynamic calculations. Familiarity with typical TBSAs and normal CO ranges can aid in recognizing incorrectly entered values. Although the CI helps to interpret CO values for patients of various sizes, it should not be viewed in isolation; that is, CO should always be considered as well.

Heart Rate

The fastest means of increasing a patient's CO is to increase the heart rate. Within seconds, raising the heart rate can double or even triple CO in a healthy patient's system. Nevertheless, there are limits to improvements in CO driven by an increased heart rate. Rapid rates shorten ventricular filling time and, at certain thresholds that vary among patients, can significantly reduce CO.

Heart Rate Thresholds

Although formulas that utilize far-below-maximum heart rates are often used to determine exercise limits in healthy adults, the medicolegal ceiling for an acceptable heart rate in adult patients is 120 beats/min. The CCTP should endeavor to determine the cause of a sustained rate exceeding 120 beats/min in adult patients. Faster heart rates can also increase myocardial muscle oxygen consumption, adversely affecting CO. Additionally, the shortening of the diastolic period seen as the heart rate increases may decrease coronary perfusion, also leading to lower CO.

Conversely, lowered heart rates lead to increased ventricular filling time and prolonged diastolic intervals, which may then increase preload and improve coronary blood flow, with both of these effects resulting in increased CO. At heart rates of less than 50 beats/min, hemodynamic improvements are offset by decreased CO. Although some patients may tolerate heart rates in the high 40s, 50 beats/min is generally considered the lower threshold for heart rate in adults.

Heart Rate Regulation

Heart rate is regulated in three ways: by the autonomic nervous system, by receptors, and through metabolic demands.

The autonomic nervous system is divided into the sympathetic and parasympathetic branches. The sympathetic nervous system increases heart rate and contractility primarily through the release of norepinephrine, whereas the parasympathetic nervous system lowers heart rate and decreases contractility by releasing acetylcholine.

Many receptors in the body influence heart rate, the strongest of which are the baroreceptors located in the carotid bodies and the aortic arch. Baroreceptors sense pressure and, in response to decreases in BP, will stimulate an increased heart rate. In contrast, the detection of increased BP causes the baroreceptors to decrease heart rate. Historically, the baroreceptors in the carotid sinuses were used to slow supraventricular tachyarrhythmias through carotid sinus massage. This practice was abandoned in adults because it sometimes dislodged plaque deposits, which led to strokes.

Chemoreceptors play less of a role than baroreceptors but nonetheless influence heart rate in response to changes in pH and oxygen saturation. In the presence of lower pH or lowered oxygen saturations, chemoreceptors increase heart rate. When pH or oxygen saturation increases, receptors respond by lowering heart rate. Understanding this interaction can be helpful in many clinical situations. Supplemental oxygen administration, for example, may help to lower rapid heart rates while more definitive treatments are prepared.

Certain metabolic changes may also lead to increased heart rates, including fever, pain, hyperthyroidism, and exercise. Conversely, lower heart rates often result from hypothermia, analgesia or sedation, hypothyroidism, and athletic conditioning. Treatment of tachycardias and bradycardias must take these potential underlying causes into consideration; otherwise, it is likely to be ineffective.

Measurement of Heart Rate

Heart rate is a key sign of hemodynamic instability in emergency and critical care patients. Assessment of the pulse can be performed by arterial palpation; however, in the high-noise environment of an ICU or a critical care transport (CCT) vehicle, the heart rate obtained from a pulse oximeter is more reliable than manual assessment. Correlation with an ECG display or pulse oximetry plethysmographic (pleth) waveform provides additional reassurance.

Preload

Preload is the degree of myocardial fiber stretch induced by the volume in the ventricle at the end of diastole. Preload is synonymous with end-diastolic volume (EDV) and end-diastolic pressure (EDP).

Factors Affecting Preload

The three determinants of preload are total blood volume, blood volume distribution, and atrioventricular synchrony.

The relationship between preload and total blood volume is straightforward. Preload declines in patients experiencing hemorrhage and profound fluid loss from dehydration, vomiting, gastric suction, diaphoresis, diarrhea, or massive fluid shifts leading to third-space losses. Preload increases in patients in hypervolemic states such as fluid overload, renal failure, and significantly increased venous return.

Blood volume distribution is more challenging to understand and to measure. Changes in venous tone (dilation and constriction) can result from physiologic attempts to compensate for changes in total blood volume, from administration of vasoactive medications (vasodilators or vasopressors), and from environmental or metabolic influences (eg, hypothermia, fever, or exercise). These changes affect preload by altering the size of the body's "tank." When the tank's capacity is greater or less than the total volume of blood in the system, preload will increase or decline.

One significant factor affecting blood volume distribution is changes in intrathoracic pressure. The two most significant influences on venous return to the right side of the heart are respirations and skeletal muscle activity. Continued skeletal muscle movements from physical activity and breathing serve to generate some forward flow of blood through the venous system toward the right heart. Changes in intrathoracic pressure from respirations generate a pressure differential that facilitates venous blood return to the heart. The importance of intrathoracic pressure differences in venous return should not be overlooked when assessing preload. When mechanical ventilation is employed, for example, this intervention leads to changes in intrathoracic pressure. Positive-pressure ventilation and use of positive end-expiratory pressure (PEEP) can significantly decrease preload and often require volume expansion to restore a normal preload state. Intrapericardial pressure changes resulting from cardiac tamponade, pericarditis, or pericardial effusions can also decrease preload. In these circumstances, the additional pressure being applied on the heart can dramatically decrease preload. Significant volume administration can be a lifesaving intervention by maintaining adequate preload while the patient is awaiting definitive care.

AV synchrony is variously reported to contribute to 10% to 20% of CO. Although this relationship is not well studied, the mechanism by which a well-synchronized atrial–ventricular contraction facilitates CO is preload. The ejection of a small bolus of blood from the atria into the ventricles moments before ventricular contraction provides a slight increase in ventricular volume, which then leads to an increase in ventricular SV. Maintaining AV synchrony in patients with advanced heart failure has been shown to extend their lives. Hence, medications and devices that keep these patients in sinus rhythm and ensure optimal AV contraction are key elements in the treatment of heart failure.

Frank–Starling Law

The Frank–Starling law is often referenced when assessing patients' fluid volume status. The premise of the Frank–Starling law, also referred to as the Starling curve **FIGURE 15-5**, is that SV (and hence CO) increases as the volume of blood filling the heart increases until a certain point, at which output declines as volume continues to increase.

As the ventricular preload increases, the force of contraction of the myocardium also increases, as a result of the increased stretch of the myocardial fibers. This relationship between increasing contraction and increasing stretching of the myocardium immediately before systole continues until a point is reached at which the force of contraction actually begins to fall off, with subsequent detrimental increases in preload. The Frank–Starling law describes how judicious administration of fluids results in improved CO up to a certain point, which varies between individual patients. Additional fluids given beyond the preload at which optimal CO is achieved result in worsened CO; such a patient is said to have "fallen off the end of the Starling curve."

The fundamental principle of the Frank–Starling law is often lost with use of static measurements of

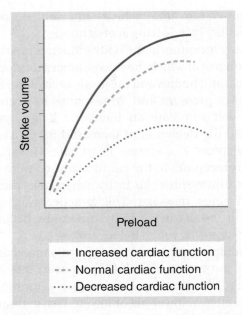

FIGURE 15-5 Frank–Starling law: the relationship between cardiac output (stroke volume) and preload.
© Jones & Bartlett Learning.

preload. The most important takeaway message from its application is that every patient has a preload point at which their CO is optimal. Should the patient's preload be less or greater than optimal, the CO will decline.

Measurement of Preload

Preload has conventionally been measured in several ways. Right ventricular preload is measured by central venous pressure (CVP), which closely matches RA pressure. LV preload is measured by pulmonary capillary wedge pressure (PCWP) or, in some patients, by pulmonary artery diastolic pressure. During cardiac operations, a left atrial pressure monitoring catheter is sometimes placed to continually monitor LV preload. In the past, the PCWP was considered the gold standard for LV preload measurement, with the definition of decompensated LV failure (heart failure) being a PCWP greater than 18 mm Hg. Today, critical care practitioners recognize that CVP and PCWP are static pressure measurements, which are significantly influenced by both vasodilation and constriction. As such, they tend to reflect circulating blood volume relatively poorly.

Controversies

Conventional assessment of preload using static pressures measured in millimeters of mercury (mm Hg) is now known to be an extremely inexact reflection of right or left ventricular volume. Historically, it was believed that a linear relationship existed between right or left heart pressures and volume. More recently, it has become understood that changes in intrathoracic pressure from respirations and PEEP significantly influence venous return and preload. Today, as a more accurate means of measuring ventricular volume is sought, there is a deliberate shift toward use of dynamic parameters that account for the fluctuations in pressures resulting from respirations and PEEP. An example of this trend can be seen in the International Guidelines of the Surviving Sepsis Campaign, which previously recommended using CVP as a fluid resuscitation parameter, but now call for use of dynamic parameters.

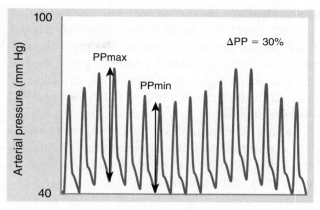

FIGURE 15-6 Respiratory changes in arterial pressure in a mechanically ventilated patient. The pulse pressure (PP; systolic minus diastolic pressure) is minimal (PPmin) three heart beats after its maximal value (PPmax). The respiratory changes in pulse pressure (ΔPP) can be calculated as the difference between PPmax and PPmin, divided by the mean of the two values, and expressed as a percentage: ΔPP (%) = 100 × (PPmax − PPmin)/([PPmax + PPmin]/2). In this case, the high value of ΔPP (30%) suggests that the patient would be potentially responsive to volume resuscitation.

Reproduced with permission from Lamia B, Chemla D, Richard C, et al. Clinical review: interpretation of arterial pressure wave in shock states. *Crit Care.* 2005;9:601. doi: 10.1186/cc3891.

Preload is increasingly being evaluated using dynamic parameters such as pulse pressure variation (PPV) **FIGURE 15-6**, stroke volume variation (SVV), and pleth variability index (PVI); all of these are proprietary algorithms that use either arterial pressure waveforms or pulse oximeter pleth waveforms to determine the percentage of change in SV resulting from respirations. The underlying premise of these dynamic parameters, which are measured over the course of a complete respiratory cycle, is that variations in blood pressure between inspiration and expiration reflect fluid volume status and fluid volume responsiveness. Normally, systolic BP (SBP) will decrease between 5 and 10 mm Hg during inspiration. Decreases exceeding 10 mm Hg are referred to as pulsus paradoxus and suggest the presence of significant hypovolemia or cardiac tamponade. Dynamic measurements calculate the percentage of change in either SBP using an arterial pressure waveform or the height of a pulse oximeter pleth waveform, with this percentage of change being displayed on a monitor.

Early studies of volume expansion in patients with sepsis demonstrated that a PPV of 13% or greater was associated with a positive response to a fluid challenge, whereas a PPV of less than 13% was associated with no improvement in CO when fluids were given. More recent studies of PPV, SVV, and PVI have arrived at various values, ranging between 13% for PPV and 15% for SVV and PVI, that can distinguish those patients with adequate preload or who will not respond to fluids from those patients with low preload who will be responsive to fluids. The mnemonic "high is dry" has been used to reflect the interpretation of these dynamic preload parameters.

One reason for caution in using PPV, SVV, and PVI as means to assess preload is that the majority of published evidence has evaluated their effectiveness in mechanically ventilated patients who are not overbreathing. Although data from spontaneously breathing patients suggest that these dynamic parameters have equal efficacy in this population, further studies are needed to confirm this finding.

A more simplistic and readily available test for fluid responsiveness is the passive leg raise (PLR). Passive leg raising evaluates the real-time effects of shifting a small amount (150 to 300 mL) of venous blood from the legs into circulating volume. To properly conduct a PLR test, the patient should initially be supine with the head elevated at a 45° angle. The head is then lowered to a flat position and the legs are elevated at a 45° angle. A response observed within 1 minute suggests that the patient is fluid responsive. PLR can also be used to confirm the reliability of PPV, SVV, and PVI measurements.

Many other variables can be observed to ascertain a response to fluid administration, including heart rate, BP, CO, and preload variables such as static or dynamic pressures.

Afterload

Afterload is the resistance the ventricles must overcome to eject blood. Afterload has an inverse relationship to ventricular function; that is, as afterload increases, ventricular function decreases. Poiseuille's law is often used to explain the determinants of afterload. It is expressed by the following equation:

$$Q = \frac{\pi P r^4}{8 \eta l}$$

where

Q = Flow rate
P = Pressure
r = Radius
η = Fluid viscosity
l = Length of tubing

Poiseuille's law states that flow varies directly with any increase in pressure. That is, as the radius (or diameter) of a tube increases, flow also increases to the fourth power of the increase in radius. When this concept is applied to IV fluid administration, it simply means that squeezing the IV bag or putting the bag into a pressure infuser will result in a faster flow. Using larger-diameter tubing or a large-size vascular access catheter, however, will increase the flow by a factor of four based on the increased-size catheter (a much greater increase than seen with pressure alone).

Poiseuille's law also states that flow varies inversely with the length of the tubing or vessel and inversely with a coefficient of the viscosity of the fluid. When this concept is applied to the human body, it means that flow decreases as blood moves farther away from the heart (length) and as the hemoglobin level increases (viscosity). It is

no wonder, then, that patients with polycythemia have decreased blood flow, whereas patients with anemia have increased CO.

Poiseuille's law was developed based on the flow of fluid through a capillary tube. When evaluating afterload in the human body, however, pulsatile blood flow and the compliant vascular walls found in the blood vessels must also be taken into account. Early physiology textbooks were at a loss to explain timing differences between central and peripheral pulses, as it was believed that LV contraction was the force responsible for forward blood flow. With the advent of more sophisticated technologies for measuring physiologic parameters, such as magnetic resonance imaging, it is now understood that the LV ejects blood into the aorta, with the vascular compliance of the aorta and the expansion and contraction of subsequent vessels then helping to propel the blood forward throughout the body. As a result of this multistep process, a carotid pulse will be felt slightly earlier than a femoral or radial pulse. Patients with significant atherosclerotic disease, for instance, have a loss of elasticity of their blood vessels; as this disease process progresses, their blood flow can become significantly decreased. Conversely, vascular surgical procedures to improve blood flow in patients with significant peripheral vascular disease utilize the blood vessel radius part of Poiseuille's law to improve flow: Dilating a blood vessel or placing a stent to increase the radius of the blood vessel reduces afterload and improves blood flow.

Factors Affecting Afterload

Four factors typically determine afterload: outflow obstructions, vascular tone, blood viscosity, and ventricular dilation.

Outflow obstructions, such as aortic valvular stenosis, hypertension, and atherosclerosis, produce greater resistance and, therefore, increase afterload.

In terms of vascular tone, as is the case with preload, both vasoconstriction and vasodilation affect afterload: Vasodilation reduces afterload, and vasoconstriction increases afterload. Although vasodilation has many potential causes that can result in decreased afterload, including fever, exercise, and vasodilating drugs, only one shock state is associated with decreased afterload: distributive shock. This state can be an important finding when attempting to determine the cause of shock in a critically ill patient. Physiologically, it is important to understand the causes of afterload increases in the right heart versus those in the LV. Two conditions lead to pulmonary vasoconstriction, which then creates increased right ventricular afterload: hypoxia and hypercarbia. A newly observed increase in right heart afterload, then, should be attributed to one or the other of these conditions and interventions taken to address that imbalance (such as increasing the fraction of inspired oxygen [Fio_2] level if hypoxia is suspected or increasing the minute volume if hypercarbia is suspected). Systemic vasoconstriction leading to increased LV afterload can result from hypothermia, administration of vasopressors, cardiogenic shock, or hypovolemic shock states.

Blood viscosity directly affects afterload. Increased afterload results from polycythemia, for example, because very viscous blood does not flow as readily as less viscous or very thin blood. This important concept explains why lowered hemoglobin levels are often tolerated and, in fact, sometimes considered beneficial in critically ill patients. Presuming that adequate hemoglobin is available to carry oxygen, values below those considered normal may well improve CO by decreasing afterload.

The relationship between ventricular dilation and afterload is a complex but important concept for the CCTP to understand. Without delving into the physics behind the interaction, suffice it to say that patients with dilated cardiomyopathies require a reasonable degree of afterload for LV ejection. Typically, heart failure is associated with elevated afterload. Indeed, almost all patients in cardiogenic shock exhibit extremely high afterload, usually requiring treatment to lower their vascular resistance. A significantly enlarged ventricle, however, has lost much of its ability to drive blood flow forward in conditions of very low resistance. This kind of disruption can occur in distributive shock states, with overzealous administration of vasodilators, or with large doses of sedatives, analgesics, or anesthetic agents.

Measurement of Afterload

LV afterload is measured by **systemic vascular resistance (SVR)**, and right ventricular afterload is measured by **pulmonary vascular resistance (PVR)**. In clinical practice, LV afterload is more often evaluated when addressing issues with CO because manipulations of SVR affect systemic circulation. Two instances when clinicians are interested in right ventricular afterload are when assessing a correlation between pulmonary artery diastolic pressure and PCWP, and when evaluating a patient for heart transplantation to determine if significant PVR is reversible. Patients with end-stage heart failure with elevated PVR that is not reversible will require heart and lung transplantation because a transplanted heart would fail in the face of significant right-side resistance.

Contractility

Contractility is defined as the inotropic state of the heart or the force with which the heart muscle contracts. Contractility is not directly measurable using conventional hemodynamic monitoring technology, but it can be assessed with the newer Doppler and ultrasonography devices that are increasingly being used to evaluate critically ill patients. Six factors influence contractility: myocardial muscle health, the autonomic nervous system, metabolic states, the ion environment, pharmacologic agents, and heart rate.

Myocardial muscle injury or ischemia can decrease contractility temporarily or permanently, although conditioning in a supervised cardiac rehabilitation program will normally improve contractility following injury. The parasympathetic and sympathetic arms of the autonomic nervous system responsible for increasing and decreasing heart rate simultaneously affect contractility. Metabolic states such as acidosis, hypoxemia, and sepsis decrease contractility.

Three ions have significant influence on contractility: calcium, sodium, and potassium. Hypocalcemia, hyponatremia, and hyperkalemia all decrease contractility, although the opposite changes in these ion levels do not seem to boost contractility above normal. In the critical care patient with suspected low CO, blood levels of ionized calcium are measured and treated as necessary with calcium replacement. Hyperkalemia has such a dramatic influence on contractility that IV potassium is used during cardiac operations to arrest cardiac motion after the patient is placed on cardiopulmonary bypass. This process allows the surgeon to sew grafts and valves. Potassium is also used in chemical executions to induce pulseless electrical activity.

Multiple pharmacologic agents influence myocardial contractility. Agents that increase contractility are referred to as positive inotropic agents; they include digoxin, dopamine, dobutamine, milrinone, calcium, epinephrine, and glucagon. Negative inotropic agents, or those that decrease contractility, include beta blockers, quinidine, procainamide, and calcium channel blockers.

Heart rate can influence contractility through its effect on diastolic filling time and coronary artery perfusion. Slower heart rates are associated with a longer diastolic time than are faster heart rates, allowing more time for coronary artery filling compared with very rapid heart rates. The shorter diastolic time seen with rapid heart rates may potentially diminish coronary artery perfusion and lower myocardial perfusion below the level needed for adequate contractility.

Contractility is inferred from the values for the stroke volume index, left ventricular stroke work index, and right ventricular stroke work index. When assessed using echocardiography, contractility is reported as the ejection fraction, representing the average percentage of blood ejected from the LV.

Blood Pressure

BP is one of the most often used, yet perhaps least understood assessments. Direct monitoring of BP is accomplished by the use of an arterial line. Indirect monitoring of BP is accomplished with a device that senses pulsatile flow, most commonly using a sphygmomanometer (BP cuff) to measure the systolic and diastolic pressures. Systolic blood pressure (SBP) is the measure of pressure on the arterial walls during systole, whereas diastolic blood pressure (DBP) is the measure of pressure on the walls of the arteries during diastole. The formula for BP is CO multiplied by SVR: $BP = CO \times SVR$. Other methods that indirectly measure BP include assessment of pulses, electronic BP cuffs (also called noninvasive blood pressure [NIBP] units), and Doppler ultrasonography machines. It is extremely important to note that these indirect measurements assess flow, whereas direct monitoring devices (ie, arterial lines) measure pressure. Because pressure and flow are entirely different parameters,

readings obtained by indirect and direct methods cannot be expected to correlate exactly.

Incorrect use of a monitoring device is the leading cause of erroneous measurements, whether the provider is using an indirect monitoring device such as a BP cuff or a direct monitoring device such as an arterial line or pulmonary artery catheter (PAC). The CCTP should be careful to avoid errors in measurement. BP cuff size and the position of the extremity during the measurement process are the two factors that most commonly contribute to inaccuracies.

The cuff bladder size should be matched to the size of the patient's extremity where BP is measured. Determining the bladder size is often difficult in the critical care setting; many practitioners instead choose a cuff that covers two-thirds of the extremity being measured. Using a cuff that is too large will result in readings that are lower than the actual pressures; a cuff that is too small will yield readings higher than the actual levels. The significant potential for error mandates that the transport unit carry various sizes of BP cuffs appropriate for the ages and sizes of the patient populations most commonly transported.

Depending on the patient's size and age, the CCTP may choose to measure BP in the lower arm, thigh, or leg. Regardless of the location used, an appropriate-size cuff should span two-thirds of the distance between the joints of the extremity where the cuff is applied. When using the lower arm, for example, the cuff should cover two-thirds of the area between the elbow and wrist. A cuff selected for an upper arm would be the proper size if it covered two-thirds of the distance from the elbow to the shoulder. On the lower leg, the cuff should cover two-thirds of the distance between the knee and ankle.

One exception to the two-thirds rule arises when using a conical radial artery BP cuff. These recently marketed cuffs, which are designed for patients with obesity, are applied to the forearm and cover a relatively smaller area. Because of their conelike shape, they can obtain BP values with accuracy similar to that achieved with conventional-size rectangular cuffs.

Positioning of the extremity in which BP is measured also affects accuracy. Proper assessment requires that the extremity be located at mid-heart level when BP is measured. Elevation of an arm (or leg, if that is where the cuff is placed) above mid-heart level will yield falsely low readings, whereas placing the extremity below mid-heart level will yield false high readings. This issue can be particularly problematic when measuring BP in side-lying patients or when measurements are taken in the lower leg of a patient who is seated or lying with the leg elevated above the heart.

Often, NIBP units are incorporated into transport monitors and used to obtain indirect BP measurements at predetermined intervals automatically. The NIBP units measure heart rate and mean arterial pressure (MAP) only. (MAP is discussed later in this chapter.) The NIBP software then calculates the patient's SBP and DBP values by using the measured parameters to determine the amount of time spent in systole and diastole computed against the MAP. If the NIBP unit fails to obtain an accurate heart rate, then an erroneous calculation will occur. Additionally, the formulas used by different manufacturers of NIBP devices vary. Notably, systolic and diastolic values calculated by different NIBP monitors for the same patient will vary, sometimes significantly. Because MAP is actually measured by the NIBP unit, this value should be used in making patient care and treatment decisions.

Outdated textbooks and literature suggest that pulses could be correlated with SBP. Current studies have failed to find any consistent correlation between SBP and the presence or absence of central or peripheral pulses. At present, the only setting where pulses may have some utility is in an austere environment such as the battlefield, where radial pulses help with decision making regarding fluid resuscitation.

Arterial Lines

Arterial lines (sometimes called A-lines) include a catheter that is inserted into the patient's arterial vascular system and connected to a transducer. The transducer is a biomedical device that converts the pressure waveform into an electrical signal. The electrical output of the transducer is connected by a proprietary electrical cable to the transport (or bedside) monitor, which then displays the waveform and its corresponding values. In the United States, pressure waveforms are usually measured in millimeters of mercury (mm Hg).

Arterial lines may be inserted in the radial, brachial, femoral, axillary, and dorsalis pedis arteries **FIGURE 15-7**. The radial artery is the preferred site because it is easily accessed and because the patient's hand can receive collateral circulation from the ulnar artery. It is best to use the patient's nondominant hand.

In addition to offering the benefit of a continuously displayed BP reading while titrating vasoactive agents, the arterial line confirms the presence of pulsatile blood flow and allows access for arterial blood samples for arterial blood gas analysis. Commercial arterial line kits designed for insertion into the brachial artery have been gaining popularity in

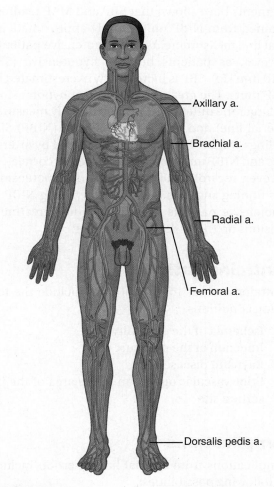

FIGURE 15-7 The radial artery is the preferred site for placing an arterial line. Other possible sites are the brachial, femoral, axillary, and dorsalis pedis arteries.

© Jones & Bartlett Learning.

Labels on figure: Axillary a., Brachial a., Radial a., Femoral a., Dorsalis pedis a.

adult ICUs in recent years, because these lines are somewhat easier to insert and stabilize and may have longer patency than do radial catheters.

Indications

Direct BP measurement using an arterial line is indicated for patients who require constant BP measurement. The current indication for an arterial line is any patient in shock who is not rapidly responsive to therapy, including not only patients who are hypotensive, but also patients who are hypertensive and require powerful vasodilator therapy to reduce their vascular resistance. Arterial lines are also used routinely in patients receiving continuous vasoactive or antihypertensive infusions.

Studies comparing direct and indirect BP measurements have shown that SBP and MAP readings obtained from NIBP units closely approximate arterial line measurements in normotensive patients. However, as patients become hypotensive (SBP <110 mm Hg), SBP is increasingly overestimated by NIBP units. The greater the degree of hypotension, the larger the difference between directly measured (arterial line) and indirectly measured (NIBP) SBP readings will be. MAP readings obtained by arterial lines and NIBP units remain consistently correlated, however, regardless of the degree of hypotension. This finding suggests that clinicians using NIBP in hypotensive patients should base their treatment decisions on the NIBP-obtained MAP.

Contraindications

Contraindications to arterial lines include the following conditions:

- Ischemia of the extremity
- Infection at the puncture site
- Raynaud disease
- Prior vascular operation in the area of the insertion site

Complications

Complications from arterial line insertion include the following possibilities:

- Arterial line thrombosis
- Embolization
- Hematoma
- Insertion-site infection

- Median nerve neuropathy (radial artery insertion)
- Pseudoaneurysm of the artery
- Ischemic necrosis
- Digit, hand, leg, or foot ischemia
- Hemorrhage
- Arterial air embolism
- Arteriovenous fistula
- Arterial aneurysm

Arterial Line Placement

Although some CCTPs may be trained and credentialed to insert central venous catheters, they generally do not place arterial lines. They may, however, need to assist in the procedure. For the reader's background knowledge, this section explains how arterial lines are placed. While traditional arterial line placement is performed blindly, using landmarks and tactile sensation, ultrasound-guided placement is increasingly common.

Allen Test

The Allen test can be used to assess extremity perfusion and ulnar artery function. With this technique, the patient's radial and ulnar arteries are compressed while the fist is clenched **FIGURE 15-8A**. The fist is then opened **FIGURE 15-8B**. Pressure is kept on the radial artery, whereas ulnar pressure is released. After ulnar pressure is released, the color should return to the hand within 6 seconds.

Prior to insertion of a radial artery arterial line catheter, it is common practice to perform an Allen test to ensure collateral flow to the hand from the ulnar artery should the radial catheter occlude blood flow. Regardless of whether this test is conducted, development of signs of ischemia in any extremity following placement of an arterial catheter mandates immediate removal of the catheter.

Equipment

The following equipment is needed to insert an arterial line:

- 20-gauge radial over-the-needle catheterization kit with guide wire
- 18- to 20-gauge 6-inch (15-cm) femoral artery catheterization kit with guide wire
- Tape

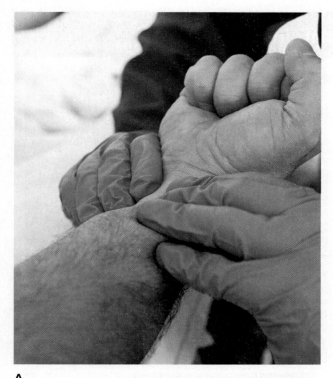

A

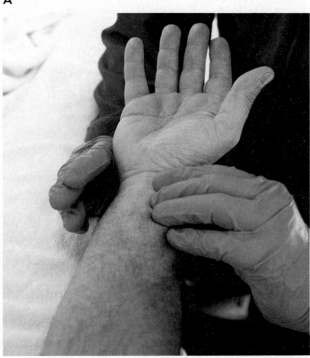

B

FIGURE 15-8 The Allen test. **A.** The patient raises their hand above their head with the fist clenched. The CCTP compresses the radial and ulnar arteries. **B.** The patient lowers their hand with the fist open and the CCTP releases ulnar pressure while keeping pressure on the radial artery.

- Sterile 2 × 2–inch (5.1 × 5.1–cm) gauze sponges
- Sterile 4 × 4–inch (10.2 × 10.2–cm) gauze sponges
- Local anesthetics
- Analgesic medications
- Sterile gloves, gown, mask, and drapes
- Chlorhexidine solution
- Pressure transducer
- Pressure tubing
- Pressure monitor
- Suture material or commercial suture kit

Steps

SKILL DRILL 15-1 outlines the steps for inserting an arterial line using the modified Seldinger technique (note that ultrasonography to assist with insertion is becoming commonplace):

1. Take standard precautions.
2. Prepare all equipment using a sterile technique.
3. Position the patient by placing rolled gauze under the wrist area, hyperextending the wrist **STEP 1**.
4. Select and clean the insertion site; ensure IV access. Use sterile drapes to reduce infection risk **STEP 2**.
5. Palpate the artery at the distal radius **STEP 3**.
6. Anesthetize the area **STEP 4**.
7. Insert the needle over the radial artery approximately 0.5 inch (1 cm) distal to the wrist joint **STEP 5**.
8. Advance the needle at an approximately 20° to 45° angle. Entry into the artery will be indicated by pulsating arterial blood.
9. Immobilize the needle with your free hand.
10. Advance the guide wire, and then remove the needle, leaving only the guide wire in the artery **STEP 6**.
11. Place the arterial catheter over the guide wire **STEP 7**.
12. Remove the guide wire, leaving only the cannula in place **STEP 8**.
13. Connect the tubing to the pressure transducer **STEP 9**.
14. Secure the catheter to the skin with sutures and apply a sterile dressing to the insertion site. It is imperative that line placement be radiographically confirmed before departing with the patient.

Skill Drill 15-1 Inserting an Arterial Line

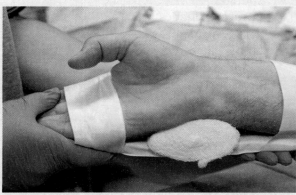

Step 1

Place rolled gauze under the wrist area, hyperextending the wrist.

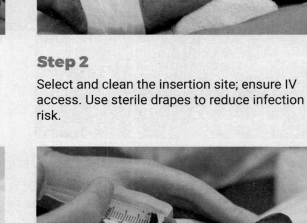

Step 2

Select and clean the insertion site; ensure IV access. Use sterile drapes to reduce infection risk.

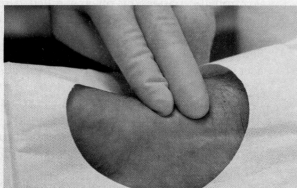

Step 3

Palpate the artery at the distal radius.

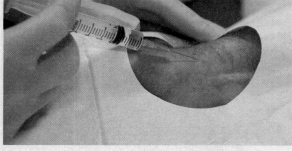

Step 4

Anesthetize the area.

Step 5

Insert the needle over the radial artery approximately 0.5 inch (1 cm) distal to the wrist joint. Advance the needle at an approximately 20° to 45° angle, watching for entry into the artery, indicated by pulsating arterial blood.

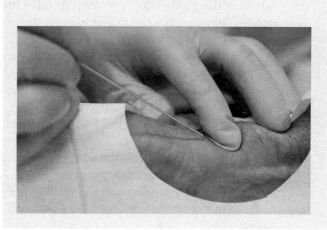

Skill Drill 15-1 Inserting an Arterial Line (continued)

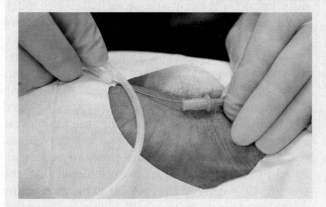

Step 6

Immobilize the needle with your free hand. Advance the guide wire, and then remove the needle, leaving only the guide wire in the artery.

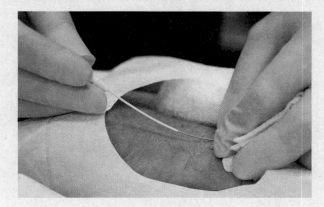

Step 7

Place the arterial catheter over the guide wire.

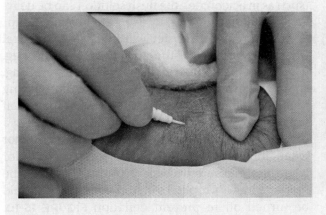

Step 8

Remove the guide wire, leaving only the cannula in place.

All images © Jones & Bartlett Learning.

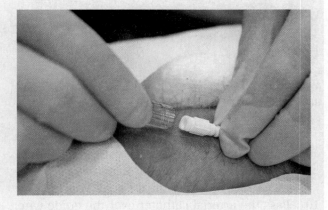

Step 9

Connect the tubing to the pressure transducer. Secure the catheter to the skin with sutures and apply a sterile dressing to the insertion site.

The steps for femoral artery cannulation are also listed here for reference:

1. Prepare the equipment.
2. Use a complete aseptic technique.
3. Ensure IV access.
4. Palpate the femoral artery below the inguinal ligament.
5. Anesthetize the area.
6. Enter the skin over the femoral artery approximately 0.5 to 0.75 inch (1 to 2 cm) below the inguinal ligament **FIGURE 15-9**.
7. Advance the needle at an approximately 45° angle. Entry into the artery will be indicated by pulsating arterial blood.

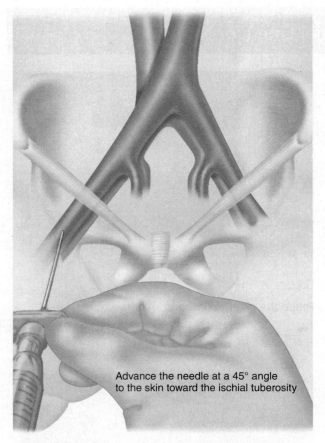

Advance the needle at a 45° angle to the skin toward the ischial tuberosity

FIGURE 15-9 Femoral artery cannulation toward ischial tuberosity.

© Jones & Bartlett Learning.

8. Immobilize the needle with your free hand.
9. Advance the guide wire through the needle. Remove the needle, leaving the guide wire in place.
10. Pass the arterial catheter over the guide wire; remove the guide wire.
11. Connect the tubing to the pressure transducer.
12. Secure the catheter with sutures and apply a sterile dressing. Line placement must be radiographically confirmed before departing with the patient.

Obtaining Invasive Hemodynamic Measurements

After an arterial line is placed, it is connected to a pressure-monitoring transducer by using rigid pressure-monitoring tubing. This tubing is filled with an isotonic solution, usually normal saline. Historically, heparinized saline was used, but its lack of demonstrated benefit and the potential for harm to patients have all but eliminated its use as a flush solution. The difference between pressure-monitoring tubing and IV extension tubing is important because the latter will absorb much of the pressure waveform generated by the patient before it reaches the transducer.

To maintain the patency of the pressure-monitoring line and fluid-filled system, a continuous flush solution system is used. Most often, the flush solution used to fill the monitoring system is placed into a disposable pressure bag. After the monitoring system is connected to the patient, free of bubbles, and functioning properly, the pressure bag is inflated to 300 mm Hg, or a pressure higher than the patient's BP. Whenever the pressure in the monitoring system exceeds the patient's BP, each transducer will flow 3 mL/h of flush solution into the patient. Such a continuous flush system maintains the catheter's patency and prevents blood backflow into the catheter and monitoring system. In cases in which less than 3 mL/h of flow through each transducer is necessary (such as in a neonate), the flush solution can be delivered to the transducer(s) by using an infusion pump.

If the patient transfer will involve air medical transport, then all of the air left in the fluid bag, which has been placed inside the pressure bag, should be expelled to prevent its expansion during flight. As mentioned earlier, the pressure bag itself must remain at 300 mm Hg; in fact, it may have a pressure indicator that will display a green color when inflated near 300 mm Hg and a red color when the pressure exceeds 300 mm Hg. After the pressure bag is properly inflated, the air to it should be turned off to prevent deflation **FIGURE 15-10**. The pressure bag should be periodically checked during transport to verify that it is still inflated.

Before moving a patient with hemodynamic monitoring equipment already in place, the CCTP should examine the equipment, note the values currently being displayed, and trace the tubing from each transducer to the pressure-monitoring catheter to which it is connected. The catheter site should be examined and documented to be visibly clean, dry, and covered by an occlusive dressing. The CCTP should be familiar with the operation of the stopcocks and catheters in use or should ask the clinician at the bedside for a review of their proper use.

A CCTP may elect to transfer a patient to the transport stretcher before connecting transducers to the transport monitor or may make the connections

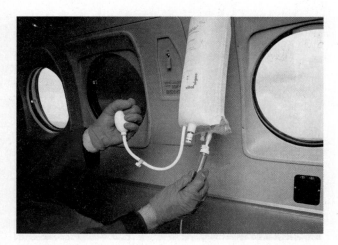

FIGURE 15-10 An inflated pressure bag with proper inflation.

© Jones & Bartlett Learning.

to the transport monitor before moving the patient. In either case, one pressure cable is moved at a time to the transport monitor, with the CCTP ensuring that waveforms and values similar to those displayed on the hospital monitor appear on the transport equipment before transferring additional lines and pressure channels. Proceeding in such a deliberate, stepwise manner avoids periods in which the patient is not connected to any monitoring equipment, when changes may not be readily detected.

Extra caution is needed when moving a patient with hemodynamic monitoring equipment in place because catheters can easily become dislodged or pulled out if they are not adequately secured. Agency or service policy for securing monitoring lines and catheters during transport should be followed. The most reliable hemodynamic waveforms and pressure readings will be obtained from tubing that spans less than 48 inches (122 cm) from transducer to invasive catheter, with no more than one stopcock between the transducer and the invasive catheter.

The best protection against accidental dislodgement or dislocation of invasive monitoring catheters is to carefully set monitoring alarms. The transport environment is no exception to the need for monitoring alarm parameters designed to alert the CCTP if hemodynamic parameters are outside of reasonable thresholds. Disconnected catheters will invariably register less than physiologic levels that can be readily detected if alarms are properly set by the CCTP. Despite the provider's singular focus on the patient, care of a critically ill patient is a task-intensive

endeavor, meaning the CCTP cannot continuously observe the transport monitor for changes. Consequently, alarms must be set for each parameter being monitored during transport. Failure to do so increases the risk of missing sudden or transient events with important patient safety implications.

Leveling and Zeroing the Pressure Transducer

The most common cause of error in obtaining direct hemodynamic pressure measurements is incorrect leveling of the transducer. The fluid used to fill the rigid pressure tubing that connects the monitoring catheter between the patient and the transducer will interfere with pressure readings if the pressure transducer is lower or higher than mid-heart level, commonly located at the patient's atrium. This reference point, which is referred to as the **phlebostatic axis**, is located at the fourth intercostal space, mid-chest position **FIGURE 15-11**. **Leveling** is the process

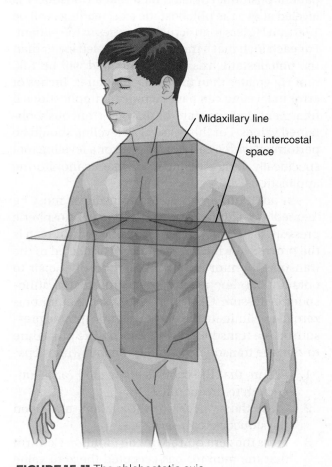

Midaxillary line

4th intercostal space

FIGURE 15-11 The phlebostatic axis.

© Jones & Bartlett Learning.

of ensuring that the hemodynamic pressure transducer is at the level of the atrium, which also corresponds to the level of the aortic root. Having the transducer at this level eliminates the influence of hydrostatic pressure from the fluid in the tubing from the measured pressures. The transducer must be releveled with every change in the patient's position; therefore, this point is often marked on the patient's skin. The simplest way to ensure proper placement during transport is to secure the transducer at the phlebostatic axis, although this step is not always practical in the critical care setting. The point on the transducer that is leveled is the air–fluid interface, or the location that was opened to air so as to perform the zeroing procedure described later in this section.

The phlebostatic axis moves with the patient, and transducers can be adjusted to obtain accurate readings in almost any sitting or lying position. Transducers must be releveled with any change in patient position. For each inch that a transducer is leveled above the phlebostatic axis, readings will be 1.86 mm Hg less than actual pressures in the patient. For each inch that a transducer is leveled lower than the phlebostatic axis, values obtained will be 1.86 mm Hg greater than the actual pressures. Inches of error in leveling can have significant implications if treatment decisions are based on erroneously obtained values. For this reason, all leveling should be performed with a carpenter's level or a leveling tool specifically designed for hemodynamic monitoring applications.

In addition, any pressure transducer must be "zeroed" to eliminate the effects of atmospheric pressure on the measurements obtained. **Zeroing** is the process in which a transducer connected to the transport monitor is opened to atmospheric air to obtain a baseline reading of environmental atmospheric pressure. Once opened to air, the monitor is zeroed to eliminate the effects of atmospheric pressure on the transducer **FIGURE 15-12**. The procedure to zero the transducer includes the following steps:

1. Ensure that the cable is connected (or reconnected) to the monitor.
2. Close the stopcock to the patient, and open the stopcock to the air.
3. Press the zero button on the monitor. Confirm that the monitor has accepted the zero value and actually indicates zero on the pressure and waveform displays.

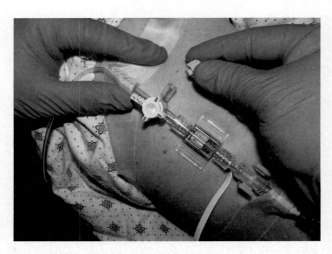

FIGURE 15-12 Zeroing the transducer.

© Jones & Bartlett Learning.

Zeroing should be performed in the following circumstances:

- Immediately after connecting the transducer to the transport monitor
- Once the transducer is reconnected to the monitor following any disconnection
- Whenever displayed values are in question

Depending on flight patterns and altitudes, zeroing is often performed at the initial connection of the transducer to the transport monitor, at cruising altitude, and again on arrival at the destination.

Transducers and Cables

Several transducer brands are available, each of which has its own fast-flush system. The two most commonly encountered types are the squeezable style and the pull style. The squeezable-style device includes two pieces of plastic on either side of the transducer that, when squeezed, will fast-flush the closed fluid-filled system **FIGURE 15-13A**. The pull-style (or pigtail) device has a small piece of rubber that resembles a pigtail **FIGURE 15-13B**. To flush the system, the CCTP pulls the tail straight out (away from the transducer).

Fast flushing overrides the normal delivery of 3 mL/h of flush solution through the transducer into the patient and allows free flow of the pressurized flush solution through the system for as long as the fast-flush assembly is activated. It is useful as an initial technique to troubleshoot a **dampened waveform** or absent waveform in a system that had previously been functioning normally.

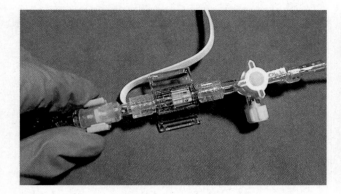

A

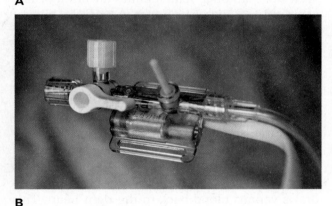

B

FIGURE 15-13 The two most common transducer flush system devices. **A.** Squeezable style. **B.** Pull style.

© Jones & Bartlett Learning.

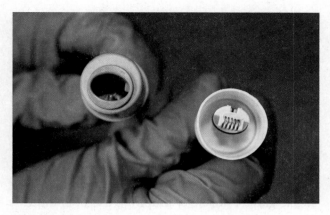

FIGURE 15-14 Two types of cables that connect the transducer to the monitor are a phone line–type connection and a half-moon connection (shown here).

© Jones & Bartlett Learning.

The CCTP should become familiar with transport monitors and the cables needed to connect them to pressure-monitoring equipment and transducers. Transport monitors are often limited to monitoring two pressure channels; thus, it may be necessary to decide which pressures will be observed during transport. Any patient with a PAC must have the distal port (pulmonary artery) continuously monitored in case the catheter spontaneously wedges (ie, migrates into a wedged position without manipulation by a clinician). Unmonitored or undetected spontaneous wedging can result in pulmonary infarction.

The cables that connect patient transducers to the monitor that an agency uses must be compatible with the equipment in use at both the referring and receiving hospitals. Two main cable types are available. In the most commonly used version, one end of the cable that attaches to the transducer resembles a phone line connection; the other is best described as a half-moon connection **FIGURE 15-14**. All patient monitors have a standard pressure cable receptacle. Because the transducer end of the monitoring cable is specific to the transducer manufacturer and the cables are extremely costly, many transport services elect to carry several spare transducers in case the transferring facility transducers are from a different manufacturer than those ordinarily used by the transport service.

Asepsis

The importance of asepsis cannot be overemphasized as an element of care for patients with central lines and hemodynamic monitoring equipment. The Centers for Disease Control and Prevention's National Healthcare Safety Network uses the term central line–associated bloodstream infection (CLABSI) to describe and track primary bloodstream infections (meaning that there is no infection present or suspected at another site) that develop in a patient who had a central line in place within the 48-hour period prior to the onset of the bloodstream infection. Preventing CLABSI is a major focus of critical care practitioners worldwide. Because central venous catheters disrupt the integrity of the skin, they provide a pathway for bacteria and fungi to enter the bloodstream. Critically ill patients are at greater risk for such infection. CLABSIs have serious implications for patients, typically causing prolonged hospital stays and increased costs and risk of mortality. Although the incidence of CLABSIs declined in US hospitals from 2008 through 2019, they continue to occur in ICUs and wards of acute care facilities. Notably, increased volumes of critically ill patients and the complexities born of the COVID-19 pandemic were associated with a 28% increase in CLABSIs in US hospitals in 2020 versus 2019.

With application of evidence-based practices, all CLABSIs are considered preventable. Indeed, several key practices can assist the CCTP in preventing such infections. If the CCTP is involved in catheter insertion, then CLABSI prevention includes meticulous hand hygiene, strict adherence to aseptic technique, use of maximal sterile barrier precautions (eg, removal of any unnecessary people from the room; wearing of masks, caps, gowns, and sterile gloves; full-body draping), use of chlorhexidine for skin antisepsis, site selection to minimize infections, and use of an appropriate dressing after the catheter has been inserted.

When central line placement is implemented, the patient's skin should be prepared with a chlorhexidine antiseptic using a back-and-forth friction scrub lasting at least 30 seconds. The antiseptic solution should not be wiped off or blotted from the skin, but rather must be allowed to dry completely (for approximately 2 minutes) before puncturing the site. Older antiseptic solutions, such as povidone–iodine solution, are no longer considered effective skin antisepsis.

CCTPs caring for patients with previously established central lines should strictly adhere to hand hygiene requirements, using an alcohol-based hand gel or other appropriate hand sanitizer frequently during transport. They should scrub the catheter hub or access port immediately before each use with an appropriate antiseptic, and use only sterile devices to access the catheter or fluid path. In addition, they should replace any wet, soiled, or damaged central line dressings using aseptic technique, including wearing clean or sterile gloves and placing face masks on the patient (unless intubated) and all providers in the vicinity.

The frequency with which central lines are accessed is directly related to the risk of CLABSIs. Interventions that reduce the need to connect, disconnect, and reconnect IV tubing and medication syringes help to reduce this risk. Such measures include use of tubing with multiple ports and adding multiple port adapters to catheter hubs that allow tubing to remain connected continuously, thereby eliminating the need to repeatedly connect and disconnect tubing when infusions are started and stopped. Prompt removal of unnecessary central lines is also a key practice in CLABSI prevention, and the CCTP should discuss the need to remove unnecessary central lines with referring staff.

Central Venous Lines

Central venous lines are invasive catheters placed inside the central venous system that provide access to the core vessels of the body. The right internal jugular vein **FIGURE 15-15** is the easiest site to access and in which to insert a central venous line because of the desirable surrounding anatomy and a relatively low rate of complications. Subclavian sites are preferred because they best minimize infection risks. Femoral and brachial veins are also commonly used sites, although femoral lines are strongly discouraged in adults because they have the highest risk for infection of any central venous line location.

The catheter of a central venous line is inserted until the tip resides just outside the RA (in the superior vena cava). This position allows for CVP readings (also known as right atrial readings). CVP reflects right ventricular preload, intravascular volume status, and right heart function. The normal range for CVP is 2 to 6 mm Hg in a critically ill patient. In healthy patients, CVP often ranges between 0 and –2 mm Hg, because this pressure draws venous blood back to the right heart. This phenomenon is the rationale for use of the Trendelenburg position when placing a central line in a

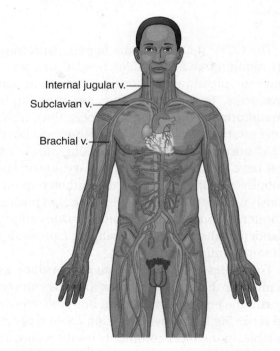

Internal jugular v.
Subclavian v.
Brachial v.

FIGURE 15-15 The right internal jugular vein is the easiest site to access and insert a central venous line. The subclavian, brachial, and femoral veins are also common sites.

patient with an unknown CVP. It also explains why a laceration of a jugular vessel is likely to be more lethal than a similarly lacerated carotid artery: The former injury carries a greater risk of air embolism.

The CVP waveform is subject to fluctuations during spontaneous and assisted respirations. For this reason, the CCTP should obtain a CVP measurement during end expiration to ensure its accuracy. Most monitors designed for use with critical care patients measure the CVP with a presumption that the patient is being mechanically ventilated.

Indications

In addition to their role in hemodynamic monitoring, central venous lines often include ports for obtaining blood specimens and for delivery of IV fluids and medications. These lines are frequently used when providers are unable to establish adequate peripheral vascular access or require access to the patient's central circulation to administer medications that cannot safely be given through peripheral sites. In summary, central venous lines provide a means to perform the following care:

- Rapid fluid replacement
- Medication administration
- Rapid access to central circulation
- Invasive monitoring

Contraindications

Some of the relative contraindications to central venous access include the following:

- Significant coagulopathy
- Local trauma to the site of insertion
- Infection at the site of insertion

Complications

Insertion of a central line carries some risks to the patient, including infection or bleeding at the insertion site. The most common complication is pneumothorax or hemothorax from an unsuccessful attempt at subclavian insertion. Additional complications include the following:

- Air embolism
- Infection
- Thrombosis
- Phlebitis
- Limb ischemia
- Arterial puncture
- Improper placement

- Myocardial perforation (resulting in tamponade)
- Thoracic duct injury (with left internal jugular or subclavian approaches)
- Nerve injury
- Catheter occlusion
- Sluggish infusion
- Catheter damage with resultant air embolism or infection
- Blood withdrawal problems (inability to obtain specimens)
- Retained guide wire

Types of Central Venous Catheters

The most commonly used central line in critical care has three lumens and is simply referred to as a **triple-lumen catheter FIGURE 15-16**. All three lumens can be used for phlebotomy or fluid and drug administration; alternatively, two lumens can be used for fluid administration and the other for CVP monitoring. In some cases, one port of a triple-lumen catheter may be reserved for total parenteral nutrition and should not be used during transport, except in

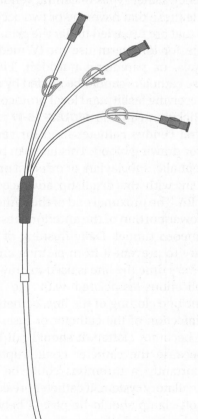

FIGURE 15-16 Hickman triple-lumen catheter.
© Jones & Bartlett Learning.

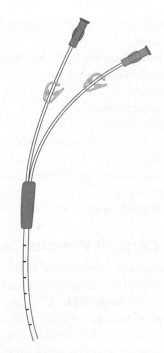

FIGURE 15-17 Hickman catheter.

© Jones & Bartlett Learning.

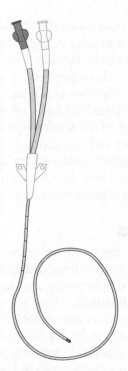

FIGURE 15-18 Groshong catheter.

© Jones & Bartlett Learning.

an emergency. Other types of central venous catheters include those that have one or two access ports and those that are tunneled under the skin, a design appropriate for long-term use for IV medications, hemodialysis, or parenteral nutrition. Emergency use of these catheters should be guided by direction from the receiving facility and local protocols.

The Hickman catheter **FIGURE 15-17** is a long-term central venous catheter used for venous access and for drawing blood. This line can be placed into the cephalic, subclavian, or external or internal jugular vein, with the distal tip advanced to just above the RA. The proximal end of the catheter exits from the lower portion of the anterior chest wall via a subcutaneous tunnel. Daily flushing of this line is necessary to prevent it from clotting and is also required every time the line is used to draw blood.

Complications associated with the Hickman catheter include clotting of the line, catheter breakage, and infection of the catheter or insertion site. If the line becomes clotted, it should not be force-flushed because the catheter could rupture and, more importantly, a thrombus could be released into the circulatory system. If catheter breakage does occur, a soft clamp should be placed between the break and the patient's skin until repair of the catheter can be accomplished. If a soft catheter clamp

is unavailable, the CCTP should fold the distal end of the catheter over itself several times and wrap it with a rubber band. Infection at the insertion site is evidenced by erythema, edema, or discharge. Catheter infection is often apparent as bacteremia, with fever and chills progressing to septic shock if not recognized and promptly treated. All complications should be reported to the receiving facility on arrival.

The Groshong catheter **FIGURE 15-18** is thinner, is more flexible, can have up to three lumens, and is equipped with a subcutaneous cuff. This catheter usually exits the skin near the nipple. A pressure-sensitive, two-way valve on its adjacent lateral wall allows for the tip of the catheter to be closed. Because venous pressure maintains the valve in the closed position, minimal backflow of blood into the catheter occurs. The advantages of this design are that clamping and frequent flushing are not necessary, although a saline flush is needed after each use or once daily.

The Port-A-Cath is a titanium chamber with a catheter that threads under the skin into the subclavian vein to the RA **FIGURE 15-19**. The titanium chamber is $1 \times 1 \times 0.5$–inch ($2.5 \times 2.5 \times 1$–cm) in dimension and has a self-sealing rubberlike top, which is implanted under the skin of the anterior

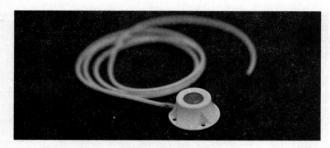

FIGURE 15-19 Port-A-Cath.

© NINUN/Shutterstock.

part of the chest in the pectoral region. This kind of catheter can be used for the infusion of fluid or medications and for blood draws. It is accessed using a Huber needle, which is inserted through the skin and into the rubber top of the portal. A Huber needle is a specially designed noncoring needle that minimizes damage to the port and bends at a 90° angle, allowing it to be secured to the chest wall after its insertion into the port. The advantages of a Port-A-Cath are that it may remain in place for years with proper care, it allows the patient to be active, and it does not require daily care. The catheter must be flushed with saline (or heparin) once every 4 to 6 weeks if not in use. The risks of the Port-A-Cath are similar to those associated with external catheters and include kinks, ruptures, and, rarely, infections.

A peripherally inserted central catheter (PICC) **FIGURE 15-20** is used when medium-duration, long-term access is needed (usually limited to several months). This catheter can be used in ways similar to other centrally placed lines. It is inserted via the brachial or other arm vein and is advanced to the superior vena cava, with the tip of the line located just outside the atrium. The PICC requires regular flushing with saline solution to prevent clotting. Low-dose warfarin may be added to the patient's daily medications to augment line patency if clotting problems have occurred in the past. The disadvantages of a PICC include limited arm mobility and limitations on aggressive exertion (eg, swimming), in addition to other risks associated with placement of centrally placed catheters.

Central Venous Catheter Placement

Although central venous catheters are rarely placed by CCTPs, the steps are useful to understand as background knowledge. This section explains how such lines are placed.

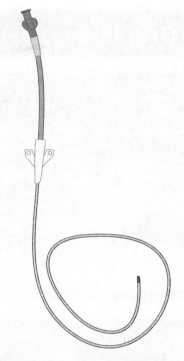

FIGURE 15-20 Power-injectable peripherally inserted central catheter.

© Jones & Bartlett Learning.

Equipment

The following equipment is needed to insert a central venous line:

- Catheters (various sizes and lengths)
- 5- and 10-mL syringes
- Saline flush solution
- Chlorhexidine solution
- J-tipped guide wire
- IV tubing
- IV fluids
- Suture materials
- Occlusive dressing
- Sterile drapes
- Tape
- Local anesthetic

Steps

The most common technique for line insertion is the Seldinger technique. **SKILL DRILL 15-2** outlines the steps for inserting a central venous line using this technique (note that ultrasonography to assist with insertion is becoming commonplace):

1. Take standard precautions.
2. Prepare all equipment and flush all lumen ports.

Skill Drill 15-2 Inserting a Central Venous Line

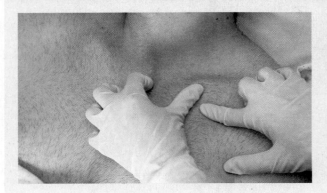

Step 1

Locate the appropriate landmarks.

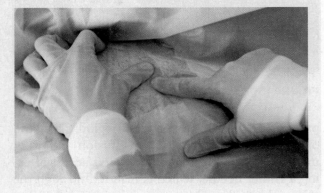

Step 2

Palpate for the entry location.

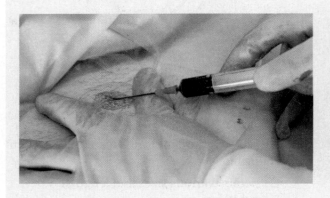

Step 3

Insert the needle with the connected syringe at the site, aspirating until blood is drawn into the syringe.

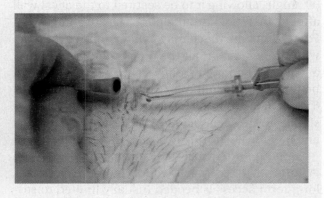

Step 4

Remove the syringe, insert the guide wire into the needle, and feed the guide wire into the vein.

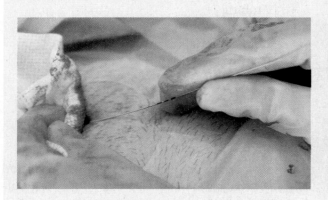

Step 5

Remove the needle while holding the guide wire in place.

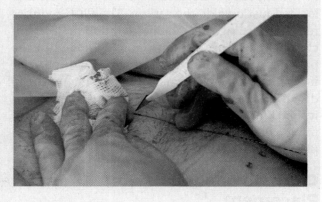

Step 6

Pass the dilator over the guide wire to the skin. Use a scalpel to make a small (approximately 0.25- to 0.5-inch [0.5- to 1-cm]) incision in the skin.

Skill Drill 15-2 Inserting a Central Venous Line (continued)

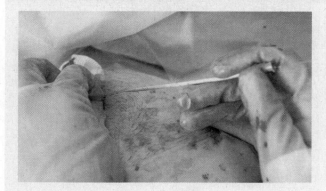

Step 7

Remove the dilator, while maintaining contact with the guide wire.

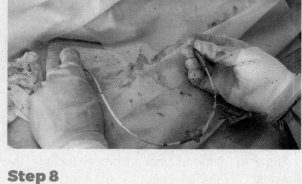

Step 8

Insert the catheter over the guide wire and into the vessel, removing the guide wire as the catheter advances.

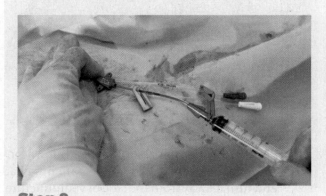

Step 9

Aspirate blood and flush all ports to ensure patency.

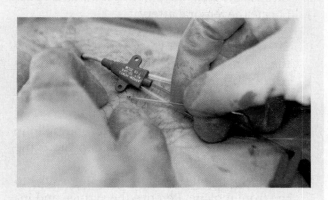

Step 10

Secure the line to the patient's skin using sutures or staples.

3. Locate the appropriate landmarks **STEP 1**.
4. Palpate for the entry location **STEP 2**.
5. Clean and prepare the site using a sterile technique.
6. Administer a local anesthetic.
7. Insert the needle with the connected syringe at the site, aspirating until blood is drawn into the syringe **STEP 3**.
8. Remove the syringe and insert the guide wire into the needle. Feed the needle into the vein, while continually maintaining contact with the guide wire **STEP 4**.
9. Remove the needle while holding the guide wire in place **STEP 5**.
10. Pass the dilator over the guide wire to the skin. Use a scalpel to make a small (approximately 0.25- to 0.5-inch [0.5- to 1-cm]) incision in the skin to facilitate passing of the dilator **STEP 6**.
11. Remove the dilator, while maintaining contact with the guide wire **STEP 7**.

12. Insert the catheter over the guide wire and into the vessel, removing the guide wire as the catheter advances **STEP 8**.
13. Aspirate blood, and flush all ports to ensure patency **STEP 9**.
14. Secure the line to the patient's skin using sutures or staples **STEP 10**.
15. Dress the site, and follow up with a radiograph to ensure proper line placement. It is imperative that line placement be radiographically confirmed before departing with the patient.

The following lists outline specific procedures for insertion of central lines in the femoral, internal jugular, and subclavian veins.

Steps for femoral vein insertion include the following:

1. Prepare the equipment.
2. Clip hair from the area, and, if necessary, drape the area.
3. Cleanse the area with chlorhexidine antiseptic.
4. Locate the femoral artery.
5. Numb the area using a local anesthetic.
6. Puncture the area two fingerbreadths below the inguinal ligament, medial to the artery, directing the needle cephalad at a 45° angle with the skin until the needle can no longer be advanced **FIGURE 15-21**.
7. Maintain suction on the syringe, and pull the needle back slowly until blood appears in the syringe.
8. Lower the needle so that it is more parallel to the frontal plane. Remove the syringe and insert the catheter.

Steps for internal jugular vein insertion include the following:

1. Prepare the equipment.
2. Determine the depth of catheter placement by measuring from the point of insertion to the following surface markers on the chest wall **FIGURE 15-22**:
   a. Sternoclavicular joint to the subclavian vein
   b. Midmanubrial area to the brachycephalic vein
   c. Manubriosternal junction to the superior vena cava
   d. 2 inches (5 cm) below the manubriosternal junction (the RA of the heart)
3. Place the tip of the catheter above the RA for administration of fluids.

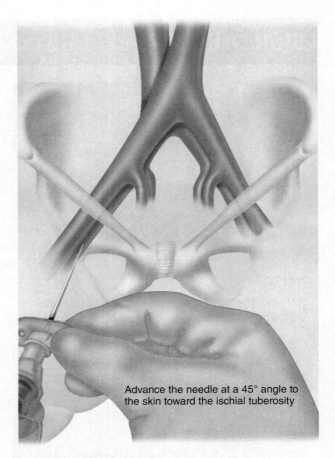

Advance the needle at a 45° angle to the skin toward the ischial tuberosity

FIGURE 15-21 Femoral vein insertion.

Data from Henretig FM, King CC, eds. *Textbook of Pediatric Emergency Procedures*. Baltimore, MD: Williams and Wilkins; 1997.

4. Place the patient in a supine, head-down position at a 15° angle. Extend the patient's head and turn it away from the side of venipuncture.
5. Cleanse the area with chlorhexidine antiseptic and drape the area. Maintain sterility.
6. Administer a local anesthetic.
7. Insert the needle at a 45° to 60° angle directed caudally **FIGURE 15-23**. Advance to a depth of 1 to 2 inches (3 to 5 cm), depending on the patient's size.
8. If the vein is not entered, then redirect the needle tip slightly more medially and repeat; do not direct the needle across the midline because the carotid artery may be punctured.
9. After entering the vein, advance the guide wire through the needle; minimal to no resistance should be met. Monitor the ECG during insertion for atrial ectopy.
10. With the guide wire in place, withdraw the needle and advance the catheter to the predetermined depth.

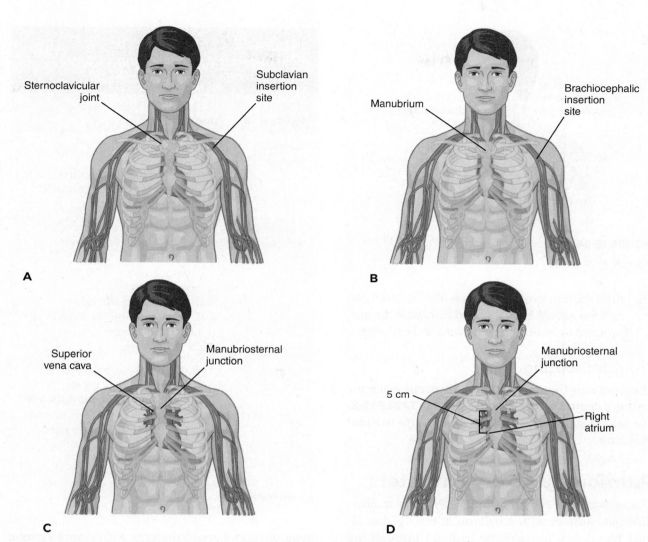

A

Sternoclavicular joint

Subclavian insertion site

B

Manubrium

Brachiocephalic insertion site

C

Superior vena cava

Manubriosternal junction

D

5 cm

Manubriosternal junction

Right atrium

FIGURE 15-22 Determine the depth of catheter placement by measuring from the point of insertion to the following surface markers on the chest wall. **A.** Sternoclavicular joint to the subclavian vein. **B.** Midmanubrial area to the brachycephalic vein. **C.** Manubriosternal junction to the superior vena cava. **D.** 2 inches (5 cm) below the manubriosternal junction (right atrium of the heart).

© Jones & Bartlett Learning.

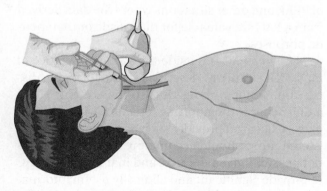

FIGURE 15-23 Internal jugular vein insertion with ultrasonographic guidance.

© Jones & Bartlett Learning.

Steps for subclavian vein insertion include the following:

1. Position the patient in a 15° angle head-down position.
2. Stand at the side of the bed.
3. Turn the patient's head away from the side to be cannulated.
4. Puncture the skin at the junction of the medial (middle of the clavicle) and middle third of the clavicle **FIGURE 15-24**.
5. Advance the needle beneath the clavicle toward the sternal notch to a depth of 1 to 2 inches (3 to 5 cm).

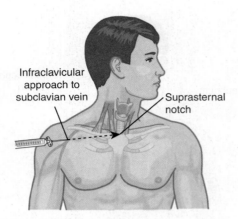

FIGURE 15-24 Subclavian vein insertion.

© Jones & Bartlett Learning.

6. After the lumen of the vein has been entered, rotate the needle cephalad and clockwise 90° and proceed to insert the guide wire and catheter.

Troubleshooting

The problems that most commonly occur when inserting a central venous line are listed in **TABLE 15-2**. The table also identifies potential solutions to these problems.

Pulmonary Artery Catheters

The **pulmonary artery catheter (PAC)** is a flow-directed catheter with a balloon at the tip that allows blood flow to carry the catheter through the heart and into the pulmonary artery, where it terminates. A PAC is also known as a Swan–Ganz catheter (or simply a "swan") after Harold Jeremy Swan and William Ganz, who invented this catheter in 1970.

Much of our current knowledge of hemodynamics came from frequent use of PACs in patients being treated in the ICU. Overuse of these catheters became a concern in the mid- to late 1990s; during that era, the majority of clinical studies suggested that routine use of PACs was not indicated, because this intervention was associated with a variety of complications, including mortality.

The PAC is a diagnostic, not therapeutic, device. Considerable knowledge and experience are required to properly interpret the hemodynamic data obtained from a PAC. Today, use of PACs is infrequent, but valuable in select situations. These cases include patients with cardiogenic shock, patients being evaluated and treated for pulmonary arterial

TABLE 15-2 Common Problems Encountered When Inserting a Central Venous Line	
Problem	**Possible Actions to Resolve the Problem**
Sluggish infusion	Check for kinks in the catheter. Reposition the catheter. Remove the injection cap and check for clots. Flush vigorously with 10 mL of normal saline.
Inability to withdraw blood	Check for kinks in the catheter. Make sure the catheter is not clamped. Flush vigorously with 10 mL of normal saline. Use repositioning maneuvers. Remove the injection cap and attach the syringe. Flush with saline.
Catheter damage	Clamp the catheter between the damaged area and the skin with a soft clamp or fold the distal end of the catheter over itself several times and apply a rubber band. Cover the damaged area with a sterile dressing. Do not attempt to repair.

© Jones & Bartlett Learning.

hypertension, certain patients with severe systolic or diastolic heart failure, patients being assessed for heart and/or lung transplantation, patients undergoing some high-risk operations such as cardiothoracic procedures, patients with acute respiratory distress syndrome (ARDS) who require high levels of PEEP, and other situations where the data derived from a PAC are valuable for diagnostic or therapeutic purposes.

Use of a PAC is outside the scope of practice of most CCTPs and, as described in the following discussion, is not without risks to the patient. When a CCT team is transporting a patient with a PAC in place, a licensed provider such as a critical care registered nurse should accompany the crew. If this is not possible, given the risks and inability of the PAC to provide significant and clinically useful information to the transport team, it may be advisable to discuss removal of this catheter from the patient prior to transport. Because PACs are placed through

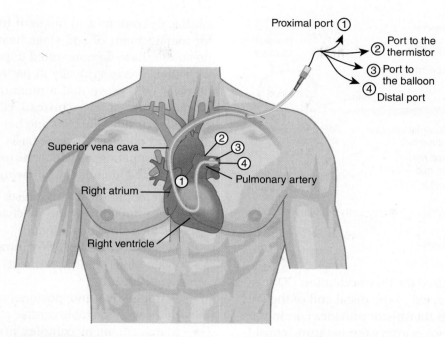

Proximal port ①
② Port to the thermistor
③ Port to the balloon
④ Distal port

Superior vena cava
② ③
④
Pulmonary artery
①
Right atrium
Right ventricle

FIGURE 15-25 Pulmonary artery catheter placement. Once in place, the tip is deflated to allow blood flow around the catheter.

© Jones & Bartlett Learning.

an introducer, inserting a new one at the destination facility is a relatively simple procedure.

A PAC uses the same access routes as any other central line and can be placed at the bedside within minutes. The catheter is fed into the vena cava and then through the RA **FIGURE 15-25**. Once past the lumen of the introducer sheath, the catheter tip balloon is inflated with as much as 1.5 mL of air to facilitate further placement. With the balloon inflated, the catheter is "floated" through the RA into the right ventricle and ultimately wedges into a proximal branch of the pulmonary artery. After the PAC is in place, the balloon is deflated to allow blood flow around the catheter.

A PAC is 43 inches (110 cm) long and contains multiple lumens that terminate at various points along the length of the catheter, corresponding to different locations in the heart. The PAC is marked at 10-cm intervals beginning at the distal tip of the catheter, with one thin black line representing 10 cm, two thin black lines representing 20 cm, three thin black lines representing 30 cm, and so on, up to one thick black line representing 50 cm, one thick black line accompanied by a thin black line representing 60 cm, one thick black line and two thin lines representing 70 cm, and so on. During the initial assessment, the CCTP should

note the centimeter measurement of the PAC at the introducer. This information will help to determine whether the catheter has moved into or out of the patient during transport.

Two of the lumens are connected to pressure transducers that continuously display measurements. The first pressure reading is the RA pressure, and the second pressure reading is the pulmonary artery pressure. The RA pressures are displayed as mean pressures, whereas pulmonary artery pressures are displayed as systolic, diastolic, and mean values. After the PAC is properly placed in the pulmonary artery, inflation of the PAC balloon results in blockage of blood flow from the right ventricle behind the balloon tip and the appearance of a PCWP waveform on the monitor. The PCWP waveform, like the RA pressure, is measured as a mean value.

Complications of PAC insertion are nearly the same as complications of central line insertion, with the addition of pulmonary artery perforation or rupture, pulmonary infarction, arrhythmias, tricuspid and pulmonic valve injury, tamponade, and knotting of the catheter. The greatest potential complication of PAC use is misinterpretation of the data by clinicians, resulting in inappropriate therapy and potentially worsening outcomes.

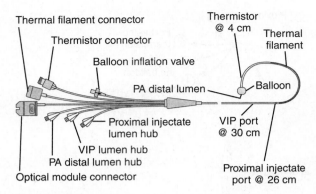

FIGURE 15-26 A pulmonary artery catheter with a thermistor.

Courtesy of Edwards Lifesciences. Used with permission.

A **thermistor** used for thermodilution CO measurement is connected to the distal end of the PAC **FIGURE 15-26**. This thermistor provides continuous readings of pulmonary artery temperature, considered the gold standard for core body temperature measurement. Some PACs also have a fiberoptic oximetric catheter at the distal tip for continuous monitoring of mixed venous oxygen saturation.

Although PACs vary in terms of their size and number of lumens, manufacturers have standardized the coloring of the primary PAC lumens. All PACs have a blue RA (proximal) port, a yellow pulmonary artery (distal) port, a red balloon inflation port, and a yellow temperature thermistor port. Some PACs have additional RA and/or right ventricular ports that can be used for infusions or pressure monitoring. Specially designed PACs with integrated pacing wires are available that can be used for transvenous cardiac pacing, as well as PACs with an integrated thermal filament that allows for continuous CO measurement using pulse-coded electrical signals.

Indications

Commonly accepted indications for pulmonary artery catheterization have little or no evidence supporting them and are largely determined by clinician experience, expertise, and preference. As mentioned earlier, a PAC may be warranted when clinicians have a specific question about a patient's hemodynamic status that has not or cannot be readily answered by noninvasive assessment. Use of bedside ultrasonography has greatly diminished the uncertainties that had previously led to insertion of a PAC. Despite common use of these catheters in

cardiac operations and frequent insertion of PACs for management of end-stage heart failure, as yet no studies have demonstrated improved outcomes with their use in critically ill patients. Conversely, no clear data prove that a moratorium should be placed on use of PACs. Instead, clinicians need to carefully consider the risks and benefits in critically ill patients on a case-by-case basis.

Some situations in which the use of a PAC might be considered include the following:

- Differentiation among causes of shock
- Determination of the mechanisms responsible for pulmonary edema
- Evaluation or diagnosis of intracardiac shunt(s)
- Evaluation and treatment of pulmonary hypertension
- Perioperative and postoperative care of patients with unstable cardiac status
- Management of complex myocardial infarction (MI)
- Care of patients undergoing cardiac operations
- Guidance for titration of inotropic, vasopressor, or vasodilator therapy
- Complex fluid volume status management
- Assessment of cardiac performance
- Evaluation of patients for heart, lung, or heart and lung transplantation

Contraindications

As with central venous catheterization, few absolute contraindications exist to pulmonary artery catheterization, although the risks of PAC use are greater than those associated with the use of central venous catheters alone. Relative contraindications to the use of PACs include the following:

- Significant coagulopathy
- Local trauma to the site of insertion
- Infection at the site of insertion
- Inability to float the PAC into the pulmonary artery

Pulmonary Artery Catheter Placement

Equipment

The following equipment is needed to insert a PAC:

- The PAC
- A PAC introducer kit (must be 0.5F to 1F larger than the PAC)

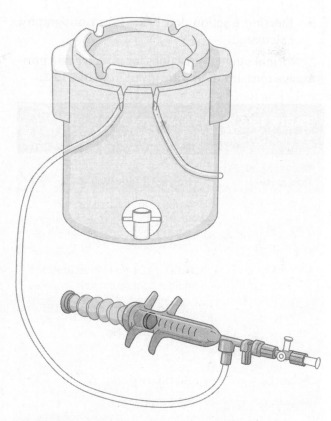

FIGURE 15-27 A thermodilution cardiac output set.

© Jones & Bartlett Learning.

- Sterile gowns and drapes for complete draping of the patient and bedside area
- ECG and pulse oximetry monitoring
- Transducer setup
- Patient monitor and cables to connect to transducers
- Thermodilution CO set **FIGURE 15-27**
- Appropriate antiseptic solution (usually chlorhexidine)
- 2% lidocaine and atropine (to treat arrhythmias during the procedure)

Steps

Although the CCTP would not insert a PAC, the steps are listed here to provide useful background knowledge:

1. Assemble and connect the transducers to the monitor.
2. Zero the transducers (described previously in the section "Leveling and Zeroing the Pressure Transducer").
3. Assemble the equipment.

4. Position the patient in reverse Trendelenburg (head-down) position, arms by their side, with their head turned in the opposite direction of the intended cannulation site.
5. Ensure that cardiac and pulse oximetry monitoring devices are in place and functioning.
6. Establish a sterile field. Open the introducer supplies.
7. Prepare the insertion site.
8. Administer a local anesthetic agent.
9. Prepare the introducer equipment while awaiting the onset of anesthetic effects.
10. Cannulate the vein at the selected insertion site using an 18-gauge or larger needle that is attached to an empty 10-mL syringe.
11. After the vein has been entered and the IV position of the needle has been confirmed, pass a Seldinger wire (included in the introducer insertion supplies) through the needle.
12. Remove the needle.
13. Widen the skin opening using a scalpel.
14. Using a dilator, pass the PAC introducer over the wire into the vein. Remove and discard the wire.
15. Aspirate and flush the side port of the introducer with sterile saline.
16. Secure the introducer to the skin with suture(s).
17. Prepare the PAC by flushing the ports. Connect it to the transducer(s) and slide the sterile sleeve over the catheter.
18. Test the PAC balloon and distal port to ensure that the waveform appears on the monitor.
19. Advance the PAC through the introducer.
20. Inflate the balloon after the PAC is past the distal end of the introducer (usually 6 inches [15 cm]).
21. Advance the PAC to the wedge position, by observing the waveforms on the monitor, through the RA, right ventricle, and pulmonary artery.
22. If arrhythmias occur while the PAC is in the right ventricle, quickly advance the PAC into the pulmonary artery.
23. After the pulmonary artery wedge tracing is observed, deflate the balloon to check for return of the pulmonary artery pressure waveform.
24. With the balloon deflated, pull back the catheter 0.5 to 0.75 inch (1 to 2 cm) and recheck wedge function.
25. Wedging the catheter should require 1 to 1.5 mL of air. If the catheter wedges with less

than 1 mL of air, it has been inserted too far and should be pulled back slightly.

26. Secure the sterile sheath to the introducer and attach the PAC to the patient to prevent accidental dislodgement.

27. Obtain an anterior–posterior chest radiograph to check for pneumothorax and proper catheter position.

Invasive Pressure Measurements

By placing invasive catheters into the vasculature, several hemodynamic parameters can be continually monitored, and others can be periodically assessed. Pressure measurement in hemodynamic monitoring is measured in millimeters of mercury (mm Hg) in the United States; outside the United States, the units for these measurements are torr and kilopascals.

Common hemodynamic parameters are listed here. The line from which the measurement is obtained is shown in parentheses after each item, and the values that are calculated by a provider (rather than obtained from the device) are noted.

- CVP (central line, large-bore antecubital line, or PAC)
- SVV, PPV, PVI (arterial line or pulse oximeter pleth, measured)
- SBP (arterial line, calculated when using an electronic cuff)
- DBP (arterial line, calculated when using an electronic cuff)
- MAP (arterial line or electronic cuff, calculated or computed if using a manual cuff measurement)
- Pulse pressure (arterial line, calculated)
- Pulmonary artery pressure (systolic, diastolic, and mean) (PAC)
- PCWP (PAC)
- CO (PAC)
- PVR (PAC, calculated)
- SVR (PAC, calculated)
- SV (PAC, calculated)
- Mixed venous oxygen saturation (PAC)
- Central venous oxygen saturation (central line)
- TBSA (calculated using height and weight)
- CI (PAC, calculated)

- Ejection fraction, left heart (ultrasonography, calculated)

Normal ranges and values for invasive and non-invasive measurements are given in **TABLE 15-3**.

TABLE 15-3 Normal Ranges and Values for Hemodynamic Measurements

Assessment Parameter	Normal Range/Value
CVP	2 to 6 mm Hg
PPV	9% to 13% (>13% suggests fluid responsiveness)
SVV/PVI	10% to 15% (>15% suggests fluid responsiveness)
SBP	100 to 120 mm Hg
DBP	60 to 80 mm Hg
MAP	70 to 105 mm Hg
Pulse pressure	40 to 60 mm Hg
Heart rate	60 to 100 mm Hg
Pulmonary artery pressure, systemic	15 to 30 mm Hg
Pulmonary artery pressure, diastolic	8 to 15 mm Hg
PCWP	4 to 12 mm Hg
CO	4 to 8 L/min
CI	2.2 to 4 L/min/m^2
PVR	100 to 250 dyne-sec/cm^{-5}
SVR	800 to 1,200 dyne-sec/cm^{-5}
SV	60 to 100 mL/beat
Svo$_2$	60% to 80%
Scvo$_2$	70% to 90%
SV index	30 to 50 mL/beat/m^2
EF	55% to 75% (mean normal 65%)

Abbreviations: CI, cardiac index; CO, cardiac output; CVP, central venous pressure; DBP, diastolic blood pressure; EF, ejection fraction; MAP, mean arterial pressure; PCWP, pulmonary capillary wedge pressure; PPV, pulse pressure variation; PVI, pleth variability index; PVR, pulmonary vascular resistance; SBP, systolic blood pressure; Scvo$_2$, mixed central venous oxygen saturation; SV, stroke volume; Svo$_2$, mixed venous oxygen saturation; SVR, systemic vascular resistance; SVV, stroke volume variation

Measurements From an Arterial Line

Pressure Waveforms

The following pressure changes occur in the LV during the cardiac cycle:

1. At the beginning of the cardiac cycle, aortic pressure is at its lowest (ie, diastolic) level. The elastic state and vascular resistance of the arteries determine this pressure. During diastole, the AV valves are open and blood flows passively from the atria into the ventricles. The pressures in the ventricles and atria are nearly equal and significantly lower than the pressure in the aorta.

2. The SA node depolarizes, causing the atria to contract. This contraction causes the pressure in the atria and ventricles to rise. As the impulse is conducted through the ventricles, the pressure rises sharply.

3. When the pressure in the LV exceeds that in the LA, the mitral valve snaps closed. The pressure continues to rise until the pressure in the aorta is exceeded, causing the aortic valve to open. As the aortic valve opens and blood enters the aorta, the pressure rises to the peak systolic level and then begins to fall as ventricular ejection tapers.

4. The aortic pressure begins to decrease. As the pressure in the LV drops, the pressure in the aorta becomes greater than that in the LV. This change in pressure causes a slight backward flow of blood into the ventricle, and the backward flow causes the aortic valve leaflets to be forced outward and into the closed position, much like the opening of a parachute.

5. As the aortic valve leaflets are forced outward into place, the pressure gradient across the valve increases significantly because the ventricle continues isovolumetric relaxation. The valves bulge slightly under the pressure of the blood from the aorta and then spring back slightly. This springing back causes a slight bump in the aortic pressure waveform, referred to as the dicrotic notch, signaling the onset of diastole. With the valve closed and the ventricles continuing to relax, the ventricular pressure decreases rapidly **FIGURE 15-28**.

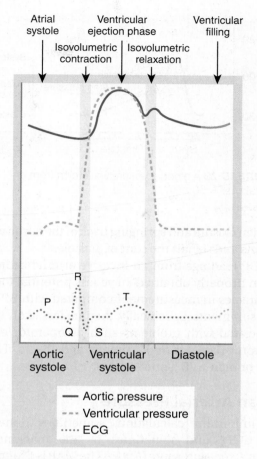

FIGURE 15-28 Aortic pressure waveform.

Illustration from source material by Maquet Cardiovascular. Used with permission.

6. When the pressure in the ventricle is less than the pressure in the atrium, the mitral valve opens and blood begins to flow passively into the ventricle from the atrium.

Arterial BP

Direct BP measurement using an arterial line provides continuous assessment of arterial (or systemic) pressure. Because hemodynamic status can change by the minute, continual BP monitoring can help the CCTP more closely observe patients during transport. An arterial line connected to the transport monitor provides constantly updated SBP, DBP, and MAP values and an arterial waveform **FIGURE 15-29**. Components of the arterial waveform include the dicrotic notch, mean pressure, systole, diastole, systolic pulse pressure, and diastolic pulse pressure. The dicrotic notch represents a brief increase in aortic pressure reflected as a notching of the wave. It is caused by the

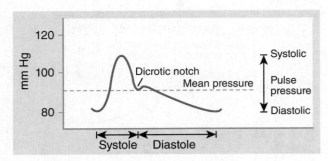

FIGURE 15-29 A blood pressure waveform from an arterial line.

© Jones & Bartlett Learning.

sudden closure and springing back of the aortic valve leaflets and signals the start of diastole.

BP readings from an invasive arterial catheter, when properly obtained, have less potential for inaccuracies in measurement compared with BP cuff measurements. Specifically, they are less likely to be associated with problems such as operator error, inappropriate size or placement, and effects of low-flow or high-SVR (shock) states.

Mean Arterial Pressure

An important calculation, sometimes done by the CCTP and sometimes by the machine, is mean arterial pressure (MAP). The MAP is a function of heart rate, SBP, and DBP. It represents the average (ie, constant) pressure that the arterial vasculature feels from the pulsatile nature of the heartbeat.

The MAP is calculated by the transport monitor software, which measures the mean area under the arterial pulse pressure waveform. The reverse calculation is used by NIBP software to derive the SBP and DBP for display. If precisely one-third of the cardiac cycle was spent in systole and two-thirds was spent in diastole, then the MAP could be calculated by using the following formula:

$$MAP = DBP + 1/3 \ (SBP - DBP)$$

Because a heart rate of 70 beats/min is typically required to spend one-third of the cardiac cycle in systole and two-thirds of the cycle in diastole, this formula is relatively inaccurate in practice. In contrast, the MAP measured by a transport monitor connected to an arterial line or by an NIPB is the most precise of the pressure measurements available to CCTPs.

The location of an arterial line's placement significantly affects the SBP. The farther out from the heart that an arterial line is placed, the more pressure that will be needed to flow blood and, therefore, the higher the SBP will be. The MAP, however, is unaffected by the location of line placement and is the best parameter to use when making treatment decisions. Usually, a person needs a MAP between 70 and 105 mm Hg to satisfactorily perfuse the tissues. The organs most sensitive to hypotension are the kidneys, which typically require a MAP of 60 mm Hg or higher and are likely to sustain irreversible injury when faced with a MAP of less than 60 mm Hg for more than 20 minutes. For that reason, most medical orders for BP parameters require titration of drugs or administration of fluids to maintain a MAP of 70 mm Hg or greater.

A long-standing debate in critical care has focused on the accuracy of NIBP-obtained BP measurements versus those obtained using an arterial line. Clearly, the NIBP measures flow, whereas the arterial line measures pressure. Nevertheless, there are times, especially when critically ill patients become hypotensive, when clinicians have questioned the accuracy of the arterial line, choosing instead to rely on NIBP readings.

A large study published in 2013 examined data from 4,957 patients in a university teaching hospital whose BP measurements were taken from both an arterial line and an NIBP. When 27,022 simultaneous readings were compared, the researchers found that the NIBP overestimated SBP in patients with hypotension. Moreover, beginning at systolic pressures less than 100 mm Hg, the more hypotensive the patient became, the greater the overestimation by the NIBP was. Despite the difference in SBP, measured MAPs by both arterial line and NIBP consistently correlated down to a MAP of 40 mm Hg. This very large study and many smaller studies like it have fairly conclusively demonstrated that, regardless of whether direct monitoring with an arterial line or indirect monitoring with an NIBP is performed, the MAP is the value that should be used to make treatment decisions. One additional finding in the large 2013 study was that a MAP of less than 60 mm Hg closely correlated with increased incidence of acute kidney injury and death.

Pulse Pressure

Pulse pressure is the mathematical difference between the SBP and the DBP. Values of 40 to 60 mm

Hg are seen in healthy people, but may be altered in critically ill patients.

Both SV and vascular compliance affect the pulse pressure. An elevated pulse pressure can be indicative of high SV states (eg, hypervolemia) or low vascular compliance (eg, arteriosclerosis). In these states, SBP increases. If a concomitant rise in DBP is not present, then an elevated pulse pressure develops. Bradycardia can also cause an elevated pulse pressure. In this instance, lower DBP develops because of an extended diastole, which can lead to diastolic runoff. Low SV states (eg, hypovolemia) and high vascular compliance (eg, shock) will cause a decrease in SBP and, therefore, a decrease in pulse pressure (barring a proportional decrease in DBP). Tachycardia may cause a decreased pulse pressure by the reverse of the bradycardia mechanism.

The fast-flush feature previously discussed can also be used to test the accuracy of an arterial line or any transduced pressure. At times, it may appear to the CCTP that a monitoring system may not be accurately reproducing the pressures being measured inside the patient. The ability to reliably reproduce the actual pressures being measured is referred to as dynamic response. Two components make up the dynamic response: the frequency response (FR) and the damping coefficient. The FR is the speed of oscillation or the frequency with which the monitoring device samples the pressure being measured. Modern computers running hemodynamic monitoring software all but ensure sufficient FR. The damping coefficient refers to how quickly the system comes to rest or the shock-absorbing capability of the transducer. A system with too little shock-absorbing capability will not come to rest in between cardiac cycles, causing it to include part of the previous pressure waveform in the next one. This effect, which is called underdamping, often results in the display of falsely high systolic pressure values (ie, overshoot) and sometimes in the display of falsely low diastolic pressures. Often a "ringing" type of artifact is observed in the waveform tracings. In contrast, a system with too much shock-absorbing capability will not be sufficiently responsive so that it can accurately display the pressure waveforms. This effect, which is called overdamping, commonly results in poorly defined waveform tracings, slurred upstrokes, decreased systolic pressures, and increased diastolic pressures.

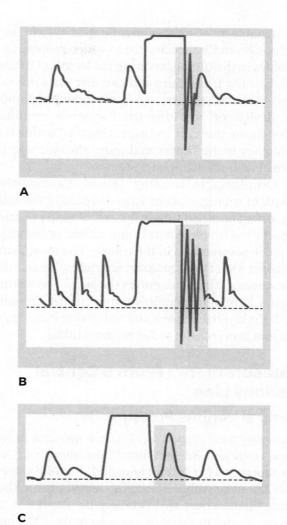

FIGURE 15-30 The square wave test. **A.** Normal test. **B.** Underdamped system. **C.** Overdamped system.

Reproduced from Tintinalli J, Stapczynski J, Ma OJ, Yealy D, Meckler G, Cline D. *Tintinalli's Emergency Medicine: A Comprehensive Study Guide*. 8th ed. New York, NY: McGraw-Hill; 2015.

The fast-flush activator can be used to conduct a test of dynamic response, known as the square wave test or fast-flush test **FIGURE 15-30**. This test is performed by quickly activating and releasing the fast-flush activator, which produces a sharp upstroke on the waveform trace that peaks and flatlines at the maximal point on the monitor and then rapidly descends. The resultant waveform has the appearance of a square wave. Following its descent, the waveform should exhibit one or two oscillations (bounces) and then return to a normal waveform. If multiple oscillations or bounces (more than two) are present, then the system is underdamped. If only one or no oscillations appear following the fast flush, then the system is overdamped.

Troubleshooting an underdamped system may include carefully checking for so-called pinpoint air bubbles in the tubing, assuring the length of tubing between the transducer and catheter does not exceed 48 inches (122 cm), using a commercial damping device, or adjusting the frequency response through the monitor software. Often adjusting the frequency is the fastest and most efficient way to correct an underdamped system.

Overdamping is often caused by excessive length of tubing, clots or large bubbles in the tubing, use of nonrigid tubing instead of rigid pressure monitoring tubing, kinks in the tubing or catheter, or loose connections in the tubing. The most likely place for a kink to occur in an arterial catheter is the site where the catheter enters the skin. Discovering such a kink often requires removing the dressing from the arterial line site and redressing it in a fashion that prevents the catheter from kinking.

Measurements From a Central Venous Line

Central Venous Pressure

Central venous pressure (CVP) is a measure of the vena caval and RA pressures. Even though a CVP waveform tracing has systolic and diastolic values, only the mean value is used in clinical practice because the numbers are extremely low **FIGURE 15-31**. Three positive deflections are seen in the CVP tracing: the *a* wave, which represents atrial contraction; the *c* wave, which represents closure of the tricuspid valve; and the *v* wave, which represents passive atrial filling during diastole. Some textbooks suggest that the components of the CVP waveform can be identified by the corresponding location in an ECG tracing, but this technique is impractical given the varied lengths of tubing used and the differences in ECG monitor display timing between manufacturers.

The absence of *a* waves in a CVP tracing suggests that atrial contractions are not occurring or, as in atrial fibrillation, they are so rapid that there is no meaningful output. In fact, when atrial fibrillation is suspected, a CVP tracing showing only *v* waves can be helpful in confirming the rhythm.

The normal range for CVP in a critically ill patient was previously listed as 2 to 6 mm Hg. Historically, CVP was considered a reflection of fluid volume status, with patients being given fluid boluses when their CVP fell below 5 to 8 mm Hg. Today, it is understood that as a static parameter, CVP must be interpreted in the context of other information when assessing fluid volume status. Elevated CVP may be suggestive of right-side heart failure, cardiac tamponade, massive pulmonary embolus, significant pulmonary vasoconstriction, or hypervolemia. Healthy patients typically have a CVP ranging from 0 to –2 mm Hg. This negative pressure facilitates a significant percentage of blood return to the heart.

Additional Measurements From a Pulmonary Artery Catheter

Right Ventricular Pressure

Although not routinely monitored or measured, the right ventricular pressure is important during insertion and use of a PAC. The right ventricular pressure has three components **FIGURE 15-32**:

- Systolic pressure, usually 20 to 30 mm Hg
- Diastolic pressure, usually 0 to 5 mm Hg
- Mean pressure, usually 10 to 20 mm Hg

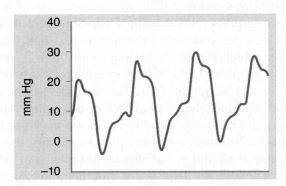

FIGURE 15-32 A right ventricular pressure waveform has a systolic pressure comparable to the pulmonary artery systolic pressure.

© Jones & Bartlett Learning.

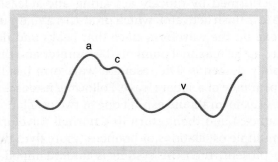

FIGURE 15-31 A central venous pressure waveform.

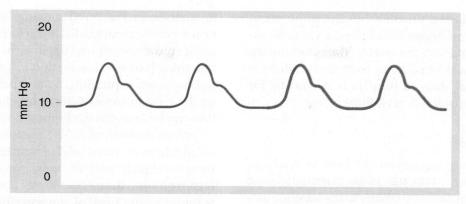

FIGURE 15-33 A pulmonary artery pressure waveform, which is similar to the arterial pressure waveform (ie, systolic, dicrotic notch, and diastolic components).

© Jones & Bartlett Learning.

Ventricular ectopy is common when the tip of the PAC is in the right ventricle. For this reason, it is important for the CCTP to be able to recognize a right ventricular waveform and its characteristic low diastolic pressure, which distinguishes it from a pulmonary artery pressure waveform.

Pulmonary Artery Pressure

Like the arterial BP waveform, the pulmonary artery pressure has three components **FIGURE 15-33**:

- Systolic pressure, usually 15 to 30 mm Hg
- Diastolic pressure, usually 8 to 15 mm Hg
- Mean pulmonary artery pressure, usually 10 to 20 mm Hg

Pulmonary artery pressures are a function of right ventricular health and the vascular resistance of the pulmonary circuit. Although patients with significant heart failure or pulmonary obstructive disease can have chronically elevated pulmonary artery pressures or pulmonary hypertension, acute elevations in pulmonary artery pressures are unlikely to stem from causes other than hypoxemia or hypercarbia. An astute CCTP who observes a sudden and sustained increase in pulmonary artery pressures will immediately assess and correct any issues with oxygen saturation or ventilation (as reflected by end-tidal carbon dioxide readings or point-of-care blood gas testing).

Elevations in the pulmonary artery pressure can result from conditions that increase pulmonary blood flow, such as atrial and ventricular septal defects or hypervolemia. Elevations in the pulmonary artery diastolic pressure can result from tachycardia (usually greater than 120 beats/min in adults) or pulmonary emboli. Decreased pulmonary artery diastolic pressure can be seen with hypovolemia.

If pulmonary artery diastolic pressures suddenly drop, then the catheter position should be re-evaluated to determine if the PAC has migrated into the right ventricle (see the earlier section "Right Ventricular Pressure").

Pulmonary Capillary Wedge Pressure
Definition

The pulmonary capillary wedge pressure (PCWP) reflects LA pressure and was previously considered the gold standard for LV preload assessment. This measurement is also called pulmonary artery occlusion pressure and pulmonary artery wedge pressure. A function of a PAC, PCWP is an intermittent assessment performed by inflating a small balloon on the distal tip of the PAC, which causes the catheter to shift forward to wedge against the opening of the proximal branch of the pulmonary artery. This action occludes the pulmonary artery from any antegrade blood flow. With the tip inflated, the transducer reads a pressure that is equivalent to the left atrial pressure. The left atrial pressure is closely related to and often parallels the left ventricular end-diastolic pressure, which is indicative of LV health.

The normal range for PCWP is 4 to 12 mm Hg. A properly obtained PCWP will normally be slightly less than the pulmonary artery diastolic pressure (≤4 mm Hg). A PCWP of 10 to 12 mm Hg had previously been used to differentiate hypovolemia from euvolemia in clinical practice, but as a static measurement, it is no longer considered a valuable assessment of fluid volume status. More commonly, PCWP is followed in patients with heart failure. A PCWP of greater than 18 mm Hg is diagnostic for acute decompensated heart failure.

Interpretation

The CCTP needs to understand how to read the PCWP waveform **FIGURE 15-34**. Hemodynamic waveforms often show variations in the baseline as a result of respiratory-induced intrathoracic pressure fluctuations. Atmospheric and pleural pressures are most closely approximated at end expiration. To eliminate the effects of intrathoracic pressure on PCWP values, they must be measured at end expiration.

Like the CVP waveform, a typical PCWP has three positive deflections: the *a* wave represents atrial contraction, the *c* wave represents closure of the mitral valve, and the *v* wave represents passive atrial filling during diastole. In practice, the *c* wave is rarely seen in a PCWP tracing, as the additional distance of the catheter often interferes with transmission of this part of the waveform.

One clinically significant condition that is readily seen in the PCWP waveform is mitral regurgitation. The greater the regurgitation, the greater the height of the *v* waves will be. The term "cannon *v* waves" refers to significant mitral regurgitation.

Depending on whether the patient is mechanically ventilated or spontaneously breathing, end expiration will be observed in different locations on the PCWP baseline. In mechanically ventilated patients, positive-pressure inspiration elevates intrathoracic pressure and results in a positive fluctuation in the PCWP tracing baseline. Expiration is passive; end expiration is found at the lowest point in the waveform baseline. In spontaneously breathing patients, inspiration is induced by negative pressure. Expiration in these patients produces an increase in the waveform baseline; end expiration can be found at the highest point.

When measuring PCWP, a helpful mnemonic to recall where to locate end expiration on the waveform baseline is "patient—peak; ventilator—valley." End expiration in spontaneously breathing patients is found at the peak of the waveform baseline. In contrast, in mechanically ventilated patients, end expiration is found in the valley of the waveform baseline.

After the proper position on the waveform is located, measurement of the PCWP waveform is done by locating two sequential positive deflections on the waveform immediately before the point where the baseline changes. In spontaneously breathing patients, this point would be immediately before the baseline begins to fall; in mechanically ventilated patients, it would be immediately before the baseline starts to rise. The two sequential deflections are averaged to determine the mean pressure **FIGURE 15-35**.

The PAC balloon typically holds up to 2 mL of air. Syringes included with the PAC normally allow the operator to inject only 1.5 mL of air to inflate the balloon. Regardless of the balloon's maximum capacity of 2 mL of air, it is recommended to inflate the balloon with only 1.5 mL, as overinflation may result in rupture of the pulmonary artery or damage to the balloon. This injection should be done slowly, over 2 to 3 seconds. It is common to feel some initial resistance during inflation (similar to the resistance one needs to overcome when blowing up a

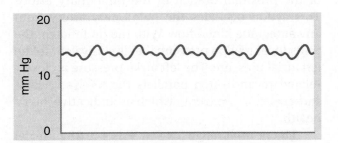

FIGURE 15-34 The waveform of a normal pulmonary capillary wedge pressure.
© Jones & Bartlett Learning.

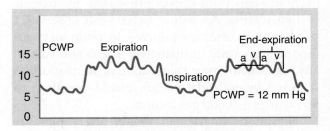

FIGURE 15-35 Respiratory-related variations in the pulmonary capillary wedge pressure (PCWP).
© Jones & Bartlett Learning.

toy balloon by mouth). After a PCWP waveform is observed, the tracing can be "frozen" on the monitor screen, and the balloon should be allowed to passively deflate. Maximum inflation times should not exceed 10 to 15 seconds.

If less than 1 mL of air is needed to produce a PCWP tracing, then the PAC is likely inserted too far into the patient and is at risk for spontaneously wedging. Prolonged inflation or spontaneous wedging can result in pulmonary infarction. Manual flushing of a wedged catheter may cause pulmonary artery perforation.

Causes of elevated PCWP are numerous and difficult to resolve definitively. Often, elevated PCWP results from the LV not being able to clear the antegrade blood flow. If the LV cannot clear increased flow from the right side of the heart (as in heart failure), then an elevated PCWP will result. Left-side heart dysfunction (as in LV failure and mitral valve disease) will cause retrograde blood accumulation within the pulmonary vasculature, thereby creating an increased PCWP. A PCWP level greater than 18 mm Hg often suggests the potential for pulmonary edema, especially with a normal colloidal osmotic pressure (ie, normal serum albumin level).

High levels of PEEP used with mechanical ventilation can also cause an elevated PCWP. When PEEP levels greater than 10 cm H_2O are used, correction of the measured PCWP may be requested. This correction is done by subtracting 1.5 mm Hg from the measured PCWP for every 5 cm H_2O of PEEP. For example, if the PEEP is 15 cm H_2O and the measured PCWP is 22 mm Hg, the corrected PCWP would be 17.5 mm Hg. When correcting a measured PCWP for PEEP, both the measured PCWP and the corrected PCWP values should be recorded. This documentation eliminates potential confusion that might result if some clinicians correct their measured values and others do not.

In a patient with pulmonary edema, the CCTP may use the PCWP to differentiate between its possible causes. If pulmonary edema is the result of left-side heart failure (cardiogenic), the PCWP will be elevated. If the pulmonary edema results from increased pulmonary capillary permeability (as in pneumonia or ARDS), the PCWP may not be elevated. Care must be exercised with patients diagnosed as having ARDS because they often have elevated MAP levels and high levels of PEEP, so PCWP readings may be elevated as well. PCWP has increasingly been seen as a less reliable way to differentiate causes of pulmonary edema as the understanding of hydrostatic pulmonary pressures has evolved.

Between the transducer on the tip of the PAC and the LV lie three major anatomic components that may interfere with an accurate PCWP reading: the mitral valve, the LA, and the pulmonary venous vasculature. Furthermore, the PCWP is a pressure often used to reflect volume. Although this relationship sometimes holds, it fails if the distensibility of the LV has been affected (such as in a LV MI) or if the size of the tank changes as a result of vasoconstriction or vasodilation.

Like CVP, PCWP is a static measurement. While useful in guiding heart failure therapies, PCWP must be interpreted in the context of other data to accurately judge the patient's fluid volume status.

Cardiac Output

Measurement of CO rounds out the basic assessments performed by a PAC. Like PCWP, CO is an intermittent assessment that involves some action by the CCTP. Normal CO ranges between 4 and 8 L/min. Investigation of low or higher than normal CO requires a stepwise approach considering each of the elements that compose the CO formula ($CO = HR \times SV$).

Typical CO assessment using a PAC is based on the thermodilution method. This method involves injecting 5% dextrose in water (D_5W) at a known temperature (iced or room temperature) into the proximal port (usually the CVP port) of the PAC. Note that D_5W is the solution with the precise osmolarity on which the PA catheter and monitor software are programmed to base the calculations. Other solutions should not be used, although the level of error introduced with these solutions is negligible (less than 1%).

As the injectate moves past the thermistor on the distal end of the catheter, the temperature is recorded by the monitoring system. A curve is plotted comparing the temperature change over time between the injectate sensor and the distal end of the catheter. The monitor then calculates the CO. This procedure is repeated several times (three to six times, depending on local protocol), and the mean of these results is used to interpret the patient's CO. Curves that suggest erroneous injection technique or faulty temperature measurement are not included in the averaging strategy.

Most transport monitors do not have the capability of performing thermodilution CO measurements during transport. Because thermodilution measurement of CO relies on the measured temperature change between blood and the injectate, rapid infusions of blood or medications into central catheters can potentially interfere with CO calculations.

Variations on CO Measurement

Various volumes of injectate can be used (3, 5, or 10 mL), different ports can be chosen, and either iced or room-temperature solutions can be used during CO measurements. Each requires a different computation constant to be entered into the monitor for performing the CO computations. The constants, which are specific to each manufacturer and each PAC, are available on the PAC package insert or on the manufacturer's website.

Continuous cardiac output (CCO) PACs continuously calculate and display CO by emitting a coded thermal energy signal from an element wrapped along the catheter. The CCO computer uses the thermodilution principle to calculate CO as often as every few minutes. Interference from infusions and other temperature variations is eliminated by downstream analysis of only the coded thermal signal. Although the greater accuracy and seeming simplicity of CCO catheters might appear attractive, troubleshooting the CCO technology requires considerably more experience and education than does the same task with thermodilution PACs.

Fick Principle

CO can also be calculated or estimated by using the Fick principle. First described by Adolph Fick in 1870, this method divides oxygen consumption based on the difference between the oxygen content of arterial versus venous blood. The formula uses assumed values for oxygen consumption derived from basal metabolic studies on healthy subjects, which may or may not be valid in critically ill patients. Nevertheless, the Fick principle is commonly used in cardiac catheterization laboratories and critical care units. The formula is as follows:

$$CO = \frac{\text{Oxygen Consumption}}{\text{Arteriovenous Oxygen Content Difference}}$$

The following data are needed to calculate CO with this equation:

- TBSA
- Hemoglobin level
- Arterial oxygen saturation (from a pulse oximeter or blood gas–measured oxygen saturation)
- Mixed venous oxygen saturation (from a blood gas sample drawn from the pulmonary artery port of a PAC or Svo_2 reading from a fiberoptic PAC)

TBSA is expressed in square meters, oxygen saturation is expressed as a decimal (eg, 98% would be expressed as 0.98), and hemoglobin is expressed in grams per deciliter (g/dL).

The estimated Fick CO is calculated as follows:

1. Calculate the oxygen consumption based on a presumed 125 mL of oxygen consumed per square meter of TBSA (ie, 125 × TBSA).
2. Calculate the arteriovenous oxygen content difference. Each gram of hemoglobin can carry 1.36 mL of oxygen. Hence, the difference is expressed as follows: 1.36 × Hemoglobin × (Arterial saturation – Venous saturation) × 10.
3. Divide the calculated oxygen consumption by the calculated arteriovenous oxygen content difference to produce the estimated CO in liters per minute.

Assuming the following values, here is an example of the calculation:

- TBSA = 1.33 m^2
- Hemoglobin (Hgb) = 12 g/dL
- Spo_2 (pulse oximeter) = 0.98 (98%)
- Svo_2 (saturation of blood gas sample drawn from pulmonary artery port) = 0.70 (70%)

$$CO = \frac{125 \times \text{BSA } 1.33}{\text{Hgb } 12 \times 1.36 \times (0.98 - 0.70) \times 10}$$

$$CO = \frac{166.25}{16.32 \times (0.28) \times 10}$$

$$CO = \frac{166.25}{45.696} = 3.64 \text{ L/min}$$

A simplified version of the formula can also be used. This version calculates the constants (here, 125 has already been divided by 1.36 and 10), so that fewer calculations are needed overall:

$$CO = \frac{9.19 \times BSA\ 1.33}{Hgb\ 12 \times (0.98 - 0.70)}$$

Pulmonary Vascular Resistance

PVR is calculated with the following equation:

$$PVR = \frac{(Mean\ Pulmonary\ Artery\ Pressure - PCWP)}{CO} = 80$$

PVR represents the resistance of the pulmonary vascular circuit that opposes flow out of the right ventricle and pulmonary artery, commonly referred to as right-side heart afterload. The normal value is 100 to 250 dyne-sec/cm^{-5}. As mentioned previously, PVR is not commonly used when determining the treatment plan for critical care patients. The CCTP may see an elevated PVR in patients with pulmonary hypertension or mitral valve stenosis.

Systemic Vascular Resistance

If a patient's MAP, CVP, and CO are known, then the CO computer will calculate the SVR by using the following equation:

$$SVR = \frac{(MAP - CVP)}{CO} \times 80$$

In a manner similar to PVR, a patient's SVR represents the total impedance to blood flow felt by the LV, commonly referred to as afterload. Calculation of SVR, which has a normal range of 800 to 1,200 dyne-sec/cm^{-5}, is extremely useful in helping to differentiate among the possible causes of shock. If SVR is elevated, the patient has vasoconstriction, suggesting hypovolemia or pump failure. If SVR is low, a distributive shock state such as neurogenic or septic shock is likely. Obviously, the effects of vasodilating or vasoconstricting agents can affect SVR values. Also, note that SVR is a calculated (not measured) value. As such, changes or errors in measuring any of the components included in the calculation could alter the results and lead to decisions based on inaccurate information.

The ideal SVR is thought to be slightly less than 1,000 dyne-sec/cm^{-5}. When a PAC is used to titrate vasodilator therapy (usually angiotensin-converting enzyme inhibitor agents) in patients with heart failure, the goal is to achieve an SVR of 900 to 1,000 dyne-sec/cm^{-5}.

Stroke Volume

The amount of blood ejected in each stroke of a ventricle is measured in milliliters and recorded as the SV. A normal SV is 60 to 100 mL/beat. The familiar equation that relates SV to CO and heart rate is as follows:

$$SV = \frac{CO}{Heart\ Rate}$$

As explained previously, ventricular performance is affected by the contractility (health) of the heart muscle and the preload and afterload for the respective ventricle. Any pathophysiologic factor that affects one of the performance determinants will either augment or depress the SV.

The stroke volume index is calculated by dividing SV by TBSA:

$$Stroke\ Volume\ Index = \frac{SV}{TBSA}$$

The normal stroke volume index is between 33 and 47 mL/beat/m^2.

An estimation of contractility can be made by calculating the left and right ventricular stroke work indexes.

Left ventricular stroke work index:

$$= \frac{Stroke\ Volume}{Index\ (MAP - PCWP) \times 0.0136}$$

Right ventricular stroke work index:

$$= \frac{Stroke\ Volume\ Index}{(Mean\ Pulmonary\ Artery\ Pressure - CVP) \times 0.0136}$$

The normal left ventricular stroke work index is 40 to 75 g-m/m^2/beat. (Note: g-m represents grams per meter.) The normal right ventricular stroke work index is 5 to 10 g-m/m^2/beat.

Mixed Venous Oxygen Saturation

If a fiberoptic oxygen saturation probe is attached to the distal end of the PAC, then a mixed venous oxygen saturation (Svo_2) measurement can be recorded. This measurement is constant and requires no action by the clinician after the catheter is placed. In PACs without fiberoptic oximetry capability, a blood gas specimen can be obtained from the distal (pulmonary artery) port of the catheter to determine the Svo_2 value.

In effect, the Svo_2 value reflects the global balance between oxygen delivery and consumption. The measurement is performed at the distal end of the PAC because the pulmonary artery is the most appropriate place to sample a mixture of all blood returning from the body. When obtaining a blood gas specimen from the pulmonary artery port of a PAC so as to determine the mixed venous oxygen saturation, the speed of withdrawal of the blood specimen does not affect the results. Historically, it was believed that rapid withdrawal from the very small lumen led to falsely elevated Svo_2 values.

When evaluating an Svo_2 value outside the normal range (0.60 to 0.80 [60% to 80%]), the CCTP should consider each of the four components that contribute to this parameter: total hemoglobin level, arterial oxygen saturation, CO, and oxygen consumption. Three of these factors pertain to oxygen delivery, with the other being related to oxygen consumption in the body. Oxygen delivery is affected by total hemoglobin levels, arterial oxygen saturation, and CO. Increases or decreases in any of these factors can affect the Svo_2 value. Changes in oxygen consumption (also called oxygen demand) can also affect the Svo_2 value. Oxygen consumption is increased with conditions that increase metabolic rate or muscle activity, such as fever, seizures, shivering, and increased work of breathing. Oxygen consumption may decrease when maldistribution of blood is present, which most commonly occurs in sepsis as a result of microcapillary obstruction that leads to arterial blood being shunted past the capillaries into the venous blood. Supranormal values can also be seen with exposure to certain poisons that impair tissue oxygen delivery, such as septic, carbon monoxide, and cyanide poisonings. Normally, when oxygen demand increases and threatens to exceed oxygen supply, the body compensates by increasing CO and/or oxygen extraction.

The mixed central venous oxygen saturation ($Scvo_2$) measurement is similar to mixed venous oxygen saturation. Like the Svo_2 value, the $Scvo_2$ value reflects the balance between oxygen supply and delivery. Measurements of $Scvo_2$ are obtained from a central venous catheter by drawing a blood gas specimen or using a fiberoptic oximetric tip connected to a specially designed monitor that displays the oxygen saturation. Because the location of the central venous line is more proximal than the pulmonary artery, blood sampled from a central venous line reflects extraction of oxygen by the brain and upper body rather than global extraction of oxygen from the blood; therefore, the $Scvo_2$ values are approximately 8% to 10% higher than the Svo_2 values. A normal $Scvo_2$ value is considered to be 0.70 to 0.90 (70% to 90%).

Heart Failure

Myocardial oxygen supply must balance myocardial oxygen demand (myocardial oxygen consumption [MVo_2]) to meet the myocardial metabolic requirements or ischemia will result. Factors that can affect myocardial oxygen supply include coronary artery pathology or pathoanatomy, diastolic pressure, diastolic time, and oxygen extraction. Because the majority of blood flow to the coronary arteries occurs during diastole, when the ventricle is at rest and the aortic valve is closed, diastolic pressure and time spent in diastole (diastolic time) profoundly affect the blood flow to the coronary arteries and, therefore, myocardial oxygen supply. Because the time required to complete systole is fixed, any increases in heart rate result in decreased diastolic time and, therefore, less time to perfuse the coronary arteries. The MVo_2 varies with heart rate, preload, afterload, and contractility; any increase in these factors increases oxygen demand.

Heart failure is a cyclic phenomenon. Injury to the myocardium, such as might occur with an acute myocardial infarction (AMI), results in a series of physiologic and hemodynamic changes that can affect the balance between oxygen supply and demand. The injury (from whatever cause) decreases pumping efficiency, CO, and arterial pressure. As discussed previously, CO depends on stroke volume (SV) and heart rate: CO = SV × Heart rate. In this equation, for CO to remain the

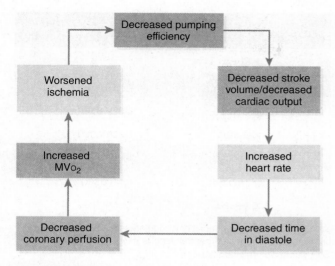

FIGURE 15-36 The cycle of heart failure.

© Jones & Bartlett Learning.

same, a decrease in either SV or heart rate must be compensated for by an increase in the other component. Therefore, if the ability of the heart to pump effectively were to become impaired (such as might occur with an MI), causing a drop in the SV, then the heart rate must increase for CO to remain the same. Coronary perfusion occurs only during diastole, and any increase in heart rate results in less diastolic time and, in turn, less time for coronary perfusion. Because the heart rate is increased, the MVo_2 also increases, worsening the mismatch of oxygen supply and demand. The decreased coronary perfusion, coupled with the increased MVo_2, leads to worsened ischemia. Ischemia causes the heart to pump less effectively, leading to a greater decrease in SV. The heart rate increases to maintain CO, and the cycle of heart failure continues **FIGURE 15-36**.

The treatment of cardiac failure is aimed at restoring normal cardiac function and the balance between myocardial oxygen supply and oxygen demand. If the initial intervention fails to restore the balance among these factors, then the intra-aortic balloon pump (IABP) offers a mechanical means of rebalancing them.

Shock

Shock is a common cause of morbidity in the critical care setting. Because shock is characterized by reduced systemic tissue perfusion, the end result is decreased tissue perfusion. Prompt recognition and reversal of shock can help avoid the otherwise rapidly irreversible sequence of cell death, end-organ damage, and lactic acidosis resulting from anaerobic metabolism, multisystem organ failure, and death.

The three recognized shock states are hypovolemic, cardiogenic, and distributive. Each of these shock states is associated with classic hemodynamic findings that help differentiate among them. Specifically, two hemodynamic parameters distinguish the different types of shock: CO and SVR. Hemodynamic monitoring can help the CCTP to differentiate between the various types of shock and assess the effectiveness of treatment during transport.

Hypovolemic shock includes volume loss from acute or chronic hemorrhage, excessive diuresis, third-space losses, and any other condition that depletes intravascular volume. In this type of shock, preload is decreased as a consequence of depleted intravascular volume. Decreased preload leads to a decline in SV, which results in decreased CO. To maintain end-organ perfusion, SVR increases to compensate for the declining CO.

Cardiogenic shock causes are diverse and include myocardial depression from ischemia and/or infarcts, cardiomyopathies, stunning following cardiac operations, arrhythmias that decrease flow, mechanical abnormalities leading to pump failure, and obstructive conditions such as massive pulmonary embolism, tension pneumothorax, pericardial tamponade, and aortic clots. This type of shock involves a complex cascade of events resulting from pump failure leading to decreased CO. The SVR typically increases in an effort to maintain CO, which further exacerbates pump failure and leads to increased preload and a relative total hypervolemic condition.

Distributive shock states include sepsis, systemic inflammatory response syndrome, toxic shock syndrome, anaphylaxis, poisonings, neurogenic conditions such as spinal cord injury, narcotic overdoses, and other vasodilatory etiologies. In this type of shock, vasodilation is often the primary culprit and is manifested as a significantly decreased SVR. When afterload declines dramatically, CO increases.

TABLE 15-4 summarizes the findings expected with each of the three shock states.

TABLE 15-4 Relationship Between Shock Type and Invasive Hemodynamic Measurements

Measurement	Shock Type		
	Hypovolemic	**Cardiogenic**	**Distributive**
Preload (SVV, PPV, PVI, CVP, PCWP)	Decreased	Increased	Decreased
Afterload (SVR, PVR)	Increased	Increased	Decreased
Cardiac output	Decreased	Decreased	Increased
Svo_2 or $Scvo_2$	Decreased	Decreased	Increased
Blood pressure (MAP)	Decreased	Increased	Decreased

Abbreviations: CVP, central venous pressure; MAP, mean arterial pressure; PCWP, pulmonary capillary wedge pressure; PPV, pulse pressure variation; PVR, pulmonary vascular resistance; PVI, pleth variability index; $Scvo_2$, mixed central venous oxygen saturation; Svo_2, mixed venous oxygen saturation; SVR, systemic vascular resistance; SVV, stroke volume variation.

© Jones & Bartlett Learning.

Flight Considerations
Effects of Altitude Changes on Hemodynamic Monitoring

Concerns pertaining to flight physiology include the hypoxic effects of altitude and gas expansion. Even in pressurized cabins, oxygen saturation in healthy people at normal cruising altitudes above 20,000 feet declines by a mean of 5.5%, and it often approaches 0.90 (90%). Patients with reduced oxygen saturation on the ground can be expected to experience further declines during flight. Close monitoring of oxygen saturation will enable the CCTP to respond to changes in the patient's condition and maintain sufficient levels of inspired oxygen to ensure adequate saturation.

Physiologic changes that may be evident in the patient in response to lowered oxygen levels at high altitude include a chemoreceptor-induced increase in tidal volume and, if respiratory compensation is inadequate, an increased CO achieved mainly through an increased heart rate. Hypoxia and increased sympathetic nervous system tone predispose patients to arrhythmias.

Gas expansion in flight occurs in accordance with Boyle's law, which states that the volume to which a given quantity of gas is compressed is inversely proportional to the surrounding atmospheric pressure. Pneumothoraces may become tension pneumothoraces with significant hemodynamic compromise. Air should be removed from IV bags before takeoff because it will expand at altitude, potentially increasing infusion rates. Pumps should be used for medication infusions. Zeroing of transducers is recommended when cruising altitude is reached, and once again following landing. The CCTP may see changes in transduced pressures with changes of altitude of 1,000 feet; if these variations appear clinically significant, then re-zeroing of the transducer is recommended prior to initiating treatment.

Summary

Hemodynamic monitoring provides CCTPs with multiple measures of the cardiovascular status of their patients. Proper use of these clues to guide patient care requires technical skill in the correct use of the equipment and an understanding of the meaning of the data it provides. Experienced CCTPs will use multiple methods (such as physical assessment findings and laboratory test results) to confirm that the hemodynamic measurements obtained accurately reflect perfusion. Hemodynamic monitoring provides one piece of the clinical picture needed to form an overall impression and diagnosis. The most important tool for hemodynamic monitoring will always be the CCTP's own knowledge and experience.

Perfusion deficits are the primary pathology that require critical care, both in hospital and during transport. Assessing perfusion should be the ultimate goal of hemodynamic monitoring and requires an understanding of oxygenation, circulation, preload, afterload, and cardiac performance. The plethora of monitoring devices, blood tests, and tools available to the CCTP all contribute to the ability to assess perfusion and correct deficits.

Case Study

A 68-year-old man with pulmonary edema was brought to the emergency department of a community hospital by emergency medical services responders. Paramedics found the patient with acute shortness of breath and intubated him in the field when he failed to respond to high-dose nitroglycerin and continuous positive airway pressure. The patient is now in the ICU of the community hospital awaiting your arrival for ground transport to a heart failure program at a tertiary center located 2 hours away. The referring hospital personnel advise that an arterial line and PAC have been placed and that they are attempting to lower the patient's BP while they await your arrival. No evidence of an AMI is present. A chest radiograph revealed diffuse interstitial edema consistent with pulmonary edema. The results of all laboratory tests, including cardiac markers, electrolytes, and renal function tests, were normal.

On arrival, you confirm the information previously reported. You note the patient is ventilating well on a fraction of inspired oxygen of 0.4, a tidal volume of 7 mL/kg, a respiratory rate of 14 breaths/min in the synchronized intermittent mandatory ventilation mode, and a PEEP of 5 cm H_2O. Continuous infusions of propofol, fentanyl, and nitroglycerin are running. The nitroglycerin is infusing at 200 µg/min. The registered nurse reports that escalating doses of furosemide have not resulted in any increased urine output. The following hemodynamic readings were taken 5 minutes before your arrival at the bedside:

- Pulse rate: 100 beats/min
- BP (systolic/diastolic/mean): 220/110/135 mm Hg
- Pulmonary artery pressure (systolic/diastolic/mean): 57/34/40 mm Hg
- PCWP: 28 mm Hg
- CVP: 20 mm Hg
- CO: 3.9 L/min
- CI: 1.7 L/min/m^2
- SVR: 2,359 dyne-sec/cm^{-5}

1. What are the implications of these hemodynamic values?
2. Which interventions would help stabilize this patient's condition for transport?
3. Are other hemodynamic data available that would be helpful?

Analysis

Familiarity with the hemodynamic findings associated with various forms of shock would immediately point to cardiogenic shock in this patient. An initial decline in myocardial pumping efficiency from an as yet undetermined cause triggered a cascade of events beginning with vasoconstriction and progressing to hypervolemia, which ultimately resulted in pulmonary edema. Vasoconstriction is seen in the elevated afterload (SVR) and hypertension; hypervolemia is evidenced by elevated preload values (CVP and PCWP). The CO is likely low because the patient's heart is unable to pump against the incredibly high afterload. Urine output is likely compromised by renal retention of sodium and water in response to the low CO. The values seen in this case example are, in fact, classic values seen in patients with cardiogenic shock. As this patient's condition deteriorates, he will ultimately become hypotensive and acidotic and will die if untreated.

The first intervention suggested by the values obtained with the PAC is use of an agent to reduce the high afterload state. Staff reported attempting to lower the patient's BP with nitroglycerin, but the current dosing is generally considered maximal. Nitroglycerin is primarily a venodilating agent with minimal arterial-dilating properties except at extremely high doses. Given the patient's degree of hypertension, which persists even with the nitroglycerin infusion, achieving a significant reduction in afterload will require an agent with more potent arterial-vasodilating properties. The transport crew consulted with providers caring for the patient and decided to initiate an infusion of sodium nitroprusside. Nitroprusside has venous- and arterial-dilating properties and is a potent antihypertensive agent. Following initiation of a nitroprusside drip, gradually titrated up to 3 μg/kg/min, the patient's MAP declined to 95 mm Hg, CVP to 14 mm Hg, and PCWP to 24 mm Hg. The CO doubled to 7.8 L/min. The calculated SVR was then 831 dyne-sec/cm^{-5}. With the improved CO, the patient's urine output immediately increased.

Had CO remained low after afterload reduction was achieved, the transport crew would likely have sought to initiate an inotropic infusion. Dobutamine is the inotropic agent of choice for first-line treatment of low CO associated with heart failure.

Not all hemodynamic parameters discussed in this chapter were used in evaluating this patient. The patient's specific problems and the potential treatment options under consideration guide the hemodynamic measurements and calculations used. With the data used by the CCTPs receiving this patient, a clear picture of pump failure with low CO emerges. One question not apparent from these data is whether the perfusion needs of the patient are being met by the present CO. If the oxygen demand exceeds the oxygen supply, then the patient's condition will deteriorate, and most likely will continue to do so with the additional stress of transport.

Clearly, the patient's CO is low. The Svo$_2$ value would indicate whether the present CO is meeting the patient's perfusion needs. Some PACs have a fiberoptic oximetric tip that continuously displays the mixed venous oxygen saturation. Because this PAC did not, the transport crew requested that the hospital staff send a blood specimen from the pulmonary artery port of the PAC for blood gas analysis. The results showed an Svo$_2$ of 0.49 (49%), well below the normal range of 0.60 to 0.80 (60% to 80%). The result for a repeated specimen drawn after hemodynamics appeared more stable (ie, following initiation of the nitroprusside infusion) at 0.64 (64%), a dramatic improvement reflecting adequate tissue perfusion.

Prep Kit

Ready for Review

- Invasive hemodynamic monitoring is used to assess the heart, vascular network, and fluid volume status. It is used in conjunction with (not as a replacement for) physical assessment techniques such as capillary refill, skin color, skin turgor, body temperature, heart and lung sounds, and mental status.
- The atrioventricular (AV) valves (mitral and tricuspid) lie between the atria and the ventricles, and the semilunar valves (aortic and pulmonic) are the exits from the ventricles. The purpose of the cardiac valves is to prevent the backward flow of blood in the heart.
- The AV valves have chordae tendineae, which attach the edge of the valve to the papillary muscles attached to the endocardium; they hold the AV valves in place in the closed position and prevent them from prolapsing into the atria during systole or ventricular contraction. The semilunar valves do not have chordae tendineae; their opening and closing are related to the pressure changes in the heart, aorta, and pulmonary artery.
- Systole and diastole include five phases: atrial systole, isovolumetric contraction, ventricular ejection, isovolumetric relaxation, and ventricular filling.
- In atrial systole, the pressure in the ventricles increases. The atria contract, extra blood is ejected from the atria into the ventricles, the mitral and tricuspid valves are open, and the pulmonary and aortic valves are closed.
- Isovolumetric contraction occurs between the closure of the AV valves and the opening of the semilunar valves (in which no change in ventricular blood volume occurs) immediately before the blood is ejected through the semilunar valves. The pressure in the ventricles rises abruptly.

Prep Kit Continued

- During ventricular ejection, the pressure in the left ventricle exceeds the pressure in the aortic root, resulting in the aortic valve opening.
- During isovolumetric relaxation, the pressure in the ventricles is less than the arterial pressure. The ventricles are no longer contracting, the mitral and tricuspid valves are closed, and the pulmonary and aortic valves are closed.
- Ventricular filling occurs after the mitral and tricuspid valves open.
- Cardiac output (CO) is the product of stroke volume (SV) and heart rate: CO = SV × Heart rate. SV is determined by preload, afterload, and contractility of the heart. Because SV is determined by three components, heart rate contributes more to and has a more immediate effect on CO than any one component of SV. When confronted with a patient who has low CO, critical care transport professionals (CCTPs) should investigate the heart rate before evaluating the components of SV.
- Some hemodynamic values are indexed to account for differences in body size; for example, the cardiac index is the patient's CO divided by the total body surface area.
- Heart rate is a key sign of hemodynamic instability in the emergency or critical care patient. A heart rate obtained from a pulse oximeter is more reliable than manual assessment by the CCTP, particularly in the noisy environment of an intensive care unit or a CCTP vehicle.
- Preload is the degree of myocardial fiber stretch induced by volume in the ventricle at the end of diastole. Hypovolemia, venodilation, intrathoracic pressure changes, and intrapericardial pressure changes result in decreased preload. Hypervolemia and vasoconstriction result in increased preload.
- The Frank–Starling law states that a relationship exists between the distention of the ventricular myocardium and the force of the contraction. As the ventricular preload increases, the force of contraction of the myocardium also increases due to the increased stretch of the myocardial fibers. The Frank–Starling law describes how administration of fluids can improve CO to a certain point, which varies among individual patients. Additional fluids given beyond that point worsen CO.
- Right ventricular preload is measured by central venous pressure. Left ventricular preload is measured by pulmonary capillary wedge pressure (PCWP) or pulmonary artery diastolic pressure.
- Afterload is the resistance the ventricles must overcome to eject blood. Four factors typically determine afterload: outflow obstructions, vascular tone, blood viscosity, and ventricular dilation. Outflow obstructions, vasoconstriction, and polycythemia increase afterload. Vasodilation reduces afterload. Lowered hemoglobin levels are often tolerated in critically ill patients because CO may be improved by decreasing afterload. Left ventricular afterload is measured by systemic vascular resistance, and right ventricular afterload is measured by pulmonary vascular resistance (PVR).
- Contractility is the inotropic state of the heart or the force with which the heart muscle contracts. Contractility is assessed with newer Doppler and ultrasonography devices. Six factors influence contractility: myocardial muscle health, autonomic nervous system, metabolic states, the ion environment, pharmacologic agents, and heart rate.
- BP is measured directly through the use of an arterial line or indirectly through the use of a device that senses pulsatile flow such as a sphygmomanometer, which measures systolic and diastolic pressures. Indirect measurements assess flow, and direct monitoring devices measure pressure. Pressure and flow are different parameters, so readings obtained

Prep Kit Continued

using indirect and direct methods cannot be expected to correlate exactly.

- Direct pressure measurements are affected by changes in intrathoracic pressure. To obtain accurate measurements, readings should be taken at end expiration (the lower portions, or valleys, of the rise-and-fall pattern for mechanically ventilated patients; and the peaks of the rise-and-fall pattern for spontaneously breathing patients).
- Systolic BP (SBP) is the measure of pressure on the arterial walls during systole; diastolic BP (DBP) is the measure of pressure on the walls of the arteries during diastole. The formula for BP is CO multiplied by systemic vascular resistance (SVR): BP = CO × SVR.
- To avoid errors when using indirect monitoring devices to measure BP, CCTPs should be careful to use the correct BP cuff size for the patient and to position the patient's extremity in which BP is measured at mid-heart level.
- Transport monitors often include noninvasive BP (NIBP) units, which automatically measure indirect BP at predetermined intervals. The NIBP units measure heart rate and mean arterial pressure (MAP) only. Computer software then calculates SBP and DBP.
- CCTPs should evaluate the heart rate obtained from the NIBP unit against the actual patient pulse, the heart rate displayed on a pulse oximeter, or an ECG heart rate display to determine the accuracy of the NIBP measurements. If the NIBP heart rate differs significantly from the actual patient heart rate, then the calculated SBP and DBP should be considered unreliable.
- Invasive hemodynamic measurements are obtained via a closed catheter system, which is typically placed in the patient by a physician. Catheter placement is usually outside the scope of practice for CCTPs. Measurements are read on a monitor that is connected to a transducer on the catheter.

- Direct BP measurement using an arterial line is indicated for patients who require constant BP measurement, particularly patients who are in shock and are not responding to therapy. In addition, arterial lines are used for patients receiving vasoactive or antihypertensive infusions. The arterial line also confirms the presence of pulsatile blood flow and enables access for arterial blood samples for arterial blood gas analysis.
- Contraindications to the use of an arterial line include ischemia of the extremity, infection at the puncture site, Raynaud disease, and a prior vascular operation in the area of the insertion site.
- CCTPs generally do not place arterial lines, but they may need to assist in the procedure; therefore, they should be familiar with the insertion procedure.
- The Allen test is used to assess extremity perfusion and test ulnar artery function.
- Before moving a patient with hemodynamic monitoring equipment in place, CCTPs should examine the equipment in use, note the values displayed, and trace the tubing from each transducer to the pressure-monitoring catheter. The catheter site should be examined to ensure that it is visibly clean, dry, and covered by an occlusive dressing and its condition documented. A CCTP who is unfamiliar with the operation of the stopcocks and catheters in use should ask the clinician at the bedside to explain their operation.
- The patient can be transferred to a stretcher before or after transducers are connected to the transport monitor. A deliberate, orderly manner is needed when moving connections from the hospital monitor to the transport monitor to avoid periods when the patient is not connected to any monitor. Agency or service policy should be followed for securing monitoring lines and catheters during transport. Monitoring alarms need

Prep Kit Continued

to be set to protect against accidental dislodgement or dislocation of invasive monitoring catheters.

- The most common cause of error in obtaining direct hemodynamic pressure measurements is incorrect leveling of the transducer. To ensure accurate pressure readings, the transducer must be at mid-heart level. The transducer must be releveled with each position change of the patient. Because errors in leveling can significantly impact treatment decisions, all leveling should be performed using a carpenter's level or a leveling tool specifically designed for the hemodynamic monitoring application.

- Pressure transducers must be "zeroed" to eliminate the effects of atmospheric pressure on the measurements obtained. Depending on flight patterns and altitudes, transducers may be zeroed at initial connection to the transport monitor, at cruising altitude, and at the destination.

- CCTPs should become familiar with transport monitors, cables, and transducers. Cables must be compatible with the equipment used at the referring and receiving hospitals.

- Asepsis is critical in the care of patients with central lines and hemodynamic monitoring equipment. Key practices that decrease the incidence of catheter-related bloodstream infections include hand hygiene, strict adherence to aseptic technique, maximal sterile barrier precautions, chlorhexidine skin antisepsis, optimal catheter site selection, and use of an appropriate dressing after the catheter has been inserted.

- Central venous lines provide access to the core vessels of the body. The right internal jugular vein is the easiest site to access. Other common insertion sites are the subclavian, brachial, and femoral veins. Subclavian sites have the lowest infection risk; femoral sites have the highest risk for infection, and their use is strongly discouraged in adults.

- Central venous pressure (CVP) monitoring is used to determine right ventricular preload and intravascular volume status and to assess right-side heart function. The normal range for the CVP is 2 to 6 mm Hg. To ensure accuracy, CVP measurement should be obtained during end expiration.

- Central venous lines often include outlet ports, which are used for rapid fluid replacement, medication administration, rapid access to central circulation, and invasive monitoring.

- Only a few contraindications to central venous access exist. They include significant coagulopathy, local trauma to the site of insertion, and infection at the site of insertion.

- The most common complication associated with the insertion of a central line is pneumothorax or hemothorax from an unsuccessful attempt at subclavian line insertion. Other complications range from bleeding, to infection, to blood withdrawal problems.

- The triple-lumen catheter is the most commonly used central line. The lumens can be used for fluid and drug administration and for CVP monitoring. For some patients, one port may be reserved for total parenteral nutrition; that port should not be used during transport.

- Some central venous catheters have one or two access ports, and some are installed under the skin (tunneled). CCTPs should consult the receiving facility and local protocols for direction in using tunneled central lines.

- CCTPs should be familiar with the placement, use, and maintenance required for different types of catheters, including the Hickman catheter, the Groshong catheter, the Port-A-Cath, and the peripherally inserted central catheter. They should understand the possible complications and advantages and disadvantages of each catheter. All complications should be reported to the receiving facility as soon as possible.

Prep Kit Continued

- Although central venous lines are rarely placed by CCTPs, knowledge of how they are placed will help CCTPs care for patients who have a central venous line.
- The Seldinger technique is the technique most commonly used for line insertion. Specific procedures are used for femoral, internal jugular, and subclavian vein insertion.
- Common problems that occur when inserting a central venous line include sluggish infusion, inability to withdraw blood, and catheter damage.
- A pulmonary artery catheter (PAC), also known as a Swan–Ganz catheter or "swan," is inserted into the patient's venous system. Although CCTPs do not insert PACs, knowledge of the insertion procedure is useful in providing care.
- PACs have multiple lumens that terminate at different points along the catheter and correspond to different locations in the heart. PACs are marked at 10-cm intervals beginning at the distal tip of the catheter. CCTPs should note the centimeter measurement of the PAC at the introducer when initially assessing a patient. This information will help to determine whether the catheter has moved into or out of the patient during transport.
- The PAC measures right atrial (RA) and pulmonary artery pressure. The RA pressures are displayed as mean pressures; pulmonary artery pressures are displayed as systolic, diastolic, and mean values. Inflation of the PAC balloon blocks blood flow from the right ventricle behind the balloon tip and results in the appearance of a PCWP waveform on the monitor. The PCWP waveform is measured as a mean value.
- Complications with PAC insertion are nearly the same as those with central line insertion. Probably the greatest potential complication of PAC use is misinterpretation of the data by clinicians, resulting in inappropriate therapy and potentially worsening outcomes.
- A thermistor is connected to the distal end of the PAC. The thermistor measures thermodilution CO and provides a continuous reading of the pulmonary artery temperature, which is considered the gold standard for core body temperature measurement.
- Indications for the use of PACs are based on clinician experience, not outcome studies. Clinicians are advised to consider the risks and benefits for critically ill patients on an individual basis.
- Contraindications to the use of a PAC include significant coagulopathy, local trauma to the site of insertion, infection at the site of insertion, and inability to float the PAC into the pulmonary artery.
- CCTPs should be familiar with normal hemodynamic ranges and values, as well as the lines from which these measurements are obtained.
- Continuous BP monitoring through an arterial line provides CCTPs with constantly updated SBP, DBP, and MAP values and an arterial waveform. Components of the arterial waveform include the dicrotic notch, mean pressure, systole, diastole, systolic pulse pressure, and diastolic pulse pressure.
- The MAP is a function of the SBP and DBP. It is calculated by the transport monitor software or the CCTP. A MAP between 70 and 105 mm Hg is needed to satisfactorily perfuse the body's tissues; most medical orders require titration of drugs or administration of fluids to maintain a MAP of 70 mm Hg or greater.
- Regardless of whether direct monitoring with an arterial line or indirect monitoring with an NIBP is performed, the MAP is the value that should be used to make treatment decisions.
- Pulse pressure is another value calculated using SBP and DBP readings. It is the mathematical difference between these values. Normal values are 40 to 60 mm Hg.
- Central venous pressure (CVP) is a measure of the vena caval and right atrial pressures.

Prep Kit Continued

It is measured from a central venous line or pulmonary artery catheter. A CVP waveform tracing has systolic and diastolic values, but only the mean is used in clinical practice because the numbers are extremely low.

- The normal range for CVP is 2 to 6 mm Hg. Fluids are often administered to patients with CVP values below 5 to 8 mm Hg to increase their preload.
- Pulmonary artery catheter measurements include right ventricular pressure, pulmonary artery pressure, PCWP, and CO. CCTPs should know the normal values for each of these measurements and how to evaluate each of the measurements.
- CCTPs should be able to recognize a right ventricular waveform and its characteristic low diastolic pressure, which distinguishes it from a pulmonary artery pressure waveform.
- A CCTP who observes a sudden elevation in pulmonary artery pressures should immediately assess and correct any issues with oxygen saturation or ventilation. If pulmonary artery diastolic pressures suddenly drop, then the catheter position should be reevaluated to determine if the PAC has migrated into the right ventricle.
- CCTPs should also know how to read a PCWP waveform. When a PCWP waveform is observed, the tracing can be frozen on the monitor screen, and the balloon should be allowed to passively deflate.
- The thermodilution method is typically used to assess CO with a pulmonary artery catheter. Most transport monitors are not capable of performing thermodilution CO measurements during transport.
- CO can be calculated or estimated by using the Fick principle. The formula used is as follows:

$$CO = \frac{\text{Oxygen Consumption}}{\text{Arteriovenous Oxygen Content Defference}}$$

- PVR is the resistance of the pulmonary vascular circuit that opposes flow out of the right ventricle and pulmonary artery. It is commonly referred to as right-side heart afterload. PVR may be elevated in patients with pulmonary hypertension or mitral valve stenosis.
- SVR is the total impedance to blood flow felt by the left ventricle, commonly referred to as afterload. Calculation of SVR is helpful in determining the cause of shock.
- The amount of blood ejected in each stroke of a ventricle is measured in milliliters and recorded as the SV. A normal SV is 60 to 100 mL/beat.
- Mixed venous oxygen saturation (Svo_2) reflects the global balance between oxygen delivery and consumption. It is measured at the distal end of the PAC because the pulmonary artery is the most appropriate place to sample a mixture of all the blood returning from the body. Four components contribute to Svo_2: total hemoglobin level, arterial oxygen saturation, CO, and oxygen consumption.
- Mixed central venous oxygen saturation ($Scvo_2$) reflects the balance between oxygen supply and delivery in the brain and upper body.
- Myocardial oxygen supply must balance myocardial oxygen demand to meet the body's myocardial metabolic requirements; otherwise, ischemia will occur.
- Prompt recognition and reversal of shock can help avoid a rapidly irreversible sequence of events that can result in the patient's death. Understanding the relationship between hemodynamic measurements and the different types of shock can help CCTPs recognize the type of shock and assess the effectiveness of treatment during transport.
- Oxygen saturation and gas expansion are concerns during flight. CCTPs should closely monitor the patient's oxygen saturation level so they can quickly respond to changes in the patient's condition and maintain sufficient levels of inspired oxygen. Gas expansion should be addressed by removing air from IV bags, using pumps for medication infusions, and zeroing transducers.

Prep Kit Continued

Vital Vocabulary

afterload The tension or stress that develops in the ventricles during systole; measured by pulmonary and systemic vascular resistance.

Allen test A technique in which the patient's hand is initially held above the head while the fist is clenched and the radial and ulnar arteries are compressed; the hand is then lowered and the fist is opened, ulnar pressure is released, and radial pressure is maintained. After the ulnar pressure is released, color should return to the hand within 6 seconds.

arterial lines Catheters inserted into the patient's arterial vascular system for the purpose of producing a waveform with pressure measurements; also called A-lines.

atrioventricular (AV) valves The valves (mitral and tricuspid) that separate the atria from the ventricles.

cardiac index (CI) A hemodynamic value that adjusts a patient's cardiac output to take into account the total body surface area.

cardiac output (CO) The amount of blood pumped out of the heart in 1 minute; the product of the stroke volume (average = 70 mL) and the heart rate (average = 60 to 100 beats/min).

caudal Pertaining to or in the direction of the feet.

central line–associated bloodstream infection (CLABSI) A primary bloodstream infection that develops in a patient who had a central line in place within the 48-hour period prior to the onset of the bloodstream infection.

central venous lines Intravenous access catheters that terminate in the central circulation, usually just proximal to the right atrium.

central venous pressure (CVP) The pressure in the superior vena cava (average = 2 to 6 cm H_2O), which reflects the pressure in the venous system when the blood is returned to the right atrium. It

is indicative of a patient's fluid volume status and right-side heart performance.

cephalad Pertaining to or in the direction of the head or front.

chordae tendineae Tendons that connect the papillary muscles to the tricuspid and mitral valves.

dampened waveform A hemodynamic pressure waveform that appears to have lost crisp deflections.

diastole The relaxation phase of the heart cycle, in which the ventricles are dilated and filling with blood.

diastolic blood pressure (DBP) The trough or resting pressure in the arterial system that occurs during ventricular diastole.

dicrotic notch The brief increase in aortic pressure reflected in a notching of the wave; it is caused by the sudden closure and springing back of the aortic valve leaflets, and signals the start of diastole.

ejection fraction The average percentage of blood ejected from the left ventricle with each heartbeat.

Fick principle A method of indirectly determining cardiac output, in which the amount of oxygen uptake of blood as it passes through the lungs is equal to the oxygen concentration difference between mixed venous and arterial blood. The formula uses assumed values for oxygen consumption derived from basal metabolic studies on healthy subjects, which may or may not be valid in critically ill patients.

Frank–Starling law The principle that the force of the cardiac muscle contraction is proportional to the amount of stretch placed on the muscle fibers (meaning that the more the heart is stretched by the incoming blood, the more forcefully the ventricles contract and the more blood that is ejected); it demonstrates how changes in

Prep Kit Continued

ventricular preload lead to changes in stroke volume. Also called the Starling curve.

invasive hemodynamic monitoring Methods for assessing the physiologic condition of the three principal components of the cardiovascular system: heart, vascular network, and fluid volume. It mainly assesses the capability of a patient's heart to pump the requisite amount of blood to the body, but also can assess compliance, tone, resistance of the vascular network, and fluid status; it includes a variety of pressure values and other measurements.

isovolumetric contraction The early stage of ventricular contraction during which ventricular blood volume is unchanging because all valves are closed (the semilunar valves have not yet opened).

isovolumetric relaxation The early stage of ventricular relaxation during which ventricular blood volume is unchanging because all valves are closed (the atrioventricular valves have not yet opened).

left ventricular end-diastolic pressure The pressure exerted on the left ventricle at the end of diastole; the normal value is 4 to 12 mm Hg and is measured by using a pulmonary artery catheter.

left ventricular stroke work index A calculation of the contractility of the left ventricle indexed to the patient's body surface area; equivalent to the stroke volume index.

leveling The process of ensuring that the hemodynamic pressure transducer is at the level of the atrium, which also corresponds to the level of the aortic root.

mean arterial pressure (MAP) The average (ie, constant) pressure in the arterial vasculature; a function of the systolic and diastolic blood pressures.

microcirculation Blood circulation provided to the tissues by the terminal end of vascular blood distribution: the capillaries, arterioles, postcapillary venules, and subunits.

mixed central venous oxygen saturation (Scvo$_2$) The percentage of oxygen bound to hemoglobin in blood returning to the right side of the heart from the head and upper body, which is representative of oxygen extraction from the blood by the head and upper extremities.

mixed venous oxygen saturation (Svo$_2$) The percentage of oxygen bound to hemoglobin in blood returning to the right side of the heart, which is representative of global oxygen extraction from the blood.

myocardial oxygen consumption (MVo$_2$) The volume of oxygen that the heart muscle consumes; an expression of the level of oxygen demand in the heart.

papillary muscles A type of muscle in the ventricle from which the chordae tendineae extend and attach to the cusps of the atrioventricular valves.

perfusion The circulation of oxygen and nutrients at the cellular level and removal of waste products of metabolism for elimination.

phlebostatic axis An imaginary point located at the fourth intercostal space, mid-chest level, which serves as an external landmark for the right atrium.

preload The end-diastolic stretch of the muscle fibers of the ventricle; measured by right atrial pressure or central venous pressure and wedge pressure.

Poiseuille's law The relationship that flow varies directly with any increase in pressure.

pulmonary artery catheter (PAC) A catheter with a balloon near its tip that is passed through a vein into the right side of the heart, through the right ventricle, and into the pulmonary artery; it records the pressure transmitted back from the left atrium. Also called a Swan–Ganz catheter.

pulmonary artery pressure The pressure measured in the pulmonary artery, usually displayed with a pressure waveform and digital systolic, diastolic, and mean values.

Prep Kit Continued

pulmonary capillary wedge pressure (PCWP) The mean pressure measured while occluding the pulmonary artery with a balloon-tipped catheter proximal to the site of measurement; it reflects left atrial pressure. Also called pulmonary artery wedge pressure or pulmonary artery occlusion pressure.

pulmonary vascular resistance (PVR) The resistance or impedance to ejection of the right ventricle of the heart.

pulse pressure The difference between the systolic and diastolic blood pressures.

pulsus paradoxus A decrease of more than 10 mm Hg in systolic blood pressure during inspiration.

right ventricular pressure The pressure in the right ventricle, which consists of the systolic, diastolic, and mean pressures; it is important during insertion and use of a pulmonary artery catheter.

right ventricular stroke work index A calculation of the contractility of the right ventricle indexed to the patient's body surface area.

Seldinger technique The technique most commonly used for inserting a central venous line. It involves inserting a needle with a syringe, then inserting a guide wire into the needle. After the guide wire is in place, the needle is removed, an incision is made, and a catheter is inserted over the guide wire; the guide wire is then removed.

semilunar valves The valves (aortic and pulmonic) that are the exits from the left and right ventricles into the aorta and the pulmonary artery, respectively.

stroke volume (SV) The amount of blood ejected by the ventricles during each contraction; it varies between 60 and 100 mL/beat, with the average being 70 mL.

stroke volume index A calculation of the contractility of the left ventricle indexed to the patient's body surface area; equivalent to the left ventricular stroke work index.

systemic vascular resistance (SVR) The resistance or impedance to ejection of the left ventricle of the heart.

systole The contraction phase of the heart cycle in which the ventricles pump blood out of the heart through the aorta and the pulmonary artery into the systemic and pulmonary circulatory systems.

systolic blood pressure (SBP) Peak pressure in the arterial system, which occurs during ventricular ejection or systole.

thermistor The apparatus used for quickly determining very small changes in pulmonary artery temperature.

triple-lumen catheter A type of catheter consisting of three distinct continuous tubes that allow for pressure monitoring, blood sampling, and fluid and drug administration.

zeroing The process of calibrating a pressure transducer to eliminate extraneous atmospheric and hydrostatic pressures from the data being measured.

References

Ahrens T. Continuous mixed venous (Svo$_2$) monitoring: too expensive or indispensable? *Crit Care Nurs Clin North Am.* 1999;11(1):33-48.

Ahrens T. Hemodynamic monitoring. *Crit Care Nurs Clin North Am.* 1999;11(1):19-31.

Ahrens T, Penick JC, Tucker MK. Frequency requirements for zeroing transducers in hemodynamic monitoring. *Am J Crit Care.* 1995;4(6):466-471.

Bridges EJ. Monitoring pulmonary artery pressures: just the facts. *Crit Care Nurse.* 2000;20(6):59-80.

Centers for Disease Control and Prevention. Bloodstream infection event (central line–associated bloodstream infection and non-central line–associated bloodstream infection. http://www.cdc.gov/nhsn/pdfs/pscmanual/4psc _clabscurrent.pdf. Published January 2021. Accessed November 11, 2021.

Prep Kit Continued

Chang D. *Clinical Application of Mechanical Ventilation*. 4th ed. Clifton Park, NY: Delmar; 2014.

Darovic DO. *Hemodynamic Monitoring: Invasive and Noninvasive Clinical Application*. 3rd ed. St. Louis, MO: Saunders; 2002.

DeBacker D, Durand A. Monitoring the microcirculation in critically ill patients. *Best Pract Res Clin Anaesthiol*. 2014;25:441-451.

Hall JE. *Guyton and Hall Textbook of Medical Physiology*. 13th ed. Philadelphia, PA: Elsevier; 2015.

Haupt MT, Kaufman BS, Carlson RW. Fluid resuscitation in patients with increased vascular permeability. *Crit Care Clin*. 1992;8(2):341-353.

Hersh LT, Sesing JC, Luczyk WJ, Friedman BA, Zhou S, Batchelder PB. Validation of a conical cuff on the forearm for estimating radial artery blood pressure. *Blood Press Monit*. 2014;19(1):38-45.

Hinkle JL, Cheever KH, Overbaugh K. *Brunner and Suddarth's Textbook of Medical–Surgical Nursing*. 15th ed. Philadelphia, PA: Lippincott Williams and Wilkins; 2021.

Jaschke K, Brown D, Clark A, et al. Speed of blood withdrawal and accurate measurement of oxygen content in mixed venous blood. *Am J Crit Care*. 2014;23(6):486-493.

Lanken P, Manaker S, Kohl BA, Hanson CW III. *The Intensive Care Unit Manual*. 2nd ed. Philadelphia, PA: WB Saunders; 2013.

Lehman LW, Saeed M, Talmor D, Mark R, Malhotra A. Methods of blood pressure measurement in the ICU. *Crit Care Med*. 2013;41(1):34-40.

Lough ME. *Hemodynamic Monitoring: Evolving Technologies and Clinical Practice*. St. Louis, MO: Mosby; 2016.

Marik PE, Monnet X, Teboul J-L. Hemodynamic parameters to guide fluid therapy. *Ann Intens Care*. 2011;1:1.

Mermel LA. Prevention of intravascular catheter–related infections. *Ann Intern Med*. 2000;132(5):391-402.

Michard F, Boussat S, Chemla D, et al. Relation between respiratory changes in arterial pulse pressure and fluid responsiveness in septic patients with acute circulatory failure. *Am J Respir Crit Care Med*. 2000;162(1):134-138.

Monnet X, Rienzo M, Osman D, et al. Passive leg raising predicts fluid responsiveness in the critically ill. *Crit Care Med*. 2006;34(5):1402-1407.

Monnet X, Saugel B. Could resuscitation be based on microcirculation data? We are not sure. *Intens Care Med*. 2018;44:950-953.

Parsons P, Wiener-Kronish J, Stapleton RD, Berra L. *Critical Care Secrets*. 6th ed. Philadelphia, PA: Elsevier; 2018.

Patel P, Weiner-Lastinger L, Dudeck M, et al. Impact of COVID-19 pandemic on central-line–associated bloodstream infections during the early months of 2020, National Healthcare Safety Network. *Infect Control Hosp Epidemiol*. 2021:1-4. doi:10.1017/ice.2021.108.

Senzaki H, ed. *Hemodynamics: Monitoring, Theory and Applications*. New York, NY: Nova Science Publishers; 2013.

Shoemaker WC, Velmahos GC, Demetriades D. *Procedures and Monitoring for the Critically Ill*. Philadelphia, PA: Saunders; 2002.

Soufir L, Timsit JF, Mahe C, Carlet J, Regnier B, Chevret S. Attributable morbidity and mortality of catheter related septicemia in critically ill patients: a matched, risk-adjusted, cohort study. *Infect Control Hosp Epidemiol*. 1999;20(6):396-401.

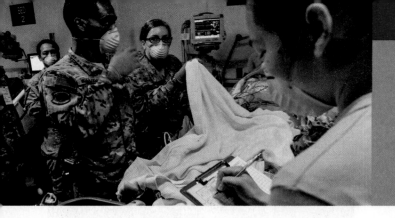

Chapter 16

Mechanical Circulatory Support

W. David Sadler, MS, BSN, CCRN, CFRN, NRP

Johnnie Peoples, BSN, CCRN, CFRN, NREMT-P

William Hallinan, MSBA, RN

OBJECTIVES

After completing this chapter, you will be able to:
1. Describe the technical considerations in transporting a patient receiving mechanical circulatory support (MCS) (pp 841–842).
2. Explain how MCS systems interact with native circulation (p 841).
3. Discuss the considerations a provider should address when caring for a patient receiving MCS (pp 841–842).
4. Discuss how a team should approach and organize a transport involving MCS (p 842).
5. Discuss the principles of and indications for intra-aortic balloon pump therapy (p 842).
6. Discuss the principles of and indications for extracorporeal membrane oxygenation (p 860).
7. Discuss the principles of and indications for a microaxial catheter pump system (pp 866–868).
8. Discuss the principles of and indications for implantable left ventricular assist devices (pp 869–886).

Introduction

Mechanically assisted circulation, mechanical circulatory systems, and ventricular assist devices all describe means of augmenting or replacing the native cardiac output (CO) from the heart. The general term used for these interventions in this chapter is mechanical circulatory support (MCS). MCS may be used to treat both acute and chronic conditions and may apply either a univentricular or biventricular approach, where the circulatory system's pumping mechanism may be external to the body (ie, extra-corporeal) or internal to the body (*intracorporeal*). MCS may be complemented by gas exchange, temperature control, or renal replacement therapy.

MCS may occur in the prehospital, community hospital, or specialty hospital setting. As patient volume grows, the critical care transport provider (CCTP) will, in turn, be called upon to transport these patients with increasing frequency. Given the advanced medical technology and rapidly progressing nature of this field, CCTPs will need to stay current and competent on the procedures and equipment used to support and care for patients receiving MCS.

Safe transport should focus on detailed assessment and patient monitoring, balanced with high-quality patient care and technical proficiency with the pump system. Critical care transport (CCT) teams should include members who have been adequately trained and have demonstrated competency working in this transport environment. Team members should have a strong understanding of the interdependence of the pump system and the patient, including how the patient interacts with the pump.

This chapter addresses the commonly seen pump platforms: the intra-aortic balloon pump (IABP), the microaxial percutaneous pump, extracorporeal membrane oxygenation, and left ventricular (LV) assist systems.

Intra-aortic Balloon Pump

The earliest and perhaps best-known cardiac-assist device is the IABP. Intra-aortic balloon pump (IABP) therapy involves use of a balloon connected to a pump via a catheter that has been inserted into the aorta to provide temporary assistance to a failing heart. IABP counterpulsation is a therapy used worldwide to assist patients with LV failure.

IABP units have benefited from miniaturization, such that some IABP models will fit easily into a helicopter for transport. The intra-aortic balloon (IAB) catheters have also become smaller, with multiple-lumen designs allowing for arterial pressure monitoring, IAB inflation and deflation, and, in current models, fiberoptic sensors.

Important responsibilities of the CCTP include securing the patient to prevent movement of the balloon (which can create significant problems or injuries) and ensuring that all equipment has the necessary power supply to continue operating during transport **FIGURE 16-1**. Although the transport of a patient during IABP therapy can be a daunting task for even IABP-trained transport professionals, CCTPs can obtain the knowledge and skills necessary to comfortably assist in this situation, and in some programs may actually transport patients receiving IABP therapy themselves. IABP therapy is an advanced skill. This section discusses maintaining IABP therapy, recognizing and

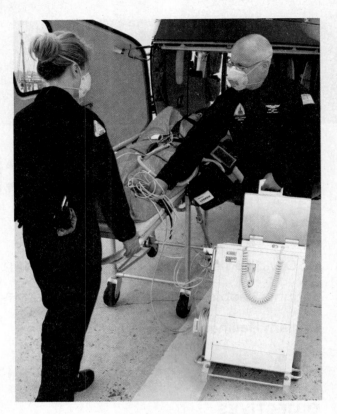

FIGURE 16-1 An important CCTP responsibility when transporting a patient with an intra-aortic balloon is to secure the patient to prevent balloon movement.

© Jones & Bartlett Learning.

correcting problems, and performing emergency procedures during IABP failure. It is not intended to be an all-inclusive guide to IABP therapy.

Most CCT programs require that a CCTP be accompanied by a certified perfusionist or critical care registered nurse knowledgeable about the IABP. Thus, CCTPs will be working with a colleague with additional training in this area on calls that involve a patient receiving IABP therapy.

Mechanics of IABP Function

IABP therapy begins with the insertion (by a trained and credentialed provider, physician, or surgeon) of a balloon, typically via the femoral artery, into the descending thoracic aorta. The tip of the balloon catheter is located just distal (approximately 0.75 inch [2 cm] below) the takeoff of the left subclavian artery. After it is in place, the balloon is connected to a console to shuttle helium gas; the balloon is inflated with this gas at the onset of diastole and then deflated just before systole (ventricular ejection).

Inflation and deflation are timed to the cardiac cycle, resulting in significant augmentation of flow to the coronary and renal arteries during diastole (increased supply) and substantially reduced afterload during systole (decreased demand).

Balloon Structure and Position

The IAB catheter consists of a long, narrow balloon mounted on a thin catheter. Older catheters had two lumens: a central lumen and a gas lumen. Newer catheters have a third, fiberoptic lumen.

- The **central lumen** is used to guide catheter insertion into the femoral artery and through the arterial system, positioning the IAB tip in the descending thoracic aorta just below the origin of the left subclavian artery **FIGURE 16-2**. After the catheter is in place, the central lumen also allows monitoring of aortic blood pressure (BP) through a setup much like a standard arterial line.
- The **gas lumen** carries helium gas from the pump console to the IAB to control balloon inflation.

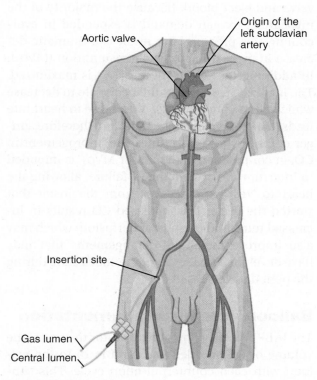

FIGURE 16-2 Intra-aortic balloon placement.

Illustration from source material by Datascope Corp. and Maquet Cardiovascular. Used with permission.

- The fiberoptic lumen contains fiberoptic strands used to measure aortic pressure and (in some models) aortic oximetry.

Typically, the IABP catheter is threaded into the descending aorta through the femoral artery. Alternative placement strategies for these catheters include access through the axillary artery and, rarely, transthoracic placement, which is typically reserved for critically ill patients unable to be weaned from cardiopulmonary bypass following cardiac operations in whom femoral access is not possible or is contraindicated.

Insertion can be accomplished through a sheath (a large-diameter catheter placed into a vessel to allow smaller catheters or devices to be inserted through the catheter lumen into the vessel) or by using a catheter designed for sheathless insertion. When access to the femoral artery has already been obtained using a sheath (such as in a cardiac catheterization laboratory), a practitioner inserting an IABP catheter may decide to insert the device through the existing sheath rather than making a separate puncture. When IABP placement is elective or planned, or when significant concerns about leg ischemia exist, sheathless insertion offers the advantage of an overall smaller-diameter device in the access vessel. Sheathless insertion, then, may reduce complications of limb ischemia by reducing the size of the obstruction in the femoral artery.

Counterpulsation Sequence

Following placement of the catheter, it is connected to the IABP console. The IABP console pump inflates and deflates the balloon with helium in conjunction with the mechanical cardiac cycle. Helium is used because of its low molecular weight, which allows it to be pumped rapidly without much turbulence from the flow of the gas. Helium also enhances the safety of this therapy because it is less likely to cause an air embolus if the balloon ruptures. Correct IABP timing inflates the balloon during diastole when the LV is relaxed and the coronary arteries are filling with oxygenated blood **FIGURE 16-3**.

During IABP therapy, the balloon deflates during systole and inflates during diastole. An electrocardiography (ECG) machine determines when the balloon should be inflated and deflated. If a ECG signal is unavailable, then timing can be triggered based on an arterial pressure waveform or at a fixed rate.

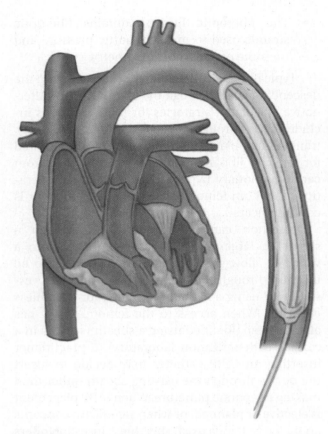

FIGURE 16-3 Intra-aortic balloon inflation.

Illustration from source material by Datascope Corp. and Maquet Cardiovascular. Used with permission.

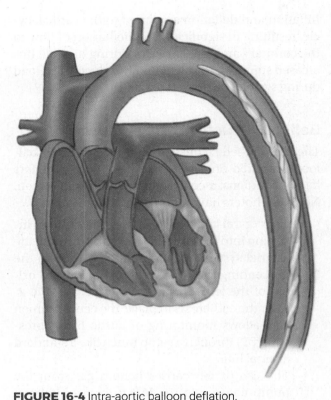

FIGURE 16-4 Intra-aortic balloon deflation.

Illustration from source material by Datascope Corp. and Maquet Cardiovascular. Used with permission.

Physiologic Effects of IABP Therapy

For patients in cardiogenic shock, IABP therapy lowers systolic blood pressure (SBP) as the balloon deflates at the onset of systole and raises diastolic pressure when the balloon inflates during diastole. Mean arterial pressure (MAP) will also rise as a result of the diastolic augmentation. Diastolic augmentation may be best thought of as a "second systole" because it occurs during diastole, but the rapid inflation of the balloon augments the diastolic pressure and effectively creates a second pressure wave to perfuse the heart and tissues. This sudden increase in pressure improves the flow to the coronary arteries and systemic circulation.

The balloon deflates at the end of diastole, just before the next ventricular ejection **FIGURE 16-4**. The sudden deflation of the balloon causes a drop in aortic pressure because the space that was occupied by the balloon is suddenly gone. This dramatic drop in pressure reduces the resistance against which the ventricle has to work to open the aortic valve and eject blood. Because the majority of the myocardial oxygen demand is expended in overcoming this pressure, the result is a dramatic decrease in myocardial oxygen consumption (MVo_2). In addition, the stroke volume (SV) is maximized. The increase in SV allows the heart rate to decrease while still maintaining CO. A decrease in heart rate leads to increased diastolic time and, therefore, longer coronary perfusion time. The improvement in CO, in conjunction with a lower MVo_2, is intended to interrupt the cycle of heart failure, allowing the heart to "rest" and recover from the insult that started the cycle. The increased CO results in increased renal and peripheral perfusion, which may also improve metabolic derangements that may have developed as a result of the shock state during the period of decreased CO.

Balloon Volume or Augmentation

The IABP console allows the operator to control the volume of gas shuttled back and forth to the balloon with each counterpulsation cycle. This control is referred to as either augmentation or balloon volume. Typically, when IABP therapy is initiated immediately after the IABP catheter is inserted, software in the console begins shuttling gas at the lowest volume possible, gradually increasing the volume over several inflation–deflation cycles to allow the balloon to unfurl from the compressed condition in which it is packaged.

During routine use or during transport, little reason exists to adjust the balloon volume or augmentation to less than maximal or full volume. This control is used with nonstandard balloon catheters, such as might be inserted in pediatric patients or, in some settings, to wean the patient from IABP therapy before removing the balloon. Given that a fully inflated balloon rarely occupies more than one-half the total diameter of the average aorta, weaning is more efficiently accomplished by reducing the assist ratio or frequency (discussed later in this chapter) rather than the inflation volume.

Waveform Changes and Triggers

The **timing** of the balloon's inflation and deflation is crucial; if inflation and deflation do not occur at the proper time in the cardiac cycle, then the device will not only fail to yield the desired results, but also could harm the patient. In earlier-model IABP consoles, it was necessary to ensure that timing occurred at the proper points in the cardiac cycle. Modern consoles use complex computerized algorithms to continually monitor the patient's ECG and pressure waveforms, optimizing timing with a level of accuracy that exceeds the capabilities of human operators. Although it is possible for the CCTP to modify IABP timing, this modification is almost never necessary except in emergency situations. However, because improper timing can be detrimental to the patient, it is important for clinicians to be able to recognize incorrect timing and understand the implications for the patient. Not only does poor timing fail to maximize IABP therapy, but errors in timing, such as late deflation of the balloon, can actually worsen heart failure and early inflation can damage the aortic valve.

The console constantly monitors the arterial pressure waveform, the patient's ECG, and the balloon gas pressure waveform during pumping to evaluate and adjust the timing and effectiveness of the therapy. The arterial pressure waveform that the IABP console monitors may come from the central lumen of the IAB catheter, from the fiberoptic

catheter, or from a peripheral arterial catheter **FIGURE 16-5** and **FIGURE 16-6**. IAB inflation and deflation can be set to respond to the ECG, a pressure waveform, a pacemaker, an internally preprogrammed rate, or combinations of these factors. The most reliable triggering mechanism, however, is based on the ECG. Triggering the IABP from the ECG provides the optimal timing for inflation and deflation while still permitting the IAB to immediately deflate if the console senses an increase in pressure indicating ventricular ejection (such as with a premature ventricular or atrial contraction), a paced beat, or another signal that systole has begun. Most modern IABP console computers are able to track irregular arrhythmias and tachyarrhythmias (eg, atrial fibrillation) and adjust the timing as needed to protect the patient. The provider caring for the patient chooses the trigger best suited to the patient's condition.

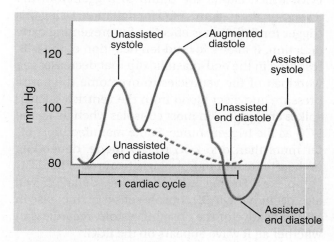

FIGURE 16-5 Arterial pressure waveform during intra-aortic balloon pump therapy.

Illustration from source material by Datascope Corp. and Maquet Cardiovascular. Used with permission.

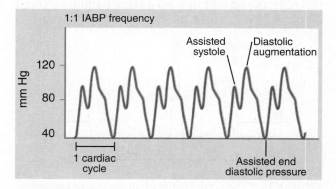

FIGURE 16-6 Diastolic augmentation.

Illustration from source material by Datascope Corp. and Maquet Cardiovascular. Used with permission.

Trigger Selection

Trigger signals available to initiate balloon inflation and deflation vary by manufacturer, although all IABP consoles usually default to using the QRS complex from the ECG to locate each cardiac cycle **FIGURE 16-7**. Current-generation IABP consoles have sophisticated computer software capable of not only recognizing changes in heart rate, balloon pressure, patient BP, tubing dead space, and console pneumatic rate of response, but also instantly making changes in timing to inflate and maintain balloon inflation throughout diastole. So-called real timing using sophisticated computer software offers greater afterload reduction and improved MAP by extending the inflation period into the early isovolumetric contraction period.

ECG Triggering

The safest trigger on most IABP consoles is the ECG, which allows the pump to trigger from the R wave on the patient's ECG for deflation. Using this trigger for deflation is effective for preventing early deflation. It allows for sudden deflation of the IAB, resulting in the end-diastolic dip that decreases the workload of the ventricles to overcome the aortic pressure and eject blood from the ventricles. Pacer spikes are ignored in most consoles when using the ECG as the trigger source. Some manufacturers offer more than one ECG trigger mode, depending on heart rate and morphologic features of the ECG complexes. During ECG triggering, deflation will also occur if the IABP console senses an increase in SBP indicative of the onset of systole, regardless of whether an R wave appears on the ECG.

Pressure Triggering

Pressure can also be selected as a trigger source. In this case, the systolic upstroke of the patient's arterial pressure waveform is used as the trigger source. Using pressure as a trigger source is not as desirable as using the ECG because pressure delays deflation until systolic ejection has already begun, reducing the beneficial effects of deflation simultaneously with ventricular ejection. With pressure selected as the trigger, most IABP consoles ignore the ECG signal. Pressure is the preferred trigger mode during cardiopulmonary resuscitation (CPR) because it works synchronously with compressions to improve diastolic perfusion. This mode can be useful when the ECG signal is unavailable, excessive artifact exists, or ECG voltage is too low to produce a recognizable R wave. Excessive movement of ECG wires, very active patients, and procedures such as operations that involve considerable staff contact with ECG lead areas or electrocautery interference with ECG signals may make pressure a desirable trigger mode.

Pacemaker Triggering

Most IABP consoles also offer a pacemaker trigger, which may be set based on either atrial-paced or ventricular-paced rhythms. The only time that pacemaker triggers are useful is when the patient rhythm is 100% paced and the QRS complex has such poor morphologic features that the IABP console cannot use it when operating in the ECG trigger mode. For patients with an AV-paced rhythm, the ventricular-paced trigger should be selected if pacer triggering is required. Most IABP consoles also offer an internal trigger mode that works completely asynchronously with the patient's ECG and arterial pressure. This internal trigger mode should never be used in any patient with a cardiac output, including patients undergoing CPR. Situations when internal triggering may be used are generally limited to cardiac surgical procedures where no ECG and external circulatory support is available. Internal triggering can prevent thrombus formation on the IABP catheter in such cases.

Evaluation of an IABP Waveform

The IABP device has the option to pump in several modes called **assist ratios** or IABP frequency. These modes are as follows:

- 1:1 assist ratio, in which the pump inflates with each heartbeat
- 1:2 assist ratio, in which the pump inflates with every other heartbeat

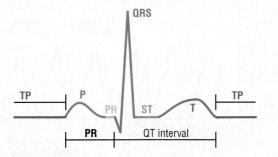

FIGURE 16-7 The components of an electrocardiographic strip.

Data from *12-Lead ECG: The Art of Interpretation*, courtesy of Tomas B. Garcia, MD.

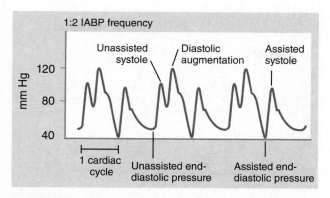

FIGURE 16-8 Pressure waveform augmented with a 1:2 assist ratio.

Illustration from source material by Datascope Corp. and Maquet Cardiovascular. Used with permission.

- 1:3 assist ratio, in which the pump inflates with every third heartbeat
- 1:4 assist ratio, in which the pump inflates with every fourth heartbeat
- 1:8 assist ratio, in which the pump inflates with every eighth heartbeat

The CCTP should assess several parameters of the waveform. The evaluation of the IABP waveform is most easily accomplished by placing the IABP into the 1:2 assist ratio, which allows comparison of pressure waves of the unassisted cycle with the assisted one. In this mode, every other contraction is augmented by the IABP. In a strip of 1:2 augmentation waveforms, the peaks created by the inflation of the IAB are easily identified because they should be the highest pressure peaks **FIGURE 16-8**. Because the IAB inflates during diastole, these pressure waveforms are referred to as the diastolic augmentation waveforms. The pressure waveform that follows the diastolic augmentation peak (IAB inflation) is referred to as the assisted systole waveform because the deflation of the IAB assists the ventricle in ejecting blood, thereby reducing the ventricular afterload (the resistance that must be overcome to eject the blood from the ventricles). The third pressure waveform is referred to as unassisted systole because the balloon pump is not moving and the waveform reflects what would normally occur without IABP intervention.

To evaluate for correct IABP timing, the pressure peaks, slopes, and inflation and deflation points of each of these pressure waveforms must be evaluated in a systematic manner. The parameters of the IABP waveform that should be evaluated are as follows:

- **Systole and diastole of each pressure waveform.** Although it may seem confusing at first, it is critical to identify systole and diastole in the pressure waveforms. The balloon inflation gives an appearance of systole as the pressure peaks are high; however, it is important to remember that the heart is in diastole. It may help to think of balloon inflation as a second systole that occurs in diastole.
- **Diastolic augmentation, assisted systole, and unassisted systole.** When looking at a 1:2 augmentation strip, this step can be done easily by identifying the balloon inflation. This pressure waveform will be the diastolic augmentation. Immediately before this waveform is the unassisted systole. The pressure waveform that occurs immediately after the diastolic augmentation is the assisted systole.
- **The point of inflation.** Inflation should occur at the dicrotic notch, which signals the closure of the aortic valve **FIGURE 16-9A**. In the rare case in which the operator might need to adjust the timing, the dicrotic notch can be visualized by manually moving the IAB inflation point to a later time in the cardiac cycle. After the dicrotic notch is located, the inflation should be adjusted to an earlier time until the notch created by the inflation of the balloon on the dicrotic notch forms a crisp *V* **FIGURE 16-9B**. The balloon inflation point should be reflected on the pressure waveform as a sudden increase in pressure during diastole. A crisp *V* with no evidence of the dicrotic notch reflects inflation of the balloon immediately at the onset of diastole. If the dicrotic notch is visible, then inflation is likely occurring too late. If inflation occurs too early, then the *V* will open slightly as the slope of the diastolic augmentation decreases slightly (less steep slope).
- **End-diastolic dip in pressure created by balloon deflation.** The end-diastolic dip should dip below the baseline end-diastolic pressure (EDP) occurring with unassisted systole. This dip should be followed by a straight-line slope to the next systolic peak. If a diastolic dip is created, followed by a plateau and then the beginning of the systolic peak, then deflation is occurring too early. If no end-diastolic dip is present, but rather an EDP that is above the baseline of the unassisted systole and a straight slope up to the next systolic peak, then

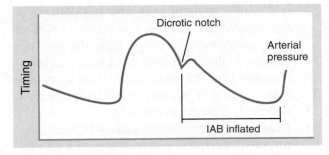

A

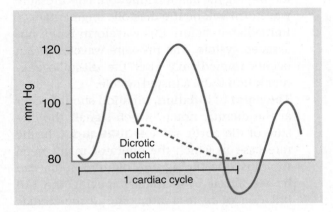

B

FIGURE 16-9 Pressure waveform showing the point of inflation. **A.** Dicrotic notch. **B.** A crisp *V* after adjusting the console for inflation to occur earlier.

Illustration from source material by Datascope Corp. and Maquet Cardiovascular. Used with permission.

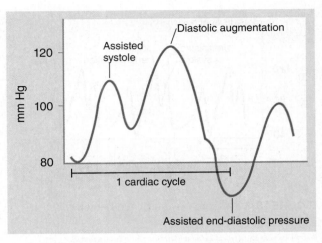

FIGURE 16-10 Pressure waveform with the slopes of diastolic augmentation and assisted systole marked.

Illustration from source material by Datascope Corp. and Maquet Cardiovascular. Used with permission.

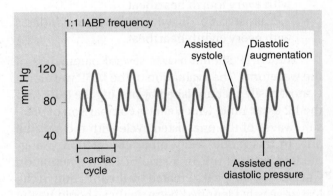

FIGURE 16-11 Pressure waveform showing the peak pressures of assisted systole and unassisted systole.

Illustration from source material by Datascope Corp. and Maquet Cardiovascular. Used with permission.

deflation is occurring late. Ideally, the IABP software will optimize deflation by adjusting it (earlier or later) to obtain the lowest possible assisted EDP while not reducing diastolic augmentation. CCTPs will find it helpful to be familiar with the expected waveforms; however, it is important to remember that deflation is best optimized to achieve the most favorable pressures indicative of reduction in afterload (assisted EDP) without impinging on ventricular ejection (reduced diastolic augmentation).

- **Slope of diastolic augmentation pressure and slope of assisted systole.** The slopes of the diastolic augmentation peak (balloon inflation) and the slope from the end-diastolic dip to the assisted systolic peak should be straight lines and nearly parallel **FIGURE 16-10**.
- **Diastolic augmentation peak pressure.** With effective IABP therapy, the diastolic augmentation peak pressure will be higher than (or at least equal to) the systolic pressures.

- **Comparison of the peak pressure of assisted systole with the peak pressure of unassisted systole.** With effective IABP therapy, the peak pressure of assisted systole will be lower than the systolic peak of unassisted systole **FIGURE 16-11**. This reflects that the IABP is reducing the peak pressures and, therefore, decreasing the workload of the heart and reducing the MVo_2.

Evaluation of IABP Timing

Software algorithms work effectively and efficiently to monitor and adjust IABP timing in virtually any situation. Nonetheless, although this knowledge is far less important today than with earlier IABP technology, the CCTP should be familiar with

TABLE 16-1 IABP Timing Errors

Error	Definition	Waveform Characteristics	Physiologic Effects
Early inflation	Inflation of the IAB before aortic valve closure	IAB inflation before the dicrotic notch; diastolic augmentation encroaches onto systole (may be unable to distinguish the two)	Possible premature aortic valve closure; possible increase in LV, EDV, EDP, or PCWP; increased LV wall stress (afterload); aortic regurgitation; increased MVo_2
Late inflation	IAB inflation occurs markedly later than aortic valve closure	IAB inflation after the dicrotic notch; absence of sharp *V*	Suboptimal coronary artery perfusion
Early deflation	Premature IAB deflation, during the diastolic phase	Sharp drop following diastolic augmentation; suboptimal diastolic augmentation; assisted aortic EDP may be equal to or less than unassisted aortic EDP; assisted systolic pressure may rise	Suboptimal coronary artery perfusion; potential for retrograde coronary and carotid blood flow; suboptimal afterload reduction; increased MVo_2
Late deflation	Balloon deflation late in the cardiac cycle	Assisted aortic EDP may be equal to unassisted aortic EDP; prolonged rate of rise of assisted systole; diastolic augmentation may appear widened	Afterload reduction essentially absent; increased MVo_2 because of prolonged isovolumetric contraction and greater resistance to LV ejection; increased afterload if IAB impinges on LV ejection

Abbreviations: EDP, end-diastolic pressure; EDV, end-diastolic volume; IAB, intra-aortic balloon; LV, left ventricular; MVo_2, myocardial oxygen consumption; PCWP, pulmonary capillary wedge pressure

© Jones & Bartlett Learning.

potential timing errors, waveform characteristics, and physiologic effects associated with this therapy **TABLE 16-1**. Today, most timing errors result from operators overriding the IABP software.

Early Inflation

The IAB should inflate at the dicrotic notch, which signals the closure of the aortic valves. Inflation that occurs too early is reflected on the waveform by a shortened normal pressure decrease that follows diastole. Because the aortic valves have not closed, this error in timing can be detrimental to the patient by decreasing pumping efficacy. On the pressure waveform, this is reflected as an "opened *V*" and with a lessened slope on the diastolic augmentation waveform. The pathophysiologic effect of early inflation is that the ejection of blood from the LV is impaired by the sudden increase in aortic pressure while the aortic valve is open, forcing premature closure of the aortic valves and decreasing the SV **FIGURE 16-12**. It is also possible for early inflation to result in damage to the aortic valve.

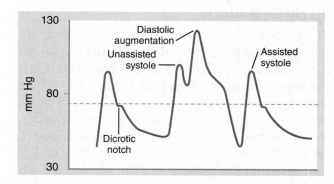

FIGURE 16-12 Early inflation.

Illustration from source material by Datascope Corp. and Maquet Cardiovascular. Used with permission.

Late Inflation

If the dicrotic notch is visible on the pressure waveform, then inflation of the IAB is late. The late inflation of the IAB, although causing little harm to the patient, does not maximize the benefits of IABP therapy because the pressure in the aorta has decreased before the IAB inflates. Therefore, the profound increase in diastolic pressure that maximizes coronary and systemic circulation is not realized **FIGURE 16-13**.

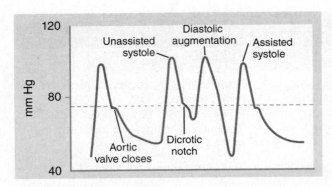

FIGURE 16-13 Late inflation.

Illustration from source material by Datascope Corp. and Maquet Cardiovascular. Used with permission.

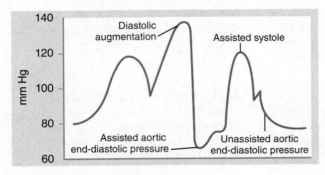

FIGURE 16-14 Early deflation.

Illustration from source material by Datascope Corp. and Maquet Cardiovascular. Used with permission.

Early Deflation

If deflation occurs too early, then the pressure in the aorta will equalize and rise slightly to plateau before systole, meaning that a higher EDP must be overcome for the ventricles to eject blood. The waveform will exhibit a sharp drop from diastolic augmentation with a characteristic prolongation of the assisted aortic end-diastolic period. This lack of inflation through to the end of diastole means not only that the benefits of IABP therapy are not realized by assisting the next systole, but also that the duration of increased pressure during diastole (which benefits the coronary arteries and systemic circulation) is decreased **FIGURE 16-14**.

Late Deflation

Late deflation of the IAB can be extremely detrimental to the patient. Late deflation is characterized by a widened appearance of the diastolic augmentation waveform base and a prolonged rate of rise in the assisted systolic waveform **FIGURE 16-15**. Because the balloon is still inflated while the heart is

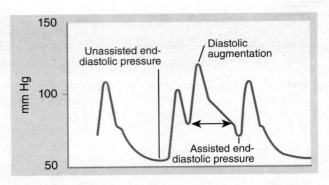

FIGURE 16-15 Late deflation.

Illustration from source material by Datascope Corp. and Maquet Cardiovascular. Used with permission.

trying to eject blood from the LV, the pressure in the aorta never drops to the baseline or dips below it. This increased pressure at which the aortic valves can open and eject blood from the ventricles increases the afterload and significantly increases the MVo_2 of the LV because the majority of MVo_2 is used to overcome the pressure in the aorta to eject the blood. Thus, late deflation of the balloon worsens myocardial ischemia and needs to be avoided.

IAB Insertion

Indications

IABP therapy can be used effectively to treat a variety of conditions resulting in heart failure. Conditions or situations that benefit from IABP therapy are listed in **TABLE 16-2**. Whatever the indication for its use, the IABP fulfills basic roles: reducing the workload of the myocardium, improving coronary and systemic flow, and restoring the balance between the metabolic demands of the heart and body and the supply of oxygen available. **TABLE 16-3** summarizes the potential benefits of IABP therapy.

Indications for IABP therapy include the following:

- Refractory ventricular failure
- Cardiogenic shock
- Unstable refractory angina
- Impending infarction
- Mechanical complications caused by acute myocardial infarction (AMI), ventricular septal defect (a hole in the wall between the ventricles), mitral regurgitation, or papillary muscle rupture
- Ischemia-related intractable ventricular arrhythmias

TABLE 16-2 Conditions or Situations That Benefit From IABP Therapy

Chest pain from unstable angina

Severe arrhythmias

Cardiogenic shock

Heart failure

Myocardial ischemia from unstable angina

Myocardial infarction

Ventricular irritability

Ventricular septal defect (before surgical intervention)

Papillary muscle dysfunction (before surgical intervention)

Papillary muscle rupture (before surgical intervention)

Impaired cardiac function (before surgical intervention)

Support during diagnostic and interventional procedures (eg, coronary angiography and angioplasty)

Weaning from cardiopulmonary bypass

Failed angioplasty (until the patient undergoes surgical intervention)

Unsuccessful valvuloplasty (until the patient undergoes surgical intervention)

During cardiopulmonary bypass

Cardiac support during noncardiac operations

Prophylactic support while awaiting cardiac operations

Myocardial contusion

Mechanical bridge to other assist devices or heart transplantation

Abbreviation: IABP, intra-aortic balloon pump

© Jones & Bartlett Learning.

TABLE 16-3 Benefits of IABP Therapy

Improves coronary artery perfusion

Increases cardiac output

Maintains peripheral perfusion

Reduces myocardial ischemia

Decreases myocardial oxygen demand

Improves hemodynamic stability

Decreases afterload

Abbreviation: IABP, intra-aortic balloon pump

© Jones & Bartlett Learning.

infarction, and intractable ventricular arrhythmias related to ischemia, the IAB can be beneficial in maintaining adequate coronary artery perfusion, relieving myocardial ischemia, and decreasing myocardial oxygen demand. If cardiac catheterization and further interventions are necessary, then the patient can undergo these procedures while in a more hemodynamically stable condition. The IAB can also be used in conjunction with cardiopulmonary bypass pumps to provide pulsatile flow.

Patients who experience severe chest pain accompanied by ECG changes or arrhythmias and who do not obtain relief from drug therapy are at great risk of developing a myocardial infarction (MI). Improving coronary blood flow and reducing LV work will minimize chest pain and the ECG changes associated with the MI. IABP therapy is often considered when symptoms persist despite maximal medical therapy. If cardiac catheterization and further interventions are indicated, then the IABP can improve the patient's hemodynamic status before these procedures are performed.

Depending on the area of an AMI, mechanical complications can occur from the heart damage. Although these complications arise in only a small percentage of MIs, the resulting hemodynamic compromise can have lethal consequences, especially if not treated immediately. Ventricular septal defects, papillary muscle dysfunction, and papillary muscle rupture usually require surgical interventions, often on an emergency basis. If the patient undergoes cardiac catheterization or surgical intervention in a hemodynamically compromised state, then the potential for mortality and morbidity increases significantly. The IABP provides temporary

- Cardiac support during high-risk general surgical or coronary angiography or angioplasty procedures
- Weaning from cardiopulmonary bypass
- Intraoperative pulsatile flow generation
- Support for failed angioplasty and valvuloplasty

In patients with myocardial ischemia and chest pain associated with unstable angina, impending

support to achieve hemodynamic stability before undertaking definitive treatment measures.

Ventricular irritability, a frequent complication of an AMI, can lead to severe arrhythmias and further hemodynamic compromise. In most patients, conventional drug therapy and supportive measures are sufficient to reverse the irritability and arrhythmias. However, those patients who do not respond to conventional medical therapy are at high risk for further myocardial damage and death. IABP therapy has proved effective in stabilizing the hemodynamic condition of patients with ventricular irritability or arrhythmias by increasing coronary artery perfusion, reducing ischemia, and maintaining adequate peripheral perfusion.

In the already compromised heart, a decrease in arterial pressure can reduce the myocardial oxygen supply and cause a loss of functional myocardial tissue. To prevent worsening of their heart failure and cardiogenic shock, these patients require prompt treatment of any signs of hemodynamic instability. Treatment aims at relieving LV workload and restoring the balance between myocardial oxygen supply and demand, allowing the myocardium time to heal and recover its maximal function. IABP therapy assists in this effort by decreasing LV workload and increasing coronary artery perfusion.

LV failure following an AMI may progress to cardiogenic shock. As with LV failure, the objectives of cardiogenic shock treatment are decreased cardiac work, increased myocardial oxygen supply, and a lowered MVo_2. The combined effects of IABP therapy (ie, increased oxygen supply, decreased afterload, and improved systemic perfusion) allow the heart to rest and help halt the subsequent vicious cycle that often occurs in an AMI.

Patients with impaired cardiac function are considered high-risk candidates for general surgical procedures. Anesthetic agents and the procedure itself can place increased oxygen demands on the weakened heart. IABP therapy provides hemodynamic stability by helping balance myocardial oxygen supply and demand preoperatively, intraoperatively, and during the critical postoperative period when demands on the heart are particularly high.

The IABP works in conjunction with coronary angiography and angioplasty to support and stabilize the condition of high-risk patients undergoing these procedures. Overall, IABP therapy can provide increased coronary artery perfusion and a reduction in cardiac work, thereby lowering the risk of hemodynamic compromise caused by reduced coronary flow during IAB inflation or acute coronary occlusion.

Weaning a patient from cardiopulmonary bypass may be difficult when support of the heart and lungs on the cardiopulmonary bypass machine is prolonged, surgical revascularization (placement of bypass grafts around blocked coronary arteries) is only partially achieved, or the patient has preexisting myocardial dysfunction. Termination of cardiopulmonary bypass may result in hypotension and a low CO, despite administration of inotropic and vasoactive drugs. IABP therapy in this setting decreases LV resistance, improves CO, and increases coronary artery and systemic perfusion pressures, facilitating the patient's removal from the cardiopulmonary bypass machine.

IABP therapy can support and stabilize patients with severe LV failure resulting from failed angioplasty (ie, an attempt to open an occluded coronary artery in an interventional cardiac catheterization laboratory). In this setting, it can provide increased coronary artery perfusion and decreased cardiac work, thereby reducing the risk of hemodynamic compromise because of reduced coronary flow or acute coronary occlusion. When valvuloplasty (a procedure in which a balloon-tipped catheter is used to dilate a stenotic heart valve) is unsuccessful, however, it may produce cardiac dysfunction. The IABP helps support cardiac function until the patient can undergo definitive valve repair or replacement.

Contraindications

Although CCTPs do not insert the IAB, they may arrive before or during consideration of IAB insertion. It is useful to understand the contraindications to IABP therapy, which include the following:

- Severe aortic valvular insufficiency
- Abdominal or aortic aneurysm
- Severe calcific aortic or iliac arterial disease or severe peripheral vascular disease

These contraindications are discussed individually in the following sections.

Severe Aortic Insufficiency

IABP therapy is contraindicated in patients with severe aortic valve insufficiency. For the benefits of

IABP therapy to be realized, the aortic valve must be competent. Balloon inflation in the setting of aortic valve insufficiency would force blood from the aorta across the valve into the ventricle. This aortic regurgitation, in turn, would increase cardiac work by overloading the ventricle with additional blood volume. In essence, the ventricle would have to pump the same blood back and forth, paradoxically increasing the workload. An incompetent aortic valve is also more likely to sustain damage from an improperly inserted IAB or poorly timed inflation and deflation of the IAB.

Aortic Aneurysm or Dissection

Use of the IABP is contraindicated if the patient has an abdominal or thoracic aortic aneurysm or aortic dissection. During insertion, the IAB catheter could become misdirected into the aneurysm itself or tear the weakened wall of the aorta. The increased pressure generated with counterpulsation could worsen the aneurysm or dissection.

Aortoiliac or Severe Peripheral Vascular Disease

Severe, calcific arterial or peripheral vascular disease is also a contraindication to IABP therapy, although some sources view it as a relative contraindication. The physician must decide whether the benefits of IABP therapy outweigh the risk of further compromise of the arterial blood flow. Peripheral vascular disease may limit the ability to advance the catheter through the atherosclerotic vessel. In addition, the presence of the catheter could cause plaque rupture or vessel occlusion, resulting in leg ischemia. This information is important to the IABP operator (usually a CCTP) because blood flow to the extremity distal to insertion must be monitored for evidence of circulation compromise.

Insertion Site Factors

Using a catheter without a sheath (ie, sheathless insertion) is not recommended if the patient has any of the following conditions:

- A large amount of fatty tissue at the insertion site over the common femoral artery, because the excessive distance between the skin and the femoral artery is likely to trap the catheter in the subcutaneous tissue

- Extensive scarring or fibrosis at the insertion site
- Other contraindications to percutaneous insertion

Side Effects and Complications

Side effects and complications of IABP therapy include the following:

- Limb ischemia (compartment syndrome may develop after the IAB is removed)
- Excessive bleeding from the insertion site
- Thrombocytopenia (owing to platelet destruction)
- Immobility of the balloon catheter
- Balloon leak
- Infection
- Aortic dissection
- Thrombosis

Note that anticoagulation is no longer routinely prescribed specifically to prevent IABP-associated clotting or thrombus, although some patients who receive IABP therapy may be anticoagulated for reasons unrelated to the IABP. Management of specific complications is discussed later in this chapter.

Equipment

The following equipment should be gathered before working with an IABP during transport:

- IABP with transport module
- Appropriate-size balloon catheters with insertion kit
- Spare helium tank (200 psi)
- Operator's manual
- Stopcocks
- 60-mL syringe (Luer tip)
- Skin electrodes
- IABP extension tubing
- Doppler ultrasonography device (to assess distal pulses)
- Extra ECG cables
- 2-inch (5-cm) cloth tape to secure the IABP ECG electrodes and catheter to the patient
- Arterial pressure monitoring transducer and setup
- Pressure transducer cables
- Arterial flush solution (normal saline)
- Adapters to fit other brands of balloon catheters to the IABP console
- Knee splint
- Soft restraints

Steps for Using the IABP

SKILL DRILL 16-1 describes the steps when beginning a call involving a patient receiving IABP therapy. These steps are summarized here:

1. When entering the facility to transport a patient receiving IABP therapy, visually assess the surroundings to ensure that hallways, elevators, and routes of travel will accommodate the necessary equipment and personnel **STEP 1**.
2. Obtain the patient care report **STEP 2**.
3. Determine the current battery status of the IABP console (it should be fully charged and connected to a power outlet). Ascertain the current IABP settings and note typical pressures (console systolic, diastolic, augmentation, and mean arterial pressures) **STEP 3**.
4. Determine IABP catheter model, size, and insertion depth (measured at the insertion site) **STEP 4**.
5. Ascertain that the balloon tip's location has been verified by chest radiograph **STEP 5**.
6. Conduct an assessment **STEP 6**. The focus of assessment for a patient attached to an IABP includes inspection of the insertion site for active bleeding, peripheral pulses in both lower extremities (may require Doppler ultrasonographic confirmation), and a radial pulse in the left upper extremity (to ensure subclavian blood flow).
7. Attach new ECG leads and secure each lead over the electrode with 2-inch (5-cm) cloth tape **STEP 7**. This step will prevent lead disconnection and potential loss of trigger during transport.
8. Ensure that the IAB catheter is taped securely to the patient's leg **STEP 8**.
9. Apply a knee immobilization splint to the leg in which the IAB was inserted to prevent leg flexion during transport **STEP 9**.
10. Ensure that the appropriate connectors to attach the IABP to the transport console are available. Determine the console that will be used at the receiving facility, and be certain to take any necessary adapters or connectors (usually included in the IAB insertion kit).
11. Move the patient to the transport stretcher **STEP 10**. Connect and secure all pumps, monitors, ventilators, and other equipment.
12. Transfer the IABP to the transport console at the bedside or in the transport vehicle (if the IABP console is mounted in the vehicle) **STEP 11**.
13. Establish power to the transport IABP console. Ensure that the console screen indicates that the battery is charging **STEP 12**.
14. Open the helium tank, and verify its pressure **STEP 13**.
15. Follow the IABP console instructions for start-up (on the console help screens or in the manufacturer-provided user manual) **STEP 14**:
    • Establish the ECG and pressure waveforms from the patient.
    • Confirm the initial pump settings.
    • Ascertain the appropriate timing.
    • Initiate IAB pumping.
    • Set the console alarms.
    • Confirm all pump settings.

Special Populations

Always immobilize the knee of the patient's leg to which the IABP is attached prior to transport. This step helps avert sudden leg movement, which may lead to bleeding or dislodgement of the IABP catheter. This step is especially relevant with geriatric patients, whose tissues are less elastic and therefore more susceptible to damage from sudden movement.

Patient Assessment

Among all patients who are admitted to a community hospital with an AMI, cardiogenic shock develops in 7% to 10%. Because the IABP can be an effective means of support for patients in LV failure and cardiogenic shock, personnel in these facilities may initiate IABP therapy. Unfortunately, such hospitals may not be equipped with cardiac surgery or cardiac catheterization laboratories or have the ability to perform interventional cardiology procedures. When the choice is made to transfer a patient with such a condition to a tertiary facility for further evaluation and treatment, early insertion of an IAB may make transport safer by promoting hemodynamic stability. Some IABP-related considerations need attention before transport.

Assessment of a patient receiving IABP therapy revolves around two questions:

• Is the therapy effective for the patient?
• Are there any complications as a result of the therapy?

Skill Drill 16-1 Operating the IABP During Transport

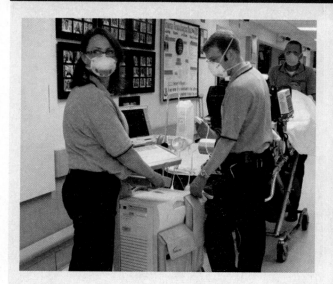

Step 1

Visually assess the surroundings to ensure that hallways, elevators, and routes of travel will accommodate the necessary equipment and personnel.

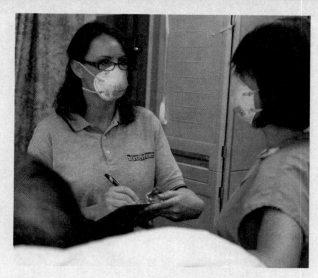

Step 2

Obtain the patient report.

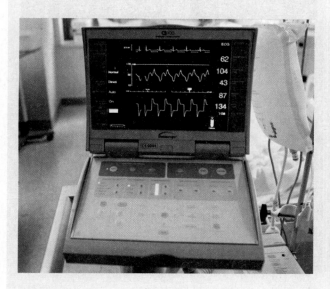

Step 3

Determine the current battery status (it should be fully charged and connected to a power outlet). Ascertain the current IABP settings and note typical pressures.

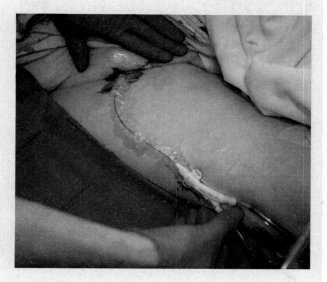

Step 4

Determine the IAB catheter model, size, and insertion depth.

Continues

Skill Drill 16-1 Operating the IABP During Transport (continued)

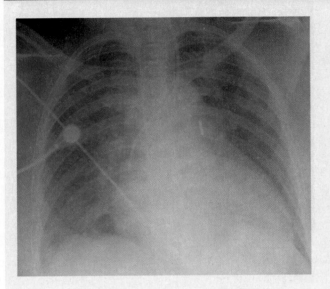

Step 5
Ascertain that the balloon tip's location has been verified by chest radiograph.

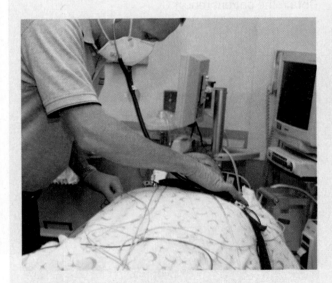

Step 6
Conduct an assessment.

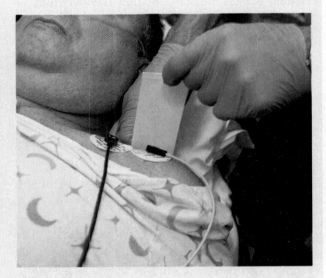

Step 7
Attach new ECG leads and secure each lead over the electrode with 2-inch (5-cm) cloth tape.

Skill Drill 16-1 Operating the IABP During Transport (continued)

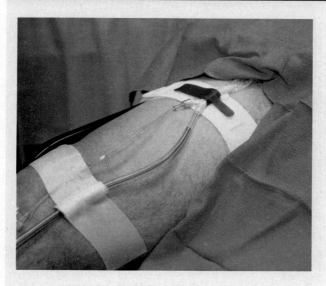

Step 8

Ensure that the IAB catheter is taped securely to the patient's leg.

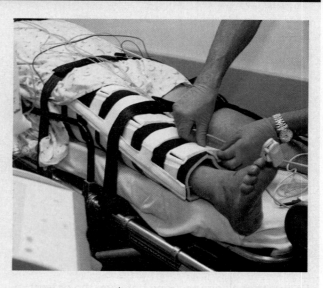

Step 9

Apply a knee immobilization splint to the leg in which the IAB was inserted to prevent leg flexion during transport. Ensure that the appropriate connectors to attach the IABP to the transport console are available. Take any adapters that will be necessary at the receiving facility.

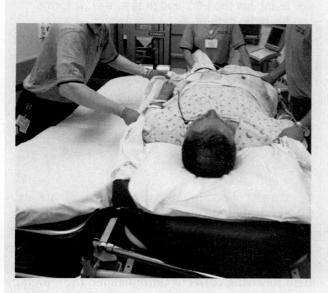

Step 10

Move the patient to the transport stretcher. Connect and secure all pumps, monitors, ventilators, and other equipment.

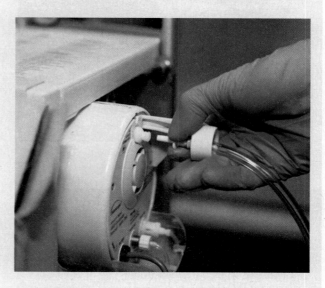

Step 11

Transfer the IABP to the transport console at the bedside or in the transport vehicle (if the IABP console is mounted in the vehicle).

Continues

Skill Drill 16-1 Operating the IABP During Transport (continued)

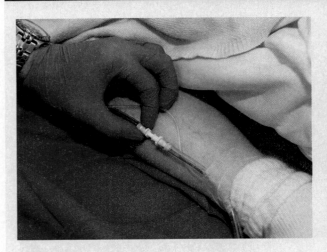

Step 12

Ensure that all connections between the patient and the console are tight and correct.

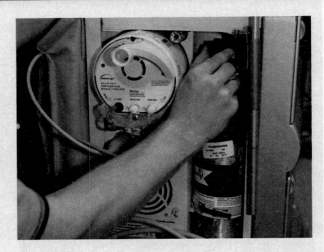

Step 13

Open the helium tank and verify its pressure.

Step 14

Follow the IABP console instructions for start-up (on the console help screens or in the manufacturer-provided user manual):
- Establish the ECG and pressure waveforms from the patient.
- Confirm the initial pump settings.
- Ascertain the appropriate timing.
- Initiate IAB pumping.
- Set the console alarms.
- Confirm all pump settings.

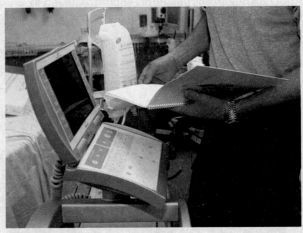

Steps 1-4, 6-14: © Jones & Bartlett Learning; **Step 5:** Courtesy of Andrew N. Pollak, MD, FAAOS.

Special Populations

Be certain to evaluate the patient's mental status and level of orientation prior to transport. IABP therapy may lead to confusion, necessitating use of physical or chemical restraints during transport. With geriatric patients, it is important to determine whether this confusion is normal behavior for the patient (such as with dementia) or the result of altered cerebral blood flow secondary to IABP counterpulsation.

Patient assessment parameters that are useful for evaluating the effectiveness of IABP therapy include vital signs, oxygenation, urine output, peripheral perfusion, the central nervous system (mentation), and overall general condition. A patient receiving correctly administered IABP therapy would be expected to experience an improvement in each of these parameters (except in the most severe cases). Improvement of the vital signs, oxygenation, urine output, peripheral perfusion, and mentation, and overall condition of the patient can be expected because of the increase in CO. Some patients develop confusion or agitation during IABP therapy, which may be attributed to alterations in cerebral circulation induced by IAB counterpulsation. In the transport environment, the CCTP should be prepared to restrain or sedate an agitated patient receiving IABP therapy to ensure the safety of both the patient and the crew. The CCTP should assess and document these parameters at least every 15 minutes or whenever a change occurs in the patient's condition.

Complications that may result from IABP therapy are most often related to the device's insertion site or impairment of circulation by the balloon or in the extremity where it is inserted. When in the proper position, the IAB lies in the thoracic aorta just distal to the takeoff of the left subclavian artery. The depth of insertion of the IAB should be monitored and documented. If the IABP were to migrate toward the patient's head (cephalad) during transport, then the distal portion of the IAB could occlude the takeoff to the left subclavian artery, which may be evidenced as a dampening or absence of the pulse in the left arm. Therefore, the CCTP should palpate or, if necessary, use a handheld Doppler ultrasonography device to assess the left radial pulse and compare it with the right radial pulse when performing vital signs or patient assessments. Placing a pulse oximeter probe on a finger of the patient's left hand would also provide an early warning of compromised circulation to the left subclavian artery. Alternatively, the IAB may potentially migrate toward the patient's feet (caudal), causing an impairment in renal function. A sudden decrease in urine output may signal this impairment in renal blood flow; therefore, urine output should be noted and documented.

As mentioned earlier, the majority of IABs are inserted using a percutaneous technique in the femoral artery. This site should be inspected for evidence of bleeding, externally or internally. Any hematomas that have developed should be noted and marked on the skin to allow the CCTP or other health care providers to assess progression of the hematoma. Care should be taken to inspect the patient's buttocks and posterior hip area, because bleeding in this area may be difficult to detect.

If the femoral artery is used as the insertion site, then the CCTP should assess and document the presence of the distal pulses and capillary refill time (CRT) in the extremity used and compare it with the distal pulses and CRT in the other leg. The CCTP should splint the knee of the leg in which the IAB was inserted to prevent excessive movement that might lead to bleeding at the site or impairment of distal circulation.

A sudden loss of pulses or decrease in CRT could signal that the IAB is occluding the femoral artery and causing ischemia in the limb. If this complication occurs, medical control should be notified immediately and consideration given to removal of the device in a facility as soon as feasible. In addition, because circulation in the extremity may be impaired, the potential for compartment syndrome is high both while the catheter is in place and after it has been removed. Compartment syndrome is heralded by the five Ps: Pain (out of proportion to what is expected), Pallor, Paralysis, Pulselessness, and Paresthesia. Also, the extremity might feel cold to the touch.

Transport Considerations

Patients receiving IABP therapy are candidates for transport in ground ambulances or in fixed- or rotary-wing aircraft. Some issues to consider when using these vehicles for transport of IABP-treated patients include battery life and vehicle power supply, space and weight constraints, and loading, unloading, and securing the pump in the vehicle. Addressing these issues when developing an IABP transport program will resolve most potential problems before the first transport occurs. Careful attention to transport-related physical and logistic considerations, well in advance of an actual transport, ensures that CCTPs will be able to focus on patient-specific needs during transport.

Transport vehicles often have an inverter capable of converting the direct current (DC) voltage generated by the engine to alternating current (AC) voltage suitable for powering the IABP. In addition to AC power, some aircraft produce 24 V of DC power. Many IABPs are capable of operating on 110 V to 120 V of AC power or 24 V of DC power, although the latter may require an adapter cable. Most IABP systems also incorporate batteries that allow for limited periods of portable operation **FIGURE 16-16**.

Ensuring a match between the IABP power requirements and the available power supply in the transport vehicle is a crucial planning step when establishing an IABP transport program. Given the electrical demands of all the medical equipment likely to accompany an IABP-treated patient, it is recommended that the crew have access to the inverter circuit breaker from inside the transport

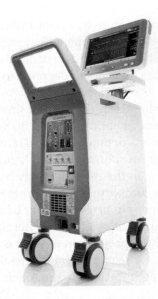

FIGURE 16-16 A portable intra-aortic balloon pump.

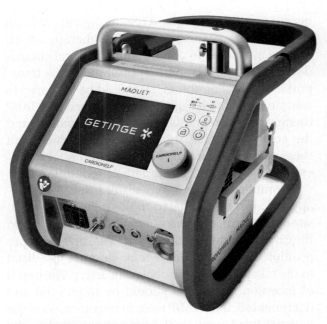

FIGURE 16-17 Extracorporeal membrane oxygenation systems provide forward blood flow and/or removal of carbon dioxide and add oxygen to venous blood.

vehicle. This access allows the crew to monitor the status of the inverter and reset the circuit breaker without having to stop the transport and disembark from the vehicle.

It is also necessary to evaluate the space and weight constraints of the transport vehicle before transport and the logistics of loading and unloading the IABP and the patient. Ground ambulances generally have minimal restrictions on weight, and the system will usually fit easily into the vehicle. In a transport aircraft, space limitations may require reconfiguration of the pump and monitor module. The additional weight of the system may also be an issue in air operations—another important planning point during transport program development.

After the IABP is placed in the transport vehicle, it is critical to secure the pump so that it remains stable for safe operation throughout transport. It may be necessary to work with the IABP manufacturer, Federal Aviation Administration representatives, and the aircraft mechanic to ensure that an adequate system is in place to secure the IABP against air turbulence.

Extracorporeal Membrane Oxygenation

Extracorporeal membrane oxygenation (ECMO), also referred to as extracorporeal life support (ECLS), is a temporizing mechanism of extracorporeal gas exchange with or without hemodynamic support **FIGURE 16-17**. Artificial extracorporeal oxygenation has held an allure for scientists and physicians throughout modern medicine. In 1869, Ludwig and Schmidt documented the first successful attempts at extracorporeal oxygenation by shaking blood inside a balloon. Research and advancements continued with surgeon John Gibbon completing the first successful extracorporeal bypass on a human in 1953. Born from the cardiopulmonary bypass machine found in the operating room, the original application of ECMO was primarily for support of severe respiratory failure where native cardiopulmonary function is pathologically decoupled. In contrast to cardiopulmonary bypass, ECMO allows for longer-term support in the intensive care unit (ICU), makes use of the patient's intravascular volume as the fluid reservoir, and ostensibly captures 80% of circulating blood volume. ECMO is not curative; rather, it is a supportive therapy for presumed reversible respiratory and/or cardiac failure and is a keystone to one of the following strategies: bridge to recovery, bridge to transplantation, destination therapy, or bridge to decision. ECMO is currently the only available therapy to functionally replace the heart and lungs, albeit imperfectly.

Calculating Uncaptured CO in the ECMO Circuit

The following equation is used to estimate the percentage of CO that is not captured by the ECMO circuit:

$$(Q \times Sao_2) + (x \times Svo_2) = Spo_2(Q + x)$$

where Q is ECMO flow, Sao_2 is arterial oxygen saturation, Svo_2 is venous oxygen saturation, and Spo_2 is oxygen saturation as measured by pulse oximetry. For example, if Q is 3.5 L/min, ECMO Sao_2 is 100%, ECMO Svo_2 is 60%, and the patient's Spo_2 is 85%, the equation would be written as follows:

$$(3.5 \text{ L/min} \times 100\%) + (x \times 60\%) = 85\%(3.5 + x)$$

$$3.5 + 0.6x = 3 + 0.85x$$

$$3.5 = 3 + 0.25x$$

$$0.5 = 0.25x$$

$$2 = x$$

Thus, $x = 2$ L/min, meaning 2 L/min of CO is not being captured by the ECMO circuit. The uncaptured or deoxygenated blood would continue through the native pulmonary circulation. (Note: This calculation assumes that the lungs do not contribute to oxygen saturation.)

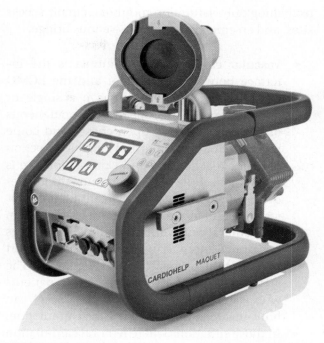

FIGURE 16-18 The circulatory function of extracorporeal membrane oxygenation systems is provided with a centrifugal pump; the pulmonary function relies on the use of an artificial lung, known as an oxygenator, to exchange gases.

ECMO Support Types and Configurations

Cannulation sites and circuit configurations vary depending on the patient and intended type of support. A common nomenclature describes the ECMO circuit configuration and support type by a combination of the letters *V* and *A*, where the letters before the *A* are referred to as the inflow/drainage cannula(s), and the *A* and all subsequent letters refer to the outflow/return cannula(s) **FIGURE 16-18**. The exception to this nomenclature is VV-ECMO. It is imperative that all members of the care team understand the locations and the vessels accessed for the *inflow* and *outflow* cannulas.

- **Venovenous-ECMO (VV-ECMO).** Blood is drained from the venous circulation, passes through the circuit where gas exchange occurs, and is returned as oxygenated and decarboxylated blood to the venous system. VV-ECMO functions in series, with the native lungs providing gas exchange without circulatory support.

- **Venoarterial-ECMO (VA-ECMO).** Blood is drained from the venous circulation, passes through the circuit where gas exchange occurs, and is returned as oxygenated and decarboxylated blood to the arterial system. VA-ECMO functions in parallel to the native heart and lungs, providing gas exchange with a degree of circulatory support.

- **Veno-veno-arterial-ECMO (VVA-ECMO) or veno-arterio-venous-ECMO (VAV-ECMO).** These configurations are colloquially referred to as *triple-cannulation*. Both support respiratory and cardiac function without the differential hypoxemia that may occur during VA-ECMO, albeit at the expense of added circuit complexity.

Circuit Components and Concepts

A basic ECMO circuit is composed of the vascular cannulas, circuit tubing, pump, heater–cooler, and oxygenator. ECMO circuits vary in configuration and may include pressure and blood flow monitors, bubble detectors, continuous arterial and venous oxyhemoglobin saturation monitors, circuit access sites, and an emergency arterial–venous bridge:

- **Vascular cannulas.** The cannula is the interface between the patient and the ECMO equipment. Cannulas can have a single or double lumen, be designed for percutaneous or central access (ie, open chest), and come in a range of diameters and lengths. Selection of cannula style, size, and cannulation site is individualized to the patient and support required. In adults, VV-ECMO cannulation typically occurs in the right internal jugular vein and femoral vein, with the cannulas' openings positioned more than 4 inches (10 cm) apart to reduce the propensity for *recirculation*. The size of the femoral vein in pediatric patients who weigh less than 33 pounds (15 kg) can limit this location's usability for cannulation. In those situations where femoral cannulation is not possible or preferred, a double-lumen catheter placed in the right internal jugular vein can serve as an alternative strategy. VA-ECMO arterial cannulation typically occurs in the right common carotid artery or femoral artery. Venous cannulation is accomplished by using the same sites listed for VV-ECMO. Central cannulation (ie, open chest) is an additional option in VA-ECMO, where the venous cannula is placed into the right atrial appendage and the arterial cannula into the aorta.
- **Tubing.** The circuit tubing is a polyvinyl chloride compound. Modern circuit tubing and components include both biocompatible coatings and materials to pacify the body's innate inflammatory and coagulative responses to the nonbiologic material of the circuit.
- **Pump.** The pump creates forward blood flow through the circuit by generating negative pressure within the inflow/drainage limb and positive pressure after the pump in the outflow/return limb. The negative pressure pulls venous blood to the pump inlet and the spinning rotor then drives the blood forward. Modern pumps are centrifugal and nonocclusive, relying on magnetic communication between a drive motor and pump head. Due to the nonocclusive design, care must be taken to ensure that the revolutions per minute are sufficient to maintain forward flow to avoid retrograde flow.

- **Oxygenator.** Located distal to the pump, the primary function of the oxygenator is to reproduce the alveolocapillary function of the lungs. The blood passes through a mesh of hollow semipermeable membrane oxygenator fibers, exchanging oxygen and carbon dioxide through diffusion with the sweep gas. A secondary function of the oxygenator is to warm the blood, serving as a heat exchanger, in conjunction with a heater–cooler device.
- **Sweep gas.** The sweep gas is 100% oxygen, although some centers make use of blenders. The 1.0 F_{IO_2} (fraction of inspired oxygen) creates a pressure gradient between the sweep gas and blood, allowing for the diffusion of oxygen into the blood and carbon dioxide into the sweep gas. The sweep gas is titrated (L/min) to achieve a specified parameter, either pH or partial pressure of carbon dioxide (P_{CO_2}), based off the arterial blood gas. Conceptually, the *sweep* is analogous to the minute ventilation of a ventilator.
- **Heater–cooler.** This thermoregulatory device sends temperature-controlled water to the oxygenator, which acts as an external heat exchanger to warm or cool the blood to achieve a specified patient temperature. The large surface area of the ECMO circuit results in significant heat loss via convective, conductive, and radiant mechanisms.
- **Revolutions per minute (rpm).** The rpm reflects the speed of the pump rotor. This setting is directly controlled by the ECMO specialist or perfusionist to achieve a desired flow.
- **Flow (L/min).** Flow is the rate of blood movement through the circuit. It is variable at a set rpm and is a function of the rpm and conditions affecting the inflow and outflow limbs of the circuit (eg, cannula diameter, length, and position; patient fluid status, native CO). The flow delivers oxygenated blood, functioning analogously to CO during VA-ECMO, and is the main contributor to oxygen delivery (D_{O_2}) in VV-ECMO. In general, target flow rates are as follows:
  - Neonates: 100 to 160 mL/kg/min
  - Children: 80 to 90 mL/kg/min
  - Adults: 50 to 70 mL/kg/min

Note, however, that the flow rate should be goal directed and individualized to the patient.

Circuit and Patient Management

ECMO is a complicated therapy that requires constant, intensive, and careful oversight. Monitoring of a patient receiving ECMO begins with the same assessment provided to any patient in the ICU. Particular focus must be paid to the ECMO device, circuit, tubing, connectors, alarms, and overall integrity of the entire circuit. Specific considerations include the following:

- **Anticoagulation.** During ECMO, patients receive systemic anticoagulative therapy to both protect the major organs from thromboembolism and maintain the patency of the ECMO circuit. Contemporary ECMO circuits generally include biocoatings to resist thrombus formation. Owing to its importance and dynamic nature, anticoagulation status is monitored at set time intervals ranging from every hour to every 6 hours, depending on the specific coagulation study. Additionally, the significant risk for uncontrolled bleeding must be acknowledged in the planning of any patient procedure.

- **Circuit assessment.** The ECMO circuit and cannulas require continual assessment to monitor their integrity and patency. A thorough, methodical approach for assessment of all components, connections, and securing points will aid in the early identification of potential issues. Throughout therapy, providers must remain vigilant, preventing or removing kinks in the cannulas and circuit tubing. Cannula sutures must be inspected for continued integrity and tautness. A flashlight should be used to inspect the inlet and outlet of the oxygenator, as well as the entirety of the circuit and cannulas for clot and fibrin accretion. Common sites for fibrin deposition and thrombus formation are those that cause a disruption to laminar blood flow leading to turbulence and stagnation of blood; such sites include connectors, pigtails, and stopcocks. A truism of ECMO is that with the increasing complexity of a circuit comes increasing turbulence and stagnation of blood, and with it a heightened risk of clot formation.

- **Monitoring of support.** Venous oxygen saturation (Svo_2) and serum lactate levels provide insight into the adequacy of systemic perfusion; generally, Svo_2 greater than 70% and serum lactate less than 2.2 mmol/L imply a balance between Do_2 and oxygen consumption (Vo_2). Pressure monitoring can help providers detect early or acute dysfunction in the ECMO circuit and also suggest clinical changes in the patient. However, pressure monitoring is not essential, and target pressures vary with the characteristics of the ECMO circuit, cannulas, and patient status. While additional pressures can be obtained, the four typical pressures monitored are P_{vein} (venous pressure), P_{art} (arterial pressure), P_{int} (oxygenator inlet pressure), and Δp (differential pressure of P_{int} and P_{art}).

- P_{vein}. A pressure measurement taken prior to the pump (which is therefore a negative pressure). Monitoring of P_{vein} provides insight into the environment of the drainage/inflow cannula (IFC). Changes in P_{vein} reflect changes in the preload of the pump. As such, a more negative P_{vein} indicates a reduction in preload, which can result from patient hypovolemia, kinked tubing/cannula, or thrombus formation restricting blood flow, among other factors.

- P_{art}. A positive-pressure measurement taken after the oxygenator and pump (which is therefore a positive pressure). Monitoring of P_{art} provides insight into the environment of the reinfusion/outflow cannula. Changes in P_{art} reflect changes in the afterload of the pump. As such, a more positive P_{art} indicates an increase in afterload, which can be a result of increased native CO and/or systemic vascular resistance (SVR) in VA-ECMO. An increased P_{art} can also result from kinked tubing/cannula or thrombus formation and is not specific to VA-ECMO.

- P_{int}. A positive-pressure measurement taken after the pump at the inlet of the oxygenator. An increase in P_{int} is nonspecific when viewed in isolation. When used to calculate Δp and trended over time, P_{int} can be useful in assessing the patency of the oxygenator.

- Δp. This differential pressure of P_{int} and P_{art}, which is viewed as the transmembrane pressure or pressure drop across the oxygenator. A rise of greater than 20 mm Hg in the Δp can be damaging to red blood cells and is also concerning for thrombus formation within the oxygenator.

- **Routine documentation.** Documentation will vary by institution, but should at a minimum include hourly notation of flow, rpm, monitored circuit pressures, trending of the preferred coagulation study, anticoagulation dose, as well as circuit and cannulation site assessments.

- **BP and pulsatility.** When in VA-ECMO, the nonpulsatile/continuous blood flow of the pump bolsters native CO, augmenting perfusion and in the process potentially weakening or obliterating native pulsatility. In this scenario, arterial lines may display only MAP. Generally, flows are titrated to maintain a pulse pressure of at least 10 mm Hg, attempting to mitigate the increased afterload on the LV.

Complications and Troubleshooting

There are inherent risks and complications specific to each mode and configuration of ECMO support. Individualized and thorough assessment of both the ECMO circuit and the patient will give practitioners the best opportunity to identify issues before clinically meaningful events occur.

Patient Hypoxemia

- **Hemolysis.** Every component of the ECMO circuit is a potential cause of hemolysis (eg, kinking of tubing/cannulas, excessive pump rpm, thrombosis formation at any point in the system). Hemolysis is monitored through routine chemistries (eg, hematocrit, serum hemoglobin, lactate dehydrogenase [LDH]) and patient assessment (eg, voiding of dark red urine) to prevent organ damage and anemia caused by massive intravascular hemolysis; serum hemoglobin of 50 mg/dL or greater is cause for source identification.

- **Pulmonary edema and LV distention.** Prolonged LV distention from the increased afterload in VA-ECMO can lead to pulmonary edema. Initial treatment of high MAPs through preload/afterload reduction and administration of inotropes can help mitigate pulmonary edema; however, LV decompression is commonly necessary. In the setting of systemic anticoagulation, if pulmonary congestion is not addressed, it can progress to fatal pulmonary hemorrhage.

- **Limb ischemia.** Distal limb perfusion should be frequently assessed. The presence of hypoperfusion may require the insertion of a reperfusion catheter to restore blood flow to distal tissue.

- **Insufficient flow.** The pump is said to be preload dependent and afterload sensitive; flow is a product of the relationship among pump preload, rpm, and afterload. Insufficient flow must be differentiated from all potential causes: cannula malpositioning, inadequate circulating volume, sepsis, increased afterload (eg, inadequate sedation, increased native CO), pulmonary congestion, kinking of circuit tubing, or accumulation of thrombi within the circuit, cannulas, or oxygenator. *Chugging*, or *chatter* (ie, visible and often rhythmic movement or vibration within the venous line), is a sign of impaired venous drainage. Highly negative pressure around the inflow/drainage access point will lead to vessel collapse and possibly cavitation. As pressures become less negative, the vessel releases and chugging is observed. Chugging results in decreased flow, cavitation, and hemolysis. To resolve chugging, the practitioner can decrease the rpm to stabilize the flow and/or replace intravascular volume.

- **Recirculation.** This condition occurs in VV-ECMO when the oxygenated outflow is recaptured by the IFC and unable to follow the native circulation. The oxygenated blood then recirculates through the ECMO circuit instead of passing through the systemic circulation to the end organs. Multiple factors can influence the severity of recirculation, including flow, rpm, and cannula type, size, or position. Classic signs of recirculation are a low Sao_2 in the presence of elevated and/or rising Svo_2. Initial reaction to a low Sao_2 or Spo_2 may be to increase flow to increase Do_2; however, increasing flow in the presence of recirculation will only exacerbate the recirculation and reduce the Do_2. A more effective approach to reducing the degree of recirculation would be to increase the distance between the cannulas' openings, ensure additional drainage cannula, or insert a dual-lumen cannula with reinfusion directed toward the tricuspid valve.

- **North–south (Harlequin) syndrome.** During VA-ECMO in patients with both cardiac and respiratory failure, perfusate from the LV (ie, deoxygenated blood) mixes in the aorta with highly oxygenated blood from ECMO; the mixing blood is referred to as a mixing cloud or watershed. With either low ECMO flows or the recovery of native CO, especially with a femoral return cannula, CO can push the mixing cloud distal, past the aortic arch, preventing delivery of oxygenated blood to the cerebral and myocardial capillary beds. Clinically, the patient will present with a sharp midline demarcation owing to the differential oxygenation of the upper and lower body.

ECMO Emergencies and Circuit Disruptions

The critical nature and instability inherent in patients requiring ECMO therapy leaves them vulnerable to interruptions in support, with decompensation assured if support is not restored. Vigilance is the most valuable tool in caring for ECMO-treated patients and must be employed by all members of the team for optimal management and safety. While all components of the ECMO circuit can fail or malfunction, routine thorough inspections in conjunction with a proactive approach can detect and remedy most problems before clinically meaningful events transpire. A coordinated and well-rehearsed approach by the entire care team is required to successfully manage the complexities of emergent situations during ECMO support.

- **Oxygenator dysfunction.** Oxygenator failure can be insidious and manifest as an increasing Δp and consumption of platelets. Oxygenator failures typically result from thrombus formation within the oxygenator, resulting in decreasing efficiency and Do_2. An acute change in oxygenation and ventilation of the patient may be due to a disconnection/depletion of the sweep gas line or source, although oxygenator failure due to thrombus or embolus formation should also be investigated.

- **Air entrainment.** Introduction of air into the circuit can range from a single microbubble to massive entrainment that causes a complete cessation of blood flow. While a microbubble may not be immediately detrimental to either the circuit or the patient (if it were to reach the patient), air within the circuit causes turbulence in blood flow, increasing the likelihood of thrombus formation. The presence of air within the circuit, which is caused by a communication with the external environment, threatens the continuity of ECMO support. Any access point or connection along the negative-pressure inflow limb (ie, from the tip of the IFC to the pump head) and oxygenator is a potential site of entrainment. Additionally, central lines and their placement, inadvertent injection of air into the circuit during medication administration, and cavitation of the right atrium during low-volume states can all serve as sources of air entrainment. Any air embolus must be removed, though the choice of a removal approach depends on the embolus's severity/volume and location within the circuit.

- **Circuit rupture.** A loss of integrity to the circuit can be a result of component failure or disconnection. In either case, the patient should be isolated from the circuit by clamping the circuit tubing to stop blood draining from and flowing to the patient. In the absence of an expeditious response to isolate the patient, circuit rupture will involve rapid blood loss from both the patient's circulating volume and the circuit. Both medical and mechanical ventilatory adjuncts (eg, volume replacement, titration of vasopressors, and/or an increase in ventilator settings) will be necessary to stabilize the patient in the absence of ECMO support. Circumstances will dictate whether the circuit can be repaired in the moment or if a new circuit must be implemented.

- **Pump failure.** A pump failure is described as the inability of the pump to create adequate flow in the setting of a patent circuit with no additional confounding factors. Potential causes of pump failure include pump head disengagement, pump motor failure, electrical power supply failure (battery or AC), and pump head failure. Obviously, with a pump failure, regardless of its cause, there will be a loss of ECMO support and possible retrograde flow through the circuit. Isolating the patient from the circuit is necessary to prevent retrograde blood flow and to allow for repair of the circuit.

- **Inadvertent decannulation.** In any scenario involving the accidental removal, either partial or complete, of an ECMO cannula, the patient must be isolated from the circuit. Furthermore, the patient will require medical and mechanical ventilatory support and intravascular volume resuscitation in the setting of blood loss. If the cannula was completely removed, providers must apply direct pressure to the cannulation site. The main cause of inadvertent decannulation is excessive tension placed on the circuit tubing or cannulas. Anchoring the circuit tubing and maintaining visualization of the cannulas and tubing at all times can help prevent inadvertent decannulation.

Transport Considerations

The Extracorporeal Life Support Organization (ELSO) distinguishes between two types of ECMO-related interfacility transport:

- **Primary transport.** The transport team cannulates and initiates ECMO support at the referring facility, transporting the patient to an ECMO center.
- **Secondary transport.** A patient who is already supported by ECMO is transported from the referring center to another facility.

The two components of ECMO transport are (1) transport of the ECMO team to the referring facility and (2) transport of the patient to an ECMO center. In the case of primary transport, expeditious arrival of the ECMO team is a priority. The time needed to stabilize a patient supported by ECMO prior to transport can be lengthy and may require additional equipment and supplies. The transport vehicle must be able to carry the ECMO team, plus all necessary supplies and equipment. An ECMO team usually includes a physician or surgeon, an ECMO specialist/perfusionist, and an ECMO-trained registered nurse. Checklists can help to ensure that all the necessary equipment and supplies are carried in the transport unit.

Microaxial Catheter Pump Systems

A **microaxial continuous-flow pump** is a means of temporary circulatory support that consists of an axial-flow pump mounted on a catheter connected to a bedside console. Generally, while under fluoroscopy or ultrasonography, the catheter tip is maneuvered in a retrograde fashion up the aorta, across the aortic valve, and into the LV. Alternatively, placement can be done surgically through a graft attached directly into the aorta or via the axillary artery. When positioned properly, the pump pulls blood into the IFC located in the LV and propels it through an outflow port into the ascending aorta, functioning like a jet pump on a jet ski.

CCT teams working within referral networks for cardiogenic shock should be prepared to conduct interfacility patient transports involving a microaxial continuous-flow pump system. Specifically, CCTPs should be familiar with Impella ventricular assist catheters **FIGURE 16-19**. The Impella is a catheter-based ventricular assist system containing a microaxial pump that is designed to provide temporary partial hemodynamic support. Like most cardiac-assist devices, the Impella device aims to reduce ventricular work and provide the circulatory support necessary to allow cardiac tissue recovery and early assessment of residual myocardial function. Impella devices have been applied in settings of cardiogenic shock, low output syndrome, ST-segment elevation MI (STEMI),

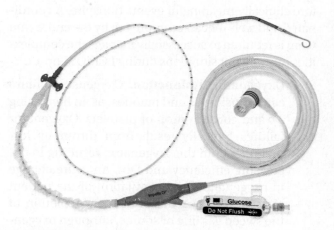

FIGURE 16-19 Impella CP with SmartAssist.

ventricular support during high-risk percutaneous coronary interventions, VA-ECMO to unload the LV, and cardiac decompensation while on VV-ECMO support.

The Impella system is not specifically designed for transport. However, with a thorough understanding of its operation, device positioning, and monitoring, safe patient transport via ground or air is possible when this system is in use.

Features and Concepts

The Impella system includes a catheter that functions in conjunction with an automated Impella controller (AIC) and purge fluid infusion pump. There are several different Impella catheters **FIGURE 16-20**. The Impella 2.5, Impella CP with SmartAssist, Impella 5.0, Impella 5.5 with SmartAssist, and Impella LD are all left-side heart devices. The Impella RP is a right-side heart device.

The Right-Side Heart Catheter

The Impella RP right-side heart catheter is the only microaxial pump device approved by the Food and Drug Administration (FDA) for use in patients with right-side heart failure. It is important to note that this device is inserted and positioned differently than the left-side heart devices previously discussed in this section. With the right-side heart device, the catheter pump is advanced antegrade under fluoroscopic guidance and positioned across the tricuspid and pulmonic valves through a sheath inserted in the femoral vein. The pump inflow is positioned in the inferior vena cava and the outflow in the pulmonary artery; thus, the pump aspirates blood from the inferior vena cava and expels it into the pulmonary artery, bypassing the right ventricle (RV).

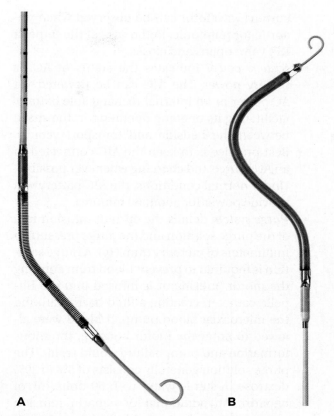

FIGURE 16-20 A. A left-side heart Impella catheter. **B.** The right-side heart Impella catheter.

The AIC allows for management and monitoring of pump operation and catheter position via multiple parameters: performance level, Impella flow, placement signal, and motor current. These parameters, as well as the system power and purge system features, are described as follows:

- *Performance level* on the AIC is analogous to pump speed or rpm in other MCS devices. Depending on the specific catheter, the performance level (P-level) will range from P-0 to P-8 or P-9. Left-side Impella catheters should never be set at less than P-2 while placed across the aortic valve; P-levels lower than P-2 can lead to aortic insufficiency. The Impella RP should never be set to less than 1.5 L/min of flow.
- *Impella flow* is a mean flow value, calculated from both the systolic and diastolic flows.
- *Placement signal* is used to determine proper placement of the catheter and should be monitored during transport. However, the specific waveform characteristics will vary with the model of catheter in use. Regardless of the waveform morphology and pressures observed, the pressure should not be used to infer the hemodynamic status of the patient.
- *Motor current* is displayed as a pulsatile waveform, which is also used to determine proper placement of the catheter and should be monitored in transport. Changes in the motor

current waveform can be observed when the aortic (or pulmonic, in the case of the Impella RP) valve opens and closes.

- *System power* indicates the status of AC or battery power. The AIC can be powered via AC power or an internal rechargeable battery, facilitating its ongoing operation in the space between the bedside and transport vehicle. Best practice is to keep the AIC connected to an AC source and charging whenever possible. Under normal conditions, the AIC battery will provide power for about 60 minutes.

- *Purge system* details the current infusion rate of the purge solution and the purge pressure in millimeters of mercury (mm Hg). A purge solution is required to prevent blood from entering the motor housing; it is infused into the Impella catheter, creating a fluid barrier around the microaxial blood pump. If blood were allowed to enter the motor housing, thrombus formation and pump failure would result. The purge solution generally consists of 5% to 20% dextrose in sterile water with 50 units/mL of heparin. An additional IV heparin infusion is often necessary to achieve adequate systemic anticoagulation to prevent clot formation within the catheter. Coagulation studies should be monitored frequently to ensure the proper continuous anticoagulation, and adjustments in anticoagulants require consideration of the contribution from the microaxial blood pump device to the total hourly anticoagulant infused.

Transport Considerations

Transport of the patient with the Impella system requires the transport team to be equipped, at a minimum, to continue the current level of patient hemodynamic support and monitoring in place at the referring facility. Changes in atmospheric pressure do not affect the ventricular assistance capability of Impella catheters, allowing for transport via ground or air.

A thorough assessment of the patient and catheter position should be performed prior to equipment exchange or manipulation of support. Special attention should be given to the catheter insertion site to assess for bleeding and hematoma, as well as perfusion distal to the insertion site. Providers should note the catheter insertion depth and ensure the catheter is locked and sutured to the patient to help prevent migration during transport. Excessive or uncontrolled bleeding from any site, waveform dampening, or motor current tracing that appears as ventricular in nature on the AIC are harbingers of instability in transport and can be sufficient reasons to defer transport. The absence of a motor current waveform or the presence of a tracing appearing as a ventricular waveform can indicate that the pump is malpositioned. Incorrect positioning of the Impella catheter must be remedied before proceeding with transport.

If the transport team will conduct an AIC swap (ie, a transfer from the referring facility's control module to the transport team's control module), the crew must complete post-transfer assessments of the patient and pump to identify any change in catheter positioning or patient stability.

When preparing the patient for transport, patient positioning and extremity immobilization should be considered to limit the possibility of catheter migration and consequential dislodgement of the pump: The head of the transport cot should remain elevated less than 30°, and the lower extremity containing the Impella catheter should be immobilized to minimize the potential for catheter migration during transport. All lines and tubing for the Impella device should be visible to facilitate quick and accurate assessment for leaks and kinking during transport. The AIC, battery, and purge fluid infusion pump must also be protected from extremes in temperature, moisture, and vibration, which could affect their continued functioning in transport.

Complications

As mentioned earlier, the potential for dislodgement or malpositioning of the catheter during transport requires ongoing attention by the CCT team. Abrupt changes in the placement signal or motor current waveform can suggest malpositioning of the Impella catheter. If malpositioning is suspected, the catheter and purge solution should be continued as a preventive measure against thrombus formation. The P-level should be decreased to P-2 (or a minimal flow of 1.5 L/min for the Impella RP catheter). With a malpositioned catheter, the supportive function of the system is lost and the patient likely will need to be supported medically. The accepting facility should be notified of the change so that its staff can prepare for immediate repositioning of the catheter on the patient's arrival. Repositioning the catheter in the transport environment should not be attempted.

A catheter motor failure is another possible complication that can arise during transport. In this situation, the patient will obviously lose the supportive function of the system and, therefore, will likely require inotropic and/or vasopressor agents to support hemodynamics. An additional complication in this scenario is caused by the catheter remaining in place across the aortic valve; aortic insufficiency should be anticipated. This caution bears repeating: *Providers should not attempt to reposition the catheter in the transport environment.*

Dysrhythmias

No adjustments to the Impella device are necessary if defibrillation or cardioversion is required. However, if the patient requires chest compressions, then the P-level should be decreased to P-2 prior to beginning compressions.

Common Alarms

The following list is not exhaustive but highlights alarms commonly encountered when transporting a patient with an Impella system.

- **Suction alarm.** Patient hypovolemia and catheter malpositioning can present with lower-than-expected flows and evolve into a suction event. Suction events occur when tissue occludes the inlet of the pump. Attempts at breaking the suction can be made by decreasing the P-level by one or two increments. If suction alarms continue to occur, the transport team can continue to lower the P-level; however, the level should not decrease below P-2. Patients experiencing suction events should be assessed for euvolemia and given additional volume if indicated. Abiomed, the manufacturer of the Impella system, recommends maintaining central venous pressure (CVP) of at least 10 mm Hg; a CVP of less than 10 mm Hg

could indicate that augmenting intravascular volume may help resolve suction alarms.
- **Purge alarm.** This alarm indicates that the purge pressure is either too low or too high. A low purge pressure generally results from a leak in the system; providers should assess for any leaks or disconnections in the system. A high purge pressure can be caused by kinking of the infusion tubing or the yellow purge sidearm. If the integrity of the infusion system is confirmed, then the low or high purge pressure can be corrected by increasing or decreasing the rate of the infusion pump, respectively.
- **Air in purge system alarm.** This alarm occurs when air is drawn into the purge fluid system, which commonly occurs when the purge fluid bag is laid on top of the AIC in transport. The CCT team should proceed with the *de-air* procedure, as instructed on the AIC, to resolve this alarm.

Implantable Left Ventricular Assist Devices

The demand for MCS has grown steadily over the past 30 years. Implantations of these devices are expected to continue to rise due to the epidemic of heart disease, particularly heart failure (HF), in the United States and worldwide. Heart transplantation remains the gold standard in the treatment of patients with end-stage HF. However, the number of patients awaiting donor hearts for transplantation significantly outnumbers the number of donor hearts available, and that gap continues to widen. Moreover, globally there has been a constant decline in the number of heart transplantations performed. An estimated 50,000 people worldwide are awaiting heart transplantation, with as many as 4,000 people awaiting transplantation in the United States at any given time.

Fortunately, continued improvements in the left ventricular assist device (LVAD) have provided increasingly more effective and longer-duration treatment for these patients in the absence of heart transplantation. According to the current Interagency Registry for Mechanically Assisted Circulatory Support (Intermacs) database, patients with HF who have undergone an implantation of a current-generation, continuous-flow LVAD have a

30-day mortality survival rate of 95%, a 1-year survival rate of 83%, a 2-year survival rate of 73%, and a 5-year survival rate of 46%. In this population, 29% will remain supported on MCS at 4 years, and 33% of those patients will have undergone cardiac transplantation. The explantation rate of LVADs at the 5-year mark is less than 5%.

History of LVAD Systems

Dr. Michael DeBakey is recognized as one of the pioneers in the development of the LVAD. In 1966, DeBakey performed a double-valve replacement in a middle-aged female, who postoperatively developed cardiogenic shock. He successfully implanted a pneumatically powered, paracorporeal LVAD from the left atrium to the right subclavian artery. On postoperative day 10 from LVAD implantation, the patient recovered and the LVAD was removed.

Dr. John Norman implanted the first LVAD as a bridge to transplantation in 1978. A young man developed "stone heart" after a double-valve replacement, leading to the implantation of the LVAD. The LVAD remained in place for 6 days until the patient underwent a heart transplantation.

Indications for LVAD Use

An LVAD can be used for a variety of reasons. If the LVAD is used as MCS until the native heart recovers its pumping ability, the indication is referred to as bridge to recovery (BTR). When myocardial recovery does not occur and the device is used for prolonging the patient's life until a heart transplant can be secured, the use is referred to as bridge to transplantation (BTT). The final indication for an LVAD is destination therapy (DT), which refers to long-term use of MCS in a patient with HF who does not meet the heart transplantation criteria.

MCS with LVAD is safe and effective for patients with end-stage HF that is refractory to medical therapy. Approximately 2,500 LVADs are implanted annually. LVADs were originally indicated as BTR or BTT therapy, but as the volume of people awaiting heart transplantation continues to increase in the United States, the number of patients receiving such a device as BTT until a donor heart is available will also continue to rise. This trend dovetails with the increasing use of the LVAD as DT.

Stratification

The American Heart Association's (AHA) Heart Failure Stages and the New York Heart Association's (NYHA) Functional Classification System are the two most widely used methods of classifying HF.

The NYHA developed its original HF classification system in 1928. This tool categorized patients into four groups, Classes I to IV, based on functional capacity. Class I patients do not demonstrate symptoms after ordinary physical activity. Class II patients have cardiac disease resulting in slight limitation of physical activity. Class III patients have marked limitation of physical activity. Class IV patients are unable to tolerate any physical activity without discomfort.

The NYHA revision in 1994 included the addition of what are now referred to as the AHA Heart Failure Stages. These stages were revised in 2001. This rating system evaluates the progression of a patient's HF symptoms, with phases designated as Stage A to Stage D. Stage A includes the presence of HF risk factors but not heart disease. These patients do not have any symptoms. Stage B patients have heart disease with structural changes, but also do not have any symptoms. Stage C patients have structural heart disease and symptoms. Stage D patients have advanced heart disease with continued HF symptoms that require aggressive medical therapy. The AHA Heart Failure Stages system uses an objective assessment method to retrieve data for classifying patients, including data from ECGs, stress tests, echocardiography, and radiology imaging.

The Intermacs registry has also developed patient profile levels to assist with selection of ideal candidates for LVAD implantations. These levels range from 1 to 7. Level 1 patients are in cardiogenic shock and require circulatory support. This level, which is often referred to as "crash and burn" status, accounts for approximately 15% of all implantations. The 1-year survival rate for these patients is 74%. Level 2 patients require inotropic support and are declining. Level 3 patients are stable while on inotropic support. Patients in Levels 2 and 3 have a 1-year survival rate of 82%. Level 4 patients take oral therapy with resting symptoms. Level 5 patients are exertion intolerant. Level 6 patients are able to participate in activities requiring limited exertion. Level 7 patients have NYHA Class III HF: They have minimal symptoms, are hemodynamically stable, and account for only 1% of all implantations. Patients in Levels 4 through 7 have a 1-year survival rate of 84%. Of note, Levels 2 through 4 account for 80% of LVAD implantations.

Generations of LVAD

There have been substantial advancements over the first three generations of LVADs **FIGURE 16-21** and **FIGURE 16-22**. These improvements include a significant decrease in the size of the device, advanced performance with improved durability, and advanced clinical applicability. In terms of patient outcomes, the current generation of LVADs has achieved decreased mortality, decreased adverse reactions, and improved quality of life.

First-Generation LVAD

The first-generation LVAD was also known as a volume displacement pump. These devices were either intracorporeal or paracorporeal membrane pumps that were driven pneumatically or electrically. They generally consisted of pump chambers with one-way valves that controlled inflow and outflow. This arrangement provided a fill to empty mode of mechanical flow, creating an augmented pulsatile flow delivery similar to that of the native heart function.

   Limitations of the first-generation LVAD included increased probability of bleeding, cerebrovascular accident (either embolic or hemorrhagic), and infectious complications. Other limitations and challenges included extensive surgical dissection, decreased mobility, venting requirement due to air pressure changes related to the pneumatic pumping mechanism, durability concerns, large size, and significant noise emission. These limitations led to the development of the second-generation LVAD.

Second-Generation LVAD

This discussion pertains to the HeartMate II, which is the only FDA-approved second-generation LVAD for BTR, BTT, and DT.

   In the second-generation LVAD, the pulsatile-flow technology of the first-generation LVAD gave way to continuous-flow technology. The Heart-Mate II's axial-flow technology is based on the Archimedes screw concept, which describes the

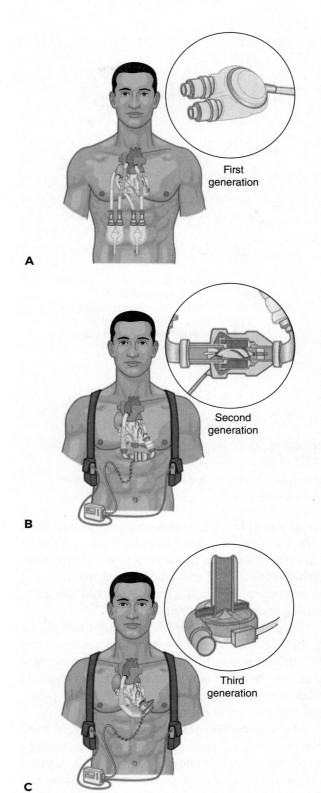

FIGURE 16-21 Comparison of the first three generations of left ventricular assist devices (LVADs). **A.** First generation. **B.** Second generation. **C.** Third generation.

© Jones & Bartlett Learning.

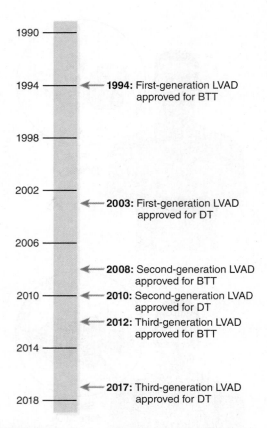

1990

1994 ← **1994:** First-generation LVAD
approved for BTT

1998

2002

2003: First-generation LVAD ← **2003:** First-generation LVAD
approved for DT

2006

← **2008:** Second-generation LVAD
approved for BTT

2010 ← **2010:** Second-generation LVAD
approved for DT

← **2012:** Third-generation LVAD
approved for BTT

2014

← **2017:** Third-generation LVAD
approved for DT

2018

FIGURE 16-22 Timeline of left ventricular assist device (LVAD) development.

Abbreviations: BTT, bridge to therapy; DT, destination therapy

© Jones & Bartlett Learning.

use of a positive-displacement pump to trap fluid from a source and then force the fluid to move to a discharge location. In the HeartMate II, the magnetized rotor spins and pulls blood from the LV through the pump until it reaches the outflow graft, leading to the arterial circulation.

Inside the rotor impeller, in order from the LV to the aorta, are the following vital components: IFC, inflow stator, inflow bearings, rotor, outflow bearings, outflow stator, and outflow cannula **FIGURE 16-23**. The motor rests within the pump housing, directly above and below the rotor.

The decrease in pump size, including a minimal number of moving parts when compared to pneumatic technology, allows for a smaller intra-abdominal pump pocket when implanted. This smaller pump also offers improved comfort, longer operating time, and possibility of use in smaller patients than those who were eligible for the larger first-generation LVADs. The rotary pump relies primarily on a single part, the internal

rotor, which is suspended by contact bearings. The pump speed of the rotor is generally set between 9,000 and 10,000 rpm. Simplifying the design of the second-generation LVAD and relying on a single moving part was crucial in providing improved durability. The combined mechanical and magnetic positioning of the rotor stretched this device's durability up to the 5-year mark.

The motor chamber of the first-generation LVAD required venting of air to safely operate the push plate pump and its valves. These components were also very loud. The second-generation LVAD no longer requires venting and is substantially less noisy. The elimination of parts that continually open and close, together with the removal of the pumping chamber, directly improved patients' quality of life and increased the longevity of the LVAD.

A limitation of the second-generation LVAD is its slightly lessened ability to prevent a disabling stroke, as compared to the pulsatile-flow LVAD. Additional major limitations that were addressed during development of the third-generation LVAD include pump thrombosis, gastrointestinal (GI) bleeding, and ventricular unloading.

Third-Generation LVAD

This discussion pertains to the HeartWare and the HeartMate III, which are the only FDA-approved third-generation LVADs for BTR, BTT, and DT.

The third-generation LVAD continues to advance the continuous-flow technology; however, the rotating elements have transitioned from an axial flow to a centrifugal-flow design to provide cardiac support. The centrifugal-flow pump consists of a blood inlet port, an outlet port, and a pump house that contains a single rotating disk impeller **FIGURE 16-24**. The impeller rapidly spins around a fixed axis, essentially "throwing" the blood off the blade tips into circulation. This design stands in contrast to the axial continuous-flow impeller, which operates like a propeller in a pipe that "pushes" the blood forward.

Depending on the type of LVAD or the patient's condition, the pump speed is generally set at a rate of 2,400 to 9,000 rpm. The centrifugal pump design allows for intrapericardial placement and enables the device to maintain lower rotor speeds. The intrapericardial placement of the smaller

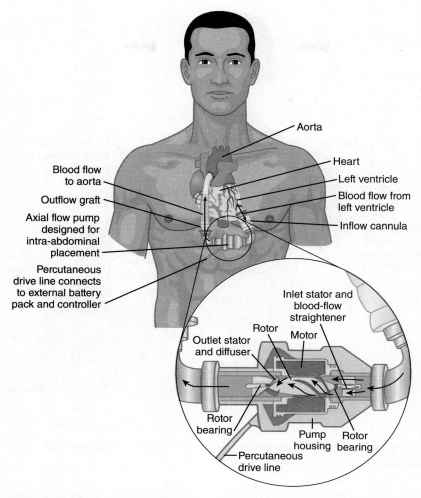

FIGURE 16-23 Design of the axial-flow pump of a second-generation LVAD.

© Jones & Bartlett Learning.

third-generation LVAD also has significant implications for reducing infection risks, minimizing surgical implantation methods, and providing MCS options for pediatric patients.

One of the key advancements of the third-generation LVAD is the introduction of the magnetically levitated rotor, which in turn provides noncontact bearings. Freeing the rotor from the pump housing allows for the near elimination of frictional wear and heat generation and minimizes the potential for thrombus formation. Advancements within the centrifugal-flow design have allowed for wider blood flow passages to help reduce shear stress on red blood cells. Furthermore, the speed modulation technology included in these devices creates an intrinsic pulsatility and reduces rpm speeds, thereby helping to reduce stasis and

minimize the formation of thrombi. These improvements addressed the nonpulsatility effects associated with the second-generation LVAD: GI bleeding, aortic insufficiency, and pump thrombosis. The benefits of these changes were measured by the MOMENTUM 3 trial: 77% of patients receiving the HeartMate III had not experienced a disabling stroke or reoperation 2 years after implantation, versus 65% of patients receiving the HeartMate II. Two-year survival was comparable but slightly better for the HeartMate III (79%) versus the HeartMate II (77%).

Both third-generation LVADs incorporate speed modulation technology, with the rpm being altered at preprogrammed intervals to promote increased ventricular mixing and "washing" of the LV and the device. The HeartMate III uses an artificial pulse

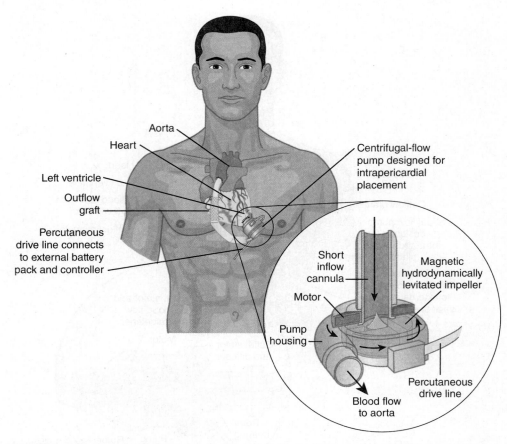

FIGURE 16-24 Design of the centrifugal-flow pump of a third-generation LVAD.

© Jones & Bartlett Learning.

algorithm where the rpm changes every 3 seconds to create an intrinsic artificial pulse. The Heart-Ware LVAD uses the Lavare cycle to create an intrinsic artificial pulse. The Lavare cycle is a pump speed modulation algorithm designed to change the set speed over 3 seconds and repeat the cycle every minute. During a 2-second low-speed phase, the set speed decreases by 200 rpm. After 2 seconds, the pump speed then increases by 400 rpm for a 1-second high-speed phase. The decrease in pump speed allows the LV preload to increase, alters the LV blood flow patterns, and mixes stagnant blood. This mixing also creates a "washing" within the LV and decreases the probability of thrombogenesis. During the period of increased rpm, there is increased pressure within the pump, which creates a "washing" of blood within the pump and impeller. After the 1-second high-speed phase, the rpm returns to the set baseline speed until the next 2-second low-speed phase is repeated the following minute.

Special Populations

In 2020, the HeartMate III was approved by the FDA for use in pediatric patients with advanced refractory LV HF. This is a tremendous step forward in providing pediatric patients with advanced HF an additional option for treatment.

LVADs in the Community

There are more than 24,000 patients with LVADs in the United States. Advancements in treating HF have increased the number of patients living in the community with a variety of LVADs. These devices have increased patients' quality of life and allowed many to return to their everyday activities of living, working, and traveling. Given the prevalence of LVADs, emergency medical services (EMS) providers must be prepared to respond to an LVAD emergency. This emergency may or may not involve the device itself. The EMS provider should have a basic knowledge of how the devices work and be aware of the types of complications that patients with LVADs may experience.

Generally, a patient with an LVAD will have substantial knowledge of the device and likely will have a designated caregiver with a working knowledge of how the LVAD functions and how to manage the device. While the patient and caregiver may be excellent sources of information, the EMS provider should also know how to troubleshoot the device, know which emergency interventions can and cannot be performed, and be aware of how to contact designated LVAD support staff. An emergency phone number can often be found on the back of the patient's controller, but the number may also be stored in the patient's or caregiver's phone, or otherwise maintained in an accessible location, such as attached to the patient's bag of LVAD equipment. This emergency phone line should promptly connect the EMS provider to a trained representative who can assist with decision making as it relates to this patient and their specific equipment.

There are an estimated 500 VAD coordinators in the world and about 155 hospitals in the United States that implant LVADs. These limited numbers make it a challenge to train all community providers in managing LVAD emergencies. Many states offer EMS providers continuing education courses on LVADs, but such education may not be a requirement at the state level. Given the increased number of patients with LVADs who lead active lives in their communities, EMS and CCT services should have a standardized, universal LVAD management training system.

Considerations for LVAD Placement

In addition to risk stratification using the NYHA and Intermacs classifications to select candidates for LVAD implantation, there are other considerations related to LVAD placement. Age, aortic valve regurgitation, RV function, infection, bleeding disorders, irreversible hepatic or renal failure not due to poor CO, metastatic cancer, cerebral accident with neurologic deficits, and psychosocial status with support are all additional factors in determining LVAD candidacy.

Many geriatric patients have multiorgan dysfunction or other comorbidities that may negatively affect outcomes. Nevertheless, many patients have received LVAD implantation well into their 70s and 80s. Carefully assessing social support and level of frailty is crucial in selecting the appropriate geriatric candidate for LVAD therapy. Untreated aortic regurgitation is a contraindication to LVAD implantation. In such a case, either the aortic valve must be repaired at the time of the implantation or the valve must be oversewn during the LVAD implantation. The RV must be able to pump strongly enough to move blood from the right side of the heart through the lungs and over to the left side of the heart. Although no consensus has been reached on the level of RV dysfunction that represents an absolute contraindication to receiving an LVAD, factors that increase the likelihood of ventricular failure after LVAD implantation include elevated CVP, severe renal dysfunction, and ventilator dependence. Systemic infections, either bacterial or fungal, are contraindications to LVAD implantation.

To avoid pump thrombosis, patients will be placed on anticoagulants, usually warfarin. International normalized ratio (INR) targets vary by the patient's condition and the LVAD program's protocols; standard LVAD INR targets are between 2.0 and 3.0. These patients are usually placed on aspirin in addition to the warfarin. Patients with preexisting conditions that involve bleeding disorders are at an unacceptably high risk for LVAD implantation. Patients with LVADs are also at a higher risk of acquiring von Willebrand disease and have an increased risk of developing arteriovenous malformations, particularly in the GI tract. Patients with chronic kidney disease who are receiving dialysis are not considered candidates for LVAD implantation because they would be at higher risk of device infection and overall risk of poor outcomes. Finally, psychosocial instability, including factors such as an ongoing alcohol or substance use disorder, lack of a care plan, and noncompliance, may also be cited as a reason to not implant an LVAD.

Adverse Events
Bleeding

Bleeding is one of the most common adverse events and causes of hospital admission after LVAD implantation. The most common source of bleeding in these patients is the GI tract. Multifactorial mechanisms may contribute to this complication, with shear stress on red blood cells leading to acquired von Willebrand deficiency, arteriovenous malformation, and anticoagulation being the major causes of GI bleeding in patients with LVADs. The combination of increased shear stress, increased intraluminal pressure, and a narrowed pulse pressure is believed to be the cause of arteriovenous malformations.

Because endothelial dysfunction and elevated baseline activity of the coagulation system, which increases the risk of thromboembolic events, have been found in patients with LVADs, prophylactic treatment with anticoagulants and antiplatelet agents may be warranted. Anticoagulant medications used generally include warfarin, heparin, and direct thrombin inhibitors. Antiplatelet medications generally include clopidogrel, aspirin, and dipyridamole. Patients with LVADs will most likely be prescribed both aspirin and warfarin. The prescribed aspirin dose may vary between 81 and 325 mg orally daily. Direct contact between their blood and the LVAD leads to a hypercoagulable state and predisposes these patients to platelet activation. There is also an increase in activated endothelial cells, leading to elevated levels of inflammatory markers, which can promote coagulopathies. As mentioned previously, patients with LVADs are generally prescribed warfarin based on INR goals between 2.0 and 3.0, although this therapy is often reduced or discontinued if the patient experiences a GI bleed.

Studies have also revealed the significant relationship between GI bleeds and subsequent thromboembolic events, with the latter being related to the alterations in anticoagulation observed after the initial GI bleed. Preventing GI bleeds may result in fewer thromboembolic events and improved outcomes. The challenge remains maintaining the appropriate balance of antiplatelet and anticoagulation therapy.

LVAD Infections

Infection remains one of the most common LVAD complications contributing to major morbidity and mortality. By the 2-year mark, the incidence of major infection related to LVADs increases to 51% for axial-flow devices, 55% for centrifugal-flow hybrid levitation devices, and 41% for centrifugal-flow full-magnetic levitation devices. Infection accounts for 7% of all LVAD-related deaths in the first year after device implantation and 15% of all LVAD-related deaths thereafter. The most commonly encountered pathogens are *Staphylococci* species, *Pseudomonas aeruginosa*, and *Enterococcus* species.

Most LVAD-specific infections are isolated to the driveline, with subsequent infection involving the pocket and internal surfaces of the pump. The driveline transmits communication between the pump and the controller. It also provides energy from an external source (ie, batteries or AC power unit). Driveline infections occur frequently because the exit site where the driveline enters through the skin and abdominal wall creates a conduit for the entry of bacteria and the prosthetic material of the driveline creates an environment that supports bacterial biofilm formation. Such an infection can affect the driveline site and continue ascending to the subcutaneous tunnel, the abdominal pocket, the implanted pump itself, and the remainder of the body.

Multiple studies have identified predisposing factors for LVAD infections. Elevated body mass index is the most commonly cited independent predictor of infection. Recent studies have also revealed that age has emerged as a strong predictor of percutaneous site infection. For every 10-year decrease in patient age, the risk of percutaneous site infection has been found to rise by 20%. It is believed that younger patients are more active and more likely to suffer trauma at the driveline exit site, further compromising the integrity of the driveline–integument barrier. Prevention includes using anchors to immobilize the driveline in all patients and using binders as determined by specific LVAD implantation programs.

A systematic multidisciplinary approach that spans the operative technique, including postoperative management, patient education, and long-term follow-up, continues to be paramount in combating driveline infections in patients with LVADs. The CCTP should be able to recognize the signs and symptoms of infection, particularly as they pertain to the LVAD driveline. During the assessment of the LVAD's driveline, both the patient and care providers should don gloves and a mask. Providers should inspect for erythema, bleeding, or purulent drainage and note any wound odor.

Ischemic and Hemorrhagic Stroke

Strokes, both ischemic and hemorrhagic, and their sequelae are major concerns for patients with

LVADs. Hypertension is a significant risk factor for stroke. The risk of stroke in patients with severe hypertension (SBP > 160 mm Hg) is four times that in normotensive patients. A MAP of greater than 110 mm Hg in patients with LVADs is considered hypertensive. Clinical management guidelines have recommended a goal MAP range of 70 to 80 mm Hg, and current International Society for Heart and Lung Transplantation (ISHLT) guidelines recommend a target MAP of less than 80 mm Hg, provided the adverse effects of hypotension can be avoided.

The mechanisms behind ischemic strokes are believed to include embolic sources such as thrombus formation at the pump, the aortic valve, and inflow or outflow grafts.

The highest priority when providing care for the patient with an LVAD and current intracerebral bleeding is a safe return to a near-normal coagulation profile. There are currently no established guidelines for the duration of cessation of anticoagulation or the timing of its resumption following resolution of a bleeding event in a patient with an LVAD. Recommendations for INR targets will vary depending on the LVAD, the patient's past medical history, and the guidelines established by the LVAD implantation program. As mentioned previously, patients are generally prescribed warfarin as their anticoagulation therapy, with INR goals between 2.0 and 3.0, and their antiplatelet therapy usually includes daily oral intake of either aspirin or a short-term alternative such as a glycoprotein IIb/IIIa inhibitor. Studies have suggested that preventing a bleed may ultimately decrease the risk of future thromboembolic events.

Providers should exercise extreme thoughtfulness when providing initial care to a patient with an LVAD who is experiencing bleeding, including in their approach toward cessation of anticoagulation during an episode of bleeding. Potential interventions, which must be carefully monitored, include (1) active reversal of INR versus observation and simple cessation of anticoagulation, (2) discontinuation of the antiplatelet medication, and (3) careful timing of anticoagulation therapy resumption after a bleeding episode.

Cardiac Arrhythmias

Atrial and ventricular arrhythmias are common in LVAD recipients, originating from the preexisting myocardial substrate or from the complex electrical remodeling that occurs after LVAD implantation. There is a high prevalence of atrial arrhythmias in these patients (21% to 54%), with 20% to 30% of patients developing new-onset atrial arrhythmias following implantation of their LVAD. Most of these patients with new-onset atrial arrhythmias will have atrial fibrillation, which is believed to be caused by the post-LVAD reduction in left atrial size and volume. Pre-LVAD atrial arrhythmias are associated with post-LVAD atrial arrhythmias as well as ventricular arrhythmias.

Postoperative atrial fibrillation is not strongly associated with an immediate risk of mortality or stroke, although persistent atrial fibrillation is associated with a combined end point of HF and increased mortality. The major concern for developing thromboembolic events secondary to atrial fibrillation applies to all patients, with or without an LVAD. Limited studies and current clinical data have yielded conflicting information on whether atrial fibrillation increases the risk of thromboembolic events in LVAD recipients. In regard to treating the patient with an LVAD and new-onset atrial fibrillation, anticoagulation is required and the patient should not have INR targets readjusted due to atrial fibrillation. Rate control has been shown to be the most effective management strategy for patients with atrial fibrillation. Beta blockers are the agents most commonly used to treat atrial fibrillation associated with a rapid heart rate. Nondihydropyridine calcium channel blockers should be used with caution because of their negative inotropic effects. Digoxin is frequently used as an adjunct when treating patients with recurrent HF post LVAD implantation and has been combined with beta blockers to achieve atrial fibrillation rate control. If the patient cannot maintain hemodynamic stability due to the atrial fibrillation, then the following medications may be prescribed for rhythm control: amiodarone, dofetilide, or sotalol. Only limited studies and guidelines are available to provide strategies for rhythm control in hemodynamically unstable patients with LVADs. In consequence, management typically follows AHA recommendation guidelines for treating atrial fibrillation in patients with a reduced ejection fraction or systolic HF.

There is also a high prevalence of ventricular arrhythmias in patients with LVADs (20% to 50%), with 20% of patients developing new-onset sustained monomorphic ventricular tachycardia after implantation of their device. The majority of these ventricular arrhythmias result from the underlying substrate. Incidence is higher immediately after LVAD implantation and in the month that follows. In the setting of documented ventricular arrhythmias, no antiarrhythmic drug has been shown to improve survival better than implantable cardioverter-defibrillator (ICD) therapy. Given the history of advanced HF noted in many LVAD recipients, an ICD may already be in place during LVAD implantation. Antiarrhythmic drugs are often used in conjunction with ICD therapy to improve symptoms, reduce ICD therapies, and help prevent hemodynamic instability associated with ventricular arrhythmias. Beta blocker use has been shown to improve ventricular arrhythmias, although LVAD recipients are generally already on a beta blocker regimen when the new onset of ventricular arrhythmia occurs. Limited studies of patients with LVADs who received beta blockers for ventricular arrhythmias have shown conflicting results with the use of these medications for secondary prevention of ventricular arrhythmias. The following medications may be prescribed to treat ventricular arrhythmias in LVAD recipients: amiodarone, sotalol, azimilide, celivarone, lidocaine, and procainamide. Conclusive evidence that antiarrhythmic therapy improves outcomes remains lacking, however. Careful assessment of the symptoms and hemodynamic changes associated with ventricular arrhythmias, balanced against the risks of side effects and drug interactions, must be undertaken when selecting the appropriate medical therapy for the patient with an LVAD and ventricular arrhythmias.

Many patients with LVADs exhibit sustained ventricular tachycardia, ventricular fibrillation, or even asystole. Cases have described patients who have demonstrated a stable presentation with sustained ventricular tachycardia or fibrillation for greater than 24 hours; however, there is concern about the potential reduction in pump flow and CO during sustained ventricular arrhythmias. There is also concern regarding the potential adverse effects on RV function or possible thrombus formation in a fibrillating RV.

The decision to implant an ICD in a patient with an LVAD is generally made on a case-by-case basis. Consideration is given to the patient with a history of ventricular arrhythmias that have been associated with hemodynamic instability or other symptoms such as syncope or impaired LVAD flow. The AHA has stated that ICD implantation can be beneficial for an LVAD recipient who is experiencing sustained runs of ventricular arrhythmias. Continued research on this topic is needed, however, as are more appropriate ICD algorithms for the patient with both an LVAD and an ICD.

LVAD recipients with ICDs are frequently admitted to the hospital for ICD firing and arrhythmia management. The majority of patients with LVADs can tolerate ventricular arrhythmias, and most of these patients are awake when their ICD fires. At the present time, cardiologists are restricted from adjusting ICD programming limits due to FDA rules. Therefore, patients with LVADs and active ICDs sometimes receive a shock while they are wide awake. As one would expect, such painful experiences can have drastic effects on patients' psychological health and quality of life. Certain patients opt to have their ICD turned off to stop the painful shocks. This decision should involve members of the LVAD team, the patient, and the patient's family.

Many tachyarrhythmias, ventricular tachycardia, and ventricular fibrillation, as previously mentioned, might be well tolerated. However, if the LVAD recipient without an active ICD is in a shockable rhythm and is hemodynamically unstable, providers should follow current advanced cardiac life support protocols for defibrillation or cardioversion. The defibrillator pads should be placed in the anterior–posterior position and not over the device.

LVAD Thrombosis

LVAD thrombosis is a potentially lethal complication that may be noted by signs of inadequate circulation. It is typically associated with sustained low LVAD flow despite normovolemia (which could be caused by partial obstruction of the LVAD blood pathway by thrombus) or thrombus formation within the pump house interface, causing increased friction of the rotor or impeller. This thrombus formation will cause increased LVAD power consumption that may be intermittent or sustained, resulting in an activated high LVAD power alarm. A thrombus that is causing excessive power consumption could produce an overestimated pump flow reading. If signs of poor circulation persist despite appropriate treatment, device thrombosis should be highly suspected. When managing this emergency, providers should consult the patient's LVAD center for guidance before transferring the patient to the appropriate LVAD center.

A number of factors contribute to the formation of a thrombus within an LVAD device, including anticoagulation therapy, surgical technique, and device engineering. The obstruction is typically attributed to a clot within the circulation path of the LVAD, including the inflow and outflow cannulas, and the pump housing itself, which includes the stators, bearings, rotor, and impeller. A thrombus located on the rotor or impeller is likely to produce power spikes or falsely elevated pump flow. A thrombus located within the IFC is likely to produce a pump flow reduction.

The thrombus can originate from within the device or from the LV, left atrium, or right side of the heart, most likely via an atrial septal defect or ventricular septal defect. The consequences vary from a small thrombus formation requiring minimal intervention to device malfunction requiring surgery and exchange of the LVAD.

Signs and symptoms of device thrombosis include HF symptoms, hemoglobinuria, an elevated LDH value greater than 2.5 times the upper limit of normal, an elevated plasma-free hemoglobin level greater than 40 mg/dL, anemia, and an elevated bilirubin level. LDH is considered the most specific biochemical indicator of pump thrombosis.

Antithrombotic management of pump thrombosis includes aggressive anticoagulation with warfarin and antiplatelet therapy with aspirin. When device thrombosis is highly suspected, the patient's LVAD center should be consulted for care management guidance until patient transport occurs. Providers should anticipate initiating a short-term parenteral anticoagulant such as heparin. Conflicting data have been collected regarding the efficacy of direct thrombin inhibitors, such as argatroban, in managing suspected pump thrombosis. Conflicting data also exist on the efficacy of thrombolytic therapy.

The current-generation LVADs, particularly the HeartMate III, have been associated with minimal levels of shear stress and reduced hemolysis due to the framework of their fully magnetically levitated impeller. This centrifugal pump has wide passages for blood flow, frictionless propulsion with magnetic levitation, and an intrinsic pulse designed to reduce blood stasis. This design, in turn, mitigates platelet activation and helps to inhibit activation of the coagulation system.

Right-Side HF

As described previously, the RV must be able to pump strongly enough to move blood from the right side of the heart through the lungs and over to the left side of the heart. Despite precautions and evaluations of RV status before an LVAD implantation, RV failure after implantation is common, occurring in 5% to 13% of patients. Approximately 4% of patients in RV failure will require support with a right ventricular assist device (RVAD) within 2 weeks of LVAD implantation. Ideally, LVAD unloading of the LV should decrease RV afterload and improve RV contractility.

Multiple factors contribute to RV failure after LVAD implantation. One or more of the following conditions may result in RV failure: the sudden increase in RV unloading, increased RV preload, increased RV afterload, and progressive cardiomyopathy. Symptoms of right-side HF will include HF symptoms and fluid overload.

Medical management remains the mainstay for treating right-side HF after LVAD implantation. There are four major areas of focus and treatment:

- RV preload: diuretics and hemofiltration
- RV afterload: pulmonary vasodilators, optimal LV unloading with LVAD
- RV contractility: inotropes
- Rhythm: optimal atrioventricular synchrony

LVAD speed adjustments may be required to help manage right-side HF after LVAD implantation. These adjustments are usually performed at LVAD centers. LVAD unloading of the LV may result in RV reshaping and septal shifting, inducing right-side HF. Leftward septal shift secondary to high LVAD speeds may result in RV distention and tricuspid regurgitation. Maintaining hemodynamic stability with LVAD support is paramount with LVAD management. Vasodilation or poor perfusion can lead to unloading of the LV, which then leads to leftward septal shift and resultant suction events. Suction events prevent adequate LVAD filling and output. They also contribute to the onset of ventricular arrhythmias.

When medical therapy in conjunction with LVAD speed adjustments is unsuccessful in treating right-side HF, right-side MCS may be indicated. Right-side MCS can be used in conjunction with an LVAD as a bridge to right-side heart recovery, bridge to heart transplantation, bridge to durable biventricular support, or bridge to the implantation of a total artificial heart.

ECMO can be another alternative for acute right-side HF support after LVAD implantation. ECMO indications include primary RV failure or RV failure secondary to primary pulmonary pathology, including the presence of systemic oxygen desaturation.

Device Malfunction

Device malfunction is not limited to pump failure; other components of the LVAD system may also be subject to failure. The controller is the most common source of LVAD malfunction, accounting for approximately 30% of instances. The battery (19%), patient cable (14%), and pump (14%) are also leading culprits. According to the FDA, malfunctions of the following LVAD components/mechanisms have resulted in product recalls: battery malfunction, loose driveline connector, malfunction of the system controller, loose power supply connector ports, malfunction of the driveline splice kit, problems with the percutaneous lead connection, disconnection of the bend relief system and outflow graft, and outflow graft occlusion. Malfunction of these components could lead to pump inactivation, and subsequently to HF symptoms, cardiogenic shock, and death. Thorough assessment of all LVAD components is essential when providing patient care.

Recognition of LVAD complications as they specifically relate to the pump, the controller, the battery, and the percutaneous lead requires a basic understanding of how these components function **FIGURE 16-25**. As discussed previously, the patient or the patient's caregiver will have a thorough understanding of those components. While these individuals may offer invaluable assistance, the CCTP is responsible for providing safe and appropriate care during prehospital and interfacility transport of the patient with an LVAD.

Mental Health

Everyday life with an LVAD presents challenges for patients. Living with an LVAD requires constant monitoring, consistent medical follow-up, and adjustment to overwhelming lifestyle changes. Depression is common in patients with HF and has been associated with increased morbidity and

mortality. Post-LVAD anxiety and depression are prevalent predictors of decreased quality of life. Depression may affect cognitive status and motivation, making it difficult for patients to understand and adhere to medical recommendations. This functional impairment may be particularly problematic given the complicated medical regimens and significant lifestyle changes required after LVAD placement. Depression and anxiety vary throughout the course of the patient's care, intensifying just before LVAD implantation, decreasing after immediate implantation, and rising again when adjustment problems overwhelm coping skills.

Studies of patients who underwent LVAD implantation as DT and BTT, where symptoms of depression were measured preoperatively, revealed that signs of clinical depression were more prevalent in the DT group. These results might reflect that patients and caregivers preparing for LVAD implantation as BTT consider this intervention to be a temporary means to achieve medical stability until heart transplantation is possible. In contrast, patients receiving an LVAD as DT know the device will be in place for the remainder of their lives.

Family members may also feel overwhelmed by the responsibility of managing the device and the fear of it malfunctioning on their watch. Studies show that caregivers experience emotional strain particularly during the first 3 months after implantation. This includes an increase in stress levels due to all of the adjustments made at home for the patient and the other family members.

Patients could benefit from psychological support before and after LVAD implantation to further improve their quality of life and mental recovery.

Respiratory Failure

Respiratory failure commonly occurs either before or after implantation of LVADs. According to Intermacs data, more than 5% of patients require respiratory support within 48 hours before implantation, and 6.1% of patients experience respiratory failure within the first week after implantation. More importantly, both intubation before and respiratory failure after LVAD implantation are independently associated with a significantly increased risk of adverse clinical outcomes, including mortality at 1 year (2.5 times increased risk of death). Studies also reveal that the risk of respiratory failure is twice

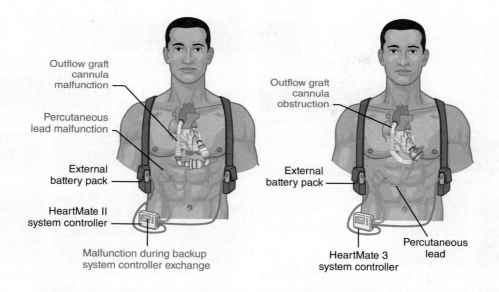

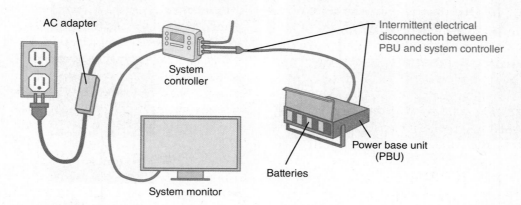

FIGURE 16-25 Causes of malfunction relating to the LVAD system.

Reproduced with permission from Baruqui DL, Maning J, Chaparro SV. Food and Drug Administration malfunction recalls of left ventricular assist devices. *ASAIO J.* 2020;66(7):739-745.

as great if the patient with an LVAD develops an infection. An LVAD recipient in respiratory failure is five times as likely to experience renal failure, and the LVAD recipient with a neurologic adverse event is most likely to experience respiratory failure.

The incidence of adverse reactions relating to respiratory failure within the first 60 days after LVAD implantation remains high, and these adverse reactions rarely occur in isolation; furthermore, an initial adverse reaction will often be followed by subsequent adverse reactions. It is therefore imperative that the CCT recognize adverse events early, and avoid inadvertently triggering a cascade of adverse events, so as to help reduce the overall morbidity and mortality of patients with LVADs.

Point-of-Care Ultrasonography

Point-of-care ultrasonography (POCUS) is a valuable tool in assessing the patient–pump balance. It can be used to determine the following:

- Native RV and LV function.
- Hypovolemia: Decreased RV size suggests low preload.
- LVAD-induced RV failure: Decreased LV size with the septum bowing toward the LV suggests a possible suction event.
- RV failure or high pulmonary vascular resistance (PVR): Large RV and small LV suggest RV failure.
- Device failure: Large RV and LV suggest pump thrombosis or obstruction.

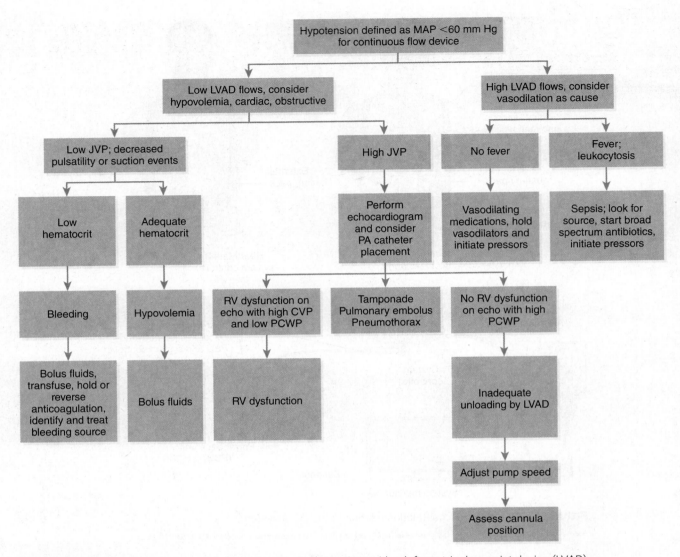

FIGURE 16-26 Algorithm for managing hypotension in the patient with a left ventricular assist device (LVAD).

Abbreviations: CVP, central venous pressure; JVP, jugular venous pressure; MAP, mean arterial pressure; PA, pulmonary artery; PCWP, pulmonary capillary wedge pressure; RV, right ventricle

Reproduced with permission from Feldman D, Pamboukian SV, Teuteberg JJ, et al. The 2013 International Society for Heart and Lung Transplantation Guidelines for mechanical circulatory support: executive summary. *J Heart Lung Transplant*. 2013;32(2):157-187.

Recognizing LVAD Dysfunction

Hypotension (Shock)

The differential diagnosis for post–LVAD implantation hypotension includes a broad range of conditions. Hypotension in the patient with an LVAD is defined as a MAP of less than 60 mm Hg **FIGURE 16-26**. Hypovolemia should be at the top of the CCTP's differential diagnosis list as an etiology of hypotension. Generally, in patients with LVADs, hypotension is secondary to hypovolemia; the CCTP should anticipate a decrease in the LVAD flows, a decrease in the pulse index, and a potential

suction event. Hypotension with decreased LVAD flows can also present with RV failure, arrhythmias, tamponade, or a device-related complication. If the pump flow falls below 2.5 L/min, the low-flow hazard alarm will be displayed, the pump running symbol will remain green, the red heart warning light will illuminate, and a steady tone alarm will sound.

Hypotension can also present secondary to vasodilatory shock resulting from either sepsis or vasoplegia. LVADs are afterload sensitive; therefore, the CCTP should anticipate an increase in LVAD flows if vasodilation is present and adequate preload exists. Hypotension will persist once the LVAD's augmented forward flow is overcome by increased systemic vascular resistance. When vasodilatory shock is suspected, appropriate fluid resuscitation and vasopressors should be administered to maintain a MAP of 65 to 80 mm Hg.

Decreased pump preload can also occur secondary to bleeding. As discussed previously, patients with LVADs are at a high risk of bleeding due to the need for anticoagulation, acquired von Willebrand disease, and arteriovenous malformations in the GI tract. Providers should assess for bleeding from the GI tract, nares, and thorax, and throughout the body. Increased pump afterload can be due to systemic hypertension, kinking of the outflow cannula, or thrombus. Pump malfunction can also result in hypotension. Arrhythmias that affect RV filling will generally affect LV filling, which could ultimately result in hemodynamic instability, although not all patients with arrhythmias will present with hemodynamic instability.

It is not uncommon for a patient with an LVAD to be in ventricular tachycardia or fibrillation and remain conscious. The LVAD may be able to provide enough forward flow despite ventricular tachycardia or fibrillation and other arrhythmias. Given this possibility, the decision to cardiovert or defibrillate should be based on the patient's mental and perfusion status. Hypotension can also result from increased PVR. Increased PVR can result from hypoxemia, hypercarbia, or obstruction of pulmonary blood flow. Pulmonary embolism is the usual culprit of obstructed pulmonary blood flow. Increased PVR will decrease LV preload, which will result in a decrease in overall LVAD flow.

Hypertension

Intermacs has defined new-onset hypertension in patients with LVAD as the presence of a MAP greater than 110 mm Hg. Clinical management guidelines recommend a goal MAP of 70 to 80 mm Hg. The current ISHLT guidelines recommend a target MAP of less than 80 mm Hg, provided the adverse effects of hypotension can be avoided. The guidelines also recommend standard HF pharmacotherapy to maintain optimal MAP control. Evidence has shown that maintaining MAP goals protects against adverse events such as stroke, pump thrombosis, and aortic insufficiency.

Ventricular Recovery

Ventricular recovery after LVAD implantation is the most desirable goal in treating the patient with end-stage HF. With the improvements in the durable LVAD, there has been a substantial increase in the number of LVAD implantations performed. There are also more patients with HF and a higher Intermacs profile who are accepting LVAD implantations. Newer minimally invasive implantation techniques, in conjunction with the overall growth in the number of MCS providers, favors an increase in the ventricular recovery of patients with LVADs. Ventricular recovery occurs in approximately 1% to 5% of these patients, allowing for explantation of their device. The type of cardiac pathology present has proved to be a determining factor in ventricular recovery. Recovery mechanisms vary due to the different etiologies of cardiac pathology, the different proportions of patients who recover, and the overall time of recovery: Patients with dilated cardiomyopathy can recover after several months of LVAD support. By comparison, research shows that patients with severe acute myocarditis or noncoronary shock can recover after only weeks of LVAD support.

Results of BTR treatment in patients with LVADs show encouraging safety and long-term survival outcomes. Studies reveal that 10-year survival outcomes after LVAD explantation in selected patients are superior to the corresponding outcomes in BTT recipients. With a careful selection process for LVAD implants and an aggressive cardiac reconditioning effort, BTR success rates should continue to rise.

Inflow Cannula Malpositioning

Ideal IFC positioning lies on a line from the apex to the center of the mitral valve. Malpositioning of the IFC includes deviations toward the superior free wall, the inferior wall, the septum, or the lateral wall.

IFC malpositioning has been associated with a number of adverse events, including ischemic stroke, suction events, low flows, speed reductions, and thromboses. Axial pumps are associated with a substantial number of IFC-malpositioning implantations as compared to the centrifugal-flow hybrid levitation pumps. Such malpositioning incidents are largely due to the axial pump's requirements for an intra-abdominal pump pocket and the relatively inflexible IFC position. The smaller centrifugal-flow pumps are designed for direct intracardial placement, which minimizes IFC movement when compared to the axial pumps.

LVAD Pump Parameters

Pump Flow

The displayed pump flow is a calculated value that is directly related to the set rpm and power. An increase in power produces an increase in calculated flow. The spinning impeller creates the pump flow and ultimately generates the forward flow of blood. The device flow is directly proportional to the rpm and inversely related to the difference in the inflow and outflow cannulas, as described by the following equation:

$$\text{Device flow} = \frac{\text{Rotor speed}}{(\text{Pump}_{\text{inflow}} - \text{Pump}_{\text{outflow}})}$$

Hypovolemia, cardiac tamponade, RV failure, thrombus, or a kink within the IFC will result in a low flow rate. A low flow rate can also result from an increase in afterload (elevated SVR). Increased afterload may result from uncontrolled hypertension, a kink, or a thrombus in the outflow cannula.

> ### Confirming Pump Function
>
> Anytime the pump is running, a green light will be illuminated on the controller and the CCTP will be able to hear and feel a hum when listening or placing a hand over the pump.

Pump rpm Setting

The rpm setting determines pump flow. This set rate is determined by either the cardiac surgeon or the physician caring for the patient with HF and is adjusted as flow needs change. Ramp studies are increasingly used to evaluate heart and LVAD function and possible malfunction of the LVAD. Ramp studies measure cardiac hemodynamics and assess changes in heart size at various rpm settings. The results help to indicate possible pump dysfunction, IFC malpositioning, appropriate or inappropriate LV unloading, hypovolemia, aortic valve function, and LV compliance.

Output from the LVAD depends on preload, afterload, and pump speed. However, it should be noted that the pump speed is fixed and does not fluctuate with loading conditions of the heart.

Pump Power

The pump power of the LVAD is the measurement of the current required to maintain the pump's rpm at a set speed. Generally, an increase in pump power is caused by formation of a thrombus within the pump. Decreases in pump power most often result from a low battery.

Pulsatility Index

With the centrifugal-flow full-magnetic levitation, the pulsatility in flow is quantified as the pulsatility index (PI). PI is calculated as follows, where PP represents pump pressure:

$$PI = \frac{\text{Maximum PP} - \text{Minimum PP}}{\text{Average PP}}$$

The PI corresponds to the magnitude of flow pulse through the pump. It fluctuates with changes in fluid status and the heart's native contractility. PI increases when preload and contractility increase; conversely, it decreases when preload and afterload decrease, such as with an obstruction that causes low flows and abnormal pump power.

Troubleshooting Abnormal LVAD Conditions

Management of specific problems and device alarms is discussed next. **TABLE 16-4** offers a brief overview of these conditions.

Suction Events

Suction event complications are generally associated with low-flow events that occur secondary to arrhythmias and hypovolemia. Decreased LV preload can cause collapse of the LV and decreased flow to the LVAD. Ventricular arrhythmias can also result from suction events, potentially further compounding decreased preload. The controller alarms will reveal low flows, low speeds, and low power **FIGURE 16-27**. Suction events will also trigger an automatic transient decrease in rpm to a set lower speed limit. Managing the underlying etiology and providing appropriate fluid resuscitation will improve preload and intravascular volume.

TABLE 16-4 Troubleshooting LVAD Events

Condition	Possible Causes	Considerations
Low LVAD flow	Right heart failure Arrhythmia Hypovolemia High pulmonary vascular resistance	Assess right ventricular function. Obtain an electrocardiogram. Interrogate the implantable cardioverter–defibrillator. Assess volume status. Assess patient's native pulse.
High LVAD flow	Vasodilation Sepsis/infection Aortic insufficiency	Treat the root cause. Obtain an echocardiogram.
High pump power	Device thrombosis Clot ingestion	Obtain an echocardiogram. Assess the native left ventricular flow. Provide patient support. Consider anticoagulation. Exchange the device.
Low pump power	Device dysfunction	Assess power cables and power sources. Change components as needed.
High pulse index	Heart recovery Arrhythmia Hypervolemia Incorrect pump speed	Obtain an echocardiogram. Assess the rhythm. Check external components.
Low pulse index	Right heart failure Hypovolemia Incorrect pump speed	Obtain an echocardiogram. Assess volume status. Optimize pump speed.
Suction event	Hypovolemia Inlet obstruction Arrhythmia Right heart failure	Obtain an echocardiogram. Assess volume status. Assess for hemolysis.

Abbreviation: LVAD, left ventricular assist device

Cable Failure and Disconnection

Consider the basic design of the modern LVAD: A miniaturized blood pump is attached to the heart and driven by an electric motor, which is powered by a cable driveline that exits the patient's body through the skin to be connected to an external power source.

Now consider the specific connections and points of attachment: Centrifugal-flow LVADs have inflow conduits that are inserted into the LV through an apical cuff. The pump is then secured to the apical cuff. The pump is connected with a power supply via a driveline cable. The driveline passes from the pump through the musculus rectus abdominis and fascial layers into the patient's abdominal region. The cable then exits the body through a small incision in the skin. The cable sheath, which is usually made of silicone or polyurethane, is covered in the implanted part with a woven or nonwoven material, which ensures optimal ingrowth. The driveline is immobilized close to

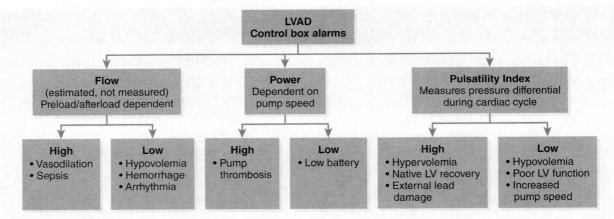

FIGURE 16-27 Left ventricular assist device (LVAD) control alarms.

Abbreviation: LV, left ventricle

Reproduced with permission from Greenwood JC, Herr DL. Mechanical circulatory support. *Emerg Med Clin North Am.* 2014;32(4):851-869.

the exit site of the skin by means of a fixing system that is designed to protect the exit site from mechanical manipulation. The exit site of the cable is protected from possible infection by a mandatory sterile dressing. The cable then connects to the LVAD controller.

LVAD System Alarms

Battery Alarm

The yellow battery icon indicates there is less than 15 minutes of power remaining, and a beep will sound every second when this alarm is activated. The red battery icon indicates there is less than 5 minutes of power remaining, and a steady tone will sound when this alarm is activated. When a battery alarm is active, the pump will default to a lower rpm speed to conserve power. It will return to the original set speed once adequate power is restored. When a battery alarm is active, check all connections and replace batteries as instructed. Do not disconnect both batteries at the same time because doing so may turn off the pump. If charged batteries are unavailable, switch to the power module.

Cable Disconnect Symbols

If the black power cable disconnect symbol is illuminated, the black side does not have power and the advisory alarm will be activated. The advisory alarm will beep and the yellow diamond will illuminate.

If the white power cable disconnect symbol is illuminated, the white side does not have power and the advisory alarm will be activated. The advisory alarm will beep and the yellow diamond will illuminate.

If the driveline cable disconnect symbol is illuminated, the driveline has been removed from the controller and the hazard alarm will be activated. The hazard alarm will emit a steady tone and the red battery icon will illuminate.

Summary

In patients with HF, MCS may be required. Although CCTPs will transport patients who rely on MCS devices to ensure adequate perfusion, the operation and management of these devices are outside of the typical CCTP's scope of practice. The CCTP's primary role is to assist in emergent care and transport of the patient or to provide interfacility transport. By preparing carefully and monitoring them diligently, the CCTP can ensure the best outcomes for these vulnerable patients.

Patients on MCS can be safely transported by ground or air and by using various team combinations when the team has the appropriate resources and skills. Frequent training and competency demonstrations should be routinely augmented with simulation and quality reviews. Medical oversight of CCT teams should be provided by professionals with experience in the care and management of patients requiring MCS.

Case Study

You are assigned to a ground CCT unit. You have just been called to a critical access hospital that operates a cardiac catheterization laboratory (catheterization lab) without on-site cardiac surgery. On arrival, you find a 56-year-old male patient who presented there 3 hours ago with an acute coronary syndrome. He has a past medical history of diabetes and hypertension. His symptoms began 72 hours ago with chest discomfort, epigastric pain, and increased work of breathing. Ground EMS handed him off with the following vital signs: heart rate, 86 beats/min; BP, 92/62 mm Hg; respiratory rate, 24 breaths/min; SpO_2, 96%. EMS administered 325 mg of aspirin and three doses of sublingual nitroglycerin without resolution of symptoms. The patient's prehospital 12-lead ECG revealed a sinus rhythm with Q waves in leads III and aVF; T-wave inversion across leads II, III, and aVF; and ST-segment depression in V_3–V_6. EMS initiated a heart team alert prior to your arrival.

In the emergency department, the patient's symptoms persisted. His skin was paler than its baseline color and his extremities were cool. Providers administered 600 mg of clopidogrel orally and initiated a heparin drip. The patient was promptly transported to the cardiac catheterization lab.

In the cardiac catheterization lab, arterial access was established via the right femoral artery. The patient was found to have triple-vessel coronary artery disease with 80% occlusion of the right coronary artery, 100% occlusion of the left anterior descending artery (resembling thrombus), and 70% occlusion of the circumflex artery. A thrombus aspiration of the left anterior descending artery was performed. During the procedure, the patient experienced transient episodes of ventricular tachycardia associated with hypotension, hypoxemia, and syncope. He was placed on high-flow oxygen by mask, and an amiodarone and phenylephrine infusion was initiated. The left ventriculogram revealed a severely depressed ventricle, and a left-side microaxial percutaneous catheter pump (Impella) was placed. The patient's

vital signs are now heart rate, 88 beats/min; sinus rhythm with frequent multiform premature ventricular complexes; BP, 98/56 mm Hg; MAP, 60 mm Hg; respiratory rate, 26 breaths/min; and SpO_2, 96%.

The Impella CP device is set to P-8 with a flow of 3.5 L/min. The device parameters show a placement signal of 108/77 mm Hg (87), LV 117/2 mm Hg, and motor current of 822/699 mA. The purge flow is 11 mL/h of D_5W with 25 units/mL of heparin with a purge pressure of 503 mm Hg.

You have initiated transport for a 45-minute drive to a quaternary care center. En route, the patient experiences more sustained episodes of ventricular tachycardia lasting 20 to 30 seconds, along with hypotension in the 70s. The Impella device begins issuing the "suction" alarm.

1. What considerations prior to transport should be considered with a patient on MCS?
2. For patients with active ventricular unloading with a heart pump, what factors can cause inadequate pump support?
3. Which troubleshooting steps can providers take to ensure adequate flow and function of the heart pump?

Analysis

This patient presented with an acute coronary syndrome with evidence of inadequate tissue perfusion and unresolved coronary artery supply–demand mismatch. This cardiogenic shock presentation places the patient at risk of worsening organ dysfunction and death. The initiation of MCS is vital to improving this patient's outcome; however, the CCT team should avoid unnecessary delays in further treatment.

Considerations for transport of a patient with cardiogenic shock receiving MCS include addressing both the patient and the pump system. Patient considerations include obtaining an adequate handoff from the sending team, ensuring adequate airway and ventilation, maintaining adequate vascular access, providing pain relief and comfort, clearly understanding the therapeutic agents and infusions involved, and formulating a plan to move the patient without causing any complications. The CCTP should be able to anticipate common adverse events related to the pathology the patient is experiencing. This patient is at increased risk of worsening cardiac arrhythmias, pulmonary edema, right-side HF, and complications related to anticoagulants. Considerations for maintaining optimal device function include maintaining adequate preload through volume and right-side heart output. Heart pumps are also sensitive to increases in afterload, and CCTPs should be aware of the target hemodynamics and have the resources needed to titrate to them. Pumps can also become malpositioned during patient transfer or movement or as a result of device migration. Externalized devices should be secured according to the agency policy and the manufacturers' instructions for their use. The power supply for transport should be deemed adequate and tested with a margin of backup before loading the patient.

Inadequate pump support can be caused by inadequate patient volume, inadequate pressure, worsening HF, pump malposition, thrombosis, ingestion of a clot, or malfunction of the pump system. Anticipating, recognizing, and treating these patient or device problems can be challenging in the transport environment. Team members should have appropriate technical resources available to them, staffing adequate to handle the situation, and the ability to communicate with experts during the transport.

Troubleshooting pump systems is best done in a systematic fashion, by following two paths. The first path is the functional path of power supply to terminal pump performance. The second is the blood flow path to and through the device. In the first path, the power source, power supply, cables, connections, gas delivery, tubing, obstructions, device settings, alarm conditions, device position, and device function should all be examined. In the physiologic blood path, patient volume status, pneumothorax, hemothorax, cardiac rhythm, vascular thrombus, right-side heart function, PVR, pulmonary vein patency, heart valves, intraventricular thrombus, mechanical heart defect, heart recovery, cardiac tamponade, and high afterload states can all result in inadequate pump support. The ability to recognize, resolve, and communicate these conditions is crucial to the patient's survival.

In this case study, several scenarios are possible:

- The patient may have primary arrhythmias that transiently reduce the right-side output and cause the pump to have a suction event.
- The pump may have migrated farther into the ventricle, causing the arrhythmias.
- The patient may have worsening right-side HF, reducing LV volume.
- The patient may be experiencing hypovolemia related to procedural or anticoagulation complications.
- The pump setting could be too high for the available right-side heart output.

This very common device condition demonstrates the challenges in caring for patients with artificial circulation.

Prep Kit

Ready for Review

- Mechanical circulatory support (MCS) encompasses all mechanical interventions aimed at augmenting or replacing the native cardiac output from the heart. It is also referred to as mechanically assisted circulation, mechanical circulatory systems, and ventricular assist devices.

- IABP therapy involves use of a balloon connected to a pump via a catheter that has been inserted into the aorta to provide temporary assistance to a failing heart.
- IABP therapy is an advanced skill. Important responsibilities of the CCTP include securing the patient to prevent movement of the balloon

and ensuring that all equipment has the necessary power supply to continue operating during transport.

- In IABP therapy, a balloon connected to a pump via a catheter is inserted into the aorta to provide temporary assistance to a failing heart. The catheter containing the intra-aortic balloon (IAB) is typically threaded into the descending aorta through the femoral artery.
- The balloon is connected to a console to shuttle helium gas, inflating the balloon at the onset of diastole and deflating it just before systole (ventricular ejection). An ECG machine determines when the balloon should be inflated and deflated.
- Inflation and deflation are timed to the cardiac cycle, resulting in significant augmentation of flow to the coronary and renal arteries during diastole (increased supply) and substantially reduced afterload during systole (decreased demand).
- One of the CCTP's main roles in transporting a patient receiving IABP therapy is to ensure proper timing by reading the patient's ECG and pressure waveforms and by continuously monitoring the patient's condition and all devices, modifying their timing if necessary. Other CCTP responsibilities include securing the patient to prevent movement of the balloon and ensuring that all equipment has the necessary power supply.
- Each IABP console allows the operator to control the volume of gas shuttled back and forth to the balloon with each counterpulsation cycle. This control is also referred to as augmentation or balloon volume.
- Inflation and deflation of the IAB can be set to trigger based on the ECG, pressure changes, a pacemaker, an internally preprogrammed rate, or combinations of these factors. The most reliable basis is the ECG. The provider caring for the patient chooses the trigger best suited to the patient.

- Pressure waveforms are one of the main variables evaluated to determine the effectiveness of IABP therapy. The dicrotic notch, a slight bump in the aortic pressure waveform that signals the onset of diastole, occurs during isovolumetric relaxation as the valves bulge under the pressure of the blood from the aorta and then spring back slightly.
- The IABP device can pump in several modes, called assist ratios or IABP frequency. IABP waveform evaluation is usually easiest with a 1:2 assist ratio, which allows for comparison of the pressure waves of the unassisted cycle with those of the assisted cycle. In this mode, every other contraction is augmented by the balloon pump.
- When evaluating a waveform in the 1:2 mode, the peaks created by the inflation of the IAB are usually the highest pressure peaks and are referred to as the diastolic augmentation waveforms. The pressure waveform that follows is referred to as the assisted systole waveform because the deflation of the IAB assists the ventricle in ejecting blood. The third pressure waveform is referred to as the unassisted systole waveform because the balloon pump is not moving and the waveform reflects what would normally occur without IABP intervention.
- To evaluate for correct IABP timing, the pressure peaks, slopes, and inflation and deflation points of each of these pressure waveforms must be evaluated in a systematic manner:
  - Identify systole and diastole of each pressure waveform.
  - Identify diastolic augmentation, assisted systole, and unassisted systole.
  - Identify and evaluate the point of inflation.
  - Identify and evaluate the end-diastolic dip in pressure created by balloon deflation.
  - Evaluate the slope of diastolic augmentation pressure and the slope of assisted systole.

Prep Kit Continued

- Evaluate the diastolic augmentation peak pressure.
- Compare the peak pressure of assisted systole with the peak pressure of unassisted systole.
- Early inflation is reflected on the waveform by a shortened normal pressure decrease that follows diastole or as an opened V, and with a lessened slope on the diastolic augmentation waveform. Early inflation can force the premature closure of the aortic valves, decrease the stroke volume, and damage the aortic valve.
- Late inflation causes little harm but does not maximize the benefits of IABP therapy. Early deflation also results in the benefits of IABP therapy not being fully realized.
- Late deflation, which can be extremely detrimental to the patient, is characterized by a widened appearance of the diastolic augmentation waveform base and a prolonged rate of rise in the assisted systolic waveform. Late deflation worsens myocardial ischemia and needs to be avoided.
- IABP therapy reduces cardiac work and myocardial oxygen consumption and improves peripheral perfusion in patients with a variety of conditions and those undergoing cardiovascular and surgical procedures.
- Patient assessment parameters useful for evaluating the effectiveness of IABP therapy include vital signs, oxygenation, urine output, peripheral perfusion, central nervous system (mentation), and overall general condition of the patient.
- If the femoral artery is used as the insertion site, the CCTP should assess and document the presence of the distal pulses and CRT in the extremity used, and compare the pulses and CRT with those in the other leg. The CCTP should splint the knee to prevent excessive movement of the leg. The sudden loss of pulses or CRT could signal that the IAB is occluding the femoral artery, causing ischemia in the limb. Medical control should be notified immediately.
- Patients receiving IABP therapy are candidates for transport in ground ambulances or in fixed- or rotary-wing aircraft. Some issues to consider when using these vehicles include space and weight constraints, battery life and vehicle power supply, and loading, unloading, and securing the pump in the vehicle.
- Many IABPs are capable of operating on 110 V to 120 V of alternating-current power or 24 V of direct-current power, although the latter may require an adapter cable. Ensuring a match between IABP power requirements and the available power supply in the transport vehicle is crucial.
- After the IABP is placed in the transport vehicle, it is critical to secure the pump so that it remains stable for safe operation throughout transport.
- Temporary circulatory support may be provided with a continuous-flow pump. This kind of device, which consists of an axial-flow pump mounted on a catheter connected to a bedside console, is inserted like an IABP through the femoral artery.
- Extracorporeal membrane oxygenation (ECMO) is a temporizing mechanism of extracorporeal gas exchange with or without hemodynamic support. ECMO is not curative; rather, it is a supportive therapy for presumed reversible respiratory and/or cardiac failure and is a keystone of one of the following strategies: bridge to recovery, bridge to transplantation, destination therapy, or bridge to decision.
- Cannulation sites and circuit configurations vary depending on the patient and intended type of support. Common nomenclature describes the ECMO circuit configuration and support type by a combination of the letters.
  - In venovenous-ECMO (VV-ECMO) configurations, blood is drained from the venous circulation, passes through the circuit

where gas exchange occurs, and is returned as oxygenated and decarboxylated blood to the venous system.

- In venoarterial-ECMO (VA-ECMO) configurations, blood is drained from the venous circulation, passes through the circuit where gas exchange occurs, and is returned as oxygenated and decarboxylated blood to the arterial system.
- Veno-veno-arterial-ECMO (VVA-ECMO) and veno-arterio-venous-ECMO (VAV-ECMO) support respiratory and cardiac function without the differential hypoxemia that may occur during VA-ECMO, albeit at the expense of added circuit complexity.

- A basic ECMO circuit is composed of the vascular cannulas, circuit tubing, pump, heater–cooler, and oxygenator. ECMO circuits vary in configuration and may include pressure and blood flow monitors, bubble detectors, continuous arterial and venous oxyhemoglobin saturation monitors, circuit access sites, and an emergency arterial–venous bridge.
- Patients undergoing ECMO therapy receive systemic anticoagulative therapy to both protect the major organs from thromboembolism and maintain the patency of the ECMO circuit.
- The ECMO circuit and cannulas require continual monitoring of their integrity and patency. A thorough, methodical approach for assessment of all components, connections, and securing points will aid in the early identification of potential issues.
- Venous oxygen saturation and serum lactate levels provide insights into the adequacy of systemic perfusion. Pressure monitoring can help providers detect early or acute dysfunction in the ECMO circuit and suggest clinical changes in the patient. While additional pressures can be monitored, the four pressures that are typically assessed are P_{vein} (venous pressure), P_{art} (arterial pressure), P_{int} (oxygenator inlet pressure), and Δp (differential pressure of P_{int} and P_{art}).

- Documentation for patients receiving ECMO therapy will vary by institution, but should at a minimum include hourly notation of flow, rpm, monitored circuit pressures, trending of the preferred coagulation study, and anticoagulation dose, along with circuit and cannulation site assessments.
- ECMO-related complications that the CCTP must be prepared to troubleshoot may relate to hypoxemia (eg, hemolysis, pulmonary edema and left ventricular distention, limb ischemia, insufficient flow, recirculation, north–south syndrome) and circuit disruptions (eg, oxygenator dysfunction, air entrainment, circuit rupture, pump failure, and inadvertent decannulation).
- A microaxial continuous-flow pump is a means of temporary circulatory support that consists of an axial-flow pump mounted on a catheter connected to a bedside console; this catheter is inserted like an IABP through the femoral artery. The most commonly used microaxial continuous-flow pumps used in the United States are Impella heart pumps.
- The Impella system includes a catheter that functions in conjunction with an automated Impella controller and purge fluid infusion pump. There are several different Impella catheters. The Impella 2.5, Impella CP with SmartAssist, Impella 5.0, Impella 5.5 with SmartAssist, and Impella LD are all left-side heart devices; the Impella RP is a right-side heart device.
- The automated Impella controller allows for management and monitoring of pump operation and catheter position via multiple parameters: performance level, Impella flow, placement signal, and motor current.
- Transport of the patient with the Impella system requires the transport team to be equipped, at a minimum, to continue the current level of patient hemodynamic support and monitoring in place at the referring facility. A thorough assessment of the patient and

Prep Kit Continued

catheter position should be performed prior to equipment exchange or manipulation of support.

- Common alarms encountered when transporting a patient with an Impella system include the suction alarm, purge alarm, and air in purge system alarm. The CCTP must recognize the meaning of these alarms and respond appropriately.

- Left ventricular assist devices (LVADs) enable circulatory function in patients with heart failure (HF), either indefinitely or until heart transplantation can occur.

- An LVAD may serve as a bridge to recovery until the native heart recovers its pumping ability, as a bridge to transplantation to prolong the patient's life until a heart transplant can be secured, or as destination therapy when long-term MCS is needed for a patient with HF who does not meet the heart transplantation criteria.

- Generally, the patient with an LVAD and/or their caregiver will have substantial knowledge of the device. While these individuals may be excellent sources of

information, the provider should also know how to troubleshoot the device, know which emergency interventions can and cannot be performed, and be aware of how to contact designated LVAD support staff.

- All patients with LVADs receive anticoagulation therapies and, therefore, are more susceptible to traumatic hemorrhage and bleeding from all causes.

- Adverse events related to LVADs can include bleeding (typically in the gastrointestinal tract), LVAD infections (typically involving the driveline), stroke, arrhythmias, thrombosis, right-side HF, and device malfunction. CCTPs should be prepared to recognize these problems and must ensure their actions do not precipitate a chain of adverse events.

- Patients with LVADs are susceptible to depression and anxiety due to the significant changes in lifestyle and possible discomforts associated with the device.

- LVAD pump parameters that CCTPs should be prepared to monitor, and potentially troubleshoot, include conditions relating to pump flow, rpm, power, and pulsatility index.

Vital Vocabulary

aortic regurgitation Backward flow of blood through the aortic valve from the aorta into the left ventricle.

assist ratios Settings on the intra-aortic balloon pump that allow the operator to determine how often the pump inflates the balloon.

assisted systole The pressure waveform that follows the diastolic augmentation peak.

bridge to recovery (BTR) A treatment objective in which a left ventricular assist device is implanted in a patient as mechanical circulatory support until the native heart recovers its pumping ability.

bridge to transplantation (BTT) A treatment objective in which a left ventricular assist device is

implanted in a patient as mechanical circulatory support to prolong life until a heart transplant can be secured.

central lumen The lumen or port of the intra-aortic balloon catheter used to guide initial catheter insertion and to monitor arterial pressure during operation.

destination therapy (DT) A treatment objective in which a left ventricular assist device is implanted in a patient with heart failure as ongoing mechanical circulatory support because the patient does not meet the heart transplantation criteria.

diastolic augmentation The increase in aortic pressure during diastole that the intra-aortic balloon inflation produces, thereby improving coronary and peripheral perfusion; it may be thought of as a "second systole."

extracorporeal membrane oxygenation (ECMO) A temporizing mechanism of extracorporeal gas exchange with or without hemodynamic support; also referred to as extracorporeal life support.

gas lumen The lumen or port of the intra-aortic balloon catheter that carries helium between the intra-aortic balloon and the pump console to inflate and deflate the balloon.

intra-aortic balloon pump (IABP) therapy A procedure involving insertion of a balloon into the descending thoracic aorta and its connection to a pump via a catheter; this therapy helps to increase blood flow to the coronary arteries during diastole (inflation) and decrease the afterload of blood from the left ventricle (deflation).

left ventricular assist device (LVAD) A means of mechanical circulatory support in which a pump is implanted in the patient's chest to help circulate blood from the left ventricle of the heart to the rest of the body.

mechanical circulatory support (MCS) Mechanical interventions aimed at augmenting or replacing the native cardiac output from the heart;

also called mechanically assisted circulation, mechanical circulatory systems, and ventricular assist devices.

microaxial continuous-flow pump A means of temporary circulatory support that consists of an axial-flow pump mounted on a catheter that is typically inserted through the femoral artery and connected to a bedside console.

pulsatility index (PI) A measurement of a left ventricular assist device's pumping power; calculated as follows: Pulsatililty index = (Maximum pump power – Minimum pump power)/Average pump power.

relative contraindication A condition that makes a particular treatment or procedure somewhat inadvisable but does not completely rule it out.

suction event An emergency in which tissue occludes the inlet of the pump in a mechanical circulatory support device.

timing In the context of intra-aortic balloon pump therapy, a method for coordinating the intra-aortic balloon inflation–deflation cycle with the cardiac cycle (inflation during diastole and deflation synchronous with systole).

unassisted systole Pressure waveform reflecting what would normally occur without intra-aortic balloon pump assistance.

References

Bartlett RH. Physiology of gas exchange during ECMO for respiratory failure. *J Intens Care Med*. 2017;32(4):243-248.

Broman LM, Dirnberger DR, Malfertheiner MV, et al. International survey on extracorporeal membrane oxygenation transport. *ASAIO J*. 2020;66(2):214-225.

Choi MS, Sung K, Cho YH. Clinical pearls of venoarterial extracorporeal membrane oxygenation for cardiogenic shock. *Korean Circ J*. 2019;49(8):657-677.

ECMO. Learn PICU website. http://www.learnpicu.com/ecmo. Accessed November 23, 2021.

Frankfurter C, Molinero M, Vishram-Nielsen JKK, et al. Predicting the risk of right ventricular failure in patients undergoing left ventricular assist device implantation. *Circ Heart Fail*. 2020;13. https://doi.org/10.1161/CIRCHEART FAILURE.120.006994.

Griffith KE, Jenkins E. Abiomed Impella 2.5 patient transport: lessons learned. *Perfusion*. 2010;25(6):381-386.

Guihaire J, Haddad F, Hoppenfeld M, et al. Physiology of the assisted circulation in cardiogenic shock: a state-of-the-art perspective. *Can J Cardiol*. 2020;36(2):170-183.

Hori M, Nakamura M, Nakagaito M, Kinugawa K. First experience of transfer with Impella 5.0 over the long distance in Japan. *Int Heart J*. 2019;60(5):1219-1221.

Interagency Registry for Mechanically Assisted Circulatory Support (Intermacs). National Heart, Lung, and Blood Institute website. https://biolincc.nhlbi.nih.gov/studies/intermacs/. Updated January 21, 2020. Accessed November 23, 2021.

Kormos RL, McCall M, Althouse A, et al. Left ventricular assist device malfunctions: it is more than just the pump. *Circulation*. 2017;136:1714-1725.

Prep Kit Continued

Lamarche Y, Cheung A, Ignaszewski A, et al. Comparative outcomes in cardiogenic shock patients managed with Impella microaxial pump or extracorporeal life support. *J Thorac Cardiovasc Surg*. 2011;142(1):60-65.

Lemaire A, Anderson MB, Lee LY, et al. The Impella device for acute mechanical circulatory support in patients in cardiogenic shock. *Ann Thorac Surg*. 2014;97(1):133-138.

Lequier L, Horton SB, McMullan DM, Bartlett RH. Extracorporeal membrane oxygenation circuitry. *Pediatr Crit Care Med*. 2013;14(5 suppl 1):S7-S12.

MOMENTUM 3 IDE clinical study protocol (HM3). ClinicalTrials .gov website. https://clinicaltrials.gov/ct2/show/NCT 02224755. Updated September 9, 2021. Accessed November 5, 2021.

Napp LC, Kühn C, Hoeper MM, et al. Cannulation strategies for percutaneous extracorporeal membrane oxygenation in adults. *Clin Res Cardiol*. 2016;105(4):283-296.

Patel A, Joong A, Lelkes E, Gossett JG. Should physicians offer a ventricular assist device to a pediatric oncology patient with a poor prognosis? *AMA J Ethics*. 2019;21(5): E380-E386. doi:10.1001/amajethics.2019.380.

Pujara D, Sandoval E, Simpson L, et al. The state of the art in extracorporeal membrane oxygenation. *Semin Thorac Cardiovasc Surg*. 2015;27(1):17-23.

Quintel M, Bartlett RH, Grocott MPW, et al. Extracorporeal membrane oxygenation for respiratory failure. *Anesthesiology*. 2020;132(5):1257-1276.

Randomized Evaluation of Mechanical Assistance for the Treatment of Congestive Heart Failure (REMATCH). Clinical Trials.gov website. https://clinicaltrials.gov/ct2/show /NCT00000607. Updated December 23, 2015. Accessed December 5, 2021.

Right heart failure and the Impella RP heart pump. Abiomed Heart Recovery website. https://www.heartrecovery.com /education/education-library/faq-what-are-the-causes -and-incidence-of-right-heart-failure. Published August 2, 2019. Accessed December 14, 2021.

Sangalli F, Patroniti N, Pesenti A. *ECMO: Extracorporeal Life Support in Adults*. Milan, Italy: Springer Verlag; 2014.

Schmack B, Seppelt P, Weymann A, et al. Extracorporeal life support with left ventricular decompression-improved survival in severe cardiogenic shock: results from a retrospective study. *Peer J*. 2017;5:e3813. doi:10.7717/peerj.3813.

Slaughter MS, Pagani FD, Rogers JG, et al. Clinical management of continuous-flow left ventricular assist devices in advanced heart failure. *J Heart Lung Transplant*. 2010;29 (4 suppl):S1-S39.

Slaughter MS, Rogers JG, Milano CA, et al. Advanced heart failure treated with continuous-flow left ventricular assist device. *N Engl J Med*. 2009;361:2241-2251.

Timpa JG, O'Meara C, McIlwain RB, et al. Massive systemic air embolism during extracorporeal membrane oxygenation support of a neonate with acute respiratory distress syndrome after cardiac surgery. *J Extra Corpor Technol*. 2011;43(2):86-88.

Yeager T, Roy S. Evolution of gas permeable membranes for extracorporeal membrane oxygenation. *Artif Organs*. 2017;41(8):700-709.

Yeo HJ, Jeon D, Kim YS, et al. Veno-veno-arterial extracorporeal membrane oxygenation treatment in patients with severe acute respiratory distress syndrome and septic shock. *Crit Care*. 2016;20:28.

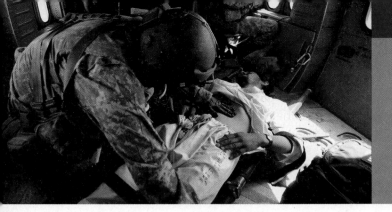

Chapter 17

Gastrointestinal and Genitourinary Emergencies

Lorenzo Albala, MD

Sean M. Kivlehan, MD, MPH

OBJECTIVES

After completing this chapter, you will be able to:

1. Describe the anatomy and physiology of the gastrointestinal system, including the alimentary canal and accessory organs (pp 896–901).

2. Describe the anatomy and physiology of the genitourinary system, including the urinary system and the male and female reproductive systems (pp 901–906).

3. Differentiate between upper and lower gastrointestinal bleeding (pp 920–922).

4. Describe the pathologies related to common disorders of the gastrointestinal system, including peptic ulcers, gastritis, esophageal varices, Mallory-Weiss syndrome, diverticulitis, appendicitis, inflammatory bowel disease, ulcerative colitis, and Crohn disease (pp 908–915).

5. Assess the signs and symptoms of the various gastrointestinal conditions (pp 924–926).

6. Describe laboratory results as they relate to specific gastrointestinal system disorders (pp 925–926).

7. Describe the management of the various gastrointestinal conditions (p 926).

8. Describe gastrointestinal system imaging, including endoscopy, colonoscopy, angiography, and scintigraphy, as well as other in-hospital assessment and management techniques (pp 918–919).

9. Describe the pathologies related to diseases of the gastrointestinal system, including intestinal obstructions, ileus, liver disease, cholecystitis and choledocholithiasis, and pancreatitis (pp 922–938).

10. Describe the pathologies related to common disorders of the genitourinary system, including kidney injury, renal failure, urinary tract infections, testicular torsion, nephrolithiasis, penile fracture, and priapism (pp 940–948).

11. Assess the signs and symptoms of the various genitourinary pathologies (pp 940–948).

12. Describe the management of the various genitourinary pathologies (pp 940–948).

13. Describe laboratory results as they relate to specific disorders of the genitourinary system (pp 942–946).

14. Describe various gastrointestinal- and genitourinary-related feeding and drainage tubes, including their assessment,

Introduction

The gastrointestinal (GI) and genitourinary (GU) systems are exquisitely tuned to process the body's waste and alimentation. Both systems are composed of a vast network of specialized cells for absorption and filtering, neutralization of infections and toxins, and excretion of waste. Harmony between the two systems maintains stability in the body's internal environment, a state known as homeostasis. Unfortunately, various disease processes and injuries can cause significant impairment to either organ system, significantly limiting the body's ability to maintain homeostasis. These conditions require a careful assessment and diagnosis followed by appropriate management—a process that is inherently difficult because the signs and symptoms that accompany abdominal conditions are often vague and nonspecific. Without prompt treatment, patients with GI or GU pathologies may experience pain, altered mental status, and shock. Critical care transport professionals (CCTPs) must possess a detailed understanding of GI and GU anatomy, physiology, and diagnostics to successfully manage a patient with a GI/GU condition, as well as any complications that may arise during transport of such a patient.

Anatomy and Physiology
Gastrointestinal System

Intricately complex yet stunningly efficient, the GI system consists of an interconnected network of organs and ducts devoted to the digestion of food and the extraction of its nutritional content. The alimentary canal (also referred to as the GI tract) consists of the mouth, pharynx, esophagus, stomach, small intestine, and large intestine; food travels through these structures and finally exits the body via the rectum. The alimentary canal is lined with continuous specialized tissues that allow for the absorption of digested nutrients from food while maintaining a protective barrier against waste and microorganisms. During mechanical and chemical digestion, food turns into the basic molecular building blocks required by the body's cells. Enzymes that aid in digestion are secreted by a variety of accessory organs, including the salivary glands, liver, gallbladder, and pancreas.

Unnecessary side products from the digestion process are either defecated or excreted by the GU system. Cooperative action by the liver and kidneys allows for safe passage of toxic nitrogen-containing compounds during their exit from the body.

GI Tract Tissues

Although the alimentary canal contains numerous specialized cells and tissues, four layers are seen almost continuously from the esophagus to the rectum: the mucosa, the submucosa, the muscularis externa, and the serosa **FIGURE 17-1**.

The mucosa forms the first and innermost layer that is exposed to the lumen, or cavity, of the canal. This moist mucous membrane consists of three sublayers: a thin layer of columnar epithelium interspersed with mucus-secreting goblet cells (surface epithelium), a loose areolar connective tissue harboring capillaries and lymph nodes (lamina propria), and a layer of smooth muscle that forms endless folds and wrinkles in the tissues underneath to maximize absorption of nutrients (muscularis mucosae).

The submucosa consists of connective tissue just beyond the mucosa. Blood and lymphatic vessels weave through this layer to connect the vessels of the mucosa to systemic circulation. The submucosal nerve plexus resides here, permitting innervation of smooth muscle and secretory cells. The elastic character of the submucosa allows for

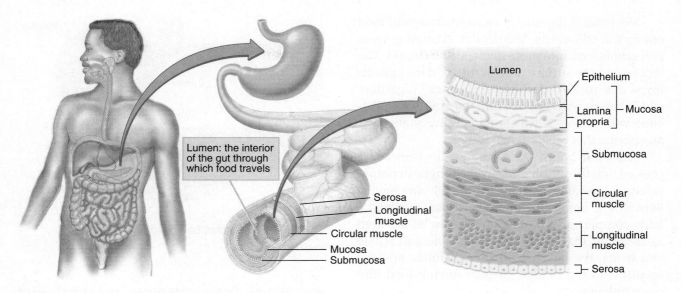

FIGURE 17-1 Gastrointestinal tract layers.

© Jones & Bartlett Learning.

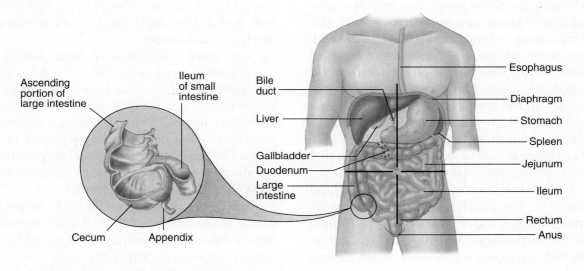

FIGURE 17-2 Overview of the gastrointestinal system.

© Jones & Bartlett Learning.

restoration of a structure's original shape after it is distended by the presence of food.

The muscularis externa forms the muscle bulk of the GI tract. It is divided into two layers of smooth muscle: an inner circular layer and an outer longitudinal layer. The arrangement of these two layers facilitates segmentation and peristalsis, the body's mechanical digestion methods (discussed in the next section).

The serosa (commonly referred to as the visceral peritoneum) consists of areolar connective tissue lined with simple squamous epithelium, called the mesothelium. The serosa is meant to be a protective layer, covering all peritoneal GI organs. In certain situations, this peritoneum can become inflamed, a condition referred to as peritonitis.

Alimentary Canal

The alimentary canal maintains a chemical environment that aids in the digestion of food, yet does not alter the environment of the rest of the body **FIGURE 17-2.**

Mechanical digestion begins the moment food enters the oral cavity. Mastication (chewing) tears and grinds food into more manageable chunks. The increase in the surface area of the food that results from this process facilitates chemical digestion, which begins when food within the mouth is moistened with saliva. Saliva contains salivary amylase, an enzyme that breaks down starch.

The food bolus, once sufficiently chewed, is pushed into the oropharynx by the tongue in preparation for swallowing. Once initiated, swallowing becomes a largely involuntary process, albeit a fairly complex one. More than 22 muscles are used to block off the nasopharynx with the soft palate and uvula, the larynx with the epiglottis, and the mouth with the tongue, thereby forcing food into the esophagus.

The esophagus is a 10-inch (25-cm) tube of muscle that connects the oropharynx to the stomach. The muscles of the esophagus receive a substantial flow of blood via several arteries, with this blood then being returned through a large network of veins in the submucosa. Peristalsis, a series of wavelike contractions of the esophagus, carries food to the stomach in less than 8 seconds. The bolus of food arrives in the stomach via the gastroesophageal sphincter, which closes following the passage of a bolus, thereby preventing backflow.

The stomach stores food while continuing chemical and mechanical digestion through the actions of a variety of enzymes and muscles. Bound superiorly by the esophagus and inferiorly by the small intestine, the stomach is a 6- to 10-inch (15- to 25-cm) J-shaped widening of the GI tract **FIGURE 17-3**. When this organ is full, it can expand to have a volume as large as 4 L. Mechanical digestion is continued and completed by the stomach muscles. A bolus of food enters the stomach at the cardia region via the cardiac sphincter. The stomach terminates at the pyloric sphincter, which regulates the exit of materials from it. The stomach is unique in that it is the only portion of the GI tract to contain a third muscle layer, which is arranged oblique to the inner and outer layers. The extra muscles aid in the mechanical digestion of food while it is in the stomach.

Throughout the stomach, glands consisting of specialized mucous neck cells secrete various substances, collectively termed gastric juice. Components of this juice include mucin, hydrochloric

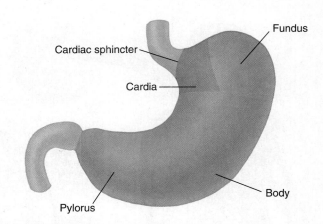

FIGURE 17-3 Anatomy of the stomach.
© Jones & Bartlett Learning.

acid, intrinsic factor, pepsinogen, and lipases, all of which aid in the digestive process. The end product of the stomach's chemical and mechanical digestion is chyme, a liquid mixture of partially digested food, gastric juice, and water that is ready for entry into the small intestine.

The small intestine is a long, 1-inch-wide (2.5-cm-wide) canal that twists throughout all four quadrants of the abdomen. Digestion is completed in this organ, and the bulk of nutrient absorption takes place here. The small intestine is divided into three areas: the duodenum, the jejunum, and the ileum. The superior mesenteric artery provides the blood supply to all three of these regions via its vast network of vessels in the mesentery.

Chyme begins its journey through the small intestine at the duodenum. The small intestine also receives bile and pancreatic juice at the duodenum, both of which aid in further digestion.

In the large intestine, chyme is transformed into feces, which is then expelled from the alimentary canal via the rectum and anus. The large intestine is divided into six regions: cecum, ascending colon, transverse colon, descending colon, sigmoid colon, and rectum **FIGURE 17-4**. The more proximal sections (cecum, ascending colon, and transverse colon) are the sites of water and electrolyte absorption, whereas the latter areas (descending colon, sigmoid, and rectum) provide storage for feces and muscles for its propulsion to the rectum.

Chyme is deposited into the cecum from the ileum of the small intestine, beginning the final leg of its journey through the body. The appendix is attached to the cecum, about 1 inch (2.5 cm) inferior

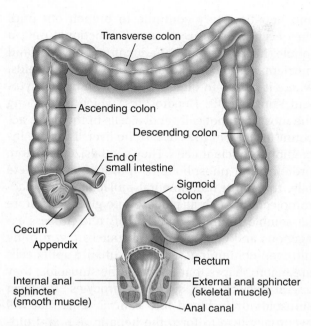

FIGURE 17-4 Anatomy of the large intestine.

© Jones & Bartlett Learning.

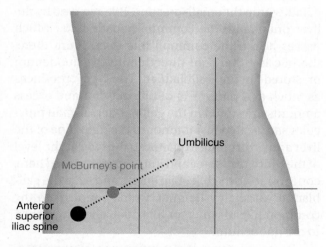

FIGURE 17-5 Location of the McBurney point.

© joshya/Shutterstock.

to the ileocecal valve. The most common location for the base of the appendix, where it attaches to the cecum, can be located topographically on the abdomen of the patient at the McBurney point **FIGURE 17-5**. From the cecum, chyme is pushed upward into the ascending colon, where water and electrolytes are reclaimed from unusable end products of digestion. Anaerobic bacteria residing here prepare a significant amount of vitamins B and K for absorption as well.

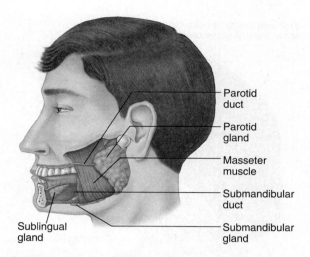

FIGURE 17-6 The salivary glands.

© Jones & Bartlett Learning.

The transverse colon proceeds across the abdomen until it makes an inferior turn, after which it becomes the descending colon. These two sections function mainly to store feces. The muscularis externa begins to thicken gradually along the length of these areas to assist with the movement of the increasingly compact feces.

The sigmoid colon starts at the level of the pelvis, taking an S-shaped path into the rectum, a 5-inch (13-cm) muscular tube. A defecation reflex is stimulated by the stretching of the rectal wall due to feces buildup, resulting in the opening of the internal anal sphincter. The external anal sphincter is voluntarily controlled.

Accessory Organs

The alimentary canal does not accomplish the feat of digestion on its own. Like any other body system, it receives support from several accessory organs—namely, the salivary glands, liver, gallbladder, and pancreas.

Three pairs of extrinsic salivary glands are found in the tissues surrounding the oral cavity; they secrete saliva to initiate the chemical digestive process **FIGURE 17-6**. This saliva not only provides enzymes that break down starches in food, but also moistens food to facilitate bolus formation. In addition, it cleanses the mouth. Tiny internal salivary glands are located throughout the oral cavity as well, supplementing the secretions of the extrinsic glands. Secretion of saliva by all of these glands is amplified by stimulation of the salivatory nuclei in

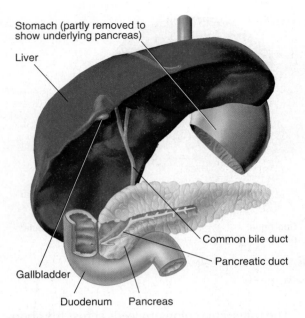

Stomach (partly removed to show underlying pancreas)

Liver

Common bile duct

Pancreatic duct

Gallbladder

Duodenum   Pancreas

FIGURE 17-7 The liver, gallbladder, and pancreas.

© Jones & Bartlett Learning.

the brainstem, whether that stimulation takes the form of the sight, smell, or taste of food.

The liver is the largest solid organ in the body, as well as the most vascular, containing more than one-fifth of a person's total blood volume at any given time **FIGURE 17-7**. It serves as a central terminal through which all blood returning to the central circulation from the alimentary canal must pass. The liver performs three functions critical to the body's functioning: metabolic regulation, hematologic regulation, and bile production. Although the liver dominates the right upper quadrant of the abdomen, the majority of its bulk actually rests within the right thoracic cage; this position allows the ribs to protect the liver from trauma to some extent. During forceful exhalation, the liver rises as high as the fourth intercostal space just below the right nipple, and sprawls past the midline approaching the left nipple. Normally, the liver can be palpated inferior to the right ribs during inspiration only, as it remains within the thoracic cage during expiration.

The porta hepatis forms the space between the stomach, duodenum, and liver, and provides the gateway into the liver for the hepatic portal vein, hepatic artery, and common hepatic duct. These three vessels bifurcate on entry, separating the liver into right and left functional lobes that are distinct from the superficial lobes. The hepatic portal vein

and hepatic artery continue to branch out until they eventually form the liver's functional unit, a lobule. Inside a lobule, the incoming oxygen- and nutrient-rich blood is drained into liver sinusoids, where it comes in direct contact with hepatocytes and Kupffer cells. Hepatocytes, which are among the most metabolically active cells in the body, account for 80% of the cells in the liver. They are incredibly proficient cells: They synthesize and store proteins and phospholipids, produce and secrete bile, transform fundamental molecules into macromolecules (such as glucose into glycogen), store fat-soluble vitamins, and detoxify and process exogenous and endogenous substances (eg, turning nitrogen-containing wastes into urea). Kupffer cells are macrophages that reside in the sinusoids; they engulf bacteria and spent erythrocytes. The liver sinusoids drain blood into central veins that will eventually fuse to form the hepatic vein and ultimately the inferior vena cava, which returns the blood to the systemic circulation.

Bile is a fat emulsifier required for the digestion of fats within the small intestine. Bile secreted by the liver drains into the common hepatic duct, which passes it into the common bile duct. From there, the bile is either sent directly into the duodenum or stored in the gallbladder. The body produces as much as 2 pints (1 L) of bile per day, and excess amounts are stored in the gallbladder, a small muscular sac located just inferior to the right lobe of the liver and protruding from under the liver at the level of the ninth rib. Water and ions are reabsorbed here, concentrating the bile. Bile enters and exits the gallbladder via the cystic duct, which connects to the common hepatic duct, or bile duct, allowing transit to the duodenum.

Pancreatic juice is a solution containing digestive enzymes secreted by the pancreas, a retroperitoneal organ found in the left upper quadrant. The head of the pancreas is framed by the duodenum, its body runs along the inferior aspect of the stomach, and finally its tail reaches the spleen. The release of pancreatic juice is an exocrine function, but the pancreas also has an equally important endocrine function—the production of insulin and glucagon.

At a microscopic level, the pancreas contains millions of acini lobules, each consisting of a ring of secretory cells around an intralobular duct through which the secreted pancreatic juice drains into the main pancreatic duct. This duct empties into the common bile duct; thus, it shares a pathway to the duodenum with bile. Zymogen granules within the acinar cells secrete trypsinogen, chymotrypsinogen, procarboxypeptidase, pancreatic amylase, lipases, and nucleases, which mix with water and bicarbonate to make up pancreatic juice. Enzymes such as trypsin within the duodenum convert the various proteins to their active forms in a process driven by the surrounding pH, preventing inappropriate self-digestion by these powerful enzymes. Collectively, these enzymes account for most of the digestion that occurs in the small intestine. The bicarbonate balances the acidity of newly arriving chyme from the stomach, and the water serves to further dilute the chyme prior to its absorption.

The pancreas can be adversely affected by mutations in the CFTR gene, which are commonly associated with the condition known as cystic fibrosis. While cystic fibrosis's detrimental effects on the lungs are well known, some of the most common symptoms of the disease actually involve the digestive tract and, in particular, the pancreas. The thick mucus associated with cystic fibrosis can obstruct the flow of pancreatic enzymes necessary for proper digestion. Scarring and damage to the pancreas may occur as well, leading to islet cell dysfunction and insulin-deficient diabetes mellitus.

Scattered throughout the acini lobules are islets of Langerhans, cells of the pancreas that secrete a variety of endocrine hormones directly into the bloodstream. Numerous insulin-secreting beta cells in the pancreas work alongside alpha cells, which produce glucagon, and delta cells, which produce somatostatin. Insulin facilitates the absorption of free glucose molecules into cells from the bloodstream. Glucagon stimulates glycogen production in the liver during times of glucose surplus. Somatostatin has numerous regulatory functions, including the inhibition of overall pancreatic function.

Genitourinary System
Urinary System

The many nutrients and ions absorbed into the bloodstream by the tissues of the alimentary canal serve a useful purpose in the body for only a finite time. Eventually, because of metabolic reactions, the molecules and atoms are either incorporated into useful products or left over as waste. The renal system provides a path for these wastes to leave the body **FIGURE 17-8**. The kidneys continuously filter blood, managing its volume, maintaining an appropriate balance between acids and bases, and discarding toxins and excessive amounts of substances by producing urine. The kidneys are extremely vascular; approximately one-fourth of the total cardiac output passes through them every minute. Although the kidneys filter approximately 200 L of fluid per day, only about 2 L is actually excreted. The remainder of the urinary system—the ureters, urinary bladder, and urethra—provides for transport and storage of urine during its journey out of the body.

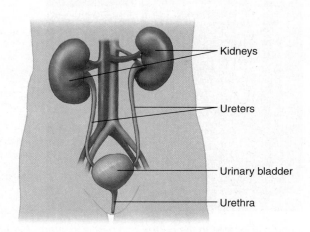

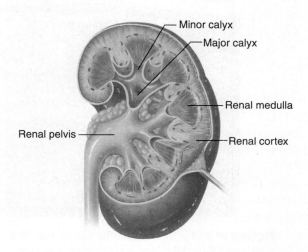

FIGURE 17-8 Organs of the urinary system.

The kidneys are a pair of retroperitoneal organs that stretch from the T12 to the L3 vertebrae. The position of the liver forces the right kidney into a slightly lower location than the left kidney's position. The adrenal glands, seated on top of the kidneys, are important in endocrine function because they produce catecholamines in response to stress. Although the 12th ribs provide the kidneys with some protection, they remain relatively vulnerable to external trauma. Three layers of tissue provide some measure of protection from such trauma:

- The renal fascia, the outermost layer, consists of dense fibrous connective tissue that encloses the kidneys and adrenal glands, securing them to the abdominal walls.
- A layer of adipose tissue directly beneath the renal fascia provides a cushion from sudden movements.

- The renal capsule, which is made up of more fibrous connective tissue, coats the kidney itself.

Internally, the tissues of the kidneys can be divided into three zones: the outermost renal cortex, the medulla, and the innermost pelvis. The functional unit of the kidney, the nephron, lies across the border between the cortex and medulla. The renal pelvis is an open space that allows for both pooling of urine and its drainage into the ureter. **FIGURE 17-9** and **FIGURE 17-10** show the nephrons of the kidney and the glomerulus, respectively.

On entering the kidney, the renal artery immediately branches off into vessels of decreasing diameter. They culminate in the afferent arterioles that feed blood into the glomerulus, a meshwork of capillaries contained within the glomerular capsule. This meshwork forms the interface between

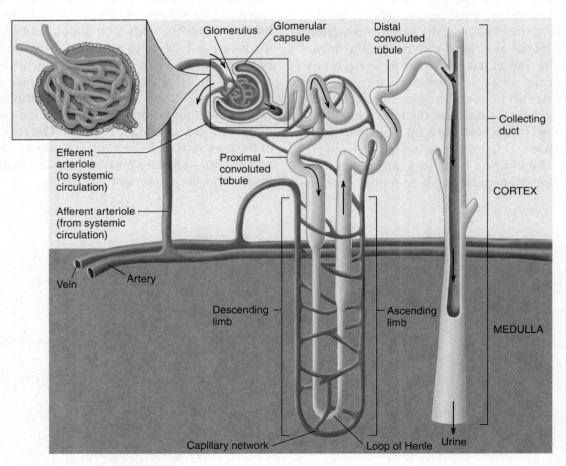

FIGURE 17-9 The nephrons of the kidney. Part of the nephron is located in the cortex, and part is located in the medulla. Insert: Close-up of the glomerulus.

© Jones & Bartlett Learning.

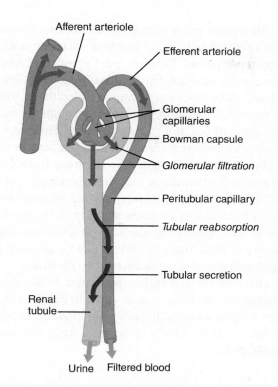

Afferent arteriole

Efferent arteriole

Glomerular capillaries

Bowman capsule

Glomerular filtration

Peritubular capillary

Tubular reabsorption

Tubular secretion

Renal tubule

Urine   Filtered blood

FIGURE 17-10 The glomerulus of the kidneys. The nephron carries out three blood-filtering processes: glomerular filtration, tubular reabsorption, and tubular secretion.

© Jones & Bartlett Learning.

arterial and venous vasculature, where an interplay between the arteriovenous (AV) pressure differential and delicate structures specialized for filtration create a gradient for fluid and solutes. These filtration structures include accessory cells (podocytes) that prevent the passage of certain macromolecules, while pores in the capillary walls prevent erythrocyte and large-protein passage into the filtrate. The filtrate is funneled from the glomerular capsule to the proximal convoluted tubule. As a consequence of this arrangement, the kidneys are extremely sensitive to vascular pressures: Any decrease in systemic arterial pressure or increased venous congestion reduces the pressure gradient and, therefore, the amount of blood the renal tissues "see." Beyond its formidable filtration function, the urinary system informs and modifies the body's vascular tone and volume status.

Once filtered, the blood exits the glomerulus by way of the efferent arterioles, which then divide into the peritubular capillaries. The filtrate-carrying proximal convoluted tubule descends into the

renal medulla, and subsequently straightens out. Within the medulla, it turns 180° to take a parallel path back to the cortex. This portion of the tubule, called the loop of Henle, is where the bulk of ion filtration and absorption occurs. A series of osmotic gradients between the lumen of the loop of Henle and the medullary tissues result in ion exchange as material moves along this pathway, which plays a significant role in the dilution and concentration of urine. Loop diuretics such as furosemide act on the loop of Henle, inhibiting solute transport systems (which reduces their reabsorption of ions) and triggering increased excretion of water.

The loop of Henle becomes the distal convoluted tubule upon its reentry to the cortex, and eventually makes its way to the collecting duct. The peritubular capillaries, which are entangled with the proximal and distal convoluted tubules as well as the loop of Henle, reabsorb water and solutes not meant to be excreted.

The effectiveness of the glomerulus in filtering blood provides a benchmark for the evaluation of overall renal function, termed the glomerular filtration rate (GFR). The normal GFR in an adult is approximately 125 mL/min. Various pathologies can affect the GFR, and a decrease in this rate will result in several metabolic alterations. Inulin is freely filtered in the kidneys, and inulin clearance is the gold-standard test for measuring the GFR in patients. However, measurement of inulin clearance entails a rigorous process that is impractical for day-to-day clinical application. As a result, numerous equations have been developed to estimate the GFR.

One such test frequently employed in assessing glomerular function, and therefore renal function, is creatinine clearance. Creatinine is the metabolized form of creatine that is eliminated through the urine. The normal elimination rate for men is 95 to 145 mL/min, and the normal rate for women is 75 to 115 mL/min. In practice, creatinine clearance is used to assess the GFR, even though it does not provide an exact measurement (it generally underestimates the GFR by 10% to 20%). A patient with low creatinine clearance is assumed to have a low GFR, and vice versa.

Specialized cells known as juxtaglomerular cells are present in the walls of the afferent and efferent arterioles. These cells secrete renin in response to stretching of the vessel walls. Renin is an enzyme that plays an important role in the activation of the renin-angiotensin-aldosterone system, which helps regulate blood pressure (BP). In between the afferent and efferent arterioles and the distal convoluted tubule is another class of specialized cells, the macula densa. These cells detect chemical changes in the concentration of the filtrate. This region, which is collectively referred to as the juxtaglomerular apparatus, is present in every nephron.

The sensors of the juxtaglomerular apparatus are the key element of a finely tuned feedback loop programmed to optimize renal perfusion pressure. As in all other organs, blood flow to the kidneys is dictated by renal perfusion pressure divided by resistance to flow through that organ. The renal perfusion pressure is the pressure differential between the arterial input and venous output. As discussed later in this chapter, any significant decrease in the pressure gradient negatively affects GFR and blood flow to the renal tissues.

The ureters, a pair of long muscular tubes running to the urinary bladder, are essentially a continuation of the renal pelvis. Through gravity and peristalsis, urine is jettisoned into the bladder. The ureters enter the base of the bladder at a region called the trigone. The ureters' distal segment tunnels through the multiple layers of bladder muscle, limiting backflow as the bladder wall stretches. The urethra also drains the bladder from the trigone, so there are three connections to the bladder at this point (hence the prefix "tri"). The bladder is a hollow, muscular organ located directly posterior to the pubic symphysis. Its layers of muscle are impressively elastic, with a urine storage capacity of more than 17 ounces (0.5 L), and can be palpated in the lower abdomen when distended.

The urethra is another muscular tube, about 8 inches (20 cm) long in men and 1 to 2 inches (3 to 5 cm) long in women. It drains the bladder, providing the route by which urine exits from the body **FIGURE 17-11**.

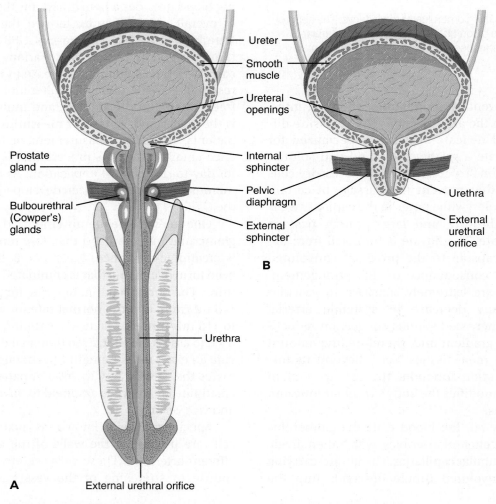

FIGURE 17-11 Structure of the urinary bladder and urethra. **A.** Male. **B.** Female.

© Jones & Bartlett Learning.

Male Reproductive System

The purpose of the male reproductive system is to generate sperm and provide a means for its delivery to a fertilizable egg in the female partner. The testes are the principal male reproductive organ; they consist of a pair of ovoid structures, suspended external to the body in a sac of skin called the scrotum **FIGURE 17-12**. This housing outside the body means that sperm production occurs in an environment at 91°F (33°C), considerably cooler than the overall body temperature. Each testis is covered by two distinct layers of tissue: the outer tunica vaginalis, which folds over itself, and the inner tunica albuginea, a tough fibrous capsule that protects the testis and penetrates it. The tunica albuginea divides the testis into hundreds of lobules. Inside these lobules, sperm are created in the seminiferous tubules. The testes receive their blood supply from the testicular arteries and drain into their complementary veins. These blood vessels branch from the abdominal aorta, and travel with autonomic nerve fibers to and from the testes through the spermatic cord.

Newly made sperm drain into the efferent ductules and then move to the epididymis, where they will mature. When stimulated by smooth-muscle contractions arising from ejaculation, sperm are forced into the ductus deferens (vas deferens), which exits the scrotum via the spermatic cord. The ductus deferens travels anterior to the pubic bone and then posterior to the bladder, finally joining with the seminal vesicle duct to form the ejaculatory duct. The two ejaculatory ducts pass through the prostate gland and terminate in the urethra, which serves as an exit route for both sperm and urine in the male.

The male reproductive system also includes five accessory glands: a pair of seminal vesicles, a pair of bulbourethral glands, and the prostate gland. Taken collectively, the secretions of the seminal vesicles, bulbourethral glands, prostate gland, and sperm are termed semen. Semen is the transport medium by which sperm enters the female's reproductive system, permitting the sperm's introduction to an egg and potential fertilization.

The final leg of the semen's journey in the male sends it through the penis, which also contains the urethra. Three vascular spaces made up of erectile tissue surround the urethra within the penis: the corpus spongiosum and a pair of corpora cavernosa.

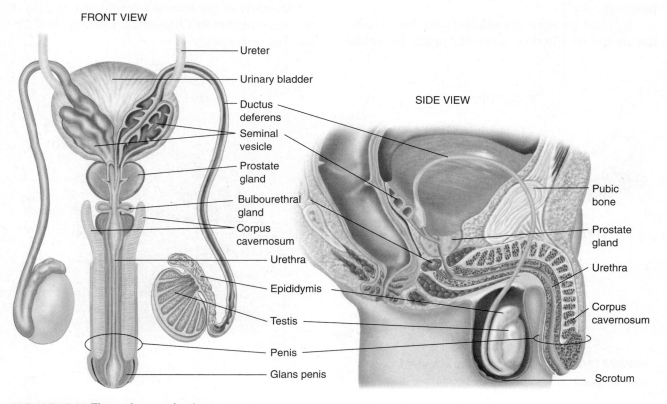

FRONT VIEW

- Ureter
- Urinary bladder
- Ductus deferens
- Seminal vesicle
- Prostate gland
- Bulbourethral gland
- Corpus cavernosum
- Urethra
- Epididymis
- Testis
- Penis
- Glans penis

SIDE VIEW

- Pubic bone
- Prostate gland
- Urethra
- Corpus cavernosum
- Scrotum

FIGURE 17-12 The male reproductive system.

© Jones & Bartlett Learning.

When the male is sexually stimulated, the parasympathetic system triggers release of nitric oxide, a potent vasodilator. As the three compartments become engorged, the normally flaccid penis becomes erect. Malfunction in this system can lead to priapism, as discussed later in this chapter.

Female Reproductive System

The female reproductive system produces and stores eggs, preparing them for fertilization by a sperm. In addition, the uterus of the female provides a home for the developing embryo during gestation. The main female reproductive organs are the ovaries, which are located on either side of the uterus within the peritoneum **FIGURE 17-13**.

Ovarian follicles within the ovary contain oocytes, or immature eggs. During the process of ovulation, an oocyte is dispelled from a vesicular follicle and the ovary each month in a female of childbearing age. This oocyte enters one of the paired fallopian (uterine) tubes, originating adjacent to the ovaries and terminating in the uterus. Cilia within the fallopian tubes project the oocyte toward the uterus. When the oocyte is fertilized and becomes implanted outside of the uterus, it can lead to a potential obstetric emergency called ectopic pregnancy.

Situated between the bladder and the rectum, the uterus is a hollow muscular organ in which embryonic development occurs following fertilization. The uterus is divided into four portions: the superior most fundus, the central body, the inferior isthmus, and the cervix. The cervix is a cylindrical structure approximately 2 to 3 cm in length with a narrow central canal that connects the uterus to the vagina. The uterus consists of three thick tissue layers: the outermost perimetrium, the muscular myometrium, and the inner endometrium. A developing embryo will lodge within the endometrium for the duration of gestation. The uterine arteries provide the uterus with its significant blood supply through a network of arcuate arteries. Every month a major portion of the endometrium of the uterus is shed and regenerated through the menstrual (uterine) cycle unless fertilization has occurred. Collectively, these structures are exquisitely sensitive to a cycle of hormones dedicated to achieving pregnancy, and they undergo impressive change and growth during pregnancy and labor.

The vagina connects the uterus to the external vaginal orifice. During intercourse, the vagina receives semen from the penis, guiding it into the uterus for possible fertilization. The vagina also serves as the birth canal during childbirth. In females, the urethra exits the body just anterior to the vagina, separating the urinary and reproductive tracts.

Anatomy of the female reproductive system is discussed further in Chapter 22, *Obstetric and Gynecologic Emergencies*.

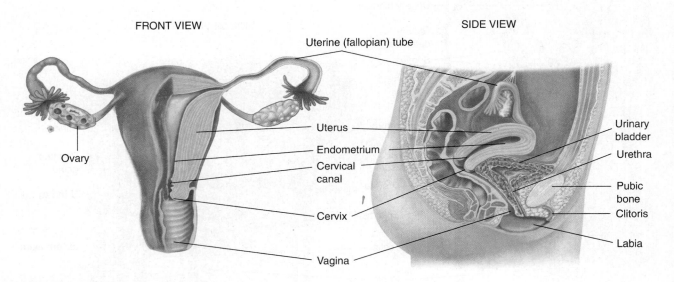

FIGURE 17-13 The female reproductive system.

Special Populations

Injuries and conditions that involve the GI and GU systems may be more difficult to diagnose in pregnant patients, individuals with psychiatric illness, and children. In the last two populations, communication is a significant barrier to localizing the disease or injury. For example, a person with decompensated schizophrenia may be unable to clearly describe pain symptoms or chronologic history. The same is true for very young children, and infants may be fussy or crying inconsolably. Obtaining collateral information (eg, trauma, eating history) and a careful exam, while keeping more common pathologies in mind (eg, appendicitis in children) will make care less daunting.

Morbidly obese patients and older adults present an additional challenge, especially in the diagnosis of abdominal emergencies. Older adults, especially those with altered mental status, may exhibit less rebound and guarding. Often, advanced imaging via computed tomography (CT) is the safer diagnostic approach in older adults and people with morbid obesity.

In pregnant patients, as the gravid uterus expands, the abdominal viscera stretches to accommodate the growing uterus. As the viscera stretches, the pain perceived by the pregnant patient may indeed be referred pain. For example, a large left lower lobe pneumonia may be "felt" by the pregnant woman in the middle of the abdomen. Keep in mind that pregnant females may develop the same abdominal problems as the general population— from appendicitis to cholecystitis to gastroenteritis. Because of the anatomic changes they have experienced, it may be difficult for females in later stages of pregnancy to pinpoint the exact source of their pain.

The abdominal/uterine area of a pregnant patient should never be painful. During your assessment of a pregnant patient, palpate the uterus and abdominal region very gently. Severe tenderness may reflect a uterine/placental or abdominal injury. During the perinatal period, it may also reflect chorioamnionitis and infection of the amniotic membranes. Such an infection can lead to profound and overwhelming sepsis in the pregnant patient. CCTPs should ask every patient in their second or third trimester the following four questions as part of the history:

- Have you noticed leakage of fluid from your vagina?
- Are you having vaginal bleeding?
- Are you having (frequent) contractions?
- Do you feel the baby moving? (Movement is expected only after 20 weeks' gestation.)

Conditions Affecting the Alimentary Canal
Epidemiology and Pathophysiology

The GI tract contains a multitude of structures operating under harsh conditions. A variety of pathologies can disrupt its normal activities, many of which reach the clinical level only after a breach of the protective layers of intestinal mucosa occurs. Disturbance of the mucosa can expose the mesenteric vasculature, nerves, lymph, and inner tissue layers to the extreme changes in pH levels and digestive enzymes found in the GI lumen. This exposure accounts for the common symptoms of GI abnormalities: abdominal pain (most common presenting symptom), tenderness, and bleeding. Depending on the etiology of GI bleeding, this symptom may lead to significant morbidity and mortality.

GI bleeding is classified into two categories based on the location of the bleeding: upper or lower GI bleeding. The source of upper GI bleeding is proximal to the ligament of Treitz, which supports the junction of the duodenum and the jejunum. Any bleeding distal to this location is referred to as lower GI bleeding. The disease process, diagnostics, and management all vary depending on the origin of the bleed.

Acute upper GI bleeding is more common than lower GI bleeding, but the two forms share a comparable mortality rate of 6% to 10% per year, with rates increasing with age and underlying comorbidities. Extrinsic factors such as alcohol and tobacco use, diet, and use of nonsteroidal anti-inflammatory drugs (NSAIDs) increase the incidence of upper GI bleeding. Recent GI surgery and critical illness increase the risk as well. In patients younger than 60 years without significant comorbidities, the mortality rate is less than 0.1%. The amount of bleeding can vary greatly depending on the etiology, from microscopic amounts of blood to massive hemorrhage.

Severe lower GI bleeding requiring hospital admission is relatively rare, accounting for fewer than 1% of hospital admissions in the United States. Differentiating between upper and lower GI bleeding can prove difficult, however, because the majority of GI bleeding presents with rectal bleeding of some kind. Lower GI bleeding may present with bright red blood at the rectum. Most upper

GI bleeding presents with dark or tarry stools from digested blood products, but brisk upper GI bleeding may also present with bright red blood at the rectum. Endoscopy is the ideal method of locating the bleeding source, although some other imaging techniques can identify active, clinically significant bleeds.

Conditions Affecting the Upper GI Tract

Gastritis

Inflammation of the gastric mucosa, termed gastritis, is a common precursor to upper GI bleeding. Causes of gastric inflammation vary widely and can be broadly separated into acute or chronic pathologies. Common causes of gastritis are listed in **TABLE 17-1**.

Mucin-producing cells, bicarbonate secretion, prostaglandins, and rapid cell turnover are some of the protective mechanisms that mitigate the corrosive effects of hydrochloric acid and pepsin in the digestive system. When this equilibrium is disturbed, inflammation and necrosis of the epithelial cells occurs because of the ensuing immune system response **FIGURE 17-14**. This process is generally consistent no matter what actually precipitates acute gastritis.

Upper GI bleeding may occur in patients with acute gastritis who experience rapid onset of mucosal inflammation or sudden breakdown of protective barriers. Ingestion of corrosive chemicals, for example, can cause chemical burns leading to sloughing of the gastric mucosa, which is often associated with pain and nausea. Depending on the chemical, these burns can cause significant inflammation and subsequent necrosis of tissues,

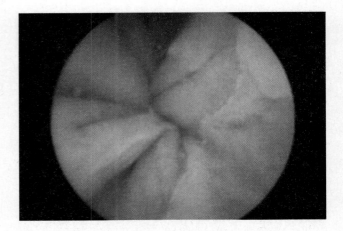

A

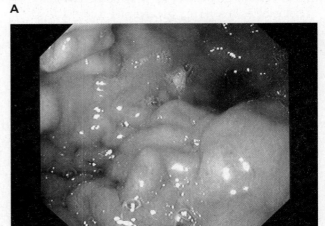

B

FIGURE 17-14 A. Normal stomach. **B.** Gastritis.

accompanied by varying degrees of hemorrhage. Chemical burns commonly affect external perioral tissues, the oral cavity, and the tongue as well. Some household cleaners, and most industrial cleaners, are potent enough to trigger this process. Blood in the vomit may be bright red or dark brown. In fact, digested blood products in the vomit may be described as coffee-ground emesis.

Many cases of acute gastritis are actually an exacerbation of a chronic GI condition. For example, extensive tissue damage is found in as many as 20% of people with chronic alcoholism. Minor bleeding occurs frequently and often goes unnoticed in these patients, but an episode of severe hemorrhage can occur suddenly after even a small intake of alcohol. The bacterium *Helicobacter pylori* causes acute gastritis during the primary period of infection. The initial immune system response to the invading

TABLE 17-1 Causes of Gastritis
Corrosive chemical ingestion
Alcohol abuse
Helicobacter pylori infection
Atrophic gastritis
Reactive gastritis
Radiation exposure

bacteria triggers an inflammation of the mucosal tissues, which is self-limiting and typically resolves within 11 to 14 days. Occasionally, the bacteria are fully eliminated from the body following the immune defense. Patients who develop ongoing symptoms of gastritis may need testing and antimicrobial treatment for *H pylori*.

Conditions involving long-term histopathologic changes to the gastric lining, such as chronic atrophic gastritis, can lead to downstream complications related to malnutrition, such as pernicious anemia. Pernicious anemia is a form of anemia resulting from malabsorption of vitamin B_{12}, an essential building block of red blood cells. Atrophic gastritis has a prevalence of 2% in older adults, but its pathogenesis remains unclear. In some cases, it has been linked to certain autoimmune disorders, as well as *H pylori* infection.

Another common etiology for epigastric discomfort and GI bleeding is reactive gastritis, which occurs when the stomach lining is chronically irritated by NSAIDs, alcohol, and bile. Patients undergoing abdominal radiation therapy may experience radiation gastritis, which resembles acute gastroenteritis and usually occurs within days of treatment. Patients with radiation gastritis may develop ulcerations, much as patients with other forms of gastritis do.

Peptic Ulcers

Peptic ulcer is the leading cause of upper GI bleeding **TABLE 17-2**. These ulcers are characterized by an erosion of the mucosal lining of the GI tract in either the stomach (gastric ulcer) or the duodenum (duodenal ulcer). Once that defensive lining becomes disrupted, exposure to the acids and pepsin in the pylorus and duodenum can cause ulceration. An ulceration that is deep enough can penetrate a blood vessel, leading to major or minor bleeding. Continued ulceration can result in perforation of the gastric or duodenal wall, causing intra-abdominal leakage of gastric juices and peritonitis. Finally, scar tissue from past ulcers can cause narrowing or obstruction in the GI tract.

Peptic ulcer disease is common in the United States, with a lifetime prevalence of 5% to 10%. Although psychological stress is commonly considered a contributing factor to ulcer formation, there is a lack of evidence to support this theory.

However, two major risk factors have been identified for peptic ulcers: the presence of *H*

TABLE 17-2 Causes of Upper and Lower GI Bleeding

Type of Bleeding	Cause
Upper GI bleeding	Aortoenteric fistula Peptic ulcers Duodenal ulcers Gastritis Esophageal or gastric varices Gastric malignancy Mallory-Weiss syndrome
Lower GI bleeding	Diverticulosis Angiodysplasia Inflammatory bowel diseases (colitis) Hemorrhoidal bleeding Malignancy

Abbreviation: GI, gastrointestinal

© Jones & Bartlett Learning.

TABLE 17-3 Causes of Peptic Ulcers

Helicobacter pylori infection
Nonsteroidal anti-inflammatory drugs
Alcohol use
Tobacco use
Stress-related erosive syndrome
Curling syndrome
Cushing syndrome
Zollinger-Ellison syndrome
Gastritis

© Jones & Bartlett Learning.

pylori and NSAID use. *H pylori* is the most prevalent cause of chronic bacterial infection globally, affecting gastric acid secretion and mucosal defense mechanisms. This pathogen is associated with both gastritis and peptic ulcers, with its presence increasing the likelihood of these conditions when combined with other risk factors **TABLE 17-3**. Patients with *H pylori* infection have a 6- to 10-fold increased incidence of peptic ulcer disease compared to uninfected individuals. A highly motile spirilla bacterium, *H pylori* colonizes the mucosa

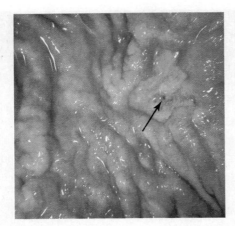

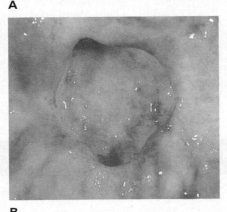

FIGURE 17-15 Peptic ulcers. **A.** Gastric ulcer, which eroded a blood vessel in the base of the ulcer (arrow) and bled profusely. **B.** Large chronic duodenal ulcer.

Courtesy of Leonard V. Crowley, MD.

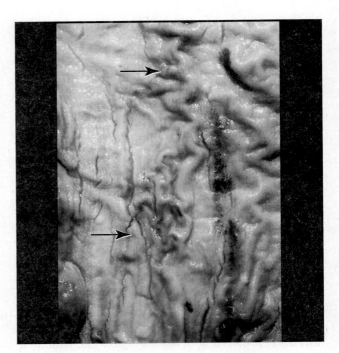

FIGURE 17-16 Mucosal surface of the esophagus illustrating varices, which appear as tortuous elevations of the mucosa (arrows).

Courtesy of Leonard V. Crowley, MD.

of the stomach and duodenum **FIGURE 17-15**. Both *H pylori* and NSAIDs such as aspirin and ibuprofen hinder the mucosa's defenses against irritation by inhibiting production of prostaglandins, the hormones that mediate the inflammatory response in tissues. When prostaglandin production is reduced, injury to the mucosal layer goes unchecked, leading to irritation (gastritis) and ulceration. Alcohol and tobacco use have deleterious effects on the mucosal barrier and are independent risk factors for peptic ulcer disease.

Stress-related erosive syndrome is believed to be a frequent cause of peptic ulcers in patients in the intensive care unit (ICU). In fact, endoscopy performed within 72 hours of the onset of illness has shown that 75% to 100% of critically ill patients exhibit gross gastric lesions. Poor mucosal perfusion because of multiple comorbidities, trauma, or burns

may be exacerbated by large-volume fluid resuscitation and gut edema, further reducing the efficiency of the mucous barrier. This general decrease in resistance to gastric juice allows numerous shallow ulcers to form throughout the esophagus, stomach, and duodenum. Ulcers associated with severe burns are termed Curling ulcers, whereas those accompanying episodes of increased intracranial pressure are called Cushing ulcers. Preventive use of histamine (H_2)-receptor antagonist or proton pump inhibitor prophylaxis has made these complications relatively rare in recent years. Less common causes of ulcers include hypersecretion of acid into the GI lumen, such as by a tumor, as seen in Zollinger-Ellison syndrome.

Esophageal Disease

Just as erosion of mucosal lining into a blood vessel will lead to GI bleeding, so will the reverse process—swelling of esophageal veins that intrudes into the lumen of the esophagus **FIGURE 17-16**. Such an exposed vein, known as an esophageal varix, is susceptible to sudden rupture, resulting in significant hemorrhage. Esophageal varices are the second-most common cause of upper GI bleeding.

Mortality following a variceal rupture approaches 30%. Unlike other causes of GI hemorrhage, in which active bleeding typically stops without intervention in most cases, esophageal varices spontaneously stop bleeding only 50% of the time.

Esophagitis is another common etiology of upper GI bleeding. It is typically a result of severe gastroesophageal reflux disease and alcohol abuse, but may also stem from irritation caused by pills (pill esophagitis) or infection.

Varices result from increased venous pressure in the hepatic portal system. When **portal hypertension** occurs, venous blood will use alternative pathways for its return to the vena cava via the **azygos system**. The azygos system drains a portion of the esophageal venous blood, and overuse of this system causes pooling and distention of these veins. The lower portion of the esophagus also drains blood into the left gastric vein, which is adversely affected by hepatic portal hypertension. Minor increases in hepatic portal venous pressure can result in varices, with the risk of rupture growing exponentially as the pressure continues to rise. Although varices can occur anywhere along the esophagus, stomach, and duodenum, ruptures leading to GI hemorrhage most frequently occur at the gastroesophageal junction.

Portal hypertension typically occurs when large swaths of hepatic cellular architecture are disrupted, which tends to result from deposition of scar tissue in cirrhosis. In **cirrhosis**, buildup of fatty acids and chronic destruction of liver tissue and fibrosis progressively obstruct venous blood flow. In the United States, liver cirrhosis is primarily caused by chronic alcohol use or hepatitis C. Patients with cirrhosis may develop classic physical findings, including abdominal ascites, jaundice, and caput medusae.

Mallory-Weiss syndrome involves a longitudinal laceration of the esophageal mucosa, typically in the distal esophagus at the gastroesophageal junction **FIGURE 17-17**. The tear develops as a result of repeated significant changes in local pressure, such as those seen with repeated forceful vomiting. These individuals may notice streaks of bright red blood in their vomitus. More significant bleeding may occur if the patient is on anticoagulant medication or has an underlying coagulopathy. Mallory-Weiss syndrome, which occurs mainly in middle-aged adults, has a mortality of less than

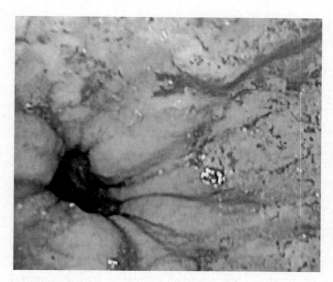

FIGURE 17-17 Mallory-Weiss syndrome.
© David M. Martin, MD/Science Source.

10%. These upper GI bleeds often cease on their own. Comorbidities that increase the likelihood of a tear include hiatal hernias, bulimia, chronic alcohol use, and increasing age.

When patients experience particularly forceful vomiting, spontaneous rupture of the esophagus, also known as **Boerhaave syndrome**, may occur. These perforations may also occur as a result of caustic ingestion or pill esophagitis; in approximately one-half of all cases, they are iatrogenic (eg, resulting from endoscopy or stricture dilation). Patients with Boerhaave syndrome can present as quite ill, with severe chest and upper abdominal pain, fever, odynophagia, and shock.

Another cause of esophageal perforation is foreign body ingestion and esophageal impaction. While foreign body ingestion typically occurs in children, it is generally associated with eating in adults (eg, fish and chicken bones, toothpicks). Foreign body ingestion and impaction of food occur more commonly in older adults and individuals with psychiatric illness or alcohol intoxication. They are usually associated with an inability to swallow liquid or solids (dysphagia) and regurgitation. Although most obstructions resolve spontaneously, patients with severe obstruction or with underlying strictures caused by anatomic anomalies or tumors may require endoscopic intervention. Patients with worsening obstruction may develop perforation, pain, and bleeding.

Conditions Affecting the Lower GI Tract

Lower GI bleeding is characterized by bleeding distal to the ligament of Treitz. It can occur in the jejunum, ileum, large intestine, rectum, and anus. Several conditions can cause bleeding, and the severity of such bleeding can vary greatly.

Diverticulosis and Diverticulitis

Diverticulosis is a common disease of the lower GI tract in older adults **FIGURE 17-18**. **Diverticula** are small outcroppings of the mucosal lining of the large intestine, typically in the descending colon and sigmoid colon **FIGURE 17-19**. These sac-like protrusions are a consequence of strong haustral muscle contractions, which push tissue against a mucosa that weakens with age. Generally painless, diverticula can be found in 50% to 70% of people older than 80 years. Lifestyle risk factors known to increase the incidence of diverticulosis include a low-fiber diet, chronic constipation, lack of physical activity, and smoking.

Diverticulitis, an inflammation of the diverticulum, occurs in as many as 15% of patients with diverticulosis. It is thought to be caused by microscopic or macroscopic perforation of the diverticulum, as a result of focal inflammation. Diverticulitis can be acute or chronic, and can lead to complications such as abscess formation, fistula, or peritonitis. **Diverticular bleeding** occurs in another 15% of patients with diverticulosis, with massive GI bleeding observed in one-third of those cases. Bleeding, which can be venous or arterial, results from structural weakness of the vessel wall as it is stretched into the herniated wall of the diverticulum.

Angiodysplasia

Angiodysplasia is a malformation of submucosal blood vessels in the GI tract **FIGURE 17-20**. Although it can occur anywhere in the alimentary canal, more than three-fourths of all cases present in the cecum and ascending colon. These thin-walled, winding vessels are highly susceptible to rupture. Angiodysplasia is the most common vascular abnormality in the GI tract, and its incidence increases with age. The most common site for angiodysplasia in the GI tract is the colon.

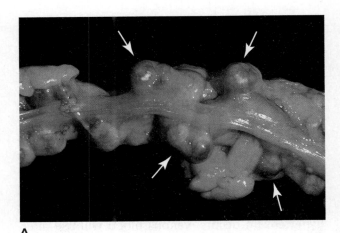

A

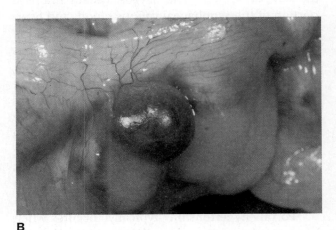

B

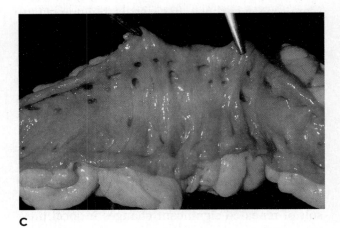

C

FIGURE 17-18 Diverticulosis of the colon. **A.** Exterior of the colon illustrating several diverticula projecting through the wall of the colon (arrows). **B.** Closer view of the diverticulum. **C.** Interior of the colon, illustrating openings of multiple diverticula. Several of the openings are well demonstrated in the mucosa just below the clamps.

Courtesy of Leonard V. Crowley, MD.

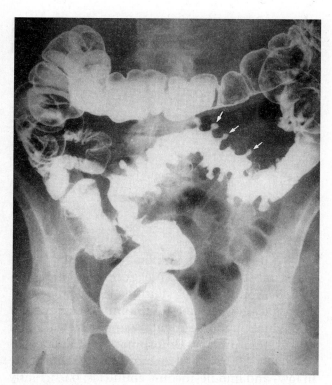

FIGURE 17-19 Diverticula of the colon demonstrated by injection of barium contrast material into the colon (barium enema). Diverticula filled with contrast material appear as projections from the mucosa (arrows).

Courtesy of Leonard V. Crowley, MD.

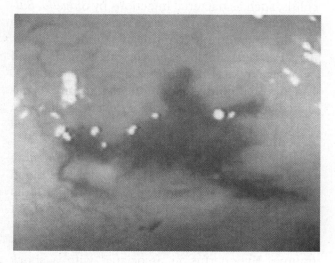

FIGURE 17-20 Angiodysplasia.

© David M. Martin, MD/Science Source.

Appendicitis

The appendix is a blind pouch, extending from the cecum, that can become inflamed and infected, causing **appendicitis**. The classic presentation is relatively rapid onset of right lower quadrant or periumbilical pain, associated with nausea, vomiting, and fever. Appendicitis is one of the most common reasons for emergency abdominal surgery in the United States and affects as much as 8% of the population over the course of their lifetime. The age range of patients who commonly develop appendicitis is bimodal, with most developing it in their teens and 40s. Advanced cases can lead to perforation, peritonitis, and sepsis.

Inflammatory Conditions of the GI Tract

Inflammatory bowel disease (IBD) is a collective term covering two colonic pathologies that are together responsible for approximately 10% of the cases of lower GI bleeding: ulcerative colitis and Crohn disease **FIGURE 17-21**. IBD is more common in white individuals, with a typical onset between 15 and 30 years of age. Common causes of inflamed colon (**colitis**) are listed in **TABLE 17-4**.

Ulcerative colitis is an inflammation of the mucosal and submucosal tissues of the rectum, commonly extending to involve the colon. In this condition, ulcers—which occasionally bleed—form throughout the colon. Patients usually present with frequent small bouts of diarrhea, which may be bloody (in as many as 50% of patients), associated with severe intermittent abdominal pain that comes and goes (colicky pain) and tenesmus. Inflammation spreads into the colon in 35% of cases, a condition termed pancolitis. Other complications may include proctitis, fistula and abscess formation, and extraintestinal complications (such as uveitis or polyarthritis).

Crohn disease is a less organized inflammation of the GI tract in which all layers of the mucosa may be affected. This inflammation is not contiguous, as in ulcerative colitis, but rather results in scattered ulcerations and fibroses throughout the GI tract. Minor bleeding occasionally occurs from these ulcers as well as from small tears that may develop in the mucosa. Cardinal symptoms include abdominal pain, diarrhea, fatigue, and weight loss. Approximately 1% to 4% of patients diagnosed with Crohn disease experience significant GI bleeding.

As ulcerative colitis and Crohn disease move into chronic stages, scar tissue formation can result in a thickening of the mucosa and create bowel obstructions. Because both diseases share similar symptoms, as many as 15% of cases are diagnosed as indeterminate colitis.

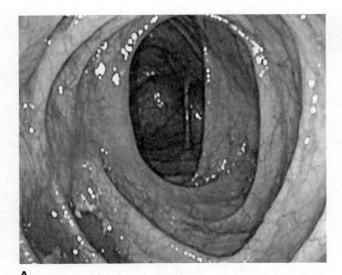

A

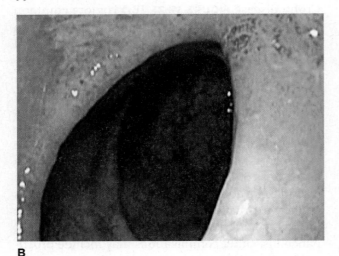

B

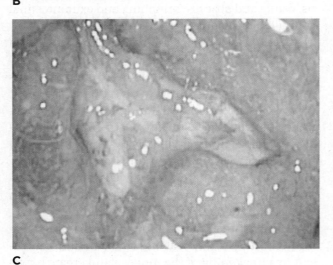

C

FIGURE 17-21 A. Normal colon. **B.** Ulcerative colitis.
C. Crohn disease.

TABLE 17-4 Causes of Colitis
Ulcerative colitis
Crohn disease
Bacterial infection
Viral infection
Ischemic colitis
Radiation colitis

Gastroenteritis is an illness caused by bacterial, viral, or parasitic infection, and characterized by vomiting and diarrhea. Such infections are typically self-limited in immunocompetent individuals, and treatment is supportive with oral rehydration therapy. Unfortunately, this illness is associated with significant morbidity and mortality in low- and middle-income countries, particularly in children. Severe dehydration or hemodynamic compromise requires not only intravenous (IV) hydration, but also careful consideration of alternative diagnoses.

A variety of infectious diseases can also cause colitis, such as bacterial infections by *Shigella*, *Salmonella*, and *Campylobacter*. These infections are self-limiting and rarely result in significant bleeding. Viral causes include the Norwalk-type virus and cytomegalovirus in immunosuppressed patients. Patients on prolonged antibiotic therapy may experience growth of *Clostridioides difficile*, which can cause profound diarrhea and dehydration, as well as permanent mucosal damage.

Ischemic colitis is a potentially life-threatening form of colitis that results from diminished blood flow to the GI tract. Etiologies range from arterial obstruction, caused by embolic events in a patient with atrial fibrillation, to severe vessel narrowing in patients with vascular occlusive diseases, to trauma. Hypoperfusion associated with a shock state can also lead to ischemic colitis. The classical presentation of a patient with an intestinal infarct is severe abdominal pain that is out of proportion to the exam; that is, the patient will not look as ill or the abdomen, at least initially, will not be as tender as the individual's pain would suggest. As bowel necrosis progresses, the patient may experience GI bleeding. This condition can progress rapidly if untreated and will lead to bowel necrosis, perforation, sepsis, shock, and death.

Radiation colitis occurs in 75% of patients who have received radiation doses of 4,000 rad (40 gray [Gy]) or more to the abdomen or pelvis. Chronic mucosal thickening can result from such therapy, as well as ulcerations throughout the colon. Although the major complication of this condition is abdominal pain and diarrhea, anemia and lower GI bleeding can occur as well.

Immune-mediated colitis is an adverse advent associated with immune checkpoint inhibitors, usually affecting the lower GI tract. Checkpoint inhibitors are monoclonal antibodies that boost the immune system's anticancer response. The incidence of colitis in patients who receive this therapy is as high as 25%. Patients usually develop mucus- or blood-tinged diarrhea and abdominal pain, and have a similar presentation and complications as patients with IBD.

Assessment

Signs and Symptoms

The signs and symptoms of patients who experience GI bleeding vary depending on the origin and severity of the bleeding. Slow, chronic bleeding that has been partially digested can result in black, tarry-appearing stool, called melena. If the bleeding in either the upper or lower GI tract is minimal, blood in the stool may be detectable only by laboratory testing.

Some ulcerative processes, such as peptic ulcer disease, will cause diffuse abdominal discomfort and will be described as a chronic stomachache or nonspecific burning and cramping. Blood products are emetogenic, meaning that even small amounts of blood may cause gastric irritation and vomiting. Emesis containing blood is known as hematemesis. In some cases, patients experience weight loss, anemia, and malnutrition as a result of poor nutrient absorption over damaged mucosa.

Complaints of dizziness and syncope are common in patients with GI bleeding. In addition, these patients may have fever, so temperature should be assessed in all patients with GI dysfunction or bleeding. GI bleeding is not a contraindication to obtaining a rectal temperature unless the patient is neutropenic.

Diarrhea is most commonly associated with lower GI disorders, as a result of reduced water absorption efficiency associated with damaged or infected mucosa. Dehydration frequently follows from diarrhea, as do electrolyte imbalances that can trigger cardiac arrhythmias.

Significant GI bleeding is usually acute and may present with hemodynamic instability and shock. Vomiting large amounts of bright red blood is suggestive of acute bleeding in the upper GI tract—for example, from ruptured varices, an ulcerated submucosal blood vessel, or Mallory-Weiss syndrome. Hematochezia, the presence of bright red blood in the stool, is usually indicative of active lower GI bleeding. However, brisk upper GI bleeding (which is too fast to be digested) may present as hematochezia as well. When it is coupled with diarrhea, the patient can experience a significant intravascular volume loss. Hypotension may or may not be immediately apparent, and testing for orthostatic changes may be helpful. Other signs of shock, such as tachycardia, diaphoresis, pallor, and altered mental status, also accompany blood loss. When paired with a decreased level of consciousness, vomiting can result in airway compromise.

When assessing for rectal bleeding, the CCTP should be aware that external sources of bleeding such as a pressure ulcer may exist around the anus. Pressure ulcers arise from prolonged pressure on body tissues and are commonly seen in patients confined to a bed. Unfortunately, pressure injuries occur disproportionately in patients at long-term care facilities, with their treatment incurring considerable costs for the health care system. Pressure ulcers are classified into stages 1 through 4 **FIGURE 17-22**. Stage 1 ulcers are reversible, characterized by warmth and nonblanchable erythema; stage 4 ulcers have full-thickness tissue necrosis, often with muscle and bone involvement. If ulcers are present, the CCTP should take care to avoid placing further pressure on the area while bandaging any exposed bleeding tissue. These ulcers are unlikely to produce life-threatening blood loss, but they do cause severe pain and place the patient at risk for infection. Other distal sources of bleeding include anal fissures and hemorrhoids, both of which tend to be associated with constipation and hard stools.

Some abdominal diseases produce distinctive pain in specific locations, aiding in their

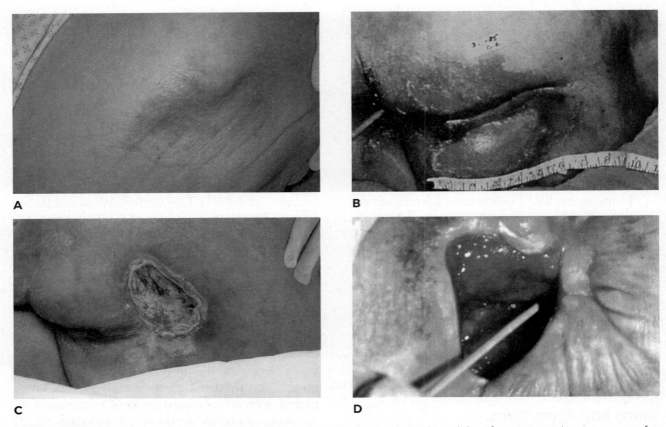

FIGURE 17-22 A pressure ulcer develops when pressure decreases blood supply, and therefore oxygenation, to an area of tissue. **A.** Stage 1. **B.** Stage 2. **C.** Stage 3. **D.** Stage 4.

diagnosis. For example, peptic ulcers cause a burning epigastric pain that is associated with eating and may be relieved by antacids. Gastric ulcer pain is exacerbated with a full stomach, whereas duodenal ulcers are more painful at night, when the stomach is empty. Gastroesophageal reflux, which is reflux of gastric acid and consequent irritation of tissues proximal to the lower esophageal sphincter, frequently accompanies peptic ulcers and gastritis. Biliary obstruction with gallstones (discussed later in this chapter) may mimic reflux and gastritis symptoms. Esophageal varices present initially with painless bleeding that evolves into a burning pain and hematemesis. Appendicitis classically leads to right lower quadrant pain and tenderness. Diverticulitis typically presents with sharp intermittent pain to the lower left abdominal quadrant, commonly referred to as left-side appendicitis. The patient's medical history and presence of risk factors for certain diseases should always be considered during the assessment to aid the prehospital provider in selecting the appropriate treatment.

Signs and Symptoms

GI Bleeding
- Diffuse abdominal pain
- Chronic stomachache
- Nonspecific burning sensation
- Vomiting, often with blood present
- Hematemesis
- Melena
- Hematochezia
- Weight loss
- Anemia
- Malnutrition
- Dizziness
- Syncope
- Fever
- Diarrhea
- Dehydration
- Hypotension

Differential Diagnosis

GI Bleeding

- Peptic ulcer disease
- Gastritis
- Esophageal varices
- Mallory-Weiss syndrome
- Zollinger-Ellison syndrome
- Gastric tumor
- Esophageal or gastric cancer
- Cirrhosis
- Angiodysplasia
- Inflammatory bowel disease
- Colon cancer
- Colitis
- Diverticulitis
- Hemorrhoids
- Abdominal aortic aneurysm
- Infectious diarrhea

Laboratory Data

Laboratory testing and monitoring are essential in the diagnosis and management of GI bleeding **TABLE 17-5**. Hemoglobin and hematocrit values may appear normal, or only mildly decreased, for several hours after acute bleeding, owing to an equivalent loss of plasma and red blood cells. Eventually, however, these values decrease as interstitial fluid shifts to blood vessels as the body attempts to maintain BP, essentially diluting the blood's oxygen-carrying capacity. Hematocrit values also fall as blood is diluted with crystalloid fluids during resuscitation. For this reason, the CCTP should avoid aggressive crystalloid resuscitation and allow for permissive hypotension. An ongoing decrease in the hematocrit value over time indicates active bleeding.

A coagulation profile is an important component of the workup, as it can identify deficiencies in clotting and platelet function requiring specific treatment. Prolonged prothrombin time (PT) and activated partial thromboplastin time (PTT) are suggestive of liver disease, and a liver function test should be performed in patients with these findings. The coagulation profile (PT, international normalized ratio [INR], and PTT) may also reflect the presence of anticoagulant medications the patient is prescribed, such as warfarin. The CCTP should make every effort to determine if the patient is taking anticoagulant medication, as some of these medications can be reversed. Thrombocytopenia may be chronic, or it may be a result of platelet loss from hemorrhage or consumption, as occurs with diffuse intravascular coagulation. Balanced transfusion of blood products, by supplementing clotting factors and platelets via infusion of fresh-frozen plasma and platelets, may be required in these patients.

TABLE 17-5 Normal Versus Abnormal Laboratory Values

Test	Normal	Abnormal
Hemoglobin	14–17.5 g/dL	↓
Hematocrit	41% to 50%	↓
Prothrombin time	10–13 s	Varies
Partial thromboplastin time	<40 s	Varies
BUN	8–23 mg/dL	↑
Creatine, serum	0.6–1.2 mg/dL	Varies (unchanged or small rise)
BUN:creatinine ratio	10:1	↑
Glomerular filtration rate	125 mL/min	↓
Blood glucose	70–110 mg/dL	↑ (early)
White blood cells (leukocytes)	4,500–11,000/μL	↑

Abbreviations: ↑, above normal values; ↓, below normal values; BUN, blood urea nitrogen

Transport Management

GI Bleeding

- Provide airway control: suction and intubation.
- Provide ventilatory support with oxygen.
- Designate the patient as being on nothing by mouth (nil per os [NPO]) status.
- Place two large-bore IV catheters.
- If the patient is in shock or extremis, place an intraosseous (IO) line, particularly if IV access is difficult.
- Provide thoughtful fluid resuscitation, with a goal of achieving permissive hypotension.
- Draw blood samples; provide blood infusion if available, preferably instead of crystalloid fluids.
- Continuously monitor BP.
- Continuously monitor pulse oximetry.
- Continuously monitor the electrocardiogram (ECG).
- Obtain lab values.
- Place a nasogastric (NG) or orogastric (OG) tube.

BUN levels increase following upper GI bleeding owing to digestion and absorption of blood proteins in the large intestine. A decreased GFR due to hypoperfusion of the kidneys secondary to hypovolemia will exacerbate this increase. A BUN-to-creatinine ratio greater than 35:1 is highly suggestive of upper GI bleeding.

The adrenergic response to GI bleeding results in hyperglycemia, whereas an insult to mucosal tissues stimulates an increase in the white blood cell (WBC) count via an inflammatory response. Serum electrolyte disturbances can occur as well, including hypernatremia and hyperchloremia from fluid resuscitation, or hypokalemia from excessive vomiting. Significant acid–base dysregulation may be present, which may portend a worsening clinical condition and indicate the need for airway management. The CCTP needs to review the most recent lab results and trends in the chart as part of the assessment before beginning the patient's transfer.

Imaging

In both upper and lower GI bleeding, the most effective method of localizing the origin of the bleeding is to search the mucosa. Endoscopy—specifically, **esophagogastroduodenoscopy (EGD)**—enables visualization of more than 90% of the upper GI tract. In addition to diagnosing the source of bleeding, endoscopists can employ various therapies to stop the bleeding, ranging from cauterization to local application of hemostatic material or vasoconstricting injections. The endoscopist may perform gastric lavage prior to endoscopy to facilitate viewing of the internal structures. Complications from endoscopy are relatively rare, with an incidence of less than 1%, and most commonly take the form of bleeding and perforation. In the past, nasogastric lavage was often performed to differentiate between upper and lower GI bleeding sources, but it is now performed less frequently due to the risk of dislodging variceal clots.

EGD is sometimes performed first in patients with undifferentiated bleeding and melena or severe hematochezia, followed by **colonoscopy** if the EGD is negative. However, results of additional testing, as well as risk stratification and clinical scenario, may affect the diagnostic approach. Visualization of the lower GI mucosa is possible via colonoscopy, although this procedure is slightly more complicated than endoscopy. A colonoscopy is usually delayed by a few hours to allow for bowel purge preparation, which both enables the physician to view the mucosa more effectively and reduces the risk of perforation. Colonoscopy allows for visualization of the entire rectum and large intestine, up to the ileocecal junction. The diagnostic yield of colonoscopy for lower GI bleeding is significantly higher than that with radiologic evaluation. Similar treatment modalities are available via colonoscopy as with EGD.

Due to ever-improving imaging technology, **CT angiography** is an increasingly convenient diagnostic tool for GI bleeding, particularly when active extravasation and bleeding are occurring. When this imaging technique is used, dye injected into blood vessels will leak into the lumen of the GI tract at the site of the bleeding. Diagnostic accuracy depends on the presence of active bleeding. Nevertheless, when it is timed correctly, angiography can rapidly localize bleeding lesions anywhere in the GI tract, obviating the need for oral contrast or bowel preparation. Angiography is more frequently used to diagnose lower GI bleeding because of the lower success rate of colonoscopy as opposed to endoscopy when brisk bleeding may hinder the endoscopist. **FIGURE 17-23** shows a normal abdominal CT scan.

Technetium-99m–labeled red blood cell **scintigraphy** is a technique in which blood cells attached

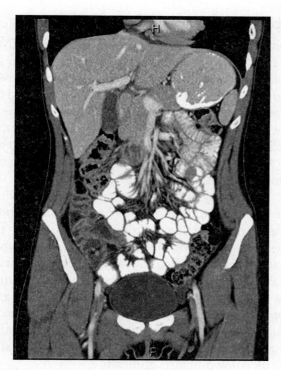

FIGURE 17-23 A normal abdominal computed tomography scan.

© Living Art Enterprises/Science Source.

to isotopes are identified as they extravasate at the source of bleeding. Once popular, this imaging modality is being rapidly abandoned in favor of CT angiography in most centers. Tagged red blood cell scans do not have the advantage of providing a vascular map, which serves as invaluable guidance for interventional radiologists or surgeons during management.

Management

The fundamentals of patient care must be ensured before any specific treatment is attempted. It is important to control and maintain the patient's airway. During acute GI bleeding, particularly with massive hematemesis, airway compromise occurs primarily by either physical obstruction or mechanical obstruction. Use suctioning to clear a physical obstruction of the airway by blood or vomit. Mechanical obstruction of the airway by the tongue or head positioning because of a decreased level of consciousness, secondary to hypovolemic shock, is managed by placement of airway adjuncts and intubation. Rapid sequence intubation is indicated in individuals with a high risk of aspiration, such as patients who are lethargic and are actively vomiting.

Administer supplemental oxygen to maintain an oxygen saturation of 92% or greater in the alert, conscious patient. Assist ventilations as necessary with a bag-mask device and high-flow oxygen.

Patients with acute GI bleeding should be designated as NPO (nothing by mouth) because of the likelihood they will undergo endoscopy and/or surgery shortly after hospital admission. Two large-bore (14- to 16-gauge) IV catheters should be placed immediately. In case of difficult IV access, IO insertion is an excellent alternative. Fluid resuscitation should begin immediately in any patient who exhibits signs of shock, although this should be done carefully. Judicious fluid administration is required because over-resuscitation can lead to hemodilution of the blood, which in turn can reduce clotting effectiveness. Increasing vascular volume too rapidly can also worsen bleeding, particularly in esophageal varices, potentially dislodging fragile clots. Aggressive fluid resuscitation in individuals without prehospital hypotension may lead to worse outcomes. Much as when treating hemorrhage caused by trauma, the CCTP should aim for permissive hypotension; that is, systolic BP (SBP) is allowed to fall low enough to avoid exsanguination, but is kept high enough to maintain perfusion. In adults with GI bleeding, boluses of 500 mL may be used to maintain a mean arterial pressure (MAP) of approximately 60 mm Hg; definitive management will entail transfusion of blood products. As in hypovolemic shock from other causes, avoiding the coagulopathy that accompanies hypothermia is paramount. Keep the transport environment warm and use warmed IV fluids, if available.

Blood samples should be drawn concurrently with IV line placement to determine a type and crossmatch, complete blood count, electrolyte levels, and PT and PTT values. Current evidence recommends withholding blood administration until the patient's hemoglobin drops below 7 g/dL, as more liberal transfusion strategies are associated with worsened outcomes. However, as discussed earlier, blood count assays may be delayed in patients with large acute bleeds; thus, transfusion based on clinical features of shock is warranted, particularly in patients with ongoing bleeding. Platelet or fresh-frozen plasma infusion may be indicated based on lab findings as well as the volume of packed red blood cells given. In patients who require massive transfusion, balanced replacement of blood products, including platelets, cryoprecipitate, or plasma, can improve outcomes by addressing the coagulopathy that occurs with dilution (eg, due to large volumes of crystalloid or packed red blood cells). Of note, the citrate preservative in blood products may cause hypocalcemia in patients with massive transfusion, and calcium must be restored accordingly. The principles of management of hemorrhagic shock are discussed in detail in Chapter 10, *Resuscitation, Shock, and Blood Products.*

Continuous BP and pulse oximetry monitoring is required to evaluate the patient's response and the effectiveness of fluid resuscitation efforts. In patients in profound shock states, pulse oximetry results may be unreliable. Care must be taken to avoid fluid overload secondary to excessive fluid administration in patients with comorbidities, specifically those with cardiac-related conditions. Arterial line placement is helpful in hemodynamically unstable patients to provide real-time visualization of their hemodynamic status. Continuous ECG monitoring should be implemented to observe patients for worsening tachycardia as a result of worsening shock, as well as a variety of arrhythmias that may develop secondary to electrolyte imbalances or hypoxia.

Controversies

Several states across the United States have been grappling with the issue of the level of training and licensure necessary to oversee administration of blood and blood products. Some states may not allow a person without specific credentialing to administer blood or blood products during transport. This restriction may force the sending facility to complete or even discontinue the administration of such products before transfer. Indeed, ground transport services rarely carry and use blood components; most services that carry blood components are helicopter-based. However, positive research findings and mortality benefits from whole blood transfusion in combat environments and the prehospital setting are prompting more EMS organizations to reconsider their position on replacing blood products. Facilities should be aware of their state regulations and the composition (ie, certified versus licensed) of their CCT teams when faced with these types of transfers. The referring physician might also confer with a transport physician or the CCT medical director to determine which resources are necessary to safely transport the patient.

Upper GI Bleeding

Some patients may have had an nasogastric (NG) or orogastric (OG) tube placed after intubation for gastric decompression (especially if they received prolonged ventilation via bag-mask device) and for evacuation of any blood or gastric contents. Due to the risk of exacerbating a bleeding varix or ulcer, as well as the risk of aspiration, NG and OG tubes are no longer routinely placed in patients who are not already intubated or during transport.

Endoscopy is performed at the hospital when the patient's condition is stable. It may serve both diagnostic and therapeutic functions. Once the bleeding site is located, *injection sclerotherapy*—that is, injection of small doses of either epinephrine or clotting factors into the site—can be performed via endoscopy. Epinephrine causes a local vasoconstriction that results in decreased blood flow to the area; human thrombin, fibrin glue, and similar products stimulate clotting, which will slow or stop the bleeding process significantly.

Endoscopic variceal band ligation can be used to control bleeding esophageal varices. This technique involves the placement of rubber bands around the varix, which shuts off its blood supply. Cauterization methods and hemostatic clip placement are alternatives to these treatments.

Of the vasoactive medications, two are quite effective at stopping active GI bleeding. If portal hypertension is suspected, these medications should be started early. Vasopressin induces vasoconstriction of the splanchnic arteries, which reduces mesenteric blood flow and, in turn, reduces portal hypertension. This effect can be beneficial to the patient with esophageal varices and undifferentiated GI bleeding because it substantially reduces blood flow to the region. Octreotide, a synthetic version of somatostatin, inhibits glucagon release and thus inhibits splanchnic vasodilation. This medication is used most commonly in the management of variceal bleeding in patients with a history of cirrhosis.

When variceal hemorrhage proves refractory to endoscopic and pharmacologic treatments, mechanical obstruction of hemorrhage via balloon inflation and shunt placement may be viable alternative therapies. Balloon tamponade of variceal bleeding is effective in controlling the hemorrhage in as many as 90% of patients. In this procedure, a **Sengstaken-Blakemore tube FIGURE 17-24** or

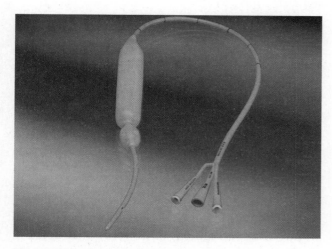

FIGURE 17-24 Sengstaken-Blakemore tube.

© 2021 Becton, Dickinson and Company. Used with permission.

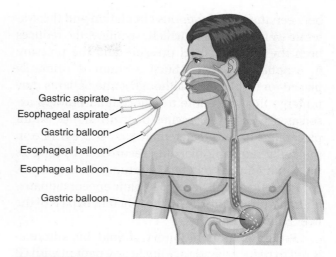

Gastric aspirate
Esophageal aspirate
Gastric balloon
Esophageal balloon
Esophageal balloon
Gastric balloon

FIGURE 17-26 Placement of a Minnesota tube.

© Jones & Bartlett Learning.

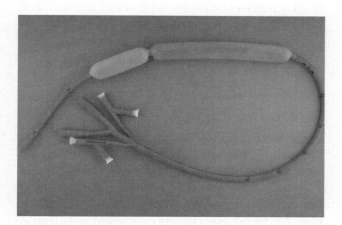

FIGURE 17-25 Minnesota esophagogastric tamponade tube.

© Mediscan/Alamy Stock Photo.

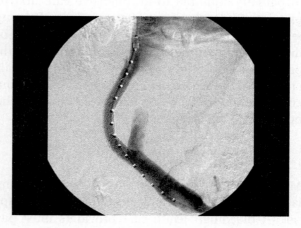

FIGURE 17-27 Transjugular intrahepatic portosystemic shunt placement.

Reprinted from Endovascular shunt reduction in the management of transjugular portosystemic shunt-induced hepatic encephalopathy: preliminary experience with reduction stents and stent-grafts by Geert Maleux, Chris Verslype, and Sam Heye. *AJR.* 2007;188(3):659-664. Copyright © 2007 American Roentgen Ray Society.

a **Minnesota esophagogastric tamponade tube FIGURE 17-25** is inserted nasally and introduced to the stomach via the esophagus.

Although insertion of the Minnesota tube is not within the scope of CCTP practice, CCTPs must understand how the tube has been placed if they are transporting a patient with such a tube. The Minnesota tube is passed through the patient's mouth, just like an OG tube, to the 50-cm mark **FIGURE 17-26** and is inflated with 50 mL of air. After placement is confirmed by obtaining a chest radiograph, the gastric balloon is inflated with an additional 200 to 250 mL of air (250 to 300 mL total). The inflated balloon is sometimes sufficient to stop the hemorrhage. Traction is applied to secure the tube and tamponade the balloon against the gastroesophageal junction. If bleeding continues, the esophageal tube is inflated. Although balloon placement has a high success rate in achieving initial bleeding control, bleeding often recurs on its removal. Thus, the gastric balloon is used only as an emergent, temporary device. Patients requiring this device will be intubated and may have traction on the tamponade tube via a 1-L bag of IV fluid hanging from the IV pole or affixed to the face shield of a football helmet.

A procedure more frequently employed to control variceal bleeding is the placement of a **transjugular intrahepatic portosystemic shunt FIGURE 17-27**. This minimally invasive procedure introduces a shunt between the hepatic venous circulation and the systemic venous return, which significantly reduces both the hepatic portal pressure and the pressure in esophageal varices. Such a shunt is primarily placed for GI bleeding, although some patients may undergo this procedure to relieve fluid buildup associated with severe ascites or hydrothorax. Shunt placement has a greater than 95% success rate in markedly reducing bleeding recurrence as long as the shunt remains patent. Unfortunately, as many as 35% of patients will develop hepatic encephalopathy after this procedure due to the inherent bypass of the liver parenchyma.

Proton pump inhibitors should be administered to reduce gastric acidity in any patient with GI bleeding. Prophylactic acid inhibition is common in patients admitted to an intensive care unit to prevent the development of stress ulcers. Patients testing positive for *H pylori* receive a combination of drugs including proton pump inhibitors, bismuth, probiotics, and antibiotics. Due to rising antimicrobial resistance to macrolide and tetracycline components, trials are ongoing to determine the optimal antibiotic regimen.

Lower GI Bleeding

Management of the patient with lower GI bleeding is similar to management of the patient with upper GI bleeding. Health care providers must pay special attention to the potential for fluid loss that can occur through water shifts in the colon and the associated dehydration and electrolyte abnormalities. Endoscopic methods of cauterization and coagulation with argon plasma are also used to terminate lower GI bleeding, and local infiltration with vasoconstrictive medication and clip placement is the first-line treatment for diverticular bleeds. As with any acute hemorrhage, acute resuscitation of the patient by administering blood and blood products to reduce coagulopathy are the key components of stabilization. Transcatheter embolization of bleeding vessels is an effective alternative approach when the approximate location of the bleed is localized. Surgical evaluation for resection is warranted (as a last resort) in patients presenting with severe hematochezia who cannot be stabilized for endoscopy or in whom endoscopic evaluation has failed to reveal a bleeding source, although this is rarely required.

Intestinal Obstructions

Blockage of the GI tract can occur in the small or large intestine through a variety of pathologies. The convoluted small intestines are far more susceptible to obstruction than are the large intestines, which have a wider diameter. Obstructions are classified as partial, complete, or strangulated. In partial and complete obstructions, fluid or gas is able to pass partially or not pass at all, respectively. Strangulated tissue is cut off from its own blood supply, which can lead to necrosis, perforation, and shock within hours. A closed-loop obstruction occurs when a segment of bowel is obstructed at two points along its course, leading to worsening dilation of that segment and increased risk of volvulus and ischemia. Although a partial intestinal obstruction can cause discomfort and malnutrition, a complete blockage stops normal GI function, resulting in significant morbidity and mortality if not treated promptly.

Epidemiology and Pathophysiology

Postoperative adhesions are the major cause of intestinal obstructions. Combined with hernias and tumors, these etiologies account for 90% of cases. Less frequent causes of intestinal obstructions include Crohn disease, volvulus, and intussusception. Among those patients diagnosed as having an intestinal obstruction, as many as 40% have bowel ischemia, which significantly increases mortality. Overall, intestinal obstructions are fairly common in the United States, accounting for as many as 15% of all acute surgical admissions to hospitals.

Mechanical Obstruction

A mechanical obstruction is the result of a physical blockage of the intestinal lumen. It can be classified into one of three categories: extrinsic, intrinsic, or intraluminal **TABLE 17-6**.

Extrinsic causes, which originate external to the intestines, include adhesions, hernias, volvulus, and masses. Adhesions are bands of connective tissue that can distort the normal anatomy of the abdomen. They are most often the result of improper healing or scar tissue growth following abdominal surgery. A hernia is a protrusion of an organ from its tissue lining. Some hernias may be readily

TABLE 17-6 Causes of Intestinal Obstruction

Type of Obstruction	Cause
Mechanical	Extrinsic • Adhesions • Hernias • Volvulus • Masses Intrinsic • Diverticula • Neoplasms • Intussusception Intraluminal • Foreign body ingestion • Fecal impaction
Nonmechanical (ileus)	Postoperative Acute colonic pseudo-obstruction Abdominal inflammation Peritonitis Heavy metal poisoning Metabolic abnormalities Spinal cord injury

© Jones & Bartlett Learning.

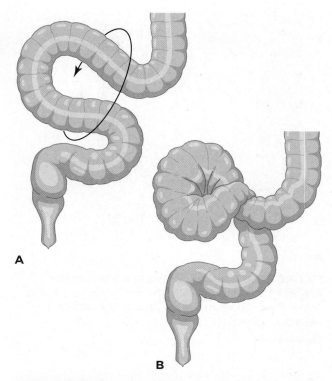

FIGURE 17-28 The pathogenesis of volvulus. **A.** Rotary twist of the sigmoid colon on its mesentery. **B.** Obstruction of the colon and interruption of its blood supply caused by volvulus.

© Jones & Bartlett Learning.

appreciated, such as umbilical or ventral hernias, while others may be wholly internal. Overall, post-surgical adhesions are the most common cause of mechanical intestinal obstruction, followed by hernias. A volvulus is a twisting of the intestine onto itself, which usually results in strangulation. Masses often originate from surrounding abdominal organs that put pressure on the intestines and may take the form of bowel hematoma (from trauma), tumors, aneurysms, or abscesses.

Intrinsic causes of intestinal obstruction arise from the intestinal lining itself; they include diverticula, neoplasms, and intussusception. An intussusception is a prolapse of the intestine into an adjacent segment. Intussusception is the most common cause of bowel obstruction in children younger than 3 years, but is a much rarer diagnosis in adults.

An intraluminal obstruction is commonly the result of an ingested foreign body or a fecal impaction. Causes of intestinal obstructions include volvulus **FIGURE 17-28**, a mass **FIGURE 17-29**, intussusception **FIGURE 17-30**, and a foreign body **FIGURE 17-31**.

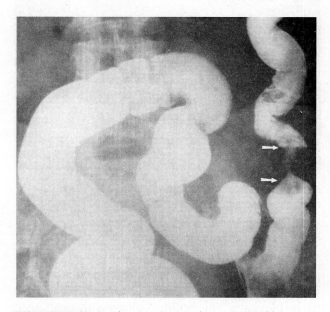

FIGURE 17-29 A colon carcinoma demonstrated by barium enema. The tumor narrows the lumen of the colon, which appears as a filling defect in the column of barium (arrows).

Courtesy of Leonard V. Crowley, MD.

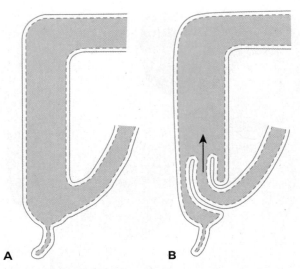

FIGURE 17-30 The pathogenesis of intussusception. **A.** Normal anatomic relationships. **B.** Vigorous peristalsis carries the distal ileum into the cecum. The dashed line indicates mucosa.

© Jones & Bartlett Learning.

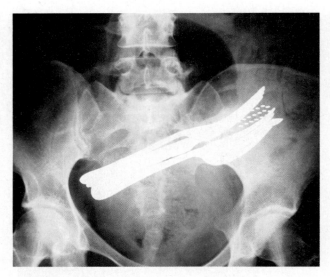

FIGURE 17-31 Radiograph of an intestinal obstruction caused by a foreign body.

© Biophoto Associates/Science Source.

Chyme, fluids, and digestive products cannot pass through or around an intestinal obstruction, so they immediately begin to accumulate proximal to the blockage. This buildup, along with swallowed air, will distend the lumen proximal to the obstruction. GI tract distention stimulates an increase in digestive juice secretion and peristalsis, worsening the situation. The continually increasing intraluminal

pressure also increases the permeability of mucosal capillary beds, allowing vascular fluid to flow into the intestinal lumen. This phenomenon, which is termed **third spacing**, can lead to dehydration, electrolyte imbalances, and hypovolemia.

Over time, the stagnation of intestinal contents facilitates significant bacterial growth. As bacteria enter the mucosal tissues, infections leading to peritonitis or sepsis may occur. If luminal distention proximal to the blockage site continues unchecked, a bowel rupture can occur. The contents of the ruptured GI tract will irritate the surrounding tissues and are likely to cause peritonitis. Of course, all of these processes are more severe in immunocompromised individuals, owing to their impaired gut mucosal defenses against bacterial translocation.

Distal to the obstruction site, tissue ischemia occurs secondary to arterial occlusion. This ischemia inhibits any residual GI functioning and eventually results in necrosis.

Ileus

Ileus is the lack of movement of GI contents through the intestines in the absence of a mechanical obstruction. This condition occurs most commonly in the postoperative period, especially when patients are receiving large doses of analgesic medications, which tend to decrease gut motility. Other factors that may contribute to postoperative ileus include direct manipulation of the GI tissues during surgery, lack of physical activity after a surgery, and use of anesthetic and paralytic medications. Postoperative ileus is transient, usually lasting 48 to 72 hours after surgery. However, it can result in significant discomfort and vomiting, and may even require bowel rest and an NG tube until it resolves. This type of ileus and other types of reversible ileus are also known as acute colonic pseudo-obstruction, or Ogilvie syndrome. Other causes of ileus include abdominal inflammation, peritonitis, heavy metal poisoning, metabolic abnormalities, and spinal cord injury. Flatulence and bowel movements typically indicate resolving ileus.

Assessment
Signs and Symptoms

Moderate to severe abdominal pain accompanies distention proximal to the intestinal obstruction, with the patient eventually vomiting as a result. Excess bacterial growth causes bad breath, along with exceptionally foul-smelling vomit. The vomit may contain large amounts of bile and have an appearance similar to feces depending on the location of the obstruction.

When an obstruction is present, the intestinal mucosa becomes inflamed secondary to ischemia and necrosis. This inflammation, along with bacterial infiltration into the tissues, can cause a fever as the patient's immune response progresses. Shock, as a result of third spacing of fluids or vomiting, manifests with tachycardia, altered mental status, cool and clammy skin, and hypotension.

In a patient with an intestinal obstruction, the abdomen is tender and distended on palpation, with diffuse pain typically being noted. If bowel perforation and peritonitis have occurred, the abdomen may become rigid to palpation. Initially, hyperactive and high-pitched bowel sounds may accompany an obstruction, followed by an eventual cessation of sound as GI function is increasingly inhibited. An incarcerated hernia occurs most commonly when gut tissue protrudes through a small defect. Although patients with hernias may be able to reduce those protrusions without incident, the herniated tissue can sometimes become inflamed and edematous, making reduction extremely difficult (and painful), if not impossible. This incarceration can lead to obstruction and strangulation of the bowel, and emergency management involves analgesia and (in some cases) procedural sedation to attempt reduction. If this fails, surgical reduction is necessary.

Laboratory Data and Imaging

Laboratory testing is performed mostly to determine the degree of dehydration and electrolyte imbalance from an intestinal obstruction. Hemoglobin and hematocrit values become elevated as the blood becomes more concentrated following excessive vomiting. Metabolic alkalosis frequently occurs as electrolyte shifts compensate for the loss of hydrogen ions through vomiting. White blood cell counts indicate inflammation as the extent of tissue ischemia and necrosis expands.

Plain radiography can provide a rapid screening tool for intestinal obstruction by detecting abnormally high air volumes proximal to the obstruction site, although this modality is only about 50% sensitive. Enteroclysis, or a small bowel series, used to be the gold standard for imaging of such obstructions, but is now being supplanted by CT. In this procedure, a barium contrast is instilled in the patient orally or via NG tube. The progression of the contrast through the intestines can be monitored with serial radiographs, allowing for observation of the blockage. Abdominal ultrasonography can also be used to diagnose an intestinal obstruction with great accuracy, although locating the transition point (the point of obstruction) is challenging.

A CT scan can be used to diagnose a bowel obstruction with exceptional specificity and is the gold-standard imaging modality for this indication. An abdominal CT scan is useful in differentiating the cause of the obstruction and potentially diagnosing additional pathology, such as intra-abdominal infection or tumor. The best results are obtained with concurrent administration of IV contrast, although an oral contrast agent may be helpful in very thin individuals or those with prior surgical history (such as gastric bypass).

Signs and Symptoms

Intestinal Obstruction

- Moderate to severe abdominal pain
- Tender, distended abdomen
- Erythematous, tense, exquisitely tender palpable mass or hernia
- Foul-smelling vomit that may contain bile or appear similar to feces
- Diarrhea
- Bad breath
- Fever
- Shock
- Tachycardia
- Altered mental status
- Cool, clammy skin
- Hypotension
- Hyperactive, high-pitched bowel sounds initially
- Eventual cessation of bowel sounds

Intestinal Obstruction

- Diverticulitis
- Cholecystitis
- Endometriosis
- Foreign body
- Gastroenteritis
- Inflammatory bowel disease
- Pancreatitis
- Appendicitis
- Urinary tract infection
- Pyelonephritis
- Pelvic inflammatory disease
- Ovarian torsion
- Cholangitis

Transport Management

Intestinal Obstruction

- Stabilize the ABCs.
- Provide fluid resuscitation.
- Provide supplemental oxygen, if needed.
- Continuously monitor the ECG.
- Designate the patient as NPO.
- Place an NG tube.
- Consider antibiotics.

Management

After addressing any life threats related to the patient's airway, breathing, or cardiac functioning, initial treatment focuses on fluid and electrolyte resuscitation, antiemetics, and analgesia. Avoid promotility agents, which may increase the patient's discomfort and risk of perforation. Administer isotonic fluid boluses as needed to maintain adequate perfusion. Provide supplemental oxygen through either a nonrebreathing mask or a nasal cannula, if the patient is hypoxemic. Monitor the patient's ECG continuously for signs of arrhythmias secondary to electrolyte imbalances.

Patients with a suspected intestinal obstruction should be placed on NPO restrictions, and an NG tube should be inserted to relieve distention proximal to the blockage, especially if the patient has ongoing vomiting. This tube may or may not be placed by the CCTP depending on regional protocols. The degree and severity of obstruction determines whether patients will require surgical management. Nonoperative management focuses on bowel rest, decompression, and fluid replacement. Patients with chronic intestinal obstruction, significant bowel dysfunction, or large resection may receive total parenteral nutrition to help them maintain adequate nutrition. Emergency surgery is required in patients with a strangulated bowel. Surgical treatment techniques are directed toward reducing the obstruction through laparoscopic lysis of adhesions or circumventing the obstruction by a bowel resection, particularly if the tissue has become necrotic. Specific treatment for ileus is aimed at correcting electrolyte disturbance.

Nasogastric Tube Insertion

The following equipment is needed to place an NG tube:

- NG tube
- 50-mL irrigation syringe
- Water-soluble lubricant
- Adhesive tape
- Saline for irrigation
- Emesis basin
- Gloves
- Stethoscope
- Low-powered suction unit

Indications for NG tube placement are as follows:

- Evacuation of stomach contents
- Dilution or lavage of poisons in the stomach
- Removal of blood in patients with GI hemorrhage

Contraindications to NG tube placement include severe facial trauma, croup, and epiglottitis. Potential complications of NG tube placement include improper positioning of the tube, which may take two forms: (1) turbinate insertion, causing bleeding and pain, or (2) tracheal insertion, causing the patient to cough and choke. If the tube cannot be advanced to its predetermined length, then it has most likely become curled in the patient's mouth, throat, or esophagus.

SKILL DRILL 17-1 shows the steps for NG tube placement, which are summarized here:

1. Take standard precautions.
2. Assemble your equipment.
3. Explain the procedure to the patient and oxygenate the patient if necessary. Position the patient in the sitting position. Ensure that the patient's head is in a neutral position and suppress the gag reflex with a topical anesthetic spray, if available **STEP 1**.
4. Examine the patient's nose for deformity or obstruction; determine the best side for insertion.
5. If the medication is available and the patient does not have severe hypertension, you may use a topical alpha agonist to constrict the blood vessels in the nares and potentially minimize epistaxis.
6. Measure the tube's insertion, following the anatomic path it will take, from the patient's nose to the earlobe, then down to the xyphoid process.
7. Note the marking on the tube at the nose; this will be the insertion depth **STEP 2**.
8. Lubricate 6 to 8 inches (15 to 20 cm) of the tube with a water-soluble gel **STEP 3**.
9. Ask the patient to flex their neck, as if attempting to touch the chin to the chest. Gently place your nondominant hand on top of the patient's head to help them maintain this position during insertion.
10. Most NG tubes will have a slight curve from the packaging; use this to your advantage when inserting the tube. With your dominant hand, insert the tube into one nostril. Gently advance the tube toward the posterior nasopharynx **STEP 4**. If you feel significant resistance within one nostril, you may pull the tube out and attempt to insert it in the other nostril.
11. When you feel the tube at the nasopharyngeal junction, rotate it 180° inward toward the other nostril if you encounter resistance.
12. Gently advance the tube until it enters the oropharynx, then instruct the patient to swallow **STEP 5**. It may help to let the patient know to swallow once they feel the tube touch the back of the throat.
13. Pass the tube to the predetermined point (nose to xiphoid) **STEP 6**. Do not force the tube if you encounter resistance. If the patient is choking or coughing excessively, the tube may be in the trachea; in such a case, you should remove the tube and try again. Note that it is not uncommon for patients to vomit during placement of an NG tube. If this happens, pull out the tube to avoid causing aspiration.
14. Check placement of the tube in two ways: auscultate over the epigastrium while injecting about 20 to 30 mL (no more than 50 mL) of air into the tube and/or observe for gastric contents in the tube. There should be no reflux around the tube **STEP 7**.
15. Apply suction (at a low setting) to the tube to aspirate the gastric contents and secure the tube in place **STEP 8**.

Orogastric Tube Insertion

Use of an OG tube is reserved for patients in whom the airway has been secured. The following equipment is needed to place an OG tube:

- OG tube
- 50-mL irrigation syringe
- Water-soluble lubricant
- Adhesive tape
- Saline for irrigation
- Emesis basin
- Gloves
- Stethoscope
- Low-powered suction unit

Indications for OG tube placement are as follows:

- Decompression of the stomach after intubation
- Pressure of the stomach on the diaphragm

Contraindications to OG tube placement include the following conditions:

- Concern for esophageal tear or rupture
- Severe facial trauma
- Esophageal obstruction

Complications include the patient biting the tube.

SKILL DRILL 17-2 shows the steps for OG tube placement, which are summarized here:

1. Position the patient's head in a neutral or flexed position **STEP 1**.
2. Measure the tube for the correct depth of insertion (mouth to ear to xiphoid process) **STEP 2**.
3. Lubricate the tube with a water-soluble gel **STEP 3**.

Skill Drill 17-1 Inserting a Nasogastric Tube in a Conscious Patient

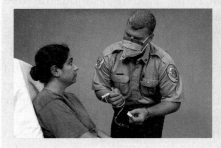

Step 1

Explain the procedure to the patient. Ensure that the patient's head is in a neutral position and suppress the gag reflex with a topical anesthetic spray.

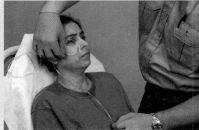

Step 2

Measure the tube for the correct depth of insertion (nose to ear to xiphoid process). Mark the correct length on the tube with adhesive tape.

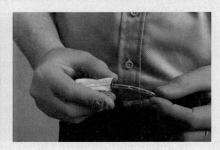

Step 3

Lubricate the tube with a water-soluble gel.

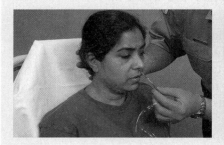

Step 4

Advance the tube gently along the nasal floor.

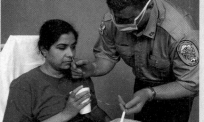

Step 5

Encourage the patient to swallow or drink to facilitate passage of the tube.

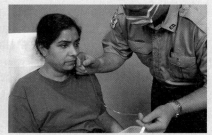

Step 6

Advance the tube into the stomach (to the predetermined point).

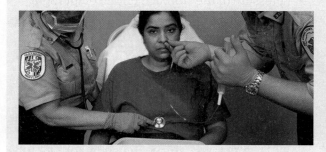

Step 7

Confirm proper placement: auscultate over the epigastrium while injecting 30 to 50 mL of air into the tube, and/or observe for gastric contents in the tube. There should be no reflux around the tube.

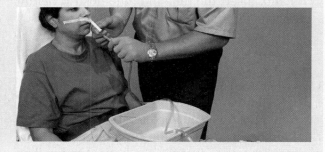

Step 8

Apply suction (at a low setting) to the tube to aspirate the gastric contents and secure the tube in place.

Skill Drill 17-2 Orogastric Tube Insertion

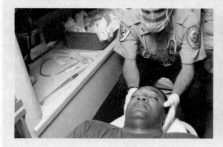

Step 1

Position the patient's head in a neutral or flexed position.

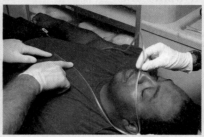

Step 2

Measure the tube for the correct depth of insertion (mouth to ear to xiphoid process).

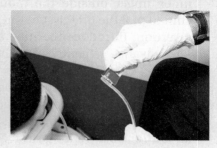

Step 3

Lubricate the tube with a water-soluble gel.

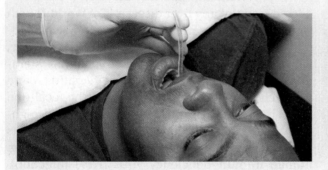

Step 4

Introduce the tube at the midline and advance it gently into the oropharynx.

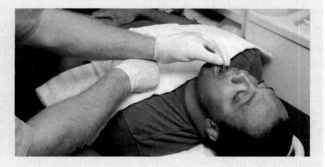

Step 5

Advance the tube into the stomach.

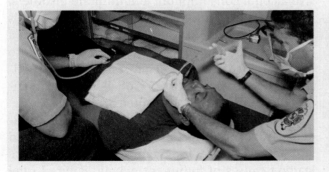

Step 6

Confirm proper placement: auscultate over the epigastrium while injecting 30 to 50 mL of air and/or observe for gastric contents in the tube. There should be no reflux around the tube.

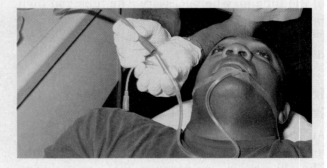

Step 7

Apply suction to the tube to aspirate the stomach contents and secure the tube in place.

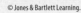

© Jones & Bartlett Learning.

4. Grasp the patient's mandible using your non-dominant hand, pinching with your thumb in the mouth behind the lower teeth and your index finger outside the mouth under the chin to pull the oral tissues out of the way for insertion. Introduce the tube at the midline and advance it gently into the oropharynx **STEP 4**.

5. Advance the tube into the stomach **STEP 5**.

6. Confirm proper placement: auscultate over the epigastrium while injecting 30 to 50 mL of air and/or observe for gastric contents in the tube. There should be no reflux around the tube **STEP 6**.

7. Apply suction to the tube to aspirate the stomach contents and secure the tube in place **STEP 7**.

An NG or OG tube may already be in place when the CCTP first encounters the patient, particularly during interfacility transports. In such cases, it is important to ensure that the tube remains properly positioned throughout the transport and to be alert for any potential complications that may arise.

Aspiration is always a concern for patients with an NG or OG tube, whether the tube has been inserted for suction or for feeding. If a patient appears to be in distress with a tube in place, first attempt to ensure the device's proper placement by injecting a small air bolus into the tube while auscultating the epigastrium. If the patient continues to gag or is vomiting, suctioning and removal of the tube may be necessary. The tube can then be reinserted if this procedure is permitted by the CCTP's regional protocols and if the patient's condition allows.

In-Flight Considerations for Intestinal Obstructions

Air transport should be postponed or avoided for any patient with a bowel obstruction if possible. The changes in gas pressure that occur during flight will distend the obstructed bowel, leading to significant pain and possible perforation. If air transport is unavoidable, measures should be taken to provide for air escape proximal to the obstruction, which may accomplished with NG tube placement.

Liver Disease

Considering the amount of vasculature that passes through the liver, it is easy to imagine the far-reaching implications that any injury to this organ could cause. In general, an insult to the liver is either infectious or noninfectious. If the problem resolves within 6 months without any permanent function deficit, it is termed acute. When symptoms persist longer, chronic liver disease has developed. Regardless of the cause, most cases of chronic liver disease have a common ending: cirrhosis.

Epidemiology and Pathophysiology

Types of Liver Disease

Hepatitis, an inflammation of the liver, is the physiologic result of any liver disease. The World Health Organization estimates that viral infection with hepatitis types B and C affects 1 in 3 people worldwide, with 90% of hepatitis-associated fatalities stemming from these infections. Unlike hepatitis A and E, which are typically contracted via the fecal-oral route, hepatitis B, C, and D are transmitted via high-risk sexual behavior or through blood products and are often comorbid with other conditions (eg, human immunodeficiency virus [HIV] infection). Fortunately, hepatitis B can be prevented via vaccination, which has significantly reduced the prevalence of this disease in high-income countries. The remaining 10% of hepatitis cases result from excessive alcohol consumption, autoimmune disorders, toxins, and drugs. Infection by hepatitis C virus is especially prominent when the disease becomes a chronic condition, with this infection evolving into chronic hepatitis in 80% of affected people. Hepatitis C accounts for 30% to 45% of all liver transplantations in Europe and the United States.

Fulminant hepatic failure is the result of a sudden significant insult to the liver and is associated with mortality rates ranging from 50% to 90%. The leading causes of fulminant hepatic failure in the United States are acetaminophen toxicity (46%), idiosyncratic drug reactions (12%), and hepatitis B (7%). This condition is characterized by the acute development of encephalopathy and impaired synthetic function (INR $\geq$1.5) in a patient without cirrhosis or preexisting liver disease.

Nonalcoholic fatty liver disease (NAFLD), the accumulation of fat in the liver in which alcohol consumption is not believed to be a contributing factor, is the most common liver disorder in Western industrialized countries. Its prevalence is on the rise given its risk factors: central obesity, type 2 diabetes mellitus, dyslipidemia, and metabolic syndrome. Although most patients with NAFLD are asymptomatic, in a subset of patients, the disease can progress to cirrhosis.

Cirrhosis is characterized by irreversible structural changes to the liver that impair its functioning. Once the disease is advanced, the only cure is liver transplantation. The leading cause of cirrhosis in high-income countries is chronic viral hepatitis (hepatitis B or C), followed by alcoholic liver disease, hemochromatosis, and NAFLD. Other causes are responsible for only 5% of cases **TABLE 17-7**. For example, hemochromatosis is a genetic disorder in which increased intestinal iron absorption results in iron overload and accumulation in hepatic tissue.

Course of Liver Disease

Inflammation of liver tissue results in damage to a variety of functional cells, including hepatocytes and Kupffer cells. As cells are destroyed, the basic acinar framework involved in blood detoxification and bile production becomes disarranged. Liver sinusoids and bile drainage canals are inflamed, creating an increased resistance to portal blood flow and bile passage. The increased portal resistance to blood flow can progress to portal hypertension, which has significant effects on the body **TABLE 17-8**. Splenomegaly can result from the initial backup of blood, decreasing the effectiveness of the spleen's metabolic processes. Collateral circulation in the mesentery increases as blood attempts to find a low-resistance route to the inferior vena cava, thereby increasing the patient's risk for esophageal or gastric varices. Abdominal ascites **FIGURE 17-32** develops as hepatic synthesis of proteins such as albumin decreases and portal hypertension worsens, leading to third spacing of fluid.

TABLE 17-8 Effects of Portal Hypertension
Splenomegaly (enlarged spleen)
Esophageal varices
Gastric varices
Increased serum bilirubin • Jaundice • Clay-colored feces • Dark urine
Azygos system overuse
Ascites
Muscle wasting

© Jones & Bartlett Learning.

TABLE 17-7 Causes of Hepatitis and Cirrhosis	
Condition	**Cause**
Hepatitis	Viral Alcohol abuse Autoimmune disorders Toxins Drugs
Cirrhosis	Hepatitis C virus Alcoholic liver disease Nonalcoholic fatty liver disease Hepatitis B virus Hemochromatosis Idiopathic

© Jones & Bartlett Learning.

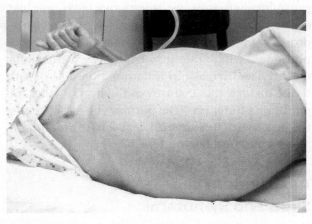

FIGURE 17-32 Marked ascites in a patient with advanced cirrhosis.
Courtesy of Leonard V. Crowley, MD.

Over time, bilirubin, which is conjugated and made water-soluble by hepatocytes and excreted via bile, begins to build up in the blood, resulting in jaundice. Pale feces are formed as bilirubin levels decrease in the GI tract. Urine darkens as excess bilirubin is excreted through the renal system.

The lack of proper nitrogen fixation by damaged hepatocytes can lead to an increased concentration of ammonia in the blood. Normally, ammonia is converted to urea by the liver, with urea then being excreted by the kidneys. Placement of an intrahepatic portal shunt in patients with varices tends to increase ammonia levels. Hyperammonemia is thought to be one of the toxic metabolites responsible for hepatic encephalopathy, although the overall mechanism is poorly understood. The cognitive deficits associated with hepatic encephalopathy fall on a spectrum, from subclinical changes in concentration to disorientation, somnolence, and ultimately, coma.

In alcoholic liver disease, the liver cells are distended from fat accumulation, disrupting their ability to perform their normal functions. Daily ingestion of more than 1 to 3 ounces (40 to 80 g) of ethanol results in excessive nicotinamide adenine dinucleotide (NADH) production from ethanol oxidation in the liver. Elevated hepatocyte NADH concentrations stimulate triglyceride synthesis; these triglycerides are stored within the cell once produced. The continued fat accumulation over time will result in an enlarged and jaundiced liver.

Cirrhosis develops once hepatocyte damage and destruction become widespread enough to cause local areas of necrotic tissue, such that liver cells attempt to regenerate themselves. During this process, fibroblasts deposit collagen at a disproportionately high rate throughout the extracellular matrix. The increase in inflammation and fibrotic tissue distorts the anatomy of the liver, further impairing its function. This permanent disruption of the liver's structure, in turn, leads to further inflammation and portal hypertension.

Assessment

Signs and Symptoms

General malaise and fatigue are the most prominent symptoms of early acute hepatitis, due to impaired metabolism and synthesis functions. Portal hypertension results in a series of problems, including ascites and weight gain from abdominal fluid retention, which leads to significant abdominal distention characterized by a "fluid wave." A combination of decreased hepatic synthesis of coagulation factors and collateral blood flow can create dangerous bleeding, particularly in the GI tract. Chronic shortness of breath can occur not only from impaired diaphragmatic expansion secondary to hepatomegaly, splenomegaly, and ascites, but also from cirrhotic cardiomyopathy (present in as many as 50% of patients with cirrhosis). A neurohormonal cascade caused by portal hypertension and mediated by nitric oxide and prostaglandins results in splanchnic and systemic vasodilation, which decreases cardiac afterload and leads to the loss of peripheral vascular resistance, causing hypotension and tachycardia, often resulting in orthostatic symptoms.

Spontaneous bacterial peritonitis, caused by infection of ascitic fluid, presents with generalized abdominal tenderness and fever. Paracentesis is required for its diagnosis.

Hair loss and gynecomastia are commonly observed as a result of improper hormone metabolism.

Hepatorenal syndrome is characterized by renal injury and renal failure in patients with cirrhosis. In this syndrome, decreased cardiac output and decreased systemic vascular resistance result in a cycle of worsening renal perfusion and renal vasoconstriction. Hepatorenal syndrome may be associated with spontaneous bacterial peritonitis in 25% of cases, a combination that carries a poor prognosis.

Laboratory Data and Imaging

Liver function is assessed by evaluating the presence of the liver's synthesized products as well as the absence of its cellular enzymes in the blood. Tests for liver function and markers of injury are not identical, however. By the time most lab values become abnormal and symptoms emerge, 60% to 80% of the hepatocytes have already been destroyed.

Albumin is a protein synthesized by the liver that assists in maintenance of osmotic fluid balance in the body. Decreased production of albumin results in the peripheral edema, ascites, and pulmonary edema observed in patients with liver failure. Elevated serum levels of bilirubin signal

TABLE 17-9 Criteria Used to Determine MELD Score

Dialysis at least twice in the last week (yes or no)
Creatinine
Bilirubin, total
INR
Sodium

Abbreviations: INR, international normalized ratio; MELD, Model for End-Stage Liver Disease

© Jones & Bartlett Learning.

TABLE 17-10 Normal Versus Abnormal Laboratory Values in Liver Disease

Test	Normal	Abnormal
Albumin	3.5–5.0 g/dL	↓
Bilirubin, serum (direct, conjugated)	0.1–0.3 mg/dL	↑
Bilirubin, total	0.3–1.2 mg/dL	↑
Prothrombin time	10–13 s	↑
Alkaline phosphatase	30–120 U/L	↑
Serum ammonia	10–80 µg/dL	↑
Blood glucose	70–110 mg/dL	↓
Blood urea nitrogen	8–23 mg/dL	↑
Creatinine, serum	0.6–1.2 mg/dL	↑
Liver Enzymes		
Aspartate aminotransferase	10–30 U/L	↑
Alanine aminotransferase	10–40 U/L	↑
Gamma-glutamyl-transferase	2–30 U/L	↑

Abbreviations: ↑, above normal values; ↓, below normal values

© Jones & Bartlett Learning.

the presence of hepatocyte insufficiency and are a reliable indicator of the severity of liver damage. A prolonged PT and INR are the result of decreased vitamin K–dependent clotting factor synthesis by the liver.

The Model for End-Stage Liver Disease (MELD) score is a validated score that predicts mortality in patients with liver disease **TABLE 17-9**. It incorporates serum sodium, bilirubin, creatinine, and INR levels. This score is often used to determine candidacy for liver transplantation.

Release of enzymes specific to hepatocytes into the bloodstream can be detected through laboratory testing and is useful as a marker of the existence and progression of liver disease. These enzymes include aspartate aminotransferase (AST), alanine aminotransferase (ALT), and gamma-glutamyltransferase (GGTP or GGT). Elevated serum levels of any of these three enzymes can suggest hepatic insult, with increases in ALT being the most specific to the liver. For example, AST may be elevated from nonhepatic causes, in cases of hemolysis or myopathy. Elevated GGT and bilirubin out of proportion with AST and ALT suggests cholestasis secondary to a biliary obstruction, particularly in conjunction with elevated alkaline phosphatase (AP). A ratio of AST:ALT greater than 2 is strongly suggestive of alcoholic liver disease.

In patients presenting with an altered mental status, a blood glucose test can reveal hypoglycemia from decreased glucose metabolism and glycogen storage secondary to hepatocyte injury. Elevated serum ammonia concentrations from decreased nitrogen fixation in the damaged liver can result in hepatic encephalopathy. Increased levels of blood urea nitrogen (BUN) and serum creatinine indicate impaired renal function and may suggest hepatorenal syndrome.

TABLE 17-10 emphasizes the many metabolic and synthetic functions that are disrupted in liver dysfunction. Although no imaging studies are necessary to diagnose hepatitis, they can prove valuable in differentiating hepatitis from similarly presenting diseases. Cirrhosis, particularly if advanced, may be visualized across various imaging modalities (CT, magnetic resonance imaging [MRI], ultrasonography). Ascites is often identified as free fluid in the abdomen **FIGURE 17-33**.

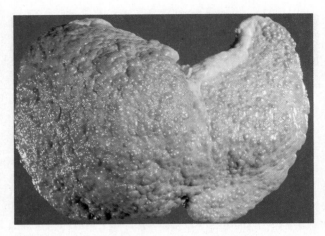

FIGURE 17-33 Advanced hepatic cirrhosis illustrating elevated nodules of liver tissue surrounded by depressed areas of scar tissue.

Courtesy of Leonard V. Crowley, MD.

Management

Treatment of hepatitis focuses on primary prevention (eg, public health and sanitation measures, vaccination programs) and prevention of further injury in an attempt to halt the progression to cirrhosis. In patients with infectious hepatitis, antiviral and interferon drugs are administered to suppress the viral load. Many of these drugs are used in the treatment of HIV infection as well. Pharmacologic treatment of hepatitis is an active topic of research, and usage of specific medications will vary between institutions.

Care for patients with fulminant hepatic failure and end-stage cirrhosis is largely supportive, mainly concentrating on preventing and correcting any complications. In more severe cases of liver disease, neurologic function and arousal may be diminished, requiring airway management. Efforts to prevent encephalopathy focus on decreasing GI absorption of ammonia or ammonia-producing bacteria with lactulose or rifaximin, respectively. Third spacing secondary to hypoalbuminemia can cause hypotension and is treated with fluid resuscitation. Severe hypotension and hepatorenal syndrome may require vasopressor therapy, along with administration of albumin. ECG monitoring enables the CCTP to observe the patient for arrhythmias from electrolyte imbalances, especially hypokalemia. Patients should also be monitored for evidence of GI bleeding, renal failure, and encephalopathy.

Avoidance of alcohol and hepatotoxic medications is essential. In many cases, dosages of common medications must be reduced in anticipation of decreased hepatic metabolism.

Prevention of ascites through a low-sodium diet, fluid restriction, and diuretics is often necessary in patients with cirrhosis, with an eye toward maintaining BP. **Paracentesis**, "tapping" of the abdomen with a needle, can be used to aspirate ascitic fluid from the abdomen as a therapeutic modality, because accumulation of this fluid can approach several liters per day. This procedure is also performed, albeit by collecting only a small quantity of fluid, to diagnose spontaneous bacterial peritonitis, which requires aggressive antimicrobial therapy.

There is no cure for hepatitis or its resultant cirrhosis other than liver transplantation. Liver transplantations have a fairly high success rate, although patients with hepatitis C commonly have graft infection and as many as 30% will have cirrhosis again within 5 years. Unfortunately, as with other organs, there is vastly greater demand for liver transplants than there is supply. In addition, individuals with cirrhotic liver disease are at increased risk of developing hepatocellular carcinoma.

Signs and Symptoms

Liver Disease
- Jaundice
- Dark urine
- Clay-colored feces
- General malaise
- Fever and chills
- Ascites
- Weight gain
- Easy bleeding
- Melena, hematochezia
- Shortness of breath
- Hypotension
- Tachycardia
- Hair loss
- Cognitive disorders
- Spider angiomas
- Hypoglycemia

Differential Diagnosis

Liver Disease

- Acute hepatitis
- Cholestasis
- Acute hepatic failure
- Chronic hepatitis
- Cirrhosis
- Hepatomegaly
- Liver mass or cancer
- Jaundice (icterus)
- Spontaneous bacterial peritonitis

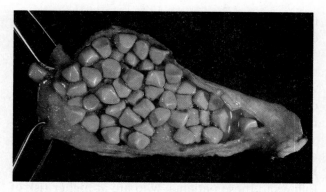

FIGURE 17-34 Open gallbladder filled with gallstones composed of cholesterol.

Courtesy of Leonard V. Crowley, MD.

Transport Management

Liver Disease

- Manage the airway.
- Provide vasopressors and fluid resuscitation as needed.
- Monitor the ECG.
- Monitor for GI bleeding, renal failure, and encephalopathy.
- Avoid medications that are metabolized by the liver.

Biliary Tract Obstructions

Blockage of the biliary system at any point will result in a backup of bile and possibly, depending on the location of the obstruction, pancreatic enzymes. These digestive juices accumulate first in the tracts, and then in the organs from which they originated. The damage caused by this type of obstruction is twofold. Distal to the obstruction, normal digestive processes of the GI system are disrupted, while proximally, the accessory organs and ducts become distended and inflamed.

Epidemiology and Pathophysiology

Most often, the biliary tract system is obstructed by a migrating gallstone. Gallstones in the gallbladder, a condition termed cholelithiasis, affect approximately 10% of Americans each year **FIGURE 17-34**. They can form one of two ways: through accumulation of excess cholesterol in the bile (cholesterol stones) or through accumulation of excess bilirubin and calcium salts in the bile (pigment stones). Both etiologies result in the crystallization of bile into stones, which may range in size from small grains to the size of a golf ball. Cholesterol stones account for the majority of gallstone cases in the United States, with the remainder accounted for by pigment and mixed stones. Notably, patients with cirrhosis are at higher risk for pigment stones.

Inside the gallbladder, stones that block the outflow of bile may cause distention and inflammation of the gallbladder itself, known as cholecystitis. When the stone becomes impacted inside the biliary ducts, the condition is termed choledocholithiasis. The stone may begin to travel into the cystic duct at any time, lacerating the inner walls as it moves. Frequently, it will lodge in either the cystic duct or the distal common bile duct. If the stone lodges in the common bile duct and fully obstructs the lumen, both bile and pancreatic juice will be unable to pass into the duodenum. As pancreatic enzymes accumulate proximal to the obstruction, they will begin to digest the tissues of both the ducts and the pancreas. This autodigestion leads to gallstone pancreatitis, a condition responsible for almost one-half of all cases of pancreatitis. As enzymes and bile leak through the compromised duct lining, peritonitis can occur and eventually lead to a systemic inflammatory response and shock.

Assessment
Signs and Symptoms

Cholecystitis causes colicky pain in the right upper quadrant of the abdomen. In some people, this pain can be localized more in the epigastrium and may mimic heartburn. Cholecystitis pain tends to emerge following ingestion of high-fat foods because fatty chyme stimulates gallbladder contraction. Due to the pain, a patient with this condition will exhibit a positive Murphy sign, or sudden arrest of inspiration when constant pressure is applied to the right upper quadrant.

Patients with choledocholithiasis have blockage of biliary outflow not only from the gallbladder, but also from the liver. Obstructive jaundice soon follows in these patients, who are at higher risk of developing a rapidly progressive infection called ascending cholangitis. This process is typically characterized by fever, jaundice, and right upper quadrant pain, which are collectively known as Charcot triad. Nausea and vomiting frequently accompany Charcot triad. As the condition progresses, these individuals develop altered mental status and shock.

Laboratory Data and Imaging

Bilirubin, a product of heme breakdown, may be elevated for a variety of reasons, ranging from hemolysis (unconjugated bilirubin) to intrahepatic cholestasis or cholelithiasis (conjugated bilirubin). A good framework for remembering how bilirubin becomes elevated is to consider whether it is accumulating before or after hepatic processing (conjugation). The effects of biliary obstruction can be observed through elevations of serum values indicating blocked secretions from the gallbladder and pancreas. Serum bilirubin levels increase, along with serum amylase and lipase, if pancreatic obstruction is also occurring. AP and GGT levels will be elevated. Over time, PT will increase as vitamin K absorption decreases owing to a lack of bile in the GI tract. If infection is present, such as in cholangitis, white blood cell levels and inflammatory markers will increase as well.

Transabdominal ultrasonography is a useful first test for evaluating patients with upper abdominal pain due to its low cost, lack of ionizing radiation, and extremely high sensitivity for cholelithiasis when a stone is visualized and the patient exhibits the Murphy sign. CT is often used as an alternative to ultrasonography, as it is also highly sensitive for cholecystitis and can be used to identify other pathologies at the same time. In addition to providing for the direct visualization of stones, ultrasonography can detect distention proximal to the obstruction, especially in the common bile duct. The presence of a dilated common bile duct is suggestive of a stone migrating beyond the gallbladder and obstructing the biliary tract more distally (choledocholithiasis). This finding may change the management from a cholecystectomy to an endoscopic retrograde cholangiopancreatography. Some patients may undergo endoscopic ultrasonography in an attempt to visualize impacted stones.

Endoscopic retrograde cholangiopancreatography (ERCP) and percutaneous transhepatic cholangiography (PTC) are two methods of cholangiography that have excellent accuracy in detecting choledocholithiasis. They are both diagnostic and therapeutic. Both involve injection of contrast into the biliary duct system to observe the obstruction. PTC is typically performed if ERCP is unsuccessful. Endoscopists are able to extract obstructing stones while using these techniques; however, these procedures are not used as an initial diagnostic strategy given the risk of complications such as perforation or pancreatitis. An alternative to ERCP, magnetic resonance cholangiopancreatography (MRCP), is noninvasive and permits visualization of stones anywhere in the biliary system. Cholescintigraphy is another modality that involves injection of radioactive dye and subsequent evaluation for cholelithiasis of the cystic duct by noting the progress (or lack thereof) of the dye into the gallbladder.

Management

Immediate treatment of gallstone disease involves pain management once general treatment has been provided. Because evidence has suggested that opioids can increase pressure at the sphincter of Oddi, NSAIDs are the treatment of choice. Providers may escalate pain relief treatment to opioids in patients with contraindications to NSAIDs and in those who do not obtain adequate relief from NSAIDs.

Definitive treatment occurs at the hospital and focuses on removal of the stone or obstruction (if it is a tumor or other structural abnormality). ERCP is frequently used to remove the stone after fulfilling its diagnostic role. Lithotripsy can break apart larger stones through external vibrations, facilitating their subsequent removal by ERCP or percutaneous transhepatic cholangiography. A sphincterotomy is often performed to allow the stones to pass into the duodenum, where they can be caught with a basket or catheter. Cholecystectomy will generally be performed in patients with cholecystitis or to prevent recurrence of choledocholithiasis.

Signs and Symptoms

Biliary Tract Obstruction

- Charcot triad
  - Fever
  - Jaundice
  - Right upper quadrant pain
- Nausea and vomiting
- Clay-colored feces
- Murphy sign: exquisitely tender right upper quadrant

Differential Diagnosis

Biliary Tract Obstruction

- Appendicitis
- Cholecystitis
- Cholangitis
- Gastritis
- Peptic ulcer disease
- Hepatitis
- Inflammatory bowel disease
- Pancreatitis
- Biliary stricture
- Choledocholithiasis
- Pancreatic tumor
- Choledochal cyst

Transport Management

Biliary Tract Obstruction

- Provide oxygen as required.
- Place an IV line.
- Monitor the ECG.
- Provide analgesia.

Pancreatic Disease

Epidemiology and Pathophysiology

Inflammation of the pancreas, known as pancreatitis, can lead to significant impairment of GI physiology depending on its level of severity and etiology. The most common causes of pancreatitis

TABLE 17-11 Causes of Pancreatitis

Gallstones
Post-ERCP or similar instrumentation
Alcohol abuse
Idiosyncratic drug reactions
Tumors
Hypertriglyceridemia
Hypercalcemia
Congenital defects
Systemic inflammatory response syndrome

Abbreviation: ERCP, endoscopic retrograde cholangiopancreatography

© Jones & Bartlett Learning.

are gallstones (40% to 70%) and alcohol abuse (25% to 35%), with the remainder of cases resulting from idiosyncratic drug reactions, ERCP, tumors, hypertriglyceridemia, hypercalcemia, and congenital defects **TABLE 17-11**. Most cases are mild, self-resolving in 3 to 4 days with a very low mortality. Pancreatic necrosis occurs in approximately 15% of patients, likely due to dysregulated caustic secretions. Approximately 20% of patients will eventually present with **systemic inflammatory response syndrome (SIRS)** and organ dysfunction, marking a shift to severe acute pancreatitis, which has a mortality rate of approximately 10%.

Chronic pancreatitis is characterized by the presence of irreversible anatomic changes to the pancreas, along with some degree of function loss. Alcohol use disorder and smoking are major risk factors for this condition, although the exact pathological mechanisms are not completely understood. Pancreatitis is more likely to develop in men than in women, and idiopathic chronic pancreatitis accounts for 10% to 30% of all cases.

The inflammatory process in pancreatitis evolves in response to autodigestion of the pancreatic tissue **FIGURE 17-35**. Pancreatic enzymes are normally produced as inactive precursors, which then become activated in the GI lumen. When these enzymes become prematurely activated inside either the pancreas or the ducts that drain the secretions, they immediately begin digesting the surrounding tissues. Because of the retroperitoneal

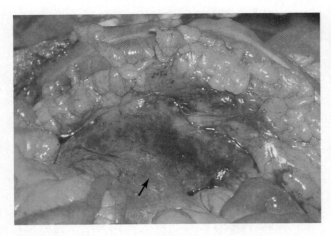

FIGURE 17-35 Acute pancreatitis. The transverse colon (upper part of the photograph) has been elevated to reveal the pancreas (arrow), which is inflamed and contains large areas of hemorrhage.

Courtesy of Leonard V. Crowley, MD.

TABLE 17-12 Normal Versus Abnormal Laboratory Values for Pancreatitis

Test	Normal	Abnormal
Amylase, serum	27–131 U/L	↑
Lipase, serum	31–186 U/L	↑
Aspartate aminotransferase	10–30 U/L	↑
Alanine aminotransferase	10–40 U/L	↑
Gamma-glutamyl-transferase	2–30 U/L	↑
Leukocytes (white blood cells)	4,500–11,000/μL	↑

Abbreviation: ↑, above normal values

© Jones & Bartlett Learning.

location of the pancreas, the activated enzymes can easily spread throughout the peritoneum as well as to other retroperitoneal organs. Once digestion of the pancreatic blood vessels begins, hemorrhaging occurs. As the disease progresses, tissue necrosis will occur. In addition to forming local fluid and necrotic collections, the resulting necrotic tissue is susceptible to bacterial infection, such that spontaneous infections of the pancreas or peritoneum frequently occur.

Pancreatic pseudocysts are walled-off aggregates of cellular debris and extracellular pancreatic enzymes that sometimes form more than 4 weeks after the onset of acute pancreatitis. The cytokine cascade that ensues following pancreatic inflammation and digestive enzyme dysregulation manifests clinically as SIRS. This condition puts patients at risk for failure of one or more organs. Pulmonary complications may include arterial hypoxemia, atelectasis, pleural effusions, pneumonia, and acute respiratory distress syndrome. Fluid shifts and enzyme-induced vasodilation can cause hemodynamic instability and shock. The resultant decrease in organ perfusion can lead to acute renal failure. Diffuse intravascular coagulation can develop, further exacerbating organ dysfunction and shock.

Assessment

Signs and Symptoms

Severe upper abdominal pain is the primary symptom of pancreatitis. This pain may radiate throughout the abdomen and to the back depending on the level of pancreatic involvement. Patients will have abdominal guarding, with rigidity if peritonitis has developed. Nausea and vomiting are common. Fever will be present secondary to the body's immune response against the infectious complications of pancreatitis. Depending on the severity of pancreatitis, patients may be tachycardic, hypotensive, and/or hypoxemic. Discoloration of the low back and flank, known as Turner sign, and periumbilical discoloration, known as Cullen sign, are both rare and nonspecific findings of the retroperitoneal hemorrhage that may occur in severe pancreatitis. If biliary tract obstruction is the cause of the pancreatitis, the patient may exhibit jaundice.

Laboratory Data and Imaging

As the pancreatic cells are destroyed or the walls of ducts are digested, pancreatic-specific enzymes are released into the bloodstream. Serum lipase and amylase levels are the most sensitive indicators; they are frequently elevated to more than three times their normal levels in acute pancreatitis **TABLE 17-12**. Serum lipase has a higher specificity and levels remain higher for longer than amylase, making it the lab test of choice for pancreatitis. Although elevated levels of these two enzymes support a diagnosis of pancreatitis, higher levels of amylase can result from several other conditions as well.

Liver function testing for ALT/AST, AP, GGT, and serum bilirubin can help rule out other causes of abdominal pain and may indicate a biliary tract origin of disease. An elevated leukocyte count indicates the presence of infection, inflammation, or both.

A CT scan with contrast can visualize pancreatic necrosis, peripancreatic abnormalities, abscesses, and the overall size of the pancreas. It has 90% specificity and is invaluable for determining disease severity. For the detection of gallstones in the bile duct, MRCP has a 90% accuracy rate. ERCP is an alternative to MRCP in patients with pancreatitis with a suspected biliary origin. In addition to supporting a diagnosis, ERCP can be used to simultaneously treat the patient if sphincterotomy and gallstone removal are necessary.

Visualization of the pancreas by abdominal ultrasonography is often obstructed by intestinal gas and adipose tissue; hence, this imaging modality performs poorly in identifying pancreatitis. When combined with endoscopy, however, it becomes a useful bedside procedure that can assist in the diagnosis of both pancreatitis and gallstones.

Management

General treatment of pancreatitis includes supportive care such as supplemental oxygen administration, analgesia, and ECG monitoring. Large-bore IV access is recommended, as fluid replacement is a priority in patients with hypotension and tachycardia. Isotonic crystalloid boluses of 20 mL/kg are recommended, with careful attention to urinary output (>0.5 to 1 mL/kg/h).

All patients with pancreatitis should be placed on NPO restrictions to prevent increased stimulation of pancreatic enzyme synthesis and secretion. In severe cases, nasojejunal tube feeding may be required. Pain management is necessary to avoid additional hemodynamic instability, and may take the form of IV opioids or IV patient-controlled analgesia devices.

Once the patient has entered the hospital, specific treatment of acute pancreatitis focuses on preventing complications and decreasing pancreatic workload. Prophylactic antibiotic administration is not recommended in patients with acute pancreatitis.

Signs and Symptoms

Pancreatitis
- Upper abdominal pain
- Tenderness and guarding of the abdomen
- Tachycardia
- Nausea, vomiting
- Fever
- Turner sign (discoloration of the low back and flank)
- Cullen sign (periumbilical discoloration)
- Jaundice
- Hemodynamic instability
- Shock

Differential Diagnosis

Pancreatitis
- Cholecystitis
- Cholangitis
- Gastritis
- Hepatitis
- Bowel obstruction
- Pancreatic cancer

Transport Management

Pancreatitis
- Administer supplemental oxygen if needed.
- Place an IV line.
- Monitor the ECG.
- Replace fluids in patients with hypovolemia.
- Monitor fluid output.
- Provide analgesia.

Urinary System Conditions

Conditions affecting the urinary system include renal failure, urinary tract infections, nephrolithiasis, testicular torsion, ovarian torsion, penile fracture, ruptured ovarian cysts, and priapism. This section discusses all of these conditions, except ovarian torsion and ovarian cysts, which are discussed in Chapter 22, *Obstetric and Gynecologic Emergencies*.

Kidney Injury

Epidemiology and Pathophysiology

The nephron, the structural and functional unit of the kidney, requires a consistent gradient of fluid flowing across its membranes to function optimally. Significant decreases in renal perfusion pressure disrupt the elimination of waste from the bloodstream by lowering the glomerular filtration rate. Furthermore, the tissues of the kidney are inherently sensitive to hypoperfusion and hypoxia. An acute decrease in glomerular filtration in a patient without preexisting renal dysfunction is termed **acute kidney injury (AKI)**. Most instances of AKI are sudden and usually reversible, and they are accompanied by a rise in serum sodium, creatinine, BUN, and other metabolic waste products. Hospitalized patients are commonly found to have some level of AKI, and this condition is especially common in patients treated in the intensive care unit. Disproportionately higher mortality rates are observed in patients with AKI in the intensive care unit compared with the general patient population. As with most disease processes, AKI exists on a spectrum of severity, with mild cases often being managed in the outpatient setting. The downstream effects of severe AKI, such as volume overload and electrolyte disturbance, tend to exacerbate the challenges of caring for a critically ill patient.

AKI is classified in terms of its location as prerenal, intrarenal, or postrenal. **TABLE 17-13** summarizes the causes and types of AKI.

Prerenal AKI is the most common type, implicated in as many as two-thirds of cases. This condition is associated with many reversible causes and, if treated promptly and appropriately, can be corrected in as many as 90% of cases. Hypovolemia and intravascular volume depletion secondary to dehydration or blood loss often cause prerenal AKI, as does hepatorenal syndrome (in patients with cirrhosis). SIRS and shock states decrease renal perfusion and are almost always associated with AKI. Conversely, increased venous congestion and hypotension from congestive heart failure will also reduce the gradient of pressure, and thus perfusion,

TABLE 17-13 Causes and Types of Acute Kidney Injury

Type	Cause
Prerenal	Hypovolemia Dehydration Congestive heart failure Hepatorenal syndrome Third spacing Systemic inflammatory response syndrome Shock of any etiology Medications
Intrarenal	Acute tubular necrosis Interstitial nephritis Glomerulonephritis Medications
Postrenal	Renal calculi Blood clots Tumors Prostate obstruction Malfunctioning urinary catheter

© Jones & Bartlett Learning.

across the nephrons. A variety of medications, including angiotensin-converting enzyme (ACE) inhibitors and diuretics, can decrease renal perfusion through both intrinsic kidney injury (intrarenal AKI) and excess volume depletion.

One of the earliest signs of prerenal AKI is oliguria, a reduction in urine volume to less than 400 mL/d. The body's attempt to conserve water results in a decreased GFR, which in turn translates to a decrease in fluid volume entering the reabsorption tubules. The kidneys attempt to increase renal perfusion pressure by increasing solute (eg, sodium) reabsorption, which draws water back into the systemic circulation. In patients with severe hypoperfusion, the body's compensatory mechanisms for maintaining BP prioritize perfusion of the heart and brain, thereby worsening the situation for the kidneys. Any vasoconstrictive effort (via vasopressors) will further decrease renal perfusion. Eventually, the decreased renal perfusion will result in tissue ischemia, injury, and necrosis. When the tubules become necrotic, they lose their ability to perform ion exchange, which prevents proper urine formation. Inflammation and extensive shedding of dead tissue will further decrease the flow rate.

In contrast to the process just described, in situations where cardiac dysfunction results in renal hypoperfusion, vasopressor medications will actually improve renal perfusion and overall kidney function. This is sometimes referred to as cardiorenal syndrome.

Intrarenal, or intrinsic, AKI is classified as a structural injury to the kidney itself. Acute tubular necrosis, the most common cause of intrarenal AKI, is usually a result of renal ischemia or the presence of a toxin. Over time, a prolonged insult, such as untreated prerenal AKI, may also transition to cellular damage and acute tubular necrosis. Interstitial nephritis commonly results from adverse reactions to medications, such as antibiotics, NSAIDs, and diuretics. Contrast-induced nephropathy has been an area of intense controversy and research. Although once thought to be nephrotoxic, modern contrast dyes have not been shown to cause clinically meaningful kidney injury.

In glomerulonephritis (another cause of intrarenal AKI), glomerular tissue becomes inflamed secondary to an immune response. Glomerulonephritis is a collective term covering approximately 20 glomerular conditions, with rapidly progressive glomerulonephritis being a severe form that impairs renal function. It is characterized by hematuria, initially on a microscopic level but progressing to visible quantities of blood in the urine and accompanied by proteinuria and hypertension. Postinfectious causes are frequently implicated in glomerulonephritis, especially group A beta-hemolytic *Streptococcus* infection following pharyngitis. Other precipitators of glomerulonephritis include immunoglobulin A nephropathy and systemic lupus erythematosus.

Postrenal AKI occurs when urine flow distal to the nephrons becomes obstructed. The least frequently observed of the three types of AKI, this condition is associated with ureteral or urethral blockage by renal calculi, blood clots, or lumen-penetrating tumors. It is also seen in prostatic hypertrophy and can occur as a result of a malfunctioning urinary catheter. Anuria (absence of any urine output) is typically a result of obstruction at the urethra or the bladder, as both ureters would require simultaneous blockage to cease all urine

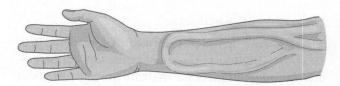

FIGURE 17-36 An arteriovenous fistula used for intermittent hemodialysis.

© Jones & Bartlett Learning.

flow. Large kidney stones tend to obstruct in the distal ureter (near the ureterovesical junction) and can cause backup of urine in the blocked kidney. This kind of total obstruction leads to severe pain, disrupts the kidney's normal architecture (termed hydronephrosis), and sometimes induces urosepsis.

A gradual decrease in renal function over a long time is known as chronic kidney disease (CKD). The hallmark of CKD is an irreversible destruction of nephrons brought about by the continuous effects of several disease processes, including diabetes mellitus, hypertension, and autoimmune disorders. Over time, CKD progresses to end-stage renal disease (ESRD), at which point dialysis is needed to replace renal function. Patients may receive dialysis via different modalities, each with its own risks and benefits. By far the most common approach is intermittent hemodialysis (IHD) **FIGURE 17-36**. These therapies are discussed later in this chapter, in the management section.

Assessment

The patient's medical history and family history are important components of the assessment for AKI. A family history of renal disease indicates a predisposition to AKI when a precursor disease of AKI is present. The incidence of AKI is increased in patients with diabetes, hypertension, congestive heart failure, or lupus. The incidence increases greatly with age as well. Taking into context the patient's environment (eg, a house with no air conditioning during a heat wave), medication list (eg, multiple antihypertensives and diuretics), and any recent illness will help facilitate accurate management of AKI. When caring for an individual with ESRD who is receiving IHD, the CCTP must confirm the days on which the patient is typically scheduled for dialysis as well as the last time the patient had a session (and whether it was a full session).

Signs and Symptoms

Signs of AKI include abnormalities in urine production. Oliguria is the most common abnormality, although an increase in urine output can occur if the nephrons cannot effectively concentrate the urine. Lack of urine production is suggestive of anuric renal failure or an obstruction. In the latter case, patients may have significant suprapubic discomfort as bladder distention worsens. Patients may have radiation of pain to the flanks and nausea as well.

Given that dehydration is often a precipitating factor for AKI, patients commonly present with dizziness, poor skin turgor, thirst, flat neck veins, dry mucous membranes, tachycardia, and orthostatic BP changes. If third spacing and fluid retention are the cause of the AKI, the patient may exhibit peripheral edema or ascites. Low back pain, suprapubic pain, and fever may be present in patients with AKI caused by urinary tract infection. With intrarenal AKI, patients may develop peripheral edema from fluid buildup from a variety of factors, mainly due to decreased urine production, inappropriate solute and protein losses, and electrolyte dysregulation. Ongoing volume overload without appropriate urinary output can lead to pulmonary edema and congestive heart failure. Accumulation of uremic toxins ultimately results in encephalopathy, while hyperkalemia can lead to fatal dysrhythmias.

Many complications of AKI overlap with CKD, and sometimes dysfunction develops more rapidly and dramatically because of already-impaired kidneys. Patients with ESRD who are completely dependent on dialysis can present with profound metabolic dysregulation because their homeostasis depends on external support. When patients miss dialysis or have a superimposed illness (eg, worsened fluid overload from heart failure), the downstream effects can overcome their body's buffer systems. These individuals can present with severe hyperkalemia and dysrhythmias, metabolic acidosis, and fluid overload. The retention of urea and other metabolic waste in the blood leads to **uremia**, a condition characterized by nausea, vomiting, fatigue, anorexia, weight loss, pruritus, and altered mental status. Elimination of uric acid through the skin in sweat causes the "uremic frost" phenomenon, which is characterized by white dust on the skin.

Laboratory Data and Imaging

The retention of wastes in the bloodstream that results from a decreased GFR provides an easy way to monitor for the existence and severity of AKI. When this disease is present, serum creatinine levels will be elevated proportionally to the decrease in GFR. The BUN level is a less reliable indicator of GFR, however, because it may be altered by numerous other metabolic functions unrelated to renal physiology. Nevertheless, it will be elevated in patients with AKI. The combination of elevated BUN level and serum creatinine is known as **azotemia**.

Urinalysis is critical for differentiating between the various types of AKI. Patients with prerenal AKI exhibit increased osmolality, specific gravity, and BUN-to-creatinine levels, along with a decreased fractional excretion of sodium and urine sodium concentration. Acute tubular necrosis is associated with nearly the opposite set of findings: Urine osmolality is decreased, with an increased urine sodium concentration and fractional excretion of sodium. **TABLE 17-14** summarizes renal laboratory values for patients with AKI.

Renal ultrasonography is the gold standard for assessing suspected postrenal AKI. This imaging modality allows for rapid visualization of hydronephrosis and bladder distention. CT can visualize and measure renal calculi, tumors, and secondary signs of inflammation (eg, perinephric fat stranding).

When they have CKD and ESRD, patients may live in a persistently anemic state due to decreased renal erythropoietin synthesis. Hyperparathyroidism can evolve from decreased renal vitamin D metabolism, causing osteoporosis and skeletal abnormalities. Although some patients may become anuric, others may exhibit polyuria as a result of the diseased nephrons' inability to concentrate urine efficiently, a phenomenon known as isosthenuria. Metabolic acidosis frequently occurs in patients with CKD from a combination of acid retention and bicarbonate wasting.

Management

Initial treatment of the patient with AKI involves maintaining the ABCs and a BP sufficient to provide for adequate perfusion of organs. Data suggest that a MAP greater than 60 mm Hg is sufficient to maintain renal perfusion and minimize AKI from hypotension.

TABLE 17-14 Normal Versus Abnormal Laboratory Values in Patients With Acute Kidney Injury

Test	Normal	Abnormal
BUN	8–23 µg/dL	↑
Creatinine, serum	0.6–1.2 mg/dL	↑
Urinalysis		
• Osmolality	275–295 mOsm/kg	↑ Prerenal
• Specific gravity	1.003–1.030	↑ Prerenal; ↓ Intrinsic
• BUN:creatinine	10:1	↑ Prerenal; ↓ Intrinsic
• Fractional excretion of sodium	1%	↓ Prerenal; ↑ Intrinsic
• Urine sodium excretion (over 24 h)	43–217 mEq/24 h	↓ Prerenal; ↑ Intrinsic

Abbreviations: ↑, above normal values; ↓, below normal values; BUN, blood urea nitrogen

© Jones & Bartlett Learning.

Once these basics are ensured, management focuses on increasing the GFR. This management goal must be factored into the choice of all treatment modalities, but particularly medication administration and fluid resuscitation. Administration of crystalloid fluid is indicated in dehydrated patients to treat oliguria, although the CCTP must be careful to avoid volume overload. Care must be taken when administering fluids in patients with prerenal AKI and congestive heart failure, as these patients may require inotropic medication to improve cardiac output and may be harmed by large volumes of crystalloid fluid. Diuretic administration is warranted in patients with signs of frank volume overload from congestive heart failure, as this treatment can reduce venous congestion and increase renal perfusion pressure and GFR. Serum electrolyte levels, especially potassium, must be monitored closely to avoid complications from hyperkalemia. Patients who develop hyperkalemia with interval widening on ECG require immediate temporizing measures (eg, calcium gluconate, insulin, dextrose) and emergent dialysis.

Renal replacement therapy (RRT) is a frequently used treatment for AKI that has resulted in significant physiologic disruption (eg, acidosis, volume overload, hyperkalemia) and has not responded to less-invasive therapies. The modality of choice remains controversial, but options include IHD, continuous venovenous hemofiltration, and peritoneal dialysis.

IHD is the most commonly used method for hemodynamically stable patients in both inpatient and outpatient settings. It involves the use of a dialysis machine, filter, extensive water supply, and tubing. The patient's blood is filtered by diffusion through an external semipermeable membrane and then returned to the body. Access to the patient's circulation can be obtained in different ways depending on the duration for which dialysis is required. A central venous catheter (CVC) is placed into either the internal jugular vein or the femoral vein for short-term access. The catheter size should allow blood flow rates of up to 300 mL/min. Subclavian access can be used but is less preferred as it can result in vessel stenosis and subsequent issues with placement of permanent AV fistulas. For long-term IHD, AV fistula is the preferred method of access: It provides for increased blood flow, superior long-term patency, and decreased likelihood of thrombosis or infection. To form an AV fistula, a vascular surgeon anastomoses an artery and a vein, most commonly in the patient's nondominant forearm. The typical patient receiving IHD is treated two to three times per week in 4-hour sessions. To avoid damaging an AV fistula, the fistula extremity should not be used for BP measurements, blood draws, or venous access.

The major indication for continuous renal replacement therapy (CRRT) instead of IHD is hemodynamic instability, which is often seen in critically ill patients. Four CRRT options are typically available, all of which require a dual-lumen hemodialysis catheter connected to a venovenous circuit using an extracorporeal pump to facilitate flow of blood through a filter. No single therapy always provides better outcomes; instead, the selection of the CRRT approach depends on hospital personnel's expertise and availability, the intended goals for removal of solutes and/or fluid volume, and acid–base control. CRRT can be run continuously or intermittently (6- to 12-hour cycles). As yet, no clear consensus statements have been published to aid in selection of therapy for patients requiring CRRT.

The most common types of CRRT include continuous venovenous hemofiltration (CVVH), continuous venovenous hemodialysis (CVVHD), continuous venovenous hemodiafiltration (CVVHDF), and slow continuous ultrafiltration (SCUF). CVVH removes solutes entirely by convection, using a high ultrafiltration rate (20 to 25 mL/kg/h), such that administering replacement fluid (usually crystalloid) is necessary to avoid hypovolemia. CVVHD adds dialysate fluid to the circuit, at flow rates of 20 to 25 mL/kg/h, and removes solutes primarily by diffusion. Ultrafiltration rates are low, typically ranging from 2 to 8 mL/min, which limits net fluid removal as well as the need for fluid replacement. CVVHDF combines convection and diffusion, uses dialysis fluid, and necessitates administration of replacement fluid to limit the net volume removed. SCUF, which is typically used for isolated volume overload, uses neither dialysate nor replacement fluid and has minimal ability to remove solutes; however, it can remove up to 8 L of fluid per day.

CRRT equipment is bulky **FIGURE 17-37**, sensitive to movement, and has power and temperature requirements that are often not compatible with transport vehicles. If a patient is leaving the ICU for a short time, blood from the CRRT machine can be returned to the patient and the machine can continuously recycle the IV fluids present until the patient returns. Alternatively, the machine can recycle the flow by using the patient's blood already in the circuit. For travel to another facility, CRRT will need to be discontinued prior to transport.

The CCTP who is caring for a patient undergoing CRRT should take the following considerations into account:

- **Access.** When connecting, disconnecting, or transferring CRRT or IHD from a temporary

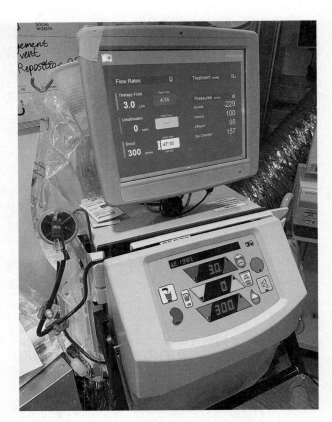

FIGURE 17-37 Continuous renal replacement therapy equipment is bulky and often not transportable.

© Jones & Bartlett Learning.

catheter, access must be preserved. Each port should be flushed with normal saline, clamped, and capped. Prior to clamping and capping, many institutions instill an anticoagulant locking solution such as 4% sodium citrate to maintain patency. Sodium citrate has several clinical advantages over concentrated heparin solution (the fluid previously used for this purpose) and is less costly. When a locking solution is not available, a temporary dialysis catheter should be periodically flushed with saline to maintain patency. Bleeding can occur at the insertion site of dialysis catheters. Should such bleeding occur during transport, the CCTP should control it with direct pressure to the site and apply a pressure or hemostatic dressing, if necessary.

- **Infection.** Large catheters are used to provide the venous access necessary for dialysis, and the presence of these devices increases patients' risk of contracting a central line–associated bloodstream infection. The CCTP should inspect IHD catheter sites to ensure the dressing is secure, clean, dry, and intact. The patient and all nearby providers should wear masks whenever such a catheter is accessed. Meticulous attention must be paid to aseptic technique.

- **Thermoregulation.** CRRT is an extracorporeal circuit, transporting the patient's blood volume external to the body for filtration. To maintain normothermia, blood heaters are used on all extracorporeal circuits. The CCTP should monitor the patient for hypothermia and compensate for lowering of the patient's body temperature by covering the patient with additional blankets or adjusting the cabin temperature.

- **Anticoagulation.** CRRT filter life may be prolonged with either systemic or regional anticoagulation. Citrate infused regionally, to facilitate anticoagulation in only the CRRT circuit, and heparin infused systemically are the two most common CRRT anticoagulation practices. When discontinuing CRRT before transport, the CCTP should determine whether the patient will still need any regional or systemic anticoagulation.

- **Volume status.** The process of initiating and discontinuing CRRT pulls and returns approximately 150 mL of blood to/from an average adult patient. Although this may seem like a small amount of fluid, the CCTP may observe significant changes in fluid volume status, particularly in hemodynamically unstable patients. Volume replacement may be necessary.

- **Laboratory abnormalities.** CRRT can remove significant quantities of small solutes and provide dramatic correction of acid–base derangements. If equipped to do so, the CCTP should monitor lab values periodically during transport, especially when CRRT is discontinued prior to the trip.

Peritoneal dialysis (PD) is infrequently initiated acutely in the hospital setting, although it can be continued in patients with CKD managed with PD in the outpatient setting. This technique involves the insertion of a rubber catheter into the abdomen and the use of the peritoneum as a semipermeable membrane. A dextrose solution is injected into the peritoneal space; from there, it moves across the membrane while wastes move in the opposite direction, thereby effecting their removal from the body. The most common complication of this form of dialysis is an increased risk of peritonitis and infection.

At times, the CCTP may encounter patients receiving dialysis who require IV access or even discontinuation of ongoing dialysis as a result of complications during transport. Patients with CKD who are on dialysis typically have poor peripheral vasculature and obtaining access may be extremely difficult. It is important to ensure that patent venous access is available prior to initiating transport. A fistula, shunt, or AV graft should never be routinely used for vascular access. An extremity with a fistula should not be used to obtain a BP reading, draw blood, obtain peripheral IV access, or obtain finger-stick blood glucose specimens. If other forms of venous access are lost during transport and the patient's condition deteriorates into extremis (a grave condition) or the patient experiences cardiopulmonary arrest, the CCTP may consider using a fistula only as a last resort. The likelihood of infection or damage to the fistula is so significant that intraosseous or central venous access (such as internal/external jugular access) should always be attempted before resorting to the use of a fistula.

Complications often arise during dialysis as well. Some of these complications can be treated during dialysis, whereas others may become so severe that dialysis must be discontinued. The most common complication is hypotension, which can usually be treated with small (100- to 250-mL) fluid boluses. Severe episodes of hypotension may necessitate that dialysis be stopped during treatment. Muscle cramping is another frequent complication and is often associated with rapid volume removal from the patient. Cramps can also be treated with small fluid boluses.

Maintenance doses of many drugs for patients on dialysis may need to be reduced, although the loading doses of drugs typically administered in the prehospital setting rarely need to be changed. Other medications, such as meperidine, NSAIDs, and oral antidiabetic agents, should be avoided in these patients. The list of medications whose dosages need to be reduced in patients on dialysis is extensive (refer to a publication on the specific topic for a complete list).

Signs and Symptoms

Acute Kidney Injury

- Dizziness
- Poor skin turgor
- Thirst
- Flat neck veins
- Dry mucous membranes
- Weight loss
- Orthostatic BP changes
- Fever
- Edema
- Ascites
- Low back pain

Differential Diagnosis

Acute Kidney Injury

- CKD
- Pyelonephritis
- Obstructing renal stone
- Glomerulonephritis
- Acute tubular necrosis
- Congestive heart failure

Transport Management

Kidney Injury

- Ensure and maintain the ABCs.
- Obtain IV access.
- Monitor the ECG.
- Maintain perfusing BP through IV fluids or vasopressor medications.
- Closely monitor serum electrolyte levels.
- Monitor the dialysis machinery (if in place) for potential complications.

Urinary Tract Infections

Bacterial flora that live symbiotically in the GI system can cause considerable damage when they are introduced into the urinary system. A urinary tract infection (UTI) develops as bacteria manage to travel up the urethra. Incidence of UTIs is significantly higher in females, owing to the shorter urethral distance needed to reach the female bladder. More than 20% of females will experience a UTI at some point in their lives. Patients with urinary retention from an obstruction or nervous system disruption are predisposed to UTIs, because regular urine flow normally prevents bacterial overgrowth and cleanses the tracts of pathogens. Patients with bladder catheters are also at a high risk for infection, as the foreign material facilitates bacterial migration.

Lower UTIs include infections of the urethra and urinary bladder, known as urethritis and cystitis, respectively. Migration of the pathogen to the ureters and kidneys results in an ascending infection called **pyelonephritis**, which can progress to urosepsis if not treated promptly. Infection can also spread into the prostate, causing prostatitis, which requires a prolonged course of antibiotics.

As many as 90% of UTIs are caused by *Escherichia coli* bacteria, which are normal inhabitants of the GI tract. The antimicrobial culprits vary in patients with frequent catheterization or chronic indwelling catheters (eg, *Enterococcus, Klebsiella*), and the rate of antibiotic resistance among these organisms continues to rise. Inflammation secondary to the infection causes bladder irritability, resulting in urinary frequency and urgency, as well as a burning pain exacerbated by urination, at times accompanied by foul-smelling urine. Pyelonephritis symptoms are more significant and include fever, chills, low back and flank pain, and nausea (with or without vomiting). Sexually transmitted infections such as gonorrhea and chlamydia may cause symptoms mimicking UTI and may be associated with urinary discharge.

The majority of both lower and upper UTIs are treated successfully with antibiotics. On occasion, surgery may be required to remove an intrarenal or perinephric abscess that forms during pyelonephritis. In more severe cases of pyelonephritis, IV antibiotics may be required, and the CCTP may have to manage their administration during interfacility transports.

Nephrolithiasis

Renal calculi, commonly referred to as kidney stones, result from mineral buildup in the renal pelvis. Most often the calculi consist of calcium-based compounds, although occasionally they are composed of struvite or uric acid. The lifetime risk of renal calculi is approximately 10%, with males being twice as likely as females to experience this condition. Family or personal history of calculi should increase suspicion for this diagnosis.

Most renal calculi pass through the urinary tract and are excreted without significant complications, although they certainly can produce excruciating pain during their travels. The crystals can cause epithelial injury, bleeding, pain, and infection. A small percentage of calculi become lodged in the lumen of either the ureter or the urethra. As the blockage worsens, these stones can cause life-threatening AKI and infections secondary to the backup of urine in the kidneys. Abnormal reflux of urine into the kidneys causes widening of renal calices and disruption of normal architecture, also known as hydronephrosis.

The classic presentation of nephrolithiasis is colicky flank pain, which may be accompanied by nausea, vomiting, and radiation of pain into the groin. Although abdominal pain may be present, these patients usually do not demonstrate a tender abdomen during palpation. Some patients may have tenderness with percussion of the costovertebral angle of the affected side. Gross hematuria is seen in only one-third of cases. Risk factors for poor outcomes include diabetes, history of renal transplant or single kidney, and urinary tract infection.

Ultrasonography is the optimal diagnostic test, as it is used to evaluate for hydronephrosis in the context of an increased pretest probability of renal calculi, while avoiding radiation. Noncontrast CT is another effective diagnostic modality; it can localize and measure a stone, as well as other pathology that may mimic the symptoms of renal calculi (eg, aortic pathology).

Toradol has excellent analgesic and antispasmodic effect in patients with this condition, with opioids being a reasonable option for breakthrough pain. Antiemetics and medical expulsive therapy with alpha-1 antagonists are often provided as well.

Testicular Torsion

Normally, the tunica vaginalis secures the testes inside the scrotum, preventing any excessive movement or rotation. In approximately 12% of the male population, this attachment is misaligned, allowing some degree of free testicular movement.

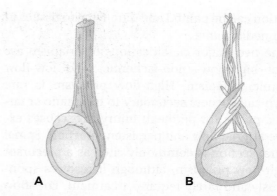

FIGURE 17-38 A. The normal testicle. **B.** Testicular torsion.

© Jones & Bartlett Learning.

These patients are susceptible to testicular torsion, a condition in which one or both testes rotate to the point of occluding their blood supply **FIGURE 17-38**. Trauma to the groin and vigorous exercise are common etiologies for torsion. A rotation of 720°—that is, two full rotations of the testicle around the axis of the testicular artery and vein—is required to fully tamponade the vessel and cause a resultant buildup of waste products within the testes and scrotal swelling. This condition is a true urologic emergency and must be addressed within 6 hours of symptom onset to maintain viability. Indeed, torsion is extremely painful, and manual detorsion followed by emergent surgical intervention may be required to salvage the testis and avoid necrosis. The CCTP must be able to recognize the symptoms and initiate rapid transport to an appropriate facility or notify the receiving facility of suspicions upon arrival. Analgesia should be administered to patients with this condition.

Patients with testicular torsion will occasionally present with nausea, vomiting, and pain. Pain may be localized to the scrotum or quite vague, radiating anywhere from the flank to the lower abdomen. In addition to nausea or vomiting, the presence of an enlarged, indurated, or high-riding testicle and an absent cremaster reflex suggest torsion. This condition is most often seen in adolescent males, with most cases occurring in males younger than 30 years.

Penile Injuries

Priapism is a penile erection lasting longer than 2 to 4 hours in the absence of sexual stimulation. This condition can be painful and damaging to tissues in the immediate area.

The two major classifications of priapism are arterial high-flow (non-ischemic) and low-flow (ischemic) priapism. High-flow priapism is rare and typically occurs secondary to traumatic or iatrogenic penile (or perineal) injury that causes excessive arterial flow and persistent erection. Spinal cord transection is commonly cited as a precursor to high-flow priapism, although it resolves spontaneously and rarely requires treatment. Low-flow priapism, which involves impaired relaxation of cavernosal smooth muscle, is the more painful of the two conditions. It is idiopathic in most cases, but is prevalent in patients with sickle cell disease or taking certain medications. Drugs that place men at risk for this condition include a number of prescription pharmaceuticals, including psychotropic medications, calcium channel blockers, and oral erectile dysfunction agents. Intracavernosal injection of drugs such as papaverine, phentolamine, and prostaglandin E_1 for erectile dysfunction are commonly implicated as well. Rarely, cases of priapism may be associated with use of the more popular selective cyclic guanosine 3′, 5′-monophosphate inhibitors such as sildenafil citrate (Viagra).

Initial treatment is application of a cold pack, followed by intracavernosal aspiration and administration of a sympathomimetic drug (eg, phenylephrine). The CCTP will rarely encounter a patient with priapism but must be prepared to treat it as a urologic emergency, with the major complication being subsequent impotence.

Some males may seek care in the aftermath of blunt injury to the penis while erect, usually during sexual intercourse. Rupture of the engorged vascular spaces within the penis results in penile fracture. Cold compresses should be applied to the area of injury. As with other urologic trauma, the CCTP should avoid inserting a urinary catheter if there is blood at the meatus or suspicion of urethral injury.

Maintenance Tubes

A variety of tubes may be encountered or placed by the CCTP while caring for a patient with a GI or GU condition. The following sections focus on two major types of these devices: feeding tubes and drainage tubes **TABLE 17-15**.

TABLE 17-15 Gastrointestinal/Genitourinary Maintenance Tubes

Type of Tube	Examples
Feeding tube	Nasogastric or Dobhoff tube Percutaneous endoscopic gastrostomy (PEG) tube Jejunostomy tube (J tube) Percutaneous endoscopic gastro-jejunal (PEG-J) tube Total parenteral nutrition
Drainage tube	Straight catheter Indwelling urinary catheter Suprapubic tube External condom catheter Colostomy Ileostomy Ileoanal anastomosis Kock pouch Ileal conduit urostomy Colon conduit urostomy Jackson-Pratt drain Hemovac drain Davol drain T tube

© Jones & Bartlett Learning.

Feeding Tubes

Proper nutrition is necessary for life, wound healing, and recovery, and must be provided enterally to patients who are extensively incapacitated by either disability or sedation. Unless total parenteral nutrition is required as a result of damage to or resection of the alimentary tract, use of the body's digestive organs is the best way to effect nutrient absorption. Enteral nutrition, commonly called tube feeding, can be administered in steps, depending on its expected duration.

Enteral Nutrition

Perhaps the largest obstacle to food intake in the incapacitated patient is the inability to swallow safely and effectively. This can be circumvented by placement of a simple NG tube, which can be used to administer food into the stomach or to remove food. These minimally invasive tubes are often inserted through the nasal orifice, with the assistance of the patient, in preparation for a short-term event during which temporary enteral feeding is required.

For longer-term situations, a gastrostomy tube (G tube) can be inserted. This type of tube is also referred to as a percutaneous endoscopic gastrostomy (PEG) tube because of the insertion technique used for its placement. PEG tubes are placed through a small, surgically created opening from the stomach, through the peritoneum, to the abdominal wall **FIGURE 17-39A**.

Alternatively, a jejunostomy tube (J tube) can be introduced directly into the jejunum through a comparable technique, known as a percutaneous endoscopic jejunostomy **FIGURE 17-39B**. J tubes possess an advantage over their PEG counterparts: Aspiration risk is much lower with J tubes because food is administered distal to the pyloric sphincter. Unfortunately, J tubes are also associated with a higher insertion complication rate because the small intestinal wall is less stable than the thicker stomach lining, which serves to anchor a PEG tube more securely.

A newer procedure known as a PEG-J tube lessens this risk while providing the benefit of decreased aspiration. During this procedure, a PEG tube is first placed through the abdominal wall, then advanced through the lumen to the duodenum and into the jejunum.

Liquid nutritional products can be administered to the patient through any of these tubes by either a rate-controlled pump or syringe boluses. Proper functioning of the tube is confirmed by a lack of pain or resistance while pushing the syringe upon food administration.

Aspiration is the most common complication from a feeding tube and could potentially develop into a life-threatening situation. To avert this complication, sit the patient upright during feeding or vomiting. Bleeding may occur at the insertion site if the tube is pulled on or traumatically removed. Significant hemorrhage from this situation is unlikely, and bleeding is typically self-limited. A third complication involves infection around the insertion site, which may be observed as a reddening or swelling in the immediate vicinity.

If the feeding tube becomes clogged, a 30- to 50-mL sterile warm water bolus can be used to clear the blockage. If the tube is removed unexpectedly, the site should be covered with an occlusive dressing until it can be properly replaced. Some

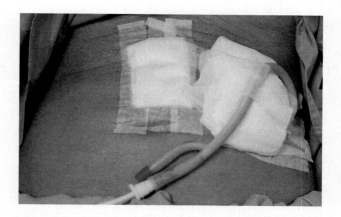

A

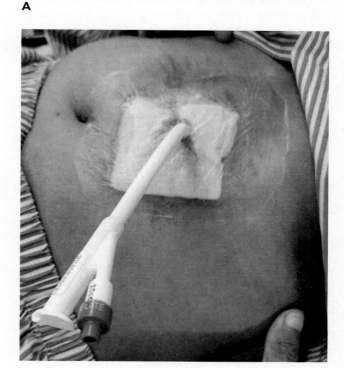

B

FIGURE 17-39 A. A percutaneous endoscopic gastrostomy (PEG) tube placed in the patient's stomach. **B.** A jejunostomy (J) tube placed in the patient's jejunum.

A: © stockphoto mania/Shutterstock; B: © Casa nayafana/Shutterstock.

protocols may allow the CCTP to replace a tube that has been removed or insert a Foley catheter to keep the tract patent. Unmanageable blockage or a removal of the PEG or J tube is not of major concern in the short-term care of the patient, as a brief lapse in feeding can be accounted for later. However, the CCTP should confirm alternative administration routes for time-sensitive medications (such as antiepileptic drugs) that are administered through an enteral tube.

Total Parenteral Nutrition

Total parenteral nutrition (TPN) is an alternative feeding method used when the GI tract is not functioning adequately. During TPN, all required nutrients are administered intravenously to the patient. Typically, central access is used for administration to prevent osmotic fluid shifts, although some preparations can be delivered through a peripheral vein. Medications are often added to the TPN solution during its creation, but they should not be introduced once that process is complete. TPN should be used when enteral feeding is not an option because of the significant GI atrophy that occurs with ongoing dormancy of the GI tract. Long-term use of TPN is associated with hypertriglyceridemia, hepatic dysfunction, and an increased risk of sepsis.

Like patients with other types of central venous lines, patients receiving TPN are at high risk for an air embolus and thrombosis. An air embolus is most likely to occur when changing a line or following an unexpected disruption of the line. This situation has a high mortality rate and must be aggressively treated with high-flow oxygen, occlusive dressing placement, and movement of the patient into a Trendelenburg position. Thrombosis is treated by removing the catheter, then administering anticoagulation and thrombolytic therapy. Continuous monitoring for metabolic abnormalities is essential when the patient is receiving TPN, as well as monitoring for electrolyte imbalances, which can easily arise with this feeding method.

Management

When transporting a patient with a feeding tube, contact medical direction if the patient develops pain at insertion site, has vomited, or develops a distended abdomen.

Transport Management

Patients With Feeding Tubes
- Examine the insertion site for signs of infection, such as redness or swelling.
- Assess for pain at the insertion site.
- Assess for any leakage or blockage of the tube.
- Keep the patient in a position of comfort.
- Provide supportive care as required.

Drainage Tubes

The digestive system has equally important input and output functions, and the tubes placed in the critically ill patient must meet both of these needs. Just as various feeding tubes exist to introduce food to the body when the patient cannot independently consume it, so drainage tubes exist to remove waste when it is being retained. Waste products of human metabolism take the form of urine and feces, which are parenterally removed through urinary catheters and ostomies, respectively. In some critically ill patients with large-volume diarrhea, rectal tubes may be placed temporarily for fecal management.

Urinary Catheters

Types of Urinary Catheters

Different methods of urine collection exist, each with its own advantages and disadvantages.

Straight catheters, often called intermittent catheters, are designed for temporary use and may be self-inserted by the patient. They enable the patient to drain residual bladder contents that might otherwise lead to infection. These catheters are associated with less inflammation than catheters intended for longer-term use, but the drainage process must be repeated three or more times per day. Intermittent catheterization is preferred if longer indwelling catheters can be avoided, in an effort to avoid catheter-associated UTIs.

Indwelling urinary catheters, also known as Foley catheters, are used as a more permanent solution for urine retention or incontinence. These may be placed in patients who require close monitoring of urine status, intubated patients, and individuals with wounds that may be soiled by incontinence, for example. These pliable rubber catheters are introduced into the bladder via the urethra. A balloon is inflated with 5 mL of saline inside the bladder to prevent inadvertent removal of the catheter.

Some urinary catheters have a slight bend at the insertion end, called a coudé tip, which allows them to pass around scar tissue or an enlarged prostate. Individuals with a history of difficult catheterization may require this type of catheter. Other patients may have a triple-lumen catheter in place to enable continuous bladder irrigation. This approach is sometimes used to remove or prevent clot formation or accumulation in the bladder, particularly in the aftermath of urologic surgery.

When surgery or trauma makes urethral catheter introduction undesirable, a suprapubic tube may be inserted instead. Patients who require permanent or semipermanent urinary drainage, such as those with neurogenic bladder or severe dementia, will benefit from this approach due to a decreased risk of infection and improved comfort. The urine collection tube is placed directly into the bladder through the abdominal wall by way of a surgically created stoma.

Some patients have the option of using noninvasive urinary devices, including suction-assisted wicks for women and condom catheters for men. Although they are less secure, they are also less susceptible to complications and are a good alternative to diapers.

Each type of urine-collection catheter functions in a similar way, draining into a bag that allows for clean collection, observation, and measurement of urine output. Two types of collection bags are frequently used: a leg bag that straps to the leg underneath clothes, allowing for greater mobility with a discreet presence, and a down-drain bag that hangs on the side of the patient's bed. Larger down-drain bags are more commonly used in hospitals and nursing homes. The drains function by gravity, so it is important to ensure they are hung below the patient.

Complications of Urinary Catheters

Common complications of urine collection catheters include clogging, infection, pain, leakage, and dislodgement. Clogging can typically be cleared with a small fluid bolus, although persistent obstruction may indicate dislodgement. Dislodgement is the largest concern during transport. Dislodgement and leakage are corrected by replacing the catheter into the bladder; they are often a result of selecting an improper size of catheter. Care must be taken to deflate the internal balloon before performing any adjustment of the catheter.

Management

It would be unlikely for urinary catheter placement to occur during transport, but the procedure is covered here in the event that the CCTP performs it prior to transport. Care should be taken when inserting urinary catheters in patients with recent GU trauma, surgery, or prior history of very difficult placement, as excessive force can cause injury to the urethra and potentially create a false passage.

When preparing to place a urinary catheter, gather the following equipment:

- Disposable sterile bladder catheter kit
- Water-soluble lubricant
- Drapes
- Cleansing solution
- Sterile gloves
- Prefilled syringe containing sterile water
- Correct size urinary catheter
- Clamp
- Connecting tubing
- Collecting bag

Indications for urinary catheter placement include drainage of the urinary bladder to precisely measure urine output and to aid fluid balance and retention. Contraindications include suspected urethral injury, as evidenced by blood at the urethral meatus (opening) of a trauma patient or significant penile or scrotal hematoma without having excluded urethral injury; postoperative urologic patients; and a history of urethral stricture (narrowing). When transporting a patient with a urinary catheter by air, air medical considerations include ensuring the balloon is filled with water.

The steps to place a female urinary catheter are shown in **SKILL DRILL 17-3** and summarized here:

1. Prepare the equipment.
2. Take standard precautions.
3. Place the patient in the supine position, with hips flexed and abducted.
4. Open the kit and prepare the equipment using sterile technique.
5. Test the balloon on the indwelling catheter by injecting it with sterile water or saline.
6. Position the drapes.
7. Lubricate the catheter.
8. Cleanse the sides of the labia and meatus with a chlorhexidine 2% solution.
9. Insert the catheter into the meatus gently until urine flow begins **STEP 1**.
10. Fill the fluid retention balloon until it is secure **STEP 2**.
11. Connect the open end of the catheter to the drainage tube and collection bag **STEP 3**.
12. Secure the catheter to the patient's leg with tape.

The steps to place a male urinary catheter are shown in **SKILL DRILL 17-4** and summarized here:

1. Prepare the equipment.
2. Take standard precautions.

Skill Drill 17-3 Placing a Female Urinary Catheter

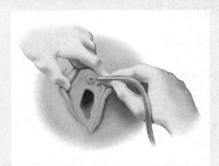

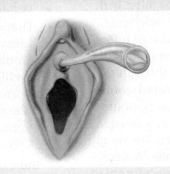

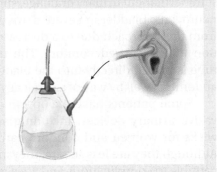

Step 1

Insert the catheter into the meatus gently until urine flow begins.

© Jones & Bartlett Learning.

Step 2

Fill the fluid retention balloon until it is secure.

Step 3

Connect the open end of the catheter to the drainage tube and collection bag. Secure the catheter to the patient's leg.

Skill Drill 17-4 Placing a Male Urinary Catheter

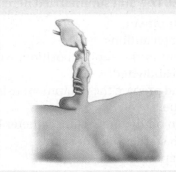

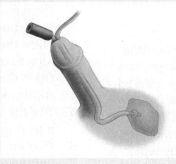

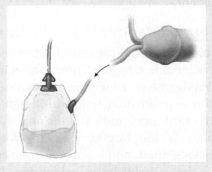

Step 1

Insert the catheter gently until urine flow begins. Once urine is observed, gently advance the catheter an additional 2 to 3 inches (5 to 8 cm).

© Jones & Bartlett Learning.

Step 2

Fill the fluid retention balloon until it is secure.

Step 3

Connect the open end of the catheter to the drainage tube and collection bag. Secure the catheter to the patient's leg.

3. Place the patient in the supine position.
4. Open the kit and prepare the equipment using a sterile technique.
5. Position the drapes.

6. Lubricate the catheter.
7. Cleanse the penis from head to base, always moving the disinfectant brush in a direction away from the meatus.

8. Insert the catheter gently until urine flow begins. Once urine is observed, gently advance the catheter an additional 2 to 3 inches (5 to 8 cm) **STEP 1**.

9. Fill the fluid retention balloon until it is secure **STEP 2**.

10. Connect the open end of the catheter to the drainage tube and collection bag **STEP 3**.

11. Secure the catheter to the patient's leg with tape.

Transport Management

Patients With Urinary Catheters

- If clogging occurs, clear the catheter with a small fluid bolus.
- If dislodgement or leakage occurs, replace the catheter. A different size of catheter may be needed.

Ostomies

Types of Ostomies

An **ostomy** is a surgically created opening of the GI tract through the abdomen that allows for waste removal. The ostomy may originate in the ileum of the small intestine (ileostomy) or anywhere in the large intestine (colostomy), depending on which segments of the GI tract must be bypassed. Urostomies may be created as well to drain urine directly from the urinary tract when a distal portion must be avoided as a result of disease or trauma. Indications for an ostomy include bowel injury or disease, bladder injury or disease, and congenital anomalies.

Colostomies **FIGURE 17-40** and ileostomies drain intestinal contents out of the GI tract and into a collection bag. The drainage from a colostomy is more solid than that from an ileostomy because the material has progressed farther through the digestive process. The drainage is collected in a bag attached to the opening and strapped to the patient's body. Sometimes a section of small intestine is surgically modified to create an internal collection site called a Kock pouch. In an ileoanal anastomosis, also known as a J pouch, the rectum is preserved, allowing it to function in fecal collection. These methods are beneficial to the patient because they allow less visible collection methods and offer more convenient waste disposal management.

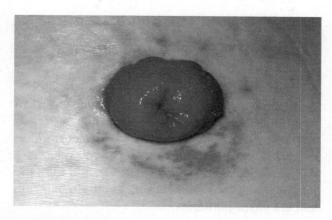

FIGURE 17-40 A colostomy.
© Medical-on-Line/Alamy Stock Photo.

Urostomies divert urine away from the urinary bladder by creating a passageway from the ureter to an abdominal stoma through a piece of ileum or large intestine that is surgically separated from the GI tract. When the ileum is used for this purpose, it is called an ileal conduit; when the large intestine is used, it is called a colon conduit. An external collection pouch is attached to the stoma and secured to the patient's body.

Management

Complications of ostomies include the following possibilities:

- Obstruction
- Constipation (with colostomies)
- Diarrhea
- Dehydration
- Leakage
- Tissue necrosis
- Detachment
- Prolapse
- Infection

The patient with an ostomy should be monitored for signs of tissue necrosis and infection, which, if detected, may warrant treatments ranging from antibiotic therapy to surgical intervention. Normal assessment findings for a patient with an ostomy include a pink, pain-free site that is free of redness or swelling. Detachment or prolapse of intestinal tissue from the abdominal wall may require bleeding control and occlusive dressings as well as surgical reconstruction. When assessing the patient with an ostomy, expose the stoma site and examine it for redness, swelling, or leakage. If any of these signs are found, notify the receiving facility upon arrival. Always ask the patient if the ostomy is functioning normally, without either leakage or obstruction.

An ileostomy pouch needs to be emptied four to six times per day; a colostomy pouch needs to be emptied one or more times per day. Laxatives should not be used by patients with ileostomies, and adequate daily fluid replacement (such as 6 to 8 glasses of water) is a necessity. In addition, the patient should not use soaps that contain baby oil, cold cream, or perfumes.

When preparing to empty or replace an ostomy, gather the following equipment:

- Stoma measuring guide or pattern
- Scissors
- New pouch
- Soft washcloth
- Soap and water
- Razor for shaving hair on abdomen
- Waste collection container
- Toilet paper

- Rubber ear (bulb)
- Biohazard bag for soiled pouch

SKILL DRILL 17-5 shows the steps for emptying an ostomy pouch. The pouch should be emptied when it is one-third to one-half full.

1. Remove the clamp that keeps the pouch closed **STEP 1**.
2. If the patient is supine, lift the pouch and position the opening over a waste collection container **STEP 2**. If possible, have the patient lie on their side with the pouch opening positioned over a waste collection container.
3. Slide your fingers down the outside of the pouch to squeeze the contents out of the pouch.
4. Clean the inside of the pouch opening with a piece of toilet paper.
5. Rinse out the pouch with room-temperature water using a rubber ear (bulb) syringe.
6. Put the clamp back onto the pouch to close it **STEP 3**.

Skill Drill 17-5 Emptying an Ostomy Pouch

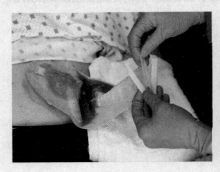

Step 1

Remove the clamp that keeps the pouch closed.

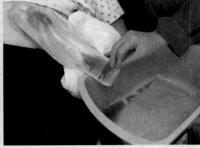

Step 2

If patient is supine, lift the pouch and position the opening over a waste collection container.

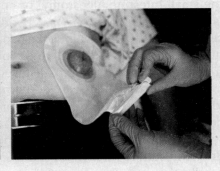

Step 3

Slide your fingers down the outside of the pouch to squeeze the contents out of the pouch. Clean the inside of the pouch opening with a piece of toilet paper. Rinse out the pouch with room-temperature water using a rubber ear (bulb) syringe. Put the clamp back onto the pouch to close it.

Although ostomy pouches typically need to be changed only every few days, the CCTP may be required to change one under certain circumstances. If a leak or rupture of the bag occurs during transport, the pouch must be removed and replaced if the equipment is available. Less-emergent reasons to change a pouch include inflammation, pain, or irritation around the insertion site. In such instances, changing the pouch can typically be delayed until arrival at the receiving facility.

SKILL DRILL 17-6 shows the steps for replacing an ostomy pouch, which are summarized here:

1. Take standard precautions.
2. Using the measuring guide or pattern, trace the correct opening onto the skin barrier of the new pouch, then cut out the opening you traced **STEP 1**.
3. Remove the paper backing that covers the adhesive on the skin barrier of the new pouch **STEP 2**.

Skill Drill 17-6 Replacing an Ostomy Pouch

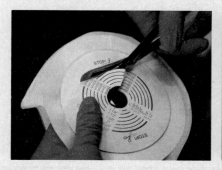

Step 1

Take standard precautions. Using the measuring guide or pattern, trace the correct opening onto the skin barrier of the new pouch, then cut out the opening you traced.

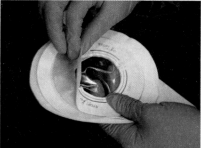

Step 2

Remove the paper backing that covers the adhesive on the skin barrier of the new pouch.

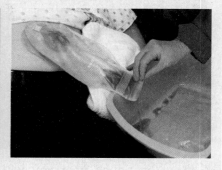

Step 3

Empty the pouch the patient is wearing.

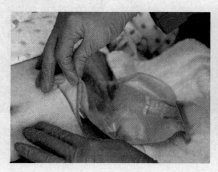

Step 4

Remove the pouch by stabilizing the skin around the pouch with your nondominant hand and peeling off the pouch with the other hand.

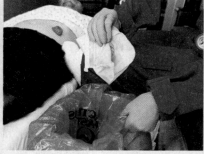

Step 5

Remove the clamp from the old pouch. Dispose of the old pouch by placing it into a biohazard bag.

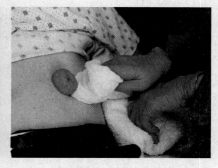

Step 6

Wash thoroughly around the stoma with mild soap and warm water. Rinse and dry the area with a soft cloth.

Continues

Skill Drill 17-6 Replacing an Ostomy Pouch (continued)

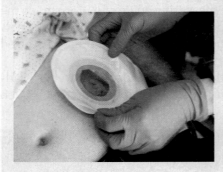

Step 7

Center the new pouch opening over the stoma.

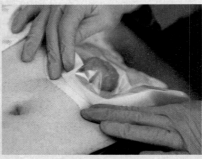

Step 8

Press the skin barrier wafer onto the abdomen, removing all wrinkles or creases in the wafer.

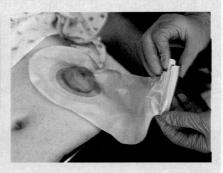

Step 9

Put the clamp from the old pouch onto the opening of the new pouch.

© Jones & Bartlett Learning.

4. Lay the pouch near you with the adhesive side up.
5. Empty the pouch the patient is wearing (see Skill Drill 17-5) **STEP 3**.
6. Remove the pouch by stabilizing the skin around the pouch with your nondominant hand and peeling off the pouch with the other hand **STEP 4**.
7. Remove the clamp from the old pouch.
8. Dispose of the old pouch by placing it into a biohazard bag **STEP 5**.
9. Wash thoroughly around the stoma with mild soap and warm water **STEP 6**.
10. Rinse and dry the area with a soft cloth. A small amount of bleeding may be normal.
11. Center the new pouch opening over the stoma **STEP 7**.
12. Press the skin barrier wafer onto the abdomen, removing all wrinkles or creases in the wafer **STEP 8**.
13. Put the clamp from the old pouch onto the opening of the new pouch **STEP 9**.

Specific Drainage Tubes

After major abdominal surgery, a number of drainage tubes are placed to both assist in and evaluate

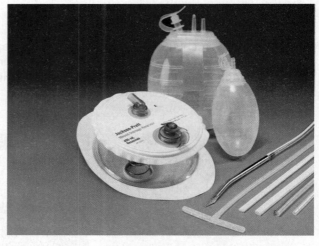

FIGURE 17-41 A Jackson-Pratt drain (in background) and a Hemovac drain (with blue connectors).

Courtesy of Cardinal Health.

the recovery process. For example, Jackson-Pratt drains are inserted to remove postoperative build-up of fluid and blood in the abdominal cavity **FIGURE 17-41**. Prevention of fluid accumulation in this way greatly decreases the risk of abscess formation and infection. The drain is controlled by the patient, who squeezes a bulb to induce suction.

A flexible tube connected to the bulb travels through the surgical incision and into the wound site.

Similar surgical drainage tubes include the Hemovac and Davol drains. Both of these draining devices operate similarly to the Jackson-Pratt drain, with the only difference being bulb design.

During liver transplantation surgery, a **T tube** is placed to monitor bile drainage from the gallbladder. After the drainage bag has been removed, the tube may remain in place to facilitate examination of the biliary tract through a T-tube cholangiogram test.

All of these drainage tubes often become obstructed by blood clots, which can usually be cleared by digitally manipulating the tube. Dislodgement can slow the healing process and greatly increase the likelihood of infection, and the drain may need to be replaced through surgical means. Bleeding may occur from the wound site after dislodgement of the tube, and should be controlled. The wound site and sutures should be monitored for any signs of infection or improper healing.

In-Flight Considerations for Maintenance Tubes

In-flight complications need to be considered when patients have any of the numerous drainage systems that include closed bags containing air. Air pressure decreases as altitude increases. Gas volume increases proportionally to the decrease in air pressure, which could lead to distention of drainage devices. Although fixed-wing aircraft typically incorporate pressure-controlling mechanisms, the CCTP should always be prepared for equipment failure and know how to handle this situation. Controlling air pressure on rotor-wing aircraft may be more difficult because the aircraft may change altitude rapidly and often.

Excess air should be vented from any drainage bag such as a colostomy or urostomy prior to flight, in anticipation of changes in air pressure. Further venting may be required during transport, and the CCTP should confirm that the specific device in use can accommodate this manipulation. Similar preparations must be made for Jackson-Pratt and other surgical drainage devices. Be sure to unclamp any feeding or drainage catheters prior to departure and ensure that they remain unclamped for the duration of travel.

Metabolic Regulation of Acid–Base Status

The human body has an amazing ability to adapt to and function in extreme environmental conditions. From the peaks of mountains to great ocean depths, arid deserts, remote arctic locations, and the weightless expanse of space, human activities continue despite the environmental challenges. Yet, even with this incredible adaptability, the human body requires a carefully controlled internal environment for cells to function, organs to perform, and life to continue.

Significant alterations of the body's oxygen and carbon dioxide levels, electrolyte concentrations, temperature, glucose levels, and acid–base status will impair cell, tissue, and organ function, eventually leading to death. CCTPs must manage any of these alterations resulting from illness, injury, or extrinsic factors to save patients' lives and improve their chances for recovery.

Acid–base status is tightly controlled by numerous organs, receptors, and buffer systems. Dysfunction of any of the body's vast array of cells, tissues, organs, and body systems threatens to disrupt this carefully maintained balance and further compromise cell, tissue, and organ function throughout the body. Although the human body can tolerate large quantities of exogenous acids and bases, widespread damage occurs when the body's capacity to sequester, neutralize, and excrete these substances is exceeded. The liver, lungs, and kidneys are central players in the body's metabolic regulation. As we discuss throughout this text, conditions that negatively impact or overwhelm any of these organs, from respiratory distress to trauma or toxicologic emergencies, will certainly affect acid–base status and lead to metabolic disarray. Detailed discussion of respiratory acidosis and respiratory alkalosis can be found in Chapter 6, *Respiratory Emergencies and Airway Management*.

Acid–Base Physiology

Hydrogen ions (H^+) are single protons released from a hydrogen atom; acids are solutions containing H^+ ions. A base (also basic or alkaline) substance can accept a free H^+. The relationship of acids to bases within the body is expressed by the pH value, which indicates the concentration of free

H^+ present. Because additional basic substances are present, they become bound with free H^+, decreasing the amount of free H^+. The normal extracellular fluid pH ranges from 7.35 to 7.45. The pH value is inversely related to the amount of free H^+ present. When the free H^+ concentration increases, the pH value decreases (acidosis). When the free H^+ concentration decreases, the pH value increases (alkalosis). Cell protein activity becomes impaired when the pH falls outside the normal range, which is approximately 7.35 to 7.45. Cell death begins to occur when the pH falls below 6.8 or increases above 7.8.

Acids and bases are both absorbed into the body from dietary sources. Additionally, H^+ ions are produced during various metabolic processes. Altered cellular metabolism, changes in excretion patterns, or exposure to various exogenous substances can lead to wide variations in extracellular fluid pH. Intracellular function is altered when excess H^+ ions from extracellular fluid enter the cells through a concentration gradient. This concentration gradient is the dominant mode of cellular exchange with extracellular fluids. Virtually every chemical process is driven by concentration gradients and the movement of protons (which acids provide) and electrons (which bases provide). Without this ceaseless activity, enzymes and cellular machinery could not function.

Intrinsic Regulation of Acid–Base Balance

Three principal mechanisms are used to maintain a physiologic acid–base status within the body. First, chemical buffers sequester excess H^+ until a rising (alkaline) pH triggers their release. Second, the respiratory system controls extracellular Pco_2 concentration, which affects carbonic acid and ultimately H^+ concentration. Finally, the kidneys can either excrete acidic or alkaline (basic) urine to balance whole-body H^+ concentrations.

Chemical Buffer Systems

The human body uses several buffer systems to mitigate the effects of acid and alkali loads. Any substance that can alternately bind or release H^+ depending on the outside conditions is a buffer. Intracellular and extracellular buffer systems are the first line of defense against changes in pH.

The bicarbonate-carbonic acid buffer system is the principal extracellular buffer system. It operates primarily in the lungs and kidneys, where carbonic anhydrase is present to facilitate the chemical reaction. Carbon dioxide (CO_2) and water (H_2O) are reversibly converted into carbonic acid (H_2CO_3), which in turn is reversibly converted into H^+ and bicarbonate (HCO_3^-). This reaction reverses itself when large quantities of H^+ are present, ultimately turning excess H^+ into water and carbon dioxide. Carbon dioxide is then eliminated via respiration.

$$H^+ + HCO_3^- \leftrightarrow H_2CO_3 \leftrightarrow CO_2 + H_2O$$

The bicarbonate–carbonic acid buffer system is linked to the lungs and kidneys because these two organs can alter the concentrations of carbon dioxide and bicarbonate, respectively, thereby affecting the concentration of the remaining components and driving the direction of these reactions **FIGURE 17-42**. This system allows the body to dampen the effects of sudden acid or alkali loads.

The phosphate buffer system operates similarly to the bicarbonate–carbonic acid buffer system, in that it allows only small pH changes following large variations of free H^+. This system functions primarily in the urine to convert strong acids or bases into weak acids or weak bases. Phosphate buffers work best in areas of the body with a normally lower pH, such as the renal tubules.

Hemoglobin, albumin, certain bone tissues, and other proteins also act as chemical buffers. Hemoglobin molecules, especially when deoxygenated (as in venous blood), can absorb a hydrogen

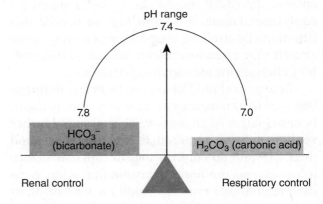

FIGURE 17-42 The balance of bicarbonate and carbonic acid shifts if either the renal or respiratory system fails, leading to an imbalance.

© Jones & Bartlett Learning.

ion, and ultimately buffer six times more H$^+$ than do other plasma proteins. Other protein buffers take several hours to resolve imbalances, but they provide the majority of total-body buffering capability. Bone buffers also contribute by absorbing and releasing excess H$^+$ when needed.

Respiratory Influence on pH

Carbon dioxide is a major determinant of the body's acid–base status. Carbon dioxide is produced during normal metabolism and must be continuously excreted. The concentration of carbon dioxide is directly related to the H$^+$ concentration and inversely related to the extracellular fluid pH. When the body is in an acidic state, alveolar ventilation automatically increases, resulting in decreased H$^+$ concentrations (and increased pH) within minutes. Conversely, any increase in alveolar ventilation above baseline will raise the pH and decrease the available concentration of free H$^+$. Such respiratory adjustments are rapid and effective to a certain point, but they will not completely resolve a primarily metabolic alteration in pH. Compensation of metabolic dysregulation ramps up over time in pulmonary and renal systems, with respiratory compensation reaching its maximum potential in 12 to 24 hours, while renal compensation reaches its optimal level after 3 to 5 days of exposure.

As mentioned previously, respiratory acidosis and respiratory alkalosis are discussed in depth in Chapter 6, *Respiratory Emergencies and Airway Management.*

Renal Influence on pH

The kidneys provide the body's last major line of defense against the catastrophic effects of large quantities of acids or bases. These organs excrete either acidic or basic urine depending on the pH of the body. In severe states, kidneys can excrete 500 mEq of H$^+$ per day. With persistent metabolic disarray, complex pathways likely involving systemic glucocorticoid and mineralocorticoid triggers uptitrate chronic renal compensation. Various types of transmembrane gates or channels exist along the nephron, through which concentration gradients and pH-dependent enzymatic reactions drive finely tuned excretion of acid or alkali loads in the urine.

To compensate for a metabolic or respiratory alkalosis, the kidneys increase bicarbonate excretion. This action decreases the available extracellular fluid bicarbonate, increasing the available free H$^+$ concentration and lowering the pH. The high bicarbonate filtration rate enables the kidneys to quickly eliminate metabolic alkali loads.

In acidic states, the kidneys reverse transmembrane flow of ions to address the imbalance. First, they directly excrete H$^+$ into the urine when excess H$^+$ ions are present. They then reabsorb previously filtered bicarbonate and return it into circulation, where the bicarbonate binds with excess H$^+$ and corrects all or part of the acidosis. Additionally, the kidneys produce additional bicarbonate to offset the excess H$^+$. Finally, of the net acid excreted, approximately one-half to two-thirds represents excretion of ammonium in the urine. It is interesting to note that Western diets high in animal protein tend to yield primarily acid loads that must then be excreted by the renal system. For this reason, patients with CKD are recommended to eat primarily vegetarian diets, as these are mainly alkali loads, to maintain acid–base homeostasis.

Hepatic Influence on pH

Although the renal and pulmonary systems deserve the limelight when it comes to acid–base regulation, it is important to acknowledge one of the most metabolically active organs in the body: the liver. Due to its role as an organ of digestion and its significant dual blood supply, hepatic tissue is both a source and a sink for hydrogen ions.

The digestion of food consumes energy and produces acids: Oxidation of consumed carbohydrates and fats yields carbon dioxide, which splits into H$^+$ and bicarbonate. During fasting states, hepatic mitochondria oxidize fatty acids and form ketones (overwhelmingly so in diabetic ketoacidosis). Hepatic tissues also convert ammonium (NH_4^+) to urea, which also yields H$^+$, but allows for excretion of nitrogenous waste.

The liver also produces albumin, a plasma protein that buffers carbon dioxide and fixed acids; furthermore, it metabolizes organic acid anions such as lactate (ie, lactic acidosis), consuming H$^+$ and turning it back to glucose (gluconeogenesis). For instance, people with liver failure often have an impressively elevated basal lactic acidosis, while decreased synthetic function (hypoalbuminemia) results in impaired ability to buffer significant acid–base fluctuations.

TABLE 17-16 Normal Arterial Blood Gas and Venous Blood Gas Values

Value	Arterial Blood Gas	Venous Blood Gas
pH	7.35–7.45	7.32–7.43
Pco₂	35–45 mm Hg	38–50 mm Hg
Po₂	80–100 mm Hg (adults)	40 mm Hg
	60–70 mm Hg (newborns)	
HCO₃⁻ (bicarbonate)	22–26 mmol/L (or mEq/L)	23–30 mmol/L

Data from Jacobs DS, DeMott WR, Oxley DK. *Laboratory Test Handbook*. Hudson, OH: Lexi-Comp; 2001.

Laboratory Analysis

The concentration of free H^+ in extracellular fluid (pH) as well as other key variables can be obtained from an arterial blood gas (ABG) or venous blood gas (VBG) sample. Results also include Pco_2, Po_2, and bicarbonate measurements. Normal values are listed in **TABLE 17-16**. Additional values such as base excess, oxygen saturation, carboxyhemoglobin, lactate, and various electrolytes or blood count values are often included in these panel results. These tests are available immediately on many transport vehicles and can be obtained in most, if not all, hospitals. Many outlying clinics, treatment centers, and offices have advanced **point-of-care testing (POCT)** capabilities.

Interpretation of Blood Gas Sample Results

ABG sample results provide the CCTP with valuable information about the existence or type of acidosis or alkalosis. First, consider the overall pH. A pH below 7.35 is considered an acidosis, regardless of any compensation (discussed later). A pH above 7.45 is considered an alkalosis, again regardless of any compensation.

Next, consider the primary source. An acidosis or alkalosis may be identified as primary metabolic, primary respiratory, or mixed (combined). Once the primary source of acidosis or alkalosis is determined, the presence of any compensation should

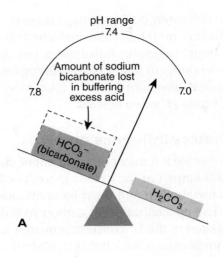

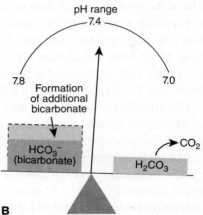

FIGURE 17-43 A. Derangement of acid–base balance in metabolic acidosis. **B.** Compensation by reduction of carbonic acid and formation of additional bicarbonate.

© Jones & Bartlett Learning.

also be evaluated. Overcompensation of a primary condition will not occur.

Metabolic acidosis is characterized by a decreased pH (less than 7.35) and a decreased bicarbonate level (less than 22 mmol/L). The latter suggests that an acid is consuming the bicarbonate. An individual may attempt to compensate for this acidic state by increasing respiratory rate and/or depth, thereby lowering the Pco_2 level. Elimination of carbon dioxide skews the equation used for the bicarbonate–carbonic acid buffer system (discussed previously) to the right, allowing for the mitigation of the excess acid. These efforts may normalize the pH but will never overcompensate **FIGURE 17-43**.

Respiratory acidosis occurs when a patient has a decreased pH (less than 7.35) and an increased

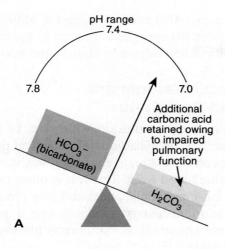

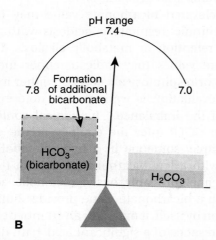

FIGURE 17-44 A. Derangement of acid–base balance in respiratory acidosis. **B.** Compensation by formation of additional bicarbonate.

© Jones & Bartlett Learning.

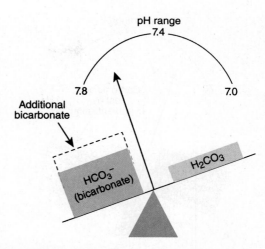

FIGURE 17-45 Derangement of acid–base balance in metabolic alkalosis. The body's compensatory mechanisms are ineffective.

© Jones & Bartlett Learning.

Pco_2 level (greater than 45 mm Hg). In this instance, the respiratory effort/exchange is inadequate to remove enough carbon dioxide to maintain a normal pH. If this condition persists, renal compensation will begin to occur via increased H^+ excretion, resulting in an elevated bicarbonate level (greater than 26 mmol/L) **FIGURE 17-44**. This finding is particularly notable in patients with conditions such as COPD.

Metabolic alkalosis occurs when a patient has an elevated pH (greater than 7.45) and an elevated bicarbonate level (greater than 26 mmol/L). The renal system is extremely effective in excreting bicarbonate. The patient's Pco_2 level may increase as a result of compensation because the alkalosis inhibits respiratory drive **FIGURE 17-45**.

Respiratory alkalosis occurs when a patient has an increased pH (greater than 7.45) and a decreased Pco_2 level (less than 35 mm Hg). This imbalance is usually the result of some type of alveolar hyperventilation (eg, resulting from anxiety or pain). Over time, renal compensation mechanisms promote the retention of H^+ and the excretion of bicarbonate **FIGURE 17-46**. Bicarbonate values will be lower if respiratory alkalosis persists for several hours to several days or longer.

Mixed acidosis involves a low pH (less than 7.35), an elevated Pco_2 level (greater than 45 mm Hg), and a low bicarbonate level (less than 22 mmol/L). This imbalance occurs when both respiratory and metabolic acidosis are present at the same time in the same patient. Severe trauma, cardiogenic shock, and drug overdose are common situations in which mixed acidosis may occur.

Mixed alkalosis involves an elevated pH (greater than 7.45), a low Pco_2 level (less than 35 mm Hg), and an elevated bicarbonate level (greater than 26 mmol/L). This imbalance may occur when two seemingly unrelated medical issues manifest at the same time in the same patient. For example, a patient with chronic respiratory alkalosis who experiences a GI emergency may have respiratory alkalosis combined with metabolic alkalosis and, therefore, demonstrate mixed alkalosis.

A patient with one of the primary conditions just described may present to the CCTP as uncompensated, partially compensated, or well compensated.

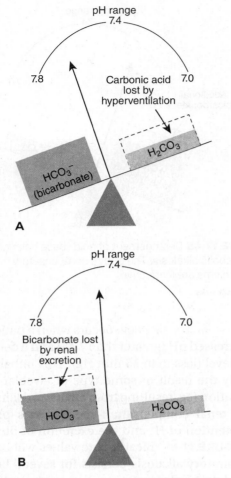

FIGURE 17-46 A. Derangement of acid–base balance in respiratory alkalosis. **B.** Compensation by excretion of bicarbonate.

© Jones & Bartlett Learning.

Practice is essential for the CCTP to become comfortable in identifying complex acid–base disorders. Various formulas exist to calculate expected compensation in different acid–base states. For instance, the Winters formula calculates the expected Pco_2 level in a metabolic acidosis:

$$Pco_2 = (1.5 \times Hco_3) + 8 \pm 2$$

VBG analysis has limitations compared to an ABG determination in certain situations. Both pH and bicarbonate levels generally remain consistent between venous and ABG measurements. The Pao_2 level does not, however, and it should not be inferred from the result of a VBG analysis. A VBG analysis can be used as a screening tool for an elevated Pco_2 level. The Pco_2 values generally correlate well between ABG and VBG analyses, although the relationship becomes less accurate as the patient's perfusion or hemodynamic status deteriorates.

Indirect Measurement of Acid–Base Status

Total blood carbon dioxide, which can be written as either Tco_2 or "bicarbonate" in clinical practice, provides an indication of an acid–base abnormality on routine blood work. This test is often included on the basic metabolic panel and may provide the information necessary to determine a patient's acid–base abnormality. The normal plasma bicarbonate value is 23 to 30 mmol/L.

An elevated bicarbonate value may indicate either chronic respiratory acidosis with carbon dioxide retention or metabolic alkalosis. Low bicarbonate values may indicate either metabolic acidosis or respiratory alkalosis. In either instance, further evaluation is warranted to determine the cause of the imbalance. The clinical context will help the CCTP infer the etiology of the change; for example, someone in a hypermetabolic state (fever) with a low bicarbonate value on the metabolic panel probably has a metabolic acidosis. Although a bicarbonate value provides limited information by itself, it may alert an attentive clinician to the presence of a significant acid–base disorder. A blood gas with pH measurement remains the definitive test, however.

Evaluation of the Anion Gap

When an acidosis is suspected, its origin can be examined using the anion gap (AG). Acidosis may be present with or without an AG, but its identification will help exclude or narrow the list of potential causes of the acidosis. The AG is a calculated value using the sodium (Na), chloride (Cl), and bicarbonate results. Many laboratory instruments automatically perform this calculation as part of the electrolyte panel. Some labs include potassium (added to sodium) in the calculation. The formula is as follows:

$$AG = Na - (Cl + HCO_3^-)$$

The normal AG is in the range of 8 to 12 mEq/L. The AG is calculated to determine the presence of unmeasured anions (eg, lactate, ketones). The normal AG is a representation of serum phosphate and albumin, the major unmeasured anion in the blood. An elevated AG can occur when the lactic acid level has become elevated as a result of trauma, shock, seizure, hypoxia, or contact with a toxic substance. Some toxic substances, including methanol, ethylene glycol, salicylates, and valproic acid, cause an elevated AG without lactic acid production. Alcoholic ketoacidosis and diabetic ketoacidosis also cause an elevated AG acidosis as a result of ketones, without increased lactic acid. Serum lactate levels greater than 4.0 mmol/L indicate lactic acidosis.

An acidosis with a normal AG results from a loss of bicarbonate or excess chloride, which happens most commonly with diarrhea, use of certain diuretics (eg, acetazolamide), and large-volume resuscitation with normal saline (chloride load). A lower than expected AG may be due to hypoalbuminemia or excess cations (hypercalcemia), for example.

Metabolic Alkalosis

When metabolic conditions create an excess of bicarbonate accompanied by a pH of greater than 7.45 on an ABG sample, the disorder is termed metabolic alkalosis. This disorder is further described as "chloride resistant" or "chloride responsive," depending on the urine chloride concentration. Metabolic alkalosis results from either H^+ losses or gains of bicarbonate, either relative or actual. Relative gains of bicarbonate occur when there is a disproportional loss of chloride, usually accompanying a sodium loss that alters electroneutrality, leading to renal bicarbonate retention.

Vomiting or gastric suction is a common cause of metabolic alkalosis. The use of certain diuretics can cause metabolic alkalosis when it leads to excretion of excess chloride ions in the urine. Various endocrine conditions, including primary aldosteronism, Bartter syndrome, Liddle syndrome, and hyperglucocorticoidism, may also produce this kind of imbalance.

Prehospital providers risk causing metabolic alkalosis when they place a patient with a previously compensated respiratory acidosis from hypercapnia or chronic obstructive pulmonary disease with an elevated Pco_2 level on a ventilator and aggressively ventilate that individual. Prior to ventilation, the body compensates for a chronically elevated

Pco_2 level through enhanced bicarbonate retention by the kidneys to maintain a neutral pH. Following aggressive ventilation, the carbon dioxide level normalizes, creating a relative bicarbonate excess, allowing a metabolic alkalosis to predominate.

Overzealous administration of sodium bicarbonate may cause significant and prolonged metabolic alkalosis. Even with renal excretion of the excess bicarbonate, reduced tissue perfusion related to persistent alkalosis can lead to serious sequelae.

Clinical Features

Patients with metabolic alkalosis demonstrate many significant clinical effects, often related to concomitant electrolyte abnormalities. Elevated blood pH increases hemoglobin's affinity for oxygen molecules, thereby inhibiting the tissues' ability to detach oxygen from the hemoglobin and leading to tissue hypoxia. Compensatory hypoventilation and hypercarbia further undermine tissue oxygenation. Expect Pco_2 levels to increase 0.7 mm Hg for every 1 mmol/L increase in bicarbonate. Seizures, altered mental status, refractory arrhythmias, and weakness may occur as well. Alkalosis will decrease ionized calcium levels and sequester potassium within cells (causing a transient hypokalemia), with both of these imbalances then causing additional symptoms. Potassium and hydrogen ions can be envisioned as moving in opposite directions. For this reason, bicarbonate is administered to patients with severe hyperkalemia to (transiently) remove potassium from the extracellular space.

Treatment

The treatment of metabolic alkalosis is directed toward the identification and correction of the cause in a specific patient. Urgent treatment should occur when the bicarbonate level exceeds 40 mmol/L or the pH exceeds 7.55. Many patients experiencing metabolic alkalosis have potentially massive hypovolemia from large GI- or renal-related fluid volume losses. These patients require volume resuscitation and electrolyte repletion with careful monitoring. Potassium, sodium, calcium, and chloride repletion are often required as well.

Specific management includes surgical management for pyloric stenosis, which causes protracted vomiting and massive GI fluid and H⁺ losses in affected children. Other GI fluid and H⁺ losses can be controlled with treatment of emesis or obstruction, or the discontinuation of gastric suction devices. Discontinuation of a diuretic medication or a change in the type of diuretic is indicated when excess renal chloride losses cause the alkalosis.

Several pharmacologic options exist for the treatment of severe metabolic alkalosis. Hydrochloric acid can be given intravenously to replete H⁺ and correct chloride losses. Potassium chloride will replete potassium and correct chloride losses. Acetazolamide (Diamox) is a diuretic and carbonic anhydrase inhibitor that can correct fluid volume excess and promote the excretion of bicarbonate in the urine. Chloride-responsive alkalosis is generally treated with the previously described medications. Chloride-resistant alkalosis often benefits from potassium chloride repletion, but also requires correction of the underlying condition to resolve the alkalosis. Certain endocrine disorders have specific treatment requirements that necessitate consultation with medical direction.

Metabolic Acidosis

Metabolic acidosis is demonstrated by a decreased serum pH (less than 7.35) accompanied by a decreased bicarbonate concentration (less than 22 mmol/L). This disorder occurs through three possible mechanisms:

- The kidneys may be unable to excrete enough of the H⁺ produced or absorbed each day.
- An increased amount of H⁺ is present because of exogenous loading or altered metabolism.
- The kidneys or GI tract excretes too much bicarbonate, causing an imbalance.

A myriad of situations cause metabolic acidosis. Cellular starvation states, such as diabetic ketoacidosis, alcoholic ketoacidosis, and profound malnutrition, lead to accumulation of acids through altered metabolism and, therefore, an increased AG acidosis. GI bicarbonate losses may occur from diarrhea, fistulas, or lower GI suctioning, causing metabolic acidosis. Many toxic chemicals (eg, iron, salicylates, toxic alcohols) produce either an AG or non-AG metabolic acidosis following exposure or absorption.

Excess accumulation or impaired excretion of lactate leads to acidosis and an elevated AG. Lactic acidosis has a large number of etiologies, including the following:

- Exposure or overdose (eg, ethylene glycol, iron, salicylates, metformin)
- Shock and inadequate tissue perfusion
- SIRS and organ dysfunction
- Infection
- Malignancy
- Exertion or exercise
- Metabolic disorders (eg, glucose-6-phosphatase deficiency)
- Liver failure

Renal Metabolic Acidosis

Kidney dysfunction may cause metabolic acidosis through a variety of mechanisms. Uremic states from the accumulation of cellular waste products directly cause a metabolic acidosis. As previously discussed, processes such as decreased bicarbonate secretion and inadequate renal ammonium production can also lead to acidosis. Certain congenital or acquired causes of acidosis are specific to the renal system.

Type 1 (distal) renal tubular acidosis (RTA) impairs the kidney's ability to excrete H⁺. This state is often characterized by plasma bicarbonate levels of less than 15 mmol/L, hypokalemia, increased urine calcium levels, and kidney stones. Urine pH remains greater than 5.5 despite the acidosis. This condition, which is relatively rare, may be hereditary, autoimmune, or linked to other diseases or chemicals.

Type 2 (proximal) RTA involves impaired bicarbonate reabsorption, which translates into increased renal bicarbonate excretion. It is characterized by an initially elevated urine pH; when plasma bicarbonate levels drop, the urine pH then decreases significantly. Glucose, protein, and phosphate are increasingly excreted in the urine in addition to bicarbonate. This condition, like type 1 RTA, is rare. It may be congenital or caused by numerous medications or various medical conditions.

Type 4 (generalized or hyperkalemic) RTA results from impaired liberation of renin by the kidneys or altered synthesis of, excretion of, or response to aldosterone by the kidneys or adrenal glands. In addition to hyperkalemia, the patient often demonstrates an elevated urine sodium level (greater than 40 mmol/L) and hyperchloremia. Type 4 RTA is the most common manifestation of RTA. It is linked with toxicity of numerous medications and genetic disorders, and may also arise as a consequence of diabetes, HIV, systemic lupus erythematosus, and sickle cell anemia.

Types 1, 2, and 4 RTA present as a metabolic acidosis without an elevated AG. Type 3 RTA is a rare classification, with characteristics of types 1 and 2, and is not clinically relevant.

Clinical Features

Metabolic acidosis is rarely a clinically isolated occurrence. Instead, the underlying pathologic conditions causing the acidosis will typically shape the patient's clinical status. Patients with metabolic acidosis may exhibit Kussmaul respirations (tachypnea with large tidal volumes) because a decreasing pH will stimulate the respiratory centers, causing an increase in alveolar ventilation. Hypotension and hypovolemia are also noted in conjunction with severe metabolic acidosis, demonstrating the progression of widespread cell, tissue, organ, and body system dysfunction. In response to acidosis, potassium ions shift out of the cell while excess H^+ moves into the cell, resulting in a pseudohyperkalemia even when the whole-body potassium presence is actually normal or perhaps decreased.

Treatment

CCTPs should resist the temptation to treat every metabolic acidosis with IV sodium bicarbonate. Certain conditions, such as RTA, hyperchloremic acidosis, and isolated GI bicarbonate losses, are amenable to treatment with IV sodium bicarbonate, but other causes of metabolic acidosis require a more specific approach. Indeed, it is usually better to correct the underlying cause of acidosis and provide supportive care. Furthermore, adequate ventilation is mandatory to allow elimination of the extra carbon dioxide produced with sodium bicarbonate administration. Sodium bicarbonate is indicated in patients with significant bicarbonate losses (eg, RTA, fistula), hyperkalemia, and sodium channel blocker overdose.

Lactic acidosis requires correction of cellular metabolism, which cannot be accomplished with administration of sodium bicarbonate. Improving cellular metabolism will cause production of excess H^+ to cease and will allow normal acid–base control mechanisms to restore a physiologic pH. Optimal

tissue oxygen delivery and adequate perfusion are the primary goals of lactic acidosis treatment, along with more specific management of potential underlying causes.

The various types of RTA are treated with agents such as sodium bicarbonate or sodium citrate, often over long periods of time. Calcium, potassium, and other electrolytes require careful monitoring and often repletion, depending on the particular type of RTA. Type 2 RTA is characterized by urine bicarbonate and potassium wasting, so it often requires potassium repletion. Type 4 RTA is characterized by hyperkalemia; it often requires volume expansion, potassium-wasting diuretics, or even mineralocorticoid replacement therapy in certain situations.

Sodium bicarbonate is not recommended for the treatment of diabetic ketoacidosis and has been shown to cause cerebral edema when administered to children with this condition. Diabetic ketoacidosis is best managed with fluid volume restoration, IV insulin, and electrolyte (especially potassium and sodium) correction.

Alcoholic ketoacidosis, another cellular starvation acidosis, is not treated with IV sodium bicarbonate unless the patient has a profound, life-threatening acidosis (pH <7.1) that is refractory to fluid repletion and dextrose supplementation. Instead, this condition is treated with IV fluids and carbohydrates to improve the patient's nutritional status and allow normal metabolic processes to resume. Crystalloid resuscitation with supplementation of dextrose and thiamine (administered before the dextrose solution to correct deficiencies and prevent Wernicke encephalopathy) are generally the only medications needed for treatment of these patients.

Other causes of metabolic acidosis, such as uremia and exposure to toxic chemicals, require specialty consultation and often complex treatment. CCTPs should seek medical direction when transporting patients with these conditions.

Diagnosis and management of patients with metabolic alterations of acid–base status can challenge CCTPs. Clinical suspicion, focused investigation, and optimal treatment of these disorders will improve patient outcomes and minimize the adverse impacts of many serious medical conditions. Providers should consider the potential for and consequences of metabolic acid–base alterations during every critical care transport.

Flight Considerations

CCTPs must take precautions and sometimes modify care-related techniques when performing air medical patient transport. Unpressurized or under-pressurized aircraft place patients with GI/GU conditions at increased risk for complications related to transport. Careful assessment and simple interventions can eliminate or minimize many of these potential adverse effects.

GU complications specifically related to air medical transport are rare. Prolonged exposure to altitude will alter urinary pH. Pneumaturia (the presence of gas within the bladder) can occur following a UTI caused by certain microorganisms, after manipulation of the GU tract, and when a fistula develops between the digestive tract and bladder (causing the bowel contents to contaminate the normally sterile bladder environment). Pneumaturia requires more specific interventions, often including an indwelling urinary (Foley) catheter for bladder and urinary tract decompression. Although placement of a catheter offers some benefits—it eliminates the need for the patient to void during transport, allows the CCTP to observe urine output, and prevents complications associated with urinary retention—the risks of infection are now considered to outweigh these benefits. Thus, routine placement of a Foley catheter is no longer a recommended practice.

Compared to GU complications, GI complications during air medical transport are much more common. Sequestered gases due to abdominal surgery, bowel obstruction, and abdominal trauma will expand significantly as cabin altitude increases. Indeed, ascending from sea level to 9,000 feet will cause any sequestered gas to expand by 50%. In severe situations, this gas expansion can lead to respiratory compromise, severe discomfort, syncope, and vasovagal episodes.

Patients with any of the previously mentioned conditions should have an NG or OG tube placed prior to any increase in cabin altitude. Once these tubes are in place, they should be either vented to ambient air or connected to suction for the duration of the transport. Patients with a colostomy should have their devices frequently monitored for excessive amounts of gas and either emptied or changed if this complication occurs. If at all possible, patients who have undergone abdominal surgery should wait 24 to 48 hours after their procedure before being transported by air.

Summary

The GI and GU systems are complex pathways through the body that support critical functions—the digestion of food and the elimination of wastes, respectively. Over the life span, these systems must withstand constant usage, leading to inevitable wear and tear. The many GI/GU pathologies that can occur require prompt recognition and treatment to preserve function. Because of the many interactions of these systems with accessory organs and other systems, local problems can quickly evolve into systemic ones. Through awareness of the possible diseases, history taking, and proper assessment, many complications can be prevented or corrected at an early stage.

The CCTP serves as the connection between the patient and the tertiary care required to manage GI/GU conditions. The continuity of care provided by the CCTP is a fundamental contributor to the treatment and recovery of the critically ill patient with such a condition. When a problem arises during transport, the CCTP is responsible for correcting it and preventing its recurrence. Being equipped with this knowledge provides the CCTP and the patient with the greatest likelihood for a safe, uneventful transfer.

Case Study

Your CCT crew is called to a community hospital ICU for transport of a 48-year-old man with a Mallory-Weiss tear and uncontrolled hemorrhage to a tertiary hospital 35 miles away. On arrival, your partner begins an assessment of the patient while you obtain a report from the patient's nurse and transferring physician.

The patient is described as having a drinking problem; he told staff that he normally consumes half a case of beer each day. The patient was admitted at 0500 hours, 14 hours before you were called, because of protracted vomiting that began the previous evening. The emesis initially appeared to the patient to be gastric contents, but after several hours it changed to have the color of bright red blood. His stools were also melanotic. The patient reported epigastric pain radiating to his back as an 8 on a scale of 0 to 10. He was hemodynamically unstable with the following values: pulse rate, 130 beats/min; BP, 80/50 mm Hg; and unlabored respirations, 26 breaths/min. He was afebrile. Past medical history included hypertension, hyperlipidemia, coronary artery disease, depression, alcohol use disorder, and obstructive sleep apnea. His medications included metoprolol, 50 mg twice daily; aspirin, 81 mg daily; and a statin. He denies having any allergies. Admission lab work revealed the following values: blood alcohol level, 160 mg/dL, hemoglobin level, 7.3 g/dL (normal, 14.0–17.5 g/dL); platelet count, 100,000/μL (normal, 150,000–350,000/μL); and clotting times (an international normalized ratio) that were 1.5 times normal. Electrolytes were normal except for a potassium level of 3.1 mEq/L (normal, 3.5–5.0 mEq/L). Cardiac enzymes and a 12-lead ECG were normal.

The patient received 1 L of normal saline while awaiting blood bank type and crossmatching for transfusion of packed red blood cells. His BP increased to 130/80 mm Hg, pulse rate slowed to 90 beats/min, and respirations slowed to 18 breaths/min. He was transfused with 2 units of packed red blood cells, and a bolus of pantoprazole was administered intravenously. Nausea was controlled by IV ondansetron, and morphine was administered for analgesia.

A gastroenterologist performed an endoscopy to determine the cause of the bloody emesis, which revealed a single, longitudinal tear in the esophagus, extending from the stomach cardia through the esophagogastric junction and upward into the esophagus. A second tear extended from the junction upward into the esophagus. Both appeared to be actively bleeding. Control of bleeding was attempted with epinephrine injections; when oozing continued, several hemoclips were applied that achieved seemingly good control of the bleeding. The patient remained in the ICU. A repeat hemoglobin level was 8.1 g/dL, and vital signs remained stable.

Serial hematocrit levels showed a gradual decline, and the patient became increasingly tachycardic and hypotensive. Three additional units of packed red blood cells and two units of fresh frozen plasma were transfused. When his BP remained low, an infusion of norepinephrine was titrated to maintain a MAP greater than 60 mm Hg. The patient had two additional episodes of hematemesis and was intubated for airway protection after he was noted to have an aspiration event. A CVC was placed in the right internal jugular vein. A Foley urinary catheter was placed for fluid monitoring. The ICU physician decided that the patient needed to be transferred for a higher level of care.

Your partner's assessment of the patient showed a sedated and mechanically ventilated 48-year-old man who appears malnourished. He has a mildly distended but soft abdomen and coarse respirations in the right lung base. His MAP is 68 mm Hg on 10 μg/min of norepinephrine infusing in one of the three lumens of a right internal jugular CVC. Assessment also reveals a heart rate of 130 beats/min and oxygen saturation of 98%. The patient is mechanically ventilated via assist-control with a tidal volume of 450 mL, respiratory rate of 20 breaths/min, FIO_2 of 60%, and PEEP of 8 cm H_2O. The most recent hemoglobin level, measured approximately 3 hours after the last transfusion but before his latest hematemesis, was 9.0 g/dL. His pH on the most recent ABG sample is 7.25, and his bicarbonate is 10 mEq/L. Per the Foley bag, his urinary output has been approximately 0.5 mL/kg/h. He had been medicated with ondansetron for his last bout of vomiting and is receiving an infusion of propofol running at 60 mg/h, with intermittent push doses of fentanyl. He appears to be adequately sedated. The patient is currently receiving a sixth unit of packed red blood cells through his peripheral IV line and just received 4 mg of calcium gluconate. The medications infusing match the doses stated in the report, and both the IV and the CVC appear to be functioning well.

During transport, the patient became aroused and was slightly agitated, so the propofol infusion was increased to 80 mg/h. His BP began to drop, and norepinephrine was titrated to 20 μg/min to maintain a MAP of 60 to 65 mm Hg, and the blood transfusion continued. No further hypotension occurred, and the patient was transferred to the ICU at the tertiary medical center.

1. Why was the initial hypokalemia not treated? Why did the patient receive a dose of calcium gluconate?
2. Did the patient have an adequate response to transfused blood products?
3. Discuss his volume status. What is his acid–base status?
4. Would a fluid bolus have been preferable to increasing the vasopressor infusion to maintain BP?

Analysis

Packed red blood cell transfusion is directly associated with hyperkalemia, especially in patients who receive multiple units of blood. Cell breakdown results in increased potassium extracellularly as intracellular stores are released. The hospital staff recognized from the admission laboratory work and patient presentation that multiple units of blood would be required. Furthermore, significant blood product transfusion is associated with hypocalcemia and cardiac dysrhythmias. In a patient with a history of cardiac disease, the staff was right in anticipating and preventing complications by administering calcium gluconate.

The patient did not have an adequate response to the transfused blood products. He received 5 units of packed red blood cells. The subsequent hemoglobin level was 9.0 g/dL, an increase from his initial level of 7.3 g/dL. Since we can expect each unit of packed red blood cells to increase the hemoglobin by 1 g/dL, it is apparent that the patient is having ongoing bleeding. He received 1 L of normal saline during initial resuscitation, as well as several units of blood products. His urine output is not optimal, likely as a result of hypotension and subsequent kidney injury. He may benefit from a small bolus of crystalloid (such as 500 mL) to determine if his urine output increases, but fluid resuscitation needs to be judicious. He has a history of cardiac disease, and is receiving a large volume of fluid in total through his infusions and carriers, and we know that his hypotension is likely the result of ongoing bleeding and hemorrhagic shock. His clinical course will improve with control of bleeding and continued replacement of blood products. Based on the overall picture and his lab values, he appears to have a metabolic acidosis, likely from a mixed picture of alcoholic ketoacidosis and lactic acidosis in the setting of tissue hypoperfusion.

Unstable patients vomiting blood originating in their esophagus or stomach can present significant airway concerns, especially if their mental status deteriorates. This patient tolerated an endoscopy and maintained his airway appropriately until he had repeat episodes of hematemesis. He was noted to have aspiration followed by oxygen desaturation, likely from a combination of altered mental status from acidosis and anemia, and lung tissue irritation from aspirated vomitus. He was appropriately intubated for airway protection.

The latest hemoglobin level was still low at 9.0 g/dL, and he had subsequent hematemesis and hypotension. He is receiving a sixth unit of blood during transport and already has norepinephrine running. His BP likely decreased from the vasodilatory effects of the increased dosage of propofol that was administered to manage his agitation. The CCTP could have opted to provide an increased amount or more frequent doses of fentanyl instead. To support the patient's BP, the CCTPs had a choice of increasing the norepinephrine infusion or the rate of the blood transfusion. They chose to increase the vasopressor dose, which served to support BP until the patient's volume status could be restored. Administration of crystalloid is an option if vasopressors and increased blood replacement rate are not effective, although a preferable alternative would have been to add a second vasopressor agent, vasopressin. Vasopressin would have the added benefit of reducing splanchnic circulation, possibly accelerating hemostasis.

Bleeding associated with Mallory-Weiss tears stops spontaneously in most cases. Factors likely responsible for the excessive bleeding in this patient include his history of alcohol use disorder and the associated liver dysfunction as evidenced by prolonged clotting times. He was also thrombocytopenic. While these factors could have resulted in the declining hematocrit, it is also possible that the patient had another source of bleeding in his GI tract.

Prep Kit

Ready for Review

- Homeostasis depends on a number of metabolic processes involving the gastrointestinal (GI) and genitourinary (GU) systems, but these processes can be affected by a number of pathologic conditions. Assessment and management of GI and GU pathologies are inherently difficult because the signs and symptoms that accompany them may be vague and difficult to recognize.
- The GI system consists of a network of organs and ducts devoted to the digestion of food and the extraction of its nutritional content.
- The alimentary canal contains numerous specialized cells and tissues. Four layers are seen almost continuously from the esophagus to the rectum: the mucosa, the submucosa, the muscularis externa, and the serosa.
- The alimentary canal maintains a chemical environment that is effective in digesting food, yet does not alter the environment of the rest of the body.
- The alimentary canal consists of the mouth, pharynx, esophagus, stomach, small intestine, and large intestine; food travels through these structures and finally exits the body via the rectum.
- The renal system provides a path for wastes to leave the body and maintains proper electrolyte parameters.
- The kidneys continuously filter blood, manage volume, maintain appropriate balances between acids and bases, and discard toxins and excesses by producing urine. The remainder of the urinary system—the ureters, urinary bladder, and urethra—provides for the transport and storage of urine during its journey out of the body.
- The purpose of the male reproductive system is to generate sperm and provide a means for its delivery to a fertilizable egg in the female partner.
- The female reproductive system produces and develops eggs. In addition, the uterus of the female provides a home for a developing embryo during gestation.

- Pregnant patients who present with an acute abdomen are considered a surgical emergency and require an appropriate diagnosis to avoid the risk of maternal and fetal mortality.
- Women of childbearing age may present with severe abdominal pain that may appear to be caused by GI or GU etiologies, although complications of pregnancy must always be considered.
- Symptoms of GI abnormalities typically include abdominal pain, tenderness, and bleeding.
- GI bleeding can be classified into two categories based on the location of the bleeding: upper GI bleeding and lower GI bleeding.
- Endoscopy is the preferred method for locating the source of GI bleeding. Vessel imaging and interventional angiographic approaches provide alternative means of localizing and treating such bleeding.
- Colonoscopy can visualize the entire rectum and large intestine, up to the ileocecal junction.
- In angiography, dye is injected into blood vessels, which will leak into the lumen of the GI tract at the site of GI bleeding.
- Peptic ulcers are the leading cause of upper GI bleeding.
- Widespread implementation of proton pump inhibitors and histamine-2 blockers have reduced the prevalence of gastric mucosal erosion.
- Acute gastritis is characterized by a rapid onset of mucosal inflammation, frequently accompanied by mild to severe upper GI bleeding.
- Alcohol and tobacco use, diet, and NSAID use are major patient-driven factors that can lead to GI bleeding.
- Reactive gastritis is a chronic mucosal edema that results from recurring contact of the mucosa with antagonistic substances such as bile, pancreatic juice, or NSAIDs.
- When portal hypertension occurs, venous blood will use alternative pathways for its return to the

Prep Kit Continued

vena cava via the azygos system. An esophageal varix occurs when the swelling of esophageal veins intrudes into the lumen of the esophagus.

- In cirrhosis, buildup of fatty acids, in combination with chronic destruction of liver tissue and fibrosis, obstructs blood flow.
- The leading cause of cirrhosis is infection with the hepatitis C virus, with alcoholic liver disease closely following as the second most common cause.
- Mallory-Weiss syndrome involves a longitudinal laceration of the esophageal mucosa as a result of repeated significant changes in local pressure, such as those seen in forceful vomiting.
- Diverticulosis is a disease of the lower GI tract that is commonly seen in older adults. Diverticula are a common source of lower GI bleeding.
- Diverticulitis, an inflammation of the diverticula, is frequently a result of infection from invading intestinal bacteria.
- Angiodysplasia is a malformation of submucosal blood vessels in the GI tract.
- Inflammation and infection of the appendix cause appendicitis. The classic presentation is a relatively rapid onset of right lower quadrant pain, nausea and vomiting, and fever.
- Inflammatory bowel disease is a collective term covering ulcerative colitis and Crohn disease.
- Ulcerative colitis is an inflammation of the rectal mucosal and submucosal tissues. Bloody diarrhea is common in patients with this condition.
- Crohn disease is a less organized inflammation of the GI tract, in which all layers of the mucosa may be affected.
- Radiation colitis and immune checkpoint inhibitor colitis may also result in lower GI bleeding.
- Symptoms of GI bleeding include melena, diffuse abdominal pain, emesis and hematemesis, fever, complaints of frequent dizziness and syncope, diarrhea, dehydration, and cardiac arrhythmias.

- Symptoms of significant GI bleeding include hemodynamic instability, shock, large amounts of bright red blood in emesis, hematochezia, hypotension, tachycardia, diaphoresis, altered mental status, and a decreased level of consciousness.
- Ongoing decreases in the hemoglobin and hematocrit values indicate active bleeding.
- Pressure ulcers can arise from prolonged pressure on body tissues; they are commonly seen in patients confined to a bed.
- During acute GI bleeding, airway compromise occurs primarily by physical obstruction or mechanical obstruction.
- Any patient with acute GI bleeding should be designated as nothing by mouth (nil per os [NPO]), and blood samples should be drawn concurrently with IV placement.
- Treatments for endoscopic- and pharmacologic-refractory variceal hemorrhage include balloon inflation (during emergent, life-threatening bleeding) and transjugular intrahepatic shunt placement.
- The introduction of a transjugular intrahepatic portosystemic shunt into the systemic venous circulation results in a significant decrease in the hepatic portal pressure and, in turn, a significant decrease in the pressure in the esophageal collateral veins.
- A mechanical intestinal obstruction results from a physical blockage of the intestinal lumen and can be classified into one of three categories: extrinsic, intrinsic, or intraluminal.
- Ileus is the lack of movement of the GI contents through the intestines in the absence of a mechanical obstruction.
- In a patient with an intestinal obstruction, the abdomen is diffusely tender and distended on palpation.
- A computed tomographic (CT) scan can be used to diagnose a bowel obstruction with exceptional specificity.
- After addressing any life threats to the patient's airway, breathing, or cardiac functioning, initial

Prep Kit Continued

treatment of a patient with intestinal obstruction focuses on fluid resuscitation and bowel rest.

- A nasogastric or orogastric tube may already be in place when the CCTP first encounters the patient, particularly during interfacility transports.
- Air transport should be postponed or avoided for any patient with a bowel obstruction, if possible.
- In general, an insult to the liver is either infectious or noninfectious. If the insult resolves within 6 months without any permanent function deficit, it is termed acute. When symptoms persist longer, the patient is diagnosed with chronic liver disease.
- Hepatitis, an inflammation of the liver, is the physiologic result of any liver disease.
- Fulminant hepatic failure is the result of a sudden significant insult to the liver, such as severe alcohol intoxication, drug overdose (eg, acetaminophen), or acute hepatitis viral infection.
- When bilirubin, which is normally conjugated by hepatocytes and excreted via bile, begins to build up in the blood as part of the hepatitis pathway, it results in jaundice and scleral icterus.
- Symptoms of early acute hepatitis include general malaise, generalized fatigue, and fever and chills. Symptoms of chronic hepatitis include portal hypertension, melena, hematochezia, shortness of breath, hypotension, tachycardia, and hair loss.
- Patients with cirrhosis and ascites are at risk of infection of the ascitic fluid, termed spontaneous bacterial peritonitis.
- Spontaneous bacterial peritonitis and hepatorenal syndrome portend poor outcomes for patients with end-stage liver disease.
- Liver function is assessed by evaluating the presence of the liver's synthesized products as well as the absence of its cellular enzymes in the blood. It is important to recognize the distinction between tests for liver function and markers of injury.

- Treatment of hepatitis focuses on preventing further injury, with a goal of avoiding progression to cirrhosis.
- Blockage of the biliary tracts at any point will result in a backup of bile and, possibly, depending on the location of the obstruction, pancreatic enzymes.
- Gallstones in the gallbladder (cholelithiasis) are a fairly common condition that causes colicky pain in the right upper quadrant of the abdomen. Patients may present with nausea and vomiting and a positive Murphy sign.
- Techniques for imaging and detecting choledocholithiasis include transabdominal ultrasonography, endoscopic ultrasonography, hepatoiminodiacetic acid scanning, magnetic resonance cholangiopancreatography, endoscopic retrograde cholangiopancreatography, and percutaneous transhepatic cholangiography.
- Immediate treatment of symptomatic cholecystitis, cholelithiasis, and choledocholithiasis focuses on pain management, antiemetics, and maintaining NPO status. Hypotension may need to be addressed with fluid resuscitation.
- Ascending cholangitis is a serious infection of the biliary system, which usually occurs after a blockage. Patients may present with right upper quadrant pain, jaundice, fever, shock, and altered mental status. IV antibiotics must be administered promptly in anticipation of interventional management of the obstruction.
- Inflammation of the pancreas (pancreatitis) can lead to significant impairment of the GI physiology depending on its level of severity and etiology.
- Upper abdominal pain is the primary symptom of pancreatitis; other symptoms include tenderness and guarding of the abdomen, tachycardia, nausea and vomiting, and a fever. Turner sign, Cullen sign, jaundice, hemodynamic instability, and shock may result from severe pancreatitis.

Prep Kit Continued

- Elevated serum amylase and serum lipase support a diagnosis of pancreatitis, with serum lipase being the diagnostic test of choice.
- A CT scan with contrast can provide a direct visual observation of pancreatic necrosis, peripancreatic abnormalities, abscesses, and overall size of the pancreas.
- General treatment of pancreatitis includes fluid resuscitation, analgesia, and antiemetics.
- Significant decreases in renal perfusion pressure disrupt the elimination of waste from the bloodstream by lowering the glomerular filtration rate (GFR). When this condition develops in the absence of preexisting renal dysfunction, it is termed acute kidney injury (AKI).
- Symptoms of AKI include dizziness, poor skin turgor, thirst, flat neck veins, dry mucous membranes, weight loss, orthostatic BP changes, fever, edema, ascites, and low back pain.
- A family history of renal disease indicates a predisposition to AKI when a precursory disease of AKI is present. The incidence of AKI is increased in patients with diabetes, hypertension, and lupus.
- The retention of wastes in the bloodstream that results from a decreased GFR provides an easy way to monitor for the existence and severity of AKI. Renal ultrasonography is the gold-standard imaging modality for assessing suspected postrenal AKI.
- A gradual decrease in renal function over a long time interval is known as chronic kidney disease (CKD).
- The results of lab studies for CKD and end-stage renal disease (ESRD) generally parallel the results seen for AKI. The most important factor in determining whether the renal failure is acute or chronic is disease duration.
- Elevations in BUN and creatinine are common in patients with kidney injury. Additional studies that evaluate excretion of electrolytes and osmolality can help determine whether injury is prerenal, intrinsic, or post-obstructive.

- Both patients with ESRD and those with acute renal failure require renal replacement therapy, which can be performed via various approaches, including IHD, continuous venovenous hemodialysis, and peritoneal dialysis.
- The bacterial flora that live symbiotically in the GI system can cause considerable damage when these organisms are introduced into the urinary system. A urinary tract infection typically begins in the urethra, because this location is the most proximal to the external environment.
- Nephrolithiasis is the condition in which the body produces renal calculi, commonly referred to as kidney stones. Kidney stones cause considerable pain during their transit through the ureters, and larger stones risk becoming impacted and causing obstruction, which may result in severe infection, hydronephrosis, and kidney injury.
- Testicular torsion, a condition in which one or both of the testes rotate to the point of occluding their blood supply, is a urologic emergency that needs to be addressed within 6 hours of symptom onset.
- Direct blunt trauma to the penis during penile erection can result in penile fracture—that is, a rupture of one or more of the vascular spaces within the penis.
- Priapism is a prolonged erection of the penis that can be painful and damaging to tissues in the immediate area. It is generally classified as either high-flow priapism or low-flow, ischemic priapism.
- A simple nasogastric tube can be used to administer food into the stomach or to remove food. For long-term situations, a gastrostomy tube (G tube) or percutaneous endoscopic gastrostomy (PEG) tube can be inserted.
- Total parenteral nutrition (TPN) is an alternative feeding method used when the GI tract is not functioning adequately.
- When transporting a patient with a feeding tube, contact medical direction if the patient

Prep Kit Continued

has vomiting, abdominal distention, or diarrhea.

- Straight catheters (intermittent catheters) are ideal for removal of urine in patients who do not have chronic urinary retention or sedation, as these devices are not associated with increased risk of urinary tract infection.
- When surgery or trauma contraindicates introduction of a urethral catheter, a suprapubic tube can be placed directly into the urinary bladder through the abdominal wall by way of a surgically created stoma.
- Common complications of urine collection catheters include clogging, infection, pain, leakage, and dislodgement.
- An ostomy is a surgically created opening of the GI tract through the abdomen that allows for waste removal.
- The patient with an ostomy should be monitored for signs of tissue necrosis and infection, which, if detected, may warrant treatments ranging from antibiotic therapy to surgical intervention.
- Jackson-Pratt drains are inserted to remove postoperative buildup of fluid and blood in the abdominal cavity. During liver transplant surgery, a T tube is placed to monitor bile drainage from the gallbladder.
- In-flight complications need to be considered for patients with any of the numerous drainage systems that include closed bags containing air. Excess air should be vented from any drainage bag such as a colostomy or urostomy prior to flight in anticipation of changes in air pressure.
- Be sure to unclamp any feeding or drainage catheters prior to departure, and ensure that they remain unclamped for the duration of travel.
- Significant alterations of oxygen and carbon dioxide levels, electrolyte concentrations, temperature, glucose levels, and acid–base status will impair cell, tissue, and organ function, eventually leading to death if not corrected.
- The relationship of acids to bases within the body is expressed by pH, which represents the concentration of free hydrogen ions (H^+) present.
- The bicarbonate–carbonic acid buffer system is the principal extracellular buffer system that operates primarily in the lungs and kidneys, where carbonic anhydrase stimulates the chemical reaction.
- The phosphate buffer system operates similarly to the bicarbonate–carbonic acid buffer system in that it allows only small pH changes following large variations in the presence of free H^+.
- The concentration of free H^+ in extracellular fluid (pH) as well as other key variables can be obtained from an arterial blood gas (ABG) or venous blood gas (VBG) sample.
- Results from an ABG sample provide the CCTP with valuable information about the existence or type of acidosis or alkalosis.
- In most cases, the VBG sample is adequate for evaluation of Pco_2 and pH when an ABG is not available. Patients in severe shock or with mechanical ventilation warrant use of an ABG sample for measuring lab values.
- Total blood carbon dioxide (written as either Tco_2 or "bicarbonate" in clinical practice) provides an indication of an acid–base abnormality on routine blood work.
- When an acidosis is suspected, its origin can be examined using the anion gap.
- When metabolic conditions create an excess of bicarbonate accompanied by a pH greater than 7.45 on an ABG sample, the disorder is termed metabolic alkalosis.
- Metabolic acidosis is demonstrated by a decreased serum pH (less than 7.35) accompanied by a decreased bicarbonate concentration (less than 22 mmol/L).
- Renal and hepatic dysfunction cause metabolic acidosis through a variety of mechanisms.
- Metabolic acidosis is rarely a clinically isolated occurrence. The underlying pathologic conditions that cause the acidosis predominantly determine the patient's clinical status.
- IV sodium bicarbonate will not provide adequate treatment of an acidosis.

Prep Kit Continued

Vital Vocabulary

acute kidney injury (AKI) Decreased renal function in the absence of preexisting renal disease. Classified into three categories: prerenal, intrarenal, and postrenal.

acute tubular necrosis Damage to the tubules of the nephron, preventing proper ion and fluid exchange in the kidneys.

adhesions Bands of connective tissue that can distort the normal GI anatomy; the result of improper healing or scar tissue growth following surgery.

alcoholic ketoacidosis A type of acidosis characterized by a buildup of ketones in the blood, caused by a large intake of alcohol and poor nutritional intake.

angiodysplasia Deformed submucosal blood vessels in the GI tract that are susceptible to bleeding.

appendicitis Inflammation and/or infection of the appendix.

ascites A buildup of fluid in the abdominal cavity.

azotemia Increased nitrogenous wastes in the blood.

azygos system A network of blood vessels that connects the superior and inferior vena cava; it also drains a portion of the esophageal venous blood.

bicarbonate–carbonic acid buffer system The principal extracellular buffer system, which operates primarily in the lungs and kidneys; in this system, carbon dioxide and water are reversibly converted into carbonic acid, which in turn is reversibly converted into hydrogen ions and bicarbonate.

bilirubin A waste product of heme formed during erythrocyte metabolism. It is moved to the small intestine within bile and then converted into urobilinogen, resulting in brown pigmented feces.

Boerhaave syndrome Esophageal rupture, associated with subcutaneous emphysema, chest pain, and vomiting.

buffer Any substance that can alternately bind or release hydrogen ions depending on the outside conditions.

Charcot triad Fever, jaundice, and right upper quadrant abdominal pain suggestive of choledocholithiasis.

cholangitis A serious ascending infection due to biliary tract obstruction that can result in fever, transaminitis, and altered mental status.

cholecystitis Inflammation of the gallbladder.

choledocholithiasis Gallstones in the biliary tract system, which put the patient at high risk for developing a biliary tract obstruction; typically initially managed with endoscopic retrograde cholangiopancreatography rather than cholecystectomy.

cholelithiasis Gallstones in the gallbladder.

chronic kidney disease (CKD) A gradual decrease in renal function resulting from irreversible damage to the nephrons. It is characterized by a glomerular filtration rate of less than 60 mL/min, and eventually progresses to end-stage renal disease.

cirrhosis Irreversible structural changes to the liver that impair its proper functioning.

colitis Inflammation of the colon.

colonoscopy An endoscopy of the lower GI tract.

concentration gradient The natural tendency for substances to flow from an area of higher concentration to an area of lower concentration, within or outside the cell.

creatinine The metabolized form of creatine that is eliminated through the urine. Increased levels indicate decreased GFR and renal function.

Crohn disease An inflammation of the GI tract in which all layers of the mucosa may be affected. It results in scattered ulcerations and fibroses throughout the large and small intestines.

CT angiography Radiographic observation of dye injected into the bloodstream.

diabetic ketoacidosis A form of acidosis observed in uncontrolled diabetes in which ketones

Prep Kit Continued

accumulate when insulin is not available; usually associated with hyperglycemia.

diverticula Small pouches of tissue that develop as outcroppings of the large intestine, typically in the descending colon and sigmoid colon.

diverticular bleeding Bleeding from diverticula that have developed in the colon.

diverticulitis Inflammation of diverticula.

diverticulosis Presence of intestinal diverticula, which may then become inflamed or bleed.

endoscopic retrograde cholangiopancreatography (ERCP) A technique combining endoscopy and fluoroscopy to diagnose and treat biliary or pancreatic ductal obstruction.

end-stage renal disease (ESRD) A loss of proper kidney functioning, with renal replacement therapy becoming a requirement for survival.

enteroclysis Infusion of barium contrast into the GI tract to observe for obstruction.

esophageal varix Swelling of esophageal veins that intrudes into the lumen of the esophagus.

esophagitis Inflammation of the tissues of the esophagus; commonly associated with severe gastroesophageal reflux disease, alcohol abuse, or irritation caused by pills or infection.

esophagogastroduodenoscopy (EGD) A technique to directly observe the GI tract in which a camera is passed into the GI tract, allowing for diagnosis and treatment of disease or injury.

fulminant hepatic failure A sudden and significant insult to the liver characterized by encephalopathy and a high mortality rate; commonly caused by toxins/overdose or viral infection.

gallstone pancreatitis A type of pancreatitis in which pancreatic enzymes accumulate proximal to a bile duct obstruction from a gallstone and digest the tissues of both the duct and the pancreas.

gastritis Inflammation of the gastric mucosa that occurs when the equilibrium of active and protective mechanisms for the lining is altered; may be accompanied by upper GI bleeding.

gastroenteritis Watery diarrhea and vomiting during inflammation of the digestive tract as a result of a viral, bacterial, or parasitic infection.

glomerular filtration rate (GFR) The amount of fluid filtered by the glomerulus per minute; a benchmark for renal function.

Helicobacter pylori A bacterium that is commonly associated with gastritis and peptic ulcers.

hematemesis Emesis containing blood, which may be bright red or partially digested (coffee-ground emesis).

hematochezia Stool streaked with bright red blood.

hepatic encephalopathy Encephalopathy secondary to hepatic disease, usually associated with hyperammonemia.

hepatitis Inflammation of liver cells that can impede proper functioning of the liver and lead to chronic conditions such as cirrhosis.

hepatitis C virus The virus that is the most common cause of cirrhosis and is especially pathogenic in causing hepatitis.

hepatorenal syndrome A condition characterized by renal injury and renal failure in patients with cirrhosis; decreased cardiac output and decreased systemic vascular resistance result in a cycle of worsening renal perfusion and renal vasoconstriction.

hernia A protrusion of an organ from its tissue lining.

homeostasis Stability in the body's internal environment.

ileus A lack of movement of GI contents in the absence of an obstruction, usually occurring post-surgery.

inflammatory bowel disease (IBD) Term covering two colon inflammation pathologies: ulcerative colitis and Crohn disease.

intussusception A telescoping of the intestine into an adjacent segment.

ischemic colitis A potentially life-threatening form of colitis that results from diminished blood flow to the GI tract.

Prep Kit Continued

Jackson-Pratt drain A surgical drain used to remove fluid buildup from the wound site during the postoperative healing process.

jejunostomy tube (J tube) A feeding tube placed through the abdominal wall into the jejunum.

lactic acidosis A form of acidosis caused by an excess accumulation or impaired excretion of lactate, leading to an elevated anion gap; it can result from exposure to various toxic substances, inadequate tissue perfusion in various shock states, dysfunction of certain organs, nutritional deficiency, infection, malignancy, diabetes, or hereditary metabolic disorders.

ligament of Treitz A small ligament supporting the small intestine at the junction between the duodenum and the jejunum. It serves as the dividing point between the upper and lower GI tract.

lithotripsy Use of external vibrations to break up gallstones.

Mallory-Weiss syndrome Laceration and bleeding of the esophagus, often following forceful vomiting.

melena Black, tarry stool containing partially digested blood, with the bleeding usually originating from the upper GI tract.

metabolic acidosis A pathologic condition (blood pH <7.35) resulting from an accumulation of acids in the body caused by any number of systems in the body, including the gastrointestinal system, or by major organ failure.

metabolic alkalosis A pathologic condition (blood pH >7.45) resulting from an accumulation of bases in the body caused by any number of systems in the body, including the gastrointestinal system, or by major organ failure.

Minnesota esophagogastric tamponade tube A tube that is placed to stop bleeding of esophageal varices. It is similar to the Sengstaken-Blakemore tube, but has a built-in suction catheter.

mixed acidosis A pathologic condition in which there is a low pH (<7.35), an elevated Pco_2 level (>45 mm Hg), and a low bicarbonate level (<22 mmol/L); it occurs when both respiratory and metabolic acidosis are present at the same time.

mixed alkalosis A pathologic condition in which there is an elevated pH (>7.45), a low Pco_2 level (<35 mm Hg), and an elevated bicarbonate level (>26 mmol/L); it occurs when both respiratory and metabolic alkalosis are present at the same time.

mucosa The outermost layer of the alimentary canal. It consists of three sublayers: surface epithelium, lamina propria, and muscularis mucosae.

Murphy sign Pain following palpation of the right upper abdomen, especially with deep inspiration.

muscularis externa The third tissue layer of the alimentary canal. It contains two levels in most places: the circular layer and the longitudinal layer.

nephrolithiasis A condition in which the body produces renal calculi (kidney stones), which are often symptomatic as they travel through the ureters; may produce impaction and infection of the urinary tract.

nonalcoholic fatty liver disease (NAFLD) Accumulation of fat in the liver, for which alcohol consumption is not believed to be a contributing factor.

ostomy A surgically created opening through which feces can be voided in the absence of some or all of the large intestine or rectum.

pancreatitis Inflammation of the pancreas leading to autodigestion, tissue destruction, and impaired function.

paracentesis Insertion of a needle into the abdomen to aspirate ascites; often done to diagnose spontaneous bacterial peritonitis.

penile fracture A rupture of one of the blood-containing sacs in the penis, resulting in deformity and possible loss of function.

peptic ulcer An erosion of the mucosal lining of the GI tract.

Prep Kit Continued

percutaneous endoscopic gastrostomy (PEG) tube A feeding tube that is placed through the abdominal wall into the stomach.

peristalsis A general term describing wavelike muscular contractions of tubular organs, which carry forward materials or liquids contained in those organs.

peritoneal dialysis (PD) Dialysate solution injected into the abdomen, using the peritoneum as a natural semipermeable membrane to separate solutes.

peritonitis Inflammation of the peritoneum; typically results in generalized abdominal tenderness and guarding.

phosphate buffer system The buffer system that functions in the renal tubules and intracellular fluids to convert strong acids or bases into weak acids or bases so that they have a minimal effect on the body's overall pH.

point-of-care testing (POCT) Laboratory testing that is performed at the patient's bedside, so that results can be obtained quickly and considered while decisions are still being made about patient care.

portal hypertension An increase in vascular resistance through the hepatic portal system. It can cause high venous pressure in the gastric and esophageal veins, leading to varices, among other problems.

pressure ulcer A sore on the skin arising from prolonged pressure. Such ulcers are classified into four stages, with stage 4 being the most severe (tissue necrosis and muscle and bone involvement); all stages are painful and susceptible to infection.

priapism Prolonged, painful erection of the penis; a urologic emergency.

pyelonephritis An infection of the kidney, typically the result of an ascending urinary tract infection.

reactive gastritis Gastric irritation that results from recurring contact of the mucosa with antagonistic substances such as bile, pancreatic juice, or nonsteroidal anti-inflammatory drugs.

renal perfusion pressure The gradient between renal arterial and venous flow. A significant decrease in this pressure results in ischemia.

renal tubular acidosis (RTA) A form of metabolic acidosis caused by dysfunction of the kidneys or renal system; it presents without an elevated anion gap.

respiratory acidosis A pathologic condition (blood pH <7.35) resulting from an accumulation of acids in the body owing to a breathing problem or insufficient function of the respiratory system.

respiratory alkalosis A pathologic condition (blood pH >7.45) resulting from an accumulation of bases in the body caused by inappropriate tachypnea.

scintigraphy An imaging technology that is similar to angiography except that the red blood cells themselves are radiologically labeled to allow greater specificity.

Sengstaken-Blakemore tube A tube with an inflatable balloon at its end that is inserted into the GI tract and inflated to tamponade bleeding.

serosa A protective layer of connective tissue over most of the alimentary canal; also called the visceral peritoneum.

spontaneous bacterial peritonitis A bacterial infection of ascitic fluid.

stress-related erosive syndrome A condition in which stress-related mucosal disease develops in critically ill patients, such as those with severe head trauma or burns.

submucosa The layer of connective tissue below the mucosa; it contains blood vessels, lymph, and nerves.

systemic inflammatory response syndrome (SIRS) An immune response to an insult that typically leads to hypotension, shock, and worsened tissue function.

Prep Kit Continued

testicular torsion Twisting of a testicle about the spermatic cord to the point of ischemia.

third spacing An abnormal increase in the amount of fluid that exits the vascular space and moves into other areas (eg, gut wall, subcutaneous tissue); it can lead to dehydration, electrolyte imbalances, and hypovolemia.

total parenteral nutrition (TPN) The IV administration of all necessary nutrients in a patient whose GI tract does not function.

transjugular intrahepatic portosystemic shunt The placement of a shunt in the abdomen that bypasses much of the hepatic portal system;

it is intended to decrease portal hypertension and its effects.

T tube A T-shaped tube used to drain bile from the gallbladder.

ulcerative colitis An inflammation of the rectal mucosal and submucosal tissues.

uremia The presence of excessive amounts of urea and other waste products in the blood; can lead to altered mental status.

volvulus A twisting of the intestine onto itself, usually causing strangulation and ischemia.

References

Aghighi M, Taherian M, Sharma A. Angiodysplasia. In: *StatPearls*. Treasure Island, FL: StatPearls Publishing; 2020.

Aycock R, Westafer L, Boxen J, et al. Acute kidney injury after computed tomography: a meta-analysis. *Ann Emerg Med*. 2018;71(1):44-53.e4. doi: 10.1016/j.annemergmed.2017.06.041.

Bardou M, Quenot J-P, Barkun A. Stress-related mucosal disease in the critically ill patient. *Nat Rev Gastroenterol Hepatol*. 2015;12(2):98-107.

Barrett KE. Functional anatomy of the GI tract and organs draining into it. In: Barrett KE, ed. *Gastrointestinal Physiology*. 2nd ed. New York, NY: Lange Medical Books/McGraw-Hill Education; 2014.

Bass NM, Mullen KD, Sanyal A, et al. Rifaximin treatment in hepatic encephalopathy. *N Engl J Med*. 2010;362(12):1071-1081.

Bono M. Esophageal emergencies. In: Tintinalli JE, Stapczynski J, eds. *Tintinalli's Emergency Medicine: A Comprehensive Study Guide*. 9th ed. New York, NY: McGraw-Hill; 2019.

Brown JB, Cohen MJ, Minei JP, et al. Goal-directed resuscitation in the prehospital setting: a propensity-adjusted analysis. *J Trauma Acute Care Surg*. 2013;74(5):1207-1212.

Calvert JH, Cline DM. End-stage renal disease. In: Tintinalli JE, Stapczynski J, eds. *Tintinalli's Emergency Medicine: A Comprehensive Study Guide*. 9th ed. New York, NY: McGraw-Hill; 2019.

Connor MJ Jr, Karakala N. Continuous renal replacement therapy: reviewing current best practice to provide high-quality extracorporeal therapy to critically ill patients. *Adv Chronic Kidney Dis*. 2017;24(4):213-218.

Davis JE. Male genital problems. In: Tintinalli JE, Stapczynski J, eds. *Tintinalli's Emergency Medicine: A Comprehensive Study Guide*. 9th ed. New York, NY: McGraw-Hill; 2019.

Ding X, Zhang F, Wang Y. Risk factors for post-ERCP pancreatitis: a systematic review and meta-analysis. *Surgeon*. 2015;13(4):218-229.

Ehrmann S, Quartin A, Hobbs B, et al. Contrast-associated acute kidney injury in the critically ill: systematic review and Bayesian meta-analysis. *Intens Care Med*. 2017;43(6):785-794.

Ferris M, Quan S, Kaplan BS, et al. The global incidence of appendicitis: a systematic review of population-based studies. *Ann Surg*. 2017;266(2):237-241.

Fisher AD, Dodge M, Nealy W, et al. Whole blood in EMS may save lives. *JEMS*. https://www.jems.com/patient-care/whole-blood-in-ems-may-save-lives/. Published February 1, 2018. Accessed June 16, 2021.

Frohlich LC, Paydar-Darian N, Cilento BG Jr, et al. Prospective validation of clinical score for males presenting with an acute scrotum. *Acad Emerg Med*. 2017;24(12):1474-1482.

Fujiwara N, Friedman SL, Goossens N, et al. Risk factors and prevention of hepatocellular carcinoma in the era of precision medicine. *J Hepatol*. 2018;68(3):526-549.

Ghassemi KA, Jensen DM. Lower GI bleeding: epidemiology and management. *Curr Gastroenterol Rep*. 2013;15(7):333.

Gore RM, Silvers RI, Thakrar KH, et al. Bowel obstruction. *Radiologic Clinics*. 2015;53(6):1225-1240.

Grudzinski L, Quinan P, Kwok S, Pierratos A. Sodium citrate 4% locking solution for central venous dialysis catheters: an effective, more cost-efficient alternative to heparin. *Nephrol Dial Transplant*. 2007;22(2):471-476.

Hall P, Cash J. What is the real function of the liver "function" tests? *Ulster Med J*. 2012;81(1):30-36.

Hamm LL, Nakhoul N, Hering-Smith KS. Acid-base homeostasis. *CJASN*. 2015;10(12):2232-2242.

Prep Kit Continued

Hoffman RS, Nelson LS, Howland MA, et al., eds. *Goldfrank's Manual of Toxicologic Emergencies*. 11th ed. New York, NY: McGraw-Hill; 2019.

Holleran RS, Wolfe AC, Frakes MA, eds. *Air and Surface Patient Transport Principles and Practice*. 5th ed. St. Louis, MO: Mosby; 2017.

Jacobs DS, DeMott WR, Oxley DK. *Laboratory Test Handbook*. 5th ed. Hudson, OH: Lexi-Comp; 2001.

Jefferies M, Rauff B, Rashid H, et al. Update on global epidemiology of viral hepatitis and preventive strategies. *World J Clin Cases*. 2018;6(13):589-599.

Kamboj AK, Hoversten P, Leggett CL. Upper gastrointestinal bleeding: etiologies and management. *Mayo Clin Proc*. 2019;94(4):697-703.

Kaufman DC, Kitching AJ, Kellum JA. Acid-base balance. In: Hall JB, Schmidt GA, eds. *Principles of Critical Care*. 4th ed. New York, NY: McGraw-Hill; 2015.

Lamontagne F, Richards-Belle A, Thomas K, et al. Effect of reduced exposure to vasopressors on 90-day mortality in older critically ill patients with vasodilatory hypotension: a randomized clinical trial. *JAMA*. 2020;323(10):938-949.

Lanas A, Chan FKL. Peptic ulcer disease. *Lancet*. 2017; 390(10094):613-624.

Levy I, Gralnek IM. Complications of diagnostic colonoscopy, upper endoscopy, and enteroscopy. *Best Pract Res Clin Gastroenterol*. 2016;30(5):705-718.

Lin KJ, García Rodríguez LA, Hernández-Díaz S. Systematic review of peptic ulcer disease incidence rates: do studies without validation provide reliable estimates? *Pharmacoepidemiol Drug Saf*. 2011;20(7):718-728.

Lo B. Lower gastrointestinal bleeding. In: Tintinalli JE, Stapczynski J, eds. *Tintinalli's Emergency Medicine: A Comprehensive Study Guide*. 9th ed. New York, NY: McGraw-Hill; 2019.

Long B, Robertson J, Koyfman A. Emergency medicine evaluation and management of small bowel obstruction: evidence-based recommendations. *J Emerg Med*. 2019;56(2):166-176.

Makris K, Spanou L. Acute kidney injury: diagnostic approaches and controversies. *Clin Biochem Rev*. 2016;37(4):153-175.

Mansoor E, Jin-Dominguez F, Cheema T, et al. Epidemiology of indeterminate colitis in the United States between 2014 and 2019: a population-based national study. *Off J Am Coll Gastroenterol*. 2019;114:S1594.

Manthey DE, Nicks BA. Urologic stone disease. In: Tintinalli JE, Stapczynski J, eds. *Tintinalli's Emergency Medicine: A Comprehensive Study Guide*. 9th ed. New York, NY: McGraw-Hill; 2019.

Manthey DE, Story DJ. Acute urinary retention. In: Tintinalli JE, Stapczynski J, eds. *Tintinalli's Emergency Medicine: A Comprehensive Study Guide*. 9th ed. New York, NY: McGraw-Hill; 2019.

Marieb E, Hoehn K. *Human Anatomy and Physiology*. 11th ed. New York, NY: Pearson; 2019.

McEvoy C, Murray PT. Electrolyte disorders in critical care. In: Hall JB, Schmidt GA, eds. *Principles of Critical Care*. 4th ed. New York, NY: McGraw-Hill; 2015.

Merck Manual Professional Version. Renal tubular acidosis (RTA). Merck Manuals website. http://www.merckmanuals.com/professional/genitourinary-disorders/renal-transport-abnormalities/renal-tubular-acidosis. Accessed June 16, 2021.

Minalyan A, Benhammou JN, Artashesyan A, et al. Autoimmune atrophic gastritis: current perspectives. *Clin Exp Gastroenterol*. 2017;10:19-27.

Mohammed SEA, Abdo AE, Mudawi HMY. Mortality and rebleeding following variceal haemorrhage in liver cirrhosis and periportal fibrosis. *World J Hepatol*. 2016;8(31):1336-1342.

Munie ST, Nalamati SPM. Epidemiology and pathophysiology of diverticular disease. *Clin Colon Rectal Surg*. 2018;31(4):209-213.

Nickson C. Diabetic ketoacidosis. Life in the Fastlane website. https://litfl.com/diabetic-ketoacidosis/. Accessed June 16, 2021.

Nickson C. VBG versus ABG. Life in the Fastlane website. https://litfl.com/vbg-versus-abg/. Accessed June 16, 2021.

Olson KR, Vohra R. Comprehensive evaluation and treatment. In: Olson KR, ed. *Poisoning and Drug Overdose*. 7th ed. New York, NY: Lange Medical; 2018.

O'Mara SR, Wiesner L. Hepatic disorders. In: Tintinalli JE, Stapczynski J, eds. *Tintinalli's Emergency Medicine: A Comprehensive Study Guide*. 9th ed. New York, NY: McGraw-Hill; 2019.

Osman D, Djibré M, Da Silva D, et al. Management by the intensivist of gastrointestinal bleeding in adults and children. *Ann Intensive Care*. 2012;2:46.

Paumgartner G, Greenberger NJ. Gallstone disease. In: Greenberger NK, Blumberg RS, Burakoff R, ed. *Current Diagnosis and Treatment: Gastroenterology, Hepatology, and Endoscopy*. 3rd ed. New York, NY: Lange Medical; 2016.

Perelló MP, Mur JP, Vives MS, et al. Long-term follow-up of transjugular intrahepatic portosystemic shunt (TIPS) with stent-graft. *Diagn Interv Radiol*. 2019;25(5):346-352.

Podugu A, Tandon K, Castro FJ. Crohn's disease presenting as acute gastrointestinal hemorrhage. *World J Gastroenterol*. 2016;22(16):4073-4078.

Rangaswami J, Bhalla V, Blair J, et al. Cardiorenal syndrome: classification, pathophysiology, diagnosis, and treatment strategies: a scientific statement from the American Heart Association. *Circulation*. 2019;139(16):e840-e878. doi: 10.1161/CIR.0000000000000664.

Scheiner B, Lindner G, Reiberger T, et al. Acid-base disorders in liver disease. *J Hepatol*. 2017;67(5):1062-1073.

Simon TG, Ma Y, Ludvigsson JF, et al. Association between aspirin use and risk of hepatocellular carcinoma. *JAMA Oncol*. 2018;4(12):1683-1690.

Sinert R, Peacock PR. Acute kidney injury. In: Tintinalli JE, Stapczynski J, eds. *Tintinalli's Emergency Medicine:*

Prep Kit Continued

A Comprehensive Study Guide. 9th ed. New York, NY: McGraw-Hill; 2019.

Singh A, Gelrund A. Acute pancreatitis. In: Hall JB, Schmidt GA, eds. *Principles of Critical Care*. 4th ed. New York, NY: McGraw-Hill; 2015.

Som A, Mandaliya R, Alsaadi D, et al. Immune checkpoint inhibitor-induced colitis: a comprehensive review. *World J Clin Cases*. 2019;7(4):405-418.

Sperry JL, Guyette FX, Brown JB, et al. Prehospital plasma during air medical transport in trauma patients at risk for hemorrhagic shock. *N Engl J Med*. 2018;379(4):315-326.

Spinella PC, Pidcoke HF, Strandenes G, et al. Whole blood for hemostatic resuscitation of major bleeding. *Transfusion*. 2016;56(suppl 2):S190-S202.

Suhocki PV, Lungren MP, Kapoor B, et al. Transjugular intrahepatic portosystemic shunt complications: prevention and management. *Semin Intervent Radiol*. 2015;32(2):123-132.

Tanagho EA, Lue TF. Anatomy of the genitourinary tract. In: Tanagho E, McAninch J, eds. *Smith and Tanagho's General Urology*. 19th ed. New York, NY: McGraw-Hill; 2020.

Todd NV. Priapism in acute spinal cord injury. *Spinal Cord*. 2011;49(10):1033-1035.

Tsay FW, Wu DC, Yu HC, et al. A randomized controlled trial shows that both 14-day hybrid and bismuth quadruple therapies cure most patients with *Helicobacter pylori* infection in populations with moderate antibiotic resistance.

Antimicrob Agents Chemother. 2017;61(11). doi: 10.1128/AAC.00140-17.

Wiles MD. Blood pressure management in trauma: from feast to famine? *Anaesthesia*. 2013;68(5):445-449.

Wise R, Faurie M, Malbrain MLNG, et al. Strategies for intravenous fluid resuscitation in trauma patients. *World J Surg*. 2017;41(5):1170-1183.

Xanthopoulos A, Starling RC, Kitai T, et al. Heart failure and liver disease: cardiohepatic interactions. *JACC Heart Fail*. 2019;7(2):87-97.

Zarrinpar A, Busuttil RW. Liver transplantation: past, present and future. *Nat Rev Gastroenterol Hepatol*. 2013;10(7):434-440.

Zhao M, Yue Z, Zhao H, et al. Techniques of TIPS in the treatment of liver cirrhosis combined with incompletely occlusive main portal vein thrombosis. *Sci Rep*. 2016;6(1):33069.

Zia Ziabari SM, Rimaz S, Shafaghi A, et al. Blood urea nitrogen to creatinine ratio in differentiation of upper and lower gastrointestinal bleedings: a diagnostic accuracy study. *Arch Acad Emerg Med*. 2019;7(1):e30. PMCID: PMC6637801.

Ziebell CM, Kitlowski AD, Welch J, et al. Upper gastrointestinal bleeding. In: Tintinalli JE, Stapczynski J, eds. *Tintinalli's Emergency Medicine: A Comprehensive Study Guide*. 9th ed. New York, NY: McGraw-Hill; 2019.

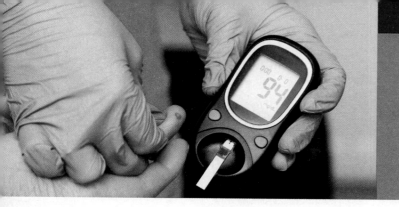

Chapter 18

Endocrine Emergencies

Eric Silverman, MD, MPH

OBJECTIVES

After completing this chapter, you will be able to:

1. Describe the anatomic structures and physiology of the endocrine system (p 981).
2. Discuss the pathophysiology, assessment, and critical care transport management of conditions related to diabetes, including hypoglycemia, hyperglycemia, diabetic ketoacidosis, and hyperosmolar hyperglycemic state (pp 985–991).
3. Discuss the pathophysiology, assessment, and critical care transport management of pituitary disorders, including central diabetes insipidus, pituitary lesions, acromegaly, and gigantism (pp 991–993).
4. Discuss the pathophysiology, assessment, and critical care transport management of adrenal abnormalities, including adrenal insufficiency, Addison disease, Cushing disease, pheochromocytoma, aldosteronism, and amyloidosis (pp 993–998).
5. Discuss the pathophysiology, assessment, and critical care transport management of thyroid abnormalities, including hyperthyroidism, hypothyroidism, myxedema coma, thyrotoxicosis and thyroid storm, and Hashimoto disease (pp 998–1001).
6. Discuss the pathophysiology, assessment, and critical care transport management of lipid disorders, including antiphospholipid syndrome and metabolic syndrome (p 1002).

Introduction

Patients with an endocrine disorder may present with overt or subtle signs and symptoms that require a thorough knowledge of the history of the present illness or injury, the patient's past medical history, and a detailed physical exam. In addition, the critical care transport professional (CCTP) will need to consider disorders that involve the endocrine system when assessing a patient's overall condition. For example, adrenal insufficiency after surgery can easily be overlooked during the unstable postoperative period. If not quickly identified and treated, this condition can result in refractory hypotension leading to death.

Anatomy and Physiology

As a CCTP student, you are likely already familiar with the components of the endocrine system, which are reviewed in **FIGURE 18-1**. **FIGURE 18-2** provides a review of substances secreted by the pituitary gland and their destinations in the body.

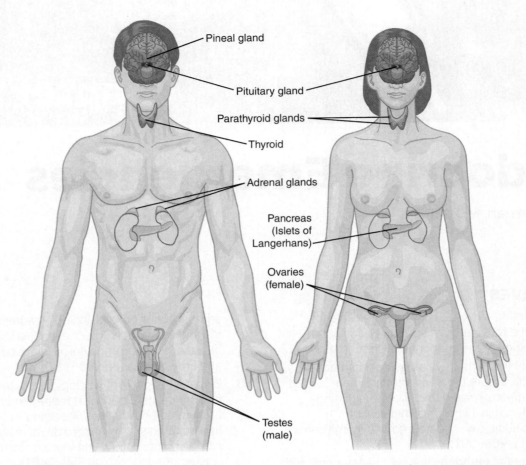

FIGURE 18-1 The endocrine system uses various glands to deliver chemical messages to organ systems throughout the body.

© Jones & Bartlett Learning.

Thyroid

The thyroid gland is the largest gland in the neck and is situated anteriorly below the skin and muscle layers. It resembles the shape of a butterfly, with the left and right thyroid lobes wrapping around the trachea. The function of the thyroid gland is to regulate the body's metabolism by secreting thyroxine (T_4) when the body's metabolic rate decreases. Thyroxine—the body's major metabolic hormone—stimulates energy production in cells, which increases the rate at which cells consume oxygen and use carbohydrates, fats, and proteins. When the body's temperature drops, for example, this increased cellular metabolism creates heat. Iodine is an important component of thyroxine. Without the proper level of dietary iodine intake, thyroxine cannot be produced, which results in physical and cognitive impairments.

The thyroid gland also secretes calcitonin, which helps maintain normal calcium levels in the blood. This hormone is secreted directly into the bloodstream when the thyroid detects high levels of calcium. Calcitonin travels to the bones, where it stimulates the bone-building cells to absorb the excess calcium. It also stimulates the kidneys to absorb and excrete excess calcium.

It is important to correctly identify the anatomic location of the thyroid gland because it is highly vascularized. If this gland is inadvertently injured during an emergency cricothyrotomy, it can hemorrhage uncontrollably.

Parathyroid Glands

The parathyroid glands are small, ovoid glands located on the posterior lobes of the thyroid gland. There are usually four parathyroid glands, each about the size of a grain of rice, which secrete parathyroid hormone (PTH). PTH plays an important role in calcium and phosphate homeostasis by

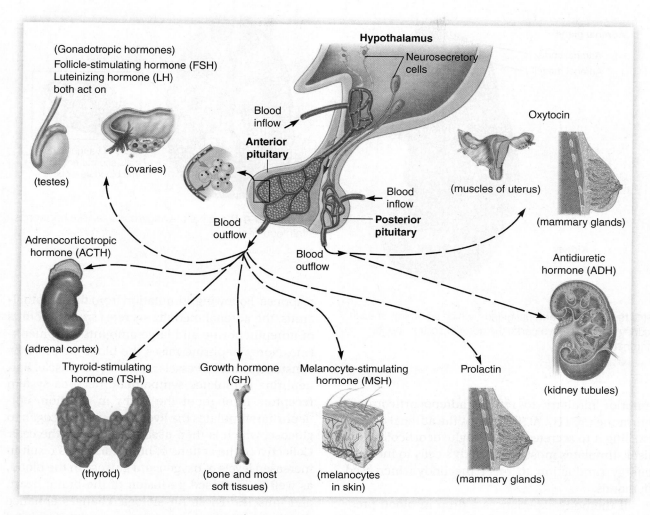

FIGURE 18-2 The pituitary gland secretes hormones from its two regions: the anterior pituitary lobe and the posterior pituitary lobe.

© Jones & Bartlett Learning.

working antagonistically to the calcitonin secreted by the thyroid gland.

Hyperparathyroidism is a disease characterized by oversecretion of PTH by the parathyroid glands, leading to increased bone resorption and hypercalcemia. Hypoparathyroidism can be caused by damage to the parathyroid glands during thyroid surgery or removal (ie, thyroidectomy). This condition can lead to hypocalcemia, which is usually treated with calcium and vitamin D supplementation.

Adrenal Glands

The adrenal glands, which are located at the superior portion of each kidney, produce several types of hormones. Each of these glands has an outer portion called the adrenal cortex and an inner portion called the adrenal medulla **FIGURE 18-3**. The adrenal cortex manufactures corticosteroids—hormones that regulate metabolism, the immune system, and sexual function. They also contribute to maintaining the balance of salt and water within the body. The adrenal medulla produces the catecholamines epinephrine and norepinephrine. These catecholamines are involved in regulating autonomic functions, such as increasing heart rate, respiratory rate, and blood pressure as needed when responding to stress.

During times of physiologic stress, the hypothalamus secretes a hormone that stimulates the

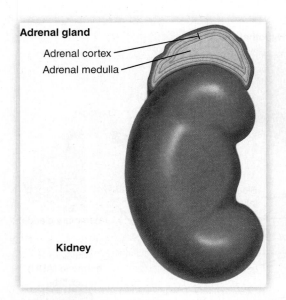

FIGURE 18-3 The adrenal glands, which sit on top of each kidney, consist of two parts: the adrenal cortex and the adrenal medulla.

© Jones & Bartlett Learning.

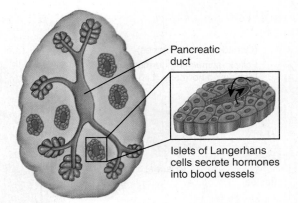

FIGURE 18-4 The islets of Langerhans secrete hormones into blood vessels.

© Jones & Bartlett Learning.

anterior pituitary to release adrenocorticotropic hormone (ACTH). ACTH targets the adrenal cortex, causing it to secrete cortisol, a glucocorticoid. Cortisol stimulates most of the body's cells to increase energy production to meet the body's increased demands.

If the body experiences a drop in blood pressure or cardiac preload, a decrease in serum sodium concentration, or an increase in serum potassium concentration, the zona glomerulosa (outer zone) of the adrenal cortex is stimulated to secrete aldosterone, a mineralocorticoid that acts primarily at the distal renal convoluted tubes. Aldosterone prompts the kidneys to reabsorb sodium from the urine and excrete potassium by altering the osmotic gradient in the blood. This adjustment indirectly leads to increases in blood volume and blood pressure. This mineralocorticoid is vital for the management of sodium in the kidneys, salivary glands, sweat glands, and colon; it reduces the loss of salt and water through the sweat and salivary glands. Abnormal overproduction of aldosterone, resulting from either primary or secondary disorders, is common in the general population and is a substantial cause of morbidity and mortality.

The body's reaction to physical or emotional stress is commonly referred to as the "fight-or-flight"

response. Following stimulation from the hypothalamus, the adrenal medulla secretes small amounts of norepinephrine and large amounts of epinephrine. Norepinephrine raises the blood pressure by constricting blood vessels and skeletal muscle. Epinephrine stimulates sympathetic nervous system receptors throughout the body. In addition, epinephrine stimulates the liver to convert glycogen to glucose, which is then used as energy in the cells. Collectively, the actions of both hormones result in increased levels of oxygen and glucose in the blood, as well as increased perfusion of the brain, heart, and muscles. These physiologic changes enhance the body's ability to rapidly respond to stressful situations.

Pancreas

The pancreas is a digestive gland that is considered both an endocrine and an exocrine gland. In its role as an endocrine organ, it secretes digestive enzymes into the duodenum through the pancreatic duct. The endocrine component comprises the islets of Langerhans, which are cell groups within the pancreas that act like "an organ within an organ." The main hormones that are secreted—glucagon and insulin—are responsible for the regulation of blood glucose levels **FIGURE 18-4**.

When the body's blood glucose level falls, such as between meals, the pancreas secretes glucagon to raise the glucose level and bring the body's energy back to normal. On entering the bloodstream, this hormone stimulates the liver to convert glycogen (a storage starch form of the sugar glucose, made up of thousands of glucose units) into glucose. This glucose then enters the bloodstream, and the blood carries it to the cells for use as energy.

Insulin is responsible for the removal of glucose from the blood for storage as glycogen, fats, and protein; in fact, it is the only hormone that decreases the blood glucose levels. When blood glucose levels are elevated, the islets of Langerhans secrete insulin, which is carried by the bloodstream to the cells. The cells then take in more glucose to produce energy. Insulin also stimulates the liver to convert glucose to glycogen for later use by the body. Once blood glucose levels have returned to normal, the islets of Langerhans discontinue the secretion of insulin.

Diabetes

The term diabetes mellitus refers to a metabolic disorder in which the pancreas's ability to metabolize simple carbohydrates (glucose) is impaired because of a lack of insulin or a decreased sensitivity of the cells to insulin. As mentioned earlier, the pancreas is the primary regulator of blood glucose levels. Production of digestive enzymes and the hormones insulin and glucagon takes place in the islets of Langerhans. Beta cells in the islets of Langerhans (65% to 80% of the islet cells) produce insulin and amylin, alpha cells (15% to 20%) release glucagon, and delta cells (3% to 10%) produce somatostatin. Insulin and glucagon are the hormones responsible for keeping the blood glucose level within the normal range, 70 to 100 mg/dL. Diabetes is characterized by abnormally elevated blood glucose concentration, which can result in the passage of large quantities of urine containing glucose (polyuria), increased thirst (polydipsia), and significantly impaired immune function.

Glucose that is not used immediately for energy is stored in the liver and muscles as glycogen, or converted by adipose tissue into fat. The liver releases glucose back into the bloodstream when the levels there decrease, and it removes glucose from the blood when the levels are too high. Only glycogen in the liver can be converted back to glucose; the glycogen stored in muscle can be used only by the muscle for energy.

Insulin is essential for glucose to be taken up and used by cells. This hormone is secreted by the beta cells of the pancreas in response to increased blood glucose levels. After eating a meal, blood glucose levels in the body rise. Glucose in the blood then triggers the release of more insulin from the pancreas. Insulin transports glucose into the cells via facilitated diffusion, a process in which the glucose is converted into energy. Insulin also has an effect on many cells that play a part in absorbing the glucose, causing the blood glucose concentration to return to normal.

Glucagon, which is secreted by the alpha cells, has the opposite effect. When blood glucose levels are low, the pancreas releases more glucagon. The presence of glucagon stimulates the release of glucose stored in liver cells, making energy available to the tissues between meals.

Diabetes mellitus results from an impairment of the body's ability to produce or use insulin. Traditionally, the two predominant types of diabetes mellitus are known as type 1 and type 2. Functionally, many clinicians categorize diabetes mellitus as either insulin-dependent or non–insulin-dependent.

Pathophysiology

Type 1 diabetes generally affects children and has historically been referred to as juvenile diabetes, although this form of diabetes is now appearing in adulthood as well. Type 1 diabetes has a hereditary predisposition, but environmental factors may be partly responsible for its development; for example, an infection may trigger an autoimmune response, causing antibodies to destroy the islets of Langerhans.

Most people with type 1 diabetes do not produce insulin. Consequently, they require daily injections of supplementary insulin throughout their lives to control their blood glucose levels. In addition to daily replacement of insulin through injections or a continuous infusion pump, and careful balancing of dietary intake of carbohydrates and simple sugars, physical activity is important to achieve optimal glucose control. This can be a particular challenge in young children, performance athletes, people with alcoholism, and patients with multiple medical comorbidities.

Type 2 diabetes (previously called adult-onset diabetes) traditionally develops later in life, usually when the patient is middle-aged, although the disease is becoming more common in younger people.

Approximately 90% of all people with diabetes in the United States have type 2 diabetes. In many people with type 2 diabetes, the pancreas actually produces enough insulin; however, for reasons not fully understood, the body cannot effectively use it—a condition known as insulin resistance. One hypothesis proposed for this phenomenon is that insulin receptor cells become altered and are no longer able to use the insulin when it arrives at the target cell. Type 2 diabetes can also be caused by a deficiency in insulin production.

The distinction between type 1 and type 2 diabetes has become less important to emergency and critical care providers due to the frequent overlap in treatments and potential complications between both types.

Special Populations

Gestational diabetes is diabetes first diagnosed during pregnancy. Its prevalence in the United States is 2% to 10%. Risk factors include prior episodes of gestational diabetes, family history of diabetes, and prepregnancy obesity. Symptoms generally present after 20 weeks' gestation and most commonly between weeks 24 and 30. Treatment consists of insulin or certain oral agents. These patients are considered to have high-risk pregnancies and require close monitoring. Patients with gestational diabetes also have a higher lifetime risk of the development of diabetes than the general population.

Hypoglycemia

Hypoglycemia in patients with diabetes most commonly occurs from taking too much medication, not eating enough food, engaging in intense or unexpected physical activity, or drinking excessive amounts of alcohol. The tissues of the central nervous system (including the brain) depend primarily on glucose as their source of energy; in contrast, other tissues can metabolize fat or protein in addition to glucose. In severe hypoglycemia, cerebral dysfunction can progresses quickly to irreversible neuronal death.

The normal blood glucose level is approximately 70 to 100 mg/dL; hypoglycemia is diagnosed when blood glucose drops below the normal level and, in people without diabetes, when

accompanied by corresponding signs and symptoms. Generally, mild hypoglycemia can be treated with oral glucose, with rapid intravenous (IV) dextrose infusions reserved for patients with blood glucose levels less than 60 mg/dL or signs of clinical instability. In emergency situations or when IV or intraosseous (IO) access is not readily available, glucagon can be administered via the intramuscular, subcutaneous, or intranasal routes to treat severe hypoglycemia. Hypoglycemia can develop rapidly, within a span of minutes to a few hours. It should be suspected in any patient with altered mental status or new neurologic deficits.

Signs and Symptoms

Hypoglycemia

- Headache
- Altered mental status
- Memory loss
- Blurred or double vision
- Lack of coordination
- Slurred speech
- Stroke like symptoms
- Seizure
- Hypertension
- Tachycardia
- Diaphoresis
- Chest pain
- Abdominal pain
- Tremor
- Anxiety
- Confusion
- Paranoia
- Hunger
- Coma

Hyperglycemia and Diabetic Ketoacidosis

Hyperglycemia is the hallmark sign of diabetes mellitus, which is typically diagnosed by a fasting blood glucose level of 126 mg/dL or higher, hemoglobin A1c of 6.5% or greater, or random blood glucose level of 200 mg/dL or higher with symptoms of hyperglycemia. Hyperglycemia can be caused by excessive food intake, insufficient medications, infection or illness, injury, recent surgery, or physiologic stressors. Onset may be rapid (within minutes) or gradual (hours to days), depending on the cause. For example, excessive food intake may cause blood glucose levels to rise quickly, whereas an infection or illness may result in gradually worsening hyperglycemia over the course of several days.

If left untreated, hyperglycemia in a patient with diabetes can progress to diabetic ketoacidosis (DKA), a life-threatening condition characterized by hyperglycemia, metabolic acidosis, and elevated serum ketone levels. DKA usually evolves rapidly (over a 24-hour period). Patients with DKA tend to be younger, with type 1 diabetes. In DKA, an insulin deficiency prevents cells from taking up the extra glucose. Because the body cannot use glucose, it turns to other sources of energy—principally, fat. The metabolism of fat generates acids and ketones as waste products. The ketones, which are exhaled as acetone, can cause the breath of a patient with DKA to have a characteristic fruity odor. High blood glucose concentrations lead to glucose being excreted in the urine, osmotically pulling excessive amounts of water and electrolytes (sodium and potassium) with it. This diuresis, together with the vomiting and the rapid, deep respirations (Kussmaul respirations) that patients may exhibit, leads to progressive dehydration and metabolic acidosis, ultimately progressing to shock, coma, and death. Blood glucose levels in DKA rarely exceed 800 mg/dL; in fact, they are most often observed to range from 350 to 500 mg/dL. In patients with DKA who are unresponsive (comatose), blood glucose levels can exceed 900 mg/dL.

Hyperosmolar Hyperglycemic State

Hyperosmolar hyperglycemic state (HHS), also known as hyperosmolar hyperglycemic nonketotic syndrome (HHNS), is characterized by hyperglycemia and hyperosmolarity (serum osmolality exceeding 320 mmol/kg) without significant metabolic acidosis or ketonemia. Blood glucose levels in patients with HHS are commonly 600 mg/dL or greater and may exceed 1,000 mg/dL. The hyperglycemia and hyperosmolarity lead to osmotic diuresis and an osmotic shift of body fluid to the extracellular space, resulting in further intracellular dehydration. Unlike DKA, HHS is not characterized by significant ketoacidosis. However, in clinical

Special Populations

Caring for pediatric patients with DKA can pose a greater challenge than caring for adult patients with this condition. Children are more susceptible to rapid shifts in fluid volume and osmolarity, which puts them at much greater risk for cerebral edema as a result of treatment. Although fluid resuscitation is the mainstay of therapy for both children and adults with DKA, a more cautious approach must be used with the pediatric patient. The CCTP must meticulously monitor the inputs and outputs for the patient. The initial fluids administered should be limited to a 10 to 20 mL/kg bolus of 0.9% saline over the first 1 to 2 hours, repeated up to two times as necessary to maintain hemodynamic stability. Subsequent fluid resuscitation using 0.45% to 0.9% saline or lactated Ringer solution should be titrated to replete total estimated fluid losses over the next 48 hours. Additionally, an insulin infusion should be initiated at a dose of 0.05 to 0.1 unit/kg/h after 1 to 2 hours of fluid resuscitation, with a goal of lowering the glucose at a rate of about 50 mg/dL/h.

Signs and Symptoms

Diabetic Ketoacidosis

- Polydipsia (excessive thirst)
- Polyuria (excessive urination)
- Polyphagia (excessive hunger)
- Nausea and vomiting
- Abdominal pain
- Deep, rapid (Kussmaul) respirations
- Dehydration
- Hypotension
- Tachycardia
- Warm, dry skin and mucous membranes
- Confusion
- Gradual deterioration of consciousness
- Fruity-smelling breath (rare)

practice, the syndromes associated with DKA and HHS often overlap, resulting in a mixed clinical picture. HHS can result in a significant mortality rate, as high as 20%, which is approximately tenfold higher than the mortality rate linked to DKA.

Although most patients diagnosed with HHS have a known history of diabetes mellitus (usually type 2), approximately 30% will have no previous diagnosis of diabetes. The onset of HHS is usually more insidious than the emergence of DKA. It is marked by polydipsia (excessive thirst), polyuria (excessive urination), and polyphagia (excessive hunger), which progress over several days before the patient seeks medical attention.

HHS often develops in patients with diabetes who have some secondary illness that leads to reduced fluid intake. Although infection (in particular, pneumonia and urinary tract infection) is the most common cause, many other conditions can lead to altered mentation or dehydration. The physiologic stress response to any acute illness tends to increase the levels of hormones that favor elevated glucose levels—cortisol, catecholamines (epinephrine and norepinephrine), glucagon, and many others.

Signs and Symptoms

Hyperosmolar Hyperglycemic State

- Severe dehydration
- Drowsiness
- Lethargy
- Delirium
- Coma
- Focal or generalized seizures
- Visual disturbances
- Hemiparesis
- Sensory deficits
- Acute myocardial infarction (AMI)

Assessment

Patients with diabetes mellitus may present with varied physical findings and vital signs on examination, depending on their current blood glucose concentration. The overall patient assessment, the history of present illness or injury, and a thorough review of the patient's medical history will help the CCTP determine whether a diabetes-related condition is influencing the patient's vital signs and symptoms.

Signs and Symptoms

The assessment of the patient with hypoglycemia may reveal fatigue, headache, altered mental status,

lack of coordination, stroke like symptoms, and even seizures. Hypertension, tachycardia, diaphoresis, chest pain, upper abdominal pain, and anxiety may be present as well because of the release of epinephrine caused by stimulation of the sympathetic nervous system.

It is important to rule out the possibility of hypoglycemia in patients presenting with signs of intoxication, including slurred speech, lack of coordination, paranoia, confusion, and behavioral emergencies. These signs may be the direct result of cerebral hypoxia, rather than use of alcohol or drugs.

Hyperglycemia and DKA typically present with the three Ps: polyuria, polydipsia, and polyphagia. Polyuria results from osmotic diuresis, polydipsia is caused by dehydration, and polyphagia is believed to stem from the body's inefficient use of nutrients. Patients, especially young individuals, may also experience abdominal pain; vomiting, which increases the degree of dehydration and can even result in hypotension; tachycardia; warm, dry skin; and dry mucous membranes. The two hallmark signs of DKA are hyperglycemia and acidosis. Acidosis can be indirectly inferred using capnography; a lower than expected end-tidal carbon dioxide (ETCO$_2$) level—that is, respiratory alkalosis—may develop as a compensatory mechanism to significant metabolic acidosis.

Laboratory Assessment

Testing for hypoglycemia or hyperglycemia is a rapid, point-of-care procedure that a CCTP can perform during transport. Administration and/or titration of existing medications or fluids may then follow based on the results of this biochemical analysis.

Because glucose is one of the three major energy sources for the body, it is important to routinely monitor the patient's blood glucose level during transport. Most commonly, this is accomplished via a portable blood glucose monitor (glucometer) **FIGURE 18-5**, similar to the one the patient may use at home. Portable blood glucose monitors measure the glucose level in whole blood using either capillary or venous samples. In contrast, blood glucose testing performed in a laboratory measures the blood glucose concentration in the plasma, which is typically about 10 mg/dL higher than that in a whole blood sample.

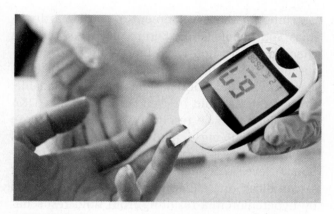

FIGURE 18-5 A portable glucometer used in the critical care transport environment.

© megaflopp/Shutterstock.

It is important to read and understand the operator's manual prior to using the glucometer because of differences in manufacturers' specifications. Some glucometers will read "Lo" when the glucose reading is less than 20 mg/dL, whereas others will display "Lo" when the reading is less than 30 mg/dL. The same variations may apply with a "Hi" reading; some glucometers read "Hi" at 550 mg/dL, and others read "Hi" at 600 mg/dL. Thus, it is important to know both the upper and lower ranges of the specific glucometer model.

The normal lab value for glucose in whole blood in nonfasting adults and children is 70 to 100 mg/dL. In a neonate, blood glucose levels should be maintained at greater than 65 mg/dL.

Venous blood gas monitoring should also be used in patients with DKA. Monitoring commonly reveals metabolic acidosis with a pH less than 7.30, a bicarbonate level less than 15 mEq/L, and a $Paco_2$ level less than 30 mm Hg.

Laboratory testing for diabetes may also include urine and/or serum ketone tests, which can identify the presence of dehydration and DKA. Generally, blood chemistry analysis and blood testing for ketones are indicated to detect elevations in blood urea nitrogen (BUN) and creatinine that may result from significant dehydration, to detect electrolyte abnormalities (which can be profound), and to calculate the anion gap, which, in the presence of serum ketones (β-hydroxybutyrate), is used to diagnose DKA and guide ongoing insulin infusion therapy.

A person with diabetes may also have had a hemoglobin A1c (glycohemoglobin) test completed prior to transport—although this test is typically not performed during an acute emergency. When a person experiences prolonged hyperglycemia, the red blood cells become saturated with glucose. The percentage of saturation can then be measured in an attempt to estimate the patient's blood glucose level during the previous 3 to 4 months. Typically, patients *without* diabetes will have a hemoglobin A1c level between 4% and 6%.

Management

Patients presenting with hypoglycemia should be treated prior to initiating transport. However, if the CCTP is called to transport a patient with persistent hypoglycemia, then a continuous infusion of a dextrose-containing solution may be needed. If IV/IO access is not readily available, glucagon can be administered via the intramuscular, subcutaneous, or intranasal routes to rapidly correct severe hypoglycemia.

Hyperglycemic patients (with DKA and HHS) who present in hypovolemic shock from dehydration should receive an initial fluid bolus with an isotonic or 0.9% saline solution via an IV, IO, or central line at a volume of 20 mL/kg in an effort to restore intravascular volume. Following the initial fluid bolus, the optimal maintenance fluid rate and type of crystalloid solution will depend on the patient's clinical condition. Patients without evidence of heart failure, renal failure, advanced liver disease, or pulmonary edema should be rehydrated at 250 to 500 mL/h for several hours. The 0.9% saline should be changed to 0.45% saline or PlasmaLyte solution once the corrected serum sodium concentration has increased to normal or above normal. Proceed with fluid administration cautiously if the patient requires more than 50 mL/kg during the first 4 hours of rehydration.

As the intravascular volume is repleted, any potassium and magnesium deficits should be corrected. Insulin therapy should be withheld and 10 to 20 mEq/h of potassium chloride should be administered until the serum potassium is at least 3.3 mEq/L, due to the risk of iatrogenic hypokalemia and cardiac dysrhythmia. Once the serum potassium concentration is between 3.3 and 5.2 mEq/L, 20 to 40 mEq of potassium chloride should be added to each liter of subsequent IV fluid to maintain the serum potassium concentration between 4 and 5 mEq/L. If the serum potassium concentration is greater than 5.2 mEq/L, potassium supplementation should be withheld. Patients with end-stage renal disease are at particularly high risk for hyperkalemia; in these patients, potassium supplementation should not begin until serum concentrations are less than 3.3 mEq/L.

Regular IV insulin is less expensive and equally as effective as the more costly rapid-acting insulin analogs; hence, most experts and institutional protocols initiate continuous insulin infusions with an IV bolus of 0.1 unit/kg of regular insulin, followed immediately by a continuous infusion of 0.1 unit/kg/h. In both DKA and HHS, this rate of infusion is expected to decrease serum glucose by 50 to 70 mg/dL/h. Larger doses do not typically produce greater reductions in serum glucose, although CCTPs should be aware that volume replacement often results in an additional lowering of serum glucose by 35 to 70 mg/dL/h due to hemodilution and improved renal function. Once the serum glucose level reaches 200 to 250 mg/dL in a patient with DKA or 250 to 300 mg/dL in a patient with HHS, the IV fluids should be switched from 0.9% or 0.45% saline to a dextrose-containing solution, typically 5% dextrose with 0.45% sodium chloride, to maintain serum glucose between 150 and 200 mg/dL. The insulin infusion may need to be reduced to 0.02 to 0.05 unit/kg/h as well. Lowering serum glucose below 150 to 200 mg/dL with a continuous insulin infusion may increase the risk of severe hypoglycemic episodes and cerebral edema. In DKA, insulin infusions should be continued until the anion gap is 12 or lower and serum pH is greater than 7.3.

Considerable controversy surrounds the practice of administering bicarbonate to correct the metabolic acidosis often seen in DKA. Most experts suggest that bicarbonate administration is warranted when the arterial pH is less than 6.90. Typically, 100 mEq of bicarbonate is added to the IV fluids infusing to run over 2 hours; this treatment is repeated until the pH rises above 7.00. Little evidence of improved outcomes exists for correcting pH beyond 7.00, and the risks may outweigh any additional benefits. Of note, if the patient does not have an arterial line, then venous blood sampling can be used to measure pH: Venous pH is typically 0.03 lower than arterial pH.

Patients being treated for hyperglycemia should have continuous cardiac monitoring, with the CCTP watching for the development of cardiac arrhythmias and hypokalemia. Serum glucose should be checked at least hourly, and more often during resuscitation. Venous blood pH should be checked at least every 2 hours; if this capability is unavailable, $ETCO_2$ values should be trended continually. DKA is considered to be resolved when blood glucose is less than 200 mg/dL and either the anion gap is 12 or lower, pH is greater than 7.3, or serum bicarbonate level is greater than 15 mEq/L. Note that serum bicarbonate measurements can be affected by hyperchloremia resulting from fluid resuscitation with 0.9% saline infusions. HHS is considered to be resolved when serum osmolality has normalized and the patient's mental status has returned to baseline (if it was found to be altered during the initial assessment). Once DKA or HHS has resolved, subcutaneous insulin can be started and insulin infusions discontinued 1 to 2 hours later. Patients not previously taking insulin can be transitioned to subcutaneous insulin at 0.5 to 0.8 unit/kg/d.

In patients with uncomplicated hyperglycemia or mild DKA (awake and alert, tolerating oral fluids without vomiting, pH > 7, bicarbonate ≥ 10 mmol/L), subcutaneous short-acting insulin can be considered instead of IV infusions. The recommended subcutaneous dosing of short-acting insulin typically includes an initial bolus of 0.3 unit/kg, followed by 0.2 unit/kg every 2 hours until the blood glucose level reaches 250 mg/dL, then 0.05 to 0.1 unit/kg every 2 hours until the DKA has resolved. If the patient is already taking a long-acting basal insulin, it may be coadministered to prevent rebound hyperglycemia.

As with all patients whom the CCTP will encounter, definitive airway management and ventilatory assistance may be required for patients with hyperglycemia. Due to the potentially severe metabolic acidosis and risk of cardiac arrest resulting from the loss of respiratory compensation, extreme caution should be taken when performing endotracheal intubation or other airway management, should it become necessary. If aspiration is possible because of the patient's decreased level of consciousness, then consider inserting a nasogastric tube. If urine output must be monitored during transport and the patient is unresponsive, then insert an indwelling (Foley) catheter. Neurologic status should be continuously monitored as well. Correction of serum glucose that is too rapid can lead to cerebral edema, which has a mortality of

20% to 40% when it occurs during DKA treatment. Early identification (headache and obtundation are the earliest signs) and aggressive treatment of this condition can improve outcomes.

Numerous studies in patients who have recently undergone cardiac surgery demonstrate that these patients have fewer infections and improved survival when tight glycemic control is achieved, yet data from the NICE-SUGAR study suggest these values cannot be applied to the rest of the critically ill patient population (ie, noncardiac surgery patients). This is not to say that insulin infusions are unhelpful in noncardiac surgical patients, but rather that standard guidelines for glycemic control can be used. Standard glucose management practices should not be abandoned in critically ill patients; in fact, CCTPs can expect to see continuous insulin infusions in many patients admitted to an intensive care unit who subsequently require transfer to another hospital. When insulin infusions are used in some critically ill patients, there appears to be a decrease in both mortality and morbidity.

Controversies

The use of continuous insulin infusions in critically ill patients has been questioned and is becoming less frequent due to two largely unresolved issues:

- Whether the increased survival results from the insulin infusion or the control of the blood glucose level
- What the optimal blood glucose target is to ensure improved outcomes in critically ill patients

Most institutions have established their own protocols for insulin infusions. These protocols may differ substantially, as does the incidence of hypoglycemia associated with the various protocols. Research has shown that hypoglycemic episodes significantly increase morbidity and mortality, and may negate the benefits of the insulin infusion in some patient populations.

In summary, the CCTP should understand that insulin infusions are a routine part of care for many patients. They require vigilance in monitoring during transport, including frequent (hourly or more often) checks of blood glucose levels using a blood glucometer, and careful management of the

insulin infusion rate to maintain blood glucose at the optimal level.

Transport Management

Hypoglycemia

- Test for hypoglycemia/hyperglycemia.
- Administer a continuous dextrose infusion, if required, and titrate the infusion to the patient's blood glucose level.
- If IV/IO access is not readily available, administer intramuscular, subcutaneous, or intranasal glucagon.

Transport Management

Hyperglycemia (DKA and HHS)

- Initiate fluid resuscitation with 0.9% saline via an IV, IO, or central line.
- Correct electrolyte derangements, including potassium and magnesium deficits.
- Administer a regular IV insulin bolus, followed immediately by a continuous insulin infusion.
- Administer sodium bicarbonate if pH is less than 6.90.
- Provide continuous cardiac and ETCO$_2$ monitoring.
- Provide airway management and ventilatory assistance if required.
- Insert an indwelling (Foley) catheter to measure urine output if the patient is critically ill or unresponsive.
- Check blood glucose at least hourly, and more often if the patient is receiving fluid resuscitation or insulin treatment.
- Measure the arterial or venous pH every 2 hours (if unable to do so, monitor the ETCO$_2$ trend).
- Monitor the patient's neurologic status for signs and symptoms of cerebral edema (eg, headaches, obtundation).

Pituitary Disorders

Pituitary disorders often present with signs and symptoms common to other disease processes, requiring the CCTP to perform a thorough medical history and physical exam to correctly identify the underlying pathology. Although these disorders are typically not acutely life threatening, they can result in significant morbidity and mortality if left untreated.

Pathophysiology

The pituitary gland, commonly referred to as the "master gland," secretes hormones that regulate the secretions of other endocrine glands. Located at the base of the brain, and approximately the size of a grape, it is attached to the hypothalamus. The pituitary gland is divided into two lobes:

- The anterior pituitary, which produces and secretes six hormones: growth hormone (GH), thyroid-stimulating hormone (TSH), ACTH, and three gonadotropic hormones
- The posterior pituitary, which secretes two hormones—antidiuretic hormone (ADH; also known as vasopressin) and oxytocin—but does not produce them

Central Diabetes Insipidus

Central diabetes insipidus occurs when the posterior part of the pituitary gland no longer secretes ADH. This condition may result from a traumatic head injury, neurosurgery, or autoimmune disease, or it may be genetic. Because of the lack of ADH, patients with this disease frequently experience free water loss from the kidneys, leading to severe dehydration and hypernatremia.

Signs and Symptoms

Central Diabetes Insipidus
- Polyuria with dilute urine
- Polydipsia
- Dehydration

Pituitary Lesions

Pituitary lesions can be classified into two types: nonfunctioning adenomas and functioning adenomas. A nonfunctioning adenoma is a tumor that does not secrete hormones. A functioning adenoma, in contrast, does secrete hormones. Depending on the type of hormone and the amount produced by the lesion, different diseases may result:

- ACTH-secreting adenomas are responsible for Cushing disease. Cushing disease is the cause

of Cushing syndrome (discussed later in this chapter).
- Growth hormone–secreting adenomas are responsible for acromegaly and gigantism.
- Prolactin-secreting adenomas are responsible for reproductive disorders.

The majority (approximately 70%) of pituitary lesions are functioning adenomas.

Acromegaly and Gigantism

Acromegaly is a syndrome that results from the secretion of excessive growth hormone by the pituitary gland *after* the epiphyseal plate has closed. Commonly affecting middle-aged adults, acromegaly can result in progressive enlargement of the face, hands, and feet; diabetes and hypertension; and ultimately, premature death if left untreated. Because of the slow progression of the syndrome, this condition often goes undiagnosed for many years.

Acromegaly is often associated with gigantism. Gigantism results from the secretion of excessive growth hormone by the pituitary gland *before* the epiphyseal plate has closed.

Regardless of the onset (childhood or adulthood), both acromegaly and gigantism are characterized by the growth of bones, muscles, and many internal organs at an abnormally fast rate. Acromegaly and gigantism are almost always caused by a benign pituitary tumor.

Signs and Symptoms

Acromegaly and Gigantism
- Abnormally fast growth of bones, muscles, and internal organs
- Onset of diabetes and hypertension

Assessment

Follow the same assessment steps for patients presenting with acromegaly or gigantism as you would for any other patient. Obtain a detailed medical history and information about weight gain as well as excessive and rapid growth.

Laboratory Assessment

Patients with acromegaly and gigantism typically present with elevated creatinine levels (greater than

1.2 mg/dL). Because acromegaly and gigantism are a result of excessive growth hormone production, GH levels will be elevated (more than 18 ng/mL).

Management

TABLE 18-1 lists medications used to treat acromegaly and gigantism. Bromocriptine (Parlodel), a dopaminergic agonist, is used to decrease growth hormone secretion. Octreotide (Sandostatin) and lanreotide (Somatuline), synthetic forms of the hormone somatostatin, stop growth hormone production entirely. Pegvisomant (Somavert), a growth hormone receptor antagonist, is used to treat acromegaly and gigantism. Pegvisomant can control acromegaly and gigantism in virtually all patients because of its ability to block the action of the endogenous growth hormone molecules.

Adrenal Abnormalities

Many abnormalities of the adrenal glands are possible. Some are hereditary (familial adrenal hypoplasia syndromes), others involve steroid resistance and hypersensitivity abnormalities such as glucocorticoid resistance syndromes and states, and some are genetic in origin, such as adrenal insufficiency as a result of X-linked adrenoleukodystrophy.

Pathophysiology

Conditions associated with a pseudo-Cushing state are a mixed group of disorders related to increased cortisol production. The physiologic conditions that cause increased cortisol production include stress associated with a recent surgery, severe illness, emotional stress, intense aerobic exercise, and caloric restriction. Nonphysiologic conditions that may elevate cortisol production include chronic alcoholism and alcohol withdrawal syndrome, poorly controlled diabetes mellitus, and obesity.

Endocrine hypertension is a result of hormonal disorders that cause clinically significant hypertension. The most common causes of endocrine hypertension are excess production of mineralocorticoids, such as aldosterone; catecholamines, such as epinephrine, norepinephrine, and dopamine; and glucocorticoids, such as cortisol. The cause of endocrine hypertension often relates to excess hormone produced by a tumor. Endocrine hypertension can be treated with surgery or antihypertensive therapy.

Adrenal Insufficiency

Underproduction of cortisol and aldosterone caused by decreased functioning of the adrenal cortex is called adrenal insufficiency (AI). When at least 90% of the adrenal cortex has been damaged, AI occurs. Cortisol helps the body respond to stress, including stress caused by surgery, illness, or infection. This hormone also aids in maintaining normal blood pressure and cardiovascular functions and regulating the metabolism of proteins, carbohydrates, and fats. AI may affect the adrenal gland (idiopathic AI) or other glands (polyendocrine deficiency syndrome).

Primary causes of AI include the following:

- Autoimmune disorders (eg, Hashimoto disease)
- Illness or increased stress
- Genetic disorders
- Renal injuries
- Radiation therapy
- Surgery
- Infections
- Pituitary and hypothalamic lesions

Adults of all ages are equally affected by AI. Causes of permanent AI include Addison disease, congenital adrenal hyperplasia, and complete surgical removal of the pituitary gland or the adrenal glands. Temporary AI can be caused by physical stress, infections, surgery, or medication noncompliance.

In the patient with chronic AI, signs and symptoms of addisonian crisis may appear suddenly as a result of an increased period of stress, trauma, recent surgery, or severe infection. The primary

TABLE 18-1 Medications Used to Treat Acromegaly and Gigantism	
Medication Class	**Examples**
Dopaminergic agonist	Bromocriptine (Parlodel)
Somatostatin analog	Octreotide (Sandostatin) Lanreotide (Somatuline)
Growth hormone receptor antagonist	Pegvisomant (Somavert)

© Jones & Bartlett Learning.

clinical manifestation of addisonian crisis is shock. Other symptoms include weakness, altered mental status, hyperthermia, and severe pain in the lower back, legs, or abdomen. Severe vomiting and diarrhea may precipitate dehydration in these patients.

The ACTH stimulation test is the most specific test for diagnosing AI; this test measures blood cortisol levels (normal range, 10 to 60 ng/L). When it goes undiagnosed, AI is a potentially fatal disease owing to hypotension or cardiac arrhythmias as a result of hyperkalemia. Acute AI may present in postsurgical or trauma patients.

Approximately 50% of patients with moderate or severe traumatic brain injury present with some form of AI. Patients with traumatic brain injury receiving high-dose pentobarbital or propofol as well as patients with vasopressors used to manage lower blood pressures should be carefully monitored for AI.

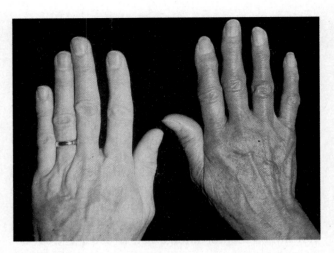

FIGURE 18-6 The hand of a patient with Addison disease (right) compared with the hand of a healthy patient (left).

Courtesy of Leonard V. Crowley, MD, Department of Laboratory Medicine and Pathology, University of Minnesota Medical School, Minneapolis, Minnesota.

Signs and Symptoms

Addisonian Crisis
- Shock
- Weakness
- Altered mental status
- Hyperthermia
- Severe pain in the lower back, legs, or abdomen
- Severe vomiting and diarrhea
- Dehydration

Addison Disease

Addison disease is a chronic hormonal or endocrine disorder that occurs in patients of all age groups; it is caused by a deficiency in cortisol and/or aldosterone. Addison disease is characterized by weakness, fatigue, hypotension, unexplained weight loss, and darkening of the skin **FIGURE 18-6**. Although other AI conditions can occur acutely, Addison disease is chronic.

Most cases of Addison disease are caused by the slow destruction of the adrenal cortex. Addison disease affects about 1 in 100,000 people.

Treatment of Addison disease is the same as that of acute AI conditions. The prognosis is good for well-managed adult-onset Addison disease, as these patients have a normal average mortality rate. In contrast, recent studies show that young patients with Addison disease are at risk for premature death. In patients diagnosed at a young age, Addison disease is still a potentially lethal condition, with excess mortality owing to acute adrenal failure, infection, and sudden death.

Signs and Symptoms

Addison Disease
- Weakness
- Fatigue
- Hypotension
- Unexplained weight loss
- Darkening of the skin

Cushing Syndrome

Cushing syndrome, also known as hypercortisolism, is caused by prolonged exposure to elevated levels of cortisol in the body. This syndrome, which is relatively rare, affects people between age 20 and 50 years. Risk factors for Cushing syndrome include obesity, poorly controlled type 2 diabetes, and hypertension. Patients taking glucocorticoids, such as prednisone for inflammatory diseases, are also at risk for developing Cushing syndrome.

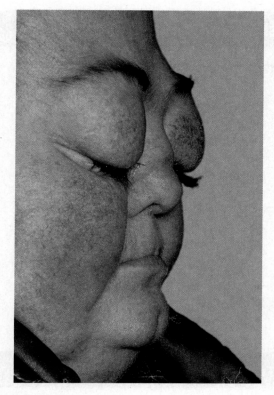

FIGURE 18-7 Weight gain in the face as a result of Cushing syndrome.

© Biophoto Associates/Science Source.

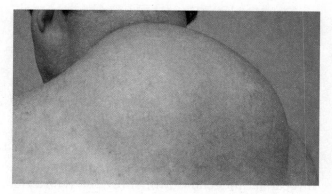

FIGURE 18-8 Weight gain in the upper part of the back as a result of Cushing syndrome.

© BSIP/Contributor/Universal Images Group/Getty Images.

Signs and Symptoms

Cushing Syndrome
- Hyperglycemia
- Weakness and fatigue
- Depression and mood swings
- Increased thirst and urination
- Weight gain (especially on the abdomen, face, neck, and upper back)
- Thinning of the skin; easy bruising and pink or purple stretch marks on the abdomen, thighs, breasts, and shoulders
- Increased acne, facial hair growth, and scalp hair loss; in women, menstrual irregularities
- Darkening of skin on the neck
- Obesity and poor growth in height in children

Regardless of the cause, excess cortisol causes characteristic changes in many body systems. The metabolism of carbohydrates, protein, and fat is disturbed, causing hyperglycemia. Protein synthesis is impaired so that body proteins are broken down, which leads to a loss of muscle fibers and muscle weakness. Bones become weaker and more susceptible to fracture. Other common signs and symptoms include the following:

- Weakness and fatigue
- Depression and mood swings
- Increased thirst and urination
- Weight gain, especially on the abdomen, face ("moon face") **FIGURE 18-7**, neck, and upper back ("buffalo hump") **FIGURE 18-8**
- Thinning of the skin, with easy bruising and pink or purple stretch marks (striae) on the abdomen, thighs, breasts, and shoulders
- Increased acne, facial hair growth, and scalp hair loss; in women, menstrual irregularities
- Darkening of skin (acanthosis) on the neck
- Obesity and restricted growth in children

Pheochromocytoma

A **pheochromocytoma** is a catecholamine-producing benign tumor of chromaffin cells, located in the center of the adrenal gland. The effects of such a tumor can manifest either sporadically or chronically. The catecholamines produced include epinephrine, norepinephrine, and occasionally dopamine. These catecholamines stimulate alpha-adrenergic receptors, resulting in severe hypertension, increased cardiac contractility, glycogenolysis, gluconeogenesis, and intestinal relaxation. Stimulation of the beta-adrenergic receptors increases the heart rate and contractility.

Although the majority of the pheochromocytomas are found in the adrenal glands, these tumors can arise anywhere there is chromaffin tissue. Approximately 95% occur in the abdomen, with the remaining 5% being found in other parts of the body.

Investigation of sustained hypertension leads to a diagnosis of pheochromocytomas in 0.05% to 0.2% of patients. Pheochromocytoma can be corrected in approximately 90% of cases if identified. If left untreated, fatal events such as catecholamine-induced malignant hypertension, heart failure, myocardial infarction (MI), stroke, or ventricular arrhythmias can occur.

Although patients may be temporarily treated with antihypertensive and cardiac rate-control medications, definitive treatment for pheochromocytoma consists of surgical removal of the tumor. Patients with pheochromocytoma should be treated with appropriate preoperative medical management to block the effects of released catecholamines.

Patients can experience a hypertensive crisis as a result of the rapid increase in catecholamines released from the tumor. They may present with varying symptoms, including severe headaches or diaphoresis, visual disturbances, palpitations, epistaxis, AMI, congestive heart failure, or stroke. Treatment of a hypertensive crisis triggered by a pheochromocytoma should be initiated immediately and commonly includes IV alpha blockers (phentolamine), beta blockers (esmolol or labetalol), and/or calcium channel blockers (nicardipine). Phentolamine is typically administered as a 5 mg IV bolus and may be repeated every 10 minutes to achieve target blood pressure. During the first hour, blood pressure targets are typically a systolic blood pressure of 140 mm Hg, not to exceed a 25% reduction in systolic blood pressure over the first hour.

Immediately following surgery for pheochromocytoma removal, some patients remain hypertensive, although the majority present with hypotension that requires treatment with fluids. Hypoglycemia is another postoperative complication that can be prevented by infusion of 5% dextrose started immediately after tumor removal and continuing for several hours thereafter. Postoperative hypoglycemia is transient, whereas hypotension may continue for several days or more after surgery.

The long-term prognosis of patients after pheochromocytoma excision is excellent. However, nearly one-half of these patients will experience resultant lifelong hypertension.

Signs and Symptoms

Pheochromocytoma

- Hypertension
- Increased heart rate
- Severe headache
- Diaphoresis
- Visual disturbances
- Palpitations
- Chest pain
- Upper abdominal pain
- Epistaxis
- Anxiety
- Acute myocardial infarction
- Congestive heart failure
- Stroke

Transport Management

Pheochromocytoma

- Administer IV boluses of phentolamine to achieve the target systolic blood pressure.

Aldosteronism

Aldosteronism is a syndrome of high blood pressure and low blood potassium levels caused by an excess of aldosterone. Two main types of aldosteronism are distinguished: primary and secondary.

Primary aldosteronism (also known as Conn syndrome) is usually caused by a tumor of a single adrenal gland that overproduces aldosterone. More than 95% of such cases are benign. On rare occasions, however, these tumors may be malignant.

Secondary aldosteronism results from other conditions not associated with the adrenal gland. It can be caused by obstructive renal artery disease, renal vasoconstriction, and edematous disorders, and occurs as a result of reduced renal blood flow. The reduced blood flow stimulates hypersecretion of aldosterone.

Aldosteronism should be suspected in patients with hypertension and hypokalemia because aldosterone normally functions to increase sodium and fluid in the bloodstream as well as potassium excretion by the kidney. Elevated aldosterone levels can be measured via blood or urine chemistry. A special blood test that measures plasma renin activity is performed to distinguish between primary aldosteronism (low plasma renin activity) and secondary aldosteronism (high plasma renin activity). Once blood chemistry testing is completed, a computed tomography (CT) scan of the abdomen may be performed to confirm the location of the disease.

Surgery is the appropriate treatment for aldosteronism if the primary cause is a single adenoma. When the cause does not lie within the adrenal gland, treatment is to correct the underlying condition that led to the elevated aldosterone levels.

Signs and Symptoms

Aldosteronism
- Hypertension
- Low blood potassium levels
- Alkalosis
- Muscular weakness
- Polyuria
- Polydipsia
- Edema
- Heart failure
- Hepatic cirrhosis

Amyloidosis

Amyloidosis comprises a group of diseases that result from abnormal deposits of the protein amyloid in various tissues of the body. This protein can be deposited in a localized area, or it may affect tissues throughout the body in a systemic fashion. Systemic amyloidosis can lead to serious changes in virtually any organ of the body and can cause the affected organs to fail.

Primary amyloidosis—the most common form of amyloidosis—affects the heart, kidneys, tongue, nerves, and intestines. This condition is associated with multiple myeloma, a form of bone marrow cancer, in a minority of cases. The form of amyloid deposited in primary amyloidosis is classified as an apolipoprotein.

Secondary amyloidosis occurs as a result of another illness, such as multiple myeloma, chronic infection, or chronic inflammatory disease. The form of amyloid deposited in secondary amyloidosis is classified as an amyloid A protein. This disease mostly affects the kidneys, spleen, liver, and lymph nodes, although other organs may be involved. Treatment of the underlying disease may help mitigate this form of amyloidosis.

There is no known cure for amyloidosis. Therapies are directed at managing symptoms and limiting the production of amyloid protein.

Signs and Symptoms

Amyloidosis
- Pedal edema
- Weight loss
- Dyspnea
- Weakness
- Diarrhea
- Fatigue
- Cardiac arrhythmias

Assessment

Patients with adrenal abnormalities may present with variable physical findings and vital signs on examination. The patient assessment, the history of present illness or injury, and a thorough review of medical history will aid in determining whether adrenal abnormalities are influencing the patient's vital signs and symptoms. It is also important to be aware of the possibility of adrenal complications in a patient's differential diagnosis. Treatment of adrenal abnormalities may not be commonly recognized as necessary, contributing to increased morbidity and mortality for patients with these conditions.

Signs and Symptoms

In addition to the medical history and physical exam, diagnosis of Cushing syndrome or Cushing disease requires laboratory studies showing elevated levels of blood cortisol.

The assessment of the patient with pheochromocytoma may reveal hypertension and other symptoms associated with catecholamine release, such as tachycardia, diaphoresis, chest pain, upper abdominal pain, and anxiety.

Primary aldosteronism typically presents with hypokalemia, alkalosis, muscular weakness, polyuria, polydipsia, and hypertension. Secondary aldosteronism is commonly associated with edematous states, heart failure, hepatic cirrhosis, and malignant hypertension.

Signs and symptoms of amyloidosis depend on the organ system affected, but typically include pedal edema, weight loss, dyspnea, weakness, diarrhea, fatigue, and cardiac arrhythmias.

Laboratory Assessment

Laboratory testing is required to definitively diagnose these underlying health conditions and will vary with the disease process.

The ACTH stimulation test, along with the cortisol test, is the most specific combination of tests for diagnosing Addison disease. In these tests, a synthetic form of ACTH is injected into the patient, with blood and urine cortisol measurements obtained before and after the injection. In a healthy patient, blood and urine cortisol levels will rise after an injection of ACTH. In contrast, patients with AI will exhibit less of an increase or no increase at all. The normal range for cortisol levels in adults is 5 to 25 µg/dL; the normal range for aldosterone levels in adults is 2 to 9 ng/dL.

No increase in blood and urine cortisol levels after injection of ACTH indicates the pituitary gland is the likely origin of the condition, whereas a delayed increase indicates the hypothalamus is the likely source. Specifically, patients with primary AI have high ACTH levels but do not produce cortisol. Patients with secondary AI have decreased cortisol responses but absent or delayed ACTH responses.

Unlike adults, children are more likely to have absolute AI, defined by a basal cortisol level of less than 18 µg/dL and a peak ACTH-stimulated cortisol concentration of less than 18 µg/dL. Patients at risk of inadequate cortisol or aldosterone production in the setting of shock include those who previously received corticosteroid therapies for chronic illness, those with pituitary or AI, and children with purpura fulminans and Waterhouse-Friderichsen syndrome.

Management

Treatment of adrenal diseases usually involves replacing or substituting the deficient adrenal gland hormones. The details vary with the underlying cause, the clinical presentation, and the severity of symptoms.

The initial treatment of acute adrenal crisis focuses on correcting hypovolemic shock via fluid resuscitation. Fluid resuscitation (500 to 1,000 mL) with an isotonic crystalloid solution should be given by the IV or IO route. For a patient diagnosed with glucocorticoid deficiency, IV steroids such as dexamethasone or hydrocortisone may be administered. Dexamethasone has a long duration of action and does not interfere with serum or urinary steroid testing; therefore, it is preferred for this indication.

TABLE 18-2 lists medications used to treat adrenal conditions. Although treatment of patients with pituitary disorders in the acute setting is rare, the CCTP should appreciate the impact that these disease processes have on a patient's day-to-day life, and should maintain a high index of suspicion when encountering a patient who may be presenting with these signs and symptoms.

Thyroid Abnormalities

Although transport of a patient with a life-threatening thyroid condition may be uncommon, a CCTP with a high index of suspicion and understanding of laboratory studies may be in a position to appreciate and better manage these conditions.

Pathophysiology

The thyroid gland, which serves as the primary controller of the body's metabolism, produces the hormones T_3 (triiodothyronine) and T_4 (thyroxine). These hormones stimulate an increase in organ function in all organs that are exposed to them.

Hypothyroidism

Hypothyroidism is caused by a deficiency of T_3 and T_4, both of which are secreted by the thyroid gland. Because of the decreased production of these hormones, the body's organ function slows, causing the patient to feel a decrease in body temperature, to have gradual weight gain, and to have an increased risk for AMI and stroke. In the critical care patient, a careful history will help with the diagnosis of hypothyroidism.

TABLE 18-2 Medications Used to Treat Adrenal Conditions	
Medication Class	**Examples**
Adrenal Insufficiency Synthetic glucocorticoids	Fludrocortisone acetate (Florinef), taken once per day.
Cushing Syndrome Synthetic cortisol	Ketoconazole (Nizoral), mitotane (Lysodren), metyrapone (Metopirone), prednisone, hydrocortisone, dexamethasone; dosages depend on the cause of the syndrome and the treatment plan.
Pheochromocytoma Antihypertensives	Phentolamine: IV bolus of 5 mg; nicardipine: 5 mg/h IV, increase by 2.5 mg/h every 5 min to a maximum of 15 mg/h; esmolol (rate-control): IV bolus of 1 mg/kg over 30 seconds followed by 150 mcg/kg/min infusion to a maximum of 200 mcg/kg/min.
Aldosteronism	Treatment for primary aldosteronism depends on the underlying cause.
Amyloidosis	Treatment is directed at managing symptoms and limiting the production of amyloid protein; it includes melphalan (Alkeran or Alkeran IV), a chemotherapy agent, and dexamethasone. New drugs being tested for use in amyloidosis include bortezomib (Velcade), thalidomide (Thalomid), and lenalidomide (Revlimid).

© Jones & Bartlett Learning.

Signs and Symptoms

Hypothyroidism

- Decrease in body temperature
- Gradual weight gain
- Lethargy
- Constipation
- Muscle aches and weakness
- Joint pain, stiffness, or swelling
- Facial swelling
- Pale, dry skin
- Brittle fingernails and hair
- Hoarse voice
- Depression

Hyperthyroidism

Hyperthyroidism is caused by increased production of T_3 and T_4. Because the excess hormones increase the body's metabolism, patients with hyperthyroidism experience an increase in body temperature and gradual weight loss, even if they are eating the same amounts of food as they did before this condition occurred. Other side effects of hyperthyroidism include increased and/or irregular heart rate, sweating, and irritability.

Signs and Symptoms

Hyperthyroidism

- Increase in body temperature
- Gradual weight loss
- Increased and/or irregular heart rate
- Hypertension
- Sweating
- Irritability

Thyrotoxicosis and Thyroid Storm

Thyrotoxicosis and thyroid storm are rare but severe, life-threatening conditions that can occur in patients with long-term, untreated or undertreated hyperthyroidism. However, they are most commonly precipitated by an acute physiologic stressor such as a surgical procedure, trauma, infection, administration of large doses of iodine such as in the cardiac catheterization lab, or abrupt discontinuation of thyroid medications. Thyrotoxicosis is sometimes referred to as "impending thyroid storm," while severe thyrotoxicosis is considered "thyroid storm," although there are no universally accepted criteria defining either condition.

Even a minor trauma, such as a laceration, can cause a patient with hyperthyroidism to experience thyrotoxicosis. It is unclear why thyroid storm develops, but the mortality from this condition is high, ranging from 10% to 20%. Patients typically exhibit severe symptoms of hyperthyroidism, including hyperpyrexia (body temperature greater than 103°F [39°C], often ranging from 104°F to 106°F [40°C to 41°C]), altered mental status, and myocardial depression. Significant tachycardias and atrial fibrillation are common as well. Treatment includes the use of beta blockers, thionamides (ie, propylthiouracil or methimazole), iodine, glucocorticoids, and, in some patients, bile acid sequestrants.

Myxedema Coma

Myxedema coma is a rare, life-threatening clinical condition in patients with long-standing, severe, untreated hypothyroidism. Most commonly seen in older adult female patients, this condition has an extremely high mortality rate if left untreated. Myxedema coma is characterized by three key features:

- Altered mental status and lethargy (including lengthy sleeping patterns)
- Failure of the thermoregulatory system (hypothermia or the absence of fever despite infectious disease)
- A precipitating event (eg, cold exposure, infection, drugs [diuretics, tranquilizers, sedatives, or analgesics], trauma, stroke, heart failure, or gastrointestinal bleeding)

A person who initially presents with myxedema coma is usually hypothermic and may be experiencing both auditory and visual hallucinations, seizures, or depressed mental status.

Signs and Symptoms

Myxedema Coma
- Hypothermia
- Auditory and visual hallucinations
- Seizures
- Depressed mental status

Hashimoto Disease

Hashimoto disease, also known as chronic lymphocytic thyroiditis, occurs when the immune system attacks the patient's thyroid gland. The resulting

inflammation leads to hypothyroidism. In fact, Hashimoto disease is the leading cause of hypothyroidism, most commonly affecting women between ages 30 and 50 years.

Assessment

A patient with a thyroid-related condition may present with signs and symptoms of hypothyroidism (general weakness, cold intolerance, altered mental status, abdominal pain, and lethargy) or hyperthyroidism (heart-related complications that can include rapid heart rate, congestive heart failure, atrial fibrillation, and hypertension). The physical exam may reveal thyroid enlargement (goiter) **FIGURE 18-9**. In cases of hyperthyroidism, thyrotoxicosis may occur. Although hypothyroid emergencies are rare, they require urgent evaluation and treatment.

Laboratory Assessment

Laboratory tests that evaluate thyroid function include serum TSH, T_3, and T_4. The normal range of serum TSH is 0.4 to 4.2 mIU/L for persons with no symptoms of abnormal thyroid function. However, people without signs or symptoms of hypothyroidism who have a TSH value greater than 2.0 mIU/L but normal T_4 levels may experience hypothyroidism in the future; this condition is called subclinical hypothyroidism (mildly underactive thyroid) or early-stage hypothyroidism. Patients being treated for a thyroid disorder should have a TSH level between 0.5 and 3.0 mIU/L. Low levels of TSH indicate

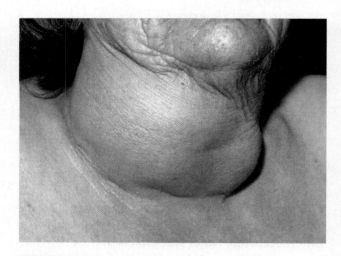

FIGURE 18-9 Thyroid enlargement.
© Dr. P. Marazzi/Science Source.

possible hyperthyroidism or pituitary gland failure, and above-normal values indicate thyroid gland failure or a pituitary gland tumor.

TABLE 18-3 describes common laboratory studies for thyroid-related conditions.

Management

Treatment of thyroid conditions depends on the cause of the condition and the severity of symptoms. As with most conditions discussed in this chapter, transport management is mainly supportive.

Hypothyroidism is typically treated with hormone replacement therapy. Complications may sometimes arise related to replacement of the thyroid hormones. If too little hormone is given, then symptoms of hypothyroidism can occur, including fatigue, increased cholesterol levels, mild weight gain, depression, and slowing of mental and physical activity. If too much hormone is given, then the symptoms of hyperthyroidism will occur.

Hyperthyroidism is usually treated with antithyroid medications, radioactive iodine (which destroys the thyroid and stops the excess production of hormones), or surgical removal of the thyroid. Beta blockers, such as propranolol, are indicated to treat the resultant tachycardia, and anxiety may be treated with diazepam, lorazepam, or midazolam until the hyperthyroidism can be controlled. If the thyroid must be removed through radiation therapy or surgery, then replacement thyroid hormones must be taken for the rest of the person's life.

Thyroid storm is a life-threatening condition with extremely high mortality if it is not promptly recognized and treated. Initial treatment consists of a beta blocker, which blocks the increased adrenergic tone that is caused by excessive thyroid hormone secretion and that results in tachycardia, tremor, hyperthermia, and arrhythmias such as atrial fibrillation. Propranolol is the most commonly used beta blocker for this purpose, as it can be given intravenously or orally and is widely available. Initial dosing is 0.5 to 1.0 mg IV over 10 minutes, followed by 1 to 2 mg IV every 15 minutes. Alternatively, 60 to 80 mg can be given orally every 4 hours.

Once adequate beta blockade is achieved, a thionamide, such as propylthiouracil or methimazole, is administered. These agents block synthesis of new thyroid hormone, and propylthiouracil also inhibits conversion of T_4 to T_3. Typical doses are a 500 to 1,000 mg loading dose of propylthiouracil, followed by 250 mg every 4 hours, or 60 to 80 mg of methimazole per day. Next, iodine is administered at least 1 hour after a thionamide is given to block thyroid hormone conversion. Additionally, glucocorticoids

TABLE 18-3 Common Laboratory Studies for Thyroid-Related Conditions

Laboratory Study	Normal Range	Causes of Low Levels	Causes of High Levels
Thyroid-stimulating hormone (TSH)	0.4–4.2 mIU/L	Hyperthyroidism, or pituitary gland failure	Thyroid gland failure, or pituitary gland tumor
T_3 (triiodothyronine)	60–180 ng/dL	Hypothyroidism	Hyperthyroidism
Total T_4 (thyroxine)	5.5–12.5 µg/dL	Hypothyroidism	Hyperthyroidism
Free T_4 (thyroxine)	0.9–2.3 ng/dL	Hypothyroidism	Hyperthyroidism
RT_3U (triiodothyronine reuptake)	24%–37%	Hypothyroidism	Hyperthyroidism
Triglycerides	<160 mg/dL	Clinically irrelevant with respect to thyroid disorders	Possible hypothyroidism
Radioactive iodine uptake	8%–25%	Hypothyroidism	Hyperthyroidism
Glucose tolerance test	Fasting: 70–1,100 mg/dL	Clinically irrelevant with respect to thyroid disorders	Hyperthyroidism
Thyroglobulin antibody	<2 ng/mL	Clinically irrelevant with respect to thyroid disorders	Hyperthyroidism

TABLE 18-4 Medications Used to Treat Thyroid Conditions	
Medication Class	**Examples**
Antithyroid medications	Methimazole (Tapazole) or propylthiouracil
Thyroid hormone	Levothyroxine (L-Thyroxin, Levolet, Levo-T, Levothroid, Levoxyl, Novothyrox, Synthroid, Thyro-Tabs, or Unithroid), liothyronine (Cytomel), or liotrix (Euthroid or Thyrolar)
Beta blockers	Acebutolol (Sectral), atenolol (Tenormin), betaxolol (Kerlone), bisoprolol (Zebeta), carteolol (Cartrol), carvedilol (Coreg), labetalol (Normodyne or Trandate), metoprolol (Lopressor or Toprol-XL), nadolol (Corgard), nebivolol (Bystolic), penbutolol (Levatol), pindolol (Visken), propranolol (Inderal), sotalol (Betapace), or timolol (Blocadren)

© Jones & Bartlett Learning.

can be given to prevent adrenal suppression and help decrease conversion of T_4 to T_3. Ultimately, the patient will require thyroidectomy.

Myxedema coma is a rare, life-threatening condition marked by severe hypothyroidism. It requires aggressive treatment, as mortality may otherwise approach 40%. Initial therapy consists of IV T_4 (levothyroxine) and T_3 (triiodothyronine). This therapy must be administered carefully and in a closely monitored setting (such as an intensive care unit), as side effects may include arrhythmia and MI. Additional treatments consist of supportive measures including management of hypothermia, fluid resuscitation and electrolyte repletion, and empiric antibiotics for an underlying precipitant infection.

TABLE 18-4 lists medications used to treat thyroid conditions.

Lipid Disorders

Lipid disorders cause a change in the production or use of cholesterol. They may also alter the way cholesterol is circulated or processed in the body. As a result, patients with lipid disorders experience very high total cholesterol levels; very low high-density lipoprotein (HDL), or "good," cholesterol levels; or high triglyceride levels.

A lipid disorder increases the patient's risk for atherosclerosis and heart disease, but is rarely a true medical emergency.

Antiphospholipid Syndrome

Antiphospholipid syndrome (APS) is an autoimmune disorder in which antibodies block certain phospholipid-binding proteins that normally protect the body from excessive coagulation. It was first recognized in patients with systemic lupus erythematosus (SLE), as the lupus anticoagulant is an antiphospholipid autoantibody. Now, however, APS is more commonly recognized as a primary condition. Patients with APS may experience venous or arterial thrombosis or fetal demise during pregnancy, and have laboratory evidence of antiphospholipid antibodies. Treatment focuses on preventing thrombotic events through the use of anticoagulants.

Metabolic Syndrome

Metabolic syndrome is a group of risk factors (hypertension, dyslipidemia, insulin resistance, hyperinsulinemia, glucose intolerance, and obesity, particularly central obesity) that together may lead to coronary artery disease, stroke, and type 2 diabetes. Although this syndrome is not widely understood, patients display the risk factors and predisposition for lipid disorders and, consequently, for heart disease.

Flight Considerations

Patients experiencing endocrine-related disorders require the same management in flight as during ground transport. No special management considerations apply when flying at altitude.

Summary

Although endocrine disorders are not a common cause for a critical care transport, an understanding of endocrine-related conditions and their pathophysiology will help the CCTP care for patients with these conditions. As always, it is important to ensure patients maintain appropriate blood glucose levels and hemodynamic parameters. An appreciation of AI, in particular, can help prevent patient death.

Case Study

You are just finishing up your dinner after a relatively quiet shift when your dispatch center advises that you are being dispatched to Pondera Medical Center, approximately 95 miles (183 km) away. A patient there has been diagnosed with DKA and requires transport to your base hospital, Northern Rockies Medical Center, for further treatment in the intensive care unit. You and your partner, an EMT, depart for the rural hospital.

When you arrive at Pondera Medical Center, you are met by the attending physician. He advises you that the patient is a 28-year-old, 84-kg man who had been complaining of general malaise and increasing thirst for the past 3 to 4 days. The patient's family called 9-1-1 this morning when they found him with altered mental status. He was subsequently transported to Pondera Medical Center via BLS ambulance with a Glasgow Coma Scale (GCS) score of 8 (eye-opening score, 2; verbal score, 2; motor score, 4). On arrival, the patient's GCS score had increased to 12 (eye-opening score, 3; verbal score, 3; motor score, 6) and he was able to answer some questions appropriately but with difficulty. According to the family members, the patient is generally healthy, has no medical conditions, takes no medications, and has no allergies. They tell you it seems as if he has been drinking "a lot" of water over the past couple of days and has had to urinate excessively.

Treatment in the emergency department included a bedside glucose test that revealed high serum glucose concentration, laboratory studies including a complete blood cell count and comprehensive metabolic panel, and an electrocardiogram that was unremarkable. The patient has a 16-gauge IV catheter in his left forearm, currently running normal saline to keep the vein open. The patient has received two boluses of normal saline, with each bolus based on a rate of 20 mL/kg, and 10 units of IV regular human insulin, which decreased the blood glucose level to 580 mg/dL on recheck.

On admission, vital signs included the following: blood pressure, 89/42 mm Hg; heart rate, 132 beats/min; sinus tachycardia with no ectopy; clear respirations, 36 breaths/min with a Kussmaul respiration pattern; and oxygen saturation as measured by pulse oximetry, 96% on room air. Laboratory studies revealed the following abnormalities: glucose, 789 mg/dL; blood urea nitrogen, 60 mg/dL; creatinine, 2.0 mg/dL; chloride, 116 mEq/L; potassium, 5.5 mEq/L; and sodium, 151 mEq/L. A urinalysis was positive for ketones and glucose. Venous blood gases showed metabolic acidosis with a pH of 7.04; $Paco_2$, 19 mm Hg; bicarbonate, 4 mEq/L; and base deficit of 12.

As your partner is securing the patient onto the stretcher and connecting him to your transport monitoring equipment for the return transport, you contact your base hospital physician to advise her of the patient's status, obtain any additional orders, and give an estimated time of arrival. The receiving intensivist has requested a continuous insulin infusion be initiated at 8.4 units/h, which she expects will decrease the blood glucose level by 50 mg/dL/h.

Once en route back to Northern Rockies Medical Center, you prepare an insulin infusion by adding 100 units of regular insulin to a 100-mL bag of normal saline and begin the infusion at 8.4 units/h, based on a rate of 0.1 unit/kg/h. Because of the patient's altered mental status, you elect to administer 4 mg of ondansetron IV as prophylaxis against vomiting and insert a 16 F nasogastric tube in the left nare. After approximately 20 minutes, you recheck the patient's blood glucose level using your glucometer and obtain a reading of 550 mg/dL. Once you arrive at Northern Rockies Medical Center, the patient is taken directly to the intensive care unit for continuing treatment.

1. How was the diagnosis of DKA determined?
2. Why was the patient given 3,360 mL of normal saline?
3. What are the potential complications that you may experience while en route with this patient?

Analysis

Because of your critical care training, you are able to recognize that this patient is experiencing DKA based on the presence of Kussmaul respirations, an elevated blood glucose reading, and arterial blood gas abnormalities. Symptoms of DKA include an elevated blood glucose level, acidosis, and an altered mental status. Signs include polydipsia, polyphagia, polyuria, and Kussmaul respirations.

This patient was given 3,360 mL of normal saline (20 mL/kg) in an attempt to hydrate him because of excessive fluid losses; the hypovolemia led to his tachycardia and hypotension. Short-acting insulin was administered in an attempt to decrease the blood glucose level. It is imperative not to decrease glucose levels too quickly in cases of DKA because of the possibility of cerebral edema. In an attempt to gradually decrease the glucose level, a continuous infusion of insulin was initiated, allowing the CCTP to accurately titrate the amount of insulin based on glucose level. Ondansetron (Zofran) was given prophylactically to minimize the risk of aspiration resulting from decreased mental status.

This patient has the potential to experience several complications en route. The ground transport was 95 miles (183 km); with the patient's decreased level of consciousness, the possibility of aspiration must be considered. Insertion of a nasogastric tube minimizes this risk, but the CCTP must still carefully monitor the patient's airway. With any patient presenting with an altered mental status in the transport environment, CCTPs need to be aware of the possible need to perform definitive airway management, which is often difficult in the confined space of an ambulance. Furthermore, with continued administration of insulin, the possibility of inadvertent hypoglycemia may develop. Hypoglycemia can be recognized through vigilant monitoring of the patient's blood glucose level and subsequently corrected by reducing the insulin infusion and administering dextrose-containing fluid based on local protocols. Close monitoring of the ECG, capnography, and pulse oximetry also provides rapid and early warning of changes in the patient's condition.

Prep Kit

Ready for Review

- CCTPs should be familiar with the endocrine system and its function.
- The thyroid gland secretes thyroxine to regulate the body's metabolism and calcitonin to maintain normal calcium levels in the blood.
- The adrenal glands consist of the adrenal cortex, which produces corticosteroids, and the adrenal medulla, which produces catecholamines (the hormones epinephrine and norepinephrine).
- During stress, adrenocorticotropic hormone causes the adrenal cortex to secrete cortisol, which stimulates the body's cells to increase energy production.
- The adrenal cortex secretes aldosterone if blood pressure or volume drops, sodium level decreases, or potassium level increases. The aldosterone increases the reabsorption of sodium and water and releases potassium into the kidneys, thereby increasing circulating blood volume and, in turn, blood pressure.
- During the "fight-or-flight" response, the adrenal medulla secretes small amounts of norepinephrine and large amounts of epinephrine to enable the body to respond to a short-term emergency.
- The pancreas is both an endocrine gland and an exocrine gland. The exocrine component secretes digestive enzymes; the

Prep Kit Continued

endocrine component comprises the islets of Langerhans.

- The main hormones secreted by the pancreas are glucagon and insulin, which regulate blood glucose levels. Insulin is the only hormone that decreases blood glucose levels; it is essential for glucose to enter and nourish the cells.
- Diabetes is a metabolic disorder in which the body's ability to metabolize glucose is impaired as a result of either insufficient production or inadequate utilization of insulin.
- There are two major types of diabetes mellitus: type 1 and type 2. Type 1 diabetes generally occurs in children, whereas type 2 diabetes commonly occurs in adults.
- Most patients with type 1 diabetes do not produce enough insulin. In patients with type 2 diabetes, the pancreas produces adequate insulin, but the body is not able to use it—a condition known as insulin resistance. Type 2 diabetes can also be caused by a deficiency in insulin production.
- Hypoglycemia, a drop in the blood glucose level, can develop rapidly in patients with diabetes, with alcoholism, following an ingested poison or certain drugs, or with other medical conditions such as cancer, liver disease, or kidney disease. If hypoglycemia persists, it can lead to seizure, coma, and death.
- Hyperglycemia, an increase in the blood glucose level to above the normal range, can have either a rapid or gradual onset. If left untreated, hyperglycemia may progress to diabetic ketoacidosis (DKA) or hyperosmolar hyperglycemic state (HHS), both of which are life-threatening conditions.
- Patients with DKA tend to be young—teenagers to young adults. The development of DKA usually progresses slowly, over a period of 12 to 48 hours, and can lead to dehydration and shock.
- HHS occurs principally in patients with type 2 diabetes. It is characterized by hyperglycemia,

hyperosmolarity, and an absence of significant ketones.

- Signs of hypoglycemia may mimic those associated with intoxication. Patients presenting with signs of intoxication, such as slurred speech and lack of coordination, should be evaluated for hypoglycemia.
- Hyperglycemia and DKA typically present with the three Ps: polyuria, polydipsia, and polyphagia. The two hallmark signs of DKA are Kussmaul respirations and fruity-smelling breath.
- Signs of HHS are similar to those of DKA, except that patients with HHS do not typically present with Kussmaul respirations or fruity-smelling breath.
- CCTPs may test for hypoglycemia or hyperglycemia during transport. Knowledge of the glucometer being used is important for accurately interpreting the readings.
- Insulin infusions are routinely used in critically ill patients. The CCTP should check the patient's blood glucose levels frequently using a blood glucometer and adjust the insulin infusion rate to maintain the blood glucose targets prescribed for the patient.
- Signs and symptoms of pituitary disorders commonly mirror those associated with other disease processes; a careful medical history and physical exam are key to identifying an underlying condition.
- The pituitary gland is divided into two lobes: the anterior pituitary and the posterior pituitary. The anterior pituitary produces and secretes six hormones; the posterior pituitary secretes two hormones, which it does not produce.
- Central diabetes insipidus, caused by a decrease in ADH secretion from the posterior pituitary gland, is characterized by polyuria and polydipsia, which lead to dehydration.
- Pituitary lesions are classified into two types: nonfunctioning adenomas and functioning adenomas. Nonfunctioning adenomas do not

secrete hormones; with functioning adenomas, overproduction of hormones may occur.

- Acromegaly results from excessive secretion of growth hormone by the pituitary gland after the epiphyseal plate has closed. Gigantism results from excessive secretion of growth hormone by the pituitary gland before the epiphyseal plate has closed. Both conditions are characterized by growth of bones, muscles, and many internal organs at an abnormally fast rate, and both are usually caused by a benign pituitary tumor.
- Acromegaly and gigantism are managed with medications.
- Disorders of the adrenal glands may stem from genetic disorders, corticosteroid resistance, or hypersensitivity abnormalities.
- Pseudo-Cushing states comprise a mixed group of disorders related to increased cortisol production. They may be caused by physiologic conditions, such as severe illness or intense aerobic exercise, or by nonphysiologic conditions, such as chronic alcoholism and obesity.
- Endocrine hypertension is a result of hormonal disorders that cause clinically significant hypertension. This condition is often related to overproduction of hormones by a tumor.
- Adrenal insufficiency (AI) is characterized by underproduction of cortisol and aldosterone, caused by decreased functioning of the adrenal cortex. This condition may be temporary or permanent, and it affects adults of all ages.
- In patients with chronic AI, signs and symptoms of addisonian crisis may appear suddenly as a result of an increased period of stress, trauma, surgery, or severe infection. If it goes undiagnosed, AI is potentially fatal.
- Addison disease is a chronic disorder caused by a deficiency in cortisol and/or aldosterone. Although it occurs in all age groups, young patients with Addison disease are at higher risk for premature death from this condition.
- Cushing syndrome is caused by prolonged exposure to elevated levels of cortisol in the

body. A relatively rare condition, it typically affects patients ages 20 to 50 years. Excess cortisol affects many body systems, leading to hyperglycemia, muscle weakness, and bone weakness, among other signs and symptoms.

- A pheochromocytoma is a catecholamine-producing benign tumor of chromaffin cells. Most (95%) arise in the abdomen; the remaining 5% are found in other parts of the body. Most pheochromocytomas can be treated successfully by surgery to remove the tumor; if untreated, they can be fatal.
- Aldosteronism is a syndrome of high blood pressure and low blood potassium levels caused by an excess of aldosterone. Two types are distinguished: primary and secondary.
- Primary aldosteronism (Conn syndrome) is caused by a tumor; most cases are benign. Secondary aldosteronism occurs as a result of reduced renal blood flow, which stimulates hypersecretion of aldosterone.
- A low plasma renin activity blood test indicates primary aldosteronism; high plasma renin activity indicates secondary aldosteronism. Treatment for either condition consists of surgery or treatment of the underlying condition.
- Amyloidosis results from abnormal deposits of the protein amyloid in various tissues of the body. Primary amyloidosis is the most common form; secondary amyloidosis occurs as the result of another illness. There is no cure for amyloidosis, so treatments focus on managing the symptoms and limiting production of the amyloid protein.
- Transport of patients with a life-threatening disorder resulting from a thyroid abnormality is rare. Transport management for patients with thyroid conditions is mainly supportive.
- The thyroid gland is the primary controller of the body's metabolism; it produces the hormones T_3 and T_4.
- Hypothyroidism is caused by a deficiency of the hormones T_3 and T_4. Patients with

Prep Kit Continued

hypothyroidism are at increased risk for acute myocardial infarction and stroke.

- Hyperthyroidism is caused by increased production of the hormones T_3 and T_4, or ingestion of exogenous thyroid replacement medication. Abnormal vital signs will commonly be more pronounced in the hyperthyroid patient compared to the hypothyroid patient, including tachycardia and hypertension.
- Thyrotoxicosis and thyroid storm are rare but severe, life-threatening events that can occur in patients with long-term, untreated hyperthyroidism. However, they are more commonly precipitated in hyperthyroid patients by an acute physiologic stressor.
- Myxedema coma is a rare, life-threatening clinical condition in patients with long-standing, severe, untreated hypothyroidism. It occurs most often in older female patients and can be fatal if untreated.
- Hashimoto disease, the leading cause of hypothyroidism, arises when the immune system attacks the patient's thyroid gland. It most commonly affects women ages 30 to 50 years.
- Laboratory tests that evaluate thyroid function include serum thyroid-stimulating hormone, T_3, and T_4.
- Lipid disorders cause a change in the production or use of cholesterol. Such disorders rarely cause a true medical emergency, but do increase the patient's risk for atherosclerosis and heart disease.
- Antiphospholipid syndrome (APS) is an autoimmune disorder in which antibodies block certain phospholipid-binding proteins that normally prevent excessive coagulation. Patients with APS may experience venous or arterial thrombosis, or fetal demise during pregnancy.
- Metabolic syndrome is a group of risk factors (hypertension, dyslipidemia, insulin resistance, hyperinsulinemia, glucose intolerance, and obesity, particularly central obesity) that together may lead to coronary artery disease, stroke, and type 2 diabetes.

Vital Vocabulary

ascromegaly A syndrome that results from excessive secretion of growth hormone by the pituitary gland after the epiphyseal plate has closed; characterized by the growth of bones, muscles, and many internal organs at an abnormally fast rate.

Addison disease A chronic hormonal or endocrine disorder caused by a deficiency of cortisol and/or aldosterone; characterized by weakness, fatigue, hypotension, unexplained weight loss, and darkening of the skin.

addisonian crisis The sudden appearance of symptoms, especially shock, in a patient with chronic adrenal insufficiency; it may appear suddenly as a result of an increased period of stress, trauma, surgery, or severe infection. Other symptoms include weakness, altered mental status, hyperthermia, and severe pain in the lower back, legs, or abdomen.

adrenal insufficiency (AI) Underproduction of cortisol and aldosterone caused by a decreased function of the adrenal cortex; it occurs when at least 90% of the adrenal cortex has been damaged.

aldosterone The main hormone responsible for adjustments to the final composition of urine; it increases the rate of active resorption of sodium and chloride ions into the blood and decreases the resorption of potassium.

aldosteronism A syndrome of high blood pressure and low blood potassium levels caused by an excess of aldosterone; there are two main types—primary and secondary.

amyloidosis A group of diseases that result from abnormal deposits of the protein amyloid in various tissues of the body; can occur in a localized area or may be systemic.

Prep Kit Continued

antiphospholipid syndrome (APS) An autoimmune disorder in which antibodies block certain phospholipid-binding proteins that normally protect the body from excessive coagulation.

central diabetes insipidus A condition caused by a decrease in ADH secretion from the posterior pituitary gland; characterized by polyuria and polydipsia, which lead to dehydration.

Cushing syndrome A condition caused by overproduction of cortisol by the adrenal glands or by excessive use of cortisol or other similar steroid (glucocorticoid) hormones; also known as hypercortisolism.

diabetes mellitus A metabolic disorder in which the pancreas's ability to metabolize simple carbohydrates (glucose) is impaired because of either inadequate production of insulin or insensitivity to circulating insulin.

diabetic ketoacidosis (DKA) A form of acidosis in uncontrolled diabetes in which certain acids accumulate in the body when insulin is not available.

endocrine hypertension Significant high blood pressure caused by a hormonal disorder; often related to excess hormone produced by a tumor.

functioning adenoma A type of pituitary lesion in which overproduction of hormones occurs.

gigantism A syndrome that results from excessive secretion of growth hormone by the pituitary gland before the epiphyseal plate has closed; characterized by the growth of bones, muscles, and many internal organs at an abnormally fast rate.

Hashimoto disease A condition that occurs when the immune system attacks the patient's thyroid gland and that is the leading cause of hypothyroidism; also known as chronic lymphocytic thyroiditis.

hyperglycemia A condition in which the blood glucose concentration exceeds the normal range (70 to 100 mg/dL).

hyperosmolar hyperglycemic state (HHS) A metabolic disorder that occurs principally in patients with type 2 diabetes, and is characterized by hyperglycemia, hyperosmolarity, and the absence of significant ketosis; also known as hyperosmolar hyperglycemic nonketotic syndrome (HHNS).

hyperthyroidism A condition caused by increased production of T_3 (triiodothyronine) and T4 (thyroxine) from the thyroid gland, resulting in an increase in the body's organ function; characterized by an increase in body temperature, gradual weight loss, increased and/or irregular heart rate, sweating, and irritability.

hypoglycemia A condition in which blood glucose drops below the normal range (70 to 100 mg/dL) and, in people without diabetes, is accompanied by signs and symptoms.

hypothyroidism A condition caused by a deficiency of T_3 (triiodothyronine) and T_4 (thyroxine) from the thyroid gland, resulting in a slowing of the body's organ function; characterized by a decrease in body temperature, gradual weight gain, and increased risk for acute myocardial infarction and stroke.

insulin resistance A condition in which the pancreas produces enough insulin but the body cannot effectively use it.

lipid disorders A group of disorders that cause a change in the production or use of cholesterol and may also alter the way cholesterol circulates or is processed in the body.

metabolic syndrome A group of risk factors that together may lead to coronary artery disease, stroke, and type 2 diabetes; usually related to a predisposition to a lipid disorder.

myxedema coma A rare, life-threatening condition that can occur in patients who have severe, untreated hypothyroidism, and that is characterized by altered mental status and lethargy, failure of the thermoregulatory system, and a precipitating event; may be accompanied by auditory and visual hallucinations, seizures, or unresponsiveness.

nonfunctioning adenoma A type of pituitary lesion in which the tumor does not secrete any hormones.

Prep Kit Continued

pheochromocytoma A catecholamine-producing benign tumor of chromaffin cells located in the center of the adrenal gland, which can occur either sporadically or chronically as a result of genetic risk factors; it causes stimulation of alpha-adrenergic and beta-adrenergic receptors, resulting in hypertension, increased cardiac contractility, glycogenolysis, gluconeogenesis, intestinal relaxation, and increased heart rate.

polydipsia Excessive thirst, resulting in excessive intake of fluid.

polyphagia Excessive desire to eat, resulting in overconsumption of food.

polyuria Frequent and plentiful urination.

primary aldosteronism A type of aldosteronism usually caused by a tumor on a single adrenal gland that overproduces aldosterone; also known as Conn syndrome.

primary amyloidosis The most common form of amyloidosis, affecting the heart, kidneys, tongue, nerves, and intestines; the form of amyloid deposited in this disease is classified as apolipoprotein.

pseudo-Cushing state A condition in which a person has higher cortisol levels from a cause other than actual Cushing syndrome—for example, depression, alcoholism, malnutrition, or panic attack.

secondary aldosteronism A type of aldosteronism that occurs as a result of reduced renal blood flow, which stimulates hypersecretion of aldosterone; it can be caused by obstructive renal artery disease, renal vasoconstriction, and edematous disorders.

secondary amyloidosis A form of amyloidosis that occurs as a result of another illness, and that primarily affects the kidneys, spleen, liver, and lymph nodes; the form of amyloid deposited in this disease is classified as amyloid A protein.

thyroid storm A rare but severe, life-threatening form of thyrotoxicosis that can occur in patients with long-term, untreated hyperthyroidism, but is more commonly precipitated in hyperthyroid patients by an acute physiologic stressor such as a recent surgery, trauma, infection, administration of large doses of iodine, or abrupt discontinuation of thyroid medications.

thyrotoxicosis An excess of thyroid hormones resulting in a hypermetabolic crisis, including tachycardia, hyperthermia (sometimes with a body temperature greater than 103.9°F [39.9°C]), coma with agitation, nausea, vomiting, diarrhea, unexplained jaundice, pulmonary edema, and elevated thyroxine level; severe cases are known as thyroid storm.

type 1 diabetes An endocrine disease that usually starts in childhood and requires daily injections of supplemental insulin to control blood glucose; sometimes called juvenile or juvenile-onset diabetes.

type 2 diabetes An endocrine disease that usually starts later in life and often can be controlled through diet and oral medications; sometimes called adult-onset diabetes.

References

Addison's disease. National Organization of Rare Disorders website. https://rarediseases.org/rare-diseases/addisons-disease/. Accessed March 22, 2021.

Akamizu T, Satoh T, Isozaki O, et al. Diagnostic criteria, clinical features, and incidence of thyroid storm based on nationwide surveys. *Thyroid*. 2012;22(7):661-679.

American Diabetes Association. Standards of medical care in diabetes—2020. *Diab Care*. 2020;43(suppl 1):S1-S212.

American Heart Association. Complementary and incremental mortality risk prediction by cortisol and aldosterone in chronic heart failure. *Circulation*. 2007;115(13):1754-1761.

Angell TE, Lechner MG, Nguyen CT, et al. Clinical features and hospital outcomes in thyroid storm: a retrospective cohort study. *J Clin Endocrinol Metab*. 2015;100(2):451-459.

Carroll R, Matfin G. Endocrine and metabolic emergencies: thyroid storm. *Ther Adv Endocrinol Metab*. 2010;1(3):139-145.

Prep Kit Continued

Centers for Disease Control and Prevention. Gestational diabetes. https://www.cdc.gov/diabetes/basics/gestational.html. Reviewed May 30, 2019. Accessed March 23, 2021.

Cervera R. Update on the diagnosis, treatment, and prognosis of the catastrophic antiphospholipid syndrome. *Curr Rheumatol Rep*. 2010;12(1):70-76.

Chiha M, Samarasinghe S, Kabaker AS. Thyroid storm: an updated review. *J Intens Care Med*. 2015;30(3):131-140.

Cohan PM, Wang CM, McArthur DL. Acute secondary adrenal insufficiency after traumatic brain injury: a prospective study. *Crit Care Med*. 2005;33(10):2358-2366.

Douglas SR, Burch HB, Cooper DS, et al. 2016 American Thyroid Association guidelines for diagnosis and management of hyperthyroidism and other causes of thyrotoxicosis. *Thyroid*. 2016;26(10):1343-1421.

Erkan D, Espinosa G, Cervera R. Catastrophic antiphospholipid syndrome: updated diagnostic algorithms. *Autoimmun Rev*. 2010;10:74.

Karslioglu French E, Donihi AC, Korytkowski MT. Diabetic ketoacidosis and hyperosmolar hyperglycemic syndrome: review of acute decompensated diabetes in adult patients. *BMJ*. 2019;365:l1114. doi: 10.1136/bmj.l1114.

Kitabchi AE, Umpierrez GE, Miles JM, Fisher JN. Hyperglycemic crises in adult patients with diabetes. *Diab Care*. 2009;32(7):1335-1343.

Kraut JA, Madias NE. Treatment of acute metabolic acidosis: a pathophysiologic approach. *Nat Rev Nephrol*. 2012;8(10):589-601.

Kumar RM, Gandhi SK, Little WC. Acute heart failure with preserved systolic function. *Crit Care Med*. 2008;36 (1 suppl):S52-S56.

LeRoith D, Taylor SI, Olefsky JM. *Diabetes Mellitus: A Fundamental and Clinical Text*. 3rd ed. Philadelphia, PA: Lippincott Williams & Wilkins; 2004.

Malone ML, Gennis V, Goodwin JS. Characteristics of diabetic ketoacidosis in older versus younger adults. *J Am Geriatr Soc*. 1992;40(11):1100-1104.

Merry WH, Caplan RH, Wickus GG, et al. Postoperative acute adrenal failure caused by transient corticotropin deficiency. *Surgery*. 1994;116(6):1095-1100.

NICE-SUGAR Study Investigators. Intensive versus conventional glucose control in critically ill patients. *N Engl J Med*. 2009;360:1283-1297.

Nyenwe EA, Kitabchi AE. Evidence-based management of hyperglycemic emergencies in diabetes mellitus. *Diab Res Clin Pract*. 2011;94(3):340-351.

Pizarro CF, Troster EJ, Damiani DM, Carcillo JA. Absolute and relative adrenal insufficiency in children with septic shock. *Crit Care Med*. 2005;33(4):855-859.

Plouin PF, Chatellier G, Fofol I, Corvol P. Tumor recurrence and hypertension persistence after successful pheochromocytoma operation. *Hypertension*. 1997;29(5):1133-1139.

Swee DS, Chng CL, Lim A. Clinical characteristics and outcome of thyroid storm: a case series and review of neuropsychiatric derangements in thyrotoxicosis. *Endocr Pract*. 2015;21(2):182-189.

UCLA Pituitary and Skull Base Tumor Program. Pituitary adenomas. UCLA Health website. http://pituitary.ucla.edu/pituitary-adenomas#PituitaryAdenomasPhysiology. Accessed March 22, 2021.

Umpierrez G, Korytkowski M. Diabetic emergencies: ketoacidosis, hyperglycaemic hyperosmolar state and hypoglycaemia. *Nat Rev Endocrinol*. 2016;12(4): 222-232.

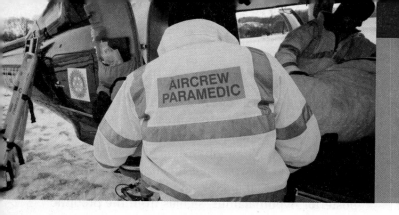

Chapter 19

Environmental Emergencies

David Fifer, MS, NRP, FAWM

Michael Murphy, RN, CEN, EMT-P

OBJECTIVES

After completing this chapter, you will be able to:

1. Discuss risk factors for environmental emergencies (p 1012).
2. Describe the process of thermoregulation, including the concepts of thermogenesis and thermolysis (p 1012).
3. Explain the process of heat transfer, including radiation, conduction, convection, evaporation, and absorption (p 1014).
4. Discuss signs, symptoms, and transport management of heat cramps (p 1016).
5. Discuss signs, symptoms, and transport management of heat syncope (p 1018).
6. Discuss signs, symptoms, and transport management of heat exhaustion (p 1019).
7. Discuss signs, symptoms, and transport management of heatstroke (p 1020).
8. Discuss signs, symptoms, and transport management of frostbite (p 1024).
9. Discuss signs, symptoms, and transport management of hypothermia (p 1026).
10. Discuss signs, symptoms, and transport management of drowning (p 1028).
11. Discuss signs, symptoms, and transport management of diving injuries (p 1029).
12. Explain the purpose of hyperbaric therapy and when it might be used (p 1030).
13. Discuss signs, symptoms, and transport management of altitude illness (p 1032).
14. List flight considerations relating to environmental emergencies (p 1034).

Introduction

Environmental emergencies are medical conditions caused or worsened by the weather, terrain, or unique atmospheric conditions. People may experience severe illness from environmental conditions in a vast array of locations and situations. Heat, cold, submersion, and decompression illnesses can occur in remote wilderness locations, major urban metropolitan areas, and any place in between. People who are used to harsh environmental conditions frequently survive environmental extremes far better than at-risk people (such as older adults, homeless individuals, and people with substance use disorders). The list of potential scenarios creating an environmental emergency is seemingly endless, regardless of geographic region.

The critical care transport professional (CCTP) often sees patients who have experienced environmental emergencies during critical care transports between facilities. Many preexisting medical and social factors predispose patients to critical illness created or exacerbated by environmental stressors. The challenge for CCTPs is to recognize those patients who are more susceptible to environmental exposure in unexpected conditions. To provide patients with the optimal chance for recovery, it is essential that CCTPs continue or initiate many critical interventions during patient transport.

Risk Factors

Risk factors that predispose people to environmental emergencies include extremes of age (young and old), taking certain medications, and being in a poor state of health. Specifically, environmental factors can be worsened in people with diabetes, cardiovascular disease, restrictive lung disease, thyroid disease, and psychiatric illnesses.

Thermoregulation

The body's ability to acclimatize—that is, to adjust to a changing environment—is part of the homeostatic process. Thermoregulation refers to the body's natural ability to ensure and maintain a balance between heat production (thermogenesis) and heat elimination (thermolysis). This process is governed by the brain.

The hypothalamus is located in the most inferior portion of the diencephalon, making up the portion of the brain between the cerebrum and the brainstem. Through the hypothalamo-hypophysial portal system, the hypothalamus sends stimulating or inhibiting factors to the pituitary gland. This interaction, which is referred to as the hypothalamic-pituitary axis, results in, respectively, an increase or a decrease in metabolism throughout the body.

The hypothalamus serves as the body's "master thermostat" through negative feedback control. A rise in the core body temperature elicits signals to shut off thermogenesis pathways and increase the activity of heat loss mechanisms; a fall in the core body temperature prompts heat production and limits the actions of thermolysis mechanisms **FIGURE 19-1**. In the preoptic area of the hypothalamus, heat-sensitive neurons fire more rapidly when the body senses an increase in temperature. In the posterior hypothalamus, signals from the preoptic area combine with signals from the remainder of the body to cause a compensating heat loss, which seeks to restore the body's temperature to a tolerable range.

This hypothalamus-driven negative feedback system cannot work properly without input from a network of complementary detectors that are sensitive to temperature changes. Cold sensors are located predominantly in the skin, spinal cord, and other areas that are sensitive to the cold end of the temperature spectrum. They respond to excess cooling by transmitting neural action potentials to the hypothalamus; these halt the heat-reducing signals. The goal is to maintain a constant core body temperature within one degree of 98.6°F (37°C).

The negative feedback system has three major components:

- Temperature receptors
- Effector organ systems
- Integrator or controller

The majority of temperature receptors are found in the papillary layer of the dermis, throughout widespread areas of the body. These exteroceptors respond to external stimuli affecting the skin directly. Areas populated by nerves (spots) respond to hot or cold stimuli, with cold spots being more numerous. Receptors are nerve endings that act as transducers, converting one form of energy into nerve impulses. These impulses are then sent along afferent nerves, including the lateral spinothalamic tract, to the diencephalon. The subsequent neural processing stimulates motor nerves and peripheral pathways to activate the effector organ systems. Based on the types of messages they receive, muscles may then contract or relax, blood vessels may constrict or dilate, and glands may secrete hormones. These impulses are coordinated as necessary by the specific integrator or controller based on information already stored in that integrator or controller (such as the "normal" body temperature of 98.6°F [37°C]).

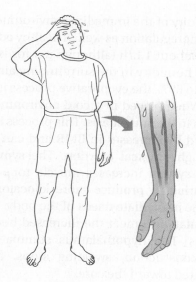

Hot Environment

- Hypothalamus stimulated
- Blood vessels dilate, maximizing heat loss from skin
- Body sweats, causing evaporation and cooling

Body temperature *decreases*

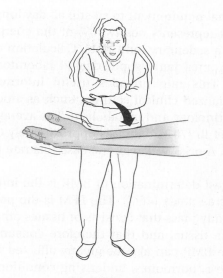

Cold Environment

- Hypothalamus stimulated
- Blood vessels constrict, minimizing heat loss from skin
- Muscles shiver, generating heat

Body temperature *increases*

FIGURE 19-1 The hypothalamus notes a rise or fall in core body temperature and elicits responses to regulate it.

© Jones & Bartlett Learning.

Through these collective actions, the hypothalamic "thermostat" reduces excesses in body heat. Three major mechanisms play key roles in the heat-reducing process:

- Blood vessels in the skin dilate, resulting in eight times as much heat transfer to the skin's surface.
- Perspiration is increased at a ratio of 10 times the normal perspiration for each degree of temperature increase.
- Increases in muscle activity, including shivering, are inhibited.

In contrast, in response to cold, three other regulatory processes increase body heat:

- Stimulation of the posterior hypothalamus causes a constriction of blood vessels.
- Hypothalamic stimulation of the primary motor center in the posterior hypothalamus stimulates the brainstem, spinal cord, and motor neurons to ultimately cause muscle activity, including shivering.

- The hypothalamic stimulation of piloerector muscles causes minimal production of heat and the visible sign of goosebumps and prompts the body hair to "stand on end."

CCTPs should consider the specific needs of their patients and how the dynamics of the transport environment, such as flight altitudes, may impact thermodynamics. Neonates and pediatric patients in particular pose unique challenges, as discussed in Chapter 23, *Neonatal Emergencies*, and Chapter 24, *Pediatric Emergencies*.

Basal Metabolic Rate

At rest, the body's chief source of heat production is the metabolism of nutrients. The heat produced at rest from normal metabolic reactions, including breathing, circulation, and digestion, is referred to as the **basal metabolic rate (BMR)**. It represents the number of calories metabolized per square inch of body surface area per hour and can be thought of as the minimal requirement to sit still all day long. In fact, BMR represents nearly 70% of the energy demands of a sedentary individual. Calculation of the BMR requires fairly sophisticated laboratory equipment. This rate provides useful information in specialized clinical settings, such as studies in endocrinology and metabolism. The average BMR of a 154-lb (70-kg) adult is approximately 60 to 70 kcal/h. A brisk walk can increase this rate to 300 kcal/h.

The largest determination of BMR is the individual's **fat-free mass (FFM)**. The FFM is the proportion of body mass that consists of tissues other than adipose tissue, and that therefore consume calories. The BMR can also be greatly affected by age, sex, stress, hormones, underlying conditions, pharmaceuticals, supplements, and body surface area. As the ratio of body surface area to body volume increases, heat loss increases. Thus, the shorter of two persons with the same weight will lose heat at a faster rate. This relationship is most relevant to pediatric patients, who have a very high surface area to body volume ratio and are most susceptible to heat loss.

Heat Transfer

Heat produced by metabolism and glycogen breakdown is used to warm the body and maintain the core body temperature. Excess heat must be eliminated. Usually this elimination is accomplished through the temperature gradient between the body and the immediate surrounding environment. The body transfers heat to the surrounding environment through five primary mechanisms:

- **Radiation**—the transfer of heat through electromagnetic waves
- **Conduction**—the transfer of heat through direct contact with a cooler object
- **Convection**—the loss of heat carried away from the body by currents of air or water
- **Evaporation**—the loss of heat carried away as a liquid is converted to a gas
- **Respiration**—the loss of heat as warm air in the lungs is exhaled into the atmosphere and cooler air is inhaled

If the surrounding environment is hotter than the body, the body gains heat through **absorption**. Convection and radiation cease as ambient temperatures reach or exceed skin temperatures. The

humidity of the immediate environment can affect thermoregulation as well. A healthy adult can sweat up to about 1 L/h (although not for very long), but if the humidity in the surrounding air is more than 75% to 80%, the evaporative process is impaired.

When placed in a cold environment, the body shifts to thermogenesis. This process is mainly controlled by increases in BMR and can be enhanced through physical exertion. The sympathetic nervous system increases muscle tone and initiates shivering to produce more kilocalories per hour for the immediate needs of the body. The thyroid is stimulated to meet the increased heat-production needs. The hypothalamus stimulates peripheral vasoconstriction, sweating stops, and blood is shunted toward the core.

In very cold temperatures, heat loss occurs through the process of respiration. When cold air is inhaled, it is warmed by the body and then exhaled, causing heat loss.

Expecting the Unexpected

A patient need not be found in the desert or a snowbank to have a temperature-related emergency. For example, patients with a spinal cord injury may have a disruption in the negative feedback loop and, therefore, a disruption of thermoregulation. CCTPs must be cognizant of these patients' inability to self-regulate body temperature and take the necessary external steps to maintain warmth or prevent overheating.

Heat Emergencies

Heat illness occurs when core body temperature increases as a result of inadequate thermolysis. According to the US Centers for Disease Control and Prevention, heat-related illness is a major public health concern, with the United States averaging more than 700 heat-related deaths each year from 2004 to 2018. CCTPs in all geographic regions should be prepared to transport patients experiencing heat-related illnesses.

Risk Factors

Factors that contribute to how heat affects the body **TABLE 19-1** include the person's general state of health, age, use of certain medications **TABLE 19-2**, amount of clothing, mobility, and surroundings.

TABLE 19-1 Factors That Predispose Individuals to Heat Illness

Factors That Increase Internal Heat Production	Factors That Interfere With Heat Dissipation
Physical exertion	High ambient temperature
Response to infection (fever)	High humidity
Hyperthyroidism	Obesity (insulation effect, and less efficient dissipation)
Agitated and tremulous states (eg, Parkinson disease, psychosis, mania, drug withdrawal—opiate and alcohol)	Impaired vasodilatation
Drug overdoses (eg, sympathomimetics, cocaine, caffeine, lysergic acid diethylamide, phencyclidine hydrochloride, methamphetamine, and 3,4-methylenedioxy-amphetamine)	Diabetes
	Alcoholism
	Drugs: diuretics, tranquilizers, beta blockers, antihistamines, and phenothiazines
	Impaired ability to sweat (as in cystic fibrosis, skin diseases, and healed burns)
	Heavy or tight clothing

Factors That Increase Heat Absorption	Factors That Impair the Body's Response to Heat Stress
Confined, unventilated, hot living quarters	Dehydration
Working in hot conditions (eg, bakeries, steel mills, and construction sites)	Prior heatstroke
Being in parked motor vehicles in the summer	Hypokalemia
	Cardiovascular disease
	Previous stroke or other central nervous system lesion

© Jones & Bartlett Learning.

Medications can cause or contribute to heat illness through a variety of mechanisms. Medications that depress the central nervous system (CNS), such as alcohol and barbiturates, impair a person's ability to properly dissipate heat generated within the body. Many CNS depressant medications can cause heat illness or hyperthermia.

Stimulant medications promote increased muscle activity and metabolism, causing increased thermogenesis. Cocaine, amphetamines, and other sympathomimetic medications may lead to hyperthermia through this mechanism. When heat dissipation mechanisms cannot compensate for the increase in heat production, the result will be hyperthermia.

Any medication that interferes with cardiovascular performance will undermine the body's ability to dissipate heat. Beta blockers, calcium channel blockers, and diuretics all interfere with heat loss, causing or worsening hyperthermia. Diuretics further complicate heat illness by limiting the fluid volume available for evaporative cooling (sweating).

Medications that impair sweating, such as antihistamines, tricyclic antidepressants, and other anticholinergics, compromise this essential thermoregulatory mechanism—another factor leading to heat illness. Other specific medication-related causes of hyperthermia or heat illness include neuroleptic malignant syndrome and malignant hyperthermia, which are discussed further in Chapter 21, *Toxicologic Emergencies*.

If thermoregulation mechanisms fail or become taxed beyond their limits, the core body temperature will rise dramatically and quickly. Indeed, it can rise to 106°F (41.1°C) or more in less than 15 minutes. Older persons are particularly at risk for rapid increases in body temperature. As a result of underlying illness and other metabolic changes, they often do not acclimatize well. Specifically, they may perspire less, feel thirst more slowly, have difficulty swallowing, and have decreased mobility

TABLE 19-2 Substances That Contribute to Heat Illness

Alcohol
Alpha agonists
Amphetamines
Anticholinergic medications (eg, atropine sulfate, scopolamine, benztropine mesylate, belladonna, and synthetic alkaloids)
Antihistamines
Antiparkinsonian agents
Antipsychotics (such as haloperidol)
Beta blockers
Calcium channel blockers
Cocaine
Diuretics (eg, furosemide, hydrochlorothiazide, and bumetanide)
Heroin
Laxatives
Lithium
Lysergic acid diethylamide
Monoamine oxidase inhibitors
Phencyclidine hydrochloride
Phenothiazines (eg, prochlorperazine, chlorpromazine, and promethazine)
Sympathomimetic medicines (eg, amphetamines, epinephrine, ephedrine, cocaine, and norepinephrine)
Thyroid agonists (eg, levothyroxine)
Tricyclic antidepressants (eg, amitriptyline, imipramine, nortriptyline, and protriptyline)

© Jones & Bartlett Learning.

(making it more difficult just to reach a glass of water). They are also more likely to be taking medications that can alter or impede thermoregulation.

Among young and healthy populations, children exposed to hot environments are most vulnerable to heat stressors. Compared with adults, children have higher rates of metabolism and do not dissipate heat as well. Infants and young children are completely dependent on others to provide the proper thermal environment. Covering them with excessive blankets or bedding, prolonged confinement in hot vehicles, and other lapses in environmental control place infants and young children at serious risk for heat-related injury.

Physical exertion in a warm environment can lead to hyperthermia, including a serious thermoregulatory emergency called exertional heatstroke. Exertional heatstroke is influenced by exercise intensity, environmental conditions, clothing, equipment, and individual health factors. It is normal for body temperature to rise during exercise when muscle-generated heat accumulates faster than heat dissipates. Heat production during intense exercise is 15 to 20 times greater than at rest, and can raise core body temperature by 1.8°F (1°C) every 5 minutes if no heat is removed from the body. Exertional heatstroke is a life-threatening condition with a high mortality rate if not promptly recognized and treated with aggressive whole-body cooling.

Adolescent athletes are at high risk for heat-related illness, and exertional heatstroke is a leading cause of death among high school athletes in the United States. Older children may elect to continue strenuous activities in hot or humid environments without understanding the risks or symptoms of heat-related illness or the importance of adequate hydration.

Heat Cramps

Heat cramps are involuntary muscle pains, usually in the abdomen, lower extremities, or both. Although the cause is not well understood, they are thought to result from electrolyte depletion caused by profuse sweating. They usually affect healthy persons who are overexerting their bodies in a hot environment. Generally, people recognize this problem and instinctively move to a cooler place and replenish fluids. However, if the person sweats profusely and drinks only water, the electrolyte loss has not been resolved, and cramps may continue. In addition, a person may attempt to quench thirst by drinking excessive amounts of water without appropriate sodium replacement, leading to dilutional hyponatremia.

Heat cramps result from an imbalance of water and sodium, and may not always be accompanied by hyperthermia. If a patient also has some degree of heat exhaustion, heatstroke, or significant hyperthermia, additional cooling measures may be required.

Treatment

The treatment for heat cramps is largely supportive: Patients should be removed from the hot environment, lie supine if they feel faint, and be instructed to drink a salt-containing liquid or electrolyte drink (if not at risk for aspiration) **FIGURE 19-2**. As the patient's salt balance is restored, the symptoms will abate. If symptoms continue, the underlying cause should be sought, and the patient should be rapidly transported to the emergency department (ED).

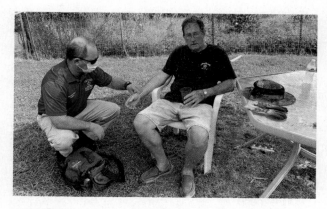

FIGURE 19-2 Give the patient experiencing heat cramps one or two glasses of a salt-containing solution if the person is not nauseated and there is no risk of aspiration.
Courtesy of Rhonda Hunt.

It is unlikely that patients will require critical care transport for heat cramps unless they have a significant degree of hyponatremia or some form of hyperthermia accompanies the heat cramps. Significant heat cramps, refractory to oral electrolyte replacement, may be managed with the administration of 1 to 2 L of intravenous (IV) isotonic fluid. To avoid contributing to hyponatremia, CCTPs should use caution before administering large volumes of IV fluids in these patients, especially in the absence of thorough patient evaluation or laboratory studies.

Signs and Symptoms

Heat Cramps
- Involuntary muscle pain, usually in the abdomen or lower extremities
- Profuse sweating

Differential Diagnosis

Heat Cramps
- Heat exhaustion
- Heatstroke
- Musculoskeletal trauma (such as sprains or strains)
- Electrolyte abnormality
- Autoimmune disease
- Medication side effect or medication withdrawal symptoms

Transport Management

Heat Cramps
- Remove the patient from the hot environment.
- Place the patient in a supine position.
- If there is no risk of aspiration, give the patient a drink containing salt.
- Consider administering 1 to 2 L of IV isotonic fluid; use caution if there is a possibility of hyponatremia.

Dilutional Hyponatremia

The normal process of homeostasis enables the body to balance intake against output. In general, an average adult takes in about 0.5 to 1 gallon (2 to 3 L) of fluid, from both food and beverages, throughout an average day. Human kidneys can excrete up to 15 to 20 L of free water (water that is not bound to molecules in the body) each day or up to 800 to 1,000 mL/h. When a euvolemic patient (one with normal blood volume) consumes or receives more hypotonic free water than the kidneys can excrete, the conditions for hyponatremia (abnormally low serum sodium) are present.

Dilutional hyponatremia—sometimes called overhydration or, colloquially, water intoxication—occurs when the normal osmotic balance of sodium in the body is pushed outside of safe limits by overconsumption of hypotonic free water. Due to its hypotonicity, the excessive quantity of water diffuses across the cellular membrane in tissues throughout the body, causing cells to swell as sodium levels are diluted.

Of particular concern is exercise-associated hyponatremia (EAH), which is defined clinically as a serum sodium concentration of less than 135 mmol/L occurring within 24 hours of sustained physical activity, typically lasting 4 hours or longer. This condition is commonly experienced by participants in physically demanding activities, often in combination with an environmental factor, such as endurance competitions, hiking, or climbing. For example, various studies have found that the incidence of EAH among marathon runners is as high as 28%, and as high as 38% among triathletes.

While much more common in hot weather, EAH can also occur in cold climates, as its primary mechanism is simply fluid consumption that exceeds fluids lost. It can occur during cooler weather and short durations of activity as individuals drink to quench thirst while not necessarily losing significant amounts of fluid through perspiration or exhalation.

The secretion of arginine vasopressin, also known as antidiuretic hormone (ADH), is believed to play a role in EAH. Stimuli resulting from exertion (eg, pain), psychological stress, hypoglycemia, and elevated temperatures can all trigger the secretion of ADH, which inhibits urination, leading to retention of water. Nonsteroidal anti-inflammatory drugs such as aspirin, ibuprofen, and naproxen also stimulate ADH production and are often consumed by individuals who engage in physical activities. The loss of sodium through sweat may play a role in EAH as well, though this mechanism is controversial.

Fortunately, most cases of EAH are asymptomatic. Generally, individuals do not exhibit significant signs or symptoms until serum sodium concentration falls below 130 mmol/L, or decreases 7% from their normal baseline. Symptoms, when they occur, are typically mild and include weakness, dizziness, peripheral edema, headache, lethargy, and nausea and vomiting. A key sign of EAH in the context of extended endurance activities is a significant weight gain (ie, typically exceeding 6.6 pounds [3 kg]) from the start of the event until its completion. Severe signs and symptoms may include mental status changes and seizures stemming from cerebral edema, as well as pulmonary edema. Deaths are rare but do occur.

Treatment

Patients suffering from mild hyponatremia are generally treated with restriction of hypotonic fluids and consumption of salty oral solutions. Patients with moderate to severe hyponatremia typically receive infusions of IV hypertonic saline, such as 3% sodium chloride. In some instances, 8.5% sodium bicarbonate may be used. For severe hyponatremia, 3% hypertonic saline is typically administered in 100-mL aliquots bolused over 10 minutes and titrated to clinical improvement (up to 300 mL total), because overcorrection of serum sodium can itself have devastating effects on the brain. For moderate hyponatremia, an infusion of 3% sodium chloride at 0.5 to 3 mL/kg/h may be administered. Generally, an increase of only 4 to 6 mmol/L serum sodium will correct symptoms.

CCTPs may be involved in the maintenance or administration of these fluids. They may also need to administer benzodiazepines to patients

experiencing seizures secondary to EAH or provide supportive care to patients in a coma resulting from especially profound cases. In addition, CCTPs may be called on to obtain point-of-care blood samples using i-STAT or similar devices to determine treatment end points.

Signs and Symptoms

Dilutional Hyponatremia
- Weakness
- Dizziness
- Peripheral edema
- Headache
- Lethargy
- Nausea and vomiting
- Mental status changes
- Seizures
- Pulmonary edema
- Weight gain

Differential Diagnosis

Dilutional Hyponatremia
- Heat exhaustion
- Hyperglycemia
- Mannitol overdose
- Hyperlipidemia
- Hyperproteinemia

Transport Management

Dilutional Hyponatremia
- Restrict hypotonic fluids and encourage consumption of salty oral solutions.
- For more severe hyponatremia, consider administration of IV hypertonic saline.

Heat Syncope

Heat syncope is an episode of collapse or near collapse, followed by immediate return to complete consciousness, that typically occurs in a non-acclimatized person. It is often seen at outdoor events where crowds are standing for long periods. Heat syncope is also common in outdoor settings when a person stands suddenly after sitting or lying on the ground for an extended period. Peripheral vasodilation, possibly exacerbated by some degree of dehydration, is theorized to be the cause of this condition.

To treat a person with heat syncope, place the patient supine and elevate the legs to autotransfuse blood volume from the lower extremities; this effect is brief and transient, but effective if the person's volume status is normal. Move the patient to a cooler environment and allow fluid intake. If the patient does not recover rapidly, suspect heat exhaustion. If the patient exhibits CNS dysfunction, suspect heatstroke. Many other conditions can cause syncope, so the CCTP should consider a wide range of differential diagnoses and rule out underlying conditions such as cardiac arrhythmias.

Signs and Symptoms

Heat Syncope
- Postural hypotension from vasodilation
- Volume depletion
- Syncopal episode
- Subjective or documented hyperthermia

Differential Diagnosis

Heat Syncope
- Heat exhaustion
- Heatstroke
- Vasovagal syncope
- Cardiovascular dysfunction
- Psychogenic syncope
- Seizure
- Dehydration
- Pseudosyncope

Transport Management

Heat Syncope
- Place the patient supine and elevate the legs.
- Provide fluids.
- Remove the patient from the hot environment.
- Manage the ABCs (airway, breathing, and circulation) as clinically indicated.

Heat Exhaustion

Heat exhaustion is a clinical syndrome representing a moderate form of heat illness on the heat emergencies continuum. Two classic forms of this syndrome are recognized: water depleted and sodium depleted.

Water-depleted heat exhaustion primarily occurs in older adults. Age-related immobility, decreased thirst sensitivity, and medications that contribute to dehydration are suspected culprits. This condition may also occur in active younger workers and in athletes who do not adequately replenish fluids during activities in a hot environment.

Sodium-depleted heat exhaustion results from excessive losses of sodium through sweating and may take hours to days to develop. When a person sweats but replenishes their internal fluids only with water, the sodium is not replaced. This condition shares many characteristics with dilutional hyponatremia but is associated with excessive consumption of hypotonic water in a short time.

Symptoms of heat exhaustion include weakness, headache, fatigue, dizziness, nausea, vomiting, and abdominal cramps. Transient syncope may also be present, but any true alteration in neurologic status would be considered heatstroke. Profuse sweating and pale, clammy skin are generally seen. Heart rate and respirations are typically elevated. Tachypnea may lead to signs of hyperventilation syndrome: carpopedal spasm, perioral numbness, and a lowered end-tidal carbon dioxide ($ETCO_2$) level. In heat exhaustion, the patient's core body temperature typically ranges from 100.4°F (38°C) to 104°F (40°C), although it is also possible for core body temperatures to remain normal. The blood pressure (BP) may be low owing to peripheral pooling or volume depletion. Orthostatic hypotension will generally be present. The patient may report having darker, brown urine, which suggests rhabdomyolysis. If left untreated, heat exhaustion may completely compromise a patient's thermoregulatory ability and may progress to heatstroke.

Treatment

Treatment of heat exhaustion is aimed at rehydrating the patient, replacing electrolytes, and, most importantly, facilitating physical rest and heat dissipation. Move the patient to a cooler environment, remove excess clothing, and place the patient supine with the legs elevated. Oral rehydration with sports drinks may be appropriate if nausea is not present.

Consider obtaining blood samples for electrolyte analysis, as well as administering IV fluids to patients who appear volume depleted and who cannot tolerate oral rehydration due to nausea or vomiting. As cooling occurs, fluids distributed throughout the body may return to the intravascular space, improving intravascular fluid volume. Administer fluids based on measurable signs of volume status, such as BP, heart rate, skin turgor, and urine output.

Closely monitor the electrocardiogram (ECG) for signs of electrolyte-induced arrhythmia. Heat illness can cause multiple electrolyte disturbances, including hyponatremia, hypocalcemia, and hypomagnesemia, which may result in ECG changes. Rhabdomyolysis, if present, may cause the release of excess potassium as muscle tissue is destroyed. Hyperkalemia may result in tall, peaked T waves on the ECG. Exertional hyponatremia may lead to a relative increase in the calcium level. Finally, monitor vital signs, body temperature, and ETCO$_2$.

Techniques such as misting the patient with water, covering the patient with sheets soaked in ice water, and immersing the patient in cold water can effectively dissipate heat (to varying extents) but are not necessary unless the patient is experiencing CNS impairment. If such signs are present, the condition is more likely to be heatstroke, not heat exhaustion, and aggressive whole-body cooling would then be indicated. In general, simply allowing patients with heat exhaustion to rest and cool down, using intuitive methods while rehydrating orally, is sufficient.

Signs and Symptoms

Heat Exhaustion

- Headache
- Fatigue
- Dizziness
- Nausea
- Vomiting
- Abdominal cramps
- Profuse sweating
- Pale, clammy skin
- Elevated heart rate and respirations
- Carpopedal spasm
- Perioral numbness
- Lowered ETCO$_2$ level
- Normal or elevated skin temperature
- Low BP
- Darker, brown urine

Differential Diagnosis

Heat Exhaustion

- Cardiac insufficiency
- Influenza
- Heatstroke

Transport Management

Heat Exhaustion

- Move the patient to a cooler environment.
- Remove excess clothing.
- Place the patient in a supine position with the legs elevated.
- Rehydrate the patient with sports drinks if nausea is not present.
- Obtain blood samples for electrolyte analysis, and consider IV administration of isotonic fluids.
- Administer fluid based on assessment of volume depletion.
- Monitor the ECG, vital signs, temperature, and ETCO$_2$.
- Consider external cooling measures.
- Care for patients receiving specialized cooling techniques initiated prior to the CCTP's arrival, such as cooling blankets; cold-water peritoneal, rectal, thoracic, or gastric lavage; cold IV fluids; or cold humidified oxygen. Determine if these measures are still necessary.
- Avoid giving antipyretic medications, which may cause severe complications in patients with heat exhaustion and which have no role in treating environmental heat stress.

Heatstroke

Heatstroke is the least common but most deadly of the heat illnesses. It is a severe disturbance in the body's thermoregulation, defined as a core body temperature of 104°F (40°C) or higher (typically, but not always) and associated CNS dysfunction. Only core body temperatures are reliable in diagnosing heatstroke; oral, axial, skin, and tympanic readings are not relevant. Heatstroke is a profound emergency, with mortality as high as 80% in untreated patients and significant sequelae and rates of morbidity among patients who initially survive the heatstroke: Two-year mortality is approximately 71%. Death occurs in as many as 10% of treated patients.

The critical thermal maximum is reached when the core body temperature exceeds 109.4°F (43°C). At this point, cellular respiration becomes impaired, cell membranes have increased permeability, denaturation of proteins begins, and tissue necrosis results. When heatstroke is suspected or confirmed, immediate and aggressive whole-body cooling is required.

Two distinct syndromes have been identified: classic and exertional **TABLE 19-3**.

TABLE 19-3 Classic Versus Exertional Heatstroke

Characteristic	Classic Heatstroke	Exertional Heatstroke
	Older	**Younger**
General health	Chronic diseases or schizophrenia	Healthy person
Medications	Beta blockers, diuretics, or anticholinergics	Often none; consider stimulant abuse
Activity	Very little to bedridden	Strenuous
Sweating	May be absent	Usually present
Skin	Hot, red, and possibly dry	Moist and pale
Blood glucose level	Normal	Hypoglycemic
Rhabdomyolysis	Rare	Common
Acute renal failure	Rare	Common

© Jones & Bartlett Learning.

- *Classic heatstroke* usually occurs during heat waves and is associated with prolonged time spent in hot dwellings with poor climate control and ventilation. Populations with poor physiologic compensatory mechanisms, such as persons who are very old, very young, or bedridden, are more vulnerable to this condition. Patients with chronic illnesses (eg, diabetes and heart disease), people taking certain medications (eg, anticholinergics, diuretics, and beta blockers), and people with alcoholism are also more susceptible, as these factors can impair normal thermoregulatory mechanisms. As high environmental temperatures elicit dissipation of body heat, the previously mentioned conditions impair heat loss and the core body temperature continues to rise unchecked.

- As discussed previously, *exertional heatstroke* typically affects younger healthy persons who are exposed to high heat and humidity during a period of strenuous activity. When the core body temperature matches the ambient temperature, radiation and convection are interrupted and heat dissipation is no longer effective. Evaporative cooling through sweating may be further impaired when the relative humidity is more than 75%. Note, however, that ambient air temperature does not have to be high for this form of heatstroke to occur; it can occur when endogenous heat production is sufficiently high or heat dissipation is sufficiently impaired. For example, heatstroke has been documented in marathon runners and firefighters despite mild ambient temperatures. As the body continues to generate heat without a mechanism for its removal, the core body temperature continues rising toward the critical thermal maximum. In addition to the heat emergency, patients may have depleted glucose and electrolytes. Their conditions may progress to rhabdomyolysis or acute renal failure. Temperature-mediated activation of the clotting cascade and damage to endothelium may contribute to coagulopathies.

Both types of heatstroke present with similar signs and symptoms, but the cardinal sign is neurologic dysfunction. The earliest signs of neurologic dysfunction may include mental status changes, such as irritability, bizarre behavior, or combativeness, or more subtle cues, such as slurred speech or altered gait. In other cases, the patient may appear briefly unwell and then suddenly collapse, or the patient may have a seizure. These symptoms often mislead bystanders, who may attribute the problem to causes other than the environment, such as substance abuse or psychiatric disorders. Notably, however, individuals who are intoxicated or who are experiencing a psychiatric crisis are especially susceptible to heatstroke. The presentation of extreme hyperthermia mimics vascular stroke or head injury, which should remain part of the initial differential diagnosis.

Dry skin from anhidrosis is often cited as an important sign of heatstroke, but this commonly taught presentation is actually an inconsistent finding and therefore diagnostically unreliable. Anhidrosis may be more common in the setting of classic heatstroke, as the patient's body temperature rises somewhat gradually and compensatory mechanisms fail, but many patients experiencing this form of heatstroke will continue to sweat. In case of exertional heatstroke, 50% of patients continue to sweat persistently. Thus, the patient's skin condition should not be used to arrive at a diagnosis of heatstroke.

Given these potentially misleading signs and symptoms, the CCTP must attend closely to the diagnostic signs of heatstroke: a markedly elevated core body temperature coupled with CNS disturbance. Tachycardia and tachypnea are common. ETCO$_2$ values may be less than 20 mm Hg as a result of hyperventilation. BP may be normal or decreased, depending on volume status and the degree of vasodilation that may be occurring as a compensatory mechanism. Most patients with exertional heatstroke, however, are euvolemic.

Heatstroke is an easy diagnosis to miss. CCTPs must keep the possibility of this condition constantly in mind during heat waves and in the context of exertional activities when presented with a patient exhibiting signs of neurologic impairment.

Treatment

Treatment of heatstroke focuses on lowering core body temperature as rapidly as possible. CCTPs should evaluate the patient's ABCs and consider controlling the airway. Immediate attempts to decrease the core body temperature begin with removing the patient's clothing and moving the patient to a cool environment.

Cold-water immersion, which involves covering the patient up to their neck in ice water, is the preferred method to treat heatstroke in all settings. If this method is unavailable or impractical based on the situation, then evaporative cooling can be started and continued during transport with relative ease. Sponging or spraying water over the patient and fanning to promote evaporation is key. Placing bags of ice or commercial ice packs at the nape of the neck, armpits, groin, and palms and soles further assists in cooling but is ineffective as a stand-alone treatment. In high-humidity environments, evaporative cooling methods are less effective.

Applying rubbing alcohol to the skin is not an effective way to reduce core body temperature. In the context of environmental etiologies, antipyretic medications also have no benefit in treating heatstroke.

Cooling should be continued until the core body temperature falls below 102°F (38.8°C) and should be sustained as a matter of priority. If this target is achieved within 30 minutes of heatstroke presentation, immediate mortality decreases dramatically. Shivering need not be a concern, as the thermogenesis it produces is insufficient to raise body temperature back to dangerous levels from the point at which it begins. Cooling promotes peripheral vasoconstriction and may raise the BP.

Treatment also includes the following steps:

- Initiate an IV line of isotonic fluid, and obtain blood samples for glucose and electrolyte analysis.
- Watch the patient closely for signs indicating development of pulmonary edema.
- Closely monitor the ECG, vital signs, and ETCO$_2$, and be prepared to treat a seizure with a benzodiazepine; keep a close eye on the ECG for indications of hyperkalemia and arrhythmia.

Monitor the patient for changes in central venous pressure, pulmonary wedge pressure, systemic vascular resistance, and cardiac index. If rhabdomyolysis is present, treatment should include aggressive hydration and administration of crystalloid fluid. Closely monitor the patient's fluid status and contact medical control about administration of additional medications (eg, mannitol and sodium bicarbonate) if the patient's condition continues to deteriorate. Additional efforts, such as dialysis, may be needed in patients with elevated potassium levels or uremia.

Signs and Symptoms

Heatstroke

- Altered mental status
- Confusion
- Irritability
- Bizarre behavior
- Combativeness
- Hallucinations
- Elevated core body temperature
- Tachycardia
- Tachypnea with $ETCO_2$ less than 20 mm Hg
- Hot, red skin
- Normal or decreased BP
- Seizure

Differential Diagnosis

Heatstroke

- Intracranial hemorrhage
- Ischemic stroke
- Diabetic ketoacidosis
- Malignant hyperthermia
- Neuroleptic malignant syndrome
- Sympathomimetic toxicity
- Salicylate toxicity
- Phencyclidine toxicity
- Encephalopathy
- Withdrawal syndrome

Expecting the Unexpected

A heat emergency can occur in any season of the year, especially in older adults who have difficulty acclimatizing, and who often have inadequate hydration and take multiple medications, which may affect the negative feedback loops in thermoregulation. CCTPs should give particular attention to

Transport Management

Heatstroke

- Evaluate the ABCs.
- Administer supplemental oxygen if the pulse oximetry reading is less than 92%.
- Consider endotracheal intubation.
- Remove the patient's clothing.
- Move the patient to a cooler environment.
- Prioritize cold-water immersion. Consider options to initiate or sustain cold-water immersion in transit, such as packaging the patient in a fluid-impervious material filled with ice water, such as a tarp, body bag, or MegaMover-like device.
- If cold-water immersion is not possible:
  - Sponge or spray water over the patient.
  - Fan the patient.
  - Place ice packs at the nape of the neck, armpits, groin, and palms and soles.
- Initiate an IV line of crystalloid fluid, and obtain blood samples for glucose and electrolyte analysis.
- Watch closely for signs of pulmonary edema.
- Closely monitor the ECG, vital signs, and $ETCO_2$.
- Be prepared to treat a seizure with antiepileptic drugs (eg, benzodiazepines).

signs of poor skin turgor during transport of older adults with an elevated temperature.

Fever and other conditions may mimic heatstroke and, therefore, increase the challenge for clinicians. The patient's history may provide important clues as to the appropriate diagnosis. For example, a recent complaint of cough or dyspnea, an obvious skin rash, a change in urine color, and intermittent shaking "chills" are more likely to be associated with infection rather than with an environmental cause. When a patient has an infection, pyrogens (proteins excreted as the body fights an infection) act on the hypothalamus to increase the body temperature. Fever in children may result in seizure. Fever is most often treated with antipyretic medications, which can prove dangerous in patients who actually have heat-related illness because of their harmful effects on the kidneys and clotting process.

Anticholinergic and organophosphate exposure and poisoning can also cause hot, red, dry skin; mental status changes; and tachycardia. Exposure to these agents usually causes dilated pupils, whereas a heat emergency generally would not. In addition, **neuroleptic malignant syndrome** is caused by some antiemetic and antipsychotic medications, and **malignant hyperthermia** may occur with use of common anesthesia agents (most notably suc-cinylcholine). These conditions may present with hyperthermia, a hyperdynamic state, and altered mentation.

Cold Emergencies

Most cold-related injuries are localized to exposed body parts, especially the face, where there are fewer cold receptors in the skin compared with areas of the body covered by clothing. The tip of the nose, ear lobes, fingers, and toes—all areas where periph-eral circulation is weakest and body temperature is the lowest—are most susceptible to such injuries.

Frostbite

Frostbite is a form of cold injury that develops slowly and generally without a lot of pain. People with frostbite may be unaware of its occurrence, and its major signs and symptoms may not manifest until after the patient has been removed from the cold environment and the affected tissue warms.

Frostbite is classified similarly to burns, using four degrees of injury. The precise nature of the injury, and thus the degree of injury, may not be evident prior to warming. First-degree frostbite is characterized by numbness, erythema, and capil-lary leakage resulting in localized edema. Second-degree frostbite involves superficial blistering. Third-degree frostbite involves deep hemorrhagic blistering, and fourth-degree frostbite involves damage to deep subcutaneous tissues such as mus-cle and bone. In severe frostbite that is still frozen, tissue may appear white and waxy **FIGURE 19-3**. Par-esthesia that results during warming may persist for weeks following the event.

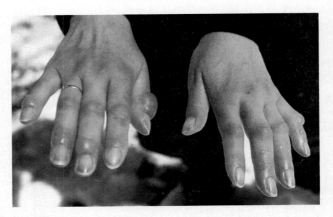

FIGURE 19-3 Frostbitten parts are hard and usually waxy to the touch.
Courtesy of Neil Malcom Winkelmann.

Severe frostbite involves the freezing of tissues exposed to temperatures below the freezing point (32°F [0°C]). When subjected to such low, freez-ing temperatures, the fluid within cells becomes ice crystals, which damage the cells. Rubbing these frozen tissues, which may be done in a well-intentioned attempt to improve circulation or to create warmth via friction, should be avoided be-cause it will cause the frozen crystals to crack and lacerate surrounding tissue. This condition is fur-ther complicated by the "sludge" effect of cooled blood, which results in increased viscosity, poor flow, capillary leakage, poor perfusion, thrombus, and ischemia. Frozen tissues appear hard and cold, are without sensation, and take on a yellow-white or mottled blue-white appearance.

The most serious complication of frostbite is seen during gradual thawing or refreezing. When tissues thaw slowly, the residual effect of this tis-sue damage becomes apparent and profound edema and third spacing can occur. If thawing is not conducted mindfully, or is not sustained and the freezing conditions eliminated, partial re-freezing may occur. Because the newer ice crystals formed at this point are larger (due to the presence of increased interstitial fluid), they cause greater tissue damage. During thawing, as circulation returns, the area becomes purple and excruciat-ingly painful. CCTPs should be prepared to pro-vide generous pain management to these patients and to safely manage that analgesia by thoroughly understanding the drugs selected for administra-tion. Gangrene, a result of permanent cell death, may set in within a few days, requiring amputation **FIGURE 19-4**.

Frostnip

Frostnip has traditionally been classified as a form of mild frostbite. It is a nonfreezing, superficial cold injury easily treated by placing a warm hand over the chilled ear, nose, or fingers. The return of warmth to the affected part is accompanied by some degree of redness and tingling. For clinical classification purposes, frostnip is not included among the degrees of frostbite.

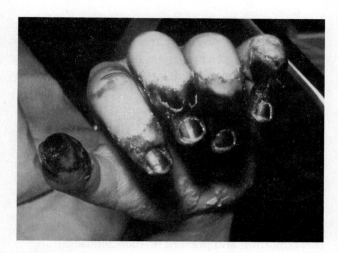

FIGURE 19-4 Gangrene can occur when tissue is frozen and permanent cell death occurs.

Courtesy of Dr. Jack Poland/CDC.

Treatment

Treatment of severe frostbite by the CCTP depends on two factors:

- The distance to the receiving hospital or burn center
- The degree of thawing before arrival at the hospital

If the part is still frozen or the transport time is less than 1 hour, do not attempt to warm the part, as rapid warming is difficult. Pad the part with dry dressings to protect it from further injury. Instruct the patient not to rub or massage the area because, as noted earlier, the ice crystals in the cells will lacerate delicate tissues.

If the tissue is partially thawed or transport will be prolonged, contact medical control for advice on field warming. Field warming can be difficult to accomplish in an effective and controlled manner, however, and the risk of incomplete thawing and refreezing may outweigh its benefits.

Should the CCTP be called to undertake this process, the general approach is to completely immerse the affected tissue in water between 98.6°F and 102.2°F (37°C and 39°C). The water must be maintained at this temperature. The frozen tissue will cool water that is not exchanged or that does not have an active heat source, so monitor the water temperature to maintain it in the therapeutic range. This treatment procedure typically takes 30 minutes or more. Establish an IV line for the administration of pain control medication (eg, fentanyl or ketamine). The patient should not consume nicotine products, because nicotine causes vasoconstriction that would further interfere with the thawing process. Once circulation has returned and the part is thawed, dry it thoroughly and apply a dry dressing to further protect the tissues during transport. Do not allow the tissues to refreeze.

Ibuprofen may be administered, chiefly to reduce inflammation. Tissue plasminogen activator may be initiated within 24 hours of thawing, typically as a 3-mg bolus followed by an infusion of 1 mg/mL at 10 mg/h. Heparin may be administered concurrently at 500 units as an adjunct treatment. Other vasodilators, such as iloprost, nitroglycerin, and nifedipine, may be infused under some protocols, although research on their efficacy is inconclusive.

Signs and Symptoms

Frostbite
- Hard, cold, waxy, and yellow-white or mottled blue-white skin

Differential Diagnosis

Frostbite
- Arterial or venous occlusion
- Hypoxia or cyanosis
- Dermal exposure to corrosive chemicals
- Vasospasm

Transport Management

Frostbite
- Do not warm, rub, or massage the area.
- If transport time is less than 1 hour, leave the part frozen.
- If transport time is expected to be prolonged, contact medical control to discuss field warming.
- If medical control advises field warming:
  - Immerse the affected tissue completely in water between 98.6°F and 102.2°F (37°C and 39°C). Monitor the water temperature to maintain it.
  - Establish an IV line; administer pain medication.
  - Dry the part thoroughly once it has thawed.
  - Apply a dressing.
- Take great care to prevent refreezing.

Hypothermia

Hypothermia is defined as a decrease in core body temperature to 95°F (35°C) or less. This condition may result from impaired thermogenesis, excessive heat loss, or excess environmental cold stress. Any environmental temperature below an individual's physiologic core body temperature can result in hypothermia, and this emergency may occur in any season. Alcohol use has been identified as a factor contributing to hypothermia. Likewise, hypothyroidism, liver disease, and malnutrition may predispose a person to this cold emergency. Trauma is the other most important factor contributing to hypothermia. Additionally, hypovolemia and hypotension interfere with normal thermoregulation.

The classification and treatment of hypothermia depend chiefly on the patient's mental status and motor function, including shivering. In general, hypothermia is considered more severe as mental status and motor function decline; this type of progression requires more assertive warming measures. Many patients exposed to cold may simply be experiencing cold stress, a nonhypothermic condition in which patients complain of being cold but remain conscious and completely alert and have mostly normal motor function, including shivering. Simple, intuitive warming methods, such as increasing the ambient temperature in the patient care environment and adding insulating layers to the patient, will likely remedy cold stress. Patients who are shivering, and therefore producing endogenous heat, often improve quickly once sources of heat loss are corrected and adequate insulation is applied.

Various methods of categorizing hypothermia exist. In the United States, a three-tiered scale of mild, moderate, and severe hypothermia is prevalent. In Europe, the five-tiered Swiss Staging System of hypothermia has gained acceptance and offers greater precision.

Mild hypothermia is defined as a core body temperature between 90°F and 95°F (32.2°C and 35°C). At these temperatures, the body usually compensates with increased thermogenesis and interrupted thermolysis. Shivering is in full force and will generally be an effective form of thermogenesis if adequate insulating layers are provided. The "umbles" (stumbles, mumbles, fumbles, and grumbles) are present, indicating impaired motor function and declining mental status. The heart rate, BP, and cardiac output may rise. These processes continue until either the core body temperature returns to normal or glycogen stores are exhausted and compensation begins to fail. If left unchecked, more serious conditions will result.

Moderate hypothermia is defined as a core body temperature between 82°F and 90°F (27.7°C and 32.2°C). Mental status is markedly decreased, although the patient is likely to still be conscious, in the absence of other contributing factors. Shivering may still be present but is less vigorous and unlikely to be an effective from of thermogenesis. Warming with an external heat source is necessary to correct this condition and prevent further deterioration.

Severe hypothermia begins as the core body temperature drops below 82°F (27.7°C). At these temperatures, the body reacts by slowing things down. This slowed metabolism decreases thermogenesis, and the heart rate, BP, and cardiac output decrease. Shivering ceases. As peripheral vasoconstriction occurs to shunt warm blood to the core, the volume receptors interpret this change as an increase in blood volume and stimulate the kidneys to produce more urine (cold diuresis). Simultaneously, a shift of fluids from the intravascular space to the extravascular space increases the blood's viscosity. Shivering ceases at a body temperature less than 91°F (32.7°C). Tracheobronchial secretions increase and bronchospasm may occur. At a core body temperature of less than 90°F (32.2°C), hypoventilation is profound.

The Swiss Staging System includes additional categories and relies more heavily on patient appearance. In stage 1, which correlates to mild hypothermia, the patient exhibits clear consciousness and shivering. In stage 2, which correlates to moderate hypothermia, the patient demonstrates decreased consciousness without shivering. In stages 3 and 4, which correlate to severe hypothermia, the patient is unconscious. In stage 4, however, the patient *appears* to be dead.

The relevance of stage 4 in the Swiss scale is that the patient may not be dead at all, despite having a core body temperature between 56.6°F and 75.2°F (13.7°C and 24°C). The oft-repeated mantra in medicine of "They're not dead until they're warm and dead," while crude, is an important reminder that severely hypothermic patients may survive even if vital signs cannot be detected, and resuscitation should be initiated unless it cannot physically be performed. ECG leads may have to be amplified for organized electrical activity to be detected in these patients. ETCO$_2$ monitoring is helpful in detecting the output of cellular respiration, even if chest rise and fall are not evident.

In stage 5 of the Swiss system, hypothermia is irreversible, and death is indeed imminent or has occurred. The core body temperature of these patients is less than 56.6°F (13.7°C).

In severe hypothermia (Swiss stages 3 and 4), the heart rate plummets, the cardiac cycle elongates, and the action potential threshold of the myocytes is greatly reduced. Bradycardia is common, and cardiac arrhythmia may be seen. An Osborn or J wave may be seen on the ECG tracing, indicating an uneven voltage gradient through the myocardium caused by the cooling of those tissues **FIGURE 19-5**. Abnormal cardiac conduction and hypothermia-induced arrhythmias may lead to ventricular fibrillation, especially as the core body temperature falls below 82.5°F (28°C). When Osborn or J waves are seen, the risk of ventricular fibrillation or pulseless ventricular tachycardia is very high. Repeated defibrillation may not be effective until the patient has been warmed to a core body temperature of more than 86°F (30°C). When giving shocks to these patients, the defibrillator's maximum energy should be used. If defibrillation of a patient with a core body temperature less than 86°F (30°C) is not successful, further shocks should not be attempted until the core body temperature rises.

Many of the usual advanced cardiac life support (ACLS) medications may be less effective in patients with severe hypothermia. Although the American Heart Association guidelines do not recommend departure from the normal ACLS regimen, the Wilderness Medical Society's Clinical Practice Guidelines for hypothermia recommend administering ACLS medications at twice the normal intervals (ie, waiting twice as long between doses) in patients with core body temperatures less than 35°C (95°F) and withholding them entirely if the core body temperature is less than 30°C (86°F).

Treatment

Treatment is based on warming the patient, which involves removing cold, wet clothing; drying the patient if necessary; and wrapping the patient in layers that retain radiant heat, minimize conductive heat loss, and protect the patient from ambient moisture such as rain or snow. This form of warming, known as passive warming because it does not involve the introduction of exogenous heat sources, will generally be effective if the patient is still shivering vigorously. Typically, this patient package, sometimes called a "hypothermia wrap," should be constructed beginning with the outermost layer (the moisture barrier), followed by insulating layers, and then a reflective inner layer. The CCTP can use materials such as tarp, cloth, or Mylar blankets for this purpose, but many lightweight, highly effective commercial products are also available that achieve the same result. In addition, the patient should be placed in a warmed environment.

Active warming involves the introduction of exogenous heat sources to the patient. This method is necessary when the patient is not shivering adequately or has ceased to shiver. Active warming may involve infusing warmed IV fluid (102°F to 105°F [38.8°C to 48.5°C]); delivering warm, humidified oxygen; or administering a peritoneal lavage of a potassium chloride–free solution or nasogastric/orogastric lavage with warmed fluids. When placing heat sources (such as heat packs) into the patient package to actively warm the person, place them around the trunk rather than along the extremities. This placement helps to avoid core afterdrop, a warming-related phenomenon in which vasodilation in the extremities returns relatively cooler blood to the warmed core of the body, causing a rebound hypothermic effect. Warm the patient compartment of ambulances or aircraft to a temperature 28°C (82.4°F) if possible, and if tolerable to the transport crew. Administration of IV dextrose

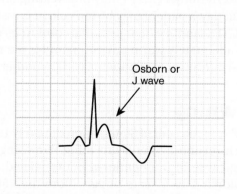

FIGURE 19-5 Osborn or J wave as it appears on electrocardiogram.

may be required to treat depleted glucose stores in patients who have experienced prolonged shivering or who are no longer shivering.

Severely hypothermic patients should be handled gently to avoid inducing cardiac arrest; these patients may be experiencing a prolonged relative cardiac refractory period, predisposing the heart to rhythm irregularities if physically jolted. ECG leads should be placed to assess for Osborn or J waves and arrhythmias, and the CCTP should consider placing defibrillation/pacing pads during transport.

Special Populations

Older adult patients are more susceptible to hypothermia compared to their younger adult counterparts. Even in warm weather or inside a heated transport unit, older patients are susceptible to significant heat losses. Monitoring temperature is as important in the older population as it is in neonates.

Signs and Symptoms

Hypothermia
- Decrease in core body temperature to less than 95°F (35°C)
- Shivering or lack of shivering
- The "umbles": stumbling, mumbling, fumbling, and grumbling
- Increased or decreased heart rate
- Increased or decreased BP
- Increased or decreased cardiac output
- Cardiac arrhythmias
- Osborn or J waves on the ECG

Differential Diagnosis

Hypothermia
- Drowning
- Profound shock
- Cardiac arrest
- Toxic chemical exposure
- Overdose

Transport Management

Hypothermia
- Remove cold, wet clothing.
- Dry the patient.
- Apply patient packaging that insulates and retains warmth.
- Move the patient to a warmed environment.
- Consider administration of warmed IV fluid, dextrose, humidified oxygen, or peritoneal lavage of a potassium chloride–free solution or nasogastric/orogastric lavage with warmed fluids.
- Monitor the ECG for arrhythmias and Osborn or J waves, and be prepared to defibrillate.
- Consult with medical direction and consider modifications to standard ACLS regimens as appropriate based on the patient's core body temperature.

Expecting the Unexpected

Hypothermia can occur in any season of the year, especially in older adults who have difficulty acclimatizing and are often prescribed multiple medications that affect the negative feedback loops of thermoregulation. CCTPs should pay particular attention during transport of both older and very young people. The transport environment creates numerous opportunities to cause or worsen preexisting hypothermia. Even brief episodes of exposure to cold temperatures while moving to or from a transport vehicle can significantly undermine warming efforts. Even when the ambient temperature is room temperature, young or older patients can be hypothermic. Although CCTPs may be sweating on a hot summer day, a patient may be too cold. It is essential that CCTPs sacrifice their personal comfort by creating an adequately warm environment for the resuscitation or transport of patients with hypothermia.

Drowning

Every day in the United States, approximately 10 people die from unintentional drowning. Drowning is the leading cause of unintentional injury-related death for children 1 to 4 years of age. More than 50% of drowning patients treated in EDs require hospitalization or transfer for further care (compared with a hospitalization rate of 6% for all unintentional injuries).

Treatment

Treatment begins with spinal motion restriction of patients witnessed diving into the water and when alcohol use is suspected. Initiate ventilation immediately if warranted, and advanced airway management where necessary. Widespread atelectasis and pulmonary shunt may be present in a drowning patient. The use of 10 cm H_2O of positive end-expiratory pressure (PEEP) may aid in keeping the alveoli open and driving fluid into the interstitial or capillary spaces. A nasogastric tube may be used, after airway control, to decompress the stomach. Bronchospasm and tracheobronchial irritation may be treated with a beta-2 adrenergic agonist.

Acute respiratory distress syndrome is a common complication of submersion incidents. Chemical or bacterial pneumonitis and renal failure are other complications that can occur days after resuscitation.

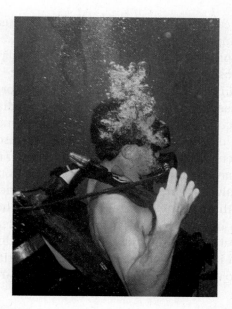

FIGURE 19-6 Decompression sickness affects divers who ascend to the surface too quickly.

Courtesy of Mass Communication Specialist 2nd Class Rebecca J. Moat/US Navy.

Transport Management

Drowning

- Provide spinal motion restriction for patients witnessed to have dived into the water and when alcohol use is suspected.
- Provide supplemental oxygen.
- Consider endotracheal intubation.
- Provide PEEP.
- Consider inserting a nasogastric or orogastric tube to decompress the stomach.
- Consider administering a beta-2 adrenergic agonist to treat bronchospasm and tracheobronchial irritation.

Diving Injuries and Decompression Sickness

Injuries associated with recreational and professional scuba diving activities can occur regardless of the diver's level of experience. All divers are subject to pressure effects. For each 33.9 feet (10.3 m) of depth, the pressure on the body increases by 1 atmosphere (atm), or 14.7 lb/in^2 (1 kg/cm^2).

The most common effect of increasing depth relates to the amount of nitrogen present within the body. Nitrogen dissolves from the gas inhaled by divers into the body's fatty tissues. It readily displaces oxygen in the brain, resulting in feelings of euphoria and disorientation known as nitrogen narcosis. The effects of nitrogen narcosis vary among divers. Some divers are affected at 30 meters, but all divers are significantly impaired at depths of 60 to 70 meters. The effects do not develop in proportion to time at a particular depth; rather, symptoms progress and new symptoms develop as a diver descends deeper to greater pressures. If the nitrogen forms gas bubbles in the blood, a condition known as decompression sickness, the person may experience excruciating pain when the bubbles become trapped in body cavities such as joints or in the folds of the intestinal tract; the resulting pain is often referred to as the "bends" **FIGURE 19-6**. In addition to the bends, patients with decompression sickness may experience respiratory disturbances (the "chokes"; discussed later), neurologic impairment (the "staggers"), and skin sensation abnormalities (the "creeps" or "skin bends").

Barotrauma may occur during either ascent or descent in a dive, depending on the situation. With changes in elevation, gases stored in confined spaces within the body may either expand or contract. As the diver travels to a higher elevation, trapped gases attempt to expand, causing increased pressure within a particular body cavity. As the diver descends, the pressure of the outside environment exceeds the pressure of various gases within the body, resulting in inward pressure. The patient's lungs, ears, and gastrointestinal tract are susceptible to injury from barotrauma.

Rapid ascent is also responsible for pulmonary overpressurization syndrome (POPS), in which gases in the lungs expand rapidly as the pressure decreases, leading to pneumothorax or mediastinal or subcutaneous emphysema. Simply holding one's breath during the last 6 feet (2 m) of the ascent is sufficient to cause these injuries. Arterial gas embolism may occur when air bubbles escape from ruptured alveoli, enter the pulmonary capillaries, and travel through the pulmonary veins to the heart. If the air bubbles end up in the coronary arteries or cerebral vasculature, they will result in acute myocardial infarction or stroke. The vast majority proceed to the cerebral arteries, resulting in a stroke.

Treatment

Treatment for decompression sickness in the prehospital setting includes rapid transport and oxygenation. Providers should administer 100% oxygen to promote nitrogen washout from the lungs. PEEP and continuous positive airway pressure (CPAP) should not be applied to patients with pressure-related diving injuries or decompression sickness unless necessary to maintain oxygenation.

A valuable resource when managing dive-related injuries is the Divers Alert Network (DAN), which provides a 24-hour hotline (919-684-9111). The DAN staff can guide CCTPs through a variety of complex decisions about treatment, transport, and patient disposition.

CCTPs should closely monitor patients with decompression sickness, even if they begin to show signs of improvement or recovery. Relapses of symptoms are possible and may be associated with an overall deterioration in the patient's condition.

The use of a pure Trendelenburg position or the combination of a head-down with left lateral decubitus (Durant) position is not currently recommended for arterial air embolisms (as seen in decompression sickness) because these positions increase intracranial pressure. Instead, transport patients in a supine position and, in aircraft, at the lowest cabin altitude pressure possible. Depending on the topography of the transport route, even ground ambulance transport may subject patients to increased physiologic stressors and worsen their conditions. Trendelenburg or Durant positioning continues to be recommended for venous air embolisms (as may be seen during central line insertion or removal).

Other potential interventions for decompression sickness may include the following: (1) administering aspirin to prevent thrombus formation, (2) managing tension or simple pneumothorax with a thoracostomy (chest) tube, (3) aggressively administering IV fluid resuscitation, and (4) following ACLS protocols for profound cardiopulmonary dysfunction. Patients with decompression sickness are likely to require analgesics, sedatives or anxiolytics, and antiemetics during transport. These patients may also have other medical concerns, such as trauma or hypothermia, that require additional resuscitative measures. In particular, hyperbaric oxygen therapy is often necessary to minimize the morbidity and mortality from decompression sickness.

> ### Transport Management
>
> **Diving Injuries**
> - Provide rapid transport.
> - Provide oxygenation.
> - Do not use PEEP or CPAP.
> - Consider hyperbaric therapy.

Hyperbaric Oxygen Therapy

Hyperbaric oxygen therapy (HBOT) is generally accomplished by placing the patient in a specially constructed chamber designed to withstand high internal pressures, well in excess of normal atmospheric pressures **FIGURE 19-7**. The chamber is filled with compressed air to a desired level, typically expressed in units of atmospheres or feet of seawater. The patient receives pure or blended oxygen via a mask or endotracheal tube.

Chambers are configured to handle one patient or multiple patients. In larger chambers, a trained medical provider typically accompanies the patient into the chamber to monitor equipment and intervene if the patient's condition begins to deteriorate.

Most patients will receive 100% inspired oxygen while undergoing HBOT. In addition to saturating the blood hemoglobin, this oxygen, which is under greater than atmospheric pressure, becomes dissolved into the circulating plasma.

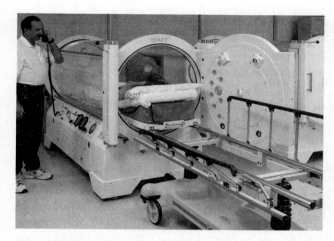

FIGURE 19-7 A hyperbaric chamber, usually a small room, is pressurized to more than atmospheric pressure. It is used in the treatment of decompression sickness and air embolism.

Courtesy of Perry Baromedical.

TABLE 19-4 Indications for Hyperbaric Oxygen Therapy
Air or gas embolism
Carbon monoxide poisoning
Carbon monoxide poisoning complicated by cyanide poisoning
Clostridial myositis and myonecrosis (gas gangrene)
Crush injury, compartment syndrome, and other acute traumatic ischemias
Decompression sickness
Enhancement of healing in selected problem wounds
Exceptional blood loss (anemia)
Intracranial abscess
Necrotizing soft-tissue infections
Osteomyelitis (refractory)
Delayed radiation injury (soft-tissue and bony necrosis)
Skin grafts and flaps (compromised)
Thermal burns

Reprinted with permission from the Undersea and Hyperbaric Medical Society (www.uhms.org).

HBOT produces a number of interesting effects that can benefit a variety of patients. An example, the localized vasoconstriction that results from hyperoxygenation decreases tissue edema following crush injuries, burns, and other types of trauma. This vasoconstriction is offset by improved blood flow at the capillary level. HBOT also creates oxygen free radicals and alters other components of a patient's inflammatory response, leading to enhanced wound healing and improvement of a pathologic inflammatory response. In specific situations, nitrogen and helium can be blended into the inspired oxygen. The Committee on Hyperbaric Oxygenation of the Undersea and Hyperbaric Medical Society established the indications for HBOT **TABLE 19-4**.

Treatment tables are used to determine the length of HBOT and treatment steps. In case of decompression sickness, these tables take into account the depth of the dive, the duration of the dive, decompression stops, and previous dives performed. A hyperbaric specialist can recommend which table to use. Patients with severe illness often require several HBOT sessions. HBOT may prove beneficial even several days or longer after the incident in selected situations, such as for patients with carbon monoxide poisoning. Whenever HBOT is considered, CCTPs or medical providers should seek consultation with a specialist in hyperbaric medicine.

Hyperbaric chambers can be facilities in a fixed location, or they may be portable units that are transported to be near high-risk diving activities. To identify HBOT facilities in North America and the Caribbean, contact the DAN at Duke University at 919-684-9111. The Undersea and Hyperbaric Medical Society also maintains a database of US and international hyperbaric chambers. Given the wide variety of indications for HBOT, it is quite possible that hyperbaric chambers may be found in locations not typically associated with underwater activities.

Transport to these special facilities often requires air medical evacuation. In cases of barotrauma, the flight should be planned to take place at low-level altitude (the lowest altitude safely possible) or in a pressurized aircraft cabin set to 1 atm or 1 ata (total ambient pressure). The sending medical providers, in conjunction with CCTPs, must carefully weigh the risks and potential benefits to the patient when selecting the appropriate transport vehicle for a patient requiring transfer to an HBOT facility. The DAN recommends that cabin altitude not exceed 800 feet (244 m) for aircraft transport of patients with decompression sickness. This altitude limit may not always be possible owing to terrain or topography, weather, aircraft limitations, or other factors.

Flight Considerations

As just noted, according to the DAN, if air evacuation is used for patients requiring treatment of decompression sickness, cabin pressure must remain near sea level and the aircraft should not travel at an elevation greater than 800 feet (244 m) unless the captain is required to do so for safety precautions. The patient should be placed in the lateral recumbent position, or the recovery position: with the patient on their side, the head supported at a low angle, and the upper leg bent at the knee. Gravity will help to keep the patient's airway clear. Other experts recommend that patients be transported in a supine position. Additional discussion of this subject is found in the Controversies box.

Controversies

Although many training materials may not reflect the evolution of thinking regarding the ideal position for an injured diver, the trends have shifted over the years. Currently, use of the Trendelenburg position is not believed to provide the best outcomes for these patients. Research suggests that a head-down position creates limitations when performing resuscitation, increased cephalic venous volumes, and compromised subsequent middle ear equalization, as well as difficulty in distinguishing cerebral arterial gas embolism from cerebral decompression sickness. Likewise, significant arterial gas emboli most likely form in decompression sickness through the arterialization of venous bubbles. In the Trendelenburg position, venous return is increased, sending these bubbles back to the heart. Finally, studies show that brain function recovery time is longer for patients who are placed in a head-down position.

Ultimately, although there may occasionally be some benefit to placing specific patients in a head-down position, many practitioners prefer keeping these patients supine.

Altitude Illness

High altitude can affect the body negatively, usually owing to a lack of acclimatization. Hypoxia from low atmospheric pressure is the main culprit in altitude sickness. In the most dramatic examples, extremes of altitude pose life-threatening hazards for experienced mountain climbers who are pushing the limits of human exploration on remote peaks throughout the world. More prosaically, scores of other people experience similar, potentially catastrophic effects of altitude illness when they travel from lower elevations to higher elevations in the course of everyday life. People with preexisting

medical conditions, extremes of age, sedentary lifestyles, and poor health choices are at increased risk of altitude-related illness following even modest changes in elevation. The severity of altitude-related illness can range from mild symptoms, such as imperceptible tachypnea or sleep disturbances, to life-threatening manifestations, such as pulmonary edema, cerebral edema, and hypoxia.

Altitude sickness is most commonly associated with mountain climbing and alpine skiing, in which case it is often called acute mountain sickness. Acute mountain sickness can occur at altitude changes of 3,000 feet to 6,000 feet (914 to 1,800 m), but generally occurs at elevations of 8,000 feet (2,438 m) or higher. The Lake Louise criteria are useful for identifying acute mountain sickness **TABLE 19-5**.

TABLE 19-5 Lake Louise Criteria for Identifying Acute Mountain Sickness (AMS)

- Headache
  - 0—No headache
  - 1—Mild headache
  - 2—Moderate headache
  - 3—Severe, incapacitating headache
- Gastrointestinal symptoms
  - 0—Good appetite
  - 1—Poor appetite or nausea
  - 2—Moderate nausea or vomiting
  - 3—Severe, incapacitating nausea and vomiting
- Fatigue/weakness
  - 0—Not tired or weak
  - 1—Mild fatigue/weakness
  - 2—Moderate fatigue/weakness
  - 3—Severe, incapacitating fatigue/weakness
- Dizziness/light-headedness
  - 0—No dizziness/light-headedness
  - 1—Mild dizziness/light-headedness
  - 2—Moderate dizziness/light-headedness
  - 3—Severe, incapacitating dizziness/light-headedness
- AMS clinical functional score (how did symptoms affect person's activities)
  - 0—Not at all
  - 1—Did not force change in activities
  - 2—Forced to stop ascent or to descend under own power
  - 3—Required evacuation to lower altitude

Suggested interpretation:
- Mild AMS: 3–5 points
- Moderate AMS: 6–9 points
- Severe AMS: 10–12 points

Data from Ho M, Siu AY. High altitude medicine. *Hong Kong Med Diary*. 2010;15(6):32-34. http://www.fmshk.org/database/articles/05sa.pdf.

More serious conditions, known as **high-altitude pulmonary edema (HAPE)** and **high-altitude cerebral edema (HACE)**, are likely to occur at higher elevations.

Treatment of Altitude Illnesses

The best and most effective treatment for all forms of altitude illnesses is descent.

High-Altitude Pulmonary Edema

HAPE is a noncardiogenic form of pulmonary edema that develops within 24 to 72 hours of reaching higher altitudes. Patients may demonstrate a variety of symptoms, including cough, respiratory distress, chest tightness, fatigue, and fever. The presence of fever may mislead clinicians and delay diagnosis.

The pathophysiologic features of HAPE are poorly understood. Pulmonary hypertension from alveolar hypoxia, localized inflammation, and capillary or arterial thromboses are implicated in patients with this condition. People who make frequent changes in altitude are at increased risk of HAPE.

Rapid descent is the preferred treatment for HAPE. Patients should also receive supplemental oxygen during the descent. Nifedipine, salmeterol, and portable hyperbaric bags are effective for this indication, and should be used, if available, for the management of HAPE. CPAP may also play a role in the care of these patients.

High-Altitude Cerebral Edema

HACE is a life-threatening emergency that should prompt immediate descent when recognized. Any patient who has recently experienced a significant increase in altitude and who now has mental status changes or ataxia should be evaluated for HACE. Either of these symptoms is presumed to be diagnostic for HACE if the person already has signs or symptoms of acute mountain sickness. If ataxia *and* mental status changes are present, HACE is presumed even if other signs or symptoms of acute mountain sickness are not present.

HACE is thought to result from cerebral vasodilation brought on by hypoxia, although the precise mechanism has not been identified. This enhanced blood flow produces cerebral edema, leading to the previously mentioned mental status changes and ataxia.

Once HACE is recognized, initiate immediate descent while providing the patient with supplemental oxygen. In addition, administer dexamethasone. Diuretic medications are not indicated and have the potential to produce harmful alterations in fluid volume.

Signs and Symptoms

Altitude Illness

- Hypoxia
- Fatigue
- Weakness
- Near-syncope
- Headache
- Dyspnea
- Cough
- Pulmonary edema
- Chest tightness
- Tachycardia

Differential Diagnosis

Altitude Illness

- Any other possible cause of respiratory distress (eg, asthma, chronic obstructive pulmonary disease, pneumonia, and bronchitis)
- Any other possible cause of altered mental status or ataxia (eg, stroke, toxic exposure, encephalitis, and traumatic brain injury)
- Unrelated cardiovascular dysfunction (eg, cardiogenic shock, cardiogenic pulmonary edema, and acute myocardial infarction)
- Unrelated gastrointestinal condition (eg, gastroenteritis, gastritis, and pancreatitis)
- Labyrinthitis
- Electrolyte or hematologic abnormality

Transport Management

Altitude Illness

- Provide oxygenation.
- Evacuate the patient and begin descent.
- Consider hyperbaric therapy.

Flight Considerations

Patients with various altitude-related illnesses pose a significant challenge for CCTPs. It is quite conceivable that CCTPs may be asked to perform a rescue or evacuation from a remote area with a high elevation. These locations are particularly hazardous for ground transport vehicles and aircraft. When requested to perform a rescue or evacuation mission, CCTPs should carefully consider safety issues, such as training and experience of the personnel, capabilities of the particular transport vehicle, and weather and environmental concerns, as well as the severity of illness and capabilities of a potential patient. Numerous emergency responders have been killed or severely injured while attempting rescue or evacuation of a patient from mountainous terrain.

During the transport, CCTPs must minimize the effect of environmental conditions on the patient. For patients with altitude-related illnesses, CCTPs must balance capabilities and safety concerns related to the particular transport vehicle employed with the patient's clinical needs. Ideally, descent should occur rapidly for patients with severe manifestations of altitude illness. Rapid or prompt descent may not be possible when weather, topography, and terrain complicate the transport.

Indwelling devices with inflated balloons, such as endotracheal tubes and laryngeal mask airways, are also affected by changes in altitude. CCTPs should closely monitor these devices during ascent and descent.

Patients with altitude illness may have other issues, such as hypothermia, dehydration, trauma, or a preexisting medical condition that requires additional interventions. CCTPs must balance their needs for warmth, privacy, and protection against patient care needs such as exposure, thorough assessment, and patient access for monitoring or procedures. It may be advisable in many situations to defer a thorough visual assessment or invasive interventions in the interest of keeping a patient clothed, covered, and warm during extreme environmental conditions.

Prolonged evacuation of a patient with altitude illness may also exceed the supplies, equipment, and capabilities of a particular transport team. When performing such transports, CCTPs should be mindful of critical supplies, such as oxygen, that may become rapidly depleted during the patient's care. Monitoring equipment, ventilator, and infusion pump batteries may not have the longevity to continue functioning during a prolonged evacuation or transport from remote locations.

Summary

Patients with medical conditions related to environmental emergencies can pose a significant challenge to CCTPs. These conditions are often difficult to diagnose and manage while in the transport environment, so there is a risk of further deterioration in the patient's condition during movement from one location or facility to another. CCTPs need to keep these conditions in mind when caring for patients in a coma or those who have collapsed suddenly as a result of unknown causes. Knowing the risk factors that predispose a patient to environmental emergencies can aid in recognizing these conditions early in the patient encounter.

Case Study

You have just arrived for your regularly scheduled rotor-wing shift, when your dispatch center advises that you are being dispatched to the Rocky Mountain Rural Clinic, situated at 8,200 feet (2,500 m) above sea level, for a patient diagnosed as having probable HAPE. The patient needs to be transported to Mercy Hospital for HBOT. After your flight team (the pilot, flight nurse, and you, a critical care paramedic) completes the safety briefing, you depart for the rural clinic.

On arrival, the attending physician meets your flight team. She advises you that the patient is a 42-year-old, 233-lb (106-kg) man who had been climbing in the local national park for the past 2 or 3 days with three other people when he started to report fatigue and severe dyspnea. The party began its descent from approximately 12,000 feet (3,700 m), which took approximately 9 hours, and then drove a vehicle to the local clinic. On arrival, the patient's dyspnea was mildly resolved; however, he had a decreasing level of consciousness.

Treatment in the clinic included oxygen via nonrebreathing mask at 15 L/min to treat central cyanosis, a chest radiograph that showed patchy bilateral infiltrates, and an ECG that indicated a right-side heart strain pattern. The patient has an IV line with an 18-gauge needle in his left wrist running normal saline to keep the vein open; he also has an indwelling urinary catheter, with minimal urine output. Medications that were given at the clinic include 10 mg of nifedipine (Procardia) by mouth and 80 mg of furosemide (Lasix) IV. The patient is presently resting but is in moderate distress and has a Glasgow Coma Scale score of 13 (eye opening score, 3; verbal score, 4; motor score, 6). Vital signs are a BP of 142/81 mm Hg, a heart rate of 132 beats/min, sinus tachycardia with no ectopy, respirations of 28 breaths/min with rales bilaterally, and an SpO_2 of 86% despite aggressive oxygen therapy. After a positive Allen test result, an arterial line was inserted into the right radial artery. Arterial blood gas readings show acute respiratory alkalosis with a pH of 7.49; $PaCO_2$, 30 mm Hg; PaO_2, 88 mm Hg; HCO_3^-, 22 mEq/L; and base excess, 1. All available laboratory values are unremarkable.

As you are preparing to secure the patient onto your litter for the flight, he coughs up a small amount of blood-tinged sputum. Rather than electively intubating the patient for the flight, you decide to apply CPAP in an effort to decrease his work of breathing. CPAP is applied initially at 5 cm H_2O, which seems to have no effect. You subsequently titrate the CPAP up to 7.5 cm H_2O, which decreases his work of breathing and decreases his anxiety level. Your partner contacts your base hospital physician to advise of the patient's status, obtain any additional orders, and give an estimated time of arrival. The base hospital physician requests that 8 mg of dexamethasone (Decadron) and 250 mg of acetazolamide (Diamox) be administered en route. As your partner transfers the patient's IV line to your pump and calibrates the arterial line to your monitor, you speak to the pilot and advise him that owing to the patient's condition, it is imperative to fly at a lower altitude to minimize the effects of altitude on the patient.

Once airborne, 8 mg of dexamethasone and 250 mg of acetazolamide are given IV, and all hemodynamic parameters are monitored throughout the 48-minute flight. When you arrive at the Mercy Hospital helipad, the patient is taken directly to the hyperbaric chamber for definitive treatment.

1. How was the diagnosis of HAPE determined?
2. Why was the patient given nifedipine, furosemide, dexamethasone, and acetazolamide?
3. What are the potential problems that you may experience en route with this patient?

Analysis

Because of your critical care training, you are able to recognize that this patient is experiencing severe HAPE based on the Lake Louise acute mountain sickness criteria (described in Table 19-5).

Although you realize that HAPE usually resolves with descent from altitude, this patient was experiencing a severe case that did not resolve. In fact, the patient's condition appeared to be deteriorating.

Nifedipine is given to patients with HAPE to promote vasodilation of the pulmonary vessels, and furosemide is given to promote diuresis. Acetazolamide is administered to increase the amount of bicarbonate excreted in the urine, making the blood slightly acidic; this effect, in turn, stimulates ventilation, increasing the amount of oxygen in the bloodstream. Dexamethasone is given to treat pulmonary edema and to minimize cerebral edema.

This patient has the potential to experience several problems en route. Owing to the 48-minute flight to the receiving hospital and the fact that the patient is receiving CPAP, there is a risk that the crew might run out of oxygen; however, during your thorough preflight check of the aircraft, oxygen cylinders that are almost depleted should have been noted and replaced before the mission began. In any patient with an altered mental status in the flight environment, CCTPs need to be aware of the possible need to perform definitive airway management, which is often difficult to achieve in the confined space of a helicopter. Finally, this patient was experiencing an acute case of HAPE, and, depending on the altitude required during the flight, his pulmonary edema could progressively worsen. Good communication between the crew and the pilot will help to minimize the effects of pressurization, thereby minimizing the risk of complications en route.

Prep Kit

Ready for Review

- Very young and very old people, people taking certain medications, and people in a poor state of health are predisposed to environmental emergencies. The challenge for CCTPs is to recognize patients who are susceptible to environmental exposure in conditions that are not extremely hot or cold. CCTPs must also initiate or continue critical interventions during transport of these patients.
- The hypothalamus acts as the body's master thermostat, using negative feedback control. The three major components of the negative feedback system are temperature receptors, effector organ systems, and an integrator or controller.
- To reduce excess body heat, blood vessels in the skin dilate, perspiration increases, and muscle activity is inhibited.
- To increase body heat, the posterior hypothalamus is stimulated to constrict blood vessels, increase muscle activity (shivering), and activate the piloerector muscles.
- The heat produced at rest by normal metabolic reactions is referred to as the basal metabolic rate (BMR). Fat-free mass, age, sex, stress, hormones, and body surface area can all affect the BMR.
- Heat produced by metabolism and glycogen breakdown warms the body and maintains the core body temperature.
- The body transfers excess heat to the environment through radiation, conduction, convection, and evaporation. If the environment is hotter than the body, the body gains heat through absorption. Humidity can affect thermoregulation by impairing the evaporative process.
- The body shifts to thermogenesis when the environment is cold. In very cold temperatures, a fair amount of heat loss occurs through respiration, and the BMR and physical exertion are increased to produce more kilocalories per hour.

- Heat illness occurs when core body temperature increases to a point that exceeds the body's ability to dissipate the excess heat. CCTPs in all geographic regions of the United States should be prepared to transport patients with heat-related illnesses.
- CCTPs should be familiar with medications that contribute to heat illness, as well as medication-related causes of hyperthermia or heat illness such as neuroleptic malignant syndrome and malignant hyperthermia.
- Older adults are particularly at risk of heat illness as a result of underlying illness and other metabolic changes. Specifically, they may perspire less, feel thirst more slowly, have difficulty swallowing, have decreased mobility, or take medications that can alter or impede thermoregulation.
- Among the young and healthy population, children exposed to hot environments are most vulnerable to heat stressors. Compared with adults, children have higher rates of metabolism and do not dissipate heat as well.
- Prolonged hyperthermia, such as may occur during athletic or recreational activity, may lead to exertional heatstroke. This life-threatening condition has a high mortality rate if not promptly recognized and treated with body cooling.
- Heat cramps are thought to result from an imbalance of water and sodium, and are often not accompanied by hyperthermia. The patient with heat cramps should be removed from the hot environment, lie supine if feeling faint, and be instructed to drink a salt-containing liquid or electrolyte drink. CCTPs should use caution when administering IV fluids to correct presumed hyponatremia.
- Dilutional hyponatremia may occur if the person tries to replenish fluids by drinking excessive amounts of free water in a very short time.

Prep Kit Continued

- Additional cooling measures may be needed if the person has heat exhaustion, heatstroke, or significant hyperthermia.
- Treatment of heat syncope—an episode of collapse or near collapse that typically occurs in a non-acclimatized person—focuses on placing the patient supine or in the recovery position and allowing fluid intake if mental status permits. If the patient does not recover quickly, suspect heat exhaustion or heatstroke.
- Two forms of heat exhaustion exist: water-depleted exhaustion, which primarily occurs in older adults, and sodium-depleted exhaustion, which results from excessive losses of sodium through sweating and may take hours to days to develop. If left untreated, heat exhaustion may progress to heatstroke.
- Heatstroke is a severe disturbance in the body's thermoregulation, resulting in CNS dysfunction and a core body temperature of more than 104°F (40°C). The critical thermal maximum is reached when the core body temperature exceeds 109.4°F (43°C).
- CCTPs should be aware of the differences between classic and exertional heatstroke and remain alert for the possibility of heatstroke during heat waves, especially when caring for patients with coma of unknown origin.
- Treatment of heatstroke focuses on lowering the core body temperature as quickly as possible. Evaporative cooling can be started and continued during transport.
- Heat emergencies can occur at any time of year, especially in older adults. CCTPs should pay attention to signs of poor skin turgor and lack of sweating when transporting an older patient with a fever. The patient's history is also an important source of information in diagnosing heatstroke.
- Most cold-related injuries are localized to exposed body parts. The most susceptible parts are the tip of the nose, the ear lobes, and the fingers and toes.

- Frostbite is classified similarly to burns, using four degrees of injury:
  - First-degree frostbite is characterized by numbness, erythema, and capillary leakage resulting in localized edema.
  - Second-degree frostbite involves superficial blistering.
  - Third-degree frostbite involves deep hemorrhagic blistering.
  - Fourth-degree frostbite involves damage to deep subcutaneous tissues such as muscle and bone.
- Hypothermia is a decrease in core body temperature to less than 95°F (35°C), which may result from impaired thermogenesis, excessive heat loss, or excess environmental cold stress.
- Mild hypothermia is defined by a core body temperature between 90°F and 95°F (32.2°C and 35°C). The body usually compensates for mild hypothermia with increased thermogenesis and interrupted thermolysis.
- Moderate hypothermia is defined by a core body temperature between 82°F and 90°F (27.7°C and 32.2°C).
- Severe hypothermia occurs when the core body temperature drops below 82°F (27.7°C). The body reacts by slowing metabolism, which decreases thermogenesis, heart rate, BP, and cardiac output and has many other effects. Treatment focuses on warming the patient.
- Hypothermia can occur at any time of year, particularly in older adults. CCTPs should sacrifice their personal comfort to create an adequately warm environment for the resuscitation or transport of patients with hypothermia.
- Treatment of drowning patients begins with spinal motion restriction of patients witnessed diving into the water and when alcohol use is suspected. Ventilation should be initiated immediately if warranted, and advanced airway management where necessary.

Prep Kit Continued

- Divers may experience nitrogen narcosis, caused by nitrogen dissolving from inhaled gas into fatty tissues. Nitrogen gas bubbles expanding rapidly on ascent from depth may cause the "bends," the "chokes," the "staggers," and the "creeps" or "skin bends."
- Barotrauma may occur during either ascent or descent in a dive, as gases stored in confined spaces within the body either expand or contract during these changes in elevation. The patient's lungs, ears, and gastrointestinal tract are susceptible to injury from barotrauma.
- Pulmonary overpressurization syndrome is caused by rapid ascent during a dive; it occurs when gases in the lungs expand rapidly as the pressure decreases and pneumothorax or mediastinal or subcutaneous emphysema results. Arterial gas embolism may occur, which can result in acute myocardial infarction or stroke.
- CCTPs can consult the Divers Alert Network (DAN) hotline for guidance on treatment, transport, and patient disposition in cases of diving injury and decompression sickness.
- CCTPs should closely monitor patients with decompression sickness, even if they show signs of improvement or recovery. Relapses are possible.
- Hyperbaric oxygen therapy may be indicated for patients with decompression sickness and some other conditions, such as tissue edema following crush injuries, burns, and other types of trauma.
- If air evacuation is used for an injured diver, cabin pressure must be kept near sea level and the aircraft should not fly above 800 feet (244 m) unless necessary for safety precautions. Many experts recommend that patients with diving injuries be transported in a supine position.
- Hypoxia from the low atmospheric pressure found at high altitude is the main culprit in altitude sickness, also called acute mountain sickness. The Lake Louise criteria are useful for identifying this condition.
- High-altitude pulmonary edema (HAPE) may develop within 24 to 72 hours of reaching higher altitudes. Symptoms include cough, respiratory distress, chest tightness, fatigue, and fever. Rapid descent is the preferred treatment for HAPE, along with supplemental oxygen.
- High-altitude cerebral edema (HACE) is a life-threatening condition; when it is recognized, immediate descent should be initiated. Mental status changes and ataxia are symptoms of HACE.
- CCTPs may be asked to rescue or evacuate patients from remote areas at high elevation. These locations are very hazardous, and safety issues such as training and experience of personnel, capabilities of the transport vehicle, weather and environmental concerns, and the severity of illness and capabilities of the patient must be considered before accepting the assignment.
- Capabilities and safety concerns related to the transport vehicle must be balanced with the patient's clinical needs. Although rapid descent is ideal for patients with severe altitude illness, it may not be possible owing to environmental factors. A thorough visual assessment or invasive interventions may have to be deferred because of environmental conditions. Critical supplies and equipment must be monitored closely.

Vital Vocabulary

Absorption Acquisition of additional heat, radiation, or other energy from the environment; or, movement of a substance's molecules from the site of entry on the body into the systemic circulation.

active warming A method of warming a hypothermic patient that involves the introduction of exogenous heat sources to the patient; measures may include infusing warmed IV fluid, delivering warm, humidified oxygen, or administering a

Prep Kit Continued

peritoneal lavage of a potassium chloride–free solution or nasogastric/orogastric lavage with warmed fluids.

atelectasis Collapse of all or part of a lung.

barotrauma Injury to tissues, organs, or structures within the body, resulting from rapid or significant changes in environmental air pressure.

basal metabolic rate (BMR) The heat energy produced at rest by normal body metabolic reactions, determined mostly by the liver and skeletal muscle.

conduction Transfer of heat to a solid object or a liquid by direct contact.

convection The mechanism by which heat (body heat, in the context of this chapter) is picked up and carried away by moving air currents.

dilutional hyponatremia A condition caused by excessive intake of fluids in which serum sodium concentration is less than 135 mmol/L; sometimes referred to as water intoxication.

evaporation The conversion of a liquid to a gas.

exercise-associated hyponatremia (EAH) A condition occurring within 24 hours of sustained physical activity in which fluid consumption exceeds fluids lost, resulting in dilution of serum sodium levels. Signs and symptoms may include nausea, vomiting, and, in severe cases, mental status changes and seizures.

exertional heatstroke A thermoregulatory emergency that occurs during activities that require physical exertion in warm environments. This condition is defined by an excessive core body temperature, typically greater than 104°F (40°C), and associated CNS impairment.

fat-free mass (FFM) The proportion of body mass that consists of tissues other than adipose tissue, and that therefore consumes calories; typically the largest determinant of the basal metabolic rate in a healthy person.

free water Water that is not bound to molecules in the body.

frostbite Localized damage to tissues resulting from prolonged exposure to extreme cold.

heat cramps Acute and involuntary muscle pains, usually in the lower extremities, the abdomen, or both, that occur because of profuse sweating and subsequent sodium loss in sweat.

heat exhaustion A clinical syndrome characterized by volume depletion and heat stress that is thought to be a milder form of heat illness on the continuum leading to heatstroke.

heatstroke The least common and most deadly heat illness, caused by a severe disturbance in thermoregulation, usually characterized by a core body temperature of more than 104°F (40°C) and altered mental status.

heat syncope An orthostatic or near-syncopal episode that typically occurs in non-acclimated people who may be under heat stress.

high-altitude cerebral edema (HACE) An altitude illness characterized by a change in mental status and/or ataxia in a person with acute mountain sickness, or the presence of mental status changes and ataxia in a person without acute mountain sickness.

high-altitude pulmonary edema (HAPE) An altitude illness characterized by dyspnea at rest, cough, severe weakness, and drowsiness that may eventually lead to central cyanosis, audible rales or wheezing, tachypnea, and tachycardia.

hyperbaric oxygen therapy (HBOT) A treatment for decompression sickness and certain other conditions that involves placing the patient in a specially constructed chamber designed to withstand high internal pressures, well in excess of normal atmospheric pressures.

hypothalamic-pituitary axis An interrelationship between the hypothalamus and the pituitary gland in which a releasing or inhibiting factor is sent from the hypothalamus to the pituitary, resulting in, respectively, an increase or decrease

Prep Kit Continued

in metabolism and other functions throughout the body.

hypothalamo-hypophysial portal system The venules between the capillaries in the hypothalamus and pituitary gland by which the hypothalamus sends releasing or inhibiting factors to the pituitary gland, thereby increasing or decreasing metabolism, respectively.

hypothalamus The most inferior portion of the diencephalon; it is responsible for control of many body functions, including heart rate, digestion, sexual development, temperature regulation, emotion, hunger, thirst, and regulation of the sleep cycle.

hypothermia A condition in which the core body temperature decreases to less than 95°F (35°C).

malignant hyperthermia A condition that can result from commonly used anesthesia medications (notably succinylcholine); it presents with hyperthermia, muscular rigidity, altered mental status, and a hyperdynamic state.

mild hypothermia A condition in which the core body temperature is between 90°F and 95°F (32.2°C and 35°C); at this stage of hypothermia, the body usually compensates with increased thermogenesis and interrupted thermolysis.

moderate hypothermia A condition in which the core body temperature is between 82°F and 90°F (27.7°C and 32.2°C); mental status is markedly decreased, and shivering may still be present but is less vigorous and unlikely to be an effective from of thermogenesis.

neuroleptic malignant syndrome A condition caused by antipsychotic and antiemetic medications that presents with hyperthermia, muscular rigidity, altered mental status, and a hyperdynamic state.

nitrogen narcosis A state resembling alcohol intoxication, which is produced by nitrogen gas dissolved in the blood at high ambient pressure.

passive warming A method of warming a hypothermic patient without the introduction of exogenous heat sources. It involves removing cold, wet clothing; drying the patient if necessary; and wrapping the patient in layers that retain radiant heat, minimize conductive heat loss, and protect from ambient moisture such as rain or snow.

pulmonary overpressurization syndrome (POPS) A diving emergency that can occur during ascent and cause pneumothorax, mediastinal and subcutaneous emphysema, alveolar hemorrhage, and the lethal arterial gas embolism; also called burst lung.

radiation Emission of heat from an object into surrounding, colder air.

respiration The loss of heat as warm air in the lungs is exhaled into the atmosphere and cooler air is inhaled.

severe hypothermia A condition in which the core body temperature drops to less than 90°F (32.2°C).

thermogenesis The production of heat in the body.

thermolysis The liberation of heat from the body.

thermoregulation The process by which the body maintains temperature through a combination of heat gain by metabolic processes and muscular movement and heat loss through respiration, evaporation, conduction, convection, and perspiration.

water intoxication A condition in which the normal balance of electrolytes in the body is pushed outside safe limits by the overconsumption of water.

Prep Kit Continued

References

American Academy of Orthopaedic Surgeons. *Nancy Caroline's Emergency Care in the Streets*. 9th ed. Burlington, MA: Jones & Bartlett Learning; 2022.

American Heart Association. *2020 American Heart Association Guidelines for Cardiopulmonary Resuscitation and Emergency Cardiovascular Care*. https://cpr.heart.org/en/resuscitation-science/cpr-and-ecc-guidelines/adult-basic-and-advanced-life-support. Accessed August 2, 2021.

Basit H, Wallen TJ, Dudley C. Frostbite. *StatPearls*. https://www.ncbi.nlm.nih.gov/books/NBK536914/. Updated July 1, 2021. Accessed August 5, 2021.

Bennet BL, Hew-Butler T, Rosner M, Myers T, Lipman G. Wilderness Medical Society clinical practice guidelines for the management of exercise-associated hyponatremia: 2019 update. *Wilderness Environ Med*. 2020;31(1):50-62.

Chun SM, Kim HR, Shin HI. Estimating the basal metabolic rate from fat free mass in individuals with motor complete spinal cord injury. *Spinal Cord*. 2017;55:844-847.

Dow J, Giesbrecht GG, Danzl DF, Zafren K, Bennet BL, Grissom CK. Wilderness Medical Society clinical practice guidelines for the out-of-hospital evaluation and treatment of accidental hypothermia: 2019 update. *Wilderness Environ Med*. 2019;30(4):S47-S69.

Drowning and injuries associated with swimming and boating: the scope of the problem. Maryland.gov website. https://health.maryland.gov/phpa/OEHFP/CHS/Pages/DrowningPrevention.aspx. Accessed August 2, 2021.

Facts and stats about drowning. Stop the Drowning website. https://www.stopdrowningnow.org/drowning-statistics/. Accessed August 2, 2021.

Ganio MS, Casa DJ, Armstrong LE, Maresh CM. Evidence-approach to lingering hydration questions. *Clin Sports Med*. 2007;26:1-16.

Giesbrecht G. "Cold card" to guide responders in the assessment and care of cold-exposed patients. *Wilderness Environ Med*. 2018;29(4):P499-P503.

Goforth CW, Kazman JB. Exertional heat stroke in Navy and Marine personnel: a hot topic. *Crit Care Nurse*. 2015;35:52-59.

Goldberg S. *Clinical Physiology Made Ridiculously Simple*. 2nd ed. Miami, FL: MedMaster; 2010.

Heneghan C, Gill P, O'Neill B, Lasserson D, Thake M, Thompson M. Mythbusting sports and exercise products. *BMJ*. 2012;345. https://doi.org/10.1136/bmj.e4848.

Heneghan C, Howick J, O'Neill B, et al. The evidence underpinning sports performance products: a systematic assessment. *BMJ Open*. 2012;2:4. https://bmjopen.bmj.com/content/2/4/e001702.

Hew-Butler T, Loi V, Pani A, Rosner MH. Exercise-associated hyponatremia: 2017 update. *Front Med*. 2017;4:21.

Hifumi T, Kondo Y, Shimizu K, Muake Y. Heat stroke. *J Intens Care*. 2018;6:30.

Jardine DS. Heat illness and heat stroke. *Pediatr Rev*. 2007;28(7):249-258.

Krabak BJ, Lipman GS, Waite BL, Rundell SD. Exercise-associated hyponatremia, hypernatremia, and hydration status in multistage ultramarathons. *Wilderness Environ Med*. 2017;28(4):291-298.

Lindell W, ed. *Hyperbaric Oxygen Therapy Indications*. 13th ed. North Palm Beach, FL: Best Publishing; 2014.

McIntosh SE, Free L, Grissom CK, Pandey P, Dow J, Hackett PH. Wilderness Medical Society clinical practice guidelines for the prevention and treatment of frostbite: 2019 update. *Wilderness Environ Med*. 2019;30(4):S19-S32.

Morris A, Patel G. Heat stroke. *StatPearls*. https://www.ncbi.nlm.nih.gov/books/NBK537135/. Updated June 25, 2021. Accessed August 2, 2021.

Musi ME, Sheets A, Zafren K, Paal P, Hoizl N, Pasquier M. Clinical staging of accidental hypothermia: the Revised Swiss System: recommendation of the International Commission for Mountain Emergency Medicine (ICAR MedCom). *Resuscitation*. 2021;162:182-187.

Porter RS, Kaplan JL. *The Merck Manual of Diagnosis and Therapy*. 20th ed. Whitehouse Station, NJ: Merck Research Laboratories; 2018.

Rodrigues R, Baroni BM, Pompermayer MG, et al. Effects of acute dehydration on neuromuscular responses of exercised and nonexercised muscles after exercise in the heat. *J Strength Cond Res*. 2014;28(12):3531-3536.

Rogers IR, Hew-Butler T. Exercise-associated hyponatremia: overzealous fluid consumption. *Wilderness Environ Med*. 2009;20(2):139-143.

Rosner MH, Hew-Butler T. Exercise-associated hyponatremia. UpToDate website. https://www.uptodate.com/contents/exercise-associated-hyponatremia. Updated September 28, 2020. Accessed August 2, 2021.

Sahay M, Sahay R. Hyponatremia: a practical approach. *Indian J Endocrinol Metab*. 2014;18(6):760-771.

Sterns RH, Nigwekar SU, Hix JK. The treatment of hyponatremia. *Semin Nephrol*. 2009;29(3):282-299.

Vaidyanathan A, Malilay J, Schramm P, Saha S. Heat-related deaths—United States, 2004–2018. *MMWR*. 2020:69(24):729-734.

Weinman M. Hot on the inside. *JEMS*. 2003;32(7):34.

Wexler RL. Evaluation and treatment of heat-related illnesses. *Am Fam Physician*. 2002;65(11):2307-2315.

Zafren K, Mechem CC. Accidental hypothermia in adults. UpToDate website. https://www.uptodate.com/contents/accidental-hypothermia-in-adults/print. Updated May 5, 2021. Accessed August 2, 2021.

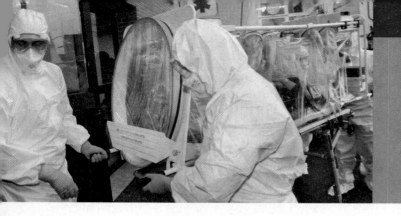

Chapter 20

Infectious and Communicable Diseases

Robert P. Holman, MD

Ryan B. Gerecht, MD

OBJECTIVES

After completing this chapter, you will be able to:

1. Describe the types of immunity and the components of humoral and cell-mediated immunity (pp 1048, 1050–1051).

2. Describe the types of anaphylaxis and the signs, symptoms, and treatment of anaphylaxis (pp 1052–1053).

3. Discuss the implications of transporting patients with immunodeficiencies (p 1054).

4. Discuss the differences between normal, opportunistic, and pathogenic organisms (p 1055).

5. Explain the virulence factors found in pathogenic organisms, including how they can spread from bacterial cell to bacterial cell (p 1055).

6. Describe the portals of entry for infectious organisms and the process of infection once entry is gained (p 1056).

7. Compare the effects of bacterial endotoxins and exotoxins (p 1056).

8. Describe viral pathogenesis (p 1057).

9. Discuss epidemiology, including reservoirs of infection and transmission of infectious disease (p 1057).

10. Discuss the etiologic agents, mode of transmission, signs and symptoms, and treatment of the following:
    - Meningitis (bacterial and viral)
    - Respiratory syncytial virus
    - Cellulitis
    - Necrotizing fasciitis
    - Epiglottitis
    - Tuberculosis
    - Pneumonia
    - Fungal diseases
    - Influenza
    - Various herpesviruses
    - Viral hepatitis
    - Human immunodeficiency virus
    - Rickettsial diseases such as Rocky Mountain spotted fever
    - COVID-19 (caused by SARS-CoV-2)
    - *Escherichia coli* O157:H7
    - West Nile virus
    - Methicillin-resistant *Staphylococcus aureus* and vancomycin-resistant *S aureus*
    - Vancomycin-resistant enterococci
    - Carbapenem-resistant gram negative bacilli (pp 1062–1095)

Introduction

The word **immunity** comes from the Latin word *immunis* and the 14th-century French word *immunité*, referring to a person who has an exemption or inviolability from something. In the modern medical sense, this term retains some of this meaning, in that it refers to protection from infection. Immunity is provided by a complex system of substances, cells, and tissues that exist to protect the human body from infection. While the function of the immune system is to protect against infection, it is also capable of causing damage.

The relationship between humans and infectious disease is an important one to understand. Perhaps it is this relationship, more than anything else, that has determined where we are today as a species.

One example of the countless outbreaks of disease and pandemics that have afflicted humans is the Black Death of the 14th century. This outbreak of bubonic plague, caused by infection with the bacterium *Yersinia pestis*, was the deadliest pandemic recorded in human history. It spread through Europe, Asia, and North Africa, killing an estimated one-third of the European population. The Black Death created religious, social, and economic turmoil.

The social impacts of disease are sometimes more dangerous than the diseases themselves. The threat of disease instills fear, oftentimes leading to irrational behaviors. In our time, the COVID-19 pandemic, caused by the SARS-CoV-2 virus, has demonstrated the dramatic effects of a serious, worldwide contagious disease.

With each outbreak, we learn more about keeping ourselves safe. Better knowledge of diseases and how they spread, consistent use of personal protective equipment (PPE), and a mix of appropriate responder behaviors and organizational policies can all improve the safety of health care providers.

Medical professionals who are involved in critical care and transportation of patients are at high risk for exposure to a multitude of pathogens during the course of their work. An understanding of infectious disease, the ways in which the body responds to disease, and the methods used to reduce the spread of disease will help critical care transport professionals (CCTPs) keep themselves—and consequently their families, coworkers, and communities—safe.

Fundamental Principles of Infectious Disease
Complexity of the Spread of Disease

The spread of infectious disease is a complex process that results from interactions between the host, the infectious agent, and the environment. It is important that all health care professionals know and understand that the spread of disease is dynamic and does not adhere to the strict models used to describe how pathogens are spread—for example, "airborne" or "airborne droplet." Additionally, the ecology of each pathogen is not always completely understood.

As an example, consider the 2004 outbreak of Nipah virus (NiV) in Siliguri, India, near the border of India and Bangladesh. People within the community started to become ill from an unknown disease. It was later discovered that their illness was somehow connected to a popular drink made from date palm sap. Further investigation revealed that fruit bats were contaminating the sap with NiV. This virus, like many zoonoses, causes disease in both humans and animals. While the natural reservoir for NiV is a type of fruit bat, this virus, like many diseases, can also exist in intermediate hosts such as pigs, cows, and goats. NiV was first recognized as a disease in humans in Malaysia in 1998. During that and other outbreaks, there were no documented cases of human-to-human spread. During the 2004 Bangladeshi outbreak, however, human-to-human spread was well documented. This factor is important because human-to-human transmission significantly increases the threat that a disease poses to a population.

NiV infection can be asymptomatic in some people, yet cause acute respiratory failure or fatal encephalitis in others. Some human-to-human spread of the disease has occurred through contact with an infected person's saliva, urine, or other body fluids. Spread throughout hospitals has occurred even when the index patient was previously unrecognized. Researchers have estimated the mortality rate to be 40% to 75% depending on local capabilities for surveillance and disease response.

Pinpointing the nature of disease spread can be complex. During the Bangladeshi outbreak, most people who became ill had contact with another ill person, yet two of the people who were infected had no known contact with other people who became ill. Adding to the puzzle, one study revealed that 57 environmental specimens were taken from the residences of people who became ill, but none tested positive for the virus. Additionally, while significant spread occurred within the hospital (although no health care workers became ill), only 11 of 498 environmental samples from that venue tested positive for the disease. This was true despite the aggressive spread and course of the disease, which often killed people.

The Nipah virus outbreaks provide an excellent example of the emergence of a deadly disease and the dynamic spread of disease that does not adhere strictly to common models.

Classification

A formal classification scheme for microorganisms was developed in the late 1960s, when Carl Woese devised a system that classified microorganisms according to their physical properties and cellular components. **TABLE 20-1** lists the major classes of microorganisms and their properties.

The same physical properties and components that are used to determine the classification of microorganisms also affect how they invade the host, turn into an infection, and cause disease. Microorganisms possess properties that are unlike the properties possessed by human cells. These differences not only allow the immune system to recognize foreign invaders, but can also be exploited by researchers who seek to develop agents that can kill pathogens or otherwise inhibit their growth and spread. Well before Woese developed his classification system, Robert Koch and Louis Pasteur proved the germ theory of disease. Later, Paul Ehrlich pursued the idea that if an invading organism could be targeted and killed, the disease could be cured. Ehrlich wrote:

> If we picture an organism as infected by a certain species of bacterium, it will be easy to effect a cure if substances have been discovered which have a specific affinity for these bacteria and act on these bacteria alone. [If] they possess no affinity for the normal constituents of the body, such substances would then be magic bullets.

In 1909, Ehrlich discovered one such silver bullet—a chemical that killed *Treponema pallidum*, the microorganism responsible for the disease syphilis. Ehrlich realized that if he could manipulate a chemical so that it would fit into the "lock" of the offending organism but not into the "locks" on any human cells, he would be able to cure disease. In 1935, based on this idea, Bayer developed sulfanilamide, a drug that was found to be somewhat effective against staphylococcal and streptococcal infections. Sulfanilamide was derived from a coal tar compound.

This "magic bullet" archetype is still used in medicine today. All antibiotic, antiviral, and antifungal drugs are designed to target (1) specific proteins, macromolecules, cellular organelles, and

TABLE 20-1 Classification of Organisms

Organism	General Information	Cell Wall/Cell Membrane Components	Drug Classes, Groups of Actions (Use)	Medications
Bacteria	Prokaryote versus eukaryote bacteria: prokaryotes Cellularity: unicellular Reproduction: binary fission	Peptidoglycan cell wall No sterols in the membrane (except *Mycoplasma*) Mycolic acid in the cell wall of mycobacteria	Cell wall synthesis inhibitors • Beta-lactams • Glycopeptides Protein synthesis inhibitors • Tetracyclines • Aminoglycosides • Macrolides DNA/RNA synthesis inhibitors • Quinolones or fluoroquinolones Alter cell membrane permeability Antimetabolites • Sulfonamides	Penicillins and cephalosporins Vancomycin Doxycycline Amikacin and gentamicin Erythromycin (many brand names) Ciprofloxacin Polymyxin B Sulfamethoxazole
Viruses	Prokaryote versus eukaryote: neither Cellularity: acellular Reproduction: N/A	None (lack cells)	Viral attachment inhibitor Viral uncoating inhibitor (influenza) Neuraminidase inhibitors (influenza) DNA/RNA synthesis inhibitors (HIV, herpes, cytomegalovirus) Protease inhibitors (HIV) Interferon (hepatitis)	Enfuvirtide Amantadine (Symmetrel) and rimantadine Zanamivir and oseltamivir Acyclovir, ganciclovir and zidovudine Indinavir and saquinavir Interferon
Protozoa	Prokaryote versus eukaryote: eukaryotes Cellularity: unicellular Reproduction: asexual or sexual	No cell wall	Antimetabolites DNA synthesis inhibitors • Nitroimidazoles (unknown mode of action) • Quinolines	Trimethoprim-sulfamethoxazole combination Metronidazole Chloroquine and quinacrine
Helminths	Prokaryote versus eukaryote: eukaryotes Cellularity: multicellular Reproduction: complex	No cell wall	Antimetabolites • Benzimidazole	Mebendazole and praziquantel

Organism	General Information	Cell Wall/Cell Membrane Components	Drug Classes, Groups of Actions (Use)	Medications
Fungi	Prokaryote versus eukaryote: eukaryotes Cellularity: unicellular (yeasts) or multicellular (molds) Reproduction: asexual or sexual	Chitin cell wall Unique sterols (ergosterol) in the membrane	Ergosterol synthesis inhibitors • Azoles • Allylamines Alters cell membrane permeability • Polyene Mitotic inhibitor (prevents cell replication)	Ketoconazole (Nizoral) and miconazole (Monistat, Micatin) Terbinafine (Lamisil) Amphotericin B Griseofulvin
Prions	Prokaryote versus eukaryote: neither Cellularity: acellular Reproduction: N/A	None (lack cells)	N/A	N/A

Abbreviations: DNA, deoxyribonucleic acid; HIV, human immunodeficiency virus; N/A, not applicable; RNA, ribonucleic acid

© Jones & Bartlett Learning.

enzymatic pathways or (2) reproductive strategies unique to the infectious agent that are not shared by their human host.

The Human Immune System

For people to contract a disease, they must be susceptible to that illness. Susceptibility is determined by numerous factors, such as nutritional status, immune status, genetic makeup, living conditions, and exposure. Diseases can be transmitted directly through inhalation, ingestion, or direct contact with infectious agents, or they can be spread indirectly via a vector (people, animals, and microorganisms), a fomite (an inanimate object such as clothing and furniture), or some other complex cycle of interactions.

Within the human body, there is a constant struggle between the host and would-be invaders, with both competing for nutrients, energy, and control of cellular synthetic mechanisms. The perpetual struggle between host and microbe pits the human immune defenses against microbes' ever-evolving ability to adapt to our defenses. These adaptations are often termed virulence factors, reflecting their contribution to the ability of the microbe to evade defenses and cause disease.

For the immune system to protect the body from invading microorganisms, it first must be able to recognize "self" components or cells and distinguish them from non-self components or cells. The immune system must be both highly specific (keeping watch for specific antigens) and general (able to keep up with numerous assaults without sending the body into a perpetual state of inflammation). The protection it provides must consist of several layers so that once one level of immunity has been breached, additional defenses against infection are launched and continue the assault. This multilayered system allows for a gradation of response, appropriate for the current threat. Additionally, the immune system must include cells that are designed to respond to many types of pathogens ("diversity") while recognizing the difference between the body's many cells and those that are non-self (tolerance). Finally, the immune system must be capable of "remembering" previous interactions so that it can mount a response to the same agent or a closely related agent sometimes years after the initial exposure—a feature called memory. All of these components must work in a coordinated effort, providing protection from infection and malignancy, without self-destruction.

Types of Immunity

Immunity can be either innate or adaptive. Innate immunity is immunity that an individual is born with. It provides protection from invading pathogens despite a lack of prior exposure to them. The skin and mucous membranes and their secretions provide mechanical and chemical barriers to invasion and are the primary components of innate immunity. Innate immunity is nonspecific, is activated immediately upon detection of invasion, and has no memory. The components of the innate immune system work to eliminate invading organisms through various methods, including activating the adaptive immune response and preventing the entry of the microorganisms into the body. In addition, nonspecific factors of the immune system help limit the growth of microorganisms within the body:

- Macrophages, a type of white blood cell, ingest and destroy microbes.
- Neutrophils, the most abundant innate immune cells, act as phagocytes.
- Natural killer cells, another type of white blood cell, have the job of recognizing and killing host cells that are infected with a virus.
- The complement system is a group of proteins that, when activated, begin a cascade of events that aid in the clearing of bacterial cells.
- Transferrin is a carrier protein that sequesters iron, keeping that vital element from being available to the invading microbes.

These parts of the innate system, in combination with the body's general responses to invasion such as fever or inflammation, react whenever the body perceives itself to be under assault by an invader.

Adaptive immunity (also referred to as acquired immunity) comes into play when the body's innate defenses are unable to stop the invading pathogen. Adaptive immunity develops as a result of interactions between components of the immune system and the invading microbe, thereby providing improved protection with repeated exposures to the same or a similar agent—a concept referred to as immunologic memory. The two main types of adaptive immunity are humoral and cell-mediated immunity. Humoral immunity is provided by B cells through the production of antibodies and by complement; cell-mediated immunity is provided by T cells. Cytokines and macrophages are modulators of both cell-mediated and humoral immunity, providing signals to the players—revving up or toning down the immune response as appropriate.

Adaptive immunity can be either active or passive.

- Active immunity refers to an ongoing process of developing antibodies and activating T cells in response to invading agents. It is activated either when an individual is exposed to microbes through the natural process of infection or when this process is artificially stimulated through a vaccine.
- Passive immunity is the process of giving an individual a preformed antibody (from a donor) in the event of an exposure to which the individual has not yet developed immunity. (There is some level of risk of contracting bloodborne infectious diseases from the use of preformed or pooled human immunoglobulin.) For example, if a provider were exposed to a patient known to have hepatitis B, the provider could be given hepatitis B immunoglobulin (HBIG) during the incubation period to prevent infection. Before the development of the hepatitis A vaccine, travelers to countries highly endemic for hepatitis A were administered preventive depot injections of standard immune globulin (formerly called gamma globulin), a concentrated solution of antibodies prepared from pooled human plasma. Passive immunity also occurs when antibodies from a mother are passed to her fetus by crossing the placenta into the fetal circulation, or to an infant through breast milk.

Active immunity, once developed, provides long-lasting protection against invading microbes, but is initially slow to develop. Passive immunity is immediate but does not confer a lasting effect. Moreover, because it does not originate with the individual, it must be continually boosted. Vaccination schedules were created for precisely this purpose: Passive immunity in the infant lasts up to 1 year depending on the pathogen, so vaccines are given to ensure continued protection.

Antigens

An antigen is anything that can cause an immune response, but typically takes the form of a protein or sugar that is anchored into the cell membrane and displayed on the cell's surface. The word *antigen* is an abbreviation for *anti*body *gen*erator. An antigen is recognized by the immune system as either self or non-self. All cells display antigens, including humans' own cells. If an antigen is identified by the body as foreign or "non-self," the body initiates either a humoral or cell-mediated response to eliminate it.

Organs and Cells of the Immune System

The highly complex immune system is composed of many organs and cell types. The organs of the immune system are categorized by anatomic location, either central or peripheral.

The lymphatic system comprises the network of capillaries, vessels, ducts, nodes, and organs that

produces and conveys lymph through the body **FIGURE 20-1**. The central lymphoid organs are the thymus and the bone marrow, which serve as the site of synthesis and differentiation of immune cells. The thymus is located in the mediastinal cavity anterior and superior to the heart. It weighs 15 to 35 g at birth and continues to increase in size until puberty, when it begins to shrink. The thymus is where the T lymphocytes differentiate from naïve, nonspecific T cells into T cells with specific purposes. In contrast, the bone marrow is the site of B-cell synthesis.

The peripheral lymphoid organs are where much of the immune cells' work is done; these organs include the spleen, lymph nodes, tonsils, intestinal Peyer patches, and mucosa. For example,

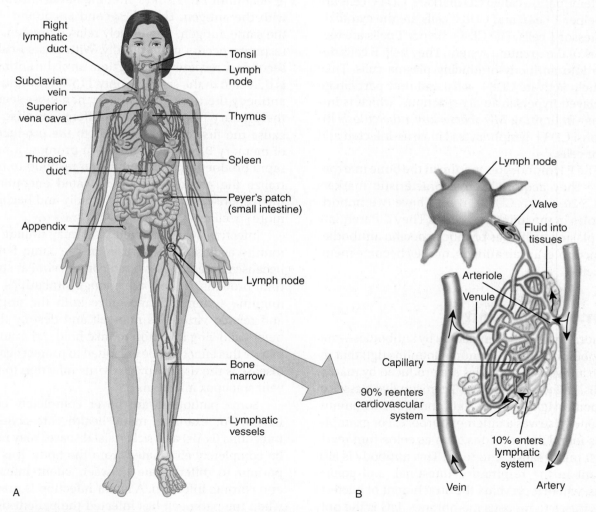

FIGURE 20-1 The lymphatic system. **A.** The lymphatic system consists of vessels that transport lymph and excess tissue fluid back to the circulatory system. **B.** Lymph is picked up by lymphatic capillaries that drain into larger vessels. Like the veins, the lymphatic vessels contain valves that prohibit backflow. Lymph nodes are interspersed along the vessels and filter the lymph.

the spleen is where encapsulated bacteria are encountered and destroyed. Removal of this organ leaves the patient more susceptible to infection, especially from *Streptococcus pneumoniae* and *Haemophilus influenzae*.

Lymph nodes are made up of lymphoidal tissue located throughout the body; they are especially prominent in the neck, axilla, mediastinum, and groin. Lymphadenopathy, an increase in the size of a lymph node or lymph nodes, indicates a high level of immunologic activity. Thus, lymphadenopathy is a clinical sign commonly seen in patients fighting infection or cancer.

The T lymphocytes acquire their distinctive characteristics while maturing in the thymus. The mature cells express phenotypic markers or clusters of differentiation called CD markers. CD4+ cells are the helper T cells, and CD8+ cells are the cytotoxic suppressor T cells. The CD4+ helper T cells are regulators of the immune system. They help B cells develop into antibody-producing plasma cells. They also help activate CD8+ cells, and they participate in delayed hypersensitivity reactions, which is important in limiting *Mycobacterium tuberculosis* infections. CD8+ lymphocytes kill virus-infected and tumor cells.

The B lymphocytes mature in the bone marrow, where they acquire their characteristic markers (eg, CD20, CD21, CD37). B cells have two important roles in the immune system: They differentiate into plasma cells that produce specific antibodies on encountering an antigen, or they become memory cells.

Humoral Immunity

Humoral immunity is mediated by antibodies—that is, globulin proteins (immunoglobulins [Ig]) that react to antigens. Antibodies are produced by mature B cells, called plasma cells. There are five classes of antibodies: IgA, IgM, IgG, IgE, and IgD. Each immunoglobulin serves a different purpose. For example, IgA is found in secretions such as colostrum (early breast milk), saliva, and tears. This antibody is also present in the respiratory, intestinal, and genital tracts, where it prevents the attachment of bacteria and viruses to mucous membranes. IgG is the only immunoglobulin that crosses the placental barrier. IgG and IgM are the only two immunoglobulins that

activate complement. IgE is important in protecting the body against certain parasitic infections, such as helminths or worms, and it mediates the immediate hypersensitivity reaction. IgE recognizes parasites; thus, an allergic reaction is actually the body believing it has been invaded by parasites. Antibodies and complement protect against infection by neutralizing toxins and viruses, and they make microorganisms more easily phagocytized (a process called **opsonization**).

The humoral (antibody-mediated) response is effective against agents that produce toxins, against bacteria that have polysaccharide capsules, and against some viral infections. The primary response occurs when the immune cells encounter a specific antigen for the first time. Antibodies do not appear until 7 to 10 days after the initial encounter with the antigen. Upon a second encounter with the same antigen, or a closely related antigen, the response occurs more rapidly. With this so-called secondary response, the lag time until the antibody is detected in the serum is only 3 to 5 days, and the antibody titers are much higher than those seen in the primary response. These differences arise because the first encounter leads to the production of memory B cells, which in turn promote a more rapid production of cells that can respond to neutralize the pathogen. With repeated encounters, the response is elicited more rapidly and becomes more specific.

Infection with a related virus may impart immunity against other viruses in the same family, because related viruses often contain similar structural proteins. If there are enough similarities, the immune system will recognize both the original and related viruses as non-self and destroy them before allowing infection to take hold. An example of how this effect can be exploited to protect against disease is the use of cowpox virus infection to prevent smallpox infection.

Some pathogens are never completely eliminated. For example, many health care–acquired infections (HAIs) and rickettsial diseases may never be completely eliminated from the body. It is important to differentiate between latent infection and chronic infection. A latent infection is present when the pathogen has infected the patient but is not reproducing or causing disease. A chronic infection is caused by a pathogen that the body has not successfully fought off and is accompanied by a reduced immune response.

Cell-Mediated Immunity

Cell-mediated immunity (CMI) plays an important role in defending against intracellular infections, such as tuberculosis or gonorrhea, as well as viral infections, fungal infections, parasites, and tumors. The strongest evidence of its importance is illustrated in acquired immunodeficiency syndrome (AIDS), a condition in which the destruction of cell-mediated immunity results in overwhelming infections and unusual tumors. Cells involved in CMI include the following:

- *CD4 helper T cells*: Help with antigen recognition and immune response by activating CD8 cytotoxic T cells, B cells, and macrophages.
- T_{reg} (*regulatory T cells*; formerly called suppressor T cells): Regulate the immune response to prevent over-response to a pathogen.
- *CD8 cytotoxic T cells*: Kill other infected or endogenous cells by producing perforins (proteins that cause holes to form in cell membranes, which lead to cell death through loss of the osmotic gradient) or by inducing apoptosis (programmed cell death).
- *Macrophages*: Ingest or destroy foreign cells, viruses, or debris (phagocytosis); present antigens (by activating T cells that can recognize foreign antigens); and produce cytokine (namely, interleukin 1 and tumor necrosis factor). The process of phagocytosis is carried out by macrophages, neutrophils, and monocytes, which engulf and destroy bacteria, foreign antigens, and cellular debris. These cells process the bacteria, breaking them down by specialized cell processes.
- *Natural killer (NK) cells*: Large granular lymphocytes that do not express T-cell antigen receptors. NK cells destroy tumor cells or virus-infected cells by recognizing that those cells are not expressing "self" markers or do not appear abnormal; these cells kill any cells that appear different. Although NK cells are regulated by other proteins in the immune response, they do not require specific activation to produce perforin and granzymes that cause apoptosis or necrosis of target cells.

- *Cytokines*: Proteins produced by immune cells that modify the immune response. Chemokines are a type of cytokine that attract macrophages or neutrophils to the site of an infection.

Monoclonal Antibodies

Most naturally produced antibodies are polyclonal, meaning they are produced by many different types of B lymphocytes. Each of these antibodies has a slightly different specificity for the target antigen. For example, antibodies may bind different epitopes or may bind the same epitope with different affinities. However, large quantities of an antibody from a single B-cell clone can be produced to protect against a specific pathogen. These antibodies are called monoclonal antibodies.

Approximately 100 monoclonal antibodies have been developed and designated as drugs. These drugs, whose names all end with the suffix *mab*, are directed against various antigens and used to treat immunologic diseases and cancer and to reverse drug effects. They may target a plasma protein, an IgG receptor, an infectious organism, hematologic malignancies, solid tumors, autoimmune disorders, hypercholesterolemia, inflammatory bowel disorder, and even drug overdose (digitalis overdose). Use of monoclonal antibodies is particularly important in treating active disease or providing prophylaxis in people who have not been vaccinated but require protection against pathogens such as the SARS-CoV-2 virus (which causes COVID-19), the Ebola virus, or the Zika virus. For example, monoclonal antibody therapy may be given to pregnant women residing in Zika virus–endemic areas.

Hypersensitivity Reactions

The immune response can be harmful to the host when it is inappropriate or exaggerated. These types of harmful reactions, which are called hypersensitivity or allergic reactions, occur when people are exposed to a specific antigen. The first encounter sensitizes the person to the antigen and induces an antibody response. Subsequent encounters with the same or a closely related antigen then elicit the allergic response. This process explains why the first exposure to an allergen rarely induces an immune response, but subsequent exposures lead to progressively stronger reactions.

There are four major types of hypersensitivity reactions. Types I, II, and III are antibody-mediated responses, whereas type IV is a cell-mediated response.

Type I Reactions

Type I is an immediate hypersensitivity reaction involving IgE. The term *immediate hypersensitivity* reflects the fact that these reactions occur within minutes of exposure to the antigen. There are two categories of type I reactions: (1) atopy, which is a localized reaction, and (2) anaphylaxis, which is a systemic reaction.

In a type I reaction, excessive amounts of IgE are synthesized and bind to mast cells or basophils, which activates these cells and causes them to release their contents. The degranulation of mast cells releases histamine, leukotrienes, and tryptase, and stimulates the production of cytokines. In turn, the cytokines play roles in various reactions, including inducing rapid contraction of smooth muscle, increased vascular permeability, hypotension, and changes in the coagulation pathway. Localized histamine release causes urticaria, whereas systemic histamine release causes dose-dependent hemodynamic and cardiovascular changes, such as an increased heart rate, hypotension, and shock, which can be life threatening. Tryptase is an enzyme found in mast cells that, when released, activates complement proteins and the coagulation pathway; it has the potential to cause angioedema, clotting, and clot lysis, leading to disseminated intravascular coagulation in severe cases.

Anaphylaxis is defined as a serious systemic allergic reaction that has a rapid onset and a variable clinical presentation. If unrecognized, it can lead to respiratory arrest, circulatory collapse, and death. Common triggers for anaphylaxis include foods, medications, insect venom (particularly *Hymenoptera* venom), and some environmental agents such as latex. Anaphylaxis is frequently unrecognized and underreported. In fact, as many as 57% of anaphylaxis incidents related to food do not receive a diagnosis of anaphylaxis. For the CCTP, then, it is important to understand what anaphylaxis is and how to recognize it.

While anaphylaxis is a systemic event, the body systems involved vary from patient to patient and even from episode to episode in some patients. Most patients with anaphylaxis (as many as 90%) will have cutaneous involvement, including flushing, itching, urticaria, or angioedema. Upper airway involvement occurs in as many as 70% of patients, with signs and symptoms including changes in phonation, the sensation of throat closure or choking, cough, wheezing, and shortness of breath. As many as 45% of patients experience gastrointestinal conditions; cardiovascular involvement occurs in 45% of these patients.

Anaphylaxis may be difficult to diagnose if the patient does not develop the commonly discussed symptoms. While death from anaphylaxis is uncommon, a patient history of chronic obstructive pulmonary disease (COPD), asthma, or cardiovascular diseases should alert the caregiver that the patient is at greater risk of life-threatening anaphylaxis. The same is true for patients who have a history of severe eczema or severe allergic rhinitis. The use of beta blockers or angiotensin-converting enzyme (ACE) inhibitors may also increase the severity of anaphylaxis.

Anaphylactic symptom progression might take minutes to hours. Biphasic anaphylaxis occurs in as many as 20% of reactions. In a biphasic reaction, the initial resolution of symptoms is followed by a reappearance of symptoms; if this resurgence is not anticipated, it can be the cause of a life-threatening recurrence. In some rare cases, the reaction can last for many hours to days in patients with protracted anaphylaxis.

Some unique circumstances may place patients at increased risk for unrecognized anaphylaxis. For example, wheezing patients with a known history of asthma may be treated for an acute asthma exacerbation without taking into account any cutaneous symptoms, thereby placing them at greater risk for unrecognized anaphylaxis. Their wheezing may be mistakenly attributed to asthma, when it is actually occurring secondary to the respiratory symptoms associated with anaphylaxis. Having asthma puts patients at a high risk of death from anaphylaxis simply because the hypersensitivity reaction may not be recognized until much later in the presentation, delaying appropriate treatment. Patients with underlying neurologic impairment and psychiatric illnesses that interfere with cognition or impair judgment may not be able to express symptoms of pruritus or throat closure. Additionally, sedated patients are unable to recognize or communicate the presence of early symptoms; thus, it is incumbent upon the health care provider to recognize any subtle changes in the skin or vital signs that may signal the emergence of an allergic reaction.

Prompt assessment and treatment are critical for all patients with anaphylaxis. The first step in its management focuses on removal of the inciting antigen. Intramuscular epinephrine should be injected, and, if symptoms persist, an epinephrine drip should be established. As with all successful resuscitations, begin with airway management. If the patient shows any evidence of stridor, significant airway edema, or impending respiratory arrest, perform intubation immediately. Maintain breathing, and support circulation with supplemental oxygen and volume resuscitation. Place two large-bore intravenous (IV) lines for rapid fluid administration and place the patient on continuous cardiac/respiratory monitoring until the episode has resolved. All patients with anaphylaxis require fluid resuscitation, and those with hypotension or signs of shock should receive large-volume resuscitation. Adjunctive agents such as H_1 blockers (antihistamines) can be used for the treatment of itching or hives that fails to resolve after the administration of epinephrine. Patients who are wheezing can be treated with an inhaled beta-2 agonist if the wheezing does not resolve after treatment with epinephrine. The use of glucocorticoids does not appear to be helpful in acute anaphylaxis but may offer some protection against biphasic or protracted reactions.

A patient who is discharged from the hospital after an anaphylactic episode should be educated about their allergy. Such a patient should have an emergency action plan for any recurrence, including a prescription for and instruction in the proper use of an epinephrine auto-injector.

Controversies

The term *anaphylactoid* is no longer in favor, although many providers continue to use this term. The difference between anaphylaxis, anaphylactoid, or pseudoanaphylaxis is not clinically significant.

Type II Reactions

Type II or cytotoxic hypersensitivity reactions are antigen-antibody reactions in which antibodies directed against an antigen on the surface of the host cell membrane cause activation of complement

Signs and Symptoms

Anaphylaxis (Type I Hypersensitivity Reaction)

Cutaneous involvement:
- Flushing
- Itching
- Urticaria
- Angioedema

Airway involvement:
- Changes in phonation
- Sensation of throat closure or choking
- Cough
- Wheezing or stridor
- Shortness of breath

Cardiovascular involvement:
- Tachycardia
- Hypotension

Transport Management

Anaphylaxis (Type I Hypersensitivity Reaction)

- Remove the antigen.
- Inject intramuscular epinephrine.
- If symptoms persist, establish an epinephrine drip.
- If there is any evidence of stridor, significant airway edema, or impending respiratory arrest, intubate the patient immediately.
- Provide oxygen supplementation and volume resuscitation.
- Place two large-bore IV lines for rapid fluid administration.
- Place the patient on continuous cardiac/respiratory monitoring including end-tidal carbon dioxide ($ETCO_2$) and pulse oximetry.
- In case of hypotension or signs of shock, provide large-volume resuscitation.
- Give H_1 blockers for ongoing itching or hives.
- Give an inhaled beta-2 agonist for ongoing wheezing.
- In case of a biphasic or protracted reaction, give glucocorticoids.

and subsequent lytic and osmotic damage to the host cells. They are seen in transfusion reactions, hemolytic disease of the newborn (erythroblastosis fetalis), and some autoimmune diseases. Either IgM or IgG antibodies are involved in this type of reaction.

Type III Reactions

In type III hypersensitivity reactions, circulating antigen-antibody complexes are deposited in tissue or on the endothelium of blood vessels. There, they cause damage by activating complement proteins, releasing chemotactic and clotting factors, and attracting other immune cells to the area. Examples of this type of reaction include serum sickness, polyarteritis nodosa, glomerulonephritis, and systemic lupus erythematosus.

Type IV Reactions

In type IV (delayed-type) hypersensitivity reactions, tissue damage results from excessive activation of macrophages. Such reactions involve the interaction of macrophages and T cells, but the response is delayed from hours to days after the antigen is encountered. This hypersensitivity reaction is cell mediated and is not a humeral response, unlike types I, II, and III. Type IV reaction is exemplified by contact hypersensitivity, like that seen with exposure to poison ivy or poison oak.

Immunodeficiency

Immunodeficiency occurs when dysfunction in one or more of the components of the immune system leaves an individual vulnerable to disease. Immunodeficiency can be genetic or can occur secondary to environmental factors, medical interventions, or other diseases such as HIV/AIDS or malignancies. The specific component of the immune system that is not fully functional predisposes the patient to certain types of infection or disease. Patients with B-cell deficiencies, for example, are susceptible to recurrent infections with pyogenic bacteria such as *S pneumoniae* and *H influenzae*. A deficiency in T cells allows for recurrent infections with viruses, fungi, or protozoa.

Critically ill patients have few reserves to fight infections as a result of their diminished host defenses and loss of innate immunity. Features of chronic illness that decrease innate immunity include stress, malnutrition, invasive procedures, loss of physical barriers (eg, skin and mucosal surfaces), and pathogenic bacterial overgrowth or bacterial growth in normally sterile tissue. In addition, patients who are maintained on immunosuppressive therapy for the management of autoimmune diseases or to prevent rejection of a transplanted organ are at increased risk for a variety of infections and cancers.

Immunosuppression
Transplant Patients

Treatment of the transplant patient is an important aspect of critical care transports. Management of illnesses and injuries in such patients may be complicated by the side effects of medications or by their immunosuppressed condition. Immunosuppressive agents, such as cyclosporine, tacrolimus, azathioprine, and prednisone, are routinely prescribed to transplant patients in an effort to prevent rejection of the donor tissue. These medications can have serious side effects, including hypertension, hyperglycemia, hyperkalemia, nephrotoxicity, and neurotoxicity, so it is important to discuss the care plan with a transplant team representative prior to initiating transport.

In addition to surgical complications or manifestations of acute rejection, prevention and detection of infection are important when transporting transplant patients. For example, the presence of a life-threatening infectious illness may not become apparent until the diagnostic evaluations have been completed. In addition, mild symptoms that may be overlooked in routine transports could indicate serious conditions in transplant patients.

Rheumatology and Cancer Patients

More common than transplant recipients are patients with rheumatologic diseases or cancers whose treatment renders them significantly immunosuppressed. For conditions such as rheumatoid arthritis, vasculitis, or lupus, patients will often receive steroids (eg, prednisone) and additional immunosuppressive medications. A range of cancer therapeutics also cause various immune deficiencies. Often an infection in these immunosuppressed patients will manifest in more subtle ways because they lack the full immune reaction of healthy hosts.

Pathogenicity
Normal Bacteria

Not all bacteria are pathogenic; in fact, most bacteria have either beneficial or neutral effects. The presence of normal bacteria (commensal bacteria) in and on the body plays an important role in disease prevention through competition for space and nutrients. Nonpathogenic bacteria assist the immune system by preventing the overgrowth of pathogenic strains; they achieve this feat by using up available nutrients, maintaining a certain pH, and creating bacteriocins (antibacterial toxins).

A good example of this beneficial relationship is found in the normal microbiota of the adult vagina. Lactobacilli normally present in the vagina produce acid and keep the pH of the adult vagina between 3.5 and 4.5. This creates a hostile environment for *Candida albicans*, the causative agent of vaginal yeast infection. If the commensal bacteria of the vagina are reduced in numbers by extended use of antibiotics or excessive douching, the pH increases and *C albicans* can dominate, leading to fungal vaginitis.

Opportunistic Bacteria

Opportunistic infections are diseases caused by normally nonpathogenic agents in patients with an abnormally functioning immune system. The normally harmless organisms that cause these infections are termed *opportunistic bacteria*. In patients who are immunocompromised, the normal balance between host and microbe is upset by a weakness in the immune system—a deficiency caused by a genetic defect, specific medications, and/or chronic diseases. When the host defense system is compromised, microbes that are otherwise harmless may replicate unchecked.

In fact, AIDS is defined by the unusual infections found in patients who have compromised immune systems as a result of human immunodeficiency virus (HIV) infection. These rare and unusual opportunistic illnesses are called indicator conditions or AIDS-defining illness because they are rarely, if ever, seen in people without severe immune dysfunction. For example, the fungus *Pneumocystis jirovecii* (formerly *P carinii*) is a common environmental fungus that usually does not cause disease in healthy people, but is the most common opportunistic infection in HIV-infected people. *P jirovecii* is not responsive to antifungal treatments.

Many patients who require critical care transport are immunocompromised. CCTPs need to be keenly aware that these very sick patients can be inadvertently infected during the course of their care. To avoid this complication, CCTPs must adhere scrupulously to proper technique, keeping their equipment sanitized or sterile and using standard precautions such as masks and gloves when appropriate. Even a mild dermatitis on the hands of a healthy person or a few bacteria left on respiratory equipment can translate into a lethal infection in the immunocompromised patient.

Pathogenic Bacteria

A pathogen is simply defined as a microorganism capable of causing disease. Pathogenic organisms cause disease because they possess unique factors that help them gain entry into the body, colonize and overcome host defenses, produce toxins that cause cytopathic effects, or do mechanical damage to the body. Some pathogens may evade immune system destruction by producing capsules, slime layers, or specialized cell walls. Others may mount preemptive strikes by destroying phagosomes or by preventing phagocytosis.

Virulence Factors

The degree of pathogenicity is called the virulence of an organism. The following properties of microbes, known as virulence factors, may influence their virulence:

- Host and tissue specificity (the ability of the organism to gain entry into a host)
- Adherence to specific host cells
- Invasion of host tissues
- Evasion of host defenses
- Toxicity
- Development of a polysaccharide capsule (encapsulation)

Pathogenic organisms may possess one or more virulence factors. A common example of a virulence factor is the long, threadlike fimbriae of *Escherichia coli*, which allow adherence to host uroepithelial (bladder) cells. This adherence is a crucial step during the infection that allows uropathogenic *E coli* to colonize the urinary tract and prevents removal of the bacteria during urination.

Virulence can be experimentally quantified by two measures: the infective dose of an organism (ID_{50}) and the lethal dose of an organism (LD_{50}). The ID_{50} measures the number of organisms required to infect a susceptible test animal. The LD_{50} measures the number of organisms required to kill 50% of the infected test animals inoculated with the microbe. The lower the ID_{50} or the LD_{50}, the more virulent

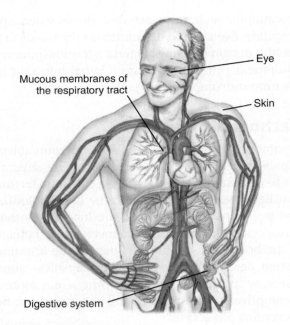

FIGURE 20-2 Portals of infection.

© Jones & Bartlett Learning.

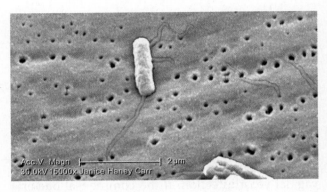

FIGURE 20-3 Pili (fimbriae) on a bacterium.

Courtesy of Janice Haney Carr/CDC.

the organism is. For example, the infective dose of *Shigella* is about 10 to 100 organisms, whereas the infective dose of *Salmonella* is approximately 1 million organisms. Thus, it takes a larger quantity of *Salmonella* to produce an infection than it does *Shigella*; that is, *Shigella* is more virulent. By contrast, Ebola requires only a single **plaque-forming unit** to cause infection.

Host and Tissue Specificity

The portal of entry **FIGURE 20-2** is important because it can influence how the pathogen manifests disease, or if it is capable of causing disease at all. For example, various *Staphylococcus* species can cause localized skin infections such as an abscess. They can also cause toxic shock syndrome when present in large numbers in sites such as the vagina or sinuses and can release the exotoxin TSST (toxic shock syndrome toxin) into the bloodstream. Other organisms are extremely site specific in terms of their portal of entry and infectivity. For example, *Salmonella typhi* causes no infection when inhaled, but does cause infection if it enters the digestive tract. Conversely, *S pneumoniae* does not cause disease if it is ingested but does cause pneumonia if it is inhaled.

Adherence

Once inside the body, the pathogenic organism must be able to adhere to specific cells to begin reproduction. Most bacteria attach themselves to cell surfaces using specialized structures that project out of the cell wall, called pili or fimbriae **FIGURE 20-3**. Gram-negative bacteria possess a common type of pili that allow them to adhere to surfaces in the gastrointestinal tract. Other bacteria produce unique pili that bind to specific tissues.

Most organisms can begin to reproduce as soon as they have adhered to the host tissue. While these microbes reproduce, they remain bound to the surface of the host cells and spread along the tissue surface or are disseminated throughout the body.

Invasion

Once inside the host cell, the organisms multiply and easily invade neighboring cells through pores connecting the cells. This cell-to-cell infection also allows bacteria to evade destruction by the immune system. Other microbes invade tissues by producing enzymes that break down the molecules that hold cells together.

Toxicity

Bacteria are capable of producing two types of toxins: exotoxins or endotoxins. An **exotoxin** is produced inside the cell and secreted into surrounding tissues or fluids. An **endotoxin**, in contrast, is a structural component of the bacterial cell and is not released until the bacterium is destroyed. *Salmonella, Pseudomonas aeruginosa, E coli*, and other well-known bacteria produce medically important endotoxins.

Exotoxins are generally specified by genetic information carried on plasmids (small pieces of deoxyribonucleic acid [DNA] that are not part of the bacterial chromosome) or on bacteriophages (viruses capable of infecting bacterial cells). These toxins are highly specific and have differing modes of action. They are produced mostly by gram-positive bacteria but can be made by a few gram-negative organisms. Exotoxins can be grouped according to the tissue type affected:

- Neurotoxins damage nervous tissue. Botulinum toxin is a potent neurotoxin, produced by *Clostridium botulinum*, which inhibits the release of acetylcholine and results in paralysis.
- Enterotoxins affect the digestive tract and disrupt the epithelial lining of the gut, leading to severe diarrhea such as that caused by *Vibrio cholerae*, the causative agent of cholera.
- Erythrogenic toxins specifically target capillaries and produce a red skin rash. For example, such a rash is seen in scarlet fever, which is caused by *Streptococcus pyogenes*.
- Cytotoxins damage a variety of host tissues. *Corynebacterium diphtheriae* (the bacterium that causes diphtheria), *Shigella*, and a number of other pathogens produce cytotoxins. For example, *Shigella* cytotoxins damage the cells of the digestive tract.

Encapsulation

Some organisms produce polysaccharide layers and surround themselves with capsules or slime layers. These polysaccharide layers inactivate proteins essential for the immune system's phagocytic mechanism to operate correctly. This activity not only makes ingestion of the pathogen by macrophages impossible, but also allows some bacteria to start reproduction within the macrophage or lymph nodes.

Still other microbes form biofilms, which are accumulations of bacteria and other organisms embedded in a matrix of polysaccharide along the surface of tissues. These microcolonies tend to be highly resistant both to antibiotics and to the host immune system.

Viral Pathogenicity

Viruses must gain entry into the body to cause disease. Some viruses simply enter through broken skin, such as a puncture wound, an insect bite, or the entry portal created by insertion of a hypodermic needle. Others enter the body through the respiratory or digestive tract and bind to the host's cell surface receptors using viral proteins found on the surface of the virion. The binding of these protein "spikes" induces receptor-mediated endocytosis that brings the virus directly into the cell. Once inside, the virus particle can be "uncoated," releasing the viral nucleic acid. The viral DNA or ribonucleic acid (RNA) then begins to direct synthesis of viral-encoded protein and nucleic acid molecules, and the process of new virion assembly begins.

The illness caused by a virus may result from the production of viral-specific molecules that deplete the host cell's resources and eventually lead to cell death. Other viruses cause illness by inducing apoptosis, even when they do little harm to the cell during their active growth cycle. Another pathogenic mechanism used by some viruses is the induction of large inflammatory responses, even with little or no actual damage to the host cell.

Epidemiology

Epidemiology is the study of how disease is distributed within populations and the factors that influence this distribution. It has several specific objectives:

- Identify the etiology (cause of disease)
- Determine the extent of disease within a given community
- Understand the natural history of disease
- Evaluate the effectiveness of therapeutic methods
- Identify sources of disease outbreaks
- Identify modes of disease transmission
- Develop methods of disease prevention

When discussing disease and the impact it has on the population, the incidence and prevalence of the disease must be quantified. The terms *incidence* and *prevalence* are often confused. The incidence of a disease is the number of new cases of that disease within a defined population over a defined period of time. The prevalence of a disease is the total number of cases of that disease within a population; it includes both old and new cases of the disease. For example, if in a population of

100 people there are 5 existing cases of a type of cancer, and 5 more cases are then diagnosed, the total number of people with cancer would be 10; therefore the prevalence is 10 in 100. Prevalence is preferred when you want to understand the total burden of a disease on a population, whereas incidence is preferred when you want to know how quickly a disease is spreading in a community. Both concepts are used for understanding the patterns of disease occurrence, for utilization planning of health services and facilities, and for determining the training of future providers.

The pattern of disease occurrence is another important element in understanding how populations are affected by disease. If a disease occurs only occasionally, it is called sporadic. If some cases of a disease are always present within a given population, and the numbers are expected and predictable, the disease is said to be endemic. Thus, an endemic disease is a disease that is always present

and whose incidence is stable. If the number of cases of a disease clearly rises (above a threshold level) in a given time or geographic area, the disease is said to be epidemic. An epidemic is not specific to whether the disease is communicable, but rather refers to an outbreak of a disease that either is usually absent or has an incidence that has grown beyond the expected range. The term pandemic refers to a worldwide epidemic.

The detection of emerging or reemerging infectious diseases is possible through the systematic collection of data and constant surveillance of the incidence of disease. The Centers for Disease Control and Prevention (CDC) continually identifies certain "notifiable" diseases that require reporting to the health department as part of its effort to monitor and track the incidence of contagious diseases **TABLE 20-2**. New diseases can be recognized as such only when the normal background cases of infectious disease are well understood.

TABLE 20-2 Infectious Diseases Designated as Notifiable at the National Level

Anthrax	Coronavirus disease 2019 (COVID-19)
Arboviral diseases, neuroinvasive and non-neuroinvasive	Cryptosporidiosis
• California serogroup virus diseases	Cyclosporiasis
• Chikungunya virus disease	Dengue virus infections
• Eastern equine encephalitis virus disease	• Dengue
• Powassan virus disease	• Dengue-like illness
• St. Louis encephalitis virus disease	• Severe dengue
• West Nile virus disease	Diphtheria
• Western equine encephalitis virus disease	Ehrlichiosis and anaplasmosis
Babesiosis	• *Anaplasma phagocytophilum* infection
Botulism	• *Ehrlichia chaffeensis* infection
• Botulism, foodborne	• *Ehrlichia ewingii* infection
• Botulism, infant	• Undetermined human ehrlichiosis/anaplasmosis
• Botulism, wound	Giardiasis
• Botulism, other	Gonorrhea
Brucellosis	*Haemophilus influenzae*, invasive disease
Campylobacteriosis	Hansen disease
Candida auris, clinical	Hantavirus infection, non-hantavirus pulmonary syndrome
Carbapenemase-producing carbapenem-resistant *Enterobacteriaceae* (CP-CRE)	Hantavirus pulmonary syndrome
• CP-CRE, *Enterobacter* spp.	Hemolytic uremic syndrome, postdiarrheal
• CP-CRE, *E coli*	Hepatitis A, acute
• CP-CRE, *Klebsiella* spp.	Hepatitis B, acute
Chancroid	Hepatitis B, chronic
Chlamydia trachomatis infection	Hepatitis B, perinatal virus infection
Cholera	Hepatitis C, acute
Coccidioidomycosis	Hepatitis C, chronic
Congenital syphilis	Hepatitis C, perinatal infection
• Syphilitic stillbirth	HIV infection (AIDS has been reclassified as HIV Stage III)

Influenza-associated pediatric mortality

Invasive pneumococcal disease

Legionellosis

Leptospirosis

Listeriosis

Lyme disease

Malaria

Measles

Meningococcal disease

Mumps

Novel influenza A virus infections

Pertussis

Plague

Poliomyelitis, paralytic

Poliovirus infection, nonparalytic

Psittacosis

Q fever

• Q fever, acute

• Q fever, chronic

Rabies, animal

Rabies, human

Rubella

Rubella, congenital syndrome

Salmonella Paratyphi infection (*Salmonella enterica* serotypes Paratyphi A, B [tartrate negative], and C [*S Paratyphi*])

Salmonella Typhi infection (*Salmonella enterica* serotype Typhi)

Salmonellosis

Severe acute respiratory syndrome–associated coronavirus disease

Shiga toxin–producing *E coli*

Shigellosis

Smallpox

Spotted fever rickettsiosis

Streptococcal toxic shock syndrome

Syphilis

• Syphilis, primary

• Syphilis, secondary

• Syphilis, early nonprimary, nonsecondary

• Syphilis, unknown duration or late

Tetanus

Toxic shock syndrome (other than streptococcal)

Trichinellosis

Tuberculosis

Tularemia

Vancomycin-intermediate *Staphylococcus aureus* and Vancomycin-resistant *S aureus*

Varicella

Varicella deaths

Vibriosis

Viral hemorrhagic fever

• Crimean-Congo hemorrhagic fever virus

• Ebola virus

• Lassa virus

• Lujo virus

• Marburg virus

• New World arenavirus—Guanarito virus

• New World arenavirus—Junin virus

• New World arenavirus—Machupo virus

• New World arenavirus—Sabia virus

Yellow fever

Zika virus disease and Zika virus infection

• Zika virus disease, congenital

• Zika virus disease, noncongenital

• Zika virus infection, congenital

• Zika virus infection, noncongenital

Abbreviations: AIDS, acquired immunodeficiency syndrome; HIV, human immunodeficiency virus; spp, multiple species

Data from Centers for Disease Control and Prevention, National Notifiable Diseases Surveillance System (NNDSS). 2020 National notifiable infectious diseases (historical). https://wwwn.cdc.gov/nndss/conditions/notifiable/2020/infectious-diseases/. Accessed February 11, 2021.

Other important epidemiologic concepts to understand include the R_0 ("R naught") value, which represents the basic reproduction number of a disease. It indicates how many people typically become infected by each infected individual in the absence of public health interventions. For example, R_0 for measles is 12 to 17—a range determined by the number of contacts that infected people are likely to make during a specific period, the probability of transmission, and the amount of time an infected individual will be infectious. R_0 historically is central to disease forecasting models. Although it is influenced by biologic factors, such as mode of transmission, that remain fairly constant throughout a disease outbreak, it also depends on less-fixed dynamics, such as the frequency with which members of a population interact. In comparison to previous disease outbreaks, COVID-19 uniquely revealed the limitations of R_0, with estimates of R_0 during the pandemic ranging from 1.4 to 5.7 at different times and in different places.

The R_0 value also influences the level of "herd immunity" necessary to halt spread. For measles, 83% to 94% of the population needs to be immune to extinguish the disease. For the COVID-19 pandemic, the different R_0 led epidemiologists to predict that 70% to 80% of the population would need immunization to achieve herd immunity.

Another variant of R, called R_t, describes disease transmission as an outbreak progresses. It is useful in understanding why some people become immune to a disease, whether by surviving infection or by becoming vaccinated. For epidemiologic purposes, when a new virus, such as SARS-CoV-2, begins to spread, everyone may be considered susceptible to infection. At that stage, epidemiologists may use R_0 to build models of how the disease might spread. Over time, the focus shifts to R_t (ie, how more people may survive). As with R_0, epidemiologists must take social dynamics into account when calculating R_t. R_t represents only an average across a region, so it can miss regional clusters of infection, or "superspreader" events.

The effective rate of spread, designated as R or R_e, is similar to the basic reproductive number, but determines the number of people who will become infected in the presence of public health interventions such as vaccination programs. A reproductive rate (R_0) of less than 1 suggests that disease progression is controllable, whereas a rate greater than 1 suggests it will continue to spread.

An infectious disease can be either communicable or noncommunicable. A communicable disease can be transmitted from person to person, whereas a noncommunicable disease, such as tetanus, cannot be transmitted from person to person. A contagious disease is one that is highly communicable.

The prevalence or incidence of disease within a population accounts for only clinical illness or disease that produces symptoms. Disease without symptoms is *not* equivalent to no disease or no risk of spreading disease. For example, some people have subclinical manifestations and can still transmit the disease, while others can be carriers without ever expressing symptoms. Factors such as the incubation period of the disease and the presence

Controversies

Prior to the creation of the childhood vaccination schedule, childhood infectious diseases were responsible for a significant number of deaths. Despite the widespread availability of effective vaccines, many vaccine-preventable diseases are now reemerging.

While the reemergence of these diseases is not always completely understood, we do know that over the past few decades some parents have made a decision not to vaccinate their children out of fear that the vaccines will cause autism. This fear is often based on a fraudulent study conducted by Andrew Wakefield, whose medical license was revoked following the discovery of his fraud. Wakefield's research, which was published in *The Lancet* in 1998, was subsequently retracted in 2010, but it remains perhaps the most damaging medical fraud in modern history.

Another concern held by parents, albeit to a lesser extent, is that some of the preservatives in vaccines, especially aluminum, may be toxic to the recipient. However, the body burden of aluminum remains below the minimal risk levels even when an infant is formula fed and receives all first-year vaccines. Aluminum has been used in vaccines for more than six decades, with no scientific evidence indicating it raises safety concerns.

Yet another argument against vaccinations is that the diseases really are not so bad—that is, that a child who becomes sick with a mild illness actually boosts their immune system. Quite the opposite happens with measles. Measles infections appear to weaken the immune system. In children not vaccinated for measles who develop measles, their mortality from infections other than measles can be higher.

In 2015, Spain experienced its first case of diphtheria since 1986; the affected child died. The parents had not vaccinated their child because of the antivaccine movement. Diphtheria historically carries a 10% mortality rate among children and is so severe in its impact that one outbreak in the 1600s was termed the "year of strangulations." As evidence of the positive impact of vaccination, worldwide incidence of measles decreased by 73% from 2000 to 2018; in that time, vaccine rates among children younger than 1 year rose from 72% to 86%. The World Health Organization (WHO) estimates that measles vaccination campaigns saved 23.2 million lives in this time. These mortality rates directly contradict the argument that "childhood illnesses" are benign.

Some parents use herd immunity as an excuse to exclude their own children from vaccination: If everyone else is vaccinated, why should my child be? This logic has contributed to many recent outbreaks. In 2019, 1,282 cases of measles were confirmed in the United States, most of them in people who were not vaccinated. Since 2015, several mumps outbreaks have been reported, the largest of which occurred in a community in Arkansas in 2016–2017, resulting in nearly 3,000 cases. As these cases suggest, when a significant portion of the "herd" remains unvaccinated, their status puts the vaccinated individuals at risk as well. For example, mumps immunity diminishes over time, a factor that often contributes to outbreaks.

of different carrier states may allow the disease to go undetected and unaccounted in an individual, yet place others at risk for contracting the disease because prevention and disease control efforts are not employed. This concept is a critical one in the safe transport of patients. CCTPs are at risk for contracting disease from each patient transported; therefore, the use of disease control and prevention practices must be evaluated and employed as appropriate every time that care is provided to patients, regardless of whether the patient is or is not currently exhibiting symptoms.

Reservoirs of Infection

For a microorganism to infect and reinfect other organisms, it must have the ability to survive, duplicate or reproduce, and spread to new hosts. A reservoir of infection provides a supply of nutrients and an environmental niche that supports long-term microbial survival. Bacteria have developed some unique systems that enable them to withstand hostile environments. For example, the spore-forming bacterial species anthrax is resistant to drying and environments with low nutrients, and can exist in soil as a spore for decades. Encapsulated bacteria are resistant to changes in pH levels and can live outside the host for long periods.

Both wild and domestic animals can act as reservoirs of infection. A disease that occurs in animals and can also be transmitted to humans is called a zoonosis. Once it has spread to humans, such a disease might stay with the infected person (as is the case with bubonic plague) or be transmitted from person to person (as is the case with pneumonic plague).

Influenza is the prototypic zoonosis. This virus jumps from an animal host to a human, who can then infect other humans. In this case, the virus's transmissibility between the animal reservoir and the human host provides selective pressure to the virus that supports its long-term survival. The influenza virus will alter its surface proteins so that it can then reinfect and cause illness in people who have developed immunity to the old strain. The new strain is just different enough to escape activation of immune memory.

In the same way that animals can serve as reservoirs of infection, humans can act as reservoirs of infection. A person who is colonized by pathogenic species but does not have symptoms of the infection is called asymptomatic or a latent carrier.

These individuals have important roles in perpetuating diseases such as diphtheria, AIDS, hepatitis, gonorrhea, and amoebic dysentery.

It is important to differentiate between a reservoir and a carrier. A reservoir refers to something that leads to the long-term survival of the organism. A broader concept is "disease ecology," which refers to the totality of all components of the disease–environment–host system. When an Ebola epidemic struck in West Africa in 2014, scientists struggled to understand the ecology of the disease and determine its natural reservoir. They tested plants, insects, bats, and animals indigenous to the areas of the outbreak. While the reservoir was not discovered during the outbreak, the researchers determined a certain type of fruit bat was an intermediate host and was, at minimum, very important to the ecology of Ebola.

Finally, the health care environment itself may serve as a reservoir of infection. Some organisms are remarkably resistant to the effects of drying and, therefore, can survive on inanimate objects (fomites) for an extended period of time. Durable medical equipment, even when treated with antimicrobial solutions, can harbor bacteria several days to several weeks after inoculation.

Modes of Transmission

Understanding the different modes of transmission of microorganisms is the first step in developing effective infection prevention measures. The unique properties and characteristics of the infectious agents determine how the disease is spread and how the infection is contracted. Infectious diseases can be transmitted directly, indirectly, or mechanically.

Direct transmission can occur vertically or horizontally. Types of direct horizontal transmission include sexual transmission, exchange of respiratory droplets or secretions, and transmission by contact. Vertical transmission is the exchange of an infectious agent between mother and fetus in utero. Perinatal transmission, another form of direct transmission, occurs when the pathogen is transmitted from mother to newborn during the birthing process. The risk of vertical transmission of HIV can be greatly reduced by initiating therapy in a pregnant woman with zidovudine (AZT), a nucleoside reverse transcriptase inhibitor, between 14 and 34 weeks' gestation.

Indirect transmission occurs when there is an intervening step in the transmission from reservoir to susceptible host. This intermediate step involves an inanimate object or fomite such as towels, bedding, thermometers, contaminated syringes, or even doorknobs. Prevention of infection via indirect transmission can be as simple as properly disposing of contaminated materials and cleaning equipment between patients, or it may require thorough decontamination of the entire patient area and caregiver materials.

Many infectious diseases are transmitted through the use of a medium, such as water, food, air, or contaminated body fluids. Water can be either the reservoir of disease or a vehicle for the disease's transmission. Water that contains raw or poorly treated sewage is the perfect vehicle for the fecal-oral route of cholera transmission. *Vehicle* transmission can usually be prevented by good hygiene, proper food preparation and storage, and a reliable water supply or the prolonged boiling of questionable water.

Vector transmission is the movement of a pathogen from an infected organism to a susceptible host via an animal or insect. The method of vector transmission can be either mechanical or biological.

- *Mechanical* transmission is the passive transport of pathogens on the body of the animal to the susceptible host. Typhoid, while most commonly associated with the fecal-oral route of spread, is an example of an infectious agent that can be transmitted on the feet of houseflies.
- *Biologic* transmission involves the vector, usually an arthropod, ingesting a blood meal from an infected organism and transmitting it after the pathogen has multiplied in the digestive tract of the vector, increasing the likelihood of transmission to a new host. Biologic transmission is seen in malaria, bubonic plague, and African sleeping sickness.

Selected Diseases

As noted earlier, CCTPs are exposed to deadly agents on a daily basis. When providing care for sick patients, contracting their diseases is an inherent risk of the job, as is the risk of passing the diseases on to other patients, fellow providers, or even family members. Knowledge of common infectious diseases and the appropriate responses can prevent the spread of disease. Many such diseases initially present as influenza like illness (ILI), which makes their diagnosis more challenging. Moreover, whenever a person has a fever and a rash, there is a strong likelihood that the individual is contagious.

Meningitis

Meningitis is an umbrella term that refers to five types of inflammation of the leptomeninges, the membranes that cover and enclose the spinal cord and brain. The meninges are organized into three distinct layers: the dura mater (external layer), the arachnoid mater (middle layer), and the pia mater (internal layer). Meningitis is a serious medical condition that may be caused by bacterial, viral, parasitic, or fungal pathogens. The fifth type, which is noninfectious, results from medications, cancer, or other injury.

Bacterial Meningitis

Bacterial meningitis occurs when a bacterial infection migrates to the meninges. It may occur after cranial trauma in which the normal barriers to infection are damaged. Bacterial meningitis may also result from septicemia if it spreads bacteria to the meninges. This life-threatening illness has an acute onset and is considered a medical emergency requiring prompt diagnosis and treatment to preserve life and neurologic function. Bacterial meningitis is fatal in as many as 30% of patients and causes permanent neurologic impairment in 10% of surviving patients.

Signs and Symptoms

The classic triad of symptoms observed in patients with bacterial meningitis consists of fever, nuchal rigidity, and altered mental status, although these symptoms are seen together in fewer than 50% of patients. Most patients (as many as 95% at presentation) have fever, usually greater than 100.4°F (38°C), and almost all patients with meningitis have at least one of the other classic triad of symptoms. Other symptoms of meningitis include headache, significant photophobia, and cutaneous manifestations such as petechiae or palpable purpura.

Additionally, neurologic complications may be present early in the disease course or occur as a late complication. Seizures and neurologic deficits, such as an altered mentation or oculomotor nerve palsies, have been described in as many as 30% of patients. Hearing loss is a late neurologic complication seen especially among children with meningitis. Treatment with dexamethasone, given at the same time as or before the first dose of antibiotics, may reduce the risk of mortality and adverse neurologic deficits in meningitis caused by *S pneumoniae*.

Patients may not specifically complain of a stiff neck, but nuchal rigidity can be demonstrated clinically by a few simple maneuvers. If the patient is unable to touch the chin to the chest by either active or passive flexion, the CCTP should suspect nuchal rigidity. While not very sensitive, the Brudzinski and Kernig signs are often used to determine whether neck signs are present.

- The *Brudzinski sign* is positive when spontaneous involuntary flexion of the hips occurs during attempted passive flexion of the neck. This sign may be elicited by having the patient look down at the feet while laying supine; if the legs draw up, it is considered positive.
- The *Kernig sign* is elicited by straightening a patient's flexed legs. The inability to allow full extension of the knees when the hips are flexed is interpreted as a positive result.

Management

When meningitis is suspected, the patient should undergo a lumbar puncture to obtain cerebrospinal fluid (CSF), unless this procedure is contraindicated. If the collection of CSF is delayed, blood culture results are often reliable and can be useful for diagnosis in the event that CSF cannot be obtained prior to the administration of antibiotics. Some physicians will delay the lumbar puncture until a computed tomography (CT) scan has been obtained to exclude the possibility of increased intracranial pressure that may lead to cerebral herniation during the removal of CSF. It is not normally necessary to obtain a CT scan prior to a lumbar puncture except in the following circumstances:

- History of immunosuppression (eg, a patient with HIV infection or a patient who has received a transplant)
- Seizure (new onset, within 7 days of presentation)
- History of central nervous system disease (tumor, stroke, or focal infection)

- Abnormal level of consciousness
- Focal neurologic deficit
- Papilledema

If for any reason the collection of CSF is delayed, the administration of antibiotics should not be withheld. Empirical antibiotic treatment is warranted when bacterial meningitis is suspected clinically.

Infecting Organisms

Clinicians use epidemiologic knowledge to predict the infecting organism by understanding which bacterium (or virus) is the most likely pathogen, given the patient's age, medical history, immune status, and presenting symptoms. The organisms that cause community-acquired bacterial meningitis are quite different from those that cause meningitis in hospitalized patients or in immunosuppressed patients. The major causes of community-acquired bacterial meningitis in adults are *S pneumoniae* and *Neisseria meningitides*. *Listeria monocytogenes* is a major cause in patients older than 55 years.

The epidemiology of bacterial meningitis underwent a major change after the introduction of the *Haemophilus influenzae* type b (Hib) conjugate vaccine in 1987. Before the 1990s, most cases of meningitis were seen in infants and children, and were caused by *H influenzae*, a gram-negative bacterium. Today, most cases of bacterial meningitis are observed in adults and can be caused by a variety of bacterial species, including *N meningitidis*, *S pneumoniae*, and *H influenzae*.

Haemophilus influenzae type b is a small bacterium that can colonize the respiratory tract of humans. Individuals colonized with *H influenzae* may be asymptomatic, and most isolates of this bacterium are not pathogenic. Hib is the most virulent form, and it is encapsulated, which enables it to evade destruction by phagocytic cells. This pathogen spreads from one individual to another via airborne droplets or direct contact with contaminated secretions. *H influenzae* is most commonly found in the nasopharynx of healthy asymptomatic children ages 2 to 5 years. When *H influenzae* meningitis is encountered in the adult population, the patient often has a predisposing medical condition such as paranasal sinusitis, otitis media, alcoholism, head trauma, asplenia, or immunocompromised states. For this reason, the *H influenzae* vaccine is recommended for both children and susceptible adults.

Neisseria meningitidis can cause meningitis, though this disease is rare in the United States. This bacterium is pathogenic only in humans and is spread during prolonged close contact with infected people through direct contact with respiratory secretions. Thus, outbreaks of this type of meningitis typically occur in prisons, military barracks, and college dormitories. The bacterium can be isolated from 10% to 30% of healthy adults, but the disease is not common. When a case of *N meningitidis* infection is reported, all close contacts of the infected individual are treated prophylactically with a short course of antibiotics.

The *N meningitidis* pathogen enters the body through the epithelial surfaces of the nasopharynx. If the bacteria reach the bloodstream, they can cause gram-negative sepsis, extensive tissue damage, and death. The onset of symptoms is abrupt (ie, fever, headache, and other systemic symptoms). Patients with *N meningitidis* meningitis often develop a characteristic rash that starts as petechial lesions (1- to 2-mm purple hemorrhagic spots that do not blanch with pressure) and advances to palpable purpura (larger areas of bleeding under the skin) within a short time. Caregivers should maintain a high index of suspicion, because this rash is considered a classic presentation. The mortality rate for untreated *N meningitidis* meningitis is nearly 100%.

Streptococcus pneumoniae is the most common cause of community-acquired bacterial meningitis. This bacterium possesses several pathogenic properties that make infection with *S pneumoniae* a serious medical event. Its polysaccharide capsule prevents this organism from being opsonized and phagocytized. It is able to adhere to the surface of epithelial cells, which allows *S pneumoniae* to colonize these cells, and it produces toxins that directly inhibit the body's cell-mediated phagocytic activity.

In healthy people, *S pneumoniae* is commonly isolated from the nasopharynx. The rate of colonization is estimated to be as high as 70% in the winter and spring. Patients with chronic bronchitis are frequently colonized by this bacterium.

The development of *S pneumoniae* meningitis is often preceded by a mild upper respiratory tract infection. People at highest risk for contracting *S pneumoniae* infection include those with sickle cell anemia, chronic alcoholism, multiple myeloma, functional or anatomic asplenia, and general disability. The mortality rate of *S pneumoniae* meningitis in older adults and people who are immunocompromised is quite high, even when treatment is initiated promptly. Therefore, vaccination against *S pneumoniae* is strongly encouraged for at-risk populations and is now included in the routine childhood vaccination schedule.

Signs and Symptoms

Bacterial Meningitis
Classic triad of symptoms:
- Fever
- Nuchal rigidity
- Altered mental status

Possible other symptoms:
- Headache
- Photophobia
- Focal neural deficits
- Seizures

N meningitidis meningitis:
- Fever
- Headache
- Meningismus
- Petechial lesions (1- to 2-mm purple hemorrhagic spots that do not blanch with pressure), progressing to palpable purpura (larger areas of bleeding under the skin)

Differential Diagnosis

Bacterial Meningitis
- Viral meningitis
- Brain tumor
- Subarachnoid hemorrhage
- Herpes simplex encephalitis
- Febrile seizure
- Delirium tremens
- Hepatic encephalopathy
- Brain abscess

Viral Meningitis

Cases of viral meningitis are reported each year in the United States, although the specific number cannot be verified. Although all age groups are affected, this type of meningitis is more commonly seen in young adults. Viral meningitis can be acute, subacute, or relapsing. The peak incidence occurs in summer.

A variety of species can cause viral meningitis, including Coxsackie A and B viruses, echovirus, adenovirus, lymphocytic choriomeningitis virus, cytomegalovirus, poliovirus, and Epstein-Barr virus. Enteroviruses are the most common cause of aseptic meningitis; all enterovirus species are transmitted through the fecal-oral route. The meningitis will often originate from structures close to the brain, such as the middle ear, sinuses, or respiratory tract, which can be colonized by pathogenic species.

Viral meningitis presents with the same symptoms as bacterial meningitis and is also considered a serious medical condition; however, it typically resolves without intervention within 7 to 10 days. Because it is difficult to distinguish between bacterial

and viral meningitis at the onset of symptoms, all cases should be treated as bacterial in origin until this possibility has been ruled out.

Generally, when providing care for a patient suspected of having viral meningitis, careful handwashing should be employed to prevent the spread of the disease.

Respiratory Syncytial Virus

Respiratory syncytial virus (RSV) causes seasonal outbreaks of acute respiratory infections. Its clinical manifestations depend on the age and health of the affected individual. RSV season in the United States occurs in the winter months, with the peak incidence of this disease occurring in January and February.

Each year in the United States, RSV infections account for 58,000 hospitalizations in children younger than 5 years. In infants 1 year or younger, the virus usually causes a lower respiratory tract infection, either bronchiolitis or pneumonia. Apnea is a risk for 20% of all infants hospitalized with the infection and may put the child at risk for sudden death.

People older than 1 year may also be infected with RSV. In fact, most children test positive for RSV by the time they reach the age of 2 years. Older children and adults may present with a mild ILI. Persons at risk for severe infections or complications from infections include those with a history of prematurity and those who are immunocompromised. RSV detected in adults usually does not cause long-term pulmonary dysfunction, but infection does result in 177,000 hospitalizations each year in older adults.

Currently, no vaccine exists to prevent respiratory tract infections caused by RSV. A monoclonal antibody called palivizumab does confer passive immunity to recipients; it can be used prophylactically in premature infants at risk for severe infections.

Transmission is known to occur via respiratory droplets and via direct contact with hands that have been contaminated with mucus from the nose or mouth of an infected individual. To avoid contracting this disease, CCTPs should employ droplet and contact precautions when transporting patients with a suspected or a confirmed case of RSV. Diagnosis is made by testing the respiratory secretions of the infected individual using polymerase chain reaction technology.

Signs and Symptoms

Respiratory Syncytial Virus

- Runny nose
- Congestion
- Cough
- Sore throat
- Headache
- Malaise
- In infants and young children: listlessness, decreased appetite, fever, wheezing, tachypnea, and cyanosis

Differential Diagnosis

Respiratory Syncytial Virus

- Asthma
- Bronchiolitis/bronchitis
- Pneumonia
- Foreign body aspiration
- Pertussis

Transport Management

Respiratory Syncytial Virus

- Provide supportive care.
- Administer fluids.
- Administer oxygen.
- Administer a nebulized bronchodilator for wheezing, if indicated by protocols.
- Monitor mechanical ventilator, if applicable.

Skin and Soft-Tissue Infections

Cellulitis and abscess are common skin and soft-tissue infections. Cellulitis presents as an area of skin with indistinct borders and is characterized by erythema, edema, and warmth (**FIGURE 20-4**). It is most commonly seen in middle-aged and older adults. Erysipelas, a specific type of cellulitis, is more common in young children and older adults (**FIGURE 20-5**). A skin abscess is a collection of pus within the dermis or subcutaneous space. These conditions are commonly misdiagnosed, and providers should carefully consider possible alternative diagnoses.

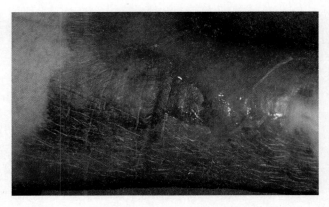

FIGURE 20-4 Cellulitis presents as an area of skin with indistinct borders and is characterized by erythema, edema, and warmth.
© Biophoto Associates/Science Source.

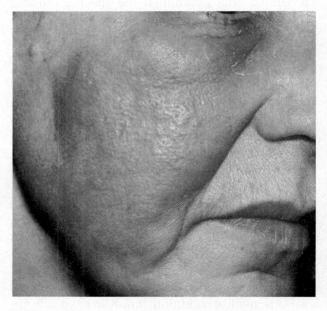

FIGURE 20-5 Erysipelas lesions are raised above the level of surrounding skin, and there is a clear line of demarcation between involved and uninvolved tissue.
© BSIP/Universal Images Group/Getty Images.

Risk factors for cellulitis and skin abscess include the following:

- Traumatic disruption of the skin barrier (eg, penetrating wound, pressure ulcer, insect bite, injection drug use)
- Skin inflammation (eg, eczema, radiation therapy, psoriasis)
- Edema caused by impaired lymphatic drainage
- Edema caused by venous insufficiency
- Obesity
- Immunosuppression

- Skin breaks between the toes (toe web intertrigo)
- Preexisting skin infection (eg, tinea pedis, impetigo, varicella)
- Close contact with someone infected with or carrying methicillin-resistant *S aureus* (MRSA)

The most common cause of cellulitis is infection with beta-hemolytic streptococci. These bacteria are classified as group A, B, C, G, or F. The most common source of infection is group A *Streptococcus* or *S pyogenes*. *S aureus* (including methicillin-resistant strains), a less common cause, should also be considered. Most cases of erysipelas are caused by beta-hemolytic streptococci.

Necrotizing Fasciitis

First noted by Hippocrates, **necrotizing fasciitis** is a limb-threatening and life-threatening infection of the soft tissue that affects the subcutaneous tissues, fat, and fascia, but initially spares the skin and the muscle. Prompt diagnosis and treatment with antibiotics and complete surgical debridement are important to reduce the high mortality rate associated with this disease.

Two main types of necrotizing fasciitis are distinguished. Type I is polymicrobial, meaning that the infection results from a mixture of aerobic and anaerobic microorganisms. This type is commonly seen in postoperative patients with comorbid conditions such as diabetes and peripheral vascular disease. The microorganisms seen in type I necrotizing fasciitis may be a mixture of *S aureus*, *Streptococcus* species, *Enterococcus* species, *E coli*, *Peptostreptococcus* species, *Bacteroides* species, *Vibrio vulnificus*, and *Clostridium* species.

Type II is a monomicrobial infection caused by the group A streptococci (GAS) known as *Streptococcus pyogenes*. This infection was previously known as "streptococcal gangrene." Breaching of the skin barrier during surgery is thought to create the portal of entry for GAS infection.

Fournier gangrene is a specific type of necrotizing fasciitis that occurs in the skin and fat of the perineum, usually associated with genital, urinary, anal, or abdominal infections. It typically occurs in men older than 50 years and people with diabetes. In men, it creates an infected perineal site that initially spares the testes.

Initial symptoms of necrotizing fasciitis include warmth, erythema, or edema at the site, with no distinct borders. The initial site is often an extremity. Occasionally fever or hypotension will begin early. As symptoms progress, the patient may develop bullae, crepitus, and restricted limb movement (secondary to pain). As with compartment syndrome, the pain is disproportionate to the visible injury. Fever, tachycardia, and hypotension may evolve as the infection worsens. Gas, as evidenced by crepitus on exam, may develop under the skin. Often this gas can be detected on radiographic imaging as air along the fascial planes. Vomiting, fatigue, and nerve involvement are later signs. Visible skin necrosis is a very late sign; fat and fascia are much more involved than the skin, such that exploratory surgery is often required to make the diagnosis.

When necrotizing fasciitis is recognized in the field, the area should be covered with sterile gauze. Aggressive fluid replacement should also be initiated. Treatment using antibiotics alone, without surgical intervention, is associated with a nearly 100% mortality rate. Time is of the essence when dealing with a patient with necrotizing fasciitis. Any delay in surgical diagnosis and treatment may increase mortality and cause extension of the disease. Sometimes hyperbaric oxygen therapy, nutritional support, skin grafting, or amputation is used in the treatment of patients with necrotizing fasciitis.

Signs and Symptoms

Necrotizing Fasciitis

- Unexplained pain that increases over time and is out of proportion to the exam
- Mild erythema that develops into a dark red to purple color within 24 to 48 hours
- Blisters or bullae
- Fever or tachycardia
- Hypotension
- Gas, as evidenced by crepitus on exam

Differential Diagnosis

Necrotizing Fasciitis

- Cellulitis
- Gas gangrene
- Toxic shock syndrome

Necrotizing Fasciitis
- Provide supportive care.
- Apply sterile gauze over the site.
- Provide aggressive fluid replacement.
- Continue IV administration of antibiotics that have been started by the sending facility.
- Perform cardiac monitoring.
- Monitor urine output to the indwelling catheter, if one has been placed at the sending facility.
- Provide rapid transport (to be followed by surgical intervention).

CCTPs may be called on to transport patients to facilities that have the resources needed to care for these patients. In any case of suspected or known necrotizing fasciitis, contact precautions must be maintained at all times, and all equipment must be thoroughly disinfected after the transport is complete.

Epiglottitis

Epiglottitis is caused by an infected and inflamed epiglottis, aryepiglottic folds, and/or surrounding tissues. In the past, most cases were caused by infection with Hib. Since the introduction of the Hib vaccine in 1991 in the United States, however, the epidemiology of this disease and others caused by Hib has been changing. The incidence of epiglottitis has been drastically reduced in vaccinated children, but because of its severity and rapid progression to airway obstruction and continued infection patterns in adults, it remains important for health care providers to be familiar with this disease's clinical presentation.

Epiglottitis can occur at any age, although most cases in the past occurred in children ages 1 to 5 years. The causative agent and median age at presentation have now shifted to adult forms of the disease as the population continues to be immunized against Hib. Today, causes of epiglottitis may include *Haemophilus parainfluenzae*, *S pneumoniae*, *S aureus*, and beta-hemolytic *S pyogenes*. Hib epiglottitis still may occur, but is most likely to affect children who are incompletely immunized or those who are noncompliant with vaccinations. There is no predominant bacterial species found in adults with epiglottitis.

An abrupt onset of symptoms is the common theme in the presentation of epiglottitis. Symptoms include high fever, severe sore throat, dysphasia, and dysphonia. Often, a child will start drooling as a result of painful or difficult swallowing. The child's speech or voice may be altered so that it is muffled, and has been described classically as the "hot potato voice." As the symptoms progress, the child may assume a distinctive posture: While sitting, the arms are outstretched to support the forward-leaning trunk, and the chin is thrust forward to maximize the diameter of the hypopharynx. Unlike in croup, stridor is not a predominant sign and increased respiratory effort with use of accessory muscles may not be present; thus, the severity of the disease may be underestimated. The symptoms of epiglottitis can rapidly progress to airway obstruction, hypoxia, and cardiopulmonary arrest.

The diagnosis of epiglottitis can be made by visualization of a fiery-red and edematous epiglottis. The optimal method of visualization is under controlled conditions via direct laryngoscopy by an otolaryngologist. Radiographs are not usually necessary to make the diagnosis of epiglottitis; however, if direct visualization cannot be achieved and doubt remains, a lateral soft-tissue neck radiograph may aid in diagnosis. If a radiograph is obtained, the patient should not go to the radiology department unaccompanied. An advanced airway cart should always be readily available, and a person trained in advanced airway management should accompany the patient if the patient leaves the emergency department prior to placement of a secure airway.

Epiglottitis is a potentially life-threatening infection; as such, patients with epiglottitis must be promptly treated with empirical antibiotics. The antibiotic regimen should be selected to provide coverage for streptococci, pneumococci, staphylococci, and Hib.

CCTPs must maintain a high level of suspicion for epiglottitis in any patient who presents with the abrupt onset of fever, sore throat, muffled voice, and drooling. Agitation of the patient should be minimized, as it may lead to worsening of the patient's condition and hasten the progression to complete airway obstruction. Interactions with children should be conducted in a manner that minimizes their anxiety, because agitation only makes the situation worse.

If airway intervention is necessary in the prehospital environment, it should be performed by the most experienced team member, as orotracheal intubation can be difficult secondary to edema and anatomic distortion. Patients with epiglottitis often require advanced airway management. Providing rapid transport to the nearest, most appropriate level of care/facility is a must.

Signs and Symptoms

Epiglottitis

- High fever
- Severe sore throat
- Dysphasia
- Dysphonia
- Drooling as a result of painful or difficult swallowing
- Alteration of speech or voice so that it is muffled—"hot potato voice"
- Sitting with the arms outstretched to support the forward-leaning trunk, with the chin thrust forward to maximize the diameter of the hypopharynx

Differential Diagnosis

Epiglottitis

- Anaphylaxis
- Foreign body aspiration
- Laryngotracheobronchitis
- Mononucleosis
- Pertussis
- Pharyngitis
- Pneumonia
- Caustic ingestion

Transport Management

Epiglottitis

- Support the airway.
- Continue IV administration of antibiotics if they have been started by the sending facility.
- Note: When epiglottitis is strongly suspected, transfer of a patient without an artificial airway (endotracheal tube or tracheostomy) is unsafe.

Tuberculosis

Tuberculosis (TB) is caused by the acid-fast bacterium called *Mycobacterium tuberculosis*. The genus *Mycobacterium* includes other ominous organisms such as the pathogen that causes leprosy (*Mycobacterium leprae*) and *Mycobacterium avium-intracellulare* complex (MAC), which causes a tuberculosis-like pneumonia usually seen only in immunocompromised patients such as those with advanced HIV/AIDS. MAC is particularly insidious because these organisms are very resistant to antibiotics and are becoming even more resistant at an alarming rate.

Tuberculosis causes more deaths globally than any other single microbial agent, killing 1.4 million people in 2019. The risk of contracting this highly infectious disease is increased in people who live in poor housing conditions, those who are usually malnourished, and those who are coinfected with HIV. Owing to better recognition of TB and appropriate treatments for this disease, the United States saw only 8,916 cases in 2019, roughly one-tenth the yearly total seen in the early 1950s. The case rate of TB continues to steadily decrease in the United States as a result of education and quick actions taken to control the spread of the disease.

Pathophysiology

The *M tuberculosis* bacterium is transmitted via respiratory droplets from the cough of an infected person, which then contact the respiratory epithelium of a susceptible person. The first site of infection is the lungs. The bacterium, being an obligate aerobe, has a propensity to set up infection in the upper lobes of the lungs because that tissue is highly oxygenated. TB can also spread to the kidneys or spine.

After a person recovers from a primary infection, the immune system resists secondary infection and reactivation through cell-mediated immunity. (Reactivation of a previously contained infection may occur in an immunocompromised or debilitated patient.) Antibodies to tuberculin are formed, and their existence is exploited in tuberculin skin testing (TST) with the purified protein derivative (PPD). In TST, the tuberculin antigen is injected into the skin; if positive, it indicates a previous infection, but does not necessarily indicate active disease. If the reaction is large enough (more than 15 mm in diameter in healthy patients not from a country highly endemic for TB), then the person is considered to be actively infected and should receive treatment. As with some other infectious diseases, there is a delay between the primary infection and a positive PPD test result: It takes approximately 6 weeks for the TB skin test to be reactive. The induration seen following injection of PPD is a type IV delayed hypersensitivity reaction, used for diagnostic advantage in TST. Interferon-gamma release assays (IGRAs) can help detect *M tuberculosis* infection but do not differentiate latent tuberculosis infection from tuberculosis disease.

A vaccine is available for the prevention of TB. The bacillus Calmette-Guérin (BCG) vaccine is made from a related bacterium, *Mycobacterium bovis*, which usually infects bovines (cows). The BCG vaccine is not used in the United States because it is effective only 70% of the time, but is used in countries highly endemic for TB. Inoculation with the BCG vaccine causes a person to have a weakly positive PPD test result.

Diagnosis and Management

Most people infected with *M tuberculosis* are asymptomatic. The immune status of the patient, in large part, determines the clinical symptoms of an infection with this bacterium. Persons with active pulmonary TB typically have five symptoms: cough, fever, weight loss, night sweats, and fatigue.

Infection with *M tuberculosis* can be difficult to diagnose because it is a slow-growing bacterium, taking weeks to culture. Because treatment must begin as soon as possible, diagnosis is based on clinical signs and confirmed via positive acid-fast staining of three sputum samples from patients suspected of being infected **FIGURE 20-6**.

The emergence of drug-resistant strains of TB has precipitated the use of a multidrug regimen for curing patients with this disease. The individual drugs used may vary slightly according to known sensitivities, but the mainstay of therapy is isoniazid. The drugs are typically given for many months.

Multidrug-resistant tuberculosis (MDR-TB) is TB that is resistant to at least two of the standard anti-TB medications, isoniazid and rifampin. Extensively drug-resistant TB (XDR-TB) is TB that is resistant to isoniazid, rifampin, any fluoroquinolone, and at least one second-line IV drug. Because XDR-TB is resistant to many first- and second-line drugs, treatment options are limited for patients

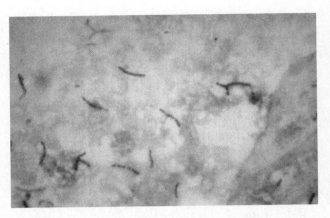

FIGURE 20-6 Acid-fast staining technique to diagnose tuberculosis.
Courtesy of Dr. George P. Kubica/CDC.

with this form of the disease. Both MDR-TB and XDR-TB are contracted via the same mechanism as TB—that is, through the inhalation of infected droplets from a person who is already infected when that person coughs, sneezes, or spits into the environment. These infected droplets can exist in the air for several hours, and anyone who breathes in these particles is at risk for contracting the disease.

When transporting a patient with a history of fever, weight loss, and night sweats, and anyone with a cough, take proper precautions for airborne pathogens by placing a mask on the patient (if tolerated); the CCTP should also wear an N95 mask. CCTPs should comply with yearly TST or IGRA testing to determine their personal exposure history. If care was provided for a patient known to have TB and exposure was a possibility, providers should undergo PPD or IGRA testing 6 weeks after exposure to assess their own status. If the test result is negative, the CCTP can resume routine TB screening tests. If the TB screening test result is positive, a chest radiograph will be required to determine whether signs of active or previous TB infection exist.

Signs and Symptoms

Tuberculosis

- Cough
- Fever
- Weight loss
- Night sweats
- Fatigue

Pneumonia

Pneumonia is a leading cause of death in the United States, with approximately 50,000 people dying from this cause in 2017. Most patients affected with pneumonia are adults.

Pneumonia is an infection of the lung parenchyma that is caused by bacterial, viral, or fungal agents. Physicians normally classify pneumonia as either community acquired or nosocomial (contracted in a medical facility) because the differential acquisition of pneumonia influences the most likely infecting agent, treatment, and prognosis. The mortality rate for community-acquired pneumonia ranges from 5% to 14%, whereas the mortality rate for nosocomial pneumonia is as high as 40%.

Pneumonia is generally diagnosed in a patient presenting with symptoms of sudden-onset fever, chest pain, or dyspnea, and leukocytosis. Patients may also have a cough, either dry or productive, depending on the causative agent. Plain chest radiographs, posteroanterior and lateral, are the gold standard for diagnosing a consolidated or infiltrative lesion.

Community-Acquired Pneumonia

The most common pathogen in all age groups of patients with community-acquired pneumonia is *S pneumoniae*. This bacterium gains entry to the respiratory tract following aspiration into the lungs from previously colonized nasopharyngeal mucosa. Older adult patients and those with other comorbidities are at a higher risk for succumbing to pneumonia infections. A history of tobacco use, COPD, immunosuppression, and obesity are independent risk factors for developing community-acquired pneumonia.

Many different bacterial species cause pneumonia, with the most common being *S pneumoniae*, *H influenzae*, *S aureus*, *Chlamydia pneumoniae*, and *Legionella pneumoniae*. Symptoms of bacterial pneumonias include high fever, productive cough, and pleuritic chest pain.

Mycoplasma pneumoniae and viruses cause atypical pneumonias. These infections are considered atypical because patients usually present with a slower onset of symptoms, low-grade fever, and a dry cough. *Mycoplasma* pneumonia is often misdiagnosed as viral because of its less severe presentation. The clinical lung exam result may be normal, but the chest radiograph will demonstrate infiltrates. *Mycoplasma* pneumonias are often preceded by a flulike prodrome consisting of headache, malaise, and fever.

Viral pneumonia is more common in infants and young children. RSV and parainfluenza virus are the most common causes of viral pneumonia in pediatric patients. The incidence of these viral infections peaks in the fall and winter. Viral pneumonia is often preceded by an upper respiratory tract infection. As with atypical pneumonias, its onset can be slower than the onset of bacterial pneumonia.

Nosocomial Pneumonia

Hospitalized patients, particularly older adults, are susceptible to nosocomial pneumonias. The definition of nosocomial or hospital-acquired pneumonia (HAP) is a pneumonia that occurs in a hospitalized patient at least 48 hours after admission. (In other words, this type of pneumonia was not apparent at the time of admission.) Among all nosocomial infections, HAP is the leading cause of death, with a mortality rate as high as 50%. Ventilator-associated pneumonia (VAP) is a type of HAP that occurs in ventilated patients and that appears more than

48 hours after endotracheal intubation. **Health care–associated pneumonia (HCAP)** is a pneumonia that occurs in nonhospitalized patients who have contact with health care facilities or personnel, such as residents of long-term health care facilities, those undergoing hemodialysis, and those who have had a recent admission to an acute care facility.

HAP, VAP, and HCAP can be caused by a number of pathogenic bacteria and can be polymicrobial in origin. Commonly implicated pathogens include *E coli*, *Klebsiella pneumoniae*, *Enterobacter*, *Pseudomonas*, *S aureus*, and *Streptococcus*. Nosocomial bacterial pneumonias secondary to viral or fungal infection are much less common except in patients with severe immunosuppression.

Pneumocystis jirovecii (previously *P carinii*) pneumonia (PCP) is a fungal infection that is seen in patients with immunosuppression, such as those taking immunosuppressive therapy for solid-organ transplantation and those infected with HIV. It is included in the list of AIDS-defining illnesses. In fact, a patient whose CD4 cell count is less than 200 cells/μL is placed on trimethoprim-sulfamethoxazole prophylactically to prevent the development of PCP. The classic radiographic findings for PCP are bilateral interstitial infiltrates.

Management

As with all patients who have respiratory illnesses, CCTPs should use standard precautions when caring for patients suspected of having pneumonia and those diagnosed as having pneumonia. If a patient is actively coughing, place a mask on the patient (if tolerated) and on yourself, wear gloves, and use good handwashing technique between transports. Thoroughly clean and decontaminate your equipment, including the transport vehicle, before undertaking further transports.

Signs and Symptoms

Pneumonia
- Sudden-onset fever
- Chest pain
- Dyspnea
- Leukocytosis
- Cough, either dry or productive

Differential Diagnosis

Pneumonia
- Asthma
- Bronchiectasis
- COPD
- Lung cancer
- Pulmonary edema
- Pulmonary emboli

Transport Management

Pneumonia
- Provide supportive care.
- Continue administration of IV antibiotics or other medications if they have been started by the sending facility.

Fungal Diseases

Over the past 20 years, the incidence of serious fungal infections has been increasing. These infections are not particularly contagious to healthy people, but their presence in patients is an indication of serious immunosuppression. It is especially important to decontaminate equipment, such as laryngoscopes and suction equipment, after transporting patients with oral candidiasis (thrush) or patients infected with *P jirovecii*.

Influenza

Influenza virus causes an acute upper respiratory illness lasting between 7 and 14 days depending on the severity of symptoms. The causative agent is an orthomyxovirus that has three variants (A, B, and C).

Influenza has an incubation period of about 1 to 3 days and is spread by droplet or fomite transmission. Complications in older adults and the very young can include the development of primary or secondary pneumonia.

An influenza epidemic may potentially cause illness in 10% to 20% of the population. Influenza viruses are responsible for as many as 36,000 deaths and more than 100,000 hospitalizations per year **TABLE 20-3**.

TABLE 20-3 Influenza Landmarks in Humans

Year	Colloquial Name (Subtype)	Source	Impact
Pandemics			
1918	Spanish flu (H1N1 viruses such as swine flu)	Possible emergence from swine or an avian host of a mutated H1N1 virus	Pandemic with more than 50 million deaths globally
1957	Asian flu (H2N2)	Possible mixed infection of an animal with human H1N1 and avian H2N2 virus strains in Asia	Pandemic; H1N1 virus disappeared
1968	Hong Kong flu (H3N2)	High probability of mixed infection of an animal with human H2N2 and avian H3Nx virus strains in Asia	Pandemic; H2N2 virus disappeared
1977	Russian flu (H1N1)	Source unknown but virus is almost identical to human epidemic strains from 1950; reappearance detected at almost the same time in China and Siberia	Benign pandemic, primarily involving people born after the 1950s; H1N1 virus has cocirculated with H3N2 virus in humans since 1977
Incidents With Limited Spread			
1976	Swine flu (H1N1)	United States/New Jersey; virus enzootic in US swine herds since at least 1930	Localized outbreak in military training camp, with one death
1986	(H1N1)	The Netherlands; swine virus derived from avian source	One adult with severe pneumonia
1988	Swine flu (H1N1)	United States/Wisconsin; swine virus	Pregnant woman died after exposure to a sick pig
1993	(H3N2)	The Netherlands; swine reassortant between old human H3N2 (1973/1975-like) and avian H1N1	Two children with mild disease; fathers suspected of transmitting the virus to the children after being infected by pigs
1995	(H7N7)	United Kingdom; duck virus	One adult with conjunctivitis
1997	Avian flu (H5N1)	Hong Kong; poultry virus	Outbreak in 2003 resulted in 774 deaths worldwide
2009	Novel H1N1	Mexico	From April 12, 2009, to April 10, 2010, approximately 60.8 million cases, 274,304 hospitalizations, and 12,469 deaths

Modified from H1N1 flu. Centers for Disease Control and Prevention website. https://www.cdc.gov/h1n1flu/estimates_2009_h1n1.htm. Updated June 24, 2014. Accessed May 28, 2021; Taubenberger JK, Morens DM. The pathology of influenza virus infections. *Annu Rev Pathol.* 2008;3:499-522; Severe acute respiratory syndrome (SARS): SARS basic fact sheet. Centers for Disease Control and Prevention website. https://www.cdc.gov/sars/about/fs-sars.html. Accessed April 23, 2021.

Evolution of New Influenza Strains

Influenza type A is divided into subgroups based on the presence of two surface proteins (also called envelope spikes): hemagglutinin and neuraminidase. Unlike influenza B and C, this form of influenza is subject to antigenic drift, which is caused by small genetic changes in the virus. This process alters the virus just enough that antibodies generated during previous infections no longer recognize the viral epitope or surface protein and, therefore, do not protect the body from the symptoms of a new infection. Influenza A is also subject to more drastic changes called antigenic shift, in which the protein structure of one or both of the spike proteins changes. Antigenic shift typically occurs only once in several years, whereas antigenic drift occurs more frequently. The phenomenon of antigenic drift is what precipitates the need for yearly preparation of influenza vaccine and, therefore, annual immunization.

The influenza virus can infect species of animals other than humans. In fact, waterfowl are the natural reservoir for the influenza A virus. Influenza A is an avian virus that has "jumped species" to infect humans and other mammals. Humans, pigs, ducks, chickens, and other animals are susceptible to influenza A. This variability of hosts causes mutations to occur in the virus that facilitate antigenic drift. When animals are infected with swine, human, and avian influenza simultaneously, mixing of the genes that encode the neuraminidase and hemagglutinin proteins can occur. Many different variations of these proteins are possible because there are 9 known variations of neuraminidase and 16 known variations of hemagglutinin.

Variations in influenza A are closely monitored by WHO, the CDC in the United States, and other global health associations. The subtypes of influenza A are categorized and tracked each year. The predominant subtypes of influenza A circulating throughout the world in 2014–2015 were H3N2 (a designation indicating that the hemagglutinin is type 3 and the neuraminidase is type 2) and H1N1. The highly pathogenic forms of avian influenza are H5 and H7. When influenza undergoes a major antigenic drift or a novel combination of hemagglutinin and neuraminidase emerges (antigenic shift), people have little or no antigenic protection based on their prior infections. Pandemics of influenza may then break out and spread quickly, causing major illness around the world.

Historically, new strains of influenza A virus have arisen in Asia, likely because of socioeconomic and geographic factors there. It is common for farmers in southeast China to live in close proximity with pigs and ducks. This sets up a perfect environment for the avian and human strains to recombine in pigs, and then jump species back into humans with an antigenic shift. Each year, WHO and the CDC collect samples from Asia to use as sentinel viruses when preparing the influenza vaccine subsequently offered in the United States and other countries.

Management

Treatment for influenza is mostly supportive. When an individual is diagnosed within the first day of symptoms, however, treatment with an antiviral medication may reduce the severity and duration of symptoms.

CCTPs should be aware of the signs and symptoms of influenza infection and should use standard and respiratory precautions to avoid infection and spread of infection.

Signs and Symptoms

Influenza
- High fever
- Runny nose or congestion
- Cough
- Sore throat
- Muscle aches
- Fatigue
- Headache
- Nausea, vomiting, or diarrhea

Differential Diagnosis

Influenza
- Bacterial infection
- Fungal infection
- Parasitic infection
- Viral infection
- Typhoid

Transport Management

Influenza
- Provide supportive care.

Herpesviruses

The herpesvirus family is a group of double-stranded DNA viruses, all of which share the characteristic of being surrounded by a lipoprotein envelope. Herpesviruses are noted for their ability to cause latent infections when the acute viral syndrome is followed by a symptom-free period during which the virus is quiescent (inactive). Depending on the species, reactivation of the virus can occur when the patient is immunosuppressed or through inciting agents.

Six pathogenic herpesviruses cause significant disease in humans:

- Herpes simplex types 1 and 2
- Varicella zoster virus
- Cytomegalovirus
- Epstein-Barr virus
- Human herpesvirus 8

Both Epstein-Barr virus and human herpesvirus 8 are associated with the development of cancer, Burkitt lymphoma, and Kaposi sarcoma.

Herpes simplex virus type 1 (HSV-1) and type 2 (HSV-2) cause lesions, but the lesions differ in their location. HSV-1 is transmitted in saliva, whereas HSV-2 is transmitted via sexual contact. Therefore, it follows that HSV-1 causes lesions above the waist, whereas HSV-2 causes lesions below the waist. However, either virus can be isolated from either location after oral-genital contact.

HSV-1 causes an acute gingivostomatitis in children and recurrent *herpes labialis* in adolescents or adults, commonly known as cold sores. It can also cause keratoconjunctivitis and encephalitis in immunocompromised hosts. HSV-2 commonly causes genital herpes.

HSV-1 and HSV-2 can cause infection of the fingers with recurring painful blisters, a condition called herpetic whitlow (**FIGURE 20-7**). This condition is seen commonly in health care professionals such as respiratory therapists and dentists following a break in barrier protections (eg, gloves). It can also develop with exposure to genital secretions.

Viral Hepatitis

Hepatitis is the inflammation of the liver. This disease can be caused by exposure to infectious agents (usually viral), toxins (eg, alcohol), or drugs (eg, acetaminophen). The course and severity of the illness range from acute to chronic and from mild to life threatening, respectively. Signs and symptoms of liver disease can range from subclinical symptoms and nonspecific malaise to jaundice, hepatomegaly, bleeding dyscrasias, altered mental status, and multiple organ failure. Damage to the liver can be caused by direct injury to the hepatocytes caused by the agent, or it may result indirectly from an inflammatory response or an autoimmune attack.

There are six known hepatotropic viruses (hepatitis A, B, C, D, E, and G), each of which has its own characteristic causative agent, mode of transmission, incubation period, associated risk factors, and sequelae. Viral hepatitis is first classified by the duration of the illness as either acute or chronic. Acute viral hepatitis is defined as the presence of signs or symptoms of liver inflammation for less than 6 months duration, whereas chronic viral hepatitis is defined as the presence of persistent liver inflammation for 6 months or longer. Liver inflammation can also be described by histologic and pathologic findings, which allows for the grading and staging of liver disease. The grade of liver disease describes the severity of the inflammatory process and cell necrosis, and the stage of liver disease describes the severity of the scarring of the liver tissue.

Elevation of liver enzyme levels in the serum is considered evidence of damage to the liver, and the pattern of their elevation provides insight into the nature and probable cause of the insult. An acute viral hepatitis will have an acute onset and be accompanied by marked elevations in aspartate aminotransferase (AST) and alanine aminotransferase (ALT); by comparison, a chronic viral hepatitis produces more moderate and persistent elevations in these same enzymes. The ratio of serum AST to ALT is commonly greater than 2 in patients with liver disease caused by alcohol abuse, whereas the ratio is characteristically less than 1 in patients with liver disease caused by viral agents.

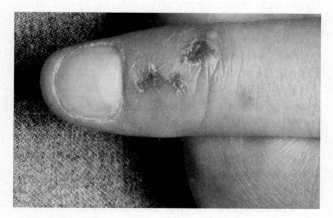

FIGURE 20-7 Herpetic whitlow can produce painful blisters on the finger.

Alkaline phosphatase (AP) is an enzyme that is present in many different tissues within the body, such as the bones, intestine, kidney, liver, and placenta. When a rise in AP levels is accompanied by a rise in gamma-glutamyl transferase (GGT) levels, this condition is assumed to have a hepatic origin. Elevations in levels of AP and GGT are seen with damage to the bile canaliculi—the cells that line the intrahepatic bile ducts. Such damage can occur acutely when bile ducts are blocked by an obstructive process, such as an impacted gallstone, or it can develop more slowly from a chronic process.

Chronic viral hepatitis may produce swelling within the liver that results in compression of the pericanalicular cells, leading to a marked rise in the so-called cholestatic enzyme levels, with the rise in the levels of hepatocellular enzymes being more moderate. The elevation of GGT and AP levels that results from a viral process then occurs later in the course of the disease, and the elevation is more moderate.

Signs and Symptoms

Hepatitis
- Nonspecific malaise
- Jaundice
- Abdominal pain
- Loss of appetite
- Intermittent nausea and diarrhea
- Scleral icterus
- Hepatomegaly
- Bleeding dyscrasias
- Altered mental status
- Multiple organ failure

Differential Diagnosis

Hepatitis
- Alpha-1 antitrypsin deficiency
- Biliary obstruction
- Drug-induced liver disease
- Sclerosing cholangitis
- Wilson disease

Transport Management

Hepatitis
- Provide supportive care.

Hepatitis A

Hepatitis A virus (HAV), previously known as infectious hepatitis, is a positive single-stranded RNA virus of the Picornaviridae family. Sexual and parenteral transmission of HAV is possible; however, because the period of viremia is brief, fecal-oral transmission is more common. Large-scale outbreaks can occur, usually as the result of contaminated food or drinking water.

Incidence of HAV cases decreased by more than 95% from 1995 to 2011, but since 2016 there has been a dramatic increase in incidence due to person-to-person outbreaks. In 2018, 12,474 cases were reported in the United States, though the actual number of cases was probably twice as high; many HAV infections are asymptomatic and likely go unreported. Vaccination of all children 12 to 23 months of age remains crucial to preventing the spread of infection.

The clinical features of HAV include jaundice, fatigue, abdominal pain, loss of appetite, and intermittent nausea and diarrhea.

People at highest risk of HAV infection are household/sexual contacts of already-infected people, international travelers, and people living in American Indian reservations, Alaskan Native villages, and other regions with endemic HAV. During localized outbreaks, people at greatest risk include children who attend day-care centers and such centers' employees, men who have sex with men, and IV drug abusers.

The incubation period for HAV infection ranges from 2 to 6 weeks. The period of greatest infectivity is the last 2 weeks of incubation, just before the onset of clinical symptoms. Nevertheless, the infected individual remains infectious by shedding virus in the feces for 2 to 3 weeks after the onset of clinical symptoms.

The diagnosis of HAV is made by detection of anti-HAV IgM antibody. Anti-HAV IgG antibody is detected in the blood after exposure and recovery or immunization, which provides lifelong immunity.

HAV infection can be prevented by active immunization with the HAV vaccine or by passive immunization with immune globulin administered before or after a known exposure. The vaccine is highly effective and is recommended for children starting at age 1 year and for people at high risk of HAV infection, such as those planning to travel abroad, people living in HAV-endemic areas, and children and caregivers at day-care centers. The prevention of infection can also be accomplished by improving sanitation and by employing good personal hygiene and handwashing.

Hepatitis B

Hepatitis B virus (HBV) is a double-stranded DNA virus of the Hepadnaviridae family. It is transmitted through parenteral routes (non-oral transmission) and has an incubation period of 1 to 6 months. Transmission can occur by sharing needles, having sex with an infected person, or accidental medical exposures, such as needlesticks, blood spray, or touching bloody items with unprotected hands. Although blood is the most effective fluid of transmission, the virus lives in all human body fluids and is present in semen, saliva, urine, and breast milk.

In the United States, 3,322 acute HBV infections were reported in 2018. The actual case number, accounting for underreporting, was likely closer to 21,600. Persons at highest risk for contracting HBV include people who participate in high-risk behaviors; live in or travel to disease-endemic areas such as parts of Greenland, northern Canada, southeast Asia, China, and all of Africa; and those exposed to infected body fluids through their lifestyles or occupations. They include IV drug users, sexually active heterosexuals, men who have sex with men, people of low socioeconomic status, children of immigrants from disease-endemic areas, infants born to infected mothers, and patients receiving hemodialysis. In addition, because health care providers routinely come into contact with patients who are infected with HBV, they are considered an at-risk group for viral infection and should receive the HBV vaccine series, with immunity subsequently confirmed by titer.

The clinical features of HBV are similar to those of HAV, including jaundice, scleral icterus, fatigue, abdominal pain, loss of appetite, and intermittent

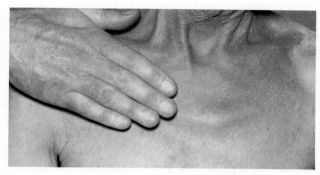

A

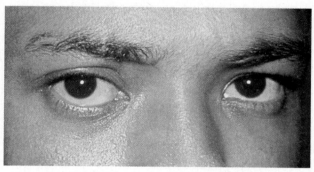

B

FIGURE 20-8 A. Jaundice. **B.** Scleral icterus.

A: © SPL/Science Source; **B:** Courtesy of Dr. Thomas F. Sellers, Emory University/CDC.

nausea or vomiting **FIGURE 20-8**. However, unlike HAV, HBV can induce other disease states in addition to causing acute infections. Specifically, it can cause acute hepatitis, fulminant hepatitis, and chronic hepatitis. Fulminant hepatitis is a severe inflammation of the liver that is accompanied by rapid destruction of the liver, leading to liver failure. The liver damage is accompanied by encephalopathy within 8 weeks of the onset of the symptoms. Coagulopathy, electrolyte disturbances, and cerebral edema are common in the setting of fulminant hepatitis, and death is likely if the patient does not receive an urgent liver transplant.

Chronic HBV can take several forms. A patient can be chronically infected, yet remain symptomless—that is, a chronic asymptomatic carrier. Such an individual never develops immunity to the virus, but harbors the virus and is infectious to others without actually sustaining liver damage. There were an estimated 257 million carriers of HBV worldwide in 2015. In contrast, chronic-persistent hepatitis is infection with HBV that "smolders": it is a persistent low-grade infection from which the patient eventually recovers. In chronic-active hepatitis, the patient has an active hepatitis state for more than 6 months, but neither recovers nor experiences a severe decline in liver function during this period. The identification and treatment of people with chronic infections and asymptomatic carriers is important for preventing the spread of the disease.

The key to understanding HBV serology, infectivity, and immunity begins with knowledge of the structure of this enveloped DNA virus. Immunity to HBV is acquired after exposure to the surface antigen through exposure either to the natural virus or to viral surface components in the vaccine. In either case, immunity is acquired through the development of antibodies to the surface antigen (anti-HBs). Antibodies to the core proteins (anti-HBc) do not confer immunity because, for an individual to ward off the virus, antibodies must attack the intact virion before the virus has a chance to replicate and before the individual is exposed to the core antigen. If the person has only anti-HBc, an immune response will not be mounted until the core protein is unmasked, which is too late to prevent infection. Therefore, antibodies to the core antigen (anti-HBc) are not protective and do not confer immunity; rather, their presence in the serum is considered a marker of previous exposure. Only anti-HBs will develop in response to the hepatitis B vaccine.

This information helps a provider determine how immunity to HBV was acquired. For example, if an individual has both anti-HBs and anti-HBc, then they have been exposed to the wild-type virus (because of the presence of anti-HBc) and are now immune (because of the presence of anti-HBs). The subtype of immunoglobulin yields information about the duration of infection. If the anti-HBc consists of IgM-type immunoglobulin, then the infection is acute or from a recent exposure. The presence of anti-HBc IgG indicates that the exposure occurred more than 3 months prior and the infection is resolving or is chronic.

Measures to prevent HBV infection include screening the blood supply and removing HBV-contaminated units and donors from the blood donation pool. The HBV vaccine is recommended for all infants at birth and for children up to age 18 years. It is also recommended that adults with a high risk of exposure be vaccinated. All pregnant women should be screened for the disease, and infants born to infected mothers should receive treatment with HBIG at birth, in addition to completing the vaccination series during the first 6 months of life. The vaccine is given in three separate doses at 0, 1, and 6 months. Passive immunity can be conferred by giving HBV immunoglobulin to people who experience known exposures within 24 hours of the exposure.

Primary hepatocellular carcinoma is a known complication of chronic HBV infection. The risk of its development is 200 times greater for those people with chronic HBV infection relative to those people who are not infected. In the United States, 20% of people with hepatocellular carcinoma are hepatitis B surface antigen–positive. Other potential complications of HBV infection include cirrhosis and fulminant liver failure (in fewer than 1% of cases).

Hepatitis C

Hepatitis C virus (HCV) is an enveloped RNA virus of the Flaviviridae family, which was originally known as non-A, non-B hepatitis. HCV causes both acute and nonacute or chronic hepatitis. The virus is transmitted parenterally through transfusion or IV drug use, through sexual contact with infected people, and from mother to infant; however, the vertical transmission rate of HCV is significantly lower than that of HBV. The incubation period of HCV varies from 2 weeks to 6 months.

In 2018, 3,621 cases of acute HCV infection were reported in the United States, although the actual case number, accounting for underreporting, was likely more than 50,000. In cases of acute hepatitis, the symptoms usually consist of nausea, vomiting, and jaundice. In most cases (more than 85% of infections), acute infection leads to chronic infection; spontaneous clearance of the virus is rare once chronic infection is established. Chronic infection typically begins with a long period in which the patient has no symptoms. The natural history of HCV has been difficult to determine because the disease is so often silent and goes undetected during the early stages, and the interval from infection to the development of cirrhosis can exceed 30 years. Most chronic infections lead to hepatitis and fibrotic liver disease. Cirrhosis develops in 5% to 25% of infected people. HCV cirrhosis is the major cause of liver transplantation.

The risk factors most strongly associated with HCV infection include IV drug use and a history of blood transfusion before 1990. Others at risk for HCV infection include patients receiving hemodialysis, health care workers, sexual contacts of infected people, hemophiliacs, and infants born to infected mothers.

Anti-HCV antibodies develop after exposure to the virus but do not confer immunity. Their presence in the blood is exploited by serologic assays that screen for contaminated blood products and seek to identify the carriers of infection. The antibody is detected through an enzyme-linked immunosorbent assay, a technique that has a sensitivity of 97%, but only a 25% positive predictive value in low-risk populations. Other screening techniques, such as a recombinant immunoblot assay, have been developed and are more useful for testing low-risk populations.

While cures for HCV disease caused by genotypes 1 and 4 have been recently developed, no vaccine is available to prevent infection. Patients with chronic active HCV infections are candidates for treatment. The goal of treatment is to prevent the development of cirrhosis and liver failure, but its success is limited and the side effects of treatment with interferons and antivirals can be difficult to tolerate. Most clinicians agree that treatment should be offered to those patients who have detectable levels of HCV RNA with persistently elevated liver transaminases and who demonstrate evidence of liver damage on biopsy.

Hepatitis D

Hepatitis delta virus (HDV) is another RNA virus that is transmitted parenterally, but it can replicate only with the aid of HBV. HDV is endemic in the Mediterranean region, the Middle East, and parts of South America. Outside of these areas, most HDV infections are a result of transfusion with tainted blood products or IV drug use.

Hepatitis E

Hepatitis E virus (HEV) is rare in the United States and is limited to travelers to endemic areas of India, Southeast Asia, Africa, and Mexico. The virus is transmitted via the fecal-oral route through the ingestion of contaminated food or water sources. Its transmission and course are similar to those of HAV, but HEV is associated with a high fatality rate in pregnant women.

Hepatitis G

Hepatitis G virus (HGV) is another RNA virus of the Flaviviridae family and is transmitted through parenteral routes. It has frequently been detected in patients with chronic liver disease, but a causative link has not yet been established.

Human Immunodeficiency Virus

Human immunodeficiency virus causes HIV disease, which in turn can lead to AIDS.

Epidemiology

The first reported case of AIDS occurred in 1981 in Los Angeles. Although the disease was first encountered in homosexual men, it was also seen in IV drug users, transfusion recipients from Haiti, female sexual contacts of infected men, prisoners, and Africans. In the beginning, many theories were proposed regarding the causative agent of the disease, but the observation that the epidemiology of AIDS was similar to that of hepatitis B infection persuaded researchers to search for a viral component. The cause of AIDS, a novel retrovirus that belongs to the human T-lymphotropic virus group, was isolated in 1983; it was positively identified as the primary cause of AIDS in 1984. At the end of 2018, the estimated prevalence of HIV in the United States—that is, the total number of people living with HIV infection—was estimated at 1.2 million, with 14% of these individuals believed to be unaware of their infections. AIDS is now pandemic: According to recent estimates, nearly 38 million people around the globe are infected with HIV, with 770,000 people dying from AIDS-related illnesses in 2018.

Transmission of HIV infection occurs by the transfer of infected cells or free virus from one individual to another. Transmission occurs horizontally via sexual contact or by exposure to infected blood, and vertically from mother to neonate across the placenta or during delivery. An infant can also contract HIV from an infected mother through breast milk. The transmission rate of HIV during pregnancy or delivery is 5% to 10%, versus 10% to 20% while breastfeeding. The transmission rate can be reduced to less than 1% if the mother is treated adequately with AZT during her pregnancy, the infant is delivered by cesarean section, and the mother does not breastfeed. The HIV transmission rate increases in people who also have other sexually transmitted infections (STIs), especially STIs that disrupt the mucous membrane barrier.

The risk of contracting HIV from a blood transfusion has been reduced through aggressive screening of donated blood; this risk is now extremely low but cannot be completely eliminated, because there is a small window of time when the virus is not detected in people with new infections. The CDC, in partnership with 14 countries in Africa and the Caribbean and under the President's Emergency Plan for AIDS Relief, has worked to reduce the risk of transmitting HIV through blood transfusions. The goal is to deliver an adequate supply of safe blood to these participating countries by collecting blood from low-risk, voluntary, nonremunerated donors and strengthening laboratory and screening capacity.

Prevention of exposure (ie, needlesticks) is the most important method of protecting health care workers against HIV transmission. The incidence of needlesticks has been reduced by advances in needleless devices, safety education, and emphasis on proper sharps disposal. Even so, needlestick injuries continue to occur. Fortunately, the risk of becoming infected with HIV after a significant exposure to body fluids from a patient infected with HIV is low. The estimated risk of transmission is 0.33% for hollow-bore needlesticks and 0.09% for mucosal contact; there are no known cases of HIV transmission with intact-skin exposures.

Pathophysiology

HIV is a retrovirus that infects T lymphocytes and other cells that display the CD4 surface protein **FIGURE 20-9**. It belongs to a subgroup of retroviruses called the lentiviruses, which cause "slow" infections with long incubation periods.

Three essential enzymes are enclosed in the retroviral capsid of the virus:

- *Reverse transcriptase* is an RNA-dependent DNA polymerase that gives the retrovirus its name. This enzyme is responsible for converting the RNA viral genome into a DNA provirus.
- *Integrase* is the enzyme that catalyzes the integration of the newly transcribed proviral DNA into the host cell genome.
- *Protease* is the enzyme that is responsible for producing functional viral proteins.

Understanding these specific retroviral enzymes is important for understanding how antiretroviral therapy was designed for the treatment of HIV/AIDS.

HIV infects CD4+ helper T cells and kills them, resulting in the suppression of cell-mediated immunity. There are three stages in HIV infection: acute, latent, and late (or the period of immunodeficiency). The stage of the illness is largely determined by the CD4 cell count and symptoms of the disease **TABLE 20-4**. The disease classification is based on the lowest CD4 cell count, not the current count. Once a patient has a CD4 count of less than 200 cells/µL, the patient is diagnosed with AIDS regardless of whether the T cells rebound with therapy.

The initial exposure to the virus triggers a sequence of events that generally goes unnoticed by the individual but allows the virus to become permanently established in the immune system. Thereafter, HIV infection can be divided into two phases: acute infection and chronic **TABLE 20-5**.

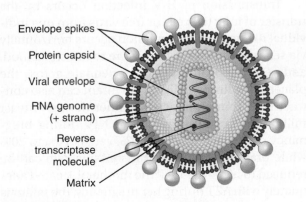

Envelope spikes
Protein capsid
Viral envelope
RNA genome (+ strand)
Reverse transcriptase molecule
Matrix

FIGURE 20-9 The human immunodeficiency virus.

© Jones & Bartlett Learning.

TABLE 20-4 HIV/AIDS: Classification of Disease Stage

Stage	Classification	CD4 Cell Count (cells/µL)
1	Asymptomatic	≥500
2	AIDS-related complex	200–499
3	AIDS	<200

Abbreviations: AIDS, acquired immunodeficiency syndrome; HIV, human immunodeficiency virus

© Jones & Bartlett Learning.

TABLE 20-5 Stages of HIV Infection

Stage	Description
Acute	Also called primary HIV infection or acute seroconversion syndrome, among other terms
Chronic	Further subdivided into the following stages: • Chronic infection, without AIDS • AIDS, characterized by a CD4 cell count <200 cells/μL or the presence of any AIDS-defining condition • Advanced HIV infection/AIDS, characterized by a CD4 cell count <50 cells/μL

Adapted from Sax PE, Wood BR. The natural history and clinical features of HIV infection in adults and adolescents. *UpToDate*. https://www.uptodate.com/contents/the-natural-history-and-clinical-features-of-hiv-infection-in -adults-and-adolescents?search=aids%20definition&source=search_result&selectedTitle=1~150&usage _type=default&display_rank=1. Updated November 21, 2019. Accessed February 12, 2021.

The initial infection begins in the immune cells of the genital tract, and the virus quickly spreads to localized CD4+ helper T cells. However, the virus is not detected in the blood until 4 to 11 days after the initial infection.

The acute phase of the disease occurs 2 to 6 weeks after the initial exposure. The patient may present with mononucleosis-like symptoms of fever, lethargy, generalized lymphadenopathy, pharyngitis, and arthralgias. A maculopapular rash on the trunk, arms, and legs, sparing the palms and soles, may also be seen during this time. The acute phase of the disease usually resolves within 2 weeks.

Antibodies to HIV are not detected in the blood until 2 to 4 weeks after the initial infection. Once antibodies are detected in the serum, the patient is said to have seroconverted. The inability to detect antibodies in the blood prior to seroconversion results in false-negative serologic test results. This has important implications for transmission of the virus and for screening of the blood supply. The HIV-infected person is capable of spreading the disease through sexual or blood contacts during this window of time, even though the HIV antibody test result might be negative.

After the initial viremia, a viral set point is reached. The viral set point represents the amount of virus present in the blood (the viral load) and tends to remain fairly constant for many years. The lower the viral set point at the end of the initial infection, the more likely the patient is to remain in the latent stage of the disease. The latent stage usually lasts for years (the median duration is 10 years), and the patient is generally asymptomatic during this period. While the patient may be asymptomatic and the symptoms are latent, the virus is *not* truly "latent," but rather is actively replicating within the patient's lymph nodes. The most important effect of HIV infection is viral entry into the CD4+ lymphocytes, which leads to slow depletion of the patient's CD4+ lymphocytes or cells. The depletion of these CD4+ cells leads to loss of cellular immunity.

AIDS is defined as the late stage of HIV infection. The criteria for AIDS diagnosis include HIV infection with a CD4+ helper T cell count of less than 200 cells/μL and/or the presence of an AIDS-defining condition. The presence of an AIDS-defining condition supersedes any CD4 cell count **TABLE 20-6**.

Patients with HIV often present many years after the initial infection or the acute stage of the disease because in the initial stages, the disease is often mild and the symptoms are nonspecific. In many patients with HIV, the illness is noticed only when the patient begins to experience symptoms such as generalized lymphadenopathy, weight loss, fatigue, fevers, or night sweats. As the disease progresses, the patient may experience frequent severe herpes infections of the mouth or anus and/or recurrent or persistent yeast infections. The loss of cell-mediated immunity predisposes the host to many opportunistic infections. Symptoms of opportunistic infections commonly seen in patients with AIDS include cough, dyspnea, headache, altered mental status, memory loss, seizures, ataxia, dysphagia, nausea, vomiting, severe persistent diarrhea, and marked weight loss.

The viral load is estimated by determining how much viral RNA is present in the blood. The viral load indicates the magnitude of HIV replication and its associated rate of CD4 cell destruction. This measure is the most accurate indicator of the risk for disease progression and is used in planning and monitoring antiretroviral therapy. The CD4 cell count is used to evaluate the extent of HIV-induced immune damage, to estimate the patient's immunologic status, and to predict the patient's likelihood of developing opportunistic infections. In the past, antiretroviral therapy was formally initiated based on the viral load, the CD4+ T cell count, and the patient's clinical condition. Today, however,

TABLE 20-6 AIDS-Defining Conditions
Bacterial infections, multiple or recurrent[a]
Candidiasis of the bronchi, trachea, or lungs
Candidiasis of the esophagus
Cervical cancer, invasive[b]
Coccidioidomycosis, disseminated or extrapulmonary
Cryptococcosis, extrapulmonary
Cryptosporidiosis, chronic intestinal (>1 month duration)
Cytomegalovirus disease (other than in the liver, spleen, or nodes), onset at age >1 month
Cytomegalovirus retinitis (with loss of vision)
Encephalopathy attributed to HIV
Herpes simplex: chronic ulcers (>1 month duration) or bronchitis, pneumonitis, or esophagitis (onset at age >1 month)
Histoplasmosis, disseminated or extrapulmonary
Isosporiasis, chronic intestinal (>1 month duration)
Kaposi sarcoma
Lymphoma, Burkitt (or equivalent term)
Lymphoma, immunoblastic (or equivalent term)
Lymphoma, primary, of the brain
Mycobacterium avium complex or *Mycobacterium kansasii*, disseminated or extrapulmonary
Mycobacterium tuberculosis of any site, pulmonary,[b] disseminated, or extrapulmonary
Mycobacterium, other species or unidentified species, disseminated or extrapulmonary
Pneumocystis jirovecii pneumonia
Pneumonia, recurrent[b]
Progressive multifocal leukoencephalopathy
Salmonella septicemia, recurrent
Toxoplasmosis of brain, onset at age >1 month
Wasting syndrome attributed to HIV

Abbreviations: AIDS, acquired immunodeficiency syndrome; HIV, human immunodeficiency virus

[a] Only among children younger than 6 years.

[b] Only among adults, adolescents, and children ages 6 years or older.

Selik RM, Mokotoff ED, Branson B, et al. Revised surveillance case definition for HIV infection—United States, 2014. *MMWR Recomm Rep*. 2014;63:1.

most clinicians initiate therapy as soon as HIV infection can be confirmed.

Management

Six general classes of antiretroviral drugs are currently available for the treatment of HIV infection:

- Nucleoside (and nucleotide) reverse transcriptase inhibitors (NRTIs)
- Nonnucleoside reverse transcriptase inhibitors (NNRTIs)
- Protease inhibitors (PIs)
- Integrase strand transfer inhibitors (INSTIs)
- Entry inhibitors: CCR5 antagonists
- Entry inhibitors: fusion inhibitors

Each class of drugs attacks HIV in a different way.

NRTIs target the enzyme known as reverse transcriptase (RT). They act to block the transcription of the viral RNA to the proviral DNA by competing with physiologic nucleosides for the enzyme-binding sites. Once they are added to the growing DNA sequence, they block the addition of the next nucleoside, thereby interrupting the synthesis process and causing chain termination. The prototype of the NRTIs is AZT.

NNRTIs are similar to the NRTIs in that they target the same viral enzyme, reverse transcriptase. In contrast to the NRTIs, NNRTIs are not competitive inhibitors of the enzyme, but rather noncompetitive inhibitors of reverse transcriptase. They bind to the enzyme near the binding site for the nucleoside substrate and alter the configuration of the enzyme, thereby preventing it from carrying out its catalytic function. The two classes of RT inhibitors are considered the backbone of anti-HIV treatment.

PIs target the viral enzyme protease that cuts the viral polyprotein into functional individual proteins. Inhibiting this protease prevents the processing of viral proteins, which then prevents the construction of the mature virion. Indinavir is an example of a typical PI. Because the step that the PIs inhibit occurs late in the viral replication process, these therapies are most often used in combination with other agents.

Integrase inhibitors target a protein in HIV called integrase, which is essential for viral replication. Integrase is responsible for inserting viral genomic DNA into the host chromosome. The integrase enzyme binds to the host cell's DNA, prepares an area on the viral DNA for integration, and then transfers this processed strand into the host cell's genome.

Entry inhibitors stop HIV from entering human cells. There are two types: CCR5 inhibitors and fusion inhibitors.

To enter a host cell, HIV must bind to two separate receptors on the cell's surface: the CD4 receptor and a co-receptor (CCR5 or CXCR4). Once HIV has attached to both, its envelope can fuse with the host cell membrane and release viral components into the cell. CCR5 inhibitors prevent HIV from using the CCR5 co-receptor by binding to it, blocking viral entry. CCR5 inhibitors do not work in all patients, however, and are very rarely used as first-line treatments. A test is required to determine if this type of treatment would be effective before it is initiated.

A fusion inhibitor (enfuvirtide) is available by injection only and is used in patients who have no other treatment options. It works by stopping the fusion of the HIV envelope protein with the CD4 cell.

The goal of current therapies for HIV infection is to prolong life, while maintaining the best possible quality of life. Achieving this goal requires weighing the benefits from preventing opportunistic infections and malignancies, and slowing the rate of virus production, against the side effects of therapy. In addition, therapy must be delivered to the patient in a manner that promotes compliance. Although the PIs are highly effective at reducing HIV viral load, their serious side effects (ie, fat redistribution with facial wasting, insulin resistance with hyperglycemia, high cholesterol, and liver problems) and the improved effects of other classes of antiretrovirals have limited their usefulness for initial therapy. Initial antiretroviral regimens should typically be based on tenofovir and have a high barrier to resistance. This treatment is very effective in prolonging life and reducing the viral load, but ensuring patient compliance can be challenging because the regimens are often complicated and the side effects can be debilitating. Viral resistance to the antiretroviral drugs increases when patients use the drugs intermittently or incorrectly. Patient adherence to uninterrupted HIV treatment has been greatly assisted by fixed-dose pills that combine two or three antiretroviral drugs from more than one class into a single pill that is taken once per day.

The risks of occupational exposures and post-exposure prevention protocols are discussed later in this chapter.

Signs and Symptoms

HIV Infection/AIDS

Early symptoms:
- Generalized lymphadenopathy
- Weight loss
- Fatigue
- Fevers
- Night sweats

Symptoms associated with disease progression:
- Frequent, severe herpes infections of the mouth or anus
- Recurrent or persistent yeast infections

Symptoms associated with opportunistic infections:
- Cough
- Dyspnea
- Headache
- Altered mental status
- Memory loss
- Seizures
- Ataxia
- Dysphagia
- Nausea
- Vomiting
- Severe persistent diarrhea
- Marked weight loss

Transport Management

HIV Infection/AIDS
- Provide supportive care.

Rickettsial Diseases

Rickettsial diseases are transmitted via tick bite. In consequence, patients with these diseases are not considered infectious by human-to-human contact, although transmission is known to have occurred via blood transfusion from an infected but asymptomatic donor. Three major diseases are classified as tick-borne rickettsial diseases: Rocky Mountain spotted fever, ehrlichiosis, and anaplasmosis.

Of these diseases, the highest mortality rate is seen with Rocky Mountain spotted fever. Early signs and symptoms of these tick-borne diseases are generally mild and nonspecific, making diagnosis problematic; however, Rocky Mountain spotted fever should be considered a possible diagnosis in all patients presenting with fever and having suspected or known tick exposure (through outdoor activities during April through September in North America). In particular, children and young adults are at risk because of their increased outdoor activity. Despite its name, Rocky Mountain spotted fever is seen mostly in the southeastern United States (especially North Carolina), followed by two midwestern states (Missouri and Tennessee). **TABLE 20-7** compares initial signs and symptoms of anaplasmosis, ehrlichiosis, and Rocky Mountain spotted fever.

Rocky Mountain spotted fever begins acutely with fever accompanied by one or more of the following: headache (usually severe), rash, muscle aches, nausea and vomiting, and malaise. Patients may also exhibit neurologic symptoms resembling those associated with meningitis. Children may present with abdominal pain, altered mental status, and conjunctival injection (bloodshot eyes). Within a few days after the initial fever, a petechial rash develops on the hands and feet, which then spreads to the rest of the body in approximately half of all adults and most children. The skin on the hands and feet of some patients will slough off about a month after a severe petechial rash occurs. Of patients with tick-borne rickettsial diseases, 50% or more require hospitalization, and some patients will experience long-term complications such as renal failure, myocarditis, meningoencephalitis, hypotension, adult respiratory distress syndrome, thrombocytopenia, and multiple-organ failure.

Diagnosis is determined by using a serum antibody test or polymerase chain reaction test, or by obtaining a biopsy specimen of the rash. If rickettsial disease is suspected, treatment with doxycycline (or a similar antibiotic) should be initiated immediately and not delayed by waiting for results from diagnostic tests.

Prevention of tick-borne diseases includes using insect repellents that contain N,N-diethyl-meta-toluamide (DEET) and wearing light-colored clothing (to make ticks more visible). If possible, individuals should wear long sleeves and long pants, and tuck their pants into their socks when outside, particularly when walking through grassy areas.

TABLE 20-7 Initial Signs and Symptoms of Tick-Borne Rickettsial Diseases

Anaplasmosis		Ehrlichiosis		Rocky Mountain Spotted Fever
Anaplasma phagocytophilum	*Ehrlichia chaffeensis* (Ehrlichiosis)	*Ehrlichia ewingii* (Infection)		*Rickettsia rickettsii*
Fever	Fever	Fever		Fever
Headache	Headache	Headache		Headache
Malaise	Malaise	Malaise		Malaise
Muscle aches	Muscle aches	Muscle aches		Muscle aches
Vomiting		Vomiting		Vomiting
		Nausea		Nausea
				Loss of appetite
Rare rash	Rash in <30% of adults and approximately 60% of children	Rare rash		Maculopapular rash approximately 2–5 days after onset of fever in 35%–60% of adults (and <90% of children); might involve the palms and soles

Centers for Disease Control and Prevention. Symptoms of tickborne illness. http://www.cdc.gov/ticks/symptoms.html. Reviewed January 10, 2019. Accessed February 12, 2021.

They should also inspect their body for ticks after being outdoors.

Embedded ticks should be removed with tweezers or gloved hands; avoid removal with bare hands. Grasp the tick as close to the skin as possible and lift the tick with enough force to "tent" the skin surface. Hold the tick in this position for a minute or until the tick lets go. Then, either save the tick for analysis (in a plastic bag placed in the freezer) or dispose of the tick by flushing it down a drain. To avoid contamination from body fluids, do not crush or squeeze the tick. After removal, thoroughly wash the area of the tick bite with soap and warm water and apply rubbing alcohol. Wash hands with soap and water.

Emerging Infectious Diseases

The influenza pandemic of 1918–1919, which caused more than 20 million deaths, was thought to be a phenomenon of historic interest. With the advent of effective vaccinations and antibiotics, the death rate from infectious disease declined dramatically during the 20th century, but these successes should not lead to complacency. Hantavirus, West Nile virus, SARS, and avian influenza have emerged as new threats on the medical landscape. The emergence and reemergence of drug-resistant infectious agents, such as methicillin-resistant *S aureus*, vancomycin-resistant enterococci, and MDR-TB, have increased dramatically in the past two decades.

The term *emerging infectious disease* refers to both new and reemerging diseases caused by infectious agents that have recently increased in incidence or those that threaten to increase in the near future. The CDC has identified several major factors that contribute to the development or reemergence of infectious disease—namely, changes in human behaviors or ecology, changes in economic and technologic advances, and adaptive changes of the infectious agents. The high mobility of modern society has greatly facilitated the movement of people, animals, and other commodities across countries and continents; unfortunately, this population on the move also includes carriers of disease. The triangle of transmission between microbe, vector, and host is exacerbated when microbes and vectors have access to naïve populations who lack immunity (herd immunity). Selective pressures from overuse of antibiotics have precipitated the development of resistant microbes, and abuse of antimicrobials has allowed the reemergence of more deadly infections.

Additionally, infectious agents are now thought to be important in the etiology of many diseases previously classified as noninfectious. *Helicobacter pylori* has long been found in association with peptic ulcer disease, but it is now known to have a causative association. Human papillomavirus (HPV) is the major cause of cervical cancer (an HPV vaccine is now available). Hepatitis C virus is a leading cause of chronic liver disease and cirrhosis in the United States and is a major risk factor for the development of hepatocellular carcinoma.

Emerging infectious diseases can be particularly damaging to immunocompromised people, such as those with HIV disease, those receiving immunosuppressive therapy (eg, recipients of organ transplants), and those who are immunosuppressed as a result of their treatment for cancer. Public water supplies that are contaminated by emerging infectious agents put entire communities at risk. In 1993, *Cryptosporidium* contaminated a municipal water supply in Wisconsin; 4,400 people were ultimately hospitalized with infections. Large segments of populations may also be exposed to emerging infections through contaminated food sources. For example, *E coli* O157:H7 in contaminated beef cooked in fast-food restaurants caused a multistate outbreak of hemorrhagic colitis and serious kidney disease and resulted in the deaths of at least four children. Emerging diseases include HIV infections, SARS CoV-1, SARS-CoV-2, Lyme disease, *E coli* O157:H7, *Cryptosporidium*, hantavirus, dengue fever, West Nile virus, and Zika virus. In addition, multidrug-resistant bacterial infections can be considered emerging diseases.

To effectively detect and ward off the threat of emerging infections, the public health sector, health care providers, and emergency medical services must cooperate to control any potential outbreaks and prevent the spread of potentially deadly diseases. Such cooperation can have a significant impact when emergency medical services (EMS) is involved in surveillance and education of the community. As part of this effort, all health care workers should follow the recommendations for using standard precautions **TABLE 20-8** and PPE **TABLE 20-9**.

TABLE 20-8 Recommendations for the Application of Standard Precautions for the Care of All Patients in All Health Care Settings

Component	Recommendations
Hand hygiene	After touching blood, body fluids, secretions, excretions, and contaminated items; immediately after removing gloves; and between patient contacts
Personal protective equipment	Gloves, mask, and gown
Gloves	For touching blood, body fluids, secretions, excretions, and contaminated items; for touching mucous membranes and nonintact skin
Mask, eye protection, and face shield	During procedures and patient care activities likely to generate splashes or sprays of blood, body fluids, and secretions; N95 mask to prevent respiratory transmission
Gown	During procedures and patient care activities when contact of clothing/exposed skin with blood/body fluids, secretions, and excretions is anticipated
Soiled patient care equipment	Handle in a manner that prevents transfer of microorganisms to others and to the environment; wear gloves if visibly contaminated; and perform hand hygiene
Environmental control	Develop procedures for routine care, cleaning, and disinfection of environmental surfaces, especially frequently touched surfaces in patient care areas
Textiles (linen and laundry)	Handle in a manner that prevents transfer of microorganisms to others and to the environment
Needles and other sharps	Do not recap, bend, break, or hand-manipulate used needles; use safety features when available; and place used sharps in a puncture-resistant container
Patient resuscitation	Use a mouthpiece, resuscitation bag, or other ventilation device to prevent mouth contact
Patient placement	Prioritize admission to a single-patient room if the patient is at increased risk of transmission, is likely to contaminate the environment, does not maintain appropriate hygiene, or is at increased risk of acquiring infection or developing an adverse outcome following infection
Respiratory hygiene/cough etiquette (source containment of infectious respiratory secretions in symptomatic patients, beginning at the initial point of the encounter)	Instruct symptomatic people to cover their mouths/noses when sneezing/coughing; use tissues and dispose in a no-touch receptacle; observe hand hygiene after soiling of hands with respiratory secretions; and place a surgical mask on the patient if tolerated, wear an N95 mask, or maintain spatial separation, greater than 3 feet (1 m) if possible

Data from Centers for Disease Control and Prevention (CDC), Department of Health and Human Services, 2004. Severe acute respiratory syndrome: public health guidance for community-level preparedness and response to severe acute respiratory syndrome (SARS)—Version 2, January 8, 2004. http://www.cdc.gov/sars/guidance/core/downloads/core-full.pdf. Accessed February 12, 2021.

Severe Acute Respiratory Syndrome

Severe acute respiratory syndrome (SARS) is an emerging lower respiratory tract illness caused by a coronavirus. A coronavirus causes infection in the nose, sinuses, or upper throat. Most coronaviruses are not dangerous. However, SARS first appeared as a highly contagious, deadly virus early in 2003 in the Guangdong Province of China. The virus quickly disseminated via person-to-person droplet transmission to people in Hong Kong and Vietnam, and subsequently to people in Singapore and Canada.

TABLE 20-9 Personal Protective Equipment Recommended (by Infectious Disease)

Disease	Airborne		Droplet	Standard Precautions	
	Negative-Pressure Transport	N95 Mask	Surgical Mask	Contact Gloves Face and Gown	Eye Protection Goggles or Mask/Shield
Respiratory Infections					
Respiratory syncytial virus			Required	Required	Recommended
Influenza			Required	Required	Recommended
Novel respiratory infection (such as SARS or avian flu)	Required	Required	Required if N95 is not available	Required	Required
SARS-CoV-2		N95 or higher[a] (respirator) required	Face mask required of the patient	Gown, gloves	Face shield or goggles[a]
Pulmonary TB	Recommended	Recommended	Required if N95 is not available	Required	
Meningitis			Surgical mask	Required	
Hepatitis				Required	Recommended
MDR diseases					
MRSA or VRSA			Recommended	Required	Recommended
VRE			Recommended	Required	Recommended
MDR TB	Recommended	Recommended	Required if N95 is not available	Required	Recommended
Clostridioides difficile				Required	
Human immunodeficiency virus		Required	Required if N95 is not available	Required	Required
Necrotizing fasciitis			Required	Required	
Hemorrhagic fevers of unknown etiology	Recommended	Recommended	Required if N95 is not available	Required	Required
Any contact with blood, body fluids, or feces, especially if aerosolized			Required	Required	Required

Abbreviations: MDR, multidrug resistant; MRSA, methicillin-resistant *Staphylococcus aureus*; SARS, severe acute respiratory syndrome; SARS-CoV-2, severe acute respiratory syndrome coronavirus 2; TB, tuberculosis; VRE, vancomycin-resistant enterococci; VRSA, vancomycin-resistant *Staphylococcus aureus*
[a]Each EMS agency should follow the CDC recommendations closely, paying attention to guidance for aerosol-generating procedures and changes relative to the level of community spread.

Special Populations

Zika virus (ZIKV) was first recognized in humans in 1954, but caused only sporadic infections and outbreaks. Thus, this disease attracted little attention until an outbreak occurred in Yap in 2007. The disease was originally thought by some to cause nothing more than a rash and a fever. As ZIKV infection spread throughout Latin America and the Caribbean, however, scientists began to observe far more troubling effects: microcephaly and brain damage in infants born to mothers who became infected during pregnancy, as well as an increased incidence of Guillain-Barré syndrome. Although strong evidence suggests a connection between the virus and these conditions, researchers are still working to clearly describe the pathophysiologic mechanisms and establish a definitive link.

The Zika virus is a mosquito-borne pathogen; specifically, it is carried by the *Aedes* species. The mosquito obtains the virus from the blood of an infected human and spreads it to others who are not infected. In some cases, the disease has been spread sexually from a recently infected man to others. This mode of transmission is possible because, like Ebola, ZIKV can persist in immunologically protected areas, including where semen is produced and stored. While individuals infected with Zika fever usually present with little more than an ILI, there is growing concern over the newly recognized connection to microcephaly and other previously unrecognized neurologic effects.

Those at highest risk during the early stages of the epidemic were health care workers. Ultimately, the epidemic spread to 29 countries, resulting in more than 8,000 infected people and 780 deaths. The cooperative efforts of scientists and physicians in WHO and the CDC as well as in China, Canada, Hong Kong, and other countries led to quick identification of the etiologic agent and isolation and prevention of the spread of the disease. Because of the high morbidity and mortality associated with SARS, the CDC has included it on its list of notifiable diseases to ensure careful monitoring of the US population for further outbreaks.

COVID-19

In early 2020, after a December 2019 outbreak in China, WHO identified SARS-CoV-2 as a new type of coronavirus. Coronaviruses cause most of the colds that affect populations during the year. Most strains are not a serious threat to otherwise healthy people, but SARS-CoV-2, along with the strains of coronavirus that cause Middle East respiratory syndrome (MERS) and SARS, poses a greater threat to humans.

The disease caused by SARS-CoV-2 was named COVID-19, an abbreviation for "CoronaVirus Infectious Disease discovered in 2019." COVID-19 can affect the upper respiratory tract, lower respiratory tract, gastrointestinal tract, and heart. The virus spreads the same way as other coronaviruses do, mainly through person-to-person contact. Transmission is principally by airborne droplets within 6 feet, but airborne transmission has been demonstrated at greater than 6 feet when there is inadequate ventilation or when people are exposed to respiratory particles generated with expiratory exertion, such as singing, shouting, or exercising.

Effects of infection range from mild symptoms to death. Associated symptoms reported to the CDC in the United States include the following:

- Cough in 50% of patients
- Fever (subjective determination or temperature great than 100.4°F [38°C]) in 43%
- Myalgia in 36%
- Headache in 34%
- Dyspnea in 29%
- Sore throat in 20%
- Diarrhea in 19%
- Nausea/vomiting in 12%
- Loss of smell or taste, abdominal pain, and rhinorrhea in fewer than 10% each

Within 1 year after the first report of SARS-CoV-2, the COVID-19 pandemic had spread around the world, with more than 70 million people infected globally and more than 16 million people infected in the United States. The global mortality was more than 1.6 million, including more than 300,000 deaths in the United States.

Two key characteristics increase the likelihood that severe illness will develop in a person infected with SARS-CoV-2: older age and comorbidities. In an analysis from the United Kingdom, the risk of death among people 80 years and older was

20 times higher than among people 50 to 59 years old. The following comorbidities place a patient at higher risk of severe illness:

- Cardiovascular disease
- Diabetes mellitus
- Hypertension
- Chronic lung disease
- Cancer
- Chronic kidney disease
- Obesity
- Smoking

Several complications of COVID-19 have been described, including the following:

- Respiratory failure
- Cardiac and cardiovascular complications
- Thromboembolic complications
- Neurologic complications
- Inflammatory complications
- Secondary infections

During the COVID-19 pandemic, health care workers have been encouraged to adhere strictly to PPE guidelines and infection control policies when interacting with patients, even those who do not seem to be sick with COVID-19. By September 1, 2020, at least 7,000 health workers had died worldwide after contracting COVID-19. For the health care community and the general population alike, measures to reduce transmission, such as social distancing and wearing face masks, have been crucial in controlling the spread of this disease. Development of improved treatments and COVID-19 vaccinations, the first of which were approved for use in the United States in December 2020, have provided hope that the pandemic may be controlled in the same manner as past global diseases.

Escherichia coli O157:H7

E coli is a family of microorganisms found in the intestinal tract of humans and other mammals. Hundreds of different strains of *E coli* exist, most of which are harmless. A few strains are pathogenic, however. These strains often have specialized fimbriae (finger-like borders), allowing them to adhere to certain intestinal epithelial cells and produce toxins that cause gastrointestinal conditions. Several specific pathogenic groups of *E coli* are distinguished, including enterotoxigenic, enteroinvasive, enteroaggregative, enteropathogenic, and enterohemorrhagic variants. *E coli* O157:H7, which causes hemorrhagic colitis, is emerging as a particularly virulent strain.

E coli O157:H7 is found in the intestinal tracts of ruminant animals, especially cattle. People have become infected with these bacteria after eating undercooked, contaminated ground beef; drinking unpasteurized milk and fruit drinks; eating unwashed lettuce or sprouts; eating salami; and swimming in or drinking sewage-contaminated water. Transmission can also occur via person-to-person contact, usually from infected people who have poor hygiene or handwashing technique. It takes fewer than 10 *E coli* bacteria to cause the onset of symptoms.

The Shiga-like toxins produced by these microorganisms are responsible for causing hemorrhagic colitis, an inflammation of the colon with bleeding and abdominal cramps. Most episodes are self-limiting and last only 5 to 10 days. A small number of infected people, usually those younger than 5 years or older than 65 years, experience hemolytic uremic syndrome. This syndrome is manifested when the toxin affects the kidneys, leading to kidney failure and end-stage renal disease that necessitates dialysis or transplant to sustain life.

Diagnosis of *E coli* infection relies on stool cultures performed using a specialized growing medium such as sorbitol-MacConkey agar plates. Treatment is difficult because of emerging antibiotic resistance.

Transport Management

COVID-19

- All crew members don proper PPE.
- Place a mask on the patient.
- Keep the patient in respiratory isolation.
- Monitor the mechanical ventilator, if applicable.
- Use noninvasive means of oxygenating patients with hypoxemic respiratory failure.
- Avoid all aerosol-generating procedures.
- Minimize suctioning of the patient's airway.
- Continue IV administration of any medications if they have been started by the sending facility.
- Perform high-level disinfection of all equipment after transport.

Thoroughly cooking beef, avoiding unpasteurized drinks, and washing hands after handling raw meat can prevent infection with *E coli* O157:H7.

West Nile Virus

West Nile virus (WNV) is an arthropod-borne virus that was first isolated in Uganda's West Nile district in 1937. A single-stranded RNA *Flavivirus* of the Flaviviridae family, WNV is a member of the Japanese encephalitis virus serocomplex that contains other medically important viruses, such as the St. Louis encephalitis virus. The close antigenic profiles of the flaviviruses, especially those of the Japanese encephalitis group, cause serologic cross-reactions in the diagnostic laboratory.

Epidemiology

In 1999, the first US cases of WNV–associated encephalitis were reported in New York City. Evidence suggests that international travel and commerce have played a significant role in this pathogen's introduction into the Western hemisphere. In Africa and Asia, disease outbreaks caused by WNV were infrequent and were not associated with serious morbidity or mortality. Since the virus's introduction in the United States, however, the frequency and apparent severity of WNV cases have increased, spiking in 2012 with more than 5,674 cases before settling down to an annual average of approximately 2,000 cases per year. The WNV epidemic of 2002, the largest meningoencephalitis epidemic recorded to date, resulted in more than 4,000 cases and 200 deaths.

In 2015, an outbreak in the United States led to more than 1,900 people becoming infected and 111 deaths. The majority of these cases occurred in California (including 100 cases in Orange County), where there is an ongoing drought. Without rain to flush them away, mosquitoes were able to lay and hatch their eggs in stagnant pools of water in drainage systems, resulting in an explosion in the mosquito population. WNV is a mosquito-borne pathogen. Adult mosquitoes emerge in the spring. Viral amplification occurs through mosquito–bird–mosquito cycling until early fall, when female mosquitoes begin diapause and infrequently bite humans or other animals (typically horses) to gain protein for egg development from a blood meal **FIGURE 20-10**. The virus is found in the salivary

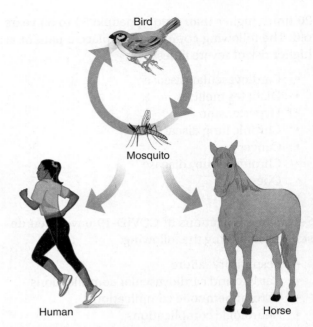

FIGURE 20-10 Transmission cycle of the West Nile virus.
© Jones & Bartlett Learning.

glands of the mosquito and is transferred during the bite. Mosquitoes are the bridge vectors that maintain the cycle of infection by feeding off both humans and birds.

In temperate climates, human disease outbreaks peak in late summer and continue into fall; however, year-round transmission is possible in the more southern states. WNV is endemic in all of the continental United States and in the District of Columbia (as well as in Canada and Mexico). The mosquito responsible for transmission to humans is primarily the *Culex* species; however, other types of mosquito can carry the disease as well.

Diagnosis and Management

The incubation period of WNV ranges from 3 to 14 days. Most infections are subclinical, and patients remain asymptomatic. A febrile viral syndrome develops in approximately 20% of infected people; only 50% of those infected will seek medical attention. The signs and symptoms of WNV infection vary, but frequently include sudden onset of fever with malaise, anorexia, nausea, vomiting, eye pain, headache, and myalgia, which last 3 to 6 days. Symptoms may also include rash, lymphadenopathy, fatigue, and arthralgias. Approximately 1 in 100 infections results in meningitis or encephalitis. Advanced age is the most significant risk factor associated with severe neurologic sequelae following infection.

A high index of clinical suspicion is required for prompt diagnosis. Arboviral disease should be included in the differential diagnosis in any older adult who presents with a sudden onset of unexplained encephalitis or meningismus in the late summer or early fall. The presence of local WNV enzootic activity or other human cases should amplify the level of suspicion. Because WNV infections have occurred in people of all ages and because year-round transmission is possible in southern states, any person presenting with unexplained encephalitis or meningismus should trigger suspicion of WNV infection.

WNV is most efficiently diagnosed by detection of IgM antibody to WNV in the CSF via antibody-capture enzyme-linked immunosorbent assay. The presence of WNV-positive IgM antibody in the CSF strongly suggests WNV infection of the central nervous system, because IgM antibody does not cross the blood–brain barrier. The CSF may reveal normal to elevated leukocyte levels, with lymphocytes predominating; an elevated protein level; and normal glucose levels. Serum samples also have a high rate of positive results for WNV IgM antibody.

There is no cure for WNV encephalitis. Infections are treated symptomatically, and supportive therapy is important for patients with more severe illnesses.

Prevention of Infection

WNV encephalitis has been added to the list of nationally notifiable arboviral encephalitides. The timely identification of acute WNV has substantial public health implications, and case reports will likely prompt a vigorous public health response to reduce the risk of additional human infections.

Integrated vector management programs are the best way to control mosquito populations and prevent human infection. Mosquito control measures should emphasize the elimination of standing water. Mosquito development consists of three aquatic stages: egg, larva, and pupa. Therefore, elimination of this environmental niche is an effective way to reduce mosquito populations without resorting to insecticides.

CCTPs working outdoors should apply an insect repellent while engaging in prolonged extraction or search-and-rescue activities. The CDC recommends repellents containing the active ingredient DEET for this purpose. Increasing the concentration of DEET in the repellent does not increase its strength, but does increase the duration of effect. DEET concentrations of 50% or more do not increase the duration of protection significantly, so little benefit is gained by using them. DEET does not kill mosquitoes, but rather prevents them from detecting human skin odors and, therefore, finding a blood meal.

Peak mosquito biting times are dawn, dusk, and early evening. Long pants and long-sleeve clothing provide an added measure of protection.

Signs and Symptoms

West Nile Virus Infection
- Sudden-onset fever
- Malaise
- Anorexia
- Nausea
- Vomiting
- Eye pain
- Headache
- Myalgia
- Rash
- Lymphadenopathy
- Fatigue
- Arthralgias

Differential Diagnosis

West Nile Virus Infection
- *Borrelia burgdorferi* infection
- Brain abscess
- Brain tumor
- Dengue fever
- Guillain-Barré syndrome
- Leptospirosis
- Meningitis
- Paraspinal epidural abscess
- Stroke
- Tick paralysis
- Eastern equine encephalitis
- Other infectious encephalitis

Strategies for the Treatment of Infectious Disease

As discussed earlier in this chapter, microorganisms possess unique properties that allow them to invade their human hosts, evade immune detection, and establish infection. These same properties are exploited when developing agents to inhibit their growth or eliminate them from the body. The goal of any such therapy is to eradicate the pathogen without causing undue harm to the host. This section explores how antibiotics, antivirals, and antifungal agents are designed to target the unique organelles of each class of organism.

Antibiotics

Antibiotics are compounds that are produced by bacteria or fungi and that inhibit the growth of or kill other bacterial organisms. Compounds that inhibit bacterial growth are called bacteriostatic, whereas compounds that kill bacteria are termed bactericidal. Synthetic antimicrobials are designed using the "magic bullet" concept, exploiting the differences between human and microbial cells. The beta-lactam antibiotics include penicillin, ampicillin, amoxicillin, and carbenicillin, among others. These bactericidal drugs act on gram-positive bacteria by competitively inhibiting transpeptidase, the enzyme that catalyzes peptidoglycan cell wall synthesis.

Different families of bacterial cells have unique components that are targeted by different classes of antibacterial drugs. All antibacterial agents follow the same basic principle of targeting bacterial proteins, processes, or cellular components that are not found in human cells. Even though human cellular components are not the targets of antimicrobial therapies, these agents may have some adverse effects that must be considered when choosing the appropriate therapy. For example, quinolones such as ciprofloxacin can cause tendon rupture, particularly in people older than 60 years; alternative antibiotics may be selected for members of this age group.

Antivirals

Viruses account for millions of severe illnesses every year worldwide. The common seasonal influenza viruses alone account for 3 to 5 million severe illnesses annually and 290,000 to 650,000 deaths from respiratory illness. Despite these staggering numbers, relatively few treatment modalities have been developed to care for patients with viral illnesses. The difficulty lies in isolating the steps of the viruses' replication, which are intimately involved with the normal synthetic processes of the human host cell. The medications that are effective against viral diseases focus on interrupting the viral replication cycle at a specific step. Virus replication takes place during an incubation period, when the patient is asymptomatic and, therefore, not likely to be taking any antiviral medication. A virus can also become latent within the body, rendering it almost impossible to eradicate.

Three classes of antiviral medications have been developed: nucleoside analogs, enzyme inhibitors, and interferon. Nucleoside analogs such as acyclovir and AZT are used to treat herpesviruses and HIV infection, respectively. Enzyme inhibitors are used to treat influenza; they include drugs such as indinavir and zanamivir. Alpha-interferon is used to treat viral hepatitis.

Because of the limited number of medications available to treat active viral infections, prevention of viral infections in health care workers is best achieved through vaccination, when available. Meanwhile, biochemists continue working to create novel medications to treat both viral and bacterial infections.

Antifungals

Human and fungal cells are similar in that both are eukaryotic. Because of their similar makeup, finding agents that affect the fungal cell without harming the human cell can be challenging. Indeed, many antifungal agents can produce toxic results when used systemically. A primary difference between human and fungal cells is their membrane components. The fungal cell membrane contains ergosterols, whereas the human cell membrane contains cholesterol. This structure is different enough for the fungal cell membrane to be a target of antifungal therapy. Polyene compounds bind with the sterols in this membrane, making the membrane less fluid and more susceptible to rupture. As a result of the change in fluidity, the cell membrane leaks and loses its integrity, which leads to cell death. Other antifungal therapies are available, but all represent a variation on this theme; that is, they all target pathways or enzymes that are specific to fungal cells.

The Post-Antibiotic Era

Before the advent of antibiotic agents, bacterial infections were the cause of significant morbidity and mortality. In 1900, the three leading causes of death in the United States were infectious diseases. In 2019, the leading causes of death were noninfectious diseases: heart disease, cancer, and unintentional injuries. Even so, many scientists worry that we are entering a "Post-Antibiotic Age" because of the emergence of antibiotic-resistant bacteria. Almost all important pathogenic bacteria have demonstrated resistance to current Food and Drug Administration (FDA)–approved antibiotics. Antibiotic resistance has become one of the world's most pressing public health problems in the 21st century.

Antibiotic resistance can cause significant morbidity and mortality in people infected with previously easily treatable infections. Staphylococci, for example, are one of the most common causes of community- and hospital-acquired infections. *Staphylococcus* commonly colonizes the skin and nares of healthy people. If this bacterium causes a simple infection, most people can be successfully treated with beta-lactam antibiotics. However, staphylococci also cause serious infections, such as postoperative infections or pneumonia; treatment of these infections becomes increasingly difficult as resistance develops.

Three important factors contribute to the emergence of resistant bacteria within a given population or community:

- Misuse or overprescription of antibiotics
- Poor infection control
- Importation or intrusion of already resistant strains

The continual use of antibiotics paradoxically leads to declining effectiveness through selective pressures and the development of resistance, because increasing resistance causes a concomitant decrease in the therapeutic options for eliminating infections. In the critical care environment, there are many opportunities for contamination and subsequent cross-transmission of resistant bacteria. Infection control measures—for example, handwashing, patient isolation, and proper disposal of contaminates—are important in breaking this cycle of transmission. It is important for CCTPs to be keenly aware of how their actions can either hinder or hasten the spread of disease.

Antibiotic Resistance
Causes of Resistance

Antibiotic resistance occurs when the bacteria acquire new properties through mutation, protein alteration, or conjugative transfer of plasmid-encoded resistance factors. Resistant organisms coexist with healthy skin or gastrointestinal flora. When antibiotics are used to treat infection or used inappropriately for viral infections, the normal, protective flora is eliminated, allowing the resistant strains to dominate. This relative decrease in the sensitive strains and increase in the resistant strains leads to selective pressure on the weaker protective bacteria. The bacteria that are not eliminated are stronger (ie, more resistant to antibiotics), making it more difficult to cure the patient, and these resistant strains move on to cause infection in the next host. When this theme is applied on a grander scale to the critical care setting, where the use of antibiotics is routine and infectious sources are plentiful, the true magnitude of the problem becomes apparent.

Another emerging concern related to transferrable antimicrobial resistance is extended-spectrum beta-lactamase (ESBL). ESBL is an enzyme produced by some bacteria and is an urgently important mechanism of resistance to beta-lactams such as penicillin and third-generation cephalosporins, including ceftriaxone and cefotaxime. A particularly troubling aspect of ESBLs is that they can be transferred between strains of a single microbial species, and even between species. Complicating the problem is the difficulty in detecting which bacterial species possess the enzyme. A large percentage of *E coli* and *K pneumoniae* species are now known to express these enzymes. Infection with ESBL-expressing bacteria has resulted in treatment failures, and the prevalence of such disease is clearly increasing worldwide.

Prevention of Resistance

Infection control is critically important in thwarting the development of new resistant strains and preventing the spread of currently resistant strains. Unfortunately, health care workers are a major source of cross-infection between critically ill patients. Handwashing is the single most important act that a health care provider can perform to reduce the spread of infection. However, even under the best circumstances, compliance with handwashing is low. It is even more difficult to accomplish in the critical care transport environment, but is incumbent upon CCTPs as part of their role: If CCTPs do not practice proper hand sanitation methods when providing care, their hands may become vectors for transmission of infectious disease.

Another important method for reducing the spread of resistant bacteria is the isolation of infected patients. Methods of isolation include geographic isolation, negative-pressure isolation, contact precautions, and barrier isolation.

Antibiotics should be prescribed only when they are likely to be beneficial. The choice of antibiotic should be appropriate—using a drug that will eliminate the pathogen most likely to be causing the infection or, better yet, using definitive culture and sensitivity testing to identify the infecting bacterial strain and then combating it with the correct drug. The prescription should be written for the appropriate dose and duration of treatment. Using a drug for longer than is required to eliminate the offending bacteria does not offer any additional benefit to the patient.

Each year in the United States, an estimated one-third of all antibiotics prescribed are unnecessary, a trend that has contributed to increasing antibiotic resistance. Members of the public must be made aware of the role they play in promoting the emergence of resistant strains and, in turn, educated to reduce their demands for inappropriate prescriptions. Even though these agents are completely ineffective against viral infections, tens of millions of antibiotic prescriptions are written each year for viral illnesses. Time pressure on physicians and patients alike, diagnostic uncertainty, and demand from uninformed patients all contribute to the continued inappropriate use of antibiotics. To ensure that patients return to their practice, physicians are often under pressure to prescribe, but prescribing just for the sake of convenience and to satisfy a patient's demand is never appropriate.

Patients, for their part, must take appropriately prescribed antibiotics as directed and for the full duration of the intended treatment. All too often, once symptoms of the illness are relieved, patients stop taking the drug, even though the infection may not be completely eradicated. When infections are treated incompletely, the weaker strains of bacteria are killed, but the stronger or antibiotic-resistant strains may be left unharmed; their survival then contributes to the emergence of resistance by selection.

Patients should also be warned against the dangers of using "leftover" antibiotics prescribed from prior infections to treat their current ailments. First, their symptoms may not be caused by a bacterial infection. Second, if they do truly have a bacterial infection, the drug may be completely ineffective against the particular causative bacterial strain and may cause the patient to become sicker. Also, partially treating bacterial infections with antibiotics may make it more difficult to isolate, identify, and perform sensitivity testing on the culprit microbe, making treatment decisions all the more difficult for the health care provider.

Methicillin-Resistant *Staphylococcus aureus*

Methicillin-resistant *S aureus* (MRSA) is a gram-positive, coagulase-positive, nonmotile coccus that produces an altered penicillin-binding protein that confers resistance to beta-lactam antibiotics, including methicillin. Most strains of MRSA are also resistant to multiple classes of antibiotics, making these infections difficult to control. MRSA can colonize a variety of tissues, causing infections such as cellulitis, cutaneous abscesses, wound infections, osteomyelitis, septic arthritis, endocarditis, pneumonia, and septicemia.

MRSA was first detected in Europe and Australia in the 1960s, and it was identified in the United States 10 years later. It has gradually become a major player in resistant nosocomial infections. Humans are the major reservoir of MRSA. Most carriers are colonized in the nares, pharynx, and skin. High rates of MRSA are found among residents of long-term care facilities, but serious infections with MRSA are more prevalent in acute care settings. Risk factors for colonization include dialysis, diabetes, use of injectable drugs, chronic skin conditions such as decubitus ulcers, and a history of prior antibiotic use. MRSA is also emerging as a community-acquired pathogen; that is, MRSA may be acquired by people who have not been hospitalized recently and have not undergone a recent medical procedure.

Transient contamination of the hands of health care providers often results in the transmission of resistant organisms to other patients. MRSA may be spread by direct contact with patients who are infected, or by contact with contaminated objects. Given this risk, patients with known MRSA infections should be placed on contact precautions until they have been successfully treated and the results of their nasal and rectal swabs are negative. As always, CCTPs should avoid direct contact with wounds by wearing gloves during all dressing changes and avoiding direct contact with any patient with a known MRSA infection.

Vancomycin is the drug of choice for treating MRSA infection. An alternative to vancomycin for the treatment of MRSA skin infections and nosocomial pneumonia is linezolid. Linezolid's key advantage is that it is available in an oral form, whereas vancomycin is not absorbed in the gastrointestinal tract. Until recently, all strains of MRSA had been sensitive to vancomycin; however, vancomycin-resistant *S aureus* has also emerged and resulted in deaths in the United States.

The emergence of vancomycin-resistant MRSA poses a serious threat to patients and health care workers; if it is encountered, the patient should be isolated and the infection should be reported to public health authorities. Implement contact precautions, minimize the number of people with access to the colonized/infected patient, and provide dedicated one-on-one care to minimize exposure. Avoid transferring infected patients between or within facilities. If a transfer is necessary, fully inform the receiving institution of the patient's status.

Vancomycin-Resistant Enterococci

Enterococcus is a gram-positive bacterium normally found in the intestinal tract (ie, it is part of the normal flora); however, antibiotic-resistant species of *Enterococcus* have become a major cause of nosocomial infection in the United States. These bacteria rarely cause illness in healthy people, but can cause serious infections in immunocompromised, postoperative, and other seriously ill people. Because enterococcal bacteria colonize the intestinal tract, transmission is largely the result of direct person-to-person contact or indirect contact (eg, doorknobs and toilet seats) from inadequate handwashing after evacuation of feces.

Two types of antibiotic resistance are found in enterococci: intrinsic and acquired. Intrinsic resistance, a natural resistance found in the bacteria, is caused by the vanC gene. Acquired resistance is genetically transferred from another resistant organism. The two responsible genes are transmissible to other bacteria by plasmids and transposons, and they confer resistance to much higher levels of vancomycin. Another critical consideration is that the vancomycin-resistant genes present in vancomycin-resistant enterococci (VRE) have the potential to be transmitted to other gram-positive organisms, such as *S aureus*.

For these reasons, health care facilities should test all people at high risk for VRE; if found to be positive, patients should be isolated and standard precautions should be used during their care. Because patients can carry VRE organisms for long periods of time, particularly in their stool, the CDC and the Hospital Infectious Control Practices Advisory Committee recommend that isolation should continue until the patient has three sets of negative cultures from all appropriate sites taken at least 1 week apart.

In the critical care environment, there are many opportunities for contamination and subsequent cross-transmission of resistant bacteria. When transporting VRE-positive patients, infection control measures such as handwashing, patient isolation, use of protective barriers such as gloves and gowns, and proper disposal of contaminated materials are important in breaking the cycle of transmission.

Carbapenemase-Producing Gram-Negative Bacilli

Carbapenem antibiotics are unique in their ability to act against the gram-negative pathogens that are resistant to beta-lactam antibiotics such as cephalosporins. In recent decades, however, the clinical efficacy of these antibiotics has been threatened by the emergence of carbapenem-hydrolyzing beta-lactamases, increasing the threat of extreme drug resistance in gram-negative bacilli.

The *K pneumoniae* carbapenemase (KPC) is the most common carbapenemase in the United States. It was first described in a clinical isolate of *K pneumoniae* in the late 1990s in North Carolina and has since been identified in isolates from most other states. These organisms can easily spread by person-to-person transmission.

Carbapenemase-producing organisms can cause bloodstream infections, ventilator-associated pneumonia, urinary tract infection, and central venous catheter infections, as well as asymptomatic colonization. These organisms have been isolated from respiratory tract specimens, abdominal swabs, catheters, abscesses, urine, and surgical wounds. They have caused sporadic hospital-acquired infections, and outbreaks have been reported in both tertiary and community hospitals.

Bioterrorism

Bioterrorism (biologic weapons) is an emerging threat to the health and safety of the community. Many countries currently have or are developing offensive biologic weapons programs. Since the terrorist events of September 11, 2001, and with the continued threat of terrorism in the United States, there is increasing concern over the possibility of terrorists using biologic agents against civilian populations. To prepare for potential intentional biologic disasters, local, state, and federal officials have implemented education and training of first responders related to these threats **FIGURE 20-11**. The biologic agents that might potentially be used for bioterrorism are considered "the poor man's nuke," because just a small amount of agent can cause a large number of infections. For example, if 110 pounds (50 kg) of anthrax spores was released from a low-flying aircraft along a 1.25-mile (2-km) line above a population base of 500,000, it is estimated that there would be 125,000 people infected and 95,000 deaths. Anthrax spores can travel more than 12 miles (20 km).

The goals of a bioterrorism emergency response should be to contain the agent, protect critical personnel, and manage the health consequences of the event. Containment of a contagious disease resulting from deliberate release of an infectious agent requires that the incident

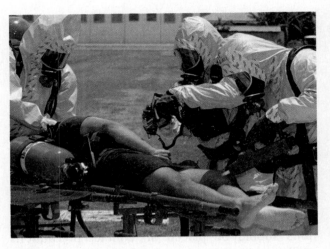

FIGURE 20-11 Homeland security and other government agencies training responders working to prepare for bioterrorism.

Courtesy of Photographer's Mate 1st Class William R. Goodwin/US Navy.

be recognized as a non-natural event based on a disease presentation that differs from the usual background of endemic infectious diseases that affect the community. The first cases are likely to go unrecognized, because most agents likely to be used for bioterrorism purposes present with initial nonspecific flulike symptoms such as fever, malaise, and headache; these types of findings make the biologic attack difficult to recognize during the initial stages of infection.

The covert release of a biologic agent could take place over a period of days to weeks, and it might be even longer before the initial cases of infection are identified, depending on the mode of transmission and the agent's incubation period. As the span of time between exposure and symptoms increases, so does the likelihood that the agent will become distributed over a wide geographic area and result in an epidemic.

It is also possible that the deliberate release of a biologic agent would be publicly announced by the attacker(s)—a possibility that poses a different set of problems for the emergency response system. Such an announcement would likely trigger large-scale panic, with many people calling for emergency services without actual need, overwhelming health care systems and preventing the efficient use of medical resources. The challenge would then be to differentiate those people who were actually exposed to the agent from those whose fear of the agent has caused them to seek care. A number of bioterrorism events have been publicly announced in the United States since 1998, though they were later determined to be hoaxes.

The CCTP must be prepared to deal with either scenario. Knowledge of epidemiologic principles is crucial in differentiating between the presentation of a naturally occurring disease and an unusual, non-natural event that should raise concern that a bioterrorist event has been initiated and that local emergency response systems should be activated.

The CCTP must maintain an index of suspicion regarding a potential threat because early symptoms may be nonspecific, but early treatment will be required to prevent severe injury or death. Before approaching a patient, CCTPs must always take steps to protect themselves first, using the standard precautions and additional precautions outlined in Table 20-9. In addition, immunologic protection is the responsibility of the CCTP. All CCTPs must stay current on required and recommended vaccines, keeping in mind what is appropriate for a particular patient population, and consider the appropriateness of being vaccinated against agents that may be exploited in bioterrorism attacks. For the most updated information, visit the CDC's website (www.cdc.gov) and search for the Infection Control Guidelines.

Exposure and Protection

CCTPs have unique occupational exposures to a variety of biologic, chemical, and physical hazards. These professionals are routinely in contact with critically injured and very sick patients, often in uncontrolled settings under emergent conditions. Resuscitating critically ill patients is associated with being in contact with potentially infected body fluids 31% of the time. CCTPs also care for trauma patients with open wounds that may be actively bleeding. Managing trauma patients is associated with exposure to body fluids 80% of the time. In the chaos of providing care for life-threatening diseases or injuries in unpredictable or dangerous conditions, adhering to well-established exposure prevention procedures is essential to protect the health of the CCTP.

The health risks associated with being a CCTP are not simply limited to blood or body fluid exposures; infectious agents also pose a significant risk. The greatest risks come from patients who are actively infectious but undiagnosed. Activities and tasks during which exposure may take place include the following:

- Patient assessment
- Airway management
- Establishing IV access
- Cleanup of the vehicle and equipment
- Assisting in childbirth
- Contact with blood or body fluids

CCTPs must take prophylactic measures to prevent infection prior to their exposure. Several effective strategies may be used to reduce the risk of contracting an infectious agent or transmitting infections to patients, but disease prevention is best achieved when the CCTP is fully prepared and properly equipped.

The use of PPE reduces exposure risks. Employers are required to provide their employees with PPE at no cost to the employee. Proper handling of contaminated medical devices, such as sharps, soiled bandages, linens, and reusable medical equipment, is also essential in reducing the risk of indirect transmission of infectious diseases **FIGURE 20-12**. In addition, the consistent implementation of isolation precautions is required to control the spread of infections to others.

Immunizations

The CDC recommends that all emergency medical care providers be vaccinated against preventable infectious diseases. The specific immunization

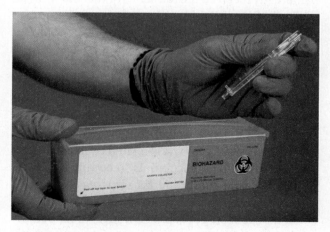

FIGURE 20-12 All sharps must be placed into containers that are puncture-resistant, closable, and leakproof, and that are labeled with the biohazard symbol.

© Jones & Bartlett Learning.

recommendations are based on the risk of exposure. Any new employees should not begin taking an active role in caring for patients until their immunization status is reviewed and up-to-date.

The current recommendations for emergency medical care providers call for them to obtain (and maintain) the following vaccinations:

- Measles
- Mumps
- Rubella
- Varicella (immunization or proof of prior infection)
- Hepatitis B
- Annual influenza
- SARS-CoV-2
- Pertussis
- Tetanus
- Polio
- Diphtheria
- Pneumococcal vaccine
- Meningococcal vaccine

If health care providers may be exposed to blood or other infectious materials during the course of performing their work-related duties, their employers are required to provide the hepatitis B vaccine to those employees at no cost. Ideally, the vaccination should start during the training period, before patient contact is initiated. The HBV vaccine is administered at 0, 1, and 6 months, with 95% of healthy adults developing protective titers on completion of the three scheduled immunizations. If an employee has already received the full series of vaccinations, an antibody titer should be drawn to verify immunity. The duration of the HBV vaccine's protection is unknown, but it has been shown to last at least 7 years in healthy young adults. If the CCTP has a medical contraindication to the vaccine, this issue should be documented and readdressed if the medical condition changes. Any employee who declines the HBV vaccine must sign a waiver releasing the employer from responsibility for work-related exposures.

The influenza vaccine is recommended for CCTPs because the influenza virus easily spreads through close contact with infected people via small aerosolized particles. Although most healthy adults are able to recover from influenza without significant morbidity, sick and older patients do not have the same immunologic reserves. On that basis, the influenza vaccine is recommended for CCTPs to prevent spread of the virus to their patients, thereby preventing significant morbidity and mortality.

Measles, mumps, and rubella—although now rare—can cause significant disease in susceptible people. The risk of contracting such infections is increased 13 times for the CCTP compared to the general public. Most adults in the United States have been immunized for these diseases, but immunity should be confirmed via a serologic titer. This is especially important for women of childbearing age to prevent the development of rubella syndrome in pregnancy.

The varicella vaccine is important for CCTPs for two main reasons. First, varicella is highly contagious, and varicella infection can cause serious complications in normally healthy adults. Second, vaccination of CCTPs is important to prevent the transmission of the disease to their patients. People with a positive history of chickenpox as children are considered immune, but if CCTPs' medical history of varicella is in doubt, they should undergo immunologic confirmation of serologic status. If an individual is seronegative and has no contraindications to the vaccine, the vaccine should be administered.

The FDA approved two SARS-CoV-2 vaccines under its emergency use authorization in December 2020. Since then, more vaccines have been developed and made available for public use. All of these vaccines are highly effective, are safe, and possess a favorable side-effect profile. Based on current understanding of the infectivity of SARS-CoV-2, it is believed that approximately 70% to 80% of the population must develop immunity to achieve the herd immunity required to end the COVID-19 pandemic.

Vaccines are considered a safe and effective way to prevent contagious diseases. All CCTPs are encouraged to discuss immunizations with their employer's health personnel or their own private physicians before vaccinations are given to ensure that there are no contraindications to receiving specific vaccines.

Needlestick Injuries

Needlestick injuries continue to occur, despite efforts to curtail these events. By law, all needlesticks and other injuries involving sharps contaminated by blood must be reported to the employer. Reporting sharps injuries is necessary when the injury occurs in the course of performing work-related duties and when the object causing the injury is contaminated with blood or other potentially infectious materials. It is not necessary to report sharps injuries that occur with clean objects. When reporting the injury, it is important to characterize it by type of injury (ie, splash, spill, stick, or cut) and by the type and amount of contaminating fluid (eg, saliva, semen, ascites, or blood). It is also important to determine the infectious status of the source patient. The Ryan White Act of 1990 mandated that all EMS personnel could request testing of a source patient to determine if they have been exposed to a life-threatening disease, with the results then being given to the affected employee. When the act was renewed in 2006, the clauses protecting emergency personnel were removed by Congress, making it much more difficult for the CCTP to gain access to this critical information.

The risk of a CCTP acquiring an infectious disease from a contaminated sharps exposure depends on the infectivity of the source and the type or severity of the exposure (**TABLE 20-10**). The larger the number of viral particles encountered during the exposure, the greater the risk is. The estimated risk of HIV transmission is 0.33% for hollow-bore needlesticks and 0.09% for mucosal contact; there are no known cases of HIV transmission for intact-skin exposures.

The following factors increase the risk of acquiring HIV after a needlestick injury:

- Deep injury
- Needle placed directly in a vessel (artery or vein)
- Visible contamination with source patient's blood
- Terminal illness in the source patient

Universal, Standard, and Transmission-Based Precautions

Universal precautions are the isolation precautions taken when dealing with all patients regardless of disease status. At a minimum, they require using gloves to prevent direct contact between the provider and the patient. The use of gloves, mask, goggles, gown, and shoe covers when handling body fluids or tissues of a patient who is not suspected of having a transmissible disease is called standard precautions. Think of a field childbirth: While the mother may be perfectly healthy, a health care provider would not think of assisting the delivery without wearing a gown, gloves, mask, goggles, and shoe covers.

More specific transmission-based precautions are used when the patient is suspected to have a specific illness. The type of PPE used is generally determined by the perceived means of spread of the pathogen—airborne, droplet, or contact. This logic actually is flawed, because few pathogens will fall neatly into these categories. Some pathogens spread by droplets may be small enough to travel via the airborne route in the right circumstances, whereas some pathogens spread by direct contact may be aerosolized into a droplet form.

Isolation Precautions

Two levels of isolation precautions are distinguished. The first level is designed for the care of all patients, regardless of their diagnoses, presumed infections, or immune status. The main goal of this level is to control nosocomial infection by facilitating the safe

TABLE 20-10 Risk of Infection and Required Postexposure Prophylaxis for the Three Most Commonly Transmitted Pathogens

Pathogen	Infection Risk After Needlestick	Postexposure Prophylaxis (PEP)	When to Act
Human immunodeficiency virus	0.3%	A 4-week course of a combination of either two or three antiretroviral drugs determined on a case-by-case basis	As quick as possible; preferably within hours
Hepatitis B virus	Approximately 0% with PEP; 6% to 30% without PEP	Hepatitis B immune globulin alone or in combination with vaccine (if not previously vaccinated)	Preferably within 24 hours; no later than 7 days
Hepatitis C virus	1.8%	No recommendation	Not applicable

Adapted from Centers for Disease Control and Prevention. Exposure to blood: what healthcare personnel need to know. https://www.cdc.gov/HAI/pdfs/bbp/Exp_to_Blood.pdf. Updated July 2003. Accessed February 13, 2021.

and proper handling of blood and other potentially infectious materials. The major features of these standard precautions are designed to reduce the risk of transmission of bloodborne pathogens from both known and unknown sources of infection. These precautions should be universally applied to all patients. They protect against contact with blood, body fluids, and secretions, regardless of the presence of visible blood, and contact with nonintact skin and mucous membranes.

The second level of isolation precautions comprises transmission-based precautions, which consist of isolation precautions designed to be employed during the transport of all patients with documented infections or those suspected to be infected with highly transmissible or epidemiologically significant infectious agents for which additional precautions above the first tier of standard precautions are warranted. The three means of providing transmission-based precautions are airborne, droplet, and contact precautions. These recommendations are intended to be used over and above the standard precautions and can be used singly or in conjunction, as the circumstances require.

It is likely that during the transport of critically ill patients from the scene to the tertiary facility, the etiology of any infectious disease will not be known. The risk of transmission is greatest before definitive diagnoses are made. Standard precautions should be implemented without fail on all transported patients. The use of transmission-based precautions should be implemented if the patient has any known risk factors or demonstrates suspicious symptoms or syndromes. It is much better to err on the side of prevention, until the definitive diagnosis can be determined, than to try to contain an infectious disease outbreak after the fact.

Certain clinical syndromes and conditions are red flags that indicate the empiric use of the second layer of precautions is warranted. Moreover, in the case of interfacility transfers, the infectious agent may have already been identified. If so, it is imperative that this information be known and contact precautions implemented accordingly.

Airborne Precautions

Airborne precautions include use of an N95 mask by CCTPs, a negative-pressure room (airborne infection isolation room) or transport vehicle, and an exhaust fan during transport. These precautions are designed to reduce the risk of transmitting infectious agents that are contained in airborne droplet nuclei or dust particles. Examples of agents carried in droplets (equal to or less than 5 μm) are tuberculosis (either pulmonary or laryngeal), measles, chickenpox, viruses that cause hemorrhagic fevers, and smallpox. Microbes found in droplet nuclei can remain viable when suspended in the air for long durations, and can be dispersed over a wide area, where they may be inhaled by susceptible hosts. Specialized air-handling equipment is required to provide airborne precautions.

Droplet Precautions

Droplet precautions include isolation of the patient and use of surgical masks by CCTPs. These precautions are designed to reduce the risk of transmitting infectious agents that are found in large-particle droplets (larger than 5 μm). Transmission via large-particle droplets requires close contact between the source of the infection and the susceptible recipient. Droplets are generated from infectious people during coughing or sneezing, and during invasive procedures such as suctioning of the airway, intubation, or bronchoscopy. Unlike airborne droplet nuclei, large-particle droplets travel only short distances and remain airborne for just a short time after being generated. Examples of infectious agents found in large-particle droplets include *S pneumoniae*, *C diphtheriae*, *Bordetella pertussis*, *N meningitidis*, *H influenzae*, and *Yersinia pestis* (pneumonic plague).

Droplet precautions should be implemented when caring for patients suspected or known to be infected with epidemiologically important pathogens that may be transmitted by infectious droplets. Eye protection (goggles, face shields, and safety eyeglasses) is recommended for use while transporting patients known to be infected with agents that can spread via the mucous membranes of the eye (conjunctiva), including *S aureus*, rhinovirus, adenovirus, herpes simplex virus, and any bloodborne agents (eg, HBV, HCV, HIV). These pathogens can be spread via respiratory droplets or by touching the patient and then touching the eyes with the contaminated hands or fingers. Eye protection prevents introduction of infectious agents into the conjunctiva. (Note: Full-face respirators also provide eye protection.)

Contact Precautions

Contact precautions for CCTPs include isolation of the patient, use of a gown (or uniform) and gloves, and, if warranted, face protection. These precautions are designed to decrease the risk of spread of infectious agents that can be transmitted by direct or indirect contact.

Direct contact transmission is defined as skin-to-skin contact and subsequent transfer of an infectious agent from an infected person to a susceptible host. It can occur during any patient care activity that requires physical contact between the CCTP and the infectious patient. Direct contact transmission can also occur between two patients, and between a patient and a family member.

Indirect transmission is the transfer of infectious agents from an infected patient through an intermediate (most often inanimate) object touched by or used during the care of the infected patient (ie, fomites). Examples of epidemiologically important infectious agents that can be transmitted via contact include MRSA, VRE, *Clostridioides difficile*, scabies, smallpox, and viruses that cause hemorrhagic fevers, and *Bacillus anthracis*.

Contact precautions must be employed during the transfer of patients known or suspected to be infected with microorganisms that can be transmitted through direct or indirect contact. Any equipment used on these patients during the course of a transport must be discarded or disinfected to interrupt the cycle of indirect transmission.

In addition, CCTPs must follow the regimen for donning and removing PPE that has been established by their agency's infection control staff **FIGURE 20-13**. In general, you should never touch your eyes, nose, or mouth with contaminated gloves or hands. After handling contaminated equipment, always wash your hands. If handwashing is not possible, use a waterless hand sanitizer and then wash your hands as soon as it is practical.

Handwashing

As noted repeatedly throughout this chapter, handwashing is the single most important measure employed to reduce the person-to-person transmission of infectious agents **FIGURE 20-14**. For the CCTP, washing hands between patient transports is logistically difficult because sinks are not available on transport units. Therefore, the conscientious CCTP must make a concerted effort to wash between patients and after touching any body fluid. Waterless antiseptic agents can be used as a substitute for washing until soap and water are available. The use of alcohol-based waterless handwashing antiseptic has been shown to improve rates of handwashing among health care workers. Therefore, transport units should be equipped with easily accessible dispensers of hand antiseptic to facilitate compliance in handwashing.

Alcohol-based hand antiseptics are not effective against all infectious agents. *C difficile*, for example, is not killed by hand sanitizers. Consequently, handwashing with soap and water between transports is of paramount importance. Handwashing should take at least 1 minute and should incorporate the often-neglected areas under the fingernails, the sides of the fingers and hands, and the wrists.

Personal Protective Equipment

PPE is specialized clothing or equipment worn by an individual that provides protection from a potentially hazardous agent. The employer is required to provide PPE at no cost to the employee. Such equipment should be readily available and used consistently by the CCTP. However, it is important to understand that PPE itself is not enough; it must be accompanied by a culture of safety within the organization. Training and practice are essential to the safe donning and doffing of PPE.

Clean, nonsterile, disposable gloves are standard equipment on critical care transport units. They must be donned by all personnel prior to initiating patient care. Gloves are worn by CCTPs for three important reasons:

- Gloves provide a protective barrier that can prevent gross contamination of the hands when exposed to blood and body fluids, and while working on patients with open injuries or nonintact skin.
- Gloves protect patients from the microbial agents that exist on the hands of the CCTP while the health care provider is performing invasive procedures.
- Gloves decrease the likelihood of transmission of microorganisms between patients or from fomites to patient—albeit only if the gloves are changed for each new patient encounter.

SEQUENCE FOR DONNING PERSONAL PROTECTIVE EQUIPMENT (PPE)

1. GOWN

- Fully cover torso from neck to knees, arms to end of wrists, and wrap around the back
- Fasten in back of neck and waist

2. MASK OR RESPIRATOR

- Secure ties or elastic bands at middle of head and neck
- Fit flexible band to nose bridge
- Fit snug to face and below chin
- Fit-check respirator

3. GOGGLES OR FACE SHIELD

- Place over face and eyes and adjust to fit

4. GLOVES

- Extend to cover wrist of isolation gown

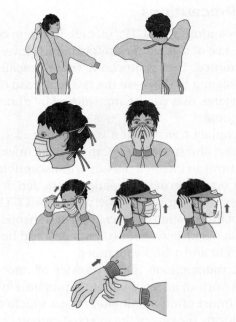

SEQUENCE FOR REMOVING PERSONAL PROTECTIVE EQUIPMENT (PPE)

1. GLOVES

- *Outside of gloves is contaminated!*
- Grasp outside of glove with opposite gloved hand; peel off
- Hold removed glove in gloved hand
- Slide fingers of ungloved hand under remaining glove at wrist
- Peel glove off over first glove
- Discard gloves in waste container

2. GOGGLES OR FACE SHIELD

- *Outside of goggles or face shield is contaminated!*
- To remove, handle by head band or ear pieces
- Place in designated receptacle for reprocessing or in waste container

3. GOWN

- *Gown front and sleeves are contaminated!*
- Unfasten ties
- Pull away from neck and shoulders, touching only inside of gown
- Turn gown inside out
- Fold or roll into a bundle and discard

4. MASK OR RESPIRATOR

- *Front of mask/respirator is contaminated—**do not touch!***
- Grasp bottom, then top ties or elastics and remove
- Discard in waste container

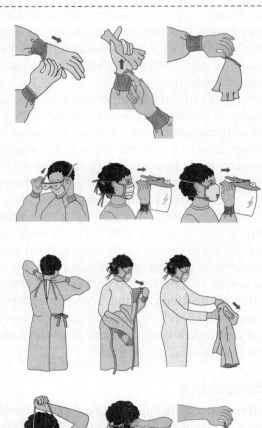

FIGURE 20-13 An example of a regimen for donning and removing personal protective equipment.

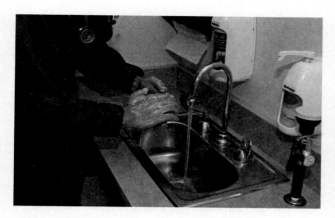

FIGURE 20-14 Handwashing is crucial to preventing the spread of infection.
© Jones & Bartlett Learning.

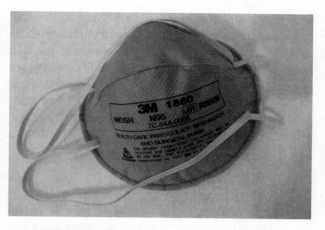

FIGURE 20-15 An N95 mask.
© The Venusian One/Shutterstock.

Gloves should be removed if torn, punctured, or contaminated with gross blood. They should be promptly discarded after each use and before touching noncontaminated objects or surfaces. After removing their gloves, CCTPs should wash their hands or sanitize them with an alcohol-based waterless handwashing antiseptic.

Masks, face shields, and eye protection are worn to protect the mucous membranes of the eyes, nose, and mouth during procedures and patient care activities that are likely to generate splashes or sprays of blood, body fluids, or excretions. Not all masks offer sufficient protection from airborne infectious agents. The N95 (or P100) mask must be worn when patients are known (or suspected) to be infected with agents that are transmitted by droplet nuclei. The N95 and P100 masks require proper fitting, so the CCTP should be fit tested before the need to use this equipment arises **FIGURE 20-15**. Studies have shown that the seals created by these masks, rather than the filters, are responsible for the protection created. A surgical mask alone is never sufficient in these situations.

Gowns are intended to protect the skin and prevent the soiling of clothing during procedures that are likely to generate splashes of blood or body fluids. They may not always be appropriate for the CCTP, however. Specifically, they may increase the risk of injury to the provider if that person tries to don the gown while in a moving vehicle. Also, when working in a small space, the gown may catch on equipment. If clothing or the gown becomes soiled, it should be removed as quickly as possible and disposed of properly,

and the provider should then wash their hands promptly to avoid the transfer of contaminants to the patient or the environment.

PPE donning and doffing procedures should be detailed on workplace checklists that are consistent with CDC guidelines. These procedures should be practiced to prevent skill deterioration over time.

Other Exposure Prevention Practices

It is important to notify the accepting institution of the nature of the patient's illness or potential infectious disease so that the receiving facility can arrange for proper isolation. This information should be communicated by the transferring facility, but it is always a good policy for the CCTP to also notify the receiving facility. Patients with epidemiologically important infections should be sufficiently isolated from other patients.

Patients themselves should be enlisted in the effort to prevent transmission by educating them on methods to prevent the spread of infectious organisms to other vulnerable people. Patients can wear masks while being transported between or within medical facilities. They can cover their mouths while coughing, frequently wash their hands, and refrain from sharing drinking cups or utensils with family and friends.

During the Ebola outbreaks, it was learned that health care provider behaviors can either help limit the spread of disease or increase the chances of spread. For example, many nurses in West Africa felt great compassion for infants and children infected with Ebola and would often pick them up to console them. This practice led to transmission of the virus to health care workers. The lesson learned was that health care providers should remain more than 3 feet (1 m) away from the patient except when necessary. The interview, for example, can be conducted from this distance. Other lessons learned from this epidemic included the following points:

- Enter the patient area only when you have a specific task to perform.
- Do not sit on the bed of an infected patient.
- When working with infected people and infectious environments, keep your hands in front of you to prevent unintentional contact with contaminated surfaces.
- Avoid walking backward in a contaminated environment to minimize potential contact with contaminated surfaces.
- When cleaning grossly contaminated surfaces, avoid spraying cleaners to avoid secondary aerosolization of the infectious agent.

During the 2003 SARS outbreak in Toronto, Canada, more than 850 paramedics had 1,166 reported potential exposures to this virus. Of these personnel, 436 were quarantined at home, where they were required to wear an N95 mask and take their temperatures twice daily. To limit the spread of the disease throughout the EMS community, the following measures were implemented:

- Headquarters and offices were closed to field personnel during the outbreak.
- All personnel were required to screen themselves before reporting to work.
- Any EMS worker showing symptoms was told to stop working in an EMS capacity.

Additional advice includes EMS workers limiting physical contact between themselves and emergency department personnel. Affectionate behaviors such as handshakes, hugging, and pats on the back, for example, should stop.

Dr. Gavin Macgregor-Skinner, a biosafety and disease containment expert at Penn State University, offered several thoughts with regard to the rationale for such steps:

1. Disease spread, unlike storms or some other natural disasters, is unpredictable.
2. The most devastating impact is often financial.
3. A virus is more nimble than your disaster plan.

4. If hospitals are your only battleground, then you have lost.
5. The experts will be wrong (often).
6. Your advice will have to sound certain when the facts and science are not.
7. In the absence of advice, your community will react.

Work Practice Controls

Control of the work environment and practices, when used consistently, can decrease the risk of contamination and subsequent transmission of infectious agents. Prohibitions against eating, drinking, smoking, applying cosmetics or lip balm, and handling contact lenses in the patient work areas, for example, help reduce the risks of uncontrolled exposures. Actions that cause splattering of fluids should be avoided. All single-use items should be disposed of immediately after they are used. Contaminated gloves must be removed before driving the ambulance and touching the steering wheel.

The proper handling of sharps is another method for controlling exposure risk in the work environment. Do not bend, remove, or recap needles. If you have no choice except to recap a needle (ie, no sharps receptacle is available, which in practice should never occur), use the one-handed "scoop" technique to do so. Shearing or breaking of needles should never occur. Dispose of sharps in an appropriate container as soon as possible after use. Sharps containers should be easily accessible, puncture-resistant, labeled or color-coded, and leakproof. They should not be filled beyond capacity and should be considered medical waste for disposal purposes.

Contaminated work surfaces must be decontaminated with an Environmental Protection Agency (EPA)–registered disinfectant on completion of the transport. All equipment used during the course of the transport must also be decontaminated. All bins, cans, and reusable receptacles must be decontaminated on a regular schedule and emptied after each use. Contaminated laundry should be placed into leakproof bags, labeled, and stored until proper disposal is possible. Regulated waste must be placed in closeable, leakproof containers designed for disposal. Regulated wastes include semiliquid blood or other potentially infectious materials, contaminated items that would release blood if compressed, and items that are caked with dried blood, contaminated sharps, and biological wastes. If droplet precautions are required, the transport vehicle should be equipped with a negative-pressure exhaust in the patient compartment. If this is not possible, the transport vehicle windows should remain open with the ventilation system set on "high" to move the air from within the vehicle to the outside.

TABLE 20-11 lists resistance of infectious organisms to disinfectants. Low resistance to disinfectant does not mean the organism is not dangerous;

rather, it simply means some organisms can be killed more easily than other organisms. CCTPs should assume that *all* patients transported carry infectious pathogens, and take the necessary steps to decontaminate the equipment and vehicle prior to the next transport. There are three levels of disinfection:

- **High-level disinfection** is used on inanimate objects to kill all microorganisms. It does *not* kill bacterial spores.

TABLE 20-11 Resistance of Infectious Organisms to Disinfectants

Resistance to Disinfection	Class of Organism	Organism Example	Class of Disinfectant	Example of Disinfectant
Most resistance	Spore formers	*Clostridioides difficile*	EPA-registered sporicidal	Glutaraldehyde; household chlorine bleach (1:10 dilution)
High resistance	Mycobacteria	TB	EPA-registered tuberculocidal	Combinations of high-percentage hydrogen peroxide (*not* household hydrogen peroxide) and peracetic acid; chlorine dioxide; various phenolics
Medium resistance	Nonenveloped viruses	Norovirus, poliovirus, adenovirus, papillomaviruses	EPA-registered effective agent against norovirus	Household chlorine bleach; Quats; high-percentage hydrogen peroxide (*not* household hydrogen peroxide)
	Cationic detergent (Quats)–resistant bacteria	*Pseudomonas aeruginosa* and *Acinetobacter baumannii*		Household chlorine bleach; high-percentage hydrogen peroxide (*not* household hydrogen peroxide) Note: Do not use Quats (Pseudomonads are resistant to Quats)
Low resistance[a]	Fungi	*Trichophyton* and *Aspergillus*	EPA-registered fungicidal	Quats
	Vegetative bacteria	*Staphylococcus aureus* (including MRSA, VRSA, and VRE)	Germicidal, EPA-registered anti-MRSA and anti-VRE	Quats; high-percentage hydrogen peroxide (*not* household hydrogen peroxide); various phenolics
Least resistance[a]	Enveloped viruses	Influenza, hepatitis B, and HIV	EPA-registered anti-hepatitis B and anti-HIV	Most environmental cleaning agents, including bleach; Quats; phenolics

Abbreviations: EPA, Environmental Protection Agency; HIV, human immunodeficiency virus; MRSA, methicillin-resistant *Staphylococcus aureus*; Quats, quaternary ammonium compounds; TB, tuberculosis; VRE, vancomycin-resistant enterococci; VRSA, vancomycin-resistant *Staphylococcus aureus*
[a] Low resistance to disinfectant does not mean the organism is not dangerous; it simply means some organisms can be killed more easily than other organisms. Assume all patients transported carry infectious pathogens and take necessary steps to decontaminate the equipment and vehicle prior to the next transport.

US Environmental Protection Agency. Selected EPA-registered disinfectants. https://www.epa.gov/pesticide-registration/selected-epa-registered-disinfectants. Accessed February 13, 2021.

- **Intermediate-level disinfection** is used on inanimate objects to kill *M tuberculosis*, vegetative bacteria, most viruses, and most fungi. It does *not* kill bacterial spores.
- **Low-level disinfection** is used on inanimate objects to kill most bacteria, some viruses, and some fungi. It does *not* kill *M tuberculosis* or bacterial spores.

CCTPs should strictly and properly decontaminate vehicles and equipment, change uniforms (including shoes/boots) or don new protective gowns over their uniforms and shoe covers, and perform handwashing between patient transports. Do not allow time constraints between transports to deter you from performing proper disinfection. Improper, cursory, or no **decontamination** of equipment and vehicles allows for transfer of organisms to susceptible hosts and spreads disease. Transport equipment, PPE, and personnel can all become reservoirs for disease organisms. To guard against this risk, ambulance and aircraft decontamination procedures in the presence of certain highly infectious agents should be included in organizational operations plans. The CDC has published specific guidelines for decontaminating EMS vehicles after exposure to a patient potentially infected with SARS-CoV-2 and similar guidelines for hospital facilities after potential exposure to the Ebola virus. The list of approved disinfectants differs for the two pathogens. Ebola virus is classified as a Category A infectious substance regulated by the US Department of Transportation's Hazardous Materials Regulations (49 CFR, Parts 171–180). Any item transported off-site for disposal that is contaminated or suspected of being contaminated with a Category A infectious substance must be packaged and transported in accordance with these regulations.

Use barrier protection (eg, plastic wrap) for surfaces of equipment touched frequently with gloved hands or those that are difficult to clean with disinfectants (eg, computer keyboards) or more likely to be contaminated with blood or body fluids. Do not attempt to clean and reuse disposable materials. Instead, place contaminated disposable materials (eg, dressings, gloves, syringes, tubing, gowns, surgical masks, and disposable N95 respirators) into appropriately marked biohazard containers. Always place reusable contaminated PPE (eg, eye protection, uniforms, and shoes/boots) into appropriately marked storage containers until it can be decontaminated; do not reuse contaminated PPE until it has been disinfected. All biohazardous waste and uniforms should be handled with gloved hands. Uniforms should first be autoclaved and then laundered after transporting patients with highly virulent and communicable diseases, such as SARS or avian influenza (H5N1); alternatively, they may be disposed of along with biohazardous waste. CCTPs should decontaminate the transport vehicle, shower and scrub with antibacterial soaps, and don street clothes prior to leaving for home after they transport patients with highly virulent and communicable diseases.

It is important to consider treatment of footwear worn during transport or to cover shoes during transport. Shoes should be considered part of the uniform and treated with disinfectant. Uniforms and shoes or boots should not be worn home routinely after patient transport.

Postexposure Risks and Protocols

After a blood exposure, the appropriate actions differ depending on the type of exposure. Generally, the appropriate actions taken should be immediately employed: Wash the area with soap and water, flush mucous membranes with copious amounts of water, and irrigate the eyes with sterile solutions of saline or water. Exposure should be reported immediately to supervisory personnel and those charged with managing blood exposures. Prompt reporting is paramount to ensure that any applicable postexposure treatment begins as soon as possible.

Hepatitis B

CCTPs who have received the hepatitis B vaccine are protected against contracting HBV from a blood exposure. Those who have not been vaccinated or have not yet achieved full immunity have a 6% to 30% risk of contracting HBV from exposure to HBV-infected blood. The precise level of risk depends on the severity of exposure and the hepatitis B antigen status of the source. Blood that is positive for the antigen is more likely to transmit infection.

Postexposure prophylaxis (PEP) is available for the prevention of seroconversion after a known exposure to HBV. HBIG is effective against HBV infection after an exposure has occurred, but its use is not without risk; therefore, the risks and benefits of treatment should be considered. Treatment is appropriate for unvaccinated

CCTPs who have been exposed to a source individual known to be positive for the hepatitis B antigen. If the exposed worker has not been immunized against hepatitis B, they should receive HBIG within 24 hours, followed by the hepatitis B vaccine within 7 days of the exposure. For this regimen to be effective, treatment should begin within 24 hours of exposure. HBV immunity should be confirmed by drawing an HB antibody titer (IgG). Any person whose antibody titer is negative and who has a blood exposure, regardless of the source person's HBV status, should receive the hepatitis B vaccine.

If the CCTP has been vaccinated against hepatitis B, but the anti-HB titer is unknown, an assay for anti-HB antibodies should be drawn to determine the person's immune status. This step should be followed by administration of HBIG and a booster dose of hepatitis B vaccine, if necessary.

Follow-up after PEP for HBV is not recommended because the treatment is highly effective. However, any symptoms associated with hepatitis should be reported to the CCTP's health care provider.

Hepatitis C

The risk of infection after direct nonintact skin exposure to blood infected with HCV is approximately 1.8%.

If the CCTP is exposed to HCV, no prophylactic treatment is available. Immune globulin is not recommended for exposures to HCV-tainted blood. As soon as possible after exposure, baseline laboratory studies should be performed, including liver function tests, and an HCV antibody titer should be drawn. These tests should be repeated at 4 to 6 months after exposure.

If and when signs of an acute infection develop, the HCV-exposed individual should receive interferon, unless the exposure involves a curable subtype of the virus. Acute infection is diagnosed based on increasing liver enzyme levels and detection of the viral RNA in the serum.

Human Immunodeficiency Virus

The average risk of contracting HIV after a percutaneous exposure to HIV-infected blood is 0.3%, or approximately 1 in 300. The risk after mucous membrane exposure is approximately 0.09%.

If the source patient is HIV negative, nothing needs to be done. If the patient's status is unknown,

the risks and benefits of PEP should be discussed with the employer's health personnel, and the exposed CCTP should be informed of the options available.

An individual exposed to the blood of a patient known to be HIV positive should be tested immediately following the injury, and again at 6, 12, and 24 weeks after exposure. CCTPs should be aware of and report any febrile illnesses that occur during the 12 weeks following such an exposure. They should also refrain from blood donation and unprotected sexual encounters during that same postexposure 12-week period, until their negative HIV status can be confirmed.

Providers should begin PEP medication regimens as soon as possible if exposed to HIV. Treatment should be continued for 4 weeks. These medication regimens should contain at least three antiretroviral drugs. Exposed providers should receive expert medical consultation and close follow-up, including counseling, baseline and follow-up HIV testing, and monitoring for drug toxicity. Follow-up appointments should begin within 72 hours of an HIV exposure.

Recommended Vaccines for Health Care Workers

During the course of their routine activities, health care workers may be exposed to serious, and possibly even deadly, diseases. They should remain current on all appropriate vaccines to reduce their risk of contracting or spreading vaccine-preventable diseases. They must take whatever actions are under their control to protect themselves, their patients, and their family members; vaccination is a simple and effective action toward this goal.

The CDC recommends that health care workers remain up-to-date on the following vaccines:

- Hepatitis B
- Annual influenza (flu)
- Measles, mumps, rubella (MMR)
- Varicella (chickenpox)
- Tetanus, diphtheria, pertussis (TDaP)
- SARS-CoV-2 (COVID-19)

Flight Considerations

There are no special patient care considerations specific to air medical transport of patients with infectious diseases. Follow the same precautions and management strategies discussed in this chapter. One important air medical service consideration when receiving a transport request is the length of out-of-service time required to properly disinfect or decontaminate the aircraft after completing the transport.

Summary

CCTPs must be aware of their risk of exposure to a variety of infectious agents. Their job inherently puts them at risk of contact with both contagious agents and those transferred by needlesticks or body fluids. A solid knowledge of microorganisms and the diseases they cause is necessary to ensure CCTPs' protection. An understanding of the fundamental principles of the immune system and infectious disease is an essential tool for medical care professionals. This knowledge, when applied to the critical care arena, will enable the CCTP to assess risks, minimize exposures, and prevent transmission of infection.

Case Study

You are dispatched to a rural hospital intensive care unit (ICU) for an emergency transfer to a tertiary hospital facility located approximately 90 miles away. En route to the transferring hospital, dispatch relays the following limited patient information. Your patient is a 37-year-old male with a past medical history of a kidney transplantation requiring lifelong treatment with immunosuppressant medications. He presented to the rural hospital emergency department 2 days ago with a fever of 102.2°F (39°C) and a mild nonproductive cough. He was diagnosed with COVID-19 following a positive reverse transcriptase polymerase chain reaction (PCR) result for SARS-CoV-2. The patient was admitted for observation to a general medical floor bed; however, last night he was transferred to the ICU and intubated for respiratory failure. The patient weighs 248 pounds (112 kg) and is 5 feet 10 inches tall. The patient is being transferred to the tertiary hospital for consideration of initiating veno-venous extracorporeal membrane oxygenation (V-V ECMO). Air transport is not available due to inclement weather. Once at the referring hospital, you anticipate a ground transport time of approximately 2 hours to the receiving facility.

On your arrival to the referring hospital ICU, you find a staff nurse and the referring physician at the patient's bedside. Both are dressed in full PPE and are attempting to suction the patient's endotracheal tube with assistance from the respiratory therapist. You and your partner note the droplet precaution signage posted on the patient's door and the isolation cart placed outside the patient's room.

After you and your partner don the appropriate PPE (gown, N95 mask, full-face shield, and gloves), the referring physician reports to you that the patient has been admitted for approximately 48 hours and has severely decompensated during that time. In the emergency department, his chest radiograph was normal; however, he was admitted to the hospital for observation given his immunosuppressed state and a new 2 L/min low-flow nasal cannula oxygen requirement. During the first 24 hours, the patient was maintaining his oxygen saturation on low-flow nasal cannula. He has been treated with IV dexamethasone daily. However, in the past 24 hours the patient complained of increasing shortness of breath and developed gradually worsening hypoxia, requiring the use of high-flow nasal cannula oxygen and a trial of awake prone positioning. A repeat chest radiograph last night showed extensive bilateral air space consolidations consistent with multifocal pneumonia. The patient was intubated early this morning for worsening hypoxic respiratory failure and increasing agitation using rapid-sequence intubation medications. The intubation was extremely challenging, requiring three attempts and the use of a hyperangulated video laryngoscopy blade.

In addition to his history of a kidney transplantation 7 years ago, the patient has a history of type 2 diabetes mellitus, hypertension, gastroesophageal reflux disease, and depression. He has no known drug allergies, smokes occasional marijuana, and drinks three to four beers per week. According to the patient's wife, he is compliant with his daily prescription regimen for his kidney transplant but does not like taking his other medications.

Your initial assessment of this patient reveals that he awakens briefly, for less than 10 seconds, to voice, which is consistent with a Richmond Agitation and Sedation Scale (RASS) score of negative 2. The patient appears comfortable and adequately sedated on a continuous fentanyl infusion at 100 µg/h IV (0.9 µg/kg/h) and midazolam 4 mg/h IV (36 µg/kg/h). His airway is secured with an 8.0 endotracheal tube at the 24-cm mark (teeth). The patient is being ventilated with synchronized intermittent mandatory ventilation (SIMV) with the following settings:

- Tidal volume: 440 mL (6 mL/kg based on a predicted ideal body weight of 73 kg)
- Rate: 24 breaths per minute
- Positive end-expiratory pressure (PEEP): 10 cm H_2O
- F_{IO_2}: 1.0
- Pressure support: 10 cm H_2O

The patient has a right internal jugular vein triple-lumen central line catheter in place and two peripheral IV lines in his bilateral antecubital fossa. The fentanyl and midazolam drips are infusing via the central line catheter, and normal saline is infusing at 150 mL/h in the right antecubital fossa peripheral IV. The second of two units of convalescent plasma has just finished infusing in the left antecubital peripheral IV. Prior to placing the transport monitoring equipment on this patient, the following vital signs are noted on the patient's ICU monitor: ECG, sinus tachycardia with occasional unifocal premature ventricular contractions; heart rate, 118–126 beats/min; blood pressure, 104/62 mm Hg; respiratory rate, 24 (SIMV); SpO_2, 83%; $ETCO_2$, 54 mm Hg; and rectal temperature, 101°F (33.3°C).

When you receive the transfer chart, you note the following laboratory values and radiology reports: WBC count, 17,000/mm³; BUN, 66 mg/dL; creatinine, 3.3 mg/dL; Na+, 133 mEq/L; K+, 5.0 mEq/L; Cl⁻, 104 mEq/L; glucose, 262 mg/dL;

D-dimer, 1.6 mg/L; pH, 7.26; PCO_2, 62 mm Hg; PaO_2, 50 mm Hg; and HCO_3^-, 22 mEq/L. Blood cultures show no growth to date, and a urinalysis is negative for infection. You verify on the patient's PCR that he is positive for SARS-CoV-2 and negative for influenza A and B. A CT scan performed this morning was negative for acute pulmonary embolism but did show bilateral multifocal ground-glass opacities, with notable consolidation in the bilateral lung bases consistent with COVID-19 pneumonia.

On completion of your assessment of this patient, you note the following findings. His skin is "hot" to the touch, dry, and pale. His pupils are equal and reactive to light at 3 mm. The trachea is midline, with no evidence of jugular venous distention. The remainder of the head/eyes/ears/note/throat examination is within normal limits for this patient. The chest wall has an equal symmetric rise and fall that is synchronous with mechanical ventilations. The breath sounds reveal bilateral coarse rhonchi, and the abdomen is soft with no distention noted. The pelvis is within normal limits, with an indwelling urinary catheter that provides for gravity drainage. There is no swelling, redness, or signs of infiltration noted with the central line or peripherally inserted IV lines.

Before you move the patient to the transport stretcher, your partner transfers the fentanyl, midazolam, and normal saline infusions to your transport pumps. The patient is placed on your unit transport monitor, with the ECG, SpO_2, $ETCO_2$ and noninvasive blood pressure alarms on and functioning. The patient remains on the hospital ventilator while your partner replicates the ventilator settings from the referring hospital. You then move the patient to your stretcher without incident as the transport ventilator is attached (alarms are on and functioning).

You depart the ICU with the transfer documentation and radiology studies to your awaiting ground unit. The patient is loaded and secured with all power and oxygen requirements transferred to the ground unit source. You depart the referral hospital and head to the receiving facility with routine traffic due to the weather conditions.

While en route to the receiving hospital, the patient's condition remains the same without any change in his hemodynamic or neurologic status. The SpO_2 remains in the range of 82% to 86% on the transport ventilator despite an FIO_2 of 1.0 and increasing his PEEP from 10 to 12 cm H_2O. Your partner contacts your dispatch center to relay an updated report and an estimated time of arrival to the receiving hospital. No orders are received from the receiving facility. You will be following your standing protocols for this patient's care.

1. When transporting a patient with a highly infectious disease, what procedural steps can you take to protect yourself, your partner, other health care workers, and bystanders from exposure?
2. When transporting a patient with a highly infectious disease, what equipment can be utilized to protect yourself, your partner, other health care workers, and bystanders from exposure?

Analysis

This is a complex scenario involving COVID-19 and severe acute respiratory distress syndrome (ARDS) in an immunosuppressed patient. Safe transportation of critically ill patients is always challenging; however, the COVID-19 pandemic has frequently highlighted some important considerations when transporting patients with a highly contagious disease. In this scenario, you must successfully manage the tenuous oxygenation and ventilation status of a patient in fulminant ARDS while also controlling for potential viral transmission. Careful execution of infection control measures to minimize nosocomial spread to other patients, health care workers, and bystanders is mission critical. Haphazard transportation resulting in breaches in infection control practices can compromise your health and that of countless others long after the transportation is complete.

The following interventions are infection control practices commonly used for the transport of patients with COVID-19. Many of these precautions are also directly applicable to the transport of other highly contagious infectious diseases:

- The transfer center should coordinate the timing of transport and the final location of patient placement within the receiving hospital to minimize use of and potential unnecessary contamination of holding areas.
- You should coordinate the route of transport within the hospital (eg, from ICU to ambulance bay or helipad) with infection control and public relation officers/hospital security. Ensure that the transport route is clear of bystanders and other nonessential staff before patient movement begins.
- Limit the number of personnel for patient transport as much as possible.
- Isolate the ambulance driver from the patient compartment and keep pass-through doors and windows tightly shut.
- When possible, use vehicles that have isolated driver and patient compartments that can provide separate ventilation to each area.
- If a vehicle without an isolated driver compartment and ventilation must be used, open the outside air vents in the driver area and turn the rear exhaust ventilation fans to the highest setting to create a pressure gradient toward the patient area.
- Before entering the driver's compartment, the driver (if involved in direct patient care) should remove their gown, gloves, and eye protection and perform hand hygiene to avoid soiling the compartment. They should continue to wear their respirator.
- Use single-use disposable or sterilizable medical equipment as much as possible (eg, intubation equipment).
- Wrap nondisposable transport equipment in transparent covers whenever possible. Ensure functionality of the wrapped transport equipment after attaching it to the patient.
- Use infusion pumps with extended tubing when available.
- When available and tolerated by the patient, use biocontainment measures (eg, IsoPod, IsoArk, plastic transparent patient drapes).
- Intubated patients should have a high-efficiency particulate absorbing (HEPA) filter inserted between the patient and the bag-mask device.
- A HEPA filter can also be placed on ventilators just prior to the exhalation valve to

prevent unfiltered expired gases from entering the transport vehicle.

- Nonintubated patients should don a surgical face mask in addition to other biocontainment efforts.
- Ensure use of a closed suction system.
- The transport team should don appropriate PPE (N95 mask or higher-level respirator, gloves, gown, and full-face shield) outside the patient room before beginning transport.
- The transport team must adhere to contact/droplet precautions throughout the transport.
- During transport, confirm that closed-loop communication can be conducted between all team members to ensure medical care and proper infection control practices are completed.
- Limit use of aerosol-generating procedures during transport. If possible, discontinue these procedures prior to entering the receiving facility or communicate clearly prior to arrival that these procedures are being performed.
- After transporting the patient, leave the rear doors of the transport vehicle open to allow for enough air changes to remove potentially infectious particles. The time needed to complete transfer of patient care and all documentation at the receiving facility should allow enough time for this to occur.

- After patient delivery to the designated COVID-19 unit, remove all protective equipment coverings.
- Doff PPE in the nearby designated area, taking care not to self-contaminate. An observer is recommended to overlook donning and doffing of PPE when possible.
- Perform hand hygiene immediately after transfer of patient care and doffing of PPE.
- Wear new PPE for the return trip to the station.
- Return all transport equipment to the station by the same ambulance for decontamination.
- When cleaning the vehicle, personnel should wear a disposable gown and gloves, as well as their respirator or face mask. A face shield or goggles should also be worn if splashes or sprays during cleaning are anticipated.
- Decontaminate the transport vehicle in accordance with standard operating procedures. All surfaces that may have come in contact with the patient or materials that became contaminated during patient care (eg, stretcher, rails, control panels, floors, walls, work surfaces) should be thoroughly cleaned and disinfected using an EPA-registered hospital-grade disinfectant in accordance with the product label.

Prep Kit

Ready for Review

- The immune system protects the human body from infection, and removes cells that are past the end of their life cycle, abnormal cells (eg, cancer cells), and damaged cells. While the function of the immune system is to protect against infection, it is also capable of causing damage.
- Better knowledge of diseases and how they spread, consistent use of personal protective equipment (PPE), and a mix of appropriate

responder behaviors and organizational policies can improve the safety of health care providers.

- An understanding of infectious disease, the ways in which the body responds to disease, and the methods used to reduce the spread of disease will help CCTPs keep themselves and their families, coworkers, and communities safe.
- For an organism to contract a disease, the host must be susceptible. Susceptibility is

Prep Kit Continued

determined by factors such as nutritional status, immune status, genetic makeup, living conditions, and exposure.

- The transmission of disease is a complex process. Disease can be transmitted directly through inhalation, ingestion, or direct contact with infectious agents, or indirectly via vectors, fomites (eg, contaminated fluids or equipment), or some other complex cycle of interactions.
- For the immune system to protect the body from invading microorganisms, it must be able to distinguish "self" components from "non-self" components or cells; it must be both highly specific and general; and it must provide protection that consists of several layers so that once one level of immunity has been breached, additional methods of fighting infection remain available.
- Immunity can be either innate (the type of immunity one is born with, which provides protection from invading pathogens despite a lack of prior exposure) or acquired (the type of immunity that develops as a result of interactions between components of the immune system and the invading microbe, which provides improved protection with repeated exposures to specific agents).
- Innate immunity is nonspecific, is activated immediately on invasion, and has no memory. The primary components of innate immunity are the skin, the mucous membranes, and their secretions, which provide mechanical and chemical barriers to invasion.
- Nonspecific factors of the immune system help limit growth of microorganisms within the body. They include cells such as natural killer cells, neutrophils, and macrophages; proteins such as complement or transferrin; and the body's general responses to invasion with actions such as fever or inflammation.
- Acquired (adaptive) immunity includes both humoral and cell-mediated immunity. Humoral immunity is provided by B cells through the production of antibodies and complement, whereas cell-mediated immunity is provided by T cells.

- Cytokines and macrophages are modulators of both cell-mediated and humoral immunity.
- Adaptive immunity results from the interaction of the agent with the host, is specific, improves with repeated interactions, allows for the development of immunologic memory, and can be either active or passive.
- Active immunity, an ongoing process of developing antibodies and activating T cells in response to invading agents, occurs either when an individual is exposed to microbes through the natural process of infection or when the immune system is artificially stimulated through a vaccine.
- Passive immunity is the process of giving an individual a preformed antibody (from a donor) in the event of an exposure to a pathogen to which the individual has not yet developed immunity.
- Antigens are a complex of proteins and/or sugars that are anchored into the cell membrane and displayed on the cell's surface. An antigen is recognized by the immune system as either self or non-self; in the latter case, it will induce a humoral or cell-mediated response.
- The immune system includes the central lymphoid organs (the thymus and the bone marrow), which are the site of synthesis and differentiation of immunocompetent cells.
- The peripheral lymphoid organs are where immunocompetency is expressed; they include the spleen, lymph nodes, tonsils, intestinal Peyer patches, and mucosa.
- Lymph nodes are made up of lymphoid tissues located throughout the body as single units or in chains of units; these nodes are especially prominent in the neck, axilla, and groin.
- T lymphocytes mature to express phenotypic markers or clusters of differentiation called CD markers. CD4+ cells (helper T cells) are regulators of the immune system; CD8+ cells

Prep Kit Continued

(cytotoxic suppressor T cells) kill virus-infected and tumor cells.

- B cells may differentiate into plasma cells that produce specific antibodies on encountering an antigen, or they may become memory cells.
- Antibodies are globulin proteins (immunoglobulins) that react to an antigen. There are five classes of antibodies: IgA, IgM, IgG, IgE, and IgD.
- The humoral (antibody-mediated) response is effective against agents that produce toxins, against bacteria that have polysaccharide capsules, and against some viral infections.
- In the primary immune response, antibodies do not appear until 7 to 10 days after the initial encounter. Upon a second encounter with the same antigen or a closely related antigen, a more rapid secondary response occurs, with antibody being detected in the serum in only 3 to 5 days, and antibody titers being produced that are much higher than those seen in the primary response.
- Cell-mediated immunity plays an important role in defending the host against intracellular infections, such as tuberculosis and gonorrhea, as well as viral infections, fungal infections, parasites, and tumors.
- Phagocytosis is performed by macrophages, neutrophils, and monocytes, which engulf and destroy bacteria, foreign antigens, and cellular debris.
- The targets of monoclonal antibodies can be a plasma protein, an IgG receptor, or an infectious organism. These therapies can be used to treat hematologic malignancies, solid tumors, autoimmune disorders, hypercholesterolemia, inflammatory bowel disorder, or even a drug overdose (digitalis overdose).
- An inappropriate or exaggerated immune response known as hypersensitivity (allergic) reaction occurs when a first encounter sensitizes an individual to an antigen and induces an antibody response, and then subsequent encounters with the same or a closely related antigen elicit the allergic response.

- Four major types of hypersensitivity reactions are distinguished: Types I, II, and III are antibody-mediated responses, whereas type IV is a cell-mediated response.
- Anaphylaxis is a serious allergic reaction that features a rapid onset of symptoms, has a variable clinical presentation, and, if unrecognized, can lead to respiratory arrest, circulatory collapse, and death. Common triggers for anaphylaxis include foods, drugs, antibiotics, and *Hymenoptera* venom.
- Most cases of anaphylaxis have cutaneous involvement, including flushing, itching, urticaria, or angioedema. Upper airway involvement may include changes in phonation, the sensation of throat closure or choking, cough, wheezing, and shortness of breath.
- The treatments for anaphylaxis focus on early recognition and the use of epinephrine to prevent progression to life-threatening symptoms. Airway management—including intubation, if necessary—and fluid resuscitation are key components of care for a patient experiencing anaphylaxis.
- In biphasic anaphylaxis, the initial resolution of symptoms is followed by a reappearance of symptoms that, if not anticipated, can pose a life threat.
- Immunodeficiency occurs when one or more of the components of the immune system become damaged or are nonfunctioning as the result of illness or lack of functioning immune cells, or when the immune system is intentionally suppressed by various immunosuppressant therapies.
- Critically ill patients have few reserves to fight infections as the result of a decrease in their host defenses and a loss of innate immunity.
- Features of chronic illness that decrease innate immunity include stress, malnutrition, invasive procedures, loss of physical barriers of skin and mucosal surfaces, and pathogenic bacterial overgrowth or bacterial growth in normally sterile tissue.

Prep Kit Continued

- Management of illnesses and injuries during transport of a transplant patient may be complicated by the side effects of immuno-suppressive medications (eg, hypertension, hyperglycemia, hyperkalemia, nephrotoxicity, and neurotoxicity) or by the patient's immuno-suppressed condition.
- The body's normal flora is composed of colonies of nonpathogenic species that assist the immune system by preventing the over-growth of pathogenic strains by using up avail-able nutrients, maintaining a certain pH level, and creating bacteriocins (antibacterial toxins).
- Many people requiring critical care transport are immunocompromised. CCTPs need to be keenly aware that these very sick patients can be inadvertently infected with opportu-nistic infections (ie, diseases caused by nor-mally nonpathogenic agents in patients with an abnormally functioning immune system).
- Pathogenic organisms cause disease because they possess unique factors that help them gain entry into the body, colonize and overcome host defenses, produce toxins that cause cytopathic effects, or do mechanical damage to the body.
- Properties of microbes that influence their virulence (ie, degree of pathogenicity) include host and tissue specificity (the ability of the organism to gain entry into a host), adherence to specific host cells, invasion of host tissue, evasion of host defenses, toxicity, and other characteristics of the pathogen such as anti-phagocytic properties.
- Virulence can be experimentally quantified by two measures: ID_{50} and LD_{50}.
- Typical portals of entry into the body for pathogens are broken skin, hair follicles, or sweat glands; the mucous membranes of the respiratory, digestive, and genitourinary tracts; and the conjunctiva of the eye.
- Once inside the body, the pathogenic organism must be able to adhere to specific cells to begin colonization.

- Bacteria are capable of producing two types of toxins: exotoxins, which are produced inside the cell and are released into surrounding tis-sues or fluids, and endotoxins, which are part of the gram-negative cell wall and are released when the bacteria are destroyed.
- Some organisms produce polysaccharide lay-ers and surround themselves with capsules or slime layers, which protect them against phagocytosis; others form biofilms, which are accumulations of bacteria and other organisms embedded in a matrix of polysaccharide along the surface of tissues.
- Viruses that enter the body bind to host cell surface receptors using viral proteins found on the surface of the virions; the resulting receptor-mediated endocytosis brings the virus directly into the cell.
- Once inside a cell, the virus particle may release its viral nucleic acid, allowing the viral DNA or RNA to direct synthesis of viral-encoded pro-tein and nucleic acid molecules and stimulate the process of new virion assembly.
- Viruses cause illness through three mecha-nisms: (1) production of viral-specific mole-cules that deplete the host cell's resources and lead to eventual cell death; (2) induction of programmed cell death (apoptosis); and (3) in-duction of large inflammatory responses.
- Epidemiology is the study of how disease is distributed within populations and the factors that influence that distribution.
- The incidence of a disease is the number of new cases of disease within a defined popula-tion over a defined period of time.
- The prevalence of a disease is the number of cases of disease detected in a specified period of time, regardless of when the illness was contracted.
- Factors such as the incubation period of a dis-ease or the presence of different carrier states may cause the disease to go undetected in an individual but can place others at risk for con-tracting the disease. For this reason, CCTPs

Prep Kit Continued

must use appropriate disease control and prevention practices when providing care to all patients, regardless of whether the patient is currently exhibiting symptoms.

- For a microorganism to infect and reinfect a host, it must have the ability to survive, duplicate or reproduce, and spread to new hosts. Reservoirs of infection provide a supply of nutrients and an environmental niche that support long-term microbial survival.

- Persons who are colonized by pathogenic species but do not have symptoms of the infection (ie, asymptomatic or latent carriers) can serve as sources of infection during extended hospital admissions.

- A reservoir refers to something that leads to the long-term survival of the organism. A broader concept is disease ecology, which refers to the totality of all components of the disease, environment, and host system.

- The health care environment itself may serve as a reservoir of infection. Some organisms can survive on inanimate objects, including durable medical equipment, for an extended duration of time.

- Direct contact involves person-to-person transmission of a pathogen (ie, no intermediate carrier is involved in the transfer).

- Horizontal transmission may occur through sexual transmission, exchange of respiratory droplets or secretions, and transmission by contact.

- Vertical transmission is the exchange of an infectious agent between mother and fetus in utero or during the birthing process.

- Indirect transmission occurs when there is an intervening step in the transmission from reservoir to susceptible host. The intermediate step involves an inanimate object (fomite), such as towels, bedding, thermometers, and contaminated syringes.

- Many infectious diseases are transmitted through the use of a medium such as water, food, air, or contaminated body fluids. Water can be either the reservoir of disease or a vehicle for the transmission of that disease.

- Vector transmission is the movement of a pathogen from an infected organism to a susceptible host via an insect or other animal.

- Meningitis (ie, the inflammation of the leptomeninges) is a serious medical condition that can be caused by bacterial, viral, or fungal infectious agents.

- Bacterial meningitis has an acute onset and is a medical emergency that requires prompt diagnosis and treatment to preserve life and neurologic function. The classic triad of symptoms observed in patients with this disease consists of fever, nuchal rigidity, and altered mental status.

- Most cases of bacterial meningitis are observed in adults and can be caused by a variety of bacterial species, including *Neisseria meningitidis*, *Streptococcus pneumoniae*, and *Haemophilus influenzae*.

- The severity of the symptoms and the disease is less serious with viral meningitis than with bacterial meningitis, and complete recovery can occur in 2 to 7 days without medical intervention.

- Respiratory syncytial virus causes seasonal outbreaks of acute respiratory tract infections.

- The most common cause of cellulitis is beta-hemolytic streptococci, most commonly group A *Streptococcus* or *S pyogenes*; *S aureus* (including methicillin-resistant strains) is a notable but less common cause.

- The vast majority of erysipelas (a specific type of cellulitis) cases are caused by beta-hemolytic streptococci.

- Necrotizing fasciitis is a limb- or life-threatening infection of the soft tissue that affects the subcutaneous tissues, fat, and fascia but usually spares the skin and muscle. Prompt diagnosis and treatment with antibiotics and complete surgical debridement are important to reduce the high mortality rate associated with this disease.

Prep Kit Continued

- Epiglottitis (the result of an infected and inflamed epiglottis, aryepiglottic folds, and/or surrounding tissues) can occur at any age. Since the introduction of the Hib vaccine, the incidence of epiglottitis has been drastically reduced in vaccinated children. Because of its severity and rapid progression to airway obstruction as well as the continued infection patterns in adults, CCTPs should be familiar with this disease's clinical presentation and treat patients promptly with empiric antibiotics.

- Tuberculosis (TB) is caused by infection with *Mycobacterium tuberculosis*, which is transmitted via respiratory droplets from the cough of an infected person to the respiratory epithelium of a susceptible person.

- In patients with TB, the first site of infection is the lungs, but the pathogen can also spread to the kidney or spine.

- Most people infected with *M tuberculosis* are asymptomatic. Patients with full-blown pulmonary tuberculosis typically exhibit five symptoms: cough, fever, weight loss, night sweats, and fatigue.

- The emergence of drug-resistant strains of TB has precipitated the use of a multidrug regimen for cure of this disease. The individual drugs used may vary slightly, but the mainstay of therapy is isoniazid.

- Multidrug-resistant TB is TB that is resistant to at least two of the standard anti-TB medications, isoniazid and rifampin. Limited treatment options are available for patients with this form of the disease.

- When transporting a patient with suspected or known TB, CCTPs should place a mask on the patient (if tolerated) and wear masks themselves.

- CCTPs should comply with yearly purified protein derivative (PPD) testing, which identifies antibodies to TB, to determine their personal history of exposure to TB.

- If care was provided for a patient known to have TB and exposure was a possibility, providers should get a PPD test 6 weeks after that exposure to assess their health status.

- Pneumonia is an infection of the lung parenchyma that may be caused by bacterial, viral, or fungal agents; it is a major cause of death in the United States.

- Many different bacterial species cause pneumonia, including *Streptococcus pneumoniae*, *Haemophilus influenzae*, *Staphylococcus aureus*, *Chlamydia pneumoniae*, and *Legionella pneumoniae*. *Mycoplasma pneumoniae* and viruses cause atypical pneumonias.

- Nosocomial or hospital-acquired pneumonia is a pneumonia that occurs in a hospitalized patient 48 hours or more after admission to the hospital, but that was not apparent at the time of admission.

- Ventilator-associated pneumonia is a type of hospital-acquired pneumonia that occurs in ventilated patients and appears more than 48 hours after endotracheal intubation.

- Health care–associated pneumonia is pneumonia that occurs in nonhospitalized patients who have contact with health care facilities or personnel, such as residents of long-term health care facilities, patients undergoing hemodialysis, and patients who have had a recent admission to an acute care facility.

- *Pneumocystis jirovecii* pneumonia is a fungal infection that is seen in patients with immunosuppression, such as those taking antirejection therapy for solid-organ transplantation or those infected with HIV. It is included in the list of AIDS-defining illnesses.

- CCTPs should use standard precautions when caring for patients suspected of or diagnosed as having pneumonia. If a patient is coughing, place masks on both the patient (if tolerated) and the CCTP; wear gloves; use good handwashing technique between transports; and clean and decontaminate equipment, including the transport vehicle, prior to undertaking further transports.

Prep Kit Continued

- It is especially important to decontaminate equipment such as laryngoscopes and suction equipment after transportation of patients with oral candidiasis (thrush) or patients infected with *P jirovecii*.
- When influenza undergoes a major antigenic drift or a novel combination of hemagglutinin and neuraminidase emerges (antigenic shift), people have little or no antigenic protection from prior infections; pandemics of influenza may then break out and spread quickly.
- Few treatments are available for influenza except supportive therapy; however, when this disease is diagnosed within the first day of symptoms, treatment with an antiviral medication may reduce the severity and duration of symptoms.
- Herpesviruses are noted for their ability to cause latent infections: The acute viral syndrome is followed by a symptom-free period during which the virus is inactive. Reactivation of the virus can occur when the patient is immunosuppressed or through inciting agents.
- Six pathogenic members of the herpesvirus family cause disease in humans: herpes simplex types 1 and 2, varicella zoster virus, cytomegalovirus, Epstein-Barr virus, and human herpesvirus 8. Epstein-Barr virus and human herpesvirus 8 are associated with the development of Burkitt lymphoma and Kaposi sarcoma, respectively.
- HSV-1 and HSV-2 can cause infection of the fingers with recurring painful blisters, a condition called herpetic whitlow.
- Hepatitis (inflammation of the liver) can be caused by exposure to infectious agents (usually viral), toxins (eg, alcohol), or drugs (eg, acetaminophen). The course of the illness ranges from acute to chronic, and the severity ranges from mild to life threatening.
- Hepatitis A virus (HAV) is usually transmitted via the fecal-oral route, although sexual and parenteral transmissions are possible. Large-scale outbreaks can occur, usually as the result of contamination of food or drinking water.

- HAV infection can be prevented by active immunization with the HAV vaccine or by passive immunization with immune globulin administered before or after a known exposure.
- Hepatitis B virus (HBV) is transmitted through parenteral routes (ie, non-oral transmission). Health care providers are considered an at-risk group for this infection and should receive the HBV vaccine series, with their immunity subsequently being confirmed by titer.
- Unlike HAV, HBV can induce other disease states in addition to causing acute infections—specifically, acute hepatitis, fulminant hepatitis (severe inflammation of the liver, accompanied by rapid destruction of the liver leading to liver failure), and chronic hepatitis (chronic asymptomatic carriers).
- Prevention of HBV infection involves screening the blood supply and removing HBV-contaminated units and donors from the blood donation pool.
- Hepatitis C virus (HCV) is transmitted parenterally through transfusion or IV drug use, through sexual contact with infected people, and from mother to infant. In most cases, acute infection leads to chronic infection, with the disease eventually progressing to hepatitis and fibrotic liver disease (cirrhosis).
- There is no cure for HCV, nor is a vaccine available to prevent infection; the goal of treatment is to prevent the development of cirrhosis and liver failure.
- Hepatitis delta virus (HDV) is transmitted parenterally, but can replicate only with the aid of HBV. All patients with severe HBV infections should be tested for HDV coinfection or superinfection.
- Human immunodeficiency virus causes HIV disease, which in turn can lead to AIDS. This retrovirus infects T lymphocytes and other cells that display the CD4 surface protein and is notable for causing "slow" infections with long incubation periods.
- Transmission of HIV infection occurs through the transfer of infected cells or free virus from

Prep Kit Continued

one individual to another. Transmission can occur both horizontally (via sexual contact or by exposure to infected blood) and vertically (from mother to neonate across the placenta or during delivery and from an infected mother through breast milk).

- For CCTPs, exposure to patients with HIV infection is a potential risk for disease contraction. Prevention of exposure (eg, through needlesticks) is the most important method of protection for health care workers.

- HIV infection can be divided into two stages: acute infection and chronic infection Chronic HIV infection can be further subdivided into the following stages:
  - Chronic infection, without AIDS
  - AIDS, characterized by a CD4 cell count <200 cells/µL or the presence of any AIDS-defining condition
  - Advanced HIV infection/AIDS, characterized by a CD4 cell count <50 cells/µL

- Antibodies to HIV are not detected in the blood until 3 to 4 weeks after the initial infection. The person is capable of spreading the disease through sexual or blood contacts during this window of time, even though the HIV antibody test result will be negative prior to seroconversion.

- Criteria for the diagnosis of AIDS include HIV infection with a CD4+ helper T cell count of less than 200 cells/µL and/or the presence of an AIDS-defining condition.

- Although an HIV-infected patient might be asymptomatic and symptoms remain latent, the virus continues actively replicating within the lymph nodes.

- Patients with HIV often present many years after the initial infection or acute stage of the disease, because in the initial stages the disease is often mild and the symptoms are nonspecific.

- For many patients with HIV, the illness is noticed when the patient begins to experience symptoms; eventually, loss of cell-mediated immunity predisposes the host to many opportunistic infections.

- In HIV-infected patients, the viral load is estimated by determining how much viral RNA is present in the blood. The viral load indicates the magnitude of HIV replication and its associated rate of CD4 cell destruction. This measurement is the most accurate indicator of the risk for disease progression and is used in planning and monitoring antiretroviral therapy.

- Six classes of antiretroviral drugs are currently used to treat HIV infection: nucleoside analog reverse transcriptase inhibitors, protease inhibitors, non-nucleoside reverse transcriptase inhibitors, integrase strand transfer inhibitors (INSTIs), and the two entry inhibitor classes—CCR5 antagonists and fusion inhibitors.

- The goal of current therapies for HIV infection is to prolong life—by preventing opportunistic infections and malignancies, and slowing the rate of virus production—while maintaining the best possible quality of life.

- Rickettsial diseases are transmitted via tick bite; they include Rocky Mountain spotted fever, ehrlichiosis, and anaplasmosis.

- Rocky Mountain spotted fever should be considered a possible diagnosis in all patients presenting with fever and having suspected or known tick exposure. It begins acutely with fever accompanied by one or more of the following: headache (usually severe), rash, muscle aches, nausea and vomiting, and malaise. Treatment is with doxycycline (or a similar antibiotic).

- Emerging infectious diseases (diseases whose incidence has increased dramatically in the past 20 years) are particularly damaging to older adults and immunocompromised people, such as those living with HIV disease, those receiving immunosuppressive therapy (eg, recipients of organ transplants), and those who are immunosuppressed as a result of their treatments for cancer.

- Severe acute respiratory syndrome is an emerging lower respiratory tract illness that is associated with high morbidity and mortality.

Prep Kit Continued

- Infection with *E coli* O157:H7 may occur after eating undercooked, contaminated ground beef; drinking unpasteurized milk and fruit drinks; eating unwashed lettuce or sprouts; eating salami; swimming in or drinking sewage-contaminated water; or having person-to-person contact.

- West Nile virus is a mosquito-borne pathogen that occasionally leads to meningitis or encephalitis; there is no cure for West Nile virus encephalitis.

- Antibiotics are compounds that are produced by bacteria or fungi that inhibit the growth of bacteriostatic organisms or kill other bacterial organisms (ie, are bactericidal).

- All antibacterial agents follow the same basic principle in their actions: They target bacterial proteins, processes, or cellular components that are not found in human cells.

- The relatively few antiviral treatments available work by interrupting the viral replication cycle at a specific step.

- Antifungal therapies typically bind with components in the fungal cell wall, making the membrane less fluid and more susceptible to rupture, which leads to cell death.

- Almost all important pathogenic bacteria have demonstrated resistance to currently available FDA-approved antibiotics.

- Three important factors that contribute to the emergence of resistant bacteria within a given population or community are misuse use of antibiotics, poor infection control, and importation or intrusion of already resistant strains.

- Antibiotic resistance occurs when bacteria acquire new properties through mutation, protein alteration, or conjugative transfer of plasmid-encoded resistance factors.

- Health care workers are a major source of cross-infection between critically ill patients, and handwashing is the single most important step that they can take to reduce the spread of infection.

- Methicillin-resistant *Staphylococcus aureus* (MRSA) can colonize a variety of tissues,

causing infections such as cellulitis, cutaneous abscesses, wound infections, osteomyelitis, septic arthritis, endocarditis, pneumonia, and septicemia.

- High rates of MRSA are found among residents of long-term care facilities, but serious infections with MRSA are more prevalent in the acute care setting.

- Risk factors for colonization with MRSA include dialysis, diabetes, use of injectable drugs, chronic skin conditions such as decubitus ulcers, and a history of prior antibiotic use.

- The emergence of vancomycin-resistant MRSA poses a serious threat to patients and health care workers. Any patient with this type of infection should be isolated, and the infection should be reported to public health authorities.

- Although antibiotic-resistant species of *Enterococcus* rarely cause illness in healthy people, they can cause serious infections in immunocompromised, postoperative, and other seriously ill people.

- When transporting patients infected with vancomycin-resistant enterococci, providers should implement infection control measures such as handwashing, patient isolation, use of protective barriers such as gloves and gowns, and proper disposal of contaminants.

- Knowledge of epidemiologic principles is crucial in differentiating between the presentation of a naturally occurring disease and an unusual, non-natural event that should raise concern that a bioterrorist event has occurred and that local emergency response systems should be activated.

- In bioterrorism scenarios, the CCTP must maintain an index of suspicion regarding a potential threat because early symptoms of exposure may be nonspecific, but early treatment will be required to prevent severe injury or death. Providers must always take steps to protect themselves before approaching patients and should take responsibility for implementing immunologic protection.

Prep Kit Continued

- The health risks associated with the CCTP's job are not limited to blood or body fluid exposures; rather, the greatest risk comes from patients who are actively infectious but undiagnosed.
- Steps to reduce exposure risks include using appropriate PPE; properly handling contaminated medical devices; and implementing isolation precautions to control the spread of infection to others.
- The Centers for Disease Control and Prevention recommends that all emergency medical care providers be vaccinated against the following preventable infectious diseases: measles, mumps, rubella, varicella, hepatitis B, influenza (annual), pertussis, tetanus, polio, diphtheria, pneumococcal vaccine, and meningococcal vaccine.
- By law, all needlesticks and other injuries with sharps contaminated by blood must be reported to the CCTP's employer.
- Universal precautions are recommended to prevent transmission of bloodborne pathogens such as HIV and hepatitis B and C; they stipulate use of gloves, gowns, or aprons (or uniforms) and masks or other eye protection to reduce exposure of the skin (especially abraded or broken skin) and mucous membranes.
- After a significant exposure, both the source patient and the health care worker should be tested for baseline values, and the exposed health care worker should receive follow-up testing at 6 and 12 weeks and at 6 months.
- Standard precautions are used with all patients; they protect against contact with blood, body fluids, and secretions, regardless of the presence of visible blood, and against contact with nonintact skin and mucous membranes.
- Transmission-based precautions are isolation precautions that are designed to be employed during the transport of all patients who have documented infection or who are suspected to be infected with highly transmissible or epidemiologically significant infectious agents.

- Airborne precautions include use of an N95 mask by CCTPs, use of a negative-pressure room (airborne infection isolation room) or transport vehicle, and use of the exhaust fan during transport.
- Droplet precautions include isolation of the patient and use of surgical masks by CCTPs (or keeping at a distance of 3 feet [1 m]).
- Contact precautions include isolation of the patient, use of a gown (or uniform) and gloves, and, if warranted, face protection by CCTPs.
- Clean, nonsterile, disposable gloves are standard equipment on critical care transport units and must be donned by all personnel prior to initiating patient care.
- Masks, face shields, and eye protection are worn to protect the mucous membranes of the eyes, nose, and mouth during procedures and patient care activities that are likely to generate splashes or sprays of blood, body fluids, or excretions.
- Gowns are used to protect the skin and to prevent the soiling of clothing during procedures that are likely to generate splashes of blood or body fluids.
- Proper handling of sharps includes not attempting to bend, remove, or recap needles; not shearing or breaking needles; and disposing of sharps into an appropriate container as soon as possible after use.
- Contaminated work surfaces and all equipment used during the course of the transport must be decontaminated with an EPA-registered disinfectant on completion of the transport.
- Contaminated laundry should be placed into leakproof bags, labeled, and stored until proper disposal is possible. Likewise, regulated waste must be placed in closeable, leakproof containers designed for disposal.
- Do not allow time constraints between transports to deter proper disinfection.
- In case of a blood exposure, wash the area with soap and water, flush the mucous membranes

Prep Kit Continued

with copious amounts of water, irrigate the eyes with sterile solutions of saline or water, and report the exposure immediately to supervisory personnel and those assigned to manage blood exposure issues.

- Postexposure prophylaxis is available for the prevention of seroconversion after a known exposure to hepatitis B or HIV, but not after exposure to hepatitis C.

Vital Vocabulary

active immunity Production of a specific antibody in response to an infection or antigen.

adaptive immunity The immunity the body develops as part of exposure to an antigen or through vaccination; also called acquired immunity.

anaphylaxis A serious systemic allergic reaction that has a rapid onset and a variable clinical presentation.

antigen An agent that stimulates the formation of specific protective proteins called antibodies.

antigenic drift A series of small genetic changes in a virus that alter the virus just enough that antibodies generated in previous infections no longer recognize the viral epitopes or surface proteins and, therefore, do not protect the body from the symptoms of a new infection.

antigenic shift More drastic genetic changes in a virus, in which the protein structure of one or both of the spike proteins undergoes changes.

apoptosis Programmed cell death.

bactericidal Capable of killing bacteria.

bacteriostatic Capable of inhibiting bacterial growth.

carrier A person or animal that is infected with a disease, but does not express symptoms of that disease.

decontamination Use of chemical, physical, or other means to remove, inactivate, or eradicate harmful microorganisms from people, surfaces, or objects.

dyscrasia In hematology, a disorder of the cellular elements of blood.

endemic A pattern of disease occurrence in which some cases of a disease are always present within a given population, and their numbers are expected and predictable.

endotoxin A toxin that is a structural component of bacterial cells and is not released until the bacteria are destroyed.

epidemic A pattern of disease occurrence in which the number of cases of a disease clearly rises (above a threshold level) in a given time or geographic area.

epidemiology The study of disease distribution within populations and the factors that determine that distribution.

epitope The specific portion of the antigen that is recognized by the antibody or B cell.

etiology The cause of a disease.

exotoxin A toxin produced by a bacterium inside the cell and secreted into surrounding tissues or fluids.

fecal–oral route A route of transmitting infectious organisms from one individual to another; commonly, enteric bacteria or viruses are shed in the feces, spread via contamination of food or water sources, and ingested by other people.

fomite An inanimate object that is capable of transmitting infectious organisms from one individual to another.

health care–associated pneumonia (HCAP) Pneumonia that occurs in nonhospitalized patients who have contact with health care facilities or personnel.

Prep Kit Continued

high-level disinfection Treatment used on inanimate objects that kills all microorganisms, but does *not* kill bacterial spores.

hospital-acquired pneumonia (HAP) Pneumonia that occurs in a hospitalized patient 48 hours or more after admission to the hospital, but that was not apparent at the time of admission.

hypersensitivity A reaction consisting of an exaggerated or inappropriate immune response that occurs after a person comes in contact with a substance the body perceives as harmful.

immunity Protection from infection, provided by a complex system of substances, cells, and tissues that exist to protect the human body from infection.

immunocompromised Unable to mount a normal immune response as the result of disease (eg, AIDS), chemotherapy treatment, or certain other medical treatments.

immunodeficiency An abnormal condition in which some part of the body's immune system is inadequate, such that resistance to infectious disease is decreased.

incidence The number of new cases of a disease within a defined population over a defined period of time.

indicator conditions Rare or unusual diseases associated with an immunocompromised state; also called AIDS-defining diseases.

innate immunity The type of immunity that an individual is born with, such as that provided by the skin and mucous membranes.

intermediate-level disinfection Treatment used on inanimate objects that kills *Mycobacterium tuberculosis,* vegetative bacteria, and most viruses and fungi, but does *not* kill bacterial spores.

isolation precautions Measures taken to prevent contact with pathogens, including airborne, droplet, and contact precautions.

low-level disinfection Treatment used on inanimate objects that kills most bacteria, some viruses, and some fungi, but does *not* kill *Mycobacterium tuberculosis* or bacterial spores.

meningitis An umbrella term referring to five types of inflammation of the leptomeninges, the membranes that cover and enclose the spinal cord and brain.

monoclonal antibodies Antibodies in which large quantities of an antibody from a single B-cell clone are produced to protect against a specific pathogen.

necrotizing fasciitis A limb- or life-threatening infection of the soft tissue that affects the subcutaneous tissues, fat, and fascia.

nosocomial Infections acquired during hospitalization or a nursing home stay.

opsonization The process of making bacterial cells more susceptible to the action of phagocytosis by the action of binding an antibody to the pathogen's cell membrane.

palpable purpura Relatively large (greater than 3 mm) areas of bleeding under the skin.

pandemic A worldwide epidemic.

passive immunity Short-lived immunity acquired from placental transfer, antibodies in the mother's milk, or antiserum administered intravenously.

pathogen Any microbe capable of causing a disease state.

petechial lesions Small areas of bleeding under the skin (pinpoint).

phonation The process by which the vocal cords create sound.

plaque-forming unit The number of viral particles capable of forming plaques per a certain volume.

prevalence The total number of cases of a disease within a population, including both old and new cases of the disease.

prodrome Early symptoms indicating the development of disease.

Prep Kit Continued

prophylaxis Treatment of disease before it occurs (ie, to prevent the disease).

pruritus Itching.

quiescent A latent state, as occurs with a dormant virus or bacterium, in which an infected patient will exhibit few to no symptoms.

reservoir of infection A host that provides a supply of nutrients and an environmental niche that enable long-term microbial survival.

respiratory syncytial virus (RSV) A labile paramyxovirus that produces a characteristic fusion of human cells in a tissue culture known as the syncytial effect; it can affect both the upper and lower respiratory tracts but is more prevalent with the lower respiratory tract, causing pneumonia and bronchiolitis.

rickettsial diseases Diseases transmitted via tick bite; the three major diseases in this class are Rocky Mountain spotted fever, ehrlichiosis, and anaplasmosis.

seroconversion Development of antibodies, measured in the serum, in response to an infection or vaccine.

severe acute respiratory syndrome (SARS) A highly contagious, potentially life-threatening lower respiratory tract illness that usually starts with flulike symptoms, including fever, headache, and muscle aches, followed within 2 to 7 days by a dry cough and pneumonia.

sporadic A pattern of disease occurrence in which a disease manifests only occasionally.

standard precautions The use of gloves, mask, goggles, gown, and shoe covers when handling body fluids or tissues of a patient who is not suspected of having a transmissible disease.

tolerance In immunology, the ability to distinguish between self and non-self cells.

transmission-based precautions Specific precautions used when a patient is suspected to have a particular illness.

universal precautions The isolation precautions taken when dealing with all patients regardless of their disease status.

vector An organism that carries a disease-causing microorganism from one organism to another.

ventilator-associated pneumonia (VAP) A type of hospital-acquired pneumonia that occurs in ventilated patients and that appears more than 48 hours after endotracheal intubation.

viremia The presence of viruses in the blood.

virion The complete viral particle, including DNA or RNA enclosed in a capsid, that is capable of infecting another cell.

virulence Physical or biochemical properties of a disease agent that determine its pathogenicity.

virulence factors Adaptations of microbes that enable them to penetrate the immune defenses.

West Nile virus (WNV) An arthropod-borne *Flavivirus* that is spread to birds and humans by mosquitoes; it may be characterized by sudden onset of fever with malaise, anorexia, nausea, vomiting, eye pain, headache, myalgia, rash, lymphadenopathy, fatigue, and arthralgias.

zoonosis A disease that occurs in animals and can also be transmitted to humans.

References

Adam D. A guide to *R*—the pandemic's misunderstood metric: what the reproduction number can and can't tell us about managing COVID-19. *Nature.* https://www.nature.com/articles/d41586-020-02009-w. Published July 3, 2020. Accessed February 15, 2021.

Ahya SN, Flood K, Paranjothi S, eds. *The Washington Manual of Medical Therapeutics.* 30th ed. Philadelphia, PA: Lippincott, Williams and Wilkins; 2001.

Bischoff WE, Reynolds TM, Sessler CN, et al. Handwashing compliance by health care workers: the impact of introducing an accessible, alcohol-based hand antiseptic. *Arch Intern Med.* 2000;160:1017-1021.

Bolyard EA, Tablan OC, Williams WW, et al. Hospital Infection Control Practices Advisory Committee. Guidelines for infection control in healthcare personnel, 1998. *Infect Control Hosp Epidemiol.* 1998;19:407-463. [Published

Prep Kit Continued

correction appears in *Infect Control Hosp Epidemiol.* 1998;19:493].

Bolyard EA, Tablan OC, Williams WW, et al. Hospital Infection Control Practices Advisory Committee. Guideline for infection control in health care personnel. *Am J Infect Control.* 1998;26:289-354.

Brocato CE, Miller GT. The next agent of terror? Understanding smallpox and its implications for prehospital crews. *JEMS.* 2002;27:44-50, 52-55.

Burnet M. *Natural History of Infectious Disease.* Cambridge, UK: Cambridge University Press; 1962.

Cardo DM, Culver DH, Ciesielski CA, et al. Centers for Disease Control and Prevention Needlestick Surveillance Group. A case-control study of HIV seroconversion in health care workers after percutaneous exposure. *N Engl J Med.* 1997;337:1485-1490.

Centers for Disease Control and Prevention. COVID-19: first responders. https://www.cdc.gov/coronavirus/2019-ncov /hcp/guidance-for-ems.html. Updated July 15, 2020. Accessed May 28, 2021.

Centers for Disease Control and Prevention. Epidemiology of HIV/AIDS: United States, 1981-2005. http://www.cdc .gov/mmwr/preview/mmwrhtml/mm5521a2.htm. Accessed July 27, 2009.

Centers for Disease Control and Prevention. *Epidemiology and Prevention of Vaccine-Preventable Diseases.* Hamborsky J, Kroger A, Wolfe S, eds. 13th ed. Washington, DC: Public Health Foundation; 2015.

Centers for Disease Control and Prevention. Hepatitis A questions and answers for health professionals. https://www .cdc.gov/hepatitis/hav/havfaq.htm#general. Reviewed July 28, 2020. Accessed February 14, 2021.

Centers for Disease Control and Prevention. Hepatitis B questions and answers for health professionals. https://www .cdc.gov/hepatitis/hbv/hbvfaq.htm#overview. Reviewed July 28, 2020. Accessed February 14, 2021.

Centers for Disease Control and Prevention. Hepatitis C questions and answers for health professionals. https://www .cdc.gov/hepatitis/hcv/hcvfaq.htm#section1. Reviewed August 7, 2020. Accessed February 14, 2021.

Centers for Disease Control and Prevention. HIV: statistics overview. https://www.cdc.gov/hiv/statistics/overview/index .html. Reviewed June 8, 2020. Accessed February 14, 2021.

Centers for Disease Control and Prevention. Immunization of health-care workers: recommendations of the Advisory Committee on Immunization Practices (ACIP) and the Hospital Infection Control Practices Advisory Committee (HICPAC). *MMWR Recommend Rep.* 1997;46(RR-18):1-42.

Centers for Disease Control and Prevention. Leading causes of death. https://www.cdc.gov/nchs/fastats/leading-causes -of-death.htm. Reviewed January 12, 2021. Accessed February 15, 2021.

Centers for Disease Control and Prevention. Measles cases and outbreaks. https://www.cdc.gov/measles/cases -outbreaks.html. Reviewed February 5, 2021. Accessed February 15, 2021.

Centers for Disease Control and Prevention. Meningococcal disease. http://www.cdc.gov/meningococcal/about/index .html. Reviewed May 31, 2019. Accessed February 15, 2021.

Centers for Disease Control and Prevention. Mumps cases and outbreaks. https://www.cdc.gov/mumps/outbreaks.html. Reviewed February 11, 2020. Accessed February 15, 2021.

Centers for Disease Control and Prevention. Notifiable diseases and mortality tables. *MMWR.* 2015;64(4):ND56-ND73.

Centers for Disease Control and Prevention. Pneumonia can be prevented—vaccines can help. https://www.cdc.gov /pneumonia/prevention.html?CDC_AA_refVal =https%3A%2F%2Fwww.cdc.gov%2Ffeatures %2Fpneumonia%2Findex.html. Reviewed October 22, 2020. Accessed February 15, 2021.

Centers for Disease Control and Prevention. Progress toward strengthening blood transfusion services: 14 countries, 2003–2007. *MMWR.* 2008;57(47):893-897.

Centers for Disease Control and Prevention. Recognition of illness associated with the intentional release of a biologic agent. *MMWR.* 2001;50(41):1273-1277.

Centers for Disease Control and Prevention. Respiratory syncytial virus infection (RSV). https://www.cdc.gov/rsv /research/us-surveillance.html. Reviewed December 18, 2020. Accessed February 15, 2021.

Centers for Disease Control and Prevention. TB incidence in the United States, 1953–2019. https://www.cdc.gov/tb /statistics/tbcases.htm. Reviewed October 24, 2020. Accessed February 14, 2021.

Centers for Disease Control and Prevention. Ticks. http://www .cdc.gov/ticks/index.html. Reviewed January 7, 2021. Accessed February 11, 2021.

Centers for Disease Control and Prevention. Tuberculosis: facts sheets; interferon-gamma release assays (IGRAs—blood tests for TB infection. https://www.cdc.gov/tb /publications/factsheets/testing/igra.htm. Reviewed May 4, 2016. Accessed February 11, 2021.

Centers for Disease Control and Prevention. Vaccine information for adults. https://www.cdc.gov/vaccines /adults/rec-vac/hcw.html. Reviewed May 2, 2016. Accessed May 28, 2021.

Centers for Disease Control and Prevention. Vaccine recommendations and guidelines of the ACIP. https://www .cdc.gov/vaccines/hcp/acip-recs/vacc-specific/covid-19. html. Reviewed May 17, 2021. Accessed May 28, 2021.

Centers for Disease Control and Prevention. Vancomycin-resistant enterococci (VRE) and the clinical laboratory. http://www.cdc.gov/hai/settings/lab/vreclinical -laboratory.html. Reviewed November 24, 2010. Accessed February 11, 2021.

Prep Kit Continued

Centers for Disease Control and Prevention. West Nile virus: final cumulative maps and data for 1999–2019. https://www.cdc.gov/westnile/statsmaps/cumMapsData.html. Reviewed November 24, 2020. Accessed February 15, 2021.

Centers for Disease Control and Prevention, Department of Health and Human Services. Severe acute respiratory syndrome (SARS): in the absence of SARS-CoV transmission worldwide: guidance for surveillance, clinical and laboratory evaluation, and reporting version 2. http://www.cdc.gov/sars/surveillance/absence.html. Reviewed May 3, 2005. Accessed February 15, 2021.

Centers for Disease Control and Prevention, Department of Health and Human Services. Severe acute respiratory syndrome (SARS): public health guidance for community-level preparedness and response to severe acute respiratory syndrome (SARS) version 2: supplement I: infection control in healthcare, home, and community settings. IV. infection control for prehospital emergency medical services (EMS). http://www.cdc.gov/sars/guidance/I-infection/prehospital.html. Reviewed May 3, 2005. Accessed February 15, 2021.

Centers for Disease Control and Prevention, Department of Health and Human Services. Severe acute respiratory syndrome (SARS): SARS basic fact sheet. http://www.cdc.gov/sars/about/fs-SARS.html. Reviewed December 6, 2017. Accessed February 15, 2021.

Chapman AS, Bakken JS, Folk SM, et al. Diagnosis and management of tickborne rickettsial diseases: Rocky Mountain spotted fever, ehrlichioses, and anaplasmosis—United States. A practical guide for physicians and other health care and public health professionals. *MMWR Recommend Rep*. 2006:55(RR04):1-27.

Chaudhary U, Aggarwal R. Extended spectrum lactamases (ESBL): an emerging threat to clinical therapeutics. *Indian J Med Microbiol*. 2004;22:75-80.

Craven R, Roehrig J. West Nile virus. *JAMA*. 2001;286:651-653.

Dailey MW, Dunn T. The prehospital needlestick. *Emerg Med Serv*. 2000;2968-2976.

Dayan GH, Rubin S, Plotkin S, eds. Mumps outbreaks in vaccinated populations: are available mumps vaccines effective enough to prevent outbreaks? *Clin Infect Dis*. 2008;47:11:1458-1467.

de Gans J, van de Beek D; for European Dexamethasone in Adulthood Bacterial Meningitis Study Investigators. Dexamethasone in adults with bacterial meningitis. *N Engl J Med*. 2002;347:1549-1556.

Dorevitch S, Forst L. The occupational hazards of emergency physicians. *Am J Emerg Med*. 2000;18:300-311.

Drazen J. SARS: looking back over the first 100 days. *N Engl J Med*. 2003;349:319-320.

Durand ML, Calderwood SB, Weber DJ, et al. Acute bacterial meningitis in adults: a review of 493 episodes. *N Engl J Med*. 1993;328:21-28.

Ellis AK. Priority role of epinephrine in anaphylaxis further underscored: the impact on biphasic anaphylaxis. *Ann Allergy Asthma Immunol*. 2015;115:165.

Ellis JS, Alvarez-Aguero A, Gregory V, et al. Influenza AH1N2 viruses, United Kingdom, 2001–2002 influenza season. *Emerg Infect Dis*. 2003;9:304-310.

English JF, Cundiff MY, Malone JD, et al. APIC Bioterrorism Task Force, and CDC Hospital Infections Program Bioterrorism Working Group. Bioterrorism readiness plan: a template for healthcare facilities. http://emergency.cdc.gov/bioterrorism/pdf/13apr99apic-cdcbioterrorism.pdf. Published April 13, 1999. Accessed February 15, 2021.

Flaherty DK. The vaccine–autism connection: a public health crisis caused by unethical medical practices and fraudulent science. *Ann Pharmacol*. 2011;45(10): 1302-1304.

Fleming-Dutra KE, Hersh AL, Shapiro DJ, et al. Prevalence of inappropriate antibiotic prescriptions among US ambulatory care visits, 2010–2011. *JAMA*. 2016;315(17):1864-1873.

Flowers LK, Mothershead JL, Blackwell TH. Bioterrorism preparedness, II: the community and emergency medical services system. *Emerg Med Clin North Am*. 2002;20: 457-476.

Foster DA, Heller ST, Young JK. Multidrug-resistant *Streptococcus pneumoniae* [Letter]. *N Engl J Med*. 2001;344:1329.

Fridkin SK. Increasing prevalence of antimicrobial resistance in intensive care units. *Crit Care Med*. 2001;29(4 suppl): N64-N68.

Fridkin SK, Gaynes RP. Antimicrobial resistance in intensive care units. *Clin Chest Med*. 1999;20:303-316.

Frith J. The history of plague: Part 1. The three great pandemics. *History*. 2012;20:11-16.

Gates RH. *Infectious Disease Secrets*. 2nd ed. Philadelphia, PA: Hanley and Belfus; 2003.

GBD 2013 Mortality and Causes of Death Collaborators. Global, regional, and national age–sex specific all-cause and cause-specific mortality for 240 causes of death, 1990–2013: a systematic analysis for the Global Burden of Disease Study 2013. *Lancet*. 2014;385(9963):117-171.

Gerberding JL. Occupational exposure to HIV in health care settings. *N Engl J Med*. 2003;348:826-833.

Gladwin M, Tattler B. *Clinical Microbiology Made Ridiculously Simple*. 3rd ed. Miami, FL: MedMaster; 2001.

Gurley ES, Montgomery JM, Hossain MJ, et al. Person-to-person transmission of Nipah virus in a Bangladeshi community. *Emerg Infect Dis*. 2007;13:1031-1037.

Hasman H, Mevius D, Veldman K, et al. β-Lactamases among extended-spectrum β-lactamase (ESBL)–resistant *Salmonella* from poultry, poultry products and human patients in the Netherlands. *J Antimicrob Chemother*. 2005;56:115-121.

Prep Kit Continued

Henderson DK, Fahey BJ, Willy M, et al. Risk for occupational transmission of human immunodeficiency virus type 1 (HIV-1) associated with clinical exposures: a prospective evaluation. *Ann Intern Med.* 1990;113:740-746.

Herbert S, Halvorsen DS, Leong T, Franklin C, Harrington G, Spelman D. Large outbreak of infection and colonization with gram-negative pathogens carrying the metallo-beta-lactamase gene blaIMP-4 at a 320-bed tertiary hospital in Australia. *Infect Control Hosp Epidemiol.* 2007;28(1):98-101.

Hoffmann C, Rockstroh JK, Kamps BS, eds. *HIV Medicine 2007.* 15th ed. Paris, France: Flying Publisher; 2007.

Jain S, Self WH, Wunderink RG, et al. Community-acquired pneumonia requiring hospitalization among U.S. adults. *N Engl J Med.* 2015;373:415-427.

Kamps BS, Hoffmann S, eds. *SARS Reference.* 3rd ed. http://www.sarsreference.com. Published October 2003. Accessed February 15, 2021.

Keith LS, Jones DE, Chou C-HSJ. Aluminum toxicokinetics regarding infant diet and vaccinations. *Vaccine.* 2002;20(suppl 3):S13-S17.

Kemp SF, Lockey RF, Simons FE; World Allergy Organization Ad Hoc Committee on Epinephrine in Anaphylaxis. Epinephrine: the drug of choice for anaphylaxis: a statement of the World Allergy Organization. *Allergy.* 2008;63:1061-1070.

Komar N, Panella N, Burns J, et al. Serologic evidence of West Nile virus infection in birds in the New York City vicinity during an outbreak in 1999. *Emerg Infect Dis.* 2001;7:621-625.

Ksiazek TG, Erdman D, Goldsmith CS, et al. SARS Working Group. A novel coronavirus associated with severe acute respiratory syndrome. *N Engl J Med.* 2003;348:1953-1966.

Kuhar DT, Henderson DK, Struble KA, et al.; US Public Health Service Working Group. Updated US Public Health Service guidelines for the management of occupational exposures to human immunodeficiency virus and recommendations for postexposure prophylaxis. *Infect Control Hosp Epidemiol.* 2013;34(9):875-892.

Lane MC, Mobley HLT. Role of P-fimbrial–mediated adherence in pyelonephritis and persistence of uropathogenic *Escherichia coli* (UPEC) in the mammalian kidney. *Kidney Int.* 2007;72(1):19-25.

Lauer GM, Walker BD. Hepatitis C virus infection. *N Engl J Med.* 2001;345:41-52. [Published correction appears in *N Engl J Med.* 2001;345:1425].

Lehman DA, Farquhar C. Biological mechanisms of vertical immunodeficiency virus (HIV-1) transmission. *Rev Med Virol.* 2007;17:381-403.

Levinson W, Jawetz E. *Medical Microbiology and Immunology.* 7th ed. New York, NY: Lange Medical Books/McGraw-Hill; 2002.

Ligon BL. Robert Koch: Nobel laureate and controversial figure in tuberculin research. *Semin Pediatr Infect Dis.* 2002;13:289.

Louie JP, Bell LM. Appropriate use of antibiotics for common infections in an era of increasing resistance. *Emerg Med Clin North Am.* 2002:20.

Macgregor-Skinner G. Personal communication. Penn State University; January 26, 2015.

Manis J. Overview of therapeutic monoclonal antibodies. *UpToDate.* https://www.uptodate.com/contents/overview-of-therapeutic-monoclonal-antibodies/print-. Updated December 16, 2020. Accessed February 15, 2021.

Morse DL. West Nile virus: not a passing phenomenon. *N Engl J Med.* 2003;348:2173-2174.

Morse SS. Factors in the emergence of infectious diseases. *Emerg Infect Dis.* 1995;1:7-15.

Murphy K. *Janeway's Immunobiology.* New York, NY: Garland Science/Taylor and Francis Group; 2012.

Nash D, Mostashar F, Fine A, et al. The outbreak of West Nile virus infection in the New York City area in 1999. *N Engl J Med.* 2001;344:1807-1814.

National Institute for Occupational Safety and Health. What every worker should know: how to protect yourself from needlestick injuries. NIOSH publication 2000-135. July 1997. http://www.cdc.gov/niosh/docs/2000-135. Reviewed June 6, 2014. Accessed February 15, 2021.

Nipah virus. World Health Organization website. https://www.who.int/news-room/fact-sheets/detail/nipah-virus. Published May 30, 2018. Accessed August 24, 2021.

Nordmann P, Cuzon G, Naas T. The real threat of *Klebsiella pneumoniae* carbapenemase-producing bacteria. *Lancet Infect Dis.* 2009;9(4):228-236.

Ong SWX, Tan YK, Chia PY, et al. Air, surface environmental, and personal protective equipment contamination by severe acute respiratory syndrome coronavirus 2 (SARS-CoV-2) from a symptomatic patient. *JAMA.* 2020;323(16):1610-1612.

Petersen L, Marfin A. West Nile virus: a primer for the clinician. *Ann Intern Med.* 2002;137:173-179.

Petersen L, Roehrig J. West Nile virus: a reemerging global pathogen. *Emerg Infect Dis.* 2001;6:611-614.

Peterson JW. Bacterial pathogenesis. In: Baron S, ed. *Medical Microbiology.* 4th ed. http://www.ncbi.nlm.nih.gov/books/NBK8526/. Accessed February 15, 2021.

Pumphrey RSH. Lessons for management of anaphylaxis from a study of fatal reactions. *Clin Exp Allergy.* 2000;30:1144-1150.

Rollins DM, Briken V, Joseph SW. Pathogenic microbiology: the study of disease-causing bacteria. NSCI home page. http://life.umd.edu/classroom/bsci424. Published September 2006. Accessed February 15, 2021.

Prep Kit Continued

Roos KL. Acute bacterial meningitis. *Semin Neurol*. 2000;20:293-306.

Rosenstein NE, Perkins BA, Stephens DS, et al. Meningococcal disease. *N Engl J Med*. 2001;344:1378-1388.

Rupe ME, Fey PD. Extended spectrum β-lactamase (ESBL)–producing Enterobacteriaceae. *Drugs*. 2003;63(4):353-365.

Salinas JL, Mindra G, Haddad MB, et al. Leveling of tuberculosis incidence—United States, 2013–2015. *MMWR*. 2016;65:273-278.

Sax PE, Wood BR. The natural history and clinical features of HIV infection in adults and adolescents. *UpToDate*. https://www.uptodate.com/contents/the-natural-history-and-clinical-features-of-hiv-infection-in-adults-and-adolescents?search=aids%20definition&source=search_result&selectedTitle=1~150&usage_type=default&display_rank=1. Updated November 21, 2019. Accessed February 12, 2021.

Schrag SJ, Brooks JT, Beneden CV, et al. SARS surveillance during emergency public health response, United States, March–July 2003. *Emerg Infect Dis*. 2004;10:185-194.

Schultz CH, Mothershead JL, Field M. Bioterrorism preparedness, I: the emergency department and hospital. *Emerg Med Clin North Am*. 2002;20(2):437-455.

Sepkowitz KA. AIDS: the first 20 years. *N Engl J Med*. 2001;344:1764-1772.

Silverman A, Simor A, Loutfy MR. Toronto Emergency Medical Services and SARS. *Emerg Infect Dis*. 2004;10:1688-1689.

Simons FER, Frew AJ, Ansotegui IJ, et al. Risk assessment in anaphylaxis: current and future approaches. *J Allergy Clin Immunol*. 2007;120(1 suppl):S2-S4.

Small PM, Fujiwara PI. Management of tuberculosis in the United States. *N Engl J Med*. 2001;345:189-200.

Snacken R, Kendal AP, Haaheim KR, et al. The next influenza pandemic: lessons from Hong Kong, 1997. *Emerg Infect Dis*. 1999;5:195-203.

Spelman D. Cellulitis and skin abscess: epidemiology, microbiology, clinical manifestations, and diagnosis. *UpToDate*. https://www.uptodate.com/contents/cellulitis-and-skin-abscess-epidemiology-microbiology-clinical-manifestations-and-diagnosis. Updated October 7, 2020. Accessed February 11, 2021.

Stockman LJ, Curns AT, Anderson LJ, Fischer-Langley G. Respiratory syncytial virus–associated hospitalizations among infants and young children in the United States, 1997–2006. *Pediatr Infect Dis J*. 2012;31:5-9.

Stokes EK, Zambrano LD, Anderson KN, et al. Coronavirus disease 2019 case surveillance—United States, January 22–May 30, 2020. *MMWR*. 2020;69(24):759.

Suerbaum S, Michetti P. *Helicobacter pylori* infection. *N Engl J Med*. 2002;347:1175.

Talbot HK, Belongia EA, Walsh EE, Schaffner W. Respiratory syncytial virus in older adults: a hidden annual epidemic. *Infect Dis Clin Pract*. 2016;24(6):295-302.

Thomas KE, Hasbun R, Jekel J, et al. The diagnostic accuracy of Kernig's sign, Brudzinski's sign, and nuchal rigidity in adults with suspected meningitis. *Clin Infect Dis*. 2002;35:46-52.

Todar K. Todar's online textbook of bacteriology. http://www.textbookofbacteriology.net. Accessed February 11, 2021.

Tortora GJ, Funke BR, Case CL. *Microbiology: An Introduction*. 10th ed. San Francisco, CA: Benjamin Cummings; 2009.

Tyler KL. West Nile virus encephalitis in America [Editorial]. *N Engl J Med*. 2001;344:1858-1859.

Update: West Nile virus activity: United States, 2001. *MMWR*. 2002;51:497-501.

U.S. Army Medical Research Institute of Infectious Diseases. *USAMRIID's Medical Management of Biological Casualties Handbook*. 7th ed. Fort Detrick, Frederick, MD: USAMRIID; 2011.

Vu HT, Leitmeyer KC, Le DH, et al. Clinical description of a completed outbreak of SARS in Vietnam, February–May 2003. *Emerg Infect Dis*. 2004;10:334-338.

Wakefield AJ, Murch SH, Anthony A, et al. Retracted: ileal–lymphoid–nodular hyperplasia, non-specific colitis, and pervasive developmental disorder in children. *Lancet*. 1998;351:9103:637-641.

Warren DK, Fraser VJ. Infection control measures to limit antimicrobial resistance. *Crit Care Med*. 2001;29(4 suppl):N128-N134.

Webster RG. Influenza: an emerging disease. *Emerg Infect Dis*. 1998;4:436-441.

Weir E. West Nile fever heads north. *CMAJ*. 2000;163:878.

Wenzel RP. Airline travel and infection [Editorial]. *N Engl J Med*. 1996;334:981-982.

Wenzel RP, Edmond MB. Managing antibiotic resistance [Editorial]. *N Engl J Med*. 2000;343:1961-1963.

Wenzel RP, Edmond MB. Managing SARS amidst uncertainty. *N Engl J Med*. 2003;348:1947-1948.

West K. AIDS update: occupational exposure and post-exposure treatment of HIV/AIDS. *JEMS*. 2002;27:48-60, 62-63.

Whitaker R. *Anatomy of an Epidemic*. New York, NY: Broadway Books; 2011.

Willams WW, Preblud SR, Reichelderfer PS, et al. Vaccines of importance in the hospital setting: problems and developments. *Infect Dis Clin North Am*. 1989;3:701-722.

Williamson EJ, Walker AJ, Bhaskaran K, et al. Factors associated with COVID-19–related death using OpenSAFELY. *Nature*. 2020;584(7821):430-436.

Wong RSM, Hui DS. Index patient and SARS outbreak in Hong Kong. *Emerg Infect Dis*. 2004;10:339-341.

World Health Organization. Hepatitis B. https://www.who.int/news-room/fact-sheets/detail/hepatitis-b. Published July 27, 2020. Accessed February 14, 2021.

World Health Organization. Influenza (seasonal). https://www.who.int/news-room/fact-sheets/detail/influenza-(seasonal). Published November 6, 2018. Accessed February 14, 2021.

Prep Kit Continued

World Health Organization. Measles. https://www.who.int/news-room/fact-sheets/detail/measles. Published December 5, 2019. Accessed February 14, 2021.

World Health Organization. Tuberculosis: key facts. https://www.who.int/news-room/fact-sheets/detail/tuberculosis. Published October 14, 2020. Accessed February 14, 2021.

Zimmer K. Why R_0 is problematic for predicting COVID-19 spread. *The Scientist*. https://www.the-scientist.com/features/why-r0-is-problematic-for-predicting-covid-19-spread-67690. Published July 13, 2020. Accessed February 11, 2021.

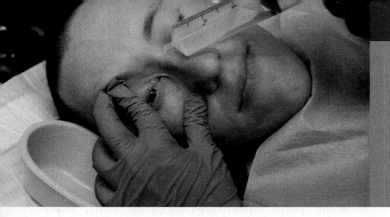

Chapter 21

Toxicologic Emergencies

Jason Chu, MD

Theodore C. Bania, MD, MS

OBJECTIVES

After completing this chapter, you will be able to:

1. Identify issues that may adversely affect the health and safety of critical care transport professionals during the treatment and transport of patients experiencing a toxicologic emergency (p 1131).
2. Describe assessment of and considerations common to all patients following a poisoning or overdose (p 1130).
3. Discuss the assessment findings associated with the various toxidromes and medication reaction syndromes encountered in the critical care environment (p 1138).
4. Discuss situations in which various means of decontamination are required or indicated following a toxic exposure or overdose (p 1141).
5. Identify those chemicals or medications that require enhanced elimination (removal of absorbed toxins) from the body (p 1145).

6. Identify the clinical presentation, mechanism of toxicity, and treatment of poisoning or overdose situations involving pharmaceutical and abuse agents (p 1146).
7. Identify the clinical presentation, mechanism of toxicity, and treatment of poisoning or overdose situations involving chemical agents (pp 1160–1161).
8. Recognize especially toxic substances that pose extreme risks to patients and providers (p 1170).
9. Discuss hazardous materials response and critical care transport considerations in such incidents (p 1171).
10. Discuss radiation emergencies and critical care transport considerations (p 1173).

Introduction

Critical care transport professionals (CCTPs) may be asked to transport patients experiencing a toxicologic emergency following a vast array of possible events. Poisons, chemicals, medications, and other toxic substances are found in dangerous quantities in homes, schools, agriculture, industry, and commercial establishments; on all modes of transportation; and naturally in the environment. As a result of accidents, carelessness, intentional misuse, abuse, or intentional acts of others, such as terrorism, people may be exposed to these toxins and experience potentially lethal consequences. CCTPs can dramatically improve patient outcomes through prompt recognition and effective treatment of such toxicologic emergencies.

The safety of the transport team and other health care or emergency responders is the highest priority when the CCTP encounters a poisoned or overdosed patient. Patients may present hazards to rescuers in a variety of ways. Bizarre, aggressive, or violent behavior may accompany or follow a medication overdose. Suicidal patients may jeopardize the safety of others during a suicide attempt. Patients exposed to hazardous chemicals may contaminate and injure unprotected rescuers if thorough decontamination is not performed before they initiate treatment.

Management of toxicologic emergencies includes many interventions common to other areas of critical care transport. For example, care for a patient who has been poisoned or one with an overdose is based on the ABCs—maintaining a patent airway, supporting respirations, and promoting effective circulation. Additional steps involve protecting the patient from additional injury through decontamination, prevention of absorption, antidote administration, enhanced elimination, and general patient safety and comfort measures. In many toxicologic emergencies, decontamination, enhanced elimination, and antidote administration will not become effective rapidly enough to correct immediately life-threatening problems with the ABCs, with a few notable exceptions (eg, naloxone given for opioid overdose and atropine given for anticholinesterase toxicity). CCTPs are strongly discouraged from delaying basic ABC interventions while locating, administering, or waiting for a possible antidote to work. Wasted time will prove fatal in many cases. Interventions to maintain and enhance the ABCs are discussed in greater depth in Chapter 6, *Respiratory Emergencies and Airway Management*.

Two types of decontamination are distinguished in this text, each with a unique purpose. **Primary decontamination** usually is done at the scene or outside a health care facility or transport vehicle; it is intended to protect rescuers and health care providers from exposure to a toxic substance during patient care or transport. **Secondary decontamination**, in contrast, requires health care providers to use personal protective equipment (PPE) but is directed at minimizing patient absorption or injury from a toxic substance. The risk to health care providers

during secondary decontamination is typically much less than that posed before or during primary decontamination. Gastric decontamination or eye irrigation should be performed well after the ABCs are addressed. Decontamination of a hazardous chemical should occur before an unprotected health care provider makes any contact with it. Both primary and secondary decontamination are beneficial to patients, but each must be considered separately to avoid confusion. Enhanced elimination is the practice of augmenting the body's removal of a toxic substance (or metabolite) once systemic absorption has occurred.

The term *antidote* also requires clarification. Certain substances have an identified antidote, which counteracts toxicity through a mechanism clearly related to the particular toxic substance (eg, acetylcysteine [Mucomyst, Acetadote] for acetaminophen overdose). Other toxic exposures cause signs and symptoms amenable to treatment with a variety of medications used to treat these symptoms in other situations (eg, benzodiazepines may be used to treat seizures whether they are caused by toxic chemicals or something else). The line between antidote and other pharmacologic interventions is not important to the outcome but is mentioned here to avoid confusion in terminology. For many toxic substances, there is a preferred medication to treat a particular sign or symptom, but the term *antidote* implies a complete reversal of toxicity, which does not usually occur.

General Toxicologic Emergency Management
Assessment

Assessment of a patient after poisoning or an overdose should ideally begin well in advance of the first face-to-face contact with the patient. In many situations, if rescuers or health care providers do not use the correct PPE before initial patient contact, it will be too late for this equipment to provide adequate protection **FIGURE 21-1**.

Once the safety concerns for health care providers and emergency responders have been adequately addressed, the transport team should evaluate and manage any problems with the patient's ABCs. The overall patient assessment should focus on identifying immediate threats to life and

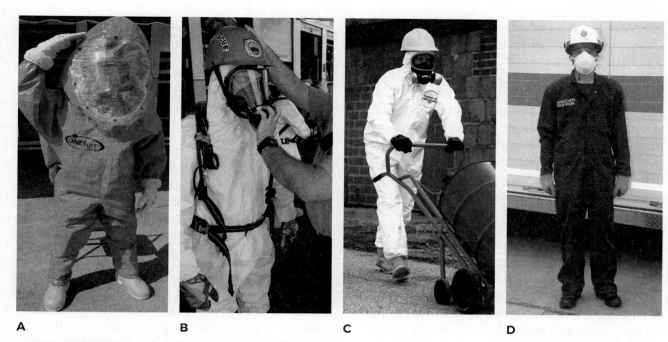

FIGURE 21-1 Adequate use of PPE during contact with patients limits the risk to rescuers and health care providers. The four levels of protection are identified as levels A through D. **A.** Level A protection is fully encapsulating, and includes self-contained breathing apparatus (SCBA). **B.** Level B protection is worn with an SCBA but is not fully encapsulating. **C.** Level C protection is geared toward a known agent. **D.** Level D protection is sometimes worn in the cold zone, an area where no environmental hazards should be present.

A & B: © Jones & Bartlett Learning. Photographed by Glen E. Ellman; **C:** Courtesy of DuPont Personal Protection; **D:** © Jones & Bartlett Learning.

health, yet be comprehensive enough to disclose the subtle cues that may assist in the diagnosis of a specific type of toxic exposure.

Safety

When the transport team receives the initial dispatch or patient report, they should consider the safety precautions and potential hazards suggested by that information. CCTPs may encounter hazardous situations during anticipated patient transports between health care facilities, while responding to an emergency in the community, or by happening upon a vehicular crash without any warning.

Cues to the presence of toxic substances may include the following:

- The presence of unusual odors, smoke, or vapors
- Signs, placards, or markings indicating chemicals or hazardous materials
- Vehicles known to carry chemicals (such as tank cars and fuel trucks)

- Industrial, manufacturing, agricultural, or laboratory facilities
- Bystanders or rescuers becoming unexpectedly ill or unconscious
- Multiple patients with similar unexpected signs and symptoms

The transport of a patient exposed to a toxic substance should not pose an increased risk to CCTPs if safety considerations are adequately addressed.

CCTPs risk illness or injury if they do not use PPE and adequate decontamination has not occurred before they treat patients exposed to toxic substances. Depending on the profile of the critical care transport agency, providers may or may not be actively involved in extrication and decontamination at hazardous material scenes. Nevertheless, all transport providers must assess the adequacy of PPE and decontamination before making patient contact or placing the patient in the transport vehicle. Contaminated patients may expose health care providers to potentially lethal substances or incapacitate a pilot or driver, leading to a possible crash. Decontamination is discussed in greater depth later in this chapter. Crew members should consult a Poison Control Center at the nationwide number, 1-800-222-1222; CHEMTREC at 1-800-262-8200; or a reliable reference source before approaching or transporting a patient exposed to suspected hazardous materials.

In addition to chemical hazards that pose a risk to health care providers and emergency responders, patients may exhibit violent, bizarre, or aggressive behavior. Hospital security staff, law enforcement personnel, or a sufficient number of trained health care providers may be necessary to restrain an aggressive or confused patient before any real assessment or treatment can begin. Intoxicated patients and patients with psychological or emotional disorders can pose a significant risk to health care providers and emergency responders. Potentially suicidal, combative, aggressive, violent, intoxicated, and confused patients should be restrained before transport. Physical restraint includes a spectrum of options, ranging from soft limb restraints, to four-point leather or nylon restraints with additional cross-straps, to handcuffs and shackles for transport of prisoners (prisoners are almost always handcuffed even when they are sedated, intubated, or paralyzed). CCTPs should follow their local and agency policies when applying or transporting patients with physical restraints. It is also imperative for CCTPs to monitor ventilation, make provisions to ensure crew safety, and have a means to release restraints if warranted by acute changes in patient condition.

In addition to physical restraints, CCTPs should consider medical therapy for patients who pose a physical risk to providers. Medical therapies may range from a mild oral sedative to an intravenous sedative, paralysis, and intubation for extremely high-risk patients. Local guidelines should be followed for the use of pharmacologic treatments. Air medical crews should consider alternative ground transport if patients cannot be adequately restrained. Ground transport crews should consider taking extra personnel or delaying transport if crew safety cannot be ensured. Note, however, that patients should not be intubated solely for the purpose of making it safe to transport them.

All patients should be evaluated for the presence of weapons before transport begins. CCTPs should also be aware of family members, visitors, and prospective passengers who might be carrying weapons or are exhibiting dangerous behavior. CCTPs should not approach an unsecured scene without law enforcement involvement when there is an increased likelihood of aggression or violence.

The following cues suggest there is an increased risk of aggression or violence:

- Reported suicide attempt or mental illness
- History of violent behavior
- Involvement of alcohol, illicit drugs, or medication or chemical abuse
- Altered or confused mental status
- Patients with escape risk (eg, prisoners and inpatient psychiatric patients)

Airway

Once safety concerns have been addressed, maintaining or establishing a patent airway is the top priority in the management of a patient with a toxic exposure. Transport team members must evaluate whether the patient currently has a patent airway and is at significant risk for developing airway compromise during the transport. Patients who are awake, alert, and speaking without difficulty demonstrate a patent airway. Unusual sounds from the airway, such as stridor, snoring respirations, and gurgling noises, indicate that the airway is at least partially compromised. In addition, visual signs such as secretions, blood, edema, and foreign substances in the airway indicate a potentially compromised airway. CCTPs should continually monitor all patients—but especially patients who have been exposed to caustic liquids (eg, acids or alkali) or gases (eg, chlorine gas or anhydrous ammonia). Caustic agents continue to react and may produce progressive airway occlusion over the course of several minutes.

A previously patent airway may become compromised during patient transport for a number of reasons. Any subsequent alteration in mental status or seizure activity may compromise the airway in a poisoned patient or a patient with an overdose. Evolving structural abnormalities from trauma or increasing edema may also jeopardize a previously patent airway. Obstructions may occur from emesis (especially unrecognized), secretions, a foreign body, or an airway that becomes displaced during the transport, leading to airway compromise.

Sometimes CCPTs may encounter patients who received activated charcoal, which presents an unusual risk of subsequent airway compromise. In supine or sedated patients, aspiration may easily occur. Aspiration of activated charcoal from an inadequately protected airway will increase morbidity and may be lethal. In patients with unprotected airways who have been given charcoal, some protection from aspiration can be afforded by maintaining a minimum 30° angle elevation of the head of the stretcher at all times. Aspiration is often a silent event, so if any doubt arises about the patient's ability to protect the airway during transport, the CCTP should secure the airway with an endotracheal (ET) tube.

Breathing

Breathing is second only to the airway in importance during patient assessment. Patients require effective oxygen delivery and ventilation to supply the body with oxygen and to remove carbon dioxide. Without effective oxygenation and ventilation, tissue hypoxia, acidosis, and cell death will occur.

The CCTP must evaluate whether a patient's oxygenation and ventilation are adequate to meet the body's metabolic needs. In addition, the CCTP must identify patients who are at risk for subsequent respiratory compromise so that appropriate interventions may begin. Despite breathing spontaneously, patients may not be oxygenating and ventilating adequately to meet their physiologic needs following a poisoning or overdose. Patients with apnea require total extrinsic ventilatory support. In either case, oxygenation and ventilation need to be supported externally with positive-pressure ventilation and/or supplemental oxygen. It is important to provide the correct oxygen concentration and ventilator settings for each patient and clinical situation. For example, patients with carbon monoxide poisoning should receive 100% oxygen despite normal oxygen saturation readings. Conventional pulse oximetry devices can only differentiate between oxyhemoglobin and deoxyhemoglobin; consequently, carbon monoxide that is bound to hemoglobin is misinterpreted as oxyhemoglobin by these devices.

A patient's intrinsic or ventilator-controlled rate and tidal volume must provide adequate gas exchange for the patient's clinical status. Physiologic stress, acidosis, hypermetabolic states (such as in pediatric patients), and many toxic substances require greater oxygenation and ventilation than would normally be required. In turn, the CCTP must consider these factors when evaluating a patient's respiratory status. Conventional ventilator settings are often inadequate for a patient's needs following a poisoning or an overdose. Indeed, catastrophic consequences may occur if a patient who is hyperventilating to compensate for severe metabolic acidosis is pharmacologically paralyzed and conventional ventilator settings are used. When such treatment is applied, respiratory compensation no longer protects the body from the devastating effects of the metabolic acidosis, leading to widespread organ, tissue, and cell dysfunction. Alterations in pH will also occur if a patient has underlying metabolic alkalosis and receives aggressive mechanical ventilation, further disrupting the essential pH balance. Any deviations from normal pH impair the performance of body systems.

Pulmonary edema, hypoxia, cardiovascular dysfunction, and hypermetabolic states all require special consideration when initiating and adjusting positive-pressure ventilation. Hypermetabolic states require greater ventilation for removal of carbon dioxide than would otherwise be required. Cardiovascular dysfunction, persistent hypoxia, pulmonary edema, and acute respiratory distress syndrome may benefit from precise adjustment of positive end-expiratory pressure. Chapter 6, *Respiratory Emergencies and Airway Management*, provides a more in-depth discussion of ventilator settings.

Clues in the patient's history of present illness and physical examination will alert the CCTP to the increased likelihood of impending respiratory compromise. Many toxic exposures will affect a patient's respiratory status either directly or indirectly. Direct toxins, including asphyxiants, organophosphates, and neuromuscular blockers, affect gas exchange, airway diameter, lung tissue, and ventilation. Indirect toxins, such as opioids, benzodiazepines, tricyclic antidepressants (TCAs), and ethanol, inhibit a patient's central respiratory drive. Hypoxia may occur when gases displace oxygen in the lungs, substances block cellular oxygenation, and agents cause cardiogenic or noncardiogenic pulmonary edema. In addition, respiratory compromise may develop as a result of associated trauma, burns, or aspiration. Cyanosis, fatigue, and dyspnea all indicate that a patient's respiratory status may be compromised. Wheezing, pulmonary edema, and

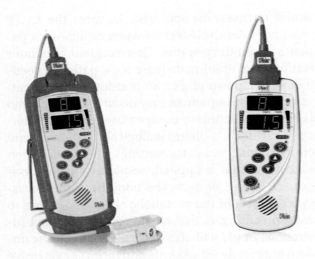

FIGURE 21-2 The Masimo Rad-57 Pulse CO-Oximeter allows clinicians to noninvasively measure oxygen saturation (Spo$_2$), carboxyhemoglobin (Spco), and methemoglobin (SpMet) levels in the blood, as well as total hemoglobin (SpHb) and the pleth variability index (PVI; a measure of perfusion) for fluid responsiveness using a finger sensor.

decreased, absent, or coarse breath sounds found during lung auscultation further indicate unstable respiratory status.

Oxygen saturation, blood gas analysis, and end-tidal carbon dioxide (ETCO$_2$) provide valuable information when the CCTP is assessing the adequacy of oxygenation and ventilation. Changes in breath sounds, patient appearance, and cardiovascular function (as shown by electrocardiogram [ECG] and assessment of perfusion) may indicate either improving or worsening respiratory functioning during transport. **Pulse CO-oximetry** is a technology that provides for noninvasive screening and monitoring for methemoglobinemia and carbon monoxide exposure **FIGURE 21-2**.

Circulation

The evaluation of a patient's circulation requires assessment of end-organ tissue perfusion and overall cardiovascular functioning. Previously healthy people may experience vast alterations in hemodynamic parameters without losing end-organ tissue perfusion. Conversely, patients with longstanding cardiovascular disease may experience devastating consequences from modest hemodynamic alterations that are normally well tolerated in healthier people.

In patients with intact circulatory functioning, adequate end-organ tissue perfusion is demonstrated by normal mental status and adequate urine output for their ages or weights. Such patients will have strong distal pulses and "normal" heart rate, blood pressure (BP), and other hemodynamic values for their age and weight. Their skin will be warm and dry, with a capillary refill time of less than 2 seconds. The ECG will show a normal sinus rhythm (or the patient's baseline rate and rhythm) without signs of conduction abnormalities, unusual ectopy, or ischemia. Any deviation from these findings suggests that the patient's circulation may potentially be compromised.

Numerous mechanisms may impair a patient's cardiovascular functioning after an exposure to a toxic substance. During the evolution of a toxic exposure, a patient's circulatory status may decline because of any of the following factors:

- Direct exposure to cardiotoxic or vasoactive substances
- Fluid volume loss or redistribution
- Electrolyte disturbance
- Airway or respiratory compromise with secondary cardiac dysfunction
- Manifestations of preexisting cardiovascular disease
- Altered oxygen-carrying capacity

A history of exposure to agents with the potential to cause any of these events provides a clue that a patient's circulatory status may become impaired before, during, or after transport.

Circulatory support for critically ill patients includes managing cardiac function, fluid balance, and vascular tone. Unfortunately, toxic exposures may adversely affect all of these components simultaneously. Sometimes impaired circulation is caused by an airway or breathing problem, resulting in hypoxia and/or ischemia. In such a case, the impaired airway or breathing condition may also be resolved by a cardiovascular intervention, such as for pulmonary edema.

Cardiac function is managed by administering medications that increase or decrease the heart rate or contractility. The therapy provided to an individual patient may be guided entirely by the patient's response or tailored specifically to the toxic substance involved. CCTPs should consult a reliable toxicology reference, a physician, or a Poison Control Center for specific guidance.

Fluid balance is closely related to vascular tone, kidney function, and electrolyte concentrations. Toxic exposures may cause alterations in any of these factors, requiring corrective action. CCTPs should anticipate the need for fluid volume replacement in hypovolemic patients or for diuresis of fluid-overloaded patients when managing circulatory function. In addition, they may need to remove excess electrolytes, replace them, or change their distribution.

Vascular tone is often managed with intravenous (IV) vasodilator or vasoconstrictor medications. Beta blockers, calcium channel blockers, catecholamines, and nitrates are used along with agents required for specific toxic substances to optimize vascular tone. For guidance in choosing the appropriate medications, CCTPs should consult a toxicology reference, a physician, or a Poison Control Center.

Additional Assessment

Patient assessment is not limited to just safety and the ABCs. Ideally, every patient transported will be assessed with a thorough history and physical examination. The depth and detail of the additional assessment should be balanced against the needs for prompt transportation and immediate clinical interventions.

The history of present illness should include the following details:

- The medication(s) or substance(s) involved (including multiple substances, particularly with intentional poisonings)
- Time, quantity, and duration of exposure
- Route(s) of exposure
- The patient's initial and subsequent clinical status
- Initial decontamination, stabilization, and treatment performed before arrival of the transport team
- Other contributory information, such as accidental versus intentional event, multiple patients, and the presence of environmental hazards

Interviews of patients, family, and bystanders may provide valuable clues to the nature and severity of a toxic exposure. Through interviews, the CCTP may become aware of prodromal symptoms not otherwise discoverable during the physical examination (eg, nausea, headache, and dizziness). An interview may be abbreviated or completed during the transport if interventions or transport cannot be delayed.

Knowing a patient's medical and social history, prescribed medications, and allergies will assist health care providers when they are treating and transporting a patient. Preexisting medical conditions may have a profound effect on the severity of a toxic exposure or overdose. Long-term exposures to various substances often present much differently from a single, brief, acute exposure to the same substance. Other factors, such as a history of a psychiatric disorder or substance abuse, may affect the present treatment plan and the discharge and follow-up options.

The physical examination performed by the CCTP must be appropriate for the clinical situation. Transport teams must balance the usefulness of a complete head-to-toe physical examination with concerns for patient thermoregulation (hyperthermia or hypothermia), privacy, patient access in confined transport vehicles, and the patient's clinical needs. Do not delay transport of a critically ill patient by performing a time-consuming comprehensive history and head-to-toe examination; conversely, do not initiate rapid transport before adequately assessing the patient.

Some patients may require only minimal intervention following a suspected poisoning or drug overdose. A toddler who possibly ingested a limited amount of a minimally toxic substance is often managed with only observation for a prescribed period of time. Other patients may become critically ill immediately following a toxic exposure, requiring immediate invasive therapy and exhaustive critical care resources. CCTPs must evaluate the details of each situation and weigh the indications, risks, and benefits of each intervention considered for the specific patient. They must also provide continuous assessment and monitoring of any patient being transported. Such monitoring must be within the skills of the transport team and adequate given the patient's clinical status. It is far better to perform excess monitoring (eg, ECG monitoring after exposure to a minimally toxic substance) than inadequate monitoring (eg, no capnography on an intubated patient).

CCTPs should establish vascular access sufficient for administering emergency medications and fluids in any patient who was exposed to a potentially harmful substance. Intraosseous access can be used as an alternative route of administration for fluids and most antidotes. Intubated patients require a nasogastric or orogastric tube for stomach decompression and protection from aspiration. Note that gastric tubes should not be used in patients who have ingested caustic substances, as they might cause additional injury. Caution is also warranted if an ingested toxin is present in the stomach and decompression will expose the CCTP to this substance **FIGURE 21-3**. Patients who are unresponsive and those who require urine output monitoring should have an indwelling urinary catheter inserted and attached to a urine collection device.

All patients who require paralytic drugs must receive adequate sedation and analgesia. If the patient is at risk of seizure activity, as many poisoning and overdose patients are, then seizure prophylaxis must be administered. Vital signs, especially following a poisoning or overdose, are *not* a reliable method of measuring patient sedation or comfort. CCTPs frequently encounter unwarranted administration of antihypertensive medications to patients who are medically paralyzed but have not received adequate analgesia or sedation. Discomfort is a common cause of unexplained hypertension and tachycardia in an intubated and paralyzed patient. Analgesia and sedation should be administered frequently enough to avoid subtherapeutic levels. In addition, patients with increased drug tolerance or hypermetabolic states require significantly more sedation and analgesia while paralyzed. Modern noninvasive commercial devices that permit monitoring of sedation in intubated and medically paralyzed patients, such as the bispectral index monitor, are available.

All patients should receive treatment that provides for their maximum comfort, privacy, and dignity, within the context of the clinical situation. Patients should also be protected from unintentional temperature alterations. Environmental exposure (eg, to heat, cold, moisture, or noise) during transport, while loading or unloading patients, and in health care facilities can adversely impact patient care. Moreover, patients experience the same stressors of flight as do air medical crew members, but are frequently more susceptible to their negative effects and lack sufficient reserves to avoid their detrimental consequences. Patients in ground transport units traveling through significant altitude changes will experience physiologic stressors similar to those encountered in flight.

Nonintubated patients may require anxiolysis and analgesia following many toxicologic exposures. Psychiatric and other at-risk patients may require sedative medications to facilitate care and promote comfort. Family members and friends should be assessed for dysfunctional coping during any crisis situation.

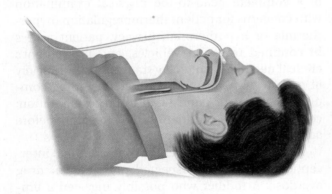

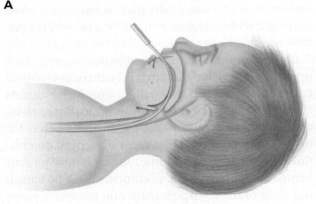

FIGURE 21-3 A nasogastric (**A**) or orogastric (**B**) tube is required for stomach decompression and protection from aspiration in intubated patients.

© Jones & Bartlett Learning.

Vital Signs

A vast array of toxic substances will cause altered vital signs in an exposed patient. Hemodynamic and respiratory alterations occur from direct action of these substances on various organs and tissues or through effects on the central nervous system (CNS), which regulates the cardiovascular and respiratory systems. The examples that follow identify only a few of the many medications and substances that can lead to changes in patients' vital signs.

Tachycardia may occur following a toxic exposure to several different classes of medications and chemicals. Sympathomimetics, such as amphetamines, caffeine, and cocaine, produce an increase in sympathetic tone and atrioventricular (AV) node conduction, increasing the heart rate. Medications with anticholinergic effects (eg, atropine, TCAs, and antihistamines) antagonize acetylcholine and enhance sinus node discharge, causing sinus tachycardia. In addition, any substance that causes cellular hypoxia (eg, carbon monoxide and cyanide) will produce responsive tachycardia in the patient. Various medications and chemicals may also induce ventricular tachyarrhythmias or myocardial ischemia with related tachycardia. The list of chemicals and medications with the potential for causing tachycardia is extensive.

Bradycardia may occur early following exposure to a toxic substance or immediately preceding asystole as the exposure evolves into a fatal event. CNS depression causing bradycardia occurs with toxicity from ethanol, benzodiazepines (eg, lorazepam, diazepam, and midazolam), clonidine, gamma-hydroxybutyric acid, and opioids, to name a few agents. Cardiac glycosides (digoxin) delay conduction through the AV node, leading to bradycardia and heart block. Organophosphates and carbamates cause bradycardia by increasing vagal tone. Bradycardia may also be triggered by direct action on myocardial cell membranes by calcium channel blockers, beta-adrenergic blockers, tricyclic antidepressants, household poisons, and other substances.

Hypertension accompanies tachycardia and bradycardia following exposure to some medications and chemicals. The sympathomimetic agents and anticholinergic agents described earlier, for example, result in hypertension with tachycardia. For instance, norepinephrine and phenylephrine can cause hypertension with bradycardia or an AV block.

Hypotension may also be accompanied by tachycardia or bradycardia. Hypotension with tachycardia may result from fluid loss, third spacing, or blood vessel dilation. Cell membrane depressant agents and agents that depress the CNS can cause hypotension and bradycardia. These medications include opioids, sedative-hypnotic agents, beta blockers, calcium channel blockers, and various others.

Many chemicals and medications can affect temperature regulation. Hyperthermia may occur from increased muscle activity or seizures, an increased metabolic rate, impaired heat dissipation, and disrupted thermoregulation. Drug withdrawal and reactions to medications at therapeutic doses may also precipitate hyperthermia in specific high-risk populations. Examples of medications that may cause *hyperthermia* include cocaine, salicylates, and phenothiazines. Examples of medications that may cause *hypothermia* include beta blockers, benzodiazepines, ethanol, and hypoglycemic agents. In addition to alterations in metabolism, vasodilation, and impaired shivering response, a patient exposed to CNS depressants may lose consciousness in a cold environment, leading to exogenous hypothermia.

Laboratory Assessment

Laboratory analysis can assist the CCTP during diagnosis and treatment of a patient with an actual or potential toxic exposure. Analysis of blood and urine samples is routinely available at sending hospitals and clinics. Advances in point-of-care testing technology also allow CCTPs to measure blood chemistry values, arterial and venous blood gases, and other assorted values during the transport and receive almost immediate results. Be aware, however, that not all chemicals are included in standard toxicology screens.

Certain toxic exposures require a specific approach to laboratory evaluation once the diagnosis is made. In these circumstances, the toxic substance has a predictable effect on various laboratory values. Such tests are used to guide treatment or monitor patient status. CCTPs do not often have the luxury of a definitive diagnosis before transport and must use available laboratory testing as a screening or an assessment tool.

Laboratory testing may also provide evidence that patients are not able to provide owing to their current condition. Patients who are exposed to a chemical or medication and who arrive unresponsive or with an altered mental status cannot provide a reliable history and require a thorough screening for life-threatening conditions. In addition, suicidal and psychiatric patients may intentionally provide misleading or incomplete information to health care providers.

The laboratory assessment should include the following elements:

- Acetaminophen level: 4 hours after exposure when the time of ingestion is known, or immediately when the time of ingestion is not known
- Salicylate level: drawn immediately for a baseline and then repeated at least 1 to 2 hours after exposure; repeated testing is needed for a positive value or a possibility of delayed absorption
- Serum electrolytes, including glucose and potassium (particularly if paralysis with succinylcholine [Anectine] is a possibility)
- Evaluation of acid–base status through arterial or venous blood gas or serum bicarbonate testing
- Ethanol level
- Serum levels of any chemicals and medications known to be available to the patient for which tests can be done (eg, digoxin, lithium, phenytoin [Dilantin], and valproic acid [Depakote])
- Anion gap: serum sodium level minus the sum of chloride and bicarbonate; normal level, 8 to 16 mEq/L
- Osmolar gap if toxic alcohol poisoning is suspected
- Urine drug screen

The tests listed here are performed for screening purposes. If they yield any abnormal or positive results, further investigation is essential. Known exposure to a particular medication or chemical or profound clinical instability may require a more comprehensive laboratory assessment.

Toxic Syndromes and Medication Reaction Syndromes

Exposure to certain classes of chemicals and medications will produce a readily identifiable pattern of clinical signs and symptoms, called a toxidrome.

TABLE 21-1 Toxidromes and Medication Reaction Syndromes

Toxidromes
Anticholinergic syndrome
Cholinergic syndrome
Opioid syndrome
Sedative-hypnotic syndrome
Sympathomimetic syndrome
Medication Reaction Syndromes
Malignant hyperthermia
Neuroleptic malignant syndrome
Serotonin syndrome

© Jones & Bartlett Learning.

These patterns aid in diagnosis when the exact nature of the exposure is unclear and permit health care providers to initiate the correct life-saving interventions. CCTPs should be careful not to overlook other possible causes when making treatment decisions based solely on identification of a toxidrome.

In some cases, patients may experience life-threatening reactions to medications taken at therapeutic doses. Prompt recognition of these rare events is essential and will happen only if health care providers recognize the unusual clues or at-risk patients. Misdiagnosis of these events will adversely affect patient care, with possibly lethal consequences.

TABLE 21-1 lists some of the most common toxidromes and medication reaction syndromes.

Toxic Syndromes (Toxidromes)

Anticholinergic syndrome occurs following excessive exposure to medications such as antihistamines, atropine, benztropine (Cogentin), TCAs (amitriptyline [Elavil]), and some other substances, such as jimson weed. Poisoning results in muscarinic receptor blockade within the CNS and various other organs. In anticholinergic syndrome, patients demonstrate tachycardia, hyperthermia, dilated (mydriatic) pupils, warm (or hot) dry skin, ileus, delirium, seizures, hallucinations, and urinary retention. Seizure activity is treated with benzodiazepines (eg, lorazepam, diazepam, and midazolam) and phenobarbital if the patient does not respond to benzodiazepines. Severe toxicity may be treated with physostigmine (Antilirium, Isopto Eserine), though it should be administered only after consultation with a toxicologist.

Cholinergic syndrome (cholinesterase inhibitor toxicity) typically occurs following exposure to organophosphate and carbamate insecticides or to certain chemical nerve agents. Cholinesterase inhibitors may affect nicotinic receptors, muscarinic receptors, or both, and alter the function of the neurotransmitter acetylcholine. Patients may have two distinct patterns of toxicity, depending on which receptors are involved. Nicotinic receptor toxicity produces tachycardia, hypertension, fasciculations, weakness, hyperglycemia, and dilated pupils. Muscarinic receptor toxicity produces the classic SLUDGEM syndrome (Salivation, Lacrimation, Urination, Diarrhea, Gastroenteritis, Emesis, and Miosis) plus bronchorrhea, bronchospasm, sweating, and bradycardia. The mnemonic DUMBELS (Diaphoresis/diarrhea, Urination, Miosis, Bradycardia/bronchospasm/bronchorrhea, Emesis, Lacrimation, and Salivation) can also be used to remember these symptoms. Nicotinic and muscarinic toxicity leads to altered mental status, coma, and seizure activity in patients with severe exposures to cholinesterase inhibitors. It is essential that health care providers and rescuers use adequate PPE during evaluation and treatment of these exposed patients. Atropine, in doses much higher than are used in typical Advanced Cardiac Life Support protocols, and pralidoxime are the antidotes for cholinesterase inhibitor toxicity. Seizure activity is treated with benzodiazepines. In addition to antidotal therapy, airway and ventilation management should be a high priority due to the bronchorrhea and bronchospasm associated with these exposures.

Both prehospital and emergency department health care providers frequently encounter patients with opioid syndrome. This toxicity commonly develops following illicit use or abuse of opioids in the community, or as an adverse consequence of a therapeutic error or accidental ingestion of opioids (eg, morphine, heroin, and fentanyl [Duragesic]). Signs include lethargy, sedation, hypoventilation, apnea, pinpoint pupils, and noncardiogenic pulmonary edema. Treatment focuses on airway and ventilation support and the prompt administration of an opioid antagonist such as naloxone (Narcan).

CCTPs should be aware that administration of an opioid antagonist may precipitate severe, violent withdrawal symptoms. In addition, many opioids may exert effects that last much longer than the duration of opioid antagonists, which means that life-threatening symptoms may return after the medication wears off. It is often necessary to use repeated doses of opioid antagonists in severe overdose situations.

Sedative-hypnotic syndrome occurs following exposure to any medication or chemical that can cause CNS sedation, lethargy, or coma. The most common cause is ethanol, but other potential causes include benzodiazepines, gamma-hydroxybutyric acid, sleep aids (diphenhydramine [Benadryl], zolpidem [Ambien]), barbiturates, selective serotonin reuptake inhibitors (SSRIs), and trazodone (Desyrel). Signs can include lethargy, sedation, hypoventilation, apnea, bradycardia, and hypotension. Opioid syndrome, in fact, can be viewed as a subset of sedative-hypnotic syndrome. Treatment of sedative-hypnotic syndrome is, therefore, similar to treatment for opioid syndrome, focusing on airway, ventilation, and circulatory support. Unlike for opioid syndrome, there is not a good antidote for most of the causes of sedative-hypnotic syndrome.

Sympathomimetic syndrome involves overstimulation of the adrenergic nervous system, which results in tachycardia, hypertension, agitation, seizures, hyperthermia, dilated pupils, and diaphoresis. An isolated alpha-adrenergic or beta-adrenergic syndrome may cause bradycardia or hypotension, respectively, but the classic (mixed) syndrome involves the listed symptoms. Amphetamines, caffeine, cocaine, MDMA, synthetic cathinones, and synthetic cannabinoids may all cause sympathomimetic syndrome. Treatment is primarily supportive, involving benzodiazepines for sedation and aggressive cooling measures. Hypertension should be treated with direct-acting vasodilators. Beta blocker drugs should be avoided or used with extreme caution in patients with sympathomimetic syndrome because of the risk of unopposed alpha-adrenergic stimulation worsening the hypertension.

Signs and Symptoms

Anticholinergic Syndrome

- Tachycardia
- Hyperthermia
- Dilated (mydriatic) pupils
- Warm (or hot) dry skin
- Ileus
- Delirium
- Seizures
- Hallucinations
- Urinary retention

Nicotinic Receptor Toxicity

- Tachycardia
- Hypertension
- Fasciculations
- Weakness
- Hyperglycemia
- Dilated pupils

Muscarinic Toxicity

- SLUDGEM symptoms: Salivation, Lacrimation, Urination, Diarrhea, Gastroenteritis, Emesis, and Miosis
- DUMBELS symptoms: Diaphoresis/ diarrhea, Urination, Miosis, Bradycardia/ bronchospasm/bronchorrhea, Emesis, Lacrimation, and Salivation

Opioid Toxicity

- Lethargy and sedation
- Hypoventilation or apnea
- Pinpoint pupils
- Noncardiogenic pulmonary edema

Sedative-Hypnotic Toxicity

- Lethargy and sedation
- Hypoventilation or apnea

Sympathomimetic Toxicity

- Tachycardia
- Hypertension
- Agitation
- Seizures
- Hyperthermia
- Dilated pupils
- Diaphoresis

Medication Reaction Syndromes

Malignant hyperthermia is a condition that occurs following administration of succinylcholine or certain inhaled anesthetic agents to genetically susceptible patients. CCTPs may encounter this condition following a rapid sequence intubation (RSI) procedure in the prehospital setting or when responding to a health care facility to perform a patient transport. Affected patients exhibit muscle spasms, profound muscle rigidity, acidosis (metabolic or respiratory), hypercarbia, hyperthermia, tachycardia, tachypnea, myoglobinuria, rhabdomyolysis, and hyperkalemia, beginning up to 12 hours after exposure. Treatment involves aggressive cooling, correction of acidosis, and administration of dantrolene sodium, 2.5 mg/kg initially. Larger patients may require massive quantities of dantrolene for severe reactions; some reports have described the need for more than 36 vials, each containing 20 mg of dantrolene, with 3 g of mannitol. The Malignant Hyperthermia Association of the United States recommends that facilities stock 36 vials of dantrolene to provide initial treatment for a patient weighing 100 to 110 kg, who may require 8–10 mg/kg for stabilization.

Neuroleptic malignant syndrome (NMS) is a potentially fatal reaction to antipsychotic and neuroleptic medications (eg, haloperidol [Haldol], prochlorperazine [Compazine], promethazine [Phenergan], and risperidone [Risperdal]) as a result of excessive blockade of central dopamine receptors or abrupt withdrawal of dopamine agonists (eg, carbidopa/levodopa [Sinemet]). It is not dose dependent and has a 5% to 11% mortality rate overall. Affected patients often demonstrate hyperthermia, profound muscle rigidity, autonomic dysfunction, metabolic acidosis, and confusion. Severe manifestations include renal failure, respiratory failure, arrhythmias, and cardiovascular collapse. Treatment involves good supportive care, aggressive cooling, and muscle relaxation. Prompt, effective muscle relaxation with benzodiazepines, dantrolene, and nondepolarizing neuromuscular blocking agents will prevent many catastrophic consequences of NMS. Dopamine agonists (bromocriptine [Parlodel], ropinirole [Requip], amantadine [Symmetrel], levodopa) can be given as well.

Serotonin syndrome is an unusual response to serotonin-altering medications that produce hyperserotoninergic symptoms. SSRIs (eg, fluoxetine [Prozac], sertraline [Zoloft], and paroxetine hydrochloride [Paxil]), meperidine (Demerol), and monoamine oxidase inhibitors (eg, phenelzine sulfate [Nardil] and tranylcypromine [Parnate]) are the usual culprits. Amphetamines, TCAs, serotonin and norepinephrine reuptake inhibitors (SNRIs), and lithium are implicated less frequently. Serotonin syndrome may occur following an SSRI (or similar) overdose or when the medications mentioned earlier are inadvertently combined. Affected patients demonstrate irritability, muscle rigidity, increased lower extremity rigidity compared to upper extremity, clonus, myoclonus, hyperthermia, diaphoresis, headaches, seizures, coma, tachycardia,

Signs and Symptoms

Malignant Hyperthermia
- Muscle spasms
- Profound muscle rigidity
- Acidosis (metabolic or respiratory)
- Hypercarbia
- Hyperthermia
- Tachycardia
- Tachypnea
- Myoglobinuria
- Rhabdomyolysis
- Hyperkalemia

Neuroleptic Malignant Syndrome
- Hyperthermia
- Profound muscle rigidity
- Metabolic acidosis
- Autonomic dysfunction
- Confusion

Serotonin Syndrome
- Irritability
- Muscle rigidity
- Hyperthermia
- Diaphoresis
- Headaches
- Seizures
- Coma
- Tachycardia
- Hallucinations

and hallucinations. Treatment includes aggressive cooling, IV hydration, and seizure control. Muscle relaxation is achieved by providing sedation with benzodiazepines and nondepolarizing neuromuscular blocking agents. **Rhabdomyolysis** is treated with aggressive IV fluid administration. Serotonin antagonist medications (cyproheptadine [Peritol]) and atypical antipsychotic medications with serotonin antagonist activity (olanzapine [Zyprexa], chlorpromazine [Largactil]) have been used to counteract this syndrome but are not currently recommended for widespread use.

Decontamination

Patient decontamination following exposure to a toxic substance is directed at minimizing the quantity of that substance absorbed by the patient and the extent of any local damage. Decontamination may be as simple as providing the patient with fresh air for several minutes or as complicated as whole-bowel irrigation, which takes many hours to perform. Prompt, effective decontamination has the potential to prevent the fatal consequences of an otherwise lethal overdose. As the following topics relate to the CCTP, decontamination will be completed on scene prior to transport.

Skin Decontamination

Caustic agents and acetylcholinesterase inhibitors (such as pesticides and chemical weapons) can cause systemic toxic effects from dermal absorption. Numerous other chemicals cause severe local reactions or burns when placed in contact with skin. Given these risks, it is essential that health care providers use the correct PPE during skin decontamination. Skin decontamination, like all other methods of decontamination, is most effective if initiated immediately following exposure and may have no benefit if significantly delayed. Certain agents, such as lime (calcium oxide) and elemental metals, react violently with water and require a specialized approach to skin and eye decontamination.

To perform skin decontamination, remove any potentially contaminated clothing. Gently brush dry powders away, and then flush the affected area with copious amounts of water or saline **FIGURE 21-4**. During irrigation, pay particular attention to the patient's ears and groin, the area between the fingers and toes, and any skin folds. Hydrocarbon-based products often require a mild soap or shampoo for more effective removal.

No attempt should be made to neutralize chemicals on the skin. Such a reaction often generates heat and causes additional injury.

Other chemicals recommended for topical treatment beyond irrigation include calcium for hydrofluoric acid exposure, calcium for oxalic acid exposure, and low-molecular-weight polyethylene glycol (PEG 400) or isopropyl alcohol for phenol exposure. Treatment with 1% copper sulfate solution for white phosphorus exposure is no longer recommended because of the risk of hemolysis and increased mortality from the copper. Consult a reliable reference before administering any topical treatment for chemical exposure.

Ocular Decontamination

Many agents that cause toxicity to skin will also damage the eyes. In particular, the cornea is extremely sensitive to hydrocarbons and corrosive agents.

Each affected eye should be flushed with copious amounts of water, saline, or other approved solution. Local ocular anesthetic drops, along with a commercially available irrigation adjunct (Morgan Lens), may be used as well **FIGURE 21-5**. Before beginning irrigation, remove the patient's contact lenses, if they are still in place **FIGURE 21-6**.

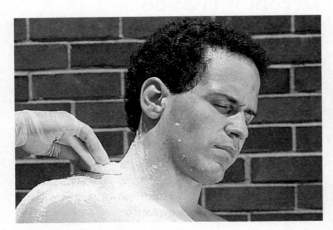

FIGURE 21-4 To decontaminate skin, gently brush away any dry powders before flushing the area with water or saline. Always ensure patients are protected against hypothermia after decontamination, because patients get cold quickly.

© American Academy of Orthopaedic Surgeons.

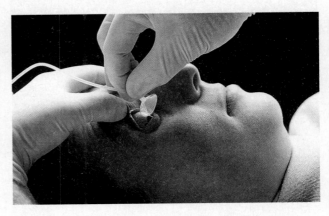

FIGURE 21-5 An irrigation adjunct, like the Morgan Lens, can help flush toxins away from the eye.

The Morgan Lens courtesy of MorTan, Inc.

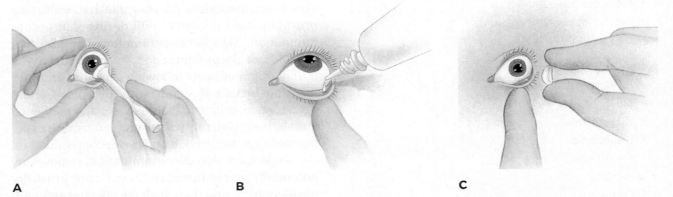

A   **B**   **C**

FIGURE 21-6 Remove contact lenses, if still in place, before beginning irrigation. **A.** To remove hard contact lenses, use a specialized suction cup moistened with sterile saline solution. **B.** To remove soft contact lenses, instill 1 or 2 drops of saline or irrigating solution. **C.** Pinch off the lens with your gloved thumb and index finger.

© Jones & Bartlett Learning.

Following exposure to an acid or base, each eye needs to be irrigated with at least 1 L of water until the ocular pH is normal. (Ocular pH is tested by touching the pH paper to the moist surface of the conjunctival cul-de-sac of the affected eye. The pH paper is then compared with the shades on the package.) No attempt should be made to neutralize chemicals in the eye. Such a neutralization reaction often produces heat, which then causes devastating injury. Once irrigation is complete, consult a Poison Control Center about definitive treatment or arrange for a thorough ophthalmology exam for any significant exposures.

Gastric Decontamination

Patients who have ingested toxic chemicals or dangerous amounts of otherwise therapeutic medications may benefit from gastrointestinal (GI) decontamination. GI decontamination is accomplished through gastric lavage and emptying, activated charcoal administration, and whole-bowel irrigation. In each case, the goal is to prevent systemic absorption of a toxic chemical or medication.

Orogastric Lavage

Pills, pill fragments, and liquid toxins can be removed from the stomach by gastric lavage. While once widely accepted, use of this procedure is now limited to a very small number of clinical situations. It is not performed in the transport setting. Patients who go to a health care facility within 1 hour of taking a life-threatening ingestion are candidates for gastric lavage. Indications include the following:

- Highly toxic ingestion, likely to remain unabsorbed in the stomach
- Substances poorly adsorbed by activated charcoal
- No effective antidote or treatment therapy currently available

Despite its potential for preventing harmful stomach contents from being absorbed, gastric lavage has several disadvantages. Notably, it is a time-consuming, invasive procedure that will delay administration of activated charcoal or oral antidote medications. The amount of actual pills (or fragments) that is removed is limited. Moreover, this procedure requires cooperation from awake, alert patients. Resistance is common, and use of sedative medications—given to counteract resistance—places patients at increased risk of aspiration. In addition, gastric lavage may propel toxic substances farther into the digestive tract and limit the effectiveness of other treatments.

The role of gastric lavage following a caustic ingestion is controversial. Contraindications include the following:

- Minimally toxic ingestion
- Significant time since ingestion and absorption has likely occurred
- Availability of a highly effective antidote
- Inability of the patient to protect the airway during the procedure (ET intubation may be required before gastric lavage)

In terms of complications, aspiration is the main risk during gastric lavage. Injury to the airway, stomach, and esophagus is also possible.

Highly toxic liquids can be evacuated from the stomach using a common orogastric or nasogastric tube much more quickly than they are removed by the conventional gastric lavage procedure.

Emesis induced by syrup of ipecac is no longer a routine treatment for toxic ingestions and is very rarely administered. Ipecac has many contraindications and side effects, almost completely eliminating its usefulness in toxic ingestions. Any patient who is sedated, is obtunded, or has a history of seizure activity is not a candidate for ipecac. Ingestion of any medication with the potential to induce CNS depression or seizures, any hydrocarbon, or any corrosive agent is an absolute contraindication to ipecac. Aspiration is a potentially lethal consequence of inappropriate administration of ipecac. Side effects of ipecac include sedation, vomiting-related trauma (including Mallory-Weiss tear), and delay in the administration of activated charcoal or oral antidote.

Activated Charcoal

Activated charcoal can often be administered to prevent absorption of medications and chemicals in the digestive tract. **Activated charcoal** is a carbon-based liquid with an incredible absorptive ability **FIGURE 21-7**. It is typically administered orally or via a nasogastric or orogastric tube to decrease the available quantity of a toxic substance. This therapy also has the novel ability to remove certain toxic

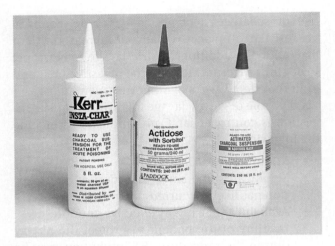

FIGURE 21-7 Activated charcoal.

© American Academy of Orthopaedic Surgeons.

substances from circulating blood by "gut dialysis." Orally administered activated charcoal can reduce the available quantity of a purely IV overdose of certain medications (eg, theophylline and phenytoin) or decrease serum drug levels of some medications (eg, carbamazepine, salicylates, digoxin) long after systemic absorption has occurred. This ability is limited to selected chemicals, however.

Activated charcoal is administered as a single dose for routine ingestions and in repeated doses for certain severe exposures. Adults usually receive 1 g/kg, and children receive 0.5 to 1 g/kg. This treatment is most effective immediately following oral ingestions (within 1 hour of ingestion), but may have no benefit once systemic absorption of the toxin has occurred. It is indicated in the following situations:

- Ingestion of a harmful amount of a substance known to be adsorbed by activated charcoal within a time frame in which adsorption by charcoal is likely to take place (varies dramatically by substance and situation)
- Unknown substances ingested or presumption of toxic ingestions in high-risk patients

Toxicology reference sources are vague regarding the outer time limits for single-dose activated charcoal administration. Several factors, however, extend the usefulness of activated charcoal beyond the 1-hour window of optimal efficacy:

- Evidence of continued medication absorption demonstrated by increasing serum levels or unexplained continued deterioration in the patient's clinical status
- Ingestion of enteric-coated or sustained-release preparations
- Ingested drug packets with likelihood of rupture
- Exposure to substances removed through gut dialysis
- Other conditions that delay toxin absorption (eg, food in the stomach and delayed GI motility)

Massive overdoses may require several doses of activated charcoal to adsorb a sufficient amount of toxin in the intestines.

Sedated patients with an unprotected airway are not candidates for activated charcoal treatment. Unresponsive patients needing activated charcoal require definitive airway protection with an ET tube. Aspiration can cause significant morbidity and may be a lethal complication. Vomiting and constipation are frequent side effects of administration.

Activated charcoal is also contraindicated following caustic ingestions, because these chemicals are not adsorbed by activated charcoal and it obscures the views in diagnostic imaging procedures. Likewise, it is contraindicated for patients with hydrocarbon ingestions because of its high aspiration potential. Numerous substances (eg, lithium, iron, certain heavy metals, hydrocarbons, and alcohols) are not well adsorbed by activated charcoal. If these substances are taken simultaneously with toxins that can be adsorbed, however, use of activated charcoal may still confer some benefits. A careful risk-benefit analysis is essential in such cases.

Activated charcoal is often combined with a saline or magnesium-containing cathartic agent to decrease the likelihood of constipation. Consult a Poison Control Center or a reliable toxicology reference to determine the appropriateness of using activated charcoal in unusual poisoning situations.

Multiple-Dose Activated Charcoal

Multiple-dose activated charcoal should be used for substances with delayed absorption. In addition, because of its unique ability to remove chemicals and medications already absorbed into the body, multiple-dose activated charcoal can reduce the elimination half-life of various chemicals, theoretically improving clinical outcomes. Typically, a reduced dose of activated charcoal is administered every 1 to 6 hours for several doses, or for up to 12 hours total. A toxicologist should be consulted for specific dosing recommendations.

Whole-Bowel Irrigation

One additional option exists for treating ingestions of toxic substances that are not amenable to treatment with activated charcoal. Whole-bowel irrigation (WBI) requires the patient to drink (or receive via orogastric or nasogastric tube) large quantities of a nonabsorbable, electrolyte-balanced liquid that propels stomach and intestinal contents through the digestive system. WBI is indicated for significant ingestions of potentially toxic substances, substances not well adsorbed by activated charcoal (eg, iron, heavy metals), and substances with delayed absorption. It can be given in combination with activated charcoal when patients have ingested large quantities of sustained-release or enteric-coated medications (eg, calcium channel blockers and theophylline). It is also indicated when patients have swallowed packages containing illicit drugs, as is done by body stuffers and body packers. This procedure is performed in the intensive care unit.

Body packers (people who swallow prepared packages of illicit substances for smuggling purposes) and body stuffers (people who hastily swallow packets of illicit substances, often to avoid impending arrest) pose a challenge to health care providers. Body packers are at increased risk because they have ingested large amounts of very concentrated substances. Body stuffers are at increased risk because their swallowed packages are often poorly prepared with unreliable materials and marginal technique. Patients may appear completely asymptomatic, but rapid, unexpected, catastrophic clinical instability will develop if the packaging fails and the chemicals are rapidly absorbed by the digestive tract.

Commercial products for WBI are widely available and are used for other purposes, such as preparation for intestinal surgery and diagnostic procedures. Adult patients receive 1.5 to 2 L/h for 4 to 6 hours or until the rectal effluent is clear. Clinicians may use radiography to assist in the diagnosis or monitoring of radiopaque materials.

Enhanced Elimination

In certain poisoning and overdose situations, treatment with enhanced elimination is appropriate. This process replaces or augments the body's normal method of eliminating, modifying, or breaking down toxic substances. Enhanced elimination should be considered when the ordinary route of elimination from the body is impaired by the overdose or other pathology, or if the patient cannot tolerate the adverse effects of the poisoning because of a preexisting medical condition. Substances that become heavily concentrated in the blood or extracellular fluids and only minimally concentrated in body tissues are more likely to respond to enhanced elimination. In contrast, this process is less likely to successfully remove highly protein-bound medications. Options to enhance elimination of certain toxins may include multiple-dose activated charcoal (discussed previously), urinary manipulation, and various modes of dialysis. A toxicologist or nephrologist should be consulted when considering these interventions.

Urinary Manipulation

Alkalinization of urinary pH promotes the increased excretion of weak acids such as salicylates and phenobarbital. Sodium bicarbonate is added to IV fluids to maintain a urinary pH of 7 to 8.5, usually in amounts of 1 to 2 mEq/kg every 3 to 4 hours. During therapy, fluid volume status, serum pH, and electrolytes (especially potassium and sodium) must be carefully monitored. Hypokalemia is extremely common, so frequent point-of-care testing and/or potassium replenishment during transport, if available, should be considered. Continuous cardiac monitoring is also indicated.

Peritoneal Dialysis, Hemodialysis, Hemoperfusion, and Continuous Renal Replacement Therapy

These modes provide additional options for clinicians in managing a severe poisoning or overdose. CCTPs may be called to transport patients who are receiving these treatments. Such treatments generally cannot be continued during transport and will need to be discontinued or interrupted to safely transport the patient. Specialized training and equipment are required in such cases, and their description is beyond the scope of this text. Patients requiring these services may be transported to tertiary care centers from smaller community facilities and clinics.

Specific Toxicologic Emergencies
Pharmaceutical and Abuse Agents

As noted earlier, patients may experience life-threatening reactions to medications (both prescription-only and over-the-counter agents) and drugs of abuse.

Acetaminophen

Acetaminophen (Tylenol, Paracetamol, APAP) is the drug whose ingestion most commonly results in overdose. This medication is used widely as an analgesic and antipyretic, and it is often found combined with narcotic analgesic and cold-symptom ingredients in prescription and over-the-counter preparations. The presence of these other agents may complicate toxicity from acetaminophen when they are ingested together.

Acetaminophen toxicity is insidious. Toxic signs and symptoms may not manifest until well after the optimal time to administer the known antidote,

acetylcysteine. Untreated acetaminophen toxicity can lead to liver failure, liver transplantation, or death.

The diagnosis of acetaminophen poisoning is based on patient history and laboratory analysis. Documentation of time, duration, and nature of exposure is essential. The acetaminophen (Rumack-Matthew) nomogram is useful only for single, acute ingestions; it is not reliable for exposures that have occurred over several hours or days **FIGURE 21-8**. A serum acetaminophen level should be obtained at least 4 hours (but less than 24 hours) following ingestion, and the level and time plotted on the nomogram. The nomogram will indicate whether toxicity is anticipated and treatment is indicated. *Once toxicity is established, measurement of future acetaminophen levels will not assist in clinical management.* The serum acetaminophen level will continue to decline regardless of toxicity. A metabolite actually causes hepatotoxicity, but the decreasing acetaminophen level may mislead providers into discontinuing antidote administration prematurely. A toxicologist should be consulted for situations not covered adequately by the nomogram or if treatment questions persist.

Nausea and vomiting are quite common during acetaminophen toxicity. In addition, patients have anorexia, dehydration, diaphoresis, and elevated

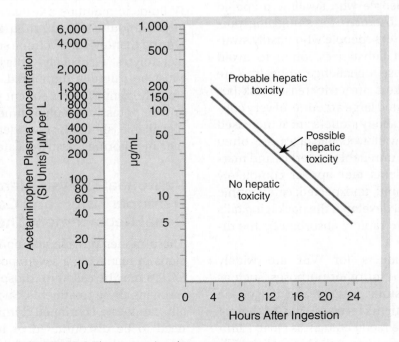

FIGURE 21-8 The acetaminophen nomogram.

liver function test results. During subsequent days, abdominal pain (usually in the right upper quadrant), oliguria, hepatomegaly, coagulopathy, and eventual liver failure may develop. A patient who presents with abdominal pain, nausea, or vomiting following a probable acetaminophen overdose should be assumed to have toxicity until proven otherwise.

Acetaminophen toxicity is treated with activated charcoal for initial GI decontamination. Acetylcysteine is the antidote for acetaminophen toxicity and can be given orally or intravenously. This medication decreases the risk of hepatotoxicity to less than 5% when given within 8 hours of ingestion. Although the risk of hepatotoxicity increases if acetylcysteine is started beyond 10 hours after ingestion, it still has benefit for delayed presentations or even in liver failure.

Treatment with acetylcysteine should begin immediately for symptomatic patients presenting more than 8 hours after ingestion. Patients with uncomplicated acetaminophen poisoning are often administered IV acetylcysteine over 21 hours of treatment. A loading dose of 150 mg/kg in 200 mL D_5W (dextrose 5% in water) is administered over 15 to 60 minutes, followed by an IV infusion of 50 mg/kg in 500 mL D_5W over 4 hours, and then a final IV infusion of 100 mg/kg in 1,000 mL D_5W over 16 hours. Fluid and electrolyte abnormalities are possible when pediatric patients receive IV acetylcysteine. Consult a toxicologist or a Poison Control Center for specific IV dosing recommendations beyond 21 hours.

Oral acetylcysteine is given with a 140 mg/kg loading dose, followed by 70 mg/kg every 4 hours for 17 additional doses. Acetylcysteine has a sulfur like odor and is irritating to the GI tract. Even when it is diluted with juice or soda, patients often require aggressive treatment with antiemetics during oral acetylcysteine therapy. Refractory vomiting, from toxicity or related to oral administration of acetylcysteine, often requires IV acetylcysteine.

Amphetamines

Amphetamines are available as therapeutic medications (such as methylphenidate [Concerta], amphetamine-dextroamphetamine combination [Adderall], and dextroamphetamine [Dexedrine]); used as illicit stimulants for personal, academic, or professional enhancement; and abused in society

---

Signs and Symptoms

Acetaminophen Toxicity

- Early (0 to 24 hours):
  - Nausea and vomiting
  - Anorexia
  - Dehydration
  - Diaphoresis
- Late (24 to 96 hours):
  - Abdominal pain (usually in the right upper quadrant)
  - Elevation of liver function test results
  - Oliguria
  - Hepatomegaly
  - Coagulopathy
  - Liver failure
  - Renal failure (rare)
- Longer than 4 days:
  - Resolution of symptoms or multiple organ failure

Transport Management

Acetaminophen Toxicity

- Manage the ABCs.
- Perform GI decontamination with activated charcoal.
- Administer acetylcysteine (oral Mucomyst or IV Acetadote).

---

for euphoric properties (eg, MDMA [Ecstasy, Molly], methamphetamines). Newer drugs of abuse with similar stimulant effects as amphetamines include synthetic cathinones (bath salts) and synthetic cannabinoids (K2, Spice). These drugs produce many desirable and adverse effects through central and peripheral nervous system stimulation. Frequent users develop tolerance to the psychological effects but not to the physiologic effects, thereby placing them at higher risk for toxicity when they increase their dosage.

Patients who overdose on amphetamines have classic sympathomimetic symptoms (discussed earlier in the chapter). Acute amphetamine toxicity produces hypertension, tachycardia, hyperactivity (although amphetamines are often used in the treatment of hyperactivity disorders), restlessness, anxiety, diaphoresis, tremors, fasciculations, and rhabdomyolysis. Severe toxicity causes seizures, organ ischemia (including but not limited to the cardiovascular, gastrointestinal, renal, and nervous systems), and cerebral hemorrhage. Prolonged use of large quantities of amphetamines may cause a stimulant washout syndrome (similar to cocaine washout syndrome, sometimes referred to as a meth crash). In this syndrome, amine stores within the body become depleted following prolonged amphetamine use, leading to excessive sleep, hunger, and depression. Stimulant washout syndrome is completely the opposite of the typical effects of amphetamine use and has features similar to a sedative-hypnotic toxidrome (discussed earlier in the chapter).

Urine drug screening may identify patients taking amphetamines and possibly methamphetamines but often will not detect synthetic analogs (ie, MDMA, synthetic cathinones, synthetic cannabinoids). Serum drug levels are not clinically useful. The patient's urine output and results of blood tests should be monitored for signs of dehydration and rhabdomyolysis.

Gastrointestinal decontamination with activated charcoal or WBI should be considered when clinically appropriate. Treatment of amphetamine overdose is supportive and based entirely on presenting signs and symptoms. Benzodiazepines are used initially for sedation or seizure control. Phenobarbital can be added for prolonged seizures or status epilepticus. Patients with significant hyperthermia should be cooled aggressively. Typical antipsychotics (haloperidol) should not be given because they inhibit cooling and decrease the seizure threshold. Fluids should be replaced by the IV route as clinically indicated. Hypertension that does not respond to sedative medications is treated with vasodilators (IV nicardipine, clevidipine, phentolamine, labetalol). Tachyarrhythmias can be treated with IV esmolol.

Benzodiazepines

Benzodiazepines (eg, diazepam [Valium], midazolam [Versed], and lorazepam [Ativan]) are a group of medications used therapeutically for anxiolysis, sedation, muscle relaxation, and seizure control. Toxicity occurs following therapeutic error, accidental or intentional ingestion, and illicit misuse

Signs and Symptoms

Amphetamine Overdose

- Hypertension
- Tachycardia
- Hyperactivity, restlessness, and anxiety
- Diaphoresis
- Tremors
- Fasciculations
- Rhabdomyolysis
- Seizures
- Myocardial ischemia
- Cerebral hemorrhage

Transport Management

Amphetamine Overdose

- Manage the ABCs.
- Perform GI decontamination with activated charcoal if needed.
- Administer benzodiazepines for sedation seizure control.
- Administer phenobarbital for additional seizure control, if needed.
- Provide aggressive cooling for significant hyperthermia.
- Replace IV fluids.
- Administer IV vasodilators for refractory hypertension.
- Administer IV esmolol for tachyarrhythmias.

and abuse in the community. Judicious administration of these agents by health care providers may prevent serious adverse effects when the medications are used therapeutically. Benzodiazepines, even in toxic doses, exert sedative and seizure-protective effects, which are desirable during clinical treatment.

Deaths due to pure benzodiazepine overdoses are rare. Overdoses are often easy to manage conservatively, although sedation and respiratory depression may persist for several days with certain preparations. Benzodiazepine exposure becomes problematic when multiple agents with sedative properties are combined. When benzodiazepines are taken with ethanol, opioids, or other sedative agents, for example, profound CNS and respiratory depression occurs. Toxic effects also include hypothermia, ataxia, and slurred speech. Most urine drug screen tests can detect benzodiazepines that are metabolized to oxazepam (ie, diazepam, chlordiazepoxide [Librium], temazepam [Restoril]) but not benzodiazepines with different metabolites (ie, alprazolam [Xanax], lorazepam, clonazepam [Klonopin], flunitrazepam [Rohypnol]).

Activated charcoal adsorbs orally ingested benzodiazepines, but it is often contraindicated in nonintubated patients with decreased levels of consciousness. Intubation should be considered whenever significant concern arises about a patient's ability to protect the airway, especially during transport. The majority of patients with benzodiazepine toxicity require only conservative management and careful observation.

Flumazenil (Romazicon), a benzodiazepine antagonist, is an appropriate treatment only for a small minority of overdose situations. Reversal with flumazenil places patients at risk for increased intracranial pressure, sedative withdrawal, increased agitation, and potentially untreatable seizure activity. This medication is contraindicated in patients with poisoning or overdose by unknown substance(s); in patients with a history of seizures; in patients with toxic exposures to chemicals known to cause seizures, increased intracranial pressure, agitation, or CNS stimulation; and in patients taking benzodiazepine medications on a long-term basis. The vast array of situations where flumazenil is contraindicated severely limits its usefulness following benzodiazepine overdose.

Flumazenil is useful when a therapeutic error during procedural sedation requires benzodiazepine reversal in patients without known benzodiazepine dependence. The toxic effects of many benzodiazepines last much longer than the reversal achieved with flumazenil. Thus, unrecognized resedation may occur if patients are not monitored adequately. The adult dose of flumazenil is 0.2 mg IV, increased to 0.3 mg and 0.5 mg at 30-second intervals, up to a maximum dose of 3 mg. Pediatric doses start at 0.01 mg/kg and are titrated up to a maximum of 1 mg total. Flumazenil may be safely used in situations where CCTPs are confident of the patient's clinical status and the substances being treated, such as with overmedication during procedural sedation. Nevertheless, these types of

situations may not occur frequently enough in critical care transport to justify routine use of flumazenil by CCTPs.

Signs and Symptoms

Benzodiazepine Overdose
- CNS and respiratory depression
- Hypothermia
- Ataxia
- Slurred speech

Transport Management

Benzodiazepine Overdose
- Manage the ABCs.
- Intubate the patient for airway control and ventilatory support.

Beta-Adrenergic Blocking Agents

Beta-adrenergic blocking agents (beta blockers) are used therapeutically for a wide variety of medical conditions. Toxicity may occur from an intentional or accidental overdose in the community or a profound therapeutic error in a health care facility. Atenolol (Tenormin), propranolol (Inderal), and metoprolol (Lopressor) are widely used beta blockers. These medications inhibit catecholamines both centrally and peripherally. Beta-1 blockers decrease heart rate, myocardial contractility, myocardial conduction, and myocardial oxygen consumption. Beta-2 blockers relax blood vessel walls, constrict bronchi in the lungs, and block catecholamines in the GI and genitourinary tracts. Both beta-1 and beta-2 blockers cause hypoglycemia through inhibition of **glycogenolysis** and **gluconeogenesis**. These medications are prescribed based on their beta-1 or beta-2 blocking actions. During overdoses, beta selectivity is lost, resulting in both beta-1 *and* beta-2 blocking effects.

Patients' responses to overdose with beta blockers largely reflect their preexisting cardiovascular status. The effects of an overdose will be significantly worse if beta blockers are combined with other cardiotoxic substances. In adults, two to three times the therapeutic dose has the potential to be fatal. Importantly, one normal dose for an adult may have catastrophic effects in a small child.

In addition to hypotension, bradycardia, and hypoglycemia, patients with beta blocker toxicity may exhibit bronchospasm, pulmonary edema, conduction disturbances, tachycardia, mental status depression, and even seizures. Gastric lavage may be considered for recent (within 1 hour), significant ingestions, though it is not performed in the transport setting. Activated charcoal should also be considered for recent toxic ingestions (within 1 hour). Atenolol and acebutolol, but not other beta blockers, can be removed by dialysis for enhanced elimination.

Glucagon is a good choice for initial treatment of a beta blocker overdose. When given at increased doses, it exerts positive inotropic and chronotropic effects, although these effects are often transient. An initial dose of 5 to 10 mg IV is followed by an infusion at 1 to 5 mg/h in adults. This treatment requires a significant amount of glucagon—often more than is available to transport teams.

Bradycardia can be treated with IV atropine (0.01 to 0.03 mg/kg) or cardiac pacing but may prove refractory in patients with severe toxicity. Catecholamines, including dopamine, norepinephrine, and epinephrine, are given for refractory hypotension and bradycardia. **Phosphodiesterase** inhibitors (eg, milrinone) have an **inotropic** effect in beta blocker overdoses but should be used only when invasive monitoring technology is available, because they often result in hypotension from peripheral vasodilation. High-dose insulin therapy (given with IV glucose to prevent hypoglycemia) and intravenous lipid emulsions have been reported to improve survival in beta blocker overdoses. Some medical centers have the facilities and personnel available to place these patients on extracorporeal membrane oxygenation (ECMO). A toxicologist or a Poison Control Center should be consulted for guidance in managing these patients during complicated transports.

Calcium Channel Antagonists (Calcium Channel Blockers)

Calcium channel blockers are used clinically to treat hypertension, migraines, cardiomyopathy, and other conditions. These medications include

Signs and Symptoms

Beta-Adrenergic Blocking Agent Overdose

- Hypotension
- Bradycardia
- Hypoglycemia
- Bronchospasm
- Conduction disturbances
- Pulmonary edema
- Possibly seizures, mental status depression, and tachycardia

Transport Management

Beta-Adrenergic Blocking Agent Overdose

- Manage the ABCs.
- Administer activated charcoal (if within 1 hour of ingestion).
- Consider enhanced elimination (for atenolol ingestions).
- Administer IV fluids.
- Administer glucagon.
- Administer IV atropine or use cardiac pacing for bradycardia.
- Administer catecholamines, including dopamine, norepinephrine and epinephrine, for refractory hypotension and bradycardia.
- Administer high-dose insulin (given with glucose).
- Administer intravenous lipid emulsions.
- Consider milrinone when invasive monitoring technology is available.

diltiazem (Cardizem), verapamil (Calan), and dihydropyridines (ie, amlodipine [Norvasc], nifedipine [Procardia XL]). They act by blocking the L-type calcium channels to decrease intracellular calcium levels, which results in vasodilation, decreased myocardial contractility, slowed conduction, and decreased heart rate. Other effects associated with calcium channel blocker toxicity include nausea, vomiting, metabolic acidosis, and hyperglycemia. Management of calcium channel blocker overdoses is complicated by the widespread availability of sustained-release preparations.

Gastrointestinal decontamination with activated charcoal should be considered for recent toxic ingestions (within 1 hour). Repeated doses of activated charcoal may also be considered for severe ingestions. Gastric lavage may be an option for recent (within 1 hour) significant ingestions, though it is not performed in the transport setting. WBI may be appropriate when the overdose involves enteric-coated or sustained-release preparations but, again, this procedure is not done by CCTPs.

Hypotension and bradycardia are the most common signs of overdose with calcium channel blockers. These clinical features may evolve as additional medication is absorbed from sustained-release preparations. One tablet is often enough to cause serious toxicity or death in a small child. Any medication taken beyond the therapeutic dose should be considered potentially toxic.

Intravenous calcium salts are the initial antidotes to an overdose with a calcium channel blocker. Adult patients are given calcium chloride 10% (10 mL) or calcium gluconate 10% (30 mL) every 5 to 10 minutes as needed. In severe cases, patients have been given more than 15 g of calcium safely. Intravenous calcium use is controversial in the setting of concurrent cardiac glycoside medication (ie, digoxin) toxicity. Although the older literature describes increased cardiac dysrhythmias and mortality associated with this treatment, the more recent literature does not report the same adverse effects.

Glucagon and catecholamines (dopamine, norepinephrine, epinephrine) are useful in the management of refractory hypotension and bradycardia from calcium channel blocker overdoses. Other therapies may include high-dose insulin therapy, intravenous lipid emulsions, or methylene blue (for amlodipine toxicity). In addition, cardiac pacing may be required for patients with severe, symptomatic bradycardia. Selected phosphodiesterase inhibitors (such as milrinone) improve contractility but often result in systemic vasodilation, limiting their usefulness. Atropine may improve the bradycardia early in the toxicity, but is not generally effective as the calcium channel blocker toxicity progresses further.

Cardiac Glycosides

Cardiac glycosides (digoxin, digitoxin [not available in the United States]) are used therapeutically to

---

Signs and Symptoms

Calcium Channel Antagonist Overdose

- Hypotension
- Bradycardia
- Nausea and vomiting
- Metabolic acidosis
- Hyperglycemia

Transport Management

Calcium Channel Antagonist Overdose

- Manage the ABCs.
- Perform GI decontamination with activated charcoal.
- Administer IV fluids.
- Administer IV calcium chloride or calcium gluconate.
- Administer glucagon and catecholamines (dopamine, norepinephrine, epinephrine) for hypotension and bradycardia.
- Administer high-dose insulin (given with glucose).
- Consider intravenous lipid emulsions for refractory hypotension.
- Perform cardiac pacing for bradycardia.
- Consider milrinone when invasive monitoring technology is available.

---

achieve heart rate control, for treatment of supraventricular arrhythmias, and to increase contractility in heart failure. Cardiac glycosides are also found naturally in plants such as foxglove, oleander, and lily of the valley.

Peak effects from oral ingestion of cardiac glycosides occur in 6 to 12 hours. Potentially toxic ingestions require 12 to 24 hours of observation before discharge of the patient from the health care facility.

In acute ingestions, patients often have an initial asymptomatic period ranging from minutes to hours due to the delay in peak effects; this period is followed by the development of nausea, vomiting, abdominal pain, lethargy, or confusion. Hyperkalemia is common after acute cardiac glycoside toxicity. Symptoms of chronic cardiac glycoside toxicity are often vague, frequently resulting in misdiagnosis of this condition. Patients may experience nausea, vomiting, and abdominal pain, possibly accompanied by lethargy, confusion, weakness, and/or yellow-green visual disturbance. Hypokalemia predisposes patients who are taking digoxin or digitoxin on a chronic basis to the drug's toxicity.

Almost any ECG change (with the exception of supraventricular tachycardia) may be present with cardiac glycoside toxicity. Bradycardia and conduction disturbances are common. Serum drug levels are extremely valuable in the diagnosis and management of cardiac glycoside poisoning. The therapeutic level of digoxin is 0.5 to 2 ng/mL, whereas that for digitoxin is 10 to 30 ng/mL. These levels become falsely elevated after patients receive digoxin immune Fab (ovine) (DigiFab) treatments.

Cardiac glycosides are adsorbed in the intestines by activated charcoal. Severe exposures can benefit from administration of multiple-dose charcoal (discussed earlier in the chapter). Gastric lavage is not usually indicated.

The symptomatic bradycardia associated with cardiac glycoside poisoning may respond to atropine early in the toxicity. Transcutaneous or transvenous cardiac pacing increases the incidence of ventricular arrhythmias and is not indicated unless DigiFab is not available.

The hyperkalemia linked to this condition must be corrected promptly, but without the use of calcium. Cardiac glycosides increase the level of intracellular calcium, which in turn increases myocardial contractility (a beneficial effect), but this pathway also leads to the development of digitalis toxicity. Intravenous calcium use is controversial in the setting of concurrent cardiac glycoside medication (ie, digoxin) toxicity. The older literature describes increased cardiac dysrhythmias and mortality with such treatment, but the more recent literature does not report the same adverse effects. Lidocaine and phenytoin may be considered in the management of ventricular arrhythmias.

DigiFab is the antidote for cardiac glycoside overdoses and the preferred treatment for symptomatic bradycardias, ventricular arrhythmias, and hyperkalemia. Dosing is based on the serum drug level and the patient's weight. Severe hyperkalemia, arrhythmias, and renal disease are indications for antidote administration. Consult a toxicologist or a Poison Control Center for specific treatment and dosing recommendations.

Signs and Symptoms

Cardiac Glycoside Overdose
- Nausea and vomiting
- Abdominal pain
- Bradycardia and conduction disturbances
- Hyperkalemia
- Possibly lethargy, confusion, and/or weakness

Transport Management

Cardiac Glycoside Overdose
- Manage the ABCs.
- Perform GI decontamination with activated charcoal (single dose or multiple doses).
- Administer atropine for bradycardia.
- Administer DigiFab for bradycardia, ventricular arrhythmias, or hyperkalemia.
- Administer lidocaine and phenytoin for ventricular arrhythmias.
- Perform cardiac pacing for bradycardia if DigiFab is not available.

Cocaine

Cocaine shares many toxic properties with amphetamines and other sympathomimetics. This potent drug is used therapeutically for anesthesia and vasoconstriction of the mucous membranes, but toxic exposures most often occur following illicit use and abuse. Cocaine is rapidly absorbed via all mucous membranes: the GI tract, lungs, rectum, and vagina. Depending on the route and method of administration, the effects of cocaine peak in 1 to 30 minutes, and the drug has a duration of action up to 140 minutes. Cocaine handlers may hide cocaine internally for smuggling purposes (body packers) or rapidly conceal cocaine internally when arrest is believed to be imminent (body stuffers); thus, their care poses a particular challenge to health care providers.

Diagnosing cocaine toxicity involves obtaining a patient history and performing urine drug screens and a clinical examination. Chest pain is the most common symptom of cocaine intoxication. In addition to myocardial ischemia and infarction, chest pain may stem from cocaine-induced aortic dissection, pneumothorax, and pneumomediastinum.

Young patients without a cardiac history, who have an acute myocardial infarction or acute coronary syndrome, should be assessed for the possibility of cocaine use.

Other symptoms of cocaine intoxication involve many body systems. Ventricular and supraventricular tachycardias are common. Hypoxia, acidosis, and sympathetic stimulation contribute to the development of tachycardias. Bradycardia also occurs from vagal stimulation in some situations. Most cocaine-related deaths are ultimately caused by arrhythmias. Additional vascular effects include hypertension and renal or intestinal vasospasm.

Cocaine has significant effects on the CNS. Patients may have cerebral hemorrhage or infarction, coma, anxiety, agitation, delirium, and psychosis. Seizures occur following exposure, but status epilepticus suggests continued absorption or concomitant toxicity.

Other harmful effects from cocaine include hyperthermia, muscle rigidity, various movement disorders, rhabdomyolysis, acidosis, pulmonary edema, and exacerbation of asthma. Patients may exhibit skin alterations such as tissue necrosis, ulcerations, and scratches, sometimes because of scratching imaginary insects. (These signs and symptoms are far from a complete list of the effects of cocaine intoxication.) Heavy cocaine users may experience **cocaine washout syndrome**, which manifests as profound exhaustion due to depletion of their neurotransmitters, but they maintain the ability to regain normal mental status and orientation when aroused.

Activated charcoal and WBI are useful for patients who have orally ingested cocaine-containing packages (ie, body packers or body stuffers). The effects of orally ingested cocaine peak within 60 minutes of consumption. Activated charcoal may theoretically be of benefit if given immediately after ingestion, but any delay drastically reduces its efficacy. Cocaine-containing packages trapped in the digestive tract may require surgical removal if WBI is unsuccessful.

There is no antidote for cocaine overdose. Instead, treatment is supportive and based on the patient's clinical presentation. Benzodiazepines should be administered for agitation, anxiety, muscle rigidity, and seizure control and have a beneficial effect on hypertension. Hypertension

that does not respond to benzodiazepines should be approached with caution. Beta blockers given for hypertension may cause an increase in BP because of unopposed alpha-adrenergic stimulation, although recent evidence has challenged this theoretical caution. The use of a vasodilator medication should be considered instead of a beta blocker, or another approach should be utilized for alpha-adrenergic control.

Cocaine-induced myocardial infarction should be treated with conventional strategies, including thrombolytics (or percutaneous transluminal coronary angioplasty [PTCA] in the hospital in certain cases), with the exception that beta blockers must be withheld to avoid unopposed alpha stimulation leading to severe hypertension. Administration of benzodiazepines, phentolamine, and calcium channel blockers may also mitigate sympathetic tone or vasospasm in patients with cocaine intoxication. Care for cocaine-induced myocardial ischemia includes nitrates, oxygen, and aspirin.

Other treatments for cocaine overdose focus on providing IV hydration adequate to maintain a urine output of at least 3 mL/kg/h, monitoring for rhabdomyolysis, and active external cooling for patients with hyperthermia. Various specialists (eg, in cardiology, neurosurgery, or vascular surgery) should be consulted for any cocaine-related end-organ injury.

Signs and Symptoms

Cocaine Toxicity
- Chest pain
- Tachycardias
- Cerebral hemorrhage or infarction
- Coma
- Anxiety, agitation, delirium, and psychosis
- Seizures
- Hyperthermia
- Muscle rigidity and movement disorders
- Rhabdomyolysis
- Acidosis
- Pulmonary edema
- Exacerbation of asthma
- Skin alterations (eg, tissue necrosis, ulcerations, and scratches)

Cocaine Toxicity

- Manage the ABCs.
- Perform GI decontamination with activated charcoal if needed for oral ingestions, body packing, or body stuffing.
- Administer benzodiazepines for agitation or seizures.
- Administer IV hydration.
- Monitor for rhabdomyolysis; alkalinize the urine with IV sodium bicarbonate if evidence of rhabdomyolysis is present.
- Provide active external cooling for hyperthermia.
- Administer vasodilators for hypertension.
- Administer thrombolytics for cocaine-induced myocardial infarction or transport patients to a health care facility capable of performing percutaneous transluminal coronary angioplasty (PTCA) promptly.
- Administer benzodiazepines, phentolamine, and calcium channel blockers to mitigate sympathetic tone or vasospasm.
- Administer nitrates, oxygen, and aspirin for cocaine-induced myocardial infarction.
- Do not administer beta blockers to patients with recent cocaine ingestion.

Opioids and Opiates

Opioids are the class of chemicals that includes naturally derived opiates (eg, heroin, morphine, and codeine) and newer artificial medications with the same properties (eg, fentanyl and meperidine). These chemicals are widely used for analgesia in modern health care, but are also abused throughout the world for their euphoric properties. Absorption may occur through oral, dermal, lung, IV, and mucosal routes, resulting in a vast range of times of onset, peak effects, and duration of effects. Toxicity is highly variable and is determined by the amount, route and rate of administration, and individual tolerance.

Opioid substances may or may not be detected by routine urine drug screening tests, depending on the particular chemical involved. Prehospital and emergency department health care providers frequently encounter opioid-intoxicated patients. The diagnosis of opioid overdose is routinely made based on the patient's clinical presentation or when symptoms are reversed by an opioid antagonist such as naloxone.

In opioid intoxication, patients have profound CNS and respiratory depression. The triad of CNS depression, respiratory depression, and pinpoint pupils may lead to a presumptive diagnosis. In addition, patients may exhibit euphoria and dermatologic signs such as needle marks or subcutaneous ulcerations. Hypoxia and death occur from severe respiratory depression or noncardiogenic pulmonary edema in untreated patients. Patients may have more unusual symptoms when exposed to specific opioids, such as seizures with meperidine use and histamine release with morphine use. Manifestations of hypoxic brain injury may further complicate the clinical diagnosis in opioid-intoxicated patients.

In patients with severe opioid overdoses, the airway and breathing are frequently compromised. Consequently, initial treatment involves establishing and maintaining a patent airway while supporting oxygenation and ventilation. Naloxone, when administered promptly, can reverse the opioid effects and often reestablishes a patent airway and spontaneous breathing.

Naloxone is the most commonly used antidote for acute opioid overdose. It can be administered intravenously, intramuscularly, subcutaneously, intranasally, and via nebulization. Dosing is titrated to reverse respiratory arrest or depression without precipitating withdrawal symptoms in long-term users. Because the reversal effects of naloxone do not last as long as the effects of many opioids do, careful monitoring is needed following naloxone administration to avoid an unrecognized return of toxic effects. Naloxone can also be administered as an IV drip to maintain CNS and respiratory functioning in patients with long-acting opioid toxicity.

Treatment with activated charcoal is indicated for patients who have recent oral ingestions of opioid substances, especially when they are combined with other toxic chemicals (ie, acetaminophen), and for patients who have ingested opioid-containing packages (ie, body packers or body stuffers). Following an oral opioid overdose, patients should be evaluated for the presence of acetaminophen and salicylates.

Signs and Symptoms

Opioid Toxicity

- Profound CNS and respiratory depression
- Pinpoint pupils
- Euphoria
- Noncardiogenic pulmonary edema
- Dermatologic signs of needle marks or subcutaneous ulcerations
- Pruritus
- Bradycardia, hypotension

Transport Management

Opioid Toxicity

- Manage the ABCs.
- Administer naloxone to reestablish a patent airway and spontaneous breathing.
- Perform GI decontamination with activated charcoal if needed for oral ingestions, body packing, and body stuffing.

Salicylates

Poisoning from aspirin (acetylsalicylic acid) and other salicylate-containing compounds continues to challenge health care providers. In addition to being present in aspirin, salicylates are found in topical analgesics, liniments, and antidiarrheal agents. Toxic exposure may occur through accidental ingestion by children, due to therapeutic error, and as a suicidal gesture. Ingestion of less than 1 mL of a concentrated topical preparation can cause toxicity in small children.

Diagnosing salicylate poisoning involves obtaining a patient history, performing a clinical examination, and laboratory testing. Serum salicylate levels can be obtained at most health care facilities. Samples should be drawn as soon as possible following exposure, and serial samples should be performed for any toxic ingestions of either regular salicylates or enteric-coated preparations.

A presumptive clinical diagnosis can be made when patients report taking excessive doses of salicylate products and have tachypnea and tinnitus. Any new patient report of tinnitus, dizziness, or deafness should prompt an evaluation for possible salicylate poisoning. Salicylate toxicity can cause a spectrum of neurologic changes, ranging from mild confusion to coma. Nausea, vomiting, abdominal pain, GI bleeding, and hyperthermia may also be present. In severe cases, salicylates may cause pulmonary edema, liver or renal failure, dehydration, electrolyte abnormalities, profound metabolic acidosis (although respiratory alkalosis is also frequently present), and coagulopathy.

Patients with salicylate poisoning require careful attention to the ABCs. Initially, these patients exhibit a CNS-driven tachypnea. As the poisoning evolves, the respiratory rate and depth increase to compensate for worsening metabolic acidosis. For patients who require intubation and mechanical ventilation, their respiratory rate, tidal volume, and minute volume should be matched carefully to avoid undermining their potentially life-saving compensatory hyperventilation. Fluid volume and electrolyte status should be carefully monitored during treatment and transport. Acidosis and subsequent treatments will alter the elimination and distribution of critical electrolytes, such as potassium. Potassium replenishment should be anticipated during patient treatment and transport, especially if urinary alkalinization is performed.

There is no antidote for salicylate poisoning. GI decontamination may include gastric lavage (if the ingestion occurred within 1 hour of presentation), activated charcoal, or WBI for massive ingestions in older children, adolescents, and adults. Depending on the quantity of aspirin or salicylate ingested, patients may require repeated doses of activated charcoal to adsorb the vast quantity of available toxin.

Patients with salicylate toxicity are candidates for treatment with several modes of enhanced elimination. Urinary alkalinization is extremely effective for reducing the salicylate level. This simple procedure can easily be initiated while other interventions are performed or during transport. Salicylate toxicity is also effectively treated in the hospital with hemodialysis or **hemoperfusion**, although hemoperfusion does not provide the same correction of electrolyte levels and acidosis as is delivered by hemodialysis. Indications for hemodialysis include a salicylate level greater than 100 mg/dL, a salicylate level greater than 90 mg/dL with impaired renal function, hypoxemia, altered mental status, and a pH of 7.2 or lower despite bicarbonate therapy. Both hemodialysis and hemoperfusion are performed in the intensive care unit. Use caution when intubating patients with salicylate overdose. A high respiratory rate is needed and blunting the respiratory drive during intubation and ventilation may abruptly worsen toxicity.

Signs and Symptoms

Salicylate Toxicity

- Tachypnea
- Tinnitus, dizziness, or deafness
- Hyperthermia
- Neurologic changes ranging from mild confusion to coma
- Nausea, vomiting, abdominal pain, and GI bleeding
- Pulmonary edema
- Liver or renal failure

Transport Management

Salicylate Toxicity

- Manage the ABCs.
- Monitor fluid volume and electrolyte status.
- Provide potassium replenishment.
- Perform GI decontamination with activated charcoal and consider multiple-dose activated charcoal.
- Perform urinary alkalinization for reduction of the salicylate level.

SSRIs (and Noncyclic Antidepressants)

This category includes medications such as fluoxetine (Prozac), paroxetine (Paxil), sertraline (Zoloft), and a host of others. These medications represent less-toxic alternatives to TCAs for the treatment of depression and anxiety and for smoking cessation.

In general, the toxicity of SSRIs is limited, although severe exposures can cause seizures, serotonin syndrome (discussed earlier in the chapter), cardiovascular alterations, and rarely death. No clear toxic dose has been established. Neither urine nor serum drug screening is widely available to assist in diagnosis or management of SSRI toxicity.

Sedation, ataxia, dizziness, and coma are CNS complications of toxicity seen after SSRI ingestions. Nausea, vomiting, diarrhea, headache, restlessness, shivering, diaphoresis, and sinus tachycardia may also occur. Large ingestions of citalopram (Celexa) and escitalopram (Lexapro) can cause seizures and QTc prolongation leading to torsades de pointes.

There is no antidote for SSRI poisoning or overdose. Gastric lavage and WBI are not typically indicated unless SSRIs are taken in combination with more toxic substances. Activated charcoal is effective for adsorption in the GI tract if given promptly following ingestion (within 1 hour). In SSRI overdose situations in which serotonin syndrome occurs, the treatment is supportive and is based on the patient's symptoms. Hypotension is treated initially with volume resuscitation. Seizures are treated initially with IV benzodiazepines. Patients' ABCs need to be carefully monitored in severe overdoses.

Signs and Symptoms

SSRI Toxicity

- Sedation, ataxia, dizziness, and coma
- Nausea, vomiting, and diarrhea
- Headache, restlessness, shivering, and diaphoresis
- Hypotension, QTc prolongation, and sinus tachycardia
- Muscle rigidity, tremors, and hyperreflexia
- Seizures

Transport Management

SSRI Toxicity

- Manage the ABCs.
- Perform GI decontamination with activated charcoal if needed.
- Provide volume resuscitation for hypotension.
- Administer IV benzodiazepines for seizures.

Toxic Alcohols (Ethylene Glycol and Methanol)

The toxic chemicals ethylene glycol and methanol are commonly available in the community and present a significant challenge to health care providers following accidental or intentional ingestion.

Each can cause profound, lethal metabolic acidosis following ingestion of even very small quantities. Ethylene glycol is the primary component in vehicle antifreeze; methanol is the primary component in windshield washer fluid and other solvents. Accidental exposure to these chemicals occurs when they are mislabeled or placed in a beverage container. Children may be drawn to the sweet taste of ethylene glycol. People with alcoholism may consume either chemical while searching for an ethanol substitute.

Serum methanol or ethylene glycol levels are usually available only in larger health care facilities. Even in larger tertiary centers, obtaining results for quantitative serum levels may take many hours or several days. The long delay tends to undermine the clinical utility of these tests for diagnosis and management of toxicity.

Clinicians have additional options to assist with diagnosis of ethylene glycol toxicity. Oxalate crystals in the urine are highly suggestive of ethylene glycol poisoning in the right setting. Some laboratory lactate analyzers can cross-react with the ethylene glycol metabolite glycolate to produce falsely elevated lactate levels, sometimes markedly so. If a laboratory has some lactate analyzers that cross-react and other analyzers that do not cross-react with glycolate, the resultant difference in the measured lactates, or lactate gap, can help in the diagnosis of ethylene glycol toxicity. Vehicle antifreeze often has fluorescein added and was previously thought to be visible in urine when viewed under a Wood's (ultraviolet) lamp. However, several studies have shown that using urinary fluorescence is an unreliable technique for diagnosing ethylene glycol ingestion.

Both methanol and ethylene glycol cause an elevated serum osmolar gap—a finding that is very useful for timely diagnosis in outlying facilities. Osmolality is calculated as follows (BUN = blood urea nitrogen):

$$2 \times (\text{Serum sodium}) + \frac{\text{Glucose}}{18} + \frac{\text{BUN}}{2.8} = \frac{290 \text{m Osm/kg}}{(\text{Normal})}$$

By comparing the calculated serum osmolality with the measured serum osmolality, clinicians can determine the osmolar gap. For a rough estimation of the serum level (mg/dL), the osmolar gap is multiplied by the appropriate conversion factor **TABLE 21-2**.

TABLE 21-2 Osmolar Gap Conversion Factors

Substance	Conversion Factor
Ethanol	4.6
Ethylene glycol	6.2
Methanol	3.2
Isopropyl alcohol	6.0

Data from Olson KR, ed. *Poisoning and Drug Overdose.* 5th ed. New York, NY: McGraw-Hill; 2007:32.

When hospital laboratories measure, rather than estimate, serum osmolality, it is essential that they use the "freezing-point method." Other analysis methods, which may lead to evaporation of alcohols in the specimen, will give inaccurate results. The serum osmolar gap is adjusted for the presence of serum ethanol and is unreliable when the patient has alcoholic ketoacidosis. It is not an exact test, because at least 12 other chemicals or conditions will cause an elevated osmolar gap. Even so, when serum methanol or ethylene glycol levels are not available, this test can assist with diagnosis and guide initial treatment.

Patients who have ingested ethylene glycol initially exhibit ataxia, slurred speech, and lethargy. These signs, which are characteristic of ethanol intoxication 3 to 4 hours after ingestion, are sometimes accompanied by nausea and vomiting. During this time, laboratory analysis will reveal an elevated serum osmolar gap. As the toxicity progresses (4 to 12 hours after ingestion), profound anion-gap metabolic acidosis develops in conjunction with a drop in the serum bicarbonate level. Seizures, cerebral edema, and coma are common. Respiratory manifestations include tachypnea, hyperventilation, and pulmonary edema. Severe exposures lead to renal failure, cardiac arrhythmias, and conduction disturbances. See Chapter 17, *Gastrointestinal and Genitourinary Emergencies*, for a further discussion of acid–base balance.

Patients with methanol poisoning have signs and symptoms somewhat different from those associated with ethylene glycol exposure. During the first several hours, patients exhibit signs of classic ethanol intoxication, which may be accompanied by gastritis, nausea, and vomiting. An elevated serum osmolar gap is also present. Toxicity progresses into a severe anion-gap metabolic acidosis. Some patients can have a latent period ranging from 6 to 30 hours during which the inebriation and GI symptoms resolve. As toxicity progresses, however, patients may report a "snowfield" in their vision, hazy visual disturbance, or blindness. Severe untreated exposures can lead to further CNS depression, seizures, cerebral edema, coma, hypotension, respiratory arrest, and death.

Gastric emptying with gastric lavage (or gastric suctioning) is the only effective method of decontamination for ethylene glycol and methanol poisoning. Unfortunately, gastric lavage or suctioning is often not effective because the toxic alcohols are absorbed very rapidly. Patients require aggressive treatment for the ABCs following severe exposures.

Two equally effective antidotes are available for the treatment of methanol and ethylene glycol poisoning: ethanol and fomepizole (Antizol). Ethylene glycol and methanol need to be metabolized to cause toxicity, and alcohol dehydrogenase is the first step in their metabolism. Both of the antidotes effectively block alcohol dehydrogenase metabolism of ethylene glycol or methanol into their toxic metabolites.

Ethanol, given either orally or intravenously, promotes methanol and ethylene glycol excretion through an alternative metabolic pathway, drastically reducing the metabolic acidosis. Serum levels are titrated to approximately 100 mg/dL (which may be measured in serum or tested at the bedside using a breathalyzer device). Hospital pharmacies may stock IV ethanol preparations. Patients who receive ethanol therapy require close monitoring. Administration of ethanol may cause abnormal behavior, CNS depression, gastritis, pancreatitis, hyponatremia, and hypoglycemia.

Fomepizole, a commercial antidote for ethylene glycol and methanol poisoning, creates the same alternative metabolic excretion pathway that ethanol does. It is significantly more expensive than ethanol but does not require the same depth and frequency of monitoring as ethanol therapy. Fomepizole does not cause CNS sedation and does not require specific serum monitoring. In selected cases, this treatment may cause headache, nausea, vomiting, dizziness, fever, or rash.

Both of these antidotes—ethanol and fomepizole—not only block toxic alcohols' metabolism into their toxic metabolites, but also increase the elimination half-life of the toxic alcohols. When untreated, methanol is metabolized at a rate of 10 mg/dL/h, such that the elimination half-life is 1 to 3 hours for small ingestions and up to 24 hours for large ingestions. Ethylene glycol's elimination half-life ranges from 3 to 9 hours. With antidotal treatment and normal kidney function, the elimination half-life of methanol increases to 30 to 54 hours and that of ethylene glycol increases to 11 to 18 hours.

Enhanced elimination by hemodialysis is the most effective way to rapidly remove the toxic alcohols and toxic metabolites. Hemodialysis will also normalize the patient's acid–base status and electrolyte levels. Indications for hemodialysis include worsening clinical condition, signs of end-organ toxicity (renal failure, vision loss, coma, seizures), severe metabolic acidosis (arterial pH <7.3), and methanol or ethylene glycol level greater than 50 mg/dL. Hemodialysis also removes the antidotes, so ethanol and fomepizole doses will need to be increased after hemodialysis sessions.

Several adjunct therapies can be given to help enhance metabolism of toxic alcohols via normally minor pathways to nontoxic metabolites. Thiamine and pyridoxine can shift ethylene glycol metabolism away from oxalic acid and toward ketoadipic acid and hippuric acid, respectively. Folate or leucovorin (folinic acid) can increase the clearance of methanol's toxic metabolite, formic acid.

Tricyclic Antidepressants

TCAs are highly toxic medications that are frequently prescribed as last-resort antidepressants. These agents are also prescribed to patients for the treatment of chronic pain, neuropathy, and

Signs and Symptoms

Ethylene Glycol Toxicity
- Ataxia, slurred speech, and lethargy
- Nausea and vomiting
- Seizures, cerebral edema, and coma
- Hyperventilation
- Pulmonary edema
- Renal failure
- Cardiac arrhythmias and conduction disturbances

Signs and Symptoms

Methanol Toxicity

- Ataxia, slurred speech, and lethargy
- Possible gastritis, nausea, vomiting
- "Snowfield," hazy visual disturbance, or blindness
- Hypotension
- Seizures
- Respiratory arrest
- Coma

Transport Management

Ethylene Glycol and Methanol Poisoning

- Manage the ABCs.
- Administer fomepizole (Antizol) or ethanol (oral or IV).
- Consider enhanced elimination with hemodialysis in patients with a worsening clinical condition, renal failure, vision loss, coma, seizures, severe metabolic acidosis (arterial pH <7.30), and methanol or ethylene glycol levels greater than 50 mg/dL.

migraines. Toxicity usually occurs from accidental ingestions by young children and intentional overdoses in patients attempting self-harm. The toxic dose is approximately 10 to 20 mg/kg. Any TCA overdose should be considered potentially life threatening.

Any patient admitted to a health care facility for an intentional overdose should be screened for the presence of TCAs. A 12-lead ECG is more sensitive than serum levels and should be performed on any patient with a suspected TCA overdose. A terminal R wave in lead aVR and a terminal S wave in leads I and aVL are indicative of TCA effects **FIGURE 21-9**. Prolongation of the QRS to greater than 100 milliseconds indicates serious TCA toxicity and increases the patient's risk of seizures and arrhythmias. Patients with TCA toxicity also often exhibit sinus tachycardia. In severe exposures, they can develop ventricular tachycardia or fibrillation, torsades de pointes, and asystole. Hypotension and cardiogenic shock are possible as well.

Patients exhibit many anticholinergic signs and symptoms following TCA overdose, but these are usually mild (discussed earlier in the chapter). They should not be treated with physostigmine, as this agent may result in worsening cardiac toxicity.

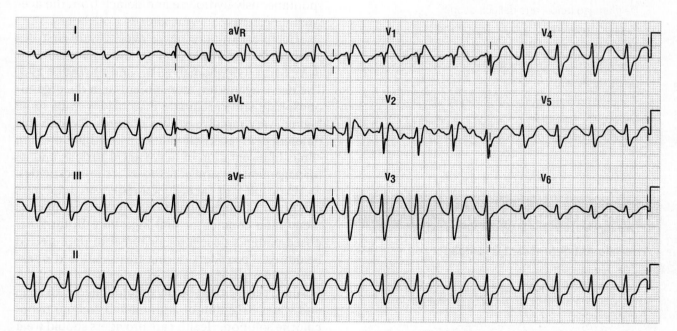

FIGURE 21-9 A 12-lead electrocardiogram for a patient experiencing tricyclic antidepressant overdose. Note the terminal R wave in lead aVR and the terminal S wave in leads I and aVL.

Ipecac is contraindicated following TCA exposure. Gastric lavage is appropriate for recent large ingestion (within 1 hour). Use of activated charcoal can be considered, but its benefits must be weighed against the risk of aspiration due to concomitant CNS depression.

Patients require aggressive supportive treatment following a TCA overdose. QRS widening or ventricular arrhythmia is treated with IV sodium bicarbonate. Initial boluses of 1 to 2 mEq/kg every 3 to 5 minutes are followed by a maintenance infusion of 150 mEq in 1 L of D_5W to maintain serum pH in the range of 7.50 to 7.55. Hypotension should be treated with 0.9% sodium chloride, sodium bicarbonate, and catecholamines (dopamine, norepinephrine, epinephrine). Seizures are usually brief and are treated with IV benzodiazepines. Status epilepticus is uncommon.

Signs and Symptoms

Tricyclic Antidepressant Overdose

- Dry mouth and skin
- Dilated pupils
- Seizures
- Delirium, agitation, and hallucinations
- Rhabdomyolysis
- Muscle tremors
- Hyperthermia
- Sinus tachycardia
- Conduction disturbance (QRS widening)
- Ventricular arrhythmias
- Hypotension

Transport Management

Tricyclic Antidepressant Overdose

- Manage the ABCs.
- Administer IV sodium bicarbonate for conduction disturbance, ventricular arrhythmia, or refractory hypotension.
- Administer IV benzodiazepines for seizures.
- Administer IV fluids and/or catecholamines (dopamine or norepinephrine) for hypotension.

Chemical Agents

Acetylcholinesterase Inhibitor (Organophosphate, Carbamate, and Chemical Warfare Nerve Agents) Toxicity

Acetylcholine is a neurotransmitter that is metabolized by acetylcholinesterase. Organophosphates, carbamates, and the chemical warfare nerve agents all block the acetylcholinesterase enzyme, resulting in excess acetylcholine and excessive activation of nicotinic, muscarinic, and CNS receptors. The presence of excessive acetylcholine at muscarinic receptors produces a constellation of symptoms that can be remembered with the mnemonic DUMBELS. Excessive acetylcholine at the nicotinic receptors results in tachycardia, hypertension, dilated pupils, muscle fasciculation, weakness, and paralysis. Excessive acetylcholine in the CNS leads to altered mental status, agitation, coma, and seizure activity.

Both organophosphates and carbamates are used as insecticides. The main difference between these chemicals is that the organophosphates' binding to acetylcholinesterase becomes irreversible over time by a process called "aging," which prevents the regeneration of acetylcholinesterase by the antidote pralidoxime. In contrast, carbamates spontaneously hydrolyze and detach from the acetylcholinesterase enzyme after 24 to 48 hours.

Chemical warfare nerve agents were first developed during World War II and include Tabun (GA), Sarin (GB), Soman (GD), and VX **TABLE 21-3**. The nerve agents are more potent than the organophosphate and carbamate insecticides, with some "aging" very rapidly—within minutes. Despite this difference in acetylcholinesterase inhibition, the clinical presentation of nerve agent toxicity and its management are similar to those for the insecticides.

Exposure to acetylcholinesterase inhibitors can occur through inhalation, dermal and mucous membrane contact, or oral ingestion. In turn, exposed patients pose a major threat to unprotected health care providers during treatment and transport. When patients have experienced dermal exposures, they should be decontaminated with soap and water irrigation or with diluted sodium hypochlorite solution. Health care providers should wear appropriate PPE during decontamination. Any potentially contaminated clothing and jewelry should be removed and secured in a container, as it may

TABLE 21-3 Chemical Warfare Terrorist Agents

Nerve Agents/Acetylcholinesterase Inhibitors
Tabun
Sarin
Soman
VX
Blister Agents
Sulfur and nitrogen mustards
Lewisite
Phosgene oxime
Pulmonary Agents
Phosgene
Diphosgene
Chlorine
Incapacitating Agents
3-Quinuclidinyl benzilate (BZ)
Kolokol-1

© Jones & Bartlett Learning.

carry the toxin and contaminate health care providers or result in continued exposure to the patient. Following an oral exposure, gastric lavage and activated charcoal may be considered to remove acetylcholinesterase inhibitors—but only after securing the patient's airway with intubation because of the high potential for seizures and aspiration. Gastric contents from gastric lavage or vomiting should be secured in a container, because contact with them may result in exposure to health care providers.

Diagnosis of acetylcholinesterase inhibitor toxicity is based on patient history, similar illnesses experienced by multiple people at the same location, and a physical exam that confirms the cholinergic toxidrome. Laboratory measurement of red blood cells' acetylcholinesterase level is preferred over plasma cholinesterase measurement, but is usually not available rapidly following an acute exposure. M8 and M9 chemical detection paper can be used by responders with special training to identify chemical warfare nerve agents, but have poor sensitivity and specificity for organophosphate toxins.

In general, symptoms (DUMBELS or SLUDGEM) are more sensitive indicators of exposure, especially when the patient also develops miosis.

Atropine, pralidoxime (2-PAM, Protopam), and benzodiazepines are the antidotes for acetylcholinesterase inhibitor toxicity. Benzodiazepines are used to control seizures.

Atropine decreases airway secretions. Its initial dose is 0.5 to 2 mg IV, with the dose then being doubled every 5 minutes until the patient's bronchial secretions decrease and adequate oxygenation is achieved. Severe exposures require vast quantities of atropine, which potentially deplete the hospital's and transport team's supplies. Tachycardia is not an indication to withhold additional atropine doses.

Pralidoxime can regenerate acetylcholinesterase activity on enzymes where "aging" has not occurred and will decrease the amount of atropine required as an antidote. The preferred dosing is a bolus of 1 to 2 g administered over several minutes, followed by an IV infusion of 500 mg/h. Pralidoxime can also be administered as 600 mg IM every 15 minutes up to three times if symptoms persist.

Atropine, pralidoxime, and benzodiazepines can be administered intramuscularly in mass-casualty events following a chemical warfare or terrorist exposure. They are stockpiled for these disasters and supplied as auto-injectors.

Signs and Symptoms

Acetylcholinesterase Inhibitor Toxicity

- Nicotinic receptors:
  - Tachycardia
  - Hypertension
  - Fasciculations
  - Weakness
  - Paralysis
  - Dilated pupils
- Muscarinic receptors:
  - SLUDGE: Salivation, Lacrimation, Urination, Diarrhea, Gastroenteritis, Emesis
  - DUMBELS: Diaphoresis/diarrhea, Urination, Miosis, Bradycardia/bronchospasm/bronchorrhea, Emesis, Lacrimation, and Salivation
- CNS:
  - Severe exposures: altered mental status, agitation, coma, and seizure activity

Other Chemical Warfare and Terrorist Agents

Blistering Agents

Blistering agents include sulfur mustard, nitrogen mustard, lewisite, and phosgene oxime. Blistering agents were first developed and used in World War I; more recently, they have been used in Iraq and Syria. These toxicants have a low mortality rate but cause a high number of casualties. Specifically, they create blisters and severe tissue damage and burns on the skin and exposed areas such as the eyes and, if inhaled, cause airway and pulmonary damage. Sulfur mustard causes immediate tissue damage, but its clinical effects may be delayed. Lewisite and phosgene oxime have immediate clinical effects.

Sulfur mustard has a garlic, onion, or mustard odor; exposure to it may be diagnosed with M8 and M9 paper. Lewisite has a geranium-like odor.

Patients who are exposed to blistering agents should be decontaminated with soap and water irrigation. Health care providers should wear PPE suits while decontaminating patients. There is no antidote for the mustards and phosgene oxime, but British anti-lewisite can be used for lewisite exposure. Treatment is supportive, including analgesia, IV fluids, and wound care for chemical burns.

Pulmonary Agents

Pulmonary agents include phosgene, diphosgene, and chlorine. Chlorine has a yellow-green color and carries a "bleach" odor. It was used in World War I and, more recently, in Iraq and Syria. Phosgene and the more potent diphosgene have an odor of freshly mowed hay or green grass.

Chlorine causes immediate pulmonary irritation and can result in acute or delayed pulmonary edema. Pulmonary irritation can be treated with inhaled bronchodilators, corticosteroids, and an inhaled solution of sodium bicarbonate (4 mL of 3.75% to 4.2% solution). Phosgene and diphosgene are less irritating and lead to a delayed onset of pulmonary edema, ranging from 2 to usually 48 hours.

Incapacitating Agents

Incapacitating agents are aerosolized and designed to temporarily prevent normal functioning of the target.

- 3-Quinuclidinyl benzilate (BZ) is a centrally acting anticholinergic agent; exposure to it results in confusion and hallucinations. Physostigmine is a potential antidote.
- Kolokol-1 is a fentanyl analog. It was used by Russian forces during the Moscow theater siege, in which Chechen rebels held patrons hostage. Although naloxone can reverse the opioid effects, overexposure to kolokol-1 can be fatal.

Carbon Monoxide

Carbon monoxide (CO) is a colorless, odorless, tasteless gas that causes serious toxicity and is the number one cause of poisoning deaths. Carbon monoxide is created during the incomplete combustion of carbon-based materials. The most common exposure to CO occurs from motor vehicles, small gasoline engines, stoves, lanterns, burning charcoal and wood, gas ranges, heating systems, and industrial settings where CO from these sources can build up in enclosed or semi-enclosed spaces. Carbon monoxide exposure also occurs intentionally by people attempting self-harm.

CO has an affinity for hemoglobin 200 to 270 times greater than that of oxygen, so its presence in large amounts in the body decreases the amount of oxygen carried by hemoglobin. CO displaces oxygen that is normally bound to hemoglobin, which shifts the oxygen-hemoglobin dissociation curve to the left, decreasing oxygen delivery and resulting in profound tissue and organ hypoxia. In addition, CO exerts direct adverse effects on internal cellular functioning, binding to myoglobin and cytochrome oxidase, preventing the utilization of oxygen, and producing free-radical formation and cellular damage. The decreased oxygen delivery and utilization associated with CO poisoning forces cells into anaerobic metabolism in an attempt to supply the body's energy needs. Those organs that are highly dependent on the supply of oxygen are the first to exhibit signs of CO poisoning. Specifically, the brain and heart are the primary sites of CO toxicity owing to their large oxygen requirements. The heart may manifest ischemia as chest pain, shortness of breath, arrhythmias, a drop in cardiac output, and, in severe cases, cardiac arrest. The brain may demonstrate its dysfunctional state through headache, mild confusion, altered mental status, seizures, and coma.

CO poisoning should be suspected in any survivor of a fire in a confined space. It can be diagnosed by an elevated CO level in an arterial or a venous blood gas sample. Victims who have been removed after being in a CO-toxic environment for several hours may show low or normal CO levels, despite serious CO poisoning, owing to the half-life of CO on hemoglobin. Measured CO levels do not directly correlate with the severity of symptoms.

The oxygen saturation value is accurate only if it is directly measured in an arterial or venous blood gas sample using CO-oximetry. Values calculated from the arterial partial pressure of oxygen dissolved in the serum or obtained from conventional standard bedside pulse oximetry devices are inaccurate in the setting of CO toxicity and should not be used. Multiwave CO pulse oximetry, however, uses various wavelengths of light to measure carboxyhemoglobin and other values through a noninvasive skin sensor, similar to a pulse oximeter. This device rapidly determines both the CO level and methemoglobinemia (a condition in which the hemoglobin molecule contains a ferric iron [Fe^{3+}] ion) at the bedside and can be used to screen multiple patients following CO exposures. If any doubt exists regarding possible CO exposure, aggressive treatment with 100% oxygen via nonrebreathing face mask should be started before laboratory results are obtained.

Mild CO toxicity results in headache, nausea, vomiting, abdominal pain, and dizziness. Patients without a clear history of CO exposure are at risk of misdiagnosis as having a gastrointestinal virus or colic. Moderate CO toxicity produces confusion, dyspnea, ataxia, tachycardia, and chest pain. Patients with severe CO toxicity have seizure activity, coma, syncope, cardiac arrhythmias, hypotension, and myocardial ischemia. Cherry red skin, a late finding, is usually seen only postmortem. Delayed

neurologic signs and symptoms may occur in as many as 20% of CO-poisoned patients; they present 4 days to 4 weeks after exposure with cognitive and emotional deterioration, personality changes, and diffuse demyelination of white matter. Delayed neurologic signs and symptoms are seen more often in older patients and patients with hypotension, coma, or loss of consciousness.

Patients should be removed from any toxic environment before treatment is administered, and precautions need to be taken to prevent exposure of first responders. When CO poisoning is suspected, fresh air should be provided to patients until supplemental oxygen is available. CO has a half-life of 3 to 4 hours in room air, 60 to 90 minutes if 100% oxygen is administered, and 23 minutes in an environment at 3 atmospheres of hyperbaric oxygen. All symptomatic and confirmed patients should continue on 100% oxygen until their symptoms resolve.

Hyperbaric oxygen is usually needed for all symptomatic patients. Continued treatment is indicated in symptomatic patients who have low CO measurements, as hyperbaric oxygen may prevent the development of delayed neurologic sequelae by decreasing cerebral edema and inhibiting leukocyte activation.

Special Populations

Fetal hemoglobin interacts differently with CO than maternal hemoglobin does, and its higher binding affinity for CO places a fetus at greater risk of CO poisoning. Although maternal blood levels of CO will begin to decline immediately after exposure to CO ceases, elimination of CO in fetal blood takes 3.5 times longer to complete. Fetuses are at increased risk of fetal demise and low birth weights when the mother experiences CO exposure. Pregnant patients with CO poisoning are often referred to hyperbaric oxygen therapy.

The airways of patients with altered mental status or seizures in the setting of CO poisoning or patients with airway burns should be actively managed by ET intubation. In preparation for hyperbaric therapy, patients who require ET intubation and have CO poisoning should have the ET tube cuffs filled with water to prevent the cuffs from decreasing in size.

Cyanide poisoning may complicate CO poisoning as a result of fire exposure, because fires that burn polyurethane, acrylonitrile, nylon, wool, and cotton release cyanide. Cyanide poisoning should be suspected in addition to CO poisoning when the patient has an elevated lactate level; treatment in such a case begins with hydroxocobalamin. The nitrites in the cyanide antidote kits should not be used in patients with both CO and cyanide poisoning, because they will induce methemoglobinemia and decrease the amount of oxygen that hemoglobin can carry.

The remaining treatment for CO exposure is supportive. Airway and ventilator support is needed for comatose patients. Seizures should be controlled with IV benzodiazepines. Exposure to other drugs and toxins should be considered in intentional exposures.

The CCTP should consider the source of CO poisoning in any patient, inasmuch as other family members or coworkers may have remained in a poisoned environment. The insidious nature of CO poisoning has prompted safety-conscious prehospital response services to attach personal CO monitors to first-in bags so providers are alerted immediately when they enter a potentially CO-poisoned atmosphere.

Controversies

Carbon monoxide is the leading cause of poisoning in every industrialized country, yet as many as 50% of cases continue to be misdiagnosed. Long-term consequences of CO poisoning include a significantly increased incidence of neurologic changes ranging from decreased intelligence, to cognitive, emotional, and personality changes, to Parkinson like syndromes. Because symptoms have little correlation to carboxyhemoglobin (blood CO levels), providers must maintain a high index of suspicion and use noninvasive screening technologies whenever available.

Signs and Symptoms

Carbon Monoxide Toxicity
- Mild: headache, nausea, vomiting, abdominal pain, and dizziness
- Moderate: confusion, dyspnea, ataxia, tachycardia, and chest pain
- Severe: seizure activity, coma, cardiac arrhythmias, hypotension, myocardial ischemia, syncope

Transport Management

Carbon Monoxide Toxicity
- Remove the patient from the toxic environment.
- Provide fresh air.
- Perform CO oximetry.
- Give 100% oxygen immediately; if ventilating, also give 100% oxygen.
- Manage the ABCs.
- Perform ET intubation and provide 100% oxygen; fill the ET tube cuffs with water if hyperbaric treatment is anticipated.
- Administer IV benzodiazepines for seizures.
- Assess for other possible causes of altered mental status or cardiovascular dysfunction.
- Consider concomitant poisoning with cyanide if the patient's lactate level is elevated.

Caustics and Corrosives

Patients may be exposed to caustic agents through occupational and industrial exposures, household contacts, and a vast array of other scenarios. Caustics include acids, alkalis, and many other chemicals, all of which may cause mucosal, skin, or internal organ damage following exposure.

The duration of exposure, concentration, pH, particular substance, and site exposed are all factors that influence the degree of toxicity. Exposure can occur through inhalation, ingestion, or dermal or eye exposure. Systemic toxicity is also possible following exposure through any of these routes. Acidic substances cause coagulation necrosis, which limits the depth and extent of injury, although the acid can still be absorbed. Alkali substances form liquefactive necrosis, allowing for extensive tissue penetration. Hydrocarbons and hydrofluoric acid are discussed separately in this chapter.

Diagnosis is often aided by the patient's reported history or description of the setting where the exposure occurred or the symptoms began. Material Safety Data Sheets and other documents may indicate the particular chemical involved and provide suggestions for treatment, decontamination, and PPE needed for rescuers.

Eye and skin exposures to caustics and corrosives require copious irrigation with saline or water. Prolonged eye irrigation is usually best achieved using a Morgan Lens and topical anesthetic. Irrigation of the eye should continue until the pH is normal or at least 2 L of fluid has been used. Skin exposure is best treated by removing clothing and solid materials first, then using a shower to wash off any remaining materials.

Patients with an inhalation exposure require immediate fresh air. Symptomatic patients may require supplemental oxygen, bronchodilator medications, humidified oxygen or air, or assisted ventilation in severe exposures.

The ingestion of caustic agents has the potential to cause devastating injury. Close monitoring for airway compromise, gastrointestinal bleeding and perforation, and free air in the thorax or abdomen is needed. Immediately after oral exposure, patients should be given a small amount of water or milk to drink to remove the caustic agent from the upper airway. Do not induce vomiting or make any attempt at neutralization. Secure the airway with an ET tube early if the patient has signs of airway injury, because such an injury may progress quickly. The patient should be monitored and evaluated for complications and esophageal or gastric perforation for several days following a significant exposure, if such injuries are not immediately apparent.

Consult a toxicologist or Poison Control Center for treatment recommendations for specific exposures. For example, iodine is a caustic and cytotoxic agent and is more toxic than iodide. Dilution with starch (eg, cornstarch, flour, or milk) will convert iodine to the less toxic iodide and may be recommended.

Phenols cause painless caustic burns and coagulation necrosis, but can also produce systemic symptoms such as bradycardia, hypotension, seizures, and movement disorders. They are sticky, oily, and lipid soluble—characteristics that increase skin penetration. Application of water may spread phenols to other areas, so soapy water, vegetable oil, or low-molecular-weight polyethylene glycol may be recommended as means of decontamination.

Hydrogen peroxide is a very mild mucosal irritant. When concentrations greater than 9% are ingested, however, they can produce large amounts of gas that can be absorbed and result in systemic air embolisms.

Anionic and nonionic detergents can result in minor gastrointestinal irritation if ingested. Cationic detergents are more toxic, resulting in severe gastrointestinal distress. In recent years, the introduction of brightly colored single-use laundry packets or laundry "pods" has created an increased risk of poisoning among children, who may mistake these containers for candy. Biting into these pods delivers a concentrated amount of detergent and has resulted in vomiting, respiratory distress requiring intubation, coma, and seizures.

Transport Management

Caustic and Corrosive Exposure

- Perform decontamination: irrigate the eyes or skin with water or saline (combined with a mild soap or detergent if these chemicals are combined with hydrocarbons).
- Check the mucosal eye pH; ensure the pH is normal before discontinuing irrigation.
- Manage the ABCs.
- For inhalation exposure:
  - Provide fresh air.
  - Administer supplemental oxygen.
  - Administer bronchodilator medications if the patient is wheezing.
  - Administer humidified oxygen or air.
  - Provide assisted ventilation in severe exposures.
- For ingestion:
  - Monitor closely for airway compromise, gastrointestinal bleeding and perforation, and free air in the thorax or abdomen.
  - Immediately provide water or milk to drink.
  - Do not induce vomiting or attempt neutralization.

Chlorine, Ammonia, and Asphyxiate Gases

Various gases have the potential to damage or irritate the mouth, nose, and airway; to displace oxygen in a patient's lungs; or to otherwise disrupt effective respiration. These substances exist in gas form or become gases through chemical reactions or when a liquid or solid container is somehow compromised. Exposures occur during a hazardous materials release or when adequate safety precautions are not implemented during the use or storage of these chemicals. The toxicity of such gases is highly variable, depending on the gas, its concentration, the duration of exposure, the preexisting health of the exposed people, and myriad environmental factors.

Chlorine gas is used in the production of a variety of industrial and commercial products, as a disinfectant, and to kill bacteria in public drinking water supplies and swimming pools. As noted earlier, chlorine is also used as a chemical warfare/terrorist agent. In addition, chlorine can be produced inadvertently in the home by mixing an acid cleaner with bleach; a similar compound, chloramine, is produced by mixing ammonia cleaner with a bleach cleaner. Chlorine has the odor of bleach and, when present in concentrated amounts, is yellow-green in color. This water-soluble chemical forms hydrochloric acid on contact with water. Upon dissolving in the water in the eyes, mucous membranes, and airway, it immediately causes irritation. Patients present with airway irritation, coughing, burning, and, in severe cases, wheezing, shortness of breath, and pulmonary edema. Nebulized beta agonists and steroids can be used to counteract these effects. Severe symptoms often respond to neutralization of the hydrochloric acid using a half-strength preparation of sodium bicarbonate (4 mL of 3.75% to 4.2% solution) administered by nebulizer

Ammonia is also a water-soluble irritant gas with a unique, pungent odor. It is used in a variety of industrial processes, released from fertilizer tanks and animal waste, found in household cleaners, and commonly used in the illicit manufacture of methamphetamine. Ammonia dissolves in water in the mucous membranes, thereby forming an alkali solution that results in irritation of the eye, nose, and throat; coughing; and shortness of breath. Treatment is primarily supportive, consisting of oxygen and beta agonists.

Nitrogen oxides are produced by burning fossil fuels, but acute toxicity can occur from ice-making (Zamboni) machines on ice rinks, gas stoves, welding, and farm silos. Nitrogen oxides are water-soluble and penetrate deep into the lungs, resulting in injury there. Care for acute exposure is supportive, but be aware that symptoms may be delayed.

Asphyxiate gases displace oxygen; they include nitrogen, helium, neon, argon, methane, propane, and carbon dioxide. These gases are relatively inert, and exposure to them does not result in tissue damage, metabolic effects, or systemic toxicity. Nevertheless, toxicity-related symptoms may include fatigue, increased rate of breathing, nausea and vomiting, loss of consciousness, seizures, and death. Treatment consists of removing the person from the environment, providing oxygen, and offering other supportive measures.

Hydrogen sulfide gas is produced from the decomposition of organic matter. It can be encountered in oil wells and petroleum refineries, is commonly released in wastewater treatment plants, and collects in enclosed septic systems. This gas smells like rotten eggs and is a respiratory irritant. Like cyanide, it combines with Fe^{3+} on cytochrome AA3, inhibiting cellular energy use. Patients who are exposed to hydrogen sulfide are usually overcome by the gas and present with CNS depression and acidosis. Frequently, first responders are also overcome when they enter the enclosed area. To avoid becoming casualties, rescuers should wear SCBA when entering the area. Treatment for patients exposed to hydrogen sulfide gas consists of high-concentration oxygen—a measure that can reverse the binding of hydrogen sulfide to cytochrome AA3. Depending on the duration of exposure, patients may develop pulmonary edema and sustain permanent anoxic injury.

Cyanide

Cyanide is used in several manufacturing processes, such as paper, textiles, and plastics manufacturing; it is also used for electroplating, cleaning metal, developing photographs, and fumigating or exterminating rodents. This gas is released from some plants, such as almonds, apricot pits, and cassava. In addition, cyanide is produced when synthetic materials such as wool and plastics are burned. Artificial nail removers containing acetonitrile release cyanide as well. German authorities used cyanide in World War II concentration camps to exterminate prisoners; this poison has also been used by other combatants as a chemical warfare agent. Finally, cyanide has been used in both homicides and suicides.

Signs and Symptoms

Chlorine, Ammonia, and Asphyxiate Gases Toxicity

- Lacrimation, coughing, and drooling
- Airway discomfort, swelling, and irritation
- Labored, rapid, or absent breathing
- Wheezing
- Pulmonary edema

Transport Management

Chlorine, Ammonia, and Asphyxiate Gases Toxicity

- Manage the ABCs.
- Provide fresh air.
- Administer supplemental oxygen.
- Administer bronchodilator medications for wheezing.
- Administer humidified oxygen or air.
- Provide assisted ventilation in severe exposures.
- Chlorine exposure: administer a half-strength preparation of sodium bicarbonate by nebulizer (half-strength or 3.75% sodium bicarbonate mixed with saline).
- Administer IV corticosteroids in refractory cases.

Cyanide is a rapid-acting cellular poison that exists as either a colorless gas (hydrogen cyanide) or a solid form (sodium cyanide or potassium cyanide). Although it may have an odor of "bitter almonds," 40% of people cannot detect this odor. Moreover, rescuers should not attempt to identify any exposures through smell and risk their exposure to hazardous materials.

Cyanide exposure can occur though inhalation, ingestion, or transdermal routes. Toxicity is very fast, occurring within seconds to minutes after inhalational exposure, though it may be more delayed with exposure via other routes. Cyanide exposure should be considered in any survivor of smoke inhalation, especially one who has an elevated lactate level.

Cyanide has a high affinity for Fe^{3+}. It causes toxicity by blocking normal energy utilization in the mitochondria. Cyanide binds to Fe^{3+} on cytochrome AA3, blocking this last step in the electron transport chain. Normal cellular energy use is then prevented, efficient production of adenosine triphosphate (ATP) is blocked, and the cells are forced to rely on the relatively inefficient use of anaerobic energy, which generates lactic acid as a by-product. Overall, this process results in clinical signs of hypoxia but without any decreases in pulse oximetry (Po_2). Initial symptoms of cyanide poisoning include dizziness, headache, nausea and vomiting, rapid breathing and heart rate, restlessness, and weakness. They are followed by seizures, loss of consciousness, hypotension, bradycardia, respiratory failure, and death.

When cyanide toxicity is suspected, rescuers should wear appropriate protective suits and SCBA during extrication operations. Copious irrigation with soap and/or shampoo and water should be performed to decontaminate patients. Rescuers should also protect themselves against oral exposures, because the emesis of patients may contain cyanide and contaminate rescuers.

Cyanide poisoning is confirmed by measurement of serum cyanide and thiocyanate levels. These results are not routinely available, however, and treatment should not be delayed for a confirmatory test. Rather, treatment should be started immediately upon recognition of the first signs of toxicity.

Several kits to counteract cyanide exposure are available **FIGURE 21-10**. Nithiodote contains sodium

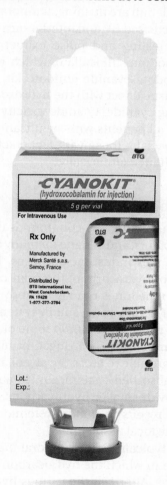

FIGURE 21-10 Cyanide antidote kits are available commercially and may already be present at industrial, laboratory, and manufacturing settings.

CYANOKIT is a registered trademark of SERB Sàrl, licensed to BTG International Inc.

nitrite and sodium thiosulfate. The sodium nitrite induces methemoglobinemia. The methemoglobin is able to bind cyanide, pulling it off cytochrome AA3 and reversing toxicity. Sodium thiosulfate complexes with the cyanide on the methemoglobin, removing the cyanide and helping to eliminate the cyanide in a nontoxic form into the urine.

Nithiodote has now been mostly replaced as a cyanide exposure treatment by the Cyanokit, which contains hydroxocobalamin. Cyanide has a high affinity for cobalt (Co^{2+}), which is found on hydroxocobalamin. Cyanide binds to the Co^{2+}, forming cyanocobalamin and removing it from the Fe^{3+} on cytochrome aac3, which reverses the cyanide toxicity. The dose in adults is 5 g given over 15 minutes; in pediatric patients, it is 70 mg/kg given intravenously over 15 minutes. The main adverse effects of hydroxocobalamin are flushing, temporary red skin and urine, increased BP, and interference with some colorimetric testing and pulse oximetry. Administration of sodium thiosulfate, which is included in the Nithiodote cyanide antidote kit, may have some synergistic effect with the hydroxocobalamin in eliminating cyanide. Cyanide toxicity should be suspected in all patients with significant smoke inhalation, especially those with lactic acidosis, and treatment initiated empirically.

Hydrocarbons

Hydrocarbons are organic compounds used in solvents, fuels, paints, and oils and for many household, commercial, and industrial purposes. Depending on the type of hydrocarbon, they can cause toxicity directly in the lungs or may be absorbed across the lungs or GI tract and result in systemic toxicity. Inhalation is the most common route of absorption for these compounds. The ringed or aliphatic hydrocarbons are able to cross the alveoli in the lungs and can be absorbed systemically. GI absorption is more likely with smaller hydrocarbons. Skin exposure usually results in minor systemic absorption but can cause local tissue injury.

Toxicity typically follows an oral ingestion of a hydrocarbon in which the hydrocarbon also enters into the lungs. Although the various hydrocarbons have different properties, those with high volatility, low surface tension, and low viscosity are most likely to enter the lungs following an oral ingestion. Most toxicity occurs in children who ingest lamp oil, kerosene, lighter fluid, or paint thinner.

Signs and Symptoms

Cyanide Poisoning
- Dizziness
- Weakness
- Headache
- Air hunger
- Acidosis
- No decrease in pulse oximetry or Po_2
- Hyperventilation
- Respiratory depression
- Pulmonary edema
- Complete respiratory failure
- Confusion
- Anxiety
- Seizures
- Complete cardiovascular collapse
- Hypertension or hypotension
- ST-segment and T-wave ECG changes
- Asystole or other conduction blocks and arrhythmias

Transport Management

Cyanide Poisoning
- Perform skin decontamination: copious irrigation with soap and/or shampoo and water.
- Manage the ABCs.
- Administer hydroxocobalamin (Cyanokit).

Hydrocarbons alter the lipid surfactant, a substance that is important to keep the alveoli of the lungs open. Thus, following an oral exposure, a patient may present with cough, shortness of breath, wheezing, and hypoxia. Systemic absorption through the lungs and GI tract can result in CNS depression. Induced vomiting or gastric lavage should be avoided, as both may increase the exposure to the lungs. Treatment is primarily supportive, including oxygen, bronchodilators, and steroids for wheezing and intubation for hypoxia and CNS depression.

Dermal or ocular exposure to hydrocarbons will cause local irritation, burns, or corneal injury. Patients may experience profound chemical burns when hydrocarbon-saturated clothing or footwear is not promptly removed and skin decontaminated. A mild soap or shampoo should be used when irrigating hydrocarbon-contaminated skin.

Solvent abuse is the sniffing of volatile hydrocarbons. Common commercial products such as glues, gas, paint thinners, nail polish removers, adhesives, and cleaning products may contain hydrocarbons and are easily obtained by solvent abusers. These hydrocarbons, when introduced to the lungs, cause dizziness, drowsiness, slurred speech, and unsteady gait.

Trichloroethylene is a halogenated hydrocarbon associated with sudden sniffing deaths. It sensitizes the myocardium to catecholamines, resulting in arrhythmias. Consequently, administration of catecholamines should be avoided in patients who have experienced such exposures. Chronic toluene use results in a renal tubular acidosis, hypokalemia, and severe muscle weakness. Potassium supplementation may be needed for chronic toluene users. Otherwise, treatment for solvent abuse is primarily supportive, consisting of oxygen and intubation for hypoventilation and CNS depression.

The most common types of mothballs are hydrocarbons; they include paradichlorobenzene, naphthalene, and camphor. Paradichlorobenzene is considered nontoxic and is the form most commonly used in households. Naphthalene can cause hemolysis in patients with glucose-6-phosphate dehydrogenase deficiency but is nontoxic in most other patients. Camphor can cause seizures. Although camphor has been removed as an ingredient of mothballs from the US market, it is still found in some imported products.

Transport Management

Hydrocarbon Toxicity

- Manage the ABCs.
- For oral exposures, avoid inducing vomiting, as it may increase pulmonary exposure and toxicity.
- Intubation may be required for patients with CNS depression.

Hydrofluoric Acid

Hydrogen fluoride (HF) is used in semiconductor manufacturing and glass etching, and as a rust remover, vehicle wheel cleaner, and stain remover to clean metal and remove graffiti on walls. Toxicity and time of onset of symptoms from HF poisoning depend on the concentration and duration of exposure. Highly concentrated formulations cause rapid onset of symptoms, while symptoms from low prolonged exposures may present several days later. HF is a relatively weak acid, but it penetrates into the skin; there, the fluoride ion complexes with cations such as calcium and magnesium, resulting in local tissue damage and, in some cases, systemic hypocalcemia.

The fluoride in HF leaches calcium and magnesium from body tissues, resulting in profound and often lethal hypocalcemia and hypomagnesemia. Fluoride also poisons many cellular transport systems, including the Na^+/K^+-ATPase transporter, leading to massive release of intracellular potassium into the systemic circulation. In turn, rapid clinical deterioration of HF-exposed patients may occur unexpectedly. Poisoning by ammonium bifluoride has a presentation and treatment approach similar to that of HF.

Many interventions following HF poisoning are quite unusual and require individualized guidance. Consult a toxicologist or a Poison Control Center for specific treatment decisions about HF exposure.

HF may cause throat discomfort, bronchospasm, stridor, and local airway injury following inhalation. Lung auscultation reveals wheezes, rhonchi, or rales. Serious inhalation exposures can cause delayed chemical pneumonitis or pulmonary edema. Some sources suggest using a nebulized calcium gluconate solution for treatment.

Eye exposure requires thorough and copious irrigation. Early ophthalmologic consultation and evaluation is essential following ocular HF exposure.

Dermal exposure also requires copious irrigation. Potentially contaminated clothing should be removed. Rescuers must use adequate PPE to protect against accidental contact with HF during decontamination.

The ingestion of HF may cause vomiting, abdominal pain, and gastritis, in addition to profound systemic toxicity. Ingestions of large amounts or concentrated solutions of HF are often lethal. If available, immediate stomach evacuation with a nasogastric tube or an orogastric tube should take place. Patients should also immediately ingest a calcium- or magnesium-containing substance such as milk, antacids, magnesium citrate, or magnesium hydroxide. Do not induce vomiting. Likewise, there is no benefit to using activated charcoal, and its presence may obscure a subsequent endoscopic evaluation of the gut.

Most exposures occur on extremity digits when low-concentration HF solutions are used without gloves or there is a break in a glove during industrial or commercial uses. Prolonged low-concentration exposure usually results in a delayed presentation of pain and tissue injury. Patients present with severe throbbing pain at the sites of exposure, with such pain often arising before evidence of local tissue injury becomes apparent.

Treatment for local toxicity includes immersion of the extremity in a high-concentration calcium chloride solution, or application of such a solution to the affected area. Patients may be treated with local IV, intra-arterial, subcutaneous, or dermal calcium administration. This solution is made by dissolving 10% calcium gluconate solution in three times the volume of a water-soluble lubricant (eg, K-Y Jelly). For exposures to the fingers, place the solution into a glove and then put the filled glove over the hand. If this treatment is ineffective, intra-arterial calcium gluconate can be used to perfuse a high concentration of calcium to the affected extremity. Calcium chloride should not be used for subcutaneous or intra-arterial administration. Distal extremity involvement should prompt consultation with a hand surgeon or other appropriate specialist.

High-concentration HF exposure results in immediate severe pain, but the tissue destruction and burns may not become evident for several hours. Large exposures or small exposures with highly concentrated formulations may result in systemic toxicity from hypocalcemia. This may present as tetany, Chvostek sign (facial twitching with tapping of the facial nerve) or Trousseau sign (muscle contraction with inflation of a BP cuff), prolonged QT interval, or cardiac arrhythmias.

Systemic clinical manifestations and arrhythmias from hypocalcemia are treated with intravenous calcium and magnesium. Systemic toxicity requires aggressive replenishment of calcium. Administer calcium gluconate or calcium chloride to any patients with impending or documented hypocalcemia or hyperkalemia, and repeat this treatment as necessary. Multiple grams of IV calcium or a calcium infusion may be required. Monitor serum magnesium levels, and replenish magnesium as indicated. Treat hyperkalemia as necessary with calcium, insulin, dextrose, sodium bicarbonate, and inhaled beta-2 agonists.

Signs and Symptoms

Hydrogen Fluoride Toxicity
- Severe throbbing pain at the site of exposure
- Tissue damage, which may present late
- Hypocalcemia (often severe)
- Hypomagnesemia
- Hyperkalemia

Transport Management

Hydrogen Fluoride Toxicity
- Perform eye and skin decontamination: copious irrigation.
- Manage the ABCs.
- For ingestion exposure:
  - Provide immediate stomach evacuation with a nasogastric or orogastric tube.
  - Administer a calcium- or magnesium-containing substance such as milk, antacids, magnesium citrate, or magnesium hydroxide.
- For skin exposure:
  - Administer calcium gluconate or calcium carbonate gel.
- Administer calcium gluconate or calcium chloride for impending or documented hypocalcemia or hyperkalemia.
- Monitor serum magnesium levels and replenish as necessary.
- Administer calcium gluconate or calcium chloride, insulin, dextrose, sodium bicarbonate, and inhaled beta-2 agonists for hyperkalemia.

Highly Toxic Substances

A vast array of toxic medications and chemicals are discussed throughout this chapter. The topics in this chapter may appear random, but each substance has been included for one of three reasons:

1. The substance may be frequently encountered in the critical care transport environment.
2. Exposure to the substance may require a specialized or unusual approach to treatment.
3. The substance may be highly toxic in very small quantities, requiring greater attention when exposure is suspected.

TABLE 21-4 Substances Highly Toxic to Children (One-Pill Killers)
Prescription Medications
Calcium channel blockers
Tricyclic antidepressants (TCAs)
Antimalarials
Opiates (eg, codeine, hydrocodone, methadone, fentanyl patch)
Sulfonylureas
Class 1 antiarrhythmic agents
Over-the-Counter and Household Products
Camphor
Oil of wintergreen and other topical salicylates Liquid nicotine
Selenium dioxide

Data from Karb R. Toxicology: one pill (or sip) can kill. American College of Emergency Physicians website. https://www.acep.org/how-we-serve/sections/toxicology/news/march-2016/one-pill-or-sip-can-kill/. Accessed April 29, 2021.

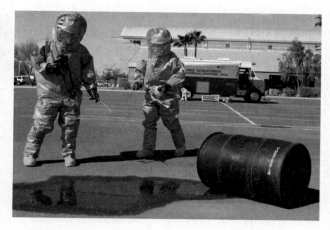

FIGURE 21-11 Hazardous materials scenes pose challenges to providers because of the substances involved and the potential effects on the community.

© Jones & Bartlett Learning.

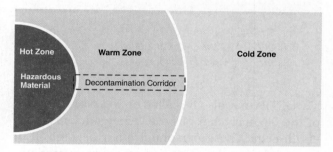

FIGURE 21-12 Configuration of a hazardous materials scene.

© Jones & Bartlett Learning.

CCTPs should be aware that a variety of substances could cause serious illness or death in very small quantities, especially in children **TABLE 21-4**.

Hazardous Materials Response

Hazardous materials (hazmat) incidents pose challenges to emergency responders and health care providers for a variety of reasons **FIGURE 21-11**. These scenes may be in remote, almost inaccessible, locations or in dangerous proximity to major population centers, posing an immediate threat to the health and safety of a community. In many cases, numerous chemicals are released simultaneously. Identification, isolation, and mitigation of a hazardous materials release is often hampered by inadequately prepared responders or a limited number of trained and available emergency responders. In addition, weather, terrain, and other environmental factors may complicate conventional disaster response plans. CCTPs should expect involvement in these incidents as emergency responders, through inadvertent contact, or while performing evacuation and interfacility patient transports.

CCTPs' Role at Hazardous Materials Scenes

Unless CCTPs receive specific training in hazmat response, their role on the scene may be quite limited. Hazmat scenes often involve mechanical extrication, fire suppression, chemical spill containment, population evacuation, crowd and traffic control, the use of complicated PPE, comprehensive primary decontamination, and so forth—skills that CCTPs may be ill prepared to perform without specialized training and equipment. These skills are well beyond the scope of this text.

CCTPs without specialized training or equipment should remain well outside the "hot" and "warm" zones **FIGURE 21-12**, where provider exposure to toxic substances is possible. The areas and shapes of these zones will vary dramatically based on the chemicals involved, wind direction, topography, and other factors. CCTPs can quickly switch roles from rescuer to patient if the wind changes and they are not appropriately positioned and wearing the necessary PPE.

CCTPs should be prepared to evaluate decontaminated patients delivered by hazmat team personnel. It is imperative that CCTPs collaborate with hazmat team personnel to determine which substances are potentially involved and which PPE is appropriate for health care providers during treatment and transport. Poison Control Centers and CHEMTREC can provide invaluable assistance to responders if reliable on-site reference materials are not available.

Hazardous Materials Contact Information

- American Association of Poison Control Centers: 1-800-222-1222, www.aapcc.org
- CHEMTREC: 1-800-262-8200, www.chemtrec.com

CCTPs may also be called on to assist members of the hazmat team or other emergency responders directly. These personnel often become ill or injured during the course of on-scene operations. For example, wearing comprehensive PPE can easily cause heat-related illnesses and dehydration, especially during unfavorable environmental conditions, such as on a hot day with a long walking distance from the staging area to the working area. Fires, falls, traffic incidents, and equipment-related activities all create the potential for trauma to emergency responders. Inadequate PPE for hazmat personnel and incorrect decisions related to the staging area or evacuation can place anyone on the scene at increased risk of toxic chemical exposures.

The main objective of CCTPs at hazmat scenes should be to assess and ensure personnel safety during patient care and transportation. Patient assessment and treatment must occur only after personnel safety has been addressed. Rescuers may needlessly place themselves at risk while attempting to resuscitate a patient who has no chance of being revived. As stated earlier in the chapter, inadequate decontamination on the scene exposes CCTPs to toxic chemicals and compromises the safety of the transport vehicle.

Transport Considerations

Once adequate patient decontamination has been performed and other safety concerns have been addressed, patients should be transported to the closest appropriate health care facility. A small community hospital may be the facility closest to a hazmat incident, but often cannot provide adequate treatment for a critically ill patient requiring complex interventions. For example, a small community health care facility may not have sufficient quantities of antidotes or many of the infrequently used antidotes. CCTPs should consider bypassing such a facility in favor of a larger tertiary center when the risks of a longer transport time are outweighed by the benefits of access to greater health care resources.

CCTPs should carefully monitor for the following situations during patient transport:

- Deterioration in the patient's clinical condition as the toxic exposure evolves
- Signs of inadequate decontamination
- Any interventions appropriate for the patient's clinical situation, within the ability of the transport team, that have not been already performed

Any indications of inadequate primary decontamination warrant prompt correction of that condition. Unusual smells or fumes in the transport vehicle, unexplained symptoms experienced by transport personnel, and new knowledge about the suspected toxic chemical may require immediate aircraft landing, vehicle evacuation, or donning of additional provider PPE.

During patient transport, CCTPs should provide an adequate report to the receiving facility, including the aforementioned elements. In addition, they should thoroughly and accurately document the patient's condition, the interventions performed, and patient status or events during transport. Crews should weigh the benefits of providing a hazmat container to the receiving facility staff (for substance identification purposes) against any additional risks posed by transporting this container. A common gasoline container provides minimal benefit but poses a high risk; in contrast, a tightly sealed container of an unusual substance that is not highly toxic may greatly improve subsequent patient care while posing negligible increased risk. Every situation requires special consideration.

Radiation Emergencies

The threat of radiation exposure or a nuclear incident is ever present in our modern society. Ionizing radiation is capable of causing injury from the release of heat generated by a controlled or uncontrolled reaction. It is important to evaluate the nature of a particular radiation event to determine if it poses any risk to emergency responders and health care providers. Radiation releases may occur in health care, industrial, or laboratory settings; during transportation and disposal of radioactive materials; and following a military or terrorist event.

The approach to the treatment of a potentially exposed patient hinges on the distinction between irradiation and contamination. Health care providers and emergency responders are not placed at any risk by irradiated patients. In contrast, patients with radioactive contamination are likely to spread this material and expose others to radiation. Irradiation will continue to occur until the contaminating materials are contained or otherwise removed. The use of a radiation detection device **FIGURE 21-13** can help responders identify which patients are contaminated with radioactive particles.

Further radiation exposure occurs during incorporation. Devastating individual patient toxicity develops when radioactive materials enter the body, causing ongoing internal exposure.

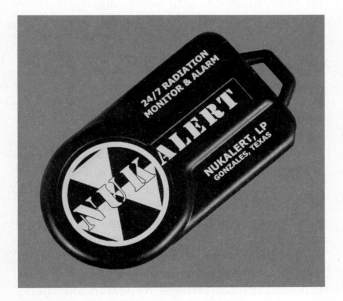

FIGURE 21-13 A radiation detection device.

NukAlert courtesy of Ki4u, Inc.

Clues to the diagnosis of radiation exposure may be obtained through a number of methods. A history of radiation exposure through patient report of an isolated event or widespread knowledge of a large-scale event will greatly assist in diagnosis. The military, health care facilities, emergency responders, laboratories, and industrial settings have various radiation detection devices available. Radioactive particles may be present in a patient's mucous membranes or body fluids and tissues. Acute radiation syndrome (radiation poisoning) may also be diagnosed clinically in potentially exposed people.

Emergency responders should develop a formal radiation response plan. Providers working in proximity to a radiation release need appropriate protective clothing for the situation and must use respirators to avoid inhaling contaminated material. There is little to no risk to the health care provider when caring for a patient who has been removed from the source of contamination. All exposed patients should be decontaminated before care is initiated, unless immediate life threats exist. Once patients are decontaminated, no risk exists to the health care provider from radiation.

Patient decontamination involves removing contaminated clothing and jewelry and providing copious irrigation and thorough washing of the skin with soap and water. Providers should also be checked and decontaminated if necessary. Patients who are exposed to only electromagnetic radiation do not require decontamination. Following decontamination, patients should be reassessed for the presence of persistent radiation by using a handheld or similar device. Persistent radiation requires repeated decontamination.

Patients who experience a massive radiation exposure may die within several hours of that event. Early symptoms include nausea, vomiting, diarrhea, abdominal pain, fever, mental status changes, shock, and coma. In the first 1 to 2 days after exposure, patients may have a brief recovery period. Subsequent toxic effects include multisystem organ dysfunction, bone marrow depression, sepsis, hair loss, dermatologic injury, and eventual death.

Initial treatment focuses on removing any accessible radioactive substances in the body. Chelating agents may bind and remove certain radioactive substances. Potassium iodide can block the uptake of radioactive iodine into the thyroid gland. Water can be given to dilute tritium, and sodium bicarbonate may be used to alkalinize the urine in uranium exposures. Additional treatments depending on the patient's presenting symptoms and are directed toward minimizing the potential for catastrophic infection.

Vehicle Decontamination

Providers must decontaminate the transport vehicle (including aircraft) after the call. This process includes the following steps:

1. Strip used linens from the stretcher immediately after use and place them in a plastic bag or the designated receptacle in the destination facility.
2. In an appropriate receptacle, discard all disposable equipment used for care of the patient that meets your state's definition of medical waste. Most items will be considered general trash.
3. Wash all contaminated areas with soap and water. Scrub blood, vomitus, and other substances from the floors, walls, and ceilings with soap and water. Cleaning must be done first for disinfection to be effective.
4. Disinfect all nondisposable equipment used in the care of the patient. For example, the ECG leads and cables should be cleaned after each patient use as recommended by the manufacturer.
5. Clean the stretcher with an Environmental Protection Agency–registered germicidal/virucidal solution or with bleach and water at 1:100 dilution.
6. If any spillage or other contamination occurred in the transport vehicle, clean it up with the same germicidal/virucidal or bleach/water solution.
7. Clean the outside of the transport vehicle as needed.
8. Replace or repair broken or damaged equipment without delay.
9. Replace any other equipment or supplies that were used.
10. Refuel the vehicle if the fuel tank is below required reserves. Other fluid levels should be checked each time the vehicle is refueled or as your service's standard operating procedure requires.

Restock any supplies you did not get at the receiving facility. Finally, have a written policy/procedure for cleaning each piece of equipment. Refer to the manufacturer's recommendations as a guide.

Radiation burns appear the same way as other burns, and their management varies only by the need to decontaminate the wound of radioactive particles. In addition, for massive doses of radiation, the systemic effects of radiation exposure should be considered and treated. Wounds should be dressed with clean, dry dressings.

Flight Considerations

The importance of safety during air medical transport cannot be overstated when transporting patients following a poisoning, overdose, or toxic exposure. Affected patients pose a serious risk to the lives and health of the transport team.

As stated repeatedly throughout this chapter, patients should not be placed into any transport vehicle, but especially a helicopter or airplane, until an effective initial decontamination has been completed. Whereas ground transport vehicles can stop almost anywhere when conditions in the transport vehicle become unsafe owing to the presence of toxic substances from a contaminated patient, helicopters and airplanes require safe areas to land, which are often unavailable on short notice. In many cases, effective decontamination requires the removal of all contaminated clothing and adequate cleansing and irrigation for a particular substance before air transport can begin.

Air medical crews are also at risk from patients (or family members) with bizarre, aggressive, combative, or violent behavior. It is essential to screen patients (and family members) before transport and to use sedation and restraints as appropriate. At least one fatal air medical crash has been attributed to a patient interfering with aircraft operation. The risk from patients or family members interfering with safe aircraft or transport vehicle operation should not be underestimated.

During air medical transport, access to patients is often limited. In the confined space of an aircraft, with its environmental variables and loud noises, it may be impossible to perform an adequate patient assessment and many therapeutic interventions. Noise and vibration are likely to undermine the accuracy of patient monitoring. The low light conditions found in many aircraft make it difficult to detect skin color changes, respiratory alterations, and even subtle emesis. Air medical crews must be especially prepared to anticipate and manage changes during the flight.

Summary

The management of patients after poisoning or overdose is often a challenging, complicated endeavor. CCTPs must ensure transport team safety while optimizing the chances for patient recovery following a toxic exposure. This chapter serves only as a general overview of various toxicologic emergency situations. During actual patient care, early consultation with a toxicologist, a Poison Control Center, or a reliable toxicology reference will provide invaluable assistance. CCTPs must never lose focus on safety and the ABCs when treating or transporting patients experiencing a toxicologic emergency.

Case Study

You are a member of a helicopter flight crew. You have been called to a rural facility to transport an 18-year-old man who reportedly took his mother's amitriptyline (a TCA) after his girlfriend broke up with him.

On arrival, you receive a report from the attending physician. He states that the patient took an unknown amount of amitriptyline 1 hour before his arrival at the emergency department. The patient has been in the hospital for approximately 45 minutes. He was administered 60 g of activated charcoal when he arrived. The physician reports that all of the patient's laboratory values were normal, and he recently received the patient's arterial blood gas measurements, which were as follows: pH, 7.37; $Paco_2$, 43 mm Hg; Pao_2, 80 mm Hg; and oxygen saturation, 96%. On an ECG, the only other finding was sinus tachycardia at a rate of 118 beats/min with a prolonged QRS interval of 120 ms. The patient has a 20-gauge antecubital IV line in place.

When you obtain the patient's history from his mother, she tells you that she takes 75 mg of amitriptyline at bedtime for depression. She said she receives 2 weeks' worth of medication at a time, and she just filled her prescription. She found her son asleep on his bed with an empty pill bottle beside him. She was able to wake him up and then called 9-1-1. The mother states that her son told her that his girlfriend just broke up with him and that he just wanted to "end it all."

On your arrival at the patient's bedside, you find an 18-year-old man who appears lethargic and is currently lying on his side vomiting black charcoal. His vital signs are as follows: BP, 92/60 mm Hg; temperature, 97°F (36.1°C); pulse rate, 118 beats/min; respiratory rate, 24 breaths/min; and oxygen saturation, 92%. His Glasgow Coma Scale score is 11. The patient opens his eyes to pressure and is able to localize pain. His conversation is confused. The patient has scattered rhonchi throughout, consistent with probable aspiration. You are unable to auscultate bowel sounds, and he has diminished reflexes.

1. What are your priorities with this patient prior to transport?
2. Which other priorities would be important for the treatment of this patient?

Analysis

One of your most important priorities prior to transport is airway management. Depending on their transport vehicle, some providers might elect to rapidly transport the patient and secure the airway en route; however, this patient is already at high risk for aspiration and it would probably be more effective to manage his airway in the more controlled environment of the emergency department prior to transport. This patient needs rapid sequence intubation with both sedative and short-term paralytic medication. Long-term paralysis with a nondepolarizing paralytic should be avoided (unless your service has continuous electroencephalographic monitoring). Patients who overdose with TCAs are at high risk for seizures. Patients whose QRS interval is greater than 100 ms have up to a 34% chance of having seizures and up to a 14% chance of having a life-threatening arrhythmia. If the patient has been paralyzed with a long-term paralytic, you would be unable to tell if he is seizing.

Sedation is required to allow the patient to tolerate the ET tube. An anxiolytic agent such as lorazepam or midazolam should be used for this purpose, as these agents also protect against seizures. The typical sedative dose for midazolam is 0.025 to 0.05 mg/kg IV. If you are administering midazolam for seizures, the usual loading dose is much higher—0.1 mg/kg IV or greater. Propofol, a short-acting sedative, can be used if your service carries it or the sending agent stocks the medication. The ET tube should be secured prior to transport, and a nasogastric tube should be placed. You would also want to instill 60 g of charcoal into the nasogastric tube and then clamp it prior to transport because the patient vomited the first dose. Once BP allows it, elevating the head of the bed by 30° would further reduce the risk of continued aspiration.

Lastly, you need to secure one or two additional large-bore IV lines. Because of the anti-alpha-adrenergic effect of TCAs, this patient is at high risk for further hypotension. He will probably require aggressive fluid resuscitation to stabilize his BP during transport. If the patient remains hypotensive despite administration of fluids, you should administer vasopressors with an alpha-agonist effect (norepinephrine) to maintain an adequate BP. The additional IV lines should be started in the emergency department.

Serum alkalinization with sodium bicarbonate is important in treating patients who have taken a TCA overdose. Most Poison Control Centers recommend serum alkalinization if the QRS duration is 100 ms or greater, if the pH is less than 7.1, or if the patient is hypotensive or having arrhythmias. Alkalinization protects patients from the cardiotoxic effects of TCAs. Correction with sodium bicarbonate promotes protein binding of TCAs and improves myocardial contractility. The goal of therapy is to achieve a pH in the range of 7.5 to 7.55.

Sodium bicarbonate is initially given as a bolus of 1 to 2 mEq/kg IV. You then can begin an IV drip with 150 mEq of sodium bicarbonate per liter of 5% dextrose in water and titrate to keep the patient's pH within the goal range (1 to 3 mL/kg/h). Frequent pH determinations are needed. Obtaining this information is difficult during transport, unless you have point-of-care testing in the helicopter. If the sending institution has started this therapy, it is usually maintained during the flight and it is not titrated until the patient's pH is checked at the receiving facility. If the sending institution has not initiated this treatment, typically the bolus dose is given and the drip is started at the receiving institution.

Prep Kit

Ready for Review

- Poisons, chemicals, medications, and other toxic substances are found in dangerous quantities in homes, schools, agriculture, industry, and commercial establishments; on all modes of transportation; and naturally in the environment.
- Interventions to maintain and enhance the ABCs should not be delayed in favor of interventions specific to toxicologic emergencies (decontamination, enhanced elimination, and antidote administration), which will not become effective rapidly enough to correct immediately life-threatening problems with the ABCs.
- Primary decontamination usually occurs at the scene or outside a health care facility or transport vehicle. It is undertaken to protect rescuers and health care providers from exposure to toxic substances during patient care and transport.

Prep Kit Continued

- Secondary decontamination, which is directed at minimizing patient absorption of or injury from a toxic substance, poses much less risk to health care providers than does primary decontamination.
- Decontamination of a hazardous chemical should occur before an unprotected health care provider makes any contact with the material.
- If rescuers or health care providers do not use the correct PPE before initial patient contact, it may be too late for the equipment to provide adequate protection.
- CCTPs may encounter hazardous situations during anticipated patient transports between health care facilities, while responding to an emergency in the community, or by happening on a vehicular crash.
- Patients may sometimes exhibit violent, bizarre, or aggressive behavior, such that medical or physical restraints may be necessary before effective assessment or treatment can begin.
- Potentially suicidal, combative, aggressive, violent, intoxicated, and confused patients should be restrained, using physical restraints or medical sedation, before transport.
- All patients should be evaluated for the presence of weapons before transport.
- Once the safety concerns have been addressed, maintaining or establishing a patent airway is the top priority in the management of a patient with a toxic exposure.
- A previously patent airway may become compromised during patient transport owing to alteration in the patient's mental status or seizure activity, evolving structural abnormalities from trauma or increasing edema, or obstructions from emesis, secretions, or a foreign body that becomes displaced during the transport.
- Patients who received activated charcoal or syrup of ipecac have an unusual risk of subsequent airway compromise.
- If any doubt arises about the patient's ability to maintain the airway during transport, the airway should be secured with an ET tube.

- Breathing is second only to the airway in importance during patient assessment. Without effective oxygenation and ventilation, tissue hypoxia, acidosis, and cell death will occur.
- Patients with physiologic stress, acidosis, hypermetabolic states (such as occur in pediatric patients), or exposure to many toxic substances require greater oxygenation and ventilation than would usually be required.
- Conventional ventilator settings are often inadequate to meet a patient's needs following a poisoning or overdose.
- Cyanosis, fatigue, and dyspnea indicate that a patient's respiratory status may be compromised.
- Lung auscultation findings of wheezing, pulmonary edema, and decreased, absent, or coarse breath sounds indicate the patient has an unstable respiratory status.
- Oxygen saturation, blood gas analysis, and ETCO$_2$ provide valuable information about the adequacy of oxygenation and ventilation; ongoing monitoring of respiration focuses on changes in breath sounds, patient appearance, and cardiovascular function (as shown by an ECG and assessment of perfusion).
- Evaluation of a patient's circulation requires assessment of end-organ tissue perfusion and overall cardiovascular functioning.
- During the evolution of a toxic exposure, a patient's circulatory status may decline because of the following factors:
  - Direct exposure to cardiotoxic or vasoactive substances
  - Fluid volume loss or redistribution
  - Electrolyte disturbance
  - Airway or respiratory compromise with secondary cardiac dysfunction
  - Manifestations of preexisting cardiovascular disease
  - Altered oxygen-carrying capacity
- Toxic exposures may cause alterations in vascular tone, kidney function, and electrolyte concentration, thereby disrupting fluid balance.

Prep Kit Continued

- The patient, family, and bystander interviews may provide valuable clues about the nature and severity of a toxic exposure, including information about prodromal symptoms and preexisting medical conditions.
- Transport teams must balance the usefulness of a complete head-to-toe physical examination with concerns for patient thermoregulation, privacy, patient access in confined transport vehicles, and the patient's clinical needs.
- Vascular access or intraosseous access sufficient for administering emergency medications and fluids should be established in any patient exposed to a potentially harmful substance.
- Every patient must receive adequate sedation and analgesia while medically paralyzed and should be prophylactically medicated against seizures.
- Patients with increased drug tolerance or a hypermetabolic state require significantly more sedation and analgesia while chemically paralyzed.
- Nonintubated patients require anxiolysis and analgesia following many toxicologic exposures.
- Psychiatric and other at-risk patients may require sedative medications to facilitate patient care and promote patient comfort.
- Hemodynamic and respiratory alterations (eg, tachycardia, bradycardia, hypertension or hypotension, and hyperthermia or hypothermia) may occur as a result of direct action on organs and tissues or through effects on the CNS.
- Advances in point-of-care testing technology allow CCTPs to measure blood chemistry values, arterial or venous blood gases, and other assorted values during transport and obtain results almost immediately.
- Exposure to certain classes of chemicals and medications produces a readily identifiable pattern of clinical signs and symptoms (toxidrome), which aids in diagnosis when the exact nature of the exposure is unclear.

- Some patients may experience life-threatening reactions even when medications are taken at therapeutic doses.
- Anticholinergic syndrome occurs following excessive exposure to medications such as antihistamines, atropine, and benztropine, resulting in muscarinic receptor blockade at the CNS and various other organs.
- Cholinergic syndrome (cholinesterase inhibitor toxicity) occurs following exposure to organophosphate and carbamate insecticides or to certain chemical nerve agents. Cholinesterase inhibitors may affect nicotinic receptors, muscarinic receptors, or both, and alter the function of the neurotransmitter acetylcholine.
- Opioid syndrome commonly develops following illicit use or abuse of opioids in the community or as an adverse consequence of a therapeutic error or accidental ingestion of opioids (eg, morphine, heroin, and fentanyl).
- The administration of an opioid antagonist (naloxone) as a treatment for opioid syndrome may precipitate severe, violent withdrawal symptoms. Many opioids also exert effects much longer than the duration of opioid antagonists, meaning that life-threatening symptoms may return after administration of therapy.
- Sympathomimetic syndrome involves overstimulation of the adrenergic nervous system, resulting in tachycardia, hypertension, agitation, seizures, hyperthermia, dilated pupils, and diaphoresis.
- Malignant hyperthermia occurs following the administration of succinylcholine or certain inhaled anesthetic agents to genetically susceptible patients; it is characterized by muscle spasms, profound muscle rigidity, acidosis, hypercarbia, hyperthermia, tachycardia, tachypnea, myoglobinuria, rhabdomyolysis, and hyperkalemia.
- Neuroleptic malignant syndrome is a potentially fatal reaction to antipsychotic medications; it is characterized by hyperthermia, profound muscle rigidity, metabolic acidosis,

Prep Kit Continued

autonomic dysfunction, confusion, and, in severe cases, renal failure, respiratory failure, arrhythmias, and cardiovascular collapse.

- Serotonin syndrome is an unusual response to serotonin-altering medications that cause hyperserotoninergic symptoms (eg, irritability, muscle rigidity, clonus, myoclonus, hyperthermia, diaphoresis, headaches, seizures, coma, tachycardia, and hallucinations).

- Patient decontamination following exposure to a toxic substance is directed toward minimizing the quantity of the substance absorbed by the patient and the extent of any local damage. Decontamination may be as simple as providing the patient with fresh air or as complicated as whole-bowel irrigation.

- Chemical warfare nerve agents can cause systemic toxic effects from dermal absorption; other caustic chemical warfare agents cause severe local reactions or burns when they come in contact with skin.

- Flushing with water or saline (if the chemical is not water-reactive) is the recommended approach for removal of chemical agents from the patient's skin or eyes.

- Methods for gastrointestinal decontamination include activated charcoal administration, gastric lavage and emptying, and whole-bowel irrigation; however, gastric lavage and whole-bowel irrigation are not done in the transport environment.

- Enhanced elimination methods such as dialysis and urinary alkalinization may be considered if the patient is exposed to lethal quantities of a toxic substance, the ordinary route of elimination from the body is impaired by the overdose or other pathology, or a pre-existing medical condition suggests that the patient will not tolerate the adverse effects of the poisoning.

- Acetaminophen toxicity, which can result in liver failure in severe cases, is treated with initial gastrointestinal decontamination with activated charcoal, followed by oral or IV acetylcysteine (Mucomyst, Acetadote).

- In the field, treatment of an amphetamine overdose—which presents with classic sympathomimetic symptoms—is largely supportive, but may also include sedation with benzodiazepines.

- The majority of patients who experience benzodiazepine overdose require only conservative management and careful observation.

- Glucagon is the initial treatment of choice for a beta blocker overdose. In large ingestions, however, multiple therapies are required.

- One tablet of a calcium channel blocker is often enough to cause serious toxicity or death in a small child. Intravenous calcium is the initial antidote to an overdose of a calcium channel blocker. However, in large ingestions, multiple therapies are required.

- Symptoms of chronic cardiac glycoside toxicity are often vague, frequently leading to misdiagnosis.

- There is no antidote for cocaine toxicity; the treatment for overdose of this illicit drug is supportive, including sedation, and is based on the patient's clinical presentation.

- Patients who experience an opioid overdose can have profound CNS and respiratory depression. Naloxone—which may be administered intravenously, intramuscularly, subcutaneously, via ET tube, nebulized, or intranasally—will reverse the opioid effects and often reestablish a patent airway and spontaneous breathing.

- Any new patient report of tinnitus, dizziness, or deafness should prompt an evaluation for possible salicylate poisoning. There is no antidote for salicylate poisoning, but this condition is a candidate for enhanced elimination with urine alkalinization and hemodialysis. Intubation without adequate ventilation may acutely worsen the toxicity.

- In selective serotonin reuptake inhibitor (SSRI) overdose situations accompanied by serotonin syndrome, the treatment is supportive and based on the patient's presenting symptoms.

- Ethylene glycol and methanol can cause profound, lethal metabolic acidosis following

Prep Kit Continued

ingestion of even very small quantities of these chemicals. Two antidotes are available for the treatment of methanol and ethylene glycol poisoning: ethanol and fomepizole.

- Any patient admitted to a health care facility for an intentional overdose should be screened for the presence of tricyclic antidepressants (TCAs) with an ECG and given aggressive supportive treatment following a TCA overdose.

- The potential for rescuer exposure is high when the incident involves acetylcholinesterase inhibitors, such as during unintentional contact with certain pesticides or as part of a chemical weapon release. Rescuers or health care providers using the appropriate PPE should promptly initiate skin and eye decontamination.

- The brain and heart are the primary sites of carbon monoxide (CO) toxicity owing to their large oxygen requirements. If CO exposure is suspected, aggressive treatment with high-dose oxygen should be started before laboratory results are obtained.

- Exposure to caustic agents can occur through inhalation, ingestion, dermal exposure, or eye exposure; ingestion of these agents has the potential to cause devastating injury.

- Chlorine, ammonia, and asphyxiate gases have the potential to displace oxygen in a patient's lungs; damage or irritate the mouth, nose, and airway; and otherwise disrupt effective respiration. Symptomatic patients may require supplemental oxygen, bronchodilator medications, humidified oxygen or air, or assisted ventilation in severe exposures.

- Although cyanide poisoning can be confirmed with serum cyanide and thiocyanate levels, these measurements are often not readily available. Patients with such toxicity will experience a multitude of neurologic, cardiovascular, and respiratory symptoms. Any exposure to cyanide should be considered potentially lethal. Patients should be treated with hydroxocobalamin (Cyanokit)

or sodium nitrite and sodium thiosulfate (Nithiodote).

- Hydrocarbons can cause toxicity directly in the lungs or may be absorbed across the lungs or GI tract and result in systemic toxicity.

- Hydrocarbons such as gasoline, kerosene, and petroleum may pose a risk of chemical pneumonitis following their aspiration. The care of patients who have toxic exposures to these substances is largely supportive and includes oxygen, bronchodilators, and steroids for wheezing and intubation for hypoxia and CNS depression.

- Hydrofluoric acid is a potent caustic substance that can cause devastating local and systemic toxicity from exposure to even a small amount of concentrated liquid. The treatment for hydrogen fluoride poisoning includes administering a calcium- or magnesium-containing substance such as milk, antacids, magnesium citrate, or magnesium hydroxide.

- A variety of substances can cause serious illness or death in very small quantities, especially in children. The top three culprits in such pediatric poisonings are calcium channel blockers, beta blockers, and TCAs.

- At a hazardous materials incident, CCTPs without specialized training or equipment should remain well outside the "hot" and "warm" zones, where provider exposure to toxic substances is possible.

- Poison Control Centers and CHEMTREC may provide invaluable assistance to health care providers at incidents involving hazardous materials.

- The main objective of CCTPs at hazmat scenes is to assess and ensure personnel safety during patient care and transportation; only when these concerns are addressed can patient assessment and treatment begin.

- Once adequate patient decontamination has been performed and other safety concerns have been addressed, patients involved in hazmat incidents should be transported to the closest appropriate health care facility.

Prep Kit Continued

- CCTPs should carefully monitor for the following situations during patient transport:
  - Deterioration of the patient's clinical condition as the toxic exposure evolves
  - Signs of inadequate decontamination
  - Any interventions appropriate for the patient's clinical situation, within the ability of the transport team, that have not been already performed
- Radiation release may occur in health care, industrial, or laboratory settings; during transportation and disposal of radioactive materials; and following a military or terrorist event. Patients may die within several hours of a massive radiation exposure. The use of a radiation detection device will help identify which patients are contaminated with radioactive particles.
- Radiation burns appear the same way as other burns; their management varies only by the need to decontaminate the wound of any radioactive particles.
- In the flight environment, effective initial decontamination before takeoff is extremely important. Other flight considerations for critical toxicologic emergencies include thoroughly screening patients and family members to prevent violence and behavioral problems during flight and anticipating changes in the patient's condition that may be difficult to detect during flight.

Vital Vocabulary

activated charcoal A carbon-based liquid with an incredible adsorptive ability that is typically administered orally or via nasogastric or orogastric tube to decrease the available quantity of a toxic substance.

acute radiation syndrome Radiation poisoning.

adsorption The process of attracting molecules of a substance to the surface of that substance.

anticholinergic syndrome A syndrome that occurs following excessive exposure to medications such as antihistamines, atropine, and benztropine (Cogentin), or other substances such as jimson weed, resulting in muscarinic receptor blockade at the CNS and various other organs; characterized by tachycardia, hyperthermia, dilated pupils, warm (or hot) dry skin, ileus, delirium, seizures, hallucinations, and urinary retention.

anxiolysis The reduction of anxiety by the administration of an antianxiety agent.

body packers People who swallow carefully prepared packages of illicit substances for smuggling purposes.

body stuffers People who hastily swallow poorly packaged illicit substances (often to avoid impending arrest).

cholinergic syndrome Cholinesterase inhibitor toxicity.

cocaine washout syndrome Profound exhaustion with the ability to regain normal mental status and orientation when aroused; commonly seen with heavy cocaine users.

contamination A state in which a certain substance, such as blood, infectious material, or a toxic substance, is present on an item or surface. In the case of radiation, it is important to distinguish between contamination and irradiation.

DUMBELS Mnemonic for symptoms of anticholinesterase inhibitor toxicity: Diaphoresis/diarrhea, Urination, Miosis, Bradycardia/bronchospasm/bronchorrhea, Emesis, Lacrimation, and Salivation.

enhanced elimination A process that replaces or augments the body's normal method of eliminating, modifying, or breaking down toxic substances.

gluconeogenesis Glucose formation.

glycogenolysis The breakdown of glycogen to glucose.

Prep Kit Continued

hemoperfusion A treatment in which a patient's blood is filtered outside the body through a substance that removes toxic substances from it; a method of removing toxic substances from the blood.

hepatotoxicity Damage to the liver.

incorporation In the radiation context, a process in which radioactive materials enter the body during radiation exposure, causing ongoing internal exposure and creating devastating individual patient toxicity.

inotropic Affecting the contractility of muscle tissue, especially cardiac muscle.

irradiation Exposure to radiation. It is important to distinguish between irradiation and contamination because health care providers and emergency responders are not placed at any risk by patients who have been irradiated but are not contaminated.

malignant hyperthermia A condition that may occur after administration of certain inhaled anesthetics; characterized by muscle spasms, rigidity, acidosis, hypercarbia, hyperthermia, tachycardia, tachypnea, myoglobinuria, rhabdomyolysis, and hyperkalemia.

neuroleptic malignant syndrome (NMS) A potentially fatal reaction to antipsychotic and neuroleptic medications; characterized by patient hyperthermia, profound muscle rigidity, autonomic dysfunction, metabolic acidosis, and confusion.

opioids The class of chemicals that includes naturally derived opiates and newer synthetic medications with the same properties.

opioid syndrome Toxicity that develops following illicit use and abuse of opioids or as an adverse consequence of a therapeutic error or accidental ingestion of opioids and characterized by CNS and respiratory depression.

phosphodiesterase An enzyme that helps break phosphodiester bonds, creating smaller nucleotides.

point-of-care testing Laboratory testing that is performed at the point of care—for example, at the bedside—so that results can be quickly obtained and considered while decisions are being made about patient care.

primary decontamination A form of decontamination that usually occurs at a scene or outside a health care facility or transport vehicle; intended to protect rescuers and health care providers from exposure to a toxic substance during patient care and transport.

prodromal Referring to the early signs and symptoms that occur before a disease or condition, such as a toxic exposure, fully appears—for example, dizziness before fainting.

pulse CO-oximetry A noninvasive screening and monitoring method for methemoglobinemia and carbon monoxide exposure.

rhabdomyolysis The destruction of muscle tissue.

secondary decontamination A form of decontamination directed at minimizing patient absorption or injury from a toxic substance; it occurs after initial decontamination has occurred outside a health care facility or transport vehicle.

sedative-hypnotic syndrome A syndrome characterized by lethargy, sedation, hypoventilation, apnea, bradycardia, and hypotension that occurs following exposure to any medication or chemical that can cause central nervous system sedation, lethargy, or coma.

serotonin syndrome An unusual response to serotonin-altering medications causing hyperserotoninergic symptoms.

SLUDGEM Acronym for symptoms of anticholinesterase inhibitor toxicity: Salivation, Lacrimation, Urination, Diarrhea, Gastroenteritis, Emesis, and Miosis.

stimulant washout syndrome Excessive sleep, hunger, and depression as a result of excessive amphetamine use.

Prep Kit Continued

sympathomimetic syndrome A syndrome that involves overstimulation of the adrenergic nervous system, resulting in tachycardia, hypertension, agitation, seizures, hyperthermia, dilated pupils, and diaphoresis.

toxidrome A group of symptoms, or syndrome, associated with toxicity of a given substance.

whole-bowel irrigation (WBI) A gastric decontamination method that involves the patient drinking or receiving via a nasogastric tube large quantities of a nonabsorbable, electrolyte-balanced liquid that propels stomach and intestinal contents through the digestive system.

References

Ables AZ, Nagubilli R. Prevention, recognition, and management of serotonin syndrome. *Am Fam Physician.* 2010;81(9):1139-1142.

Alapat PM, Zimmerman JL. Toxicology in the critical care unit. *Chest.* 2008;133(4):1006-1013.

American Academy of Clinical Toxicology; European Association of Poisons Centres and Clinical Toxicologists. Position statement and practice guidelines on the use of multi-dose activated charcoal in the treatment of acute poisoning. *J Toxicol Clin Toxicol.* 1999;37(6):731-751.

Bartkus A. Toxicologic emergency transport. In: Clark DY, Stocking J, Johnson J, eds. *Flight and Ground Transport Nursing Core Curriculum.* Denver, CO: Air and Surface Transport Nurses Association; 2005:593-633.

Benson BE, Hoppu K, Troutman WG, et al.; American Academy of Clinical Toxicology; European Association of Poisons Centres and Clinical Toxicologists. Position paper update: gastric lavage for gastrointestinal decontamination. *Clin Toxicol.* 2013;51(3):140-146.

Beuhler MC, Gala PK, Wolfe HA, Meaney PA, Henretig FM. Laundry detergent "pod" ingestions: a case series and discussion of recent literature. *Pediatr Emerg Care.* 2013;29(6):743-747.

Borron SW, Bebarta VS. Asphyxiants. *Emerg Med Clin North Am.* 2015;33(1):89-115.

Boyer EW. Management of opioid analgesic overdose. *N Engl J Med.* 2012;367(2):146-155.

Brooks DE, Levine M, O'Connor AD, French RNE, Curry SC. Toxicology in the ICU. Part 2: specific toxins. *Chest.* 2011;140(4):1072-1085.

Carvalho M, Carmo H, Costa VM, et al. Toxicity of amphetamines: an update. *Arch Toxicol.* 2012;86(8):1167-1231.

Christensen DM, Iddins CJ, Sugarman SL. Ionizing radiation injuries and illnesses. *Emerg Med Clin North Am.* 2014;32(1):245-265.

Chyka PA, Seger D, Krenzelok EP, Vale JA; American Academy of Clinical Toxicology; European Association of Poisons Centres and Clinical Toxicologists. Position paper: single-dose activated charcoal. *Clin Toxicol.* 2005;43(2):61-87.

Frommer DA, Kulig KW, Marx JA, Rumack B. Tricyclic antidepressant overdose: a review. *JAMA.* 1987;257(4):521-526.

Furtado MC, Walter FG, Klein R. Personal protective equipment and decontamination. In: Walter FG, Klein R, Thomas RG, eds. *Advanced Hazmat Life Support Provider Manual.* 3rd ed. Tucson, AZ: University of Arizona; 2003.

Goldfarb DS, Ghannoum M. Principles and techniques applied to enhance the elimination of toxic compounds. In: Nelson LS, Howland MA, Lewin NA, Smith SW, Goldfrank LR, Hoffman RS, eds. *Goldfrank's Toxicologic Emergencies.* 11th ed. New York, NY: McGraw-Hill; 2019:90-100.

Hodgman MJ, Garrard AR. A review of acetaminophen poisoning. *Crit Care Clin.* 2012;28:499-516.

Hoegberg LCG. Techniques used to prevent gastrointestinal absorption of toxic compounds. In: Nelson LS, Howland MA, Lewin NA, Smith SW, Goldfrank LR, Hoffman RS, eds. *Goldfrank's Toxicologic Emergencies.* 11th ed. New York, NY: McGraw-Hill; 2019:48-70.

Hoffman RS, Burns MM, Gosselin S. Ingestion of caustic substances. *N Engl J Med.* 2020;382(18):1739-1748.

Holstege CP, Borek HA. Toxidromes. *Crit Care Clin.* 2012;28:479-498.

Huzar TF, George T, Cross JM. Carbon monoxide and cyanide toxicity: etiology, pathophysiology and treatment in inhalation injury. *Expert Rev Respir Med.* 2013;7(2):159-170.

Jang DH, Spyres MB, Fox L, Manini AF. Toxin-induced cardiovascular failure. *Emerg Med Clin North Am.* 2014;32:79-102.

Kant S, Liebelt E. Recognizing serotonin toxicity in the pediatric emergency department. *Pediatr Emerg Care.* 2012;28(8):817-821.

King AM, Aaron CK. Organophosphate and carbamate poisoning. *Emerg Med Clin North Am.* 2015;33(1):133-151.

Kruse JA. Methanol and ethylene glycol intoxication. *Crit Care Clin.* 2012;28:661-711.

Lugassy DM. Salicylates. In: Nelson LS, Howland MA, Lewin NA, Smith SW, Goldfrank LR, Hoffman RS, eds. *Goldfrank's Toxicologic Emergencies.* 11th ed. New York, NY: McGraw-Hill; 2019:555-566.

Mack E. Focus on diagnosis: CO-oximetry. *Pediatr Rev.* 2007;28:73-74.

Prep Kit Continued

Marraffa JM, Cohen V, Howland MA. Antidotes for toxicological emergencies: a practical review. *Am J Health Syst Pharm.* 2012;69:199-212.

McQuade DJ, Dargan PI, Wood DM. Challenges in the diagnosis of ethylene glycol poisoning. *Ann Clin Biochem.* 2014;51(2):167-178.

Musselman ME, Saely S. Diagnosis and treatment of drug-induced hyperthermia. *Am J Health Syst Pharm.* 2013;70(1):34-42.

National Disaster Life Support Education Consortium. *Basic Disaster Life Support (BDLS).* 2nd ed. Augusta, GA: NDLSEC; 2001.

Nelson LS, Erdman AR, Booze LL, et al. Selective serotonin reuptake inhibitor poisoning: an evidence-based consensus guideline for out-of-hospital management. *Clin Toxicol.* 2007;45(4):315-332.

Newton EH, Shih RD, Hoffman RS. Cyclic antidepressant overdose: a review of current management strategies. *Am J Emerg Med.* 1994;12(3):376-379.

O'Malley GF. Emergency department management of the salicylate-poisoned patient. *Emerg Med Clin North Am.* 2007;25(2):333-346.

Occupational Safety and Health Administration. Standard interpretations: cyanide antidotes. https://www.osha.gov /laws-regs/standardinterpretations/2020-03-31. Published March 31, 2020. Accessed January 30, 2021.

Schneiderbanger D, Johannsen S, Roewer N, Schuster F. Management of malignant hyperthermia: diagnosis and treatment. *Ther Clin Risk Manag.* 2014;10:355-362.

Smollin CG, Hoffman RS. Cocaine. Nelson LS, Howland MA, Lewin NA, Smith SW, Goldfrank LR, Hoffman RS, eds. *Goldfrank's Toxicologic Emergencies.* 11th ed. New York, NY: McGraw-Hill; 2019:1124-1134.

Stork CM. Serotonin reuptake inhibitors and atypical antidepressants. In: Nelson LS, Howland MA, Lewin NA, Smith SW, Goldfrank LR, Hoffman RS, eds. *Goldfrank's Toxicologic Emergencies.* 11th ed. New York, NY: McGraw-Hill; 2019:1054-1064.

Thanacoody R, Caravati EM, Troutman B, et al. Position paper update: whole bowel irrigation for gastrointestinal decontamination of overdose patients. *Clin Toxicol.* 2015;53(1):5-12.

Tomassoni AJ, French RN, Walter FG. Toxic industrial chemicals and chemical weapons: exposure, identification, and management by syndrome. *Emerg Med Clin North Am.* 2015;33(1):13-36.

Tormoehlen LM, Tekulve KJ, Nañagas KA. Hydrocarbon toxicity: a review. *Clin Toxicol.* 2014;52(5):479-489.

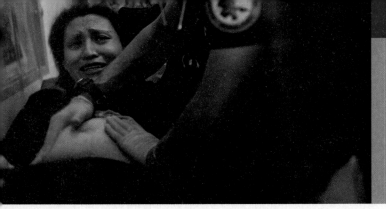

Chapter 22

Obstetric and Gynecologic Emergencies

Kathleen Kerrigan, MD

Adrianne Wurzl, DO

OBJECTIVES

After completing this chapter, you will be able to:

1. Discuss the anatomy of the female reproductive system (p 1186).
2. Recognize the physiologic changes that occur during pregnancy (p 1188).
3. Describe the changes that occur in the cardiovascular, respiratory, gastrointestinal, renal, and endocrine systems during pregnancy (pp 1188–1191).
4. Discuss dermatologic changes that occur during pregnancy (p 1191).
5. Discuss special areas of concern when performing a critical care transport of a pregnant patient (p 1191).
6. Describe the management of the pregnant patient who is in cardiac arrest (p 1192).
7. Discuss potential maternal cardiovascular complications exacerbated or induced by pregnancy (p 1192).
8. Discuss fetal oxygenation and heart rate, including conditions associated with fetal distress during labor (p 1193).
9. Discuss how to assess a fetus during a critical care transport (p 1193).
10. Describe several methods of fetal monitoring during critical care transport of a pregnant patient, including electronic fetal monitoring (p 1195).
11. Explain how to use a Doppler device (p 1197).

12. Describe the complications of pregnancy, including early pregnancy loss, ectopic pregnancy, and causes of bleeding (pp 1202–1203).
13. Discuss the signs and symptoms and treatment of abruptio placentae, placenta previa, and uterine rupture (pp 1203–1206).
14. Discuss medical conditions that can exist during pregnancy, including hypertension complicating pregnancy, preeclampsia, eclampsia, and HELLP syndrome (pp 1206–1209).
15. Explain how to manage medical conditions that can exist during pregnancy, including hypertension complicating pregnancy, preeclampsia, eclampsia, and HELLP syndrome, during critical care transport (pp 1206–1209).
16. Explain the concerns regarding preterm labor and premature delivery (p 1209).
17. Discuss the use of tocolytic agents to interrupt labor (p 1211).
18. Recognize fetal malpresentations of delivery, including frank breech, complete breech, incomplete breech, footling breech, and umbilical cord prolapse (pp 1212–1214).
19. Discuss how to manage fetal malpresentations during a critical care transport (p 1212).

Introduction

Management of the pregnant patient can challenge the critical care transport professional (CCTP). In such a scenario, the CCTP must take into account the competing concerns of the woman and the fetus, the physiologic changes induced by pregnancy, and the presence of potentially life-threatening pathologic conditions. This chapter provides an overview of the physiologic changes in pregnancy and describes specific emergency conditions associated with pregnancy, childbirth, and postpartum care. Understanding of the anatomic and physiologic changes that occur during pregnancy is essential to provide effective care to obstetric patients.

Controversies

A common concern when faced with a critically ill or injured pregnant woman is whether the mother or the fetus takes priority. In all cases, the priority is resuscitation and stabilization of the mother. The key to a viable fetus, even when a decision is made to expedite delivery, is restoration of adequate perfusion in the mother.

Anatomy and Physiology of the Female Reproductive System

Within the female reproductive system, the 28-day menstrual cycle is regulated by a series of hormonal secretions. These hormones prepare the uterus for implantation of a fertilized egg and the start of pregnancy. In the absence of pregnancy, the uterine wall sheds its inner lining, known as the endometrium. The mucosal tissues and blood are discharged through the vagina, in a process known as menstruation. Menstruation lasts approximately 3 to 7 days.

FIGURE 22-1 depicts the menstrual cycle. At the beginning of the menstrual cycle, a rise in the levels of follicle-stimulating hormone (FSH) triggers the start of the preovulatory phase, also known as the follicular phase. During the next 7 to 8 days, the uterine wall begins to swell, or proliferate, and the process of maturity begins with follicle stimulation in the ovaries. FSH stimulates the creation of an oocyte in the ovary. As the oocyte begins to mature, the ovary secretes estrogen, which causes the endometrium to swell with blood. As the follicle matures, the increased levels of estrogen cause the anterior pituitary to secrete luteinizing hormone (LH). Introduction of this hormone stimulates the release of the oocyte—called an ovum now that it is mature—from the ovaries and the start of ovulation. For the next 24 to 48 hours, as the newly formed ovum travels down the fallopian tube to the uterus, the woman's fertility is at its peak. A hard shell known as the corpus luteum, which begins to secrete more estrogen, testosterone, and progesterone, is left behind in the ovary. As progesterone levels rise over the next 14 days, the endometrium continues to swell and provides a soft shelter for the egg. If conception does not occur, the unfertilized ovum travels into the uterus. Progesterone levels drop off as the corpus luteum begins to dissolve in the ovary and menstruation begins, ending the cycle.

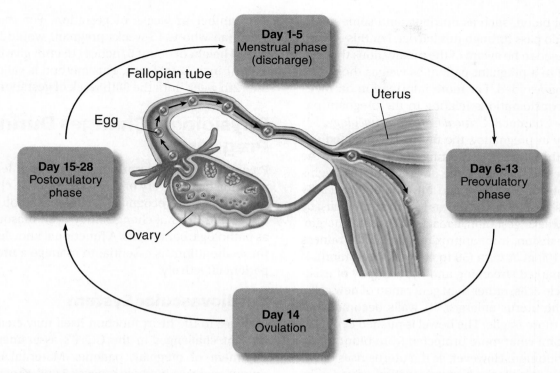

FIGURE 22-1 The menstrual cycle, based on an average 28-day cycle. The length of the cycle and the number of days in each phase vary from woman to woman, but generally fall within a range of 24 to 35 days.

© Jones & Bartlett Learning.

Conception and Gestation

If fertilization has occurred, the egg—known as the zygote—implants in the endometrium. Blastocytes inside the zygote secrete human chorionic gonadotropin (hCG), which extends the life of the corpus luteum. The placenta, which is attached to the wall of the uterus, supplies the fetus with oxygen and vital nutrients and removes waste products such as carbon dioxide. In addition, the placenta continues to secrete the progesterone needed to maintain a swollen endometrium and continue the pregnancy. The placenta and the fetus are connected by the umbilical cord, which contains two arteries and one vein that carry the blood of the fetus to and from the placenta **FIGURE 22-2**.

The placenta is an ephemeral, or transitory, organ that is formed early by the implantation of the zygote into the endometrium. The placenta grows with the fetus; it contains a thin membrane that separates maternal and fetal blood from coming into contact with each other. Nutrients, oxygen, and carbon dioxide diffuse across this membrane to nourish the placenta. It is important to understand that

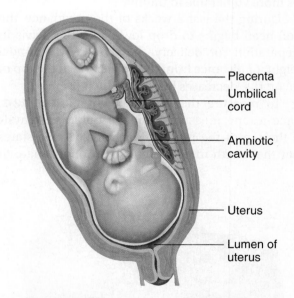

FIGURE 22-2 The umbilical cord and other structures of the uterus in a pregnant woman.

© Jones & Bartlett Learning.

maternal blood is never shared with fetal blood; a fetal barrier prevents maternal blood from entering the fetal circulation, although substances from the maternal blood, such as nutrients and some medications, do pass through this barrier. For this reason, CCTPs need to be aware of the medications that can be given to a pregnant patient as well as those that should be avoided. For more information on medication considerations relating to the pregnant patient, see Chapter 8, *Critical Care Pharmacology*.

Early in pregnancy, the uterus is contained entirely within the protective ring of the pelvis. By the 12th week of gestation, the enlarged uterus begins to rise out of the pelvis and into the abdomen. By 20 weeks' gestation, the uterus is at the umbilicus; by 34 to 36 weeks' gestation, it reaches the costal margin. This expansion, from approximately 2 to 39 ounces (50 to 1,100 g) at term (39 to 40 weeks' gestation), is due to marked stretching and hypertrophy of existing muscle cells, rather than generation of new cells.

As the uterus enlarges, its walls become thinner and more fragile. The bowel is pushed cephalad and is somewhat more protected from blunt injury to the abdomen. However, as the uterus rises out of the pelvis, it loses the bony protection provided by the pelvis and becomes more vulnerable to trauma. Also, as the fetus grows, the relative proportion of amniotic fluid to fetal size decreases, making the fetus more vulnerable to trauma.

During the last 2 weeks of the pregnancy, the fetal head begins to drop lower into the pelvis in preparation for delivery. As a result, the fundal height, or distance from the pelvic ring to the top of the uterus, decreases by about 1 inch (2 cm).

To measure the fundal height **FIGURE 22-3**, place a tape measure from the pubic symphysis to the top of the fundus. MacDonald's rule states that the length in centimeters is proportionate to the number of weeks of gestation. For example, a woman who is 15 weeks pregnant would have a fundal height of about 6 inches (15 cm), give or take 0.5 to 1 inch (1 to 3 cm). This method is valid from the 12th week until the 38th week of gestation.

Physiologic Changes During Pregnancy

Pregnancy alters the normal physiology of females, affecting nearly every organ system. These changes may mask well-recognized signs or symptoms of disease, or normal changes may even masquerade as pathologic conditions. A functional knowledge of these alterations is essential to manage a pregnant patient effectively.

Cardiovascular System

Changes to the heart function itself may create significant challenges in the CCTP's assessment and treatment of pregnant patients. Maternal cardiac output begins to increase by week 5 and remains elevated throughout the duration of pregnancy. During the first 10 weeks of pregnancy, the cardiac output increases 20% to 30%, or 1 to 1.5 L/min, and by gestational term it could be as much as 43% higher than baseline. This increase in the cardiac output is primarily due to an increase in plasma volume, a decrease in vascular resistance, and an increase in heart rate by approximately 10 beats/min. This change in hemodynamics allows for increased blood flow to the uterus. The increased baseline pulse rate must be considered when the CCTP is interpreting a pregnant woman's tachycardia in response to hypovolemia.

Cardiac arrhythmias are also quite common in pregnancy. A common finding is sinus tachycardia, with the average maternal heart rate being 60 to 104 beats/min by the third trimester. Atrial fibrillation, atrial flutter, supraventricular tachycardia (SVT), premature atrial contractions (PACs), and premature ventricular contractions (PVCs) all have an increased prevalence during pregnancy, as do ventricular tachycardia and heart failure.

Another consideration regarding the pregnant patient's heart function is the positioning of the heart. Elevation of the diaphragm during pregnancy causes a leftward and upward shift of the heart, which can present on electrocardiograms as left axis deviation, and even Q waves in leads II, III, and aVF or inverted T waves in III and V_1–V_3.

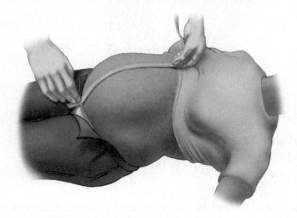

FIGURE 22-3 Measuring fundal height.

Blood Pressure

By weeks 6 to 8, blood pressure (BP) begins to drop as a result of the ongoing release of progesterone, which relaxes the walls of the blood vessels, causing a decrease in systemic vascular resistance. BP reaches its lowest point in the second trimester, decreasing by 5 to 10 mm Hg systolic and 10 to 15 mm Hg diastolic. At term, BP returns to near pre-pregnancy levels. CCTPs need to be mindful that patients may present with slightly lower BP levels than baseline when they are trying to distinguish physiologic versus pathologic hypotension in the pregnant patient.

Body positioning in the third trimester may significantly affect BP and cardiac output. When the patient is lying supine, the uterus may compress the inferior vena cava, reducing venous return from the lower extremities and causing hypotension. This phenomenon is referred to as **supine hypotensive syndrome**. Displacement of the gravid uterus off of the vena cava by manual manipulation or by placement of the patient in the left lateral position will relieve this obstruction and, in turn, restore BP.

For patients secured to a long backboard, it is important to tilt the backboard to the left to relieve the pressure on the inferior vena cava. This positioning is accomplished by placing blankets or towels under the right side of the backboard **FIGURE 22-4**. Note that these materials are placed under the backboard, not directly under the patient.

Venous Pressure

The peripheral venous pressure in the lower extremities also increases progressively during the later stages of the pregnancy. The compression of the inferior vena cava and pelvic veins by the uterus causes this increased pressure. As a result, more bleeding than expected may occur from minor wounds to the lower extremities. Increased venous pressure can also increase the patient's risk of leg edema, hemorrhoids, varicose veins, and deep venous thrombosis.

TABLE 22-1 summarizes cardiovascular system changes during pregnancy.

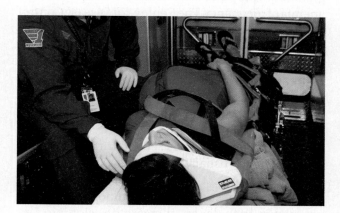

FIGURE 22-4 Place pregnant patients with spinal injuries on a backboard with blankets and towels under the right side of the backboard to tilt it toward the left and relieve pressure on the inferior vena cava.

© Jones & Bartlett Learning.

TABLE 22-1 Cardiovascular Changes in Normal Pregnancy

	Nonpregnant Patient	**Pregnant Patient**
Cardiac output	<5,000 mL/min	Up to 7,000 mL by third trimester (30% to 50% increase)
Stroke volume	65 mL	85 mL
Pulse rate	80 beats/min	10% to 20% increase
Red blood cell mass	5 million mm³	Up to 40% increase
Systemic vascular resistance	1,500 dyne-sec/cm^{-5}	25% decrease
Mean arterial pressure	85 mm Hg	Gradual decrease until 16 to 20 weeks, then return to normal
Systolic blood pressure	120 mm Hg	120 mm Hg
Diastolic blood pressure	70 mm Hg	80 mm Hg

Data from Hall ME, George EM, Granger JP. The heart during pregnancy. *Rev Esp Cardiol*. 2011;64(11):1045-1050; Sanhavi M, Rutherford JD. Cardiovascular physiology of pregnancy. *Circulation*. 2014;130(12):1003-1008.

Blood Volume and Composition

One of the most significant changes in pregnancy is the marked increase in total plasma volume. Circulating blood volume expands by an average of 40% to 45%. This greater volume provides adequate blood supply to the fetus and compensates for impaired venous return to the maternal heart and blood loss during labor. Hemoglobin and hematocrit concentrations do not, however, increase by the same amount. The increase in plasma volume is greater than the increase in the level of hemoglobin, causing dilutional anemia. The hematocrit value decreases, reaching its lowest point between 32 and 34 weeks' gestation. This point is referred to as the physiologic anemia of pregnancy. The Centers for Disease Control and Prevention (CDC) defines anemia during pregnancy as a hemoglobin level less than 11.0 g/dL in the first and third trimesters, and less than 10.5 g/dL in the second trimester. Platelet counts, however, remain stable throughout pregnancy.

The leukocyte count is generally elevated during pregnancy and may reach 25,000/µL during labor. However, beginning in the second trimester, leukocyte function is usually depressed, which can leave the pregnant patient more vulnerable to infection.

Other changes in blood components during pregnancy include an increase in clotting factors. Increased coagulation factors decrease the prothrombin time (PT) and partial thromboplastin time (PTT). Fibrinogen levels increase dramatically during pregnancy, nearly doubling by delivery. These changes predispose pregnant patients to clotting and deep vein thrombosis in the lower extremities and pulmonary embolus.

Given their larger blood volume, pregnant patients with active bleeding may experience a significant blood loss before they exhibit clinical signs and symptoms of hypovolemia, including changes in vital signs. While external bleeding may be obvious on physical exam, internal bleeding may be masked by relatively unchanged vital signs. CCTPs must be aware that these patients, especially those who have sustained known blunt trauma to the abdomen, may have significant internal bleeding with normal vital signs in the beginning but then quickly decompensate once a significant blood volume is lost. Thus, pregnant patients with blunt trauma must be considered to have internal bleeding even when they are hemodynamically stable.

Respiratory System

The respiratory system undergoes significant changes during pregnancy. The diaphragm elevates approximately 4 cm by term. Chest diameter increases, though overall the functional reserve capacity decreases. Minute ventilation increases due to an increase in tidal volume, likely secondary to increased levels of progesterone. The increased ventilation leads to a lower P_{CO_2} (partial pressure of carbon dioxide) level of approximately 30 mm Hg (normal is 40 mm Hg) and respiratory alkalosis. The body compensates for the increase in pH by creating a state of metabolic acidosis, resulting in only a mild change in the overall pH to a slightly more alkalotic state, with the average pH ranging from 7.40 to 7.47. Respiratory rate stays below 20 breaths/min, and a rate higher than 20 breaths/min should be considered abnormal.

The demand for increased oxygen created by the growing fetus results in a significantly reduced oxygen reserve for the mother. In turn, desaturation occurs more quickly in pregnant patients than in nonpregnant patients. Using the accessory muscles is also difficult for pregnant patients in respiratory distress because the diaphragm is displaced and the abdominal muscles are weakened, resulting in ineffective tripoding. CCTPs must be aware that pregnant patients in respiratory arrest are likely to become hypoxic faster than nonpregnant patients. Early oxygenation to ensure a saturation level of 92% or greater and aggressive airway management with intubation should be primary considerations. Laryngeal edema should be expected, with an average Mallampati score of 3 (discussed in detail in Chapter 6, *Respiratory Emergencies and Airway Management*). Consider use of alternative airways if you are unable to intubate a pregnant patient; use of a bag-mask device alone will increase her already high risk of aspiration.

Gastrointestinal System

The gastrointestinal system undergoes positional changes and overall relaxation during pregnancy. The uterus displaces the stomach and intestines cephalad, increasing the risk of nausea and vomiting. Gastric emptying is delayed and gastroesophageal sphincter tone is reduced, leading to gastroesophageal reflux and further nausea and vomiting. Increased nausea and vomiting can place patients at higher risk of dehydration. Administration of intravenous (IV) fluids and oxygen and patient positioning (position of comfort or on the left side) can help lessen these effects during transport.

During labor, gastric emptying time may increase further, increasing the likelihood of regurgitation and aspiration. The risk is further increased if the patient has an altered level of consciousness or if analgesics are administered. Consequently, CCTPs must consider intubation early in the pregnant patient because of the higher probability of aspiration.

Gastrointestinal changes also require consideration in pregnant trauma patients. Given the displacement of the diaphragm, a pregnant patient requires placement of a chest tube in a more cephalad location to avoid injuring the bowel. The intestines are relocated to the upper part of the abdomen during pregnancy, so they may be shielded by the uterus from blunt trauma. In contrast, the liver and spleen remain in their normal locations under the diaphragm, but are pushed cephalad somewhat in late pregnancy.

Renal and Endocrine Systems

During pregnancy, the renal system is stressed; there is a 30% increase in the glomerular filtration rate (GFR), an increase in kidney size, and relative obstruction of the ureters, leading to hydroureteronephrosis. While many women may experience only frequent urination from an increase in GFR, renal outlet obstruction by the growing uterus may cause flank pain and a decrease in urination volume. Placing the patient in a left lateral recumbent position may relieve this flank pain. Renal calculi are no more common in pregnant patients than in nonpregnant patients, and their treatment should remain the same: observation, pain control, and allowing the stone to pass. Nonsteroidal anti-inflammatory drugs (NSAIDs) should be avoided in pregnancy.

Urinary tract infections are more frequent in pregnant patients; untreated early trimester infections will lead to pyelonephritis in the third trimester of pregnancy approximately 50% of the time. Given the significant consequences for the patient and fetus, all pregnant women should be screened for bacteriuria. Patients with chronic renal failure (CRF) can undergo dialysis treatment as needed. Patients with acute renal failure will have issues

with compensation of respiratory alkalosis, as discussed earlier, so CCTPs must be aware of changes in their pH levels and treat them accordingly.

At the beginning of conception, the endocrine system goes into overdrive. The pituitary and thyroid glands enlarge, resulting in increased production of estrogen, progesterone, cortisol, and thyroxine. These hormones play important roles in fetal development and in preventing the fetus from aborting; however, in some cases, the elevated hormone levels alter the effectiveness of insulin and result in a condition known as insulin resistance. After 20 weeks' gestation, insulin resistance can lead to elevated blood glucose levels and gestational diabetes. Gestational diabetes is treated primarily by diet control and, if needed, insulin.

Thyroid conditions (hyperthyroidism or hypothyroidism) may affect fetal development, because thyroid-releasing hormone can cross the placenta. Consequently, patients with these conditions should be monitored carefully during prenatal care. CCTPs should expect complications during delivery and the possibility of a distressed neonate if a patient who has a thyroid disorder has had poor control of thyroid abnormalities.

Dermatologic Changes

The hormonal changes during pregnancy have an impact on the largest organ of the body—the skin. In addition to acne, pregnant patients can experience linea nigra, a darkened line that typically develops from the navel to the pubis, although it may extend for the entire length of the abdomen in some patients. Chloasma refers to darkened skin patches on the cheeks and forehead that appear during pregnancy. Finally, some late-term patients present with an itchy rash known as pruritic urticarial papules and plaques of pregnancy (PUPPP), which may be either isolated to one region or more widespread. Patients can be prescribed topical corticosteroid ointments to treat this condition and will occasionally require systemic corticosteroids.

Critical Care Transport of the Pregnant Patient

The role of the CCTP in any critical care transport is to safely and effectively manage, treat, and transport the patient to the facility that can best meet the needs of that patient. The pregnant patient's dynamic physiologic changes and the developing fetus can pose a challenge for any hospital, especially those without obstetric services. In addition, pregnancy can lead to exacerbation of maternal chronic diseases such as coronary heart disease, mitral valve prolapse, and aortic stenosis. Treatment must focus on maintaining the pregnant woman's hemodynamics. CCTPs need to remember that taking care of the pregnant woman means that the fetus is being taken care of as well. In critical cases, treatment of the pregnant patient is no different than that of the nonpregnant patient; for example, treatment of a pregnant patient with an existing cardiovascular condition does not differ from treatment of a nonpregnant patient with this condition. There is one exception: In a patient whose pregnancy is 20 weeks or greater, positioning during transport may be different. The gravid uterus can compress the inferior vena cava when the patient is supine. Performing a left lateral tilt or transporting the patient in the left lateral decubitus position will alleviate this compression.

The CCTP must perform a complete physical exam, including maternal and fetal hemodynamic monitoring. If the patient is in labor, perform external visualization of the perineum to assess for crowning. If delivery is imminent, the CCTP should assist in the delivery. On arrival at the facility, if delivery is imminent, assist with delivery at that facility. Do not begin transport when delivery is imminent.

Cardiac Arrest Management of the Pregnant Patient

When faced with cardiac arrest of a pregnant patient, CCTPs need to remember that the pregnant woman's health is the treatment priority. When the pregnant patient is treated appropriately, the fetus also benefits. Pregnant patients who go into cardiac arrest typically have a 30% to 80% mortality rate. Common causes of cardiac arrest in pregnancy include hemorrhage, severe hypertension, amniotic fluid embolism, peripartum cardiomyopathy, respiratory arrest, pulmonary embolism, stroke, trauma, and/or infection.

In general, management of cardiac arrest in pregnancy follows similar principles and guidelines as advanced cardiac life support (ACLS) for a nonpregnant patient. The standard rules of cardiopulmonary resuscitation (CPR) apply, with chest compressions in the traditional position and limited interruptions for ventilation. One major difference involves positioning of the uterus. At approximately 20 weeks' gestation, the uterine fundus can be palpated at the umbilicus. At this size, the uterus can cause circulatory problems by decreasing return of blood flow to the heart. If the fundus is palpated at or above the umbilicus, the following technique is recommended: One provider should manually displace the uterus to the left to relieve aortocaval compression and allow for effective venous return and maximal circulation, while another provider continues CPR per BLS/ACLS guidelines. If using an automatic CPR compression device, another option is to tilt the patient to the left lateral decubitus position while automated compressions are ongoing. Manual CPR and intubation are difficult and not as effective when the patient is tilted to the left, so this repositioning should occur only if the providers are using an automated compression device.

Standard guidelines for medication administration in cardiac arrest should be followed with pregnant patients. Epinephrine can be potentially beneficial in these patients, as in other patients in cardiac arrest, although it may harm the fetus. However, in this situation the benefits of such treatment greatly outweigh the risks. Lidocaine may be used especially in the setting of ventricular tachycardia and ventricular fibrillation and has no teratogenic effect on the fetus. Amiodarone can be quite harmful to the fetus, although the benefits outweigh the risks in pregnant patients with refractory ventricular fibrillation or tachycardia. Calcium chloride and calcium gluconate to treat hyperkalemia are both safe in pregnancy. Use the standard doses for pregnant patients. Overall, as in any adult cardiac arrest, survival depends on high-quality CPR and early defibrillation.

Defibrillation remains essential for patients in ventricular fibrillation or pulseless ventricular tachycardia and is safe for the fetus. Use the same settings and paddle positioning as you would for nonpregnant patients. Fetal monitors (discussed later in this chapter) must be disconnected prior to delivering a shock. Pregnant patients become hypoxic more rapidly than nonpregnant patients, so early oxygenation is essential. Provide airway management early; intubate if possible. Intubation should be performed as usual. The only adjustment is manual displacement of the uterus to the left, so as to avoid critical hypotension during intubation.

IV access should be obtained above the diaphragm because blood flow to the heart from below the diaphragm is reduced secondary to uterine compression of the blood vessels. Given the tasks required for performing the resuscitation, the AHA recommends that four BLS responders be present.

Transport Management

Cardiac Arrest in the Pregnant Patient
- Administer CPR.
- Provide early oxygenation.
- Manually displace the uterus to the left to relieve aortocaval compression.
- Defibrillate the patient in ventricular fibrillation and pulseless ventricular tachycardia (but remove the fetal monitor if present).
- Administer resuscitation medications.
- Obtain IV access above the diaphragm if possible.

Fetal Assessment and Monitoring

Several methods can be used to assess and monitor the fetus. Fetal circulation, oxygenation, and heart rate are reviewed first.

Fetal Circulation, Oxygenation, and Heart Rate

Fetal oxygenation depends on a well-oxygenated maternal blood flow to the placenta. Both adequate maternal oxygen saturation and adequate oxygen tension in maternal arterial blood are needed to promote adequate fetal oxygenation. Fetal circulation occurs through the umbilical vein and umbilical arteries **FIGURE 22-5**. The umbilical vein carries highly oxygenated, nutrient-rich blood from the placenta to the fetus's right atrium via the ductus venosus and the inferior vena cava, and the umbilical arteries carry arteriovenous blood back to the placenta. This system allows the fetal circulation to largely bypass the fetus's lungs until birth.

The oxygen content of fetal blood is lower than that of maternal blood, even though the rate of oxygen consumption by the fetus is nearly twice that of a pregnant woman per unit of weight. However, oxygen will bind preferentially to fetal hemoglobin, as it has a different molecular structure than adult hemoglobin does. The developing fetus obtains its oxygen from the blood of a pregnant woman that passes through the placenta and has only a small reserve of oxygen—usually only 1 to 2 minutes if the maternal supply is cut off or diminished. During uterine contractions, blood flow through the uterine arteries to the placenta is momentarily interrupted or diminished. A healthy fetus with a normal placenta can withstand the stress of labor without having hypoxia develop because sufficient oxygen exchange occurs during the interval between contractions. However, premature fetuses or fetuses under stress (small for gestational age, multiple gestation, hypertensive disorders of pregnancy) may not tolerate labor well and are at risk for hypoxia.

The fetal heart rate is sensitive to the changes in oxygen supply. Fetal monitoring is an ongoing indirect assessment of physiologic factors, both extrinsic and intrinsic to the fetus, that affect fetal oxygenation. A decrease in fetal heart rate may be a sign of fetal hypoxia.

TABLE 22-2 summarizes conditions associated with fetal distress during labor that may decrease oxygenation and cause an abnormality in fetal heart rate.

Fetal Assessment

The most difficult job that the CCTP has when transporting a critical pregnant patient is assessing the second patient—the fetus. All patient assessments start with the ABCs. Assessment and monitoring can be extremely challenging in the fetus, but they can be done effectively. Before transporting any pregnant patient, a fetal assessment needs to be performed.

Prior to physical assessment of the fetus, history can be useful in determining fetal health. "Kick counts" are one assessment method. In a pregnancy of 20 weeks' or greater gestation, fetal movement has been reported as a way to assess fetal health and can be determined by asking the patient how often fetal movements are felt. Maternal perception of 10 distinct fetal movements within a 2-hour period is considered reassuring.

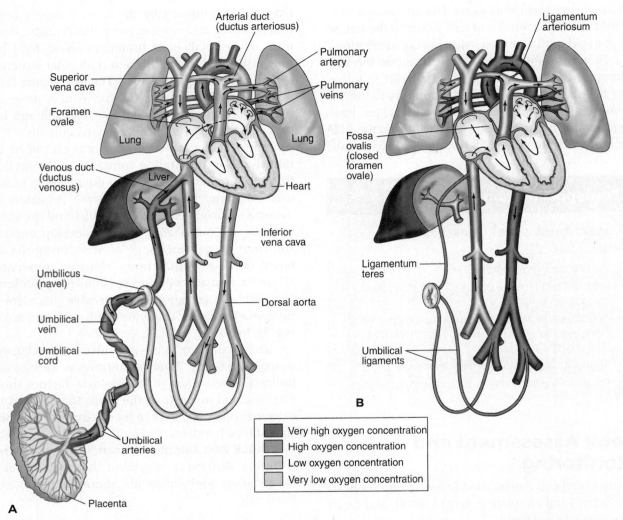

FIGURE 22-5 Fetal circulation. **A.** Oxygenated blood from the placenta reaches the fetus through the umbilical veins. Blood returns to the placenta via two umbilical arteries. **B.** Fetal circulation following transition.

© Jones & Bartlett Learning.

The next step in assessing fetal health is to evaluate the heart rate. It is not recommended to use a normal stethoscope for this purpose, especially in early-term patients; instead, CCTPs should use a Doppler ultrasonograph starting at 10 weeks' gestation or a fetal stethoscope (fetoscope) after 20 weeks' gestation to detect a heartbeat. First, palpate the abdomen to determine the uterus resting tone and assess for uterine contractions. Next, auscultate the fetal heart rate. The fetus's back is the optimal location to hear the heartbeat; feel for the most rigid part of the fundus to detect the proper location for auscultation. When using a Doppler ultrasonograph, apply conductive gel to the pregnant

patient's abdomen at this location before applying the ultrasound transducer, and then listen for the heartbeat. To confirm that you are listening to the fetal heartbeat, take the pregnant patient's radial pulse and compare the rates; the fetal heart rate should be faster.

The normal heart rate of a fetus is between 110 and 160 beats/min **TABLE 22-3**. If a patient is in labor, monitor the fetal heart tones for at least 30 to 60 seconds every 15 minutes and record the results. In a noisy environment, auscultation of fetal heart tones can be challenging, and it may be difficult to determine how the heart rate is changing over time. For this reason, continuous electronic fetal

TABLE 22-2 Conditions Associated With Fetal Distress During Labor

Source	Condition
Umbilical cord	Hematoma True knot in cord Nuchal cord Prolapsed cord Cord compression
Placenta	Infarction Abruption
Uterus	Tetanic contractions Hyperstimulation Tachysystole
Fetus	Anemia Infection
Maternal	Hypertension Hypotension Severe anemia Seizures Fever Infection Diabetic mother

© Jones & Bartlett Learning.

TABLE 22-3 Fetal Heart Rate Parameters

Rate	Beats/min
Normal	110–160
Abnormal	
Tachycardia	>160
Bradycardia	<110

© Jones & Bartlett Learning.

TABLE 22-4 Elements of a Biophysical Profile

Fetal heart rate
Fetal breathing movements
Fetal body movements
Fetal muscle tone
Amount of amniotic fluid

Note: Each characteristic of the biophysical profile is given a score of 0–2 points, with a maximum score of 10.

Data from Mayo Foundation for Medical Education and Research.

monitoring should be performed during high-risk transports. Continuous electronic fetal monitoring is discussed in the next section.

An insufficient fetal movement count or nonreassuring heart rate requires further detailed evaluation of the fetus, such as a nonstress test (NST) or biophysical profile (BPP). NST is a more practical approach for the CCTP because it takes a mere 20 minutes to perform, whereas a BPP can take from 30 minutes to an hour. **TABLE 22-4** summarizes the elements of a BPP. An NST requires the CCTP to use electronic fetal monitoring (explained later). A sign of a healthy fetus is at least two accelerations that occur in 20 minutes, where an acceleration is defined as an increase of the heart rate from the fetus's baseline by 15 beats/min for at least 15 seconds. Fewer than two accelerations in 20 minutes may be a sign of nonreassuring fetal status. NSTs require an external fetal monitor with recording capability. BPP requires an ultrasonogram as well as someone to perform and interpret the results.

Electronic Fetal Monitoring

Electronic fetal monitoring can be done externally, internally, or both, but during critical care transports it is usually done externally. **External fetal monitoring** uses ultrasonic transducers that are applied to the surface of the pregnant patient's abdomen to assess the fetal heart rate and uterine activity **FIGURE 22-6**. To perform this monitoring, first apply ultrasound gel to the ultrasound (Doppler) transducer. Place the transducer on the maternal abdomen, preferably over the fetal back. Next, palpate the maternal abdomen, and place the tocotransducer (toco) on the abdomen over the upper uterine segment where there is the least amount of maternal tissue between the pressure-sensing button and the uterus. The fetal heart rate data collected via external fetal monitoring is converted into a visual display that can appear on paper, a computer screen, or both.

Electronic fetal monitoring is recommended for all high-risk interfacility transports. Monitoring enables continuous reporting of the fetal heart rate and uterine contractions by a two-channel strip chart recorder that prints the results **FIGURE 22-7**. An alteration in fetal heart rate correlates with fetal oxygenation.

Equipment

The following equipment is needed to perform external fetal monitoring:

- Fetal monitor
- Conducting gel

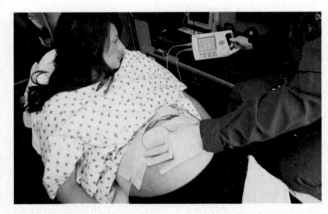

FIGURE 22-6 External fetal monitoring.

© Jones & Bartlett Learning.

- Tracing paper
- Ultrasonographic Doppler
- External uterine activity detector (tocodynamometer)

Steps

SKILL DRILL 22-1 shows the steps for performing fetal monitoring, which are summarized here:

1. Prepare all equipment prior to transport. Introduce yourself and explain the procedure to the patient **STEP 1**. Be sure to clarify that this procedure is normal for all transports and that it is essential to monitor the baby's health during the trip.
2. Connect to the power source **STEP 2**.
3. Connect the Doppler ultrasound probe to the patient and adjust the volume **STEP 3**.
4. Note that the fetal heart rate should be displayed in green.
5. Make sure that the *Auto Nonstress Test* switch is in the off position **STEP 4**.
6. Manually set the uterine Doppler ultrasonograph to zero. Wait for the alerting sound.
7. Press the recording switch.
8. Set the fetal heart tone alarms.

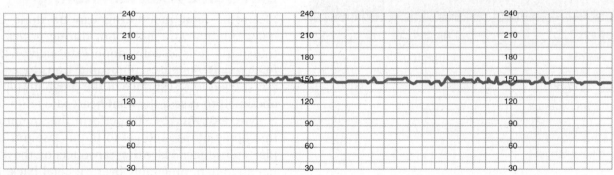

Fetal Heart Rate   Time

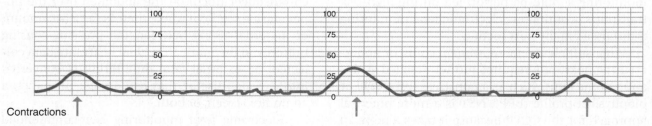

Contractions

FIGURE 22-7 A fetal monitoring strip showing uterine contractions.

© Jones & Bartlett Learning.

Skill Drill 22-1 Fetal Monitoring

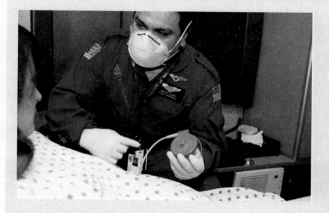

Step 1

Prepare all equipment prior to transport. Explain the procedure to the patient.

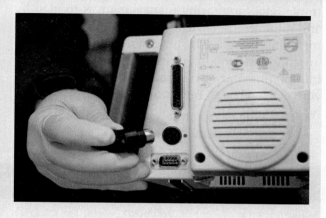

Step 2

Connect to the power source.

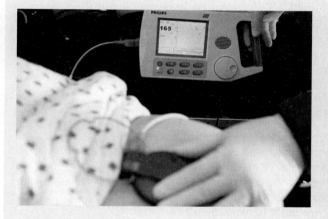

Step 3

Connect the Doppler ultrasound probe to the patient and adjust the volume. The fetal heart rate should be displayed in green.

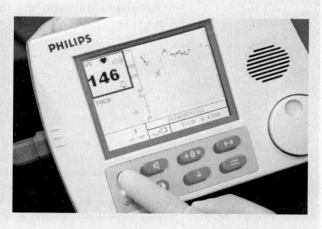

Step 4

Make sure that the *Auto Nonstress Test* switch is in the off position. Manually set the uterine Doppler ultrasonograph to zero. Wait for the alerting sound. Press the recording switch. Set the fetal heart tone alarms.

© Jones & Bartlett Learning.

Assessment of fetal monitoring strips rarely occurs during transport, although the CCTP may obtain a strip during transport if possible and needed. If internal fetal monitoring was initiated prior to transport, it may be continued en route. Nevertheless, external monitoring should be in place due to the high likelihood of displacement of the internal monitor during movement.

Electronic fetal monitoring is intended to assess the adequacy of fetal oxygenation during labor. As described earlier, oxygen is carried from the internal environment to the fetus by maternal and fetal blood along a pathway that includes the maternal lungs, heart, vasculature, uterus, placenta, and umbilical cord. Interruption of this oxygen pathway at one or more points can result in a fetal heart rate deceleration. Electronic fetal monitoring in the normal patient is expected to show an absence of metabolic acidemia. The goal of standardized electronic fetal monitoring management is to identify and minimize potential sources of preventable error when caring for the pregnant patient and fetus.

Interpretation of monitoring results involves interpreting uterine contractions **TABLE 22-5** along with five fetal heart rate components:

- Baseline heart rate
- Baseline variability
- Accelerations
- Decelerations
- Changes or trends over time

Uterine contractions are defined as the number of contractions present in a 10-minute time frame averaged over 30 minutes. The CCTP should assess for contraction frequency, duration, intensity, and resting tone between contractions **TABLE 22-6**. Assessment of contractions can be done by palpation of the abdomen, or by palpation in conjunction with use of an external tocodynamometer or intrauterine

TABLE 22-5 Five Fetal Heart Rate Components

Term	Definition
Baseline heart rate	• Mean FHR rounded to increments of 5 beats/min during a 10-min period • Baseline must be persistent for a minimum of 2 min in a 10-min segment • Normal FHR baseline: 110–160 beats/min • Tachycardia FHR baseline: >160 beats/min • Bradycardia FHR baseline: <110 beats/min
Baseline variability	• Fluctuations in the FHR baseline that are irregular in amplitude and frequency • Four types of variability: • Absent: Amplitude range undetectable • Minimal: Amplitude range detectable but ≤5 beats/min • Moderate (normal): Amplitude range 6–25 beats/min • Marked: Amplitude range >25 beats/min
Acceleration	• A visually apparent abrupt increase (onset to peak in less than 30 s) in the FHR • At 32 weeks' gestation and beyond, acceleration has a peak ≥15 beats/min above baseline, with duration of 15 s or more but less than 2 min from onset to return • Before 32 weeks' gestation, an acceleration has a peak ≥10 beats/min above baseline, with a duration of 10 s or more but less than 2 min from onset to return • Prolonged acceleration lasts ≥2 min but <10 min in duration • If an acceleration lasts ≥10 min, it is a baseline change
Early deceleration	• Visually apparent, usually symmetric gradual decrease and return of the FHR to baseline associated with a contraction • Gradual FHR decrease from onset to nadir of the deceleration associated with a contraction • Nadir of the deceleration occurs at the same time as peak of the contraction
Late deceleration	• Visually apparent, usually symmetric gradual decrease and return of the FHR to baseline associated with a contraction • Delayed onset, with nadir always occurring after peak of the contraction
Variable deceleration	• Abrupt decrease in FHR below the baseline of ≥15 beats/min lasting ≥15 s but <2 min
Prolonged deceleration	• Visually apparent decrease in FHR below the baseline • Decrease in FHR from baseline ≥15 beats/min lasting ≥2 min but <10 min in duration • Decrease in FHR lasting >10 min is considered a baseline change
Sinusoidal pattern	• Visually apparent, smooth, sine wave-like undulating pattern in FHR baseline with a cycle frequency of 3–5 cycles/min that persists for ≥20 min

Abbreviation: FHR, fetal heart rate

Data from Miller DA. Intrapartum fetal evaluation. In: Gabbe SG, Niebyl JR, Simpson JL, et al., eds. *Obstetrics: Normal and Problem Pregnancies.* 7th ed. Philadelphia, PA: Elsevier; 2017.

TABLE 22-6 Assessment of Uterine Contractions

Contraction Component Assessment	Defined
Frequency	Measured from the beginning of one contraction to the beginning of the next; has units of minutes.
Duration	The length of the contraction from start to end of the contraction; has units of seconds.
Intensity	The strength of the contraction; described as mild, moderate, or strong by palpation or measured in units of millimeters of mercury if an intrauterine pressure catheter is used.
Resting tone	Assessed in the absence of contractions or between contractions. Using direct palpation, the abdomen is described as soft or hard.

© Jones & Bartlett Learning.

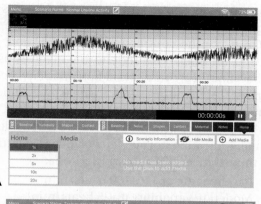

A

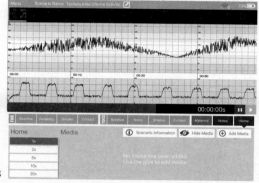

B

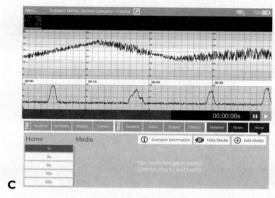

C

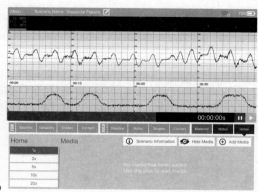

D

FIGURE 22-8 Uterine contraction patterns. **A.** Normal uterine activity. **B.** Tachysystole uterine activity. **C.** Normal Category I tracing. **D.** Sinusoidal pattern.

Courtesy iSimulate, www.isimulate.com.

pressure catheter. The tocodynamometer is part of electronic fetal monitoring and externally detects abdominal pressure of the contour changes resulting from uterine contractions. A normal contraction pattern is defined as 5 or fewer contractions in 10 minutes, averaged over a 30-minute time frame **FIGURE 22-8A**.

Tachysystole is defined as more than 5 contractions in 10 minutes, averaged over a 30-minute time frame **FIGURE 22-8B**. Tachysystole increases the amount of time that blood in the intervillous spaces remains in stasis, reducing the potential for maternal-fetal exchange of respiratory gases. The intervillous space contains the vessels that communicate between the mother and fetus. Tachysystole can occur from exogenous stimulation—for example, with use of cervical ripening medications—or from internal production of endogenous agents such as maternal oxytocin or prostaglandin. It is important to recognize and intervene when this abnormal pattern is observed.

Once uterine contractions are calculated, the next section of external monitoring involves using the baseline heart rate, baseline variability, accelerations, decelerations, and changes over time to identify tracings as Category I, II, or III.

A Category I tracing **FIGURE 22-8C** is considered normal, indicating normal fetal acid–base status at that time. It meets the following criteria:

- Baseline rate of 110–160 beats/min
- Moderate variability (6–25 beats/min)
- No late or variable decelerations
- Present or absent early decelerations
- Present or absent accelerations

FIGURE 22-9 shows some external fetal monitoring results related to fetal heart rate variability. **FIGURE 22-10** presents results related to accelerations and decelerations.

Moderate variability or accelerations in the fetal heart rate reliably predict the absence of fetal metabolic acidosis at the time they are observed. In contrast, minimal or absent variability does *not* reliably predict the presence of metabolic acidosis. Likewise, the absence of accelerations does *not* reliably predict the presence of metabolic acidemia or hypoxia.

Bradycardia is a concerning finding, as it suggests congenital heart block or serious fetal compromise. Tachycardia can be a sign of maternal

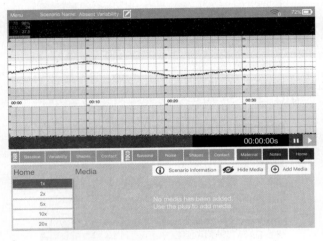

A

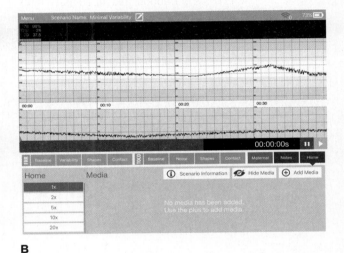

B

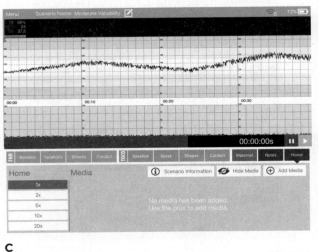

C

D

FIGURE 22-9 External fetal monitoring results: variability. **A.** Absent variability. **B.** Minimal variability. **C.** Moderate variability. **D.** Marked variability.

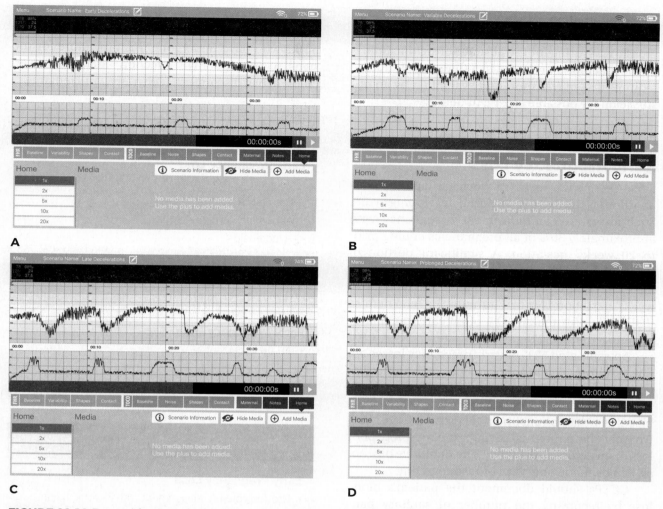

FIGURE 22-10 External fetal monitoring results: accelerations and decelerations. **A.** Early decelerations. **B.** Variable decelerations. **C.** Late decelerations. **D.** Prolonged decelerations.

Courtesy iSimulate, www.isimulate.com.

infection, cardiac arrhythmias, maternal drug administration, or fetal compromise.

A Category III tracing has at least one of the following components:

- Absent variability with any of the following:
  - Recurrent late decelerations
  - Recurrent variable decelerations
  - Bradycardia
- A sinusoidal pattern **FIGURE 22-8D**

Late and recurrent variable decelerations are considered recurrent when they are observed in at least 50% of contractions within a 20-minute period.

Category III tracings are considered abnormal and require emergent measures to improve fetal oxygenation and/or to expedite delivery to reduce neonatal morbidity and mortality. Continued Category III fetal heart rate patterns herald an increased risk of fetal hypoxia and acidosis, which can lead to cerebral palsy and hypoxic ischemic encephalopathies.

Category II tracings represent fetal heart rate patterns that do not meet the classification criteria for either Category I (normal) or Category III (abnormal); hence, they are considered indeterminate or atypical. The potential for development of fetal acidosis varies widely across the spectrum of Category II tracings. While they have an uncertain prognosis, such fetal heart rate patterns may be observed for prolonged periods of time, which make them very challenging to evaluate and manage.

In summation, if the CCTP observes a Category I tracing during external fetal monitoring, this is grossly reassuring for the absence of significant hypoxia or acidosis in the fetus. A Category III tracing requires urgent transport and evaluation by an obstetrician for possible emergent delivery.

Complications of Pregnancy
Early Pregnancy Loss

Early pregnancy loss (miscarriage, spontaneous abortion) is the loss of a fertilized developing ovum. Such losses are common in early pregnancy, with approximately 30% of all pregnancies ending prior to 20 weeks' gestation. A significant portion of those losses will occur prior to the woman becoming aware of the pregnancy. Loss of a fetus after 20 weeks' gestation is called intrauterine fetal demise (IUFD). Approximately 80% of all early pregnancy losses occur during the first trimester.

An estimated 50% of early pregnancy losses are due to chromosomal abnormalities in the fetus. Patients often present with vaginal bleeding or cramping. Assessment of the female patient with vaginal bleeding or abdominal pain focuses on identifying whether the patient is having an early pregnancy loss or an ectopic pregnancy. The definitive diagnosis can be made only with ultrasonography.

CCTPs should document the patient's blood loss by recording the number of sanitary pads soaked during transport and relay this information to the receiving facility. Vaginal bleeding that soaks more than one pad every hour is cause for concern. Hypotension is treated with isotonic fluid volume replacement such as lactated Ringer solution or normal saline. Treatment for women having an early pregnancy loss also includes providing comfort and emotional support.

If patients do not completely expel all of the products of conception, this retention puts them at higher risk of continued bleeding or infection. These patients may require a dilation and curettage (D&C). In this surgical procedure, the physician dilates the cervix with special cervical dilators and curettes the uterine lining, usually with a suction device, to remove the remaining products of conception. The goal is to reduce the risk of infection caused by tissue left behind on the uterine wall. Such patients should be transported to a facility where this procedure can be performed within 24 hours.

As with any invasive procedure, there is a risk for infection with D&C. CCTPs need to watch patients who have undergone this procedure for the signs of postoperative infection, including fever, chills, pelvic discomfort, tachypnea, and lethargy.

Signs and Symptoms

Early Pregnancy Loss
- Vaginal bleeding
- Cramping
- Abdominal pain
- Hypotension

Differential Diagnosis

Early Pregnancy Loss
- Abruptio placentae
- Ectopic pregnancy
- Placenta previa

Transport Management

Early Pregnancy Loss
- Provide volume replacement with isotonic fluids.
- Provide comfort and emotional support.
- Apply sanitary pads, and count how many become saturated.

Ectopic Pregnancy

An ectopic pregnancy is a pregnancy that implants outside of the uterus. Complications of ectopic pregnancies can be life threatening for the woman. Ectopic pregnancies represent 1% to 2% of all pregnancies and account for 9% of pregnancy-related deaths in the United States. Most ectopic pregnancies occur in the fallopian tubes, although a small percentage can implant in the peritoneum, in an ovary, in the cervix, or interstitially. When the fertilized egg attempts to implant in tissue other than the uterus, it causes bleeding and damage to the underlying tissue. Women of childbearing years with sudden onset of abdominal pain or uncommon vaginal bleeding must be considered to have an ectopic pregnancy. The greatest risk factor for the occurrence of an ectopic pregnancy is pelvic inflammatory disease. Severe pelvic inflammatory disease can cause tubule scarring, which destroys the cilia that would otherwise guide the ovum to the uterus. This scarring results in a higher risk for ectopic pregnancy. Other risk factors include tubal ligation, reversed ligation, previous ectopic pregnancy, current intrauterine device use, and smoking.

Treatment for ectopic pregnancy can be medical or surgical. For patients who meet certain criteria, medical therapy with methotrexate is possible. For those who do not meet these criteria or who have other contraindications to methotrexate, surgery is indicated.

Signs and Symptoms

Ectopic Pregnancy
- Abdominal pain (sudden onset)
- Vaginal bleeding

Differential Diagnosis

Ectopic Pregnancy
- Abruptio placentae
- Placenta previa
- Preterm labor
- Early pregnancy loss
- Ovarian cyst
- Ovarian torsion
- Appendicitis

Transport Management

Ectopic Pregnancy
- Continue supportive therapy.
- Obtain IV access.
- Administer IV fluids if the patient has hypotension.

Bleeding

Vaginal bleeding in early pregnancy may indicate an early pregnancy loss or an ectopic pregnancy. Bleeding in the second and third trimesters of pregnancy is often associated with significant pathologic conditions that may endanger the lives of both the woman and the fetus.

As the pregnant woman approaches term, as much as 30% of the maternal cardiac output is going to the uterus, fetus, and placenta. Thus, it is easy to understand how rapidly the patient can bleed and become hemodynamically unstable. Three major causes of life-threatening bleeding in pregnant patients are abruptio placentae, placenta previa, and uterine rupture. Because of the high risk of maternal and fetal death associated with any of these clinical entities, any vaginal bleeding during the third trimester of pregnancy must be regarded as a dire medical emergency until proven otherwise. The CCTP should suspect placenta previa or abruptio placentae in any patient with third-trimester abdominal pain or vaginal bleeding. The classic teaching is that placenta previa is associated with "painless" vaginal bleeding, whereas abruptio placentae is associated with "painful" vaginal bleeding.

Regardless of the cause of the vaginal bleeding, patient management is the same. Place the woman on her left side in a recumbent position to maximize blood return to the heart and prevent supine hypotensive syndrome. Administer oxygen if the saturation is less than 92%, and place at least one large-bore IV line. Lactated Ringer solution is the optimal treatment, but normal saline can be given as an alternative in 250-mL boluses and titrated to the patient's hemodynamic status. BP should be maintained at no less than 90 mm Hg systolic. Rapid transport is required, with the receiving hospital being notified of the nature of the problem as well as any changes in the patient's condition that occur en route. *Under no circumstances should the CCTP perform an internal vaginal exam.*

Abruptio Placentae

Abruptio placentae (also called placental abruption) is the premature separation of a normally implanted placenta from the uterine wall **FIGURE 22-11**. It occurs in 1% of pregnancies, leading to a neonatal death in 10% to 30% of cases. Abruptio placentae accounts for 30% of life-threatening vaginal bleeding in the second half of pregnancy. This condition can be either spontaneous or a result of trauma. Even minor trauma, such as a fall from standing, can cause an abruption.

Risk factors associated with spontaneous abruptio placentae include tobacco use, cocaine

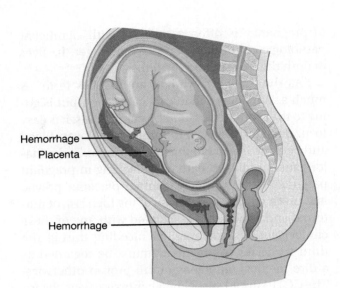

Hemorrhage
Placenta
Hemorrhage

FIGURE 22-11 Abruptio placentae is a premature separation from the uterine wall, with resultant hemorrhage between the wall and the placenta.

© Jones & Bartlett Learning.

use, chronic hypertension, preeclampsia, thrombophilias, and abruption in a previous pregnancy. Bleeding from spontaneous abruptio placentae usually occurs late in the third trimester of pregnancy, with a peak incidence at 37 weeks.

Abruptio placentae associated with trauma is less common and is usually due to direct trauma to the abdomen. However, it is a complication in 1% to 5% of minor injuries that occur during pregnancy and as many as 40% to 50% of major trauma injuries that occur during pregnancy. Because the placenta is less elastic than the uterus to which it is attached, when a pregnant woman is subjected to trauma that stretches or deforms the uterus, the relatively inelastic placenta separates from the uterine wall, causing abruption. Fetal mortality is high with traumatic abruption, ranging from 67% to 75%. Ultrasonography is useful to assess for fetal well-being; however, its ability to detect an abruption is limited.

Regardless of the cause, the presenting signs and symptoms of abruptio placentae include abdominal pain, back pain, uterine tenderness, and usually vaginal bleeding. On some occasions, an abruption may occur without any visible vaginal bleeding; that is, the abruption is concealed. The separation may occur in such a way that the bleeding is contained by the part of the placenta attached to the uterine wall. In such a case, the amount of vaginal bleeding may be small or no blood may be evident, and the patient's condition may be easily mistaken for premature labor. The amount of visible blood does not directly correlate with degree of abruption, as shock may ensue from the concealed blood loss.

On physical exam, the abdomen is usually tender and the uterus is rigid on palpation. When vaginal blood is present, it may be bright, dark, or mixed with amniotic fluid. The pregnant patient may exhibit signs of shock out of proportion to the amount of vaginal bleeding.

Important factors in the management of the pregnant patient with suspected abruptio placentae are the fetal status and the presence or absence of labor. Most women who experience abruptio placentae spontaneously go into labor. The same procedures for all vaginal bleeding in the third trimester of pregnancy should be followed, with a focus on oxygenation and administration of IV fluids to maintain hemodynamic stability. Place the patient on her left side in a recumbent position, give oxygen to maintain saturation of 92% or greater, establish at least one large-bore IV line and administer lactated Ringer solution or normal saline, and provide rapid transport. Consider administering tranexamic acid (TXA) where local protocols allow.

Signs and Symptoms

Abruptio Placentae
- Vaginal bleeding
- Abdominal pain
- Back pain
- Uterine tenderness/contractions of severe intensity
- Signs of shock
- Lack of fetal heart sounds

Differential Diagnosis

Abruptio Placentae
- Ectopic pregnancy
- Placenta previa
- Preterm labor
- Early pregnancy loss

Transport Management

Abruptio Placentae

- Place the patient on her left side, in recumbent position.
- Provide oxygenation to maintain oxygen saturation of 92% or greater.
- Administer IV fluids.
- Provide rapid transport.
- Consider TXA where permitted.

Placenta Previa

In placenta previa, the placenta is implanted low in the uterus and partially or completely covers the cervical canal **FIGURE 22-12**. Placenta previa can be seen on approximately 4% of ultrasonographic studies performed at 20 to 24 weeks' gestation but occurs at term in only 0.4% of pregnancies. Bleeding usually occurs late in the third trimester of pregnancy, as the cervix begins to dilate in preparation for delivery.

The usual presenting complaint of the woman with placenta previa is bright red vaginal bleeding. In contrast to abruptio placentae, the bleeding in placenta previa is painless and the uterus remains soft.

Treatment of the patient with suspected placenta previa is the same as for all patients with

third-trimester bleeding. CCTPs need to make the mother the priority. Maintaining her hemodynamics with IV fluids and oxygenation will benefit the fetus as well. However, CCTPs must be cautious when examining the patient with placenta previa. Because the placenta is precariously placed over the cervical opening, *no* internal examination of the vagina or cervix should be performed. Treatment should be accomplished with minimal movement. Electronic fetal monitoring should be performed, again with minimal patient movement. Administration of TXA may be appropriate if the local protocols permit it.

Signs and Symptoms

Placenta Previa

- Bright red vaginal bleeding
- Lack of abdominal pain

Differential Diagnosis

Placenta Previa

- Abruptio placentae
- Ectopic pregnancy
- Preterm labor
- Early pregnancy loss

Transport Management

Placenta Previa

- Administer IV fluids.
- Administer oxygen.
- Allow minimal movement.
- Perform electronic fetal monitoring.
- Consider TXA where permitted.

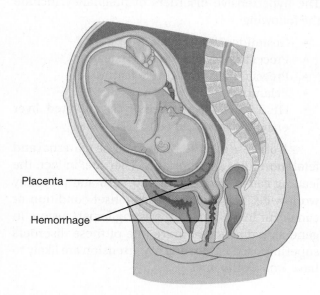

Placenta

Hemorrhage

FIGURE 22-12 Positioning of the placenta in placenta previa.

© Jones & Bartlett Learning.

Uterine Rupture

Uterine rupture is a cause of catastrophic bleeding in the second half of pregnancy. Rupture associated with trauma is relatively uncommon. Maternal mortality from trauma-induced uterine rupture is approximately 10%, whereas fetal mortality approaches 100%. Uterine rupture should be suspected in the pregnant trauma patient who has loss of palpable uterine contour, has easily palpated fetal parts, and has severe abdominal pain. As with any pregnant patient who experiences trauma, initial management is directed at the resuscitation and stabilization of the pregnant patient.

Uterine rupture can also occur without trauma, in which case it is almost always associated with labor. A weakened portion of the uterine wall is at risk for rupture at any time during the pregnancy. Women who are at highest risk for this condition are those who have had previous uterine surgery, including cesarean section.

Incomplete rupture is usually diagnosed at the time of cesarean section and is an incidental finding; however, complete ruptures can be catastrophic. Signs or symptoms of uterine rupture include abnormal maternal vital signs, sudden or worsening abdominal pain, abnormal fetal heart rate, loss of fetal station (fetus appears to be retreating back into the uterus), abnormal uterine contractions, vaginal bleeding, and hematuria (rupture extends into the bladder).

Fetal monitoring in the setting of uterine rupture will show fetal distress such as fetal bradycardia and increased uterine contractions. In some cases, the fetus and placenta may exit the uterus into the abdominal cavity.

Treatment of spontaneous uterine rupture consists of volume resuscitation and oxygen. CCTPs need to prepare the patient for surgery, because definitive care involves surgery and cesarean section. During transport, consider administering IV fluids and whole blood transfusions to ensure hemodynamic stability, in addition to optimizing oxygenation and providing advanced airway management.

Signs and Symptoms

Uterine Rupture
- Loss of palpable uterine contour
- Easily palpated fetal parts
- Sharp, tearing abdominal pain
- Hemodynamic instability
- Fetal heart rate abnormalities
- Vaginal bleeding

Transport Management

Uterine Rupture
- Perform electronic fetal monitoring.
- Provide volume resuscitation.
- Administer oxygen to maintain oxygen saturation of 92% or greater.
- Provide rapid transport.

Medical Conditions During Pregnancy

Hypertension complicating pregnancy is classified into four types: chronic hypertension, chronic hypertension with superimposed preeclampsia-eclampsia, preeclampsia-eclampsia, and gestational hypertension. Hypertensive disorders of pregnancy, including preeclampsia, complicate 10% of pregnancies. If such disorders are left untreated, dangerous—if not fatal—consequences for the woman and the fetus can ensue. Risk factors include multiple gestations (twins, triplets), first-time pregnancies, and maternal chronic hypertension.

Hypertensive Disorders of Pregnancy

The hypertensive disorders of pregnancy include the following:

- Gestational hypertension
- Preeclampsia without severe features
- Preeclampsia with severe features
- Eclampsia
- HELLP syndrome (hemolysis, elevated liver enzymes, low platelets)

All of these disorders can increase maternal and fetal morbidity and mortality. They are, in fact, the leading cause of maternal and perinatal mortality worldwide. They can be a new-onset condition or can occur in women with existing hypertension. In general, patients who have one of these disorders superimposed on existing hypertension are likely to have worse outcomes.

Gestational Hypertension

Gestational hypertension is the development of hypertension (BP of 140/90 mm Hg) after 20 weeks' gestation in a previously normotensive patient. BP returns to normal after delivery. The definition of this diagnosis includes two separate measurements of BP at least 4 hours apart. Gestational hypertension is managed in a similar fashion to preeclampsia. Fifty percent of women with gestational hypertension will progress to preeclampsia. Women with BP in the severe range (160/110 mm Hg or higher) are managed in a similar fashion to women with preeclampsia with severe features.

Preeclampsia

As mentioned earlier, preeclampsia is classified into two types, based on whether it presents with severe features. *Preeclampsia without severe features* is hypertension developing after 20 weeks' gestation, defined as a systolic blood pressure of 140 mm Hg and a diastolic blood pressure of 90 mm Hg. Preeclampsia can develop up to 12 weeks postpartum. In addition, patients may develop new-onset proteinuria (protein in the urine). In the absence of proteinuria, preeclampsia can be diagnosed as hypertension in association with thrombocytopenia (platelet count less than 100,000/μL), impaired liver function (liver transaminases elevated to twice normal values), new-onset laboratory-documented renal insufficiency (creatinine level of 1.1 mg/dL or a doubling of the patient's baseline creatinine), pulmonary edema, or new-onset visual or cerebral disturbances.

These patients may be treated with magnesium sulfate for seizure prophylaxis, depending on local practice patterns. The loading dose of magnesium is 4 to 6 g given IV over 15 to 20 minutes. High levels of magnesium can result in respiratory depression and cardiac arrest. An early sign of magnesium toxicity is the loss of deep tendon reflexes. If the patient has respiratory depression, stop the magnesium infusion, assist with ventilation, and administer calcium gluconate. If the patient goes into cardiac arrest, proceed with ACLS and give calcium gluconate.

Preeclampsia with severe features has many of the same diagnostic features as preeclampsia without severe features. However, the BP is in the severe range—160/110 mm Hg or higher. These patients are at higher risk of progressing to eclampsia and should be treated with magnesium sulfate to prevent seizures. Even more important than loading with magnesium is controlling the patient's BP. The longer the BP remains elevated, the greater the

incidence of stroke. These patients should receive antihypertensive medications. Labetalol, hydralazine, and nifedipine can all be used safely in pregnancy. The goal BP is approximately 140/90 mm Hg. BP should be reassessed every 10 to 15 minutes. If the BP is not at goal, repeat the dose of the antihypertensive medication if local protocols permit. If the maximum dose has been given, additional medication may be required.

Controversies

The use of magnesium sulfate for seizure prophylaxis for patients with preeclampsia without severe features is somewhat controversial. It is dictated by local practice patterns. Defer to your local protocols.

Signs and Symptoms

Preeclampsia
- Hypertension
- Edema or pathologic edema
- Proteinuria
- Headache
- Visual disturbances
- Abdominal pain

Differential Diagnosis

Preeclampsia
- Preexisting hypertension
- Migraine

Transport Management

Preeclampsia
- Place the patient on her left side.
- Obtain IV access.
- Control BP if in severe range.
- Prevent/control seizures.
- Administer oxygen.
- Administer magnesium sulfate if seizures occur.

Eclampsia

Eclampsia is defined as new-onset seizures in a woman at greater than 20 weeks' gestation, and who usually has one of the hypertensive disorders of pregnancy. However, eclampsia can occur without a previous diagnosis of preeclampsia or HELLP syndrome. Preeclampsia may progress rapidly to eclampsia before, during, or after delivery, especially during the first 48 hours postpartum. Both preeclampsia and eclampsia can present up to 6 weeks postpartum. Eclampsia should always be considered in any pregnant or postpartum patient who is seizing. Even in patients with a known seizure disorder, if they have a seizure and are 20 weeks' gestation or greater, they should be considered to have eclampsia until proven otherwise.

The only true treatment for eclampsia is delivery. Maternal complications from eclampsia include permanent central nervous system (CNS) damage, stroke, renal insufficiency, and death.

The management goal for the CCTP caring for a patient with eclampsia is to prevent any additional seizures. This is accomplished by administering 4 to 6 g of magnesium sulfate over 15 to 20 minutes, then continued as a drip at 2 to 4 g/h. Magnesium sulfate is the drug of choice for treating seizures due to eclampsia; it is a better choice than phenytoin, benzodiazepines, and nimodipine for this indication. The actual mechanism by which magnesium achieves its effects is poorly understood. Notably, it is a poor antihypertensive medication and should not be used in that capacity.

Seizures may occur suddenly and should be anticipated. If they occur, routine seizure management and protection of the patient should be initiated first. Ensure a patent airway and adequate oxygenation. Position the patient on the left side (if possible) and protect the patient from additional physical injury. Check glucose levels at the point of care. Consider the administration of magnesium sulfate based on the transfer orders or consultation with medical direction. This therapy should always be accompanied by clinical observation for loss of reflexes, respiratory depression, and, if the patient is not currently experiencing a seizure, CNS depression. The antidote for magnesium sulfate toxicity is calcium gluconate. Alternatively, benzodiazepines or phenytoin can be used to initially terminate the seizure, with magnesium sulfate administered immediately thereafter. Additional magnesium sulfate should first be considered for a recurrent seizure as long as no signs of magnesium toxicity are present.

If magnesium sulfate is not available, standard seizure therapy may be followed, which includes the use of diazepam or other benzodiazepines. Even though benzodiazepines are effective anticonvulsants, they are not as effective as magnesium sulfate for the treatment of eclampsia. If benzodiazepines are given, it is imperative to report this treatment to the receiving providers. Neonates can experience respiratory depression from these medications and may require additional support at the time of delivery.

Signs and Symptoms

Eclampsia

- Severe headache
- Scotomata (visual changes)
- Hyperreflexia (overactive reflexes)
- Epigastric pain
- Anxiety

Differential Diagnosis

Eclampsia

- Seizure disorder
- Hypoglycemia
- Alcohol withdrawal

Transport Management

Eclampsia

- Place the patient on her left side.
- Obtain IV access.
- Control BP if in severe range.
- Prevent/control seizures.
- Administer oxygen.
- Administer magnesium sulfate

HELLP Syndrome

HELLP syndrome occurs during the latter stages of pregnancy, usually after 20 weeks' gestation. This syndrome is named after its clinical findings—namely, hemolytic anemia, elevated liver enzyme levels, and a low platelet count.

The cause of HELLP syndrome is unknown, but it appears to be a severe form of preeclampsia coupled with activation of the coagulation system, leading to multiorgan dysfunction syndrome (discussed in Chapter 10, *Resuscitation, Shock, and Blood Products*). Patients most often present with right upper quadrant pain and generalized malaise. Fifty percent will present with nausea and vomiting. Hypertension and proteinuria are present in 85% of cases but absent in 15% of cases, making the diagnosis more elusive.

Treatment may include blood and blood products, antihypertensives, and magnesium (for seizure prophylaxis). However, definitive treatment can be accomplished only with delivery of the fetus. CCTPs need to be aware that HELLP syndrome occurs in 10% of postpartum women.

Signs and Symptoms

HELLP Syndrome
- Hemolytic anemia
- Elevated liver enzyme levels
- Low platelet count
- Abdominal pain
- Blurred vision
- Headache
- Edema

Differential Diagnosis

HELLP Syndrome
- Cholecystitis
- Hepatitis
- Idiopathic thrombocytopenia

Transport Management

HELLP Syndrome
- Consider administering blood/blood products (fresh-frozen plasma [FFP]).
- Manage BP.
- Administer magnesium sulfate (for seizure prophylaxis).

Complications During Labor

Normal labor includes a prodromal stage plus three distinct active stages, whose durations depend partly on whether it is the patient's first pregnancy (nullipara). **TABLE 22-7** reviews the stages of labor.

Transition of Fetal Circulation at Birth

Prior to birth, the fetus receives oxygenated blood from the pregnant woman via the umbilical vein, which flows into the ductus venosus and then the inferior vena cava of the fetus, which ultimately leads to the right atrium of the fetus. The fetal lung is collapsed and filled with fluid. The resistance to flow is high, and most of the fetal blood flow is diverted away from the lungs. Blood also goes from the right side of the heart to the left side of the heart through the foramen ovale. Additionally, some of the blood flowing into the pulmonary artery is diverted away from the lungs into the aorta via the ductus arteriosus.

As the baby is delivered, the fetal transition occurs; this process enables the baby to breathe. During the fetal transition, the newborn's lungs must expand with air within seconds. As the baby's lungs become filled with air, the pulmonary vascular resistance decreases and systemic vascular resistance increases. Blood begins to flow to the lungs, picking up oxygen there. The change in pulmonary pressure then results in closing of the foramen ovale.

This transition can be compromised by poor respiratory effort, airway obstruction, impaired lung function, persistent pulmonary hypertension, cardiac anomalies, and prematurity. During this period, neonates may require ventilatory support to prevent hypoxia, brain injury, or even death. This is a critical time, and timely intervention is essential.

Preterm Labor

Preterm labor, defined as the onset of labor between 20 and 37 weeks' gestation, is the leading cause of neonatal mortality in the United States. The use of tocolytics (medications to stop contractions) is one of the treatments for preterm labor. These medications are recommended for short-term use to allow for administration of corticosteroids and magnesium sulfate and for transport. The medications

		TABLE 22-7 Stages of Labor		
Stage of Labor	**Average Time (Nullipara)**	**Average Time (Multipara)**	**Frequency of Contractions**	**Characteristics**
Prodromal stage	Varies	Varies	N/A	Bloody show (mucus mixed with blood) expelled from the vagina
First stage	8–12 h	6–8 h	5- to 15-min intervals	Labor pains and contraction of the uterus begin. Pain may radiate into the small of the back. Amniotic sac often ruptures toward the end of this stage, signified by a gush of fluid from the vagina. This stage lasts until the cervix is fully dilated.
Second stage	1–2 h	30 min	2–3 min apart	Begins as the baby's head enters the birth canal. Woman's pulse rate increases; sweat appears on her face. Cervix becomes fully dilated and effaced. Crowning occurs (presenting part of baby becomes visible). Delivery is imminent. This stage concludes when the baby is fully delivered.
Third stage	5–60 min	5–60 min	N/A	Placental stage. Lasts from delivery of the baby until the placenta has been delivered and the uterus has contracted. Uterine contraction is necessary to squeeze shut all of the tiny blood vessels left exposed when the placenta separates from the uterine wall.

© Jones & Bartlett Learning.

indicated for this purpose include beta adrenergic receptor agonists (terbutaline), calcium channel blockers, and NSAIDs.

One of the most important interventions to reduce neonatal morbidity and mortality from preterm labor is the administration of corticosteroids. Both betamethasone and dexamethasone are used for this purpose; they are indicated for use between 23 and 34 weeks' gestation in pregnancies at risk for delivery. The use of these medications can reduce the risk of neonatal respiratory distress syndrome, intracranial hemorrhage, necrotizing enterocolitis, and death. Some evidence also supports the use of corticosteroids up to 37 weeks' gestation to reduce newborn respiratory morbidity.

Magnesium sulfate, once thought to be a tocolytic medication, is no longer recommended to treat preterm labor. However, it is recommended for neuroprotection in preterm labor at less than 32 weeks. The treatment has been shown to decrease the risk of cerebral palsy in infants less than 32 weeks' gestation.

Knowledgeable CCTPs provide a critical link between the local hospital and the tertiary care facility. Careful patient monitoring, readiness to manage changes in the patient's condition while in transit, and a smooth transfer of care to the receiving hospital can all improve patient outcomes. Bed rest and limiting physical activity are no longer routinely recommended to extend gestation. IV hydration,

Magnesium Sulfate

In the context of childbirth, magnesium sulfate is primarily indicated for fetal neuroprotection. While it does have tocolytic properties, this agent is no longer recommended to treat preterm labor. It is usually administered as a 4- to 6-g bolus, followed by a continuous infusion at 2 to 4 g/h. The mechanism by which magnesium inhibits uterine contraction is not completely clear, but it appears to assert its effects through the antagonism of calcium in muscle cells. The doses required to achieve this effect are close to toxic. Symptoms of magnesium toxicity include decreased reflexes and, ultimately, respiratory depression and respiratory arrest. In a patient receiving magnesium sulfate, the patellar reflexes should be monitored frequently, urine output should be at least 25 mL/h, and there should be no signs of respiratory depression. If any signs or symptoms of toxicity are noted, stop the infusion and contact medical control for further instruction.

Therapeutic levels of magnesium are between 4 and 7 mEq/L. Patellar reflexes become diminished when magnesium levels reach 8 to 10 mEq/L, and respiratory depression and failure occur when they rise above 12 mEq/L. If the patient exhibits a toxic reaction, such as respiratory depression, stop the infusion, give 1 g of calcium gluconate by *slow* IV push, and administer oxygen to maintain an oxygen saturation of greater than 90%. If the patient experiences respiratory failure, intubation is necessary.

Tocolytics (Terbutaline, Nifedipine, and Indomethacin)

Tocolytics are only marginally effective in stopping preterm labor. Terbutaline is a beta-2 agonist that, when used in sufficient doses, can successfully reduce uterine contractions. The doses used to produce this effect, however, can result in side effects by stimulating beta-2 receptors elsewhere, such as in the myocardium. Stimulation of myocardial receptors can result in tachycardia or frank myocardial ischemia in patients with underlying coronary artery disease. Thus, the patient should have continuous cardiac and fetal monitoring during transport and be frequently assessed for signs and symptoms of myocardial ischemia, such as chest pain or pulmonary edema. Terbutaline should not be administered if the maternal pulse exceeds 140 beats/min.

The effects of beta-2 stimulation of the pancreas can result in hyperglycemia, which can be monitored in the pregnant patient using finger-stick glucose checks. If the baby is delivered during transport, the baby should be checked for hypoglycemia. Fetal hypoglycemia occurs secondary to the need for increased insulin production by the fetus to compensate for high maternal glucose levels. Other, less significant side effects of terbutaline treatment may include maternal headache, tremor, vomiting, fever, and hallucinations.

Nifedipine may be the most effective tocolytic. It is typically administered as a 10- to 30-mg loading dose orally or sublingually every 15 to 20 minutes for the first hour, followed by 10 to 20 mg orally every 4 to 8 hours thereafter. Side effects are usually mild and related to peripheral vasodilation. Hypotension is more often seen with sublingual than oral administration and is typically limited to the initial few hours of dosing.

Indomethacin, an NSAID, can be used before 32 weeks' gestation as a tocolytic. It is not used beyond this point in gestation because it may cause premature closure of the ductus arteriosus, which can be catastrophic. This medication is typically used for only 72 hours, as it may cause oligohydramnios (low amniotic fluid). Indomethacin is started as a loading dose of 50 to 100 mg, followed by 25 mg every 4 to 6 hours.

once considered beneficial, has not demonstrated the ability to improve outcomes, either.

Precipitous delivery, which is delivery in less than 3 hours from the onset of regular contractions, may occur with premature labor. On presentation, inquire about the frequency and duration of contractions. Ask about any vaginal leakage of blood, fluid, or mucus. **Premature prelabor rupture of membranes (PPROM)** is the rupture of membranes before the onset of labor in a gestation of less than 37 weeks. PPROM accounts for as many as 30% of all preterm deliveries. Most women will deliver within 7 days of rupture of membranes. There is an increased risk of infection with PPROM, so antibiotics are routinely administered to patients with this condition. All prehospital deliveries are considered emergencies and, by definition, are high risk. The best way to reduce risk is to be prepared.

Prolonged Pregnancy

Prolonged pregnancy (past 40 weeks' gestation) can lead to instances of fetal hypoxia during labor, a higher percentage of meconium production, and a low amniotic fluid index. CCTPs need to be aware of these risks and have meconium suctioning equipment available prior to delivery **FIGURE 22-13**.

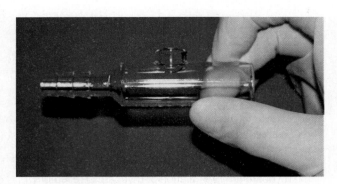

FIGURE 22-13 A meconium aspirator.

Meconium aspirator courtesy of Neotech Products, Inc.

Signs and Symptoms

Preterm Labor

Prior to 37 weeks' gestation:
- Rhythmic uterine contractions
- Cervical dilation
- Rupture of membranes
- Passage of blood-stained mucus

Differential Diagnosis

Preterm Labor
- Abruptio placentae
- Ectopic pregnancy
- Placenta previa
- Early pregnancy loss

Transport Management

Preterm Labor
- Provide or continue glucocorticoids to promote lung maturity.
- Continue antibiotics if the patient has PPROM.
- Consider administration of tocolytic agents.

Delivery

Vertex, or head-first presentation, is the ideal and most common presentation for all deliveries; crowning is observed as the second stage of labor begins. It is the CCTP's responsibility to note unexpected events and to manage them to minimize maternal and fetal mortality and morbidity.

Normal crowning and normal shoulder presentation are shown in **FIGURE 22-14** and **FIGURE 22-15**, respectively.

Malpresentations

Breech presentation is the most common malpresentation, occurring in 4% of all deliveries. This presentation is associated with an increased risk of asphyxia and fetal mortality, though one-third of these deaths are considered preventable. Breech presentations are more common with premature infants and low-birth-weight infants, although two-thirds of breech infants weigh more than 5.5 lb (2,500 g).

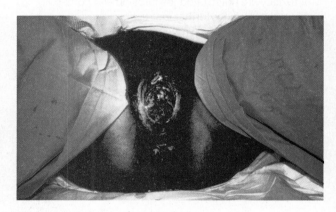

FIGURE 22-14 Normal crowning.

© American Academy of Orthopaedic Surgeons.

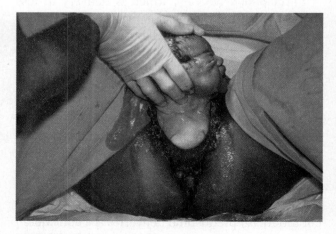

FIGURE 22-15 Normal shoulder presentation.

© American Academy of Orthopaedic Surgeons.

There are four common variants of breech presentation:

- **Frank breech**: Both of the infant's hips are flexed and the feet are near the infant's head **FIGURE 22-16**.
- **Complete breech**: The hips are flexed and the legs are flexed at the knees and oriented transversely to the birth canal; the buttocks present

with the legs flexed and the feet along the buttocks **FIGURE 22-17**.
- **Incomplete breech**: Similar to complete breech except one foot extends into the birth canal **FIGURE 22-18**.
- **Footling breech**: Both feet extend into the birth canal **FIGURE 22-19**.

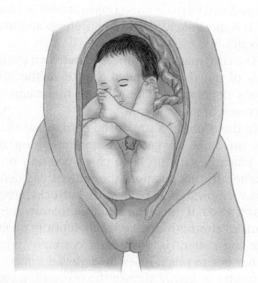

FIGURE 22-16 Frank breech presentation.

© Jones & Bartlett Learning.

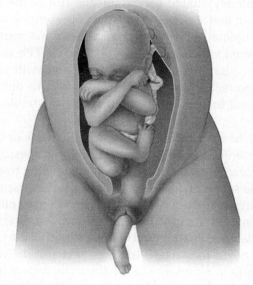

FIGURE 22-18 Incomplete breech presentation.

© Jones & Bartlett Learning.

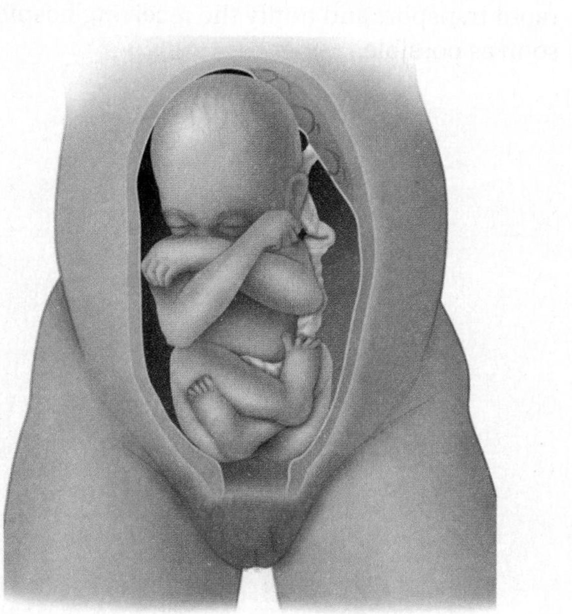

FIGURE 22-17 Complete breech presentation.

© Jones & Bartlett Learning.

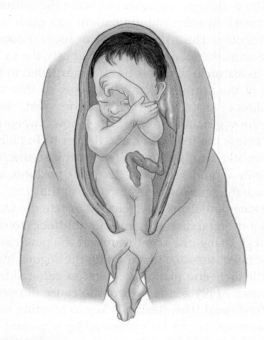

FIGURE 22-19 Footling breech presentation.

© Jones & Bartlett Learning.

In a normal vertex delivery, the head presents first and dilates the cervix. The largest part of an infant is the head, so the rest of the body usually delivers without difficulty. This is not the case in a breech delivery. In a frank breech or complete breech, the hips, thighs, and buttocks are thought to adequately dilate the cervix and vaginal delivery can be accomplished. In an incomplete or footling breech presentation, a foot can slip through an incompletely dilated cervix, but the rest of the fetus will not deliver. Therefore, fetuses presenting in the incomplete or footling breech positions must be delivered via cesarean section. The CCTP's role in these situations is to provide safe and swift transport to facilities that can accomplish this delivery. External inspection for cord prolapse should also occur.

When delivering an infant in the frank or complete breech position, the overarching message is *do not apply traction to the fetus.* Applying traction to the fetus increases the risk of head entrapment and injury to the fetus. The delivery is accomplished with maternal expulsion effort alone. Once the fetus has delivered to the level of the umbilicus, the CCTP may begin to assist. If the legs have not delivered, apply gentle pressure to the posterior aspect of the fetal knee, flexing the leg and sweeping it across the trunk, then inferiorly to an extended position.

Once the legs are delivered, wrap the buttocks in a towel. At this time the patient can push with contractions. The arms may deliver spontaneously. If the arms do not deliver spontaneously, the CCTP may assist once the fetus has been expelled to the level of the scapula. Rotate the fetus so that one shoulder is at the 12 o'clock position. Next, reach into the vagina and identify the elbow. Sweep the arm across the fetal trunk and deliver it. To deliver the second arm, rotate the fetal trunk so that the opposite shoulder is in the 12 o'clock position, and execute the same maneuver to deliver the arm.

Once both arms are delivered, rotate the trunk so that the fetal sacrum is anterior (buttocks toward the sky). Using one arm to support the now visible body, insert the second hand into the vagina. Identify the face, and place one finger in either side of the nose. Apply gentle pressure to cause flexion of the fetal head. This flexion is key to averting head entrapment. It can be enhanced by a second responder applying fundal pressure. Lastly, deliver the head in an upward arc, in contrast to a vertex delivery where the primary motion is downward. This upward movement follows the shape of the maternal sacrum.

Umbilical Cord Prolapse

Occasionally, the presenting part may be the umbilical cord **FIGURE 22-20**. This condition, in which the umbilical cord passes through the birth canal in advance of the infant, is known as a prolapsed cord and can have serious consequences for the infant. It is most likely to occur in preterm and breech deliveries.

The cord may be compressed between the bony pelvis of the mother and the head of the infant, thereby decreasing blood flow to the infant. This may result in fetal hypoxia.

In the event of a prolapsed cord, place the patient on 100% oxygen by nonrebreathing mask and place her in the knee-chest position on the stretcher. In this position, the patient is facedown on her elbows and knees with buttocks elevated **FIGURE 22-21**. If the patient cannot tolerate this position, an alternative is the Trendelenburg position. Once the patient is positioned correctly, encourage her not to push. Insert two gloved fingers into the vagina to gently elevate the presenting part to relieve pressure on the cord. *Do not push the cord back into the cervix.* Minimize manipulation of the cord to reduce the risk of vasospasm. Continue rapid transport and notify the receiving hospital as soon as possible.

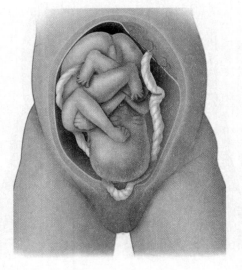

FIGURE 22-20 A prolapsed cord.

© Jones & Bartlett Learning.

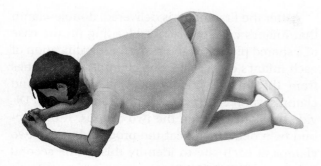

FIGURE 22-21 The knee-chest position should be used in the event of a prolapsed cord.

© Jones & Bartlett Learning.

Transport Management

Umbilical Cord Prolapse

- Administer oxygen.
- Position the patient in either the knee-chest position or the Trendelenburg position.
- Insert two gloved fingers to elevate the presenting part.
- Encourage the patient not to push.
- Avoid manipulation of the cord.
- Provide rapid transport.

Shoulder Dystocia

Shoulder dystocia occurs in approximately 1 of every 100 vertex deliveries. This condition can be recognized from the "turtle sign": The fetal head will begin to protrude and then withdraw back inside because the shoulders are too large to exit the pelvis. This is a true obstetric emergency, and recognition is key to a good outcome. CCTPs must assist the mother with the next contraction. The first intervention is to perform the McRoberts maneuver. Have the patient flex her legs against her abdomen (**FIGURE 22-22**). This maneuver increases the functional size of the pelvis. With the next contraction, have the patient push. This will successfully reduce the dystocia in approximately 40% of cases. Adding suprapubic pressure will further increase the rate of success. Apply direct pressure just above the pubic symphysis to move the anterior shoulder of the infant underneath the pubic bone. Do not apply fundal pressure, however; doing so will further impact the shoulder against the pubic bone.

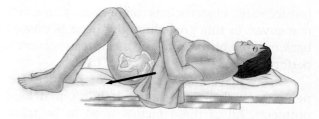

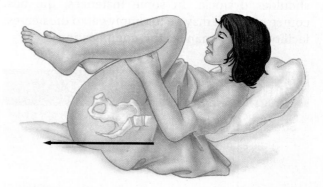

FIGURE 22-22 If the fetal head begins to protrude and then withdraws back inside (a sign of shoulder dystocia), the first step is to have the mother flex her legs to her abdomen to help enlarge the birth canal.

© Jones & Bartlett Learning.

Additional maneuvers may be required if the preceding approaches are not successful. The next maneuver is delivery of the posterior arm. (Remember to stop the suprapubic pressure during this maneuver.) Insert a gloved hand underneath the infant. Identify the humerus and sweep it across the trunk and ultimately the face. This will create more room for the anterior shoulder to slide under the pubic bone. Rotational maneuvers can also be employed if the dystocia persists. For example, the CCTP can apply pressure to either shoulder and attempt to turn the baby within the birth canal. Additionally, the Gaskin maneuver can be used. In this maneuver, the mother is placed on all fours, with hands and knees on a flat surface. The thought is that gravity will assist in the delivery.

It is imperative to not apply excessive traction on the fetal head during the delivery effort. Infants can experience fractures and brachial plexus injuries from excessive force. Timing is also crucial. Often there is compromised blood flow and thus compromised oxygenation of the fetus during a shoulder dystocia. If possible, keep a timetable of events. If the attempts to reduce the dystocia are unsuccessful, obstetricians can perform a Zavanelli maneuver. In this procedure, the head is pushed back into the birth canal and a cesarean section is performed.

CCTPs have varying scopes of practice, depending on their experience, training, and local protocols. All of these factors need to be taken into consideration when managing a complicated shoulder dystocia. In some instances, the best course of action may be to simply get to the nearest facility that can manage this complication.

Signs and Symptoms

Shoulder Dystocia

- "Turtle sign"—the infant's head protruding and withdrawing into the birth canal

---

Transport Management

Shoulder Dystocia

- Perform the McRoberts maneuver.
- Apply suprapubic pressure.
- Consider delivery of the posterior arm.
- Provide rapid transport.

Multiple Births

Single gestations are most common, but many CCTPs will encounter a multiple-gestation pregnancy and potential delivery. The incidence of twin gestation is 1 in 100 births; that of triplets is 1 in 10,000 births. The presence of a multiple-gestation pregnancy should be identified through the history obtained from the patient. Twins may share a placenta and a gestational sac, or each may have its own individual sac and placenta. Twins that share a sac should not deliver vaginally. Instead, they must be delivered by cesarean section to avoid cord accidents; umbilical cords of the two fetuses could become entangled and cut off their circulation.

The presentation of the twins is important. The first twin needs to be in a vertex presentation to allow for a safe delivery. There is a theoretical risk of interlocking chins if the first twin is breech and the second twin is vertex (**FIGURE 22-23**).

After the first infant is delivered, double-clamp that infant's cord to prevent bleeding (in the case of a shared placenta) and allow for identification of each infant's cord. Place one clamp several inches from the infant's abdominal wall and a second clamp several centimeters away from the first. Divide the cord between the two clamps. If the second twin delivers, repeat the process, but use two clamps at each site to identify this as the second twin's cord **FIGURE 22-24**.

The timing of delivery for the second twin is highly variable. During this interval, transport should continue and should be interrupted only if the next infant begins to emerge from the birth canal. Malpresentation is common in the second twin. A breech presentation, and even a footling or

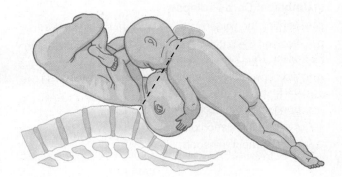

FIGURE 22-23 When assisting in the delivery of twins, be aware of the infants' presentation. Their chins may become interlocked if the first twin is breech and the second twin is vertex.
© Jones & Bartlett Learning.

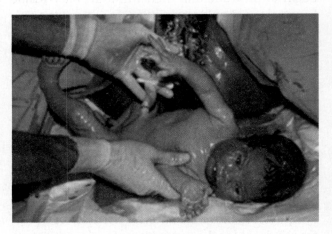

FIGURE 22-24 Tie or clamp the cord in two places. Cut the cord between the two ties or clamps.
© American Academy of Orthopaedic Surgeons.

incomplete breech, can be delivered vaginally because the cervix has already been completely dilated by the first twin. Watch for transverse lie and cord prolapse in the second twin.

Do not attempt to deliver the placenta of the first twin before delivery of the second twin. Placentas can be fused, and an attempt to deliver the first infant's placenta can disrupt the placenta of the second twin.

Delivery of the Placenta

Delivery of the placenta defines the third stage of labor. Active management of this process has been shown to reduce the risk of postpartum hemorrhage. Active management consists of administration of oxytocin 20 to 40 units in 1 L IV saline solution over 20 to 40 minutes. *Do not give oxytocin via IV push; doing so can cause profound hypotension.* The second action is to apply gentle traction to the umbilical cord. The third action is to perform fundal massage. The CCTP will be able to identify when the placenta is beginning to separate from the uterine wall by a small gush of blood and a lengthening of the umbilical cord. The patient may assist the delivery of the placenta with a push.

Postdelivery Care

Once delivery is complete, care for both the mother and the infant should continue. Determine the newborn's ABCs and Apgar score (further discussed in Chapter 23, *Neonatal Emergencies*). Examine the mother's perineum for tears. Place a large absorbent pad (to determine pad count) under the mother at the perineum. If large tears are actively bleeding, apply direct pressure. Significant postpartum hemorrhage is defined as greater than 500 mL of blood loss within 24 hours after delivery of the infant. In general, a saturated sanitary pad contains 100 mL of blood; a soiled pad is estimated to contain 30 mL. Often the source of bleeding is not easy to identify, so massage the uterus and establish one or two large-bore IV lines with a crystalloid solution running open. Administer high-flow oxygen as well.

The infant should be thoroughly dried, wrapped in warm blankets, and placed on the mother's chest with skin-to-skin contact if possible. Umbilical cord clamping should be delayed 30 to 60 seconds when the infant is vigorous. If the infant is depressed, resuscitate as indicated. The Apgar score should be obtained at 1 and 5 minutes after delivery. If the Apgar score is less than 7, repeat it every 5 minutes. Continue with any supportive measures applied as needed while transporting.

Postdelivery Complications
Postpartum Hemorrhage

Obstetric hemorrhage is the leading cause of maternal mortality worldwide. Prompt recognition and treatment of such hemorrhage, therefore, is important in lowering maternal mortality. Although bleeding is common during delivery, blood loss of more than 500 mL or any volume of blood loss that causes signs of hemodynamic instability is considered serious. Previous cesarean sections, more than four previous vaginal births, low-lying placenta, and magnesium sulfate therapy are all risk factors associated with postpartum hemorrhage. To assess the causes of postpartum hemorrhage, use the four Ts:

- Tone: uterine atony and uterus not contracting, leading to excessive bleeding
- Trauma: lacerations, hematomas, uterine rupture
- Tissue: retained placenta
- Thrombin: coagulopathy

Uterine atony is treated with fundal massage (**FIGURE 22-25**) and uterotonic agents, including oxytocin, methylergonovine, misoprostol, and

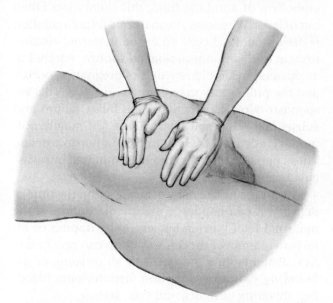

FIGURE 22-25 Fundal massage should be performed with the patient lying supine once the patient has delivered.

© Jones & Bartlett Learning.

carboprost. Direct pressure should be applied to lacerations and hematomas until the patient arrives at the definitive care location. Retained tissue is often removed manually by the obstetrician. Coagulopathy is likely to be seen after abruptio placentae or amniotic fluid embolism.

Signs and Symptoms

Postpartum Hemorrhage
- Severe bleeding after delivery

Transport Management

Postpartum Hemorrhage
- Place padding to absorb the blood.
- Perform fundal massage.
- Administer oxytocin after the placenta has delivered.

Amniotic Fluid Embolism

Amniotic fluid embolism (AFE) is a rare event, occurring in 2 to 6 of every 100,000 pregnancies. While this condition was historically believed to be a true embolism of amniotic fluid, this theory has fallen out of favor. Whenever the maternal fetal circulation is disrupted, fetal cells enter the maternal circulation. In AFE, an immunologic response, referred to as the anaphylactoid reaction of pregnancy, occurs and the pulmonary vasculature constricts. This vasoconstriction causes right-side heart failure and subsequently left-side heart failure. Ultimately, pulmonary edema and systemic hypotension occur. These patients often go into disseminated intravascular coagulation.

Although AFE usually occurs around the time of delivery, it can happen with any disruption of the maternal-fetal barrier. For example, trauma or efforts to maneuver the fetus in utero can precipitate AFE. Patients may present with all or some of the following symptoms: hypoxia, hypotension, bleeding, shivering or rigors, and even seizure.

AFE carries a significant mortality rate, ranging from 24% to 80% in developed countries. The CCTP must recognize its signs and symptoms early.

Care is supportive, as there is no "cure" for AFE. Patients will require airway management, including supplemental oxygen and progressing up to intubation. IV access should be obtained to allow for treatment of hypotension or hemorrhage with crystalloid or blood. These patients require immediate transport.

Signs and Symptoms

Amniotic Fluid Embolism
- Sudden onset of shortness of breath
- Sudden onset of hypotension
- Chest pain
- Restlessness
- Anxiety
- Coughing
- Vomiting
- Pulmonary edema with pink, frothy sputum
- Sense of impending doom
- Shivering or rigors
- Seizures
- Coma
- Sudden death

Transport Management

Amniotic Fluid Embolism
- Administer supplemental oxygen.
- Provide fluid resuscitation.
- Provide rapid transport.
- Administer positive end-expiratory pressure.
- Perform intubation if necessary.
- Administer blood.

Uterine Inversion

Uterine inversion is an obstetric emergency, which can be associated with life-threatening hemorrhage and shock. It occurs when the uterine fundus collapses into the endometrial cavity. This condition usually occurs during the third stage of labor (delivery of the placenta). Care should be taken when delivering the placenta to avoid excessive traction on the umbilical cord before the placenta is separated from the uterine wall. The CCTP should suspect uterine inversion when a smooth round mass protrudes from the introitus. The immediate treatment is replacement, which is beyond the CCTP's scope of practice. It is imperative to avoid removing the placenta from an inverted uterus, as uncontrollable hemorrhage may ensue. Surgical intervention is often required for uterine replacement.

Transport Management

Uterine Inversion
- Flush the vagina with saline (hydrostatic correction).
- Administer oxytocin.

Gynecologic Emergencies
Pelvic Inflammatory Disease

Pelvic inflammatory disease (PID) is an infection of the female reproductive tract typically caused by a sexually transmitted infection (STI)—namely, gonorrhea or chlamydia. It can occur as a result of delayed antibiotic treatment of an STI, which allows bacteria to travel from the vagina and cervix into the uterus, fallopian tubes, and/or ovaries. Initially, patients with gonorrhea and/or chlamydia may experience vague or no symptoms, or they may experience vaginal discharge, abnormal vaginal bleeding, or vaginal pain. If the patient does not receive adequate treatment with antibiotics, the bacteria may ascend up the reproductive tract. At that point, patients will begin to experience signs and symptoms of PID, including lower abdominal pain, vaginal discharge, right upper quadrant abdominal pain, abnormal vaginal bleeding, fever/chills, dysuria, nausea/vomiting, and/or pain with intercourse. The symptoms may mimic those associated with appendicitis or urinary tract infection, so a careful history and physical exam are important in diagnosing PID.

Treatment consists of IV antibiotics, which the patient may be receiving when transport is initiated. CCTPs must be aware of any drug interactions when transporting patients on an antibiotic regimen. Complications of PID can include sepsis, septic shock, or abscess formation, which may require surgical drainage. Treatment of septic shock or sepsis should follow the standard protocol.

Recurrent PID can cause formation of scar tissue, which then leads to chronic pelvic pain, increases the patient's risk for ectopic pregnancies, or impairs functionality of the reproductive system. As a result, 10% of the 1 million women diagnosed per year with PID will ultimately become infertile.

Signs and Symptoms

Pelvic Inflammatory Disease
- Back and abdominal pain
- Vaginal discharge
- Abnormal vaginal bleeding
- Pain with intercourse
- Painful urination
- Low-grade fever

Differential Diagnosis

Pelvic Inflammatory Disease
- Appendicitis
- Urinary tract infection
- Ovarian cyst or torsion

Transport Management

Pelvic Inflammatory Disease
- Continue the administration of IV antibiotics.
- Treat sepsis or septic shock per protocol.

Toxic Shock Syndrome

Toxic shock syndrome results from the release of bacterial toxins into the body, specifically following infection with *Staphylococcus aureus*, *Streptococcus pyogenes*, or *Clostridium sordellii*. While it has many potential underlying causes, historically this condition has been associated with tampon use. Toxic shock syndrome from *S aureus* was initially identified in the late 1970s. In the 1980s, when menstruating women began using superabsorbent tampons, which allowed for bacterial overgrowth, the syndrome was again seen. The composition of tampons has since changed, and the incidence of toxic shock syndrome has decreased. The CDC now reports that only 10 in every 100,000 menstruating women will develop a bacterial infection leading to toxic shock syndrome.

Signs and symptoms occur secondary to toxin release from bacteria into the bloodstream. They include high fever, malaise, headache, body rash, skin shedding, vomiting, diarrhea, and signs and symptoms of shock, including tachycardia and hypotension. Treatment includes airway management, fluid resuscitation, source control, and IV antibiotics such as clindamycin and vancomycin.

Signs and Symptoms

Toxic Shock Syndrome
- High fever
- Malaise
- Vomiting/diarrhea
- Skin shedding
- Body rash
- Headache
- Hypotension

Transport Management

Toxic Shock Syndrome
- Manage the airway.
- Treat sepsis or septic shock according to local protocols, with IV fluids and pressor support as indicated.
- Continue the administration of IV antibiotics.

Ovarian Cysts

An ovarian cyst is a pouch or sac that can grow in the ovaries. These cysts are quite common, occurring in approximately 8% to 18% of the female population. The majority are benign and resolve on their own; however, some are malignant. Ovarian cysts are categorized into four main groups:

- Functional ovarian cysts: often asymptomatic, self-resolving in 6 to 8 weeks
- Teratomas: can contain body tissue, hair, and skin, and rarely can become cancerous over time
- Cystadenomas: large but mostly benign
- Endometriomas: made up of endometrial tissue

Ovarian cysts are often undetectable and, as noted previously, may resolve on their own. Nevertheless, a small percentage may continue to grow and cause lower abdominal pain and pelvic pressure. On occasion, larger cysts can cause the ovary to twist on itself, a gynecologic emergency known as ovarian torsion. Cysts can also rupture, causing sharp, severe pain, and, if hemorrhagic, can cause bleeding into the abdomen.

Treatment typically consists of pain management with NSAIDs; however, complications such as torsion, cyst rupture, or malignancy may necessitate emergent surgical removal. During transport, ovarian cyst pain may be controlled with NSAIDs, but consider morphine or fentanyl for patients with severe pain. Also consider alternative diagnoses such as ovarian torsion, ectopic pregnancy, and appendicitis.

Diagnostic Evaluation

Most ovarian cysts are found incidentally on pelvic exam or ultrasonography. Emergent diagnosis is made through ultrasonography and Doppler flow studies that can monitor blood flow as well as cyst size and location. A computed tomography (CT) scan and magnetic resonance imaging (MRI) are useful alternatives, although usually not required, as ultrasonography is the preferred imaging modality. There is no specific laboratory technique to test for an ovarian cyst **FIGURE 22-26**.

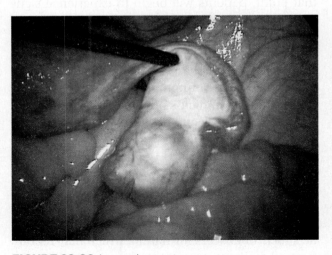

FIGURE 22-26 An ovarian cyst.

Underlying and resultant conditions related to the cyst may be detected with blood tests, which can also help determine the differential diagnosis. A complete blood count, for example, can detect leukocytosis related to an infectious process. A decreased hematocrit value may indicate anemia, and prolonged PT and PTT times can detect clotting abnormalities that may complicate the healing process. Cancer antigen 125 (CA-125) levels greater than 35 U/mL suggest carcinoma as the origin of the cyst. CA-125 is a surface protein that is found on normal ovarian tissue cells and carcinomas; its level increases with abnormal excessive tissue growth. Blood and cervical cultures should be monitored for signs of infection. Last, a urinalysis is helpful in determining whether any blood is present in the urine.

Ruptured Ovarian Cysts

Ovarian cysts may rupture spontaneously or following trauma. Hemorrhage, which may be either mild or severe, frequently occurs when a cyst ruptures. If a rupture with hemorrhage has occurred, patients may present with increased lower abdominal and pelvic pain, vaginal bleeding, and hypovolemia leading to shock. The rupture of an ovarian cyst causes pelvic pain. Corpus luteal cysts occur during the final 1 to 2 weeks of the menstrual cycle, and their rupture can lead to pelvic inflammation and hemorrhage.

Treatment for patients with a ruptured ovarian cyst includes controlling any immediate life threats. Definitive management occurs at the hospital and often involves laparoscopic surgery to control bleeding and remove the cyst.

Ovarian Torsion

In some cases, an enlarged ovary, either by itself or as a result of another condition, will twist and limit its blood supply—a condition called **ovarian torsion FIGURE 22-27**. Ovarian torsion causes lower

Differential Diagnosis

Ruptured Ovarian Cyst

- Ectopic pregnancy
- Hematuria
- Appendicitis
- Diverticulitis
- Bowel obstruction
- Ovarian tumor
- Ovarian torsion
- Salpingitis (inflammation of the fallopian tubes)
- Inflammatory bowel disease
- Pelvic inflammatory disease

Transport Management

Ruptured Ovarian Cyst

- Control any immediate life threats.
- Evaluate for hypovolemic shock; treat per protocol with IV fluids and pressors as indicated.
- Manage pain.

abdominal pain in females, which initially presents similar to appendicitis or ectopic pregnancy. The presentation typically involves acute onset of severe pelvic pain in a woman with an adnexal mass (a mass felt in the area of the uterus, ovaries, and fallopian tubes), often accompanied by nausea and vomiting. Most commonly, torsion occurs

Signs and Symptoms

Ruptured Ovarian Cyst

- Increased lower abdominal and pelvic pain
- Vaginal bleeding
- Hypovolemia leading to shock

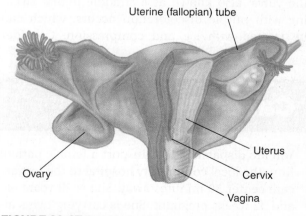

FIGURE 22-27 Ovarian torsion.

© Jones & Bartlett Learning.

as a result of ovarian cysts. Cysts larger than 5 cm are mostly likely to torse. Pregnancy is also an independent risk factor for ovarian torsion. When not treated rapidly, this condition can lead to ovarian infarction and necrosis. Pregnant, nonpregnant, and postmenopausal women are all at risk for ovarian torsion.

It is important to immediately exclude the possibility of pregnancy prior to proceeding with specific treatment for ovarian torsion. The CCTP can initiate this process by taking a thorough history, including sexual history and the date of the patient's last menstrual cycle. Pelvic ultrasonography is the preferred method of diagnosis, with an enlarged ovary typically being observed on the imaging. Laparoscopic **oophoropexy**, in which the ovary is moved out of the distorted position, is the most common treatment.

Transport Management

Ovarian Torsion
- Manage pain (administer morphine or fentanyl).

Gynecologic Trauma

Examples of gynecologic trauma include lacerations and hematomas. Lacerations can result from direct trauma to the vagina, vulva, labia minora, or labia majora. Management includes bleeding control with direct pressure and vaginal packing, as indicated, and treatment of possible hypovolemic shock.

A hematoma can result from blunt trauma to the vulva, also known as a straddle injury. Swelling with purple discoloration occurs, which can be treated with ice and compression. Consider indwelling urinary catheterization if the hematoma expands to compress the urethra, causing bladder outlet obstruction.

Signs and Symptoms

Vaginal Laceration
- Significant bleeding
- Swelling and pain

Vulvar Hematoma
- Swelling with purple discoloration of the vulva

Transport Management

Vaginal Laceration
- Apply direct pressure and/or pack with gauze as indicated.
- Treat hypovolemic shock per protocol.
- Manage pain.

Vulvar Hematoma
- Administer ice.
- Provide compression.
- Monitor the indwelling catheter, if one is placed.

Summary

The dynamic changes that occur with pregnancy can prove challenging for the CCTP who is treating a pregnant patient. For the pregnant patient, each day is different physiologically as a new life grows inside her. Gynecologic emergencies do not require significantly different treatment during critical care transport, but, as always, are important to treat properly and with sensitivity.

Case Study

You are dispatched to transport a female patient from the local community hospital to the tertiary care center 30 minutes away. She is 38 years old and 32 weeks pregnant. She is carrying twins after undergoing in vitro fertilization. The patient presented to the local hospital with complaints of headache and right upper quadrant pain.

Upon arrival, you receive a report from the nurse. Currently, the patient is hemodynamically stable. Her BP is 135/85 mm Hg, heart rate is 72 beats/min, and oxygen saturation is 97% on room air. Fetal heart rate tracings have been reassuring for both babies. Blood work drawn on arrival revealed a white blood cell count of 11,000 mm^3, a hemoglobin level of 11.2 g/dL, and a platelet count of 98,000 mm^3. The patient's electrolytes are all within normal range and her liver function tests are within normal limits. The only abnormality is a creatinine level of 1.5 mg/dL. Her initial BP on arrival to the community hospital was elevated, at 150/92 mm Hg. The hospital providers obtained IV access with an 18-gauge catheter in the antecubital fossa. Magnesium sulfate was administered starting with a 4-g load, and now continuing at 2 g/h via IV line. The patient is awake and alert and appears to be in no acute distress. You confirm the IV access is patent. You confirm the medication is running through the pump at the prescribed amount. The patient is transferred to your gurney with fetal monitors in place.

Five minutes into your transport, you notice a change in the patient's BP, which now measures 165/110 mm Hg. She complains of worsening headache. You confirm that the magnesium sulfate is being administered. You contact medical control and request recommendations. You are advised to increase the magnesium to 4 g/h. Ten minutes later, the patient reports difficulty breathing. Her BP is unchanged, but the oxygen saturation level is now in the mid-80s. You administer supplemental oxygen and continue your transport. Despite the oxygen, the patient has worsening dyspnea and is becoming less responsive. You apply nasal capnography and determine the end-tidal carbon dioxide (ETCO$_2$) is 67 mm Hg. Realizing the patient is experiencing magnesium toxicity, you turn off the magnesium and begin assisting respirations. You arrive at the tertiary care center while you are performing bag-mask ventilation.

1. What is the patient's underlying diagnosis?
2. Was increasing the magnesium the correct response?
3. What is the antidote to magnesium sulfate toxicity?
4. What would have been a better option to control the patient's BP?

Analysis

You recognize that this patient has preeclampsia, based on her elevated BP and her low platelet count. The initial treatment for the patient's preeclampsia was correct, with a magnesium load of 4 g continuing at 2 g/h. The patient's risk factors for preeclampsia were her age (older than 35 years) and multiple-gestation pregnancy. Assisted reproduction also increases the risk of preeclampsia.

Increasing the magnesium in this patient in response to her increasing headache and BP was inappropriate. This patient is at increased risk of magnesium toxicity due to her impaired renal function. A creatinine level of 1.1 mg/dL or greater indicates impaired renal function in a pregnant woman without preexisting renal disease. Magnesium is excreted via the kidneys. Because the patient was experiencing difficulty breathing, the initial response should have been to reduce the magnesium and assess respiratory status. An ETCO$_2$ level of 67 mm Hg suggests respiratory insufficiency; assisting ventilations would have been more helpful than administering oxygen. After you ultimately identified that the patient was experiencing magnesium toxicity, the decision to turn off the magnesium was correct. However, when the patient's respiratory status requires assisted ventilations, an appropriate intervention would be to administer calcium gluconate 1 g over 3 minutes to reverse the effects of the magnesium.

You received faulty advice from your medical control. The correct medical advice would have been to administer labetalol 20 mg IV, hydralazine 10 mg IV, or nifedipine 10 mg immediate release. BP would then need to be reassessed in 10 to 15 minutes. When BP is in the severe range, patients are at increased risk of stroke. This condition should be managed in a similar fashion to a hypertensive emergency. Magnesium is not indicated to manage BP; in this case it was being used to prevent seizure.

The patient was given calcium gluconate upon arrival and did not require intubation. She was taken to the operating room to undergo a cesarean section for preeclampsia with severe features. She delivered two healthy, although premature, infants who are doing well in the neonatal intensive care unit.

Prep Kit

Ready for Review

- The physiologic changes induced by pregnancy and the presence of potentially life-threatening pathologic conditions can make management of obstetric patients challenging.
- The female reproductive system, which is regulated by hormones, experiences an approximately 28-day menstrual cycle.
- The placenta provides the fetus with oxygen and vital nutrients. It grows with the fetus and includes a thin membrane that separates the maternal and fetal blood supplies.
- As the fetus grows and the ratio of fetal size to amniotic fluid decreases, the fetus becomes more vulnerable to trauma.
- Pregnancy alters the normal physiology of females, affecting nearly every organ system.
- During pregnancy, cardiac output increases, circulating blood volume expands, and peripheral venous pressure increases. BP and levels of serum albumin and serum protein decrease as pregnancy progresses.
- The growth of the fetus increases the demand for oxygen and reduces the oxygen reserves in the pregnant woman.
- Gastroesophageal reflux is more common during pregnancy, and a pregnant patient with an altered level of consciousness has a greater likelihood of aspiration.
- Pregnancy places increased strain on the renal and endocrine systems.
- Hormonal changes in the pregnant patient can cause dermatologic changes, including acne, linea nigra, chloasma, and rashes.
- Obstetric patients require a complete physical exam, including maternal and fetal hemodynamic monitoring and, if in labor, external vaginal evaluation for the presence of crowning.
- If delivery is imminent, CCTPs should seek to assist in the delivery at the hospital rather than attempt delivery during transport.
- To ease the anxiety caused by the stress and noise of transport, analgesics may be administered to patients in labor.
- When necessary, CPR should be performed on pregnant patients by following standard guidelines, with constant chest compressions and limited interruptions for ventilation and gas exchange.
- If defibrillation of the pregnant patient is necessary, fetal monitors should be removed before administering a shock.
- The developing fetus has a very small reserve of oxygen, usually only 1 to 2 minutes, if the supply from the mother is cut off or diminished. If the fetus does not receive enough oxygen, the heart rate decreases and death ensues.
- The well-being of the fetus may be assessed by auscultation for heart rate and movement, use of a hand-held Doppler ultrasonograph or fetal stethoscope, and electronic fetal monitoring.
- Electronic fetal monitoring records the fetal heart rate and uterine contractions on a fetal monitoring strip. Late or variable decelerations in the heart rate are abnormal and may indicate fetal distress.
- The normal heart rate of a fetus is between 110 and 160 beats/min. Fetal heart tones should be recorded for at least 30 to 60 seconds every 15 minutes during labor. During high-risk transports, electronic fetal monitoring should be performed continuously.
- Any vaginal bleeding during the third trimester of pregnancy must be regarded as an emergency.
- Bleeding may indicate an early pregnancy loss, ectopic pregnancy, abruptio placentae, placenta previa, or uterine rupture.
- CCTPs should be aware of the warning signs of dangerous medical conditions, such as gestational hypertension, preeclampsia, eclampsia, and HELLP syndrome, and the appropriate treatment protocols.
- Labor includes three distinct stages as the cervix dilates, the baby descends through the birth canal and is born, and the placenta is delivered.

Prep Kit Continued

- During delivery, a crucial fetal transition occurs as the baby begins to breathe independently of the oxygen supply from the mother. Anything that delays the decline in pulmonary pressure (and therefore delays breathing) during the fetal transition can lead to delayed transition, hypoxia, brain damage, and death.
- Preterm labor and fetal immaturity are the leading causes of neonatal mortality.
- Tocolytic agents may be administered to help stop preterm labor.
- A baby may present in the vertex, frank breech, complete breech, incomplete breech, or footling breech position for birth.
- In the event of a prolapsed cord, the pregnant patient should be given oxygen, placed in the knee-chest position, and transported rapidly.
- If shoulder dystocia occurs (ie, the infant is too large to travel through the birth canal unassisted), a rapid treatment plan is needed, which may include positioning the pregnant patient using the McRoberts maneuver, suprapubic pressure, or delivery of the posterior arm.
- During the interval between multiple births (such as twins or triplets), transport should continue. Transport should be interrupted only if the next infant begins to emerge from the birth canal.
- Once delivery is complete, care for both the mother and the infant should continue, to include examining the mother's perineum for tears, monitoring the infant's Apgar score, performing fundal massage, and drying and warming the infant.
- CCTPs must monitor the antepartum patient for possible postpartum hemorrhage, amniotic fluid embolism, and uterine rupture.
- Pelvic inflammatory disease is an infectious process causing inflammation in the reproductive system, including the uterus, fallopian tubes, and ovaries. If untreated, it may cause infertility.
- CCTPs should be prepared to treat gynecologic emergencies such as toxic shock syndrome, ovarian cysts, ruptured ovarian cysts, and ovarian torsion.
- Ovarian cysts are typically a result of follicular maturation during the normal female menstrual cycle and are often undetectable and self-resolving. A small percentage may continue to grow and cause lower abdominal pain.
- Symptoms of a cyst include abdominal pain, nausea, vomiting, and, with very large cysts, frequent urination from bladder pressure.
- Ovarian cyst diagnosis is made through ultrasonography and Doppler flow studies, which can monitor blood flow as well as cyst size and location. Consider alternative diagnoses such as ovarian torsion, ectopic pregnancy, and appendicitis.
- An ovarian cyst may rupture spontaneously or following trauma, resulting in hemorrhage. If hemorrhage is present, patients may present with increased lower abdominal and pelvic pain, vaginal bleeding, and hypovolemia leading to shock.
- Treatment for a patient with a ruptured ovarian cyst includes controlling any immediate life threats, including evaluation for hypovolemic shock and maintaining adequate BP with isotonic fluids if the patient is in shock.
- Ovarian torsion is often a cause of lower abdominal pain in females; it initially presents similarly to appendicitis or an ectopic pregnancy.
- Gynecologic trauma includes vulvar hematoma (straddle injury), which is treated with ice and compression.
- Gynecologic emergencies do not require significantly different treatment during critical care transport but must be treated properly and with sensitivity.

Prep Kit Continued

Vital Vocabulary

amniotic fluid embolism (AFE) A rare and poorly understood condition in which fetal tissue crosses over the placental barrier into the maternal circulation. It can occur antepartum and postpartum, and is believed to be associated with an anaphylactoid response leading to multisystem organ failure and disseminated intravascular coagulation.

breech A delivery presentation in which the presenting part is not the head.

chloasma A dermatologic condition affecting pregnant women in which darkened skin patches appear on the cheeks and forehead.

complete breech A delivery presentation in which the buttocks present first and the legs are crossed inside the uterus.

dilation and curettage (D&C) A surgical procedure in which the cervix is opened and the uterus scraped of tissue.

early pregnancy loss Expulsion of the fetus that occurs naturally; also called miscarriage or spontaneous abortion.

eclampsia The condition that exists once a patient with preeclampsia develops seizures; it causes serious maternal complications. Warning signs of the transition from preeclampsia to eclampsia include severe headache, scotomata, hyperreflexia, epigastric pain, and anxiety.

ectopic pregnancy A pregnancy in which the ovum implants somewhere other than the uterine endometrium.

endometrium The inner mucous membrane of the uterus.

external fetal monitoring Electronic heart monitoring of the fetus while in utero, performed via electrodes placed on the pregnant woman's abdomen.

footling breech A delivery presentation in which both feet extend into the birth canal.

foramen ovale The opening in the fetal heart that allows blood to flow from the right atrium to the left atrium of the fetus, bypassing the lungs prior to birth.

frank breech A delivery presentation in which the buttocks present first, both of the infant's hips are flexed, and the feet are near the fetus's head.

gestation Period of time elapsed from conception to birth. For humans, the full period is normally 40 weeks.

gestational diabetes A condition in which a woman without previous diabetes develops high blood glucose, especially during the third trimester.

gestational hypertension The occurrence of hypertension in a pregnant woman, usually after 20 weeks' gestation, defined as a blood pressure of 140/90 mm Hg or greater in a woman with a previously normal blood pressure. Also called pregnancy-induced hypertension.

HELLP syndrome A hemolytic disorder that occurs during the latter stages of gestation, usually after the 20th week, and whose clinical findings include hemolytic anemia, elevated liver enzyme levels, and a low platelet count. Patients will present with blurred vision, abdominal pain, headache, and edema.

hydroureteronephrosis Dilation and obstruction of a ureter, which results in dilation of the connected kidney.

incomplete breech A delivery presentation in which the buttocks present first and one foot extends into the birth canal.

introitus The visible opening to the vagina.

linea nigra A dermatologic condition affecting pregnant women in which a darkened line develops from the navel to the vagina.

Prep Kit Continued

metabolic acidemia A condition characterized by the body's production of excessive quantities of acid or the kidneys' inability to remove enough acid from the body.

metabolic acidosis A pathologic condition characterized by a blood pH of less than 7.35, which is caused by an accumulation of acids in the body from a metabolic cause.

oophoropexy Surgery in which the ovary is attached to the pelvic sidewall so it cannot twist on itself.

ovarian cyst A fluid buildup within an outcropping of tissue from the ovary. If such a cyst ruptures, significant bleeding can occur.

ovarian torsion Twisting of an ovary about its ligaments, resulting in ischemia and possibly necrosis.

partial thromboplastin time (PTT) A value that represents the intrinsic coagulation pathway's clotting ability; also known as activated partial thromboplastin time (aPTT).

pelvic inflammatory disease (PID) An infection of the female upper organs of reproduction—specifically, the uterus, ovaries, and fallopian tubes.

precipitous delivery Delivery in less than 3 hours from the onset of regular contractions; may occur with premature labor.

preeclampsia A condition of late pregnancy that involves onset of hypertension and proteinuria that manifests with headache, visual changes, and swelling of the hands and feet; also called toxemia of pregnancy. It may be classified as occurring with or without severe features.

premature Underdeveloped; refers to infants born before 36 weeks from the first day of the last menstrual period.

premature prelabor rupture of membranes (PPROM) A rupture of membranes in a pregnant woman signaled by a gush of fluid or constant fluid leakage; it accounts for as many as 50% of all preterm deliveries.

preterm labor Labor occurring before 36 weeks' gestation, leading to early birth.

prolapsed cord A delivery presentation in which the umbilical cord passes through the birth canal in advance of the infant.

proteinuria Protein levels detected in the urine.

prothrombin time (PT) A value that represents the extrinsic coagulation pathway's clotting ability by taking into account various clotting factors, fibrinogen, the prothrombin ratio, and the international normalized ratio.

pruritic urticarial papules and plaques of pregnancy (PUPPP) An itchy rash affecting pregnant women; it may be either isolated to one region or systemic.

shoulder dystocia A condition in which the infant's shoulders are too large to travel through the birth canal without additional clinical maneuvering of the infant.

supine hypotensive syndrome Low blood pressure resulting from compression of the inferior vena cava by the weight of the pregnant uterus when the mother is supine.

term Used to describe an infant delivered at 39 to 40 weeks' gestation.

thrombocytopenia Reduction in the number of platelets.

tocolytics A group of medications used to suppress preterm labor.

toxic shock syndrome A condition that results from the release of bacterial toxins into the body, specifically following infection with *Staphylococcus aureus*, *Streptococcus pyogenes*, or *Clostridium sordellii*.

vertex A fetal position in which the head is the lowest part of the fetus, resulting in the head presenting first during delivery; the normal delivery presentation.

Prep Kit Continued

References

American College of Obstetricians and Gynecologists. *Practice Bulletin 106: Intrapartum Fetal Heart Rate Monitoring: Nomenclature, Interpretation, and General Management Principles.* Washington, DC: American Congress of Obstetricians and Gynecologists; July 2009.

American College of Obstetricians and Gynecologists. *Practice Bulletin 171: Management of Preterm Labor.* Washington, DC: American Congress of Obstetricians and Gynecologists; January 2016 (reaffirmed 2020).

American College of Obstetricians and Gynecologists. *Practice Bulletin 200: Early Pregnancy Loss.* Washington, DC: American Congress of Obstetricians and Gynecologists; November 2018.

American College of Obstetricians and Gynecologists. *Practice Bulletin 222: Gestational Hypertension and Preeclampsia.* Washington, DC: American Congress of Obstetricians and Gynecologists; June 2020.

American College of Obstetricians and Gynecologists. *Practice Bulletin 767: Emergent Therapy for Acute-Onset, Severe Hypertension During Pregnancy and the Postpartum Period.* Washington, DC: American Congress of Obstetricians and Gynecologists; February 2019.

American College of Obstetricians and Gynecologists. *Safe Motherhood Initiative: Maternal Safety Bundle for Severe Hypertension in Pregnancy.* Washington, DC: American Congress of Obstetricians and Gynecologists; 2014: 74-126.

American Heart Association. Cardiac arrest in pregnancy. *Circulation.* 2015;132:1747-1773.

Anderson JM, Etches D. Prevention and management of postpartum hemorrhage. *Am Fam Phys.* 2007;75(6):875-882.

Association of Women's Health, Obstetric, and Neonatal Nurses. *Fetal Heart Monitoring: Principles and Practices.* 4th ed. Dubuque, IA: Kendall Hunt; 2009.

Ayres S, Grenvik A, Holbrook P, Shoemaker W. *Textbook of Critical Care.* 3rd ed. Philadelphia, PA: WB Saunders; 1995.

Beltran W. Prehospital management of obstetric bleeding. In: Dobiesz V, Kerrigan K, eds. *Manual of Obstetric Emergencies.* Philadelphia, PA: Wolters Kluwer; 2021:165-171.

Blocker W. Ovarian cysts. eMedicineHealth website. http://www.emedicinehealth.com/ovarian_cysts/article_em.htm. Accessed June 9, 2021.

Burns B, Fisher E. Resuscitation in pregnancy. In: Tintinalli JE, Stapcyzynski JS, Ma OJ, et al., eds. *Tintinalli's Emergency Medicine: A Comprehensive Study Guide.* 9th ed. New York, NY: McGraw-Hill; 2020:164-169.

Capeless E. Cardiovascular changes in early phase of pregnancy. *Am J Obstet Gynecol.* 1989;161(6):1449-1453.

Caroline N. *Nancy Caroline's Emergency Care in the Streets.* 9th ed. Burlington, MA: Jones & Bartlett Learning; 2022.

Centers for Disease Control and Prevention. Pelvic inflammatory disease: CDC fact sheet. http://www.cdc.gov/std/PID/STDFact-PID.htm. Accessed June 9, 2021.

Centers for Disease Control and Prevention. Preterm birth. http://www.cdc.gov/reproductivehealth/maternalinfanthealth/pretermbirth.htm. Accessed June 9, 2021.

Centers for Disease Control and Prevention. Progress in chronic disease prevention anemia during pregnancy in low-income women—United States, 1987. *MMWR.* 1990;39(5):73-76,81.

Chames M, Pearlman M. Trauma during pregnancy: outcomes and clinical management. *Clin Obstet Gynecol.* 2008;51: 398-408.

Chang C, Ghermezi M, Robinson N. Breech deliveries. In: Dobiesz V, Kerrigan K, eds. *Manual of Obstetric Emergencies.* Philadelphia, PA: Wolters Kluwer; 2021:322-331.

Chen T, Bittner C. Physiologic changes in pregnancy. In: Dobiesz V, Kerrigan K, eds. *Manual of Obstetric Emergencies.* Philadelphia, PA: Wolters Kluwer; 2021:3-15.

Clark SL, Cotton DB, Lee W, et al. Central hemodynamic assessment of normal term pregnancy. *Am J Obstet Gynecol.* 1989;161(6):1439-1442.

Cleary V, Wilson P, Super G. *Prehospital Care: Administrative and Clinical Management.* Rockville, MD: Aspen; 1987.

Cunningham FG, Leveno KJ, Bloom SV, et al. *Williams Obstetrics.* 25th ed. New York, NY: McGraw-Hill Education; 2018.

Deutsch A. Amniotic fluid embolism. In: Dobiesz V, Kerrigan K, eds. *Manual of Obstetric Emergencies.* Philadelphia, PA: Wolters Kluwer; 2021:398-401.

Fernandez-Frackelton M. Bacteria. In: *Rosen's Emergency Medicine: Concepts and Clinical Practice.* 9th ed. Elsevier; 2018:1573-1597.

Food and Drug Administration. *Content and Format of Labeling for Human Prescription Drug and Biological Products; Requirements for Pregnancy and Lactation Labeling.* Washington, DC: Department of Health and Human Services; 2006.

Frasure S, Kerrigan K. Emergency delivery. In: Tintinalli JE, Stapcyzynski JS, Ma OJ, et al., eds. *Tintinalli's Emergency Medicine: A Comprehensive Study Guide.* 9th ed. New York, NY: McGraw-Hill; 2020:637-647.

Gabbe SG, Niebyl JR, Simpson JL, et al. Intrapartum fetal evaluation. In: *Obstetrics: Normal and Problem Pregnancies.* Philadelphia, PA: Elsevier; 2017:317.

Gherman RB, Goodwin, TM, Souter I, et al. The McRoberts' maneuver for the alleviation of shoulder dystocia: How successful is it? *Am J Obstet Gynecol.* http://dx.doi.org/10.1016/S0002-9378(97)70565-9.

Gyetvai K, Hannah ME, Hodnett ED, et al. Tocolytics for preterm labor: a systematic review. *Obstet Gynecol.* 1999;94(5 pt 2): 869-877.

Haas DM, Benjamin T, Sawyer R, Quinney SK. Short-term tocolytics for preterm delivery: current perspectives. *Int J Womens Health.* 2014;6:343-349.

Prep Kit Continued

Hall JE, Hall ME. *Guyton and Hall Textbook of Medical Physiology*. 14th ed. Philadelphia, PA: Elsevier; 2020.

Heniff M, Fleming H. Abdominal and pelvic pain in the non-pregnant female. In: Tintinalli JE, Stapcyzynski JS, Ma OJ, et al., eds. *Tintinalli's Emergency Medicine: A Comprehensive Study Guide*. 9th ed. New York, NY: McGraw-Hill; 2020:612-615.

Hoffman BL, Schorge JO, Bradshaw KD, et al. *Williams Gynecology*. 3rd ed. New York, NY: McGraw-Hill Education; 2016.

Kaaja RJ, Greer IA. Manifestations of chronic disease during pregnancy. *JAMA*. 2005;294:2751-2757.

Kass EH. Asymptomatic infection of urinary tract. *Trans Assoc Am Phys*. 1956;69:56-63.

Kish K, Collea JV. Malpresentation and cord prolapse. In: DeCherney AH, Nathan L, eds. *Current Obstetric and Gynecologic Diagnosis and Treatment*. 9th ed. New York, NY: Lange/McGraw-Hill; 2003:369-386.

Lattanzi DR, Cook WA. Urinary calculi in pregnancy. *Obstet Gynecol*. 1980;56:462-466.

Lo JO, Mission JF, Caughey AB. Hypertensive disease of pregnancy and maternal mortality. *Curr Opin Obstet Gynecol*. 2013;25(2):124-132.

Lutfy-Clayton L, Goodrich M, Skotnicki K. In: Dobiesz V, Kerrigan K, eds. *Manual of Obstetric Emergencies*. Philadelphia, PA: Wolters Kluwer; 2021:56-72.

Mastrobattista J. Therapeutic agents in preterm labor: steroids. *Clin Obstet Gynecol*. 2000;43(4):802-808.

Moore K. *The Developing Human: Clinically Oriented Embryology*. 4th ed. Philadelphia, PA: WB Saunders; 1988.

Oxorn H. *Human Labor and Birth*. 5th ed. Norwalk, CT: Appleton-Century-Croft; 1986.

Peters CW, Layon AJ, Edwards RK. Cardiac arrest during pregnancy. *J Clin Anesth*. 2006;50:27-28.

Seifert S. Umbilical cord abnormalities. In: Dobiesz V, Kerrigan K, eds. *Manual of Obstetric Emergencies*. Philadelphia, PA: Wolters Kluwer; 2021:346-357.

Shorette AS. Uterine inversion and uterine rupture. In: Dobiesz V, Kerrigan K, eds. *Manual of Obstetric Emergencies*. Philadelphia, PA: Wolters Kluwer; 2021:382-397.

Simhan H, Caritas S. Inhibition of acute preterm labor. UpToDate website. https://www.uptodate.com/contents/inhibition-of-acute-preterm-labor. Updated October 26, 2020. Accessed June 9, 2021.

Stanton SL, Kerr-Wilson R, Grant Harris V. The incidence of urological symptoms in normal pregnancy. *Br J Obstet Gynecol*. 1980;87:897-900.

Strassmann BI. The evolution of endometrial cycles and menstruation. *Q Rev Biol*. 1996;71(2):181-220.

Vegetti W. FSH and follucogenesis: from physiology to ovarian stimulation. *Reprod Biomed Online*. 2006;12(6):684-694.

Weiss B, Shepherd S. Pelvic inflammatory disease. In: Tintinalli JE, Stapcyzynski JS, Ma OJ, et al., eds. *Tintinalli's Emergency Medicine: A Comprehensive Study Guide*. 9th ed. New York, NY: McGraw-Hill; 2020:654-658.

Whittaker P, Macphail S, Lind T. Serial hematologic changes and pregnancy outcome. *Obstet Gynecol*. 1996;88(1):33-39.

World Health Organization. Newborn death and illness. http://www.who.int/pmnch/media/press_materials/fs/fs_newborndealth_illness/en/. Accessed June 9, 2021.

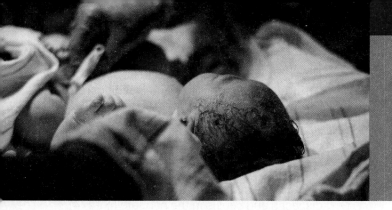

Chapter 23

Neonatal Emergencies

Patricia R. Chess, MD

Yogangi Malhotra, MD

Nirupama Laroia, MD

OBJECTIVES

After completing this chapter, you will be able to:

1. Define the terms *newborn*, *neonate*, and *term newborn* (p 1233).

2. Discuss the roles of the CCTP when caring for a neonate (p 1233).

3. Recognize anatomy and physiology unique to a neonate, including differences in thermoregulation, respiratory structure and function, oxygen transport, cardiovascular function, renal function, fluid and electrolyte balance, central nervous system, and skeletal system (pp 1233–1237).

4. Understand how problems with transitional circulation can result in neonatal emergencies (p 1236).

5. Describe developmental aspects of pain in the neonate (p 1237).

6. Discuss anatomic and physiologic differences in the premature infant, including how these relate to patient care (p 1237).

7. Discuss medical complications for which late preterm infants are at risk (p 1237).

8. Identify important antepartum and intrapartum risk factors that can affect labor, delivery, and the neonate (p 1238).

9. Understand the pathophysiology that is associated with antepartum and intrapartum factors that can affect labor, delivery, and the neonate (pp 1237–1238).

10. Identify when a CCTP would use the Apgar score in caring for a newborn (p 1238).

11. Discuss neonatal assessment, stabilization, and treatment (p 1237).

12. Discuss how to prepare for and provide neonatal resuscitation (p 1240).

13. Identify situations in which neonatal resuscitation should be performed (p 1240).

14. Describe the appropriate assessment technique when examining a neonate (p 1240).

15. Explain the initial steps in resuscitation of a neonate (p 1240).

16. Describe methods that can be used to improve airway and breathing in a neonate with inadequate respiration (p 1241).

17. Describe free-flow oxygen delivery (p 1241).

18. Explain the appropriate assisted ventilation for a neonate (p 1242).

19. Describe the appropriate endotracheal intubation technique for a neonate (p 1247).

20. Identify when an orogastric tube should be inserted in a neonate (p 1249).

21. Describe the procedure for inserting an orogastric tube in a neonate (p 1249).

22. Describe the appropriate chest compression and ventilation technique for a neonate (p 1250).

23. Discuss indications for medications, dosages, and routes of administration for a neonate (p 1252).
24. Discuss the use of ventilators during neonatal transports (p 1256).
25. Discuss the pathophysiology, assessment findings, management, and treatment plan for the following respiratory emergencies in a neonate: apnea, meconium aspiration, pneumonia, respiratory distress syndrome, pneumothorax, and respiratory acidosis (pp 1257–1260).
26. Distinguish between primary and secondary apnea (p 1257).
27. Discuss the causes, assessment, and management of primary and secondary apnea (p 1257).
28. Describe how to perform needle thoracentesis for pneumothorax decompression in a neonate (p 1259).
29. Determine when vascular access is indicated for a neonate (p 1261).
30. Recognize congenital anomalies that may lead to compromise of the neonate (p 1261).
31. Discuss the pathophysiology, assessment findings, and management of the following cardiovascular emergencies in a neonate: cyanosis, cyanotic congenital heart disease, tachyarrhythmias, bradyarrhythmias, cardiac arrest, persistent pulmonary hypertension, shock, anemia, and hyperbilirubinemia (pp 1261–1267).
32. Describe how to perform umbilical vein catheterization in a neonate (p 1264).
33. Discuss the pathophysiology, assessment findings, and management of the following gastrointestinal emergencies in a neonate: gastroschisis, omphalocele, gastrointestinal

obstruction and vomiting, acute intestinal perforation, hematemesis and bleeding from the rectum, volvulus, intussusception, and diarrhea (pp 1269–1274).
34. Explain appropriate fluid selection when vascular access is indicated for a neonate (p 1270).
35. Discuss the management of infectious diseases and sepsis in the neonate (p 1274).
36. Discuss the management of hyperthermia and hypothermia in the neonate (p 1274).
37. Discuss the management of toxic exposure in the neonate, including the appropriate treatment for the neonate with narcotic depression (p 1274).
38. Discuss the pathophysiology, assessment findings, and management of the following trauma/birth injuries in the neonate: head and neck injuries, nerve injuries, bone injuries, and abuse/maltreatment (pp 1275–1276).
39. Discuss the pathophysiology, assessment findings, and management of the following neurologic conditions in the neonate: seizures, hypoxic ischemic encephalopathy, and lethargy (pp 1276–1278).
40. Discuss the pathophysiology, assessment findings, and management of the following metabolic conditions in the neonate: metabolic acidosis, hypoglycemia, hypocalcemia, and inborn errors of metabolism (pp 1278–1279).
41. Discuss the use of an incubator (p 1280).
42. Recognize the emotional impact of a neonate's illness or injury, and the need for information, empathy, and compassion for the parent/guardian during a critical care transport (p 1280).
43. Discuss risks associated with critical care transport, including factors unique to air transport of a neonate (p 1282).

Introduction

The care of a newborn or neonate must be tailored to meet the unique needs of this population. The term **newborn** refers to an infant within the first few hours after birth; a **neonate** is an infant within the first 28 days after birth **TABLE 23-1**. A **term newborn** is one delivered between 37 0/7 and 41 6/7 weeks' **gestation**. Term can be further defined as early term (37 0/7 to 38 6/7 weeks' gestation), full term (39 0/7 to 40 6/7 weeks' gestation), and late term (41 0/7 to 41 6/7 weeks' gestation).

This chapter reviews challenges that the critical care transport professional (CCTP) may face when transporting a neonate, including recognizing the anatomic differences in a neonate and understanding the physiologic changes that occur in a newborn during the transition from fetal circulation after birth, thermoregulation, and the special needs of infants delivered prematurely, or births complicated by other factors. The steps involved in neonatal resuscitation, the pathophysiology of common congenital anomalies, medical emergencies

TABLE 23-1 Infant Age Terminology	
Term	**Age**
Newborn	Within the first few hours after birth
Neonate	Within the first 28 days after birth
Infant	Age 1 month to 1 year
Term newborn	Delivered between 37 and 42 weeks' gestation
Preterm	Delivered before 37 weeks' gestation

© Jones & Bartlett Learning.

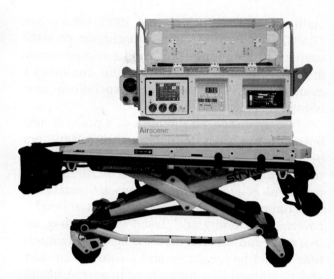

FIGURE 23-1 A transport incubator.
Used with permission from International Biomedical.

encountered during the first month after birth, and the effects of these factors on the process of transporting a critically ill infant are also discussed.

Additional skilled care interventions—such as intubation, obtaining peripheral intravenous (IV) access, placement of umbilical venous and arterial lines, needle aspiration of the chest, and chest tube placement—are needed for approximately 6% of neonates, with the rate of complications increasing as the neonate's birth weight and gestational age decrease. In the United States, approximately 80% of the 30,000 babies born each year weighing less than 3 pounds (1,500 g) require resuscitation. Because both short- and long-term outcomes in neonates have been linked to initial stabilization efforts, it is imperative that CCTPs anticipate problems with neonates, be knowledgeable about how to deal with them, have the appropriate resuscitation equipment readily available, and carefully consider the neonate's ultimate transport plan.

Anatomy and Physiology of a Neonate

Neonates are not small children. That is, newborn infants have anatomic differences and undergo unique physiologic changes at birth, placing them at special risks.

Thermoregulation

Neonates become cold easily due to a variety of factors. Their potential for heat loss is greater due to their high body surface area-to-body weight ratios and limited subcutaneous fat stores. Neonates also lose heat to the environment through the mechanisms of thermal conduction, convection, radiation, and increased evaporative heat loss through the skin. Heat production is limited because of their low glycogen stores, small supply of brown fat (brown fat is used in older people as a heat energy source), and limited capacity to generate heat by shivering. This is especially true in infants who are small for their gestational ages and prematurity. Neonates have a relatively narrow range for their **neutral thermal environment**, the temperature at which maintenance of normal body temperature requires only minimal metabolic expenditure. Although the term newborn is able to increase heat production through brown fat metabolism (nonshivering thermogenesis), this process comes at the cost of increased oxygen consumption. Hypothermia in infants is associated with hypoxia, prolonged coagulation time with reduced platelet function and increased risk of intraventricular hemorrhage, reduced drug metabolism, cerebral depression, myocardial depression, acidosis, decreased immunity, patient discomfort, and increased mortality. The preterm infant is particularly vulnerable because the immature skin is thin, allowing significant heat (and evaporative fluid) loss to occur.

To help maintain normothermia in neonates, CCTPs should use prewarmed blankets and equipment, including a prewarmed transport incubator **FIGURE 23-1**, place a cap on the infant's head, and minimize the infant's exposure to cold. It is recommended that the temperature of a newborn be maintained between 98°F and 100°F (36.5°C and 37.5°C) after birth through resuscitation or stabilization. It is important to avoid environmentally induced hyperthermia, because this condition is associated with increased energy expenditure, morbidity, and mortality.

In preparation for the birth of a preterm newborn, it is important to increase the ambient temperature of the room where the newborn will receive initial care to 73°F to 77°F (23°C to 25°C). For newborns delivered prior to 32 weeks' gestation, it is recommended that the newborn's lower body be covered with food-grade plastic wrap or a bag, and that a hat and thermal mattress be used. Temperature should be measured and recorded after birth and monitored as a measure of quality. A healthy baby can be placed skin to skin with the mother after resuscitation.

Respiratory Structure and Function

Lung development starts early in embryonic life, but the lungs are unable to sustain life ex utero until later in the canalicular stage of development, after approximately 23 weeks' gestation or 1 pound (500 g) of fetal weight. The neonatal lungs are small relative to the body size, with little respiratory reserve. Surfactant is present by 23 weeks' gestation, but surfactant deficiency is common before 32 weeks' gestation; thus, babies born prematurely may benefit from exogenous surfactant delivered endotracheally.

The neonate has a respiratory rate of 30 to 60 breaths/min with a tidal volume in the range of 5 to 7 mL/kg. The head is large in relation to the neonate's body, resulting in neck flexion and obstruction when the infant is in the supine position. Placing a rolled towel under the neonate's shoulders helps open the airway.

The infant's tongue occupies a proportionally larger intraoral volume than in older people, a difference that can lead to airway obstruction. Newborn infants are obligate nose breathers and may present with obstructive apnea when the nasal passages are blocked by a developmental defect (choanal atresia), edema of the nasal mucosa caused by vigorous suctioning, or secretions. Placing and maintaining an oral airway is often a sufficient intervention to stabilize a neonate with a fixed nasal obstruction during transport.

Another important airway anatomic feature of neonates is their relatively more cephalad and anterior larynx, a factor that needs to be considered when locating the vocal cords during intubation. When positive-pressure ventilation (PPV) is needed, attempts should be made to maintain physiologic tidal volume breaths because volutrauma, hypercapnia, and hypocapnia have been associated with bleeding in the brain (intraventricular hemorrhage), hearing loss, and chronic lung disease or bronchopulmonary dysplasia.

Oxygen Transport

Fetal hemoglobin (HbF) accounts for 70% to 80% of the total hemoglobin in the neonate. Fetal hemoglobin delivers oxygen to the fetus's tissues in the hypoxic condition found in utero, but tends to hold on to oxygen in the normal conditions after birth (ie, the oxygen dissociation curve is shifted to the left). Neonates have a high oxygen requirement (6 to 8 mL/kg/min versus 4 to 6 mL/kg/min in adults). Tissue oxygenation is achieved through a relatively high cardiac output (300 mL/kg/min versus 60 to 80 mL/kg/min in adults), high heart rate (120 to 160 beats/min), and high respiratory rate (30 to 60 breaths/min). Neonates do not tolerate interruption in oxygen delivery for any length of time, but rather become hypoxic and bradycardic quickly.

Cardiovascular Function

The heart rate, normally 100 to 205 beats/min in neonates, is an important determinant of cardiac output because the neonate's cardiac muscle is immature. Neonates respond to careful volume loading (fluid bolus of 10 to 20 mL/kg) with an increase in cardiac output, but they do not tolerate fluid overload. The two inotropic agents most commonly used in neonates are dopamine (used when an infant has cardiac compromise and is peripherally vasodilated from septic shock) and dobutamine (which also improves cardiac function but can exacerbate hypotension due to peripheral vasodilation). **TABLE 23-2** summarizes normal blood pressure (BP) for newborns through infants.

Transitional Circulation

In utero, the pulmonary vasculature has a high resistance, so most of the blood returning to the right atrium from the placenta (oxygenated blood) passes to the left atrium via the foramen ovale **FIGURE 23-2**.

TABLE 23-2 Normal Infant Vital Signs

Age	Systolic BP (mm Hg)	Diastolic BP (mm Hg)	Mean Arterial Pressure (mm Hg)[a]
Birth (12 hours, <1,000 g)	39–59	16–36	28–42
Birth (12 hours, 3 kg)	60–76	31–45	48–57
Neonate (96 hours)	67–84	35–53	45–60
Infant (1–12 months)	72–104	37–56	50–62

[a] For practical purposes, approximations may be used, where the goal is for the mean arterial pressure (MAP) to be no lower than the gestational age. For example, a 28-week infant should have a MAP of no lower than 28 mm Hg, a 36-week newborn will have a MAP of no lower than 36 mm Hg, and so on.
Abbreviation: BP, blood pressure

Adapted from American Association of Critical-Care Nurses, American Heart Association. *PALS: Vital Signs in Children.* Dallas, TX: American Heart Association; 2020.

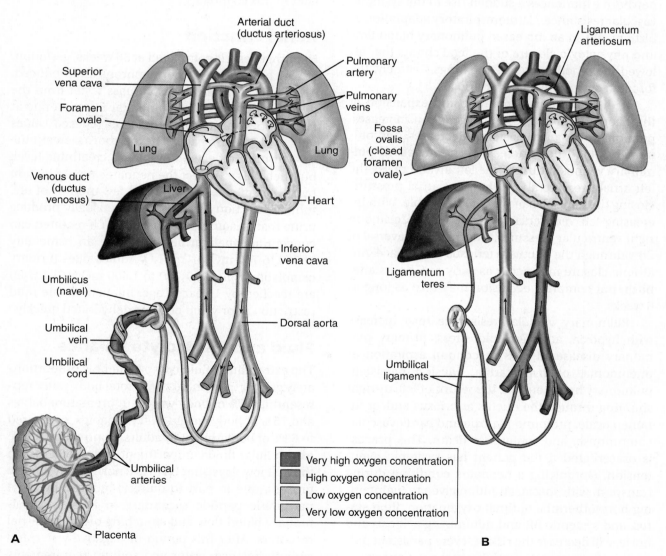

FIGURE 23-2 Fetal circulation. **A.** Oxygenated blood from the placenta reaches the fetus through the umbilical vein. Blood returns to the placenta via two umbilical arteries. Right-to-left shunts occur at the foramen ovale and the ductus arteriosus. **B.** Fetal circulation following transition.

The oxygenated blood enters the left atrium, mixes with the small pulmonary return, and is pumped via the left ventricle and the aorta to the coronary arteries and the brain. Deoxygenated blood returns from the lungs to the left atrium, where it mixes with the oxygenated blood. Of the ejected right ventricular output, most blood flows to the aorta via the ductus arteriosus, mixing with the left ventricular output. Blood carried by the descending aorta perfuses various organs and the lower body. Umbilical arteries, which branch from the internal iliac arteries, lead to the placenta where blood is oxygenated.

With the clamping of the umbilical cord at birth (ie, removal of the low-resistance placenta), the newborn experiences a sudden rise in the systemic vascular resistance. Cardiorespiratory adaptation at birth results in an increased pulmonary blood flow and physiologic closure of the fetal shunts that allowed the blood to bypass the lungs—namely, the foramen ovale and ductus arteriosus.

With extrauterine breathing and expansion of the neonate's lungs, tissue oxygenation increases, pulmonary vascular resistance decreases, and pulmonary blood flow increases. The increased pulmonary venous return to the left atrium raises the left atrial pressure above the right atrial pressure, closing the flap valve of the foramen ovale. With increasing left ventricular pressure and a decline in right ventricular pressures, a decrease or reversal of flow through the ductus arteriosus takes place. Anatomic closure may occur as early as 6 hours after birth, but complete occlusion may take as long as 6 weeks.

Pulmonary vascular resistance may increase with hypoxia, acidosis, cold stress, primary pulmonary disease such as meconium aspiration or pneumonia, or hypercarbia, causing persistent pulmonary hypertension, the return of left-to-right shunting through the ductus arteriosus and/or foramen ovale, profound hypoxia and cardiovascular compromise, and sometimes death. This process is exacerbated if the patient has systemic hypotension. Optimizing a neonate's condition during transport, with special attention given to maintaining normothermia, optimal oxygenation, fluid status, and systemic BP, and minimizing acidosis and noise, will decrease the risk of severe persistent pulmonary hypertension evolving in the patient.

Patent ductus arteriosus is seen in 50% of extremely premature infants (less than 26 weeks' gestation) and is a risk factor for intraventricular hemorrhage and necrotizing enterocolitis. Whereas immediate treatment for a patent ductus arteriosus during critical care transport is not indicated, minimizing fluid overload during transport can decrease the risk of a persistent symptomatic patent ductus arteriosus.

Some cardiac abnormalities depend on a patent ductal flow. In patients with these conditions, circulatory collapse may occur with the closure of the ductus, often at 2 to 7 days of age. Maintenance of ductal patency with prostaglandins during transport can be lifesaving and is discussed further in the section on cyanotic congenital heart disease (CHD) later in this chapter.

Renal Function

Nephrogenesis is completed at 36 weeks' gestation, at which point no further nephrons are produced. Additional increases in renal mass result from the growth of tubules. The glomerular filtration rate at term is low and reaches the adult indexed values only at 2 years of age. The newborn's creatinine level at birth reflects the mother's creatinine level, but then falls to reflect the neonate's renal function by 1 week of age. Over the first few months of life, tubular function matures; infants usually produce urine that is isotonic to plasma, but if required can concentrate their urine to achieve an osmolality of 500 to 700 mOsm/kg H_2O. Adult values (urinary osmolality, typically 1,200 to 1,400 mOsm/kg H_2O) are reached by 1 year of age. Infants tolerate fluid restriction poorly and become dehydrated quickly.

Fluid and Electrolyte Balance

The extracellular fluid compartment is proportionately greater in neonates, with total body water representing 85% of body weight in premature babies and 75% of body weight in term babies, compared to 60% of body weight in adults. Contraction of the extracellular fluid compartment and weight loss in the first few days after birth is a normal physiologic process, due in part to diuresis induced by atrial natriuretic peptide secondary to increased pulmonary blood flow and stretching of the left atrial receptors. After this period of negative water and sodium balance, water and sodium requirements increase to match those of the growing infant. For this reason, fluids should be restricted in the infant until the expected postnatal weight loss has occurred. Liberal fluid regimens in the first few days of life have been shown to be associated with worse outcomes in premature infants (eg, increased patent ductus arteriosus, necrotizing enterocolitis, and death). Fluid requirements increase incrementally from day 1 of life (60 to 100 mL/kg/d for term to extremely low-birth-weight infants, respectively) to 150 mL/kg/d at 1 week of life.

The solution 10% dextrose in water ($D_{10}W$) is commonly used for IV fluid maintenance in a newborn for the first 24 hours after birth. After 24 hours, once adequate urine output is established, 10% dextrose in 0.25% saline is used as a maintenance fluid in a neonatal transport; 10 mEq of potassium chloride in 500 mL may be added unless findings show abnormal electrolyte levels or renal function, necessitating adjustment. In general, a full-term infant needs 60 mL/kg/d of fluid, a very-low-birth-weight infant (less than 3 pounds [1,500 g]) needs 80 mL/kg/d, and an extremely low-birth-weight infant (less than 2 pounds [1,000 g]) needs 100 mL/kg/d on day 1 of life, increasing by 10 mL/kg/d each day until reaching total fluids of 150 mL/kg/d.

Central Nervous System, Nociception, and the Stress Response

The lower limit for cerebral autoregulation in neonates is not known but is thought to approximate a cerebral perfusion pressure of 30 mm Hg. In general, neonates are considered to have pressure-passive cerebral circulation: As mean arterial pressure falls, cerebral blood flow falls, and vice versa. Appropriate mean arterial BPs for extremely premature neonates have not been determined, but it is generally acknowledged that an acceptable mean arterial pressure equates to the gestational age of the newborn. It is also important to minimize stress in neonates and use appropriate sedation for procedures to minimize BP peaks in these patients that can lead to intraventricular hemorrhage.

Developmental Aspects of Pain

Neonates, including premature neonates, show well-developed responses to painful stimuli. Pain in neonates should be treated using appropriate analgesic measures, such as bundling and a pacifier dipped in $D_{10}W$ for blood draws or IV placement, or local anesthetics or opiates for more invasive procedures.

Skeletal Development

Neonates have incomplete ossification of bones, and their tissues are more fragile than those in older children and adults, making them more susceptible to both soft-tissue and bony injuries. This risk should be considered when providing cardiopulmonary resuscitation (CPR) because neonates are at higher risk of rib fractures and liver laceration during chest compressions. The optimal technique for chest compressions in neonates is reviewed later in the section on neonatal resuscitation.

Neonatal Assessment and Stabilization

The steps taken to assess, stabilize, and transport an ill neonate in an optimal manner can make a significant difference in long-term outcomes. For this reason, it is crucial for CCTPs to recognize neonatal emergencies and know how to respond to them. The CCTP should optimally review the patient's relevant history, including prenatal issues, neonatal symptoms, vital signs (including BP), physical exam findings, chest or abdominal radiographs (if obtained), and laboratory values (including glucose) as soon as the transport need is identified, or at the very latest, on arrival at the referring institution. Communication among all health care providers remains critical throughout the transport to optimize care. Specifics regarding assessment and stabilization are described in the remainder of this section.

Risk Factors for Neonates

The risks for complications in neonates increase as birth weight and gestational age decrease. They also increase in term infants when additional complications such as maternal infection, diabetes, hypertension, or meconium are present. Low-birth-weight infants are at increased risk for hypoglycemia and hypothermia, and late-gestational-age babies are at increased risk for delayed transition and persistent pulmonary hypertension. Antepartum and intrapartum risk factors for complications are listed in **TABLE 23-3** and **TABLE 23-4**, respectively.

Cord Clamping

Both the American Academy of Pediatrics (AAP) and the American College of Gynecologists (ACOG) recommend delayed cord clamping (30 to 60 seconds) for most vigorous term and preterm infants when feasible. This practice reduces the need for BP support and transfusion and may improve survival in the preterm infant. In addition, delayed cord clamping is associated with higher hematocrit and better iron levels in infancy. However, if the placental circulation is not intact, such as after abruptio placentae, bleeding placenta previa, bleeding vasa previa, or cord avulsion, the cord should be clamped immediately after birth. There is insufficient evidence at this time to recommend cord milking at delivery or an approach to cord clamping for neonates who require resuscitation at birth. It is important for the CCTP to inform the hospital whether delayed cord clamping was performed.

Apgar Score

The Apgar score is a standardized numeric expression of a baby's condition after birth **TABLE 23-5**. Traditionally, 1- and 5-minute scores are recorded, although extended scores (every 5 minutes, up to 20 minutes, if the score is less than 7) may need to be recorded if the newborn's condition remains depressed. Each of the five signs is awarded a score of 0, 1, or 2, with the total maximum score being 10.

TABLE 23-3 Antepartum (Before Birth) Risk Factors
Multiple gestation
Maternal age <16 years or >35 years
Postterm (>42 weeks') gestation
Toxemia, hypertension, diabetes
Polyhydramnios (excessive amount of amniotic fluid)
Premature rupture of the membrane and fetal malformation
Inadequate prenatal care
History of perinatal morbidity or mortality
Maternal use of drugs/medications
Fetal anemia
Oligohydramnios (decreased volume of amniotic fluid during a pregnancy)

© Jones & Bartlett Learning.

TABLE 23-4 Intrapartum (During Birth) Risk Factors
Premature labor
Rupture of membranes >24 hours before delivery
Abnormal presentation
Prolapsed cord
Chorioamnionitis
Meconium-stained amniotic fluid
Use of narcotics within 4 hours of delivery
Prolonged labor or precipitous delivery
Bleeding
Placenta previa

© Jones & Bartlett Learning.

TABLE 23-5 The Apgar Score			
	Score		
Sign	**0**	**1**	**2**
Appearance (color)	Blue or pale	Body pink, extremities blue	Completely pink
Pulse (heart rate)	0	0–100	>100
Grimace (irritability)	No response	Grimace	Cries
Activity (muscle tone)	Limp	Some flexion	Active movement
Respirations	Absent	Slow or irregular	Strong cry

Data from Apgar V. A proposal for a new method of evaluation of the newborn infant. *Curr Res Anesth Analg.* 1953;32(4):260-267.

The Apgar score is a limited indicator of the severity of hypoxic injury. The degree of correlation of the Apgar score with adverse neurologic outcome increases when the score remains 0 to 3 at 20 minutes. Factors that affect the Apgar score include physical maturity (Apgar scores are often lower in premature infants), maternal medication intake or narcotic use, and neuromuscular or cardiorespiratory conditions.

Laboratory Assessment

Neonatal laboratory values assist in managing a variety of critical conditions in these patients. Critical neonatal laboratory values are listed in **TABLE 23-6**.

Stabilization and Treatment

Stabilization of the neonate is needed if the patient has an acute airway obstruction, ineffective respiration, or insufficient cardiovascular circulation. As part of this care, the neonate must be evaluated for respiratory effort, heart rate, and color.

The first steps in stabilizing a neonate address airway management and ventilation. To optimize oxygenation and ventilation, ensure the neonate is in the appropriate sniffing position, and suction the neonate's mouth and nose if necessary. Continuous positive airway pressure (CPAP) is required if peripheral cyanosis is present despite adequate respiratory effort and a pulse rate greater than 100 beats/min. PPV is required if respiratory effort is inadequate, ineffective, or absent, or if the pulse rate is less than 100 beats/min. Gasping respirations usually indicate a significant problem and require the same interventions as absent respiratory effort or apnea.

Ventilations are provided at a rate of 40 to 60 breaths/min, with a tidal volume sufficient to expand the neonate's chest. Keep in mind that the physiologic tidal volume for a neonate is 5 to 7 mL/kg; hence, 15- to 20-mL breaths are needed for a term newborn. Resuscitation should begin with 21% oxygen (room air). PPV of newborns delivered prior to 35 weeks' gestation may begin with 21% to 30% oxygen. Free-flow oxygen may begin at a 30% oxygen level. The amount of oxygen delivered may be adjusted to meet the oxygen saturation target as determined by pulse oximetry by using the blender. Ensure that ventilation inflates and moves the chest. (See the section on neonatal resuscitation for more details.)

TABLE 23-6 Critical Neonatal Lab Values			
Name	Normal	Critically Low	Critically High
Blood Hematology and Coagulation Studies			
Hematocrit (% volume), neonate	44–64	<33	>70
Hemoglobin (g/dL), neonate	14.5–22	<9.5	>22
Chemistry			
Bilirubin (mg/dL), neonate	1–10	None	>13
Glucose (mg/dL), neonate	40–65	<40	>200
Microbiology (Qualitative Results) and Serology			
Group B *Streptococcus* antigen	None	None	Positive (delivery and nursery)
Urinalysis			
Note exceptions:	None	Urine glucose in patient <2 years	Positive
	None	Urine ketones in patient <2 years	Positive

Note: There is variance in unpublished lists—this is not an official list.

Intubation is no longer recommended for non-vigorous newborn infants born through meconium-stained amniotic fluid. Instead, the initial steps in the protocol for this condition should be performed and personnel trained in endotracheal intubation should be present at the delivery.

Use of a three-lead electronic cardiac monitor is a rapid and reliable method for continuously displaying the infant's heart rate. The pulse oximeter may have difficulty acquiring the signal if the patient has insufficient perfusion. Chest compressions are indicated if the neonate's pulse is less than 60 beats/min and shows no improvement despite effective and adequate PPV with T-piece/bag-mask ventilations (3 compressions followed by 1 breath, with 90 compressions and 30 breaths delivered each minute). Additional interventions—such as volume expansion (10 to 20 mL/kg bolus of normal saline), epinephrine (for persistent bradycardia of less than 60 beats/min despite optimal respirations and chest compressions), dextrose bolus (2 mL/kg $D_{10}W$ bolus for blood glucose levels less than 40 mg/dL), or sodium bicarbonate (for documented severe metabolic acidosis)—may be needed in some cases.

Special care needs to be taken when stabilizing and transporting a preterm neonate. Infants born before 34 weeks' gestation are at increased risk for bleeding into the brain (intraventricular hemorrhage). Avoiding rapid fluctuations in their BP, temperature, fluid volume, and pH status can help minimize this risk. Preterm infants who need oxygen therapy and mechanical ventilation are also at risk of long-term lung damage (bronchopulmonary dysplasia). Minimizing oxygen exposure and avoiding excessive pressures from assisted ventilation will decrease this risk. Of note, preterm infants (less than 37 0/7 weeks' gestation), including late-preterm infants (34 0/7 to 36 6/7 weeks' gestation), are also at increased risk of jaundice, dehydration, hypothermia, hypoglycemia, and sepsis.

It is important for the CCTP to communicate with the receiving facility as soon as possible when caring for a neonate. Important information includes relevant prenatal and birth history, vital signs, physical exam findings, resuscitation details, diagnostic studies done such as lab tests and radiographic results, relevant social issues, anticipated needs on arrival (eg, a ventilator), and estimated time of arrival.

Care of the neonate also includes emotional support of and communication with the neonate's parents. Encourage maternal bonding. Explain to the parents what is happening to their infant and which steps are being taken to optimize the infant's outcome. Do not provide false hope, and avoid discussing the neonate's chances of survival.

Neonatal Resuscitation

The neonate must be assessed using a systematic approach, as follows:

1. Begin with a rapid visual assessment of the newborn's overall appearance (muscle tone, cry), work of breathing (nasal flaring, reduced or absent respiratory effort), and abnormal breath sounds (grunting, stridor). Evaluation of circulation includes assessing for abnormal skin color (pallor, cyanosis, mottling) or bleeding. Determine whether the infant's clinical condition is life threatening. This evaluation can generally be completed within the first few seconds of the patient encounter.
2. Perform a rapid assessment to evaluate cardiopulmonary and neurologic function. This review includes measurement of vital signs and pulse oximetry.
3. Obtain a focused medical history and perform a thorough head-to-toe physical exam. Categorize the neonate's clinical condition by type and severity: respiratory, to include upper/lower airway obstruction, lung disease, or disorder of control of breathing; and cardiovascular, to include hypovolemia or cardiogenic shock.

The following is a modification of the neonatal resuscitation program and the pediatric advanced life support (PALS) protocol as applicable to newborns and neonates.

Primary Assessment: Airway, Breathing, and Circulation

The ABCs of neonatal resuscitation are as follows (after drying a wet newborn):

- **Airway.** Position and clear the airway.
- **Breathing.** Stimulate the infant to breathe and support breathing if insufficient.
- **Circulation.** Assess pulse rate and color; intervene as indicated.

The most important and effective actions in neonatal resuscitation are expanding the lungs and initiating ventilation, providing supplemental oxygen if indicated based on the CCTP's examination, and measuring pulse oximetry. In addition, it is essential to maintain normal body temperature in the neonate. The initial evaluation of the neonate begins with the evaluation of breathing, color, and pulse rate (counted for 6 seconds at the base of the cord or by auscultation and multiplied by 10).

It is essential to assess the neonate's airway for patency. In an infant who is cyanotic, ensure patency of the airway by positioning the head in the sniffing position; performing bulb suctioning of the mouth, followed by the nose if secretions are noted; and gently stimulating the infant. Tactile stimulation should be limited to drying an infant and rubbing the back and soles of the feet gently to avoid traumatic injury. It is important not to be too rough with the rubbing and to avoid slapping the infant, because these actions may lead to traumatic injury.

Look for movement of the chest and abdomen. Listen for breath sounds, and feel the movement of air at the nose and mouth. Upper airway obstruction presents as increased inspiratory effort with retractions, snoring or high-pitched stridor, and periods of absent breath sounds. Attempt to open and maintain the airway by use of the head tilt–chin lift or jaw-thrust maneuver. Suction the nose and pharynx. Intubation may be required if these measures do not work.

A respiratory rate of greater than 60 breaths/min is abnormal at any age in a child. A decreasing or irregular respiratory rate may suggest worsening of the clinical condition, especially if associated with a deterioration in the level of consciousness. A decreased respiratory rate or an irregular respiratory rate in an acutely ill child is an ominous clinical sign because it often signals impending cardiopulmonary arrest.

Alteration in neurologic function in infants may be caused by conditions other than cerebral hypoxia. Some drugs and metabolic conditions, such as rising ammonia from an inborn error of metabolism or increased intracranial pressure, may cause neurologic signs. Careful evaluation of pallor, mottling, and cyanosis may identify inadequate oxygen delivery to the tissues. Acrocyanosis (blue discoloration of hands and feet) is often seen in healthy

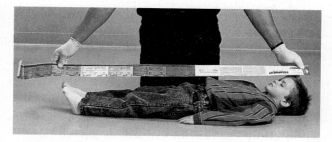

FIGURE 23-3 Use of a length-based resuscitation tape is one method to estimate a child's weight and identify the correct size for pediatric equipment and appropriate medication doses. While a child is pictured here, the tape can also be used for an infant.

© Jones & Bartlett Learning.

newborns; unlike central cyanosis, it is not associated with hypoxia.

In an emergency situation where it may not be possible to weigh the infant or child, CCTPs should be familiar with the use of a length-based/color-coded resuscitation tape (eg, the Broselow tape) to estimate body weight based on the child's crown-to-heel length **FIGURE 23-3**. Use of this tape is helpful because most neonatal and pediatric (up to 88 pounds [40 kg]) drug doses are based on body weight. Such a tape can also help the CCTP determine the appropriate size of resuscitation supplies for the patient. The sizes for pediatric supplies are organized and listed according to the length-based/color-coded classification scheme.

Airway and Breathing Management

Free-Flow Oxygen

Providing free-flow oxygen to a cyanotic newborn with inadequate respiratory effort is of little or no value and merely delays appropriate treatment. For the older neonate, however, free-flow oxygen may be used. If oxygen needs to be provided, it should be warmed and humidified if it needs to be provided for more than a few minutes.

If PPV is not indicated (ie, if the neonate has a pulse rate greater than 100 beats/min and adequate respiratory effort), oxygen can initially be delivered through an oxygen mask held close to the infant's face. Alternatively, if a flow-inflating bag is set up, the CCTP can deliver oxygen by holding the mask close to the infant's face. If a self-inflating bag is connected to an oxygen source, the CCTP can hold the oxygen reservoir close to the infant's face to provide oxygen, or the CCTP can disconnect the oxygen tubing from the self-inflating bag and hold the tubing within a hand cupped loosely over the mouth and nose to facilitate delivery of supplemental oxygen. Holding the mask over the neonate's face without squeezing the bag does not deliver oxygen from a self-inflating bag. The oxygen flow rate should be less than or equal to 5 L/min to minimize hypothermia.

Remember that a level of 5 g/dL of deoxygenated hemoglobin must be reached before clinical cyanosis is observed. A severely anemic hypoxic neonate will be pale, but not cyanotic.

Continuous Positive Airway Pressure

CPAP is the first-line option for ensuring adequate ventilation of a newborn. If the newborn is cyanotic or pale, provide supplemental oxygen using positive end-expiratory pressure (PEEP) of 4 to 6 cm H_2O using the T-piece or the flow-inflating bag. Ideally, resuscitation should be initiated with room air. Use an oxygen saturation monitor (pulse oximeter) to adjust the amount of oxygen to the target range appropriate for the patient's condition.

Studies have demonstrated that even short exposure to supplemental oxygen may be associated with adverse oxidant stress in the neonate, both directly to the lungs and indirectly to the premature neonate's eyes. Thus, CCTPs should avoid unnecessary administration of supplemental oxygen to premature infants because this practice can lead to blindness and exacerbate lung disease.

During resuscitation of the newborn, follow the chart included in the latest Neonatal Resuscitation Program guidelines to titrate oxygen to targeted preductal (right-hand) saturations **TABLE 23-7**. After the immediate newborn period, a premature infant's oxygen saturation should be maintained at 88% to 92%, and a term infant's oxygen saturation should be maintained at 95% to 98% saturation.

Oral Airways

Oral airways are rarely used in neonates, but can be lifesaving if airway obstruction leads to respiratory failure. Bilateral choanal atresia (a bony or membranous obstruction at the back of the nose that prevents airflow) can be rapidly fatal but usually improves with placement of an oral airway (or

TABLE 23-7 Target Preductal Spo$_2$ After Birth

1 min	60%–65%
2 min	65%–70%
3 min	70%–75%
4 min	75%–80%
5 min	80%–85%
10 min	85%–95%

Data from American Academy of Pediatrics, American Heart Association. *Textbook of Neonatal Resuscitation*. 8th ed. Dallas, TX: American Heart Association; 2021.

a gloved finger until an adequate-size oral airway is located). Pierre Robin syndrome comprises a series of developmental anomalies, including a small chin and posteriorly positioned tongue that frequently leads to airway obstruction. Positioning the patient prone (chest down) may relieve this obstruction. If not, an oral airway should be placed.

Positive-Pressure Ventilation Using T-Piece or Bag-Mask Ventilation

Signs of respiratory distress that suggest a possible need for PPV include gasping or periodic breathing, apnea, inadequate respiratory effort, intercostal retractions (sucking in between the ribs), nasal flaring, and grunting on expiration, or persistent pulse rate of less than 100 beats/min (which constitutes bradycardia in newborns) after clearing the airway, maintaining appropriate head position, relieving any obstructions, and providing stimulation. Respiratory distress occurs in approximately 8 in every 1,000 live births and accounts for nearly 15% of neonatal deaths. PPV is also required when the neonate exhibits persistent central cyanosis despite breathing 100% oxygen.

Adequate PPV with oxygen requires the use of appropriate-size equipment with techniques modified for the unique needs of the neonate. The face mask needs to provide an airtight seal, fitting over the infant's mouth and nose, and extending down to the chin but not over the eyes **FIGURE 23-4**. The infant needs to have a patent airway, cleared of secretions, with the neck slightly extended in the sniffing position **FIGURE 23-5**. The first few breaths of a neonate after birth frequently require higher pressures (sometimes as high as 30 cm H_2O, or even

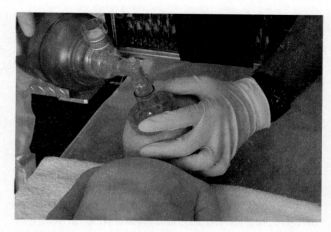

FIGURE 23-4 Bag-mask ventilation of the newborn. Hold the mask securely to the face with your thumb and index finger. Apply countertraction under the bony part of the chin with your middle finger.

Courtesy of Marianne Gausche-Hill, MD, FACEP, FAAP.

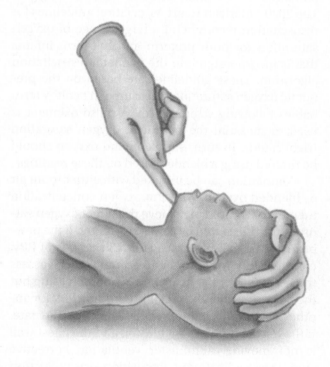

FIGURE 23-5 The sniffing position.

© Jones & Bartlett Learning.

higher for very brief periods of time) because the lungs are not yet expanded and are still filled with fluid. To deliver these initial breaths, the CCTP may need to disable the pop-off valve (usually set by the manufacturer at 30 to 40 cm H_2O) on the bag. Subsequent breaths should be delivered with sufficient pressure to result in visible but not excessive chest

rise. Assuming the newborn has normal lungs, the neonate should appear to be taking an easy breath, with a pressure of about 15 to 20 cm H_2O.

Three devices may be used to deliver PPV to a neonate. The first device is a self-inflating bag with an oxygen reservoir **FIGURE 23-6A**. With this method, an oxygen source is not necessary to provide PPV but is needed to provide supplemental oxygen. The second device is a flow-inflating bag, which requires a gas source to provide PPV **FIGURE 23-6B**. The third device is a T-piece resuscitator, which also requires a pressure source of air/oxygen; this device minimizes the risk of excessive pressures, pneumothorax, and lung injury in the neonate **FIGURE 23-6C**. The T-piece resuscitator, if available, is preferred for providing PPV to a newborn, especially if the newborn is preterm. Regardless of which piece of equipment is used, adequate pressure to achieve visible chest movement is necessary to ensure adequate ventilation. Excessive chest movement increases the risk of pneumothorax and lung injury, so it should be avoided.

CCTPs should ensure that they are familiar with the available equipment in advance and that this equipment is in working order. CCTPs will most likely use a self-inflating bag for ventilation of neonates. When providing ventilator assistance, it is important to use the infant size (240 mL) bag if available. Since the tidal volume of a neonate is only 5 to 7 mL/kg, only one-tenth the volume of a 240-mL bag is used for each breath. If a neonatal bag is not available and the infant has severe respiratory distress, apnea, or bradycardia, a bag designed for adults or older children (750 mL or greater volume) may be used if the delivered breath size is kept appropriately small. In this situation, it is even more critical to monitor chest rise to avoid an excessive volume of delivered breaths. **FIGURE 23-7** shows the algorithm for treating a distressed newborn.

The most common reasons for ineffective bag-mask ventilation are inadequate mask seal and incorrect head position. Other causes, such as mucus plugging, pneumothorax, equipment malfunction, or insufficient pressure, need to be considered as well.

The correct timing for delivering breaths in a neonate is 40 to 60 breaths/min. It is easy to deliver breaths at a much higher rate, which can increase risks such as hypocapnia, air trapping, and pneumothorax. Counting "breathe–two–three–breathe–two–three"

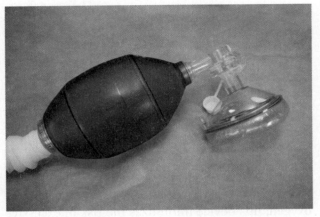

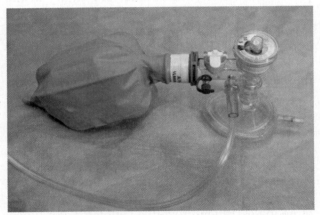

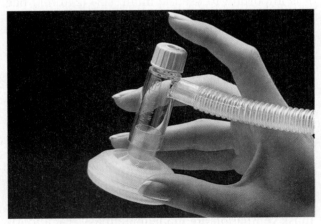

FIGURE 23-6 Three devices can be used to deliver bag-mask ventilation to a neonate. **A.** A self-inflating bag. **B.** A flow-inflating bag. **C.** A T-piece resuscitator.

A & B: © Jones & Bartlett Learning; C: Courtesy of Fisher & Paykel Healthcare, Inc.

as you ventilate (give a breath on "breathe" and release while you say "two–three") can help with timing. PPV should continue as long as the infant's pulse rate remains less than 100 beats/min or the

respiratory effort is ineffective. If prolonged PPV is needed, using a pressure manometer is important to help monitor the pressures delivered and minimize excessive pressures (usually less than 25 cm H_2O pressure in term infants, but even lower pressure in preterm infants).

Supplemental Oxygen

Initiating neonatal resuscitation with 100% oxygen is no longer recommended. As noted earlier, resuscitation (PPV) of newborns born at 35 weeks' gestation or later begins with 21% oxygen. In contrast, PPV of newborns delivered prior to 35 weeks' gestation may begin with 21% to 30% oxygen. A recent meta-analysis suggests that resuscitation initiated with room air may result in increased survival as compared with resuscitation initiated with 100% oxygen. The 2020 American Heart Association guidelines for resuscitation recommend a target range of oxygen saturation for both preterm and full-term infants that is incorporated into the neonatal resuscitation algorithm. These guidelines are based on the preductal oxygen saturations measured in healthy term babies following vaginal birth. A pulse oximeter is used to measure the preductal oxygen saturation (right hand). In turn, supplemental oxygen should be titrated using a blender based on these readings.

Ventilation can be initiated with either room air or blended oxygen, with the oxygen concentration then being titrated to achieve the target oxygen saturation as measured by a pulse oximeter. If the newborn's heart rate increases after 15 seconds of PPV, continue PPV for another 15 seconds and reassess the heart rate. If the heart rate is not increasing but the newborn's chest is moving, continue PPV for another 15 seconds before reassessing the heart rate. If the heart rate is not increasing and the chest wall is not moving, administer ventilation corrective steps (Mask adjustment, Reposition airway, Suction mouth and nose, Open mouth, Pressure increase, Airway alternative [MR SOPA]) until the newborn's chest moves with ventilation. Reassess the heart rate after 30 seconds to evaluate its stability. If the heart rate remains less than 60 beats/min despite ventilation corrective steps, consider using an alternative airway, such as an endotracheal (ET) tube or laryngeal mask airway. The laryngeal mask airway is available in one size for newborns and can be used for those weighing more than 1,500 grams. For newborns weighing less than 1,500 grams, intubation

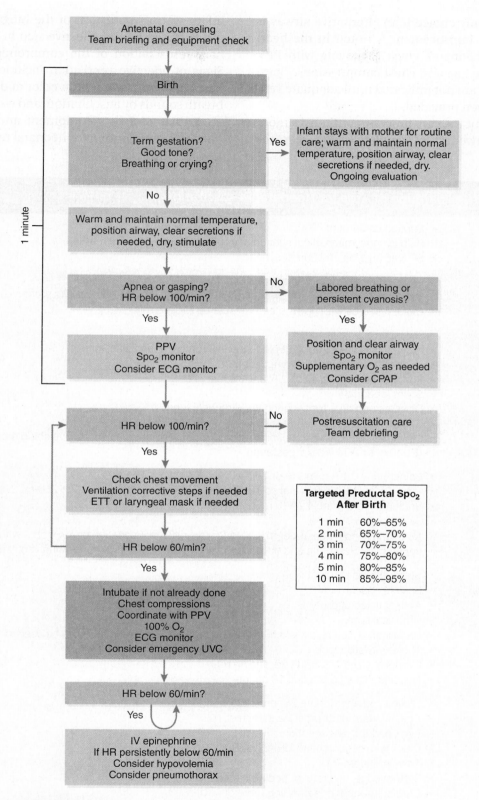

FIGURE 23-7 Resuscitation algorithm for the distressed neonate.
Abbreviations: CPAP, continuous positive airway pressure; ECG, electrocardiography; ETT, endotracheal tube; HR, heart rate; O₂, oxygen; PPV, positive-pressure ventilation; Spo₂, oxygen saturation; UVC, umbilical venous catheter

remains the only choice if an alternative airway is needed. If no improvement is noted in the heart rate but the neonate's chest is moving with PPV, begin 100% oxygen and chest compressions. Chest compressions are not indicated until adequate ventilation has been provided.

Throughout the care process, continue to monitor the effectiveness of ventilation and keep the infant warm. Ventilation of the lungs is the single most important and effective step in cardiopulmonary resuscitation of the compromised newborn. Signs of effective ventilation include rapid rise in heart rate, improvement in color and tone, audible breath sounds by auscultation, and visible chest rise.

TABLE 23-8 lists equipment and medications needed in preparation for neonatal resuscitation.

TABLE 23-8 Preparation of Area for Neonatal Resuscitation	
Resuscitation equipment and supplies	• Suction equipment • Bulb syringe, mechanical suction and tubing, 5F or 6F suction catheters • 8F feeding tube and 20-mL syringe
Bag-mask/ T-piece resuscitator equipment	• Device for delivering PPV, capable of delivering 90% to 100% oxygen • Face masks, neonatal and premature infant size (cushioned-rim masks preferred) • Oxygen source with flowmeter (flow rate up to 10 L/min)
Intubation equipment	• Laryngoscope with straight blades, size 0 (preterm) and size 1 (term) • Extra bulb, batteries for laryngoscope • Endotracheal tubes, sizes 2.5, 3.0, 3.5, and 4.0 • Stylet (optional) • Scissors and tape for securing endotracheal tube • CO_2 detectors (optional) • Laryngeal mask airway (optional): effective for ventilating newborns weighing more than 4 lb (2,000 g) or ≥34 weeks' gestation
Medications	• Epinephrine 0.1 mg/mL, 3- or 10-mL ampules • Isotonic crystalloid (normal saline or lactated Ringer solution), 100- or 250-mL bag • Sodium bicarbonate 4.2% (5 mEq/10 mL) • Dextrose 10%, 250 mL • Naloxone is no longer recommended for the initial resuscitation of newborns with respiratory depression. Heart rate and oxygenation should be restored by supporting ventilation.
Umbilical catheterization equipment	• Sterile gloves • Scalpel or scissors • Antiseptic solution • Umbilical tape • Umbilical catheters, sizes 3.5F and 5F (a sterile 3.5F feeding tube can be used in an emergency) • Three-way stopcock • Syringes, sizes 1, 3, 5, 10, 20, and 50 mL • Needles, sizes 25, 21, and 18 gauge
Miscellaneous	• Gloves and appropriate BSI protection • Radiant warmer or other heat source • Firm, padded resuscitation surface • Clock with second hand, timer optional • Towels, linens • Stethoscope, neonatal or pediatric preferred • Cardiac monitor or saturation monitor • Oropharyngeal airway (0, 00, and 000 sizes or 30-, 40-, and 50-mm long)

Abbreviations: BSI, body substance isolation; PPV, positive-pressure ventilation

Data from American Academy of Pediatrics. *Textbook of Neonatal Resuscitation.* 8th ed. Dallas, TX: American Heart Association; 2021.

Intubation

Most neonatal resuscitations can be successfully completed with bag-mask ventilation. However, intubation is indicated in the following circumstances:

- Congenital **diaphragmatic hernia** (a congenital defect in which the abdominal organs herniate into the chest cavity through an opening in the diaphragm) is suspected and respiratory support is indicated.
- The infant is not responding to bag-mask ventilation and 100% oxygen. Intubation is strongly recommended prior to beginning chest compressions. If intubation is not successful or feasible, a laryngeal mask may be used.
- Prolonged PPV is needed.

Before beginning to intubate the neonate, ensure that the appropriate equipment is at hand. Use a straight blade of size #1 for a term infant and of size #0 for a preterm infant. Endotracheal tubes for neonates are available in sizes ranging from 2.5 to 4.0 mm **TABLE 23-9**. Again, a length-based/color-coded resuscitation tape or Broselow tape can be used to estimate the appropriate ET tube size. A stylet may be used to provide rigidity to the ET tube. If a stylet is used, it is imperative to secure it in its position (bending it over at the top of the ET tube so it cannot advance) and to not allow it to extend beyond the ET tube to minimize the risk of tracheal perforation.

SKILL DRILL 23-1 shows intubation of the neonate, which is discussed in the following steps:

1. Ensure the neonate is preoxygenated by bag-mask/T-piece ventilation with oxygen as needed to maintain adequate saturation prior to an intubation attempt **STEP 1**.

TABLE 23-9 Neonatal Endotracheal Tube Sizes	
Size	**Recommended Age (weeks)**
2.5	<28
3.0	28–34
3.5	34–38
4.0	>38

© Jones & Bartlett Learning.

2. Suction the oropharynx to ensure removal of secretions if unable to visualize the vocal cords **STEP 2**. This is a vagal stimulus, so pay close attention to the infant's pulse rate; bag-mask ventilation may again be needed prior to the intubation attempt if bradycardia occurs.
3. Place the laryngoscope blade in the oropharynx and then visualize the vocal cords, keeping in mind that the vocal cords are more cephalad and anterior in neonates relative to adults **STEP 3**. Take care to avoid applying torque to the blade, which increases the risk of trauma. Place the ET tube between the vocal cords until the black line on the tube is at the level of the cords. A general rule of thumb is that the insertion depth for the ET tube is the nasal-tragus length. The following formula may also be used to calculate the initial tip-to-lip depth for the tube:

$$\text{Weight (in kg)} + 6$$

Insert the laryngeal mask airway until resistance is felt.

In an extremely low-birth-weight baby (less than 2 pounds [1,000 g]), the ET tube may need be advanced to only 6.5 to 7 cm at the lip, compared to 9 to 10 cm for a full-term newborn. Intubation attempts should be limited to 30 seconds, followed by bag-mask ventilation if unsuccessful or if significant bradycardia develops.
4. Confirm placement by observing chest rise when applying positive pressure through the ET tube, auscultating laterally and high on the chest, confirming the absence of significant air sounds over the stomach, noting mist in the ET tube (mist will be seen when the patient exhales through the tube from condensation of humidified air leaving the lungs), and observing clinical improvement of the patient **STEP 4**. A CO_2 detector should be used if available.
5. Tape the ET/laryngeal mask airway tube in place on the patient's face to minimize the risk of the tube becoming dislodged **STEP 5**. Monitor the infant closely for complications such as tube dislodgement, tube occlusion by mucus plugging, or pneumothorax.

Complications of ET tube placement may include oropharyngeal or tracheal perforation, esophageal intubation with subsequent persistent hypoxia, and right main stem intubation that can

Skill Drill 23-1 Intubation of a Neonate

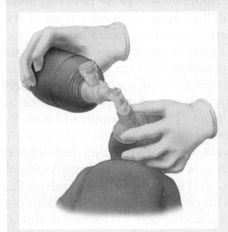

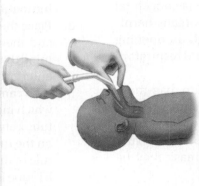

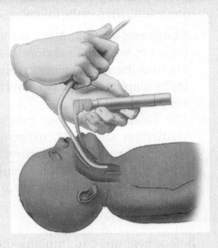

Step 1

Preoxygenate the infant by bag-mask ventilation with 100% supplemental oxygen.

Step 2

Suction the oropharynx. Provide bag-mask ventilation if bradycardia results.

Step 3

Place the laryngoscope blade in the oropharynx. Visualize the vocal cords. Place the ET tube between the vocal cords until the black line on the tube is at the level of the cords.

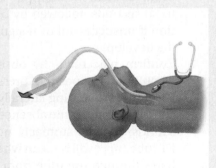

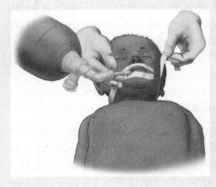

Step 4

Confirm placement. Observe chest rise, auscultate laterally and high on the chest, note the absence of significant air sounds over the stomach, note mist in the ET tube, and use a CO_2 detector.

Step 5

Tape the ET tube in place. Monitor the neonate closely for complications.

lead to atelectasis, persistent hypoxia, and pneumothorax. These risks can be minimized by ensuring optimal placement of the laryngoscope blade and by carefully noting how far the ET tube is being advanced.

Premedication is often not needed when intubating depressed neonates. Consider giving atropine to help avoid vagal-induced bradycardia. Administer sedation if agitation is present. Avoid paralytics since neonatal airways are very small and may be difficult to maintain once the neonate is paralyzed.

Gastric Decompression

Gastric decompression using an orogastric tube is indicated for infants receiving prolonged bag-mask ventilation (more than 5 to 10 minutes) to counteract abdominal distention that is impeding ventilation, or in the presence of a known or suspected diaphragmatic hernia. Many diaphragmatic hernias are diagnosed prenatally by using routine ultrasonography. They are suspected clinically if the following signs are noted: decreased breath sounds (90% of diaphragmatic hernias are left-side), a scaphoid (concave) abdomen due to the presence of abdominal contents in the chest, and increased work of breathing.

SKILL DRILL 23-2 shows neonatal orogastric tube placement, which is discussed in the following steps:

1. To determine the length of tube to insert, use an 8F feeding tube and measure the length from the bottom of the ear lobe to the tip of the nose to halfway between the xiphoid process (lower tip of the sternum) and the umbilicus **STEP 1**.
2. Insert the tube through the mouth to the appropriate depth **STEP 2**.

Skill Drill 23-2 Inserting an Orogastric Tube in the Neonate

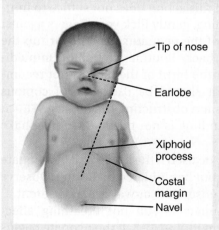

Tip of nose
Earlobe
Xiphoid process
Costal margin
Navel

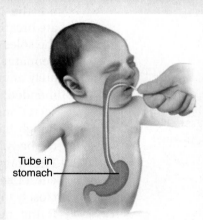

Tube in stomach

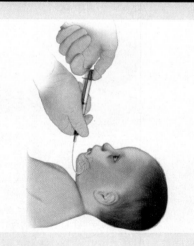

Step 1
Measure for correct depth—from the bottom of the ear lobe to the tip of the nose to halfway between the xiphoid process (lower tip of the sternum) and the umbilicus.

Step 2
Insert the tube to the appropriate depth.

Step 3
Remove the gastric contents with a 20-mL syringe. Tape the tube to the neonate's cheek. Remove the syringe from the feeding tube to allow air to vent from the stomach.

3. Attach a 20-gauge syringe and suction the stomach contents **STEP 3**. Tape the tube to the neonate's cheek. Remove the syringe from the feeding tube to allow venting of air from the stomach, and intermittently suction the feeding tube.

Circulation

Chest compressions are indicated if the neonate's heart rate remains less than 60 beats/min despite management efforts related to positioning, clearing the airway, drying and stimulation, and 30 seconds of effective PPV. Two techniques can be used to perform chest compressions: the two-thumbs, encircling-hands technique and the two-finger technique. In the two-thumbs, encircling-hands technique (the recommended technique), two thumbs are placed side by side over the sternum between the nipples, and the hands encircle the torso **FIGURE 23-8A**. The chest should be compressed one-third the anterior-posterior diameter of the chest. In the two-finger technique, the tips

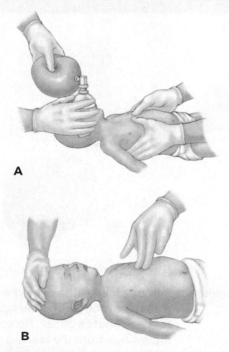

FIGURE 23-8 Chest compressions in the neonate. **A.** The two-thumbs, encircling-hands technique; this is the recommended method. **B.** The two-finger technique; use this method only if unable to use the two-thumbs, encircling-hands technique.

© Jones & Bartlett Learning.

of two fingers are placed over the sternum between the nipples, and the sternum is compressed one-third the anterior-posterior diameter of the chest **FIGURE 23-8B**. This method is used only if the provider cannot access the newborn in such a way as to perform the two-thumbs, encircling-hands technique. The two-thumbs, encircling-hands technique is preferred because it may generate higher peak systolic and coronary perfusion pressure than the two-finger technique. This technique may be performed from the head of the bed once the airway has been secured when access to the umbilicus is required during insertion of an umbilical catheter. If the infant is intubated, the two-thumbs, encircling-hands technique can be used by the CCTP who is standing at the infant's head.

SKILL DRILL 23-3 reviews the steps for resuscitating a neonate, which are listed here:

1. Lay the neonate flat (Trendelenburg position can cause intracranial hemorrhage, especially in preterm infants) **STEP 1**. Ensure that the airway is open (head in sniffing position). Add a shoulder roll to obtain the optimal position.
2. Dry the infant to stimulate the infant to breathe. If this action does not suffice to initiate breathing, gently flick your fingers against the soles of the neonate's feet and/or rub the neonate's back. Routine suctioning immediately after the birth of the baby is not recommended; it should be used only if copious secretions are obstructing the airway **STEP 2**. Rough handling is not needed. Do not shake the baby.
3. PEEP may be used if the infant had inadequate chest rise but has initiated breathing. Observe closely to ensure the airway remains patent.
4. If the neonate is still not breathing effectively, begin PPV **STEP 3**. If the neonate begins breathing on their own, support and assist respirations and recheck the airway to confirm it remains clear.
5. If the neonate is still not breathing, continue the PPV and check for an umbilical, femoral, or brachial pulse **STEP 4**. It is important to intermittently auscultate the pulse using a stethoscope.
6. If you cannot feel a pulse or if the heart rate is less than 60 beats/min, begin closed-chest cardiac compressions **STEP 5**.

Skill Drill 23-3 Resuscitating a Neonate

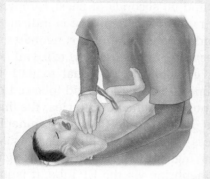

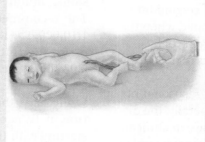

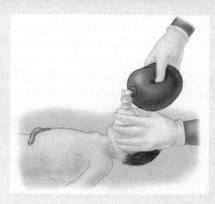

Step 1

Lay the neonate flat. Suction the mouth and nose with a bulb syringe.

Step 2

If drying and suctioning do not successfully induce breathing, gently flick your fingers against the soles of the neonate's feet.

Step 3

Begin bag-mask ventilation if the neonate is not breathing effectively.

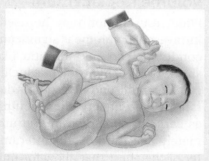

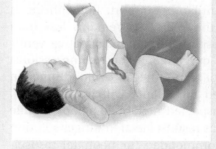

Step 4

If the neonate is still not breathing, continue bag-mask ventilation and check for an umbilical, femoral, or brachial pulse. The brachial location is shown here.

Step 5

If you cannot feel a pulse or if the heart rate is less than 60 beats/min, begin chest compressions.

© Jones & Bartlett Learning.

The depth of compression is one-third of the anterior-posterior diameter of the chest. The CCTP's fingers should remain in contact with the patient's chest at all times to minimize risk of trauma. Time the compressions in synchrony with artificial ventilation, which continues during chest compressions. (In neonates, even if respirations are being supported by PPV, the ventilation is still timed with the chest compressions.) The CCTP delivering the chest compression counts aloud, "One and two and three and breathe and. . . ." Downward strokes of chest compressions should be delivered each time a number (*one*, *two*, or *three*) is spoken. Release of the strokes should occur on the "and" that follows "three." The CCTP ventilating delivers a breath during "breathe and." This sequence results in 90 compressions and 30 breaths/min. Note that this rate applies to one-rescuer infant CPR; it is best to use two rescuers when a faster compression rate is needed. Heart rate is assessed at 30-second intervals, and chest compressions are stopped when the heart rate is greater than 60 beats/min. Liver laceration and rib fractures are possible risks of delivering chest compressions.

If the neonate is not responding to resuscitation, other causes must be considered. Generally, the difficulties relate to the following issues: technical/mechanical/equipment problems, unrecognized pulmonary complications, severe metabolic derangements, congenital abnormalities of organ systems, or severe anemia.

Pharmacologic Interventions

Medications are rarely needed in neonatal resuscitation because most infants can be resuscitated with effective ventilatory support. Epinephrine is indicated when the heart rate remains less than 60 beats/min despite intubation, effective ventilation with 100% oxygen, and chest compressions. Normal saline bolus or O-negative blood infusion may be indicated for infants with hypovolemia, blood loss, or suspected metabolic acidosis while awaiting blood gas results; lactated Ringer solution is no longer recommended for neonatal resuscitation. All fluids and medications can be infused through the umbilical venous line or into an intraosseous needle in both term and preterm newborns.

Sodium bicarbonate is no longer recommended in the initial resuscitation, though it may be used with caution when the degree of metabolic acidosis is known from a blood gas analysis. Similarly, naloxone and vasopressors are no longer recommended for the initial resuscitation, but may be useful after resuscitation.

Doses of medications in neonates are based on weight, so the CCTP may need to estimate the infant's weight for dosing purposes. A term infant usually weighs approximately 6.5 to 8.5 pounds (3 to 4 kg). An infant born at 28 weeks' gestation weighs an average of 2.2 pounds (1 kg), and an infant born at 34 weeks' gestation weighs an average of 4.5 pounds (2 kg). Medications that may be used in this patient population are listed in **TABLE 23-10**.

Epinephrine

If the infant has a pulse rate of less than 60 beats/min after 30 seconds of effective ventilation after intubation and 60 seconds of chest compressions, administration of epinephrine is indicated. The recommended concentration for neonates is 1:10,000. The recommended dose is 0.1 to 0.3 mL/kg of 0.1 mg/mL epinephrine IV, equal to 0.01 to 0.03 mg/kg, administered rapidly, and followed by a 0.5- to 1-mL normal saline flush to clear the line. While IV is the optimal route to deliver epinephrine, if IV access is not yet established, consider starting with the higher dose of 0.3 to 1.0 mL/kg of 0.1 mg/mL epinephrine via the ET tube. It is important to recheck the infant's heart rate 1 minute after administering the dose (and for longer if this medication is given endotracheally). Epinephrine dosing may be repeated every 3 to 5 minutes for persistent bradycardia.

Volume Replacement

Fluid resuscitation may be needed if the infant's intravascular volume is significantly depleted from conditions such as abruptio placentae or septic shock. Signs of hypovolemia include pallor, delayed capillary refill, and weak pulses despite a good heart rate or high-quality chest compressions—defined as compressions delivered at a depth of approximately one-third of the anterior-posterior diameter of the chest that allow for full chest recoil, at a rate of 90 compressions per minute with minimal interruptions. In the neonate, the specific depth is important because the size of the child will vary. Compressing too little leads to ineffective compressions; compressing too deeply leads to trauma.

In a newborn, a low umbilical venous catheter can be placed in the large vein in the umbilical cord by advancing the catheter just far enough to allow blood return, but not far enough to enter the liver. In an infant older than a few days, a peripheral IV or intraosseous (IO) line will need to be placed. Note that while the technique for placing an IO line in a neonate is similar to that used in older children or adults, a smaller needle should be used to avoid exiting the far side of the bone.

A fluid bolus in an infant consists of 10 to 20 mL/kg of normal saline IV over 5 to 10 minutes. More than one bolus may be needed if the patient is still clinically hypovolemic.

TABLE 23-10 Medications for Neonates

Drug Name	Dose/Route	Concentration	Indications/Comments	Side Effects
Ampicillin	50 mg/kg IV over 5–10 min		• First-line antibiotic for sepsis workup • Use with gentamicin • Use 100 mg/kg if meningitis suspected	None
Atropine	0.01–0.03 mg/kg IV/IM; may repeat every 5 min × 3 orally; 2–3 × IV dose; minimum dose of 0.1 mg in infants >5 kg		• Preintubation medication to minimize vagal-induced bradycardia • Standard dose of 0.02 mg/kg used PALS	Tachycardia, arrhythmia, fever, rash, urinary retention
Cefotaxime	50 mg/kg IV every 6–12 h depending on weight/age		• Broad-spectrum antibiotic used for suspected/documented gram-negative sepsis	Potential increased risk of fungal infection due to broad spectrum of coverage
Ceftriaxone	50 mg/kg per dose IV/IM every 24 h		• Can be used to complete antibiotic course at home • Do not use in a newborn or a neonate with total bilirubin >5 mg/dL because it displaces bilirubin from albumin and can lead to kernicterus	Cases of fatal reactions with calcium-ceftriaxone precipitates in lungs and kidneys in both term and premature neonates have been described
Dextrose	2 mL/kg IV bolus over 5–10 min		• Symptomatic hypoglycemia (blood glucose level <40 mg/dL) • May use for hydration • May repeat bolus or follow with 5 mg/kg per min • Incompatible with blood products	None
Dobutamine	3–5 μg/kg per min IV; increase 3–10 μg/kg per min to max 40 μg/kg/min		• Cardiogenic shock, hypotension, increased myocardial contractility, cardiac failure • Try volume resuscitation first • Incompatible with sodium bicarbonate	Hypoxemia, tachycardia, arrhythmia
Dopamine	5 μg/kg per min IV; increase 2–3 μg/kg per min to max 40 μg/kg/min for effect		• Nonhypovolemic shock, increased cardiac output • Try volume resuscitation first	Hypoxemia, tachycardia, arrhythmia

(Continues)

TABLE 23-10 Medications for Neonates (continued)

Drug Name	Dose/Route	Concentration	Indications/Comments	Side Effects
Epinephrine	0.01–0.03 mg/kg or 0.1–0.3 mL/kg ET or IV every 3–5 min; may titrate IV dose up to max 1 μg/kg/min for effect	Reconstitute with sterile water	• Resuscitation medication for asystole and bradycardia • Bronchodilator • Standard dose used in PALS and recommended by AAP is 0.01 mg/kg IV	Arrhythmia, hypertension, IVH, renal failure, hypokalemia
Gentamicin	4 mg/kg IV/IM (IV preferred) over 30 min OR By gestational age: >35 weeks, 4 mg/kg 30–34 weeks, 4.5 mg/kg <29 weeks, 5 mg/kg	Reconstitute with sterile water • In D_5W, $D_{10}W$, NS: infuse over 30 min • In D_5W, $D_{10}W$, NS: IV infusion given over 30–60 min • In $D_{25}W$: dilute to <12.5% to give via peripheral IV 12.5 μg/mL; reconstitute in D_5W/$D_{10}W$/NS, 40 μg/mL; reconstitute in D_5W/$D_{10}W$/NS, 0.1 mg/mL; dilute 1:1 for ET administration • Compatible with TPN, NS, D_5W, $D_{10}W$	• Part of sepsis workup • Obtain cultures before administering • Do not give with cephalosporin	None
Inhaled nitric oxide	20 ppm starting dose		• Selective decrease in pulmonary vascular resistance • Used for PPHN levels • Started with oxygenation index >25 • Needs specific delivery device	Methemoglobinemia: need daily methemoglobin levels
Morphine sulfate	0.05–0.1 mg/kg IM/IV over 15–20 min (may push over 4–5 min if needed), then every 4 h or 10–15 μg/kg/h infusion	Compatible with D_5W, $D_{10}W$, NS	• Analgesia and sedation • Do not discontinue suddenly • Do not use in shock and increased intracranial pressure • Use naloxone as antidote for respiratory depression	Respiratory depression, hypotension, bradycardia

Drug	Dose	Compatibility	Indications	Side effects
Naloxone hydrochloride	0.1 mg/kg IV push/IM; may repeat in 3–5 min 1.0 mg/mL or 0.4 mg/mL	Compatible with D_5W and NS	• Narcotic-induced respiratory depression • Avoid in newborns exposed to maternal narcotic use (may induce withdrawal seizures)	Hypertension, arrhythmia, pulmonary edema, vomiting
Normal saline–volume expander	10 mL/kg IV; may repeat × 1 if needed	Alternatives include whole blood or lactated Ringer solution, 10 mL/kg	• First line for volume resuscitation, shock, hypotension, hemorrhage	None
Phenobarbital	10–20 mg/kg IV, infuse over 10–15 min; may repeat for continued seizures	Compatible with D_5W, $D_{10}W$, NS	• Anticonvulsant • First line for seizures	Hypotension, respiratory depression, Stevens-Johnson syndrome
Prostaglandin E1	0.05 µg/kg/min infusion; may titrate down when patient is stable, with good effect	• Compatible with D_5W, NS; 1 ampule (500 µg) + 500 mL IV fluids = 1 µg/mL PGE solution • Not compatible with other solutions or medications	• Keeps ductus arteriosus patent • Recommend intubating patient for long transports and obtain second IV access prior to infusion	Apnea, hyperthermia, hypotension, bradycardia, hypoglycemia, seizures, hypocalcemia
Sodium bicarbonate	2 mEq/kg IV push over 2 min for resuscitation; repeat as needed	• 0.5 mEq/mL (4.2% solution); also available in 1 mEq/mL • Compatible with D_5W, $D_{10}W$, NS	• Resuscitation • Metabolic acidosis • Dose in mEq = base deficit on blood gas × 0.3 × weight in kg, over 15 min • When the patient has a high serum sodium level, tromethamine (Tham) may be used at a comparable dose to treat metabolic acidosis	Rapid infusion may cause IVH

Abbreviations: AAP, American Academy of Pediatrics; D_5W, 5% dextrose in water; $D_{10}W$, 10% dextrose in water; ET, endotracheal; IM, intramuscularly; $D_{25}W$, 25% dextrose in water; IVH, intraventricular hemorrhage; MI, myocardial infarction; NS, normal saline; PALS, pediatric advanced life support; PGE, prostaglandin E; PPHN, persistent pulmonary hypertension

Ventilation During Transport

Neonatal transport incubators are typically fitted with a ventilator that provides synchronized intermittent mandatory ventilation. Settings are adjusted relative to the patient's condition. Peak inspiratory pressure is adjusted to provide a comfortable breath (typically 14 to 20 mm Hg; the lower range is appropriate for more premature infants, while the higher range is appropriate for term infants with decreased lung compliance (like that seen in pneumonia). The peak end-expiratory pressure is typically 3 to 4 mm Hg, the rate is 20 to 60 breaths/min, and the inspiratory time is 0.3 to 0.4 second. If volume ventilation is used, a tidal volume of 6 to 8 mL/kg is targeted. The ventilator tubing can affect the measured tidal volume on some ventilator circuits, making close observation of chest rise and peak inspiratory pressure critical, especially when first placing a neonate on tidal volume ventilation.

For patients with very severe lung disease, a conventional ventilator may not provide adequate support. High-frequency ventilation, defined as a respiratory frequency of 400 to 800 breaths/min and optimal PEEP (usually higher than that used with conventional ventilation), relies primarily on convection and molecular diffusion of gas rather than tidal volume ventilation to exchange oxygen and carbon dioxide. Some transport incubators may be fitted with a high-frequency ventilator, in which case comparable ventilator settings can be used for transport. Frequently, however, only a conventional ventilator is available for transfer.

When switching a neonate from high-frequency ventilation back to a conventional ventilator, the neonate usually tolerates the fastest rate that the conventional ventilator can deliver; inspiratory pressures need to be kept relatively low and expiratory times long (I:E at least 1:2) to minimize the risk of air trapping. If the neonate is critically ill and the desired oxygen saturation cannot be maintained on a conventional transport ventilator, manually ventilating the child with a T-piece resuscitator or bag-mask device may provide acceptable ventilation and oxygenation until arrival at a tertiary care center.

For term infants with respiratory failure, some centers can initiate inhaled nitric oxide to optimize pulmonary vasodilation or extracorporeal membrane oxygenation to support cardiopulmonary function in the field, and then transport the neonate on inhaled nitric oxide or an extracorporeal membrane oxygenation circuit. It is important to have discussions with the regional referral center in advance to know which technology is available in the area.

Additional Transport Considerations

While PPV and chest compressions can be performed in a moving emergency vehicle, a key consideration is to secure the neonate's airway before beginning the transport. The neonate is best stabilized at the originating center.

Evaluation during air transport is especially difficult because of the vibrations, noise, and poor lighting inherent to aircraft. In this setting, CCTPs must rely on cardiorespiratory equipment to determine the stability of vital signs. Procedures such as intubation or needle aspiration of the chest can be particularly challenging in flight because of the limited space available and the inability to maintain a stable environment for needle aspiration. For all these reasons, the neonate's airway must be secured prior to a helicopter flight.

If additional interventions such as intubation or needle aspiration are needed during ambulance transport, it is recommended that the CCTP consider pulling the ambulance to the side of the road while performing the procedure. During a flight transport, the CCTP needs to rely more on nonauditory assessments (visual, tactile, electronic monitoring) to provide care and perform necessary procedures. If necessary, PPV can be performed during air transport if the ET tube becomes dislodged and cannot be readily replaced.

Respiratory Conditions

Clearing the airway and providing stimulation are sufficient to establish adequate cardiorespiratory function in most neonates. However, a small subset of these patients need assisted ventilation, as discussed earlier. Conditions that can induce respiratory compromise in the neonate include anatomic anomalies leading to obstruction, such as choanal atresia and Pierre Robin syndrome. Both of these conditions respond to placement of an oral airway. The next sections discuss specific respiratory conditions, their causes, and their management.

Apnea

Apnea is defined as a pause in respirations of more than 20 seconds. It is often associated with cyanosis, pallor, hypotonia (low or poor muscle tone), or bradycardia.

There are two types of apnea: primary and secondary apnea. Primary apnea is present at birth; it is the initial response to asphyxia at birth. This condition responds well to stimulation and oxygen supply. If asphyxia continues beyond the primary apnea period, secondary apnea sets in after a few deep gasping breaths. This condition responds only to assisted ventilation and supplemental oxygen. Although these two types of apnea might seem clinically indistinguishable, it is critically important to recognize the difference between them so as to provide appropriate management.

In the neonate, apnea may have many etiologies. Respiratory causes include fixed anatomic obstruction, positional obstruction (head on chin, obstructing the airway), secretions, and reflux with aspiration. Metabolic causes include hypoglycemia, inborn errors of metabolism that cause high ammonia levels, and hypocalcemia. Cardiovascular causes include poor tissue oxygenation from arrhythmia, CHD, shock, anemia/hemorrhage, patent ductus arteriosus, and hypotension. Infectious etiologies include necrotizing enterocolitis, pneumonia, sepsis, respiratory syncytial virus, *Chlamydia*, and pertussis. Neurologic causes include seizures, encephalopathy, intraventricular hemorrhage, congenital hypoventilation, increased intracranial pressure, stroke, and apnea of prematurity. Hypothermia or hyperthermia, trauma, child abuse, and exposure to illicit drugs or prescribed medications need to be considered as well.

Apnea is treated in the field by following a multiple-step approach:

- Stabilization: Assess and manage the ABCs as needed. Apnea is often associated with cyanosis and bradycardia. Administer free-flow oxygen at 2 L/min for cyanosis. If this measure does not improve the neonate's color and respirations, assisted ventilation may be needed. If apnea and bradycardia persist, intubate the neonate prior to transport.
- Assessment: Perform a brief history, physical exam, and lab tests.

- Check the fontanelle for a bulge, which may indicate increased intracranial pressure.
- Check the nose and oropharynx for obstruction.
- During the cardiac exam, listen for murmurs; during pulmonary auscultation, listen for crackles.
- Check capillary refill to assess perfusion.
- Obtain a set of vital signs, including temperature.
- Check the blood glucose level.
- Ensure that a complete blood count (CBC), blood cultures, chest radiograph, a blood gas analysis, and electrolyte levels are obtained, if possible.
- Further management: Keep the neonate warm except if hypoxic ischemic encephalopathy (as defined by strict criteria) is suspected. Administer 2 mL/kg of 10% dextrose as a bolus if the glucose level is less than 40 mg/dL. It may be necessary to start IV fluids for hypoglycemia. Administer antibiotics (eg, ampicillin, gentamicin) if these agents have not been started. (The sepsis workup is often started at the sending facility and antibiotics are chosen by the sending physician.) Naloxone may be indicated after the initial resuscitation and stabilization if the neonate is positive for an acute (not chronic) exposure to narcotics.

Causes of Respiratory Distress in a Neonate

Meconium-Stained Amniotic Fluid

Meconium, the first stool of an infant, is usually expelled after birth. However, it may be expelled in utero in term infants during fetal stress. Postterm infants are at even higher risk for meconium-stained amniotic fluid due to their relatively impaired placental functions. Meconium-stained amniotic fluid is present in 10% to 15% of deliveries.

Meconium aspiration occurs when infants inhale the meconium into their lungs when hypoxia or acidosis causes the infant to take a gasping breath before or during the delivery. If the infant inhales the meconium-stained amniotic fluid either in utero or at delivery, plugging of the airways and hypoxia can follow. The respiratory distress caused by meconium aspiration is termed meconium aspiration syndrome. It can lead to atelectasis in the lungs, persistent pulmonary hypertension (delayed transition from fetal to neonatal circulation), pneumonitis, and pneumothorax. The differential diagnosis for meconium aspiration syndrome includes respiratory distress syndrome, transient tachypnea of the newborn (transient respiratory distress that lasts a few hours and occurs secondary to retained fetal lung fluid), sepsis, pneumonia, and congenital respiratory or cardiac malformation. In infants who have aspirated meconium, patchy/fluffy infiltrates may be seen on the chest radiograph **FIGURE 23-9**.

If meconium is present in the amniotic fluid of a depressed newborn at birth, tracheal intubation and aspiration are no longer recommended because this intervention's efficacy is supported by only minimal evidence. Even when tracheal suctioning is performed, meconium aspiration syndrome may occur. When transporting an infant exposed to meconium-stained amniotic fluid who shows respiratory symptoms after delivery, it is important to monitor for the development of complications from meconium aspiration syndrome, such as worsening lung compliance and pneumothorax, and to intervene as necessary. Consider implementing PPV during transport if progressive hypoxia develops. A pattern of short inspiratory time and long expiratory time is commonly used to provide adequate ventilation and minimize air trapping in the neonate. High PEEP values may also be used.

A needle setup should be available in the event that the infant develops a significant pneumothorax en route to the hospital. If a significant pneumothorax develops, as suggested by acute cyanosis, increased work of breathing, and decreased breath sounds, clean the area just above the patient's nipple on the affected side. Then insert a small (22-gauge) butterfly needle in the second intercostal space, at the midclavicular line, above the rib, while pulling back on a syringe to evacuate the extrapleural air and relieve the intrathoracic pressure. This procedure is discussed further in the section on pneumothorax and illustrated in **FIGURE 23-10**.

Pneumonia

Neonates have an impaired immune response and as a result are at increased risk of developing pneumonia. Signs and symptoms of pneumonia include tachypnea (respiratory rate greater than 60 breaths/min), increased work of breathing, and hypothermia. The initial assessment for suspected pneumonia should include a chest radiograph, blood gas measurements in infants with significant respiratory symptoms, CBC, and blood culture. Management includes antibiotics (eg, ampicillin and gentamicin), maintaining the infant on nothing given by mouth (abbreviated NPO for the Latin *nil per os*) status until the respiratory symptoms resolve (because of the increased risk of aspiration), and administering IV fluids to maintain hydration

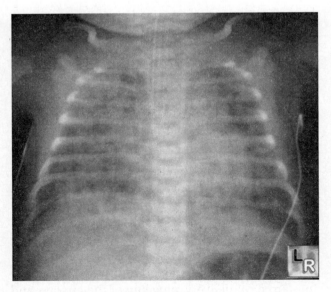

FIGURE 23-9 A chest radiograph with patchy/fluffy infiltrates, indicating meconium aspiration syndrome.

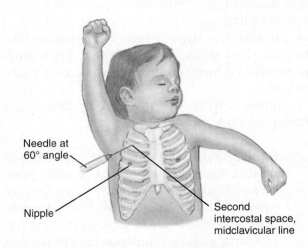

Needle at 60° angle

Nipple

Second intercostal space, midclavicular line

FIGURE 23-10 To perform needle thoracentesis to treat a tension pneumothorax or a symptomatic pneumothorax, position the child and identify the entry site.

and blood glucose levels. Respiratory support such as supplemental oxygen and PPV should be provided based on the infant's clinical condition and oxygen saturation level.

Respiratory Distress Syndrome

Infants delivered prematurely, especially at less than 32 weeks' gestation, have a high risk of experiencing respiratory distress syndrome (RDS) as the result of insufficient levels of surfactant, a surface-active agent that occurs naturally in the lungs and minimizes surface tension in the lungs. Within a few hours of birth, neonates with RDS present with grunting, retractions, nasal flaring, tachypnea, and, often, cyanosis. Male infants and infants of mothers with diabetes are at increased risk of RDS. Surfactant inactivation can also occur due to interactions with abnormal alveolar proteins such as meconium or blood or, in the case of pneumonia, albumin. Both surfactant deficiency and dysfunction may respond to exogenous surfactant, when it is administered in a controlled clinical setting by providers experienced in its delivery.

When transporting an infant after surfactant administration, the CCTP needs to recognize when lung compliance is improving and when respiratory support might need to decrease (eg, wean the patient oxygen as oxygen saturation improves, decrease peak pressure as chest excursion improves). Peak pressures and oxygen concentration should be minimized as appropriate throughout transport

to minimize the risk of pneumothorax and chronic lung disease. An oxygen saturation range of 88% to 92% should be targeted during transport of premature infants with RDS to minimize oxygen toxicity. CPAP can be helpful in neonates with mild RDS to minimize the risk of alveolar collapse during transport.

Standard nasal cannula therapy uses a maximum flow of 2 L/min to avoid drying out the mucous membranes in the nares. Special equipment that supplies humidified gas can be used to provide high-flow nasal cannula therapy, typically at gas flows between 2 and 6 L/min. Some institutions utilize high-flow therapy instead of CPAP. This therapy should be avoided during transport, however, because the high flow can provide excessive PEEP and increase the risk of pneumothorax.

In patients with suspected RDS, ensure that a sepsis workup has been performed prior to transport because pneumonia in the newborn is indistinguishable from RDS. Prevent cold stress by keeping the neonate warm and bundled.

Pneumothorax

Simple pneumothorax is a collection of gas in the pleural space that causes lung collapse. Tension pneumothorax is a life-threatening condition that involves air in the pleural space under pressure. Causes of pneumothorax include meconium aspiration, pneumonia, neonatal resuscitation, trauma, and aggressive assisted ventilation.

A pneumothorax may be treated by inserting an angiocatheter in the second intercostal space, at the midclavicular line, above the rib. The introducer needle is then removed to prevent a tension pneumothorax from developing, and the angiocatheter is attached to the extension tubing. Note that the angiocatheter may further tear the lung during its initial placement and is more likely to kink than is a butterfly needle. Remove as much air as possible with the syringe. At this point, the CCTP may briefly occlude the tubing while placing the end of the tubing that had been attached to the syringe in a small bottle of sterile water and release the tubing occlusion. This relieves the pressure buildup from the tension pneumothorax until the patient can be transferred to a facility skilled in placement of chest tubes in neonates. Intubate the infant if the respiratory distress continues.

Consider pneumothorax if the patient exhibits cyanosis, increased oxygen requirements, tachypnea, increased work of breathing, agitation, or tachycardia. If the pneumothorax is large or under pressure, life-threatening hypoxia, bradycardia, and hypotension may occur. Management of pneumothorax includes transillumination, thoracentesis (if significant cardiorespiratory compromise exists), and possibly intubation, while recognizing that PPV may cause an enlargement of the pneumothorax.

When transillumination is performed, increased transmission of light on one side of the chest suggests pneumothorax. A chest radiograph will confirm the diagnosis. Findings include an ipsilateral edge of the lung parallel to the chest wall, lucency, and a deep sulcus sign (deep lateral costophrenic angle). Mediastinal shift to the contralateral side is seen in patients with tension pneumothorax.

If a symptomatic pneumothorax is suspected, a needle thoracentesis can be lifesaving. On the side of the suspected pneumothorax, clean the area around the second intercostal space, at the midclavicular line (usually just above the nipple) with alcohol (Figure 23-10). Prepare the equipment needed: a 22-gauge butterfly needle attached to extension tubing, a three-way stopcock, and a 20-mL syringe. Insert the needle above the third rib (in the second intercostal space) as a second provider pulls back on the syringe (which is open to the patient). The nerves and blood vessels run below the ribs, so avoid piercing this area **FIGURE 23-11**. Continue to slowly advance the needle until air is recovered. The butterfly needle is rigid, so be gentle so as to avoid

further tearing of the lung. If the 20-mL syringe becomes filled with air, turn the stopcock off to the neonate, push out the air from the syringe, open the stopcock to the neonate, and continue withdrawing air. When no more air can be withdrawn, remove the needle. If the patient has a symptomatic ongoing air leak, a 22-gauge angiocatheter attached to extension tubing can be left in place, with the distal end of the tubing placed under sterile water to create a water seal.

Respiratory Acidosis

Respiratory acidosis may be caused by maternal drug use that results in respiratory depression in the neonate, or by a primary pulmonary or neurologic cause of suboptimal gas exchange. This imbalance frequently presents with visually apparent hypoventilation or increased work of breathing, and often responds to assisted ventilation.

Management of Respiratory Distress and Failure

Respiratory problems are a major cause of cardiac arrest in newborns and infants. Prompt recognition and effective management of respiratory distress and failure are fundamental to pediatric life support because clinical deterioration in respiratory function may progress rapidly. The primary goal is to restore adequate oxygenation and ventilation. **TABLE 23-11** lists measures for ensuring the airway, breathing, and circulation of a neonate with respiratory distress or failure.

Assessment of circulation includes both cardiovascular function and end-organ function. Cardiovascular function is assessed by skin color, temperature, heart rate, rhythm, BP, peripheral and central pulses, and capillary refill time. End-organ function is assessed by evaluation of mental status (brain perfusion), skin perfusion, and renal output. A systolic BP of less than 60 mm Hg in a term infant up to 1 month of age and of less than 70 mm Hg in a neonate up to 6 months of age is an ominous sign. Hypotension represents a state of shock in which physiologic compensatory mechanisms (tachycardia, vasoconstriction) have failed. Hypotension with hemorrhage is consistent with a 20% to 25% loss in circulating volume, whereas hypotension in septic shock represents inappropriate vasodilation rather than loss of circulating volume. Aggressive

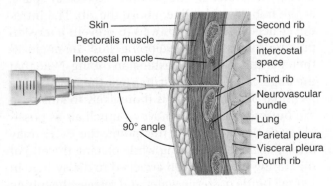

FIGURE 23-11 To perform needle thoracentesis for suspected pneumothorax in an infant, insert the needle over the top of the rib margin in the second intercostal space at the midclavicular line. Nerves and blood vessels run below the ribs, so avoid piercing this area.

Skin
Pectoralis muscle
Intercostal muscle
90° angle
Second rib
Second rib intercostal space
Third rib
Neurovascular bundle
Lung
Parietal pleura
Visceral pleura
Fourth rib

TABLE 23-11 Management of Respiratory Distress and Failure

Assessment Parameter	Action as Indicated
Airway	• Support the airway. • Clear the airway (suction the nose and mouth as needed). • Insert an oropharyngeal airway if indicated.
Breathing	• Assist ventilation (bag-mask ventilation or intubation). • Provide oxygen (humidified, if available). Begin with 100% oxygen and wean appropriately based on oximetry. • Continuously monitor oxygen saturation by pulse oximetry. • Prepare for intubation as indicated.
Circulation	• Monitor heart rate and rhythm. • Establish vascular access for fluid resuscitation and medications.

© Jones & Bartlett Learning.

fluid resuscitation, along with management of the airway and breathing, are needed to prevent cardiac arrest.

Cardiovascular Conditions

Cyanosis

Cyanosis (blue coloration of the gums and face) is caused by decreased arterial oxygenation. Acrocyanosis, or cyanosis of the extremities, with baseline skin color centrally is a benign, common condition that presents as blue coloration of the hands and feet and is often seen in newborns secondary to cold stress and peripheral vasoconstriction.

Cyanosis often presents in association with poor perfusion and congestive heart failure. It may also present with shock or result from either a pulmonary or cardiac process. Cardiac causes of cyanosis include cyanotic CHD, arrhythmia, cardiomyopathy, patent ductus arteriosus, and myocarditis. Noncardiac causes of cyanosis include persistent pulmonary hypertension (PPHN), sepsis/pneumonia, RDS, aspiration pneumonitis (meconium/blood), severe anemia, and arteriovenous malformation.

Cyanotic Congenital Heart Disease

Cyanotic congenital heart disease (CCHD) is caused by developmental anomalies of the heart or major vessels leading to abnormal blood flow. Deoxygenated blood from the right side of the heart is shunted to the left side, causing cyanosis. The cyanotic heart lesions are known as "the five Ts": truncus arteriosus, transposition of the great vessels, tetralogy of Fallot, tricuspid atresia, and total anomalous pulmonary venous return. A hypoplastic left heart also leads to cyanosis.

Management of cyanosis in a neonate suspected of having CHD includes assessing the ABCs, monitoring BP and oxygen saturation (preferably upper and lower saturations to monitor for PPHN), optimizing oxygenation to prevent acidosis, and supporting cardiovascular function. Administer oxygen to the infant, using a nonrebreathing mask if needed, to keep the oxygen saturation level at greater than 70%. Hyperoxygenation can be harmful because it reduces pulmonary vascular resistance and diverts blood from the systemic circulation to the pulmonary circulation. For the same reason, hyperventilation can be harmful to the infant. Consider intubation if the patient has severe respiratory distress.

Obtain IV access as soon as possible. Obtain a CBC with a platelet count and a differential count, and perform electrolyte and blood gas analyses. Measuring arterial blood gases helps determine the degree of oxygenation/perfusion and ventilation. Ensuring that laboratory tests for lactate and hemoglobin are performed along with blood gas measurements is a quick way of determining the extent of acidosis and anemia. Simultaneous determinations of blood gases from the preductal (right arm) and postductal (left arm) extremities are also useful. A preductal-postductal difference in Pao_2 (partial pressure of arterial oxygen) of greater than 15 mm Hg indicates that the patient has PPHN.

Sodium bicarbonate may be needed if poor perfusion has caused significant metabolic acidosis (check for base excess on the blood gas analysis). Obtain four limb BP readings to help determine the level of stenosis/obstruction to blood flow.

If possible, perform a hyperoxia test: It helps distinguish cardiac from noncardiac (lung disease) causes of cyanosis. This test is carried out by placing the infant in an oxygen hood with 100% oxygen for 20 minutes, then obtaining a blood gas measurement. A PaO_2 measurement greater than 150 mm Hg on the blood gas analysis essentially rules out cardiac causes of cyanosis, because deoxygenated blood bypasses the lungs and is shunted to the left side of the heart in the case of CHD. The exception to this rule is the condition known as total anomalous pulmonary venous return, in which oxygenated blood returns to the right side of the heart, leading to progressive pulmonary edema.

If results from a blood gas analysis are not readily available, upper and lower oxygen saturations can be obtained in their stead. A preductal saturation that is more than 10 points higher than the postductal saturation suggests pulmonary hypertension. Hyperoxia with hyperventilation supports PPHN as the cause of cyanosis. Correct any other metabolic abnormalities identified on the lab analysis.

Discuss the appropriateness of prostaglandin administration with the supervising physician. In the case of ductal-dependent congenital heart lesions (eg, transposition of the great arteries, left ventricular outflow obstruction), timely infusion of prostaglandin E1 is crucial to ensure a good outcome. This therapy keeps the ductus arteriosus open. In contrast, prostaglandin is not indicated in non–ductal-dependent lesions, but the actual diagnosis may not become clear until an echocardiogram is obtained.

An echocardiogram is used to assess the type of CHD and determine the presence of pulmonary hypertension; however, this type of study is often not available when transferring a neonate from a community hospital to a higher-level facility. If the diagnosis of CHD is suspected but uncertain during transport and the patient is severely acidotic, hypoxic, hypotensive, or poorly perfused, discuss a trial of prostaglandin with the supervising physician. The infant may need to be intubated for the infusion, as prostaglandin can cause apneas. Other side effects of this medication may include seizures, bradycardia, hyperthermia, and hypotension. Follow the patient's vital signs closely throughout the transport whenever prostaglandin is administered.

Some infants may have congestive heart failure and low BP/delayed capillary refill in addition to cyanosis. Management of hypotension includes a normal saline bolus as first-line therapy. After ensuring adequate volume expansion, consider administering inotropes or pressors. Agents for supporting BP include dobutamine and dopamine; the dose of each is 5 to 20 µg/kg/min. Administer sodium bicarbonate to treat severe acidosis.

Tachyarrhythmias and Bradyarrhythmias

Sinus tachycardia is defined as a heart rate faster than normal for the child's age. Heart rate generally varies with activity and other factors influencing oxygen demand (ie, the infant's temperature). Common pathologic causes of tachycardia include tissue hypoxia, hypovolemia, fever, metabolic stress, pain, anxiety, drugs, and anemia.

Supraventricular tachycardia (SVT) is an abnormally fast rhythm originating above the ventricles. It is the most common cause of tachyarrhythmia producing cardiovascular compromise in infancy. SVT is often caused by a reentry mechanism that involves an accessory pathway, atrioventricular nodal reentry, or ectopic atrial focus. Wolff-Parkinson-White syndrome, in which ventricular preexcitation produces a delta wave on electrocardiogram, is an example of a condition that produces SVT via an accessory pathway.

Infants often tolerate SVT quite well. They may present with symptoms of congestive cardiac failure, poor feeding, rapid breathing, irritability, pale or blue color, and vomiting. Initial management of SVT includes measuring the pulse and assessing for signs of adequate perfusion, supporting the ABCs and oxygenation as needed, obtaining an electrocardiogram to determine the rhythm, obtaining vascular access, and establishing monitoring by applying a cardiopulmonary monitor and/or pulse oximeter. Specific emergency interventions are dictated by the infant's condition and vary depending on the width of the QRS complex observed on the electrocardiogram. Vagal maneuvers, cardioversion, and pharmacologic interventions are among the options available to treat SVT, but should be performed under the supervision of a credentialed provider of such care. Children with tachyarrhythmias need to be evaluated by a pediatric cardiologist, though this assessment should not delay appropriate emergency treatment.

Bradycardia in a neonate is usually a result of tissue hypoxia and resolves when tissue oxygenation is restored. The most common neonatal bradyarrhythmia is due to maternal lupus, and results in heart block. If the resting fetal heart rate is low enough, hydrops (edema) develops. Postdelivery cardiac pacing may need to be initiated, but is usually nonurgent.

Signs and Symptoms

Supraventricular Tachycardia
- Symptoms of congestive heart failure
- Poor feeding
- Rapid breathing
- Irritability
- Pale or blue color
- Vomiting

Differential Diagnosis

Supraventricular Tachycardia
- Wolff-Parkinson-White syndrome
- Sinus tachycardia

Transport Management

Supraventricular Tachycardia
- Support the ABCs and provide oxygenation as needed.
- Monitor with a cardiopulmonary monitor and/or pulse oximeter.
- Perform vagal maneuvers, cardioversion, and pharmacologic interventions based on protocol.

Cardiac Arrest

In contrast to cardiac arrest in adults, sudden cardiac arrest in children is uncommon. Cardiac arrest in pediatric patients is more often caused by progression of respiratory distress, respiratory failure, or shock, typically associated with hypoxemia and acidosis, than by cardiac arrhythmias. In the United States, the incidence of sudden infant death syndrome has decreased significantly since the Back to Sleep campaign (now called Safe to Sleep) began in the 1990s. This initiative instructs parents to place infants on their back to sleep. Trauma is an important cause of cardiopulmonary collapse in infants older than 6 months. Details of infant resuscitation, including the importance of adequate ventilation, have already been discussed.

Persistent Pulmonary Hypertension

Persistent pulmonary hypertension (PPHN) is persistence of elevated pressures in the pulmonary vasculature after birth. It is associated with failure to transition from the fetal circulation to the postpartum or normal newborn circulation. The elevated pulmonary BP causes ineffective pulmonary perfusion, hypoxemia, and right-to-left shunting of blood via the patent foramen ovale and/or patent ductus arteriosus. PPHN presents most often in term or postterm neonates, becoming evident within the first few hours of life. It frequently co-occurs with a combination of cyanosis, tachypnea, hypoxemia (often labile/fluctuating, respiratory distress, and differential oxygen saturations [upper > lower]).

The exact cause of PPHN is not understood, but several factors are known to contribute to the failure of normal circulatory transition at birth. For example, pulmonary vasoconstriction often occurs secondary to perinatal events. The most potent vasoconstrictors of the pulmonary artery are hypoxia and acidosis. Meconium aspiration is the most common cause of PPHN, often resulting in perinatal distress. Other conditions and risk factors associated with PPHN include RDS, asphyxia, pneumonia, hypothermia, hypoglycemia, and sepsis.

Abnormal development of the pulmonary vasculature is more frequently seen if the mother has taken nonsteroidal anti-inflammatory drugs during pregnancy and in infants of mothers with diabetes. It is also common in infants with chronic fetal distress/hypoxia resulting in hypertrophy of the vascular muscles of the pulmonary artery (characterized by idiopathic or black lung PPHN; no parenchymal disease is seen on a chest radiograph), aspiration, hypoxic ischemic encephalopathy, and congenital diaphragmatic hernia.

For the CCTP caring for a neonate, it is important to have a low threshold of suspicion for PPHN. Care should be taken to optimize oxygenation, minimize stress, maintain a normal BP, and avoid or correct acidosis. Obtain a CBC, differential count, platelet count, and blood gas analysis for hyperoxia, and follow the patient's upper and lower oxygen saturations while treating the underlying cause of the PPHN.

Shock

Shock is a serious condition in which perfusion is inadequate to meet the tissue demands; it can affect all organ systems in the body. To ensure sufficient oxygen delivery to the tissues, both lung ventilation and tissue perfusion are needed. Hypovolemia is a common cause of shock in neonates, often stemming from acute blood loss or fluid losses owing to decreased intake, polyuric renal failure, or diarrhea. Cardiogenic shock can follow CHD, arrhythmias, myocardial ischemia from asphyxia, cardiac tamponade, pneumothorax, or high intrathoracic pressure from PPV combined with secondary decreased venous return. Causes of distributive shock include sepsis, cardiac depression, and vasodilation.

Mean BP is often used to assess the adequacy of perfusion in a neonate, especially in the preterm population, where the lowest acceptable mean BP is equal to the gestational age of the neonate (eg, a mean arterial pressure of 28 mm Hg in a neonate at 28 weeks' gestation and a mean arterial pressure of 38 mm Hg in a neonate at 38 weeks' gestation).

Shock presents with some, if not all, of the following signs and symptoms: hypotension, tachycardia (or bradycardia, in cases of asphyxia), poor perfusion, tachypnea, oliguria/anuria, hypothermia, acidemia, and weak pulses. Hepatomegaly, cardiomegaly, and peripheral edema are seen in cardiogenic shock. Notably, the absence of a heart murmur does not rule out cardiogenic shock. Disseminated intravascular coagulopathy may be a late presentation.

Management of shock includes managing the ABCs, checking blood glucose levels, obtaining vascular access, providing fluid resuscitation, and treating the underlying cause. If it is necessary to provide fluids to support the patient's circulation or to deliver resuscitation medications intravenously to a neonate, emergent access must be obtained. Unfortunately, it is usually difficult to establish peripheral access in an infant who needs volume or resuscitation medications. In such a case, the umbilical vein in a newborn can be catheterized by using an umbilical vein catheter and following these steps:

1. Clean the umbilical cord with alcohol or another antiseptic.
2. Place a sterile tie firmly but not too tightly around the base of the cord for control of bleeding. If available, place a sterile drape over the site. While the line needs to be placed quickly in a code situation, maintain sterile technique as much as possible.
3. Prefill a sterile 3.5F to 5F umbilical vein line catheter (a comparable-size sterile feeding tube can be used in an emergency) with normal saline using a 3-mL syringe.
4. Using a sterile technique, wrap a tie around the base of the cord to control bleeding, and then cut the cord with a scalpel below the clamp placed on the cord at birth, about 0.5 to 0.75 inch (1 to 2 cm) from the skin (between the clamp and the cord tie).
5. The umbilical vein is a large thin-walled vessel usually at the 12 o'clock position, as compared to the two thick-walled umbilical arteries usually found at 4 and 8 o'clock **FIGURE 23-12**. Insert the catheter 0.75 to 1.5 inches (2 to 4 cm), or less in preterm infants, until blood can be aspirated. If the catheter is advanced

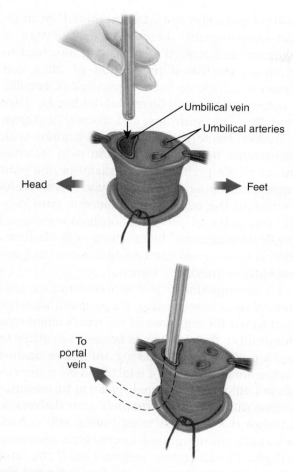

FIGURE 23-12 Location of the umbilical vein.

© Jones & Bartlett Learning.

too far, infusing hypertonic solutions directly into the liver may lead to irreversible damage **FIGURE 23-13**. If the catheter is advanced into the heart, arrhythmias may develop.

6. Once access is established, flush with 0.5 mL of normal saline and tape the catheter in place.

For an older neonate (after the first week following birth), if emergent IV access is needed but peripheral IV access cannot be obtained, an IO line can be placed, similar to the case for an older child. Take care to choose a small-size line and to avoid traversing the bone.

Signs and Symptoms

Shock

- Hypotension
- Tachycardia (or bradycardia in cases of asphyxia)
- Poor perfusion
- Tachypnea
- Oliguria/anuria
- Hypothermia
- Acidemia
- Weak pulses
- Hepatomegaly, cardiomegaly, and peripheral edema in cardiogenic shock
- Disseminated intravascular coagulopathy

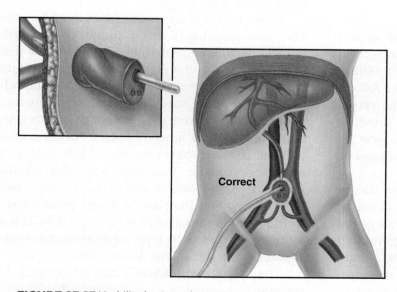
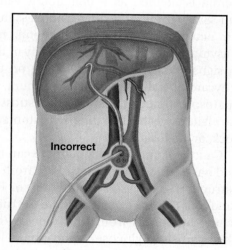

FIGURE 23-13 Umbilical vein catheterization. If the catheter is advanced too far, infusing hypertonic solutions directly into the liver may lead to irreversible damage.

© Jones & Bartlett Learning.

Anemia

Anemia is defined as a hematocrit value of less than 38% in preterm neonates and less than 42% in term neonates. A neonate with anemia may either be asymptomatic or present with any of the following signs or symptoms, depending on the cause: tachycardia, pallor, petechiae/purpura, jaundice, hepatosplenomegaly, respiratory distress, hydrops, heart failure, visible bleeding/hematoma, cyanosis, shock, or acidosis.

Causes of anemia in a neonate can be categorized based on whether they result from increased destruction, decreased production, or loss of red blood cells (RBCs). Causes of increased destruction include hemolysis from RBC defects (hereditary spherocytosis, glucose-6-phosphate dehydrogenase [G6PD] or pyruvate kinase deficiency, or thalassemia) and immune processes (Rh incompatibility, ABO incompatibility, maternal lupus,

maternal penicillin use). Disseminated intravascular coagulopathy, hemangiomas, vitamin E deficiency, and arterial stenosis can also lead to hemolysis. Decreased production of RBCs can be seen in infections such as parvovirus, rubella, or cytomegalovirus; congenital leukemia; Diamond-Blackfan syndrome; and trisomy 21 (Down syndrome). Hemorrhage can occur in utero, with fetomaternal hemorrhage or twin-twin transfusion, or in the perinatal or neonatal period with abruptio placentae, placenta previa, velamentous insertion of the cord on the placenta, cord rupture, fetomaternal bleeding, cephalohematoma, subgaleal/intracranial hemorrhage, splenic hemorrhage, intracranial hemorrhage, necrotizing enterocolitis, or traumatic injury.

Rh incompatibility is a serious situation that can have dire consequences. If a pregnant woman's blood type is Rh negative and her fetus's blood type is Rh positive, the woman can become sensitized to the Rh-positive blood, making antibodies against it, when small amounts of fetal blood enter her circulation. Rhogam is routinely given to Rh-negative mothers during and immediately after delivery to minimize this risk, but sensitization still occurs, such as after unrecognized spontaneous early miscarriages. In subsequent pregnancies, if the fetus is Rh positive, maternal antibodies can cross the placental barrier and destroy the Rh-positive fetal RBCs, leading to severe anemia and ultimately heart failure and hydrops.

Management of anemia includes managing the ABCs and obtaining IV access (optimally two sites). Initially, the following lab values should be obtained in consultation with a physician: a blood type and crossmatch, CBC, peripheral blood smear (which allows the lab to microscopically examine the structure of the blood cells), reticulocyte count, Coombs test, bilirubin level, liver function tests, a TORCH screen (a blood test that checks for several infections in a newborn, including Toxoplasmosis, Other agents, Rubella, Cytomegalovirus, and Herpes simplex), cultures of scrapings from any vesicular lesions, electrolyte levels, and coagulation factors. (TORCH is a set of infections to which pregnant women are susceptible that result in fetal deformities.)

The neonate with anemia may be in shock. In such patients, volume resuscitation with a 20 mL/kg bolus of normal saline followed by the administration of blood is crucial.

If the anemia is chronic, the infant is at risk of volume overload after transfusion. The supervising physician may need to perform an exchange transfusion to avoid cardiac collapse. If coagulopathy is suspected, use packed RBCs and fresh-frozen plasma.

Hyperbilirubinemia

Hyperbilirubinemia, a condition in which an excess of bilirubin develops in the blood, is commonly seen in newborns. Hyperbilirubinemia frequently leads to jaundice, the deposition of bile pigments in the skin. Approximately 60% to 80% of term infants and nearly 100% of preterm infants will have clinical jaundice. This condition reflects the immaturity of the bilirubin conjugating enzymes in the liver as well as the increased RBC turnover that occurs in newborns. The jaundice often appears after the first day and for the most part is self-limiting. In term infants, it usually peaks during days 3 to 5 and then slowly begins to improve. In premature infants, this process may take longer. Occasionally, bilirubin levels may be high enough to cause severe and permanent sequelae as the bilirubin becomes deposited in the brain cells, leading to bilirubin-induced neurotoxicity.

Pathophysiology

Bilirubin is produced in the reticuloendothelial system in the spleen, liver, and bone marrow; it is the end product of heme degradation. Heme is produced by the breakdown of hemoglobin and other hemoproteins. When heme oxygenase releases an equimolar amount of carbon monoxide, heme is converted to biliverdin (water soluble). Biliverdin is then converted to unconjugated bilirubin (lipid soluble) by biliverdin reductase. The unconjugated bilirubin is bound to albumin and transported to the liver, where it is conjugated with glucuronic acids by the enzyme uridine diphosphate-glucuronyl transferase (UDPGT) to form monoglucuronides and diglucuronides, or conjugated bilirubin (water soluble). The conjugated bilirubin is then excreted in the bile and metabolized by intestinal bacteria to form urobilin (excreted via the urine) and stercobilin (excreted in stools). The conjugated form can also be deconjugated by bacteria to create unconjugated bilirubin, which is reabsorbed in the intestine and transported back to the liver, thus completing the enterohepatic circulation.

Physiologic Jaundice

In most infants, the total serum bilirubin does not exceed 12 mg/dL, with levels peaking at about 3 to 5 days after birth. Breastfed babies have a higher risk for exaggerated physiologic jaundice. Breastfeeding jaundice is self-limiting and resolves as maternal milk supply increases and infant feeding becomes well established. Occasionally, jaundice may persist beyond 2 weeks of age in breastfeeding infants, a condition sometimes referred to as breast milk jaundice.

Pathologic Jaundice

Pathologic jaundice is defined as jaundice of greater than 12 to 15 mg/dL in healthy term neonates, or a rate of rise greater than 0.2 mg/dL/h or greater than 5 mg/dL in 24 hours. The etiology of pathologic jaundice must be appropriately investigated **TABLE 23-12**.

Conjugated hyperbilirubinemia, also known as cholestasis, is always pathologic. It occurs when there is impaired bile formation or interrupted bile flow in the intrahepatic or extrahepatic biliary system. Prolonged jaundice beyond 2 weeks of age or an increase in the level of direct (conjugated) bilirubin suggests cholestatic jaundice and always requires investigation. The most common cause of this condition is biliary atresia.

Acute bilirubin encephalopathy occurs when bilirubin deposition occurs in the basal ganglia, hippocampus, cerebellum, and nuclei of the floor of the fourth ventricle, leading to a loss of neurons and gliosis. It is likely to occur when bilirubin levels exceed 30 mg/dL, but rarely presents in infants with bilirubin levels less than 20 mg/dL. Evidence of bilirubin toxicity can be detected by auditory-evoked potentials. The term *kernicterus* is generally reserved for the chronic and permanent sequelae of bilirubin-induced neurologic dysfunction.

As better diagnostic and genetic tests become available, more of these conditions are being identified early.

Assessment

Serum bilirubin levels should be obtained if jaundice is suspected. Hyperbilirubinemia is one of the most common reasons for readmission of the newborn to the hospital within the first 2 weeks after birth. Because newborns are often discharged from

TABLE 23-12 Etiology of Pathologic Jaundice

Unconjugated Hyperbilirubinemia	Conjugated Hyperbilirubinemia

Increased production of bilirubin
• Physiologic jaundice
• Hemolytic process
  • Immune mediated (ABO or Rh incompatibility)
  • Non-immune mediated (spherocytosis, G6PD deficiency, disseminated intravascular coagulation)
• Polycythemia
• Cephalohematoma or bruising
	Obstruction of the biliary system
	• Biliary atresia
	• Choledochal cyst
	• Alagille syndrome
	Infections
	• TORCH
	• Sepsis, urinary tract infection
	Acute liver injury
	• Ischemia, hypoxia, acidosis

Decreased hepatocellular uptake or conjugation
• Physiologic jaundice
• Prematurity
• Breast milk jaundice
• Congenital hypothyroidism
• Enzyme deficiencies
  • Crigler-Najjar syndrome
  • Gilbert syndrome
	Parenteral nutrition–associated cholestasis
	Defect of bile acid synthesis or transport
	Metabolic liver disease
	• Tyrosinemia
	• Alpha-1 antitrypsin deficiency
	• Galactosemia
	• Mitochondrial liver disease

Abbreviations: G6PD, glucose-6-phosphate dehydrogenase; TORCH, toxoplasmosis, other agents, rubella, cytomegalovirus, and herpes simplex

© Jones & Bartlett Learning.

the hospital within 48 hours of birth, jaundice tends to be an outpatient problem.

Initial steps in evaluating a newborn with jaundice involve differentiating between unconjugated and conjugated hyperbilirubinemia. Appropriate laboratory tests and imaging studies may be used to create a differential diagnosis. A detailed history, including prenatal care, maternal blood tests, and birth history, may help identify potential risk factors. A family history, results of a newborn metabolic screening, a thorough abdominal examination (to identify an enlarged liver or spleen), and focused testing will help identify pathologic processes.

Treatment

Phototherapy

Phototherapy entails the use of a visible spectrum of light to treat hyperbilirubinemia in the newborn. It acts by transforming unconjugated bilirubin into water-soluble photo-isomers that can be eliminated by the kidney and the liver without needing to be conjugated. The dose of phototherapy is determined by the wavelength of the light (460–490 nm, blue range), the intensity of the light (irradiance), the distance of the newborn from the source of light, and the surface area of the body exposed to the light. The light transforms a bilirubin molecule into structural isomers (lumirubin) or configurational isomers. Configuration isomerization is a reversible but rapid process, whereas structural isomerization is a slower but irreversible process.

Phototherapy represents a simple measure that is effective in reducing the bilirubin levels and under most circumstances can reduce the need for an exchange transfusion. With appropriately delivered phototherapy, a significant reduction in the infant's total serum bilirubin can be achieved.

IV Immunoglobulin Therapy and Exchange Transfusion

IV immunoglobulin therapy may be used in infants with hemolytic jaundice. It has been shown to decrease the need for exchange transfusion.

When necessary, a double-volume exchange transfusion can be carried out in specialist centers to treat hemolytic jaundice. In this procedure, the baby's blood is exchanged twice, slowly for type O-negative blood. An exchange transfusion may be necessary in cases involving Rh isoimmunization or other hemolytic processes.

Gastrointestinal Conditions

Any part of the gastrointestinal tract may have congenital anomalies. The most common of these lesions noted at birth are atresia (complete absence of a lumen), stenosis (narrowing), duplication of loops of bowel, and functional obstruction.

Presenting features may include increased salivation; choking with feeding; cyanosis; vomiting, especially if bile stained; abdominal distention; blood in stool or failure to stool; lethargy; or irritability. Physical findings may include a distended, discolored (erythematous), tender abdomen; absent bowel sounds; or lethargy and poor perfusion. Important principles include the knowledge that bilious (green or yellow) vomiting is considered an indication of an obstruction until proven otherwise, passage of meconium does not rule out an obstructed bowel, and an obstructed bowel can lead to perforation and peritonitis.

Abdominal Wall Defects

Gastroschisis and omphalocele are abdominal wall defects that can be distinguished by their presentations **TABLE 23-13**.

- **Gastroschisis** is a full-thickness defect of the abdominal wall, usually to the right and adjacent to the intact umbilical cord. Variable amounts of edematous intestine and stomach tissue extrude from the defect (the liver and spleen are normally situated in the abdomen). The extruded intestine does not have a protective covering. The reported incidence of this defect is 1 in 2,000 births.
- **Omphalocele** is a herniation of the abdominal contents into the umbilical cord. A protective membrane covers the herniated contents (unless ruptured during the birth process).

Gastroschisis is usually an isolated defect, whereas omphalocele has an association with a variety of congenital defects, such as congenital diaphragmatic hernia and other anomalies.

Ideally, infants with gastroschisis or omphalocele should be delivered at a regional perinatal center that has immediate access to a neonatal intensive care unit and pediatric surgery. However, occasionally these infants are born at remote locations even when their condition may have been diagnosed prenatally. Under those circumstances, rapid newborn transport should be provided, and care coordinated between obstetricians, pediatricians, and surgeons.

Immediate care includes initial resuscitation, then placing the abdominal contents in a clear sterile bag to cover and protect the exposed contents, thereby limiting fluid and protein loss and preventing hypothermia. Handling of the bowel should be minimized to decrease vascular compromise. Hypothermia, dehydration, sepsis, and injury to the bowel will lead to a poor outcome for the neonate. With a large defect, the infant may be placed right side down to minimize stretching of the mesenteric vessels. The intestines should be visualized throughout the transport; if they begin to look dusky, they should be repositioned to optimize blood flow.

A nasogastric or orogastric tube should be maintained at low intermittent suction. A wide-bore double-lumen **Replogle tube**, if available, is

TABLE 23-13 Comparison of Gastroschisis and Omphalocele		
	Gastroschisis	**Omphalocele**
Definition	Centrally located, full-thickness abdominal wall defect	Herniation of abdominal contents into base of umbilical cord
Features	• 0.75- to 1.5-inch (2- to 4-cm) defect • Right side of cord • Intact umbilical cord • Uncovered intestine, thick, edematous, matted • Liver, spleen in normal positions	• Different sizes • Protective membrane covers the abdominal contents • Elements of umbilical cord course over the sac and come together at the top to form a normal umbilical cord • Large omphalocele may contain the liver and/or spleen
Associated abnormalities	Isolated defect	25% to 40% of infants have associated chromosomal, cardiac, neurologic, genitourinary, skeletal, or other gastrointestinal defects

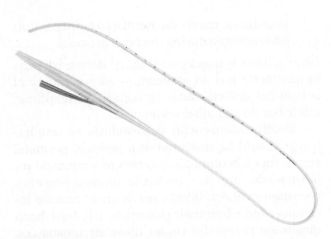

FIGURE 23-14 A Replogle tube.

Courtesy of Covidien.

ideal for this purpose **FIGURE 23-14**. A Replogle tube is used for gastric decompression in infants with gastrointestinal issues; for an infant, usually an 8F size suffices and is connected to low intermittent suction to collect gastric secretions.

Vascular access should be maintained in any infant with a gastroschisis or omphalocele. Generous IV fluids consisting of $D_{10}W$ are initiated at approximately 120 to 150 mL/kg/d because of the increased fluid loss and third space deficits associated with both of these conditions. CCTPs should provide hemodynamic support with fluids and pressors, if necessary. Broad-spectrum antibiotics should be administered before initiating the transport given the increased risk of infection in these infants.

An intact omphalocele is a less urgent surgical problem than a gastroschisis or ruptured omphalocele because the intact membrane conserves heat and protects the intestine. The sac should be carefully protected. With any of these conditions, however, surgical consultation should be obtained as soon as possible, initially by telephone, so that a surgical plan can be developed. Provide rapid transport to an appropriate pediatric surgical facility.

Gastrointestinal Obstruction and Vomiting

The causes of vomiting can be differentiated based on the presence or absence of bile, which turns the vomitus green. Presence of bile must be treated as a surgical emergency until gastrointestinal obstruction, especially **malrotation** of the intestine,

has been ruled out. Bile-stained vomiting may occasionally be seen without intestinal obstruction, such as with a septic ileus. In these situations, it may present without abdominal distention and does not continue to recur.

The differential diagnosis of bilious vomiting includes malrotation with volvulus, intestinal atresia, and annular pancreas. The differential diagnosis of nonbilious vomiting includes esophageal atresia, gastroesophageal reflux, overfeeding (excessive volume of feed), milk or formula intolerance, sepsis, and obstructive lesions above the ampulla of Vater such as pyloric stenosis or partial intestinal obstruction.

Esophageal atresia (a congenital defect in which the esophagus ends in a blind pouch) is suspected when the infant presents with increased salivation and chokes on feeding. Vomitus with esophageal atresia is never bile stained, and the infant often develops respiratory distress from aspiration. Examine the infant for other abnormalities such as anal atresia (an abnormal or absent anal opening). The diagnosis of esophageal atresia is further substantiated by inability to pass a nasogastric tube to the stomach; the tube coils in the esophageal pouch in patients with this defect. Stomach contents may be obtained when suctioning the ET tube of an intubated infant with esophageal atresia with a tracheoesophageal fistula. When trying to document an esophageal atresia, use as large a tube as will pass through the nares.

Atresia can be confirmed by obtaining a chest radiograph that includes the neck and upper abdomen. Note the presence or absence of air in the stomach: A lack of air in the stomach suggests that the patient has an esophageal atresia without a communication between the trachea and the lower esophagus, whereas the presence of air in the stomach suggests the presence of such a connection. Note the presence of other vertebral and/or rib anomalies suggesting **VATER syndrome** (Vertebral anomalies, Anal atresia, Tracheoesophageal fistula and/or Esophageal atresia, and Renal and radial anomalies). Diagnosis of atresia requires a high index of suspicion for this condition.

During transport of the neonate with esophageal atresia, position the neonate with the head elevated at a 30° angle, place a suction catheter in the upper pouch, and provide intermittent suction. Neonates often do not need to be intubated if the airway is kept clear of secretions; achieving this goal requires frequent oral suctioning.

Congenital gastrointestinal obstruction should be considered when **polyhydramnios** (extra amniotic fluid) is present. **Proximal intestinal obstruction** is an obstruction at or above the level of the jejunum. Duodenal obstruction may be complete (duodenal atresia) or partial (annular pancreas, duodenal atresia, malrotation, and midgut volvulus). The clinical presentation may include bilious vomiting, minimal dilation of the abdomen, or evidence of intestinal ischemia (bloody mucoid stools). An increased incidence of duodenal atresia is seen in neonates with trisomy 21, with prenatal ultrasonography or abdominal radiograph showing the classic "double-bubble" in which two large collections of gas are present, one in the stomach and the other in the dilated part of the duodenum **FIGURE 23-15**. The rest of the abdomen is generally gasless in complete obstruction.

The exact cause of obstruction may not be evident until laparotomy is performed. Malrotation should be considered, as midgut volvulus (twisting of the entire midgut on the superior mesenteric artery pedicle) constitutes a surgical emergency. The ensuing ischemia may result in a nonviable bowel and death, resulting in the phrase known to most pediatricians: "Never let the sun set on bilious emesis." Management includes establishing IV access, fluid resuscitation, broad-spectrum antibiotics, and urgent laparotomy. When volvulus is suspected, consult the surgeon by telephone before leaving the referring institution so as to expedite the surgical plan for the patient.

Distal intestinal obstruction refers to partial or complete obstruction of the distal small bowel (ileum) or large intestine. Its differential diagnosis includes ileal atresia, meconium ileus (obstruction of the terminal ileum by inspissated meconium), meconium plug or hypoplastic left colon, colonic atresia, and Hirschsprung disease (congenital aganglionic colon). The clinical presentation often includes a distended abdomen, failure to pass meconium in the first 24 to 48 hours after birth, and bilious or nonbilious vomiting. An abdominal radiograph often shows multiple dilated loops of bowel **FIGURE 23-16**. Management considerations include ensuring IV access, hydration, and placement of a nasogastric tube or Replogle tube if available to suction air and avoid further abdominal dilation during transport. Transfer the infant to a pediatric surgical center for specific diagnosis and treatment.

Imperforate anus is a congenital condition in which the anal opening is either absent or

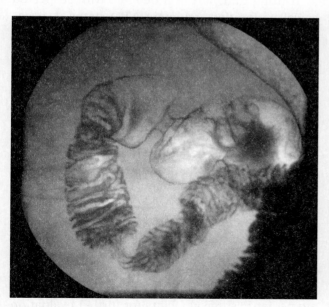

FIGURE 23-15 A fluoroscopic image showing a collection of gas in the stomach and in the duodenum.

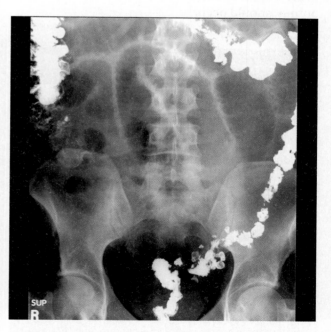

FIGURE 23-16 An abdominal radiograph after a barium enema showing multiple dilated loops of bowel.

displaced. Diagnosis requires inspection of the anal opening and should be made in the delivery room. If the condition is diagnosed shortly after birth, the infant is usually asymptomatic, but a delay in diagnosis can lead to progressive abdominal distention and perforation. After this diagnosis is made, health care providers should maintain NPO status, establish IV access, administer maintenance IV fluids, and place a nasogastric tube or Replogle tube and provide low intermittent suction to minimize abdominal distention. In addition, transfer to a surgical center for evaluation and treatment should be arranged quickly. Infants with imperforate anus also have a higher rate of CHD and other anomalies that may further complicate the transport.

Hirschsprung disease is a congenital anomaly in which a portion of the intestine lacks ganglion nerve cells. As a result, normal peristalsis does not occur, and stool backs up. If undiagnosed, this condition can lead to toxic megacolon. Signs include decreased stooling, abdominal distention, and, in later stages, shock. Fluid resuscitation and transport to a referral center with pediatric surgery capability can be lifesaving.

In each of these transports, thermoregulation of the neonate should be maintained and close monitoring of vital signs, including oxygen saturation, heart rate, respiratory rate, BP, and strict intake/output, should occur.

Differential Diagnosis

Proximal Intestinal Obstruction
- Duodenal atresia
- Annular pancreas
- Malrotation
- Midgut volvulus

Transport Management

Proximal Intestinal Obstruction
- Maintain thermoregulation.
- Closely monitor vital signs, including oxygen saturation, heart rate, respiratory rate, and BP.
- Ensure strict intake/output.

Acute Intestinal Perforation

Perforation of the bowel can be caused by an obstructed bowel; necrotizing enterocolitis (NEC), a disorder seen predominantly in premature infants; or iatrogenic perforation (may be caused by suprapubic bladder aspiration or paracentesis). Perforation may also occur spontaneously. It is sometimes seen in preterm infants in association with indomethacin use, especially when this medication is combined with hydrocortisone or dexamethasone therapy.

The clinical presentation of intestinal perforation includes progressive abdominal distention, respiratory distress, hypotension, and acidosis (mixed metabolic and respiratory). Both physical examination and laboratory tests are helpful in making this diagnosis. Radiographic studies will show free air in the abdomen, whose presence can be confirmed by a cross-table lateral or left lateral decubitus view (right side up).

NEC presents with abdominal distention, feeding intolerance, and grossly bloody stools. The infant often appears septic. The diagnosis is confirmed by an abdominal radiograph showing pneumatosis intestinalis (air in the bowel wall), and may be suspected when an abnormal gas pattern, ileus, and a fixed sentinel loop are seen on radiographs. Other features include intrahepatic portal venous gas.

During transport of a neonate with suspected bowel perforation, maintain NPO status. A nasogastric or Replogle tube should be placed and low intermittent suction provided to assist with decompression of the bowel. These infants are at high risk of shock and severe metabolic acidosis secondary to inflammation and vascular leak. Establish vascular access and provide 10-mL/kg normal saline boluses as needed to support perfusion and BP, in addition to maintenance fluids. Blood cultures and CBC should be drawn and broad-spectrum antibiotics initiated prior to leaving the referring facility. In addition, these neonates often develop apnea, so maintain a low threshold for intubation before beginning the transport. If the infant develops recurrent apnea en route, intubate the infant quickly to avoid further abdominal distention from bagmask ventilation. Provide transport to an appropriate pediatric surgical facility for further evaluation and surgical intervention. If intestinal perforation is confirmed, notify the surgeon before leaving the referring institution so a surgical plan for the patient can be expedited.

Hematemesis and bleeding from the upper gastrointestinal tract may be seen in a nasogastric tube aspirate or be associated with vomiting. Such blood is generally bright red, although brown blood may be seen if the bleeding is slow or starts high in the intestines. The differential diagnosis in such cases includes idiopathic bleeding (no clear cause; generally resolves within a few days), swallowed maternal blood (accounts for approximately 10% of cases; the infant may swallow blood during a cesarean section, and occasionally during a vaginal delivery), nasogastric trauma from a nasogastric tube, stress ulcer (often seen in sick neonates), coagulopathy (hemorrhagic disease of the newborn [vitamin K deficiency] or disseminated intravascular coagulation), bleeding Meckel diverticulum, NEC, intestinal fissure, formula intolerance (usually cow's milk protein allergy), maternal bleeding nipples in breastfed infants, or volvulus.

Volvulus is an abnormal twisting of the intestine. It can lead to gangrene and death of the affected segment of intestine, intestinal obstruction, perforation peritonitis, and death of the patient. Midgut volvulus occurs in infants with malrotation of the bowel during fetal development. Segmental volvulus can occur at any age and may be caused by abnormal intestinal contents (meconium ileus); sigmoid volvulus usually results from a dilated rectosigmoid on a narrow pedicle.

Volvulus often has a sudden onset. Its symptoms and signs may include abdominal pain, nausea, vomiting, and blood in the stool. Intestinal volvulus is a surgical emergency, requiring release of the abnormal twisting so as to ensure a normal blood supply. If this condition is suspected, keep the patient on NPO status, establish IV access, begin maintenance fluids, decompress the intestines with a nasogastric tube or Replogle tube, provide low intermittent suction, and expedite transfer to a center with pediatric surgical services.

Intussusception

Intussusception is the telescoping of one segment of intestine into another adjacent distal segment of the intestine. Intussusception is the most common cause of intestinal obstruction in children between 3 months and 6 years of age; it is extremely rare in

Signs and Symptoms

Acute Intestinal Perforation

- Progressive abdominal distention
- Respiratory distress
- Hypotension
- Acidosis (mixed metabolic and respiratory)
- Feeding intolerance
- Grossly bloody stools

Differential Diagnosis

Acute Intestinal Perforation

- Obstructed bowel
- Necrotizing enterocolitis
- Iatrogenic perforation
- Spontaneous perforation

Transport Management

Acute Intestinal Perforation

- Maintain NPO status.
- Monitor for development of apnea.
- Intubate the infant if recurrent apnea develops during transport.

children younger than 3 months of age or in older children and adults. This condition can present with passage of bloody stool, often described as currant jelly stool due to its resemblance to that food.

When intussusception is suspected, keep the patient on NPO status, establish IV access, begin maintenance fluids, decompress the intestines with a nasogastric tube or Replogle tube, provide low intermittent suction, and provide rapid transfer to a center with pediatric radiology and surgical services. An intussusception may be reduced by enema, but frequently needs open reduction to ensure its final resolution.

Diarrhea

Diarrhea in a neonate is unusual because the infant still has maternal immunoglobulins that help minimize the child's risk of contracting diarrheal illness in the first few weeks of life. When transferring a neonate with diarrhea, maintain the infant on NPO status, establish IV access, and provide fluid resuscitation as clinically indicated. Continue maintenance fluids en route to minimize further dehydration and hypoglycemia. Monitor the patient's vital signs throughout the transport, and make efforts to maintain normothermia in the infant.

Transport Management

Diarrhea
- Maintain NPO status.
- Provide maintenance fluids.
- Monitor vital signs.
- Maintain normothermia.

Infectious Diseases/Sepsis

Neonates are particularly susceptible to becoming compromised by serious infectious diseases because their immune system is not fully developed. Signs of infection in a neonate include decreased activity (lethargy), hypothermia, hypoglycemia, poor perfusion, low BP, and apnea. Neonates are at higher risk of infection with group B *Streptococcus* and gram-negative bacteria, which frequently respond to ampicillin and gentamicin. Viral illness, however, can lead to dire illness in a neonate.

Primary assessment of a neonate with a suspected infectious disease includes a blood culture, urine culture, and lumbar puncture. These measures are followed by administration of broad-spectrum antibiotics. A chest radiograph is taken if the infant has respiratory symptoms.

Regardless of the causative organism, it is important to support the infant's cardiorespiratory state and aggressively provide fluid resuscitation if signs of shock are present. Monitor vital signs and maintain normothermia while transferring the patient to a center that can care for a critically ill neonate, because the infant's condition can deteriorate rapidly.

Hyperthermia/Hypothermia

Hyperthermia (temperature greater than 99.5°F [37.5°C]) in a neonate is usually caused by overbundling or exposure to excessive heat, but it can also be seen with herpes simplex infection or dehydration. Hypothermia in the neonate, defined as a decrease in body temperature to less than 97.5°F (36.4°C), occurs in all climates, but is more common during the winter months. It can also be an early sign of sepsis.

Neonates have increased surface area-to-volume ratio relative to adults, making them extremely sensitive to environmental conditions. This is especially the case immediately after delivery, when the neonate's body is wet. An increase in metabolic function in an attempt to overcome the heat loss can cause hypoglycemia, metabolic acidosis, pulmonary hypertension, and hypoxemia. Infection should be considered as an etiology in any hypothermic neonate.

Hypothermic neonates are cool to the touch, initially in the extremities; as their body temperatures drop, however, their skin becomes cool all over. The infant may also be pale and have acrocyanosis. The hypothermic neonate may present with apnea, bradycardia, cyanosis, irritability, and a weak cry. As the body temperature decreases, the neonate may become lethargic and obtunded. In severely hypothermic infants, the face and extremities may appear bright red. Sclerema (hardening of the skin associated with reddening and edema) may be seen on the back, on the limbs, or all over the body. Thermal shock, disseminated intravascular coagulopathy, and death may occur in more serious cases.

Preventive measures include warming your hands before touching the infant, using prewarmed blankets and equipment, and placing a cap on the neonate's head (the head is the largest source of heat loss). The critically ill neonate, once stabilized, should be placed in a prewarmed incubator or, if none is available, covered with warm blankets for transport. Recent studies in neonates with hypoxic ischemic injury indicate outcomes are improved when the infant is maintained in a state of mild therapeutic hypothermia within 6 hours of birth. This approach is not recommended in the field, although it is certainly prudent to prevent hyperthermia. Maintain the infant at the lower margin of normal temperature (axillary temperature no higher than 97.5°F [36.4°C]).

Toxic Exposure

Most toxic exposures in neonates result from transplacental exposure (eg, maternal alcohol or narcotic use) or purposeful administration of a substance by another person, such as a well-meaning younger child. The most important principle in managing toxic exposure/ingestion is to stabilize the neonate. Manage the patient's ABCs. Obtain IV access as indicated based on the patient's history and physical exam. Be sure to obtain the history from the sending facility.

In the case of respiratory suppression resulting from narcotics, which is much more likely to stem from chronic maternal exposure, provide respiratory support until the infant is transferred to a tertiary hospital. If respiratory depression is suspected to reflect an acute narcotic exposure, such as when an infant delivers shortly after a dose of maternal narcotic is administered for labor pain control, naloxone 0.1 mg/kg may be administered to reverse the narcotic effect. While the IV route is preferred, intramuscular (IM) administration may be used if necessary. In case of a chronic maternal (and therefore newborn) exposure to narcotics, administering naloxone may precipitate seizures in the infant, potentially causing death; therefore, it is not recommended in this circumstance. When the maternal history is in doubt, acute narcotic intoxication in the infant can be managed by ventilator support, and naloxone administration can and should be avoided.

For additional exposures, including topical exposures, contact the local Poison Control Center. The experts at this center can guide CCTPs regarding the appropriate response to myriad exposures.

Trauma/Birth Injuries

Injuries to the infant that result from mechanical forces (ie, compression, traction) during the birth process are termed birth trauma. Significant birth injury accounts for fewer than 2% of neonatal deaths and stillbirths in the United States. It still occurs occasionally and unavoidably, resulting in an average of 6 to 8 injuries per 1,000 live births. Hypoxic injury may coexist with mechanical injury. Most birth injuries are self-limiting and have a favorable outcome.

Causes and risk factors for birth trauma include macrosomia, prolonged labor, precipitous delivery, breech presentation, instrumentation (forceps/vacuum-assisted delivery), extreme prematurity, and oligohydramnios (decreased volume of amniotic fluid during a pregnancy).

Head and Neck Injuries

Most birth injuries self-resolve with time and are not fatal. Birth injuries to the head and neck include two types of benign head and neck injuries: vacuum caput, an accumulation of fluid at the site of the vacuum extractor that usually resolves within hours, and caput succedaneum, a subcutaneous collection of fluid with poorly defined margins in the scalp, resulting from pressure on the infant's head during delivery, which usually resolves within a few days. Serious head and neck injuries include subgaleal hematoma, which can spread slowly and result in shock. A subgaleal bleed can present as an ill-defined mass in the dependent part of the head (usually the occipital region); it does not follow suture lines. Significant blood loss may occur with such a hematoma, and the infant may present with shock and acute renal failure if the condition is not promptly identified and treated. Cephalohematoma is a subperiosteal collection of blood that may be accompanied by a linear skull fracture. It is most commonly seen in the parietal region and is limited by suture lines. It resolves within a few months, with resulting calcification. A skull fracture may present with a slight depression in the skull, although this may not be obvious secondary to an overlying hematoma.

In addition to the skull findings, these birth injuries may present with anemia and jaundice. If a hemorrhage progresses, it may cause hypotension and shock. A hematoma may also become infected.

Management of head and neck injuries is based on the specific presentation. Blood transfusion may be needed for patients with hemorrhage and anemia. Phototherapy (light therapy to reduce bilirubin levels) is needed for jaundice based on the bilirubin level. If the neonate is in hypovolemic shock from excessive blood loss, manage the ABCs and treat for shock, focusing on volume resuscitation and admission to a neonatal intensive care unit (NICU).

Nerve Injuries

Nerve injuries often occur because of hyperextension or overstretching during delivery, especially with breech presentation. The nerve injuries incurred during the birth process can range from peripheral nerve branch injury to major spinal cord injury. Most nerve injuries do not require any immediate intervention.

Nerve injuries that need immediate attention and possible transfer to a facility that can provide a higher level of care include recurrent laryngeal nerve injury, which causes paralysis of the vocal cords, unilaterally or bilaterally. This injury presents with respiratory distress, stridor, or desaturation. It may be associated with intracranial bleeding. In an infant in whom such an injury is suspected, visualize the vocal cords by direct laryngoscopy. Intubate in the event of bilateral vocal cord paralysis. Do not feed the neonate to avoid the risk of aspiration during transport.

Vaginal breech delivery poses the greatest risk factor for spinal cord injury. This injury frequently presents with a loud "snap" sound at the delivery. It may be associated with epidural hemorrhage, loss of motor function distal to the injury, temperature instability, and loss of bladder and bowel function. In such a case, immobilize the head and restrain the neonate. If the nerve injury impairs spontaneous respiration, intubate and provide PPV until the infant can be transferred to an appropriate health care facility.

Bone and Other Injuries

The clavicle is the most common site of fracture in a newborn. Risk factors for such an injury include a large infant, shoulder dystocia, and use of instrumentation during delivery (especially forceps). A fractured clavicle itself does not need any urgent intervention, and should heal within 7 to 10 days as long as the motion of the arm is limited. However, a rare complication of a fractured clavicle is a pneumothorax. If the neonate presents with tachypnea or increased work of breathing, consider pneumothorax as the etiology. See the section on pneumothorax for information on management of this condition.

Fractures of the humerus or femur are uncommon birth injuries. Manage these injuries by splinting the arm or leg and transferring the neonate to a pediatric orthopaedic center.

Intra-abdominal injuries during birth are rare but often present as shock and blue discoloration of the abdominal wall. Treat the patient for shock, and ensure that a hematocrit, type and crossmatch, and, if possible, abdominal ultrasonography have been performed at the referring facility before transferring the infant to a hospital with pediatric surgical support.

Finally, soft-tissue injuries include abrasions, lacerations, and ecchymosis. These injuries mostly need routine care.

Transport Management

Bone and Other Injuries
- Monitor for pneumothorax; treat if present.
- Treat for shock.

Abuse/Maltreatment

Shaken baby syndrome is the most common cause of death in cases of child abuse. Shaking of a baby may tear bridging veins in the brain, lead to a subdural hematoma, or cause a hypoxic injury. Most often, the physical exam will not identify significant findings that indicate the presence of this condition. It should be suspected in a previously well infant who presents with nonspecific signs such as feeding intolerance, irritability, and vomiting. Severe cases may even present with seizures or apnea secondary to intracranial hemorrhage. Other maltreatment includes blunt trauma to the abdomen, burns, bruising, and skeletal injuries. The management for these injuries is again based on presentation.

Obvious extremity fractures should be stabilized, with attention given to maintaining circulation to the affected extremity. Fluid resuscitation may be needed if bleeding has occurred. Respiratory support may be needed if intracranial hemorrhage or trauma to the upper airway is present. In patients with severe burns, the affected areas should be protected with sterile material and IV fluids initiated because of the increased insensible water loss that occurs through the burned skin. The CCTP's goal is to stabilize the neonate and transport the patient safely to a health care facility where further workup and treatment may be done.

Neurologic Conditions
Seizures

Seizures represent the most distinctive sign of neurologic disease in the neonatal period. They may be identified by direct observation. A **seizure** is defined as a paroxysmal alteration in neurologic function (ie, behavioral and/or autonomic function); it often manifests with apnea in a term neonate. It is important to distinguish seizures from other motor phenomena (eg, jitteriness, myoclonic activity) that could be confused with them. Seizures represent a relative medical emergency because they are usually a sign of a serious underlying abnormality. It is critical to recognize neonatal seizures and to determine their causes because they may interfere with cardiopulmonary function, interrupt feeding, affect metabolic function, and, if prolonged, cause brain injury.

Jitteriness is often confused with a seizure **TABLE 23-14**. Jitteriness is characteristically a disorder of the newborn and is rarely seen at a later age. This condition is most commonly seen with hypoxic ischemic encephalopathy, hypocalcemia, hypoglycemia, and drug withdrawal. In addition, newborns frequently exhibit normal motor activity that could be mistaken for seizures. These myoclonic, dysconjugate eye movements, or sucking movements are often seen when the infant is drowsy or asleep.

A simple classification of seizure types suggests that four essential types can be recognized: subtle, tonic, clonic, and myoclonic. Subtle seizures are characterized by apnea, eye deviation, blinking, sucking, and pedaling movements of the legs. Tonic seizures are characterized by tonic extension of the limbs. Less commonly, with this type of seizure, flexion of the arms and extension of the legs may also occur. Tonic seizures are more common in premature infants, especially in those with intraventricular hemorrhage. Seizures characterized by clonic localized jerking are classified as focal clonic seizures; these types of seizures can occur in both term and premature infants. Lastly, myoclonic seizures are characterized by flexion jerks of the upper or lower extremities, singly or in a series of repetitive jerks.

Causes of neonatal seizures include hypoxic ischemic encephalopathy, intracranial hemorrhage, intracranial infections (meningitis), development defects, hypoglycemia, hypocalcemia, and other metabolic disturbances, frequently as the result of inborn errors of metabolism. You may observe a quiet, often hypotonic infant. The infant may be lethargic or apneic.

Hypoglycemia must be recognized quickly and treated promptly, within a few minutes, to minimize the risk of brain damage. $D_{10}W$ may be given as an IV bolus (2 mL/kg) if the blood glucose level is less than 40 mg/dL. A blood glucose measurement and administration of dextrose in an infant with hypoglycemia may be lifesaving. Recheck the blood glucose level every 30 minutes after treating an infant for hypoglycemia, until the blood glucose level is documented to be stable. An IV bolus of dextrose should be followed by an infusion of $D_{10}W$ to maintain normoglycemia during transport.

The CCTP should continue to monitor the neonate's vital signs and oxygen saturation throughout transport. Apnea, a symptom that commonly accompanies neonatal seizures, may require intubation and ventilatory support during transport. Phenobarbital (Luminal) and phenytoin (Dilantin) are the two anticonvulsants most often used in neonates. Both drugs may interfere with respiratory and cardiac function, and should be given only in consultation with the supervising physician. Because seizures may be a sign of meningitis, the referring facility should have performed a septic workup and begun antibiotics before the transfer.

Hypoxic Ischemic Encephalopathy

Hypoxic ischemic encephalopathy (HIE) is a neuronal injury caused by oxygen deprivation (hypoxia) or decreased perfusion (ischemia) to the brain.

TABLE 23-14 Jitteriness Versus Seizures		
Characteristics	**Jitteriness**	**Seizures**
Ocular phenomena (deviation or fixation of the eyes)	Not seen	Commonly associated
Stimulus sensitive (may be triggered by a stimulus)	Yes	No
Dominant movement	Tremor	Clonic jerking
Application of gentle pressure to limb	Stops jitteriness	Does not stop seizures
Autonomic phenomena	Not associated	Common association

© Jones & Bartlett Learning.

Redistribution of blood occurs during prolonged asphyxia, with more of the cardiac output being delivered to the vital organs (eg, brain, heart, adrenal glands) at the expense of the less vital organs (eg, lungs, gut, kidneys, skin). Multiple-organ dysfunction is common after HIE and may influence the infant's eventual outcome.

HIE is the single most common cause of seizures in both term and preterm infants. The time of onset for organ dysfunction from HIE, hypoglycemia, and other metabolic disturbances ranges from birth to 3 days postdelivery. In contrast, the time of onset for all other causes of seizures can be from birth to longer than 3 days postdelivery. Infants with HIE often present with decreased tone, poor perfusion, and in more severe situations, hypotension and recurrent apnea.

Management of neonatal HIE includes maintaining adequate ventilation, perfusion, and BP; maintaining adequate blood glucose levels; carefully monitoring fluid intake and output; and adjusting treatment based on the infant's renal output, oxygen saturation, and ventilation status. The infant's body temperature should be maintained in the low normal range (97.5°F [36.4°C]) to avoid hyperthermia, which is associated with a worse outcome from HIE. If a newborn with HIE arrives at the tertiary care center within 6 hours of birth, more aggressive therapeutic hypothermia may be offered as a treatment modality under controlled conditions. It is therefore critical to ensure rapid transport of these infants to a center that can provide appropriate therapy.

Lethargy

In infants, lethargy (a decreased level of consciousness during which you are unable to arouse the infant) can be caused by many conditions, but almost always implies a serious, frequently life-threatening underlying condition. Some common causes of lethargy include sepsis, severe hypoxia, severe hypoglycemia, intracranial hemorrhage, and HIE.

Management includes attention to the ABCs, obtaining IV access, ensuring normoglycemia, providing oxygen as needed, initiating antibiotics in conjunction with the supervising physician, and expediting transfer to a tertiary center skilled in dealing with critically ill neonates.

Metabolic Conditions
Metabolic Acidosis

Metabolic acidosis occurs when cations, frequently lactic acid from poor tissue perfusion or toxic by-products of inborn errors of metabolism, build up in the bloodstream. Causes of metabolic acidosis include asphyxia, CHD, sepsis, inborn errors of metabolism, hypovolemia, seizures, bradycardia, hypotension, and toxins. The presentation of metabolic acidosis may include compensatory tachypnea, mottled/gray skin with delayed capillary refill (normally less than 3 seconds), apnea, lethargy, hypertonia or hypotonia, feeding intolerance, seizures, or emesis.

Management of metabolic acidosis includes managing the ABCs; providing adequate oxygenation, ventilation, and hydration; and treating the underlying cause. If adequate ventilation and fluid resuscitation fail to clear the metabolic acidosis, sodium bicarbonate can be given at the following dose: 0.3 × the base deficit on the blood gas analysis × the neonate's weight in kilograms. If the exact deficit is not known, a dose of 2 mEq/kg can be given. In premature neonates, the dose should be administered over at least 30 minutes to minimize the risk of intraventricular hemorrhage. If an inborn error of metabolism is suspected, stop enteral feeding and initiate IV dextrose to minimize production of toxic by-products. Critically ill neonates often have a mixed metabolic and respiratory acidosis (respiratory acidosis was discussed earlier in this chapter in the respiratory conditions section).

Hypoglycemia

Hypoglycemia, defined as a blood glucose level of less than 40 mg/dL, is a medical emergency; in severe cases, it can lead to brain damage and even death. Hypoglycemia is more common in infants who are either small or large for gestational age, infants of mothers with diabetes, and infants who are stressed. Signs of hypoglycemia include decreased activity, jitteriness, and seizures.

If you suspect hypoglycemia, immediately perform a heel stick to determine the blood glucose level. If hypoglycemia is present, administer IV dextrose (2 mL/kg $D_{10}W$), followed by an infusion of glucose. First administer 60 mL/kg/d $D_{10}W$ to maintain the term neonate's blood glucose level while you contact the regional perinatal center for guidance on the rate and type of IV solution; this can vary based on the infant's gestational and chronological age.

Hypocalcemia

Hypocalcemia is most commonly seen in low-birth-weight infants and can occur after significant stress, as well as in infants whose mothers have diabetes. Significant hypocalcemia can lead to cardiac arrhythmias, seizures, and tetany. In general, calcium infusion is not indicated in an infant unless hypocalcemia is documented.

There are two time frames when hypocalcemia frequently occurs in the neonate. The first is at age 2 to 3 days. The second (late-onset hypocalcemia) is unusual in the United States but may be seen in infants who consume cow's milk or synthetic formulas that are high in phosphorus.

In an infant who has documented hypocalcemia and is younger than 24 hours, administer an IV infusion of 2 to 3 mEq/kg/d of calcium in $D_{10}W$ during transport. If an infant has documented hypocalcemia, is older than 24 hours, and has normal renal function, administer 10% dextrose in 0.25% saline with 10 mEq/kg of potassium chloride in 500 mL during transport.

Inborn Errors of Metabolism

An inborn error of metabolism is any of a class of genetic diseases mostly caused by defects in single genes that code for enzymes that facilitate conversion of various substances into others; these defects lead to accumulation of substances that are toxic or interfere with normal function. Many different inborn errors of metabolism are possible, each of which is relatively rare, so a complete review is beyond the scope of this chapter.

Common presenting features of inborn errors of metabolism include lethargy, acidosis, poor perfusion, and hypoglycemia. If such a condition is suspected, stop enteral feeding and start an IV glucose infusion before the critical care transport team begins the patient's transfer. If a neonate is lethargic and experiences tachypnea (suggesting a metabolic acidosis), start a glucose infusion even if the

neonate is normoglycemic. This infusion will help decrease the buildup of toxic by-products produced by the body when the neonate is unable to metabolize nutrients normally.

Congenital adrenal hyperplasia results from a defect in the synthesis of cortisol. An infant with this condition may have virilizing features and problems with sodium loss, depending on which enzyme is deficient. An infant experiencing sodium loss can present with dehydration and shock. Acute treatment includes normalizing electrolytes and fluid balance, and initiating hydrocortisone replacement after consultation with the supervising physician.

Transport Management

Inborn Errors of Metabolism

- If suspected, stop enteral feeding and begin an IV glucose infusion before transfer.

Congenital Adrenal Hyperplasia

- Normalize electrolytes and fluid balance.
- Consider initiating hydrocortisone replacement; consult with the supervising physician.

The Transfer Process for a Neonate

In the well-organized regional referral system, transport of a high-risk neonate proceeds through the following steps:

1. A physician at the referring hospital initiates a request for transport. A physician in the regional control center decides which facility can accommodate the patient and gives the referring physician advice on caring for the neonate until the transport team arrives.

2. A mode of transportation is chosen: ground transportation, helicopter, or fixed-wing aircraft, depending on the patient's status, distance, availability of services, and weather conditions.

3. The transport team is mobilized, the CCTP is provided with any relevant information known about the neonate to be transferred, and equipment is assembled. Optimally, the

team will consist of a health care provider with special training in caring for critically ill neonates, a respiratory therapist with similar special training, and a paramedic who has spent a period of apprenticeship or received additional training in transporting an ill neonate. With particularly critical patients, a physician may accompany the team. The equipment used by the CCTP is highly specialized, including appropriately designed ventilation and oxygenation units and an incubator meeting stringent criteria.

4. On arrival at the referring hospital, the transport team helps with further stabilization of the infant if needed, before embarking on transport. Conditions such as hypoxemia, acidosis, hypoglycemia, pneumothorax, shock, and hypovolemia must be treated before leaving the referring hospital. If the infant is suspected of having an infectious disease, appropriate cultures should be obtained prior to transport and early antibiotic therapy initiated. If a contagious disease is suspected, transport personnel should take adequate safety precautions.

5. While stabilizing the infant, the team collects information and materials, including a copy of the mother's and infant's medical records and any radiographs, lab results, and medications for the infant. Often transport teams operate on the basis of implied consent, meaning that transport is considered a part of treatment of the life-threatening emergency. Some areas require signed consent before transport is initiated. Awareness of local and state guidelines is important.

Once the infant's condition is stabilized as much as possible at the referring hospital, transport the patient to the nearest facility that can provide the appropriate level of care. Ideally, someone will contact this facility to discuss the situation and obtain advice regarding care and disposition throughout the process. Complications can arise en route, such as a dislodged breathing tube or development of a pneumothorax. Given this reality, it is critically important to remain vigilant and recognize changes in the status of the infant, such as desaturation or change in color. Quick intervention will help ensure an optimal outcome.

Using an Incubator

An **incubator** is a box with clear walls, a heat source, and portal access in which a neonate can be placed to maintain normothermia and minimize noise stress. An incubator is indicated for transport of infants who weigh less than 10 pounds (5 kg) or are younger than 30 days. When preparing to use an incubator, ensure that the oxygen tank attached to the incubator is full, and that blankets and a bulb syringe are available inside the incubator.

SKILL DRILL 23-4 shows the steps for using an incubator, which are described here:

1. Plug in the alternating current (AC) power cord **STEP 1**.
2. Set the main AC power switch **STEP 2**. The charging indicator will be a constant light if the internal batteries need charging. The light will flicker or go off when fully charged. Battery life is approximately 2 hours.
3. Depress the "controller" switch **STEP 3**. The power failure alarm and AC/DC power mode should light up. The high temperature sensor, heater temperature, and low direct current (DC) alarm should flash. A short beep will be heard at the end of the test. The set point indicator should be illuminated and the temperature reading should indicate 91.4°F (33°C) ± 0.1 for 15 seconds.
4. Check and adjust the set point temperature to 100.4°F (38°C) **STEP 4**. The maximum temperature is 104°F (40°C). It takes approximately 30 minutes to warm up.
5. Do not block or cover the end portions of the incubator.
6. Check the oxygen and air tanks **STEP 5**. All tanks should read 2,000 psi.

Family Communication and Support

Throughout the process of transporting an ill neonate, ongoing communication with the family regarding what is being done for the infant and which care is planned will help allay their fears.

Do not be specific about the infant's chances of survival. Many factors play into morbidity and mortality, and you do not want to be misleading. If family members have questions you cannot

Skill Drill 23-4 Using an Incubator

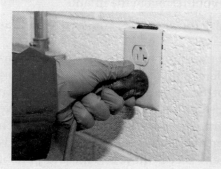

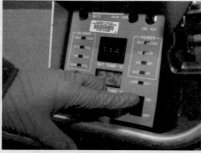

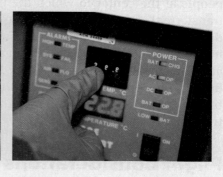

Step 1

Plug in the AC power cord.

Step 2

Set the main AC power switch. The charging indicator will be a constant light if the internal batteries need charging. The light will flicker or go off when fully charged.

Step 3

Depress the "controller" switch. Check that the power failure alarm and AC/DC power mode light up, and that the high temperature sensor, heater temperature, and low DC alarm flash. A short beep will be heard at the end of the test. The set point indicator should be illuminated and the temperature reading should indicate 91.4°F (33°C) ± 0.1 for 15 seconds.

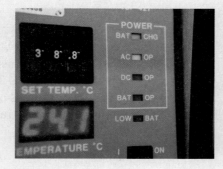

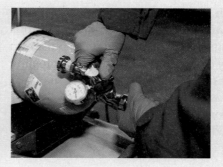

Step 4

Check and adjust the set point temperature to 100.4°F (38°C). Do not block or cover the end portions of the incubator.

Step 5

Check the oxygen and air tanks. All tanks should read 2,000 psi.

answer, be straightforward. Tell them that you do not have a definite answer, but you will help put them in touch with the people who do (most likely people at the center to which the infant is being transferred). Often, just explaining what you are doing and giving the family a realistic time frame in which they should be able to speak to someone at the receiving institution is very helpful. Families usually appreciate being told the name of the receiving physician, if it is known at the time of transfer.

Flight Considerations

Air transport, either fixed wing or helicopter, presents a new set of challenges during care of a neonate and should be managed appropriately. Some of these are listed here:

- **Airway.** It is critical to establish a secure airway before takeoff, because it is extremely difficult to intubate a neonate and assess breath sounds during flight. If this step is necessary while in flight, pay special attention to signs of adequate ventilation and ET tube position, such as condensation on the ET tube, chest rise, and change in color of the ETCO$_2$ indicator.
- **Circulation.** It can also be difficult to hear a heartbeat while in the air. Alternative methods of assessment—such as palpating pulsation on a freshly clamped umbilical cord, or feeling the cardiac movement at the point of maximal intensity—can be helpful.
- **Oxygenation.** The partial pressure of oxygen is decreased at higher altitudes, so additional

oxygen may be needed to maintain oxygen saturation in the neonate.
- **Temperature regulation.** Take measures to prevent hypothermia in the infant.

Finally, minimize the neonate's exposure to fuel vapor and noise.

Helicopter transport may be used for medium-distance transfers of up to 150 miles (241 km). This mode may not be appropriate for transporting a neonate because of limited space and the relative inability to carry the necessary equipment, such as an incubator, and additional personnel. There is restricted patient access during flight and patient evaluation may be compromised because of noise and vibrations. The cabin is not pressurized, which may lead to further hypoxic and hypothermic stress.

Fixed-wing (airplane) transport is generally reserved for long distances (more than 150 miles [241 km]). As compared to helicopter transport, the space allocated for patient care is generally adequate. Transport will involve ambulance transportation to the airport, subsequent air transport, and further ambulance transportation to the hospital. It is important to arrange not only the helicopter or airplane, but also the ambulances to and from the airports and the respective hospitals.

Summary

Neonates have a unique anatomy, physiology, and pathology, making care and transfer of such patients challenging but rewarding. The CCTP must be familiar with the special needs of this age group to provide optimal care during transfer to reduce morbidity and improve survival.

Case Study

You and your new partner have stopped for a slice of pizza after a routine transport. While ordering, you receive a call to respond to a local emergency department (ED) for a 3-week-old child with a fever. You and your partner understand that young children in febrile states do not fare well—the pizza will have to wait.

On arrival at the ED, you are met by the charge nurse and attending physician. They report to you that a 20-day-old female was brought in by her mother, who said that the infant was sleepy, refused to eat, and felt warm to the touch. Triage noted that the patient was not responding to external stimuli and presented with a weak cry and delayed capillary refill. The patient was delivered at the same hospital, and records show a normal, cephalic delivery with no complications. In addition, the mother had received prenatal care and only had a history of asthma.

Physical exam of the patient reveals diffuse congestion with mild substernal and intercostal retractions, peripheral cyanosis and mottling, a capillary refill time of 4 seconds, and a rectal temperature of 102°F (38.8°C). The child is non-responsive to verbal stimulation and grimaces when you perform tactile stimulation. Vital signs show a pulse of 180 beats/min, with atrial tachy-cardia on the monitor, a BP of 100/40 mm Hg, and an oxygen saturation of 90%. An IV line of normal saline has been established in the left antecubi-tal vein with a 24-gauge catheter, and it appears patent. You estimate the infant's weight to be 8 pounds (4 kg). A CBC was drawn, and revealed a white blood cell (WBC) count of 26,000/mm³. The serum blood glucose level was 80 mg/dL. All other blood values were normal. No arterial blood gas analysis, chest radiograph, or lumbar puncture has been performed. The attending physician advises you that he has been in contact with the NICU at University Hospital and he has the re-ceiving physician's information.

1. What is your presumptive diagnosis?
2. What are some potential causes of this pa-tient's altered mental status?
3. What are your primary concerns in caring for this patient?

You note that the patient is receiving oxy-gen by a nonrebreathing mask at a flow rate of 8 L/min. You ask your partner to switch to bag-mask ventilation at a rate of 20 breaths/min as you prepare to contact the receiving facility.

Your partner advises you that the bag-mask ventilation is compliant and there is good chest rise. The patient's oxygen saturation has in-creased to 95%, with other vital signs remaining unchanged. You contact University Hospital and speak with the receiving physician. After con-firming the bed assignment, you confer on your findings. It is agreed that bag-mask ventilation, while effective in the ED, may become a chal-lenge to maintain during the 45-minute transport. You receive an order to perform rapid sequence intubation. Your protocol for intubation includes premedication with atropine, fentanyl, and suc-cinylcholine. The patient is intubated. You are unable to obtain cultures, but due to the high sus-picion of serious infection, the referring physician instructs you to administer ampicillin and genta-micin at weight-appropriate doses per *The Harriet Lane Handbook* (a pediatric reference tool).

After administration of 160 mL of normal sa-line, you note that the infant's BP is 110/70 mm Hg, the pulse is 170 beats/min, and capillary refill is 2 seconds. During transport, your patient's ox-ygen saturation increases to 98%, the ETCO$_2$ is 43 mm Hg, and her color has improved. However, lung sounds are still diffusely congested. You ar-rive at the NICU and transfer your patient.

Analysis

Although you are somewhat convinced the infant has sepsis, your concern focuses on the patient's impending respiratory failure due to acute respira-tory distress syndrome. In addition, the ventilation-perfusion (V/Q) mismatch is causing acidosis by failing to rid the neonate's body of carbon dioxide.

In addition to hypoxia, you must be aware of other potential causes of altered mental status in neonates—namely, hypoglycemia and seizures. Once the airway is secured, the CCTPs must as-sess the infant's blood glucose level.

Overall, the most critical aspect of caring for this difficult patient is the ability to secure the airway, control oxygenation, and stabilize hemodynamics.

Two weeks later, you and your partner follow up on this case during a quality assurance (QA) meeting. On admission, the patient received a spinal tap, which was negative, but a blood cul-ture revealed *Streptococcus pneumoniae*, a very common bacterium that causes illnesses ranging from ear infections to meningitis. The patient re-ceived 7 days of IV ampicillin and gentamicin and successfully fought off the infection, remaining on a ventilator for 3 days and being discharged after 7 days. Credit was given both to the com-munity hospital, for prompt recognition that this patient was in need of more specialized care, and to the transport unit, which made the decision to aggressively manage the patient's airway.

Prep Kit

Ready for Review

- A newborn is an infant within the first few hours of life; a neonate is an infant within the first 28 days of life. Term newborns are delivered between 37 and 42 weeks' gestation.
- Because short-term and long-term outcomes in infants have been linked to initial stabilization efforts, CCTPs must be knowledgeable about problems that may occur with neonates and understand how to treat them. They must also have the appropriate equipment available to treat neonates, and must carefully consider the neonate's transport plan.
- Newborns differ anatomically and physiologically from young children, and CCTPs must be aware of those differences.
- Neonates become cold easily because of a variety of factors, ranging from their high body surface area-to-body weight ratios to increased evaporative heat loss through their skin. To avoid hypothermia, use prewarmed blankets and equipment, including a prewarmed transport incubator, place a cap on the infant's head, and minimize exposure to cold. While avoiding hypothermia, be careful to also avoid environmentally induced hyperthermia.
- The lungs of neonates are small relative to their body sizes, with little respiratory reserve. Their heads are large in relation to their bodies, resulting in neck flexion and obstruction when the infant is in the supine position. Placing a rolled towel under a neonate's shoulders helps open the airway.
- Neonates are obligate nose breathers and may require an oral airway during transport if they present with obstructive apnea. When positive-pressure ventilation is needed, attempts should be made to maintain physiologic tidal volume breaths.
- Neonates have a high oxygen requirement; they do not tolerate interruptions in oxygen delivery for any length of time, and they become hypoxic and bradycardic quickly.
- The neonate's heart rate is an important determinant of cardiac output. Neonates respond to careful volume loading with an increase in cardiac output, but they do not tolerate fluid overload. Changes in the cardiovascular circulation that take place after the umbilical cord is clamped at birth include a sudden rise in the systemic vascular resistance, increased pulmonary blood flow, and physiologic closure of the fetal shunts. With extrauterine breathing and expansion of the lungs, tissue oxygenation increases, pulmonary vascular resistance decreases, and pulmonary blood flow increases.
- Pulmonary vascular resistance may increase in the neonate, causing persistent pulmonary hypertension. During transport, give special attention to maintaining normothermia, optimal oxygenation, fluid status, and systemic BP, and minimize acidosis and noise to reduce the risk of the neonate developing severe persistent pulmonary hypertension.
- Patent ductus arteriosus is seen in 50% of extremely premature infants. Minimizing fluid overload during transport can decrease the risk of persistent symptomatic patent ductus arteriosus.
- Nephrogenesis is complete at 36 weeks' gestation. The glomerular filtration rate at term is low; the creatinine level at birth reflects the mother's level, but then falls to reflect the infant's renal function by 1 week of age. Infants tolerate fluid restriction poorly and become dehydrated quickly.
- Total body water represents 85% of body weight in premature infants and 75% of body weight in term infants, compared to 60% of body weight in adults. Contraction of the extracellular compartment and weight loss in the first few days after birth are normal. Fluids should be restricted until after the postnatal weight loss occurs.
- Liberal fluid regimens in the first few days of life have been associated with worse outcomes

Prep Kit Continued

in premature infants. $D_{10}W$ is typically used for IV fluid maintenance during the newborn's first 24 hours of life. After 24 hours and the establishment of adequate urine output, 10% dextrose in 0.25% saline is used.

- Neonates are considered to have pressure-passive cerebral circulation. An acceptable mean arterial pressure generally equates to the gestational age of the newborn. It is important to minimize stress and use appropriate sedation for procedures in these patients to minimize BP peaks that can lead to intraventricular hemorrhage.
- Neonates, including premature neonates, show well-developed responses to painful stimuli. Use appropriate analgesic measures to treat neonates for pain.
- Neonates are susceptible to soft-tissue and bony injuries, such as rib fractures, due to incomplete ossification of their bones and fragile tissues. The CCTP should be aware of this vulnerability when administering cardiopulmonary resuscitation.
- Risks for complications in neonates increase as birth weight and gestational age decrease. Complications such as maternal infection, diabetes, premature labor, and the presence of meconium also increase these risks. The CCTP should be familiar with antepartum and intrapartum risk factors.
- The Apgar score is a numeric expression of an infant's condition after birth. It measures the infant's appearance, pulse, grimace, activity, and respiration. The score is affected by the infant's physical maturity, maternal medication intake or narcotic use, and neuromuscular or cardiorespiratory conditions.
- The first steps in stabilizing a neonate with an acute airway obstruction, ineffective respiration, or insufficient cardiovascular circulation are airway management and ventilation. To optimize oxygenation and ventilation, thoroughly suction the neonate's airway. Continuous positive airway pressure,

ventilations, chest compressions, or volume expansion may be necessary. The CCTP should communicate information such as relevant history, vital signs, and physical exam to the accepting facility as soon as possible.

- General assessment of the neonate includes assessment of appearance, work of breathing, or abnormal breath sounds. Evaluation of circulation includes abnormal skin color or bleeding. Determine whether the condition is life threatening.
- The ABCs of neonatal resuscitation are the same as those applied to adults—airway, breathing, and circulation. The most important and effective action in neonatal resuscitation is getting oxygen into the infant's lungs. Maintenance of normal body temperature is also important.
- As part of the primary assessment, evaluate the airway to determine whether it is patent. Assess cardiovascular and end-organ function. Respiratory problems are a major cause of cardiac arrest in newborns and infants, and prompt recognition and effective management of such issues are fundamental to pediatric life support.
- Familiarity with the length-based, color-coded resuscitation tape allows the CCTP to estimate body weight based on the child's crown-to-heel length. Most neonatal drug doses are based on body weight, and pediatric supplies are organized according to the color-coded, length-based classification scheme.
- Free-flow oxygen, continuous positive airway pressure, oral airways, bag-mask ventilation, or intubation may be required to assist ventilation in a neonate. The CCTP should be familiar with the equipment and procedures associated with each of these interventions.
- Chest compressions and resuscitation may be necessary if the infant's heart rate remains less than 60 beats/min despite other interventions. Chest compressions should be performed using the two-thumbs, encircling-hands

Prep Kit Continued

technique; if this method is not possible, providers may use the two-finger technique.

- Medications are rarely used to resuscitate neonates, but the CCTP should be familiar with the medications that may be administered for this purpose.
- Fluid resuscitation may be required if the infant is hypovolemic. A low umbilical vein is used for this purpose in a newborn; a peripheral IV or intraosseous line is placed in an infant more than a few days old.
- Neonatal transport incubators are typically fitted with a ventilator that provides synchronized intermittent mandatory ventilation. In some areas, high-frequency ventilators are available, as well as the ability to initiate and transport infants on a nitric oxide or extracorporeal membrane oxygenation circuit. CCTPs should be familiar with the technology available in their areas.
- Two types of apnea can occur: primary and secondary. Primary apnea responds to stimulation and supplemental oxygen. Secondary apnea does not respond to stimulation and supplemental oxygen; instead, ventilation is necessary and, if delayed, can lead to further complications.
- If the infant inhales meconium-stained amniotic fluid in utero or at delivery, the airways can become plugged and hypoxia can follow. Meconium aspiration syndrome is the respiratory distress caused by meconium aspiration.
- Tracheal intubation and aspiration with a meconium aspirator are no longer recommended when meconium is present in the amniotic fluid of a depressed newborn at birth. During transport, the CCTP should monitor the infant for complications of meconium aspiration syndrome and be prepared to perform a needle thoracentesis for pneumothorax decompression if necessary.
- Neonates are at increased risk for pneumonia. Premature infants, especially those less

than 32 weeks' gestation, are at high risk for developing respiratory distress syndrome (RDS). Male infants and infants of mothers with diabetes are at increased risk of RDS.

- Providers experienced in the delivery of exogenous surfactant may administer this medication to the infant with RDS in a controlled clinical setting. During transport, following administration of exogenous surfactant, the CCTP needs to monitor the infant for improved compliance and the potential need to decrease respiratory support.
- In infants with mild RDS, continuous positive airway pressure can be helpful to minimize alveolar collapse during transport.
- A sepsis workup should be performed prior to transport because pneumonia is indistinguishable from RDS in a newborn.
- Simple pneumothorax causes lung collapse; tension pneumothorax is a life-threatening condition. Management of pneumothorax includes transillumination, thoracentesis, and possible intubation. If a symptomatic pneumothorax is suspected, a needle thoracentesis can be lifesaving.
- Critically ill neonates often have a mix of metabolic and respiratory acidosis. Respiratory acidosis often responds to assisted ventilation.
- Cyanosis is caused by decreased arterial oxygenation, which may have either a cardiac or a noncardiac origin. Acrocyanosis is a benign, common condition.
- Cyanotic congenital heart disease (CHD) is caused by developmental anomalies of the heart or major vessels leading to abnormal blood flow. The CCTP may perform tests for CHD ranging from a complete blood count to a hyperoxia test to monitor the infant's condition and determine the appropriate course of action.
- Sinus tachycardia is a heart rate faster than the norm for the child's age. Common pathologic causes of tachycardia include tissue hypoxia,

Prep Kit Continued

- hypovolemia, fever, metabolic stress, pain, anxiety, drugs, and anemia.
- Supraventricular tachycardia is an abnormally fast cardiac rhythm. To manage it, emergency interventions such as vagal maneuvers, cardioversion, and pharmacologic interventions should be performed under appropriate supervision.
- Bradycardia in a neonate is usually a result of tissue hypoxia and resolves when tissue oxygenation is restored. After the neonate's delivery, cardiac pacing may need to be initiated, but is usually nonurgent care.
- Cardiac arrest is uncommon in children. In this age group, it is typically caused by progression of respiratory distress, respiratory failure, or shock typically associated with hypoxemia and acidosis, rather than by cardiac arrhythmias.
- Persistent pulmonary hypertension (PPHN) is persistence of elevated pressures in pulmonary vasculature after birth. Meconium aspiration is the most common cause of PPHN. Care for an infant with PPHN includes optimizing oxygenation, minimizing stress, maintaining a normal BP, and avoiding or correcting acidosis.
- Shock is a serious condition that can affect all organ systems. If emergent access is necessary to provide fluids in case of shock, an umbilical vein line can be placed in a newborn, or an intraosseous line can be placed in an infant older than 1 week.
- Anemia is defined as a hematocrit value of less than 38% in preterm neonates and less than 42% in term neonates. A neonate with anemia may be asymptomatic or present with signs and symptoms, including tachycardia, jaundice, heart failure, and shock.
- Management of anemia includes managing the ABCs and obtaining IV access (optimally via two sites). Treatment may include volume resuscitation with a normal saline bolus, followed by blood if the infant is in shock, or packed red blood cells and fresh-frozen plasma if coagulopathy is suspected.

- Physiologic jaundice is common in neonates and is due to immature liver conjugation. Jaundice in the first 24 hours after birth reflects a pathogenic process and must be investigated.
- Pathologic jaundice requires investigation, close monitoring, and treatment to prevent irreversible neurologic damage. Laboratory investigations include fractionated bilirubin, blood type, direct antiglobin (Coombs) test, hemoglobin level, and peripheral smear. Other tests may be indicated based on family history, the clinical course, and the results of the physical exam.
- Therapeutic options for hyperbilirubinemia include phototherapy, IV immunoglobulin, and exchange transfusion.
- Any part of the gastrointestinal tract may be affected by congenital anomalies. Bilious vomiting is considered an indication of an obstruction until proven otherwise; passage of meconium does not rule out an obstructed bowel. An obstructed bowel can lead to perforation and peritonitis.
- Gastroschisis is a centrally located, full-thickness abdominal wall defect; it is usually an isolated defect. Omphalocele is a herniation of abdominal contents into the umbilical cord; it is often associated with congenital defects, CHD, and other anomalies.
- If an infant with gastroschisis or omphalocele is born at a remote facility, rapid transport must be provided to a facility with a neonatal intensive care unit and pediatric surgery. Precautions must be taken to cover and protect the exposed abdominal contents and to prevent infection.
- The presence of bile in the neonate's vomit must be treated as a surgical emergency until obstruction, especially malrotation, has been ruled out. The CCTP should know the signs and symptoms of esophageal atresia, proximal intestinal obstruction, distal intestinal obstruction, imperforate anus, and Hirschsprung disease. During transport

- of neonates with any of these conditions, maintain thermoregulation of the neonate and monitor vital signs closely.
- Obstructed bowel, necrotizing enterocolitis, and iatrogenic perforation can cause perforation of the bowel. Infants with acute intestinal perforation are at high risk of shock and severe metabolic acidosis secondary to inflammation and vascular leak. Hematemesis can occur with several conditions, including volvulus. Intestinal volvulus, which can be fatal, is a surgical emergency.
- Intussusception is the most common cause of intestinal obstruction in children between 3 months and 6 years of age. Intussusception may be reduced by enema, but frequently needs open reduction.
- Diarrhea in a neonate is unusual. In such a case, maintain fluids during transport, monitor vital signs, and maintain normothermia.
- Neonates are susceptible to becoming compromised by serious infectious diseases because their immune systems are not fully developed. The infant's condition can deteriorate rapidly in such a case. The CCTP must monitor vital signs and maintain normothermia while transferring the patient to a center that can care for a critically ill neonate.
- Hyperthermia is usually caused by overbundling or exposure to excessive heat. It is also seen with herpes simplex infection.
- Hypothermia is more common during the winter months. It can lead to thermal shock, disseminated intravascular coagulopathy, and death in serious cases. Once the patient's condition is stabilized, place the infant in a prewarmed incubator or cover the infant with warm blankets for transport.
- The most important principle in managing toxic exposure/ingestion is to stabilize the neonate. Be sure to obtain a history from the sending facility. Contact the local Poison Control Center for expert guidance in managing exposure to toxins.

- Most birth traumas are self-limiting and have a favorable outcome. Birth injuries can result from prolonged labor, breech presentation, and extreme prematurity, among other causes.
- Head and neck injuries include vacuum caput and caput succedaneum, which are benign, and serious head injuries such as subgaleal hematoma and cephalohematoma. Nerve injuries often occur because of hyperextension or overstretching during delivery, especially with breech presentation. Recurrent laryngeal nerve injury requires immediate attention and transfer of the neonate to a facility that can provide a high level of care.
- Vaginal breech delivery is the greatest risk factor for spinal cord injury.
- The clavicle is the most common site of fracture seen in newborns. A fractured clavicle will heal itself within 7 to 10 days, as long as the motion of the arm is limited. Pneumothorax is a rare complication of fractured clavicle. Soft-tissue injuries mostly need routine care.
- Shaken baby syndrome is the most common cause of death in cases of child abuse. Other types of maltreatment include blunt trauma to the abdomen, burns, bruising, and skeletal injuries.
- It is important to be able to distinguish between seizures and jitteriness in the neonate. Seizures are usually a sign of a serious underlying abnormality; jitteriness is characteristically a disorder of the newborn and is rarely seen at a later age.
- Hypoxic ischemic encephalopathy (HIE), caused by oxygen deprivation or decreased perfusion to the brain, is the most common cause of seizures in term and preterm infants. Multiple-organ dysfunction is common after HIE and may affect the outcome for the infant. Hyperthermia has been associated with a worse outcome for the infant with HIE.
- Lethargy is almost always a sign of a serious, frequently life-threatening underlying condition.

Prep Kit Continued

- Management of metabolic acidosis includes managing the ABCs; providing adequate oxygenation, ventilation, and hydration; and treating the underlying cause. Treatment may include administering IV dextrose and sodium bicarbonate.
- Hypoglycemia is a medical emergency that can lead to brain damage and even death in severe cases. Signs of hypoglycemia include decreased activity, jitteriness, and seizures.
- Hypocalcemia is most commonly seen in low-birth-weight infants and can occur after significant stress, as well as in infants of mothers with diabetes. Significant hypocalcemia can lead to cardiac arrhythmias, seizures, and tetany.
- An infant with congenital adrenal hyperplasia may present with dehydration and shock. Acute treatment includes normalizing electrolytes and fluid balance, and hydrocortisone replacement after consultation with the supervising physician.

- Transport of a high-risk neonate proceeds through a series of well-organized, established steps. Awareness of local and state guidelines is important, as is communication among the members of the transport team, the referring facility, and the receiving facility.
- An incubator is a box with clear walls, a heat source, and portal access, in which a neonate can be placed to maintain normothermia and minimize noise stress. An incubator is indicated for transport of infants who weigh less than 10 pounds (5 kg) or are younger than 30 days.
- Communicating with family members regarding what is being done for the infant and a time frame in which they can expect to speak to someone at the receiving facility is helpful in allaying their fears.
- The CCTP must be prepared to manage the challenges presented by different modes of air transport. Airway, circulation, oxygenation, and temperature regulation are foremost among those challenges.

Vital Vocabulary

acrocyanosis A decrease in the amount of oxygen delivered to the extremities. The hands and feet turn blue because of the lack of oxygen.

Apgar score A scoring system for assessing the status of a newborn that assigns a numerical value to five areas of assessment (the total possible score range is 0 to 10).

apnea Respiratory pause greater than or equal to 20 seconds.

atresia Complete absence of a lumen.

caput succedaneum In the newborn, a subcutaneous collection of fluid with poorly defined margins within the scalp, resulting from pressure on the head during delivery.

central cyanosis Blue coloration of the skin caused by the presence of deoxygenated hemoglobin in blood vessels near the skin surface.

cephalohematoma A subperiosteal collection of blood; it may be accompanied by a linear skull fracture.

choanal atresia A congenital narrowing or blockage of the nasal airway by membranous or bony tissue.

congenital adrenal hyperplasia A group of diseases in which the adrenal glands do not function properly and as a result do not produce a sufficient amount of the hormone cortisol.

Coombs test A test used to identify antibodies that may bind to red blood cells and cause hemolysis.

cyanosis Blue discoloration of the gums and face.

cyanotic congenital heart disease (CCHD) Heart disease caused by developmental anomalies of

Prep Kit Continued

the heart or major vessels (truncus arteriosus, transposition of the great vessels, tetralogy of Fallot, tricuspid atresia, or total anomalous pulmonary venous return) leading to abnormal blood flow. Deoxygenated blood from the right side of the heart is shunted to the left side, causing cyanosis.

diaphragmatic hernia Passage of loops of bowel, with or without other abdominal organs, through the diaphragm muscle; it occurs as the bowel from the abdomen herniates upward through the diaphragm into the chest (thoracic) cavity.

distal intestinal obstruction Partial or complete obstruction of the distal small bowel (ileum) or large intestine.

esophageal atresia A congenital defect, often associated with other anomalies such as tracheoesophageal fistula, in which the esophagus ends in a blind pouch.

gastroschisis A centrally located, full-thickness abdominal wall defect.

gestation Period of time from conception to birth. For humans, the full period is normally 9 months (or 40 weeks).

Hirschsprung disease A congenital lack of ganglion nerve cells in a portion of the distal intestines leading to poor intestinal peristalsis, constipation, and, if not diagnosed and treated, potentially death.

hyperbilirubinemia A condition commonly seen in the newborn, in which an excess of bilirubin develops in the blood; often leads to jaundice.

hypotonia Low or poor (floppy) muscle tone.

hypoxic ischemic encephalopathy (HIE) Damage to cells in the central nervous system (the brain and spinal cord) from inadequate oxygen.

imperforate anus A congenital condition in which the anal opening is either absent or displaced.

inborn error of metabolism A class of genetic diseases mostly caused by defects in single genes that code for enzymes that facilitate conversion of various substances into others; such defects lead to accumulation of substances that are toxic or interfere with normal function.

incubator An enclosed, clear plastic, heated bed that keeps the infant warm.

intussusception An event in which one part of the intestine telescopes into another part of the intestines, leading to a blockage.

jaundice The deposition of bile pigments in the skin; associated with hyperbilirubinemia.

malrotation A congenital anomaly of rotation of the midgut, in which the small bowel is found predominantly on the right side of the abdomen.

meconium A dark green fecal material that accumulates in the fetal intestines and is discharged around the time of birth.

meconium aspiration syndrome The respiratory distress caused by meconium aspiration, which can lead to atelectasis in the lungs, persistent pulmonary hypertension (delayed transition from fetal to neonatal circulation), pneumonitis, and pneumothorax.

necrotizing enterocolitis (NEC) A disorder seen predominantly in premature infants in which the bowel experiences necrosis (tissue death).

neonate An infant during the first 28 days after birth.

neutral thermal environment The temperature at which maintenance of normal body temperature requires only minimal metabolic expenditure.

newborn An infant within the first few hours after birth.

oligohydramnios Decreased volume of amniotic fluid during a pregnancy; a risk factor associated with abnormalities of the urinary tract, postmaturity (birth after a prolonged pregnancy), and intrauterine growth retardation.

omphalocele Herniation of abdominal contents into the base of the umbilical cord.

oxygen hood A tent that is placed over the head of an infant for the purpose of delivering supplemental oxygen.

Prep Kit Continued

patent ductus arteriosus A condition in which the ductus arteriosus, which assists in fetal circulation, does not transition as it should after birth to become the ligamentum arteriosum. The result is that the connection between the pulmonary artery and the aorta remains open, allowing some oxygenated blood to move back into the heart rather than all of it moving out of the aorta and into the systemic circulation.

peripheral blood smear A glass slide containing a drop of blood that can be used to microscopically examine the structure of the blood cells.

persistent pulmonary hypertension (PPHN) The persistence of elevated pressures in the pulmonary vasculature after birth, associated with failure to transition from the fetal circulation to the postpartum or normal newborn circulation.

Pierre Robin syndrome A condition present at birth marked by a very small lower jaw (micrognathia) and a cleft palate; the tongue tends to fall back and downward (glossoptosis).

pneumatosis intestinalis Air in the bowel wall as demonstrated by abdominal radiograph.

pneumothorax A collection of gas in the pleural space which causes lung collapse.

polyhydramnios An excessive amount of amniotic fluid that may cause preterm labor.

primary apnea The initial response to asphyxia at birth that responds to stimulation and oxygen therapy; it is characterized by decreased respiratory effort and a slightly decreased heart rate. If not addressed, the infant will progress to secondary apnea.

proximal intestinal obstruction Obstruction at or above the level of the jejunum.

Replogle tube A double-lumen tube used for gastric decompression in infants with gastrointestinal issues. An 8F size is typically used for an infant and is connected to low intermittent wall suction to collect gastric secretions.

sclerema Hardening of the skin associated with reddening and edema.

secondary apnea The response if asphyxia at birth continues, which is characterized by a period of gasping respirations, decreasing heart rate, and decreasing blood pressure; it does not respond to stimulation unless resuscitation is initiated immediately.

seizure A paroxysmal alteration in neurologic function (ie, behavioral and/or autonomic function).

sinus tachycardia A heart rate that is faster than normal for the patient's age.

sulcus sign A deep lateral costophrenic angle on a chest radiograph, which is associated with pneumothorax.

supraventricular tachycardia (SVT) An abnormally fast rhythm originating above the ventricles.

surfactant A substance formed in the lungs that helps keep the small air sacs or alveoli from collapsing and sticking together; a low level of this substance in a premature infant contributes to respiratory distress syndrome.

term newborn An infant born between 37 and 42 weeks' gestation.

TORCH screen A set of lab values taken to detect congenital infections, including toxoplasma immunoglobulin G and immunoglobulin M (1:1,024), rubella titers, urine cytomegalovirus titer, viral culture (for herpes), and culture of scrapings from any vesicular lesions.

total anomalous pulmonary venous return A condition in which oxygenated blood returns to the right side of the heart, leading to progressive pulmonary edema.

transient tachypnea of the newborn Transient respiratory distress that lasts a few hours in the newborn and occurs secondary to retained fetal lung fluid.

vacuum caput In a newborn, an accumulation of fluid at the site where a vacuum extractor was used to assist in delivering the newborn.

Prep Kit Continued

VATER syndrome A syndrome consisting of multiple birth defects: vertebral anomalies, anal atresia, tracheoesophageal fistula and/or esophageal atresia, and renal and radial anomalies.

volvulus Twisting of the stomach or intestine, which often has the effect of cutting off its blood supply.

Wolff-Parkinson-White syndrome A type of heart disease in which ventricular preexcitation produces a delta wave on electrocardiogram. It is one of the conditions that produces supraventricular tachycardia via an accessory pathway.

References

American Academy of Medicine, American Heart Association. *Pediatric Advanced Life Support*. Dallas, TX: American Heart Association; 2020.

American Academy of Pediatrics, American Heart Association. *Textbook of Neonatal Resuscitation*. 8th ed. Dallas, TX: American Heart Association; 2021.

American Academy of Pediatrics, Committee on Fetus and Newborn, American College of Obstetricians and Gynecologists, Committee on Obstetric Practice. Policy statement: the Apgar score. *Pediatrics*. 2006;117:1444-1447.

American Academy of Pediatrics, Subcommittee on Hyperbilirubinemia. Management of hyperbilirubinemia in the newborn infant 35 or more weeks of gestation. *Pediatrics*. 2004;114(1):297-316.

Aziz K, Lee HC, Escobedo MB, et al. Part 5: neonatal resuscitation: 2020 American Heart Association guidelines for cardiopulmonary resuscitation and emergency cardiovascular care. *Circulation*. 2020;142(16 suppl 2):S524-S550.

Bhutani VK, Johnson LH, Keren R. Diagnosis and management of hyperbilirubinemia in the term neonate: for a safer first week. *Pediatr Clin North Am*. 2004;51:843-861.

Colletti JE, Kothari S, Jackson DM, Kilgore KP, Barringer K. An emergency medicine approach to neonatal hyperbilirubinemia. *Emerg Med Clin North Am*. 2007;25:1117-1135.

Crain EF, Gershel JC. *Clinical Manual of Emergency Pediatrics*. 6th ed. New York, NY: McGraw-Hill Professional Publishing; 2018.

Davis PG, Tan A, O'Donnell CP, et al. Resuscitation of newborn infants with 100% oxygen or air: a systematic review and meta-analysis. *Lancet*. 2004;364:1329-1333.

Jaimovich DG, Vidyasagar D. *Handbook of Pediatric and Neonatal Transport Medicine*. 2nd ed. Philadelphia, PA: Hanley and Belfus; 2002.

Laroia N. Birth trauma. Medscape website. https://emedicine.medscape.com/article/980112-overview. Updated December 17, 2017. Accessed February 3, 2021.

MacDonald MG, Seshi MMK, Mullett MD, eds. *Avery's Neonatology: Pathophysiology and Management of the Newborn*. 7th ed. Philadelphia, PA: Lippincott, Williams and Wilkins; 2015.

Macononchie IK, Aickin R, Hazinski MF, et al. Pediatric life support: 2020 international consensus on cardiopulmonary resuscitation and emergency cardiovascular care science with treatment recommendations. *Circulation*. 2020;142(16 suppl 1):S140-S184.

Maisels MJ, Kring E. Length of stay, jaundice, and hospital readmission. *Pediatrics*. 1998;101:995-998.

Martin R, Fanaroff A, Walsh M. *Fanaroff and Martin's Neonatal Perinatal Medicine: Diseases of the Fetus and Infant*. 11th ed. St Louis, MO: Mosby; 2019.

Newman TB, Xiong B, Gonzales VM, Escobar GJ. Prediction and prevention of extreme hyperbilirubinemia in a mature health maintenance organization. *Arch Pediatr Adolesc Med*. 2000;154:1140-1147.

Pan DH, Rivas Y. Jaundice: newborn to age 2 months. *Pediatr Rev*. 2017;38(11):499-510.

Rabi Y, Rabi D, Yee W. Room air resuscitation of the depressed newborn: a systematic review and meta-analysis. *Resuscitation*. 2007;72:353-363.

Saugstad OD, Ramji S, Soll RF, Vento M. Resuscitation of newborn infants with 21% or 100% oxygen: an updated systematic review and meta-analysis. *Neonatology*. 2008;94(3):176-182.

Taeusch WH, Ballard RA, Gleason CA. *Avery's Diseases of the Newborn*. 8th ed. Philadelphia, PA: WB Saunders; 2004.

Volpe JJ. *Neurology of the Newborn*. 6th ed. Philadelphia, PA: WB Saunders; 2017.

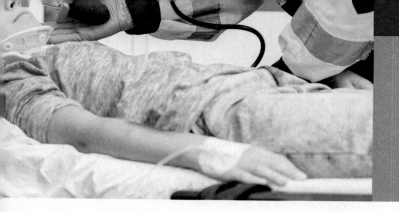

Chapter 24

Pediatric Emergencies

Matthew Harris, MD, FAAP, FAEMS

OBJECTIVES

After completing this chapter, you will be able to:

1. Explain the anatomic and physiologic differences between adult and pediatric patients (p 1294).
2. Explain the physical and psychosocial growth and development of children (pp 1299–1300).
3. Outline the differences in the general approach to critical care transport patient assessment of adult and pediatric patients (p 1300).
4. Discuss the indications, dosage, and route of administration for medication administration in pediatric patients in the critical care transport environment (p 1312).
5. Describe which special pediatric equipment may be needed in a critical care transport (p 1313).
6. Discuss interfacility transport considerations relating to pediatric critical care transport (p 1313).
7. Explain considerations when parents and caregivers accompany pediatric patients during a transport (p 1314).
8. Explain some of the common medical emergencies in the pediatric population, including their assessment and management in the critical care transport environment (pp 1310–1316).
9. Explain common pediatric trauma emergencies, including their assessment and management in the critical care transport environment (pp 1337–1338).
10. Describe the common invasive and noninvasive methods of assisting ventilation in the pediatric patient during transport (pp 1324–1325).
11. Explain critical care transport considerations for a pediatric patient with suspected abuse or neglect (p 1345).
12. Explain critical care transport considerations for a pediatric patient with hypothermia (p 1346).
13. Explain critical care transport considerations for a pediatric patient who has experienced drowning (p 1347).

Introduction

Interfacility transport of the critically ill or injured child can be challenging in many ways for critical care transport professionals (CCTPs). They may have limited clinical exposure to high-risk pediatric patients, with few opportunities to perform advanced procedures for this unique group; moreover, they may feel cognitive distress while caring for these patients. To care for pediatric patients, CCTPs must understand how they differ physiologically, anatomically, and psychosocially from adult patients, and must remain mindful of the important mantra that "Kids aren't just small adults." In fact, the unique physiology and anatomy of children make them vulnerable to pathologies that are distinct from those seen in adults, and the CCTP's ability to recognize sometimes subtle hints of decompensation is paramount in safely treating and transporting these patients.

This chapter addresses some of the special considerations that will enhance the CCTP's effectiveness in caring for ill or injured children in the critical care transport (CCT) environment. It discusses the special needs of children, the most common reasons for pediatric CCT, and CCT management for pediatric emergencies.

Anatomy and Physiology
Cardiovascular System

Outside the neonatal period, and absent known anomalies, the basic anatomy of the circulatory system in children is the same as that in adults. An important distinction, however, is the recognition that normal vital signs vary by age and condition. Parameters for pediatric vital signs are presented in **TABLE 24-1**.

Vital signs must be considered in the context of the clinical setting. A febrile child may have a heart rate and respiratory rate well outside the normal range, but resulting directly from the fever. Anxiety, crying, and pain can also markedly affect vital signs. Important physiologic phenomena in children are their significant physiologic reserves and healthy vascular tone. Children facing physiologic stressors (eg, sepsis, acute blood loss) will maintain a normal cardiac output (determined by the heart rate multiplied by stroke volume) by increasing their heart rate significantly. This means of compensation is supported by a robust catecholamine reserve; once this reserve is exhausted, acute cardiovascular collapse occurs. The clinical implications of this process are important. Adult patients deteriorate in a predictable fashion, with tachycardia, followed by hypotension, and eventually cardiovascular collapse. Children will maintain a normal blood pressure (BP) late into shock, and the presence of hypotension signals imminent and often irreversible decompensation **FIGURE 24-1**.

Respiratory System

The respiratory system in children has a number of important physiologic and anatomic differences from an adult's. Central regulation of respirations is immature in infants, which may result in an irregular

TABLE 24-1 Normal Pediatric Vital Signs	
Age[a]	**Respiratory Rate (breaths/min)**
Infant	30–53
Toddler	22–37
Preschooler	20–28
School-age child	18–25
Adolescent	12–20
	Responsive Pulse Rate (beats/min)
Infant	100–180
Toddler	96–140
Preschooler	80–120
School-age child	75–118
Adolescent	60–100
	Systolic Blood Pressure Ranges (mm Hg)
Infant	72–104
Toddler	86–106
Preschooler	89–112
School-age child	97–115
Preadolescent[b]	102–120
Adolescent	110–131

Note: Values for neonates are provided in Chapter 23, *Neonatal Emergencies*.

[a]Age categories may vary across sources and depending on the value being measured. In general, infant is 1 month to 1 year, toddler is 1 to 2 years, preschooler is 3 to 5 years, school-age child is 6 to 12 years, and adolescent is 12 to 18 years.
[b]The preadolescent category is included for blood pressure values. It includes children ages 10 to 12 years, who are normally included in the school-age category.

Data from The American Heart Association. *Pediatric Advanced Life Support.* 2012.

respiratory pattern, which may or may not be pathologic. Irregular respiratory patterns are especially likely in infants, those born prematurely, and those who sustained perinatal neurologic insults. Children achieve a more regular respiratory rate, depth, and pattern as they approach 1 year of life. Young children are obligate nose breathers, which facilitates breathing while feeding. As such, anatomic abnormalities such as choanal atresia (blockage of the nasal airway

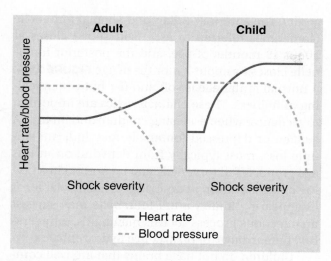

FIGURE 24-1 Blood pressure will not decline in children until they are in the late stages of shock. As cardiac output decreases, vascular resistance increases to maintain the blood pressure. Children do not become hypotensive until they lose a significant percentage of circulating blood volume.

© Jones & Bartlett Learning.

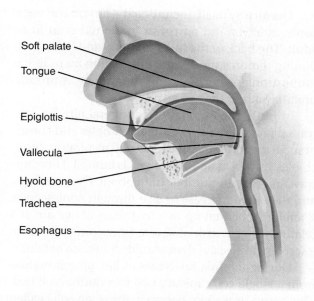

FIGURE 24-2 The child's epiglottis and surrounding structures.

© Jones & Bartlett Learning.

by tissue), as well as more benign pathologies such as nasal congestion or rhinorrhea, can lead to significant respiratory distress in young infants.

When assessing a child's airway, the CCTP should consider a number of important anatomic characteristics. As compared to adults, children have a relatively large tongue relative to the size of the oropharyngeal space. In infants and toddlers, the epiglottis is long, floppy, and narrow and tends to extend over the glottis opening more so than in adults **FIGURE 24-2**. The vocal cords are thin and angled, relatively deeper in the larynx, and more anterior than in adult patients. The narrowest part of the young child's airway is the cricoid ring, which provides a degree of anatomic subglottic stenosis. The effects of these airway differences on airway management are discussed later in the chapter.

The larynx, trachea, and bronchial tree are smaller and less rigid in children than in adults and are therefore more susceptible to obstruction and collapse **FIGURE 24-3**. Smaller airways cause greater resistance to airflow. The airway grows as the child grows, so it is logical that any disease causing narrowing of the airways, such as croup, will be more serious in younger children than in adolescents. The mucosa is less adherent to the airway in younger children and more likely to experience edema, which contributes to increased airway resistance.

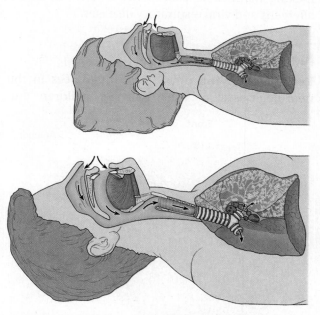

FIGURE 24-3 The anatomy of a child's airway differs in several ways compared with an adult's airway. The tongue is larger and more prominent than in most adult patients. In young children, the glottis is considerably more anterior than in older children or adult patients. There is an anatomic subglottic narrowing in young children, which resolves with growth. The trachea is smaller in diameter and more flexible. The back of the head is larger, and head positioning requires more care.

© Jones & Bartlett Learning.

The airway itself, including the larynx and vocal cords, is lower and narrower in a child than in an adult. The back of the head is larger, and head positioning requires more care. Finally, the mandible is proportionately smaller and the tongue is proportionately larger than in an adult.

At birth, the number of peripheral airways (airways that are less than 2 mm in diameter and consist of small membranous, terminal and respiratory bronchioles, as well as alveolar ducts) is limited. These airways increase in number until about 7 years of age, and they then increase in size through adolescence. Therefore, children up to 3 to 4 years of age are at a relatively higher risk of severe symptoms related to lower airway disease than are older children or adults.

During the first few years of life, alveoli mature from a single cell capillary bed to a double cell bed. The communication between these alveoli, called collateral ventilation, then increases. Because children may not be able to ventilate airways distal to an obstruction, they may be at a higher risk for experiencing **atelectasis** (complete or partial lung collapse).

Finally, infants have highly reactive airways, making them more susceptible to environmental allergens and viral respiratory diseases.

Neurologic System

Key anatomic and physiologic differences in the neurologic system exist between children and adults. The anterior or diamond-shaped fontanelle (sometimes referred to as a "soft spot") closes at about 18 months of age, and the posterior fontanelle closes by about 2 months of age **FIGURE 24-4**. A normal fontanelle is soft and flat but with a feeling of fullness. These characteristics are important to recognize when assessing children and infants. A sunken or depressed fontanelle may indicate volume loss, most typically from dehydration in this age group. A full fontanelle can be normal in a crying child. However, in an irritable, inconsolable, or ill-appearing infant, a full fontanelle may suggest an infectious process such as meningitis, intracerebral hemorrhage, or obstructive hydrocephalus.

Children do not have brains that are well compartmentalized, which means their brains have more room to move around within the skull. As a consequence, children are more susceptible to brain injuries, such as diffuse axonal injuries.

CCTPs may encounter children during transfers to a neonatal intensive care unit (NICU). Perinatal birth injuries may be noted during evaluation of the infant's head. For example, a newborn may be born with a **cephalohematoma**, a collection of blood between the bone and subperiosteal space. Although this condition is infrequently seen by the CCTP, it occurs in 1% to 2% of all live births that involve mechanical trauma (forceps or vacuum-assisted delivery). This type of hematoma can occur anywhere on the skull but is found more predominantly in

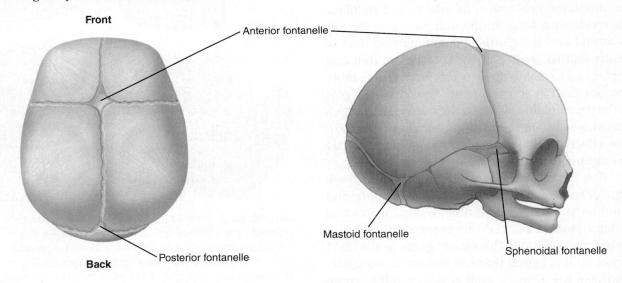

FIGURE 24-4 The fontanelles. **A.** Superior view. **B.** Lateral view.

the parietal region of the skull. The hematoma usually resolves in 6 to 8 weeks, and can be associated with linear skull fractures (in 10% to 25% of infants). The CCTP should note the size of the hematoma during the initial assessment and during transport. The swelling does not cross the suture line and may increase in size after birth. Conversely, caput succedaneum is merely soft-tissue swelling that usually resolves within 24 hours.

Musculoskeletal System

Several differences exist between the musculoskeletal system of a child and that of an adult. First, children have fewer calcified bones. The immature bones of children are more porous than those of adults and tend to respond to kinetic forces by buckling rather than fracturing. Nevertheless, children do sustain fractures, which often have a morphology distinct from that of the fractures sustained by adult patients. Unique to children, fractures that involve the growth plate (known as Salter-Harris fractures) can affect growth and, when left unmanaged, can result in limb length discrepancies. These epiphyseal–metaphyseal growth plate injuries account for 10% to 15% of fractures in children; however, with reduction and immobilization, most of these injuries have excellent outcomes. Growth plates close in a predictable manner, achieving a mature skeleton in early adolescence.

The ligaments in children are stronger and more resilient to tensile forces, thereby providing strength to the joints. As a result, dislocations are rarely found in pediatric populations compared with adult populations. However, subluxation (partial dislocation) may be seen in infants and toddlers, the classic example being nursemaid's elbow.

The pediatric spine is characterized by incomplete ossification, epiphyseal growth plates, and hypermobility. As a result, the cervical spine in children is highly flexible, such that young children tend to experience ligamentous injuries more frequently than bone fractures. When fractures occur, they are often avulsion fractures, where a small portion of bone is pulled away from the larger portion of the bone. Compression fractures can be seen with high-impact axial loading injuries. Any vertebral fracture should prompt evaluation for concomitant visceral and spinal cord injuries.

Recognizing Unusual Injuries

Vertebral fractures in the very young should raise suspicion for inflicted injury or underlying bone disorders.

Children have relatively large, heavy heads with weak neck muscles, causing the head to lean forward when they fall. As a consequence, pediatric patients are more susceptible to head injuries. Rapid deceleration injuries resulting in hyperflexion and torsion forces are most commonly seen in children.

The child's thorax is pliable, meaning it can withstand greater kinetic forces without fracturing. The chest is surprisingly resilient and can absorb a significant amount of energy compared to the child's size. Rib fractures are uncommon, and should prompt evaluation for internal injuries, especially in small children, where rib fractures are suggestive of child abuse. The pediatric pelvis is more flexible than that of adult patients. Hip laxity in the neonatal period can result in dislocation or subluxation.

Gastrointestinal System

The cardiac sphincter, which is the valve between the esophagus and the stomach, is located above the diaphragm until 6 months of age and does not completely close, which increases the risk for regurgitation. The relatively small stomach capacity combined with poor satiation may potentially result in overfeeding, which further increases the risk of reflux. Children with reflux are at risk of aspiration, though aspiration is less common in term infants and those without neurologic insult. Reflux can present with vomiting, fussiness, and irritability. Sandifer syndrome—that is, arching of the back seen with severe reflux—is often mistaken for a seizure condition.

Because young children eat frequently, the CCTP should obtain a history of recent oral intake. This information can help the CCTP prepare for vomiting that can result from positive-pressure ventilation or endotracheal (ET) intubation.

Liver function is also immature in young children, resulting in fewer glucose stores. As a result, these patients are susceptible to hypoglycemia during periods of poor oral intake or high gastrointestinal or renal losses. Therefore, an essential component of pediatric resuscitation is checking blood glucose levels.

Another key difference between adults and children is that the abdominal muscles are weaker in the younger child, providing less protection to the internal organs. The liver and spleen extend below the costal margin, which renders these organs more susceptible to blunt abdominal trauma.

Renal System

The pediatric renal system has some significant physiologic differences from the adult renal system. Notably, children have a higher percentage of body water compared to adults, making them more susceptible to dehydration. In addition, children are unable to concentrate urine as effectively as adults. They may be more susceptible to electrolyte loss because they have higher clearance rates of blood urea nitrogen (BUN), creatinine, and electrolytes. The minimum urine outputs expected in pediatric patients are as follows:

- Infant: 2 mL/kg/h
- Child: 1 mL/kg/h
- Adult: 0.5 mL/kg/h

Infants younger than 6 months cannot tolerate free water (devoid of electrolytes). Ingesting large volumes of free water in this age group, which can occur when parents dilute baby formula with the aim of making the volume last longer, can lead to life-threatening hyponatremic seizures. Urine output is an important measure of hydration status. A key component of the patient history is the number of wet diapers in the past 12 to 24 hours. Many infants urinate with each feeding and will produce 10 to 12 diapers per day. Parents often have a good sense of their child's normal urine output.

Thermoregulation

Temperature regulation in infants is not fully developed, making them highly susceptible to hypothermia. Infants have thinner skin and lack a subcutaneous layer of fat. They are unable to shiver and lose heat through the head, which is proportionally larger relative to the body. Low body temperature has numerous manifestations in young children and may be a harbinger of sepsis or hypotension. Young infants' skin may appear mottled and will feel cool to the touch.

Children have a high ratio of body surface area to mass relative to the ratio for adults. This ratio can be advantageous to children when they are exposed to mildly warm environments and during times of intense exercise in mildly cool weather, because they have an increased ability to dissipate heat. However, when this population is exposed to temperature extremes of cold and heat, their ability to dissipate heat can be a disadvantage that leads to environmental emergencies.

Metabolism

The basal metabolic rate is accelerated in the pediatric population, which means children consume glucose and oxygen at a higher rate than adults do. An infant's consumption of oxygen is, in fact, twice that of an adult. In combination with an infant's poor respiratory reserves, this relatively high oxygen demand can lead to earlier hypoxia in response to a respiratory insult. Like the rate of metabolism, the rate of onset of hypercapnia and hypoxemia, with bradypnea, is accelerated in this patient population, warranting close monitoring during transport.

While an epidemic of obesity has been noted in the pediatric population in the United States, children generally have less adipose tissue than adults. Because many emergent medications are lipophilic (eg, propofol), and because children have a higher basal metabolic rate than adults, redosing may be required in the pediatric population.

Glucose Requirements

Infants and small children have decreased glycogen reserves and an immature liver that is not capable of stimulating glycogen release when required due to metabolic stressors. When ill or injured, many children refuse to eat and drink. This refusal, coupled with the additional stress on the body from the illness or injury, can increase the risk for hypoglycemic events. The need to assess and reassess glucose levels is paramount while caring for the critical pediatric patient during a transport.

Pediatric patients with hypoglycemia present with a broad spectrum of symptoms. Newborns and young infants may be asymptomatic or may have nonspecific symptoms ranging from irritability to lethargy, pallor to cyanosis, and tremors to seizures. By comparison, older children will have a more classic presentation that mirrors adult symptoms (anxiety, diaphoresis, tachypnea, and weakness).

The treatment regimen for hypoglycemia varies depending on the patient's weight, age, and clinical status. While it is preferable to resolve hypoglycemia with enteral nutrition, critically ill or injured children should be kept on NPO (*nil per os*, Latin for "nothing by mouth") status during CCT. Children require 0.5 to 1 mg/kg/dose of dextrose when hypoglycemic. When translating this into a milliliter per kilogram dose of dextrose solution, the "rule of 50" is useful. Using this rule, the volume to be administered multiplied by the dextrose content equals 50 (Volume × Dextrose content = 50). For example, volume would be calculated as follows for a patient receiving 10% dextrose (D_{10}):

$$Volume \times 10 = 50$$
$$Volume = 50/10$$
$$Volume = 5 \text{ mL/kg}$$

Thus, a patient receiving D_5 solution would require a 10-mL/kg bolus, and a patient receiving D_{25} is typically administered a 2-mL/kg bolus. Due to the risk of extravasation, D_{50} is typically avoided in children and adults. If the hypoglycemic episode has been corrected prior to the arrival of the CCTP, then a glucose maintenance infusion should be initiated at a rate of 6 to 8 mg/kg/min or per the standing protocol.

Growth and Development

The CCTP will encounter children at various stages of physical and psychosocial development. In some of these patients, the cognitive ability to recognize and cope with the stressor of acute illness or injury will be limited. Having a foundational understanding of developmental stages can enable the CCTP to engage with the child at an appropriate level. Where young infants are incapable of verbalizing their distress, their crying pattern or their responsiveness to their caregivers can provide a great deal of information about their status. In contrast, older children and adolescents may be acutely aware of the seriousness of their ailment and may respond emotionally, such as with anxiety, fear, or anger.

Additionally, CCTPs must be attuned to the needs of these patients' parents. They are also under enormous stress. The intimate moments during transport are an opportunity to bridge the divide that many parents feel with members of the caregiving team who may be only transiently involved in their child's care.

Physical Growth and Development

One extremely important aspect of pediatric care is an understanding of normal growth and development. Failure to meet normal developmental milestones, such as the ability to walk or talk, may be a sign of an underlying illness, a family crisis, or a neurologic injury (ie, a lack of oxygen or blood flow to the brain that may permanently affect the child's ability to reach normal developmental milestones) **TABLE 24-2**. Knowledge of the child's developmental level also helps to guide safety considerations.

Ideally, the CCTP should have an understanding of the child's developmental level prior to assessment so that appropriate comparisons can be made. Parents and other caregivers are the best source for information about how the child will react under normal circumstances. The parent or primary caregiver may be able to tell you the developmental age of the child, which will guide the manner in which you communicate with the child and explain procedures. Communication techniques for children who do not have language skills include using sign language, observing facial expressions, and having the child move their eyes to the right or left or

TABLE 24-2 Developmental Milestones	
Age (months)	**Milestone**
2	Smiling
5	Rolling over
9	Crawling
10	Grasping small objects
12	Walking
24	Talking

© Jones & Bartlett Learning.

blink a specific number of times to indicate yes or no. Remember that parents are likely their child's best advocate and can be a tremendous resource in helping guide the child through the stressors of the CCT process.

Psychosocial Growth and Development

Psychosocial concerns for pediatric patients vary tremendously based on the patient's age:

- An infant's primary fear is often separation from the parents, so efforts should be made to minimize the time of separation.
- Toddlers also fear separation from parents or caregivers, and they fear loss of control. Distracting tools such as toys or electronic devices (eg, a parent's phone) can help alleviate a toddler's stress and allow the CCTP to complete the exam and interventions.
- Preschoolers also fear loss of control, in addition to bodily injury, the dark, and the unknown. Explain your actions clearly and provide plenty of reassurance.
- Like preschoolers, school-age children fear body injury, so simple and concise explanations should be used to describe procedures as ways to help the child.
- Adolescents and teenagers may fear a loss of control or an alteration to their physical appearance. Encourage the adolescent's involvement and respect the adolescent's privacy. Adolescents often demonstrate increased compliance if honest explanations are given and if they are allowed to participate in decision making regarding their health care.

Basic care strategies to address psychosocial concerns span all age groups. Foster trust by addressing the child at eye level, using their first name, and explaining medical procedures using age-appropriate words. Honesty is important, especially regarding painful procedures such as a needlestick. Preschoolers and school-age children fear the unknown. If a procedure will be uncomfortable, prepare the parents and child for this reality, and offer an age-appropriate explanation of how you will attempt to mitigate that discomfort. Encourage a sense of control by offering choices whenever possible, while keeping in mind that bargaining and negotiating may not be possible or appropriate in

some situations. At all times, maintaining a calm and confident demeanor can help reassure both the parent and the child.

Approach to Parents and Caregivers

CCTPs should do a self-assessment to ensure they are prepared—academically, technically, and emotionally—to care for pediatric patients. Children of any age may be seriously ill or injured. CCTPs may become distracted by the emotional response of a child or parent. Be mindful of your own emotions, and watch for signs of increased stress in your CCT partners.

Be sensitive to the fact that the child may not be the only person on scene who will benefit from compassionate care; you should also consider the needs of the parents, guardians, or caregivers. Their responses may include guilt for not preventing or recognizing the illness or injury, frustration related to not being the primary caregiver to the child during hospitalization (loss of parenting role), or helplessness from a perceived inability to protect the child. Parents or other caregivers often feel fearful, out of control, and uninformed, so make an effort to keep them informed and actively involved in health care decisions. This often requires that information be repeated, sometimes on numerous occasions. Whenever possible, provide parents or caregivers with written information and involve them in the plan of care.

Pediatric Assessment

Patient assessment for pediatric patients follows the same basic process as for other patients, as described in Chapter 5, *Patient Assessment*. This process begins on receipt of the referral call. CCTPs should collaborate with their call-intake center to identify the crucial clinical information needed to facilitate interfacility transport, without prolonging time from call receipt to arrival at the patient's bedside.

Your primary survey will include an assessment of the patient's airway, breathing, and circulation, using both your clinical evaluation and the available monitoring technology (eg, pulse oximetry, external or invasive cardiorespiratory monitoring). Any abnormal finding indicates a need for immediate treatment and may require deferral of the next step; for example, if the airway is not patent as the result of an airway obstruction, intervention must be immediate.

Obtaining the patient's weight, age, and vital signs can help you evaluate the patient's acuity and form your care plan. Staff at the receiving facility will determine whether a child is weighed during triage or on arrival to the treatment area. At the facility, the actual (not estimated) weight is measured and reported in kilograms. Estimating a weight or reporting it in pounds can result in drug dosing errors. In the CCT setting, you should obtain the child's weight from the parents or caregivers and use a computerized program or printout to identify resuscitation medications, doses, and equipment used in the child's care. In the prehospital setting, providers may use a tool, such as a length-based resuscitation tape, for estimating the child's weight and selecting appropriate medication doses **FIGURE 24-5**.

All pediatric assessments should begin with a general impression that can be accomplished using the **pediatric assessment triangle (PAT)** **FIGURE 24-6**. The PAT is an assessment tool based on the child's appearance, work of breathing, and circulation. Appearance can be assessed using the **TICLS** (tickles) mnemonic: Tone, Interactiveness, Consolability, Look or gaze, and Speech or cry **TABLE 24-3**. The nature of the child's airway sounds and signs of increased breathing effort characterize the work of breathing. Circulation is assessed by observing the child for pallor, mottling, or cyanosis. By combining the three parameters of the PAT, the CCTP can form a general impression of the child's stability and, in conjunction with the chief complaint, can make decisions regarding the need for acute interventions.

After using the PAT to form a general impression of the patient, perform a primary assessment by evaluating the following items, in this order:

- Airway patency
- Respiratory rate and quality
- Pulse rate and quality
- Skin temperature and capillary refill time
- BP (using age-appropriate equipment)
- Neurologic status

The child's neurologic status can be obtained by forming a general impression and assessing the level of consciousness (LOC) and pupillary reaction. In young infants, an assessment of the patient's suck reflex and axial tone (where appropriate) can often indicate the severity of the child's illness: A poor suck or a decrease in axial tone suggests serious pathology. The neurologic status in older children can be assessed by their ability to interact with the parents or caregivers in an age-appropriate way. Older children should be able to follow commands and answer questions.

All pediatric patients—even the youngest children—should be assessed for pain. The quality of pain can be assessed using a numeric scale for older children and adolescents. Younger children and infants may be assessed using pain scores,

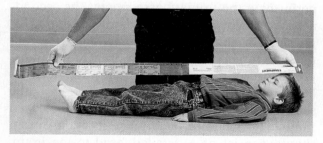

FIGURE 24-5 Using a length-based resuscitation tape helps providers estimate a child's weight and identify the correct size for pediatric equipment and medication doses when an exact weight is not available. Such equipment, due to its limited precision, is not an acceptable tool outside of emergency resuscitation settings.

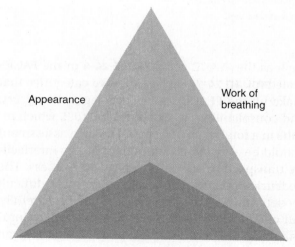

Appearance

Work of breathing

Circulation to skin

FIGURE 24-6 The pediatric assessment triangle.

TABLE 24-3 Characteristics of Appearance: The TICLS Mnemonic

Characteristic	Features
Tone	Is the child moving or resisting examination vigorously? Does the child have good muscle tone? Is the child limp, listless, or flaccid?
Interactiveness	How alert is the child? How readily does a person, object, or sound distract the child or draw the child's attention? Will the child reach for, grasp, and play with a toy or exam instrument, such as a penlight or tongue blade? Is the child uninterested in playing or interacting with the caregiver or CCTP?
Consolability	Can the child be consoled or comforted by the caregiver or the CCTP? Is the child's crying or agitation relieved by gentle reassurance?
Look or gaze	Does the child fix their gaze on a face, or does the child have a blank, glassy-eyed stare?
Speech or cry	Is the child's cry strong and spontaneous or weak and high pitched? Is the content of speech age appropriate or confused or garbled?

© Jones & Bartlett Learning.

TABLE 24-4 FLACC Scale

Category	0	1	2
Face	Disinterested, no expression	Occasional grimace, withdrawn	Frequent frown, clenched jaw
Legs	No position or relaxed	Uneasy, restless, tense	Kicking or legs drawn up
Activity	Normal position, moves easily	Squirming, tense	Arched, rigid, or jerking
Cry	No crying	Moans or whimpers	Cries steadily, screams, or sobs
Consolability	Content, relaxed	Distractible	Inconsolable

Scores add up and range from 0 to 10.

© Jones & Bartlett Learning.

such as the FLACC scale **TABLE 24-4** or the FACES scale **FIGURE 24-7**. Each of the five categories that make up the FLACC scale—face, legs, activity, cry, and consolability—is scored from 0 to 2, which results in a total score of 0 to 10. The pain assessment should be a dynamic component of any interfacility transport: Assess, intervene, and reassess. The pediatric patient's pain level can be more difficult to determine, and analgesia should be carefully, but adequately, dosed. For children who are intubated and sedated, a number of validated tools can be used to assess the depth and appropriateness of sedation.

Although physiologic abnormalities are more likely to be identified by applying the PAT and performing the primary assessment, the secondary assessment may further identify anatomic or physiologic abnormalities. Sometimes it is not possible to perform this exam prior to the transport because the patient is unstable and needs to be transported immediately. In such a case, the secondary assessment should be conducted en route to the receiving facility. The secondary exam should consist of a detailed head-to-toe exam, with a special focus on the body region or system known to be involved in the underlying pathology, but also with the express purpose of identifying other issues that may need to be addressed. Detection of additional injuries is especially important in the trauma setting.

Wong-Baker FACES® Pain Rating Scale

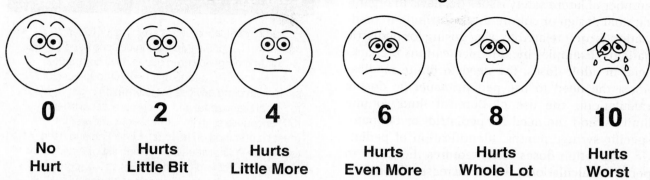

0	2	4	6	8	10
No Hurt	Hurts Little Bit	Hurts Little More	Hurts Even More	Hurts Whole Lot	Hurts Worst

FIGURE 24-7 Pictures such as the Wong-Baker FACES pain rating scale allow for self-assessment of pain in young children.

© 1983 Wong-Baker FACES Foundation. www.WongBakerFACES.org. Used with permission. Originally published in *Whaley & Wong's Nursing Care of Infants and Children*. © Elsevier, Inc.

History

As mentioned previously, the history begins with the initial referral call. While a great deal about the history of the present illness will be obtained during the report from the referring hospital staff, obtaining a baseline history before departure can help the CCT team prepare to care for the child. Once the team is at the bedside, parents or caregivers can provide extensive information regarding the child's history. The history for infants will include the perinatal history, delivery information, gestational age, and gestational weight. A history from the parents is crucial in all pediatric transports, but is especially helpful for chronically ill or technology-dependent children. Many of these children have abnormal vital signs and physical exam findings at baseline; a thorough report from the primary caregiver can help the CCTP to understand the child's acute issue in the context of the underlying medical issues.

Scene or situation information may be useful as well, especially for children with traumatic injuries after a motor vehicle accident where the mechanisms of injury or extent of damage may help providers plan for the child's needs. Scene information is also valuable if there is any concern for nonaccidental trauma or neglect. CCTPs may be able to obtain this type of information from prehospital run sheets or through direct conversation with the responding EMS providers. Information from these sources may include a description of the environment and details about the accident scene, among other important pieces of information. For example, if providers responded to the child's home, they may note that the home was inadequately heated, weapons were visible and within the child's reach, or trash had accumulated on the floor and furniture. If providers responded to a vehicle crash, they may note that the child was buckled into the front passenger seat rather than being properly secured in a car seat in the backseat.

Special Populations

Children with special needs represent a particularly vulnerable group within the pediatric population. Parents and caregivers of these children know their needs well and can contribute significantly to both the history of the present illness and the broader clinical picture. They can describe the child's medications, baseline function, and degree of technology dependence. For example, children with complex congenital heart disease often live in a hypoxic state. It is crucial that the CCTPs obtain this information, as providing too much oxygen to children with complex congenital heart disease can worsen the clinical picture. For children with severe developmental delays, or those who exist on the severe portion of the autism spectrum, parents can describe the child's functional status and suggest ways to support the child during interfacility transport.

Pediatric Medication Delivery

Safely delivering medications to critically ill or injured children is challenging. Nearly all emergent medications are administered as weight-specific doses, and some have age restrictions. There are a number of latent safety issues (ie, flaws in organizational design or culture that contribute to medication errors) related to drug dosing for pediatric patients. Examples include medications prepackaged in adult doses, the need to dilute medications, the need to use pediatric-specific dosing calculations, the use of Buretrol fluid volume limiters, and the need for pediatric- or neonate-specific syringe pumps. Identification of pediatric medication doses often requires the CCTP to perform calculations, which increases the risk of errors. Doses of high-alert medications, such as opioids, heparin, insulin, and potassium chloride, require an independent recheck before they are administered.

Several methods are available for delivery of medications to pediatric patients, including intravenous (IV) push, syringe pump, or infusion pump. Because infusion pumps include safety guards, such as a flow stop, they are routinely used for the administration of fluids and medications. When using a syringe or infusion pump, always follow the manufacturer's recommendations for flushing and maintenance. The best option for administering resuscitation medications is a vascular access device.

A pediatric resource with a formulary may be helpful in determining the amount and type of diluent required for specific medications. The formulary will also list the time frame for administration. Medications used in pediatric CCT are described in Chapter 8, *Critical Care Pharmacology*.

Most children are kept NPO during CCT. It is important to identify any oral medications that the child may be due to receive during transport, as IV alternatives are often available and can be substituted if necessary; for example, oral levetiracetam has an IV equivalent. If children lose vascular access en route, it is important to consider other methods of administration, as obtaining access during transport can be technically challenging. Many opioids and benzodiazepines, as well as naloxone, glucagon, and ketamine, among other drugs, can be administered via the intranasal route (with use of a mucosal atomizer device). This route is well tolerated, with good absorption, and avoids the pain associated with needlesticks en route. Intramuscular and subcutaneous routes can also be used.

Controversies

Pediatric medication errors are a major focus of concern in hospitals. Measuring devices used to calculate emergency drug doses have contributed to errors for hospitalized children. Although use of such measuring devices for estimation is appropriate for initial prehospital and emergency department (ED) encounters, an accurate height and weight must be obtained on hospital admission and used to prepare an individualized dosing list of emergency medications for each child. CCTPs should consider printing a patient-specific medication-dosing document before beginning transport. Using this reference reduces the cognitive stress of performing emergent medical calculations en route. Any medication errors should be reported for evaluation as part of a robust continuous quality improvement initiative for pediatric prehospital medication administration.

Airway

All infants are obligatory nose breathers, meaning they actively breathe through their mouths only if they are crying. Therefore, nasal congestion in an infant can produce significant respiratory distress. Irrigation with normal saline spray and suction with a bulb syringe are often the only interventions necessary to clear the nasal airways. Positioning the infant with the head up at a 30° to 45° angle also aids in keeping the nasal airways clear. Administration of oxygen via a nasal cannula may work well in infants with mild to moderate respiratory distress because a significant amount of tidal volume comes through their noses and they do not tolerate face masks **FIGURE 24-8**.

Anatomic considerations are important when planning airway management. As mentioned earlier, children have relatively large tongues in relation to the size of their mouths. Proper choice of blade size, proper positioning, and effective sweeping of the tongue are essential for successful intubation. It is also common to find large tonsils and copious oral secretions in pediatric patients. In most cases, spending the time to properly prepare the child will make securing the airway faster and easier. This approach prevents the tube from getting caught on the angled vocal cords, which are relatively more anterior compared to those of adults. In young children,

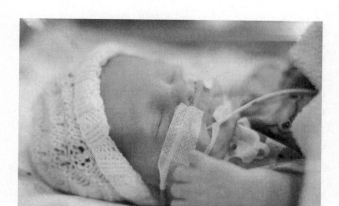

FIGURE 24-8 A nasal cannula may be the most effective way to provide oxygen to an infant in respiratory distress.

© Steve Lovegrove/Shutterstock.

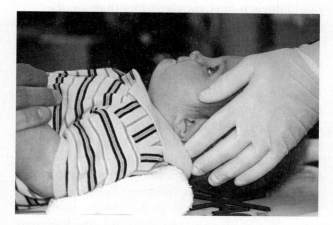

FIGURE 24-9 For an infant who has not sustained traumatic injury, a rolled towel beneath the shoulders helps to maintain the airway in a neutral position.

© American Academy of Orthopaedic Surgeons.

cartilaginous support for the trachea varies, requiring that providers be especially careful not to compress the pediatric upper airway. Further, providers must avoid hyperextending the neck. Placing the noninjured child in the sniffing position with the aid of a rolled towel provides optimal positioning **FIGURE 24-9**.

Patency of the pediatric airway may be compromised for numerous reasons, including congenital anomaly, infections, trauma, edema, foreign body airway obstruction, or loss of airway protective reflexes. Foreign body airway obstruction is a particularly high risk in children younger than 5 years. Diminished protective reflexes may result from any condition that causes a decreased LOC, including infection, trauma, neuromuscular disorder, and toxic ingestion.

Clinical signs of upper airway obstruction are those typical of respiratory distress, including tachypnea, nasal flaring, abnormal respiratory sounds, and the use of accessory muscles (retracting). Symptoms more specific for upper airway obstruction include stridor (a high-pitched, primarily inspiratory sound), snoring, poor control of secretions, and biphasic wheezing. Certain infectious upper airway etiologies, such as a peritonsillar abscess, can also present clinically as drooling, difficulty speaking, and trismus (difficulty opening the mouth).

A child with a decreasing LOC may not be able to protect their airway and may require airway management. The loss of protective reflexes occurs in ascending order: The swallowing reflex is lost first, then coughing, then the gag reflex, and finally the corneal reflex. A useful intubation suggestion is to assess the corneal reflex prior to inserting an oral airway or to assess for paralysis related to neuromuscular blocking agents. A child who does not blink when the open eyelids are stroked no longer has a gag reflex. This strategy avoids the need to test the gag reflex with a tongue blade or a suction catheter, which may cause the child to vomit and thus aspirate.

Breathing

Children with difficulty breathing present with a variety of clinical symptoms, depending in part on the child's age and the disease pathology. During the assessment of breathing, the CCT should assess for the rate and quality of breathing. Early signs of distress may include tachypnea and use of accessory muscles. It is crucial to expose children during the primary assessment to effectively assess their work of breathing. CCTPs should not be reassured by a normal or slow respiratory rate; this presentation may reflect significant fatigue and, therefore, signal the child is approaching respiratory failure. Infants and young children may have nasal flaring or pursed lips on inspection. These signs may be accompanied by grunting, which occurs when the child is trying to exhale against a partially closed glottis. Such a child is making a physiologic attempt to stent open the distal airways to improve oxygenation and ventilation, a process known as auto-PEEP (positive end-expiratory pressure). Because young infants are obligate nose breathers, the CCTP should assess for the presence of a significant nasal mucus burden, which can be a cause of significant respiratory distress.

Children having respiratory difficulties often assume a tripod position **FIGURE 24-10**, which allows the muscles of the anterior chest wall and neck to facilitate more effective ventilation. Respiratory distress rarely improves when the child is in a supine position. Moreover, as the stomach fills with excessive air (aerophagia) secondary to the increased respiratory rate, the child may be at a higher risk of vomiting and subsequent aspiration.

As part of determining the work of breathing, the CCTP may assess for stridor, snoring, retractions, head bobbing, accessory muscle use, tripoding, nasal flaring, wheezing, and grunting. In younger children, the diaphragm is the chief muscle used for ventilation; intercostal and accessory muscles are not fully developed until the child reaches

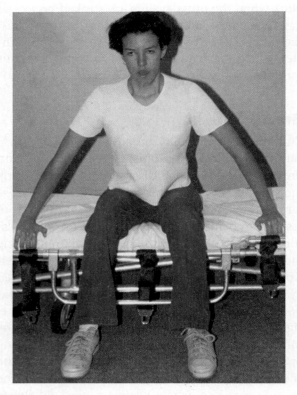

FIGURE 24-10 Children may assume a tripod position to maximize their use of the accessory muscles of respiration.

© American Academy of Orthopaedic Surgeons.

school age. If the diaphragm fails in a young pediatric patient, the child may develop paradoxical breathing. This breathing pattern is best described as a seesaw motion, in which the abdomen and the chest move in opposite directions. As respiratory distress progresses, the respiratory rate may become slower and more irregular. Bradypnea (a slow respiratory rate) is a late sign of respiratory distress and predicts impending respiratory failure. In such a case, immediate interventions are required to prevent complete respiratory and cardiac collapse.

Children have a high metabolic rate and, consequently, a high oxygen demand. Oxygen demand for infants ranges from 6 to 8 mL/kg/min, which is twice that of adults (3 to 4 mL/kg/min). Coupled with their relatively poor reserves, children are at risk of developing hypoxia sooner than adults.

Hemodynamic monitoring (heart rate, pulse oximetry, respiratory rate, and end-tidal capnography) is an important adjunct to the assessment of a child with respiratory distress. However, CCTPs should always couple this information with their findings from the clinical assessment of the child. For example, a child in status asthmaticus for a prolonged period may have a normalization of the respiratory rate during the course of their exacerbation. If the child is speaking more comfortably and is more interactive, this trend is reassuring that treatments are effective. If the child's respiratory rate is decreasing and the child remains lethargic, this may be an ominous sign of impending respiratory failure.

The PAT can be used as a dynamic tool to continuously reevaluate the child's LOC, with particular emphasis being placed on the child's appearance, work of breathing, and circulation. A child with mild to moderate hypoxia may appear agitated and anxious. As the hypoxia progresses and is likely coupled with hypercapnia, the child may become quiet and sleepy. In such a case, do not be falsely reassured that the child is better. Key assessment points include whether the child can maintain and protect the airway. In addition, determine whether the child can maintain the current respiratory effort and determine the likelihood of deterioration en route to the treatment facility. It is imperative for the CCTP to monitor the patient's respiratory rate, pattern, oxygen saturation levels, and electrocardiogram (ECG) waveform for any changes in heart rate (tachycardia or bradycardia) or increased cardiac ectopic foci (premature atrial contraction, premature junctional contraction, or premature ventricular contraction).

Auscultation is the primary tool used to assess the adequacy of a child's respiratory effort. Auscultation begins during the initial assessment, while evaluating for overt signs of respiratory distress. The CCTP should evaluate for grunting, stridor, audible wheezing, and quality of the child's cough (eg, barky, bronchospastic, staccato). Children may exhibit the same adventitious breath sounds as adults, such as fine crackles, coarse crackles, rhonchi, wheezing, or a silent chest. When caring for young children, a common clinical mistake is failure to recognize the presence of transmitted upper airway sounds during auscultation of the chest. CCTPs should auscultate in front of the patient's nose/mouth and neck, progressing downward to the lung exam. The pulmonary exam frequently offers information to guide treatment.

CCTPs should take advantage of the various technological adjuvants that, when coupled with the history and physical exam findings, support the management of critically ill children. Oxygen saturation, as measured by pulse oximetry, and end-tidal carbon dioxide ($ETCO_2$) are ubiquitous measurements in emergency medical services (EMS) practice. Pulse oximetry readings indicate the percentage of hemoglobin molecules that are bound with oxygen, abbreviated SpO_2. As useful as this information is, CCTPs must remember that in some disease states, the SpO_2 value will remain normal even in the presence of significant physiologic abnormalities. A child with profound anemia may have an SpO_2 of 100% because all the hemoglobin molecules are saturated. However, if insufficient hemoglobin molecules are available, the end-organ tissues' needs for oxygen will not be met. Similarly, carbon monoxide poisoning can yield deceptive SpO_2 values. Carbon monoxide's affinity for hemoglobin is greater than oxygen's, so it readily binds to the hemoglobin molecule. Pulse oximeters cannot distinguish between oxyhemoglobin and carboxyhemoglobin, so they will give a falsely normal reading in case of carbon monoxide poisoning. Other factors that can interfere with the reliability of SpO_2 measurements include poor perfusion and coldness of the measured extremity.

Measurement of $ETCO_2$ is the standard of care for assessing adequate respiration in ventilated patients. Measurement of carbon dioxide, the by-product of respiration, is more reliable for measuring adequate gas exchange. $ETCO_2$ monitors are available for tracheal tubes and nasal cannulas. In children with poor mentation, monitoring $ETCO_2$ levels may provide the CCTP with insight into the child's ventilatory status. Normal values for $ETCO_2$ are 35 to 45 mm Hg, similar to the values found in arterial blood gas (ABG) samples.

ABG analysis may be available to the CCT provider. Its results can provide insights into the adequacy of ventilation and oxygenation efforts. However, numerous medications and physiologic states can alter the findings of an ABG analysis, thereby creating diagnostic confusion and leading to inappropriate intervention. The partial pressure values of carbon dioxide in an ABG analysis correlate well with end-tidal values, which are more commonly used by EMS providers. ABG values should be discussed with the medical control physician. Like other adjuvant measurements, they should be assessed as part of the clinical picture and not evaluated in isolation.

Circulation and Vital Signs

Physical assessment of a child's cardiovascular system begins with observing the child's general appearance and LOC. A child who is well perfused will be watching the CCTP and other activity in the room. Observation of the chest may reveal the child's heart beating through the skin (precordial activity); this can be a normal finding in pediatric patients. Assessment of the fingers and toes should be conducted to look for evidence of clubbing. Clubbing is the broadening of a child's fingers and toes in response to chronically low oxygen levels for longer than 3 months **FIGURE 24-11**.

As with an adult patient, evaluating respiratory status in a child should include an assessment of the pulse rate and quality, blood pressure, and capillary refill. The position of a child's heart in the thoracic cage is identical to that of an adult. When auscultating the pulse rate of an infant, it may be useful to place the stethoscope over the second intercostal space at the midclavicular line. For older children, auscultation may be easiest over the fourth intercostal space at the midclavicular line. Cardiac sounds should be absent of rubs, murmurs, gallops, and secondary sounds. Keep in mind that

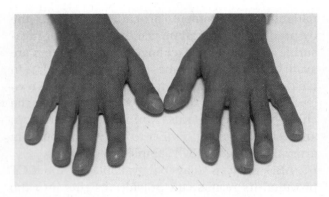

FIGURE 24-11 Clubbing.

© Mediscan/Visuals Unlimited.

heart sounds heard over the apex of the heart represent precordial activity. Patients with poor cardiac output may not have strong peripheral pulses.

In young infants, the heart rate can be palpated by identifying the brachial artery in the medial upper arm or the femoral artery. In older children, assessment of the radial pulse becomes more reliable. Tachycardia may be present in a child with fever, pain, or anxiety but may also be a sign of infection, hypervolemia, or shock. The heart rate should be evaluated in the context of the clinical picture. A fast, thready pulse, coupled with other signs of poor perfusion (eg, mottled skin, prolonged capillary refill), is a worrisome finding.

BP readings should be taken with age- and size-appropriate equipment. Recall that BP will likely be normal even in children experiencing shock until they reach the very latest stages. Children with hypotension resulting from shock are in imminent risk for irreversible deterioration. A child with significant hypoperfusion may present with altered mental status, as insufficient systolic BP (SBP) reduces the cerebral perfusion pressure.

Mean arterial pressure (MAP) [calculated as (2 × diastolic BP [DBP] + SBP) / 3] offers valuable information about the end-organ perfusion and can be measured by invasive arterial line or a noninvasive BP monitor. These parameters ultimately reflect the child's cardiac output. Cardiac output in children, as in adults, is determined by stroke volume and heart rate. Children, especially younger infants, have a limited ability to increase stroke volume; ability to compensate is especially limited in children with volume loss or dehydration. In children, the primary means of increasing stroke

volume is an increase in the heart rate. Children will maintain a normal BP because of the robust ability to increase their heart rate during times of physiologic stress. Be wary of the bradycardic child, who is likely in imminent risk for acute deterioration.

Doppler ultrasonography may be useful if the CCTP cannot palpate a pulse; however, if the pulse cannot be palpated, cardiac activity and perfusion are considered inadequate. In addition to assessing the presence and quality of pulses, compare the pulses bilaterally and in the upper and lower limbs. In a child older than 1 year, the pulse rate should be assessed in the carotid, radial, femoral, and dorsalis pedis arteries. To assess a pulse in an infant younger than 1 year, use the brachial and femoral arteries. Palpating carotid pulses in infants is difficult because of their thick, short necks. The carotid pulse is palpated only by hyperextending the child's neck.

Point-of-care ultrasonography (POCUS) is another method for assessing cardiac function and volume status in the interfacility transport setting. POCUS should be performed only after appropriate training and credentialing by the agency's medical director.

An evaluation of the child's skin can provide valuable insights into the child's circulation and may help identify hypoperfusion. Early compensatory mechanisms shunt blood from the skin to the vital organs. Skin that is well perfused should be warm, dry, and the appropriate color for that individual. As a child becomes hypoperfused, the skin becomes cool, pale, mottled, or cyanotic. If perfusion deteriorates further, the child's hands and feet will typically be affected first. Clammy or diaphoretic skin may also be present in the child with poor perfusion.

Capillary refill is also an excellent indicator of peripheral perfusion. Normal capillary refill in pediatric patients is usually immediate; however, up to 3 seconds is considered an acceptable limit in a child who otherwise appears healthy. Capillary refill of greater than 4 to 5 seconds represents a significant delay. Keep in mind that ambient temperatures may affect capillary refill time; such differences are seen with hypothermia.

Blood Pressure

Children, at least initially, can maintain a normal BP despite other indicators of shock (eg, disproportionate tachycardia, prolonged capillary refill time, signs of altered mental status). They respond to physiologic stress by releasing catecholamines that cause vasoconstriction, an increased pulse rate, and increased cardiac contractility. As a result, children will maintain a normal BP until their compensatory mechanisms are depleted. For example, in case of hypovolemia, a child can lose as much as 25% to 30% of the total blood volume before hypotension is noted.

A common error when measuring BP in a child is not fitting the cuffs correctly. A cuff that is too large and exceeds two-thirds the length of the child's arm will give a falsely low reading; a cuff that is too small or is less than half the length of the upper arm will give a falsely elevated reading. Often, providers choose to measure BP in a lower extremity, because it is well tolerated by children. BP values obtained from the lower extremities have been shown clinically to correlate well with values obtained from upper extremities; however, it is advised that both upper- and lower-extremity BP values be documented to ensure correlation. Always consider the child's normal range and clinical condition. Pain, fear, and anxiety often increase a child's BP.

Where available, invasive arterial monitoring allows for precise BP measurements and may better identify trends than intermittent BP readings. For some disease processes, such as traumatic brain injury (TBI), the MAP may be a more important measurement than BP in guiding treatment. The MAP may be a better measure of end-organ perfusion and may be measured by either an arterial line or a noninvasive BP monitor.

Fluid Volume and Access

Understanding circulating blood volumes for children is useful for quantifying volume loss and calculating fluid replacements. An estimate of 80 mL/kg of body weight for a child's circulating volume is appropriate.

In a child in critical condition, any trauma or medical condition that causes fluid losses, such as bleeding, vomiting, urination, or insensible losses (those that cannot be quantified), requires IV access for volume replacement. IV access can be obtained via a peripheral or central route. The use of intraosseous (IO) access has become common in infants and children requiring urgent interventions with fluids, blood, or medications, in whom

rapid venous access cannot be obtained. The most common site for IO insertion is the anterior tibia **FIGURE 24-12**. Alternative sites include the distal femur, medial malleolus, and anterior superior iliac spine. In adolescent patients, a humeral head location can be considered. Contraindications to IO access include, but are not limited to, osteogenesis imperfecta (also called brittle bone disease or Lobstein syndrome), osteopetrosis, evidence of infection at the potential insertion site, and fractures of the ipsilateral (same side) extremity.

Additional IO devices include the EZ-IO and the Bone Injection Gun (BIG). The EZ-IO features a hand-held battery-powered driver, to which a special IO needle is attached **FIGURE 24-13**. This device

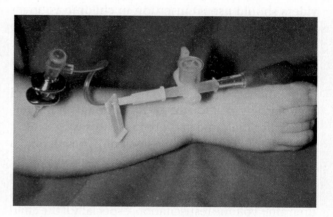

FIGURE 24-12 Standard pediatric intraosseous needle.
© American Academy of Orthopaedic Surgeons.

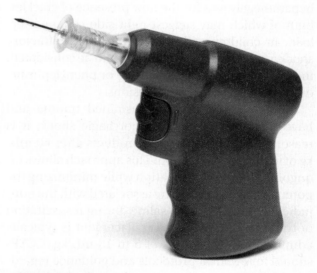

FIGURE 24-13 EZ-IO intraosseous infusion system.
Courtesy of VidaCare Corporation.

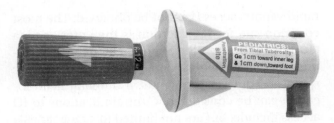

FIGURE 24-14 Pediatric Bone Injection Gun.

Used with permission of PerSys Medical and Bound Tree Medical.

is used to insert an IO needle into the proximal tibia of adults and children when IV access is difficult or impossible to obtain. The battery-powered driver of the EZ-IO is a standard piece, but different sizes of needles are available for adults and children. Providers should use IO insertion in children younger than 6 months, because higher rates of failure are associated with use of the EZ-IO in this age group.

The BIG is a spring-loaded device that is used to insert an IO needle into the proximal tibia of adult and pediatric patients. It comes in an adult size and a pediatric size **FIGURE 24-14**, although both versions offer the same operational features.

If the child shows any signs of hypovolemia, a 20-mL/kg bolus of normal saline should be given, and repeated as necessary, up to 60 mL/kg during transport. It is important to clinically reassess children after volume resuscitation, especially if the child has a history of cardiac disease or if providers suspect cardiac pathologies (eg, myocarditis, heart failure). This reassessment should include an evaluation for hepatomegaly and for the new presence of crackles, both of which may suggest right-side volume overload. In children with evidence of fluid-refractory shock, vasoactive medications should be considered, including boluses of epinephrine or phenylephrine, or initiation of vasoactive infusions.

In patients who have sustained trauma and have signs of refractory hemorrhagic shock, it is reasonable to initiate blood products after 40 mL/kg of volume resuscitation. This approach allows for ongoing volume resuscitation while minimizing the potential for coagulopathy associated with the nonjudicious use of normal saline during resuscitation of trauma patients. Blood replacement is typically administered in aliquots of 5 to 15 mL/kg. CCTPs should follow local protocols and guidance regarding the initiation of blood products during interfacility transport.

Urine output can be an objective guide when assessing pediatric circulatory status and the effectiveness of volume replacement. Signs of poor kidney perfusion include a low urine output. In children wearing diapers, low urine output is considered fewer than 4 to 6 wet diapers in a 24-hour period. In children with a urine catheter in place, it is considered less than 0.5 to 1 mL/kg/h. An adequate urine output is typically 1 to 2 mL/kg/h. An accurate assessment of urine output in the critical care setting can be made by comparing the weight of wet to dry diapers. This may be impractical in the transport environment, but attention to diapers provides information about renal perfusion.

Neurologic Assessment

As with other assessments of the pediatric patient, the neurologic evaluation will be age dependent. During the primary assessment, evaluate the infant's general appearance. Neonates' appearance can be deceptive, and a focused neurologic assessment can identify a potentially critically ill child. How is this child responding to the environment: is the child responsive or unresponsive, awake or lethargic?

Assessment of the fontanelles is important. A sunken fontanelle may indicate dehydration. A tense or bulging fontanelle may indicate increased intracranial pressure (ICP); that is, as the ICP rises above normal limits, the fontanelle allows for expansion.

Infants retain a number of intrinsic reflexes early in life. Chief among them is a strong suck. The sucking reflex can be evaluated by placing a gloved fifth digit into the infant's mouth with the palmar surface facing up. Healthy infants have a strong, well-coordinated suck. Absence of this reflex suggests a neurologic problem.

Healthy infants should have rigorous axial and peripheral tone. Axial tone can be evaluated by lifting the infant from under the armpits while supporting the head. Healthy infants will maintain this position; in contrast, children with poor axial tone will "slip like a fish" through the provider's hands, with arms extending upward. Regarding extremity tone, infants normally have flexed elbows and knees. Completely flaccid extremities are an abnormal finding. Another measure of motor function is the presence of normal reflexes, such as the

Moro reflex, which occurs when the infant jumps or is startled in response to a loud noise. The stepping reflex occurs when an infant is held up in the air and moves the legs up and down as if marching.

In a toddler or school-age child, motor function is assessed by observing gross motor function and the degree to which the patient interacts with the surrounding world. Healthy children move all four extremities, with symmetric strength and ability. Minimal movements, especially in response to a noxious stimulus, should raise a concern for neurologic impairment. The assessment of an adolescent very much parallels that of an adult patient.

Mental status in children is determined by observing for age-appropriate behaviors and thought processes. Infants 1 month or older can typically track with their eyes and will begin to have a social smile. For toddlers, providers should observe the degree to which they interact with the caregivers, make eye contact, and respond appropriately to stimuli (positive and negative). School-age children can be evaluated in a similar fashion as adults, with questions that are tailored to their age.

The Glasgow Coma Scale (GCS) is a sensitive indicator of mental status and offers providers a convenient means to communicate a patient's status to other caregivers; it can also be used to guide treatment. While this scale was originally validated for trauma patients, use of the GCS as a dynamic evaluation of pediatric patients with serious medical problems has become commonplace in the CCT setting. The GCS is modified when examining infants and children **TABLE 24-5** or children who are intubated.

Another important component of the neurologic assessment is checking the child's pupil size and response to light. As with adults, very constricted or pinpoint pupils are consistent with opioid overdose. A single dilated pupil is consistent with brain injury.

TABLE 24-5 Glasgow Coma Scale

Activity	Score	Description	Score	Description
Infants			**Children**	
Eye opening	4	Opens spontaneously	4	Opens spontaneously
	3	Opens to speech or sound	3	Opens to speech
	2	Opens to pressure	2	Opens to pressure
	1	No response	1	No response
Verbal	5	Coos, babbles	5	Oriented to person, place, and time
	4	Irritable cry	4	Confused
	3	Cries to pressure	3	Inappropriate words
	2	Moans to pressure	2	Incomprehensible words/sounds
	1	No response	1	No response
Motor	6	Normal spontaneous movement	6	Obeys verbal commands
	5	Withdraws to touch	5	Localizes pressure
	4	Withdraws to pressure	4	Withdraws to pressure or displays nonpurposeful movement
	3	Abnormal flexion (decorticate)	3	Abnormal flexion (decorticate)
	2	Abnormal extension (decerebrate)	2	Abnormal extension (decerebrate)
	1	No response (flaccid)	1	No response (flaccid)

In a child with a decreased LOC, the presence of protective reflexes can determine whether a child needs ET intubation for airway protection. The loss of protective reflexes occurs in ascending order— swallow reflex, cough reflex, gag reflex, and, finally, corneal reflexes. The cough and gag reflexes can be assessed by using a suction catheter to elicit a response.

Renal Assessment

Assessment of the renal system typically begins with evaluation of hydration status. The patient's history is key to this assessment. Parents or caregivers can offer information about the amount of intake by the child and the number of wet diapers, voids, stools, and frequency of emesis.

Physical assessment of the child may include assessment of the fontanelles (for an infant), assessment of skin turgor, the presence or absence of tears when crying, and sunken eyes. The measurement of wet diapers may be somewhat subjective because parents may change diapers that are not completely saturated. A good question to ask caregivers is whether the diapers are *different* from the normal pattern. A more objective measurement is weighing diapers: 1 mL of urine equals 1 g of weight. Daily weights are also an objective measurement because they may be an early indication of fluid loss. Acute weight loss may be an early indication of fluid loss.

Fluid overload is much less common in children than in adults; however, it may occur in patients with congenital heart defects or renal insufficiency; in children undergoing aggressive volume resuscitation, especially in the context of capillary leak secondary to sepsis; or in children with hypoalbuminemia, as is seen in the context of nephrotic syndrome or protein-losing enteropathy. Signs of fluid overload in children may be vague and initially have a more subtle presentation than in adults. For example, in children with pulmonary edema, hypoxia and grunting are two early signs. Other early signs, such as tachypnea, a cough, and increased oxygen needs, may be discounted as having other etiologies because of their vague presentations. Later signs, which are more obvious, may include crackles and pink, frothy sputum associated with pulmonary edema. Pulmonary edema can be confirmed by plain radiography of the chest or, in the hands of a skilled practitioner, by point-of-care transthoracic ultrasonography, as discussed in Chapter 9, *Laboratory Analysis and Diagnostic Studies*. Additional signs of fluid overload include weight gain, edema, and history of intake greater than output.

Exposure Considerations

Temperature regulation is a concern in all patients, but especially in children. Environmental concerns regarding hypothermia or hyperthermia need to be addressed during the assessment. Because of an infant's physiologic differences and inability to shiver, resuscitation of infants and children must include measures to maintain body temperature, while being careful not to overwarm the patient. The infant's disproportionately large head represents a large percentage of body surface area, making infants particularly susceptible to hypothermia.

Hyperthermia is related to increased oxygen consumption. Children left in vehicles during hot, humid weather for extended periods are at increased risk for hyperthermia. Other risk factors include physical exertion (ie, athletics) and intoxication with drugs and alcohol, which impair heat dissipation. Hyperpyrexia, defined as body temperature of 106.2°F (41.2°C) or greater, is associated with severe viral or bacterial disease.

To minimize heat loss, replace blankets on areas of the child that have been assessed and increase the temperature in the transport vehicle. Be sure to leave heating/cooling measures in place in transport units while the patient is being prepared for transport.

Transport Considerations

Dedicated pediatric specialty teams are ideal for transporting the ill or injured child, but they may not always be available or fiscally feasible. Essential knowledge for CCTPs caring for children includes understanding differences in pediatric physical assessment, airway management, ventilator management, vascular access, fluid and medication administration, and specific illnesses and injuries that are common in children. Essential skills include pediatric hemodynamic monitoring, ICP monitoring, mechanical ventilation, and use of thermoregulation devices. It is helpful to practice any new skills using the equipment found on the vehicle in which you will be working. In addition, although didactic education is required, it cannot substitute for hands-on pediatric experience including, but not limited to, routine pediatric care, critical pediatric care, and experience with pediatric intubations. Professionals who anticipate caring for critically ill or injured children should consider partnering with professional colleagues who care for pediatric patients on a regular basis.

Equipment

The CCT team must ensure appropriate equipment is available when transporting pediatric patients **FIGURE 24-15**. Significant variation among agencies and states has existed regarding the requirements for pediatric-specific equipment. In 2021, the National Association of EMS Physicians released a position statement and accompanying resource document describing the recommended equipment for basic life support (BLS) and advanced life support (ALS) ambulances; however specific equipment recommendations for CCT ambulances are limited. ECG monitoring with pulse oximetry and end-tidal capnography is the standard of care for all intubated pediatric patients. It is important to carry various sizes of ECG leads, pulse oximetry probes, and BP cuffs to ensure accuracy when obtaining vital signs.

IV fluid administration in pediatric patients should be done with an infusion pump that delivers medication infusions at a rate calibrated to at least one decimal place. Buretrol devices should be avoided because they are inaccurate and represent

a latent safety threat. Fluid boluses and medications for resuscitation should be delivered with a syringe and stopcock technique. Fluid and medication formulas should be standardized and calculated prior to transport. It is also important to carry equipment for thermoregulation, such as a disposable gel-heated mattress or an incubator. Finally, know the capabilities of the transport ventilator for your service. Common requirements for ventilating children include pressure modes of ventilation, capacity for pediatric ventilator settings, and pediatric circuits.

CCTPs should consider maintaining a supply of single-use toys to help reduce anxiety during transport or to distract the patient, when appropriate, during procedures. Consider also the value of tablet devices for distraction of young patients.

Interfacility Transport Considerations

When you are conducting an interfacility transport, several important pieces of information will help to determine the mode of transport, the team configuration, and any specialized equipment that is needed. This information includes the age and weight of the patient, diagnosis, reason for transfer, physical exam findings, lab and other diagnostic test results, IV access, and consent. It is helpful to develop a standardized intake form that the transfer team can use in determining the need for airway management or other procedures to stabilize the patient for transport. For example, for patients with an altered mental status, ask the sending facility for the patient's GCS score and information on the presence of cough and gag reflexes to determine the need for emergent airway management. Any treatment recommendations must be recorded on the transfer documentation.

Once the CCTPs arrive at the sending facility, it is important to assess the patient immediately to determine the need for additional procedures prior to preparing the patient for transfer. Although it is important to ensure all lines and tubes have been secured and to double-check all fluid and medication rates, a standardized team approach to the patient care handoff is best. Using communication tools such as SBAR (situation, background, assessment, and recommendation) helps to standardize the exchange of information so that each provider

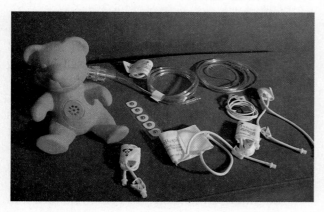

FIGURE 24-15 Appropriate-size equipment should always be accessible for transport of pediatric patients.

has an expectation for what is to be discussed, even if the transport is time critical. This method can also be used to frame the conversation with other providers. Finally, a predeparture safety checklist ensures that the CCTP team has evaluated for potential safety threats (eg, equipment failure) and has had an opportunity to discuss any concerns for transport with either the referring physician or the receiving physician.

Mode of Transport

To ensure their safe transport, pediatric patients must be adequately restrained in the event of a motor vehicle (or flight) crash. Children should *never* be transported in the arms of a parent, guardian, or provider.

Particular attention must be paid to the positioning and placement of child passenger safety restraints. Devices for restraining infants and young children include an Isolette or similar product with attached straps to maintain body temperature, a child safety seat or a similar product that can be secured to the ambulance stretcher, and a pediatric immobilization device or backboard, although pediatric immobilizers are not approved by the Federal Aviation Administration.

While there are no federally approved standards for pediatric safety equipment, the National Highway Traffic Safety Administration has provided guidance and made recommendations for the safe ground and air transport of children. For young children, five-point restraints are recommended. For children older than 4 years, the standard stretcher straps may be used. Generally, a child who requires resuscitation should be positioned supine and secured to the stretcher. If there is no likely threat to physiologic stability, the child should be transported in an upright, secured position **FIGURE 24-16**.

Accompanying Parents and Caregivers

The decision to transport parents or caregivers along with a child should be discussed, and guidelines should be put in place long before a child needs transport. In general, the presence of a parent or caregiver decreases a child's anxiety and emotional distress, which may also have a positive physiologic effect. For example, if a child in respiratory distress becomes more anxious and upset

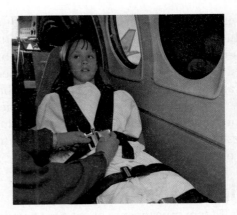

FIGURE 24-16 Transport the child in an upright, secured position if there is no likely threat to physiologic stability.
© Jones & Bartlett Learning.

because of separation from a caregiver, the child's respiratory effort may increase and their physiologic status may deteriorate. The safe transport of the child has priority, however, and the caregivers' comfort level and the potential for disruption of care during transport must be taken into account. Consideration must be given to the seating of the parent or caregiver, and guidelines should be discussed with the caregiver prior to transport—particularly the need to remain seated and restrained in a vehicle restraint. No child should ever be held on a caregiver's lap for any reason while a vehicle is in motion.

Airway Management Devices

Several oxygen delivery adjuncts are used with pediatric patients in the critical care environment. These include devices commonly used in the prehospital environment, such as the nasal cannula, simple mask, partial rebreathing mask, nonrebreathing mask, Venturi mask, oxygen tent, and bag-mask device. Flow-inflating bags, self-inflating bags, and oxygen hoods are less commonly encountered in the prehospital environment and are discussed here for that reason. Supraglottic devices and ET tubes are the advanced airway management devices most commonly used in children. Shortened tracheal tubes and blade options for children are also discussed.

The American Academy of Pediatrics (AAP), in its Pediatric Advanced Life Support course, recommends that self-inflating bags be used for resuscitation. Therefore, most of this discussion focuses

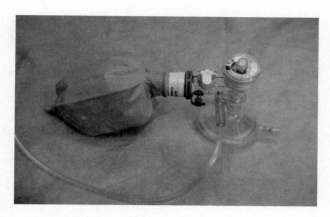

FIGURE 24-17 A flow-inflating bag.
© Jones & Bartlett Learning.

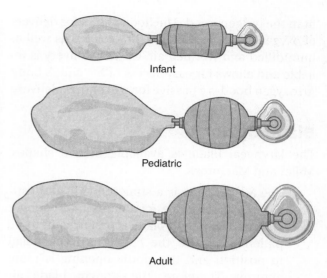

Infant

Pediatric

Adult

FIGURE 24-18 Self-inflating bags.
© Jones & Bartlett Learning.

on self-inflating bags; however, a brief review of flow-inflating bags is provided as well.

Flow-Inflating Bag

Flow-inflating bags have been routinely used for anesthesia. These devices require an outside gas source to inflate them, and they have a pressure gauge port, a flow inlet dial, and an overflow port **FIGURE 24-17**. The volume of flow-inflating bags is 500 mL for infants and 600 to 1,000 mL for children. When these bags are inflated fully, providers can provide PEEP for the patient even without ventilations.

Self-Inflating Bag

Safe and effective ventilation is possible with self-inflating bags, although they require more experience and more manipulation of the equipment to achieve adequate ventilation **FIGURE 24-18**. Consequently, these devices are not recommended for resuscitation of infants and children unless the health care professional has received extensive training in their use.

Self-inflating bags come in different sizes to accommodate the various pediatric populations. A neonatal ventilation bag has a volume of 250 mL. Be cautious when using this device because the small tidal volume may be inadequate for term newborns and infants. As an alternative, CCTPs may use a pediatric ventilation bag, which has a minimum volume of 450 to 500 mL and a maximum volume of 750 mL.

Self-inflating bags do not require a compressed gas source and can deliver a free flow of oxygen. They have a pressure release valve (pop-off valve), a safety feature that releases gas when the pressure exceeds 40 cm H_2O. This helps to prevent excessive

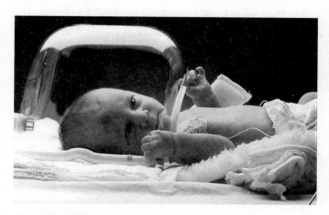

FIGURE 24-19 An oxygen hood.
Disposa-Hood™ Infant Oxygen hood. Courtesy of Utah Medical Products, Inc., Midvale, Utah.

airway pressures while ventilating children and minimizes the complication of a pneumothorax.

When providing positive-pressure ventilation with a bag-mask device, use of a PEEP valve will help augment oxygenation and limit barotrauma. Additionally, pressure-relief valves (also called pop-up valves) are available on some bag-mask devices; these valves also reduce the risk of iatrogenic barotrauma. When the clinical situation requires higher pressures (eg, pulmonary edema), the pressure-relief valve can be released.

Oxygen Hood

An oxygen hood is an oxygen delivery system used in infant populations **FIGURE 24-19**. Children older than approximately 1 year are physically too big to fit in the oxygen hood. The hood allows for delivery of oxygen concentrations of 80% to 90% as well as humidified and warmed air. Oxygen delivery is reliable and allows for easy access of the child's body. An oxygen hood is a passive form of oxygen delivery.

Blade Options

The laryngeal blade is available in two shapes: Miller and Macintosh.

- The Miller blade is a straight blade and usually the first choice for infants and younger children. A straight blade is preferred in these patients because the epiglottis is cephalad in position and the glottic opening is more anterior. Therefore, the straight blade allows better visualization for these anatomic considerations.
- The Macintosh blade is curved in shape and fits into the vallecula. This blade may be the preferred choice for older children and adolescents because it better displaces the relatively large tongue, thereby allowing better visualization of the glottic opening.

Actual blade size selection depends on the child's size, as opposed to age. **TABLE 24-6** offers some guidance on size selection.

ET Tubes

There are limited uses for uncuffed ET tubes for children. While some NICUs continue to use them in preterm infants, this practice is diminishing. It is preferable to place an appropriate-size cuffed ET tube when invasive ventilation strategies are warranted. Providers capable of advanced airway management in children during CCT should consider the following precautions:

- Where possible, secure the airway prior to departure from the referring site.
- Consider alternative airways and rescue airway devices (eg, supraglottic airway devices).
- Restrict airway attempts to the most skilled and experienced provider.

Respiratory Conditions

Respiratory illness is a common reason for pediatric transport. Respiratory compromise or failure can be caused by any airway, pulmonary, or neuromuscular disease that interferes with oxygen and carbon dioxide exchange. Respiratory conditions are often classified as either respiratory distress or respiratory failure.

Respiratory distress is characterized by a noted increase in the work of breathing. The dyspneic child is recognized by an increased rate (tachypnea) and possibly depth of breathing. Nasal flaring, retractions, and accessory muscle use are usually noted. Although the amount of effort to breathe is dramatically increased, the child may still have adequate gas exchange of oxygen and carbon dioxide. In addition, this change in the respiratory pattern may represent physiologic compensation to an underlying metabolic derangement. For example, in diabetic ketoacidosis, an increased respiratory rate and depth (Kussmaul breathing) is necessary to clear excessive amounts of carbon dioxide.

TABLE 24-6 Pediatric Laryngeal Blade Sizes

Age	Blade Size Number	Cuffed Tube Size	Insertion Depth (cm)
Premature neonate	0 straight	Not applicable	9–10
Term neonate–6 months	1 straight	3.0–3.5	11–12
1 year	1–1.5 straight	3.5	12
2 years	1.5–2 straight	4.0	13–14
5–8 years	2 straight or curved	4.5–5.5	14–18
10–12 years	2–3 straight or curved	6–6.5	18–21
15 years	3 straight or curved	6.5	20–21

Respiratory failure is characterized by inadequate oxygen intake or inadequate exchange of oxygen and carbon dioxide. No specific definition of respiratory failure exists because this diagnosis depends on the child's baseline respiratory function. Intervention to prevent respiratory and subsequent cardiac collapse is paramount for this patient population. If known risks are identified for respiratory failure in the patient prior to departing the referring facility or if the patient's signs and symptoms worsen while en route to the receiving facility, the CCTP should take all measures (per protocol) to maintain and preserve a patent airway and hemodynamic status. It is possible for a patient to experience respiratory failure without signs of respiratory distress. For example, a child who is unconscious and apneic after a traumatic head injury will not demonstrate increased work of breathing but rather inadequate or absent breathing.

Respiratory conditions that lead to respiratory failure can be classified as an upper airway condition, a lower airway condition, parenchymal disease, or disordered breathing. Upper airway obstructions are most commonly caused by foreign body aspiration or infection and are characterized primarily by inspiratory stridor. Obstructions at the level of the vocal cords may lead to biphasic stridor, and obstructions in the trachea may have an expiratory component. Partially obstructed airways cause turbulent airflow. The obstruction can be above or can include the glottis, pharynx, and trachea. In such a case, the child's voice will be muffled or hoarse. If the obstruction is subglottic or subtracheal, stridor will be present but the child's voice may sound normal.

Lower airway disease may include the trachea and main stem bronchi as well as the peripheral airways. Lower airway aspiration most commonly occurs in children younger than 3 years. A diagnosis of lower airway disease is often made after aspiration, with the presentation potentially ranging from mild coughing and wheezing to severe respiratory distress.

Peripheral airway diseases that are common indications for transport include asthma, bronchiolitis, and bronchopulmonary dysplasia.

Croup

Croup (laryngotracheobronchitis) is a common viral infection of the upper airway that affects the larynx but may also extend into the trachea and bronchi. Symptoms include a low-grade fever and a hoarse, "barking seal" cough that often becomes worse at night. Children may also present with inspiratory stridor. Stridor at rest is particularly concerning for severe disease. Croup is most common in children younger than 3 years. In these children, the diameter of the cricoid area is at its smallest, so swelling may cause severe symptoms. Children most commonly present with mild distress, but severe respiratory effects have also been reported. The CCTP should be familiar with the hallmark sign of croup—namely, the harsh, "barking seal" cough.

Management of croup depends on the severity of the child's symptoms. A child in mild distress may be best managed by maintaining a calm environment. Humidified oxygen is the initial therapy. Allow the parents to sit next to the child to hold the humidified oxygen to the child's face using a mask or blow-by method.

For children with stridor at rest, a continuous barky cough, and/or signs of respiratory distress, racemic epinephrine (2.25% with 2.0 to 3.5 mL of normal saline) administered via a nebulizer usually improves airflow. The following dosages may be given:

- Age <6 months: 0.25 mL
- Child: 0.5 mL
- Adolescent: 0.75 mL

Racemic epinephrine is subtly different in chemical makeup from epinephrine, and it stimulates both alpha and beta adrenergic receptors, with a preference for the beta-2 adrenergic receptors that cause bronchodilation. The vasoconstrictive effects of racemic epinephrine are temporary, however, and persist only until the drug is metabolized, a factor that should be considered with long transport times. Once the drug is metabolized, the swelling ("rebound worsening") may return to the same level as before or may worsen. Services that do not carry racemic epinephrine may instead use L-epinephrine (1 mg in 1 mL), dosing it at 0.5 mL/kg (maximum dose, 5 mL) and combining it with 2 mL of normal saline for nebulization.

Children with refractory croup may benefit from Heliox, a gas that combines helium and oxygen. Heliox reduces turbulent airflow through narrowed airways. It is typically delivered in one of two mixtures: 80% helium and 20% oxygen, or 70% helium and 30% oxygen. CCTPs should be aware that the 80:20 mixture is a *hypoxic* mixture and should be used with caution in patients with borderline saturations. Additionally, the CCTP should consider noninvasive positive-pressure ventilation methods, such as continuous positive airway pressure (CPAP) or bilevel positive airway pressure (BPAP), to support the patient. A special consideration with CPAP or BPAP is the ability to provide in-line nebulization for continued administration of racemic epinephrine.

Signs and Symptoms

Croup
- Low-grade fever
- Hoarse, "barking seal" cough
- Mild distress
- Stridor

Differential Diagnosis

Croup
- Acute laryngeal fracture
- Allergic reaction/anaphylaxis
- Angioneurotic edema
- Arnold-Chiari deformity
- Bacterial tracheitis
- Burns or thermal injury
- Dandy-Walker syndrome
- Diphtheria
- Epiglottitis
- Extrinsic obstruction by a vascular ring
- Foreign body
- Laryngeal papillomatosis
- Laryngomalacia
- Neoplasm or hemangioma
- Peritonsillar abscess
- Retropharyngeal abscess
- Smoke inhalation
- Subglottic stenosis
- Viral croup
- Vocal cord paralysis

Transport Management

Croup
- Administer humidified oxygen using a mask or blow-by method.
- Consider corticosteroids (if not previously administered).
- For more severe obstruction, administer racemic epinephrine via a nebulizer.
- Consider Heliox for refractory croup.
- Apply noninvasive positive-pressure ventilation strategies.
- If the child is no longer able to protect the airway, consider oral intubation.

Early administration of systemic corticosteroids reduces the severity and duration of croup. Dosing of dexamethasone is usually 0.2 to 0.6 mg/kg (maximum dose, 16 mg), and this medication can be administered orally, intramuscularly, or IV. In children with severe disease and those requiring intubation, scheduled steroids should be considered. Alternative steroids include prednisolone, prednisone, and methylprednisolone.

In the rare circumstance in which the obstruction is so severe that the child is no longer able to protect their own airway, oral intubation may be considered. When you suspect that the airway is edematous, the size of the ET tube chosen may be one-half to one size smaller than the tube typically used.

Epiglottitis

Epiglottitis (also called supraglottitis) is most commonly caused by a bacterial infection with *Haemophilus influenzae*. Historically, this infection occurred most commonly in children ages 3 to 5 years. With the approval of the *H influenzae* type b (Hib) vaccine in 1991 and its widespread administration to infants, epiglottitis is now seen primarily in adults. Symptoms include rapid onset of fever, stridor, and pronounced signs of toxicity. The patient may appear anxious, have a muffled voice, and be in a tripod position with pronounced drooling because of supraglottic swelling and excess secretions. Remember the four Ds for epiglottitis: dysphagia, dysphonia, drooling, and distress. Patients with epiglottitis are at a tremendous risk of acute and complete airway obstruction. Invasive procedures should be kept at a minimum so as not to aggravate and increase the child's work of breathing.

Management of suspected epiglottitis in the prehospital setting is controversial because this condition can worsen rapidly, leading to a complete airway obstruction. The use of racemic epinephrine with this condition is contraindicated because it can cause additional swelling of the affected inflamed tissues. There is consensus that a calm environment should be maintained so as not to precipitate complete obstruction. There is also agreement that a definitive airway should be secured prior to transport. However, children with epiglottitis are often difficult to intubate and may require specialized teams or specialized techniques, such as retrograde intubation, direct bronchoscopy, or possibly tracheostomy, if intubation is unsuccessful. Therefore, the

Signs and Symptoms

Epiglottitis

- Rapid onset of fever
- Stridor
- Pronounced signs of toxicity
- Distress
- Muffled voice
- Drooling
- Tripod position

Differential Diagnosis

Epiglottitis

- Bacterial tracheitis
- Foreign body ingestion
- Mononucleosis
- Anaphylaxis
- Croup or laryngotracheobronchitis
- Pertussis
- Pharyngitis
- Pneumonia
- Peritonsillar abscess
- Retropharyngeal abscess
- Caustic ingestion

Transport Management

Epiglottitis

- Maintain a calm environment.
- Secure a definitive airway prior to transport.
- Ensure early antibiotic therapy

decision to attempt definitive airway management in the prehospital setting is multifactorial, with key considerations including EMS protocols, the skill and experience of the CCT team, and the time and distance of the transport. If intubation needs to be performed, it should be carried out by the most skilled practitioner. Ideally, intubation will occur in the operating room by a subspecialist with the expertise to perform a surgical airway.

Foreign Body Airway Obstruction

Foreign body airway obstruction remains a significant source of morbidity and mortality in pediatric populations. Its onset may be dramatic, posing an immediate life threat or having varying severity.

Removal of the foreign body should be attempted only in the prehospital setting by following the guidelines set forth by the American Heart Association (AHA) and AAP. These guidelines include the use of chest thrusts in infants and abdominal thrusts in older children, leading to direct laryngoscopy

Controversies

Some organizations have suggested the initial use of back blows in adults with a foreign body airway obstruction and an ineffective cough. However, this recommendation is weak and supported by only low-certainty evidence. Some experts argue against the use of back blows in larger patients due to the simple impracticality of this procedure: The provider can hold an infant with the head downward while giving back blows, allowing gravity to help draw the object out of the airway. The provider cannot likely position an adult in an inverted position while giving back blows, meaning that as the back blows dislodge the object, gravity may pull it downward, deeper into the airway.

Always follow your local protocols and contact medical control for direction when needed.

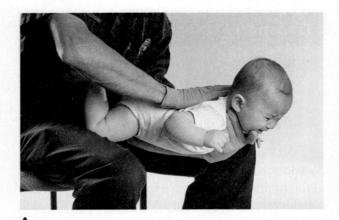
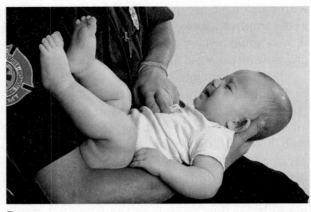

A   **B**

FIGURE 24-20 Back blows are typically recommended for infants (children younger than 1 year). **A.** Hold the infant facedown with the body resting on your forearm. Support the jaw and face with your hand, and keep the head lower than the rest of the body. Give the infant five back blows between the shoulder blades, using the heel of your hand. **B.** Give the infant five quick chest thrusts, using two fingers placed on the lower half of the sternum.

© Jones & Bartlett Learning.

Signs and Symptoms

Foreign Body Airway Obstruction

- Choking or gagging when the object is first inhaled or swallowed
- Sudden onset of coughing or cough that gets worse
- Stridor
- Wheezing
- Inability to speak
- Pain in the throat or chest
- Hoarse voice
- Blue around the lips
- Not breathing
- Unconscious

Differential Diagnosis

Foreign Body Airway Obstruction

- Asthma
- Croup
- Myocardial infarction
- Anaphylaxis
- Acute epiglottitis

Transport Management

Foreign Body Airway Obstruction

- Removal of the foreign body is attempted only following AHA and AAP guidelines: chest thrusts in infants or abdominal thrusts in older children.
- Direct laryngoscopy with Magill forceps.
- Back blows for infants younger than 1 year.
- Direct visualization of the trachea and removal of the foreign body only in the event of impending respiratory failure.

with Magill forceps to remove the foreign body. Specific algorithms should be followed **FIGURE 24-20.** Direct visualization of the trachea and removal of the foreign body should be considered only in the event of impending respiratory failure.

Inflammation

Generalized inflammation of the upper airway may be a result of inhalation burns or allergic and/or anaphylactic reactions. These airway insults are often precipitous in their presentations; early recognition and intervention are imperative to lessen morbidity and mortality. Therapeutic measures to treat all upper airway obstructions include the basics of ensuring a calm environment, administering supplemental humidified oxygen, providing a position of comfort, and preparing for deterioration of the airway status.

Bronchiolitis

Bronchiolitis is an inflammatory condition of the lower respiratory tract that results from viral infections, most commonly from the respiratory syncytial virus (RSV). Bronchiolitis begins with a viral upper respiratory tract prodrome (ie, nasal congestion, rhinorrhea, and often fever). Significant mucus production and edema in the nasal passages progress to involve the lower respiratory tract. Although wheezing is common initially in children younger than 2 years with bronchiolitis, this condition can also present with retractions, noisy breathing, and poor feeding.

The treatment for bronchiolitis is mainly supportive. Patients who are hypoxic or tachypneic may benefit from supplemental oxygen delivered via low-flow or high-flow nasal cannula and may require positive-pressure ventilation. Aggressive pulmonary toileting (ie, methods used to clear mucus from the airway) can be helpful, with saline and nasal suctioning as the mainstay treatments. Deep suctioning of the trachea or lower airways has fallen out of favor and may be harmful.

Bronchiolitis is a pathology of mucus production and inflammation. As such, the wheezing sometimes noted is not bronchospastic. Generally, there is no role for bronchodilators or steroids in patients with bronchiolitis. However, in children older than 18 months who have a strong family history of asthma or atopy, a trial of albuterol may be appropriate. If there is no significant improvement with albuterol therapy, further bronchodilators

Signs and Symptoms

Bronchiolitis
- Mild wheezing
- Tachypnea
- Noisy breathing
- Nasal flaring
- Retractions

Differential Diagnosis

Bronchiolitis
- Asthma
- Gastroesophageal reflux
- Foreign body aspiration
- Vascular ring
- Enlarged adenoids
- Heart failure
- Chronic lung disease

Transport Management

Bronchiolitis
- Administer supplemental oxygen and fluids.
- Provide aggressive pulmonary toileting.
- Suction as needed.
- Assess the child's work of breathing before and frequently during transport.

should not be attempted. Dehydration is common with bronchiolitis, and patients frequently require IV fluids.

Asthma

Wheezing is common in young children, especially those with hyperreactivity of the lower airways in response to stimuli such as allergens, exercise, infections, and exposure to cold air. This symptom, over time, may become suggestive of asthma, a chronic inflammatory condition that produces significant inflammation, bronchospasm, and edema in the lower airways. Recurring episodes present with shortness of breath, wheezing, and chest tightness. Asthma frequently occurs in parallel with eczema and allergies, a presentation known as the atopic triad.

Reactive airway disease (RAD) is a term often used synonymously with asthma in younger children. RAD occurs in children younger than 3 years; in 30% of children with RAD, the condition will progress to asthma. As of 2018, nearly 5.5 million children in the United States, or 7.5% of the pediatric population, had asthma. Asthma exacerbations are a frequent reason for EMS calls, ED visits, and admission to the hospital and intensive care unit for children.

Asthma is described as intermittent or persistent. Persistent asthma is further differentiated as mild, moderate, or severe, based on the frequency of symptoms and the need for controller medications.

Parents of children who experience chronic exacerbations of asthma are usually successful at treating the symptoms or preventing rapid deterioration while at home. Typically, when CCTPs are needed to transport a child with an exacerbation of asthma, traditional treatments have failed and more advanced therapies are required. In such a case, the CCTP should obtain a history from the child and parents or caregivers at the referring facility if they are available, and also obtain a detailed report from the transporting EMS crew (if available), the bedside nurse, and/or the referring physician. For example, if a child has a history of requiring numerous intubations for severe asthma, the child should receive all available treatments during rapid transport to the hospital.

Care for a child with an asthma exacerbation includes oxygen therapy because this condition is characterized by a significant ventilation/perfusion mismatch. Bronchodilators are the mainstay of treatment. By definition, asthma is marked by wheezing that is responsive to bronchodilators. Beta agonists such as albuterol result in the activation of sympathetic nerve receptors that act directly to stimulate bronchodilation within the smooth muscle of the bronchial tree. In contrast, ipratropium bromide works as a parasympatholytic agent that causes bronchodilation by inhibiting the typically tonic muscles that encircle the bronchi. For children in mild to moderate distress, these medications can be delivered with equal efficacy either by nebulizer or by metered-dose inhaler with an appropriate aerochamber device. Children in more severe distress may benefit from nebulizer administration earlier in the course.

Corticosteroids are the cornerstone of anti-inflammatory therapy for asthma; they are used to manage both acute and chronic episodes. The effects of corticosteroids are often not seen for approximately 4 to 6 hours, so they should be administered early in the course of an acute exacerbation

of asthma. Corticosteroid use should not replace aggressive beta-2 agonist therapy, but rather should complement it. Monitoring end-tidal capnography is useful in assessing the degree of obstruction and the response to therapy (or lack thereof).

Also available to the CCTP treating a child with an asthma exacerbation are medications that act on the bronchi and their associated musculature.

Signs and Symptoms

Asthma
- Shortness of breath
- Wheezing
- Chest tightness

Differential Diagnosis

Asthma
- Airway obstruction with a foreign body
- Bronchitis
- Pneumonia/bronchiolitis
- Cystic fibrosis
- Bronchopulmonary dysplasia (in premature infants)
- Dysmotile cilia syndrome
- Alpha-1 antitrypsin deficiency
- Heart failure
- Immunodeficiencies

Transport Management

Asthma
- Administer a bronchodilator, commonly a beta-2 agonist.
- Administer corticosteroids early in an acute exacerbation.
- Consider administering magnesium sulfate, epinephrine, and/or terbutaline.
- Consider Heliox.
- Apply noninvasive positive-pressure ventilation strategies.

These medications include magnesium sulfate, epinephrine, and terbutaline. In extreme cases, Heliox can be used to deliver nebulized medications to help improve laminar flow in the distal bronchioles.

Pneumonia

Pneumonia is a type of parenchymal lung disease that occurs in the lung itself and can result from viral infections, bacterial infections, or a combination of the two. While children with pneumonia frequently have focal physical exam findings such as diminished lung sounds and crackles, it can be clinically difficult to differentiate pneumonia from other etiologies such as viral pneumonitis. As such, the clinical diagnosis of pneumonia is typically confirmed by plain radiography or ultrasonography. Transport treatment includes a vigilant assessment of the patient's work of breathing and hydration status. Antibiotic therapy is frequently required and may have begun at the initial facility prior to transport.

Signs and Symptoms

Pneumonia
- Fever
- Grunting
- Cough
- Congestion
- Irritability
- Decreased feeding
- Shortness of breath
- Sweating
- Shaking and chills
- Pleurisy
- Headache
- Muscle pain
- Fatigue

Differential Diagnosis

Pneumonia
- Airway foreign body
- Asthma
- Bronchiolitis
- Bronchiectasis
- Bronchitis
- Cystic fibrosis
- Gastroesophageal reflux
- Heart failure
- Human immunodeficiency virus
- Pertussis

Transport Management

Pneumonia
- Be vigilant in assessing the child's work of breathing and hydration status.

Acute Respiratory Distress Syndrome

The presentation of acute respiratory distress syndrome (ARDS) is similar in children and adults. Regardless of the underlying cause, the cardinal determinant of ARDS is intrapulmonary shunting that shows minimal or no response to oxygen therapy. Typically resulting from an acute pulmonary infection, sepsis, or profound exposure to a toxic irritant, ARDS is caused by the loss of surfactant, an increase in pulmonary vascular permeability, and the loss of aerated tissue. This diagnosis also includes the presence of bilateral opacities on chest imaging **FIGURE 24-21**. In addition to treating the underlying etiology, management is primarily

Signs and Symptoms

Acute Respiratory Distress Syndrome
- Shortness of breath
- Rapid breathing
- Cough
- Fever
- Low BP
- Confusion
- Extreme tiredness

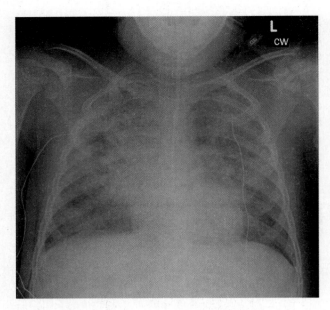

FIGURE 24-21 AP plain radiograph of the chest shows several areas of dense opacification involving multiple lung segments.

Differential Diagnosis

Acute Respiratory Distress Syndrome

- Goodpasture syndrome
- Hypersensitivity pneumonitis
- Multisystem organ failure from sepsis
- Pneumonia
- Respiratory failure
- Bacterial sepsis
- Septic shock
- Hemorrhagic shock
- Toxic shock syndrome

Transport Management

Acute Respiratory Distress Syndrome

- Provide support, including mechanical ventilation.

supportive, including mechanical ventilation with the use of judicious PEEP and cardiovascular support.

Mechanical Ventilation
Noninvasive Mechanical Ventilation

Noninvasive methods of mechanical ventilation or support have become increasingly popular in recent years. As providers have recognized the resilience of pediatric physiology and the deleterious effects of ET intubation in unseasoned hands, noninvasive strategies have become commonplace in the prehospital, hospital-based, and interfacility settings. Noninvasive methods include heated high-flow nasal cannula (HHFNC), CPAP (including "bubble CPAP" for infants), BPAP, and nasal noninvasive positive-pressure ventilation (essentially BPAP with a respiratory rate). These modalities offer a therapeutic option for children with significant hypoxic or hypercapneic respiratory failure who are maintaining their airway and for whom ET intubation is not yet warranted.

HHFNC requires the use of humidified oxygen and can provide support ranging from 2 to 60 L/min. This method can ensure a fraction of inspired oxygen (FIO_2) level of 0.21 to 1.00, and while it provides a small degree of PEEP, the amount is limited and varies between ventilators. Depending on the flow rate, limiting factors for providing ventilation via HHFNC are the type of ventilator available to the CCTP and the available oxygen supply. At high rates, HHFNC can quickly exhaust the oxygen supply on standard ambulances and air medical units. Providers can use mathematical equations to predict the available oxygen supply based on flow rate, transport time, and size of the oxygen tank, as discussed in Chapter 7, *Ventilation*. HHFNC requires specialized nasal prongs that are generally shorter and wider than those found on standard nasal cannula.

CPAP has become more ubiquitous in prehospital and interfacility protocols for managing respiratory distress. For patients with the ability to maintain their own airway but who require significant respiratory support, CPAP is the first in the array of noninvasive strategies available for children. This ventilation method provides pressure to continuously stent open distal airways. This effect is particularly helpful in patients with pneumonia, asthma/RAD, bronchiolitis, and other pathologies that cause distal airway collapse caused by bronchoconstriction, inflammation, or mucus burden. CCTPs can titrate both the FIO_2 and the flow pressure and can optimize patient oxygenation and support, to some extent, the work of breathing.

BPAP ventilation provides two levels of pressure: one during inspiration and the other during exhalation. This method provides a greater degree of ventilatory support than CPAP does. BPAP is typically triggered by a patient's respiratory effort, but a backup rate can provide a minimum number of breaths per minute. When a rate is set using BPAP, this modality is sometimes referred to as noninvasive positive-pressure ventilation.

Both CPAP and BPAP require specialized nasal prongs or face masks, which have variable degrees of tolerance by pediatric patients.

Invasive Mechanical Ventilation

The CCTP may be called upon to perform ET intubation in children who require invasive ventilation strategies. Pediatric ET intubation programs should be supported by education and clinical opportunities to manage airways in a controlled environment such as an operating room. Continuous education, supported by a robust quality improvement program, are hallmarks of high-functioning CCTP pediatric intubation programs. Skilled providers should anticipate the challenges associated with difficult airways, including the need for rescue devices and medications to facilitate rapid sequence intubation. Further, CCTPs should be familiar with different strategies for ventilating the patient, once intubated.

A target tidal volume of 7 to 10 mL/kg is recommended. Tidal volumes of less than 7 mL/kg may result in hypoventilation and atelectasis. Tidal volumes of greater than 10 mL/kg may result in overdistention of alveoli, compressing the pulmonary capillary bed and causing barotrauma.

The initial peak inspiratory pressure (PIP) should be the lowest possible value that results in adequate chest excursion. Most children should be adequately ventilated with a PIP of 20 to 30 cm H_2O, although children with lung disease may require higher PIP values—specifically, in the range of 30 to 39 cm H_2O. PIP levels greater than 40 cm H_2O increase the risk of barotrauma, especially pneumothorax. Many CCTPs will consider an alternative type of mechanical ventilator if the pediatric patient requires a PIP of more than 40 cm H_2O. **TABLE 24-7** lists age-appropriate ventilator settings.

TABLE 24-7 Age-Appropriate Ventilator Settings

Setting	Infant	Child
FIO_2	0.21–1.0	0.21–1.0
I time, s	0.5–0.8	0.6–0.8
I:E ratio	1:2 to 1:3	1:2 to 1:3
Tidal volume, mL/kg	7–10	7–10
PEEP, cm	5	5
PS, cm	5–15	5–20
Rate, breaths/min	25–30	20 (neonates: 30–50)

Abbreviations: FIO_2, fraction of inspired oxygen; I time, inspiratory time; I:E, inspiratory to expiratory; PEEP, positive end-expiratory pressure; PS, pressure support

© Jones & Bartlett Learning.

Physiologic PEEP for infants and children is 3 to 5 cm. Higher levels of PEEP may help with alveolar recruitment and improve oxygenation. Higher levels of PEEP also increase intrathoracic pressure, resulting in decreased venous return to the heart. This decreased venous return may cause hypotension in children with decreased intravascular volume status or cardiovascular instability. PEEP levels of 8 to 12 cm H_2O increase the risk of barotrauma and spontaneous pneumothorax. Many CCTPs will consider an alternative type of mechanical ventilator if the pediatric patient requires PEEP values of greater than 12 cm H_2O.

The use of pressure support is most helpful in patients who are best ventilated with a spontaneous respiratory pattern and in patients who are being weaned from mechanical ventilation. Increasing pressure support increases the tidal volume of the patient's spontaneous breaths. This intervention may be helpful in patients who have an adequate spontaneous rate but an inadequate tidal volume. A patient with status asthmaticus, for example, generally is more effectively ventilated with a spontaneous pattern such as pressure support. The initial rate is set based on age-appropriate values and then titrated based on blood gas findings and exhaled carbon dioxide values.

In infants and children with severe lung disease, an alternative for the type of ventilator is an oscillator. An oscillator delivers smaller tidal volumes with very rapid respiratory rates (60 to 1,000 breaths/min) that reduce the risk of barotrauma and pneumothorax. The availability of an oscillator may be the reason for transporting the child to another facility.

Ventilator Setting Changes

Ventilatory strategies are aimed at optimizing oxygenation and ventilation. Consultation between the referring hospital and the intensive care team at the accepting hospital will help identify the optimal strategy for the specific patient. The CCTP may be called upon to make modifications to the ventilatory settings in response to clinical changes in the patient's condition, mainly the arterial partial pressure of oxygen and $ETCO_2$.

In pressure- and volume-cycled ventilation, increasing FIO_2, inspiratory time, and PEEP will all improve oxygenation. Increasing PIP and tidal volume within the target range will also improve oxygenation. Ventilation, as assessed by the $ETCO_2$ level, is predominantly rate driven. Increasing the respiratory rate may result in the desired decrease in retained carbon dioxide, but care must be taken when implementing this change. The expiration phase of respiration must be sufficiently long to allow gas exchange to occur. Increases in the respiratory rate above a certain threshold will result in diminished expiratory times, which may worsen ventilation.

For example, consider a patient with an inspiratory time of 0.8 second and a respiratory rate of 12 breaths/min. The total time for each breath cycle is 5 seconds. This time frame is determined by dividing 60 seconds by the rate of 12. The expiratory time is calculated by subtracting the inspiratory time from the total time for each breath cycle. In this case, 5 seconds – 0.8 second = 4.2 seconds. If the rate is increased to 15, then the total time for the breath cycle is 4 seconds. The expiratory time is now 3.2 seconds, which leaves the patient plenty of time for adequate expiration.

Now consider a patient with an inspiratory time (I) of 0.8 second and a respiratory rate of 30 breaths/min. In this case, the total time for each breath cycle is 2 seconds. The expiratory time is 2 seconds – 0.8 second = 1.2 seconds. This gives the patient an I:E ratio of 1:2. If the ventilatory rate is increased to 33, then the total time for the breath cycle is 1.8 seconds. This changes the expiratory time to 1 second, and the I:E ratio changes to 1:1.25. In this case, increasing the respiratory rate would worsen ventilation because it decreases the time available for exhaling carbon dioxide. For this patient, increasing PIP or tidal volume is a better strategy. The CCTP might also consider decreasing the rate or the inspiratory time to lengthen the time available for expiration. This strategy is particularly helpful in patients with bronchospasm, in whom elevated carbon dioxide levels might be a result of air trapping.

Cardiac Conditions

Pediatric cardiac conditions that have an effect on the circulatory system are common indications for transport. These conditions range from acquired conditions, such as hypovolemia related to trauma, to congenital conditions, such as structural heart defects (addressed later in this chapter). The CCTP will routinely be involved in care of children with four types of heart disease or conditions: a known cardiac defect, an unknown or suspected cyanotic defect (based on patient presentation), a cardiac arrhythmia, and some form of shock (cardiogenic, septic, hemorrhagic, neurogenic, or anaphylactic).

Cardiac Anomalies

Some children with congenital heart defects may need immediate medical management or surgical intervention to repair the defect. These children typically have ductal-dependent lesions, meaning they rely on the patency of the ductus arteriosus for survival, as described in this section. Survival with a good neurologic outcome depends on early recognition, the initiation of IV prostaglandin to maintain the patency of the ductus, and transport to a pediatric facility with the surgical and medical expertise to manage these lesions.

Congenital cardiac anomalies may not be diagnosed until a neonate is 1 to 2 weeks of age because the ductus arteriosus remains patent and allows adequate mixing of oxygenated and deoxygenated blood. Once the ductus closes, children with ductal-dependent lesions can present with a broad spectrum of symptoms, but often exhibit an ill appearance, pallor, and poor feeding cyanosis. These symptoms can also be seen in the setting of sepsis, trauma, and inborn errors of metabolism, which may delay the diagnosis of complex congenital heart disease. In a neonate who has a relatively small lesion and a more subtle presentation, diagnosis of such an anomaly may not be made until the child reaches 2 to 8 weeks of age, when the characteristic murmur may be heard or when the child develops signs of heart failure.

The development of both palliative and curative surgical approaches has created generations of patients (both young and old) with complex repairs that include artificial shunts, single-ventricle pathology, and support from continuous medications such as milrinone and technology such as left ventricular assist devices. The depth of knowledge needed to manage these children exceeds the scope of this text. The CCTP should consult with medical control and accepting subspecialists to identify those complications that may be encountered or anticipated during interfacility transport of these medically fragile patients.

Acquired anatomic diseases are not as common as they once were. In recent years, incidence of cardiac disease related to rheumatic fever (ie, mitral valve disease) and Kawasaki disease (ie, coronary artery aneurysms) has declined.

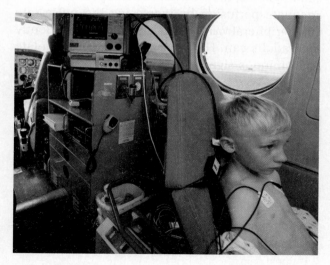

FIGURE 24-22 A pediatric critical care transport patient with ECG leads placed. A 12-lead ECG is not as commonly used in children as it is in adults.

© Jones & Bartlett Learning.

Pediatric ECG Interpretation

The interpretation of an ECG rhythm in children differs from that in adults. To decrease the amount of respiratory artifact, it is helpful to avoid placing the ECG leads at the level of the diaphragm. Specifically, the leads may be placed on the lower abdomen or on the pediatric patient's thighs. A 12-lead ECG is not as commonly used in children but may be obtained for children with abnormal findings on the rhythm strip, arrhythmias, congenital heart disease, acquired heart disease, chest trauma, or suspected cardiotoxic ingestions **FIGURE 24-22**.

The first aspect of rhythm strip interpretation is assessing whether the rate is appropriate for the child's age. The next step is evaluating the components of the rhythm, including the PR interval and the width of the QRS complex. Normal values for these components vary with age. A general guideline for children is that the PR interval should be 0.16 second or less and the QRS complex should be 0.08 second or less. A PR interval of greater than 0.20 second indicates a first-degree heart block. A QRS complex of greater than 0.08 second indicates a wide complex arrhythmia.

In patients with tachyarrhythmia, it may be helpful to increase the ECG monitor sweep speed (typically 25 mm/s) to assess for the presence of a P wave. By increasing the ECG monitor sweep speed, the CCTP can identify subtle nuances in the components of the ECG (P, QRS, T wave).

Pediatric Arrhythmias

Similar to adults, pediatric patients can have both bradyarrhythmias and tachyarrhythmias. Bradyarrhythmias are uncommon in neonates and young children. First-degree heart block is sometimes identified incidentally during the evaluation of complaints such as syncope or chest pain. As in adults, first-degree heart block in children is of little clinical consequence. Symptomatic bradycardia should raise the suspicion for sepsis, myocarditis, Lyme disease, or poisoning. Third-degree heart block has occasionally been identified in patients with Lyme carditis and infrequently in neonates born to mothers with systemic lupus erythematosus. Symptomatic children should be treated in accordance with the AHA guidelines for pediatric advanced life support.

Narrow complex tachycardias, typically supraventricular tachycardias, are more frequently encountered in children. While school-age children and adolescents may present with the more prototypical story of palpitations, younger children and infants frequently present with nondescript symptoms such as fussiness or poor eating. As young children can tolerate tachyarrhythmias longer than adults can, they may present later and often do so with signs of heart failure. Ventricular tachyarrhythmias are uncommon in children, except those with a history of cardiac surgery. A child who experiences a cardiac arrest from a ventricular arrhythmia may have familial disorders of electrolyte transport, otherwise known as channelopathies. Long QT syndrome can also precipitate torsades de pointes and other ventricular arrhythmias, although this scenario is uncommon in children.

The CCTP should be familiar with the range of normal heart rates in children. Misunderstanding what is normal for a given age group is a frequent contributor to errors in diagnosing tachyarrhythmias.

Cardiac Arrest and Death During Interfacility Transport

Cardiac arrest during pediatric interfacility transport is uncommon; nonetheless, discussion with the referring and receiving physicians may identify patients at highest risk for cardiac arrest. This consultation might lead providers to change the mode of transportation. For example, performing compressions in a helicopter is more challenging than in a ground ambulance. In children who have experienced cardiac arrest prior to transport, the CCT team should discuss both anticipated medical challenges and goals of care.

In the event of cardiac arrest during ground transport, providers should stop the ambulance in a safe location to safely facilitate high-quality cardiopulmonary resuscitation. If resuscitation does not rapidly result in return of spontaneous circulation, providers should follow preestablished agency policies that direct the ambulance to the closest hospital. Likewise, if cardiac arrest occurs during air medical transfer, all attempts should be made to resuscitate the patient prior to landing. Agencies offering helicopter or fixed-wing transport should develop contingency plans for these events; these

> ## Advance Directives for Pediatric Patients
>
> Although less common in pediatric patients than in adults, children with complex and long-standing medical problems that are known to be life limiting may have an advance directive; the CCT team will need to ascertain this information from the referring facility.

plans should designate, among other considerations, available airports and landing zones, and the resources available to intercept the patient for transfer to a hospital.

Shock

Shock is a state of poor perfusion and can result from various precipitating events. Due to their unique physiology, children will manifest the signs and symptoms of shock differently than adults do. The CCTP must understand these differences to recognize shock in a sick child and to intervene appropriately.

Shock is broadly categorized as compensated or uncompensated. A child in early or even moderate stages of shock is able to maintain perfusion. Because children typically have strong cardiovascular systems, they are able to compensate for inadequate perfusion by increasing the pulse rate and peripheral vascular resistance more efficiently than adults can. Hypotension is, therefore, a late and ominous sign in an infant or a young child,

> ## Signs and Symptoms
>
> **Shock**
> - Light-headedness
> - Tachycardia
> - Decreasing BP
> - Confusion or loss of consciousness (coma)
> - Chest pain
> - Diarrhea
> - Kidney failure
> - Pale, clammy skin

Transport Management

Shock

- Assess airway, breathing, and circulation.
- Attempt to control obvious bleeding with direct pressure.
- Obtain a finger-stick blood glucose level to ensure hypoglycemia is not present.
- Administer oxygen.
- Administer IV fluids and medications per protocols.

and urgent intervention is needed to prevent cardiac arrest. As a result, BP should not be the only parameter that the CCTP uses to assess for shock. Other indicators, such as the child's LOC, heart rate, skin temperature, respiratory rate and pattern, capillary refill time, and urinary output, are also valid markers of hemodynamic stability and fluid status.

Hypovolemic Shock

Hypovolemic shock is the most common cause of shock in pediatric populations and is characterized by inadequate intravascular volume. Young children experiencing respiratory illnesses tend to eat and drink less. Given their relatively poor fluid reserves, as compared to adults, they are susceptible to severe dehydration. Dehydration is marked clinically by poor urine output. Coupled with vomiting and/or diarrhea, the volumes of which are difficult to quantify, severe dehydration can insidiously lead to hypovolemic shock in children.

Volume loss related to blood in children is most commonly associated with trauma. Another form of fluid loss is excessive urination, like that seen in children with diabetes. Finally, shock resulting from severe allergic reactions may be related to increased capillary permeability that results in third spacing, as well as to distributive shock states that result in decreased peripheral vascular tone.

When intravascular volume falls, there is inadequate venous return and decreased cardiac output. Cardiac output is a primary factor in end-organ perfusion. Inadequate volume may be related to a deficit in the circulating fluid volume, resulting in insufficient volume for perfusion.

Hypovolemic shock is categorized into four stages **FIGURE 24-23**:

- Stage 1: The child appears asymptomatic.
- Stage 2: The child attempts to accommodate for volume losses but compensatory mechanisms are being maximized. BP may still be compensated at this time, but the child is dangerously close to decompensating if interventions are not rapidly applied.

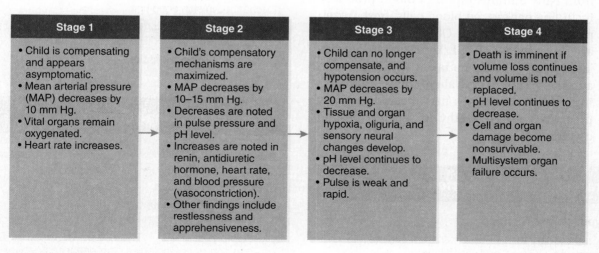

FIGURE 24-23 Progression of hypovolemic shock.
Abbreviation: ADH, antidiuretic hormone

- Stage 3: The child is no longer able to compensate and hypotension occurs. In addition to traditional signs of shock, the child demonstrates mental status changes and significantly decreased urine output. Many children require blood transfusions at this point for resuscitation to be successful.
- Stage 4: Death is imminent without cessation of the volume loss and aggressive volume replacement, including crystalloids and blood products.

Regardless of the etiology of the volume loss, the principles of resuscitation for patients are identical:

1. Stop the source of volume loss, whether it involves bleeding, vomiting and diarrhea, or vasodilation.
2. Replace the volume loss. Fluid resuscitation for children consists of 20 mL/kg of crystalloid solutions. Fluid boluses of crystalloid solution may be repeated up to three times for a total of 60 mL/kg. If losses are ongoing, such as occurs in severe gastroenteritis (ie, cholera), the child should continue to receive replacement fluids. If a child has a cardiac history or concurrent cardiogenic shock, fluid boluses should be administered at a rate of 10 mL/kg. Ultimately, the child may receive up to three boluses of 20 mL/kg but in smaller increments. Children with volume loss related to trauma will benefit from early administration of blood products, including packed red blood cells, fresh frozen plasma, and platelets. Often blood products are preceded by 40 mL/kg of crystalloid fluids. Caution should be taken with continued administration of crystalloid fluids, as emerging evidence indicates that these fluids may precipitate coagulopathy in severely injured children.

Successful resuscitation is measured by a return to a normal heart rate, respiratory rate, BP, improved mental status, and improved skin condition.

Cardiogenic Shock

Causes of cardiogenic shock include, but are not limited to, congenital cardiac defects, drug toxicity, metabolic causes, hypovolemia, myocarditis, and arrhythmias. Congenital defects are much more likely to be the cause of cardiogenic shock compared to the other etiologies. The child with cardiogenic shock will present with traditional signs of shock, including tachycardia, tachypnea, hypoxia, mental status changes, and changes in skin condition. Such a patient also often presents with pulmonary congestion resulting in crackles heard on auscultation and jugular venous distention. A chest radiograph may reveal cardiomegaly.

Treatment principles concentrate on improving cardiac function with fluid resuscitation and inotropic support, to include dopamine, dobutamine, epinephrine, milrinone, and norepinephrine. Primary pathologies or impedances are treated, and cardiac function may be supported pharmacologically until myocardial function returns.

Signs and Symptoms

Cardiogenic Shock

- Traditional signs of shock, including tachycardia, tachypnea, hypoxia, mental status changes, and changes in skin condition
- Pulmonary congestion resulting in crackles heard on auscultation
- Jugular venous distention

Transport Management

Cardiogenic Shock

- Resuscitate with fluids if needed to ensure normovolemia.
- Provide inotropic support, including dopamine, dobutamine, epinephrine, milrinone, and norepinephrine.
- Treat primary pathologies or impedances.
- Support cardiac function pharmacologically until myocardial function returns.

Transport Management

Hypovolemic Shock

- Stop the source of volume loss (ie, bleeding, vomiting, diarrhea, and vasodilation).
- Replace the volume loss with fluid boluses and blood products.

Distributive Shock

The major treatment goals for distributive shock include stopping the vasodilation, returning volume to the intravascular space, and improving tissue perfusion. Types of distributive shock include neurogenic shock, anaphylactic shock, and septic shock.

Neurogenic Shock

Neurogenic shock, also known as spinal shock, often presents with significant hypotension without tachycardia due to the loss of spinal cord–mediated vascular tone. Treatment for neurogenic shock may include administration of vasoactive medications; however, volume replacement with crystalloids must occur first. The principle of "fill the tank first and then make the container smaller" is the cornerstone of treatment. Neurogenic shock may respond to norepinephrine.

Transport Management

Neurogenic Shock
- Replace volume with crystalloids.
- Administer vasoactive medications.

Anaphylactic Shock

Children in anaphylactic shock often present with increased general body edema, hypotension, rash, urticaria, anxiety, and warm, flushed skin. Bronchospasm and laryngeal edema may also be life threatening.

Management of anaphylactic shock involves removal of the allergen, volume replacement, and epinephrine. Epinephrine dilates the bronchioles, relaxes the smooth muscle, causes vasoconstriction, and decreases vascular permeability, thereby inhibiting more volume loss. Adjuncts such as antihistamines (ie, diphenhydramine) and corticosteroids are controversial, though their use remains common practice.

Systemic Inflammatory Response Syndrome and Septic Shock

Systemic inflammatory response syndrome (SIRS) and sepsis are both distributive shock syndromes

Signs and Symptoms

Anaphylactic Shock
- General body edema
- Hypotension
- Rash
- Urticaria
- Anxiety
- Warm, flushed skin
- Bronchospasm
- Laryngeal edema

Transport Management

Anaphylactic Shock
- Remove the allergen.
- Replace fluid volume loss.
- Administer epinephrine.

characterized by inflammation, vasodilation, significantly increased microvascular permeability, and accumulation of leukocytes resulting in hypoperfusion and end-organ dysfunction. Early recognition and aggressive resuscitation are key to good outcomes with these conditions.

As in adults, SIRS in pediatric patients is an inflammatory response that may result from injury (trauma) or infection. Hallmarks of SIRS are altered thermoregulation (hyperthermia or hypothermia), tachycardia, tachypnea, and age-specific alterations in white blood cells (WBCs). WBCs may be increased (usually a WBC count greater than $20,000/mm^3$ is indicative of infection) or decreased (a WBC count less than $4,000/mm^3$, referred to as *leukopenia*, is most often due to low numbers of neutrophils, a condition called neutropenia). In addition, bandemia is often present, meaning that certain bands of immature WBCs are released into the bloodstream in excess (more than 10% of the total WBC population).

Sepsis is SIRS that occurs in tandem with a known or suspected infection. Normally, the body has a balanced immune response to infection, mounting an immune assault that results in elimination of the pathogens and full recovery. In some instances, however, the immune system becomes exhausted during the usual response, leading to impaired immunity. If the pathogens were contained prior to the onset of impairment, secondary infection may ensue, leading to increased morbidity or mortality. If the pathogens were not contained, morbidity or mortality may result from the primary infection. Alternatively, for reasons that remain poorly understood, excessive inflammation or SIRS can occur, the consequences of which are potentially more injurious than the original insult. Early and targeted antibiotic therapy should be initiated to combat the suspected infectious agent. Some evidence indicates that early and judicious administration of fluids reduces morbidity and mortality related to sepsis.

Renal Conditions

Acute kidney injury (AKI) is defined as profound deterioration of renal function associated with increasing levels of solute (BUN or creatinine). Actual urine volume in such cases can vary from normal urine output to oliguria. Causes of AKI are generally divided into three categories **TABLE 24-8**:

- Prerenal acute kidney injury is caused by decreased perfusion of an intact nephron.
- Intrarenal acute kidney injury is caused by damage of an actual nephron.
- Postrenal acute kidney injury is caused by downstream obstruction with initially intact nephrons.

Prerenal Disorders

Prerenal causes of AKI are the most common in children and are primarily related to dehydration and decreased renal perfusion. Dehydration results from fluid loss or acute blood loss. The patient may present with a range of signs and symptoms—nausea, vomiting, diarrhea, diabetic ketoacidosis, all forms of shock, and burns. A decreased circulating blood volume results in decreased renal perfusion.

Other causes of decreased renal perfusion may be related to any cardiac condition that results in decreased cardiac output, such as heart failure. In patients with sepsis or burns, there may actually be sufficient or increased extracellular fluid volume as a result of increased vascular permeability, but the intravascular volume is greatly depleted. AKI from volume loss is frequently corrected with volume resuscitation.

Intrarenal Disorders

Intrarenal or parenchymal causes of AKI are diverse; all of these etiologies, however, lead to nephron damage and loss of glomerular function as a result of damage to the glomerular basement membrane. Damage to the arterioles and glomerular capillaries may be the result of coagulation, inflammation, barotrauma, or prolonged ischemia.

The proximal tubular cells of the kidneys have high metabolic demands, which render them more susceptible to ischemic insults. Nephrotoxins cause sloughing and necrosis of cells in the proximal tubule and ascending loop of Henle, which results in obstruction of tubular blood flow and leakage of fluid into the peritubular space and plasma.

Occlusion of the renal arteries from emboli or thrombosis may cause infarction as a result of decreased renal blood flow. Vascular congestion and hemorrhagic necrosis may also occur as a result of renal vein thrombosis.

Hemolytic Uremic Syndrome

Hemolytic uremic syndrome (HUS) is one of the major causes of AKI in infants and children younger than 4 years. Its hallmarks include the classic triad of microangiopathic hemolytic anemia, thrombocytopenia, and acute injury to the kidney. Classification of HUS has traditionally been divided into diarrhea-positive and diarrhea-negative forms. Diarrhea-positive HUS is caused by Shiga toxin–producing *Escherichia coli* (STEC) infections, which are responsible for 90% of HUS cases and typically affect children 5 years or younger, and occasionally by *Shigella dysenteriae* type 1 infection. All other types of HUS are considered atypical and labeled as diarrhea-negative HUS.

The primary pathology in HUS is thought to be related to endothelial cell injury in the renal cortex that leads to localized vascular coagulation and fibrin deposits. As the red blood cells (RBCs) pass through the fibrin strands in the renal vasculature, they become fractured and cause microangiopathic anemia. Thrombocytopenia is the result of localized intravascular coagulation-consuming platelets.

The presentation of HUS typically follows a gastroenteritis-type illness, with symptoms

TABLE 24-8 Common Causes of Acute Kidney Injury

Type of Failure	Causes	Example
Prerenal (decreased perfusion of an intact nephron)	Hypovolemia	Hemorrhagic shock Dehydration (gastrointestinal losses and diabetic ketoacidosis) Insensible losses (prematurity, burns) Sodium and water losses (renal, adrenal, endocrine) Hypoproteinemia
	Hypotension	Heart failure Decompensated shock Congenital heart disease
	Renal vessel injury with obstruction	Not applicable
Intrarenal (damage of the actual nephron)	Primary parenchymal disease	Hemolytic uremic syndrome Post-strep (acute) Glomerulonephritis Lupus erythematosus Henoch-Schönlein purpura Pyelonephritis Malignant hypertension
	Acute tubular necrosis	Ischemia (prolonged prerenal acute kidney injury) Nephrotoxins (heavy metals, uric acid, nonsteroidal anti-inflammatory drugs, angiotensin-converting enzyme inhibitors, aminoglycoside antibiotics, beta blockers, diuretics, radiocontrast, myoglobin, organic solvents)
	Large-vessel occlusion	Renal vein thrombosis Renal artery stenosis Thrombosis or emboli
	Congenital abnormalities	Renal agenesis Infantile polycystic kidney disease Bilateral multicystic kidneys
	Neoplasm	Not applicable
Postrenal (downstream obstruction with initially intact nephrons)	Obstructive uropathy	Posterior urethral valves Prune belly syndrome Neurogenic bladder Ureteropelvic junction syndrome Tumor Nephrolithiasis Renal calculi Trauma to the collecting system Ureterocele

© Jones & Bartlett Learning.

including vomiting, abdominal pain, and bloody diarrhea. As the gastrointestinal symptoms subside, the child again becomes acutely ill, presenting with irritability, pallor, and a petechial rash. This presentation is often, but not always, accompanied by signs of fluid overload including peripheral edema, pulmonary edema, and hypertension.

Laboratory studies show fragmented RBCs, thrombocytopenia, and evidence of AKI, including elevated BUN and creatinine levels, hyperkalemia, and metabolic acidosis. Urine studies show proteinuria and hematuria with or without anuria.

Treatment of HUS is primarily supportive and includes fluid and metabolic balance, control of hypertension (treatment of DBP greater than 120 mm Hg with labetalol, nifedipine, or hydralazine), transfusion of packed RBCs and platelets if required, and aggressive treatment of AKI with possible dialysis or continuous renal replacement therapy (CRRT) when the BUN exceeds 80 mg/dL. The prognosis is usually excellent when aggressive treatment is initiated early.

Signs and Symptoms

Hemolytic Uremic Syndrome

- Gastroenteritis-type symptoms: vomiting, abdominal pain, and bloody diarrhea
- After the gastrointestinal symptoms subside: irritability, pallor, signs of fluid overload, including peripheral and pulmonary edema, hypertension, and petechiae

Transport Management

Hemolytic Uremic Syndrome

- Support fluid and metabolic balance.
- Control hypertension.
- Transfuse packed RBCs and platelets if required.

Acute Glomerulonephritis

Acute glomerulonephritis (AGN) is a histopathologic diagnosis that is associated with edema, hypertension, and hematuria. AGN results from the deposition of circulating immune complexes in the kidney basement membrane, which ultimately reduces the glomerular filtration rate. This syndrome can be induced by infection with a variety of organisms, but especially group A beta hemolytic streptococci.

Acute postinfectious glomerulonephritis (APIGN) or AGN following an acute infection can occur after a skin infection or a pharyngeal infection. Most typically caused by infection with group A *Streptococcus*, APIGN occurs most commonly in

school-age children and more frequently in boys than in girls. Its pathology is thought to involve activation of the complement pathway leading to inflammation, which then causes glomerular damage through immune complex deposition in the basement membrane of the glomeruli.

Symptoms of APIGN typically manifest 1 to 2 weeks after infection, with a classic symptom being gross hematuria with brown urine. The severity of presentation runs the spectrum from mild and not requiring hospitalization, to severe oliguria with symptoms of overload including heart failure, peripheral and pulmonary edema, and hypertension.

Laboratory urinalysis values in patients with APIGN reveal RBCs and proteinuria. WBCs represent glomerular inflammation in such cases, rather than pyelonephritis (inflammation of the kidney linings). In addition, expected evidence of renal insufficiency includes elevated BUN and creatinine levels, hyperkalemia, hyponatremia, and acidosis. Elevated antibody titers (ie, measurements of the presence and amount of antibodies in the blood) of streptococci confirm APIGN after streptococcal infection.

Treatment of severe APIGN is primarily supportive and includes fluid restriction of IV solutions to avoid promoting peripheral and pulmonary edema. Loop diuretics are useful in treating mild hypertension, edema, and fluid overload. The prognosis is good, and full recovery is expected in more than 98% of all children.

Signs and Symptoms

Acute Postinfectious Glomerulonephritis

- Gross hematuria with brown urine
- Heart failure
- Peripheral and pulmonary edema
- Hypertension

Transport Management

Acute Postinfectious Glomerulonephritis

- Restrict fluids.
- Administer loop diuretics.

Acute Tubular Necrosis

Acute tubular necrosis (ATN) is a condition that results in damage to the tissue of the kidneys' tubules. Like most renal pathologies, it can have numerous etiologies; however, the most common cause is renal ischemia precipitated by severe hypovolemia. Tubular damage can also occur following a toxic insult, such as heavy metal poisoning, or as a result of myoglobin or hemoglobin accumulation in the tubules following a severe crush injury, burn, or hemolytic crisis.

In patients with ATN, the renal tubular cells die when they do not get enough oxygen or if they are exposed to a toxic drug. Injury to the tubular cells is most prominent in the straight portion of the proximal tubules and in the loop of Henle. In addition to decreased filtration being noted, a buildup of casts and debris obstructs the tubule lumen, such that filtrate leaks through the damaged epithelium. In addition, decreased perfusion leads to diminished production of vasodilators such as nitric oxide, resulting in further vasoconstriction and hypoperfusion.

ATN is clinically defined as proceeding in three phases:

- *Phase 1: oliguric phase.* Severe oliguria lasts approximately 10 days. Renal recovery from ATN is highly unlikely if the oliguria or anuria persists longer than 3 to 6 weeks.
- *Phase 2: diuretic phase.* Passage of large volumes of isothenuric urine containing sodium levels of 80 to 150 mEq/L occurs.
- *Phase 3: recovery phase.* Signs and symptoms resolve rapidly as a result of regeneration of tubular epithelial cells, although polyuria may be present for days to weeks. The mechanism of this diuresis is not completely understood.

Signs and Symptoms

Acute Tubular Necrosis

- Severe oliguria lasting approximately 10 days
- Diuretic phase: passage of large volumes of isothenuric urine
- Recovery phase: signs and symptoms resolve rapidly
- Polyuria

Transport Management

Acute Tubular Necrosis

- Replace fluids and electrolytes.

Transport treatment usually consists of fluid and electrolyte replacement. Ultimately, dialysis is required to remove the toxins.

Postrenal Disorders

Postrenal or obstructive failure has numerous etiologies. In most cases, unilateral obstructive abnormalities do not result in AKI. Flank or abdominal pain is often present. Prolonged, unrelieved obstruction causes irreversible parenchymal damage because of infection and increased hydrostatic pressure. Obstruction of urine outflow in the renal system causes an increase in hydrostatic pressure at the proximal tubule and glomerulus, resulting in a decrease in glomerular filtration and renal function. Large nephrolithiases (renal stones), anatomic abnormalities, or obstruction from malignancy can all lead to postrenal disorder.

Complications of AKI

Several potentially life-threatening events can occur in patients experiencing AKI.

Electrolyte Imbalances

Electrolyte imbalances such as hyponatremia, hypocalcemia, and hyperkalemia may occur in patients with AKI.

Hyponatremia is most often dilutional (low sodium levels as a result of excessive fluid intake) secondary to volume overload, is asymptomatic, and is simply treated with fluid restrictions. Severe hyponatremia may cause seizures and is managed by infusing a hypertonic (3%) saline solution.

Hypocalcemia is caused by hyperphosphatemia and is not usually treated unless symptoms such as tetany, seizures, or decreased cardiac contractility are present. Rapid correction of hypocalcemia may result in the deposition of calcium salts in body tissues. Treatment includes oral dosing of calcium carbonate or, in emergent cases, cautious administration of IV calcium gluconate (10%) at a dose of

50 to 100 mg/kg. Hypocalcemia can manifest clinically with a prolonged QRS complex on ECG.

Hyperkalemia has the potential to cause life-threatening arrhythmias by producing membrane excitability. ECG changes may include peaked T waves, widened QRS complexes, and eventually bradycardia. An elevated serum potassium level is treated based on lab values and the presence of ECG abnormalities. Management may include careful monitoring, the removal of potassium chloride from IV fluids, pharmacologic treatments, and, in rare circumstances, dialysis. The following medications may be administered:

- Sodium polystyrene sulfonate resin: This ion-exchange resin acts in the colon or ileum. Usual dosing is 1 g/kg every 2 to 4 hours, and the medication may be mixed with sorbitol. Recent studies suggest this medication may be of questionable benefit.
- Calcium gluconate: This drug has no direct effect on the serum potassium but stabilizes the myocardial membrane and ventricular rhythm by changing the cell's action potential. When it is administered, the CCTP should monitor the patient's heart rate and stop the infusion if the child's pulse rate drops by more than 20 beats/min. In patients with cardiac arrest secondary to hyperkalemia, the CCTP should substitute calcium chloride.
- Glucose and insulin: Potassium can be moved into the intracellular space by administering insulin (usually by infusion) with a glucose infusion of 5% dextrose in water or 5% dextrose and normal saline and a concurrent insulin infusion. The goal is to maintain the glucose level between 120 and 300 mg/dL. This has the effect of rapidly lowering the serum potassium level; however, careful assessment of glucose blood levels is necessary to prevent hypoglycemia.
- Sodium bicarbonate: This drug can be used even in the absence of acidosis. Calcium gluconate is not compatible with $NaHCO_3$, however, so IV lines must be flushed prior to administering this medication.
- Albuterol: Massive doses of nebulized albuterol cause a shift of extracellular potassium into the cell and can lower the serum potassium by 1.0 to 1.5 mEq/L. Albuterol also helps to protect against insulin-induced hypoglycemia.

Hypertension and Hypertensive Encephalopathy

Hypertension that may progress to hypertensive encephalopathy is also a life-threatening complication in patients with AKI. Hypertension is usually caused by sodium and water retention. Hypertensive encephalopathy is hypertension associated with neurologic symptoms such as nausea, vomiting, headache, visual changes, seizures, and mental status changes. As with any hypertensive crisis, it is important to aim for a MAP reduction of 15% to 25%. A more precipitous or pronounced drop in MAP that returns the child to normal BP parameters may lead to hypoperfusion of the end organs.

Meningitis

The presentation of the pediatric patient with meningitis depends largely on the child's age, the type of infectious organism, and the child's current health. Bacterial meningitis is uncommon, especially among children who are fully vaccinated against this disease. The onset of symptoms is typically abrupt, with hallmark signs including fever, chills, nuchal rigidity, vomiting, photophobia, headache, back pain, and seizures in older children. Infants and young children may present with some of the same symptoms as are noted in older children, but also may experience poor feeding, marked irritability and agitation, and a characteristic high-pitched cry with bulging fontanelles.

Viral meningitis is more common than bacterial or fungal meningitis. Fungal meningitis occurs only in immunocompromised patients or in geographic areas where such infections are endemic. In young children, viruses such as enterovirus are a common cause of viral meningitis. In young infants, the toxic-appearing infant with meningitis may have an infection with herpesvirus. If unrecognized, meningitis caused by herpesvirus is frequently fatal. Bacterial meningitis in young infants can result from infections from group B *Streptococcus*, *E coli* (as the result of urosepsis/bacteremia), or, infrequently, *Listeria*. Infection with the *Neisseria meningitidis* bacterium is exceedingly rare, and vaccinations for serogroups A and B are ubiquitous around the world.

On arrival to the patient's bedside, the CCTP may inquire whether the patient with meningitis has a positive **Brudzinski sign** or **Kernig sign**. To test for the Brudzinski sign, the patient lies supine and the examiner flexes their head and neck in an attempt to touch the chin to the chest. An abnormal response includes flexion of the legs and hips during this process (positive Brudzinski sign). Testing for this condition should not be performed if a cervical spine injury is suspected. To evaluate for the Kernig sign, the patient lies supine with the legs flexed at the hip and the knees flexed at a right angle; the CCTP then tries to extend the knees. An abnormal response is present if there is pain and resistance to knee straightening (positive Kernig sign). If pain and resistance are present bilaterally, then meningeal irritation is likely present.

The neonate patient with meningitis may be extremely difficult to assess; moreover, it is difficult to make the diagnosis of meningococcal infection in a neonate because the symptoms are usually vague in nature and challenging to differentiate from other septic etiologies. The CCTP should inquire about the infant's feeding and sucking ability. The infant with meningitis may also present with a poor cry,

Signs and Symptoms

Meningococcal Infections
- Fever
- Chills
- Nuchal rigidity
- Vomiting
- Photophobia
- Headache
- Back pain
- Seizures

Infants and Young Children
- Poor feeding
- Marked irritability and agitation
- Characteristic high-pitched cry with bulging fontanelles
- Poor cry
- Decreased muscle tone
- Jaundice
- Weight loss
- Hypothermia
- Apnea
- Cyanosis
- Seizure activity

Transport Management

Meningococcal Infections
- Ensure standard universal precautions are followed.

decreased muscle tone, jaundice, weight loss, hypothermia, apnea, cyanosis, and seizure activity.

Standard universal precautions should be taken with all pediatric patients with suspected meningitis, considering the close proximity of the patient to the transport provider.

Trauma

In the United States, trauma is the leading cause of death among pediatric patients 1 year or older. Traumatic injuries in children most commonly involve motor vehicle crashes, suffocation, submersion, burns, falls, and violence. While assessment and care of pediatric trauma patients employ the same systematic approach taken for the adult population, one assessment tool, the GCS, is modified for pediatric patients. As described earlier in this chapter, the GCS can be used to assess neurologic status. This dynamic evaluation should be repeated to note changes or trends in the acutely injured child. Recent research supports the evaluation of the modified motor score in particular as a marker for acuity and for neurologic prognostication.

Another important assessment tool for the child with traumatic injury is the pediatric trauma score. Providers combine the scores for several components—weight, airway status, central nervous system status, systolic BP, pulse rate, fractures, and wounds—to arrive at a total score reflective of injury severity **TABLE 24-9**. Scores are categorized as follows:

- A score of 9 to 12 indicates minor trauma. Follow local guidelines/protocols for treatment.
- A score of 6 to 8 indicates a potentially life-threatening condition. Consider transporting the patient to a trauma center.
- A score of 0 to 5 indicates a life-threatening condition. Transport the patient to a trauma center.
- A score of less than 0 indicates a condition that is usually fatal. Transport the patient to the nearest trauma center equipped to care for critically ill children.

TABLE 24-9 Pediatric Trauma Score

Variable/Source	+2	+1	−1
Weight	>20 kg (44 lb)	10–20 kg (22–44 lb)	<10 kg (22 lb)
Airway	Patent	Maintainable	Unmaintainable
Systolic blood pressure	>90 mm Hg	50–90 mm Hg	<50 mm Hg
Pulse	Radial	Carotid	Nonpalpable
Central nervous system	Awake	Responsive	Unresponsive
Fractures	None	Closed or suspected	Multiple closed or open
Wounds	None	Minor	Major, penetrating, or burns >10%

Reprinted from Tepas JJ III, Mollitt DL, Talbert JL, Bryant M. The pediatric trauma score as a predictor of injury severity in the injured child. *J Pediatr Surg.* 1987;22(1):14-18. Copyright © 1987, with permission from Elsevier. http://www.sciencedirect.com/science/journal/00223468.

Traumatic Brain Injury

TBI is the leading cause of morbidity and mortality in children, accounting for 70% to 80% of all pediatric deaths from trauma. The death rate from TBI is five times higher than that from leukemia, the next most common cause of pediatric mortality. The main source of injury is motor vehicle crashes involving passengers, pedestrians, or bicyclists. Less common sources of head injury include sports-related injuries, falls, and abuse.

Injuries to the brain are traditionally evaluated as primary or secondary injuries. Primary injuries that result from penetrating, rapid deceleration or rotational injuries occur at the moment of impact and cause physical and mechanical destruction of brain tissue; they can include parenchymal injury, diffuse axonal injuries, and cerebral edema. In comparison with primary injuries, many factors may improve or worsen secondary brain injury, which involves a complicated cascade of cellular destruction. The primary brain injury causes a certain amount of tissue and cellular death. Some injured areas of the brain (penumbra) surrounding the dead tissue may remain viable, but are vulnerable to hypoxic, ischemic, and inflammatory responses. *Aggressive management to prevent hypoxia, hypotension, and progressive edema is required to protect this unstable brain tissue.* If these conditions are uncorrected, secondary brain injury leads to irreversible brain damage and death.

Increased ICP

Increased ICP can have numerous etiologies. The most common cause of increased ICP in pediatric populations is related to trauma or a malfunction of an existing cerebrospinal fluid shunt.

Signs and symptoms of increased ICP may include headache, irritability, fever, dizziness, nausea, projectile vomiting, lethargy, changes in vision, unsteady gait, high-pitched cry, bulging fontanelle, pupillary dilation, seizures, coma, and Cushing triad. The symptoms become more progressive and severe as the ICP rises.

The medical management of increased ICP may include the following:

- Mild hyperventilation ($Paco_2$ between 30 and 35 mm Hg). Most neurosurgeons recommend keeping the patient normocapneic.
- Administration of 3% sodium chloride (also called hypertonic saline), 4 to 6 mL/kg as a bolus, followed by a 1 mL/kg/h infusion. Alternatively, the CCTP can consider administration of mannitol (0.5 to 1 mg/kg/dose).
- Maintenance of cerebral perfusion pressure at more than 50 to 60 mm Hg (increased MAP to maintain adequate cerebral perfusion pressure).
- Elevation of the patient's head at a 15° to 30° angle to the stretcher to promote cerebral venous drainage.
- Normothermia or mild hypothermia to decrease the metabolic rate.

- Airway management as clinically indicated.
- Pain management.
- Possible induction of coma using barbiturates (decreases the cerebral metabolic rate and oxygen consumption).

Treatment modalities may include inserting a monitor to measure ICP. This treatment is more pertinent for interfacility transports as compared to prehospital transports. A ventricular catheter is placed in the ventricles connected to an external ventricular drain; this drain evacuates fluid within the ventricle and measures objective ICP.

Signs and Symptoms

Increased ICP

- Headache
- Irritability
- Fever
- Dizziness
- Nausea
- Projectile vomiting
- Lethargy
- Visual changes
- Unsteady gait
- High-pitched cry
- Bulging fontanelle
- Papillary dilation
- Seizures
- Coma
- Cushing triad

Transport Management

Increased ICP

- Maintain cerebral perfusion pressure at greater than 50 to 60 mm Hg.
- Position the patient so the patient's head is raised at a 15° to 30° angle.
- Maintain a normal or slightly elevated body temperature.
- Administer mannitol.
- Manage pain.

A subarachnoid bolt placed in the subarachnoid space can also measure ICP, but cannot drain fluid and does not sound an alarm for increased pressure.

Normal ICP is 0 to 10 cm H_2O. An acceptable ICP is usually less than 15 to 20 cm H_2O. Cerebral perfusion pressure should be, at a minimum, 50 to 60 mm Hg to ensure adequate brain perfusion.

Concussion

Concussion is the most commonly seen type of TBI in the pediatric population. It is described as an injury to the brain resulting from a force applied directly or indirectly to the head, which may potentially produce a variety of symptoms. A concussion may or may not initially involve loss of consciousness. It results in a constellation of cognitive, somatic, emotional, and sleep-related symptoms. The duration of symptoms can vary, lasting from several minutes to several days, weeks, months, or longer. Recent data indicate that high school athletes exhibiting concussive symptoms on the playing field that resolve in less than 15 minutes will often later demonstrate deficits on formal neuropsychological testing and have reemergence of active symptoms, lasting up to a week post injury.

There are several issues of importance to the CCTP regarding concussions. First, all concussions involve some degree of injury to the brain. Second, in cases of sports-related concussions, athletes must be removed from play for a mandatory medical evaluation. Last, while it is clear that athletes—particularly children—have a greater vulnerability to reinjury following a concussion, there is lack of agreement on definitions and guidelines on when and how an athlete should be allowed to return to play. Long-term sequelae following repeated head injuries can be significant. All CCTPs should be familiar with the recommendations for evaluation of young athletes following a head injury. Current guidelines and most state laws require an on-field evaluation. The Centers for Disease Control and Prevention's Heads Up campaign provides authoritative, up-to-date information on prevention and recognition of concussions; its criteria are useful for the CCTP in assessing patients with suspected concussion.

Concussion is a mild form of TBI that, by its nature, leads to brain dysfunction induced by trauma without evidence of structural injury on standard neuroimaging studies such as computed tomography (CT) or magnetic resonance imaging of the head. In turn, diagnosis of concussion is based on symptoms. Today, the decision to obtain a head CT must be balanced with the long-term risks of malignancy from the CT radiation exposure, which is higher in children than in adults. The most comprehensive and thoroughly validated decision-making tool for use of CT in pediatric patients currently available is the Pediatric Emergency Care Applied Research Network's low-risk clinical decision rules **TABLE 24-10**.

TABLE 24-10 Pediatric Emergency Care Applied Research Network's Low-Risk Clinical Decision Rules	
Age (years)	**Criteria**
Up to 2 years	Normal mental status
	Normal behavior according to caregiver
	No loss of consciousness
	No severe mechanism of injury
	No nonfrontal scalp hematoma
	No evidence of skull fracture
2 to 18 years	Normal mental status
	No loss of consciousness
	No severe mechanism of injury
	No vomiting
	No severe headache
	No signs of basilar skull fracture

© Jones & Bartlett Learning.

Transport Management

Concussion

- Provide supportive measures.
- Frequently perform and document a neurologic assessment (baseline and continuous).
- Document the patient's pain level and tolerance of transport.

Cerebral Contusion

A cerebral contusion most commonly occurs at the point of impact and/or on the side opposite the impact, such as with a coup–contrecoup injury. The resulting focal hemorrhage in the brain may be associated with a concurrent concussion.

Epidural Hematoma

Epidural hematomas typically include arterial bleeding from vascular injuries after blunt trauma, most commonly involving the middle meningeal artery. This blood vessel is located just outside the dura and may be torn when a parietal skull fracture occurs. Another potential cause of epidural bleeding is damage to the diploic veins in the posterior cranial fossa, although the most common cause is a lateral temporal fossa injury. The accumulation of blood noted in these injuries does not "touch" the brain tissue. Epidural hematomas most commonly occur after blunt trauma to the head.

The classic pattern associated with epidural hematoma is a lucid period followed by rapid neurologic deterioration. However, this pattern occurs in only a minority of pediatric patients with an epidural hematoma. Children may never have a loss of consciousness or a lucid period. Epidural hematomas frequently require surgical evacuation.

Subdural Hematoma

Subdural hematomas are 5 to 10 times more common than epidural hematomas, especially in infants. These injuries are caused by shearing forces that slide the fragile brain tissue over the rough base of the skull. The hematoma occurs just below the dura, so that blood comes into contact with brain tissue. Subdural hematomas are usually caused by a disruption of bridging veins or venous sinuses beneath the dura. They can be a result of child abuse such as shaken baby syndrome. Shaking an infant violently causes acceleration–deceleration forces that shear the bridging veins in the subdural space.

Risk Assessment and Management

Many children who experience closed head trauma may have only minor injuries. Children who have low-risk injuries are often asymptomatic, with normal neurologic findings on exam. Care at home with responsible adult supervision may be all that is necessary for these patients.

Children with moderate-risk injuries will present with an altered LOC, progressive headache, or vomiting and may have an associated injury. They often require basic trauma care, including basic wound management and spinal motion restriction with radiologic evaluation.

Children with high-risk injuries will present with a depressed LOC and possible neurologic deficits or signs of increased ICP. These children often require immediate surgical interventions. Good patient outcomes require early recognition and treatment, including an early consultation with a neurosurgeon for children with high-risk injuries.

As with any traumatic injury, initial management involves stabilization of the cervical spine, airway, breathing, and circulation. All attempts should be made to prevent secondary injury, including steps to avoid hypotension and hypoxia. If clinical conditions warrant, then ET intubation should be implemented. Proper sedation and analgesia should be administered to prevent spikes in ICP. Hyperventilation should be avoided in children who are intubated. Although routine hyperventilation is not recommended for treatment of increased ICP, it may be used emergently to transiently decrease cerebral blood flow. The benefit of creating "more room in the vault" is short-lived, however, because decreased blood flow causes hypoxia in already injured brain tissue.

Any source of bleeding in the head, including the brain, face, mandible, and scalp, can lead to significant blood loss in the pediatric patient. Hypovolemia is of great concern in children, and particularly in infants, who have a proportionally larger amount of blood volume in their heads. Even in older children, an open scalp laceration can be a significant source of blood loss that needs to be stopped while administering aggressive fluid resuscitation. The treatment goal is euvolemia, because cerebral perfusion pressure (CPP) depends on the MAP (CPP = MAP – ICP). Maintaining the patient's head at a 30° angle and midline also improves venous outflow from the head.

The child's mental status may be altered for a number of reasons. The most life-threatening situation involves herniation syndromes, in which increased pressure in the cranial vault causes the brain to shift. In such a case, the brain may be shifted laterally or down through the foramen magnum. The treatment of increased ICP, as discussed earlier, can include the use of osmotic diuretics such as mannitol or 3% saline. Elevating the head of the bed by 15° to 30° and elective airway management to maintain normocapnia can be considered. Children with intracranial injuries should be maintained in spinal motion restriction even if imaging performed at the referring center is negative.

Spinal Cord Injuries

Of all children who experience traumatic injuries, fewer than 4% have an injury to the spine and/or spinal cord. Although this is a relatively low incidence, mortality related to spinal cord injuries in children is more than double that in the adult population. Serious neurologic injuries are more common in older children and are often associated with sports injuries, diving injuries, or falls. High-grade injuries are most common in children after an axillary loading mechanism. The incidence of spinal cord injury dramatically increases in adolescents between 15 and 18 years of age. Of all sports-related injuries and reported spinal cord injuries, 30% to 50% involve the cervical spine and result in quadriplegia and/or severe disability.

Injuries in children younger than 8 years are most commonly found in the C1 (occiput) to C3 area, whereas older children and adults tend to have injuries in the lower cervical spine **FIGURE 24-24**. Because of the anatomic spine differences between adults and children, children are more susceptible to sustain cervical spine injuries of greater severity. By comparison, older children and adults incur injuries that are more evenly distributed throughout the cervical and thoracic spine.

Similar to brain injury, spinal cord injury may occur with a primary insult and then a secondary insult. The primary insult occurs from hyperflexion (most commonly), extension, rotational injury, or compression injuries. The secondary injuries occur from biochemical reactions, including oxygen free-radical production that damages endothelial cells within the brain, ion fluxes involving extracellular potassium, ischemia, and edema. No evidence supports the empiric use of IV glucocorticoids for acute spinal cord injury.

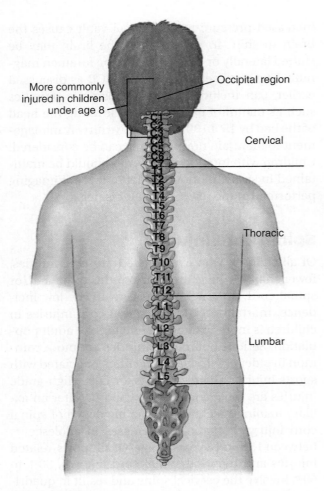

More commonly injured in children under age 8

Occipital region

Cervical

Thoracic

Lumbar

C1
C2
C3
C4
C5
C6
C7
T1
T2
T3
T4
T5
T6
T7
T8
T9
T10
T11
T12
L1
L2
L3
L4
L5

FIGURE 24-24 Injuries in children younger than 8 years are most commonly found in the occiput region to C3 area. Older children and adults tend to have injuries in the lower cervical spine.

© Jones & Bartlett Learning.

The most important intervention in the treatment of children with known or suspected spinal cord injury is prevention of further injury through appropriate use of spinal motion restriction.

Because children have relatively weak spinal ligaments and increased mobility of the spine, they may sustain damage to the spinal cord and spinal ligaments without damage to the spinal vertebrae. This damage is called **SCIWORA**: spinal cord injury without radiographic abnormalities. SCIWORA should be suspected when there are clinical signs or symptoms of spinal cord injury in the presence of normal cervical spine radiographs. This condition is often associated with a poor neurologic outcome, a high proportion of

complete neurologic injuries (no sensory or motor function below the level of injury), and a high susceptibility to delayed neurologic deficit. If a child reports pain, has difficulty with range of motion, or is unresponsive, spinal motion restriction should remain in place until additional studies can confirm there is no injury or until a skilled pediatric specialist clears the spine.

Transport Management

Spinal Cord Injuries

- Manually secure the child's cervical spine while assessing the airway.
- Immobilize the child on a pediatric or standard backboard; secure the child's body first, then the head.
- Release manual stabilization of the cervical spine.
- Reassess the child's neurologic status, and continue to reassess this status frequently during transport.

Breathing Abnormalities

Trauma and the effects of trauma may also cause upper airway obstruction. Facial trauma and soft-tissue swelling can block the upper airway. There may be direct trauma to the upper airway, such as in hanging injuries or "clothesline" injuries, or there may be secondary injury related to the trauma. Hanging injuries may occur in toddlers from crib accidents and window cords. Hanging injuries may also occur in adolescents as a method of suicide or during a "choking game," in which an individual at the point of near strangulation escapes to enjoy an altered mental state. A clothesline injury is most common in all-terrain vehicle crashes and occurs when the patient in motion is struck in the anterior neck by a stationary object (eg, a clothesline wire).

Head injury may cause a decreased LOC, which itself can depress the respiratory drive. The obtunded child's airway might be obstructed by the atonic tongue. Additionally, abnormal respiratory patterns in a child with recent head injury should raise suspicion for seizure activity.

Life threats that providers may encounter in pediatric patients with breathing abnormalities include simple pneumothorax, tension pneumothorax, open pneumothorax, hemothorax, and flail chest. Flail chest is unusual in pediatric patients because their rib calcification is poor, except in adolescents. Management of these injuries in the pediatric population is usually exactly the same as with adult patients. The following sections discuss only the differences in managing these injuries in children. For a complete discussion of these injuries, refer to Chapter 11, *Trauma*.

Tension Pneumothorax

Children with any type of pneumothorax should receive supplemental oxygen. Treatments for tension pneumothorax include a 14- to 16-gauge angio-needle decompression for older children and adolescents, with the needle being placed in the second to third intercostal space, midclavicular on the affected side **FIGURE 24-25**; alternatively, decompression may occur at the anterior axillary line, above the fifth or sixth rib. For infants, treatment is a 21- to 23-gauge butterfly needle inserted in the same location. The needle is then attached to a stopcock and a 20-mL syringe. The chest is emptied of air or fluid until the infant's condition improves. These interventions are temporizing procedures, which typically require follow-up with a larger-bore chest tube.

Transport Management

Tension Pneumothorax

- For older children and adolescents, insert a 14- to 16-gauge angio-needle in the second to third intercostal space, midclavicular on the affected side; alternatively, decompression may occur at the anterior axillary line, above the fifth or sixth rib.
- For infants, insert a 21- to 23-gauge butterfly needle in the same location. Attach to a stopcock and a 20-mL syringe. Empty the chest of air or fluid until the infant's condition improves.
- If a patient with a pneumothorax requires air medical evacuation, consider the effect of altitude on the pneumothorax. Gases expand at higher altitude where there is lower atmospheric pressure. If a chest tube is clamped, the gas can expand and create tension physiology.

Hemothorax

Treatment for a hemothorax includes inserting an appropriate-size chest tube in the fifth intercostal space, anterior and midaxillary. Ideally, the chest tube will be attached to a fluid collection or suction system that allows for autotransfusion. Large amounts of blood can accumulate within the pleural cavity; as long as this blood does not become

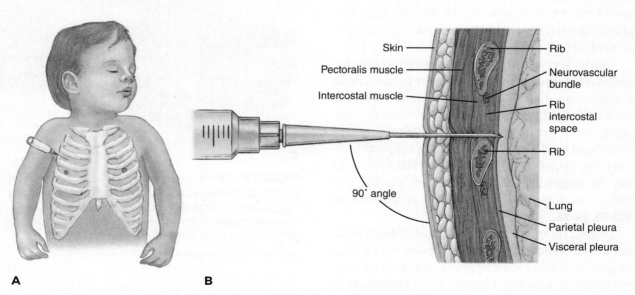

A   **B**

FIGURE 24-25 Decompression of a tension pneumothorax. **A.** The needle should be inserted into the second or third intercostal space, midclavicular on the affected side (shown here); alternatively, decompression may occur at the anterior axillary line, above the fifth or sixth rib. **B.** Insert the needle at a 90° angle and listen for the release of air.

contaminated by an open wound, it can be returned to the child's circulation. This relieves the concern about draining too much blood from the pleural space. If autotransfusion collection is an option, it should be used to reduce the risk associated with donor transfusions.

Transport Management

Hemothorax

- Insert an appropriate-size chest tube in the fifth intercostal space, anterior and midaxillary.
- If available, attach the chest tube to a fluid collection or suction system that allows for autotransfusion.
- If autotransfusion collection is not possible, follow advanced trauma life support guidelines regarding how much blood should be accumulated before clamping the thoracostomy tube.
- Fluid resuscitation with blood or crystalloids may be necessary.

Abuse and Neglect

Given the high incidence of child abuse and neglect in the United States, EMS providers, including CCTPs, are likely to be called upon to care for victims of these horrific events. The primary responsibility of the transport crew is to ensure the safety of all involved.

Abuse is any improper or excessive action that injures or otherwise harms a child or infant. Forms of abuse that the CCTP must be able to recognize while caring for pediatric patients include psychological (emotional) abuse, physical abuse, sexual abuse, and neglect. While bruises in atypical locations (eg, upper back), burns, or certain fractures may be suggestive of nonaccidental trauma, the absence of such findings does not exclude abuse **FIGURE 24-26**.

Neglect is the intentional or unintentional withholding of needed care and support, which may present as a child who appears unkempt or malnourished or who has recently been diagnosed as having failure to thrive. A key component of the physical assessment at the bedside is the child's behavior. Children younger than 6 years who have experienced neglect usually appear markedly passive

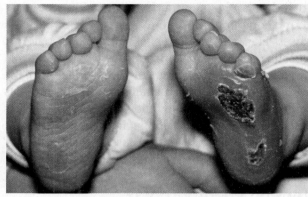

A

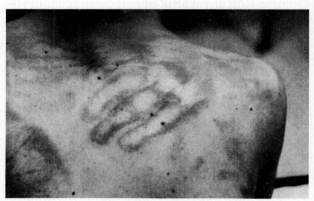

B

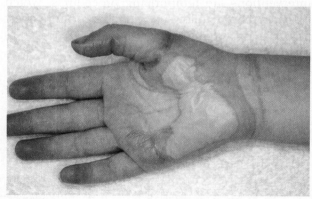

C

FIGURE 24-26 Obvious signs of abuse. **A.** Burns on the bottom of the feet, such as those shown here, are highly suggestive of abuse. **B.** Imprints of a hand on the skin suggest assault or other forms of abuse. **C.** Burns on the palm in susceptible patients can be signs of abuse.

to their environments, whereas children 6 years or older may seem aggressive on initial evaluation.

The transport crew should conduct a thorough assessment and gather all necessary transfer documentation and radiographic studies for the receiving hospital. If a detailed assessment cannot be completed based on the pediatric patient's response, then this fact should be noted in the transfer documentation. As with any patient population, if the provider's assessment and knowledge of age-appropriate behavior do not correlate with the findings for the child, and a suspicion of abuse or neglect is present, then the CCTP must adhere to agency protocol regarding the reporting of suspected abuse or neglect. In a case of confirmed abuse, all measures should be taken to preserve evidence. Transfer documentation must reflect findings from the physical exam and statements made by the victim or suspected perpetrator. CCTPs may be requested to testify in court regarding such cases, so it is imperative to document the events and transport details with the utmost completeness and clarity.

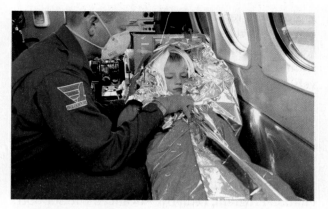

FIGURE 24-27 To manage a pediatric patient with hypothermia, remove wet clothing, place the patient under a heat lamp, and provide warm blankets and liquids.

© Jones & Bartlett Learning.

Signs and Symptoms

Neglect

- Child appears unkempt or malnourished, or has a diagnosis of failure to thrive.
- Younger than 6 years: Child is markedly passive to the environment.
- Older than 6 years: Child seems aggressive.

Transport Management

Abuse and Neglect

- Conduct a thorough assessment.
- Adhere to agency protocol regarding reporting of suspected abuse or neglect.
- Document the events and transport details.

Hypothermia During Transport

Hypothermia exists when the patient's core body temperature is 95°F (35°C) or less. It can result from a systemic disease process, prolonged environmental exposure, or a situation in which heat production is less than heat loss by convection, conduction, or radiation. Children are at an increased risk for hypothermia secondary to their relatively larger body surface areas, proportionally large heads, immature temperature-regulating mechanisms, decreased energy stores, and lesser body fluid volume and protective fat. In particular, low-birth-weight (premature) infants, newborns, and children involved in trauma are at high risk for hypothermia.

The management of these patients starts by removing them from the cold environment, removing wet clothing, placing them under a heat lamp, and providing warm blankets and liquids **FIGURE 24-27**. As with any patient, address the ABCs during the initial/primary assessment. Warm humidified oxygen and warmed IV fluids should be administered based on the level of hypothermia. Be aware that

Transport Management

Hypothermia

- Remove the child from the cold environment.
- Remove wet clothing.
- Place the child under a heat lamp.
- Provide warm blankets and liquids.
- Address the ABCs.
- Administer warm humidified oxygen and warmed IV fluids based on the level of hypothermia.
- Provide additional heat from the vehicle.
- Follow agency protocols regarding cardiac medication and defibrillation.

rapid fluid replacement in this population may cause or increase the state of hypothermia. Regardless of the outside ambient temperature, CCTPs should provide additional heat from the transport vehicle's (rotor wing, fixed wing, or ground) heater. In the event of severe hypothermia, cardiopulmonary arrest may occur in children. Cardiac medications and defibrillation may not be effective when the body core temperature is less than 82.4°F (28°C); therefore, CCTPs must adhere to their agency protocols or resuscitation guidelines (Neonatal Resuscitation Program, Pediatric Advanced Life Support).

Drowning

Drowning, also known as a fatal submersion injury, is a major cause of death for children between the ages of 1 and 14 years. Drowning rates are highest for children ages 1 to 4 years. Despite educational campaigns alerting the general public about the risk of drowning in pools and lakes for the pediatric population, a lack of awareness persists regarding the dangers posed by other hazards, including bathtubs and buckets: A child can drown in as little as 1 inch of standing water.

Most drownings are unwitnessed incidents where the victim is found floating in water. The primary insult in such cases is hypoxemia, which may or may not be attributed to aspiration. Hypoxemia as a result of aspiration begins the insult to these patients, and is followed by metabolic acidosis, hypothermia, and cardiac compromise. The key to a successful outcome is good resuscitation and a brief submersion. Secure the airway early, provide positive-pressure ventilations, and add PEEP early. Rewarm the patient and work to reverse metabolic acidosis. These patients might be on fluid restriction per their physician's orders, or at least half maintenance infusions, and furosemide might be needed. In addition, vasopressors might be needed. Antibiotics are needed only if a bacterial infection is suspected. Patients can experience a drowning incident in fresh or salt water, although the exact etiology does not change the initial treatment. Recent research suggests that the mammalian dive reflex occurs mostly with sudden submersion in extremely cold water **FIGURE 24-28**.

In approximately 10% to 20% of drowning incidents, the drowning occurs when the patient has a laryngospasm that prevents water from entering

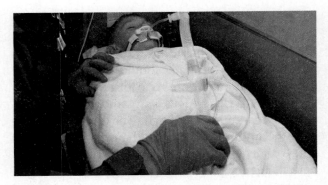

FIGURE 24-28 Early airway management with positive-pressure ventilation and PEEP should be used when treating patients with cold-water drowning.
© Jones & Bartlett Learning.

the lungs. The duration of the laryngospasm determines the extent of the hypoxemia. Death from this type of drowning is the result of asphyxiation, rather than aspiration.

Flight Considerations

There are no specific flight considerations for pediatric CCT; that is, the same flight considerations presented in other chapters apply to the pediatric patient. As mentioned previously, CCTPs can maintain a supply of single-use toys to help reduce the child's anxiety during transport. Such toys, as well as electronic devices, can help keep the patient calm and entertained during what may be a boring or uncomfortable journey.

In most circumstances, a parent or caregiver should be offered the opportunity to be transported with the child, as their presence may put the pediatric patient at ease with the environment. As with adult patients, never lie to pediatric patients. Use every opportunity to build their trust.

Summary

The emergency care of children is challenging and difficult under the best of circumstances. Well-guided, standardized preparation for the transport of a critically ill or injured child is essential. Working collaboratively with various organizations, such as Emergency Medical Services for Children and pediatric components of emergency medical professional organizations, allows the CCTP to provide appropriate care to this vulnerable population.

Case Study

It is 0100 hours when the parents of an 11-year-old boy call EMS because he is "sucking for air." EMS arrives on the scene 6 minutes later. The paramedics immediately complete an initial/primary assessment, establish that the patient has no known allergies, and begin treatment with an albuterol nebulizer. The parents acknowledge they have been noncompliant with administering their son's rescue inhalers and nebulizers. The patient is alert and cooperative but has audible wheezing with intercostal, subcostal, and substernal retractions with tracheal tugging. The cardiac monitor reveals sinus tachycardia with a rate of 118 beats/min, a BP of 110/62 mm Hg, respirations of 36 breaths/min, and an initial SpO_2 of 84% on room air. En route to the hospital, IV access is obtained. During that time, the SpO_2 rapidly increases to 94%, and the patient's work of breathing begins to decrease.

At 0118 hours, the patient arrives at the local ED and care is transferred to the ED nurse and ED physician. A physical exam reveals a patent airway, but the patient has thick secretions that he cannot cough up. Breathing is rapid and forced. He continues to have retractions and an SpO_2 of 95% while on the nebulizer. Diminished breath sounds with expiratory wheezing are auscultated. The patient's pulses are bounding, the skin is a pale pink compared to baseline and is diaphoretic, and capillary refill is 3 seconds centrally and peripherally. The patient is cooperative but very fatigued.

At 0125 hours, the patient is started on a continuous albuterol/ipratropium nebulizer to a maximum of three doses, and he is given methylprednisolone and magnesium sulfate for management of his asthma. A chest radiograph is ordered. The ED physician calls the pediatric intensivist at the children's hospital for a possible transfer as a result of the child's history of asthma and previous intubations. The children's hospital accepts the patient to its pediatric floor, and you depart for the referring facility in a critical care ground ambulance.

Thirty minutes later, the patient's work of breathing is reported as "improving" and the chest radiograph shows the hyperinflation of the lungs typically seen in children with asthma. You arrive, begin your assessment, and obtain a report from ED personnel.

At 0202 hours, the patient becomes unresponsive and has an SpO_2 of 78% and an $ETCO_2$ of 78 with a "shark fin" appearance on the waveform. You and your partner initiate bag-mask ventilation. You immediately prepare your equipment and intubate the child with a size 6.5 ET tube and insert an orogastric tube.

After successful intubation and ET tube placement, confirmation with visualization of the tube passing the cords, fogging of the ET tube, and $ETCO_2$ monitoring, the child is given adequate pain medication sedation and paralytics, and is placed on a ventilator. His SpO_2 is now 93%, $ETCO_2$ is 45 mm Hg, and his vital signs are stable. You and your partner start an in-line nebulizer and prepare to move the patient to the stretcher for transport.

At 0221 hours, the child suddenly deteriorates as his SpO_2 decreases to 81% and his heart rate increases to 150 beats/min. The alarm on the ventilator is displaying "high pressure." The ventilator is disconnected, and manual ventilation with a bag-mask device is initiated.

A few minutes later, the patient's ET tube placement is reconfirmed, he is suctioned, and all equipment is working properly. He remains difficult to ventilate as a result of increased resistance, and the $ETCO_2$ increases to 60 mm Hg. Reassessment now reveals decreased breath sounds on the right side, jugular venous distention, and a decreasing BP.

At 0230 hours, you perform needle decompression on the patient's right side. There is a rush of air and resistance to bagging decreases. The patient is then placed back on the ventilator. His vital signs are a BP of 112/61 mm Hg and a heart rate of 102 beats/min; he is being ventilated at a rate of 12 breaths/min. His SpO_2 is now 98% on an FIO_2 of 60%. He is resting comfortably under adequate sedation and pain medicine, and his condition is greatly improved.

The rest of the transport is uneventful. You and your colleagues advise the receiving physician of the changes in the patient's condition during transport. All paperwork, treatments, and medications given are reported to the pediatric intensive care unit nurse with a copy of the transport report to be left with the patient's chart.

1. How was the ET tube size calculated?
2. What is the treatment priority after the patient is intubated and placed on the ventilator?
3. What is the treatment priority after the child's SpO_2 level deteriorates to 81%?
4. Which mnemonic can be used initially to help address the acute change in this patient's status?
5. Which procedure should be performed when you observe that the child's stomach is distended with air?

Analysis

The uncuffed ET tube size is calculated with the following formula:

$$\frac{\text{Age} + 16}{4}$$

For cuffed tubes, decrease this size by 0.5. A length-based resuscitation tape, called the Broselow tape, can also be used to select the ET tube size. Remember, ET tube size formulas are only guides for ET tube selection. ET tubes that are 0.5 mm smaller and larger must be readily available.

After the child is intubated and placed on the ventilator, the treatment priority is sedation and possibly pain medication. When you observe the patient's stomach distended with air, a nasogastric or orogastric tube should be inserted to decompress the stomach and reduce the risk of aspiration.

When the child deteriorates to an SpO_2 of 81%, the treatment priority is assessment of the ABCs. At this point, the CCTP should take the patient off of the ventilator and manually ventilate the patient with a bag-mask device.

The DOPE acronym is used to help remember how to care for this deteriorating patient. It stands for Dislodgement of the tube, Obstruction of the tube, Pneumothorax, and Equipment failures.

When the crew discovers a pneumothorax, the next treatment priority is needle decompression. In pediatric populations, patients may still have an equal rise/fall of the chest and audible lung sounds on both sides of the chest. Children typically have thin chest walls and lung sounds "echo" to the affected side from the unaffected side. In addition, the inflated lung may still elevate the side of the chest with the collapsed lung, a phenomenon related to the pliable and compliant chest walls of children.

Children with asthma are at a greater risk for pneumothorax because of hyperinflation of the lungs and high airway pressures. In most cases, the air can get in, but it has difficulty getting out. Particular caution must be taken with children during bag-mask or mechanical ventilation. Slow down your expiration time for these patients. Some children may need I:E times of 1:3 to 1:5. Assess, treat, and *reassess*!

Prep Kit

Ready for Review

- The basic anatomy of the cardiovascular system is the same in children as in adults, but there are physiologic differences, such as differences in normal ranges for pulse rate and blood pressure (BP) and children's limited duration of compensatory mechanisms.
- Children's respiratory systems—lungs that continue developing through adolescence,

Prep Kit Continued

smaller lower airways, smaller number and size of peripheral airways, immature alveoli, and decreased collateral ventilation—put them at higher risk for severe symptoms caused by respiratory diseases and for atelectasis.

- Infants' highly reactive airways make them more vulnerable to environmental allergens, viral respiratory diseases, and hereditary factors.

- Children are more susceptible to brain injuries because their brains are not well compartmentalized, which means there is more room for the brain to move in the skull.

- A normal fontanelle is soft and flat but has a feeling of fullness. The posterior fontanelle closes at 2 months of age, and the anterior fontanelle closes at 16 to 18 months of age.

- Cephalohematoma occurs in 1% to 2% of live births involving mechanical trauma, and is found predominantly in the parietal region of the skull. It usually resolves in 6 to 8 weeks and can be associated with linear fractures. The critical care transport professional (CCTP) should note the size and location of the hematoma during initial assessment and during transport. Possible complications are rare but include infection, hyperbilirubinemia, meningitis, and osteomyelitis.

- Caput succedaneum is soft-tissue swelling in a neonate's head that usually resolves within 24 hours.

- Children's bones are more porous than adults' bones, and tend to buckle rather than fracture. Epiphyseal–metaphyseal growth plate injuries account for 10% to 15% of fractures in children; with reduction and immobilization, most have excellent outcomes.

- The child's thorax is pliable and able to absorb a significant amount of energy without fracturing. A small or suspected rib fracture may indicate a severe pulmonary contusion, which is more life threatening to the child than the rib fracture.

- Children's ligaments are strong and more resilient than those of adults, making their joints strong and dislocations rare.

- Because of a highly flexible cervical spine, young children tend to have avulsions rather than fractures. They are more susceptible to head injuries because they have relatively large, heavy heads with weak neck muscles.

- Children have a higher risk of aspiration as a result of an immature cardiac sphincter, are more susceptible to blunt abdominal trauma because they have weaker abdominal muscles, and are susceptible to hypoglycemia as a result of immature liver function.

- Children are more susceptible to dehydration than adults are because they have a higher percentage of body water. Minimum urine outputs are 2 mL/kg/h for infants and 1 mL/kg/h for children, compared to 0.5 mL/kg/h for adults.

- Infants and children exposed to extremes of cold are at higher risk for hypothermia compared to adults because their ability to regulate temperature is not fully developed and they have a larger body surface to mass ratios.

- Close monitoring of oxygen and medication consumption is essential with children because they have a higher rate of metabolism and consume more oxygen than adults do. The rate of onset of hypercapnia and hypoxemia is accelerated in pediatric patients.

- The CCTP should monitor the pediatric patient closely for hypoglycemia, which can manifest with a rapid onset and either an asymptomatic or classic presentation. Treatment depends on the patient's weight and age. Administration of 50% dextrose is contraindicated in the pediatric population.

- An understanding of normal growth and development, as well as the individual pediatric patient's developmental level, helps guide assessment, safety considerations, and communication techniques.

Prep Kit Continued

- Care strategies for psychosocial concerns vary with the age of the child. Speaking at eye level, using first names, and explaining medical procedures with age-appropriate words are techniques that can be used at all age levels. Maintaining a calm and confident manner also helps to reassure both the child and the parent.

- CCTPs need to be academically, technically, and emotionally prepared to care for pediatric patients. They must recognize and address the needs of the parents, guardians, or caregivers, as well as those of the patient.

- Pediatric assessment begins with the pediatric assessment triangle (PAT), which assesses the child's appearance, work of breathing, and circulation.

- After using the PAT to form a general impression of the patient, perform an initial/primary assessment. Any abnormal finding indicates the need for immediate treatment and may require deferral of the next step. Perform a secondary assessment on medical and trauma patients.

- Assess all children for pain. A numeric scale can be used for older children and adolescents; the FLACC or FACES scale can be used for infants and young children.

- The CCTP can get extensive information for the child's history from the child's parents or caregivers. Scene or situation information may also be useful.

- Pediatric medication doses often have to be calculated, which increases the possibility of errors; doses of high-alert medications require an independent recheck before they are administered.

- The CCTP should be familiar with pediatric medications used for critical care transport and the different methods of medication delivery. The best option for administering resuscitation medications is a vascular access device.

- Nasal congestion can be life threatening to an infant because infants are obligate nose breathers. Normal saline spray and a bulb syringe can be used to clear the nasal airways. Positioning the infant with the head up at a 30° to 45° angle also aids in keeping the nasal airways clear. Administration of oxygen via a nasal cannula may work as well.

- Airway differences and other factors, such as infection, trauma, or foreign body airway obstruction, can impair the patency of the child's airway. Proper choice of blade size, proper positioning, and effective sweeping of the tongue are essential for successful intubation. Assess the corneal reflex to determine if the child has a gag reflex before inserting the oral airway.

- Assessment of the work of breathing in children should include observation for stridor, snoring, retractions, head bobbing, accessory muscle use, tripoding, nasal flaring, wheezing, and grunting. The CCTP should know the parameters for normal pediatric vital signs but should remember to assess the patient, not the numbers or monitors. Assessment of the child's level of consciousness (LOC), palpation of the child's chest, and auscultation are used to assess breathing adequacy. Measurements used to determine breathing adequacy include percentage of hemoglobin molecules that are bound with oxygen (Spo_2), end-tidal carbon dioxide ($ETCO_2$), and arterial blood gas readings.

- Assessment of a child's cardiovascular system includes observing the child's general appearance and LOC, including assessing the child's fingers and toes for evidence of clubbing; obtaining vital signs; assessing the child's skin, which should be warm, dry, and the appropriate color; and measuring the child's BP. The capillary refill time is a good predictor of peripheral perfusion. For some disease processes, mean arterial pressure may be a more important measure in guiding treatment than BP.

- Any trauma or medical condition that causes fluid loss requires intravenous (IV) access

Prep Kit Continued

for volume replacement. Intraosseous (IO) insertion is recommended when rapid venous access cannot be obtained. The most common site for IO insertion is the anterior tibia. Contraindications to IO access include osteogenesis imperfecta, osteopetrosis, and fractures of the ipsilateral extremity.

- Urine output can be an objective indicator of pediatric circulatory status and the effectiveness of volume replacement. Low urine output indicates poor kidney perfusion.

- Neurologic assessment includes evaluating the child's general appearance, assessing the fontanelles, checking the child's pupil size and response to light, and evaluating muscle tone and reflexes, including the Moro reflex and the stepping reflex. Protective reflexes are lost in ascending order.

- The Glasgow Coma Scale is a sensitive indicator of mental status; it is modified when examining infants and children.

- Assessment of the renal system includes evaluation of hydration status and physical assessment, including assessment of the fontanelles in infants, assessment of skin turgor, the presence or absence of tears when crying, and sunken eyes. Daily weights are an objective measurement; acute weight loss may indicate fluid loss.

- Fluid overload is less common in children than in adults, but it may occur in patients with congenital heart defects or renal insufficiency. Hypoxia and grunting are early signs of pulmonary edema. Additional signs of fluid overload include weight gain, edema, history of intake greater than output, and pulmonary edema. Early signs of pulmonary edema may be discounted because of this condition's subtle presentation, but it can be confirmed by a chest radiograph.

- Resuscitation of infants and children must include measures to maintain body temperature because of children's physiologic differences. Measures must be taken to prevent hyperthermia and hypothermia.

- CCTPs who anticipate caring for critically ill or injured children need knowledge and skills specific to caring for infants and children as well as practice in pediatric care and mentoring from professional colleagues who care for pediatric patients on a regular basis.

- Equipment necessary for pediatric care should be available when transporting infants and children. All equipment and supplies should be secured prior to transport to reduce the possibility of injury in the event of a crash.

- A team approach to interfacility transfer is best. Communication tools such as SBAR (situation, background, assessment, and recommendation) help to standardize the exchange of information among providers. The team should have a contingency plan for resuscitating the child if necessary during transport, and the driver or pilot should be prepared to respond if changes in the patient's condition or in the weather prevent completion of the transport.

- For safe transport, pediatric patients and health care providers must be secured in the vehicle and appropriate protective gear should be used. Interventions needed to stabilize the patient should be performed before beginning transport. CCTPs need to be aware of local, regional, and national protocols for addressing the increased risks of air medical transport and be prepared to take measures to reduce them.

- Guidelines for transporting parents or caregivers with a child should be in place before a child needs transport. Safe transport of the child is the priority, and the caregiver's comfort level and the potential for disruption of care during transport must be taken into account.

- The American Academy of Pediatrics recommends that self-inflating bags be used for resuscitation of children. CCTPs who will be caring for children should be familiar with the

Prep Kit Continued

use of self-inflating bags, as well as the use of flow-inflating bags, oxygen hoods, shortened tracheal tubes, and laryngeal blade options.

- Respiratory illness is a common reason for pediatric transport. Upper airway conditions, lower airway conditions, parenchymal diseases, and abnormal control of ventilation can lead to upper airway failure.

- Respiratory distress is characterized by increased work of breathing. Although the effort to breathe is increased, the child may still have adequate exchange of oxygen and carbon dioxide. The additional effort may also occur for compensatory reasons.

- The definition of respiratory failure depends on the child's baseline respiratory function. Intervention to prevent respiratory or cardiac collapse is paramount. The CCTP should take all measures (per protocol) to maintain and preserve a patent airway and hemodynamic status before transport begins.

- Croup is a common viral infection characterized by a hoarse, "barking seal" cough that often becomes worse at night. Its management ranges from the administration of humidified oxygen, to the administration of racemic epinephrine, to oral intubation in severe cases of obstruction.

- Epiglottitis is a bacterial infection that most commonly occurs in children ages 3 to 5 years. Symptoms include the four Ds: dysphagia, dysphonia, drooling, and distress. A calm environment should be maintained, and a definitive airway should be secured prior to transport. Use of racemic epinephrine is contraindicated.

- Foreign body aspiration causes more than 90% of pediatric deaths in children younger than 5 years. Its onset may be dramatic, with an immediate life threat or with varying severity. Removal of the foreign body should be attempted only by following American Heart Association and American Academy of Pediatrics guidelines.

- Early recognition of upper airway inflammation and intervention are imperative to lessen the morbidity and mortality associated with this condition. Therapeutic measures are the same as for all upper airway obstructions: Maintain a calm environment, administer humidified oxygen, provide a position of comfort, and prepare for deterioration of the airway status.

- Bronchiolitis is a viral infection caused by respiratory syncytial virus or another virus that primarily affects infants and young children. Symptoms may vary from mild wheezing to severe respiratory distress. Treatment is supportive, with IV fluids, oxygen, and positive pressure being administered when needed. There is no role for routine use of bronchodilators or steroids in the management of bronchiolitis. Ribavirin, an antiviral drug, should be administered as prophylaxis to high-risk neonates. Diligent assessment and monitoring of the child's work of breathing before and during transport are critical.

- Asthma is a chronic inflammatory disorder of the lower airways that results in a significant number of pediatric transports. When transport is required, traditional treatments have likely failed and more advanced therapies are required. If a child has a history of requiring intubation for severe asthma, all treatments should be given during rapid transport to the hospital. Management includes oxygen therapy and the administration of a bronchodilator and corticosteroids.

- Pneumonia is a parenchymal lung disease. Infants and children may not tolerate pneumonia as well as older children and adults do. Transport treatment includes vigilant assessment of the work of breathing and hydration status. Antibiotic therapy is required and may have been started at the initial facility.

- The presentation of acute respiratory distress syndrome is similar in children and adults.

Prep Kit Continued

In addition to reversing the underlying etiology, management is primarily supportive.

- As noninvasive methods of mechanical ventilation become increasingly popular, providers must be proficient in the following methods: heated high-flow nasal cannula, continuous positive airway pressure (CPAP; including "bubble CPAP" for infants), bilevel positive airway pressure (BPAP), and nasal noninvasive positive-pressure ventilation (essentially BPAP with a rate).
- CCTPs may be asked to initiate or manage invasive methods of maintaining difficult airways, including rescue devices and medications to facilitate rapid sequence intubation. Further, CCTPs should be familiar with different ventilation strategies for the patient, once intubated.
- Pediatric cardiac conditions are common indications for transport. CCTPs will routinely be involved in transport of children with four types of heart disease or conditions: known cardiac defect, unknown or suspected cyanotic defect, cardiac arrhythmia, or some form of shock.
- Electrocardiogram (ECG) rhythm interpretation is different for children than for adults. Normal values vary with the child's age. It may be helpful to increase the ECG monitor sweep speed to identify subtle nuances in the components of the ECG.
- Depending on the severity, congenital heart defects may require immediate surgery or supportive care until the child is older and able to tolerate surgical intervention. Children with a known or new-onset cardiac condition may present with a defect in their cardiac pumps.
- Pediatric patients can experience both bradyarrhythmias and tachyarrhythmias. CCTPs should be familiar with the range of normal heart rates in children; misunderstanding what is normal for a given age group is a frequent contributor to errors in diagnosing cardiac disorders.

- In the event of cardiac arrest during ground transport, providers should stop the ambulance in a safe location to facilitate high-quality cardiopulmonary resuscitation. If resuscitation does not rapidly result in return of spontaneous circulation, providers should follow preestablished agency policies that direct the ambulance to the closest hospital.
- Shock may lead to rapid death or may be more progressive. It is categorized as compensated or uncompensated, based on the child's BP.
- Hypovolemic shock, which is characterized by inadequate intravascular volume, is the most common cause of shock in pediatric populations.
- There are four stages of hypovolemic shock: (1) The child appears asymptomatic; (2) the child maximizes compensatory mechanisms; (3) the child is no longer able to compensate and hypotension occurs; and (4) death is imminent if the volume loss is not eliminated and aggressive volume replacement is not initiated. Resuscitation is deemed successful when there is a return to normal heart and respiratory rates, normal BP, and improved mental status and skin condition.
- The child with cardiogenic shock presents with traditional signs of shock, pulmonary congestion, and jugular venous distention. Treatment focuses on improving cardiac function with fluid resuscitation, inotropic support, and pharmacologic support.
- Neurogenic shock, anaphylactic shock, and septic shock are types of distributive shock. Treatment focuses on stopping vasodilation, returning volume to the intravascular space, and improving tissue perfusion.
- Symptoms of anaphylactic shock include increased general body edema, hypotension, rash, urticaria, anxiety, and warm, flushed skin. A child in anaphylactic shock may also experience bronchospasm and laryngeal

Prep Kit Continued

edema, which may be life threatening. Management involves removing the allergen, replacing volume, and administering epinephrine.

- Systemic inflammatory response syndrome and sepsis are both clinical shock syndromes characterized by inflammation, vasodilation, significant microvascular permeability, and accumulation of leukocytes resulting in hypoperfusion and end-organ dysfunction. Early recognition and aggressive resuscitation are key to good outcomes with these conditions.
- Causes of acute kidney injury (AKI) are divided into three categories: prerenal, intrarenal, and postrenal.
- Prerenal causes of AKI are the most common in children and are primarily related to dehydration and decreased renal perfusion.
- Intrarenal or parenchymal causes of AKI are diverse, but all lead to nephron damage and loss of glomerular function. Hemolytic uremic syndrome is one of the most common causes of intrarenal AKI in infants and children younger than 4 years. Acute glomerulonephritis, acute postinfectious glomerulonephritis, and acute tubular necrosis are also intrarenal causes of AKI.
- Postrenal or obstructive failure can cause irreversible parenchymal damage if not treated.
- Potentially life-threatening complications of AKI include electrolyte imbalances such as hyponatremia, hypocalcemia, and hyperkalemia; volume loss or pulmonary edema and fluid overload; volume overload; hypertension; and hypertensive encephalopathy.
- The presentation of the pediatric patient with meningitis depends largely on the child's age, the type of organism, and the present state of the child's health. Standard universal precautions should be taken with all pediatric patients with suspected meningococcal infection.

- Trauma is the leading cause of death for all pediatric patients 1 year or older. Injuries in children most commonly involve motor vehicle crashes, suffocation, submersion, burns, falls, and violence. The two main resources for CCTPs when assessing pediatric trauma patients are the Glasgow Coma Scale, which has been altered for pediatric patients, and the pediatric trauma score.
- Head trauma is the leading cause of morbidity and mortality in children. Injuries to the brain are evaluated as primary or secondary injuries.
- Primary injuries occur at the moment of impact and cause physical and mechanical destruction of brain tissue. Secondary injuries are injured areas of the brain that may remain viable but are vulnerable to hypoxic, ischemic, and inflammatory responses. If untreated, secondary brain injury leads to irreversible brain damage and death.
- The most common cause of increased intracranial pressure in pediatric populations is related to trauma or a failed cerebrospinal fluid shunt.
- Concussion is the most commonly seen head injury in the pediatric population. If concussion is suspected, the CCTP should provide supportive measures during transport, perform and document a neurologic assessment, and document the patient's pain level and tolerance of transport.
- Other head injuries that CCTPs may encounter with children are cerebral contusion, epidural hematoma, and subdural hematoma. Subdural hematoma can be caused by child abuse, such as shaken baby syndrome.
- Spinal cord injuries in children are relatively rare, but mortality related to such injuries in children is more than double that in adult populations. As with brain injuries, spinal cord injuries may occur with a primary insult and then a secondary insult.

Prep Kit Continued

- The most important intervention with spinal cord injuries is proper spinal motion restriction. A properly fitting cervical collar and, ideally, a pediatric backboard should be used. If a pediatric backboard is not available, a standard backboard can be used with adaptations to accommodate the child.
- Children may sustain damage to the spinal cord and spinal ligaments without damage to the spinal vertebrae. This damage is called SCIWORA, which stands for spinal cord injury without radiographic abnormalities. SCIWORA is suspected when there are clinical signs or symptoms of spinal cord injury but the cervical spine radiographs are normal.
- Facial trauma, soft-tissue swelling, hanging injuries, and clothesline injuries can cause upper airway obstruction. The patient's tongue can also obstruct the airway. Simple pneumothorax, tension pneumothorax, open pneumothorax, hemothorax, and flail chest may threaten the child's life. Management of these conditions is generally the same for children as for adults. The CCTP should be aware of differences in managing these conditions in children.
- CCTPs must adhere to agency protocol regarding reporting suspected child abuse or neglect. In cases of confirmed abuse, they must preserve evidence. CCTPs may be requested to testify in court, so it is important to document findings from the physical exam, statements made by the victim or suspected perpetrator, and transport details.
- Children are at higher risk for hypothermia than adults. Hypothermia exists when the patient's core body temperature is 95°F (35°C) or less. CCTPs should adhere to agency protocols or resuscitation guidelines for treating children with hypothermia.
- Drowning is a major cause of death for children ages 1 to 14 years. Educating the public about drowning hazards remains a top priority in emergency medical services.

Vital Vocabulary

acute glomerulonephritis (AGN) A histopathologic diagnosis associated with edema, hypertension, and hematuria; results from deposition of circulating immune complexes in the kidney basement membrane, which ultimately causes reduced glomerular filtration.

acute kidney injury (AKI) Decreased renal function in the absence of preexisting renal disease. Classified into three categories: prerenal, intrarenal, and postrenal.

acute postinfectious glomerulonephritis (APSGN) A form of acute glomerulonephritis that occurs following an infection by streptococci.

acute tubular necrosis (ATN) A condition that results in damage to the tissue of the kidneys' tubules.

aerophagia A condition in which the stomach fills with excessive air secondary to increased respiratory rate.

anaphylactic shock A potentially life-threatening allergic reaction that presents with increased general body edema, hypotension, rash, urticaria, anxiety, and warm, flushed skin.

atelectasis Complete or partial lung collapse.

bandemia Release of excessive numbers of band cells from the bone marrow into the blood.

bradypnea A slow respiratory rate.

bronchiolitis A condition seen in children younger than 2 years, characterized by dyspnea and wheezing.

Brudzinski sign Passive flexion of the legs and thighs when the examiner flexes the patient's neck to the chest. If this causes pain or causes

Prep Kit Continued

the knees and hips to flex involuntarily, the sign is positive.

caput succedaneum Soft-tissue swelling in a neonate's head owing to fluid collection.

cardiogenic shock Shock caused by failure of the heart's ventricles to pump adequate amounts of blood; it may be caused by congenital cardiac defects, drug toxicity, metabolic causes, hypovolemia, myocarditis, and arrhythmias.

cephalohematoma A collection of blood between the bone and subperiosteal space.

cerebral contusion A focal brain injury in which brain tissue is bruised and damaged in a defined area.

clubbing Broadening of a child's fingers and toes in response to chronically low oxygen levels for longer than 3 months.

concussion A transient interruption of normal neurologic function.

croup A childhood viral disease characterized by edema of the upper airways with barking cough, difficult breathing, and stridor; also called laryngotracheobronchitis.

distributive shock A form of shock in which the smallest blood vessels fail to deliver adequate blood to the tissues; it includes neurogenic shock, anaphylactic shock, and septic shock.

epiglottitis Inflammation of the epiglottis.

FLACC scale A pain assessment scale that scores points for five categories, including face, legs, activity, cry, and consolability.

Glasgow Coma Scale (GCS) A scale used in neurologic assessment, which scores patients on eye opening, verbal, and motor performance.

hemolytic uremic syndrome (HUS) A serious condition in which the patient develops acute kidney injury, and which also causes anemia and thrombocytopenia; thought to be caused by several bacterial and viral infectious organisms, most often verotoxin-producing strains of *Escherichia coli*.

hyperkalemia An increased level of potassium in the blood.

hypocalcemia A low level of calcium in the blood.

hyponatremia A blood serum sodium level that is below 135 mEq/L, and a serum osmolarity level that is less than 280 mOsm/kg.

hypovolemic shock The most common cause of shock in pediatric populations, which is characterized by inadequate intravascular volume.

intrarenal acute kidney injury A type of acute kidney injury caused by damage to an actual nephron.

Kernig sign Resistance and pain elicited on extension of the leg at the knee, with the patient in the supine position and the hips flexed perpendicular to the trunk; when pain occurs as a result of this test, the test result is positive.

Moro reflex An infant reflex in which, when an infant is caught off guard, the infant opens their arms wide, spreads the fingers, and seems to grab at things.

neurogenic shock A form of shock that results in low blood pressure.

neutropenia Abnormally low concentration of neutrophils (white blood cells) in the blood.

osteogenesis imperfecta A congenital disorder in which the individual has brittle bones that are susceptible to fracture; also known as brittle bone disease or Lobstein syndrome.

osteopetrosis An inherited disorder in which the bones become extremely hard and dense.

pediatric assessment triangle (PAT) An assessment tool that allows rapid formation of a general impression of the type and level of illness or injury in an infant or child without touching the patient; consists of assessing appearance, work of breathing, and circulation to the skin.

postrenal acute kidney injury A type of acute kidney injury caused by downstream obstruction of urine flow from the kidneys, with initially intact nephrons; commonly caused by a blockage of the

Prep Kit Continued

urethra by prostate enlargement, renal calculi, or strictures.

prerenal acute kidney injury A type of acute kidney injury caused by decreased perfusion of an intact nephron; often reversible if the underlying condition can be found and perfusion can be restored to the kidney.

reactive airway disease (RAD) Any condition that causes hyperreactive bronchioles and bronchospasm.

SCIWORA Spinal cord injury without radiographic abnormalities.

sepsis A life-threatening complication of infection, in which the entire body mounts an immune response.

stepping reflex An infant reflex that occurs when the infant is held up in the air and moves the legs up and down as if marching.

systemic inflammatory response syndrome (SIRS) A clinical shock syndrome characterized by inflammation, vasodilation, significant microvascular permeability, and accumulation of leukocytes resulting in hypoperfusion and end-organ dysfunction.

tachypnea Shallow, rapid respirations.

TICLS A mnemonic used to remember the priorities during initial assessment of an infant's appearance: Tone, Interactiveness, Consolability, Look or gaze, and Speech or cry.

References

Asthma. Centers for Disease Control and Prevention website. https://www.cdc.gov/asthma/default.htm. Reviewed September 16, 2021. Accessed October 10, 2021.

Brierley J, Carcillo JA, Choong K, et al. Clinical practice parameters for hemodynamic support of pediatric and neonatal septic shock: 2007 update from the American College of Critical Care Medicine. *Crit Care Med.* 2009;37(2):666-688.

Cicero MX, Adelgais K, Hoyle JD, et al.; Pediatric Committee of NAEMSP adopted by NAEMSP Board of Directors. Medication dosing safety for pediatric patients: recognizing gaps, safety threats, and best practices in the emergency medical services setting. A position statement and resource document from NAEMSP. *Prehosp Emerg Care.* 2021;25(2):294-306.

Drowning. World Health Organization website. https://www.who.int/en/news-room/fact-sheets/detail/drowning. Published April 27, 2021. Accessed October 10, 2021.

Drowning facts. Centers for Disease Control and Prevention website. https://www.cdc.gov/drowning/facts/index.html. Reviewed June 17, 2021. Accessed October 10, 2021.

Fuchs S, Pante MD, eds. *Pediatric Education for Prehospital Professionals.* 4th ed. Burlington, MA: Jones & Bartlett Learning/American Academy of Pediatrics; 2020.

Gausche-Hill M, Fuchs S, Yamamoto L, eds. *APLS: The Pediatric Emergency Medicine Resource.* 5th ed. Burlington, MA: Jones & Bartlett Learning/American Academy of Pediatrics and American College of Emergency Physicians; 2012.

Goldstein B, Giroir B, Randolph A; International Consensus Conference on Pediatric Sepsis. International pediatric sepsis consensus conference: definitions for sepsis and organ dysfunction in pediatrics. *Pediatr Crit Care Med.* 2005;6(1):2-8.

González Valdepeña H, Wald ER, Rose E, et al. Epiglottitis and *Haemophilus influenzae* immunization: the Pittsburgh experience—a five-year review. *Pediatrics.* 1995;96(3 Pt 1):424-427.

Guskiewicz KM, Bruce SL, Cantu RC, et al. National Athletic Trainers' Association position statement: management of sports-related concussion. *J Athl Train.* 2004;39(3):280-297.

Hartman ME, Linde-Zwirble WT, Angus DC, Watson RS. Trends in the epidemiology of pediatric severe sepsis. *Pediatr Crit Care Med.* 2013;14(7):686-693.

Heads up. Centers for Disease Control and Prevention website. https://www.cdc.gov/headsup/index.html. Reviewed February 25, 2021. Accessed October 10, 2021.

Hohenhaus S, Powell S, Hohenhaus J. Enhancing patient safety during hand-offs: standardized communication and teamwork using the "SBAR" method. *Am J Nurs.* 2006;106(8):72A-72B.

Kuppermann N, Holmes JF, Dayan PS, et al. Identification of children at very low risk of clinically-important brain injuries after head trauma: a prospective cohort study. *Lancet.* 2009;374(9696):1160-1170.

Lyng J, Adelgais K, Alter R, et al. Recommended essential equipment for basic life support and advanced life support ground ambulances 2020: a joint position statement. *Prehosp Emerg Care.* 2021;25(3):451-459.

Merkel SI, Voepel-Lewis T, Shayevitz JR, Malviya S. FLACC: a behavioral scale for scoring postoperative pain in young children. *Pediatr Nurse.* 1997;23(3):293-297.

Prep Kit Continued

National action plan for child injury prevention. https://www
.cdc.gov/safechild/nap/. Centers for Disease Control and
Prevention website. Published 2012. Accessed October 10,
2021.

Pifko EL, Price A, Busch C, et al. Observational review of
paediatric intraosseous needle placement in the paediatric emergency department. *J Paediatr Child Health*.
2018;54(5):546-550.

Summary health statistics: National Health Interview Survey,
2018. Centers for Disease Control and Prevention website.
https://ftp.cdc.gov/pub/Health_Statistics/NCHS/NHIS
/SHS/2018_SHS_Table_C-1.pdf. Published 2018. Accessed
October 10, 2021.

What causes pediatric injury. Centers for Disease Control and
Prevention website. https://www.nichd.nih.gov/health
/topics/pediatric/conditioninfo/causes. Reviewed April 20,
2020. Accessed October 10, 2021.

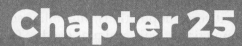

Chapter 25

Bariatric and Special Situations

Bariatric Patients:

Peter Dworsky, MPH, EMT-P, CEM, FACPE

Excited Delirium:

Eric Silverman, MD, MPH

Children With Special Health Care Needs:

Emily J. Kivlehan, MD, MS

Lindsay Riedl, MD

OBJECTIVES

After completing this chapter, you will be able to:

1. Describe the major types of bariatric procedures, including potential complications from those procedures (pp 1361–1363).

2. Discuss considerations related to oxygen consumption in bariatric patients (p 1364).

3. Describe safe methods of moving bariatric patients from the facility to the stretcher, and vice versa, and of moving the stretcher to and from the ambulance (pp 1366–1370).

4. Explain reimbursement issues related to bariatric-specialty units (pp 1371–1372).

5. Discuss excited delirium, including its risk factors, pathophysiology, signs and symptoms, and management (pp 1372–1375).

6. Discuss the elements of interfacility transport monitoring of patients with excited delirium (p 1377).

7. Describe the unique considerations that arise with the critical care transport of pediatric patients with special needs, including children with congenital heart defects; hematology–oncology pediatric patients; pediatric patients with venous access devices; and pediatric patients with respiratory, neurologic, and gastrointestinal disorders (pp 1379–1391).

Introduction

Critical care transport professionals (CCTPs), no matter where they practice, are likely to encounter diverse populations, including some special populations with unique needs. This chapter covers three of these special populations: bariatric patients, patients with acute agitation or violent behavior, and pediatric patients with special needs.

Obesity rates in the United States have more than doubled in the past 3 decades, prompting an increase in bariatric procedures. The care and transport of bariatric patients, especially when not done on a routine basis, requires careful planning to provide the best outcomes for the patient and transport crew.

Excited delirium, sometimes called agitated delirium, is a potentially fatal condition. Many patients with this syndrome have developed it as a result of substance abuse or psychiatric disorders, and their aggressiveness can put anyone at the scene, including themselves and the transport crew, at risk.

Children with special needs include those with congenital heart defects; hematologic–oncologic conditions; respiratory, neurologic, or gastrointestinal disorders; or dependency on technology for survival. To ensure optimal outcomes for these vulnerable patients, CCTPs must be able to treat the patient while communicating with parents and/or caregivers.

Bariatric Patients

A relatively new area in which critical care transport (CCT) units have become involved is the transport of patients with obesity, referred to as bariatric patients. Obesity is an unhealthy accumulation of body fat, defined as a body mass index (BMI) greater than or equal to 30 kg/m². This is a good general guideline, except in cases where body weight does not correlate to excess fat, such as in very muscular people. The Centers for Disease Control and Prevention (CDC) further defines obesity as follows:

- Class 1: BMI of 30 kg/m² to <35 kg/m²
- Class 2: BMI 35 kg/m² to <40 kg/m²
- Class 3: BMI of 40 kg/m² or higher

Health risks increase with each increase in class. In the United States, more than 40% of adults have a BMI greater than 30 kg/m² and, therefore, are considered to have obesity. More than 50% of children and adolescents in the United States have obesity.

The CDC would term class 3 obesity as **morbid obesity**. Morbid obesity includes all of the health risks associated with obesity, but also makes essential functions such as walking or breathing difficult.

People who are overweight are also at increased risk for disease, although their risk is not as high as for those persons who have obesity. Being **overweight** is defined as having a BMI of 25 to 29.9 kg/m².

It should be noted that the United States is not alone in its battle against excess body weight. According to the US Surgeon General, in the last 20 years, the prevalence of obesity has doubled, with worldwide estimates of 1.1 billion people classified as overweight and 250 million people classified as having obesity.

Obesity has widespread and diverse long-term negative effects on all organ systems in the body **TABLE 25-1**. These effects are often manifested during the transport phase, as the patient is brought into a less-than-ideal setting with uncontrollable environmental factors that place additional stressors on these systems.

TABLE 25-1 Effects of Obesity on Organ Systems	
Organ System	**Disease States**
Cardiovascular	Hypertension, coronary artery disease, heart failure, cerebral vascular accident (stroke), peripheral vascular disease
Pulmonary/respiratory	Positional apnea, asthma, chronic obstructive pulmonary disease, acute respiratory distress syndrome
Metabolic	Diabetes
Gastrointestinal	Gastroesophageal reflux disease, renal failure, liver and gallbladder disease
Musculoskeletal	Gout, back injuries

© Jones & Bartlett Learning.

Types of Bariatric Procedures

Bariatric procedures are becoming increasingly common in the United States. According to the American Society for Metabolic and Bariatric Surgery, the number of bariatric procedures increased from approximately 16,000 procedures per year in the early 1990s to approximately 252,000 procedures in 2018. Several types of bariatric procedures are currently performed, including laparoscopic adjustable banding, vertical banded gastroplasty, sleeve gastrectomy, biliopancreatic diversion with duodenal switch, Roux-en-Y ("roo-en-y") anastomosis, and intragastric balloon insertion.

Laparoscopic Adjustable Banding

Laparoscopic adjustable gastric banding (LAGB) is the least invasive bariatric surgical procedure **FIGURE 25-1**. In this procedure, one large incision site, approximately 1.5 inches (4 cm) long, is placed in the upper abdomen for the laparoscopy port. Four smaller incisions are used as insertion points for instrument trocars.

In recent years, this five-incision procedure has been modified to become a one-incision procedure. In the one-incision LAGB procedure, a single incision is placed just below the left ribs; alternatively, it can be hidden in the umbilicus. Passage and placement of the band are all conducted through this single incision.

The LAGB procedure, without complications, takes approximately 90 minutes to perform. During that time, an adjustable band is placed around the upper portion of the stomach, with an adjustment port located on the right side of the abdomen, under the skin. The band divides the stomach, creating an upper pouch that can hold approximately 0.5 cup (118 g) of food. The port, located just below the skin, can be accessed to decrease the size of the opening between the upper and lower portions of the stomach. Injecting saline into the port increases the amount of constriction the band provides.

The mortality rate for LAGB, whether it involves one incision or five incisions, is less than 1%.

Vertical Banded Gastroplasty

Vertical banded gastroplasty (VBG), also known as "stomach stapling," divides the stomach into two

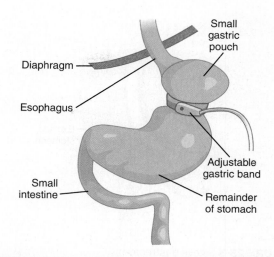

FIGURE 25-1 Laparoscopic adjustable gastric banding.
© Jones & Bartlett Learning.

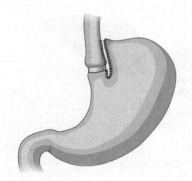

FIGURE 25-2 Vertical banded gastroplasty.
© Jones & Bartlett Learning.

parts **FIGURE 25-2**. Staples, in conjunction with a polypropylene band or Silastic ring, are used to create a small stomach pouch with a small (about the size of a dime) opening that empties into the larger, lower part of the stomach. Plastic mesh is used to strengthen the opening and keep it from stretching. During the procedure, the front wall of the stomach is stapled to the back wall. VBG is performed laparoscopically and no part of the stomach is removed.

Sleeve Gastrectomy

Sleeve gastrectomy, also known as vertical sleeve gastrectomy, is the first part of a biliopancreatic diversion with duodenal switch procedure **FIGURE 25-3**. During this procedure, the structure of the stomach is changed to a tube, restricting the amount of calories the body can absorb; specifically,

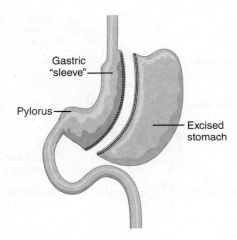

FIGURE 25-3 Sleeve gastrectomy.

© Jones & Bartlett Learning.

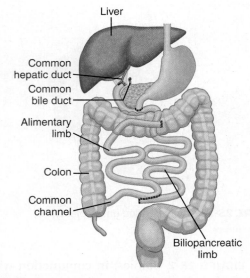

FIGURE 25-4 Biliopancreatic diversion with duodenal switch.

© Jones & Bartlett Learning.

approximately 80% of the stomach is removed. Like the VBG and LAGB, a sleeve gastrectomy is performed laparoscopically using five incisions, and the stomach is reshaped using surgical staples. This procedure is not reversible and has a higher complication rate than the LAGB procedure.

Biliopancreatic Diversion With Duodenal Switch

Biliopancreatic diversion with duodenal switch (BPD/DS) is generally used in patients who have BMI greater than 50 kg/m^2. This two-part procedure requires reshaping of the stomach and bypassing of

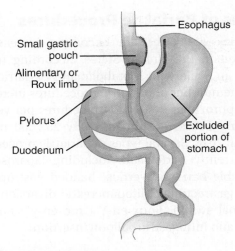

FIGURE 25-5 Roux-en-Y.

© Jones & Bartlett Learning.

a large portion of the small intestine **FIGURE 25-4**. Weight loss occurs due to decreased intake and decreased absorption of nutrients, because most of the small intestine is bypassed in the new gastrointestinal tract.

Unlike the LAGB, VBG, and sleeve gastrectomy, the BPD/DS can be performed as either open abdominal surgery or laparoscopic surgery. The lower two-thirds of the stomach is removed and the remaining, smaller upper portion of the stomach is reattached to the ileum. The risk of death with this procedure is 1 in 200, and the procedure is not reversible.

Roux-en-Y

Roux-en-Y gastric bypass, one type of gastric surgery, is the most common type of bariatric procedure and considered the gold standard **FIGURE 25-5**. Much like the BPD/DS, the Roux-en-Y is a two-part procedure that can be performed as either open abdominal surgery or laparoscopic surgery. During this surgery, the stomach, which can normally hold approximately 6 cups (1,420 g) of food, is reduced to a holding volume of approximately 30 mL, or roughly the size of a walnut. Next, the small intestines are divided, and the jejunum is connected to a small hole in the stomach pouch. Roux-en-Y is not a reversible procedure.

Intragastric Balloon

The intragastric balloon is a temporary nonsurgical procedure that involves placing a removable silicone balloon filled with 500 to 750 mL of saline in

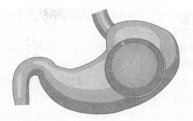

FIGURE 25-6 Intragastric balloon.
© Jones & Bartlett Learning.

the patient's stomach by endoscopy **FIGURE 25-6**. The balloon helps achieve weight loss by taking up space in the stomach and restricting food intake. The balloon can remain in place for as long as 6 months. This procedure is often an option for patients with a BMI between 30 and 40 kg/m^2. Risks associated with this procedure include overinflation of the balloon, acute pancreatitis, ulcerations leading to gastrointestinal bleeding, and sudden deflation of the balloon leading to a gastrointestinal blockage.

Complications of Bariatric Procedures

Complications of bariatric procedures that may require intervention in the form of emergency medical services (EMS) or CCT are divided into early and late complications. Early complications are those that occur within the first month after the procedure, such as deep vein thrombosis, pulmonary embolism, wound infection, sepsis, and gastrointestinal bleeding. These procedures also carry the risk of a stomach or bowel leak from a staple line or anastomosis. With gastric banding, patients can develop an obstruction at the site of the banding.

Late complications occur more than 1 month after the procedure. With all of the bariatric procedures, patients can develop obstructions from strictures, hernias, or hardware complications. Gallstones frequently form after the patient experiences a considerable weight loss. Indeed, they are such a frequent complication of bariatric procedures that the gallbladder is often removed prophylactically as part of the initial operation. Gastric bypass also carries a significant risk of development of ulcers near the area where the stomach and the jejunum are joined. With the banding procedure, a hardware malfunction may develop that results in symptoms of a leak, infection, or obstruction. Thus, undifferentiated abdominal pain is a common 9-1-1 complaint among bariatric patients.

Other specific procedural complications include band erosion, in which the band grows into the stomach and must be permanently removed. Symptoms of this condition include increased hunger and weight gain.

Band intolerance occurs when the body responds to the band as a foreign object, necessitating its removal. Symptoms associated with this complication include excessive vomiting and continuous abdominal and/or epigastric discomfort.

If the lower part of the stomach "slips" through the band, forming a larger pouch above the band, then the complication known as band slippage has occurred. Treatment may include removal of fluid from the band through the port, followed by evaluation of the patient to determine whether the lower portion of the stomach has returned to its previous position. Surgical repair may be required. Symptoms of band slippage include vomiting and reflux.

Port flip/inversion or dislodgment is the most common port-related complication. Port inversion or dislodgment occurs when the port rotates or "flips over." Port dislocation occurs when the port moves from the original placement location. Both of these complications require a simple surgical repair under local anesthesia.

General Management Considerations for Bariatric Patients

Complications also may occur when bariatric procedures are performed as open abdominal surgery. They include the following conditions:

- Significant blood loss
- Possible need for transfusion
- Allergic reaction to medications
- Anesthetic complications
- Myocardial infarction
- Stroke
- Renal failure
- Pneumonia
- Urinary tract infection
- Deep vein thrombosis
- Sepsis

Airway Management

In patients with morbid obesity or those who have undergone bariatric surgery, both oxygen consumption and carbon dioxide production are increased. As a person's obesity increases, their metabolic demands increase, as there is more tissue that needs to be oxygenated. These changes reflect the increased workload placed on the tissues and the presence of excess fat. The lungs do not proportionally grow in size, resulting in diminished lung capacity. Additionally, fat around the chest wall increases the effort needed to breathe, and the weight of the abdominal tissue restricts movement of the diaphragm, resulting in a rapid and shallow breathing pattern and decreased lung capacity. Bariatric patients also have increased breathing difficulty when in the supine position and have a higher incidence of sleep apnea, snoring, and hypercapnia—the hallmark signs of Pickwickian syndrome. Bariatric patients will desaturate faster than patients with an ideal body weight (IBW), which means CCTPs must monitor them more closely during transport and will have a shorter time period to implement interventions if they become hypoxic.

Preparation and anticipation are paramount when moving the bariatric patient between facilities. A significant consideration in patient management is ensuring the CCT team has all the needed equipment and skills to manage the airway in the less-than-ideal setting. Whenever possible, the team should transport the patient in the semi-Fowler position or the ramped position **FIGURE 25-7**, rather than the supine position. The team should also make sure they have ready access to noninvasive airway modalities, including high-flow oxygen via nasal cannula in conjunction with a nonrebreathing mask or a continuous positive airway pressure (CPAP) device. Planning includes ensuring multiple oxygen delivery ports and regulators are available in the transport vehicle.

Intubation equipment must be ready, should the need to intubate the patient arise during transport. The process of intubating the bariatric patient is the same as it is for the patient with IBW; however, CCTPs must be prepared for several possible complications:

- The patient will desaturate more rapidly.
- Placing the patient in the sniffing position may not adequately align the fields of view, allowing the CCTP to visualize the vocal cords.
- The medication dosages for a rapid sequence intubation (RSI) may be different.

Research has shown that even in the ideal setting of an operating room, intubation of bariatric patients is significantly more difficult or may require the use of additional airway adjuncts. Intubation success rates decrease by more than 10% in bariatric patients as compared to patients without obesity.

Oxygen consumption rises sharply in bariatric patients during exercise or movement, compared with patients who do not have obesity. This increase in oxygen consumption has implications for the CCTP. Specifically, it may necessitate the use of a full main oxygen cylinder or the inclusion of additional oxygen cylinders on the transport unit, depending on the patient and the length of transport or time spent on the stretcher. One of the responsibilities of the transport team is to ensure there is enough oxygen available for the transport. The necessary calculations are based on Boyle's law, which is described in Chapter 4, *Aircraft Fundamentals and Flight Physiology*.

In the CCTP setting, it is expected that many patients will be ventilator dependent. The optimal tidal volume in the bariatric patient is between 6 and 8 mL/kg of IBW, with attention to associated positive end-expiratory pressure to avoid atelectasis. Increased tidal volume has not been shown to be beneficial in bariatric patients. Calculation of tidal volume is discussed in Chapter 7, *Ventilation*.

Pharmacology

Many medications carried by transport units are weight based. Recall that IBW is calculated as follows:

- Males (kg): 50 ± (2.3 times patient's height in inches over 5 feet)
- Females (kg): 45.5 ± (2.3 times patient's height in inches over 5 feet)

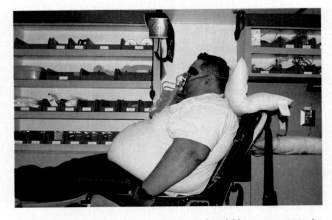

FIGURE 25-7 The bariatric patient should be transported in the semi-Fowler position or the ramped position.

Courtesy of Dr. Darren A. Braude.

Unfortunately, use of patients' IBW to calculate dosages tends to cause underdosing of bariatric patients, and using their actual body weight (ABW), if it is accurately known, tends to cause overdosing. To address these problems, an adjustment factor (usually 40%) is often used to estimate the proportion of adipose tissue that distributes a given medication. In situations where the patient's ABW is less than IBW, dosing should be based on ABW. If the ABW is greater than 125% of IBW, an adjusted body weight (AjBW) should be used. For all other patients, the IBW should be used for dose calculations. For AjBW, the following calculation can be used:

$$\text{AjBW} = \text{IBW} + 0.4(\text{ABW} - \text{IBW})$$

This calculation is especially important when transporting patients who may require intubation.

Dosing of succinylcholine, a neuromuscular blocker, is based on the patient's ABW, whereas dosing of rocuronium is based on the patient's IBW. Of the common induction agents, etomidate's dosing is based on ABW, whereas ketamine's is based on lean body mass. Of the agents commonly used to maintain analgesia and sedation of the intubated patient, dosing of fentanyl and ketamine is based on lean body mass, whereas dosing of midazolam and propofol is based on IBW.

Lean Body Mass

The patient's body composition, not just weight, is an important consideration when calculating medication doses for bariatric patients. In bariatric patients, the excess adipose weight is accompanied by a 20% to 40% increase in lean body weight. Because increased lean body weight correlates to increased drug clearance (the body's ability to metabolize and excrete a drug), drug clearance is significantly increased in patients with obesity.

Another important insight in properly dosing bariatric patients is that increased cardiac output results in more blood flow through the kidneys, resulting in quicker clearance of medications from the body. A patient with a greater body mass may require higher dosages to obtain a therapeutic level and redosing to maintain this level. Additionally, if the medication is fat soluble, a larger dose may be required, as the drug will be absorbed by the fat cells. The medication will be released slowly, potentially producing a longer-lasting effect.

Dispatch Procedures

The call intake process is crucial in initiating the bariatric transport process. The dispatch center or call center should have a detailed protocol for receiving the bariatric transport request. Training for dispatch personnel should include a standardized protocol for gathering information pertinent to the call type, whether it is a prehospital request or an interfacility transport.

Part of the call screening process should include questions about the patient's height and weight. This information is used to calculate the patient's BMI. The BMI can then be used to determine which resources are appropriate, based on the transport agency's definition. The transport agency must educate personnel in the facilities it serves about the criteria for use of the bariatric truck and balance this information against the desires of both the crews and facility staff. Having objective criteria in place in advance will aid in this endeavor.

Underestimation of the patient's weight places both CCTPs and the patient at risk for injury. Specifically designed scales for these patients can help ensure providers have an accurate knowledge of the patient's weight **FIGURE 25-8**. All too often, however, estimation is often "guesstimation," as many people are simply poor at estimating both height and weight, especially when the patient is

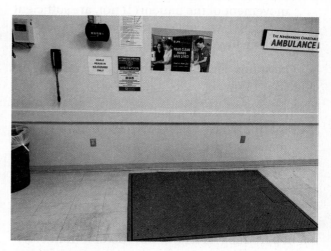

FIGURE 25-8 Some medical facilities have scales designed to accommodate patients of all sizes, including those using assistive devices or in chairs or beds.
© Jones & Bartlett Learning.

supine. Providers should become familiar with methods to quickly determine BMI. The standard way is to multiply the patient's weight in kilograms by the patient's height in meters squared (kg × m²). Another method is to measure the circumference of the patient's upper arm and the patient's height and to compare these measurements to the values shown in **TABLE 25-2**. Research has shown that this method can estimate the bariatric patient's weight within 15% of the actual weight 90% of the time.

Other patient-specific questions that need to be asked of the sending facility include the following:

- What is the patient's acuity level?
- What is the reason for transport?
- Does the patient have specific needs during the transport (eg, ventilator support and the need for pain medication or repositioning)?
- What is the patient's mobility level? Is the patient able to assist with movement from bed to stretcher?

Questions pertaining to operational issues with bariatric patients include the following:

- How long will the transport take?
- Are stairs or ramps present at both the sending and receiving facilities?
- Are the doors capable of allowing egress of the stretcher?
- Do both the sending and receiving facilities have mechanical lift devices to aid in the movement of the patient? If not, are sufficient personnel available to assist in this process at each facility?

Questions pertaining to the receiving facility include the following:

- Are they expecting a bariatric patient?
- Do they have the resources to receive and manage the bariatric patient?

One of the issues faced by transport units is lack of readiness on the part of receiving hospitals to accept bariatric patients in both the emergent and interfacility settings. This lack of preparation is often in part due to a lack of information from either the sending facility, the transfer center, or the transporting unit, depending on the process. To facilitate a smooth transfer, the receiving facility should be advised of not only the patient's weight, but also height and, when possible, abdominal girth, so as to ensure they have the necessary resources for addressing the patient's medical needs.

The diagnostic needs of the patient with obesity should be considered when selecting a receiving facility. Scan tables for computed tomography (CT) have typically been able to accommodate a higher weight than magnetic resonance imaging (MRI) tables, with CT tables typically rated to 200 kg (441 pounds) and MRI tables rated to 150 kg (331 pounds). Open MRI scanners can accommodate up to 250 kg (551 pounds), but the quality of the scan may be diminished. With the CT table, the patient's abdominal circumference can also be a limiting factor: The diameter of the CT scanner's aperture is approximately 75 to 85 cm (30 to 33 inches). Given the ever-increasing prevalence of obesity, CCTPs should consider this additional dimension when caring for bariatric patients and should not focus only on body mass. This information should be available from radiology staff; alternatively, a simple tape measure may be enough to prevent a wasted journey to the CT scanner.

When scheduling the bariatric transport, the CCTP must be aware that the time on task will be significantly increased. Operationally, the CCTP must be prepared for this extended duration and the deleterious effects it may have on the transport service's system-wide performance. Another negative impact on system unit-hour utilization will be that additional resources may be required, further affecting the system's resources and response times. Given these factors, it is recommended that whenever a request for a bariatric transport is received, the agency makes every effort to schedule the transport during a time of low call volume.

One consideration is whether the transport service maintains a staffed bariatric unit 24 hours per day or whether it must recall a crew for the transport. Additionally, what is the crew configuration for bariatric transports: two providers, three providers, or more? Will the call require extra resources?

Moving Bariatric Patients

Although vast numbers of specialty moving devices for bariatric patients are employed within treatment facilities as well as in the prehospital environment, it is important to focus on the mission of the specialty-care transport unit. Adding an excessive amount of space-consuming equipment

TABLE 25-2 Predicted Body Weight (kg) in Adult Men

Height (cm)	\ Arm Circumference (cm) 34	36	38	40	42	44	46	48	50	52	54	56	58	60	62
150				103	110	116	123	129	136	143	149	156	162	169	175
152				104	111	117	124	130	137	143	150	157	163	170	176
154				105	111	118	125	131	138	144	151	157	164	171	177
156				106	112	119	125	132	139	145	152	158	165	171	178
158				107	113	120	126	133	139	146	153	159	166	172	179
160			101	107	114	121	127	134	140	147	153	160	167	173	180
162			101	108	115	121	128	135	141	148	154	161	167	174	181
164			102	109	116	122	129	135	142	149	155	162	168	175	182
166			103	109	117	123	130	136	143	149	156	163	169	176	182
168			104	110	117	124	131	137	144	150	157	163	170	177	183
170			105	111	118	125	131	138	145	151	158	164	171	178	184
172			106	112	119	126	132	139	145	152	159	165	172	178	185
174		100	107	113	119	127	133	140	146	153	159	166	173	179	186
176		101	108	114	120	127	134	141	147	154	160	167	174	180	187
178		101	109	115	121	128	135	141	148	155	161	168	174	181	188
180		102	109	116	122	129	136	142	149	155	162	169	175	182	188
182		103	110	117	123	130	137	143	150	156	163	170	176	183	189
184		104	111	118	123	131	137	143	151	157	164	170	177	184	190
186		105	112	119	124	132	138	144	151	158	165	171	178	184	191
188		106	113	119	125	133	139	145	152	159	166	172	179	185	192
190	101	107	114	120	126	133	140	146	153	160	166	173	180	186	193
192	101	108	115	121	127	134	141	147	154	161	167	174	180	187	194
194	102	109	116	122	128	135	142	148	155	162	168	175	181	188	194
196	103	110	117	123	129	136	143	149	156	162	169	176	182	189	195
198	104	111	118	124	130	137	143	150	157	163	170	176	183	190	196
200	105	111	119	125	131	138	144	151	158	164	171	177	184	190	197

Reprinted from Crandall C, Gardner S, Braude DA. Estimation of total body weight in obese patients. *Air Med J.* 2009;28(3):139-145. Copyright © 2009, with permission from Elsevier.

to an ambulance could be counterproductive, so it is important to include only the essential equipment. Two basic moves are unavoidable and must be planned for:

- Moving the patient from the facility bed, chair, or table to the ambulance stretcher, and doing the reverse at the destination
- Loading the patient into the ambulance, and removing the patient at the destination

Several types of equipment should be considered for the transport of bariatric patients. Some devices best used for the first phase of transporting a bariatric patient (ie, facility to stretcher, and vice versa) are described next.

Slide Boards

A slide board is a basic device that is specifically used when movement of the patient from one level surface to another surface of similar height is indicated, typically from the bed to the treatment table to the ambulance stretcher. Its purpose and the common need for this type of movement means that some sort of slide board is typically readily available in most facilities. Such boards are simple and inexpensive and allow for a reduction of friction. A slide board should be used only under bed linens; it should not be in direct contact with the patient's skin. This low-tech device has multiple handles and can be used by several health care providers simultaneously to minimize the weight each provider is responsible for.

Slide boards come in many variations, such as boards that are foldable and boards with built-in rollers **FIGURE 25-9**. They are typically made of plastic but may also be made of wood. These devices can often be stored in exterior cabinets or under ambulance bench seats. Because of its one-piece construction, a slide board is easily decontaminated.

Disposable, plastic transfer sheets may also be carried in the ambulance, or even on the back of the ambulance stretcher for a simple deployment. Although a plastic transfer sheet might not be as effective as a rigid device, the underlying principle for its use is the same.

Hydraulic and Mechanical Lift Devices

Because of their size and weight, hydraulic and mechanical lift devices are not typically carried on a standard ambulance. Rather, this equipment is most often seen in hospitals, surgical centers, skilled nursing facilities, and rehabilitation facilities. Such lifts use a harness or sling that is often positioned under the patient and connected to a manual or electric-powered mechanical or hydraulic arm **FIGURE 25-10**. The patient can be raised from a bed, a wheelchair, or even the floor and wheeled to the desired location, such as the ambulance stretcher. Before making contact with the stretcher, the patient can be properly positioned and adjusted for comfort. Because of the potential danger when using this equipment, a hydraulic and mechanical lift device should be operated only by those who are properly trained in its use.

Some hospitals have installed overhead lift systems in the ambulance bays to facilitate movement of bariatric patients. Use of these devices must be coordinated with hospital staff to ensure trained personnel are available to operate the devices **FIGURE 25-11**.

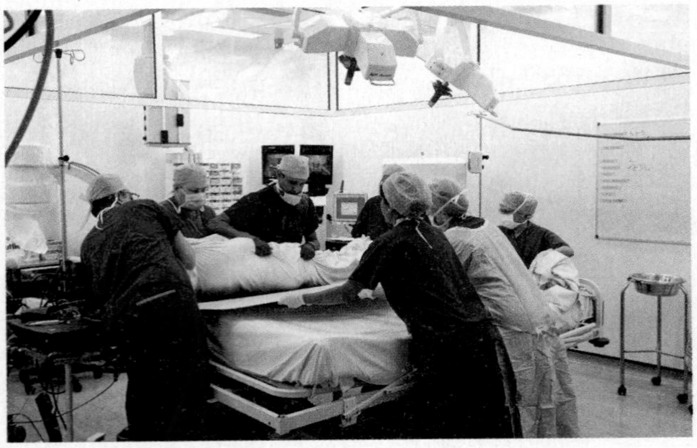

FIGURE 25-9 Slide boards are used to move a patient from one level surface to another.
© Mark Thomas/Science Source.

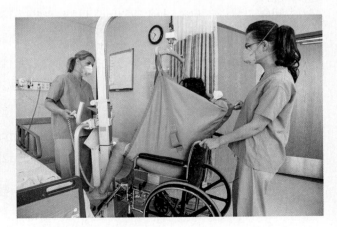

FIGURE 25-10 Hoyer lift.
© Tyler Olson/Shutterstock.

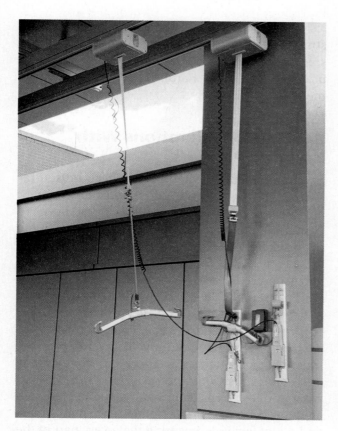

FIGURE 25-11 An overhead lift system for bariatric patients installed in a hospital's ambulance bay.
© Jones & Bartlett Learning.

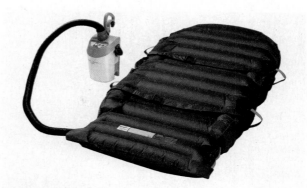

FIGURE 25-12 An air transfer mat.
© HoverTech International, 9/7/10.

Air Transfer Mats

Air transfer mats work similarly to slide boards, in that they are used to laterally transfer patients, regardless of their size, from one level surface to another at a similar height. These mats are typically constructed from vinyl or plastic covered in either a fabric or disposable plastic cover and connect to a compressor that resembles a small canister vacuum **FIGURE 25-12**. After the compressor is activated, the mat fills with air that passes through the perforated underside, making laterally sliding even the largest patient much smoother. Air transfer mats often come equipped with straps or multiple handles, allowing several providers to slide the patient on the device from one bed to the other level surface. These devices are less commonly used, and might not be as simple to store on a standard ambulance.

Stretchers

For the second phase of the transport of the bariatric patient (ie, loading the patient into the ambulance

and then unloading the patient at the destination facility), the medical transportation service must consider which type and manufacturer of commercially available bariatric ambulance stretcher it will employ. The two most commonly used stretcher manufacturers, Ferno and Stryker, produce both regular and bariatric-specialty stretchers. The bariatric versions closely resemble the standard models, with the intent of being similarly operated; thus, they require minimal extra training for use in organizations that employ both bariatric- and regular-model stretchers. The bariatric models are rated for a higher capacity and size. They are made with stronger construction and are considerably wider to ensure the patient's comfort. They come with a variety of (sometimes optional) features, such as larger, locking wheels; thicker mattresses; additional loading handles; longer belts; and a "tow package" (ie, a cable that allows the stretcher to be loaded into the ambulance via an electric winch when ramps are also used). Some bariatric ambulance stretchers have battery-powered systems that raise and lower the patient, reducing the need for the providers to do so. The addition of a low-friction slide device will also assist in the lateral movement of the large patient **FIGURE 25-13**.

Ramp and Winch Systems

In addition to the bariatric ambulance stretcher, many services have deployed a ramp and winch system in specific vehicles designated for the transportation of bariatric patients. These systems avoid the need for providers to manually load the bariatric stretcher into the ambulance. When used, the ramps are deployed as pictured in **FIGURE 25-14**. They are

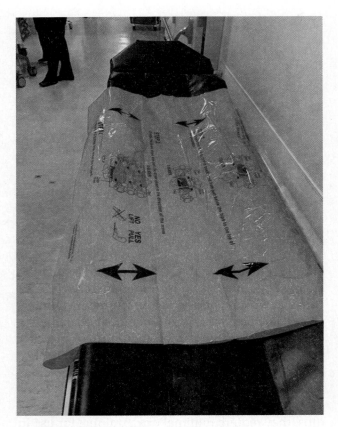

FIGURE 25-13 A low-friction slide device.

© Jones & Bartlett Learning.

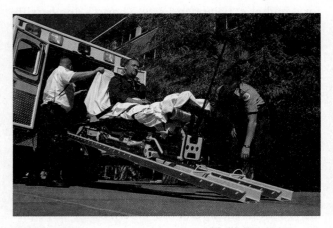

FIGURE 25-14 A crew loading a patient using a ramp and winch system.

© Lyn Alweis/*The Denver Post*/Getty Images.

connected to the rear patient compartment of the ambulance, typically via a transition plate that is easily secured and removed via heavy-duty thumb screws. The stretcher is pulled into the ambulance by using an electric winch mounted in the ambulance near the front of the patient compartment.

All providers operating the bariatric ambulance stretcher, ramps, and other equipment must be specifically trained in their use, because improper usage could lead to harm of the patient or crew members.

Special Considerations With Bariatric Patients

Bariatric patients present the medical transportation industry with some unique problems. As with any other segment of the population, the needs of bariatric patients must be accommodated. Some of these problems are related to medical treatment; others are related to the patients' emotional needs and general customer service matters.

For example, due strictly to their sizes, bariatric patients require special considerations when being prepared for transport. Often, conventional clothing and linens simply do not fit, yet the provider must be committed to ensuring the same dignity and comfort as would be accorded to the patient without obesity. One solution may be to craft specific covers for the bariatric patient when moving in and out of facilities, ensuring that every part of the body is covered and warm. Doing so may require the use of multiple layers of blankets and bed linens. Patients may be unable to comfortably adjust their position on an ambulance stretcher in the same way that smaller patients might. It is best to consider this issue while preparing for transport; at this point, more assistance is typically available to move patients in a way to ensure that they are most comfortable. By comparison, such adjustments may prove extremely challenging during a long-distance trip with only a single provider to attend to the patient. Specific attention must be paid to not only the position the patient wants to be in for comfort, but also the position the patient might need to be in to support the effort to breathe. Bariatric patients may have difficulty breathing unless they are in an upright position.

Another special consideration is that the bariatric patient's body parts often do not fit into the same spaces that a smaller patient's do. Accommodating the bariatric patient might require using less routine methods to ensure comfort, such as strategically placed pillows, rolled blankets, and other aids. In addition, bed-bound bariatric patients often have chronic skin problems such as decubitus ulcers. Providers must manage the severe pain caused by these wounds, change bandages during transport, and after the transport, thoroughly decontaminate the ambulance equipment that came in contact with wound drainage.

Often, the best way to accommodate the bariatric patient's special needs is through proper communication. Such patients, similar to those with other challenges, have likely learned ways to deal with these challenges and can assist providers in helping with moving, positioning, and other transport issues. To this point, it is of utmost importance to protect the patient's dignity and privacy. For example, although additional personnel might be needed to make the patient transfer, these needs should not be publicized. Thus, for a typical interfacility transfer of a bariatric patient, agencies should avoid sending multiple teams of providers into the facility at the same time, causing a spectacle.

Safety during bariatric transports is a paramount concern for both the providers and the patient. Such patients' weight and atypical body shape contribute to an increased risk of injury to both providers and patients during patient handling and movement tasks. Moreover, with the increase in the number of bariatric patients and the trend toward health care providers working longer at an older age, CCTPs' higher likelihood of caring for these patients translates into an increased risk of injury that can have catastrophic outcomes for provider and patient alike.

Many tools exist to reduce the risk of injury, and several states have enacted "no lift" laws that require health care facilities to use mechanical devices to move patients whenever feasible. Such devices include ceiling harnesses, emergency lifting cushions, patient boosters, and motorized wheelchair and bed movers. When these devices are present, it is incumbent upon the transport crew to ensure they are used by properly trained staff. If these devices are unavailable, then it is imperative that adequate personnel be present to facilitate the safe moving of the patient. The proper prehospital equipment must also be available, and CCTPs need to be trained in its use.

Diagnostic Tools

If the proper diagnostic tools are not available during transport of the bariatric patient, medical evaluation and monitoring may be challenging, unreliable, or

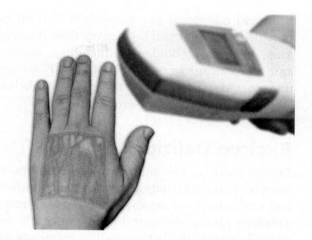

FIGURE 25-15 Using an infrared vein finder may help providers locate an appropriate vessel in the bariatric patient.
© Samunella/Alamy Stock Photo.

even impossible. Providers must have the proper sizes of blood pressure (BP) cuffs, airway adjuncts, and intravenous (IV) equipment and any specialized diagnostic tools necessary. A BP cuff that is too small will give a false reading. Standard IV catheters may not be long enough to cannulate a vein in the patient with morbid obesity. Additionally, locating an appropriate vessel will be complicated **FIGURE 25-15**. Even standard pulse oximetry can be difficult because tissue thickness will impede the light waves. CCTPs should make sure other probes, including an earlobe attachment, are available. Another option is to use nasal capnography to monitor respiratory and cardiovascular function during transport.

Point-of-care ultrasonography (POCUS) in patients with obesity can be challenging. The machine needs to penetrate additional tissue and fat before the ultrasound wave reaches its desired structure and travels back. One problem with using POCUS for these patients is the attenuation. The machine must have enough energy and the necessary hardware and software to compensate for the imperfections introduced by the additional tissue. Such capabilities may not be available with current prehospital devices.

Reimbursement Issues

Because of the intense personnel and equipment requirements, maintaining a bariatric transport program can be expensive and often represents a financial drain on a transport agency. The ability to obtain additional reimbursement beyond that provided under normal billing practices is limited. Most insurance companies, including Medicare and Medicaid programs, do not classify bariatric transport as a specialty care transport, so it is ineligible for a higher reimbursement rate.

Excited Delirium

Excited delirium, also called agitated delirium, is a complex condition that can cause severe morbidity and mortality if not rapidly identified and treated. Although excited delirium has only recently been formally recognized in the medical literature, clinically similar conditions were documented as long ago as the 19th century. Early documented cases came primarily from institutions housing patients with mental illness who demonstrated violent and aggressive behavior. The syndrome was first described by Dr. Luther Bell in 1849. Termed Bell's mania, it was noted to carry a mortality rate of 75%. In 2008, the Council of the American College of Emergency Physicians adopted a resolution to formally recognize excited delirium as a disease entity within emergency medicine, followed in 2009 by a white paper characterizing its clinical presentation, pathophysiology, and treatment. Since then, the biologic basis of excited delirium has become better understood, leading to improvements in diagnosis and treatment of this critical illness.

Delirium has long been recognized as a psychiatric diagnosis. It is described in the *Diagnostic and Statistical Manual of Mental Disorders, Fifth Edition* (*DSM-5*) as an acute disturbance in attention and awareness resulting from another condition such as substance intoxication or toxicologic exposure. Delirium, as described in the *DSM-5*, is not associated with sudden death, distinguishing it from excited delirium. Excited delirium, as a distinct diagnosis, is not included in either the *DSM-5* or the International Classification of Diseases (ICD-9, ICD-10).

The frequency with which excited delirium occurs outside of hospital settings, often involving law enforcement and paramedic restraint of highly agitated individuals, and the wide variety of causes of death issued by medical examiners in suspected excited delirium deaths have made use of the term controversial. In 2021, the American Medical Association (AMA), following a Special Meeting of its House of Delegates, adopted a policy opposing the use of excited delirium as a medical diagnosis until a clear set of diagnostic criteria has been established. Further, it reasserted the need for physician-led medical oversight in out-of-hospital situations deemed medical emergencies. The AMA has emphasized the risk posed by sedative-hypnotic and dissociative drugs when given without an adequate understanding of the patient. The AMA's policy is guided by a concern for the violent policing practices born of institutional racism. By calling for the disuse of this term, the AMA hopes to delegitimize a concept that it believes is often used as a "cover-up" for policing practices that tend to target members of marginalized and minority communities who would be better served by behavioral crisis interventions, such as de-escalation.

The Term *Excited Delirium*

Delirium, as described in the *DSM-5*, often goes unrecognized in hospitalized patients and is associated with adverse outcomes. In all areas of medicine, care of the agitated, violent, or combative patient poses some of the most challenging legal concerns and potential risks to all involved. While acknowledging the current disagreements in terminology, recognition, and actual pathophysiology of this condition, this text continues to use the term *excited delirium*, recognizing that it refers to a legitimate form of delirium that, when untreated or poorly managed, can result in death.

Symptoms of excited delirium include the acute onset of hyperactive, aggressive, and/or combative behavior, often associated with excessive physical strength. Signs include disorientation and altered mental status, tachycardia, tachypnea, heightened pain tolerance, hyperthermia, and metabolic acidosis. Frequently, excited delirium is precipitated by recent use of sympathomimetic or hallucinogenic recreational drugs (cocaine, methamphetamine, phencyclidine [PCP], phenethylamine, or methylenedioxymethamphetamine [MDMA]). Less commonly, excited delirium may occur without drug use in the context of acute decompensated psychiatric illness, such as schizophrenia or bipolar disorder.

As has been portrayed in the media, patients with excited delirium are at significantly increased risk of sudden cardiac death while restrained or in police custody. Deaths have also occurred prior to apprehension by police, during EMS transport, or in the emergency department (ED). Importantly, patients with excited delirium most frequently die within approximately 1 hour of first contact with police or EMS. The reported mortality rates for this condition are as high as 16.5%. Even with timely and appropriate treatment, mortality remains high; nevertheless, early, targeted treatment may greatly improve outcomes.

Risk Factors

Several risk factors have been identified that appear to predispose an individual to developing excited delirium. Demographically, excited delirium typically occurs in men in their 30s, commonly in the setting of cocaine use, but also frequently involving methamphetamine, PCP, or phenylethylamine. In addition, recreational drugs sold in pill form under the street name "Molly" (often a phenylethylamine variant such as 2CE or 2CT7) have been identified in excited delirium cases. Individuals who chronically use stimulants appear to have a higher risk for experiencing excited delirium, although this syndrome typically occurs after an acute binge. Additionally, underlying psychiatric disorders may be seen in patients with excited delirium, most commonly schizophrenia or bipolar disorder.

One theory for the link between stimulant drug use and psychiatric disease, as these factors relate to excited delirium, is increased activation of the dopamine pathway. This neurotransmitter is commonly implicated in the psychotic features of both conditions. While neurochemical similarities between stimulant use and psychiatric disease have been identified, they do not account for the difference in risk of sudden cardiac death noted between patients with excited delirium and those with underlying schizophrenia.

Pathophysiology

Excited delirium is thought to be the result of increased catecholamine levels in the brain. The pathophysiology of excited delirium has been studied most extensively in cocaine users. Stimulant use, including cocaine use, is known to alter brain neurochemistry and is an independent risk factor for the development of excited delirium. Cocaine produces intoxication by preventing the removal of dopamine from the synaptic cleft between adjacent neurons by dopamine transporter (DT) proteins, thereby increasing the synaptic concentration of dopamine. In individuals who chronically use cocaine, the repeated exposure to cocaine results in up-regulation of DT proteins in response to the long-term elevation in synaptic dopamine levels. In essence, the body attempts to autoregulate the chronically elevated dopamine levels associated with repeated cocaine exposure by increasing the concentration of proteins that eliminate dopamine from the synapse.

Autopsy studies examining brain tissue in patients believed to have died from excited delirium due to cocaine use have been compared with brain tissues taken from patients without excited delirium who were also intoxicated with cocaine at the time of death. These postmortem studies demonstrate that patients with cocaine intoxication and excited delirium show a lower number of DT proteins relative to patients who died of cocaine intoxication without excited delirium. These findings suggest that the brains of patients with excited delirium show distinct chemical differences: They are unable to clear dopamine from the synaptic cleft (due to decreased numbers of DT proteins), resulting in very high synaptic levels of dopamine.

Dopamine is a fundamental neurotransmitter, playing important roles in executive function, impulsivity, sensory perception, and key physiologic parameters (eg, heart rate, BP, and temperature regulation). Elevated dopamine levels have long been linked to the perceptual disturbances seen in schizophrenia, including hallucinations and paranoid delusions. Early antipsychotic agents such as haloperidol and chlorpromazine, which have been shown to improve the symptoms of schizophrenia, work by blocking dopamine receptors in the brain. Dopamine is also known to affect renal function and alter BP through multiple mechanisms, including alteration of the renal renin–angiotensin pathway and modulation of sympathetic tone, which impacts vascular smooth muscle as well as heart rate.

The clinical manifestation of excited delirium is a hypermetabolic state, which increases both consumption of energy and production of metabolic wastes. The sympathomimetic effects associated with excited delirium, including tachycardia, hypertension, and elevated temperature, increase the body's metabolic oxygen consumption. On a cellular level, oxygen supply–demand mismatch occurs, and energy generation transitions from aerobic metabolism to anaerobic metabolism. This not only decreases the efficiency of energy (ie, adenosine triphosphate) production, but also leads to production of excessive amounts of lactic acid. Accumulation of lactic acid, in turn, leads to a significant metabolic acidosis. In an attempt to compensate for the declining pH of the blood, the body increases the respiratory minute ventilation to increase exhalation of carbon dioxide and neutralize the lactic acid via its conversion to carbon dioxide and water. **Kussmaul respiration** is a typical respiratory pattern seen in patients with metabolic acidosis; it is characterized by a high respiratory rate and high tidal volume, leading to increased minute ventilation. Laboratory abnormalities in patients with lactic acidosis include an elevated anion gap and decreased bicarbonate levels (corresponding to carbon dioxide levels on a basic metabolic profile). As the metabolic acidosis becomes more profound, elevated potassium levels cause cardiac conduction problems, leading to arrhythmias and eventually sudden cardiovascular collapse. In cases of cardiac arrest, brady-asystolic cardiac arrest and pulseless electrical activity are the predominant terminal cardiac rhythms.

Psychomotor agitation is another hallmark sign of excited delirium. Elevations in cerebral dopamine levels lead to restlessness, paranoia, disorientation, decreased attention span, and hallucinations. These symptoms are similar to those observed in patients with mania but can wax and wane in intensity. When they are drug induced, their presence supports a formal diagnosis of delirium (ie, acute confusion, hallucinations, and disorientation that is rapid in onset and may fluctuate in intensity).

Similarly, the peripheral musculature (via a mechanism that is not fully understood) shows a hyperactive state in excited delirium. Repetitive muscle contractions manifest as pacing, constantly moving extremities, darting eyes, or an inability to sit still. When physically restrained, patients often struggle violently against their restraints until sedative medications are administered.

The constant muscle contractions lead to an elevation in body temperature, further worsening the metabolic demands on the body. This elevation in temperature and hypermetabolic state can lead to

muscle breakdown, triggering the release of intracellular potassium and renal toxins, including myoglobin. As myoglobin levels in the blood increase (myoglobinemia), the patient develops rhabdomyolysis, which directly injures the kidney. Acute tubular necrosis develops as the excess myoglobin damages the nephrons of the kidneys and the patient's blood urea nitrogen (BUN) and creatinine levels rapidly increase. Renal failure has a multifactorial etiology in these patients, demonstrating both a prerenal component from hypovolemia and intrarenal damage from the direct toxic effects of the myoglobin. The net increase in extracellular potassium and waste products places the patient at high risk for cardiac dysrhythmias and death.

Signs and Symptoms

As mentioned previously, excited delirium is a relatively new diagnosis. It is easily recognized as tachycardia, hypertension, psychomotor agitation, and diaphoresis. Patients with excited delirium are often aggressive or combative and may exhibit unanticipated strength with impaired pain perception; as such, they may resist painful stimuli and physical restraint attempts.

Delirium is manifested by hallucinations, paranoia, and disorganized behavior and thought processes. Frequently described manifestations include severe agitation, violent behavior often resulting in damage to property; a lack of awareness of one's surroundings, including disrobing in public; and verbal responses to internal stimuli. These behaviors often result in calls for a law enforcement response, which may be the initial patient contact. In these situations, less lethal methods to take an individual into custody, including use of pepper spray and conducted electrical weapons (eg, TASER device), are frequently ineffective.

Medical conditions other than excited delirium should be included in a provider's differential diagnosis for an agitated patient with altered mental status **TABLE 25-3**. It can be difficult to differentiate excited delirium from other diagnoses without a thorough evaluation. Unfortunately, such an evaluation may be nearly impossible to perform prior to the administration of sedative medications due to the risk of injury to the patient and health care providers. Often, only a very limited history can be obtained due to the patient's altered mental status

TABLE 25-3 Differential Diagnosis: Excited Delirium

Possible Condition[a]	Pertinent Diagnostic Evaluations
Alcohol intoxication/withdrawal, Wernicke encephalopathy	Ethyl alcohol level, thiamine level
Anticholinergic toxicity	Medication history, physical exam (patient will exhibit hypothermia, dilated pupils, dry skin and mucous membranes, flushed skin, and agitation or delirium), core temperature, bladder scan for urinary retention, CK level, basic metabolic panel, acetaminophen and salicylate levels (possible co-ingestion with nighttime formulation medications), ECG
Head injury/central nervous system lesion (consider spinal motion restriction and imaging if trauma is suspected)	Computed tomography brain noncontrast imaging; may require magnetic resonance imaging in the subacute setting
Heatstroke	History, core temperature, renal function, CK level
Hypoglycemia	Fingerstick blood glucose level
Hyponatremia	Serum chemistry
Hypoxia/hypercapnia	Pulse oximetry, venous/arterial blood gas analysis
Infection (encephalitis, meningitis, sepsis)	Physical exam, chest radiograph, urinalysis, blood cultures, lumbar puncture
Neuroleptic malignant syndrome	Medication history, muscular rigidity or tremor, core temperature, CK level, pH, lactate level, ECG, comprehensive metabolic panel
Psychiatric emergency	History and physical exam, evaluation for any precipitating factors: infection, drug ingestion (including psychiatric and recreational), ethyl alcohol, TSH
Seizure/postictal state	Past medical and medication history, lactate level, CK level, pH, electroencephalography, drug screen
Serotonin syndrome	Medication history, reflexes (clonus, lower extremity greater than upper), core temperature, CK level, pH, lactate level, ECG
Sympathomimetic toxidrome	History and physical exam (eg, diaphoresis, tachycardia, mydriasis, rotary or vertical nystagmus), drug screen
Thyrotoxicosis	TSH, free thyroxine test, evaluation for any precipitating factors
Uremia/renal failure	BUN, creatinine, electrolytes

Abbreviations: BUN, blood urea nitrogen; CK, creatine kinase; ECG, electrocardiogram; TSH, thyroid-stimulating hormone
[a]With all potential underlying diagnoses, it is imperative to first treat and control the symptoms to avoid potentially fatal deterioration.

© Jones & Bartlett Learning.

and combative behavior. When possible, obtaining a 12-lead electrocardiogram (ECG) can be useful to identify arrhythmias, QTc interval prolongation, QRS complex widening, cardiac ischemia, and evidence of hyperkalemia.

Laboratory evaluation of a patient with excited delirium typically reveals a severe anion gap metabolic acidosis, primarily due to elevated lactic acid levels from the anaerobic metabolic state. Additionally, patients may have a nonspecific leukocytosis, which is generally not helpful in narrowing the differential diagnosis. Severe tachycardia can lead to coronary underperfusion, resulting in cardiac-demand ischemia and subsequently elevated troponin levels. Rhabdomyolysis is frequently seen with excited delirium, evidenced by elevated creatine kinase (CK) levels, myoglobinuria, hyperkalemia, and eventual acute renal failure.

Treatment

Excited delirium is a dangerous and often fatal condition that requires prompt diagnosis and careful management to minimize morbidity and mortality. Given the relatively recent formal recognition of this syndrome in emergency medicine, clinical management has historically been largely anecdotal, with treatment algorithms based on ED protocols and expert opinion. In recent years, however, evidence-based guidelines have increasingly been adopted. The primary goals in treating a patient with excited delirium are to protect the patient and providers from injury while maintaining patient dignity, reduce psychomotor agitation, perform a detailed physical exam and continuous monitoring of vital signs, establish IV access, and prevent morbidity and mortality.

Initial treatment focuses on reducing the patient's agitation through the use of verbal de-escalation techniques. If these tactics are ineffective, as may occur with patients demonstrating extreme aggression, agitation, and unexpected physical strength, rapidly administering sedative medications, correcting hypovolemia with IV volume resuscitation, initiating specific therapies targeted at metabolic abnormalities, and controlling environmental conditions that increase mortality have been shown to improve outcomes. The National Association of EMS Physicians revised its position statement on excited delirium in 2020 to recommend that treatment include using appropriate verbal and environmental de-escalation techniques, using the least restrictive physical restraints and pharmacologic interventions necessary to facilitate safe patient assessment and transport, and prohibiting dangerous actions such as EMS use of handcuffs, patient transport in the prone position, and maneuvers that constrict the patient's chest or neck.

Frequently, severe restlessness or combative behavior prevents the establishment of IV access, and pharmacologic sedation must be administered via the intramuscular (IM) route. The most commonly used medications for this purpose include benzodiazepines (eg, midazolam, lorazepam), antipsychotics (eg, droperidol, haloperidol, olanzapine, ziprasidone), and ketamine. Although agents from each of these drug classes have been used effectively, they are characterized by different risk–benefit profiles.

Benzodiazepines are often used as an initial therapy to blunt the sympathomimetic component of the excited delirium, especially when stimulant drug use is present. Midazolam is typically the preferred agent because it has a rapid onset of 3 to 10 minutes, is heat-stable, and can be administered to an adult as a 1-mL injection IM or intranasally via the 5 mg/mL concentration. Lorazepam has slower IM absorption, leading to an onset of sedation in the range of 15 to 30 minutes and peak serum concentration within 3 hours. After IV access has been established, titration of additional benzodiazepines or other medications can be used to maintain adequate sedation. Caution should be used with all benzodiazepines since patients with excited delirium may have also ingested ethanol or other central nervous system (CNS) depressants, a behavior that increases the risk of respiratory depression with even a single dose of sedative medication.

Antipsychotics present an attractive pharmacologic approach to treating excited delirium because they antagonize the dopamine receptor. Unfortunately, first-generation antipsychotics, such as haloperidol and droperidol, may significantly prolong the QTc interval and can lead to extrapyramidal adverse reactions. Haloperidol, a frequently used medication in patients with acute agitation, has an onset of action of approximately 15 to 30 minutes via the IM route. In patients thought to be intoxicated with ethanol, however, antipsychotics may be less likely to potentiate the risk of respiratory depression than benzodiazepines are. Second-generation agents, such as olanzapine, offer less risk of QTc interval prolongation and extrapyramidal side effects compared to first-generation antipsychotics, and can be given via IM or rapidly dissolving tablet. Research is limited on the use of second-generation antipsychotics in patients with excited delirium, and their higher cost may be a barrier to their use in some EMS systems. If antipsychotic medications are required, the CCTP should obtain an ECG to evaluate for QTc interval prolongation and QRS complex widening as soon as possible.

More recently, the dissociative medication ketamine has been successfully used to treat acute agitation in patients with excited delirium. Ketamine, which acts primarily as an N-methyl-D-aspartate (NMDA) receptor antagonist, is widely used for procedural sedation in the hospital. Its major benefits include its rapid onset of action (less than 5 minutes), wide therapeutic window, hemodynamic stability, and relative (although not absolute) preservation of respiratory drive and airway reflexes. Ketamine does not antagonize the underlying hyper-dopaminergic state, as antipsychotics do, nor does it blunt the sympathomimetic response, as benzodiazepines do. Additionally, ketamine can cause emergence reactions, hypersalivation, and laryngospasm, which may increase the risk of aspiration. Due to its rapid onset of action, ketamine is effective in quickly achieving adequate sedation with a typical dose of 3 to 5 mg/kg IM, though it may also be effective with a dose as low as 2 mg/kg IM. Rapid sedation will limit physical struggling by the patient and allow prehospital providers to safely perform an assessment and initiate life-saving interventions (eg, IV volume resuscitation, correction of critical cardiac arrhythmias, and treatment of hyperthermia, metabolic acidosis, and hypoxia).

In studies investigating the use of ketamine in patients with excited delirium, intubation rates typically range from 23% to 39% but have been reported to be as high as 63%. Confounding variables such as coadministration of benzodiazepines and lack of hospital provider familiarity with the drug may partly account for the increased intubation rate. Overall, however, patients who receive higher ketamine doses tend to be intubated more frequently. Given this finding, keeping the initial IM dosing to approximately 3 to 5 mg/kg (200 to 300 mg IM for an average adult), with a maximum dose of 400 mg, is appropriate. If the patient has already received another medication, such as a benzodiazepine, an initial ketamine dose of 2 mg/kg IM should be considered. After preliminary sedation has been achieved and IV access has been established, additional benzodiazepines and/or antipsychotics may be required to maintain the sedated state until the patient's vital signs and mental status have improved. Since patients who receive pharmacologic sedation are at increased risk of respiratory depression, high-flow oxygen should be readily available and used to treat hypoxia.

After sedation has been achieved, providers should rapidly evaluate the patient for underlying physiologic disorders that could be driving or exacerbating the delirium. Specific considerations for patients with excited delirium include, but are not limited to, identification and treatment of trauma, hyperthermia, rhabdomyolysis, hyperkalemia, hypoxia, and metabolic acidosis.

With a prolonged state of extreme hyperactivity, patients with excited delirium often become dangerously hyperthermic, and cooling, although controversial, may be required in addition to benzodiazepine therapy. The patient's body temperature should ideally be monitored with a core temperature probe (via esophageal access, Foley bladder catheter, or rectal access), although in most situations it is not practical to do so. While less accurate, temperature should be frequently monitored via a temporal artery, tympanic, oral, or skin thermometer to detect rising body temperature and hyperthermia if core temperature assessment is not possible. Standard treatment for hyperthermia (eg, removal of clothing, misting water over a patient, adding a fan to increase convection and evaporation, ice packs to the axilla and groin) is indicated; this protocol is described in Chapter 19, *Environmental Emergencies.*

The extreme hyperactivity of excited delirium also elevates the risk of muscle breakdown, leading to rhabdomyolysis and hyperkalemia. The treatment of rhabdomyolysis emphasizes aggressive IV volume resuscitation and urine output monitoring to maintain adequate renal perfusion and reduce the risk of kidney damage. Initial treatment is 20 to 30 mL/kg (2 to 3 L) of crystalloid (normal saline or lactated Ringer solution) over the first 30 minutes. After initial fluid boluses have corrected any hypovolemia and restored the patient to a euvolemic state, IV fluids at a rate of 1.5 to 2 times the maintenance rate in the form of an isotonic sodium bicarbonate solution can be considered, because alkalization of the urine may protect the kidneys against further damage from myoglobinuria. The goal of volume resuscitation is to maintain urine output at a rate of 0.5 to 1 mL/kg/h. An ECG finding of hyperacute T waves should prompt standard advanced cardiac life support treatment for hyperkalemia

Interfacility Transport Monitoring

Patients with excited delirium who require transport should be placed on continuous cardiopulmonary monitoring, including ECG and pulse oximetry. End-tidal carbon dioxide ($ETCO_2$) monitoring should also be used, especially if sedative medications have been administered. Respiratory status and cardiac rhythm are the critical vital signs to monitor continuously for changes during transport. In addition, the CCTP should monitor the patient's body temperature and initiate aggressive cooling interventions in the event of hyperthermia.

If the patient requires physical restraints for transport, the CCTP should use the least restrictive management strategy that allows for safe evaluation and treatment. Providers should be able to quickly remove physical restraints if necessary, and handcuffs or locked restraints should not be used by CCTPs. If handcuffs are required by law enforcement, an officer should accompany the patient and the key should be immediately available at all times. The CCTP should never transport a patient in the prone position, with hands and feet tied together behind the patient's back (often referred to as "hogtied"), or in a position that constricts the chest or neck. Patients requiring physical restraints and/or pharmacologic sedation should have their airway and the neurovascular status of all restrained extremities constantly monitored.

Patient Restraint

Never restrain the patient in a prone position with neck function restricted or pressure on the chest or neck, as these positions are dangerous and can lead to asphyxiation. If the patient is already restrained in such a position when you arrive, you are responsible for safely placing the patient into an acceptable position/restraint as quickly as possible.

In an intubated patient, a properly placed esophageal temperature probe provides continuous, real-time core temperature measurements and is ideal for critically ill patients. A urine bladder thermistor catheter can also provide continuous monitoring of both temperature and urine output. Of note, ensuring the accuracy of monitoring requires the patient to have at least minimal urine output; in addition, measurements have been reported to lag behind changes in core temperature by as much as 20 minutes. If these temperature measurement devices are unavailable or contraindicated, a rectal temperature provides the next best method for intermittent or continuous core temperature monitoring, as indicated by clinical concern for worsening hyperthermia. The least invasive method is to use a temporal artery infrared thermometer; although it does not provide a core body temperature measurement, its findings can supplement the clinical exam and assist with medical management decisions. The goal of active cooling is to achieve a core temperature of less than 39°C (102.2°F).

End-tidal capnography (the graphical measurement of $ETCO_2$) monitoring is of great benefit in patients with excited delirium. First, it provides useful real-time monitoring of the patient's respiratory status. Any change in the respiratory rate, including apnea, can be immediately recognized well before the pulse oximetry value changes. Second, the quantitative $ETCO_2$ value has been shown to be helpful in screening for metabolic acidosis. The body's natural response to metabolic acidosis is to induce a compensatory respiratory alkalosis by hyperventilation, which will drive down the measured $ETCO_2$. Patients with significant metabolic acidosis often display a characteristic respiratory pattern consisting of large tidal volumes and rapid respiratory rate to generate a large minute ventilation (ie, Kussmaul respiration). An $ETCO_2$ threshold of greater than 36 mm Hg in most patients indicates that a significant metabolic acidosis is unlikely.

The relevance of this measured $ETCO_2$ value depends on the presence of spontaneous respirations and inherent functional acid–base regulatory mechanisms. With patients who are paralyzed or highly sedated and intubated, the $ETCO_2$ level more closely represents the ventilation rate and tidal volume than the underlying acid–base status. In these situations, it is critically important to understand that the ventilation rate, or more accurately the total minute ventilation volume (tidal volume × respiratory rate), should not be titrated to a normal $ETCO_2$ level (35 to 45 mm Hg), as would typically be the case. Instead, the total minute ventilation volume should be adjusted to a respiratory alkalosis (less than 35 mm Hg) to compensate for the underlying metabolic acidosis, because patients cannot spontaneously adjust their own respiratory rate to compensate for this imbalance. In patients with severe metabolic acidosis, $ETCO_2$ targets as low as 10 to 15 mm Hg may be necessary. Obtaining an $ETCO_2$ value for a spontaneously breathing patient with a patent airway prior to intubation, if possible, allows the CCTP to titrate the ventilator settings to obtain a postintubation minute ventilation that mirrors the preintubation $ETCO_2$ value.

When performing RSI, administering 1 to 2 mEq/kg of sodium bicarbonate 3 to 5 minutes before intubation may help raise the pH and prevent acute decompensation during the apneic period that occurs during intubation. Minimizing the use of postintubation sedation medications that depress the respiratory drive (eg, benzodiazepines and propofol) and avoiding the use of long-acting paralytics (eg, vecuronium and rocuronium) may allow an intubated patient to continue respiratory compensation via spontaneous breathing. Ketamine has also been used successfully to achieve postintubation sedation without inhibiting spontaneous breathing. Without respiratory compensation, the patient could become severely acidemic, leading to dangerous arrhythmias and cardiovascular collapse. If the preintubation $ETCO_2$ value is known, then it is an appropriate initial target after mechanical ventilation is initiated, so as to match the patient's inherent compensatory drive.

Ongoing ventilator management is best accomplished with the aid of arterial blood gas analysis, although this test is not routinely available during most interfacility transports. Maximal compensation may take 12 to 24 hours to achieve its full effects, but the maximally compensated arterial carbon dioxide ($Paco_2$) level can be calculated using Winter's formula (expected $Paco_2 = 1.5 \times$ (actual $[HCO_3]$) + 8 mm Hg), which gives a reasonable target $ETCO_2$ for initial ventilator settings. Generally, if the cardiac output remains sufficient, then the $ETCO_2$ value runs approximately 2 to 4 mm Hg lower than the $Paco_2$ value, and this correlation can be verified by documenting the measured $ETCO_2$ at the time the blood gas is drawn for analysis. Adequate respiratory compensation for the underlying metabolic acidosis is provided by titrating ventilator settings (respiratory rate and tidal volume) to achieve this goal $ETCO_2$ level.

Children With Special Health Care Needs

Children with special health care needs (CSHCN) are defined by the US Department of Health and Human Services as "those who have or are at increased risk for a chronic physical, developmental, behavioral, or emotional condition and who also require health and related services of a type or amount beyond that required by children generally." With advancements in medicine, more children have become able to survive with chronic conditions, and they can often be cared for in a home setting. According to the National Survey of Children's Health, CSHCN account for approximately 18.5% of the pediatric population. Thanks to the many advances in medicine and technology, many children who would otherwise spend time in the hospital and intensive care unit (ICU) can be sent home with nursing coverage and specialized equipment.

Within this population, children with medical complexity (CMC) are at particular risk of receiving lower-quality health care. CMC have chronic medical disease and significant functional limitations. The conditions affecting these children may be congenital, such as hypoplastic left heart syndrome, or acquired, such as brain injury. CMC may be dependent on medical technology. Technologies used may include respiratory supports or monitoring equipment (eg, tracheostomy, ventilator, apnea monitor), enteral feeding devices (eg, nasogastric, gastrostomy, or jejunostomy tube), indwelling IV access (eg, peripherally inserted central catheter, implanted port), colostomies, ventricular shunts (eg, ventriculoperitoneal, external ventricular drain), and baclofen pumps.

This section discusses the basic pathophysiology of common anomalies, the implications for the CCTP, and care and use of the technologies associated with these anomalies.

Congenital Heart Defects

A congenital heart defect (CHD) affects nearly 1% of live births each year in the United States, with approximately one in four of these CHDs being a critical condition that requires surgery or other procedures in the first year of life. The clinical consequences of a CHD are heart failure and hypoxemia. Commonly, symptomatic hypoxia (pallor, respiratory distress, altered mental status) or inadequate end-organ perfusion from heart failure prompts the need for medical care.

Classification of CHDs

CHDs historically were classified as cyanotic or acyanotic **FIGURE 25-16**. The newer classifications are based on hemodynamic characteristics and include four categories: (1) increased pulmonary blood flow; (2) decreased pulmonary blood flow; (3) mixed blood flow; and (4) obstructive blood flow out of the heart **TABLE 25-4**.

Acyanotic defects are usually caused by increased pulmonary blood flow and obstructive blood flow out of the heart. The increased pulmonary blood flow classification is based on defects that cause a left-to-right shunt, resulting in

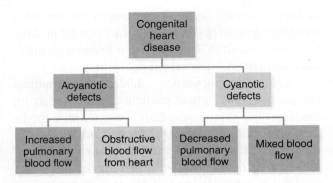

FIGURE 25-16 Classification of congenital heart defects: acyanotic versus cyanotic defects.

© Jones & Bartlett Learning.

TABLE 25-4 Classification of Congenital Heart Defects

- Increased pulmonary blood flow (acyanotic)
  - Atrial septal defect
  - Ventricular septal defect
  - Patent ductus arteriosus
  - Atrioventricular canal
- Decreased pulmonary blood flow (cyanotic)
  - Tetralogy of Fallot
  - Tricuspid atresia
- Obstruction of blood flow from the heart (acyanotic)
  - Coarctation of the aorta
  - Aortic stenosis
  - Pulmonic stenosis
- Mixed blood flow (cyanotic)
  - Transposition of the great vessels
  - Total anomalous pulmonary venous return
  - Truncus arteriosus
  - Hypoplastic left heart syndrome

© Jones & Bartlett Learning.

oxygenated blood repeatedly going through the pulmonary system. Depending on the size of the defect and the volume of blood that flows between them, acyanotic defects can cause heart failure due to volume overload. Although types of CHD are individually described, some patients may have multiple types or more unique defects.

- **Atrial septal defect (ASD)** is an opening in the septal wall of the heart between the left and right atria that allows blood flow from the left atrium to the right atrium **FIGURE 25-17A**.
- In **ventricular septal defect (VSD)**, blood flows from the left ventricle to the right ventricle through a hole in the septal wall **FIGURE 25-17B**.

- **Atrioventricular canal defect** consists of both VSD and ASD as well as a defect affecting the mitral and tricuspid valves, in which the valves are shared **FIGURE 25-17C**.
- A **patent ductus arteriosus (PDA)** is an extra blood vessel that allows blood to flow from the aorta to the pulmonary artery **FIGURE 25-17D**. In the neonate, the PDA usually closes completely within the first 12 to 24 hours of extrauterine life as the result of increased blood oxygenation and pressure, and decreased levels of endogenous prostaglandins. In some types of CHD, such as hypoplastic left heart syndrome, a PDA may act as the only route for blood to reach systemic circulation and the vessel is kept open through medications.

Acyanotic CHDs associated with obstructive blood flow are coarctation of the aorta, aortic stenosis, and pulmonic stenosis:

- **Coarctation of the aorta** is the narrowing or constriction of part of the aorta or aortic arch **FIGURE 25-18A**. Although it is considered an acyanotic defect, one sign of this disease in the neonate may be cyanosis of the lower extremities despite baseline skin color in the upper extremities, a condition known as differential cyanosis. These neonates may present with circulatory collapse. Femoral pulses may be absent but can also be present due to collaterals, so make sure to palpate for distal extremity pulses.
- **Aortic stenosis** is narrowing of the aortic valve **FIGURE 25-18B** and can be described as valvular, supravalvular, or subvalvular.
  - *Valvular stenosis*, the most common form of aortic stenosis, can be caused by development of a bicuspid valve instead of the normal tricuspid valve.
  - *Supravalvular stenosis*, the least common form of aortic stenosis, is the result of narrowing of the aorta above the aortic valve and coronary arteries.
  - *Subvalvular stenosis* can be the result of isolated lesions or other congenital heart anomalies.
- **Pulmonic stenosis**, also known as pulmonary stenosis, is obstruction of blood flow from the right ventricle to the pulmonary artery **FIGURE 25-18C**.

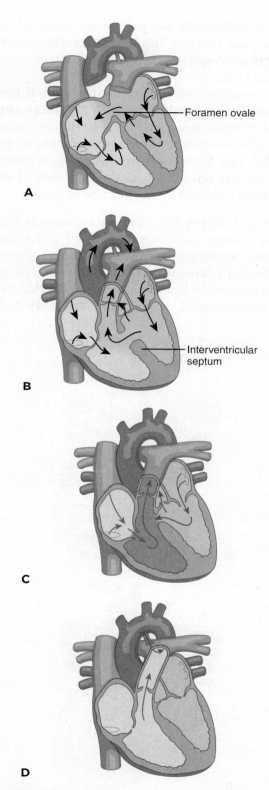

FIGURE 25-17 Acyanotic defects: increased pulmonary blood flow. **A.** Atrial septal defect. **B.** Ventricular septal defect. **C.** Atrioventricular canal defect. **D.** Patent ductus arteriosus.

© Jones & Bartlett Learning.

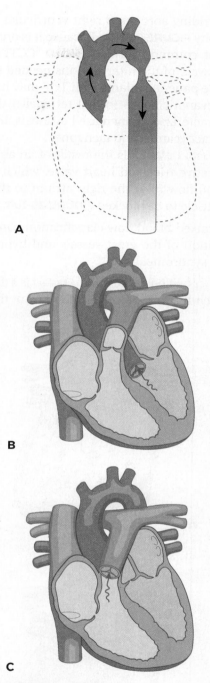

FIGURE 25-18 Acyanotic defects: obstructive blood flow. **A.** Coarctation of the aorta. **B.** Aortic stenosis. **C.** Pulmonic stenosis.

© Jones & Bartlett Learning.

Cyanotic defects consist of decreased pulmonary blood flow and mixed blood flow. Decreased pulmonary blood flow includes the following two defects:

- **Tetralogy of Fallot (TOF)** is the combination of four anomalies: VSD, pulmonary stenosis, overriding aorta, and right ventricular hypertrophy **FIGURE 25-19A**. Because it is one of the most common forms of CHD, CCTPs must be aware of the interventions needed to treat these patients. Infants with TOF may have hypercyanotic spells (called tet spells) that are characterized by increased cyanosis, irritability, tachycardia, and tachypnea.

- **Tricuspid atresia** is the result of an absent or defective tricuspid heart valve, which causes blood flow from the right atrium to the right ventricle to be blocked **FIGURE 25-19B**.

The mixed blood flow classification consists of transposition of the great vessels and hypoplastic left heart syndrome.

- **Transposition of the great vessels** is a defect in which the aorta receives blood from the right ventricle while the pulmonary artery leaves the left ventricle **FIGURE 25-20A**. Often these patients also have a patent foramen ovale and VSD.
- **Hypoplastic left heart syndrome** is caused by an abnormally small left ventricle **FIGURE 25-20B**. It is often associated with aortic and mitral valve stenosis or atresia. Obstruction to the left side of the heart results in heart failure, whereas obstruction to the right side of the heart results in hypoxemia and cyanosis.

Heart failure is defined as a set of clinical signs and symptoms indicative of myocardial dysfunction and cardiac output that is inadequate to meet the metabolic demands of the body. Common signs and symptoms of heart failure can be divided into four classifications, as shown in **TABLE 25-5**. In

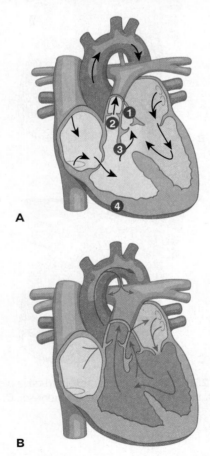

FIGURE 25-19 Cyanotic defects: decreased pulmonary blood flow. **A.** Tetralogy of Fallot. The numerals indicate (1) overriding aorta, (2) pulmonary stenosis, (3) ventricular septal defect, and (4) right ventricular hypertrophy. **B.** Tricuspid atresia.
© Jones & Bartlett Learning.

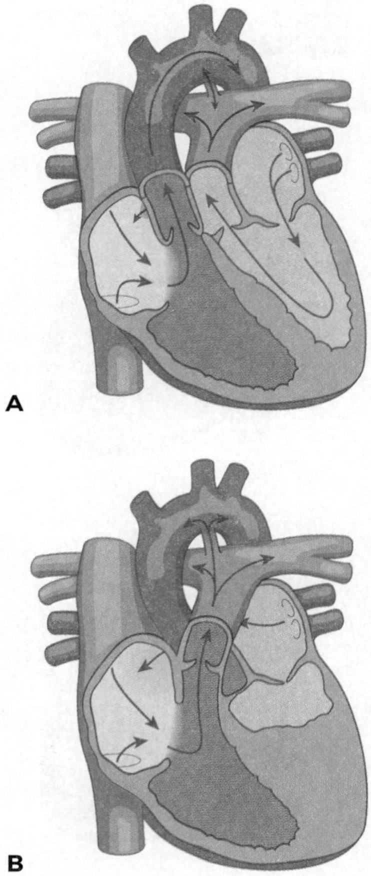

FIGURE 25-20 Cyanotic defects: mixed blood flow. **A.** Transposition of the great vessels. **B.** Hypoplastic left heart syndrome.
© Jones & Bartlett Learning.

TABLE 25-5 Signs and Symptoms of Heart Failure in Children

Adrenergic Response
- Tachycardia
- Tachypnea
- Cool skin
- Diaphoresis
- Oliguria

Systemic Venous Congestion
- Hepatomegaly
- Periorbital edema
- Pulmonary effusion, ascites (rare)

Pulmonary Venous Congestion
- Tachypnea
- Retractions
- Nasal flaring
- Pulmonary edema

Cardiorespiratory Distress
- Irritability
- Altered mental status
- Fatigue
- Poor feeding
- Sweating with feeds
- Failure to thrive
- Gray skin coloration

© Jones & Bartlett Learning.

infants, some of the common signs of heart failure are often apparent during their feedings: tachycardia, nasal flaring, irritability, diaphoresis, sweating with feeds, and easily becoming fatigued. However, tachypnea may also be the only sign of heart failure in children.

Assessment

A diagnostic tool that CCTPs can use to determine if a critical CHD is present is pulse oximetry. Placing one pulse oximetry probe on the child's right wrist and another probe on a foot can allow the CCTP to identify any difference in preductal and postductal oxygen saturation (SpO_2) levels, which would be indicative of right-to-left shunting as well as coarctation of the aorta.

Another simple monitoring tool that can be used in an infant or child with CHD is measurement of BP in the upper and lower extremities. If the systolic BP reading in the right upper extremity is substantially higher than the reading in the lower extremity,

then an obvious obstruction of blood flow is present, such as coarctation of the aorta. Another finding in patients with coarctation of the aorta may be diminished or weak pulses in the lower extremities compared with the upper extremities.

Many patients with CHD may require cardiac surgeries, which are often staged into multiple procedures over years. Some degree of hypoxemia may be expected in these patients, such as those with hypoplastic left heart syndrome, before definitive operative repair or transplant. Family or other caregivers who are present may act as a source of information on their baseline oxygen level and clinical status.

Treatment

It is important for the CCTP to have a basic understanding of CHDs and to obtain accurate histories from the parents and/or caregivers of these patients. Some of these defects, such as coarctation of the aorta and hypoplastic left heart syndrome, require patency of the ductus arteriosus for survival. Administration of oxygen must be approached cautiously in these infants, as it will accelerate PDA closure, which could be fatal. Some of these patients have normal SpO_2 levels in the range of 70% to 90%; if the SpO_2 level goes any higher, it may increase their risk of PDA closure, which may then lead to heart failure.

Ductal-dependent conditions may require administration of prostaglandin, which will help maintain the patency of the ductus arteriosus. Conversely, indomethacin is a medication that is administered to facilitate closure of the PDA.

Intravenous fluid administration must be used cautiously in pediatric patients with CHD. Although most children can handle an IV bolus of 20 mL/kg, these vulnerable patients must be closely monitored and given only 10 mL/kg to prevent fluid overload or pulmonary edema.

Infants with TOF often present with irritability, decreased feeding, and hypercyanotic spells (tet spells), which are a medical emergency. Tet spells present with tachypnea and agitation, and can result in loss of consciousness, altered mental status, and death. Initial interventions for tet spells include placing the patient in the knee-to-chest position or having an older child squat. If these measures do not work, administer IV morphine and IV fluid bolus (5–10 mL/kg). If these interventions do not work, you can give a phenylephrine continuous infusion or propranolol, but use caution with the latter medication, as it may cause hypotension.

Hematology-Oncology Pediatric Patients

When caring for the hematology–oncology population in pediatrics, it is important to remember that these patients have weakened immune systems. Fever, even the slightest low-grade fever, is an emergency in this population. This section discusses the most common hematologic–oncologic pediatric conditions seen by CCTPs: neutropenia, sickle cell anemia, and hemophilia. These children often have specific devices in place, such as peripherally inserted central catheters **FIGURE 25-21A**, central venous access devices (CVADs) **FIGURE 25-21B**, or central venous catheters **FIGURE 25-21C**. For the most part, CCTPs must be specially trained by different facilities to access these devices, owing to the high risk of infection. CCTPs should follow their agency's policies and procedures for using these devices.

Pediatric patients with hematologic–oncologic conditions are a vulnerable population. As critical care providers, CCTPs must protect these children from opportunities for infection. Because such patients are immunocompromised and often have neutropenia, strict isolation techniques are required in their care. Neutropenia is a decrease in the number of neutrophils in the body; neutrophils are essential in the body's immune response system. Strict isolation techniques to reduce the chance of infection include strict hand hygiene, limiting invasive procedures, and having patients wear a mask when out of their room or going for a procedure. Parents and/or caregivers are taught to call the oncologist or hematologist and bring their child into the ED when the child begins to have even the slightest fever at home. These children are at increased risk for sepsis and shock.

Sickle Cell Anemia

Sickle cell anemia affects 1 in 365 black or African American infants born in the United States and approximately 100,000 Americans overall. Children with sickle cell anemia have inherited two sets of recessive genes that produce an abnormal hemoglobin protein, known as Hgb S. When the child's

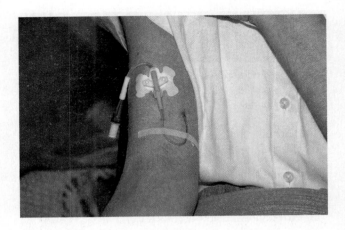

A

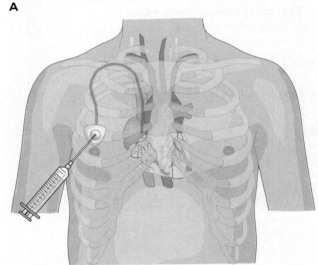

B

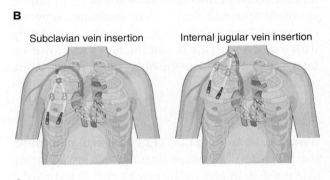

Subclavian vein insertion   Internal jugular vein insertion

C

FIGURE 25-21 Devices used in pediatric patients with hematologic–oncologic conditions. **A.** Peripherally inserted central catheter. **B.** Central venous access device. **C.** Central venous catheter.

oxygen level decreases, it affects the hemoglobin (Hgb); in turn, the red blood cell (RBC) becomes deformed. Specifically, instead of being circular in shape, the RBC assumes more of a sickle shape

FIGURE 25-22. The RBCs also become "sticky," so that they occlude vessels, clot, and cause great pain in patients. Children with sickle cell anemia often present with chest pain, extremity pain, and difficulty breathing. In the worst-case scenario, these children may have a cerebral vascular accident.

When children present in sickle cell crisis, aggressive treatment is necessary. Sickle cell crisis or vaso-occlusive crisis is associated with clinical signs of anemia, pallor, weakness, fatigue, and severe pain. These patients require oxygenation, an IV fluid bolus of isotonic crystalloids, or, if tolerated, oral rehydration. In severe cases, children may require blood transfusions. Pain management is extremely important, because these patients will be in severe pain. A life-threatening emergency in patients with sickle cell anemia is acute chest syndrome, which can be due to pneumonia or infarction. This condition typically presents as chest pain, hypoxia, tachypnea, fever, and crackles. As noted previously, these patients are at high risk for stroke, so providers should assess for classic stroke signs such as unilateral weakness, altered speech, and blown pupils. The CCTP must follow local policies, procedures, and protocols when managing these patients.

Hemophilia

Patients with hemophilia have a recessive gene trait that causes excessive bleeding. This disorder is caused by factor VIII or factor IX deficiency, which prevents blood from clotting properly. In the United States, factor VIII deficiency (also called hemophilia A or classic hemophilia) is the most common form of hemophilia. It affects 12 in every 100,000 males and is four times as prevalent as factor IX deficiency (also called hemophilia B or Christmas disease).

Children with hemophilia are at increased risk of bleeding from even the slightest injury. For example, something as simple as falling from a standing position and bumping the head on the floor or table can cause serious bleeding issues. Serious, life-threatening injuries for these children are injuries that occur to the head, neck, chest, and abdomen.

When faced with an injury to a child with hemophilia, first and foremost the CCTP must treat any obvious bleeding. These children require immediate IV administration of factor VIII for hemophilia A, or factor IX for hemophilia B.

Pediatric Patients With Venous Access Devices

Venous access devices include tunneled catheters, implanted ports, and peripherally inserted central catheters. Tunneled catheters can have single, double, or triple lumens and are inserted in the right or left subclavian vein. Several different types of long-term CVADs are available, such as Hickman, Broviac, and Groshong catheters **FIGURE 25-23**.

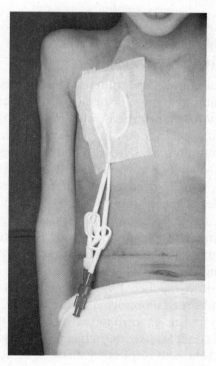

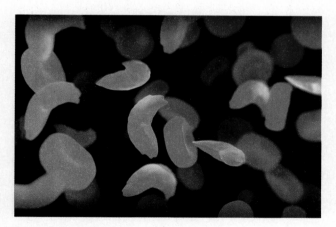

FIGURE 25-22 Red blood cells with a sickle shape.

FIGURE 25-23 Long-term central venous access devices.

Implanted ports require specific Huber needle infusion sets to access the device; the various types of implanted ports are known as Mediport, Port-A-Cath, and Infusaport devices.

Depending on the specific catheter, the smallest syringe that may be used with these devices might be a 10-mL syringe. Using anything smaller than a 10-mL syringe to aspirate fluid from the device may damage the catheter. It may also cause the catheter to collapse while aspirating the blood.

Prior to children being discharged to home with a venous access device, parents are given training and hands-on experience in accessing the device, performing dressing changes, flushing the device, and administering medication through the device. Home health infusion nurses may visit the family and patient once per week to deliver medications and supplies, and to inspect the sites. Changing the dressings for all devices and accessing the implanted ports require sterile technique. These techniques are specific, and are based on the manufacturer's guidelines. Depending on their agency's policies or protocols, CCTPs may or may not be able to use these devices for blood draws, medication administration, or IV fluid infusions. Like all indwelling devices, long-term CVADs and ports may act as a source for infection as well.

Pediatric Patients With Respiratory Disorders

Two commonly encountered respiratory disorders that may require or be the result of long-term ventilation, endotracheal tube placement, or tracheostomy placement in pediatric patients are bronchopulmonary dysplasia and tracheomalacia.

Bronchopulmonary dysplasia, or chronic lung disease, usually occurs in premature infants who weigh less than 3 pounds (1,500 g) at birth, approximately 25% of whom have respiratory distress syndrome. These neonates have long-term fibrosis and scarring sustained from oxygen toxicity, often requiring mechanical ventilation. These children may require tracheostomies, mechanical ventilation, and ETCO$_2$ monitoring. Acute bronchopulmonary dysplasia exacerbations are often triggered by viral illnesses, weather changes, or crying, and can present with respiratory distress, decreased air entry, apnea, desaturations, coarse breath sounds, wheezing, and crackles.

Tracheomalacia is a weakening or softening of the tracheal cartilage/rings that causes the trachea to become floppy and collapse during expiration. It can be due to compression from surrounding structures or intrinsic defects of the trachea, or it can occur in patients who have been on prolonged positive-pressure ventilation. Affected children are noisy breathers and often sound as if they have a continuous stridor. The stridor will worsen with crying, irritability, and lying supine. It is important to obtain an accurate history to ascertain if the child with stridor has a history of tracheomalacia because the administration of bronchodilators, such as albuterol, can worsen the symptoms by causing the airway to become more floppy and even cause the airway to collapse. Positioning of these patients plays an important role in alleviating the symptoms. Placing infants and children with tracheomalacia in a prone position allows gravity to assist in opening the airway; the supine position would be dangerous due to narrowing of the weakened trachea or even airway collapse.

Tracheostomy tubes are used in pediatric patients who require long-term mechanical ventilation, are unable to manage their secretions, or have physical or anatomic barriers to their native airway (stenosis, tracheomalacia, radiation scarring, laryngectomy). These devices are made of materials that soften when exposed to body temperature, which allows the tracheostomy tube to conform with the trachea. The tracheostomy tube may be a complete set with an obturator, or it may consist of an obturator, inner cannula, and outer cannula **FIGURE 25-24**.

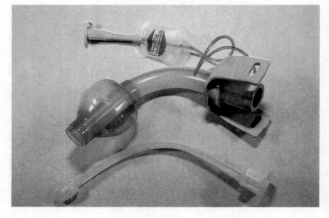

FIGURE 25-24 Tracheostomy tubes.
© Mediscan/Alamy Stock Photo.

The obturator is used to guide the tracheostomy tube into the stoma, much like the stylet is used for an endotracheal tube. The tube is then secured with the cuff inflated, and tracheal ties are placed around the patient's neck to secure the tube.

During ventilation, the cuff remains inflated to allow for a closed circuit. However, many patients with tracheostomies do not require around-the-clock ventilation. In patients who do not require pressure support, the tracheostomy may remain open with a tracheostomy collar providing moisture, or a heat moisture exchanger may allow for humidity to prevent overdrying of secretions. In other patients, a one-way valve (ie, a speaking valve or Passy Muir valve) may be in place. These valves allow the patient to inhale through the tracheostomy, but the one-way design allows exhalation through the native airway (and through the vocal cords, allowing for speech). Because of the one-way function of these valves, they can be used only with the cuff deflated. If the cuff is inflated, there would be no way to exhale the air, creating a life-threatening situation. The pilot balloon allows providers to know if the cuff is inflated or deflated. If the pilot balloon is full, the cuff is inflated; if it is not full, the cuff is deflated.

Because damage to the trachea can occur easily, it is important to ensure that the cuff is not overinflated. It is also important to remember that because the tracheostomy tube bypasses the normal "warmth and filtration" system that the nasal passages provide, the CCTP must administer only warmed, humidified oxygen via an oxygen warming device or a humidivent attachment.

Children who require tracheostomy tubes have weakened airways, so they may not be able to fully cough up secretions. Some children are dependent on intermittent suctioning of these secretions. Mucus plugging can obstruct the tube, causing respiratory arrest; thus, suctioning is an important part of the assessment. Alternatively, in some patients, suctioning may cause a vagal response, inducing bradycardia, so CCTPs must closely monitor the clinical response to suctioning interventions.

When caring for a child with a tracheostomy tube, the CCTP should ensure that an obturator, an extra tracheostomy tube of the same size, and a tracheostomy tube of a size smaller are readily available in case the tube is accidentally pulled out

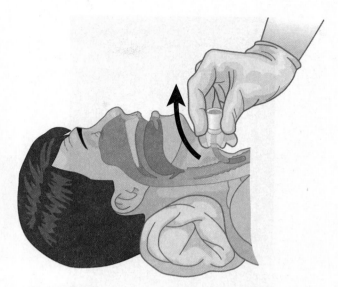

FIGURE 25-25 When changing the tracheostomy tube, place a towel roll under the patient's shoulders to ensure the patient is in the sniffing position.

© Jones & Bartlett Learning.

of place. Common complications encountered with tracheostomy tubes are the same as those linked to endotracheal tubes.

When changing the tracheostomy tube, it is important to place a towel roll under the patient's shoulders **FIGURE 25-25**. This step puts the child into the "sniffing" position and allows for easier insertion of the tracheostomy tube.

Children with respiratory disorders who are being cared for at home often have a "go-bag" with them. The go-bag will contain extra tracheostomy tubes of the same size and one size smaller, suction catheters, portable suction, a bag-mask device (Ambu bag), oxygen administration sets, nebulizers, and other emergency medications that these children may require, along with a binder containing a list of emergency contacts (physician, hospital numbers, home health care agency), medication administration record, past medical history, and allergy information. When transporting the child from home, providers should ask the family to bring this bag with them.

Pediatric Patients With Neurologic Disorders

Hydrocephalus is the result of accumulation of cerebrospinal fluid (CSF) due to an imbalance between

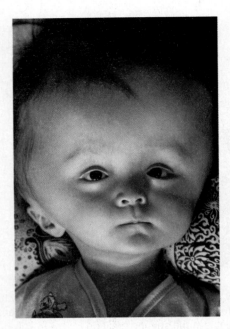

FIGURE 25-26 In hydrocephalus, the ventricles become enlarged due to buildup of cerebrospinal fluid.

© Donal Husni/NurPhoto/Getty Images.

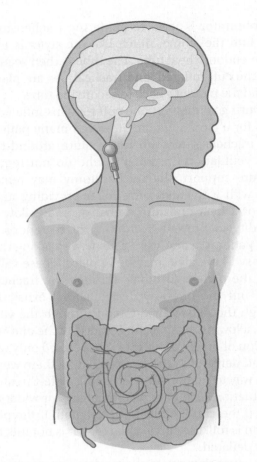

FIGURE 25-27 A ventriculoperitoneal shunt.

© Jones & Bartlett Learning.

production and reabsorption of CSF. Hydrocephalus can be differentiated into two types:

- *Congenital hydrocephalus* can be the result of a myelomeningocele, cytomegalovirus infection, or aqueduct stenosis.
- *Acquired hydrocephalus* can be the result of intraventricular hemorrhage, tumor, meningitis, or head injury.

Essentially, in hydrocephalus, CSF is unable to reach the subarachnoid space due to a blockage or injury and builds up in the ventricles **FIGURE 25-26**. As a result, these children will present with abnormally large heads, poor feeding, restlessness, bulging fontanelles, shrill or shrieking cry, upward gaze paralysis (the "sunset sign"), and inconsolability; they may also have dilated scalp veins.

Children with symptomatic hydrocephalus require surgical intervention and often have a ventriculoperitoneal (VP) or ventriculoatrial (VA) shunt placed, or undergo endoscopic third ventriculostomy. A VP shunt consists of a ventricular catheter that is inserted into a lateral ventricle; the distal end of the catheter then runs down to the peritoneal cavity via a flush pump and unidirectional-flow valve **FIGURE 25-27**. Older children who have finished going through so-called growth spurts or

somatic growth may have a VA shunt. A VA shunt consists of a catheter going from a lateral ventricle into the right atrium. VA shunts may also be placed in children with abdominal issues that contraindicate a VP shunt.

The CCTP will often encounter these children when they have a shunt malfunction or infection. VP shunts are susceptible to malfunction or may need revisions during growth spurts. Indeed, 40% of VP shunts usually need to be revised after 1 year, and 50% require revision at 2 years. Infection rates are especially high within the first 6 months of placement. Signs and symptoms of VP shunt malfunction or infection include fever, vomiting, altered mental status, dizziness, restlessness, irritability, headache, neck pain, and seizures.

Children with malfunctioning VP shunts or shunt-related infections must be monitored closely and transported with their heads elevated to a 30° angle. The head should be maintained in a neutral

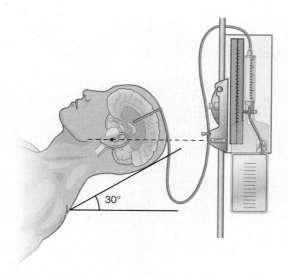

FIGURE 25-28 An external ventricular drain.

© Jones & Bartlett Learning.

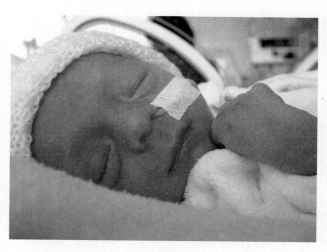

FIGURE 25-29 A nasogastric tube.

© Mediscan/Alamy Stock Photo.

position, and the child should be kept as calm as possible. Monitor the pulse oximetry as well as the ETCO₂ level (if available). Maintaining a slightly decreased ETCO₂ level and increased oxygenation can aid in decreasing cerebral blood flow.

In the event of a VP shunt infection or malfunction in which intracranial pressure (ICP) must be decreased and monitored closely, an external ventricular drain (EVD) may be inserted via a surgical procedure **FIGURE 25-28**. Such a device presents several risks—namely, worsening infection, CSF overdrainage or underdrainage, inadvertent disconnection, or bleeding. The chamber of the EVD must be hung at a specific level (measured in millimeters of mercury [mm Hg]). The zero point is placed at the level of the foramen of Monro. The drainage system is then opened as directed by the neurosurgeon and as needed to maintain a normal ICP of approximately 10 to 20 mm Hg. The CCTP must monitor any patient with an EVD closely for signs and symptoms of increased or even decreased ICP. Close monitoring of vital signs, especially BP, pulse oximetry, and ETCO₂ level, is essential. CCTPs must follow their agency's policies and procedures regarding the care of patients with shunts and EVDs.

Pediatric Patients With Gastrointestinal Disorders

Gastrointestinal disorders that may afflict children and create the need for medical technology include failure to thrive, craniofacial abnormalities, esophageal atresia, burns, strictures, chronic malabsorption, and even gastroesophageal reflux disease (GERD). Infants and children with Hirschsprung disease, Crohn disease, necrotizing enterocolitis, or imperforate anus may require colostomy or ileostomy placement.

GERD is defined as the complications associated with the reflux of gastric contents into the esophagus. This reflux can cause discomfort, and infants can present with excessive crying, irritability, emesis, and regurgitation. Causes of this condition include obesity, neurologic impairment, prematurity, and hiatal hernia, among others. Severe complications of GERD include esophageal stricture, failure to thrive, aspiration pneumonia, and acute life-threatening events. It is important for the CCTP to transport these patients in a sitting position or upright position to help prevent regurgitation. In severe cases, children with GERD may require gastric tube placement for feedings until the Nissen fundoplication surgical procedure can be performed.

CCTPs may also come in contact with children who have gastrointestinal disorders that render them unable to take in food or formula by mouth. These children may have gastric, gastrostomy, or jejunostomy tubes in place.

- *Gastric tubes* consist of nasogastric or orogastric tubes that pass through the nose or mouth into the stomach **FIGURE 25-29**. They are temporary due to the irritation they cause

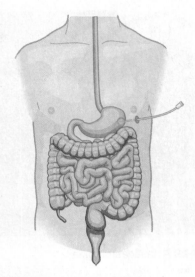

FIGURE 25-30 A gastrostomy tube.

© Jones & Bartlett Learning.

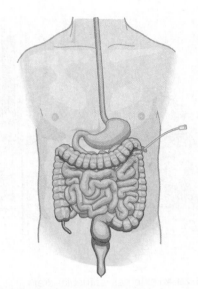

FIGURE 25-31 A jejunostomy tube.

© Jones & Bartlett Learning.

to the nasal and mucous membranes, but will remain in place for several weeks.

- *Gastrostomy tubes* are inserted directly into the stomach surgically via a tube or button **FIGURE 25-30**. Percutaneous endoscopy gastrostomy tubes are similar but are inserted endoscopically.
- *Jejunostomy tubes* are surgically placed through the stomach and into the small intestine **FIGURE 25-31**. These tubes may be necessary for children who are unable to tolerate feeds through their gastrostomy tube due to reflux, malabsorption, or other reasons. For the same reason, a small-bore nasal feeding tube may be placed into a post-pyloric position. Because they bypass the stomach and go into the small intestine, jejunostomy tubes can take in volumes only at a very low rate.
- A combination of the gastrostomy and jejunostomy tubes, called a GJ tube, is often the tube used in children. It will have two ports: Medications go through the stomach to be appropriately activated and absorbed, and larger volumes, such as feeds and fluids, go through the jejunostomy portion.

Complications that may be encountered with these devices include the accidental removal of the

gastrostomy tube. In such a case, if protocols allow, an indwelling urinary (Foley) catheter may be placed into the abdominal stoma to maintain the patency of the stoma until the gastrostomy tube can be replaced. This complication is of particular urgency if the surgical tract is "immature," typically meaning the tube was placed less than 6 weeks earlier. It is classically thought that these tracts can close in as little as 4 hours, so it is important to immediately maintain their patency. For this reason, caregivers often will have an extra tube on hand to replace the dislodged tube until definitive replacement can be performed in the hospital. Proper position of the tube should be radiographically confirmed before restarting feeds or delivering medications into a tube that has been replaced. The insertion sites of gastrostomy and jejunostomy tubes must be closely monitored for signs of infection, redness, excoriation, foul drainage, and inflammation.

Children who have colostomy or ileostomy drainage bags in place must be closely monitored for skin infection and breakdown. Colostomy and ileostomy placement increases the risk for skin breakdown due to proteolytic enzymes in the liquid stool coming in contact with skin. The ostomy bags must be well fitted to protect the skin from contact, yet loose enough to not constrict the exposed intestines.

Special Considerations With Pediatric Patients

CCTPs often come in contact with patients who have developmental or cognitive disabilities. The illness or injury that prompted the dispatch may not be a direct result of the patient's disability, but CCTPs must be able to communicate effectively with the parents and/or caregivers, and understand that the patient may or may not be able to communicate effectively with them. The parents and/or caregivers will be the best source of information in regard to how the patient normally responds. Obtaining an accurate history is vital in determining a baseline for these patients. Providers should not assume that a patient cannot understand language or communicate simply because they are not producing normal speech. Many patients communicate with communication boards or devices.

Patients with Down syndrome also warrant special consideration. These children are often difficult to intubate due to their disproportionately large tongue. Additionally, any patient with a congenital anomaly that results in a small jaw should be considered to have a difficult airway.

Considering that nearly 1 in every 10 births in the United States is premature, CCTPs are likely to encounter infants on apnea monitors. Because apnea monitors record data on events that can later be uploaded into a database at the pediatrician's office, these devices should be transported with the patient and not removed unless they impede direct patient care.

CSHCN account for approximately 18.5% of all children in the United States. It is important that CCTPs be familiar with these children, who require special attention in the CCT setting. It cannot be overemphasized that the parents and/or caregivers of such patients are the greatest resource that CCTPs have. They will know not only the child's history, but also the child's norms, which may be unique. They are the experts in their children's illnesses, and CCTPs must respect and take into consideration any input they have. As with any pediatric patient, family-centered care is a definite requirement when attending to CSHCN.

Summary

A relatively new area in which CCT units have become involved is the transport of bariatric patients, including those who have undergone bariatric procedures. Following these procedures, patients may require EMS intervention or CCT for either early or late complications. In such cases, the dispatch center or call center should have a detailed protocol for receiving the bariatric transport request, because such transports require specialized equipment and additional personnel, owing to these patients' weight and size. Two basic moves must be carefully planned: (1) moving the patient from the facility bed, chair, or table to the ambulance stretcher, and doing the reverse at the destination; and (2) loading the patient into the ambulance, and removing the patient at the destination. The challenges related to such moves require the CCTP to ensure the safety of both the crew and the patient, while simultaneously guarding the patient's privacy and maintaining good communication.

Excited delirium is a complex condition that can cause severe morbidity and mortality if not rapidly identified and treated. Patients with excited delirium experience symptoms including acute onset of hyperactive, aggressive, and/or combative behavior often associated with excessive physical strength. These symptoms present challenges for CCTPs and may necessitate assistance from law enforcement to maintain safety. Excited delirium is frequently associated with stimulant substance abuse, but may also be linked to underlying psychiatric disease. The primary goals in treating a patient with excited delirium are to protect the patient and providers from injury while maintaining patient dignity, reduce psychomotor agitation, perform a detailed physical exam and continuous monitoring of vital signs, establish IV access, and prevent morbidity and mortality. Treatment of excited delirium focuses on reducing agitation through verbal and environmental de-escalation techniques, administering sedative medications if necessary, correcting hypovolemia with IV volume resuscitation, employing specific therapies targeted at metabolic abnormalities, and preventing unsafe conditions such as transporting the patient in the prone position while handcuffed, or in a position that constricts the chest or neck.

Thanks to the many advances in medicine and technology, some children who would otherwise spend time in the hospital and ICU can be discharged to home with nursing coverage and specialized equipment. These pediatric patients often have congenital illnesses such as heart defects or may have acquired illnesses such as respiratory compromise related to bronchopulmonary dysplasia. Many of them are dependent on technology such as ventilators, tracheostomies, VP shunts, central venous catheters, colostomies, apnea monitors, or gastric tubes. When addressing the needs of these vulnerable patients, CCTPs should recognize that parents and/or caregivers are often the best sources of information.

Case Study

Your ground-based CCT service has been called to a community hospital to transport a 28-year-old man to a tertiary medical center for a higher level of care. The initial dispatch information is vague but suggests that the patient was acting oddly at a community gymnasium, so police were called. A struggle ensued and police requested EMS when they were unable to effectively restrain the patient. On your arrival at the sending facility, you learn that the patient weighs 187 pounds (85 kg) and was sedated in the field by local EMS with 350 mg of ketamine administered IM, followed by several doses of IV midazolam.

Your initial assessment reveals a muscular, incoherent, and profusely diaphoretic 28-year-old man in four-point restraints with a nonrebreathing oxygen mask in place. Despite an oxygen flow of 15 L/min, the oxygen reservoir is completely collapsing with each breath. EMS has established a large-bore IV, currently set at a TKO (to keep open) rate with the initial liter of normal saline, of which approximately 200 mL has been delivered. A second IV is in place, through which an infusion of midazolam is being delivered at 10 mg/h. SpO_2 is 98%; BP is 150/94 mm Hg; heart rate is 155 beats/min with somewhat peaked T waves on the ECG monitor; respirations are 36 breaths/min and deep; and rectal temperature is reported at 102.8°F (39.3°C). Your partner presents you with venous blood gas results that have just been reported, showing pH, 7.0; Po_2, 58 mm Hg; carbon dioxide, 23 mm Hg; bicarbonate, 12 mEq/L; and potassium, 6.1 mEq/L. Lactate is later reported as 16 mg/dL.

The patient is making incomprehensible sounds but is not struggling against the restraints. Your physical exam reveals multiple recent bruises and abrasions consistent with a significant struggle but no major deformity, trauma, or head wounds. A Foley catheter is in place and is draining a scant amount of dark-colored urine.

Following discussion with your partner, you initiate cooling with your transport cooling pads and apply nasal $ETCO_2$, noting a respiratory rate of 38 breaths/min and carbon dioxide of 21 mm Hg. You administer 100 mEq/L of sodium bicarbonate, add 15 L/min of nasal oxygen, and prepare for RSI. Using ketamine and rocuronium, your partner successfully intubates the patient, discontinuing the midazolam infusion in favor of a ketamine infusion for continued sedation. Ventilator settings are adjusted to maintain an end-tidal pressure of 20 mm Hg, an esophageal temperature probe is placed that now reads 102.4°F (39.1°C), and transport is begun. Restraints are double-checked to assure safety and adequate distal perfusion.

During transport, you closely monitor the ECG for changes, add bicarbonate to the normal saline infusion, and increase the fluids to 800 mL/h, which markedly improves the patient's urine output. After 50 minutes, the patient's BP is 140/85 mm Hg; heart rate is 140 beats/min; SpO_2 is 97% on a fraction of inspired oxygen (FIO_2) of 0.3; esophageal temperature is 101.8°F (38.8°C);

the patient is breathing spontaneously at 34 breaths/min (with the ventilator now set at 32 breaths/min in pressure control mode); ETCO$_2$ is 18 mm Hg; and urine output for the hour appears to be approaching 80 mL. You deliver the patient to the ED staff at the tertiary hospital and deliver your patient care report.

1. What was the rationale for RSI and why was ketamine selected for induction?
2. How was the end-tidal target determined?

Analysis

Excited delirium is a life-threatening syndrome with a high mortality rate, even when recognized and promptly treated. Metabolic acidosis associated with the hypermetabolic state of excited delirium results in compensatory Kussmaul respirations with increased minute volume. Hyperthermia, lactic acidosis, and excess myoglobin result in renal damage and require volume replacement to correct hypovolemia, correction of acidosis via respiratory and pharmacologic therapies, and rapid treatment with sedatives to reduce agitation. IM and/or intranasal sedative medications are commonly used initially to ensure patient and provider safety, followed by active cooling and additional sedation to lessen agitation.

Rhabdomyolysis and profound metabolic acidosis require early and aggressive IV fluid resuscitation as well as administration of IV bicarbonate. Hyperthermia should be treated with cooling measures and benzodiazepines if agitation persists. RSI and mechanical ventilation should be used only if all other interventions have failed and the patient either becomes apneic after sedative medications have been administered or has signs of impending respiratory failure. Caution must be exercised not to reduce the native minute volume being used to compensate for the underlying metabolic acidosis. Hence, after the drive to breathe is eliminated with RSI, providers must attempt to match or slightly surpass the preintubation ETCO$_2$ level. Failure to do so risks worsening the metabolic acidosis, which can rapidly lead to sudden cardiac collapse and death.

Ketamine is effective as both a sedative in excited delirium and an induction agent for intubation because it can be administered by either the IM or IV route and has a rapid onset without the hypotensive or negative inotropic effects often seen with benzodiazepines or narcotics.

Prep Kit

Ready for Review

- In the United States, more than 40% of adults have obesity. The trend toward greater levels of obesity has been accompanied by a rise in the number of bariatric (weight-loss) procedures performed.
- Several types of bariatric procedures are currently performed, including laparoscopic adjustable banding, vertical banded gastroplasty, sleeve gastrectomy, biliopancreatic diversion with duodenal switch, Roux-en-Y anastomosis, and intragastric balloon.

- Laparoscopic adjustable gastric banding is the least invasive bariatric surgical procedure; it may be performed using either five incisions or one incision.
- Vertical banded gastroplasty, also known as vertical sleeve gastrectomy, is the first part of a biliopancreatic diversion with duodenal switch procedure.
- Biliopancreatic diversion with duodenal switch is a two-part procedure that requires reshaping of the stomach and bypassing of a large portion of the small intestine.

Prep Kit Continued

- Roux-en-Y, one type of gastric bypass, is the most common type of bariatric procedure. In this two-part procedure, the stomach is reduced to a holding volume of approximately 30 mL (or the size of a walnut), and then the small intestines are divided and the jejunum is connected to a small hole in the stomach pouch.
- Early complications of bariatric procedures are those that occur within the first month after the procedure, such as deep vein thrombosis, pulmonary embolism, wound infection, sepsis, and gastrointestinal bleeding.
- Late complications of bariatric procedures occur more than 1 month after the procedure, such as obstruction from strictures, hernias, or hardware complications.
- Other specific bariatric procedural complications include band erosion, band intolerance, band slippage, port flip/inversion or dislodgement, and port dislocation.
- In patients with morbid obesity and those who have undergone bariatric surgery, both oxygen consumption and carbon dioxide production are increased. The increase in oxygen consumption may necessitate the use of a full main cylinder or the inclusion of additional oxygen cylinders on the transport unit, depending on the patient and the length of transport or time spent on the stretcher.
- The dispatch center or call center should have a detailed protocol for receiving bariatric transport requests, including obtaining information on the patient's height and weight.
- In bariatric transports, time on task will be significantly increased. Operationally, the agency must be prepared for this extended duration and the deleterious effects it may have on the transport service's system-wide performance and availability of resources.
- Two basic moves must be planned for when transporting bariatric patients:
  - Moving the patient from the facility bed, chair, or table to the ambulance stretcher, and doing the reverse at the destination
  - Loading the patient into the ambulance, and removing the patient at the destination
- A slide board is a basic device that is specifically used when movement of the patient from one level surface to another surface of similar height is indicated, typically from the bed to treatment table to the ambulance stretcher.
- Hydraulic and mechanical lift devices are most often seen in hospitals, surgical centers, skilled nursing facilities, and rehabilitation facilities.
- Air transfer mats work similarly to slide boards, in that they are used to laterally transfer patients, regardless of their size, from one level surface to another at a similar height.
- Bariatric-model stretchers are rated for a higher capacity and size; they are made with stronger construction and are considerably wider to ensure the patient's comfort.
- Many transport services have deployed a ramp and winch system in specific vehicles designated for the transportation of bariatric patients.
- Strictly because of their sizes, bariatric patients require special considerations when being prepared for transport. Covers will need to be larger, and patient adjustment on an ambulance stretcher may be difficult.
- Accommodating bariatric patients requires special considerations and proper communication. The patient has likely learned ways to deal with these challenges and can assist providers in helping with moving, positioning, and other transport issues.
- When transporting a bariatric patient, it is of utmost importance that the patient's dignity and privacy are protected.
- Safety during bariatric transports is a paramount concern for both providers and patients. Special devices such as ceiling harnesses, emergency lifting cushions, patient boosters, and motorized wheelchairs and bed movers may be available to reduce the

Prep Kit Continued

risk of injury, and additional personnel may be needed.

- Patients with excited delirium, also called agitated delirium, experience both delirium (acute confusion, hallucinations, and disorientation that is rapid in onset and may fluctuate in intensity) and an excited or agitated state. Symptoms include acute onset of hyperactive, aggressive, and/or combative behavior often associated with excessive physical strength.

- Patients with excited delirium have high rates of recent sympathomimetic or hallucinogenic recreational drug use, but may also present with or without drug use in the setting of acute decompensated psychiatric illness, such as schizophrenia or bipolar disorder.

- Even with prompt and appropriate treatment, excited delirium has a high mortality rate; nevertheless, rapid, targeted treatment greatly improves outcomes, decreasing both morbidity and mortality.

- Risk factors that appear to predispose an individual to developing excited delirium include male sex, use of stimulant drugs, and underlying psychiatric disease.

- Excited delirium is characterized by abnormal neurotransmitter physiology in the brain, including increased concentrations of the catecholamine dopamine.

- In the hypermetabolic state associated with elevated dopamine levels, sympathomimetic effects associated with excited delirium include tachycardia, hypertension, and elevated temperature. Oxygen supply–demand mismatch can occur, leading to severe lactic metabolic acidosis from anaerobic metabolism.

- Renal failure in patients with excited delirium results in accumulation of waste products in the blood, hyperkalemia, and metabolic acidosis. The combination of these factors places the patient at high risk for cardiac arrhythmias and death.

- It can be difficult to differentiate excited delirium from other diagnoses without a thorough evaluation, but such an evaluation can be nearly impossible to perform prior to pharmacologic sedation due to the risk of injury to health care providers and the patient. Often, only a very limited history can be obtained due to the patient's altered mental status.

- In suspected excited delirium, a 12-lead ECG can be useful to detect QTc interval prolongation, QRS complex widening, cardiac ischemia, and evidence of hyperkalemia.

- Laboratory evaluation of a patient with excited delirium may reveal a severe anion gap metabolic acidosis, a nonspecific leukocytosis, elevated troponin levels, elevated creatine kinase levels, myoglobinuria, hyperkalemia, and potentially acute renal failure with an elevated creatinine level.

- The primary goals of treatment of a patient with excited delirium are to protect the patient and healthcare providers from injury while maintaining patient dignity, reduce psychomotor agitation, facilitate a detailed physical exam and continuous monitoring of vital signs, establish intravenous (IV) access, and prevent morbidity and mortality. Treatment of excited delirium focuses on reduction of agitation through verbal and environmental de-escalation techniques, the use of sedative medications if necessary, correction of hypovolemia with IV volume resuscitation, specific therapies targeted at metabolic abnormalities, and the prevention of environmental conditions that increase mortality.

- It is frequently not possible to safely establish IV access during the primary assessment of a patient with excited delirium, and initial sedation must be achieved via the intramuscular route. The most commonly used medications for this purpose include benzodiazepines, antipsychotics, and ketamine. Rapidly dissolving

Prep Kit Continued

- second-generation antipsychotics, such as olanzapine, are another effective option.
- When they experience a prolonged state of psychomotor agitation, patients with excited delirium may become dangerously hyperthermic, and cooling may be required.
- The treatment of rhabdomyolysis emphasizes aggressive IV volume resuscitation and urine output monitoring to maintain adequate renal perfusion and reduce the risk of kidney damage.
- Patients being transported with excited delirium should be placed on continuous cardiopulmonary monitoring, including electrocardiogram, pulse oximetry, end-tidal carbon dioxide, and body temperature readings. Critical care transport professionals (CCTPs) should not use handcuffs or other locked physical restraints unless required by law enforcement, in which case a key and the law enforcement officer should accompany the patient at all times. Patients should never be transported in the prone position, with hands and feet tied together behind their back, or in a position that constricts the chest or neck.
- Children with special health care needs (CSHCN) are defined by the US Department of Health and Human Services as "those who have or are at increased risk for a chronic physical, developmental, behavioral, or emotional condition and who also require health and related services of a type or amount beyond that required by children generally."
- Many children who would otherwise spend time in the hospital and intensive care unit are now able to be discharged to home with nursing coverage and specialized equipment (eg, ventilators, tracheostomies, ventriculoperitoneal shunts, central venous catheters, colostomies, apnea monitors, or gastric tubes). These children often have congenital illnesses such as heart defects or may have acquired illnesses such as respiratory compromise related to bronchopulmonary dysplasia.
- The clinical consequences of congenital heart defects (CHDs) are heart failure and hypoxemia.
- Classification of CHDs is currently based on hemodynamic characteristics and consists of four categories: (1) increased pulmonary blood flow; (2) decreased pulmonary blood flow; (3) mixed blood flow; and (4) obstructive blood flow out of the heart.
- Acyanotic defects are usually caused by increased pulmonary blood flow and obstructive blood flow out of the heart; cyanotic defects consist of decreased pulmonary blood flow and mixed blood flow.
  - The increased pulmonary blood flow classification for acyanotic defects includes defects that cause a left-to-right shunt and can cause heart failure: atrial septal defect, ventricular septal defect, atrioventricular canal defect, and patent ductus arteriosus.
  - Acyanotic defects associated with obstructive blood flow include coarctation of the aorta, aortic stenosis, and pulmonic stenosis.
  - Cyanotic defects associated with decreased pulmonary blood flow include tetralogy of Fallot and tricuspid atresia.
  - The mixed blood flow classification of cyanotic defects consists of transposition of the great vessels and hypoplastic left heart syndrome.
- Some CHDs, such as coarctation of the aorta and hypoplastic left heart syndrome, require patency of the ductus arteriosus for survival. Administration of oxygen must be approached cautiously in infants with CHDs, as it may be fatal by promoting closure of the patent ductus arteriosus.
- IV fluid administration must be used cautiously in pediatric patients with CHDs. While most children can handle an IV bolus of 20 mL/kg, these vulnerable patients must be closely monitored and given only 10 mL/kg to prevent fluid overload or pulmonary edema.

Prep Kit Continued

- Pulse oximetry and blood pressure readings from both the upper and lower extremities can yield valuable clues to the presence of a CHD in pediatric patients.
- Children with sickle cell anemia often present with chest pain, extremity pain, and difficulty breathing. In the worst-case scenario, they may have a cerebral vascular accident.
- When children present in sickle cell crisis, aggressive treatment is necessary. These patients require oxygenation, an IV fluid bolus of isotonic crystalloids, or, if tolerated, oral rehydration. In severe cases, children may require blood transfusions.
- Pain management is extremely important for patients in sickle cell crisis, as is monitoring of respiratory status to assess for pneumonia.
- When faced with an injury to a child with hemophilia, first and foremost the CCTP must treat any obvious bleeding. These children require immediate administration of factor VIII intravenously.
- Venous access devices include tunneled catheters, implanted ports, and peripherally inserted central catheters. Depending on the specific catheter, the smallest syringe the CCTP may be able to use with these devices might be a 10-mL syringe.
- Bronchopulmonary dysplasia and tracheomalacia are commonly encountered respiratory disorders that may require or be the result of long-term ventilation, endotracheal tube placement, or tracheostomy placements in pediatric patients.
- Children with bronchopulmonary dysplasia may require tracheostomies, mechanical ventilation, and end-tidal carbon dioxide monitoring.
- Placing infants and children with tracheomalacia in a prone position allows gravity to assist in opening the airway; the supine position is dangerous in these patients due to the risk of narrowing of the weakened trachea or even airway collapse.
- When changing the tracheostomy tube, the CCTP should place a towel roll under the patient's shoulders (which puts the child into the "sniffing" position and allows for easier insertion of the tracheostomy tube), ensure that the cuff is not overinflated, and administer only warmed, humidified oxygen via an oxygen warming device or a humidivent attachment.
- When caring for children with a tracheostomy tube, the CCTP should ensure that an obturator, an extra tracheostomy tube of the same size, and a tracheostomy tube of a size smaller are readily available in case the tube is accidentally pulled out of place.
- Children with hydrocephalus will present with abnormally large heads, poor feeding, restlessness, bulging fontanelles, shrill or shrieking cry, and inconsolability; they may also have dilated scalp veins. The CCTP will often encounter these children when they have a ventriculoperitoneal shunt malfunction or infection.
- Children with malfunctioning ventriculoperitoneal shunts or shunt-related infections must be monitored closely and transported with their heads elevated to a 30° angle. The head should be maintained in a neutral position, and the child should be kept as calm as possible.
- Children with gastrointestinal disorders who have special devices or needs may have such issues as failure to thrive, craniofacial abnormalities, esophageal atresia, burns, or strictures, or they may experience chronic malabsorption or gastroesophageal reflux disease. Infants and children with Hirschsprung disease, Crohn disease, necrotizing enterocolitis, or imperforate anus may require colostomy or ileostomy placement.
- In case of the accidental removal of a gastrostomy tube, if protocols allow, an indwelling urinary catheter may be placed into the abdominal stoma to maintain the patency of the stoma until the gastrostomy tube can be replaced.

Prep Kit Continued

- The insertion sites of gastrostomy and jejunostomy tubes must be closely monitored for signs of infection, redness, excoriation, foul drainage, and inflammation.
- With pediatric patients who have developmental or cognitive disabilities, CCTPs must be able to communicate effectively with their parents and/caregivers, and understand that the patient may or may not be able to communicate effectively with them. The parents and/or caregivers will be the best source of information regarding how the patient normally responds.
- Patients with Down syndrome are often difficult to intubate due to their abnormally large tongues.
- Apnea monitors should be transported with the patient and not removed unless they impede direct patient care.

Vital Vocabulary

acyanotic defects Congenital heart defects in which blood is shunted from the left heart to the right heart; usually caused by increased pulmonary blood flow and obstructive blood flow out of the heart.

aortic stenosis Narrowing of the aortic valve, which can be described as valvular, supravalvular, or subvalvular.

atrial septal defect (ASD) An opening in the septal wall of the heart between the left and right atria, allowing blood flow from the left atrium to the right atrium.

atrioventricular canal defect An acyanotic heart defect that consists of both ventricular and atrial septal defects as well as a defect affecting the mitral and tricuspid valves, in which the valves are shared.

bariatric procedures Weight-loss procedures that typically involve reconfiguring the stomach and sometimes other portions of the gastrointestinal tract.

biliopancreatic diversion with duodenal switch (BPD/DS) A two-part bariatric surgical procedure that involves reshaping the stomach and bypassing a large portion of the small intestine.

bronchopulmonary dysplasia A chronic lung disorder that usually occurs in premature infants who weigh less than 3 pounds (1,500 g) at birth.

children with special health care needs (CSHCN) As defined by the US Department of Health and Human Services, those children "who have or are at increased risk for a chronic physical, developmental, behavioral, or emotional condition and who also require health and related services of a type or amount beyond that required by children generally."

coarctation of the aorta The narrowing or constriction of part of the aorta or aortic arch of the heart.

cyanotic defects Congenital heart defects that lead to low oxygen saturation, owing to either decreased pulmonary blood flow or mixed blood flow.

delirium Acute confusion, hallucinations, and disorientation that is rapid in onset and may fluctuate in intensity.

dopamine A neurotransmitter that plays important roles in executive function, impulsivity, sensory perception, and key physiologic parameters (eg, heart rate, blood pressure, and temperature regulation).

excited delirium A complex, life-threatening syndrome including both delirium and an excited or agitated state; also called agitated delirium.

heart failure A set of clinical signs and symptoms indicative of myocardial dysfunction and cardiac output that is inadequate to meet the metabolic demands of the body.

hemophilia A disease caused by inheritance of a recessive gene trait that causes excessive bleeding. The resulting factor VIII or factor IX deficiency leaves the blood unable to clot properly.

Prep Kit Continued

hydrocephalus The result of an obstruction that causes an excessive accumulation of cerebrospinal fluid.

hyperkalemia Abnormally high potassium concentration in the blood.

hypoplastic left heart syndrome A cyanotic heart defect that is caused by an abnormally small left ventricle; it is often associated with aortic and mitral valve stenosis or atresia.

Kussmaul respiration A typical respiratory pattern seen in patients with metabolic acidosis; it is characterized by a high respiratory rate and high tidal volume, leading to increased minute ventilation.

laparoscopic adjustable gastric banding (LAGB) The least invasive bariatric surgical procedure, in which an adjustable band is placed around the upper portion of the stomach, with an adjustment port located on the right side of the abdomen, under the skin.

morbid obesity A body mass index of 40 kg/m^2 or higher. Morbid obesity includes all of the health risks associated with obesity, but also makes essential functions such as walking or breathing difficult.

neutropenia A decrease in the number of neutrophils in the body; neutrophils are essential in the body's immune response system.

obesity A body mass index greater than or equal to 30 kg/m^2.

overweight A body mass index of 25 to 29.9 kg/m^2.

patent ductus arteriosus (PDA) An acyanotic heart defect in which blood flows from the aorta to the pulmonary artery.

Pickwickian syndrome A hypoventilation syndrome associated with obesity in which the person may experience increased breathing difficulty when in the supine position and have a higher incidence of sleep apnea, snoring, and hypercapnia.

pulmonic stenosis An acyanotic heart defect caused by obstruction of blood flow from the right ventricle to the pulmonary artery; also called pulmonary stenosis.

rhabdomyolysis A condition in which muscle fibers break down and release their contents (proteins) into the bloodstream.

Roux-en-Y The most common type of bariatric surgery, in which the size of the stomach is reduced, the small intestines are divided, and the jejunum is connected to a small hole in the stomach pouch; also known as gastric bypass.

sickle cell anemia A disease caused by inheritance of two sets of recessive genes that produce an abnormal hemoglobin protein, known as Hgb S. The red blood cells become deformed (have a sickle shape) and occlude vessels, clot, and cause great pain in patients.

sleeve gastrectomy A bariatric surgical procedure that is the first part of a biliopancreatic diversion with duodenal switch procedure, in which the structure of the stomach is changed to a tube; also known as vertical sleeve gastrectomy.

tetralogy of Fallot (TOF) A cyanotic heart defect characterized by four anomalies: ventricular septal defect, pulmonary stenosis, overriding aorta, and right ventricular hypertrophy.

tracheomalacia A weakening or softening of the tracheal cartilage/rings that leads to respiratory disease.

transposition of the great vessels A cyanotic heart defect that results from the aorta receiving blood from the right ventricle while the pulmonary artery leaves the left ventricle.

tricuspid atresia A cyanotic heart defect that results from an absent or defective tricuspid heart valve, which causes blood flow from the right atrium to the right ventricle to be blocked.

ventricular septal defect (VSD) An acyanotic heart defect in which blood flows from the left ventricle to the right ventricle through a hole in the septal wall.

vertical banded gastroplasty (VBG) A bariatric surgical procedure that divides the stomach into two parts; also known as stomach stapling.

Prep Kit Continued

References

Adams JP, Murphy PG. Obesity in anaesthesia and intensive care. *Br J Anaesth*. 2000;85(1):91-108.

Adult obesity facts. Centers for Disease Control and Prevention website. https://www.cdc.gov/obesity/adult/defining.html. Reviewed June 7, 2021. Accessed October 17, 2021.

Albert MS, Dell RB, Winters RW. Quantitative displacement of acid−base equilibrium in metabolic acidosis. *Ann Intern Med*. 1967;66(2):312-322.

American College of Emergency Physicians Clinical Policies Subcommittee (Writing Committee) on the Adult Psychiatric Patient, Nazarian DJ, Broder JS, et al. Clinical policy: critical issues in the diagnosis and management of the adult psychiatric patient in the emergency department. *Ann Emerg Med*. 2017;69:480.

Barras M. Drug dosing in obese adults. *Aust Prescr*. 2017;40(5):189-193.

Barton C, Wang ES. Correlation of end-tidal CO_2 measurements to arterial $Paco_2$ in nonintubated patients. *Ann Emerg Med*. 1994;23(3):560-563.

Bhat R, Rockwood K. Delirium as a disorder of consciousness. *J Neurol Neurosurg Psychiatry*. 2007;78:1167-1170.

Blazer DG, van Nieuwenhuizen AO. Evidence for the diagnostic criteria of delirium: an update. *Curr Opin Psychiatry*. 2012;25:239-243.

Bone HG, Freyhoff J, Utech M. The obese patient in the intensive care unit: what is different? [in German]. *Anasthesiol Intensivmed Notfallmed Schmerzther*. 2014;49(5):288-296.

Braude D, Dixon DR. Bariatric airway management is about more than intubation. JEMS website. https://www.jems.com/patient-care/bariatric-airway-management-is-about-more-than-intubation/. Published August 17, 2015. Accessed October 17, 2021.

Burnett AM, Peterson BK, Stellpflug SJ, Engebretsen KM, Glasrud KJ, Frascone RJ. The association between ketamine given for prehospital chemical restraint with intubation and hospital admission. *Am J Emerg Med*. 2015;33(1):76-79.

Burnett AM, Salzman J, Griffith K, Kroeger B, Frascone RJ. The emergency department experience with pre-hospital ketamine: a case series of 13 patients. *Prehosp Emerg Care*. 2012;16:1-7.

Burnett AM, Watters BJ, Barringer KW, Griffith KR, Frascone RJ. Laryngospasm and hypoxia after intramuscular administration of ketamine to a patient in excited delirium. *Prehosp Emerg Care*. 2012;16(3):412-414.

Cattano D. Airway management and patient positioning: a clinical perspective. *Anesthesiol News*. 2011:17-23.

Children with special health care needs. Heath Resources and Services Administration website. https://mchb.hrsa.gov/sites/default/files/mchb/Data/NSCH/nsch-cshcn-data-brief.pdf. Published July 2020. Accessed October 17, 2021.

Clark DY, Stocking J, Johnson J. *Flight and Ground Transport Nursing Core Curriculum*. 2nd ed. Denver, CO: Air & Surface Transport Nurses Association; 2006.

Cohen E, Kuo DZ, Agrawal R, et al. Children with medical complexity: an emerging population for clinical and research initiatives. *Pediatrics*. 2011;127(3):529-538.

Cole JB, Moore JC, Nystrom PC, et al. A prospective study of ketamine versus haloperidol for severe prehospital agitation. *Clin Tox*. 20016;54(7):556-562.

Crandall CS, Gardner S, Braude DA. Estimation of total body weight in obese patients. *Air Med J*. 2009;28(3):139-145.

Data and statistics on congenital heart defects. Centers for Disease Control and Prevention website. https://www.cdc.gov/ncbddd/heartdefects/data.html. Reviewed December 9, 2020. Accessed October 17, 2021.

Data and statistics on sickle cell disease. Centers for Disease Control and Prevention website. https://www.cdc.gov/ncbddd/sicklecell/data.html. Reviewed December 16, 2020. Accessed October 17, 2021.

Dean BV, Stellpflug S, Burnett AM, Engbretsen KM. 2C or not 2C: phenethylamine designer drug review. *J Med Toxicol*. 2013;9(2):172-178.

Defining adult overweight and obesity. Centers for Disease Control and Prevention website. https://www.cdc.gov/obesity/adult/defining.html. Reviewed March 3, 2021. Accessed October 17, 2021.

De Jong A, Chanques G, Jaber S. Mechanical ventilation in obese ICU patients: from intubation to extubation. *Crit Care*. 2017;21:63.

Drug dosing in obesity reference table. ClinCalc website. https://acphospitalist.org/archives/2011/10/obesity.htm. Accessed October 17, 2021.

Estimate of bariatric surgery numbers, 2011−2019. American Society for Metabolic and Bariatric Surgery website. https://asmbs.org/resources/estimate-of-bariatric-surgery-numbers. Accessed October 17, 2021.

Fearon DM, Steele DW. End-tidal carbon dioxide predicts the presence and severity of acidosis in children with diabetes. *Acad Emerg Med*. 2002;9(12):1373-1378.

Fighting premature birth. March of Dimes website. https://www.marchofdimes.org/mission/prematurity-campaign.aspx. Accessed October 17, 2021.

Fursevich DM, LiMarzi GM, O'Dell MC, Hernandez MA, Sensakovic WS. Bariatric CT imaging: challenges and solutions. *Radiographics*. 2016;36:1076-1086.

Garcia E, Thomas J, Abramo TJ, et al. Capnometry for noninvasive continuous monitoring of metabolic status in pediatric diabetic ketoacidosis. *Crit Care Med*. 2003;31(10):2539-2543.

Gonin P, Beysard N, Yersin B, Carron PN. Excited delirium: a systematic review. *Acad Emerg Med*. 2018;25(5):552-565.

Prep Kit Continued

Hall CA, Kader AS, McHale AM, Stewart L, Fick GH, Vilke GM. Frequency of signs of excited delirium syndrome in subjects undergoing police use of force: descriptive evaluation of a prospective, consecutive cohort. *J Forensic Legal Med.* 2013;20(2):102-107.

Hazinski MF. *Nursing Care of the Critically Ill Child.* 3rd ed. St. Louis, MO: Elsevier Mosby; 2013.

Hemophilia A. National Hemophilia Foundation website. https://www.hemophilia.org/bleeding-disorders-a-z/types/hemophilia-a. Accessed October 17, 2021.

Ho JD, Dawes DM, Nelson RS, et al. Acidosis and catecholamine evaluation following simulated law enforcement "use of force" encounters. *Acad Emerg Med.* 2010;17(7):e60-e68.

Ho JD, Smith SW, Nystrom PC, et al. Successful management of excited delirium syndrome with prehospital ketamine: two case examples. *Prehosp Emerg Care.* 2013;17:274.

Hockenberry MJ, Wilson D. *Wong's Nursing Care of Infants and Children.* 10th ed. St. Louis, MO: Elsevier Mosby; 2015.

Holleran RS, ed. *ASTNA Patient Transport Principles and Practice.* 4th ed. St. Louis, MO: Mosby Elsevier; 2010.

Hopper AB, Vilke GM, Castillo EM, et al. Ketamine use for acute agitation in the emergency department. *J Emerg Med.* 2015;48:712.

Jefferies S, Weatherall M, Young P, Beasley R. A systematic review of the accuracy of peripheral thermometry in estimating core temperatures among febrile critically ill patients. *Crit Care Resusc.* 2011;13(3):194-199.

Kartal M, Eray O, Rinnert S, Goksu E, Bektas F, Eken C. ETCO$_2$: a predictive tool for excluding metabolic disturbances in nonintubated patients. *Am J Emerg Med.* 2011;29(1):65-69.

Keidar A, Carmon E, Szold A, Abu-Abeid S. Port complications following laparoscopic adjustable gastric banding for morbid obesity. *Obes Surg.* 2005;15(3):361-365.

Keseg D, Cortez E, Rund D, Caterino J. The use of prehospital ketamine for control of agitation in a metropolitan firefighter-based EMS system. *Prehosp Emerg Care.* 2015;19(1):110-115.

Kuo DZ, Goudie A, Cohen E, et al. Inequalities in health care needs for children with medical complexity. *Health Aff.* 2014;33(12):2190-2198.

Kupas D, Wydro GC, Tan DK, Kamin R, Harrell AJ IV, Wang A. Clinical care and restraint of agitated or combative patients by emergency medical services practitioners. National Association of EMS Physicians website. https://naemsp.org/NAEMSP/media/NAEMSP-Documents/Clinical-Care-and-Restraint-of-Agitated-or-Combative-Patients.pdf. Published October 2020. Accessed October 17, 2021.

Lin J, Figuerado Y, Montgomery A, et al. Efficacy of ketamine for initial control of acute agitation in the emergency department: a randomized study. *Am J Emerg Med.* 2021;44:306.

Linder LM, Ross CA, Weant KA. Ketamine for the acute management of excited delirium and agitation in the prehospital setting. *Pharmacotherapy.* 2018;38(1):139-151.

Mankowitz SL, Regenberg P, Kaldan J, Cole JB. Ketamine for rapid sedation of agitated patients in the prehospital and emergency department settings: a systematic review and proportional meta-analysis. *J Emerg Med.* 2018;55:670.

Mash DC, Duque L, Pablo J, et al. Brain biomarkers for identifying excited delirium as a cause of sudden death. *Forensic Sci Int.* 2009;190(1-3):e13-e19.

Mash DC, Pablo J, Ouyang Q, Hearn WL, Izenwasser S. Dopamine transport function is elevated in cocaine users. *J Neurochem.* 2002;81(2):292-300.

McPherson M, Arango P, Fox H, et al. A new definition of children with special health care needs. *Pediatrics.* 1998;102:137-140.

Meier ER. Sickle cell disease in children. *Drugs.* 2012;72(7):895-906.

Morgan MM, Perina DG, Acquisto NM, et al. Ketamine use in prehospital and hospital treatment of the acute trauma patient: a joint position statement. *Prehosp Emerg Care.* 2020. doi:10.1080/10903127.2020.1801920.

Nagler J, Wright RO, Krauss B. End-tidal carbon dioxide as a measure of acidosis among children with gastroenteritis. *Pediatrics.* 2006;118(1):260-267.

New AMA policy opposes "excited delirium" diagnosis. American Medical Association website. https://www.ama-assn.org/press-center/press-releases/new-ama-policy-opposes-excited-delirium-diagnosis. Published June 14, 2021. Accessed October 19, 2021.

Nieman C. Pediatric transport. In: Clark DY, Stocking J, Johnson J, eds. *Flight and Ground Transport Nursing Core Curriculum.* 2nd ed. Denver, CO: Air & Surface Transport Nurses Association; 2006:543-592.

Obesity and overweight. Centers for Disease Control and Prevention website. https://www.cdc.gov/nchs/fastats/obesity-overweight.htm. Reviewed January 11, 2021. Accessed October 17, 2021.

O'Brien ME, Fuh L, Raja AS, White BA, Yun BJ, Hayes BD. Reduced-dose intramuscular ketamine for severe agitation in an academic emergency department. *Clin Toxicol.* 2020;58(4):294-298.

O'Connor L, Rebesco M, Robinson C, et al. Outcomes of prehospital chemical sedation with ketamine versus haloperidol and benzodiazepine or physical restraint only. *Prehosp Emerg Care.* 2019;23:201.

O'Halloran RL, Lewman LV. Restraint asphyxiation in excited delirium. *Am J Forensic Med Pathol.* 1993;14(4):289-295.

Olives TD, Nystrom PC, Cole JB, Dodd KW, Ho JD. Intubation of profoundly agitated patients treated with prehospital ketamine. *Prehosp Disaster Med.* 2016;31(6):593-602.

Pollanen MS, Chiasson DA, Cairns JT, Young JG. Unexpected death related to restraint for excited delirium: a retrospective study of deaths in police custody and in the community. *CMAJ.* 1998;158(12):1603-1607.

Prep Kit Continued

Rawson R, Huber A, Brethen P, et al. Methamphetamine and cocaine users: differences in characteristics and treatment retention. *J Psychoactive Drugs*. 2000;32(2):233-238.

Razi E, Moosavi GA, Omidi K, Khakpour SA, Razi A. Correlation of end-tidal carbon dioxide with arterial carbon dioxide in mechanically ventilated patients. *Arch Trauma Res*. 2012;1(2):58-62.

Reports and publications. US Department of Health and Human Services website. https://www.hhs.gov/surgeongeneral/reports-and-publications/index.html. Reviewed July 15, 2021. Accessed October 17, 2021.

Roca RP, Charen B, Boronow J. Ensuring staff safety when treating potentially violent patients. *JAMA*. 2016;316:2669.

Ruttenber AJ, McAnally HB, Wetli CV. Cocaine-associated rhabdomyolysis and excited delirium: different stages of the same syndrome. *Am J Forensic Med Pathol*. 1999;20(2):120-127.

Samuel E, Williams RB, Ferrell RB. Excited delirium: consideration of selected medical and psychiatric issues. *Neuropsychiatr Dis Treat*. 2009;5:61-66.

Schauer PR, Kashyap SR, Wolski K, et al. Bariatric surgery versus intensive medical therapy in obese patients with diabetes. *N Engl J Med*. 2012;366(17):1567-1576.

Scheppke KA, Braghiroli J, Shalaby M, Chait R. Prehospital use of i.m. ketamine for sedation of violent and agitated patients. *West J Emerg Med*. 2014;15:736.

Schneider A, Mullinax S, Hall N, et al. Intramuscular medication for treatment of agitation in the emergency department: a systematic review of controlled trials. *Am J Emerg Med*. 2021;46:193.

Schnitzer K, Merideth F, Macias-Konstantopoulos W, et al. Disparities in care: the role of race on the utilization of physical restraints in the emergency setting. *Acad Emerg Med*. 2020;27:943.

Simpson ML. Recognition and management of hemophilia emergencies. *Clin Pediatr Emerg Med*. 2011;12(3):224-232.

Slota M. *Core Curriculum for Pediatric Critical Care Nursing*. 2nd edition. St. Louis, MO: Saunders Elsevier; 2006.

Staley JK, Welti CV, Ruttenber AJ, et al. Altered dopaminergic synaptic markers in cocaine psychosis and sudden death. *National Institute on Drug Abuse Research Monograph Series*. 1995;153:491.

Stratton SJ. Factors associated with sudden death of individuals requiring restraint for excited delirium. *Am J Emerg Med*. 2001;19(3):187-191.

Strömmer EMF, Leith W, Zeegers MP, Freeman MD. The role of restraint in fatal excited delirium: a research synthesis and pooled analysis. *Forens Sci Med Pathol*. 2020;16:680-692.

Suter M, Calmes JM, Paroz A, Giusti V. A 10-year experience with laparoscopic gastric banding for morbid obesity: high long-term complication and failure rates. *Obes Surg*. 2006;16(7):829-835.

Takeuchi A, Ahern TL, Henderson SO. Excited delirium. *West J Emerg Med*. 2011;12(1)77-83.

Vilke GM, Bozeman WP, Dawes DM, Demers G, Wilson MP. Excited delirium syndrome (ExDS): treatment options and considerations. *J Forensic Legal Med*. 2012;19(3):117-121.

Vilke GM, DeBard ML, Chan TC, et al. Excited delirium syndrome (ExDS): defining based on a review of the literature. *J Emerg Med*. 2012;43(5):897-905.

Williams AM, Estrada C, Gary-Bryan H, MacKeil-White K. The hematology and oncology pediatric patient: a review of fever and neutropenia, blood transfusions, and other complex problems. *Clin Pediatr Emerg Med*. 2012;13(2):91-98.

Witlox J, Eurelings LSM, De Jonghe JFM, et al. Delirium in elderly patients and the risk of postdischarge mortality, institutionalization, and dementia: a meta-analysis. *JAMA*. 2010;304:443-451.

Yakushiji H, Goto T, Shirasaka W, et al. Associations of obesity with tracheal intubation success on first attempt and adverse events in the emergency department: an analysis of the multicenter prospective observational study in Japan. *PLoS One*. 2018;13(4):e0195938. doi:10.1371/journal.pone.0195938.

Yosefy C, Hay E, Nasri Y, Magen E, Reisin L. End-tidal carbon dioxide as a predictor of arterial Paco$_2$ in the emergency department setting. *Emerg Med J*. 2004;21(5):557-559.

Yu J, McKernan G, Hagerman T, Schenker Y, Houtrow A. Most children with medical complexity do not receive care in well-functioning health care systems. *Hosp Ped*. 2021;11(2):183-191.

Zavarella M, Benner R, Krost W, Mistovitch J, Limmer D. Beyond the basics: bariatric emergencies. *EMS World*. 2007;36(8):78-87.

Glossary

3-3-2 rule: A method used to predict difficult intubation; a mouth opening of less than three fingers wide, a mandible length of less than three fingers wide, and a distance from the hyoid bone to the thyroid notch of less than two fingers wide indicate a possibly difficult airway.

abandonment: The termination of the patient relationship without assurance that an equal or greater level of care will continue.

Abbreviated Injury Scale (AIS): A trauma scoring system that ranks injury severity by assigning an individual injury score of 1 to 6 to six body regions, with 1 being a minor injury and 6 being an injury with a high mortality rate; does not account for multisystem injuries.

ABCDE: A mnemonic used to help providers remember the patient assessment sequence: Airway, Breathing, Circulation, Disability, and Exposure.

abdominal compartment syndrome (ACS): A condition that can result from intra-abdominal hypertension, including decreased end-organ perfusion with evidence of failure; if untreated, it can lead to death.

ablation: Removal of a pathway or function by electrocautery or radiofrequency.

ABO-incompatible transfusion reactions: Transfusion reactions in which the patient possesses antigens to a blood type and receives that blood type.

absolute refractory period: The early phase of cardiac repolarization, wherein the heart muscle cannot be stimulated to depolarize.

absorption: Acquisition of additional heat, radiation, or other energy from the environment. Also, movement of a substance's molecules from the site of entry on the body into the systemic circulation; the process by which molecules are taken up into another medium or tissue.

accuracy: A measure of the likelihood that an average of a set of test values will be similar to the true value.

acetylcholine (ACh): A chemical neurotransmitter of the parasympathetic nervous system.

acrocyanosis: A decrease in the amount of oxygen delivered to the extremities. The hands and feet turn blue because of the lack of oxygen.

activated charcoal: A carbon-based liquid with an incredible adsorptive ability that is typically administered orally or via nasogastric or orogastric tube to decrease the available quantity of a toxic substance.

activated partial thromboplastin time (aPTT): A value that represents the intrinsic coagulation pathway's clotting ability; also known as partial thromboplastin time (PTT).

active error: An error that almost always involves frontline staff and occurs at a contact point between a staff member and some aspect of a larger system.

active immunity: Production of a specific antibody in response to an infection or antigen.

active warming: A method of warming a hypothermic patient that involves the introduction of exogenous heat sources to the patient; measures may include infusing warmed IV fluid, delivering warm, humidified oxygen, or administering a peritoneal lavage of a potassium chloride–free solution or nasogastric/orogastric lavage with warmed fluids.

acute coronary syndrome (ACS): Any group of clinical symptoms consistent with acute myocardial ischemia.

acute glomerulonephritis (AGN): A histopathologic diagnosis associated with edema, hypertension, and hematuria; results from deposition of circulating immune complexes in the kidney basement membrane, which ultimately causes reduced glomerular filtration.

acute kidney injury (AKI): Decreased renal function in the absence of preexisting renal disease. It is classified into three categories: prerenal, intrarenal, and postrenal.

acute postinfectious glomerulonephritis (APIGN): A form of acute glomerulonephritis that occurs following an infection by streptococci.

acute radiation syndrome: Radiation poisoning.

acute tubular necrosis (ATN): Damage to the tubules of the nephron, preventing proper ion and fluid exchange in the kidneys.

acyanotic defects: Congenital heart defects in which blood is shunted from the left heart to the right heart; usually caused by increased pulmonary blood flow and obstructive blood flow out of the heart.

adaptive immune system: The secondary mechanism that protects the host by reacting with and eliminating specific antigens but that requires more time than the innate immune system to mobilize its defenses against unknown pathogens.

adaptive immunity: The immunity the body develops as part of exposure to an antigen or through vaccination; also called acquired immunity.

Addison disease: A chronic hormonal or endocrine disorder caused by a deficiency of cortisol and/or aldosterone; characterized by weakness, fatigue, hypotension, unexplained weight loss, and darkening of the skin.

addisonian crisis: The sudden appearance of symptoms, especially shock, in a patient with chronic adrenal insufficiency; it may appear suddenly as a result of an increased period of stress, trauma, surgery, or severe infection. Other symptoms include weakness, altered mental status, hyperthermia, and severe pain in the lower back, legs, or abdomen.

adhesions: Bands of connective tissue that can distort the normal GI anatomy; the result of improper healing or scar tissue growth following surgery.

adrenal insufficiency (AI): Underproduction of cortisol and aldosterone caused by a decreased function of the adrenal cortex; it occurs when at least 90% of the adrenal cortex has been damaged.

adsorption: The process of attracting molecules of a substance to the surface of that substance.

adventitious breath sounds: Abnormal breath sounds that are heard in addition to, or in place of, normal sounds.

adverse drug event (ADE): An adverse reaction caused by taking a medication.

aerobic metabolism: A form of energy production in which mitochondria use glucose, amino acids, and fatty acids combined with oxygen and ADP to produce ATP, carbon dioxide, water, and heat.

aerophagia: A condition in which the stomach fills with excessive air secondary to increased respiratory rate.

afferent pathways: Ascending pathways that carry sensory impulses toward the central nervous system.

afterload: The tension or stress that develops in the ventricles during systole; measured by pulmonary and systemic vascular resistance.

agonal respirations: Slow, shallow, irregular respirations, or occasional gasping breaths; result from cerebral anoxia.

agonist: A molecule (medication) that binds and activates a receptor, producing a biologic response.

Air Medical Physician Association (AMPA): An organization of physicians and air medical professionals that promotes safe patient transport.

air medical resource management (AMRM): The term used in air medical programs to denote the concept of crew resource management—an initiative designed to ensure all parties involved in an operation have decision-making input.

alanine aminotransferase (ALT): An intracellular enzyme found in large amounts in the liver and kidney, skeletal muscle, and heart; formerly known as serum glutamic-pyruvic transaminase (SGPT).

albumin: A blood product containing this specific protein found in the blood, which is prepared by the fractionation of pooled plasma; used for volume replacement in certain conditions; the most common protein in the body; acts as a transport protein, is a free radical scavenger, and serves as the main source of protein-generated oncotic pressure.

alcoholic ketoacidosis: A type of acidosis characterized by a buildup of ketones in the blood, caused by a large intake of alcohol and poor nutritional intake.

aldosterone: The main hormone responsible for adjustments to the final composition of urine; it increases the rate of active resorption of sodium and chloride ions into the blood and decreases the resorption of potassium.

aldosteronism: A syndrome of high blood pressure and low blood potassium levels caused by an excess of aldosterone; there are two main types—primary and secondary.

alkaline phosphatase: An enzyme that is essential for proper digestion and absorption through the mucous membranes in the gastrointestinal tract; it is clinically useful for testing liver function and for diagnosing a common bile duct obstruction.

Allen test: A technique in which the patient's hand is initially held above the head while the fist is clenched and the radial and ulnar arteries are compressed; the hand is then lowered and the fist is opened, ulnar pressure is released, and radial pressure is maintained. After the ulnar pressure is released, color should return to the hand within 6 seconds.

alveolar ventilation (V_a): The volume of air that comes into contact with the alveolar-capillary membrane surfaces and participates in the exchange of gases between the lung and blood.

amniotic fluid embolism (AFE): A rare and poorly understood condition in which fetal tissue crosses over the placental barrier into the maternal circulation. It can occur antepartum and postpartum and is believed to be associated with an anaphylactoid response leading to multisystem organ failure and disseminated intravascular coagulation.

amylase: A key enzyme used by the body to metabolize carbohydrates; it is produced primarily by the salivary glands and the pancreas.

amyloidosis: A group of diseases that result from abnormal deposits of the protein amyloid in various tissues of the body; can occur in a localized area or may be systemic.

anaerobic metabolism: A less efficient form of energy production in which an alternative pathway converts glucose to pyruvic acid with the simultaneous production of ATP; it also results in the production of lactate.

anaphylactic shock: A potentially life-threatening allergic reaction that presents with increased general body edema, hypotension, rash, urticaria, anxiety, and warm, flushed skin; a severe hypersensitivity reaction that involves bronchoconstriction and cardiovascular collapse.

anaphylactoid reaction: A non–IgE-mediated response that causes the rupture of mast cells and basophils, which then release histamine and other defense mediators.

anaphylaxis: A serious systemic allergic reaction that has a rapid onset and a variable clinical presentation.

anatomic dead space (V_d): Space in airway structures such as the trachea, bronchi, and bronchioles that does not participate in gas exchange. It is defined physiologically as ventilation without perfusion.

anechoic: Free from echo.

aneurysm: A weakened portion of the wall of an artery where the blood creates a localized dilation or bulge; it can involve the intact wall or be classified as dissecting, in which case the artery wall ruptures and blood pools between the inner and outer artery wall.

angiodysplasia: Deformed submucosal blood vessels in the GI tract that are susceptible to bleeding.

anion: A negatively charged ion.

anion gap (AG): A summary of the relationship among the three major contributors to the overall electrical charge (Na^+, Cl^-, and HCO_3^-); abnormal AG values may signal disturbances in the overall electrical and acid–base balance of the serum and presence of disease.

anisocoria: A condition in which the pupils are not of equal size.

anode: The electrode in a pacing circuit that is positively charged when current is flowing.

antagonist: A molecule (medication) that blocks a receptor site from being stimulated by an agonist or other chemical mediators.

antegrade conduction: Conduction in the normal direction between cardiac structures.

anterior cord syndrome: Displacement of bony fragments into the anterior portion of the spinal cord, often as the result of flexion injuries or fractures, that disrupts blood flow in the anterior spinal artery.

antiarrhythmic: A medication used to treat and prevent cardiac rhythm disorders.

anticholinergic syndrome: A syndrome that occurs following excessive exposure to medications such as antihistamines, atropine, and benztropine (Cogentin), or other substances such as jimson weed, resulting in muscarinic receptor blockade at the CNS and various other organs; characterized by tachycardia, hyperthermia, dilated pupils, warm (or hot) dry skin, ileus, delirium, seizures, hallucinations, and urinary retention.

antigen: An agent that stimulates the formation of specific protective proteins called antibodies; substance that can create an immune response in the body.

antigenic drift: A series of small genetic changes in a virus that alter the virus just enough that antibodies generated in previous infections no longer recognize the viral epitopes or surface proteins and, therefore, do not protect the body from the symptoms of a new infection.

antigenic shift: More drastic genetic changes in a virus, in which the protein structure of one or both of the spike proteins undergoes changes.

antiphospholipid syndrome (APS): An autoimmune disorder in which antibodies block certain phospholipid-binding proteins that normally protect the body from excessive coagulation.

anxiolysis: The reduction of anxiety by the administration of an antianxiety agent.

aortic regurgitation: Backward flow of blood through the aortic valve from the aorta into the left ventricle.

aortic stenosis: Narrowing of the aortic valve, which can be described as valvular, supravalvular, or subvalvular.

Apgar score: A scoring system for assessing the status of a newborn that assigns a numerical value to five areas of assessment (the total possible score range is 0–10).

aphasia: Any loss or impairment of language function as a result of brain damage.

apnea: Respiratory pause greater than or equal to 20 seconds; the absence of respiration.

apneustic breathing: A condition in which lesions in the respiratory center of the brainstem lead to a breathing pattern characterized by prolonged, gasping inspiration, followed by extremely short, ineffective expiration.

apoptosis: Programmed cell death.

appendicitis: Inflammation and/or infection of the appendix.

arachnoid mater: The middle layer of the meninges, which contains blood vessels that give it the appearance of a spider web.

arterial blood gas (ABG) panel: A collection of lab values used to analyze the following characteristics of blood: pH, partial pressure of CO_2 (in arterial blood), partial pressure of oxygen (in arterial blood), concentration of bicarbonate ion, base excess (indicating whether the patient is acidotic or alkalotic), and oxygen saturation of the hemoglobin molecule.

arterial bruits: Turbulence or "swishing" sounds heard with a stethoscope placed over the carotid arteries that signal the presence of atherosclerosis.

arterial lines: Catheters inserted into the patient's arterial vascular system for the purpose of producing a waveform with pressure measurements; also called A-lines.

arterial oxygen content (Cao_2): The total amount of oxygen in the arterial blood.

arteriovenous malformation (AVM): A cluster of abnormally formed blood vessels that have a higher rate of bleeding than average vessels.

ascites: A buildup of fluid in the abdominal cavity.

ascromegaly: A syndrome that results from excessive secretion of growth hormone by the pituitary gland after the epiphyseal plate has closed; characterized by the growth of bones, muscles, and many internal organs at an abnormally fast rate.

aspartate aminotransferase (AST): An intracellular enzyme found in large amounts in the liver and in skeletal muscle, the brain, red blood cells, and the heart; formerly known as serum glutamic-oxaloacetic transaminase (SGOT).

assault: The unlawful act of placing a person in apprehension of immediate bodily harm without their consent.

assisted systole: The pressure waveform that follows the diastolic augmentation peak.

assist ratios: Settings on the intra-aortic balloon pump that allow the operator to determine how often the pump inflates the balloon.

atelectasis: Collapse of all or part of a lung.

atmosphere: Gases that extend from the earth's surface to space; composed primarily of nitrogen, oxygen, argon, and trace gases.

atresia: Complete absence of a lumen.

atrial septal defect (ASD): An opening in the septal wall of the heart between the left and right atria, allowing blood flow from the left atrium to the right atrium.

atrioventricular (AV) valves: The valves (mitral and tricuspid) that separate the atria from the ventricles.

atrioventricular canal defect: An acyanotic heart defect that consists of both ventricular and atrial septal defects as well as a defect affecting the mitral and tricuspid valves, in which the valves are shared.

autonomic dysreflexia: A potentially life-threatening complication of spinal cord injury that results from the loss of parasympathetic stimulation. It is characterized by a massive, uninhibited, uncompensated cardiovascular response as the result of some stimulation of the sympathetic nervous system below the level of injury; also called autonomic hyperreflexia.

auto-PEEP: The nonintended increase in end alveolar pressure due to air trapping.

AVPU scale: An evaluation tool used to determine patient responsiveness; stands for Alert, responds to Voice, responds to Pain, Unresponsive.

axonal transport: The movement of organelles and proteins along a nerve cell axon into and out of the cell body.

azotemia: Increased nitrogenous wastes in the blood.

azygos system: A network of blood vessels that connects the superior and inferior vena cava; it also drains a portion of the esophageal venous blood.

bacteremia: The presence of bacterial infection in the blood.

bactericidal: Capable of killing bacteria.

bacteriostatic: Capable of inhibiting bacterial growth.

bandemia: Release of excessive numbers of band cells from the bone marrow into the blood.

bariatric procedures: Weight-loss procedures that typically involve reconfiguring the stomach and sometimes other portions of the gastrointestinal tract.

barodontalgia: A condition caused by ambient pressure changes that may result from gas bubbles trapped below the gums during restorative dental treatments, from periodontal cysts or abscesses; previously referred to as flyer's toothache.

barometric pressure: The weight per unit area of all the molecules of the gases above the point at which the measurement was taken.

barosinusitis: An inflammation of one or more of the paranasal sinuses resulting from a pressure gradient between the sinus cavity and atmosphere.

barotitis media: Inflammation and possible petechial hemorrhage in the middle ear and possible rupture of the eardrum that results from the failure of the middle ear space to ventilate when going from low to high atmospheric pressure; also known as ear block.

barotrauma: Injury to the chest or lungs as a result of increased intrathoracic pressure; injury to tissues, organs, or structures within the body, resulting from rapid or significant changes in environmental air pressure.

basal ganglia: Masses of nuclei located deep in the cerebral hemispheres that play a major role in fine motor function.

basal metabolic rate (BMR): The heat energy produced at rest by normal body metabolic reactions, determined mostly by the liver and skeletal muscle.

base excess (BE): A measure of metabolic derangement that is part of the arterial blood gas panel; also known as base deficit (BD), as the value can be either positive (excess) or negative (deficit).

basilar skull fracture: A fracture along the base of the skull.

battery: The unlawful touching of another person without their consent.

Battle sign: Migration of blood to the mastoid region, posterior and slightly inferior to the ear, resulting in discoloration; also called retroauricular ecchymosis.

Beck triad: The combination of a narrowed pulse pressure, muffled heart tones, and jugular venous distention associated with cardiac tamponade; usually resulting from penetrating chest trauma.

Benchmarking: The process of comparing an organization's processes and performance to those of the overall industry or the best practices from other companies.

bicarbonate (HCO_3^-): An ion that is present in the blood; its measurement represents the metabolic component of the arterial blood gas panel.

bicarbonate–carbonic acid buffer system: The principal extracellular buffer system, which operates primarily in the lungs and kidneys; in this system, carbon dioxide and water are reversibly converted into carbonic acid, which in turn is reversibly converted into hydrogen ions and bicarbonate.

bifascicular block: The combination of a right bundle branch block and a block of one of the fascicles of the left bundle, the left anterior or left posterior fascicle.

bilevel positive airway pressure (BPAP): The use of two separate pressures—inspiratory positive airway pressure and expiratory positive airway pressure—to raise the breathing baseline above the ambient pressure. The pressure gradient enhances ventilation, and the reduced expiratory pressure makes exhalation easier and increases patient tolerance.

biliopancreatic diversion with duodenal switch (BPD/DS): A two-part bariatric surgical procedure that involves reshaping the stomach and bypassing a large portion of the small intestine.

bilirubin: A waste product of heme formed during erythrocyte metabolism. It is moved to the small intestine within bile and then converted into urobilinogen, resulting in brown pigmented feces.

bioavailability: The amount or percentage of a medication that reaches the systemic circulation without being altered.

Biot (ataxic) respiration: Breathing characterized by three patterns: (1) slow and deep, (2) rapid and shallow, and (3) apnea. Causes include meningitis, increased intracranial pressure, and central nervous system dysfunction.

biotransformation: The process by which the body alters a medication.

biphasic: A descriptor for a wave with negative and positive components; typically used in conjunction with P and T waves.

bipolar lead: A conduction lead comprising two electrodes attached at specific body sites with different polarity, which is used to examine electrical activity by monitoring changes in the electrical potential between those sites.

bipolar system: A closed system consisting of bipolar leads and a module to generate impulses and measure response.

blood–brain barrier: A network of endothelial cells and astrocytes (neuroglia) in the brain that regulates the transport of nutrients, ions, water, drugs, and waste products to and from the brain through the process of selective permeability.

blood urea nitrogen (BUN): A test used to measure urea, which is a biomarker for adequate kidney function.

blood urea nitrogen:creatinine (BUN:CR): A calculated index used to determine the cause of increased levels of blood urea nitrogen and creatinine.

body packers: People who swallow carefully prepared packages of illicit substances for smuggling purposes.

body stuffers: People who hastily swallow poorly packaged illicit substances (often to avoid impending arrest).

Boerhaave syndrome: Esophageal rupture, associated with subcutaneous emphysema, chest pain, and vomiting.

Boyle's law: A gas law stating that the volume of a gas is inversely proportional to the pressure to which it is subjected. Gases trapped in body cavities will expand with increases in altitude and will contract with decreases in altitude.

bradypnea: A respiratory rate that is slower than normal.

brain herniation: Displacement of a portion of the brain from its correct location within the cranial cavity to a different location.

brain tissue compliance: The change in brain volume resulting from a change in pressure.

brain tissue oxygen tension ($P_{br}O_2$): A method of monitoring temperature and oxygenation via placement of a commercial probe into the brain tissue through a bolt; it can be done simultaneously with ICP monitoring placement.

breach of duty to act: A case in which a health care provider does not conform to the standard of care by providing inappropriate care, failing to act, or acting beyond the scope of practice.

breech: A delivery presentation in which the presenting part is not the head.

bridge to recovery (BTR): A treatment objective in which a left ventricular assist device is implanted in a patient as mechanical circulatory support until the native heart recovers its pumping ability.

bridge to transplantation (BTT): A treatment objective in which a left ventricular assist device is implanted in a patient as mechanical circulatory support to prolong life until a heart transplant can be secured.

Broca area: Part of the frontal lobe that is located at the inferior frontal gyrus and that participates in the formulation of words.

bronchiolitis: A condition seen in children younger than 2 years, characterized by dyspnea and wheezing.

bronchopulmonary dysplasia: A chronic lung disorder that usually occurs in premature infants who weigh less than 3 pounds (1,500 g) at birth.

bronchovesicular sounds: A combination of the tracheal and vesicular breath sounds, heard in places where airways and alveoli are found,

including the upper part of the sternum and between the scapulae.

Brown-Séquard syndrome: Loss of function as a result of penetrating trauma accompanied by hemisection of the spinal cord and complete damage to all spinal tracts on the involved side; it is characterized by loss of motor function and sensation of light touch, proprioception, and vibration on the ipsilateral side and loss of temperature and pain sense on the contralateral side.

Brudzinski sign: Passive flexion of the legs and thighs when the examiner flexes the patient's neck to the chest. If this causes pain or causes the knees and hips to flex involuntarily, the sign is positive.

B-type natriuretic peptide (BNP): A polypeptide whose value is indicative of abnormal ventricular function and congestive heart failure.

buffer: Any substance that can alternately bind or release hydrogen ions depending on the outside conditions.

bundle branch block (BBB): A disturbance in electric conduction through the right or left bundle branch from the bundle of His.

business associate: As defined under HIPAA, a person or entity, other than a covered entity, who performs activities on behalf of, or provides services to, a covered entity that involves access to protected health information.

cable: The physical wire that connects the electrode to the electrocardiography monitor.

caloric test: A method for assessing vestibular function that involves the raising and lowering of the temperature in the external auditory canal; also called Bárány test.

capillary refill time (CRT): The time it takes for baseline skin color to return to the nail bed after being pressed by the provider; serves as a window into the state of peripheral perfusion.

capnography: A method for measuring exhaled CO_2, which in most cases correlates with the CO_2 levels in arterial blood. Two different types of devices can be used—an electronic monitor that displays a waveform and a colorimetric device that should turn yellow during exhalation, indicating proper tube placement.

capnometry: A method for measuring exhaled CO_2; it is performed the same way as capnography, but provides a light-emitting diode readout of the patient's exhaled CO_2.

caput succedaneum: In the newborn, a subcutaneous collection of fluid with poorly defined margins within the scalp, resulting from pressure on the head during delivery; soft-tissue swelling in a neonate's head owing to fluid collection.

carboxyhemoglobin (COHb): A measure of the amount of hemoglobin–carbon monoxide complexes in the blood.

cardiac imaging: A broad array of modalities used to assess the cardiac system for structural disease, acute coronary syndrome, inflammatory conditions, and other conditions.

cardiac index (CI): A hemodynamic value that adjusts a patient's cardiac output to take into account the total body surface area.

cardiac monitoring: The continuous observation of the patient's condition in relation to the cardiac rhythm.

cardiac output (CO): The amount of blood pumped out of the heart in 1 minute; the product of the stroke volume (average = 70 mL) and the heart rate (average = 60–100 beats/min).

cardiogenic shock: A condition caused by loss of 40% or more of the functioning myocardium; the heart is no longer able to circulate sufficient blood to maintain adequate oxygen delivery. It may be caused by congenital cardiac defects, drug toxicity, metabolic causes, hypovolemia, myocarditis, and arrhythmias.

cardiomyopathy: A general term for diseases in which the myocardium becomes thin, flabby, dilated, or enlarged, ultimately progressing to heart failure, acute myocardial infarction, or death.

carrier: A person or animal that is infected with a disease, but does not express symptoms of that disease.

cathode: The electrode in a pacing circuit that is negatively charged when current is flowing.

cation: A positively charged ion.

cauda equina: The collection of individual nerve roots into which the spinal cord separates at the L2 vertebra.

caudal: Pertaining to or in the direction of the feet.

CBC with differential: An expanded panel of lab tests that includes counts of specific types of white blood cells in the blood, such as neutrophils, lymphocytes, monocytes, eosinophils, and basophils.

central cord syndrome: A syndrome in which cavities form in the central portions of the spinal cord, usually in the cervical area; it may be due to a tumor, a genetic mutation, or trauma. The syndrome presents along with hemorrhage or edema to the central cervical segments.

central cyanosis: Blue coloration of the skin caused by the presence of deoxygenated hemoglobin in blood vessels near the skin surface.

central diabetes insipidus: A condition caused by a decrease in ADH secretion from the posterior pituitary gland; characterized by polyuria and polydipsia, which lead to dehydration.

central line–associated bloodstream infection (CLABSI): A primary bloodstream infection that develops in a patient who had a central line in place within the 48-hour period prior to the onset of the bloodstream infection.

central lumen: The lumen or port of the intra-aortic balloon catheter used to guide initial catheter insertion and to monitor arterial pressure during operation.

central neurogenic hyperventilation: A pattern of very deep, rapid respirations at rates of 40 to 60 breaths/min, caused by a midbrain lesion or dysfunction.

central venous lines: Intravenous access catheters that terminate in the central circulation, usually just proximal to the right atrium.

central venous pressure (CVP): The pressure in the superior vena cava (average = 2–6 cm H_2O), which reflects the pressure in the venous system when the blood is returned to the right atrium. It is indicative of a patient's fluid volume status and right-side heart performance.

cephalad: Pertaining to or in the direction of the head or front.

cephalohematoma: A collection of blood between the bone and subperiosteal space; may be accompanied by a linear skull fracture.

cerebral angiography: A procedure that uses imaging and a contrast material or dye to view and find abnormalities in the blood vessels in the brain.

cerebral aqueduct: The narrowest portion of the brain's ventricular system; it provides communication with the fourth ventricle, which lies between the brainstem and the cerebellum.

cerebral blood flow (CBF): The amount of blood flow the brain requires to maintain homeostasis. In a 24-hour period, the brain requires 1,000 L of blood to obtain 71 L of oxygen and 100 g of glucose.

cerebral contusion: A focal brain injury in which brain tissue is bruised and damaged in a defined area.

cerebral cortex: The outermost layer of the cerebrum.

cerebral function analysis monitor (CFAM): A device that can provide summed, averaged, and analyzed outputs of the general state of brain activity.

cerebral function monitor (CFM): A device that can provide summed and averaged outputs, but not analysis, of the general state of brain activity.

cerebral hemispheres: The name for each half of the brain (right or left); each of these areas contains one of the paired lobes (occipital, parietal, temporal, and frontal).

cerebral metabolic rate for oxygen (CMRo$_2$): A measurement used to determine neuronal demand for oxygen. Neurons with high activity rates require greater amounts of oxygen.

cerebral perfusion pressure (CPP): The pressure gradient across the brain; it provides an estimate of perfusion adequacy: CPP = MAP – ICP.

Charcot triad: Fever, jaundice, and right upper quadrant abdominal pain suggestive of choledocholithiasis.

Charles's law: A gas law stating that when pressure is constant, the volume of a gas is very nearly proportional to its absolute temperature. Thus, the volume is directly proportional to the temperature when it is expressed on an absolute scale where all other factors remain constant.

Cheyne-Stokes respiration: A cyclic pattern of increased respiratory rate and depth with periods of apnea. Causes include increased intracranial pressure, renal failure, meningitis, drug overdose, or hypoxia secondary to congestive heart failure.

children with special health care needs (CSHCN): As defined by the US Department of Health and Human Services, those children "who have or are at increased risk for a chronic physical, developmental, behavioral, or emotional condition and who also require health and related services of a type or amount beyond that required by children generally."

chloasma: A dermatologic condition affecting pregnant women in which darkened skin patches appear on the cheeks and forehead.

choanal atresia: A congenital narrowing or blockage of the nasal airway by membranous or bony tissue.

cholangitis: A serious ascending infection due to biliary tract obstruction that can result in fever, transaminitis, and altered mental status.

cholecystitis: Inflammation of the gallbladder.

choledocholithiasis: Gallstones in the biliary tract system, which put the patient at high risk for developing a biliary tract obstruction; typically initially managed with endoscopic retrograde cholangiopancreatography rather than cholecystectomy.

cholelithiasis: Gallstones in the gallbladder.

cholinergic syndrome: Cholinesterase inhibitor toxicity.

chordae tendineae: Tendons that connect the papillary muscles to the tricuspid and mitral valves.

choroid plexus: A cluster of nerve roots at the lateral and the third and fourth ventricles of the brain that produce cerebrospinal fluid.

chronic kidney disease (CKD): A gradual decrease in renal function resulting from irreversible damage to the nephrons. It is characterized by a glomerular filtration rate of less than 60 mL/min, and eventually progresses to end-stage renal disease.

chronotropic: A medication that affects the rate of contraction of the heart; altering the heart rate.

circle of Willis: A system of arteries located at the base of the skull that (in most people) is able to compensate for reduced blood flow from any one of the major contributors to cerebral circulation.

cirrhosis: Irreversible structural changes to the liver that impair its proper functioning.

civil damages: Monetary compensation awarded to a plaintiff in noncriminal court proceedings.

claudication: A severe pain in a muscle caused by narrowing of the arteries in that muscle and leading to ischemic pain with slight exertion such as that associated with walking.

clubbing: Broadening of a child's fingers and toes in response to chronically low oxygen levels for longer than 3 months.

cluster breathing: An abnormal respiratory pattern in which a cluster of irregular respirations that vary in depth are followed by a period of apnea at irregular intervals.

coarctation of the aorta: The narrowing or constriction of part of the aorta or aortic arch of the heart.

cocaine washout syndrome: Profound exhaustion with the ability to regain normal mental status and orientation when aroused; commonly seen with heavy cocaine users.

colitis: Inflammation of the colon.

colonoscopy: An endoscopy of the lower GI tract.

comminuted fracture: A type of skull fracture in which the skull is splintered or shattered into many pieces.

Commission on Accreditation of Medical Transport Services (CAMTS): An organization dedicated to improving the quality of patient care and safety of the transport environment for both rotor-wing and fixed-wing providers. CAMTS also provides voluntary accreditation of critical care transport agencies.

common law: Case law established by prior disputes that is published to guide future proceedings.

community hospitals: Community medical centers that offer emergency medicine and inpatient facilities but with limited inpatient specialists other than hospitalists and general surgery physicians.

compartment syndrome: A condition that develops when edema and swelling result in increased pressure within soft tissues, causing circulation to be compromised, possibly resulting in tissue necrosis.

compensatory stage: A stage of hypoxia in which the physiologic adjustments that occur in the respiratory and circulatory systems are adequate to prevent the effects of hypoxia. Factors such as environmental stress and prolonged exercise can potentiate certain effects of hypoxia.

competence: A legal determination, through a statute or court proceeding, that a person is capable of making personal decisions, including about their health care.

complete breech: A delivery presentation in which the buttocks present first and the legs are crossed inside the uterus.

complete spinal cord injury: A complete disruption of all tracts of the spinal cord, with permanent loss of all cord-mediated functions below the level of transaction.

compliance: A change in volume per unit of pressure; $\Delta V / \Delta P$.

computed tomography (CT): An imaging modality in which x-rays are used in a 360° rotation around an object to generate a computed three-dimensional model that can be viewed as multiple slices through a given plane; also called computerized axial tomography (CAT) scan; provides a mathematically reconstructed view of multiple cross-sections of the body, including the brain; it should be performed on almost every patient with abnormal neurologic findings.

computed tomography angiography (CTA): A form of imaging that includes the injection of an IV contrast agent into the patient moments before CT scanning and results in improved imaging of arterial structures.

concentration: The amount of a substance present in a given volume of fluid.

concentration gradient: The natural tendency for substances to flow from an area of higher concentration to an area of lower concentration, within or outside the cell.

concussion: A transient interruption of normal neurologic function.

conduction: Transfer of heat to a solid object or a liquid by direct contact.

congenital adrenal hyperplasia: A group of diseases in which the adrenal glands do not function properly and as a result do not produce a sufficient amount of the hormone cortisol.

conjugate movement: Movement of both eyes together in the same direction.

consent: Voluntary agreement by a patient with sufficient mental capacity to capably accept or refuse assessment, treatment, or transport offered by the care provider.

contact phenomena injuries: Injuries that occur as the direct result of trauma to the head, including local effects such as scalp laceration, skull fracture, hematoma, and intracerebral hemorrhage.

contamination: A state in which a certain substance, such as blood, infectious material, or a toxic substance, is present on an item or surface. In the case of radiation, it is important to distinguish between contamination and irradiation.

continuous positive airway pressure (CPAP): A means of raising the breathing baseline above the ambient pressure. The increased pressure across the entire breathing cycle increases the mean airway pressure, stents the airway, and increases the functional residual capacity, thereby improving oxygenation.

contrecoup injury: A situation in which an impact occurs on one side of the head, causing the brain to move within the cranial vault and forcibly contact the opposite side of the skull, resulting in damage on that side of the brain; also called transitional injury.

controlled substances: Drugs whose manufacture, possession, and use are controlled by the government.

convection: The mechanism by which heat (body heat, in the context of this chapter) is picked up and carried away by moving air currents.

Coombs test: A test used to identify antibodies that may bind to red blood cells and cause hemolysis.

corpus callosum: A large tract of transverse fibers that provides a communication link between the two cerebral hemispheres.

covered entity: As defined under HIPAA, a health care provider, a health plan, or a health clearinghouse that must transmit health information in electronic form in connection with a transaction covered by HIPAA (payment or administrative) to qualify. Ambulance providers of all kinds are explicitly included in the definition of a covered entity.

crackles: A breath sound produced as fluid-filled alveoli pop open under increasing inspiratory pressure; can be fine or coarse.

cranial nerves (CN): The 12 nerves arising directly from the brain that govern many of the senses and the functions of muscles in the eyes, face, and pharynx.

C-reactive protein (CRP): An acute-phase reactant used to identify inflammatory response.

creatine: A major storehouse of intramuscular high-energy phosphate.

creatine kinase (CK): An enzyme that cleaves the high-energy phosphate from creatine in muscle tissues and transfers it to adenosine diphosphate to yield adenosine triphosphate; its measurement is used in the assessment for muscle damage.

creatinine (Cr): A chemical waste product of creatine that results from muscle metabolism and is eliminated through the urine; increased levels indicate decreased GFR and renal function.

crew resource management (CRM): A system that originated as the result of a National Aeronautics and Space Administration workshop in 1979 as a means to improve air safety. It incorporates equipment, procedures, and crew concerns to make the best decision during flight operations, focusing on interpersonal communication, leadership, and decision making.

critical-access hospitals: As defined by the Centers for Medicare and Medicaid Services, hospitals that have 25 or fewer beds, are located more than 35 miles from another hospital, have an average length of stay of less than 96 hours, and provide 24/7 emergency medicine services. Most acutely ill or injured patients treated at these hospitals require transport to higher levels of care once stabilized.

critical care: Constant, complex, detailed health care as provided in various acute life-threatening conditions; the ability to deal with such situations rapidly and with precision using various advanced machines and devices for treating and monitoring the patient's condition.

critical care patient: Any patient who experiences an actual or potential life-threatening illness or injury that requires continual monitoring and care by a specially trained physician, registered nurse, or paramedic.

critical care transport (CCT): The transport of a patient from an emergency department, critical care unit, or incident scene during which the patient receives the same level of care as was provided in the hospital or originating facility.

critical care transport professional (CCTP): A health care professional who has successfully completed a recognized critical care program and meets the minimum qualifications set forth by the employing transport program.

critical incident stress debriefing (CISD): An approach favored since the 1980s to manage the psychological aftereffects in emergency personnel after particularly distressing responses; it requires a specially trained team and has the potential to create iatrogenic harm.

critical stage: The stage of acute hypoxia in which there is almost complete mental and physical incapacitation, resulting in rapid loss of consciousness, seizures, respiratory arrest, and death.

Crohn disease: An inflammation of the GI tract in which all layers of the mucosa may be affected. It results in scattered ulcerations and fibroses throughout the large and small intestines.

cross-tolerance: A form of drug tolerance in which patients who take a particular medication for an extended period can build up a tolerance to other medications in the same class.

croup: A childhood viral disease characterized by edema of the upper airways with barking cough, difficult breathing, and stridor; also called laryngotracheobronchitis.

crush syndrome: The combination of shock and renal failure after a crush injury; it may lead to the death of an entrapped person after the patient is freed from the entrapment.

cryoprecipitate: A blood product created from plasma and in which clotting factors, especially factor VIII, are concentrated; it is used to treat patients with coagulation disorders.

CT angiography: Radiographic observation of dye injected into the bloodstream.

CT polytrauma: An imaging protocol that typically includes computed tomography (CT) of the head, cervical spine, chest, and abdomen/pelvis to generate a continuous image from the top of the head through the pelvis; also called a pan-scan.

cumulative effect: An effect that occurs when several successive doses of a medication are administered or when absorption of a medication occurs faster than its excretion or metabolism.

current: The movement of electrons through an electrical circuit over time, measured in amperes.

Cushing syndrome: A condition caused by overproduction of cortisol by the adrenal glands or by excessive use of cortisol or other similar steroid (glucocorticoid) hormones; also known as hypercortisolism.

Cushing triad: A cascade of events provoked when intracranial pressure rises to the level of the arterial pressure, vasoconstriction occurs in an effort to shift fluid volumes in the cranium, and the ensuing brain displacement puts pressure on the medulla oblongata by pushing it into the foramen magnum, resulting in disturbances in breathing, heart rate, and blood pressure.

cyanosis: Blue discoloration of the gums and face.

cyanotic congenital heart disease (CCHD): Heart disease caused by developmental anomalies of the heart or major vessels (truncus arteriosus, transposition of the great vessels, tetralogy of Fallot, tricuspid atresia, or total anomalous pulmonary venous return) leading to abnormal blood flow. Deoxygenated blood from the right side of the heart is shunted to the left side, causing cyanosis.

cyanotic defects: Congenital heart defects that lead to low oxygen saturation, owing to either decreased pulmonary blood flow or mixed blood flow.

cytokines: Chemical messengers that enhance cell growth, promote cell activation, direct cellular traffic, stimulate macrophage function, and destroy antigens. Interleukins are a type of cytokine.

Dalton's law: A gas law stating that the total pressure of a gas mixture is the sum of the individual or partial pressures of the gases in the mixture; also referred to as the law of partial pressure.

damages: In a legal context, harm that results from a breach of duty by a health care provider who is found negligent. Usually, the injury is physical.

dampened waveform: A hemodynamic pressure waveform that appears to have lost crisp deflections.

D-dimer test: A test of hypercoagulability that detects a fragment from the fibrinolysis process; the test can be used to help diagnose and monitor diseases and conditions related to inappropriate clotting, such as deep venous thrombosis.

debriefing: A powerful inquiry tool in which a concise exchange occurs to identify what happened, what was learned, and what can be done better in the future.

decision-making capacity (DMC): The determination that a patient's brain is functioning well enough to process information and make health care decisions.

decompression sickness: A condition resulting from exposure to low barometric pressure, causing inert gases normally dissolved in body fluids and tissue to come out of physical solution and form bubbles.

decontamination: Use of chemical, physical, or other means to remove, inactivate, or eradicate harmful microorganisms from people, surfaces, or objects.

deep partial-thickness burn: A burn in which the skin is blistered but not charred and is painful to the touch; it is usually the result of steam, oil, or flames and involves the deeper layers of the dermis.

delayed hemolytic transfusion reactions: Transfusion reactions that do not occur until 3 to 30 days after transfusion.

delayed traumatic intracranial hemorrhage (DTICH): Hemorrhage that occurs within the first 3 to 10 days following an injury to the occipital-parietal region via a coup–contrecoup mechanism.

delirium: Acute confusion, hallucinations, and disorientation that is rapid in onset and may fluctuate in intensity.

delta wave: The slurring of the upstroke of the first part of the QRS complex that occurs in Wolff-Parkinson-White syndrome.

depolarization: The process of discharging resting cardiac muscle fibers by an electrical impulse that causes them to contract.

depolarizing paralytic: A medication that causes neuromuscular blockade by binding and briefly activating receptor sites at the neuromuscular junction, preventing further activation of these sites and causing chemical paralysis.

depressed skull fracture: A type of skull fracture in which a portion of the skull is depressed; the scalp and dura may or may not be torn.

dermis: The layer of skin that lies beneath the epidermis; it is a dynamic layer of thick connective tissue.

destination therapy (DT): A treatment objective in which a left ventricular assist device is implanted in a patient with heart failure as ongoing mechanical circulatory support because the patient does not meet the heart transplantation criteria.

dextrocardia: A congenital cause of right axis deviation, in which the heart develops in a right-facing position, creating a mirror image of the normal left-facing heart.

diabetes mellitus: A metabolic disorder in which the pancreas's ability to metabolize simple carbohydrates (glucose) is impaired because of either inadequate production of insulin or insensitivity to circulating insulin.

diabetic ketoacidosis (DKA): A form of acidosis observed in uncontrolled diabetes in which ketones accumulate when insulin is not available; usually associated with hyperglycemia.

diagnostic peritoneal lavage (DPL): A surgical procedure to assess for bleeding or intestinal perforation in the abdomen. Classically, a liter of crystalloid is infused into the abdomen and then drawn out to examine for the presence of blood or intestinal contents.

diaphragma sellae: An extension of the dura mater that forms a roof over the sella turcica, which contains the pituitary gland.

diaphragmatic hernia: Passage of loops of bowel, with or without other abdominal organs, through the diaphragm muscle; it occurs as the bowel from the abdomen herniates upward through the diaphragm into the chest (thoracic) cavity.

diastatic stellate fracture: A fracture involving injury to a bone with separation of an epiphysis; it is prevalent in abused children.

diastole: The relaxation phase of the heart cycle, in which the ventricles are dilated and filling with blood.

diastolic augmentation: The increase in aortic pressure during diastole that the intra-aortic balloon inflation produces, thereby improving coronary and peripheral perfusion; it may be thought of as a "second systole."

diastolic blood pressure (DBP): The trough or resting pressure in the arterial system that occurs during ventricular diastole.

dicrotic notch: The brief increase in aortic pressure reflected in a notching of the wave; it is caused by the sudden closure and springing back of the aortic valve leaflets, and signals the start of diastole.

diencephalon: Portion of the cerebrum consisting of the thalamus, the hypothalamus, the subthalamus, and the epithalamus.

differential diagnosis: The process of selecting the most likely underlying cause of the patient's condition by comparing multiple potential causes of the presenting signs and symptoms.

difficult airway: An airway in which the provider anticipates complications in securing an airway.

diffuse axonal injury (DAI): A deep-brain injury in which shearing forces damage the integrity of the axon at the node of Ranvier, which consequently alters the axoplasmic flow.

digoxin: A cardiac glycoside that produces positive inotropic and negative chronotropic activity in the heart and is primarily indicated in the treatment of chronic heart failure and to control the ventricular rate in atrial tachyarrhythmias.

dilation and curettage (D&C): A surgical procedure in which the cervix is opened and the uterus scraped of tissue.

dilutional hyponatremia: A condition caused by excessive intake of fluids in which serum sodium concentration is less than 135 mmol/L; sometimes referred to as water intoxication.

diplopia: Double vision.

direct bilirubin: Conjugated bilirubin; the result of bilirubin's conjugation in the liver, which is ultimately excreted in the bile.

discordant: A descriptor for T waves that are in the opposite direction from the terminal portion of the QRS complex in bundle branch blocks.

discovery rule: A legal rule stating that the statute of limitations for filing a legal case does not begin until the injured party can reasonably be expected to know of the injury.

dispatch: The person or organization that receives the request for critical care transport and contacts the critical care transport team with the details of that request to ascertain the team's availability.

disseminated intravascular coagulation (DIC): A complex condition arising from different causes that activate coagulation mechanisms, resulting in obstructed blood flow as a result of microclots as well as fibrinolysis, while the body attempts to reopen the microcirculation. Bleeding, thrombosis, and, potentially, organ dysfunction result.

distal intestinal obstruction: Partial or complete obstruction of the distal small bowel (ileum) or large intestine.

distribution: The process by which molecules move from the body's systemic circulation to specific organs and tissues.

distributive shock: A form of shock in which the smallest blood vessels fail to deliver adequate blood to the tissues; it includes neurogenic shock, anaphylactic shock, and septic shock.

disturbance stage: A stage of hypoxia in which physiologic responses are inadequate to compensate for the oxygen deficiency, and hypoxia is evident.

diverticula: Small pouches of tissue that develop as outcroppings of the large intestine, typically in the descending colon and sigmoid colon.

diverticular bleeding: Bleeding from diverticula that have developed in the colon.

diverticulitis: Inflammation of diverticula.

diverticulosis: Presence of intestinal diverticula, which may then become inflamed or bleed.

doll's eye test: An oculocephalic reflex test that is performed on the unconscious patient by rapidly rotating the head from side to side and observing the eye movement.

do not resuscitate (DNR) order: A type of advance directive that describes which life-sustaining procedures should be performed if the patient suffers cardiopulmonary arrest.

dopamine: A neurotransmitter that plays important roles in executive function, impulsivity, sensory perception, and key physiologic parameters (eg, heart rate, blood pressure, temperature regulation).

dorsal: Toward the back surface of an object; posterior.

drag: The resistance of an aircraft to forward motion, directly opposed to thrust.

dromotropic: Influencing the conduction rate within the heart; affecting the velocity of conduction.

drug interaction: The alteration of the action or metabolism of a particular medication when combined with another medication.

dual-chamber pacemaker: An artificial pacemaker with two leads (one in the atrium and one in the ventricle) so electromechanical synchrony can be achieved.

DUMBELS: Mnemonic for symptoms of anticholinesterase inhibitor toxicity: Diaphoresis/diarrhea, Urination, Miosis, Bradycardia/bronchospasm/bronchorrhea, Emesis, Lacrimation, and Salivation.

dural venous sinuses: Endothelial-lined spaces between the periosteal and meningeal layers of the dura mater.

dura mater: The outer membrane of the meninges.

duration of action: The amount of time a medication concentration can be expected to remain above the minimum level needed to provide the intended action.

duty to act: A legal obligation of health care providers to render medical care to a certain level. When the duty to act applies varies from state to state.

dysarthria: Difficulty articulating words caused by neurologic impairment affecting the vocal apparatus.

dysbarism: A condition resulting from the effects (excluding hypoxia) of a pressure differential between the ambient barometric pressure and the pressure of gases within the body.

dysconjugate movement: Lack of symmetric movement between the two visual axes.

dyscrasia: In hematology, a disorder of the cellular elements of blood.

dysphonia: Difficulty producing intelligible speech caused by physical impairment at the level of the larynx.

early pregnancy loss: Expulsion of the fetus that occurs naturally; also called miscarriage or spontaneous abortion.

eclampsia: The condition that exists once a patient with preeclampsia develops seizures; it causes serious maternal complications. Warning signs of the transition from preeclampsia to eclampsia include severe headache, scotomata, hyperreflexia, epigastric pain, and anxiety.

ectopic pregnancy: A pregnancy in which the ovum implants somewhere other than the uterine endometrium.

Edinger-Westphal nucleus: Part of the midbrain that is responsible for mediating the autonomic reflex centers for pupillary accommodation to light.

effective performance time: The amount of time an individual is able to perform useful duties in an environment of inadequate oxygen; also known as expected performance time.

efferent pathways: Descending pathways that carry motor impulses away from the central nervous system.

ejection fraction: The average percentage of blood ejected from the left ventricle with each heartbeat.

elastance: The tendency to collapse (as in lung tissue).

electrical alternans: An electrocardiogram pattern in which the QRS vector changes with each heartbeat. This pattern is pathognomonic of cardiac tamponade.

electrode: In the context of a 12-lead electrocardiogram, an electrical sensor placed on the chest to record the bioelectrical activity of the heart. In the context of a pacemaker, a conductor in contact with cardiac tissue at the end of a pacing lead; it delivers impulses to that tissue.

electroencephalography (EEG): A procedure that records the electrical activity of the brain by measuring brain waves.

electrophysiology: The cardiac specialty that involves evaluation and management of rhythm disturbances.

embolic stroke: A condition in which a blood clot, known as an embolus, forms in one part of the body and travels through the bloodstream to the brain or neck.

emergency medical condition: A condition manifesting itself by acute symptoms of sufficient severity (including severe pain) such that the absence of immediate medical attention could reasonably be expected to result in placing the individual's health (or the health of an unborn child) in serious jeopardy, serious impairment to bodily functions, or serious dysfunction of bodily organs.

Emergency Medical Treatment and Active Labor Act (EMTALA): A federal law passed by the US Congress in 1986, with the primary goal of preventing hospitals from failing to treat patients, or transferring patients to other facilities, based on their insurance status or ability to pay for services.

empyema: An accumulation of pus in the pleural space.

endemic: A pattern of disease occurrence in which some cases of a disease are always present within a given population, and their numbers are expected and predictable.

endocardial (transvenous) leads: Pacemaker leads guided by angiography and attached to the endocardium.

endocrine hypertension: Significant high blood pressure caused by a hormonal disorder; often related to excess hormone produced by a tumor.

endometrium: The inner mucous membrane of the uterus.

endoscopic retrograde cholangiopancreatography (ERCP): A technique combining endoscopy and fluoroscopy to diagnose and treat biliary or pancreatic ductal obstruction.

endotoxins: Lipopolysaccharides that coat the outer surface of gram-negative bacteria and elicit strong immune responses in humans while providing a layer of protection for the bacterium; they can also be secreted from the cell and are released en masse when cell death occurs.

end-stage renal disease (ESRD): A loss of proper kidney functioning, with renal replacement therapy becoming a requirement for survival.

enhanced elimination: A process that replaces or augments the body's normal method of eliminating, modifying, or breaking down toxic substances.

enteroclysis: Infusion of barium contrast into the GI tract to observe for obstruction.

enzymes: Proteins that act as catalysts for biochemical reactions within the body.

epicardial leads: Pacemaker leads attached to the epicardium (outer surface of the myocardium); placement and troubleshooting of these leads are done in the hospital and require surgery and anesthesia.

epidemic: A pattern of disease occurrence in which the number of cases of a disease clearly rises (above a threshold level) in a given time or geographic area.

epidemiology: The study of disease distribution within populations and the factors that determine that distribution.

epidermis: The outer layer of the skin, which generally consists of four layers (thin skin), except on the palms, fingertips, and soles of the feet, which have five layers (thick skin).

epidural hematoma (EDH): An accumulation of blood between the inner periosteum and the dura mater; also called extradural hematoma.

epiglottitis: Inflammation of the epiglottis.

epithalamus: An area of the cerebrum that is located in the dorsal portion of the diencephalon and contains the pineal gland.

epitope: The specific portion of the antigen that is recognized by the antibody or B cell.

error: A preventable adverse event in the delivery of care, whether or not it is evident or harmful to the patient.

erythrocyte sedimentation rate (ESR): The rate at which red blood cells settle at the bottom of a tube containing a blood sample. This test is used to identify inflammatory response and is generally less specific than testing C-reactive protein.

eschar: The leathery covering of a burn injury, formed after the burned tissues dry out.

escharotomy: A surgical incision in an eschar to lessen constriction; sometimes necessary (although rarely performed in a prehospital setting) to prevent edema from building up, impairing capillary filling and causing ischemia.

esophageal atresia: A congenital defect, often associated with other anomalies such as tracheoesophageal fistula, in which the esophagus ends in a blind pouch.

esophageal varix: Swelling of esophageal veins that intrudes into the lumen of the esophagus.

esophagitis: Inflammation of the tissues of the esophagus; commonly associated with severe gastroesophageal reflux disease, alcohol abuse, or irritation caused by pills or infection.

esophagogastroduodenoscopy (EGD): A technique to directly observe the GI tract in which a camera is passed into the GI tract, allowing for diagnosis and treatment of disease or injury.

etiology: The cause of a disease.

eupnea: Normal breathing at a rate of 12 to 20 breaths/min in the adult patient.

evaporation: The conversion of a liquid to a gas.

excited delirium: A complex, life-threatening syndrome including both delirium and an excited or agitated state; also called agitated delirium.

exercise-associated hyponatremia (EAH): A condition occurring within 24 hours of sustained physical activity in which fluid consumption exceeds fluids lost, resulting in dilution of serum sodium levels. Signs and symptoms may include nausea, vomiting, and, in severe cases, mental status changes and seizures.

exertional heatstroke: A thermoregulatory emergency that occurs during activities that require physical exertion in warm environments. This condition is defined by an excessive core body temperature, typically greater than 104°F (40°C), and associated CNS impairment.

exhalation: A passive process in which gas leaves the lungs.

exotoxins: Proteins that are secreted by some bacteria and can directly cause significant damage to host cells while also triggering an immune response.

expiratory reserve volume (ERV): The amount of air that can be expelled from the lungs after a normal exhalation.

exploratory laparotomy: Surgical exploration of the abdomen.

expressed consent: A patient's voluntary verbal, nonverbal, or written agreement to consent to treatment or transport.

external fetal monitoring: Electronic heart monitoring of the fetus while in utero, performed via electrodes placed on the pregnant woman's abdomen.

extinction: A test of sensation discrimination in which the CCTP simultaneously touches opposite, corresponding areas of the patient's body and asks the patient where the touch is felt; it is intended to identify sensory inattention.

extracorporeal membrane oxygenation (ECMO): A temporizing mechanism of extracorporeal gas exchange with or without hemodynamic support; also referred to as extracorporeal life support.

extradural space: A potential space between the cranial bones and the periosteal layer of the dura that becomes a real space only when blood from torn vessels pushes the periosteum from the cranium and accumulates; also called epidural space.

extravasation: An infusion-related complication in which the drug being administered intravenously leaks outside the vein and enters the surrounding tissues; if that substance is a vesicant, it can cause blisters and tissue damage.

face-to-face intubation: Intubation in which the provider's face is at the same level as the patient's face; used when the standard position is not possible. In this position, the laryngoscope is held in the provider's right hand and the endotracheal tube in the left.

failed airway: An unsuccessful intubation attempt in a patient for whom oxygenation cannot be adequately maintained with bag-mask ventilation; three unsuccessful intubation attempts by an experienced operator but with adequate oxygenation; and failed intubation using one best attempt in the "forced to act" situation.

failure mode and effect analysis (FMEA): A process that helps identify priorities in risk mitigation and process redesign.

falx cerebelli: A fold of dura mater that forms the division between the two lateral lobes of the cerebellum.

falx cerebri: A double fold of dura mater that divides the cerebrum into right and left hemispheres by descending vertically into the longitudinal fissure that extends from the frontal lobe to the occipital lobe.

fasciotomy: A surgical incision into an area of fascia— for example, to relieve pressure between two compartments; not usually performed in a prehospital setting.

fat-free mass (FFM): The proportion of body mass that consists of tissues other than adipose tissue, and that therefore consumes calories; typically the largest determinant of the basal metabolic rate in a healthy person.

fecal-oral route: A route of transmitting infectious organisms from one individual to another; commonly, enteric bacteria or viruses are shed in the feces, spread via contamination of food or water sources, and ingested by other people.

Federal Aviation Administration (FAA): A US governmental agency within the Department of Transportation that regulates and oversees civil aviation within the United States; it established and enforces the Title 14 CFR that govern aircraft operation within the United States.

Fick principle: A method of indirectly determining cardiac output, in which the amount of oxygen uptake of blood as it passes through the lungs is equal to the oxygen concentration difference between mixed venous and arterial blood. The formula uses assumed values for oxygen consumption derived from basal metabolic studies on healthy subjects, which may or may not be valid in critically ill patients.

Fick's law: A gas law stating that the net diffusion rate of a gas across a fluid membrane is proportional to the difference in partial pressure, proportional to the area of the membrane, and inversely proportional to the thickness of the membrane.

first-order elimination: The rate of elimination is proportional to the drug's plasma concentration.

first-pass effect: A process by which the dose of an oral medication is reduced as it passes through the liver (and, for some medications, the gut as well as the liver) before it enters systemic circulation; also called first-pass metabolism.

fissures: Deep grooves between adjacent gyri of the brain.

fixed-wing aircraft: A transportation mode typically used to transport critically ill and injured patients distances of 150 miles (240 km) or greater; also called airplanes.

FLACC scale: A pain assessment scale that scores points for five categories, including face, legs, activity, cry, and consolability.

flail chest: A fracture in two or more places to two or more adjacent ribs.

flat fracture: The least common type of depressed skull fracture, in which the depressed segment does not have any connection with the cranial vault.

flexion-extension injury: A spinal cord injury that results from forward movement of the head, typically as the result of rapid deceleration, or from a direct blow to the occiput.

flicker vertigo: An imbalance in brain cell activity caused by exposure to low-frequency flickering or flashing light. Light flickering from 4 to 20 times per second can precipitate reactions including nausea, migraines, unconsciousness, and seizures.

flight following: A service in which an authorized air-traffic control facility maintains constant contact with aircraft to notify the crew about traffic in the area.

flight surgeon: A physician who specializes in flight medicine and has been trained extensively in various aspects of aviation and the effects of flight on the human body; also specializes in working with pilots and flight crew members.

flow-cycled ventilator: A positive-pressure ventilator that ends inspiration when a predetermined flow rate is achieved.

flow rate: The speed of the gas at which the tidal volume is delivered.

focal ischemic stroke: A condition in which an area of marginally perfused tissue, the ischemic penumbra, surrounds a core of ischemic cells; the cells will eventually die without medical intervention.

focused assessment with sonography for trauma (FAST): An ultrasonographic examination directed at identifying the presence of free intraperitoneal or pericardial fluids, performed by transducing four distinct areas of the abdomen.

fomite: An inanimate object that is capable of transmitting infectious organisms from one individual to another.

footling breech: A delivery presentation in which both feet extend into the birth canal.

foramen magnum: The opening at the base of the skull through which the bundle of nerve fibers constituting the spinal cord exits.

foramen of Luschka: An opening at the lateral portion of the base of the fourth ventricle that leads to the subarachnoid space and is essential for the normal flow of cerebrospinal fluid; part of the brain's ventricular system.

foramen of Magendie: An opening at the medial portion of the base of the fourth ventricle that leads to the subarachnoid space and is essential for the normal flow of cerebrospinal fluid; part of the brain's ventricular system.

foramen of Monro: An opening in the skull that connects the two lateral ventricles with the third ventricle, a central cavity; part of the brain's ventricular system.

foramen ovale: The opening in the fetal heart that allows blood to flow from the right atrium to the left atrium of the fetus, bypassing the lungs prior to birth.

Foster Kennedy syndrome: A tumor or abscess at the base of the frontal lobe that affects the olfactory nerve.

fraction of inspired oxygen (FIO_2): Percentage of inhaled oxygen expressed as a decimal. For example, 40% oxygen = FIO_2 of 0.40.

fracture: A break in the continuity of a bone.

frank breech: A delivery presentation in which the buttocks present first, both of the infant's hips are flexed, and the feet are near the fetus's head.

Frank–Starling law: The principle that the force of the cardiac muscle contraction is proportional to the amount of stretch placed on the muscle fibers (meaning that the more the heart is stretched by the incoming blood, the more forcefully the ventricles contract and the more blood that is ejected); it demonstrates how changes in ventricular preload lead to changes in stroke volume; also called the Starling curve.

free water: Water that is not bound to molecules in the body.

fresh-frozen plasma (FFP): A blood product in which uncoagulated plasma has been separated from the red blood cells; it is primarily composed of water, proteins, salts, metabolites, and clotting factors.

frontal lobe: The largest of the four lobes of the brain; it lies underneath the frontal bone of the skull and is separated posteriorly from the parietal lobe by the central fissure and inferiorly from the temporal lobe by the lateral fissure. The frontal lobe is responsible for a variety of cognitive and motor functions.

frostbite: Localized damage to tissues resulting from prolonged exposure to extreme cold.

full-thickness burn: A burn that extends through the epidermis and dermis into the subcutaneous tissues beneath, in which skin is pale, painless, leathery, and charred; also called a third-degree burn.

fulminant hepatic failure: A sudden and significant insult to the liver characterized by encephalopathy and a high mortality rate; commonly caused by toxins/overdose or viral infection.

functional residual capacity (FRC): The amount of air remaining in the lungs after normal expiration; the sum of the residual volume and the expiratory reserve volume.

functioning adenoma: A type of pituitary lesion in which overproduction of hormones occurs.

fundus: The optic disk, macula, and blood vessels on the back wall of the internal eyeball.

gallstone pancreatitis: A type of pancreatitis in which pancreatic enzymes accumulate proximal to a bile duct obstruction from a gallstone and digest the tissues of both the duct and the pancreas.

gas lumen: The lumen or port of the intra-aortic balloon catheter that carries helium between the intra-aortic balloon and the pump console to inflate and deflate the balloon.

gastritis: Inflammation of the gastric mucosa that occurs when the equilibrium of active and protective mechanisms for the lining is altered; may be accompanied by upper GI bleeding.

gastroenteritis: Watery diarrhea and vomiting during inflammation of the digestive tract as a result of a viral, bacterial, or parasitic infection.

gastroschisis: A centrally located, full-thickness abdominal wall defect.

Gay-Lussac's law: A gas law stating that the pressure of a gas when volume is maintained at a constant level is directly proportional to the absolute temperature for a constant amount of gas. Simply stated, as pressure increases, temperature increases.

gestation: Period of time from conception to birth. For humans, the full period is normally 9 months (or 40 weeks).

gestational diabetes: A condition in which a woman without previous diabetes develops high blood glucose, especially during the third trimester.

gestational hypertension: The occurrence of hypertension in a pregnant woman, usually after 20 weeks' gestation, defined as a blood pressure of 140/90 mm Hg or greater in a woman with a previously normal blood pressure; also called pregnancy-induced hypertension.

gigantism: A syndrome that results from excessive secretion of growth hormone by the pituitary gland before the epiphyseal plate has closed; characterized by the growth of bones, muscles, and many internal organs at an abnormally fast rate.

Glasgow Coma Scale (GCS): An evaluation tool used to determine level of consciousness, which evaluates and assigns point values (scores) for eye opening, verbal response, and motor response, which are then totaled; effective in helping predict patient outcomes.

global ischemic stroke: A condition in which severe hypotension or cardiac arrest produces a transient drop in blood flow to all areas of the brain.

glomerular filtration rate (GFR): The amount of fluid filtered by the glomerulus per minute; a benchmark for renal function.

gluconeogenesis: Glucose formation.

glycogenolysis: The breakdown of glycogen to glucose.

glycosuria: The presence of glucose in the urine.

Graham's law: A gas law stating that the rate at which gases diffuse is related inversely to the square root of their densities.

gravitational forces: Force changes that occur with acceleration and deceleration.

gyri: Convolutions on the surface of the cerebrum that functionally increase the cortical surface area.

half-life (T½): The time period required to eliminate one-half of the plasma concentration. During the second half-life, an additional 25% of the original plasma concentration is eliminated. After three half-lives, one-eighth of the original plasma concentration remains.

halo test: A test for leaking CSF that is accomplished by collecting and assessing fluid that drains from the nose, mouth, or ears; a dark red circle of fluid surrounded by a lighter yellow one is a positive halo sign.

handoff: The brief report that staff at the sending facility—generally the bedside nurse, physician, or care provider currently responsible for the patient—submits to the CCTP team when they arrive to accept responsibility for the patient's care.

harm: Unintended physical injury resulting from or contributed to by medical care.

Hashimoto disease: A condition that occurs when the immune system attacks the patient's thyroid gland and that is the leading cause of hypothyroidism; also known as chronic lymphocytic thyroiditis.

health care–associated pneumonia (HCAP): Pneumonia that occurs in nonhospitalized patients who have contact with health care facilities or personnel.

Health Insurance Portability and Accountability Act (HIPAA): A federal law enacted in 1996, providing for criminal sanctions and civil penalties for releasing a patient's protected health information in a way not authorized by the patient.

heart failure (HF): A set of clinical signs and symptoms indicative of myocardial dysfunction and cardiac output that is inadequate to meet the metabolic demands of the body.

heat cramps: Acute and involuntary muscle pains, usually in the lower extremities, the abdomen, or both, that occur because of profuse sweating and subsequent sodium loss in sweat.

heat exhaustion: A clinical syndrome characterized by volume depletion and heat stress that is thought to be a milder form of heat illness on the continuum leading to heatstroke.

heatstroke: The least common and most deadly heat illness, caused by a severe disturbance in thermoregulation, usually characterized by a core body temperature of more than 104°F (40°C) and altered mental status.

heat syncope: An orthostatic or near-syncopal episode that typically occurs in nonacclimated people who may be under heat stress.

Helicobacter pylori: A bacterium that is commonly associated with gastritis and peptic ulcers.

helicopter emergency medical service (HEMS): Use of a rotor-wing aircraft to deliver air medical service, for which the goals are to rapidly transport CCTPs to a patient, stabilize the patient's condition, and rapidly transport that patient to a tertiary care center.

helicopter shopping: The practice of making sequential calls to numerous air medical providers in an attempt to find a service that will accept a mission request that has been declined by other services based on safety factors such as poor weather, limited landing zone availability, exceptional distances, or other factors.

HELLP syndrome: A hemolytic disorder that occurs during the latter stages of gestation, usually after the 20th week, and whose clinical findings include hemolytic anemia, elevated liver enzyme levels, and a low platelet count. Patients will present with blurred vision, abdominal pain, headache, and edema.

hematemesis: Emesis containing blood, which may be bright red or partially digested (coffee-ground emesis).

hematochezia: Stool streaked with bright red blood.

hematocrit: The percentage of formed elements (cells) in a venous blood sample.

hematuria: The presence of red blood cells in the urine.

hemiblock: Blocking of one of the fascicles of the left bundle branch, the left anterior or left posterior fascicle.

hemoconcentration: Decreased fluid in the blood, which means that concentrations of other blood components increase.

hemoglobin: The protein responsible for carrying oxygen to the body's cells and, to a lesser extent, carbon dioxide back to the lungs.

hemoglobinuria: The presence of hemoglobin in the urine.

hemolysis: Destruction of red blood cells, sometimes following massive blood transfusions or blood transfusion reactions; results in the release of hemoglobin and cell remnants into the bloodstream.

hemolytic transfusion reactions: Transfusion reactions caused by ABO or Rh incompatibility, intradonor incompatibility, improper crossmatching, or improper blood storage.

hemolytic uremic syndrome (HUS): A serious condition in which the patient develops acute kidney injury, and which also causes anemia and thrombocytopenia; thought to be caused by several bacterial and viral infectious organisms, most often verotoxin-producing strains of *Escherichia coli*.

hemoperfusion: A treatment in which a patient's blood is filtered outside the body through a substance that removes toxic substances from it; a method of removing toxic substances from the blood.

hemophilia: A disease caused by inheritance of a recessive gene trait that causes excessive bleeding. The resulting factor VIII or factor IX deficiency leaves the blood unable to clot properly.

hemorrhagic conversion: The condition in which, after the brain tissue surrounding the stroke has died, renewed blood flow to the region (eg, triggered by medication) is no longer held in place by the tissue, resulting in hemorrhage.

hemorrhagic stroke: A condition in which bleeding in the intraparenchymal space or subarachnoid space causes direct or secondary damage to cerebral tissue.

hemothorax: An accumulation of blood in the pleural space.

Henry's law: A gas law stating that the amount of gas dissolved in solution is directly proportional to the pressure of the gas over the solution.

hepatic encephalopathy: Encephalopathy secondary to hepatic disease, usually associated with hyperammonemia.

hepatitis: Inflammation of liver cells that can impede proper functioning of the liver and lead to chronic conditions such as cirrhosis.

hepatitis C virus: The virus that is the most common cause of cirrhosis and is especially pathogenic in causing hepatitis.

hepatorenal syndrome: A condition characterized by renal injury and renal failure in patients with cirrhosis; decreased cardiac output and decreased systemic vascular resistance result in a cycle of worsening renal perfusion and renal vasoconstriction.

hepatotoxicity: Damage to the liver.

hernia: A protrusion of an organ from its tissue lining.

hexaxial system: The system developed to describe the coronal plane that is created by the limb leads (I, II, III, aVR, aVL, and aVF).

high-altitude cerebral edema (HACE): An altitude illness characterized by a change in mental status and/or ataxia in a person with acute mountain sickness, or the presence of mental status

changes and ataxia in a person without acute mountain sickness.

high-altitude pulmonary edema (HAPE): An altitude illness characterized by dyspnea at rest, cough, severe weakness, and drowsiness that may eventually lead to central cyanosis, audible rales or wheezing, tachypnea, and tachycardia.

high-flow nasal cannula (HFNC) therapy: A form of noninvasive ventilation used to treat hypoxic respiratory failure by delivering up to 100% humidified and heated oxygen at a flow rate of up to 60 L/min.

high-level disinfection: Treatment used on inanimate objects that kills all microorganisms, but does *not* kill bacterial spores.

highly reliable organization (HRO): An organization that focuses on managing its inevitable failures, so that a failure does not affect the patient or the customer.

hippus phenomenon: A pattern of pupil response to light in which rapid constriction of the pupil is followed by dilation; it can be normal or signify compression of cranial nerve III.

Hirschsprung disease: A congenital lack of ganglion nerve cells in a portion of the distal intestines leading to poor intestinal peristalsis, constipation, and, if not diagnosed and treated, potentially death.

histamine: A neurotransmitter that is released by cells in response to injury and in allergic and inflammatory reactions; it causes vasodilation and contraction of smooth muscle tissue.

histotoxic hypoxia: Hypoxia caused by the inability of the tissues to use oxygen, usually as a result of poisoning by toxins such as carbon monoxide and cyanide.

homeostasis: Stability in the body's internal environment.

hospital-acquired pneumonia (HAP): Pneumonia that occurs in a hospitalized patient 48 hours or more after admission to the hospital, but that was not apparent at the time of admission.

huddle: A communication technique and event that often takes the form of a structured, short meeting in which patient care teams come together to talk about a patient, procedure, or situation.

human leukocyte antigen (HLA): An antigen present on the cell membrane surfaces of circulating platelets, white blood cells, and most tissue cells.

humidity: The degree of moisture in the air, expressed as a percentage.

hydrocephalus: The result of an obstruction that causes an excessive accumulation of cerebrospinal fluid.

hydroureteronephrosis: Dilation and obstruction of a ureter, which results in dilation of the connected kidney.

hypemic hypoxia: Hypoxia caused by a decrease in the blood's oxygen-carrying capacity due to a reduced amount of hemoglobin in the blood or a reduced number of red blood cells; also known as anemic hypoxia.

hyperangulated blade: A video laryngoscope blade with a high degree of curvature to get around anatomic structures.

hyperbaric oxygen therapy (HBOT): A treatment for decompression sickness and certain other conditions that involves placing the patient in a specially constructed chamber designed to withstand high internal pressures, well in excess of normal atmospheric pressures.

hyperbilirubinemia: A condition commonly seen in the newborn, in which an excess of bilirubin develops in the blood; often leads to jaundice.

hypercalcemia: An increased level of calcium in the blood.

hypercapnia: Greater than normal amounts of carbon dioxide in the blood.

hyperchloremia: An abnormally high level of chloride in the blood.

hyperdynamic state: The first stage of distributive shock, which is characterized primarily by high cardiac output and low peripheral vascular resistance; also known as warm shock.

hyperemic: An increase in blood flow into a tissue or organ; congested with blood.

hyperglycemia: A condition in which the blood glucose concentration exceeds the normal range (70–100 mg/dL).

hyperkalemia: An abnormally high level of potassium in the blood.

hyperosmolar hyperglycemic state (HHS): A metabolic disorder that occurs principally in patients with type 2 diabetes and is characterized by hyperglycemia, hyperosmolarity, and the absence of significant ketosis; also known as hyperosmolar hyperglycemic nonketotic syndrome (HHNS).

hyperpnea: A breath that is deeper than normal; it can lead to low levels of CO_2.

hypersensitivity: A reaction consisting of an exaggerated or inappropriate immune response that occurs after a person comes in contact with a substance the body perceives as harmful.

hyperthyroidism: A condition caused by increased production of T_3 (triiodothyronine) and T_4 (thyroxine) from the thyroid gland, resulting in an increase in the body's organ function; characterized by an increase in body temperature, gradual weight loss, increased and/or irregular heart rate, sweating, and irritability.

hypertrophy: An increase in the size of the cells as the result of synthesis of more subcellular components, leading to an increase in tissue and organ size.

hyphema: A collection of blood in the anterior chamber of the eye.

hypoalbuminemia: An abnormally low level of albumin in the blood.

hypocalcemia: A low level of calcium in the blood.

hypochloremia: An abnormally low level of chloride in the blood.

hypodynamic state: The second stage of distributive shock, which is characterized primarily by a subnormal temperature, a low white blood cell count, profound hypotension and hypoperfusion, and a sudden drop in cardiac output; also known as cold shock.

hypoglycemia: A condition in which blood glucose drops below the normal range (70–100 mg/dL) and, in people without diabetes, is accompanied by signs and symptoms.

hypokalemia: An abnormally low level of potassium in the blood.

hyponatremia: An abnormally low level of sodium in the blood; a blood serum sodium level that is below 135 mEq/L, and a serum osmolarity level that is less than 280 mOsm/kg.

hypoplastic left heart syndrome: A cyanotic heart defect that is caused by an abnormally small left ventricle; it is often associated with aortic and mitral valve stenosis or atresia.

hypopnea: A shallow breath; it can lead to increased CO_2 levels and decreased oxygen levels.

hypothalamic-pituitary axis: An interrelationship between the hypothalamus and the pituitary gland in which a releasing or inhibiting factor is sent from the hypothalamus to the pituitary, resulting in, respectively, an increase or decrease in metabolism and other functions throughout the body.

hypothalamo-hypophysial portal system: The venules between the capillaries in the hypothalamus and pituitary gland by which the hypothalamus sends releasing or inhibiting factors to the pituitary gland, thereby increasing or decreasing metabolism, respectively.

hypothalamus: An area of the cerebrum located below the thalamus that forms the floor and the anterior walls of the third ventricle, forming the most inferior portion of the diencephalon. It is responsible for the maintenance of homeostasis and the implementation of behavioral patterns and controls many body functions, including heart rate, digestion, sexual development, temperature regulation, emotion, hunger, thirst, and regulation of the sleep cycle.

hypothermia: A condition in which the core body temperature decreases to less than 95°F (35°C).

hypothyroidism: A condition caused by a deficiency of T_3 (triiodothyronine) and T_4 (thyroxine) from the thyroid gland, resulting in a slowing of the body's organ function; characterized by a decrease in body temperature, gradual weight gain, and increased risk for acute myocardial infarction and stroke.

hypotonia: Low or poor (floppy) muscle tone.

hypovolemic shock: A condition in which the circulating blood volume is inadequate for delivering sufficient oxygen and nutrients to the body; the most common cause of shock in pediatric populations.

hypoxemia: An abnormally low oxygen level.

hypoxia: A state of oxygen deficiency in the body, which is sufficient to cause an impairment of function. Hypoxia is caused by a reduction in the partial pressure of oxygen, inadequate oxygen transport, or an inability of the tissues to use oxygen.

hypoxic hypoxia: Hypoxia caused by a decrease in the amount of oxygen in the blood due to a reduction in oxygen pressure in the lungs, a reduced gas exchange area, exposure to high altitude, or lung disease.

hypoxic ischemic encephalopathy (HIE): Damage to cells in the central nervous system (the brain and spinal cord) from inadequate oxygen.

I time: The time frame for the delivery of the tidal volume.

I:E ratio: An expression for comparing the length of expiration to the length of inspiration. The normal ratio is 1:2, which means that expiration is twice as long as inspiration. This ratio is not measured in seconds.

iatrogenic response: An adverse condition inadvertently induced in a patient by the treatment given.

idiosyncratic reaction: An abnormal (and usually unexplained) reaction by a person to a medication to which most other people do not react.

ileus: A lack of movement of GI contents in the absence of an obstruction, usually occurring postsurgery.

immediate hemolytic transfusion reactions: Transfusion reactions that usually occur soon (between 1 and 2 hours) after the transfusion of incompatible red blood cells.

immunity: Protection from infection, provided by a complex system of substances, cells, and tissues that exist to protect the human body from infection.

immunocompromised: Unable to mount a normal immune response as the result of disease (eg, AIDS), chemotherapy treatment, or certain other medical treatments.

immunodeficiency: An abnormal condition in which some part of the body's immune system is inadequate, such that resistance to infectious disease is decreased.

impedance: Resistance to the flow of current along an electrical pathway, measured in ohms.

imperforate anus: A congenital condition in which the anal opening is either absent or displaced.

implantable cardioverter-defibrillator (ICD): A small, battery-powered electrical impulse generator that is implanted in patients at risk for sudden cardiac death as the result of ventricular fibrillation or pulseless ventricular tachycardia.

implantable pulse generator (IPG): The largest implanted element in a pacemaking system, containing the battery and control circuitry.

implied consent: The legal assumption made on behalf of a person who is unable to give consent that they would give consent if able to do so.

inborn error of metabolism: A class of genetic diseases mostly caused by defects in single genes that code for enzymes that facilitate conversion of various substances into others; such defects lead to accumulation of substances that are toxic or interfere with normal function.

incidence: The number of new cases of a disease within a defined population over a defined period of time.

incomplete breech: A delivery presentation in which the buttocks present first and one foot extends into the birth canal.

incomplete spinal cord injury: A disruption of the tracts of the spinal cord in which the patient retains some degree of cord-mediated function.

incorporation: In the radiation context, a process in which radioactive materials enter the body during radiation exposure, causing ongoing internal exposure and creating devastating individual patient toxicity.

incubator: An enclosed, clear plastic, heated bed that keeps the infant warm.

indication: The reason for using a medication; it may be an official use, approved by the FDA, or an off-label use, for a purpose other than those specifically noted on the medication's label.

indicator conditions: Rare or unusual diseases associated with an immunocompromised state; also called AIDS-defining diseases.

indifferent stage: The stage of altitude hypoxia in which the body is able to compensate for the hypoxia induced by low barometric pressures.

indirect bilirubin: A by-product of the metabolism of red blood cells that is unconjugated and, therefore, not water soluble.

infection: The invasion of normally sterile tissue by a pathogen.

inflammatory bowel disease (IBD): Term covering two colon inflammation pathologies: ulcerative colitis and Crohn disease.

informed consent: The process of proposing to the patient a course of action (assessment, treatment, transport), the risks associated with that action, the benefits associated with the action, and any reasonable alternatives, and then allowing the patient to decide if they want the provider to proceed with the action.

inhibition: A condition in which the presence of one medication decreases the effect of another medication.

Injury Severity Score (ISS): A trauma scoring system that adds the squares of the three highest abbreviated injury scale scores to create a score between 1 and 75 that accounts for multiple injuries, with 1 being a minor injury and 75 being an injury with a high mortality rate.

innate immune system: The primary nonspecific antigen and immunogen defense mechanism that protects the host by eliminating microbes and other antigens in an effort to prevent infection and allergic reactions.

innate immunity: The type of immunity that an individual is born with, such as that provided by the skin and mucous membranes.

inotropic: Affecting the contractility of muscle tissue, especially cardiac muscle.

inspiration: An active process in which gas is taken into the lungs.

inspiratory capacity (IC): The maximum amount of air that can be inspired; the sum of the inspiratory reserve volume and the tidal volume.

inspiratory reserve volume (IRV): The amount of air that can be inhaled after a tidal volume is inhaled.

instrument flight rules (IFR): A mode of flight used when adverse weather conditions exist, visibility is poor, or cloud cover is low. The pilot may not be able to see outside the aircraft, must rely on instruments, and must be in constant contact with an air-traffic controller who assists in maintaining proper separation from other air traffic.

instrument meteorological conditions (IMC): Weather conditions (eg, cloudiness or low visibility) in which a pilot must fly under instrument flight rules, depending on instruments to guide the aircraft.

insulin resistance: A condition in which the pancreas produces enough insulin but the body cannot effectively use it.

interfacility transport (IFT): The transport of a patient between two health care facilities.

interference: A direct biochemical interaction between two drugs.

intermediate-level disinfection: Treatment used on inanimate objects that kills *Mycobacterium tuberculosis*, vegetative bacteria, and most viruses and fungi, but does *not* kill bacterial spores.

internal capsule: A massive bundle of efferent and afferent fibers connecting the various subdivisions of the brain and spinal cord.

International Civil Aviation Organization (ICAO): An agency of the United Nations that defines standards for international air navigation and, as part of its role in developing safe practices, requires crew resource management.

international normalized ratio (INR): A comparative rating of a patient's prothrombin time to help standardize the prothrombin time when planning treatment.

intervertebral foramen: A space in the middle of the vertebra that allows the exit of a peripheral nerve root and spinal vein as well as the entrance of a spinal artery on both sides at each vertebral junction.

intra-abdominal hypertension (IAH): Sustained increased abdominal pressure of more than 12 mm Hg.

intra-abdominal pressure (IAP): The static pressure inside the abdominal compartment; normally 5 mm Hg, with variations caused by respirations.

intra-aortic balloon pump (IABP) therapy: A procedure involving insertion of a balloon into the descending thoracic aorta and its connection to a pump via a catheter; this therapy helps to increase blood flow to the coronary arteries during diastole (inflation) and decrease the afterload of blood from the left ventricle (deflation).

intra-atrial conduction delay (IACD): Delayed conduction within one of the atria, often associated with left or right atrial enlargement.

intra-atrial pathways: The anterior or Bachman bundle, middle bundle, and posterior internodal system, through which the electrical impulse passes after the sinoatrial node; represented by the P wave on the electrocardiogram; also called intranodal pathways.

intracerebral hemorrhage: Direct bleeding into the brain parenchyma.

intracranial pressure (ICP): The pressure exerted by brain tissue, intracranial vascular contents, and cerebrospinal fluid in the closed, nondistensible cranial cavity.

intracranial temperature (ICT): Core brain temperature or homeostatic mean gradient temperature of 101.1°F (38.4°C).

intrarenal acute kidney injury: A type of acute kidney injury caused by damage to an actual nephron.

introitus: The visible opening to the vagina.

intussusception: An event in which one part of the intestine telescopes into another part of the intestines, leading to a blockage.

invasive hemodynamic monitoring: Methods for assessing the physiologic condition of the three principal components of the cardiovascular system: heart, vascular network, and fluid volume. It mainly not only assesses the capability of a patient's heart to pump the requisite amount of blood to the body but also can assess compliance, tone, resistance of the vascular network, and fluid status; it includes a variety of pressure values and other measurements.

invasive ventilation: Application of mechanical ventilation through an artificial airway such as a tracheostomy or endotracheal tube.

involuntary (autonomic) nervous system: The sympathetic and parasympathetic branches of the nervous system, whose fibers connect the structures of the CNS with smooth muscle, cardiac muscle, and glands.

ionic bond: A type of chemical bond formed between oppositely charged ions.

ionized calcium: Calcium that is not bound or chelated; also called free calcium. Its value is useful in assessing for renal failure, nephrotic syndrome, acid–base derangements, and decreases or elevations in chelating compounds.

irradiated blood products: Blood products in which lymphocyte DNA has been exposed to radiation to damage it, and thereby limit the cells' ability to replicate and cause the rare but often fatal condition of transfusion-associated graft-versus-host disease.

irradiation: Exposure to radiation. It is important to distinguish between irradiation and contamination because health care providers and emergency responders are not placed at any risk by patients who have been irradiated but are not contaminated.

ischemic colitis: A potentially life-threatening form of colitis that results from diminished blood flow to the GI tract.

ischemic stroke: A condition in which an artery to the brain becomes blocked by a thrombus, embolus, trauma, or vasospasm (often due to drugs).

isoelectric: When referring to a wave, the status of the wave as neither positive nor negative.

isolation precautions: Measures taken to prevent contact with pathogens, including airborne, droplet, and contact precautions.

isovolumetric contraction: The early stage of ventricular contraction during which ventricular blood volume is unchanging because all valves are closed (the semilunar valves have not yet opened).

isovolumetric relaxation: The early stage of ventricular relaxation during which ventricular blood volume is unchanging because all valves are closed (the atrioventricular valves have not yet opened).

Jackson-Pratt drain: A surgical drain used to remove fluid buildup from the wound site during the postoperative healing process.

jaundice: The deposition of bile pigments in the skin; associated with hyperbilirubinemia.

jejunostomy tube (J tube): A feeding tube placed through the abdominal wall into the jejunum.

joule: A unit of measurement for energy.

jugular venous bulb oximetry: A technique in which a sampling catheter is placed in the internal jugular vein and directed upward so that its tip rests in the jugular venous bulb at the base of the brain; samples of blood can then be drawn to measure mixed venous oxygen saturation (Svo_2).

just culture: A system of beliefs and practices that focuses on blamelessly identifying issues that lead to errors or unsafe behaviors, while still maintaining individual accountability for reckless behavior.

Kehr sign: Left shoulder pain that may indicate a ruptured spleen. (Right shoulder pain may indicate trauma to the liver.) This referred pain stems from diaphragm irritation by intra-abdominal bleeding.

Kernig sign: Resistance and pain elicited on extension of the leg at the knee, with the patient in the supine position and the hips flexed perpendicular to the trunk; when pain occurs as a result of this test, the test result is positive.

ketone bodies: Organic products of fat catabolism—specifically, acetoacidic acid, acetone, and beta-hydroxybutyric acid.

ketonuria: The presence of ketone bodies in the urine.

Kussmaul respiration: A typical respiratory pattern seen in patients with metabolic acidosis; it is characterized by a high respiratory rate and high tidal volume, leading to increased minute ventilation.

lactate: The form of lactic acid that is physiologically present in the body.

lactate dehydrogenase (LDH): An enzyme that catalyzes the metabolism of pyruvate (the end product of glycolysis) to lactate in the absence of a functioning citric acid cycle.

lactic acidosis: A form of acidosis caused by an excess accumulation or impaired excretion of lactate, leading to an elevated anion gap; it can result from exposure to various toxic substances, inadequate tissue perfusion in various shock states, dysfunction of certain organs, nutritional deficiency, infection, malignancy, diabetes, or hereditary metabolic disorders.

laparoscopic adjustable gastric banding (LAGB): The least invasive bariatric surgical procedure, in which an adjustable band is placed around the upper portion of the stomach, with an adjustment port located on the right side of the abdomen, under the skin.

laryngeal mask airway (LMA): A rescue airway with a basic design similar to an endotracheal tube at the proximal end, in that a standard adapter is present to allow ventilation. The distal end is equipped with an elliptical cuff, which, when inflated, covers the supraglottic area and allows ventilation.

latent error: A mistake that is likely to occur secondary to organizational or design failures that allow the inevitable active error to cause harm.

lead: In the context of the 12-lead electrocardiogram, the designated position of the electrode, or the name of the electrode placement. In the context of a pacemaker, an insulated wire that carries signals in a pacemaking system between the implantable pulse generator and the heart tissue.

Lean: A strategy that looks at all processes and attempts to reduce waste and ensure all activities add value.

Le Fort criteria: A categorization of facial fractures involving the maxilla in which the fractures are differentiated based on the location of fracture lines and the extent of mobility of facial structures on physical examination.

left anterior fascicle: The portion of the electrical conduction system responsible for innervating the anterior and superior areas of the left ventricle. It is a single-stranded cord terminating in the Purkinje cells.

left posterior fascicle: The portion of the electrical conduction system responsible for innervating the posterior and inferior areas of the left ventricle. It is a widely distributed, fanlike structure terminating in the Purkinje cells.

left ventricular assist device (LVAD): A means of mechanical circulatory support in which a pump is implanted in the patient's chest to help circulate blood from the left ventricle of the heart to the rest of the body.

left ventricular end-diastolic pressure: The pressure exerted on the left ventricle at the end of diastole; the normal value is 4 to 12 mm Hg and is measured by using a pulmonary artery catheter.

left ventricular stroke work index: A calculation of the contractility of the left ventricle indexed to the patient's body surface area; equivalent to the stroke volume index.

leukocytosis: An abnormally high number of white blood cells.

leuko-reduced blood products: Blood products in which the white blood cells and platelet fragments have been filtered from donated blood products.

leukotrienes: A class of biologically active compounds that occur naturally in leukocytes and that produce allergic and inflammatory reactions.

leveling: The process of ensuring that the hemodynamic pressure transducer is at the level of the atrium, which also corresponds to the level of the aortic root.

Lhermitte phenomenon: A condition in which forward flexion of the neck produces an electric shock feeling, usually running down the back.

lift: The upward force created by the wings moving through the air, which sustains the aircraft in flight.

ligament of Treitz: A small ligament supporting the small intestine at the junction between the duodenum and the jejunum. It serves as the dividing point between the upper and lower GI tract.

limbic lobe: Part of the temporal lobe that is the seat of emotions and instincts; also called the rhinencephalon.

limb leads: The electrocardiography lead electrodes attached to the limbs that form the hexaxial system, dividing the heart along a coronal plane into the anterior and posterior segments.

linea nigra: A dermatologic condition affecting pregnant women in which a darkened line develops from the navel to the vagina.

linear skull fracture: A type of skull fracture characterized by a single fracture line.

linear stellate fracture: A fracture with multiple linear fractures radiating from the site of impact.

lines of cleavage: Regions between interlocking collagen fibers that run in various planes, usually parallel to the skin; they run longitudinally in the skin of the head and limbs and in a circular pattern around the neck and trunk and are used when deciding where to make incisions for escharotomies and fasciotomies.

lipase: A pancreatic hormone that metabolizes lipids.

lipid disorders: A group of disorders that cause a change in the production or use of cholesterol and may also alter the way cholesterol circulates or is processed in the body.

lithotripsy: Use of external vibrations to break up gallstones.

liver function test (LFT): A test for liver damage that measures enzymes that normally appear in liver cells but may spill out into the vasculature with parenchymal damage.

long QT syndrome (LQTS): A prolonged QT interval on the electrocardiogram that is primarily caused by a congenital disorder. Under certain conditions, it tends to deteriorate into ventricular tachyarrhythmias and can lead to syncope or sudden cardiac death; the patient loses consciousness, often without warning.

low-level disinfection: Treatment used on inanimate objects that kills most bacteria, some viruses, and some fungi, but does *not* kill *Mycobacterium tuberculosis* or bacterial spores.

lumbar puncture: A procedure in which a needle is inserted first into the lumbar portion of the back and then into the subarachnoid space to obtain spinal fluid for testing or to administer drugs.

Lund-Browder chart: A detailed version of the rule of nines chart that takes into consideration the changes in body surface area that occur with growth.

magnetic resonance imaging (MRI): A noninvasive diagnostic imaging technique that uses a powerful magnet to align water molecules present in body compartments to visualize the internal structure and function of the body; a three-dimensional image is obtained from this alignment and the speed at which molecules alter or release.

major burn: According to the American Burn Association classification system, any of the following: (1) partial-thickness burns involving more than 25% of total body surface area (TBSA) in adults or 20% of TBSA in children younger than 10 years and adults older than 40 years; (2) full-thickness burns involving 10% or more of TBSA; (3) burns involving the face, eyes, ears, hands, feet, or perineum that may result in functional or cosmetic impairment; (4) high-voltage electrical injury; (5) burns complicated by inhalation injury or major trauma; and (6) burns sustained by high-risk or debilitated patients.

malignant hyperthermia: A condition that may occur after administration of certain inhaled anesthetics (notably succinylcholine); characterized by muscle spasms, rigidity, acidosis, hypercarbia, hyperthermia, tachycardia, tachypnea, myoglobinuria, rhabdomyolysis, and hyperkalemia.

Mallampati classification: A system for predicting the relative difficulty of intubation based on the amount of oropharyngeal structures visible in an upright, seated patient who is fully able to open their mouth.

Mallory-Weiss syndrome: Laceration and bleeding of the esophagus, often following forceful vomiting.

malrotation: A congenital anomaly of rotation of the midgut, in which the small bowel is found predominantly on the right side of the abdomen.

massive transfusion protocol: The rapid administration of large amounts of blood products in fixed ratios (usually 1:1:1) for the management of hemorrhagic shock.

mean airway pressure (MAP): The amount of positive pressure in the airway, averaged over the inspiratory and expiratory phases of the breathing cycle.

mean arterial pressure (MAP): The average arterial pressure during a single cardiac cycle; the mean between the systolic and diastolic blood pressures (SBP and DBP): $MAP = DBP + (SBP - DBP)$.

mean electrical axis: The sum of all electrical impulses.

mechanical circulatory support (MCS): Mechanical interventions aimed at augmenting or replacing the native cardiac output from the heart; also called mechanically assisted circulation, mechanical circulatory systems, and ventricular assist devices.

mechanical ventilation: The application of a device that provides varying degrees of ventilatory support.

mechanism of action: The way in which a medication produces the intended response.

meconium: A dark green fecal material that accumulates in the fetal intestines and is discharged around the time of birth.

meconium aspiration syndrome: The respiratory distress caused by meconium aspiration, which can lead to atelectasis in the lungs, persistent pulmonary hypertension (delayed transition from fetal to neonatal circulation), pneumonitis, and pneumothorax.

medical control: The oversight designed to ensure that actions taken by providers on behalf of patients are appropriate. It is divided into direct (online) medical control, which is available in real time via radio or mobile phone, and indirect (off-line) medical control, such as standing orders and protocols.

medical direction: Supervision of medical care by a physician empowered to authorize and review CCTPs, usually through protocols, standing orders, education, and quality improvement efforts.

medical director: A physician who provides guidance and oversight for the practice of a critical care transport service's personnel.

medical error: The failure of a planned health care action to be completed as intended, or the use of a wrong care plan to achieve an aim.

medical screening exam: An exam that is legally required when the patient is within 250 yards of the hospital, or on hospital property, and is seeking treatment for an emergency medical condition; it must be performed by a physician, physician assistant, or nurse practitioner.

medulla oblongata: The lowermost portion of the brainstem.

melena: Black, tarry stool containing partially digested blood, with the bleeding usually originating from the upper GI tract.

meningitis: An umbrella term referring to five types of inflammation of the leptomeninges, the membranes that cover and enclose the spinal cord and brain.

metabolic acidemia: A condition characterized by the body's production of excessive quantities of acid or the kidneys' inability to remove enough acid from the body.

metabolic acidosis: A pathologic condition characterized by a blood pH of less than 7.35, which is caused by an accumulation of acids in the body from a metabolic cause; can be caused by any number of systems in the body, including the gastrointestinal system, or by major organ failure.

metabolic alkalosis: A pathologic condition (blood pH > 7.45) resulting from an accumulation of bases in the body caused by any number of systems in the body, including the gastrointestinal system, or by major organ failure.

metabolic syndrome: A group of risk factors that together may lead to coronary artery disease, stroke, and type 2 diabetes; usually related to a predisposition to a lipid disorder.

microaxial continuous-flow pump: A means of temporary circulatory support that consists of an axial-flow pump mounted on a catheter that is typically inserted through the femoral artery and connected to a bedside console.

microcirculation: Circulation that occurs in the microvasculature, the body's smallest vessels (arterioles, capillaries, and venules).

midbrain: A small area of the brainstem extending between the diencephalon, the pons, and the third ventricle.

mild hypothermia: A condition in which the core body temperature is between 90°F and 95°F (32.2°C and 35°C); at this stage of hypothermia, the body usually compensates with increased thermogenesis and interrupted thermolysis.

mild TBI: Concussion; a traumatically induced physiologic disruption of brain function that occurs without structural damage.

Mini-Mental State Examination: A simple, easily applied test of higher cognitive functions.

Minnesota esophagogastric tamponade tube: A tube that is placed to stop bleeding of esophageal varices. It is similar to the Sengstaken-Blakemore tube, but has a built-in suction catheter.

minor burn: According to the American Burn Association classification system, any of the following: (1) partial-thickness burns involving less than 15% of total body surface area (TBSA) in adults or 10% of TBSA in children younger than 20 years and adults older than 50 years; and (2) full-thickness burns involving 2% or less of TBSA that do not present a serious threat of functional or cosmetic risk to the eyes, ears, face, hands, feet, or perineum.

minute volume: Total volume of air breathed in and out in 1 minute. It is calculated by multiplying the respiratory rate per minute by the tidal volume.

mistake: A situation in which an action occurs as intended but is the wrong action; it often occurs secondary to lack of experience, insufficient training, or negligence.

mixed acidosis: A pathologic condition in which there is a low pH (<7.35), an elevated Pco_2 level (>45 mm Hg), and a low bicarbonate level (<22 mmol/L); it occurs when both respiratory and metabolic acidosis are present at the same time.

mixed alkalosis: A pathologic condition in which there is an elevated pH (>7.45), a low Pco_2 level (<35 mm Hg), and an elevated bicarbonate level (>26 mmol/L); it occurs when both respiratory and metabolic alkalosis are present at the same time.

mixed central venous oxygen saturation ($Scvo_2$): The percentage of oxygen bound to hemoglobin in blood returning to the right side of the heart from the head and upper body, which is representative of oxygen extraction from the blood by the head and upper extremities.

mixed venous oxygen saturation (Svo_2): The percentage of oxygen bound to hemoglobin in blood returning to the right side of the heart, which is representative of global oxygen extraction from the blood and is normally in the range of 50% to 75%.

mobile intensive care units: Ambulances or helicopters that are used only for maintaining specialized or intensive care treatment; they are used primarily for interfacility transports.

mode: The particular way in which a spontaneous or mechanical breath is delivered.

moderate burn: According to the American Burn Association classification system, any of the following: (1) partial-thickness burns involving 15% to 25% of total body surface area (TBSA) in adults or 10% to 20% of TBSA in children younger than 10 years and adults older than 40 years and (2) full-thickness burns involving 10% or less of TBSA in patients younger than 50 years that do not present a serious threat to functional or cosmetic impairment of the eyes, ears, face, hands, feet, or perineum.

moderate hypothermia: A condition in which the core body temperature is between 82°F and 90°F (27.7°C and 32.2°C); mental status is markedly decreased, and shivering may still be present but is less vigorous and unlikely to be an effective from of thermogenesis.

monoclonal antibodies: Antibodies in which large quantities of an antibody from a single B-cell clone are produced to protect against a specific pathogen.

Monro-Kellie doctrine: A theory developed by two Scottish anatomists, who stated that the central nervous system is enclosed in a rigid compartment along with cerebrospinal fluid, whose total volume tends to remain constant; an increase in any component—whether brain, blood, or CSF—will cause an increase in pressure and decrease the volume of one of the other elements.

morbidity: An illness or an abnormal condition or quality; the rate at which an illness occurs in a particular area or population, usually expressed as the number of nonfatal injuries in a certain population in a given time period divided by the size of the population.

morbid obesity: A body mass index of 40 kg/m^2 or higher. Morbid obesity not only includes all of the health risks associated with obesity but also makes essential functions such as walking or breathing difficult.

Moro reflex: An infant reflex in which, when an infant is caught off guard, the infant opens their arms wide, spreads the fingers, and seems to grab at things.

mortality: The condition of being subject to death, caused by injury and disease; the number of deaths per unit of population in any specific region, age group, disease, or other classification, usually expressed as the number of deaths in a certain population in a given time period divided by the size of the population.

motor area: Part of the frontal lobe containing pyramidal cells that control voluntary motor function on the opposite side of the body.

mucosa: The outermost layer of the alimentary canal. It consists of three sublayers: surface epithelium, lamina propria, and muscularis mucosae.

multiple organ dysfunction syndrome (MODS): Altered organ function in acutely ill patients, which is diagnosed when two or more organs stop functioning.

Murphy sign: A painful reaction elicited by asking the patient to take and hold a deep breath as the provider palpates the right subcostal area; if pain occurs on inspiration, when the inflamed gallbladder comes in contact with the provider's hand, Murphy sign is positive. It may signal the presence of gallbladder problems.

muscularis externa: The third tissue layer of the alimentary canal. It contains two levels in most places: the circular layer and the longitudinal layer.

myocardial oxygen consumption (MVo$_2$): The volume of oxygen that the heart muscle consumes; an expression of the level of oxygen demand in the heart.

myoglobinuria: The presence of myoglobin, a respiratory pigment of muscle tissue, in the urine.

myxedema coma: A rare, life-threatening condition that can occur in patients who have severe, untreated hypothyroidism, and that is characterized by altered mental status and lethargy, failure of the thermoregulatory system, and a precipitating event; may be accompanied by auditory and visual hallucinations, seizures, or unresponsiveness.

National Transportation Safety Board (NTSB): An independent federal agency that promotes transportation safety, including aviation, railroad, highway, maritime, pipeline, and hazardous materials safety; it investigates transportation crashes to identify the cause and make safety recommendations.

NBG codes: North American Society of Pacing and Electrophysiology/British Pacing and Electrophysiology Group Generic codes; five-letter codes used to categorize pacemakers by their functions and capabilities, developed by a joint effort of North American and British electrophysiology groups.

near miss: An unplanned event that did not cause an injury, illness, or damage, but had the potential to do so; it is indistinguishable from a full-fledged adverse event in all but the outcome.

necrotizing enterocolitis (NEC): A disorder seen predominantly in premature infants in which the bowel experiences necrosis (tissue death).

necrotizing fasciitis: A limb- or life-threatening infection of the soft tissue that affects the subcutaneous tissues, fat, and fascia.

negative-pressure ventilators: Mechanical ventilators that operate using pressure that is less than the ambient (atmospheric) pressure.

negligence: Failure to provide the same quality of care (as defined by applicable standards) that is reasonably expected for a provider to give under similar circumstances. Negligence is established when the plaintiff proves four elements: duty to act, breach of the duty, injury to the patient, and the breach as the direct cause of the injury.

neonate: An infant during the first 28 days after birth.

nephrolithiasis: A condition in which the body produces renal calculi (kidney stones), which are often symptomatic as they travel through the ureters; may produce impaction and infection of the urinary tract.

neurocranium: The part of the skull that encloses and protects the brain.

neurogenic shock: Circulatory failure caused by paralysis of the nerves that control the size of the blood vessels, leading to widespread dilation and consequent hemodynamic and systemic effects; it is seen in spinal cord injuries.

neuroleptic malignant syndrome (NMS): A potentially fatal reaction to antipsychotic and neuroleptic medications; characterized by patient hyperthermia, profound muscle rigidity, autonomic dysfunction, metabolic acidosis, and confusion.

neuromuscular-blocking agents (NMBAs): Medications that bind to acetylcholine receptors, thereby inhibiting the action of acetylcholine; this effect blocks transmission at the neuromuscular junction and causes paralysis of the muscles.

neutral thermal environment: The temperature at which maintenance of normal body temperature requires only minimal metabolic expenditure.

neutropenia: An abnormally low neutrophil count.

neutrophils: A type of leukocyte (white blood cell); these numerous phagocytic microphages usually are the first of the mobile phagocytic cells to arrive at the site of injury or infection.

never event: An event that should never occur and indicates a serious underlying safety problem.

newborn: An infant within the first few hours after birth.

nicotinic receptors: Cholinergic receptors that bind with the neurotransmitter acetylcholine.

nitrogen narcosis: A state resembling alcohol intoxication, which is produced by nitrogen gas dissolved in the blood at high ambient pressure.

nonalcoholic fatty liver disease (NAFLD): Accumulation of fat in the liver, for which alcohol consumption is not believed to be a contributing factor.

nondepolarizing agent: A medication designed to cause temporary paralysis by binding in a competitive but nonstimulatory manner to part of the acetylcholine receptor; these medications do not cause fasciculations and have a longer duration of action than succinylcholine does.

nonfunctioning adenoma: A type of pituitary lesion in which the tumor does not secrete any hormones.

noninvasive ventilation: Application of mechanical ventilation through a mask, mouthpiece, or other interfaces other than an artificial airway.

normalization of deviance: A process in which a shift away from acceptable policies and practices becomes the behavioral norm.

normal-pressure hydrocephalus (NPH): An accumulation of CSF that causes the ventricles of the brain to enlarge. The enlarged ventricles of a patient with this condition may not cause increased intracranial pressure.

normal range: A range of values encompassing the results that 95% of healthy people would have for the particular test.

nosocomial: Infections acquired during hospitalization or a nursing home stay.

nuchal rigidity: Marked resistance to head movement in any direction that is suggestive of meningeal irritation.

obesity: A body mass index greater than or equal to 30 kg/m^2.

obstructive diseases: Diseases that result in difficulty with moving air out of the lungs, such as asthma, chronic obstructive pulmonary disease, cystic fibrosis, and bronchiectasis.

occipital lobe: The lobe of the brain that occupies the most posterior portion of the cerebrum; it is the primary receptive area for vision, specifically the interpretation of visual stimuli.

off-line medical direction: Medical direction given through a set of protocols, standing orders, educational programs, policies, and/or standards.

Ohm's law: The principle given by the equation $V = IR$, which states that applied voltage is equal to the current times the resistance of the circuit.

oligohydramnios: Decreased volume of amniotic fluid during a pregnancy; a risk factor associated with abnormalities of the urinary tract, postmaturity (birth after a prolonged pregnancy), and intrauterine growth retardation.

omphalocele: Herniation of abdominal contents into the base of the umbilical cord.

online medical control/consultation (OLMC): Immediate medical direction provided to critical care transport professionals in outlying locations by a physician; a system in which field personnel contact an emergency department physician via telephone or radio for a consult.

online medical direction: Medical direction in which the care provider is in direct contact with a physician, usually via two-way radio or telephone.

onset of action: The time needed for the concentration of a medication at the target tissue to reach the minimum effective level.

oophoropexy: Surgery in which the ovary is attached to the pelvic sidewall so it cannot twist on itself.

open pneumothorax: A communicating chest wound, in which air enters the pleural space from the environment; also called a sucking chest wound.

opioids: The class of chemicals that includes naturally derived opiates and newer synthetic medications with the same properties.

opioid syndrome: Toxicity that develops following illicit use and abuse of opioids or as an adverse consequence of a therapeutic error or accidental ingestion of opioids and characterized by CNS and respiratory depression.

opsonization: The process of making bacterial cells more susceptible to the action of phagocytosis by the action of binding an antibody to the pathogen's cell membrane.

optic disk: The most prominent structure visible in the eye; it represents the termination of the optic nerve.

osmolarity: The amount of dissolved substance in 1 L of water.

osmosis: The diffusion of water across membranes.

osmotic pressure: The pressure created in a space divided by a semipermeable membrane owing to differences in concentrations of solutes found in the solutions on either side of the membrane.

osteogenesis imperfecta: A congenital disorder in which the individual has brittle bones that are susceptible to fracture; also known as brittle bone disease or Lobstein syndrome.

osteopetrosis: An inherited disorder in which the bones become extremely hard and dense.

ostomy: A surgically created opening through which feces can be voided in the absence of some or all of the large intestine or rectum.

ovarian cyst: A fluid buildup within an outcropping of tissue from the ovary. If such a cyst ruptures, significant bleeding can occur.

ovarian torsion: Twisting of an ovary about its ligaments, resulting in ischemia and possibly necrosis.

overweight: A body mass index of 25 to 29.9 kg/m^2.

oxygen consumption ($\dot{V}o_2$): The amount of oxygen used by the cells and tissues.

oxygen delivery (Do_2): The amount of oxygen delivered to the tissues each minute.

oxygen extraction fraction (OEF): The fraction of oxygen extracted from the blood as it passes by to maintain normal oxygen delivery and, consequently, normal brain functions.

oxygen extraction ratio (ERo_2): The relationship between oxygen consumption and oxygen delivery; a measure of the cells' ability to use oxygen.

oxygen hood: A tent that is placed over the head of an infant for the purpose of delivering supplemental oxygen.

P mitrale: A double-humped, M-shaped P wave that is 120 ms wide or greater, with the tops of the humps 40 ms apart or greater. Found in limb leads I, II, and III, it represents left atrial enlargement.

P pulmonale: A tall P wave that is 2.5 mm high or greater. Found in leads II and III, it indicates right atrial enlargement.

pacemaker syndrome: The occurrence of symptoms relating to the loss of atrioventricular synchrony in ventricularly paced hearts or symptoms caused by inadequate timing and ventricular contractions in paced hearts.

pacing circuit: The conduction pathway along which the pacing impulse flows; formed by a power source, one or two lead–electrode pairs, and body tissue.

pacing impulse: The electrical impulse sent to the heart to stimulate the heart to beat.

packed red blood cells (PRBCs): A blood product that retains all of the characteristics of whole blood, with the exception of the extraction of approximately 250 mL of platelet-rich plasma from each unit of whole blood.

pallor: Skin presentation suggestive of reduced blood flow or oxygenation. In patients with light skin, paleness typically presents as unusual lightness compared with the person's baseline skin color. In patients with dark skin, pallor may appear as ashen or gray skin on general assessment. In general, the mucous membranes inside the inner lower eyelid and the oral mucosa will have a pink coloration in all healthy patients, regardless of skin color; thus, a white or pale appearance of these areas in any patient suggests reduced blood flow or oxygenation.

palpable purpura: Relatively large (greater than 3 mm) areas of bleeding under the skin.

pancreatitis: Inflammation of the pancreas leading to autodigestion, tissue destruction, and impaired function.

pandemic: A worldwide epidemic.

panel: Groups of related tests that are performed as a single unit; also called a profile.

papillary muscles: A type of muscle in the ventricle from which the chordae tendineae extend and attach to the cusps of the atrioventricular valves.

paracentesis: Insertion of a needle into the abdomen to aspirate ascites; often done to diagnose spontaneous bacterial peritonitis.

parietal lobe: The lobe of the brain situated directly posterior to the frontal lobe on the other side of the central fissure; it is largely responsible for sensory functions.

Parkland formula: A formula that recommends giving 4 mL of lactated Ringer solution or normal saline for each kilogram of body weight, multiplied by the percentage of body surface area burned; sometimes used to calculate fluid needs during lengthy transport times.

paroxysmal nocturnal dyspnea: Severe shortness of breath occurring at night after several hours of recumbency, during which fluid pools in the lungs; the person is forced to sit up to breathe. It is caused by left-side heart failure or decompensation of chronic obstructive pulmonary disease.

paroxysmal supraventricular tachycardia: A supraventricular tachycardia that starts and ends abruptly.

partial pressure of oxygen (arterial) (Pao$_2$): The amount of the total pressure in the blood contributed by oxygen; a value measured when analyzing the arterial blood gas level.

partial pressure of oxygen (Po$_2$): A measurement of the amount of oxygen dissolved in the blood.

partial-thickness burn: A burn that involves the epidermis and part of the dermis, characterized by pain and blistering; also called a second-degree burn.

partial thromboplastin time (PTT): A value that represents the intrinsic coagulation pathway's clotting ability; also known as activated partial thromboplastin time (aPTT).

passive immunity: Short-lived immunity acquired from placental transfer, antibodies in the mother's milk, or antiserum administered intravenously.

passive warming: A method of warming a hypothermic patient without the introduction of exogenous heat sources. It involves removing cold, wet clothing; drying the patient if necessary; and wrapping the patient in layers that retain radiant heat, minimize conductive heat loss, and protect from ambient moisture such as rain or snow.

patent ductus arteriosus (PDA): A condition in which the ductus arteriosus, which assists in fetal circulation, does not transition as it should after birth to become the ligamentum arteriosum. The result is that the connection between the pulmonary artery and the aorta remains open, allowing some oxygenated blood to move back into the heart rather than all of it moving out of the aorta and into the systemic circulation.

pathogens: Microorganisms that activate the immune system and cause disease; they include viruses, parasites, fungi, and bacteria.

patient safety: According to the World Health Organization, freedom from unnecessary harm or potential harm associated with health care.

peak airway pressure: The amount of positive pressure generated by the ventilator to deliver the tidal volume.

peak inspiratory pressure (PIP): The greatest volume of air delivered to the lungs during inhalation.

pediatric assessment triangle (PAT): An assessment tool that allows rapid formation of a general impression of the type and level of illness or injury in an infant or child without touching the patient; consists of assessing appearance, work of breathing, and circulation of the skin.

pelvic inflammatory disease (PID): An infection of the female upper organs of reproduction—specifically, the uterus, ovaries, and fallopian tubes.

penile fracture: A rupture of one of the blood-containing sacs in the penis, resulting in deformity and possible loss of function.

peptic ulcer: An erosion of the mucosal lining of the GI tract.

percutaneous endoscopic gastrostomy (PEG) tube: A feeding tube that is placed through the abdominal wall into the stomach.

perfusion: The circulation of oxygen and nutrients at the cellular level and removal of waste products of metabolism for elimination.

perfusionists: Highly trained technicians who are intimately familiar with the operation of intra-aortic balloon pumps and adult and pediatric extracorporeal membrane oxygenation machines, and who may assist during any medical situation, including critical care transports, in which it is necessary to support or temporarily replace a patient's circulatory or respiratory function.

pericardial tamponade: Impairment of diastolic filling of the right ventricle as a result of significant amounts of fluid in the pericardial sac surrounding the heart, leading to a decrease in the cardiac output.

pericardiocentesis: A procedure in which a needle or angiocatheter is introduced into the pericardial sac to relieve cardiac tamponade.

pericarditis: An inflammatory process involving the pericardium.

peripheral blood smear: A glass slide containing a drop of blood that can be used to microscopically examine the structure of the blood cells.

peristalsis: A general term describing wavelike muscular contractions of tubular organs, which carry forward materials or liquids contained in those organs.

peritoneal dialysis (PD): Dialysate solution injected into the abdomen, using the peritoneum as a natural semipermeable membrane to separate solutes.

peritonitis: Inflammation of the peritoneum; typically results in generalized abdominal tenderness and guarding.

persistent pulmonary hypertension (PPHN): The persistence of elevated pressures in the pulmonary vasculature after birth, associated with failure to transition from the fetal circulation to the postpartum or normal newborn circulation.

petechial lesions: Small areas of bleeding under the skin (pinpoint).

pharmacodynamics: The branch of pharmacology that studies reactions between medications and living structures, including the processes of body responses to pharmacologic, biochemical, physiologic, and therapeutic effects.

pharmacokinetics: The study of the metabolism and action of medications, with the particular emphasis on the time required for absorption, duration of action, distribution in the body, and method of excretion.

pharmacology: The study of the preparation, properties, uses, and actions of medications.

pheochromocytoma: A catecholamine-producing benign tumor of chromaffin cells located in the center of the adrenal gland, which can occur either sporadically or chronically as a result of genetic risk factors; it causes stimulation of alpha-adrenergic and beta-adrenergic receptors, resulting in hypertension, increased cardiac contractility, glycogenolysis, gluconeogenesis, intestinal relaxation, and increased heart rate.

phlebitis: Inflammation, swelling, and pain along the veins that can lead to the formation of blood clots and thrombophlebitis (venous inflammation associated with a thrombus).

phlebostatic axis: An imaginary point located at the fourth intercostal space, mid-chest level, which serves as an external landmark for the right atrium.

phonation: The process by which the vocal cords create sound.

phosphate buffer system: The buffer system that functions in the renal tubules and intracellular fluids to convert strong acids or bases into weak acids or bases so that they have a minimal effect on the body's overall pH.

phosphodiesterase: An enzyme that helps break phosphodiester bonds, creating smaller nucleotides.

physician orders for life-sustaining treatment (POLST): A legal document that establishes in advance what care a person wants, and does not want, in the event that they are unable to consent to care at the time.

physiologically deficient zone: The zone that extends from 10,000 to 50,000 feet. Noticeable physiologic deficits occur above 10,000 feet. A decrease in barometric pressure results in oxygen deficiency, causing hypoxic hypoxia; the manifestation of trapped and evolved gases then occurs. The use of pressurized aircraft and/or supplemental oxygen is necessary in this zone.

physiologic zone: The atmospheric zone that extends from sea level to 10,000 feet; the area of the atmosphere to which humans are well adapted. The barometric pressure is sufficient in this zone to facilitate adequate oxygenation. The changes in pressure encountered with rapid ascents or descents within this zone can produce ear or sinus trapped-gas problems.

pia mater: The innermost layer of the meninges, which rests directly on the brain or spinal cord.

Pickwickian syndrome: A hypoventilation syndrome associated with obesity in which the person may experience increased breathing difficulty when in the supine position and have a higher incidence of sleep apnea, snoring, and hypercapnia.

Pierre Robin syndrome: A condition present at birth marked by a very small lower jaw (micrognathia) and a cleft palate; the tongue tends to fall back and downward (glossoptosis).

ping-pong ball fracture: A pediatric greenstick fracture of the skull.

plaque-forming unit: The number of viral particles capable of forming plaques per a certain volume.

plasma protein fraction: A blood product that contains 83% albumin and 17% globulins.

plateau pressure: The average pressure applied to airways and alveoli at the end of inspiration during positive-pressure mechanical ventilation.

platelet count: A measurement of the number of platelets in the blood, which is useful for assessing a patient's coagulation status.

pleural friction rub: The result of an inflammation that causes the pleura to thicken, decreasing the pleural space and allowing the surfaces of the pleura to rub together.

plexus: A cluster of nerve roots that permits peripheral nerve roots to function as a group.

pneumatosis intestinalis: Air in the bowel wall as demonstrated by abdominal radiograph.

pneumocephalus: A condition in which air or gas accumulates within the cranial cavity.

pneumomediastinum: The collection of air within the mediastinum (the space within the chest that contains the heart, major blood vessels, vagus nerve, trachea, and esophagus; located between the two lungs).

pneumoperitoneum: The collection of air within the peritoneum (the membrane in the abdomen encasing the liver, spleen, diaphragm, stomach, and transverse colon).

pneumothorax: An accumulation of gas or fluid in the pleural space that causes the lung to become detached from the chest wall and collapse.

poikilothermia: Inability to regulate temperature in an extremity due to lack of perfusion, which may result in abnormally cold extremities.

point-of-care testing (POCT): Testing done outside of a traditional laboratory, usually near where care is being delivered to a patient (ie, at the patient's bedside), with the results of the testing being used for clinical decision making; also called decentralized testing, bedside testing, and ancillary testing.

Poiseuille's law: The relationship that flow varies directly with any increase in pressure.

polydipsia: Excessive thirst, resulting in excessive intake of fluid.

polyhydramnios: An excessive amount of amniotic fluid that may cause preterm labor.

polyphagia: Excessive desire to eat, resulting in overconsumption of food.

polyuria: Frequent and plentiful urination.

pons: Part of the brainstem located between the midbrain and the medulla oblongata; it relays information to and from the brain and spinal cord along fiber tracts.

poor R-wave progression: An abnormal R-wave pattern; one of the factors that may signify anterior infarction.

portal hypertension: An increase in vascular resistance through the hepatic portal system. It can cause high venous pressure in the gastric and esophageal veins, leading to varices, among other problems.

positive end-expiratory pressure (PEEP): The amount of pressure above ambient pressure present in the airway at the end of the respiratory cycle.

positive-pressure ventilators: Mechanical ventilators that operate using pressure that is greater than the ambient pressure.

positron emission tomography (PET): A functional imaging modality that uses radiotracers to visualize physiologic changes over time or distinguish various levels of physiologic activity between tissues.

posterior cord syndrome: Extension injury that produces dysfunction of the dorsal columns, presenting as decreased sensation to light touch, proprioception, and vibration.

postrenal acute kidney injury: A type of acute kidney injury caused by downstream obstruction of urine flow from the kidneys, with initially intact nephrons; commonly caused by a blockage of the urethra by prostate enlargement, renal calculi, or strictures.

potentiation: The effect of increasing the potency or effectiveness of a drug or other treatment; it may occur when two medications are administered concurrently.

PR interval: The interval of time that occupies the space between the beginning of the P wave and the beginning of the QRS complex.

precipitous delivery: Delivery in less than 3 hours from the onset of regular contractions; may occur with premature labor.

precision: A measure of how a value is likely to be the same every time a test is performed.

precordial leads: The chest leads in an electrocardiogram.

preeclampsia: A condition of late pregnancy that involves onset of hypertension and proteinuria that manifests with headache, visual changes, and swelling of the hands and feet; also called toxemia of pregnancy. It may be classified as occurring with or without severe features.

prefrontal area: Part of the frontal lobe that provides control of thought, concentration, depth and ability to think abstractly, memory, and autonomic nervous system response, concomitant to emotional change.

preload: The end-diastolic stretch of the muscle fibers of the ventricle; measured by right atrial pressure or central venous pressure and wedge pressure.

premature: Underdeveloped; refers to infants born before 36 weeks from the first day of the last menstrual period.

premature prelabor rupture of membranes (PPROM): A rupture of membranes in a pregnant woman signaled by a gush of fluid or constant fluid leakage; it accounts for as many as 50% of all preterm deliveries.

premotor area: Part of the frontal lobe that is adjacent to the motor area and helps coordinate certain movements.

prerenal acute kidney injury: A type of acute kidney injury caused by decreased perfusion of an intact nephron; often reversible if the underlying condition can be found and perfusion can be restored to the kidney.

pressure gradients: Differences in pressure, which allow for movement of gas into and out of the lung.

pressure ulcer: A sore on the skin arising from prolonged pressure. Such ulcers are classified into four stages, with stage 4 being the most severe (tissue necrosis and muscle and bone involvement); all stages are painful and susceptible to infection.

pressure ventilator: A type of positive-pressure ventilator that ends the delivery of the tidal volume based on a predetermined pressure; therefore, the volume may vary.

preterm labor: Labor occurring before 36 weeks' gestation, leading to early birth.

prevalence: The total number of cases of a disease within a population, including both old and new cases of the disease.

priapism: Prolonged, painful erection of the penis; a urologic emergency.

primary aldosteronism: A type of aldosteronism usually caused by a tumor on a single adrenal gland that overproduces aldosterone; also known as Conn syndrome.

primary amyloidosis: The most common form of amyloidosis, affecting the heart, kidneys, tongue, nerves, and intestines; the form of amyloid deposited in this disease is classified as apolipoprotein.

primary apnea: The initial response to asphyxia at birth that responds to stimulation and oxygen therapy; it is characterized by decreased respiratory effort and a slightly decreased heart rate. If not addressed, the infant will progress to secondary apnea.

primary assessment: A brief assessment of the patient's condition in which providers quickly identify any acute life threats. This survey follows a stepwise, rapid evaluation of organ systems and anatomy fundamentally necessary for life, often described as the ABCDE (Airway, Breathing, Circulation, Disability, and Exposure) approach.

primary care centers: Medical centers that offer outpatient, routine family medicine services, including obstetrics and gynecology, geriatric care, and pediatric primary care, and that coordinate patient care with outpatient specialists as appropriate.

primary decontamination: A form of decontamination that usually occurs at a scene or outside a health care facility or transport vehicle; intended to protect rescuers and health care providers from exposure to a toxic substance during patient care and transport.

primary MODS: Multiple organ dysfunction syndrome that results from a direct insult such as trauma.

primary spinal cord injury: Spinal cord injury that occurs at the moment of impact.

procalcitonin: A peptide precursor of calcitonin used to identify serious bacterial infection.

prodromal: Referring to the early signs and symptoms that occur before a disease or condition, such as a toxic exposure, fully appears—for example, dizziness before fainting.

prodrome: Early symptoms indicating the development of disease.

prodrug: A medication that, once inside the body, becomes metabolized to a physiologically active form.

prolapsed cord: A delivery presentation in which the umbilical cord passes through the birth canal in advance of the infant.

prophylaxis: Treatment of disease before it occurs (ie, to prevent the disease).

propofol-related infusion syndrome (PRIS): A constellation of symptoms, including arrhythmias (bradycardia or tachycardia), metabolic acidosis, hyperkalemia, rhabdomyolysis or creatine phosphokinase elevations, and progressive renal and cardiac failure, associated with use of propofol.

proprioception: The ability to perceive the position and movement of one's own body or limbs.

proprioceptive: Referring to information that comes from receptors located in the skin, muscles, tendons, and joints; this information helps a person know the position of their body.

protected health information (PHI): Individually identifiable information (eg, name, Social Security number, and date of birth), health information (eg, laboratory results and medical history), and demographic information (eg, address and telephone number) that is protected by HIPAA.

proteinuria: Protein levels detected in the urine.

prothrombin time (PT): A value that represents the extrinsic coagulation pathway's clotting ability by taking into account various clotting factors, fibrinogen, the prothrombin ratio, and the international normalized ratio.

proton pump inhibitors (PPIs): Medications that reduce gastric acid secretion; they are used to treat gastroesophageal reflux disease and peptic ulcers.

proximal intestinal obstruction: Obstruction at or above the level of the jejunum.

proximally caused: A legal term that describes damages that could have reasonably been anticipated before the breach of duty occurred.

pruritic urticarial papules and plaques of pregnancy (PUPPP): An itchy rash affecting pregnant women; it may be either isolated to one region or systemic.

pruritus: Itching.

pseudo-Cushing state: A condition in which a person has higher cortisol levels from a cause other than actual Cushing syndrome—for example, depression, alcoholism, malnutrition, or panic attack.

psychological first aid (PFA): An evidence-based approach to managing psychological aftereffects in emergency personnel after particularly distressing responses that relies on the concept of human resilience.

ptosis: Drooping of an eyelid.

pulmonary artery catheter (PAC): A catheter with a balloon near its tip that is passed through a vein into the right side of the heart, through the right ventricle, and into the pulmonary artery; it records the pressure transmitted back from the left atrium; also called a Swan–Ganz catheter.

pulmonary artery pressure: The pressure measured in the pulmonary artery, usually displayed with a pressure waveform and digital systolic, diastolic, and mean values.

pulmonary capillary wedge pressure (PCWP): The mean pressure measured while occluding the pulmonary artery with a balloon-tipped catheter proximal to the site of measurement; it reflects left atrial pressure; also called pulmonary artery wedge pressure or pulmonary artery occlusion pressure.

pulmonary overpressurization syndrome (POPS): A diving emergency that can occur during ascent and cause pneumothorax, mediastinal and subcutaneous emphysema, alveolar hemorrhage, and the lethal arterial gas embolism; also called burst lung.

pulmonary vascular resistance (PVR): The resistance or impedance to ejection of the right ventricle of the heart.

pulmonic stenosis: An acyanotic heart defect caused by obstruction of blood flow from the right ventricle to the pulmonary artery; also called pulmonary stenosis.

pulsatility index (PI): A measurement of a left ventricular assist device's pumping power; calculated as follows: Pulsatililty index = (Maximum pump power – Minimum pump power)/Average pump power.

pulse CO-oximetry: A noninvasive screening and monitoring method for methemoglobinemia and carbon monoxide exposure.

pulse oximetry: Measurement of arterial oxygen saturation (Spo_2) and the pulse.

pulse pressure: The difference between the systolic and diastolic blood pressures.

pulsus paradoxus: A decrease of more than 10 mm Hg in systolic blood pressure during inspiration.

pyelonephritis: An infection of the kidney, typically the result of an ascending urinary tract infection.

QRS complex: Deflections in the electrocardiogram produced by ventricular depolarization.

quality assurance and improvement (QA&I) program: A program that seeks to generate data that are then used to improve the quality of service provided.

quaternary care centers: Highly specialized tertiary care referral centers that may be dedicated to advancing clinical research in one or more areas of medicine.

quiescent: A latent state, as occurs with a dormant virus or bacterium, in which an infected patient will exhibit few to no symptoms.

raccoon eyes: Orbital fractures and hemorrhage into the surrounding tissue; also called periorbital ecchymosis.

radiation: Emission of heat from an object into surrounding, colder air.

radiography: basic imaging modality that uses x-ray radiation to generate a two-dimensional image of the internal form of an object.

rapid decompression: A condition that occurs when a large leak or hole develops in a pressurized aircraft; it can result in hypoxia and injury to people inside the aircraft and catastrophic failure of the aircraft.

rapid sequence intubation (RSI): The coadministration of both anesthetic agents and neuromuscular blocking agents to produce a state of unconsciousness and paralysis, which in turn allows for tracheal intubation.

reactive airway disease (RAD): Any condition that causes hyperreactive bronchioles and bronchospasm.

reactive gastritis: Gastric irritation that results from recurring contact of the mucosa with antagonistic substances such as bile, pancreatic juice, or nonsteroidal anti-inflammatory drugs.

receptor sites: Specialized proteins on a cell that receive chemical mediator messages.

reciprocal changes: An electrocardiogram pattern in which a lead shows a pattern that is the opposite of the one shown in the lead located 180° from the other; for example, the electrode over the area of infarction records ST-segment elevation, whereas the electrode over the lead that is 180° away records ST-segment depression.

reckless conduct: A more serious finding than typical negligence; it involves consciously disregarding the known risks of a course of action; also called gross negligence.

red blood cell (RBC) count: A measure of the total number of erythrocytes in the blood.

refractory period: A short period immediately after depolarization in which the myocytes are not yet repolarized and are unable to fire or conduct an impulse.

refractory stage: The stage of shock characterized by persistently low mean arterial blood pressure despite vasopressor therapy and adequate fluid resuscitation.

relative contraindication: A condition that makes a particular treatment or procedure somewhat inadvisable but does not completely rule it out.

relative refractory period: The period in the cell-firing cycle during which it is possible but difficult to restimulate the cell to fire another impulse.

renal perfusion pressure: The gradient between renal arterial and venous flow. A significant decrease in this pressure results in ischemia.

renal tubular acidosis (RTA): A form of metabolic acidosis caused by dysfunction of the kidneys or renal system; it produces an inability to excrete hydrogen in the urine and presents without an elevated anion gap.

Replogle tube: A double-lumen tube used for gastric decompression in infants with gastrointestinal issues. An 8F size is typically used for an infant and is connected to low intermittent wall suction to collect gastric secretions.

repolarization: A state in which the cell becomes more negative, moving away from equilibrium with the extracellular fluid; it is an active process.

reservoir of infection: A host that provides a supply of nutrients and an environmental niche that enables long-term microbial survival.

residual volume (RV): The amount of air remaining in the lungs after the expiratory reserve volume is exhaled.

resilience: A person's ability to withstand negative pressure or "bounce back" from difficulties.

resistance: The amount of force needed to move a gas or fluid through a single capillary tube.

respiration: In the context of environmental heat loss, the loss of heat as warm air in the lungs is exhaled into the atmosphere and cooler air is inhaled.

respiratory acidosis: A pathologic condition (blood pH <7.35) resulting from an accumulation of acids in the body owing to a breathing problem or insufficient function of the respiratory system.

respiratory alkalosis: A pathologic condition (blood pH >7.45) resulting from an accumulation of bases in the body caused by inappropriate tachypnea.

respiratory depression: A low respiratory rate (<2 breaths/min in adults) for a prolonged period of time; also called hypoventilation.

respiratory failure: A situation in which the respiratory system fails to meet the body's metabolic needs. If not reversed, it may lead to respiratory or cardiopulmonary arrest.

respiratory insufficiency: The inability of the respiratory system to keep up with the metabolic demands of the body.

respiratory syncytial virus (RSV): A labile paramyxovirus that produces a characteristic fusion of human cells in a tissue culture known as the syncytial effect; it can affect both the upper and lower respiratory tracts but is more prevalent with the lower respiratory tract, causing pneumonia and bronchiolitis.

respondeat superior: The legal concept that an employer is responsible for the acts of its agents.

restrictive diseases: Diseases that result in difficulty moving air into the lungs, such as occupational lung diseases, idiopathic pulmonary fibrosis, pneumonia, atelectasis, chest wall deformities and injuries, and neuromuscular diseases that affect breathing.

resuscitative endovascular balloon occlusion of the aorta (REBOA): A surgical procedure in which arterial access is gained through a femoral approach, a balloon catheter is floated into the aorta, and the balloon is inflated to occlude flow; a temporizing measure for refractory hemorrhagic shock, blunt or penetrating abdominal trauma, pelvic fractures with significant hemorrhage, and ruptured abdominal aortic aneurysms, and possibly for outlying hospitals prior to transfer of a trauma patient to a higher-level trauma center.

reticular activating system (RAS): A diffuse system that extends from the lower brainstem to the cerebral cortex; it controls the sleep-wakefulness cycle, consciousness, the ability to direct attention to a specific task, and the perception of sensory input that might alter behavior.

reticular formation (RF): A set of neurons that extends from the upper level of the spinal cord; through the medulla, pons, and midbrain; and into the thalamus and cerebral cortex. It has both excitatory and some inhibitory capabilities, and can enhance, suppress, or modify impulse transmission.

retinal detachment: Separation of the inner layers of the retina from the pigmented epithelium.

revised trauma score: A trauma scoring system that rates injury severity by comparing the Glasgow Coma Scale score, the systolic blood pressure, and the respiratory rate and assigning a score ranging from 0 to 13 based on these three values; in some cases the parameters are weighted, resulting in a score ranging from 1.0 to 7.8408.

Rh factors: Antigens found on the cell membrane of red blood cells.

rhabdomyolysis: The destruction of muscle tissue leading to a release of potassium and myoglobin, which then accumulate in the blood and urine and impair filtration; occurs most often with crush injuries, electrical burns, or large full-thickness burns.

rhonchi: Rattling vibrations produced as air flows through mucus or around obstruction in the larger airways.

Richmond Agitation–Sedation Scale (RASS): An evaluation tool used to assess both agitation and sedation.

rickettsial diseases: Diseases transmitted via tick bite; the three major diseases in this class are Rocky Mountain spotted fever, ehrlichiosis, and anaplasmosis.

right ventricular pressure: The pressure in the right ventricle, which consists of the systolic, diastolic, and mean pressures; it is important during insertion and use of a pulmonary artery catheter.

right ventricular stroke work index: A calculation of the contractility of the right ventricle indexed to the patient's body surface area.

rigid stylet: A hyperangulated intubation stylet used to facilitate endotracheal tube passage when using an hyperangulated blade.

risk-benefit ratio: An evaluation of the therapeutic benefits of a medication versus the risks associated with that medication's side effects.

root cause analysis (RCA): A systematic approach to understanding the causes of a serious adverse event and identifying system flaws that can be corrected to prevent future harm.

rotational force: An injury-producing force in which the head moves around its center of gravity.

rotation-flexion injury: A spinal cord injury to C1-C2, the only area of the spine that allows for significant rotation, in which rotation with abrupt flexion produces a stable dislocation in the cervical spine. In the thoracolumbar spine, rotation-flexion forces typically cause fracture rather than dislocation.

rotor-wing aircraft: A transportation mode used to transport critically ill and injured patients in rural settings distances of up to 150 miles (240 km); also called helicopters.

Roux-en-Y: The most common type of bariatric surgery, in which the size of the stomach is reduced, the small intestines are divided, and the jejunum is connected to a small hole in the stomach pouch; also known as gastric bypass.

rubrospinal tract: Part of the midbrain that controls the tone of flexor muscles.

rule of nines: A system that assigns percentages to sections of the body, allowing calculation of the amount of skin surface involved in the burn area.

safety culture: In an EMS organization, a system of beliefs and practices that includes acknowledging that organizations engage in high-risk activities and determining the importance of consistent safe operations to counteract these activities, supporting a blame-free environment where errors can be reported without fear of punishment, and maintaining organizational commitment to address reported errors and safety concerns.

SAMPLE: An acronym for the pertinent details of a patient's history: Signs and symptoms, Allergies, Medications, Pertinent past medical history, Last oral intake, and Events leading up to the illness or injury.

scintigraphy: An imaging technology that is similar to angiography except that the red blood cells themselves are radiologically labeled to allow greater specificity.

SCIWORA: Spinal cord injury without radiographic abnormalities.

sclerema: Hardening of the skin associated with reddening and edema.

scope of practice: The body of knowledge, skills, and therapies that CCTPs can legally apply in patient care, based on training, certification, medical direction, and applicable law.

secondary aldosteronism: A type of aldosteronism that occurs as a result of reduced renal blood flow, which stimulates hypersecretion of aldosterone; it can be caused by obstructive renal artery disease, renal vasoconstriction, and edematous disorders.

secondary amyloidosis: A form of amyloidosis that occurs as a result of another illness, and that primarily affects the kidneys, spleen, liver, and lymph nodes; the form of amyloid deposited in this disease is classified as amyloid A protein.

secondary apnea: The response if asphyxia at birth continues, which is characterized by a period of gasping respirations, decreasing heart rate, and decreasing blood pressure; it does not respond to stimulation unless resuscitation is initiated immediately.

secondary assessment: A patient assessment that occurs after completing the primary assessment and identifying and stabilizing immediate life threats and hemodynamic instability. The secondary assessment involves several components, including a detailed head-to-toe examination, a systems-based approach to specific diseases, and a complete evaluation of vital signs.

secondary care centers: Medical centers that may not only offer primary care within the same facility but also offer outpatient specialties such as cardiology, neurology, nephrology, mental health, endocrinology, or oncology.

secondary decontamination: A form of decontamination directed at minimizing patient absorption or injury from a toxic substance; it occurs after initial decontamination has occurred outside a health care facility or transport vehicle.

secondary MODS: Multiple organ dysfunction syndrome that presents a slower, more progressive insult to organs and frequently results from the sepsis cascade.

secondary spinal cord injury: Spinal cord injury in which multiple factors permit a progression of the primary spinal cord injury; the ensuing cascade of inflammatory responses may result in further deterioration.

sedative-hypnotic syndrome: A syndrome characterized by lethargy, sedation, hypoventilation, apnea, bradycardia, and hypotension that occurs following exposure to any medication or chemical that can cause central nervous system sedation, lethargy, or coma.

seizure: A paroxysmal alteration in neurologic function (ie, behavioral and/or autonomic function).

Seldinger technique: A technique for obtaining vascular or other hollow organ access that uses a hollow-bore needle inserted percutaneously, followed by placement of a soft-tipped guide wire. The needle is removed and a dilator is temporarily placed. The dilator is removed, the desired catheter is placed over the guide wire, and the guide wire is removed. The catheter is then secured. The technique is most commonly used for inserting a central venous line.

semilunar valves: The valves (aortic and pulmonic) that are the exits from the left and right ventricles into the aorta and the pulmonary artery, respectively.

Sengstaken-Blakemore tube: A tube with an inflatable balloon at its end that is inserted into the GI tract and inflated to tamponade bleeding.

sensitivity: In the context of clinical trials, the ability of a certain test to maximize the number of true positives that test positive. In the context of mechanical ventilation, the control that regulates the amount of negative pressure required by the patient to initiate, or trigger, a breath.

sentinel event: A patient safety event in which an error reaches a patient and results in death, permanent harm, or severe temporary harm such that interventions are required to sustain life.

sepsis: A condition of life-threatening organ dysfunction caused by a dysregulated host response to infection; or, a complication of infection, in which the entire body mounts an immune response.

septic shock: A subset of sepsis in which particularly profound circulatory, cellular, and metabolic abnormalities are associated with a greater risk of mortality than occurs with sepsis alone.

sequelae: Consequence of a previous disease or injury.

serious adverse event (SAE): A sentinel event.

seroconversion: Development of antibodies, measured in the serum, in response to an infection or vaccine.

serosa: A protective layer of connective tissue over most of the alimentary canal; also called the visceral peritoneum.

serotonin syndrome: An unusual response to serotonin-altering medications causing hyperserotoninergic symptoms.

severe acute respiratory syndrome (SARS): A highly contagious, potentially life-threatening lower respiratory tract illness that usually starts with flu-like symptoms, including fever, headache, and muscle aches, followed within 2 to 7 days by a dry cough and pneumonia.

severe hypothermia: A condition in which the core body temperature drops to less than 90°F (32.2°C).

shock index: An evaluation tool used to predict mortality and the need for transfusion in the trauma patient; defined as heart rate divided by systolic blood pressure.

shoulder dystocia: A condition in which the infant's shoulders are too large to travel through the birth canal without additional clinical maneuvering of the infant.

shunt: Perfusion without ventilation.

sickle cell anemia: A disease caused by inheritance of two sets of recessive genes that produce an abnormal hemoglobin protein, known as Hgb S. The red blood cells become deformed (have a sickle shape) and occlude vessels, clot, and cause great pain in patients.

side effects: Reactions that can manifest as signs or symptoms that are not desired but are expected based on how the medication works.

simulation: A training technique that allows health care providers to hone their skills in a safe environment without risk of patient harm and to work in teams to practice both procedures and communication skills.

single-chamber demand pacemaker: A pacemaker with the pacing lead placed in only one chamber of the heart, in which the generator stimulus is inhibited by a signal derived from the heart's depolarization, thus minimizing the risk of pacemaker-induced fibrillation.

sinus tachycardia: A heart rate that is faster than normal for the patient's age.

situation, background, assessment, and recommendation (SBAR): A technique that allows for a brief, yet concise and expected, handoff of information.

Six Sigma: A disciplined, data-driven approach and methodology for eliminating defects in any process.

sleeve gastrectomy: A bariatric surgical procedure that is the first part of a biliopancreatic diversion with duodenal switch procedure, in which the structure of the stomach is changed to a tube; also known as vertical sleeve gastrectomy.

slip: A lapse in concentration that occurs in the face of distractions, fatigue, or stress.

SLUDGEM: Acronym for symptoms of anticholinesterase inhibitor toxicity: Salivation, Lacrimation, Urination, Diarrhea, Gastroenteritis, Emesis, and Miosis.

somatogravic illusion: An error in perception that occurs with acceleration, as the otolith organs are displaced rearward, similar to when a person is looking up. This perception of a nose-up altitude may cause the pilot to push the nose of the aircraft down inappropriately at night or in unlit terrain.

sovereign immunity: A type of immunity often afforded EMS providers that is provided only to governmental entities. This immunity can align with the reckless or willful and wanton requirements, or it can differentiate between ministerial acts (those requiring a specific act given a set of circumstances) and discretionary acts (those in which the provider has some latitude in decision making).

space equivalent zone: The atmospheric zone that begins at 50,000 feet. In this zone, 100% oxygen is not sufficient to prevent hypoxia without the use of a pressurized aircraft or suit. Unprotected personnel may experience boiling of body fluids at a level above 66,500 feet.

spatial disorientation: An error in perception that may result from a person's inability to determine their position, altitude, and motion in relation to the surface of the earth or to a significant fixed object during flight.

specialty care transport (SCT): The interfacility ground transport of a critically ill or injured patient, including provision of medically necessary supplies and services that are beyond the scope of practice of a paramedic; a term used by the Centers for Medicare and Medicaid Services in determining whether transport charges are reimbursable.

specific gravity: The chemical property of a fluid that relates its density to the density of water.

specificity: The ability of a certain test to minimize the number of true negatives that test positive.

spinal shock: The temporary local neurologic condition that occurs immediately after spinal trauma; it is characterized by swelling and edema of the spinal cord and can lead to a physiologic transection, mechanically disrupting all nerve conduction distal to the injury.

Spo$_2$: The noninvasive pulse oximetry measurement of oxyhemoglobin saturation by means of a beam of light applied to a superficial capillary bed such as the digits or ear lobe.

spontaneous bacterial peritonitis: A bacterial infection of ascitic fluid.

sporadic: A pattern of disease occurrence in which a disease manifests only occasionally.

stagnant hypoxia: Hypoxia caused by a malfunction of the circulatory system resulting in a decrease in blood flow.

standard geometry blade: A device used during indirect (video) laryngoscopy that allows the CCTP to visualize the oral cavity on a monitor.

standard precautions: The use of gloves, mask, goggles, gown, and shoe covers when handling body fluids or tissues of a patient who is not suspected of having a transmissible disease.

status epilepticus: A life-threatening neurologic disorder in which an individual experiences prolonged (more than 5 minutes) seizure or does not recover from such seizures.

statute of limitations: The time limit within which negligence cases must be filed; it is typically 2 years but varies from state to state and may be longer if the patient is a minor.

statutes: Formal laws passed by a legislative body and signed by an executive.

steady state: A point in drug administration at which the rate of administration (frequency and dose) is equal to the rate of elimination, resulting in a constant plasma medication level.

stepping reflex: An infant reflex that occurs when the infant is held up in the air and moves the legs up and down as if marching.

stereognosis: The ability to sense an object's form through touch.

sterile cockpit: The time when unnecessary communication that could distract the pilot is banned in the cockpit—usually during takeoffs, landings, and any other critical phase of flight at the discretion of the pilot-in-command.

Stevens-Johnson syndrome: A milder form of toxic epidermal necrolysis, in which epidermal detachment involves less than 10% of the total body surface area; it causes sloughing of the skin, mucous membranes, and cells lining the respiratory system.

stimulant washout syndrome: Excessive sleep, hunger, and depression as a result of excessive amphetamine use.

strain pattern: An electrocardiogram pattern that involves ST-segment changes and flipped, asymmetric T waves associated with right or left ventricular hypertrophy.

stress: The reaction of the mind or body to a demand for change; it can have either positive or negative effects.

stress-related erosive syndrome: A condition in which stress-related mucosal disease develops in critically ill patients, such as those with severe head trauma or burns.

stridor: High-pitched sound representing air moving past fluid or mechanical obstruction within or immediately above the glottic opening.

stroke: A disruption of blood flow to the brain that results in a neurologic deficit persisting for more than 24 hours.

stroke volume (SV): The amount of blood ejected by the ventricles during each contraction; it varies between 60 and 100 mL/beat, with the average being 70 mL.

stroke volume index: A calculation of the contractility of the left ventricle indexed to the patient's body surface area; equivalent to the left ventricular stroke work index.

ST segment: The section of the electrocardiogram complex from the end of the QRS complex to the beginning of the T wave, which represents the period of inactivity between ventricular depolarization and repolarization; mechanically, it represents the time that the myocardium is maintaining contraction.

ST-segment elevation myocardial infarction (STEMI): A myocardial infarction that shows ST-segment elevation on the electrocardiogram; patients with STEMI have a high probability of coronary thrombus occlusion.

subarachnoid hemorrhage (SAH): Bleeding between the arachnoid mater and the dura mater.

subdermal burn: A severe, life-threatening burn involving the deep structures of muscle, bone, larger blood vessels, and nerves; also called a fourth-degree burn.

subdural hematoma (SDH): Bleeding that accumulates between the dura mater and the arachnoid mater.

subdural space: The dura-arachnoid junction; this potential space may develop into a real one if a blow to the head causes a loss of blood into the cranial meninges.

submucosa: The layer of connective tissue below the mucosa; it contains blood vessels, lymph, and nerves.

subthalamus: An area of the cerebrum that is located below the thalamus and is closely related to the basal ganglia in function.

suction event: An emergency in which tissue occludes the inlet of the pump in a mechanical circulatory support device.

sulci: Grooves between adjacent gyri.

sulcus sign: A deep lateral costophrenic angle on a chest radiograph, which is associated with pneumothorax.

summation effect: The process whereby administration of multiple medications can produce a response that the individual medications alone do not produce.

superficial burn: A burn involving only the epidermis, producing very red, painful skin; also called a first-degree burn.

superficial partial-thickness burn: A burn involving the epidermis and part of the dermis, but not the deeper layers of the dermis; also called a second-degree burn.

supine hypotensive syndrome: Low blood pressure resulting from compression of the inferior vena cava by the weight of the pregnant uterus when the mother is supine.

supraventricular tachycardia (SVT): An abnormally fast rhythm originating above the ventricles.

surfactant: A substance formed in the lungs that helps keep the small air sacs or alveoli from collapsing and sticking together; a low level of this substance in a premature infant contributes to respiratory distress syndrome.

Swiss cheese model: A model in which errors made by people result in consequences related to flawed systems.

sympathomimetics: Medications that mimic the body's sympathetic nervous system response (fight-or-flight response); include epinephrine and norepinephrine.

sympathomimetic syndrome: A syndrome that involves overstimulation of the adrenergic nervous system, resulting in tachycardia, hypertension, agitation, seizures, hyperthermia, dilated pupils, and diaphoresis.

synergism: An interaction of two or more medications that results in an effect that is greater than the sum of their effects if taken independently.

systemic inflammatory response syndrome (SIRS): An immune response to an insult that typically leads to hypotension, shock, and worsened tissue function.

systemic vascular resistance (SVR): The resistance or impedance to ejection of the left ventricle of the heart.

systole: The contraction phase of the heart cycle in which the ventricles pump blood out of the heart through the aorta and the pulmonary artery into the systemic and pulmonary circulatory systems.

systolic blood pressure (SBP): Peak pressure in the arterial system, which occurs during ventricular ejection or systole.

T tube: A T-shaped tube used to drain bile from the gallbladder.

T wave: The upright, flat, or inverted wave following the QRS complex of the electrocardiogram, representing ventricular repolarization.

tachyphylaxis: A condition in which the patient rapidly becomes tolerant to a medication.

tachypnea: An abnormally fast respiratory rate; marked by shallow respirations.

TeamSTEPPS: Team strategies and tools to enhance performance and patient safety; a program that embraces the principles of crew resource management and teaches tools and methods by which team members can safely raise concerns, challenge orders that are unclear, and if necessary "stop the line."

tectospinal tract: Part of the midbrain that controls reflex motor movements in response to visual and auditory stimuli.

temporal lobe: The lobe of the brain that is located beneath the temporal bone of the cranium; its primary functions relate to hearing, speech, behavior, and memory.

tension pneumothorax: A pneumothorax in which an intact chest wall allows air that has entered the thoracic space to progressively accumulate, resulting in catastrophic collapse of pulmonary and cardiac structures in the chest.

tentorium cerebelli: A fold of the dura mater that separates the occipital lobes of the cerebrum from the cerebellum and brainstem, thereby dividing the brain into upper and lower compartments.

term: Used to describe an infant delivered at 39 to 40 weeks' gestation.

termination of action: The amount of time after the medication's concentration falls below the minimum effective level until the point at which it is eliminated from the body.

term newborn: An infant born between 37 and 42 weeks' gestation.

tertiary care centers: Medical centers that offer highly specialized inpatient medical care, including advanced and complex medical interventions performed by specialty physicians.

testicular torsion: Twisting of a testicle about the spermatic cord to the point of ischemia.

tetralogy of Fallot (TOF): A cyanotic heart defect characterized by four anomalies: ventricular septal defect, pulmonary stenosis, overriding aorta, and right ventricular hypertrophy.

thalamus: The largest portion of the diencephalons. It acts as a relay station for motor and sensory activity; basic neuronal activity; and memory, thought, emotion, and complex behavior.

therapeutic index: The ratio of a drug's lethal dose for 50% (LD_{50}) of the population to its effective dose for 50% (ED_{50}) of the population; a medication's margin of safety.

thermal burn: A burn caused by heat, contact with hot objects, ignited liquids, steam, or hot liquids.

thermistor: The apparatus used for quickly determining very small changes in pulmonary artery temperature.

thermogenesis: The production of heat in the body.

thermolysis: The liberation of heat from the body.

thermoregulation: The process by which the body maintains temperature through a combination of heat gain by metabolic processes and muscular movement and heat loss through respiration, evaporation, conduction, convection, and perspiration.

third spacing: A loss of fluids from the intravascular space into the tissues caused by an increase in intravascular pressures and/or increased permeability of the cell membranes. Physical stressors of flight such as temperature, vibration, and changes in gravitational force can cause or aggravate this condition; also, an abnormal increase in the amount of fluid that exits the vascular space and moves into other areas (eg, gut wall, subcutaneous tissue); it can lead to dehydration, electrolyte imbalances, and hypovolemia.

thrombocytopenia: An abnormally low blood platelet count.

thromboelastography (TEG): A method used to assess the viscoelastic properties of whole blood that combines multiple measurements of platelet function, the coagulation cascade, and their interaction to form clots.

thrombotic stroke: A condition that occurs when the blood supply to part of the brain is disrupted by a thrombus, or blood clot.

thrombus: A blood clot.

thrust: The force exerted by the aircraft engine, which pushes air backward with the objective of causing a reaction of the aircraft in the forward direction.

thyroid storm: A rare but severe, life-threatening form of thyrotoxicosis that can occur in patients with long-term, untreated hyperthyroidism, but is more commonly precipitated in hyperthyroid patients by an acute physiologic stressor such as a recent surgery, trauma, infection, administration of large doses of iodine, or abrupt discontinuation of thyroid medications.

thyrotoxicosis: An excess of thyroid hormones resulting in a hypermetabolic crisis, including tachycardia, hyperthermia (sometimes with a body temperature greater than 103.9°F [39.9°C]), coma with agitation, nausea, vomiting, diarrhea, unexplained jaundice, pulmonary edema, and elevated thyroxine level; severe cases are known as thyroid storm.

TICLS: A mnemonic used to remember the priorities during initial assessment of an infant's appearance: Tone, Interactiveness, Consolability, Look or gaze, and Speech or cry.

tidal volume (V_t): The volume of air moved into and out of the lungs with each respiratory cycle.

time-cycled ventilator: A type of positive-pressure ventilator in which the ventilator ends inspiration after a selected inspiratory time has been achieved.

time of useful consciousness: The time between a person's sudden deprivation of oxygen at a given altitude to the point at which deliberate function is lost. With the loss of effective performance during flight, a person is no longer capable of taking proper corrective or protective actions.

timing: In the context of intra-aortic balloon pump therapy, a method for coordinating the intra-aortic balloon inflation–deflation cycle with the cardiac cycle (inflation during diastole and deflation synchronous with systole).

Title 14 of the Code of Federal Regulations (14 CFR) Part 91: A guideline established by the Federal Aviation Administration that governs the operation of all aircraft within the United States, including the waters within 3 nautical miles (6 km) of the US coast.

Title 14 of the Code of Federal Regulations (14 CFR) Part 135: A guideline established by the Federal Aviation Administration that governs the operations of all commuter or on-demand commercial operations.

tocolytics: A group of medications used to suppress preterm labor.

tolerance: Physiologic adaptation to the effects of a drug such that increasingly larger doses of the drug are required to achieve the same effect; in immunology, it is the ability to distinguish between self and nonself cells.

TORCH screen: A set of lab values taken to detect congenital infections, including toxoplasma immunoglobulin G and immunoglobulin M (1:1,024), rubella titers, urine cytomegalovirus titer, viral culture (for herpes), and culture of scrapings from any vesicular lesions.

torsades de pointes: An undulating sinusoidal rhythm in which the axis of the QRS complexes changes from positive to negative and back in a haphazard manner.

tort: A wrongful act between people or entities that gives rise to a civil lawsuit.

total anomalous pulmonary venous return: A condition in which oxygenated blood returns to the right side of the heart, leading to progressive pulmonary edema.

total lung capacity (TLC): The maximal amount of air that can fill the lungs; the sum of tidal volume, inspiratory reserve volume, expiratory reserve volume, and residual volume.

total parenteral nutrition (TPN): The IV administration of all necessary nutrients in a patient whose GI tract does not function.

total protein: The total quantity of protein in a blood sample.

toxic epidermal necrolysis (TEN) syndrome: A severe skin reaction to certain medications, environmental allergies, and other unknown toxins, in which epidermal detachment is greater than 30%.

toxic shock syndrome: A condition that results from the release of bacterial toxins into the body, specifically following infection with *Staphylococcus aureus*, *Streptococcus pyogenes*, or *Clostridium sordellii*.

toxidrome: A group of symptoms, or syndrome, associated with toxicity of a given substance.

tracheal breath sounds: Breath sounds heard by placing the stethoscope diaphragm over the trachea or over the sternum; also called bronchial breath sounds.

tracheal deviation: A late sign of a tension pneumothorax in which the trachea is tugged to one side of the neck, usually opposite the side of the pneumothorax.

tracheal tugging: Downward traction of the trachea toward the thoracic cavity during inspiration.

tracheomalacia: A weakening or softening of the tracheal cartilage/rings that leads to respiratory disease.

transcranial Doppler (TCD) ultrasonography: A noninvasive method of assessing the state of intracranial perfusion and monitoring of cerebral blood flow velocity through thinner areas of the skull. It is used in patients following rupture of an intracranial aneurysm to assess for vasospasm, to identify intracranial lesions following a stroke, and to detect cerebral blood flow changes associated with increased ICP.

transfusion reactions: Reactions resulting from an endogenous or exogenous factor related to transfused blood.

transient ischemic attack (TIA): A temporary disruption in the blood flow to the brain that lasts less than 24 hours and has temporary side effects.

transient tachypnea of the newborn: Transient respiratory distress that lasts a few hours in the newborn and occurs secondary to retained fetal lung fluid.

transjugular intrahepatic portosystemic shunt: The placement of a shunt in the abdomen that bypasses much of the hepatic portal system; it is intended to decrease portal hypertension and its effects.

translational force: An injury-producing force in which the head's center of gravity moves along a linear path.

transmission-based precautions: Specific precautions used when a patient is suspected to have a particular illness.

transposition of the great vessels: A cyanotic heart defect that results from the aorta receiving blood from the right ventricle while the pulmonary artery leaves the left ventricle.

trauma injury severity score (TRISS): A scoring system that uses the results of the Injury Severity Score, the revised trauma score, and the patient's age to calculate the survivability rate; rarely used in the transport setting.

trauma score: A score ranging from 1 to 16 that takes into account the Glasgow Coma Scale score, respiratory rate, respiratory expansion, systolic blood pressure, and capillary refill and relates to the likelihood of patient survival; not accurate for patients with severe head injuries.

traumatic asphyxia: A condition resulting from severe, sudden crushing injury to the chest and abdomen, which forces blood backward out of the right side of the heart; engorges the veins of the chest, neck, and head; and gives the chest, neck, and head an extremely cyanotic appearance.

tricuspid atresia: A cyanotic heart defect that results from an absent or defective tricuspid heart valve, which causes blood flow from the right atrium to the right ventricle to be blocked.

trifascicular block: The combination of bifascicular block (a right bundle branch block with a block in the left anterior fascicle or left posterior fascicle) that occurs with a first-degree heart block (prolonged PR interval).

triple-lumen catheter: A type of catheter consisting of three distinct continuous tubes that allow for pressure monitoring, blood sampling, and fluid and drug administration.

troponin: A key protein involved in muscle contraction that is present in the serum only after cellular necrosis releases the cellular contents of cardiac muscle (such as after myocardial infarction).

tropopause: The space between the troposphere and the stratosphere. It rises to 60,000 feet at the equator owing to the expansion of heated air masses and sinks to about 30,000 feet at the poles owing to contracting cold air masses.

troposphere: A portion of the earth's atmosphere that extends from the surface of the earth to 5 to 10 miles (26,000–52,000 feet) high depending on the relation to the equator and the poles. This layer is characterized by the presence of water vapors, a constant decrease in temperature with increasing altitude, and large-scale vertical currents.

true anaphylaxis: An anaphylactic reaction that occurs when the allergen binds to immunoglobulin E on the cell membranes of basophils and when mast cells stimulate the release of histamine from the cell.

true fracture: The most common type of closed skull fracture, in which the depressed segment has contact with the cranial vault.

tumor necrosis factor (TNF): A protein mediator that is released primarily by macrophages and T lymphocytes, and that helps regulate the immune response.

turbid: Cloudy or opaque.

two-point discrimination: A test of sensation discrimination that measures the shortest distance at which the sides of two separate points of a compass or calipers can be distinguished from each other.

type 1 diabetes: An endocrine disease that usually starts in childhood and requires daily injections of supplemental insulin to control blood glucose; sometimes called juvenile or juvenile-onset diabetes.

type 2 diabetes: An endocrine disease that usually starts later in life and often can be controlled through diet and oral medications; sometimes called adult-onset diabetes.

Type I spatial disorientation: A loss of positional awareness in which the pilot is unaware of becoming disoriented.

Type II spatial disorientation: A loss of positional awareness in which the pilot is initially unaware of spatial disorientation, but senses that something is wrong.

Type III spatial disorientation: A sudden incapacitating form of loss of positional awareness.

type-and-crossmatch: The test to determine compatibility between patient serum and donor red blood cells prior to transfusion.

ulcerative colitis: An inflammation of the rectal mucosal and submucosal tissues.

ultrasonography: A technique for mapping the echoes produced by high-frequency sound waves transmitted into the body; the denser material reflects waves back to a transducer that produces an image. It is typically used for obstetrics, gynecology, and abdominal diagnostics.

unassisted systole: Pressure waveform reflecting what would normally occur without intra-aortic balloon pump assistance.

uncal herniation: The most common type of brain herniation, in which a portion of the temporal lobe is displaced, resulting in compression of cranial nerve III, the midbrain, and the posterior cerebral artery.

uncus: The medially curved anterior part of the hippocampal gyrus.

unipolar lead: A lead in which one of the electrodes is placed in the heart and the other lead is placed in an area of zero potential.

unipolar system: A type of pacemaker system in which contact between the pacemaker itself and the body tissue forms the ground lead for the implantable pulse generator.

universal donors: Persons who have type O blood.

universal precautions: The isolation precautions taken when dealing with all patients regardless of their disease status.

universal recipients: Persons who have type AB blood.

universal time-out: A planned pause before the beginning of a procedure that improves communication among all personnel in the room; it allows time for everyone to review important aspects of the procedure.

uremia: The presence of excessive amounts of urea and other waste products in the blood; can lead to altered mental status.

urinalysis: Laboratory tests performed on a patient's urine.

$\dot{V}/\dot{Q}$ ratio: The relationship between alveolar ventilation and alveolar capillary perfusion. The normal value is 0.8.

vacuum caput: In a newborn, an accumulation of fluid at the site where a vacuum extractor was used to assist in delivering the newborn.

vasopressor: A medication that causes constriction of blood vessels, thereby causing blood pressure to rise.

VATER syndrome: A syndrome consisting of multiple birth defects: vertebral anomalies, anal atresia, tracheoesophageal fistula and/or esophageal atresia, and renal and radial anomalies.

Vaughan-Williams classification scheme: A classification system for antiarrhythmic medications.

vector: An organism that carries a disease-causing microorganism from one organism to another.

ventilation-perfusion ($\dot{V}/\dot{Q}$) mismatch: A state of inadequate ventilation, perfusion, or both, in which there is inadequate gas exchange.

ventilator-associated pneumonia (VAP): A type of hospital-acquired pneumonia that occurs in ventilated patients and that appears more than 48 hours after endotracheal intubation.

ventral: Toward the abdomen; anterior.

ventricular septal defect (VSD): An acyanotic heart defect in which blood flows from the left ventricle to the right ventricle through a hole in the septal wall.

vertebral body: The anterior weight-bearing structure within the spine.

vertex: A fetal position in which the head is the lowest part of the fetus, resulting in the head presenting first during delivery; the normal delivery presentation.

vertical banded gastroplasty (VBG): A bariatric surgical procedure that divides the stomach into two parts; also known as stomach stapling.

vertical compression: Forces transmitted through vertebral bodies and directed either inferiorly through the skull or superiorly through the pelvis or feet (eg, from a direct blow to the parietal region of the skull or rapid deceleration from a fall through the feet, legs, and pelvis).

vesicant: A substance that causes tissue injury.

vesicular breath sounds: Softer, muffled sounds in which the expiratory phase is barely audible.

vestibular: Related to the organs of equilibrium located in the inner ear.

video laryngoscopy: An orotracheal intubation technique that involves indirect visualization of the vocal cords via a video camera at the distal end of a blade that provides a video feed to a screen.

viremia: The presence of viruses in the blood.

virion: The complete viral particle, including DNA or RNA enclosed in a capsid, that is capable of infecting another cell.

virulence: Physical or biochemical properties of a disease agent that determine its pathogenicity.

virulence factors: Adaptations of microbes that enable them to penetrate the immune defenses.

viscerocranium: The bones making up the facial skeleton.

visual flight rules (VFR): A mode of flight used when weather conditions are good, meaning there is generally very good visibility and minimal cloud cover; the pilot is responsible for maintaining separation from other aircraft.

vital capacity (V_c): The maximal amount of air that can be exhaled following a maximal inspiration; the sum of tidal volume, inspiratory reserve volume, and expiratory reserve volume; approximately 80% total lung capacity.

voltage: The force that causes current to flow in a circuit, measured in volts; also called *amplitude* in a pacing system.

volume ventilator: A type of positive-pressure ventilator in which the breath ends when the predetermined tidal volume is achieved.

voluntary (somatic) nervous system: The nervous system fibers that connect the structures of the CNS with skeletal muscles and the integument.

volutrauma: Trauma caused by excessive lung inflation volumes.

volvulus: A twisting of the intestine onto itself, usually causing strangulation and ischemia.

washed blood products: Red blood cell or platelet products in which the small amount of noncellular fluid has been replaced, typically with saline.

water intoxication: A condition in which the normal balance of electrolytes in the body is pushed outside safe limits by the overconsumption of water.

weather decline: A situation in which an air medical provider is requested, but the pilot and the flight team determine that the weather does not meet established Federal Aviation Administration guidelines and therefore decline to make the flight.

weight: The downward force due to the weight (gravity) of the aircraft and its load; directly opposed to lift.

well-being: "A positive outcome that is meaningful for people and for many sectors of society, because it tells us that people perceive that their lives are going well" (Centers for Disease Control and Prevention); a state of being comfortable, healthy, and happy.

Wernicke area: Part of the temporal lobe that is responsible for comprehension of both written and spoken words.

West Nile virus (WNV): An arthropod-borne *Flavivirus* that is spread to birds and humans by mosquitoes; it may be characterized by sudden onset of fever with malaise, anorexia, nausea, vomiting, eye pain, headache, myalgia, rash, lymphadenopathy, fatigue, and arthralgias.

wheezes: A high-pitched musical sound caused by airflow through a narrowed or constricted airway.

white blood cell (WBC) count: A measure of the total number of leukocytes in the blood.

whole-bowel irrigation (WBI): A gastric decontamination method that involves the patient drinking or receiving via a nasogastric tube large quantities of a nonabsorbable, electrolyte-balanced liquid that propels stomach and intestinal contents through the digestive system.

wide complex tachycardia: A cardiac rhythm of greater than 100 beats/min with a QRS duration of 120 ms or greater; it can be of ventricular or supraventricular origin.

willful and wanton: A more serious finding than typical negligence misconduct; it usually requires an intentional act of misconduct.

Wolff-Parkinson-White (WPW) syndrome: A syndrome characterized by short PR intervals, delta waves, nonspecific ST-T wave changes, and paroxysmal episodes of tachycardia caused by the presence of an accessory pathway; one of the conditions that produces supraventricular tachycardia via an accessory pathway.

working diagnosis: An assumed decision on the medical condition of a patient based on the preliminary investigation; assists in the provision of initial treatment and projection of further diagnostic testing requirements.

zeroing: The process of calibrating a pressure transducer to eliminate extraneous atmospheric and hydrostatic pressures from the data being measured.

zero-order elimination: A process by which medications or chemicals are eliminated from the body at a constant rate, regardless of plasma concentration.

zone of coagulation: The center of a burn, which is usually the deepest and most severely affected area.

zone of erythema: The outermost area of a burn, which represents the least severely burned area; usually an area of first-degree burn.

zone of stasis: The area found just outside the zone of coagulation, which represents a burned area that is less severely damaged.

zoonosis: A disease that occurs in animals and can also be transmitted to humans.

Index

Note: Page numbers followed by *f, t* denote figures and tables, respectively.